UNDERSTANDING
TOXICOLOGY

A BIOLOGICAL APPROACH

Steven D. Mercurio, PhD

Professor of Biology
Minnesota State University
Mankato, Minnesota

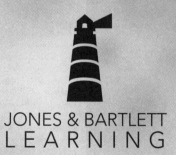

JONES & BARTLETT
LEARNING

World Headquarters
Jones & Bartlett Learning
5 Wall Street
Burlington, MA 01803
978-443-5000
info@jblearning.com
www.jblearning.com

Jones & Bartlett Learning books and products are available through most bookstores and online booksellers. To contact Jones & Bartlett Learning directly, call 800-832-0034, fax 978-443-8000, or visit our website, www.jblearning.com.

Substantial discounts on bulk quantities of Jones & Bartlett Learning publications are available to corporations, professional associations, and other qualified organizations. For details and specific discount information, contact the special sales department at Jones & Bartlett Learning via the above contact information or send an email to specialsales@jblearning.com.

Production Credits

VP, Executive Publisher: David D. Cella
Publisher: Michael Brown
Associate Editor: Nicholas Alakel
Associate Editor: Danielle Bessette
Associate Production Editor: Rebekah Linga
Senior Marketing Manager: Sophie Fleck Teague
Manufacturing and Inventory Control Supervisor: Amy Bacus

Composition: CAE Solutions Corp.
Cover Design: Kristin E. Parker
Rights & Media Specialist: Merideth Tumasz
Media Development Editor: Shannon Sheehan
Cover Image: © kgtoh/age fotostock
Printing and Binding: Edwards Brothers Malloy
Cover Printing: Edwards Brothers Malloy

Library of Congress Cataloging-in-Publication Data
Mercurio, Steven D., author.
  Understanding toxicology : a biological approach / Steven D. Mercurio.
     p. ; cm.
  Includes bibliographical references and index.
  ISBN 978-0-7637-7116-4 (paper)
  I. Title.
  [DNLM: 1. Drug-Related Side Effects and Adverse Reactions. 2. Biological Factors--toxicity. 3. Environmental Exposure. 4. Hazardous Substances--toxicity. 5. Toxicology. QV 600]
  RA1226
  615.9'02--dc23
                                    2015011989
6048

Printed in the United States of America
20 19 18 17 16   10 9 8 7 6 5 4 3 2 1

Dedication

This book is dedicated to the many students I have taught over a nearly 30-year period at Minnesota State University and to their struggles with understanding the complexity of the biological response to chemicals, biological agents, and physical stressors, including radiation. Their ability to engage in toxicology research and contribute to scientific investigation has always been a source of inspiration. I wanted to provide a tool that they could understood more logically than other sources of information. Toxicology is at the heart of the biological sciences, as toxins have been used to investigate various mechanisms of biologic action, they are taken as medications, and they are used for various other purposes. In a world and climate that has been altered by industrialization and chemical use, the study of toxicology helps us to understand the benefits and risks of humanity's ongoing experiment in the use of chemicals to enhance the economy and extend lifespan.

Contents

vi   **Contents**

Contents

Preface

This first edition of *Understanding Toxicology: A Biological Approach* is meant to serve both undergraduate and graduate students in the biological sciences who are interested in a subject that examines all levels of biological inquiry—from cellular/molecular, to complex organism, to ecosystem. This primary text will allow those students to first approach the subject from a research perspective and then from a public policy perspective, as published research reports are utilized in agencies to drive regulation.

The logical progression of the first section (Part I: Introduction) examines toxicology at all three levels of analysis—cellular, complex organism, and ecosystem. Then, students will examine common toxic mechanisms that affect cells (Part II: Toxic Reactions of Cells) from the outside to the inside, as toxicants impact various membranes, organelles, and signaling pathways. In this section, mitochondria and chloroplasts are covered, as biological impacts on plants and animals differ. Similarly, organ systems (Part III: Toxic Reactions of Tissues/Organs) start with the skin, eye, GI tract, and lung as the routes of likely entry of toxicants into a complex organism. The final organ system is the kidney, marking excretion. Each organ system is viewed from the point of entry of the toxicant to the likely exit, unless the organ is damaged beyond repair. Forensics is stressed in an introductory chapter to this section and then throughout each organ system so students can understand what the key features are of the damage that each toxicant causes to a given organ (how a pathologist might discover how complex organisms became sick or died). Environmental toxicity begins (Part IV: Toxic Reactions of Ecosystems) with a section on dispersion so that students can understand how toxicants become a concentration that is experienced by organisms in the environment. The ecosystems are based on modern land use: rural/agriculture and urban/industrial. The toxicants are then grouped into classes so students can understand how some disperse into soil, water, or air and then have their impacts. Those toxicants that biodegrade are listed together, and persistent organic chemicals have their own category within that chapter. Those that do not biodegrade (metals) are covered in their own chapter. Radiation is discussed in the chapter on toxicants that are found in the atmosphere, as these impacts are most likely based on nuclear weapons use or accidents at nuclear power plants. The inclusion of a chapter on pharmaceuticals and personal care products reflects the impact of human use of medications, musks, and antiseptic soaps and the impact of these products via sewage release into surface waters. The last section (Part V: Biological Toxicants) deals with venoms, poisonous animals, and poisonous plants. However, these sections also wrestle with the true biological origins of these toxicants, which does not always categorize them neatly into animal or plant toxins. The evolution of these biological toxicants, their roles for use by the organisms, and the metabolic cost of production and use of these toxicants are considered.

Chapter Overview and Pedagogical Features

Each chapter starts with Conceptualizing Toxicology, which gives an outline of the chapter so that the instructor and the students have a ready outline. There is also an Instructor Manual and slides in PowerPoint format with figures available for the instructor that can be made available to the students. Chapters give proper citations and websites for students to get additional information. Figures and tables in the chapter provide visual aids and summaries that aid in learning the information.

Chapter 1 sets the stage with research institutions and associations that are fully engaged in toxicology research and provide the experiments to consider throughout the course, if desired. It makes a good introductory lecture/interaction session.

Chapter 2 provides the history of the field and is provided to be thorough and indicate how dose and dosage concepts were developed along with morbidity and mortality that are toxicology concepts.

Chapter 3 focuses on toxicology terms at all three biological levels. Terms are bolded to indicate their importance. This makes a good introduction for either an introductory toxicology course or a refresher for an environmental toxicology course.

Chapter 4 is a three-level approach to risk assessment.

Chapter 5 involves absorption and damage done to cell walls or cell membranes.

Chapter 6 is an introduction to signal transductions starting with receptor-mediated toxicities on the outside of cells and downstream signaling that results in toxicity.

Chapter 7 is the biotransformation chapter. Its placement here is due to the presence of metabolic enzymes in the endoplasmic reticulum and the cytosol. Some instructors may like to cover this earlier in their courses. However, the stress up to this point is the original compound.

Chapter 8 examines cytosolic and endoplasmic reticulum damage in light of activation of some compounds by metabolism. Reactive chemical species are examined in detail as are antidotal therapies.

Chapter 9 examines how energy functions are affected by toxicants. Mitochondria and chloroplasts are examined and instructors can examine either, depending on whether herbicides will be a major focus of their course or not.

Chapter 10 examines mutagenesis, clastogenesis, and carcinogenesis. Again, some instructors like this to come earlier and it can be used that way. However, its placement here reflects the interior nature of the eukaryote nucleus. Epigenetic mechanisms are also examined, as they are important in gene expression.

Chapter 11 starts the selective toxicity/hypersensitivity discussion, as brought about by polymorphisms of genes involved in absorption, biotransformation, etc.

Chapter 12 is a chapter on nutritional toxicology and indicates how nutritional state is important in hypersensitivity.

Chapter 13 goes more thoroughly into toxicokinetics, as distribution to organs is important here. This can be a starting point if an instructor wishes to examine mainly mammalian or medical toxicity.

Chapter 14 indicates how forensic toxicity is assessed to give a sample of forensic science to students who understand that autopsies and toxicology tests are used to determine poisoning by pharmaceutical, drugs of abuse, toxic chemicals, radiation, etc.

Chapter 15 starts with the outside of the body where exposure results from spilling or misuse of chemicals.

Chapter 16 indicates toxicity to the GI tract starting with the mouth and continuing to the anus, and the digestive organs of the pancreas and liver. Accidental or intentional ingestion is how many poisonings occur.

Chapter 17 indicates the last route of exposure from the outside, inhaling particles, gases, vapors, etc. Environmental toxicity is stressed at the end of the chapter, as this route is a microcosm of how chemicals may be dispersed in an environment similar to the portion of the respiratory tract affected by different-sized agents in various chemical states.

Chapter 18 examines the cardiovascular system and how it is affected during circulation of a toxicant.

Chapter 19 is the immunotoxicology chapter and represents both blood and lymph circulation, which affecting lymph nodes, spleen, and bone marrow.

Chapter 20 is the neurotoxicology chapter and examines the peripheral and central nervous system action of toxicants including breaching the blood–brain barrier.

Chapter 21 is the endocrine organ toxicity chapter and involves discussion of endocrine disruption.

Chapter 22 gives all the reproductive indices and examines reproductive organ toxicity mechanisms.

Chapter 23 is the renal toxicity chapter and involves excretion of the metabolized toxicant. This ends organ toxicity.

Chapter 24 examines models of dispersion to show how environmental toxicology models concentrations at various distances from point sources or non-point sources.

Chapter 25 is the longest chapter, as it involves agricultural toxicants such as nutrients and pesticides (herbicides, insecticides/miticides, rodenticides, fungicides, and fumigants).

Chapter 26 involves all organic chemicals—from solvents to large, persistent highly halogenated aromatic compounds such as PCBs or TCDD.

Chapter 27 examines metal toxicity.

Chapter 28 describes compounds that are mainly atmospheric emissions, along with their direct toxicity and environmental alterations that yield indirect toxicity (e.g., CFCs' effects on the ozone layer and UV toxicity). Gases, vapors, aerosols, and radiation highlight the chapter's focus.

Chapter 29 is a chapter derived from the EPA's concerns with pharmaceutical and personal care products that have found their way into the sewage and drinking water of many communities. This ends the environmental section.

Chapter 30 classifies the biological origins and evolution of animal venoms and poisons. As all kingdoms cannot be given separate chapters, poisonings associated with consuming animals are in the animal chapter even though the origins may be from bacteria or even diatoms (plants).

Chapter 31 examines plant poisons and finishes the book.

An appendix is given that includes answers to the questions poised in each chapter for students to test their understanding.

Acknowledgments

I would like to acknowledge my colleagues at Minnesota State University who helped me comprehend the evolution of toxicants from phages to bacteria (Dr. Dorothy Wrigley) and other more complex organisms (Dr. Robert Sorensen). We all stand on the shoulders of preceding published work in our fields, and we must acknowledge the people who published scientific accounts of their work (and the easy access to this literature by the invention of the Internet). I would like to thank the people at Jones & Bartlett Learning who have guided this project forward, including Mike Brown, Chloe Falivene, Nick Alakel, Rebekah Linga, and Mary Flatley. Finally, I would like to thank my family for putting up with my writing and discussion of the writing effort over the last 7 years.

About the Author

Steven D. Mercurio is Professor of Biology at Minnesota State University, Mankato. He instituted the toxicology emphasis in the Department of Biological Sciences in 1986 and has served as the program coordinator. Dr. Mercurio has taught Introduction to Toxicology, Environmental Toxicology, Principles of Pharmacology, Industrial Hygiene, Toxicology Seminar, Methods of Applied Toxicology and Applied Toxicology Project. He has worked with many undergraduates and graduate students in a variety of research areas in toxicology. In addition to being an AAAS-EPA Fellow in 1995, his memberships include the Society for Environmental Toxicology and Chemistry, Society of Toxicology, New York Academy of Sciences, American Association for the Advancement of Science, and American Society for Nutritional Sciences. His BA, MA, and PhD were from the University of Pennsylvania and he held postdoctoral positions at University of Minnesota and Cornell University prior to his current position.

Introduction

The novel approach of this book is based on the responses of cells from the outside in—for example, moving from bacteria, fungi, or algae or cell suspensions to those of complex organisms to ecosystems exposed to foreign compounds or xenobiotics or higher than normal levels of compounds normally found in that organism. Toxicology is an "umbrella" perspective from which to view biology according to the ways compounds and physical insults stress organisms to the point of sickness or death.

CHAPTER 1

Biological Research in Toxicology

This is a chapter outline intended to guide and familiarize you with the content to follow.

Why a Three-Level Approach (Cellular, Complex Organism, Ecosystem)?

Amount (dose) of a drug you take orally, like acetaminophen →

May affect digestive structures based on the amount →

May affect the liver if the structure is altered into a more water-soluble form that may be even more toxic than the original compound you took →

Becomes a concentration in the bloodstream →

Affects other organs/cells based on the reactivity of the compound and its metabolites, concentration, time of exposure, and receptors/sensitivity →

May affect excretory organs on its way out of the system →

If you get sick due to the medicine and your system reacts, including through an allergic reaction →

Morbidity → If you die → Mortality—your excreted drug and its metabolites become part of the ecosystem and may affect other living organisms in that ecosystem

WHY IS INHALATION MORE DANGEROUS (SUCH AS CIGARETTE SMOKE)? CONCENTRATION OF GAS + SOLID PARTICLES DAMAGE AND/OR PASS THROUGH LUNG → GASES BECOME HIGH BLOOD CONCENTRATIONS IN RELATIVELY UNMETABOLIZED FORM → GO STRAIGHT THROUGH HEART TO BRAIN.

CONCENTRATIONS AND EXPOSURE TIME ARE IMPORTANT FOR CELLULAR TOXICITY AND ECOTOXICITY (STREAM ANALOGOUS TO BLOOD CIRCULATION AND INTERDEPENDENT ORGANISMS ANALOGOUS TO SPECIALIZED ORGANS). INSTRUCTORS AND STUDENTS ARE ENCOURAGED THROUGHOUT THE TEXT TO USE LOCAL EXAMPLES OF TOXICITY (MORBIDITY AND MORTALITY). OPINIONS OF AUTHOR THROUGHOUT THE TEXT ARE POINTS FOR DISCUSSION AS ONE VIEWPOINT.

B. WHY ARE THE BIOLOGICAL SCIENCES SO CENTRAL TO TOXICOLOGY AND WHY THE DETAIL

IN THE BOOK (Author's opinion for discussion)?

PHYSICAL SCIENCES ↔	BIOLOGICAL SCIENCES ↔	MEDICAL SCIENCES
Measurement/Characterization	Biological Assays	Case Reports
Environmental Fate	Biological Fate	Epidemiology
Engineering – Industrial, Environmental	Prophylactic Measures – Nutrition + Pharmacology	Treatment – Medical Assessment
Residue Analyses – Environmental Monitoring	Animal Toxicology – Animal Pathology	Poison Control – Forensics
	↕	

CONCEPTUALIZING TOXICOLOGY 1-1

RISK ASSESSMENT

Statistics/Modeling + Social Sciences/Ethics

↕

PUBLIC POLICY

Pure Food and Drug Act

Environmental Law/Regulations

Political Action

Funding for Toxicology Research

THE DETAIL IN THE BOOK IS THERE TO READ FURTHER IF STUDENTS DESIRE AND FOR INSTRUCTORS TO SELECT MATERIAL THAT THEY FIND RELEVANT OR IMPORTANT FOR THEIR COURSES. IT IS THE AUTHOR'S DESIRE THAT THE PUBLISHER MAKE INDIVIDUAL CHAPTERS DIGITALLY AVAILABLE TO INSTRUCTORS SO THAT THEY CAN ASSEMBLE THEIR OWN CUSTOMIZED BOOK, IF DESIRED, INCORPORATING THEIR OWN MATERIALS AS WELL.

CONCEPTUALIZING TOXICOLOGY 1-1 (*continued*)

The purpose of this text is to prepare future and current students for participation in toxicology research. Experimental evidence is featured throughout the text as the key to understanding discovery through design and data collection.

The historical view assumes that toxicology is the study of poisons, but in fact it is just as appropriate to consider modern toxicology as a way of determining new chemotherapies for cancer, microbial diseases, parasites, or fungal infections. One of the first treatments for syphilis was an arsenic compound. Pesticides help improve yields of crops and are used to remove lice and similar organisms from animals and humans. Even the very potent toxin of *Clostridium botulinum* treats a variety of ailments that require selective muscle paralysis. Selective toxicity may be used to harm a pathological infection or cell or group of organisms in an affected host, whether that host is a cell invaded by a virus, a patient experiencing cancer, or an ecosystem being populated by an invasive species of plant or animal.

According to the Society of Toxicology, "Toxicology is the study of the adverse effects of chemical, physical, or biological agents on living organisms and the ecosystem, including the prevention and amelioration of such adverse effects." This definition indicates that the field of toxicology encompasses antidotes, study of dose and overdose, and other research enterprises investigating the mechanisms of untoward effects exerted by a variety of chemicals, radiation, or other substances on cells, tissues/organs, complex organisms, and ecosystems (**Conceptualizing Toxicology 1-1**). Mathematical modeling of these effects in determining exposure, hazard, and risk also involves toxicology researchers.

Toxicology Research Area Specialties

Based on the large number of organizations involved and the interdisciplinary scope of modern toxicology, it is difficult to pinpoint all the research areas covered by toxicology. Rather than dissect what toxicology research may be, a listing by major organizations promoting toxicology research gives an indication of its breadth and importance to scientific research and society in general.

Society of Toxicology

The Society of Toxicology has specialty sections in biological modeling; carcinogenesis; comparative and veterinary toxicology; dermal toxicology; drug discovery toxicology; ethical, legal, and social issues; food safety; immunotoxicology; in vitro and alternative methods; inhalation and respiratory; mechanisms; metals; mixtures; molecular biology; neurotoxicology; occupational and public health; regulatory and safety evaluation; reproductive and developmental toxicology; risk assessment; and toxicologic and exploratory pathology.

Food and Drug Administration, National Center for Toxicological Research

The National Center for Toxicological Research has eight major divisions, including biochemical toxicology, genetic and reproductive toxicology, microbiology, neurotoxicology, personalized nutrition and medicine, systems toxicology, and veterinary services.

U.S. Environmental Protection Agency, Office of Research and Development

The Office of Research and Development hosts a computational toxicology center and has eight national research programs focusing on clean air, drinking water, ecological issues, global change, human health, land, pesticides and toxic substances, and water quality.

National Institute of Environmental Health Sciences

The five programs of the National Institute of Environmental Health Sciences (NIEHS) are environmental biology, environmental disease and medicine, clinical research, environmental toxicology, and the National Toxicology Program. The current areas of research for the National Toxicology Program are DNA-based products, endocrine-disrupting agents, genetic alterations in cancer, herbal medicines, hexavalent chromium, occupational mixtures and exposures, phototoxicity, radiofrequency radiation, safe drinking water, and toxicogenomics. NIEHS also houses two scientific interest groups: (1) alternate test systems and ecotoxicology faculty and (2) toxicokinetics faculty.

Hamner Institutes for Health Sciences, Chemical Industry Institute of Toxicology

The Chemical Industry Institute of Toxicology promotes a systems biology paradigm for human health research incorporating functional genomics, computational biology, and bioinformatics.

Society of Environmental Toxicology and Chemistry

According to its membership, "SETAC [Society of Environmental Technology and Chemistry] promotes the advancement and application of scientific research related to contaminants and other stressors in the environment, education in the environmental sciences, and the use of science in environmental policy and decision-making."

National Institute for Occupational Safety and Health, National Occupational Research Agenda

The National Occupational Research Agenda encompasses programs in agriculture, forestry, and fishing; construction; health care and social assistance; manufacturing; mining; oil and gas extraction subsector; services; transportation, warehousing and utilities; and wholesale and retail trade. Cross-sector programs are more directly related to toxicology issues, such as cancer, reproductive, and cardiovascular diseases; exposure assessment; health hazard evaluation; hearing loss prevention; immune and dermal diseases; musculoskeletal disorders; nanotechnology; occupational health disparities; personal protective technology; prevention through design; radiation dose reconstruction; respiratory diseases; surveillance; traumatic injury; and work organization and stress-related disorders.

Selected Research Experiments to Consider During Your Study of Toxicology

As the study of toxicology presented in this text is organized based on the various levels of biological organization, the following controversial studies should provoke some discussion as study of the toxicology field progresses.

Cellular Toxicology

Cellular toxicology involves all functions related to the cell in isolation rather than as part of a tissue, organ, or larger organism. Fields such as microbiology or cell biology deal mainly with issues of cellular toxicology. The focus of modern biology, however, is to determine the functions of the nucleus and signal transduction mechanisms. In turn, the following example uses a historically significant toxicological assay as a point for discussion and scientific controversy.

Development and Use (Misuse) of the Bacterial Mutagenesis Assay

Ames and coworkers (1973) devised a cellular method for identifying mutagenesis (i.e., alteration of DNA) that might potentially lead to oncogenesis (i.e., cancer formation) in the mid-1960s. Their test initially relied on a strain of the bacterium *Salmonella typhimurium* and mutations of the *hisT* gene. This bacterial strain required histidine for growth and experienced a small amount of spontaneous mutations back to the strain that did not require histidine

(3–4 colonies per plate). Three plates of these bacteria were kept as controls in a mutagenesis test (3 is the minimum number required to determine a mean and a standard deviation). At least three plates had a known amount of a mutagen added, which produced a high degree of revertants to the strain that did not require histidine for growth (approximately 4000 colonies per plate, which served as the positive control). The test substance was put on three other plates and tested for the chemical's innate ability to cause mutations (revertants).

This method worked well for mutagens that did not require metabolic activation, but many of the substances considered to be carcinogenic and mutagenic require activation. Thus, in the early 1970s, Ames and coworkers decided to add endoplasmic reticulum preparations (microsomes) from rat liver taken in a sterile manner to the preparation to detect those chemicals that required activation by metabolism. The rationale was that much of the metabolic activity of mammals is found in the liver cells in the microsomal fraction (**Figure 1-1**). For years, this technique served as a key test for putative carcinogens.

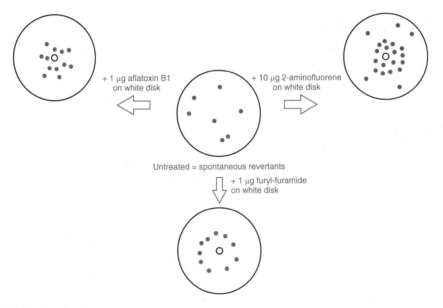

FIGURE 1-1 The Ames Spot Test

Note: The diagram shows petri plate containing a thin overlay of agar, a trace of histidine and biotin, and the bacterial tester strain *Streptococcus typhimurium* TA98 (mutant that needs histidine to grow). The middle plate shows that a small spontaneous reversion rate occurs to bacteria not requiring histidine to grow. The plate below the untreated shows the mutagenicity of a compound that does not require activation applied to the center white disk with black border. The plates to the left and right of the untreated plate show the mutagenicity of metabolites of polycyclic aromatic hydrocarbons (PAHs) to the left and right including rat liver microsomes enriched with a cytochrome P450 required for metabolic activation of PAHs (arachlor-treated rats).

In later years, Ames and Gold (1990) criticized the use of this assay by regulatory agencies. Ames, Profet, and Gold (1990) noted that the indole carbinol concentrated from broccoli and tested in the assay were as mutagenic as many of the restricted ingredients in synthetic chemicals. Ames also criticized the animal models used in such testing. A factor that would increase the growth rate of bacterial cells or animal cells was certain to increase the mutagenesis rate, leading too many chemicals to be identified as "putative human carcinogens." As Ames pointed out, the use and interpretation of a toxicological assay should adequately model the disease state in the species that interventions were being used to prevent before findings based on that assay were incorporated into government regulations.

Use of Toxicogenomics in Modern Toxicology

How do modern toxicologists propose to model the effects of mutations on cells? The abstract of the article by Gomase and Tagore (2008, p. 250) offers an excellent description of modern methods for looking for more specific information on genetic disruption via a variety of mechanisms:

Toxicogenomics is defined as an integration of genomics (transcriptomics, proteomics, and metabolomics) and toxicology. It is a scientific field that studies how the genome is involved in responses to environmental stressors and toxicants. It combines studies of mRNA expression, cell and tissue-wide protein expression, and metabonomics to understand the role of gene–environment interactions in disease. One of the important aspects of toxicogenomics research is the development and application of bioinformatics tools and databases in order to facilitate the analysis, mining, visualizing, and sharing of the vast amount of biological information being generated in this field. This rapidly growing area promises to have a large impact on many other scientific and medical disciplines as scientists could now generate complete descriptions of how

components of biological systems work together in response to various stresses, drugs, or toxicants.

This is not the only type of damage done to cells, nor is it the only way of testing for damage. An easy approach to look for gross DNA damage is the Comet assay, which will be discussed in more detail in the *Damage to Nuclear Structures/DNA: Mutagenesis and Carcinogenesis* chapter. Chemicals can also damage the membranes of cells via lipid peroxidation, alter membrane proteins in general, or abusively stimulate specific receptors. Cytosolic enzymes may be inhibited or damaged. Mitochondria or chloroplasts may be injured and the cell's ability to produce energy disrupted. The structure of the endoplasmic reticulum may be damaged by chemicals or their metabolites (recall that this structure is the major source of the cell's ability to metabolize foreign chemicals or xenobiotics). Other structures also have storage or metabolizing properties that can lead to untoward effects, such as the Golgi apparatus, peroxisomes, and lysosomes. It is the job of the toxicologist to predict the harm done by each specific insult to a part of the cell, tissue, or organs and use that information to provide data for pathologists and modelers, or develop antidotes or protective measures that can be taken to limit damage or exposure.

Organ/Complex Organism Toxicology

Organ/organism toxicology indicates that tissues, organs, and whole complex (multiple-organ) organisms may have selective toxicity or appear to be unaffected by certain toxins. European quails (*Coturnix coturnix coturnix*) have eaten hemlock (*Conium maculatum*) seeds and demonstrated no apparent toxicity, while humans consuming those birds have succumbed to the alkaloid coniine in the quails based on biblical references investigated by science (Sergent, 1941). Chocolate toxicity in dogs is another example of a species-specific toxin (Sutton, 1981). Additionally, certain toxins are more neurotoxic, others are more toxic to metabolizing organs such as the liver, and still others are more toxic to excretory organs like the kidney.

As an example of metabolic activation, Hodgson and coworkers (1980) gave an intravenous injection of the ^{14}C-labeled esophageal carcinogen *N*-nitrosomethylbenzylamine into male Wistar rats and watched for its distribution into tissue and the appearance of its metabolites. The target organ had a higher conversion rate to an activated (more carcinogenic) form than the other organs despite the route of administration. Many compounds that form active metabolites in the liver would be expected to damage the organ with the highest metabolic rate (but not for all metabolic pathways). However, at lower doses, the glutathione conjugated forms of active metabolites that are less toxic to the liver become more toxic to the excretory kidney. The kidney also has some metabolism routes that are favored more than in the liver (Monks et al., 1996).

The complexity of the organism, the proliferation of toxicology tests, and related regulatory issues in toxicology are excellent discussion topics for toxicology testing in the 21st century that have been addressed by some authors (Meek and Doull, 2009).

Ecosystem Toxicology

In ecosystems, the presence of high concentrations of industrial chemicals has caused alterations in certain microbe populations, with selected animal and plant life not being sustained. The classic example of an oil spill and its effect on soil microbes and the aquatic community of a bay area gives some idea of the type of effects expected with an accidental release of a high toxic concentration of a chemical. However, air pollution as well as pesticide and fertilizer applications are also regulated, yet have effects on ecosystems, the atmospheric composition of gases, and the radiation impact on the earth. More subtle effects have been discovered with low concentrations of mixtures that are not overtly toxic, but disrupt the early stages of development of organisms. One example of this phenomenon is found in the work of Hayes and coworkers (2002). In their study, when *Xenopus laevis* larvae were exposed to more than 0.1 parts per billion (ppb) atrazine, exposed males developed hermaphroditism (male and female organs) and less masculine features of the larynges (**Figure 1-2**).

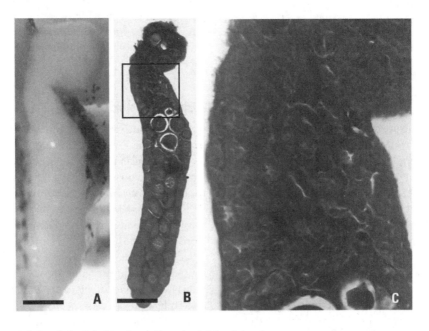

FIGURE 1-2 Left Gonad of a Male *Rana Pipiens* Treated with 0.1 ppb Atrazine

Note: A = Bouin's fixed section B = sagittal section that is almost completely converted into an ovary C = magnification indicating testicular lobules but lacking germ cells.
Reproduced from Hayes T, Haston K, Tsui M, Hoang A, Haeffele C, Vonk A. 2003. *Environ Health Perspect.* 111:568–575.

Other researchers have found feminized male fish in the Mississippi River, including the induction of egg yolk protein or vitellogenin (Folmar et al., 2001). This finding has created a controversy over whether any restriction of the use of certain chemicals would be sufficient to prevent these ultra-low concentration-induced effects. It is also important to note that these developmental anomalies are actually reduced at higher concentrations of atrazine, which are more overtly toxic to these organisms. Much higher concentrations of the herbicide atrazine appear to impact algae and other species that rely on the oxygen and food source produced by those algae, including the aquatic insect community (Dewey, 1986). These findings have been met with counterclaims from other scientists, who cite a lack of effects in their studies (Du Preez et al., 2008). These claims must be discussed and reanalyzed both in the field and in the laboratory to ascertain the validity of the research and to clarify which untoward effects can be demonstrated and which functions remain unaltered by atrazine at a given concentration in the environment.

In recent decades, amphibians have become the new "canary in the coal mine" for detection of ecosystem effects of chemicals. A rush to characterize all malformations of amphibians as related to chemical release is unwise, as various direct and indirect insults can result in malformations. For example, chlorofluorocarbons (CFCs) are not overtly toxic to amphibians. However, the increase in ultraviolet radiation in the atmosphere due to the decrease in stratospheric ozone caused by CFCs—an effect amplified by high altitude—has been recognized as an indirect toxic effect of the release of these chemicals (Blaustein et al., 1997).

Likewise, a rush to unproven conclusions led students at a Henderson, Minnesota, high school to believe they had found frog malformations consistent with the heavy agricultural use of pesticides in the Minnesota River valley. More-thorough examination proved that a trematode parasite *Ribeiroia ondatrae* had caused the malformations (Johnson et al., 2007). Nevertheless, while this case might not appear to be a toxicological problem, that conclusion is not altogether warranted. The presence of excess nitrate and phosphorus promotes the growth of snails and parasites that infest the amphibians. Thus two excess nutrients that are directly toxic to some aquatic life and that stimulate eutrophication of wetlands lead to increases in snail and parasite infestations. As this case suggests, it is not always clear where scientists should draw the line as to what is a direct toxic impact versus what may be indirect or not toxicological at all. That is the basis for this text and this discussion.

Other ecosystem problems that have been documented involve endocrine disruption of aquatic organisms. Altered serum sex steroids and vitellogenin induction in walleye (*Stizostedion vitreum*) collected near a metropolitan sewage treatment plant (Folmar et al., 2001), masculinizing effects of runoff from paper mills on female fish (Parks et al., 2001), thyroid disruption caused in amphibians (Goleman et al., 2002), and other disturbing decreases in human and animal fertility, higher rates of malformations, and other reproductive and behavioral changes (Martinovic et al., 2007) have increasingly been reported in the literature. These changes result from exposure of organisms to anthropogenic sources of chemicals such as pesticides and pharmaceuticals. Toxicity to humans or other organisms reduces the viability of those species, as they may not be able to adapt to a changing ecosystem also impacted by climate change. In addition, much higher concentrations of commonly used chemicals such as nitrate fertilizers have resulted in dramatic changes in the rivers and even impacted human populations (e.g., through nitrate oxidation of hemoglobin to methemoglobin, a form of hemoglobin that does not bind oxygen, in infants). These findings indicate that chemical releases of all types at different concentration ranges have far-reaching impacts that stress the ecosystem.

Biology as the Arbiter of Toxicology

Given that toxicological impacts are related to biological reactions to various insults, biology

CELLULAR CHAPTERS

TOXICANT CONTACTS CELL
↓
INTERACTS WITH CELL MEMBRANE
↓
ABSORBED/NOT ABSORBED/DAMAGES MEMBRANE
↓
DAMAGES MEMBRANE PROTEINS OR ABUSIVELY STIMULATES MEMBRANE RECEPTORS
↓
DETOXICATED ← ABSORBED TOXICANT → ACTIVATED
↓
CYTOSOLIC DAMAGE
↓
DAMAGES ENERGY ORGANELLES
↓
DAMAGES NUCLEUS/DNA
↓
GENETICS ALTERS CELLULAR RESPONSE
↓
NUTRIENTS ALTER CELLULAR RESPONSE

TISSUE/ORGAN/ COMPLEX ORGANISM CHAPTERS

TOXICANT CONTACTS WHOLE ORGANISM BY DIFFERENT ROUTES
↓
ORGANISM RESPONDS/DOES NOT RESPOND
↓
SKIN AND EYE MOST LIKELY ACCIDENTAL EXPOSURE ROUTES FOR DOSE OR CONCENTRATION
↓
ORGANISM INGESTS TOXICANT DOSE AND AFFECTS G.I. TRACT AND BEGINS METABOLISM
↓
ORGANISM INHALES A CONCENTRATION
↓
CARDIOVASCULAR TRANSPORT – DOSE BECOMES A DOSAGE/CONCENTRATION AND HAS EFFECTS
↓
TRAVELS VIA BLOOD AND LYMPHATIC SYSTEM AND DAMAGES MARROW, LYMPH NODES AND/OR SPLEEN
↓
CIRCULATES TO PERIPHERAL NERVOUS SYSTEM AND VIA BLOOD-BRAIN BARRIER TO CENTRAL
NERVOUS SYSTEM
↓
DAMAGES NEURAL AND NEUROENDOCRINE FUNCTIONS
↓
AFFECTS REPRODUCTIVE FUNCTIONS AND DEVELOPING ORGANISMS
↓
DAMAGES EXCRETORY ORGANS AS IT IS ELIMINATED

ECOSYSTEM CHAPTERS

CHEMICALS OR BIOLOGICAL AGENTS DISPERSE INTO ENVIRONMENT
↓
SOURCE OF CHEMICAL DETERMINES ECOSYSTEM EXPOSED
↓
AGRICULTURAL SOURCES, DISPERSIONS AND IMPACTS
↓
INDUSTRIAL ORGANIC CHEMICALS THAT BIODEGRADE
↓
INDUSTRIAL METALS THAT ARE ALTERED BUT DON'T DEGRADE
↓
VOLATILES FROM INDUSTRY, TRANSPORTATION, AGRICULTURE AND ATMOSPHERIC IMPACTS
↓
PHARMACEUTICAL AND PERSONAL CARE PRODUCTS

BIOLOGICAL AGENTS

ANIMAL PROTECTION AND DIGESTION -VENOM INJECTION AS THE USUAL ROUTE OF
ADMINISTRATION VERSUS POISON INGESTION
↓
PLANT PROTECTIVE TOXINS –
CONTACT VERSUS INGESTION

FIGURE 1-3 Flow Outline of Biological Focus of Toxicant Action

should be the crux of toxicology. Chemical modeling, dispersion modeling, and structure-activity relationships are important components of chemical toxicology. However, these models should not be a total substitute for exposing and noting the effects of the insult on the cell, organism, or ecosystem and protecting these entities from toxic action. For instance, the effect of an insecticide on nontarget species, such as bees, is important for protection of plant pollinators.

Government agencies now insist on research involving chemical models, animal testing, and finally human clinical trials for pharmaceuticals. Effectiveness with limited toxicity must be ascertained for all medicinal substances before they are approved for sale. In earlier times of U.S. history, however, prisoners and volunteers were given pesticides to test their reactions. Chemists of the past, when they synthesized new compounds, often smelled and tasted their newly synthesized structures. People exposed themselves to vectors of disease and died to prove how transmission occurred. Soldiers were marched to ground zero, where an atomic weapon had recently been exploded in the atmosphere.

Society has since determined that voluntary and involuntary testing of dangerous chemicals, radiation, and biological agents must be eliminated for safety and ethical reasons. Alternatives to animal testing are sought to eliminate inhumane treatment and avoid unnecessary retesting of cosmetics and like substances that contain reformulations of ingredients that have already been tested numerous times. The costs of testing can be exorbitant as well, especially if primates are involved.

The role of the toxicologist is to determine previously unknown effects of agents or mixtures of agents currently in use, test those agents as required by government agencies using standard methods, develop testing models for government regulation, ascertain when the use of biological species is necessary and when mathematical modeling alone should suffice, and predict effects of yet to be synthesized substances based on similar agents tested previously. A thorough knowledge of biology, chemistry, mathematics, and physics is required to understand the full gamut of these effects. The ability to communicate the information in the form of risk is important to society as well.

The outline of the study of toxicology in this text follows a logical form based on the way a cell and then an organ/complex organism is likely to be exposed to a substance and its harmful effects (**Figure 1-3**). The ecosystem is the next order of biological complexity. How ecosystems distribute, alter, and are impacted by toxicants will be examined. The chemical group is addressed based on the ability of the organism to handle or succumb to that chemical concentration by different biological mechanisms. The presentation of biological toxicants is based on the protection they provide from predators, the digestive needs of the animal, and the methods that plants use to protect themselves from predation by inclusion of toxins in seeds or other plant structures.

Questions

1. What are the three different levels of toxicological analyses, and how might concentration of a toxicant play a role in all three levels?
2. What is the future of toxicology research?
3. How does the Ames test inform scientists about the proper use of toxicology testing?

References

Ames BN, Gold LS. 1990. Too many rodent carcinogens: mitogenesis increases mutagenesis. *Science.* 249:970–971.

Ames BN, Lee FD, Durston WE. 1973. An improved bacterial test system for the detection and classification of mutagens and carcinogens. *Proc Natl Acad Sci USA.* 70:782–7866.

Ames BN, Profet M, Gold LS. 1990. Nature's chemicals and synthetic chemicals: comparative toxicology. *Proc Natl Acad Sci USA.* 87:7782–7786.

Blaustein AR, Kiesecker JM, Chivers DP, Anthony RG. 1997. Ambient UV-B radiation causes deformities in amphibian embryos. *Proc Natl Acad Sci USA.* 94:13735–13737.

Dewey SL. 1986. Effects of the herbicide atrazine on aquatic insect community structure and emergence. *Ecology.* 67:148–162.

Du Preez LH, Kunene N, Everson GJ, Carr JA, Giesy JP, Gross TS, Hosmer AJ, Kendall RJ, Smith EE, Solomon KR, Van Der Kraak GJ. 2008. Reproduction, larval growth, and reproductive development in African clawed frogs (*Xenopus laevis*) exposed to atrazine. *Chemosphere.* 71:546–552.

Folmar LC, Denslow ND, Kroll K, Orlando EF, Enblom J, Marcino J, Metcalfe C, Guillette LJ Jr. 2001. Altered serum sex steroids and vitellogenin induction in walleye (*Stizostedion vitreum*) collected near a metropolitan sewage treatment plant. *Arch Environ Contam Toxicol.* 40:392–398.

Goleman WL, Urquidi LJ, Anderson TA, Smith EE, Kendall RJ, Carr JA. 2002. Environmentally relevant concentrations of ammonium perchlorate inhibit development and metamorphosis in *Xenopus laevis. Environ Toxicol Chem.* 21:424–430.

Gomase VS, Tagore S. 2008. Toxicogenomics. *Curr Drug Metab.* 9:250–254.

Hayes TB, Collins A, Lee M, Mendoza M, Noriega N, Stuart AA, Vonk A. 2002. Hermaphroditic, demasculinized frogs after exposure to the herbicide atrazine at low ecologically relevant doses. *Proc Natl Acad Sci USA.* 99:5476–5480.

Hodgson RM, Wiessler M, Kleihues P. 1980. Preferential methylation of target organ DNA by the oesophageal carcinogen *N*-nitrosomethylbenzylamine. *Carcinogenesis.* 1:861–866.

Johnson PT, Chase JM, Dosch KL, Hartson RB, Gross JA, Larson DJ, Sutherland DR, Carpenter SR. 2007. Aquatic eutrophication promotes pathogenic infection in amphibians. *Proc Natl Acad Sci USA.* 104:15781–15786.

Martinovic D, Hogarth WT, Jones RE, Sorensen PW. 2007. Environmental estrogens suppress hormones, behavior, and reproductive fitness in male fathead minnows. *Environ Toxicol Chem.* 26(2):271–278.

Meek B, Doull J. 2009. Pragmatic challenges for the vision of toxicity testing in the 21st century in a regulatory context: another Ames test? . . . or a new edition of "the Red Book"? *Toxicol Sci.* 108:19–21.

Monks TJ, Rivera MI, Mertens JJ, Peters MM, Lau SS. 1996. The kidney as a target for biological reactive metabolites: linking metabolism to toxicity. *Adv Exp Med Biol.* 387:203–212.

Parks LG, Lambright CS, Orlando EF, Guillette LJ Jr, Ankley GT, Gray LE Jr. 2001. Masculinization of female mosquitofish in Kraft mill effluent-contaminated Fenholloway River water is associated with androgen receptor agonist activity. *Toxicol Sci.* 62:257–267.

Sergent E. 1941. Les cailles empoisonneuses daus la Bible—et en Algerie de nos jours: apercu historique et recherches experimentales. *Arch Institut Pasteur Alger.* 19:161–192.

Sutton RH. 1981. Cocoa poisoning in a dog. *Vet Rec.* 109:563–564.

CHAPTER 2

Development of the Field
of Toxicology

This is a chapter outline intended to guide and familiarize you with the content to follow.

The field of toxicology developed from defensive poisons used by plants and animals, which were adapted as means of defense for a human tribe. Poisoning, poisoners, and executions by poison subsequently gave rise to more thoughtful analyses (in early Chinese medical texts 2000 years prior to the Common Era or B.C.E. and in Western medical texts in early C.E. or A.D.). At the end of the Middle Ages, the idea that everything can be poisonous at some **dosage** (amount per body weight or body area) arose. Occupations that resulted in poisoning, such as mining, were recognized and mechanisms of toxicity first described by physiologists of the 19th century. The 20th century marked the true beginning of the scientific field of toxicology, with the passage of the Pure Food and Drug Act occurring in the United States. Mass poisoning by industrial release of mercury in Minimata Bay, Japan, compelled the founding of the Society of Toxicology. Not until 1970 did the U.S. Environmental Protection Agency (EPA) and first text in toxicology come into existence, however. Quantitative tests continue being discussed and developed, and Syria's use of chemical weapons in 2013 is only the latest indication that warfare and poisoners still exist.

CONCEPTUALIZING TOXICOLOGY 2-1

The fish of the family *Toxotidae* are known as archerfish; the family name is derived from the Greek word *toxeuma*, meaning "arrow" or "archer." The biological and Greek origins of the word *toxicology* indicate the first designed use of a toxin. Given that *toxeuma* means "arrow" or "archer" while *toxicos* means "poison or toxic substance," the combination suggests a poisoned arrow used in earliest times to target prey more effectively, with the spoils from the hunt then being eaten (Trestrail, 2000). Others suggest *toxicology* just means "toxic," simply referring to a substance that causes death (Ramoutsaki et al., 2000). Both the etymology of the word *toxicology* and its most primitive and clever use suggests a targeted poison that can incapacitate or kill one's prey, which if consumed intelligently or in the proper amount will not cause harm to the hunter. This understanding is important, because it suggests that the hunter societies employed a form of toxicology in which they weighed the size of their prey against their body size and the potency of the agent employed (**Conceptualizing Toxicology 2-1**). That distinction separates a poisoner from a toxicologist.

One of the most famous of the substances used by hunters in this way is D-tubocurarine, which, after a long search by a number of explorers and scientists, was isolated from the liana or vine of the rainforest of the species *Chrondrodendrum tomentosum* (**Figure 2-1**) (Lee, 2005). Other members of that plant species also yield similar toxic alkaloids. *Dendrobates auratus* and some other frog and toad species as well as one bird species produce a variety of defensive toxins, which vary in toxicity from bitter alkaloids that mainly induce vomiting to highly

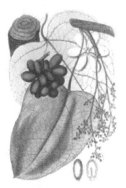

FIGURE 2-1 The Source of ᴅ-Tubocurarine Used to Paralyze or Kill Animals or Invading Spaniards in South America

Reproduced from Ruiz H, Pavon J. 1798. *Systema Vegetabilum Florae Peruvianae et Chilensis.* Madrid.

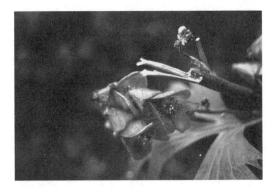

FIGURE 2-2 Monks-Hood Plant Containing the Poison Aconite

Reproduced from USDA http://plants.usda.gov/core/profile?symbol=ACONI accessed 06/10/16

toxic chemicals that can be used as deadly poisons in darts. These natural poisons will be discussed in more detail later in this text, but are recognized here as important agents for primitive toxicologists.

Earlier toxicology was more likely to be based on experience with the group of substances, taste, or aversion to certain ingested items after consuming a nonlethal but toxic dose. Animals that were poisonous or venomous and plants that were poisonous were avoided. Sour taste indicated that a food was possibly spoiled due to increased acidity. Bitter taste was associated with many toxic or medicinal herbs. However, taste cannot be relied upon as a test of toxicity. For example, Romans boiled old acidic wine in lead-lined vessels, thereby forming "sugar of lead" or lead acetate. This process turned "old" wine into "new" sweet wine—and caused significant poisoning of the Roman elite, with little warning of the toxic effects of the sweet drink.

Likewise, group avoidance is unreliable as a way to ascertain toxicity. Northern Europeans were wary of the tomato plant due to its resemblance to toxic atropine-containing members of the *Solanceae* family. Preparations of the latter plants were used to dilate the eyes to make women appear more attractive (thus deadly nightshade called *Atropus belladonna* [Cox, 2000]).

Atropus belladonna, *Aconitum napellus* (wolfsbane), *Colchicum autummale* (meadow saffron), and *Conium maculatum* (hemlock) were poisons of folklore (Holdsworth et al., 2001). *Aconitum napellus* (**Figure 2-2**) contains the cardiotoxic alkaloid aconite, which was used as an arrow poison by the ancient Chinese and has current use in homeopathy for its analgesic and anti-inflammatory properties (Guha et al., 1999). *Colchicum autummale* contains the alkaloid colchicine, which interferes with microtubule formation and was considered too toxic for ancient or medieval use. *Conium maculatum* contains several alkaloids, including coniine, which was famously used in ancient Greece for execution. Coniine causes death—or at lower concentrations, developmental deformities in cattle and other animals—by blocking the nicotinic receptor (Forsyth and Frank, 1993).

Development of the Science of Toxicology

Development Since the 20th Century

The history of toxicology has been provided elsewhere, including in a thumbnail outline on the Internet by Gilbert and Hayes (2006) and in a number of books on poisons and poisonings. The field of toxicology as it is known today is a relative newcomer to the sciences. In the past, toxicology was usually associated with pharmacology departments and was considered a subdiscipline of that field. The first textbook in the field was published in the mid-1970s. The passage of the Pure Food and Drug Act by the U.S. Congress occurred at the beginning of the 20th century (1906), and the U.S. Food and Drug Administration (FDA) was formed 24 years later (1930). The Federal Food, Drug and Cosmetics Act, which empowered the FDA to regulate those substances, took another eight years to pass. Chemical warfare became an issue in World War I (1915), and the chemicals used in that war found some peacetime uses in the treatment of cancer much later in the century.

The first journal of the Society of Toxicology was released at the end of the 1950s, a decade that also saw the mass poisoning of the Japanese population surrounding Minamata Bay, the opening of the first poison control centers, and the introduction and withdrawal of a thalidomide, a medication prescribed for nausea during pregnancy that caused limb deformities in users' offspring. The publication of Rachel Carson's book *Silent Spring* in 1962 signaled growing concerns about the carcinogenicity of industrial and agricultural chemicals. The Occupational Safety and Health Administration and the U.S. Environmental Protection Agency were founded in 1970. Only then did the first regulations on substances such as asbestos in the workplace and chemicals such as the bioaccumulating insecticide dichlorodiphenyltrichloroethane (DDT) start to come under intensive study and regulation.

Other key events that have shaped popular opinion, government oversight, and research in toxicology include the following:

- The neurotoxicity and deaths of Iraqi citizens who consumed ground seed grain coated with methyl mercury in 1971 and 1972
- The poisonings of Bangladeshi citizens due to high concentrations of arsenic in well water
- The illnesses that emerged in the late 1980s when houses were built in Buffalo, New York, on the site of an organic chemical dump known as Love Canal
- The abandonment of the town of Times Beach, Missouri, in 1983 due to high levels of the extremely toxic dioxins

- The atmospheric release of methyl isocyanate used in the manufacture of the insecticide carbaryl, which caused approximately 3800 deaths in Bhopal, India, in 1983
- The enormous radiation release and deaths resulting from the explosion of the Chernobyl nuclear plant in Ukraine in 1986
- The use of the carcinogenic respiratory agent mustard gas and neurotoxic agents sarin, tabun, and VX on the Kurdish population of Halabja, Iraq, by the country's president, Saddam Hussein
- The neurotoxic sarin gas attack launched by a terrorist group in Tokyo in 1995
- The sickness experienced by a patron in a Las Vegas, Nevada, hotel room in 2008 due to the presence of the highly toxic castor bean seed ingredient ricin

Many people are also aware of the respiratory effects of air pollution, the greater risk of melanoma attributed to increased UV irradiation caused by ozone holes, and other environmentally linked diseases. In addition, the adverse effects of some prescription drugs such as Vioxx have resulted in the highly publicized withdrawal of these medications from the market. The growth of organic, natural, and herbal products reflects the increased awareness of the effects of synthetic chemicals on humans, yet many users lack the understanding that many of the natural agents can have toxicity of their own. That is where the history of toxicology becomes important: Members of earlier previous cultures may have better understood those dangers and used these agents at some point as both poisons and medicines.

Pioneers of Toxicology

Scientists now consider which natural substances' toxic nature was well understood in earlier history and how toxicology eventually separated itself from mysticism, alchemy, and other nonscientific practices. Although reports of poisonings have been discovered in writings dating back to 1400 B.C.E. and in conjunction with the religious figure known as Gula (predates to 4500 B.C.E.), it is difficult to separate the science from the theology in antiquity.

Egyptians kings had knowledge of poisonous plants, but their knowledge was secret and forbidden as part of common instruction. They knew about a number of toxic minerals, such as copper, arsenic, and lead. They also knew how to extract the cyanogenic glycoside amygdala from peach pits (Thompson, 1875). In the 1970s, Laetril—the same compound—was marketed as a cancer cure but instead led to cyanide poisoning (of oxidative phosphorylation in mitochondria).

In 40 C.E., Dioscorides created the *Materia Medica* to characterize the animal, vegetable, or mineral origin of various toxic materials. In the Far East, Shen Nung wrote about herbal medicines and poisons as early as 2000 B.C.E. Other accounts of poisonings can be found in the literature of Homer, Aristotle, and Theophrastus. Later in the Roman era, when poisonings were rampant, many more writings on this subject appeared and "experiments" with human tasters or subjects were employed. In the Islamic world, Ibn Wahshiya wrote a book on poisons in 801 C.E. The first large treatise on poisons from insects, snakes, and infected dogs, and their antidotes, was written by Maimonides, who lived in the late 12th and early 13th century.

Theophrastus Phillippus Aureolus Bombastus von Hohenheim, known as the alchemist Paracelsus (1493-1541), is considered by many to be the first to use toxicology language and understanding. According to Paracelsus, "Medicine is not only a science; it is also an art. It does not consist of compounding pills and plasters; it deals with the very processes of life, which must be understood before they may be guided." He recognized that understanding of the biology of the organism should guide the action of remedies or poisons. Paracelsus also noted, "Poison is in everything, and no thing is without poison. The dosage makes it either a poison or a remedy." He understood that low levels of a substance may have no effect, higher levels may produce a positive result, and still higher amounts may lead to toxicity and death. Paracelsus used both the terms *dose* and *dosage*, which are now differentiated as "amount" and "amount per body weight or surface area," respectively. At the same time, his efforts cannot be considered totally scientific based on his mixture of theology, alchemy, and science in various measures.

Geogius Agricola was a contemporary of Paracelsus and described the health effects of mining. As recently as 2008, the effect of taconite on miners' lungs was being investigated by the Minnesota Department of Health, so these issues remain pertinent today.

A number of infamous poisoners who used human subjects, such as Catherine Medici, Hieronyma Spara, Marchioness de Brinvillier, and Catherine Deshayes, can be traced back to the late 1600s. The 1700s and early 1800s brought more scientific analyses from Richard Mead (book of poisons), Percivall Pott (scrotal cancer of chimney sweeps), Felice Fontana (venomous snakes), Philip Physick and Baron Guillaume Dupuytren (orogastric lavage to remove poisons), and Bonaventure Orfila (modern toxicology writings on *Traite de Poisons*). In the same time period as Orfila, Robert Christison wrote a *Treatise on Poisons* and described how acute renal failure could result from poisoning. Francois Megendie discovered the protein synthesis inhibitor of eukaryotes known as emetine and studied the neurotoxic action of strychnine and cyanide. His contemporary James Marsh developed a test for arsenic.

In the 1800s, the famous French physiologist Claude Bernard determined the mechanisms of carbon monoxide and tubocurarine poisoning. Two French scientists of that period self-demonstrated the effectiveness of activated charcoal as an antidote to ingested arsenic (M. Bertrand), and strychnine (P. Tourney). Similar demonstrations with animals (A. Garrod) and other humans (B. Howard Rand) were done in the mid-1800s. O. H. Costill wrote a book on treatments for poisonings, while Theodore Wormley published *Microchemistry of Poisons*. Qualitative tests for arsenic and mercury (Hugo Reinsch) and a quantitative test for small quantities of arsenic (Max Gutzeit) emerged in this period as well.

During the late 1800s and the beginning of the 1900s, cocaine was isolated (Albert Nieman). The cardiotoxin and medication digitalis and the gangrenous and neurotoxic ergot alkaloids, from which LSD was later synthesized by Albert Hofmann (1943), were studied by Rudolf Kobert (1854-1918). His contemporary, Louis Lewin, studied various biological toxins. Alice

Hamilton (1869–1970) made contributions to the industrial hygiene side of toxicology by working to improve working conditions. A number of infamous poisoners were active during this time as well (but will not be recognized here), but an important turning point in stopping anyone from dispensing medicines and poisons was the 1914 Harrison Act, which added penalties for nonmedical uses of these substances.

The science of toxicology experienced exponential growth in the 20th and 21st centuries, as enormous synthetic chemical and pharmaceutical manufacturing operations emerged in Europe and the United States after the 1930s. The environmental effects of these agents started to become apparent and the number of chemicals in common use expanded during the 1950s. Standard methods were developed with greater rigor and more options became available in the latter half of the 1960s, which allowed for the detection and mitigation of some of the impacts of these chemicals.

The field of toxicology continued to expand with the discovery of endocrine disruptors in the mid-1980s. Agreement among researchers and regulatory agencies about which standard assays to use when testing for these effects and which concentrations of individual chemicals, mixtures of chemicals, or chemicals plus radiation are safe has not yet been reached.

It is clear from history that toxicology has moved from a focus on poisoning or induction of death (mortality) to sickness (morbidity) to therapeutic agent versus adverse (side) effects to cancer risk posed by chronic exposure to developmental disruption of what used to be considered trace concentrations. In general, it appears that the field is moving toward analysis of more subtle effects, combinations of agents, and molecular actions of toxins.

Questions

1. What were the earliest uses of toxic agents?
2. What was the key feature that compelled philosophers to think of toxicology as a quantitative science in the Middle Ages?
3. What role did science and catastrophic events play in the development of toxicology in the 20th and 21st centuries?

References

Carson R, Darling L, Darling L. 1962. *Silent Spring*. Cambridge, MA: Houghton Mifflin.

Cox S. 2000. I say tomayto, you say tomahto . . . . http://lamar.colostate.edu/~samcox/Tomato.html.

Forsyth CS, Frank AA. 1993. Evaluation of developmental toxicity of coniine to rats and rabbits. *Teratology*. 48:59–64.

Gilbert SG, Hayes T. 2006. A small dose of toxicology: history of toxicology milestones and discoveries. http://www.asmalldoseof.org/historyoftox/index.php.

Guha S, Dawn B, Dutta G, Chakraborty T, Pain S. 1999. Bradycardia, reversible panconduction defect and syncope following self-medication with a homeopathic medicine. *Cardiology*. 91:268–271.

Holdsworth T, Tasker K, Thompson A, Thomson L, Wiles L, Willis J. 2001. Poisoning through the ages. http://www.portfolio.mvm.ed.ac.uk/studentwebs/session2/group12/index.htm.

Lee MR. 2005. Curare: the South American arrow poison. *J R Coll Physicians Edinb*. 35:83–92.

Ramoutsaki IA, Ramoutsakis YA, Tsikritzis MD, Tsataskis AM. 2000. The roots of toxicology: an etymology approach. *Vet Hum Toxicol*. 42:111.

Thompson CJS. 1875. *Poisons and poisoners*. London: J & A Churchill.

Trestrail, JH. 2000. *Criminal poisoning: investigational guide for law enforcement, toxicologists, forensic scientists, and attorneys*. Totowa, NJ: Humana Press.

CHAPTER 3

Toxicology Terms and How They Relate to Organisms

This is a chapter outline intended to guide and familiarize you with the content to follow.

Cellular Toxicity

[Toxicant]$_{external}$ + time exposed →→ Affects membrane and receptors, or is absorbed → [Toxicant]$_{internal}$ → Affects organelles or metabolites affect organelles →

Threshold [toxicant] = lowest observable effects

Morbidity toxicant concentrations = levels of illness; determines I$_{50}$ (50% inhibition), EC$_{50}$ (50% affected by a defined illness)

Mortality = death (apoptosis = programmed cell death, which is better for surrounding cells; necrosis = releases inflammatory mediators, which is worse for surrounding cells); determines LC$_{50}$ (lethal concentration for 50% of population of cells), LT$_{50}$ (time it takes a given concentration to kill 50% of cells)

Progression occurs as the logarithm of the concentration of toxicant and the standard deviation units response from 50% of the population affected

Complex Organisms

Toxicant dose or dosage → Coupled with route of administration (dermal, oral, intravenous, intraperitoneal, intrathecal, intramuscular, subcutaneous) → TD$_{50}$ (morbidity in 50% of population at a given dose) → LD$_{50}$ (mortality in 50% of population at a given dose)

[Toxicant]$_{external}$ + time exposed → Inhaled or continuously infused intravenously → Affects lung or circulatory structures → Absorbed into organs → Similar to cellular toxicity → EC$_{50}$ → Can be used occupationally to determine threshold limit value (TLV) over an 8-hour work day) → Action level → Permissible exposure limit (PEL) → Immediately dangerous to life or health (IDLH)

Environmental Toxicity

[Toxicant]$_{environmental}$ + time exposed → Determine sensitive organisms in environment by comparing EC$_{50}$ values or LC$_{50}$ values → Model-estimated environmental concentration; determine no observed effect level (NOEL) and lowest observed effect level (LOEL)

CONCEPTUALIZING TOXICOLOGY 3-1

The terms used to describe toxicology are related the organism and how it responds to the chemical, physical, or biological agent. This response reflects the likely route of exposure, the type of insult and the pressure the insult puts on the organism, and the ability of the organism to adapt to the insult. Toxicologists traditionally have focused on the chemical, physical, or biological agent, and only then indicated the effects on organisms for those agents.

This section first addresses the organism, then explains its responses.

The Cell

The cell responds to the environment that surrounds it, which usually takes the form of a water medium. The concentration or amount that causes the first observable effect is called the **threshold** (**Conceptualizing Toxicology 3-1**). Cells respond to concentrations of chemical or biological agents or effects of radiation (by absorption of radiation). The cell may not respond at all to ultra-low concentrations, may become dysfunctional (called sickness or **morbidity**), may be induced into **apoptosis** (programmed cell death), or become necrotic (death, **mortality**, or lethality).

Many responses are receptor mediated or mediated by pH. Both receptors' binding affinities and pH are logarithmic functions; thus log [toxin], ln [toxin], and $e^{-[toxin]}$ are all logarithmic functions that indicate the response to the concentration that appears in the brackets. The last function, $e^{-[toxin]}$, suggests that the response of a substance put into a medium may decline exponentially in three-dimensional space. This is important because the cell is a sphere or similar shape, rather than the two-dimensional object depicted in most diagrams in textbooks.

The use of cells in assessing toxicologic effects is used only with microbial populations, algae, or other single-cellular organisms and is considered an alternative to whole-species testing in vertebrate or other cell cultures (Schirmer, 2006). Some considerations that become less problematic in whole organisms versus cells include (1) static versus flow-through exposure (flow-through creates more sensitivity); (2) viability of cells (individual cells appear more sensitive than whole tissues or organisms); and (3) inability to use different exposure routes.

LC$_{50}$

The toxicology of cells mostly examines the concentration of a substance that kills 50% of the cells or **LC$_{50}$** (lethal concentration 50%) over a defined time period of hours. To determine this value, at least five different concentrations of the substance that cause between 10% and 90% lethality are applied over the determined time period—for example, 2 hours or 96 hours. The reason for using five concentrations and a control group is that any two points make a line and three points are not considered significant in a linear regression ($P < .05$ or 95% confident about the data represented by that line), even if the regression coefficient squared (R^2) = 1.0 (100% of the data fall on that line perfectly). It is better to use five concentrations that cause between 20% and 80% lethality, because the low and high ends then have a floor value of 0% and a ceiling value of 100% dead that cannot be plotted on a logarithmic function and can represent a variety of concentrations.

Zero percent mortality occurs at all concentrations below a certain lowest observed effect concentration (**LOEC**); if lethality is the only function observed, it should actually reflect any adverse effect. In contrast, 100% mortality occurs at all concentrations exceeding the organism's capacity to survive that insult (**Figure 3-1**).

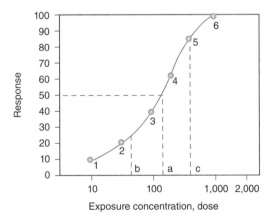

FIGURE 3-1 The Dose-Response Curve for Cellular or Ecotoxicology

Reproduced from Evenden AJ, Depledge MH. 1997. Genetic susceptibility in ecosystems: the challenge for ecotoxicology. *Environ Health Perspect.* 105:849–854.

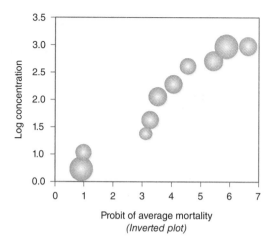

FIGURE 3-2 The Average Percent Mortality Has Been Transformed to a Probit Value and Plotted Against Log Concentration

Data from Paradise CJ. 2001. A standardized soil ecotoxicological test using red worms (Eisenia fetida). *Am Biol Teach.* 63:662–668.

Probits

The response in Figure 3-1 is not linear if viewed as a percent mortality versus log concentration. In contrast, **Figure 3-2** shows what happens if the response is given as a **probit**, or probability versus log concentration, as developed by Miller and Tainter (1944), Litchfield and Wilcoxon (1949), Weil (1952), and Finney (1978). It turns into a straight line because the responses of populations of cells (like organisms) follow a bell curve, with most dying or being otherwise affected at the LC_{50}.

The lethality percentages are spaced about the 50% point based on probit units or standard deviations from the LC_{50}. Based on a probit analysis, one standard deviation above the LC_{50} (probit 5) would be LC_{84} (probit 6), and one standard deviation below the LC_{50} would be LC_{16} (probit 4; both probit 4 and probit 6 are 34% different from the LC_{50}). Thus, one standard deviation on each side of the LC_{50} represents 68% of the population of cells. Two standard deviations would represent 95% of the population, spanning from $LC_{2.5}$ to $LC_{97.5}$.

Concentration–Response Relationship

Another way of determining a toxicity index based on concentration is the LT_{50}—that is,

based on the concentration, the time it takes 50% of the cells to die. For cells, sometimes the lethality or toxicity is related to inhibition of a specific enzyme or binding of an important receptor **agonist** (which produces the normal physiological function at that receptor). For example, the inhibition of cytochrome a_3 by cyanide causes toxicity or death of cells depending on the IC_{50} (or I_{50}; inhibitory concentration 50%), meaning the concentration that inhibits 50% of an enzyme's normal activity or antagonizes binding at a receptor by 50% (an **antagonist** blocks a receptor). Since many of these cells are also used for ecotoxicology analysis, the EC_{50} (exposure concentration 50%, which causes a toxic effect in 50% of the population) is used to estimate toxic endpoints rather than lethal endpoints. The problem with these assays is that cells are likely exposed to pulses of toxicants in the real world, and stochastic modeling and pulse exposures are rarely employed in toxicity testing (Dubinsky, 1995; Neubert et al., 1981).

Tissues, Organs, and Complex Organisms

FDA and Therapeutic Tests

When toxicology moves to tissues and organs, concentration is the factor that usually determines the impact on the organs in an animal. Although the LC_{50} is still an appropriate measure for respiratory exposures, the beagle dog is now the preferred testing organism to model human toxicity in a 4-hour exposure protocol due to its respiratory structure (Takenaka et al., 1998). However, much of the focus of tissue and organ toxicity studies has now moved to therapeutic agents (medicines) and their safety, pesticides' effects on nontarget species, and those agents that are not designed to affect animal or plant species. Therapeutic analysis relies on well-defined tests that must conform to FDA standards.

The FDA has developed standards that apply to cosmetics, food additives, foodborne illness, human biologics, medical devices, nutritional supplements, and veterinary pharmaceuticals. The toxicological information required by the

FDA can be found at http://alttox.org/ttrc/us/regulatory-research-agencies/fda.html.

Toxicological Information Required for Food Additives

- Acute oral toxicity
- Short-term (28 days) toxicity in rodents and non-rodents
- Subchronic (90 days) toxicity in rodents and non-rodents
- Chronic (1–2 years) toxicity in rodents and non-rodents
- Mutagenicity and genotoxicity
- Carcinogenicity (including possible in utero exposure phase)
- Reproductive toxicity
- Developmental toxicity
- Neurotoxicity
- Immunotoxicity
- Metabolism and pharmacokinetics
- Human clinical and/or epidemiology

Toxicological Information Required for Human Pharmaceutical Development

- Toxicokinetics and pharmacokinetics in rodents and/or other species
- Single-dose studies in rodents, and occasionally dogs and primates
- Subacute (14–28 days), subchronic (90 days), and/or chronic (90 or more days) studies in rodents, dogs, and occasionally primates
- Reproduction segment I—fertility studies in rodents
- Reproduction segment II—prenatal developmental toxicity in rodents and rabbits
- Reproduction segment III—postnatal development in rodents
- Mutagenicity and genotoxicity studies of at least two varieties
- Carcinogenicity studies in rats and transgenic mice
- Immunotoxicity in rodents
- Triggered specialized studies (e.g., phototoxicity and pyrogenicity)

Toxicological Information Required for Veterinary Pharmaceuticals

- Subchronic (90 days) and chronic (2 years) toxicity in rodents and/or dogs

- Reproductive toxicity in two or more generations of rodents
- Developmental toxicity in rodents and/or rabbits
- Genotoxicity studies of at least three varieties
- Testing for effects on human intestinal flora
- Pharmacological effects
- Immunotoxicity
- Neurotoxicity
- Carcinogenicity studies in rats and mice
- Triggered "special" studies

Cosmetics (e.g., shampoos, soaps, perfumes, makeup, moisturizers, lipsticks, nail polish, hair colors, toothpastes, and deodorants) are not subject to such extensive testing protocols but instead carry a warning that the agency will not tolerate any improperly labeled or contaminated products that "bears or contains any poisonous or deleterious substance which may render it injurious to users under the conditions of use prescribed in the labeling thereof, or under conditions of use as are customary and usual."

Dose, Dosage, and Response (LD$_{50}$, LD$_{LO}$)

Based on these parameters, the substance must be given in a measured amount (**dose**) to an animal or in a given amount per body weight or amount per surface area (**dosage**). The dose that people take for over-the-counter (OTC) medications may be the same, but the effect may be different based on their age, body weight, sex, genetics, nutritional state, medical conditions, and other medications taken. Note that most OTC medications given to adults are in a dose form—that is, a standard amount in a pill (tablet, capsule, or caplet). Most OTC medications given to children are in liquid dosage form to adjust for age/body weight.

Which compounds are toxic when given as a dose? Acetylsalicylic acid (aspirin) is certainly toxic as a dose to the stomach; it may induce bleeding and ulcers. The amount of drug taken is more important than the body weight in this case. The same medication may be toxic as a dosage when one considers whether aspirin has disturbed the acid–base balance of the blood or cerebrospinal fluid—it must become distributed into the volume of the animal or person to have that deleterious effect. Eye medications are therapeutic as a dose, but are toxic as a dosage. For example, the cat, the baby, and the adult human have large, similarly sized eyes. Atropine would dilate them all. However, based on the size of the brain and the body size, this chemical is more toxic as a dosage to the brain of the cat than to the human baby, and more toxic as a dosage to the baby than to the adult human.

When a toxicologist or pharmacologist wants to identify a similar effect within a species and the effect is due to the concentration in the plasma of that species, then it is appropriate to use dosage in mg/kg or units/kg (amount or activity per body weight) for those members of the species with approximately the same age, body weight, sex, and other characteristics. However, if switching between species or ages, the metabolic rate of the animal tested must be considered. The smaller the animal, the higher the surface area/volume ratio; thus the approximate dosage should be related to the organism's relative surface area rather than its weight to determine which dosage might be appropriate in another species.

For example, the dosage of the OTC analgesic acetaminophen that causes liver toxicity in the mouse is 500 mg/kg (Fischer et al., 1981). The **LD$_{50}$** (lethal dose 50%) is the appropriate measure of danger to life here and is 338 mg/kg orally in mice. For a 0.02-kg mouse, that represents a dose of 10 mg. A dose of 10 mg to a human would have little effect, as two extra-strength acetaminophen pills would contain 1000 mg and be distributed over approximately 70 kg (154 lb; an assumed weight). The same dosage of 500 mg/kg for a 70-kg human would equate to a dose of 35,000 mg! The **LD$_{LO}$** (lethal dose low), or minimum dose that might cause mortality, in humans is 143 mg/kg. Clearly, 500 mg/kg would be a very toxic dose in humans.

In terms of body surface area, the surface area of a mouse is 46 cm^2 while that of a human is 18,000 cm^2. The 10-mg mouse dose yields a 0.217 mg/cm^2 dosage on this basis. The same mg/cm^2 dosage in a human would yield a dose of 3913 mg, which is still approximately four times the recommended dose, so it might cause toxicity. For a 70-kg human, that dose would yield a dosage of 55.9 mg/kg, or almost one-tenth of the mouse dosage. Since toxicity is logarithmic, a factor of 10 difference is significant. Not accounting for metabolic differences, it is clear, might prove fatal.

Effectiveness, Potency, and Therapeutic Safety Measures

Effectiveness is the percentage of the population that responds positively to increased doses or dosages. Some medications improve the status of 100% of the population. Others do well in only certain genetically defined groups; for example, targeted anticancer medications are effective in only a small percentage of the population.

Potency is the entire curve for the substance, such as the LD$_{50}$ curve. If this curve is shifted to the left (i.e., low doses cause large responses), then the substance is considered potent. If the curve is shifted to the right (i.e., high doses cause responses), then the agent has low potency.

Therapeutic agents must show effectiveness, so they must have an **ED$_{50}$** (effective dose 50%) determined. The **TD$_{50}$** or dose of a drug that causes a toxic response in 50% of the tested species (morbidities not causing death) should exceed the ED$_{50}$. The therapeutic index, or **TI = LD$_{50}$/ED$_{50}$**, should be a large number, such as three log units or 1000, for OTC medications. **Figure 3-3A** illustrates these comparisons.

Small numbers (i.e., lower effectiveness) are allowed only for medications that treat terminal diseases, such as treatments for human immunodeficiency virus (HIV) infection or cancer chemotherapies. A safety measure based on the notion that a medication is effective in only half the population or may kill half the population is not very useful, however, so the **margin of safety = LD$_1$/ED$_{99}$**. This ratio assumes a bounded group from "effective in 99% of the population" to "kills 1% of the population." It still can be calculated from the LD$_{50}$ curve, so it does not represent a statistical guess about the shape of the curve at ultra-low doses (assessing a 1 in 10^6 risk is a statistical determination that may be off by a considerable degree by being overprotective or underprotective, depending on the agent).

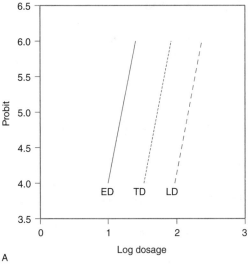

A

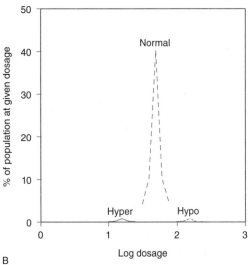

B

FIGURE 3-3 A. ED_{50}, TD_{50}, and LD_{50} for Therapeutic Compounds. B. The Graphical Respresentation of Hypersensitivity and Hyposensitivity. This Graph Is Not a Cumulative Percentage of the Population Responses as in A, but Rather the Percentage of the Population Responding at a Given Dosage.

The LD_{50} is a controversial value as well. Just consider the data for acetaminophen. Even the mouse's LD_{50} for this medication varies from 250 to 400 mg/kg depending on the researcher, the mouse species, and other factors mentioned earlier. The rat oral LD_{50} for acetaminophen has

been listed at 1944 mg/kg (definitely greater than 1000 mg/kg). This would translate to a much higher estimate of the LD_{50} for humans.

Note that the FDA requires testing in multiple species to determine the efficacy or safety of a new agent. Also, the LD_{50} gives only a single value, not a range. The $LD_{50} \mp 1$ S.D. (standard deviation) would be a better measure, since the whole curve would be calculable. For example, two curves with the same LD_{50} would have lower toxicity on the low end for a steep curve, but much higher toxicity with doses above the LD_{50}. Any chemical following this pattern would be a dangerous substance, because it would give little warning prior to killing much of the population. For a toxin or medication with a low slope, there would be some lethality at doses far below the LD_{50}. Sensitive individuals would need to guard against contact with this substance, but the majority of the population would not be affected at those low doses.

Factors That Determine the Lethality/ Toxicity Curve

Although some suggest the LD_{50} is antiquated and should be entirely eliminated, lower doses may not indicate which organs are affected in single or repeated doses, as the animal or human usually has **reserve functional capacity**. An example is a person with chronic alcoholism, who does not show the progressive signs of cirrhosis of the liver. Only a biopsy of the liver at various times and plasma liver enzyme monitoring will indicate liver damage prior to the time that a liver transplant becomes necessary. The lethality curve represents a variety of factors in which reserve functional capacity has been overcome by excessive concentrations.

Genetic variation in a population gives a distribution that, if not plotted as cumulative percent lethality, but rather as the percentage of the remaining population that responds at that dose or concentration, yields a curve on which most people die at the LD_{50}. The curve will be broader in a wild population, but much narrower in a cloned or selectively bred population. Some genetic factors lead to accumulation of the toxin, prolongation of its action, or increased sensitivity to the effects of the chemical.

The increased sensitivity at the far left portion of the lethality curve identifies the **hypersensitive** population. There are two types of hypersensitivity—one in which the hypersensitive individual has the same symptoms experienced by other organisms at a higher dose, and the other in which the individual demonstrates an immune hypersensitivity. For example, mice expressing the CD9 antigen are more sensitive to the diphtheria toxin (Brown et al., 1993). The immune type of hypersensitivity can range from the usual immediate hypersensitivity of an allergic reaction mediated by immunoglobulin E (IgE) and histamine release (e.g., in the reaction to penicillin), to the delayed-type hypersensitivity of a T-cell reaction, to an autoimmune reaction due to modification of cell surface molecules.

On the right extreme end of the lethality curve is the hyposensitive population. **Hyposensitivity** may result from prior exposure and adaptation (e.g., to drugs of abuse or toxin-induced resistance, as reported by Salles et al. [2003]) or a genetic variant with extra protective factors. An example of hyposensitivity involves the decrease in response to androgens such as testosterone in human males with long CAG repeats on their androgen receptor gene; these males are more sensitive to estrogenic influences and breast cancer formation (Backe, 2006). **Figure 3-3B** illustrates the hypersensitive and hyposensitive populations.

The **nutritional state** of an organism can also play a key role in the sensitivity to toxins. Nutritional curves are biphasic toxicity curves, with undernutrition and overnutrition having different influences on the distributions. The curve's lowest toxicity results from adequate nutrition in these two mirror-image toxicity curves. For example, undernutrition in the form of iron (Fe) deficiency causes anemias because less ferritin iron is available for hemoglobin synthesis, while excess iron is stored in the hepatotoxic hemosiderin form. This case shows the direct influence of nutrition on function. Other factors may also impact sensitivity. For example, selenium deficiency causes a decrease in the formation of the antioxidant enzyme glutathione peroxidase, but increases the production of the conjugation enzyme glutathione-S-transferase and the rate of glutathione synthesis. The lack of peroxidase activity makes selenium-deficient animals and humans more prone to lipid peroxidation, renal tubular damage, cardiomyopathies, and other oxidative toxicities from compounds such as the antibiotic nitrofurantoin, diquat, and other oxidation–reduction (redox) cycling compounds. At the same time, the increase in glutathione conjugating ability reduces the toxicity of metabolites of the activated forms of iodipamide, acetaminophen, and aflatoxin B_1 (Burk and Lane, 1983). Molybdenum toxicity may be prevented by excess copper intake (Underwood, 1959), but may cause copper deficiency and reductions in the ability to fight viral infections (Arthington et al., 1996).

Selective toxicity separates toxic action by species. For example, the guinea pig shows an extreme toxicity response to 2,3,7,8-tetrachlorodibenzodioxin (TCDD), which is much less acutely toxic to humans even when considering the differences in these organisms' body surface area ratios. Some differences are even more pronounced, such as the cocoa powder toxicity in dogs and the congenital malformations in rodents caused by prenatal dosing with salicylates (Warkany and Takacs, 1959), which do not appear to be shared with humans. An example of a toxicant that is toxic to humans if it is absorbed is dichlorodiphenyltrichloroethane (DDT). However, DDT is selectively toxic to insects if applied externally, because it is well absorbed through the exoskeleton of the insect (Hayes, 1971) but not the skin of the human. Another example of selective toxicity is the conversion of malathion or parathion to the oxon active form in insects, which inhibits acetylcholinesterase as the preferred rapid route of metabolism (Heath, 1961).

Route of Administration

The route of administration (**Figure 3-4**) is always given with the LD_{50}. This route is important for an intact animal.

The intravenous (IV) and inhalation routes allow the chemical to reach its peak concentration most quickly and, therefore, lead to the highest toxicity for the chemical. Drug abusers

A. FAST HIGH PEAKS (such as used by drug abusers) – LEADS TO OVERDOSE, THRESHOLD TOXICITY

   INHALATION → LUNG → BLOOD → HEART → BRAIN

   INTRAVENOUS (PARENTERAL = INJECTION ROUTE) → BLOOD → GOES TO ORGANS PRIOR TO LIVER METABOLISM

   INTRATHECAL (DIRECT INJECTION INTO CEBROSPINAL FLUID) → BRAIN

B. DELAYED ABSORPTION

   1. PARENTERAL ROUTES (ONLY DELAYED FOR HYDROPHOBIC COMPOUNDS)

      INTRAMUSCULAR → BINDS TO MUSCLE PROTEIN → SLOW RELEASE TO BLOOD

      SUBCUTANEOUS → BINDS TO FAT UNDERLYING SURFACE SKIN CELLS → SLOW RELEASE TO BLOOD

      INTRAPERITONEAL → ABSORBED BY INTESTINAL CELLS FROM ABDOMINAL CAVITY → IF IRRITATES ABDOMEN, WILL GET IMMUNE RESPONSE → PORTAL CIRCULATION TO LIVER → METABOLITES FROM "FIRST PASS" THROUGH LIVER CELLS → BLOOD

   2. USUAL ACCIDENTAL ROUTES OF EXPOSURE

      ORAL (Per Os or p.o.) →

      → DEGRADED IN STOMACH → BIOAVAILABILITY BASED ON CHARGE AND SIZE IN INTESTINE → PORTAL CIRCULATION TO LIVER → METABOLITES FROM "FIRST PASS" THROUGH LIVER CELLS → BLOOD → DELAYED LOWER PEAK PUT EXTENDED TIME IN BODY

      DERMAL → BIOAVAILABILITY BASED ON CHARGE AND SIZE, HYDRATION OF SKIN, CRACKS OR OTHER PERFORATIONS OR HAIRS IN SKIN → BLOOD

FIGURE 3-4 Routes of Administration Summarized

appreciate this fact and use these routes to get the most profound effect, though these routes are also associated with a very high danger of overdose. The IV route is guaranteed to be 100% in the circulation, so it also serves as a reference route to calculate the **bioavailability** of the substance via other routes.

The sublingual route also results in a fast peak concentration for compounds that are absorbed unusually rapidly through the oral mucosa such as nitroglycerin. The oral (per os or PO) and intraperitoneal (IP) routes require intestinal absorption (in the oral route, from the luminal side) and pass through the liver first. Any chemical that is not well absorbed, is inactivated by the liver, or is activated by liver xenobiotic metabolism will be profoundly affected by these routes. There is also a lag phase for absorption by these routes. The subcutaneous (SC) and intramuscular (IM) routes lead to slow release of lipophilic or fat-soluble toxins due to the binding to subcutaneous fat or muscle protein, respectively.

Skin exposure (percutaneous route) is difficult to model, as not all skin is equivalent. Human skin is a good barrier to hydrophilic chemicals that are not corrosive, metallic substances, such as mercury and compounds such as DDT. Children used to play with inorganic mercury (not recommended) with little acute toxicity as long as it was not ingested, they had no cracks in their skin, and the mercury did not vaporize in contact with a hot surface. Little acute toxicity was noted in the 1950s when children used to run behind DDT-spraying trucks or were deloused (in some countries) by DDT being sprayed directly on the heads of infested children, although future cancer rates were elevated in these populations. In contrast, the highly hydrophobic dimethylmercury can and has been absorbed through the wrong type of glove and/or through the skin, causing a tragic fatality to an academic researcher of heavy metals. The absorption of hydrocortisone in humans increases in areas of the skin with high hydration (e.g., underarms and genital area), while the palms and soles of the feet show lower absorption.

A number of studies have been done to examine the differences in percutaneous absorption of chemicals since the 1960s. One study transplanted grafts of human and pig skin to athymic nude mice and used a hairless dog and a weanling Yorkshire pig to determine percutaneous absorption differences between species (Reifenrath et al., 1984). Caffeine was used as the hydrophilic compound, while lindane served as the hydrophobic agent. This situation is modeled in general by partitioning into the hydrophobic solvent octanol and hydrophilic water and taking logarithm of this ratio, known as **log K_{ow}** or **log P** (the higher the value, the more hydrophobic is the compound). The percentage of the applied dose of caffeine (log K_{ow} = −0.07) that was recovered in the urine was measured as 60 ± 5% for the athymic nude mice, 35 ± 7% for the human skin–grafted mice, 26 ± 6% for the pig skin–grafted mice, and 14% (± 2–3%) for the pig and the dog. The percentage of the lindane (log K_{ow} = 3.72) recovered in the urine was 48 ± 3% for the athymic nude mice, 16 ± 4% for the human skin–grafted mice, 19 ± 3% for the pig skin–grafted mice, 6 ± 1% for the pig, and 7 ± 4% for the dog.

These findings indicate that animal models vary widely in their ability to absorb hydrophilic versus hydrophobic compounds. Clearly, only the human skin grafts were satisfactory in modeling the true human response and the calculated skin absorption values for human fell in line with this experimental model for caffeine: benzoic acid (log K_{ow} = 1.87), malathion (log K_{ow} = 2.75), diethyltoluamide (log K_{ow} = 2.02), testosterone (log K_{ow} = 3.32), fluocinolone acetonide (log K_{ow} = 2.48), progesterone (log K_{ow} = 3.87), and lindane.

Studies prior to the one cited here indicated that animals with dense hair (usual animal models such as the mouse, rat, guinea pig, and rabbit) had much higher skin permeability than the dog, the pig, and the primates (human and monkey).

Number of Doses and Time of Exposure

The other variable specified with a LD_{50} is the exposure time. **Acute** exposure means exposed once and observed for effects over a 14-day period. The acute LD_{50} in rats is defined as very toxic, 25 mg/kg; toxic, 25–200 mg/kg; harmful, 200–2000 mg/kg; and low toxicity, more than 2000 mg/kg.

Subacute exposure (a strange outdated historical term, since it is longer than acute) is a 14- or 28-day, or slightly longer, daily exposure following various parameters. The subacute test is meant to model injuries caused by repeated exposure or possible effects of **bioaccumulation** depending on the **half-life** ($t_{1/2}$) of the toxin. The lowest dose in the acute study should be used to design the upper doses of the subacute test.

Subchronic exposure usually involves daily exposure for 90 days. Many studies end here except those designed to satisfy FDA regulations.

The **chronicity index = 1 dose LD_{50}/ 90-day dose LD_{50}** may also be determined. This value should ideally be as low a number as possible, meaning that the acutely lethal dose is as close as possible to the dose that causes mortality in multiple doses. A high number signals a low 90-day LD_{50}, which means that low repeated doses of a putative medicine are very carcinogenic, represent an extreme allergen, or lead to another problem. A **NOAEL** or **NOEL** outcome (no observed adverse effect level or no observed effect level) may be established from these data. However, for carcinogenicity studies, it is more appropriate to assess a significant portion of the life cycle of an animal. For a rat or mouse with a lifespan of approximately 2 years before some dying- or age-related effects occur, a chronic study can extend from the length of a subchronic exposure (usually 6 months) upward to the full 2-year lifespan.

Toxicity is determined not only by the relative LD_{50}s but also by the **reversibility** of effects. A review of biochemistry reveals that binding of a competitive inhibitor such as carbon monoxide to hemoglobin may be reversed by increasing the amount (or in this case the pO_2) of the substrate for the enzyme or the physiological ligand for the receptor. This relationship is also the basis of antidotal therapy in pharmacology, such as use of the antagonist naloxone to reverse the overstimulation of opiate receptors in overdose. Noncompetitive inhibitors may bind at allosteric sites; their binding cannot be reversed by the ligand to the active site, but only by those substances that bind to that allosteric site. Uncompetitive inhibitors are thought to bind to the enzyme–substrate complex and may be even more difficult to reverse. All of these effects are theoretically reversible as long as covalent bonds to the sites are not formed and the correct chemical can be found to antagonize the action of the inhibitor without itself blocking the receptor or inhibiting the enzyme.

Acetylcholinesterase has been heavily studied and can be inhibited through these means by reversible agents used in the treatment of Alzheimer's disease, Parkinson's disease, myasthenia gravis, and the development of insecticides. Military uses have employed such chemicals as VX or sarin gas, which form fast and stable phosphonyl groups (Millard et al., 1999). The carbamates, such as physostigmine, have been used as medications (rapid reversal of carbamylated enzyme); the organophosphates are less reversible depending on their structure (a moiety that may stabilize the phosphorylated enzyme) and have pesticide and military applications; while the quaternary ammonium compounds also inhibit the enzyme (Fukoto, 1990). Natural irreversible inhibitors of acetylcholinesterase also exist—for example, onchidal, a defensive secretion of the mollusc *Onchidella binneyi* (Abramson et al., 1989).

Another aspect of the relative toxicity is the ability of the organism to adapt to or repair the toxic damage.

Responses with Repeated Dosing

When repeated dosing yields effects, a number of assays should be considered.

Skin Sensitization: Allergic and Cumulative Irritation

A good discussion of this issue can be found in the article by Kimber and colleagues (2001). Certain chemicals such as laundry and dishwasher detergents contain substances that, following consistent use or contact, may trigger irritation that will generate an immune response. Other substances work through the release of histamine, as in the development of a hapten-allergic reaction.

Guinea pig exposures involved the guinea pig maximization test (Magnusson and Kligman, 1969) and the occluded patch test developed by Buehler (1965). In these tests, the number of animals showing reactions to potent sensitizers such as 2,4-dinitrochlorobenzene versus weak sensitizers were determined. However, potency may also be indicated by the ability of a chemical to generate a 100% response in an individual animal as well as the number of animals that show a response. Another test for the guinea pig is the open epicutaneous test, which involves a 20-dose regimen given over a 4-week period; surface skin exposure without occlusion is assessed in this test.

Local lymph node assays in exposed mice and human skin exposure have been other testing alternatives used in the past.

Currently, the 7th amendment of the European Union does not allow for animal testing of sensitization. This ban has sparked the development of human cell line alternatives using known allergens, such as $NiSO_4$, versus detergent agents, such as Tween 80 (Sakaguchi et al., 2006).

Phototoxicity and Photosensitization

Similar issues arise and similar methods are used with the skin sensitization test, with the addition of ultraviolet radiation. Phototoxicity and photosensitization occur with chemicals such as the antipsychotic agent chlorpromazine, the sulfa antibiotics, and other agents that either color the skin (e.g., high levels of beta-carotene) or become more toxic or allergenic in the presence of UV irradiation. Again, toxicologists are under pressure from animal welfare advocates and government agencies to develop alternative models for these tests (Horio, 1981).

Eye Tests

Eye tests are some of the most controversial in the toxicology area, along with the skin tests and the LD_{50} assays. The Draize test introduced chemicals and toxins directly into the rabbit's conjunctiva. This test is considered highly variable and it is not clear how well it models the contact made by cosmetics, chemicals that accidently come in contact with the eye, or agents that are taken by other routes of administration. Many cosmetics companies advertise that they do no animal testing to avoid customer disgust with the Draize test. The alternatives of isolated eye preparations and other preparations have been called into question as well (Prinsen, 2006).

Developmental/Reproductive Assays, and Other Genotoxicity Assays (Mutagenic/Carcinogenic)

The FDA and the U.S. EPA have combined their efforts in the area of genotoxicity, which is now defined as also encompassing damage to the developing organism (developmental toxicity). Reproductive toxicities (which hinder males' and females' ability to reproduce via damage to reproductive structures) and carcinogenesis are determined through rodent studies. Genetic toxicology is determined with in vivo and in vitro tests that test for mutations, **clastogenesis** (breakage of chromosomes or loss or rearrangement of chromosomal pieces), and direct DNA damage. Since these toxicities are related, the FDA has developed a genetic toxicity, reproductive and developmental toxicity, and carcinogenicity database (http://www .fda.gov/Cder/Offices/OPS_IO/genrepcar .htm; Matthews et al., 2006). It reveals that 14 composite endpoints (taken from 32 individual endpoint data sets) are correlated with carcinogenesis in rodents: gene mutation assays in *Salmonella*, *Escherichia*, other microbes, fungi, plant mutations, *Drosophila*, Hgprt (hypoxanthine-guanine phosphoribosyl transferase), and rodent mutation in vivo; clastogenesis as indicated by chromosome aberrations in vivo, micronucleus formation in vivo, and DNA damage in unscheduled DNA synthesis (UDS); reproductive toxicity as exhibited by sperm effects; and male and female rodent impacts. Note, however, that 13 composite endpoints assembled from 31 individual endpoints were not well correlated with carcinogenicity in rodents, but provided other toxicology information: gene mutation from two different mouse lymphoma models; clastogenicity from fungal aneuploidy, plant cytogenetics, *Drosophila* aneuploidy, chromosome aberrations in

vitro, micronucleus formation in vitro, sister chromatid exchanges (SCE) in vitro or in vivo; cell transformation; developmental toxicity in rodents; fetal toxicity in rodents; and behavioral toxicity in rodents.

Much of the research into carcinogenesis was based on the **maximum tolerated dose (MTD)**. The MTD is the maximum dose that elicits toxicity without affecting survival of the organism or population. It is a highly controversial measurement, as it has been defined a number of ways over the years, and its predictive value in toxicology or medicine has been called into question based on the degree of irreversibility of the toxic effects elicited. Developers of medications, especially those that are employed in the treatment of cancer, still determine the MTD and use 1/10 of the MTD or the LD_{10} as a way of establishing a ratio useful for the development of human safety guidelines for the introduction of chemotherapeutic agents first developed in rodents (Newell et al., 1999). Unfortunately, a rodent will not vomit, so some of the important human toxicity is not modeled adequately by rodent testing.

Mutagenicity is determined by the Ames test (an in vitro test for point mutations) utilizing *Salmonella typhimurum* and *Escherichia coli*. The mouse lymphoma tests for forward mutations at the thymidine kinase (TK) locus. Other tests include determination of chromosome aberrations, in vitro human peripheral lymphocyte tests, in vivo mouse micronucleus assays, and the dominant lethal test in rodents (male mice are given a sublethal dose [$1/5LD_{50}$] and then mated with untreated females; mutagenic index = early fetal deaths/total implantations $\times$ 100, according to Epstein and Rohrborn [1981]).

Only a subset of developmental and reproductive tests elucidates cancer pathways or genetic damage leading to cancer. Some tests cause other toxicity that manifests itself in reproductive damage or abnormal development. The FDA set the following goals in 1997:

1. Develop improved methods and new strategies for detection and prediction of developmental toxicity in laboratory animals and the human

population, focusing on reproductive tract development, central nervous system development, whole embryo development, pharmacokinetics during development, and the molecular biology aspects of development.

2. Develop new concepts on how xenobiotics produce developmental toxicant effects.

3. Develop a knowledge base for the estrogenic action of xenobiotics during development. (http://www.fda.gov/nctr/science/96-97%20 Research%20Plans/organizations/ reproductive.htm)

This direction was provoked by increased understanding of the various synthetic and natural estrogens and antiestrogens, and their effects on both reproduction and development. The FDA noted that 20% of infant deaths are attributable to birth defects and that states spend more money on developmental disabilities than on any other category of chronic disease.

Reproductive testing is divided into three segments:

- Segment I (rats) measures mating, cohabitation, implantation, and maternal and paternal fertility. Males are dosed 14 days prior to mating and mated with undosed females. Females are dosed 14 days prior to mating with undosed males and up to day 8 of gestation.

- Segment II employs rats, mice and/ or rabbits and determines birth defects (**teratology**) and embryotoxicity. Pregnant females are dosed starting at implantation (day 6) and continuing through organogenesis (day 16 for rats and mice, day 18 for rabbits). Females are sacrificed on day 22 (rats and mice) or day 28 (rabbits) just prior to parturition. Skeletal and visceral evaluations of fetuses/neonates are performed.

- Segment III (rats) is concerned both with prenatal and postnatal development and measurements of length of gestation (look for delays), parturition, and ability to nurse. Dosing starts on day 16 of gestation and continues throughout weaning. Some medications require evaluation through a second generation.

Immunotoxicity/Allergy

According to the FDA,

An effect is considered adverse or immunotoxic if it impairs humoral or cellular immunity needed by the host to defend itself against infectious or neoplastic disease (immunosuppression) or it causes unnecessary tissue damage (autoimmunity, hypersensitivity, or chronic inflammation). This definition incorporates the concept that the immune system is in a complex balance that includes interactions with other systems (e.g., nervous and endocrine) that may utilize or be affected by the same biological mediators (e.g., neuropeptide and steroid hormones). (http://www.fda.gov/ cdrh/ost/ostggp/immunotox.html)

The histopathology is examined via cell surface markers and morphology. Humoral responses are examined via immunoassays (e.g., enzyme-linked immunosorption assay [ELISA]) for antibody response to antigen plus adjuvant, plaque-forming cells, lymphocyte proliferation, antibody-dependent cell-mediated cytotoxicity, passive cutaneous anaphylaxis, and direct anaphylaxis. Cellular responses are subdivided into T cells, natural killer cells (tumorcytotoxicity), macrophages (phagocytosis, antigen presentation), granulocytes (degranulation, phagocytosis), host resistance (to viruses, bacteria, and tumors), and signs of illness (allergy, skin rash, urticaria, edema, lymphadenopathy). T-cell responses are determined through the guinea pig maximization test, mouse local lymph node assay, mouse ear swelling test, lymphocyte proliferation, and mixed lymphocyte reaction.

Tolerance, Dependence, and Cross-Tolerance

Tolerance is defined as requiring a higher dose to achieve the same effect with repeated exposures. **Cross-tolerance** means more than one ligand can bind to a receptor and add to the creation of tolerance. This effect can occur by **down-regulation** of receptors, increases in metabolism, or changes in the firing rate of cells with receptor occupancy. **Dependence** causes an organism to require a certain receptor occupancy by the substance with repeated exposures of receptors and other cellular adjustments (such as expression of proteins that modify neuron firing rates); otherwise, **withdrawal** occurs and may result in lethality. This is a powerful influence. Many of the drugs of abuse are toxic to the developing organism, and the hypoxia and neurochemical changes associated with withdrawal during pregnancy must be considered as well.

Behavioral Toxicity

Changes in behavior are clearly evident when an animal is given a psychoactive chemical such as lysergic acid diethylamide (LSD) or amphetamine. Changes in locomotor activity, rearing behavior, grooming, feeding behavior, and other measures or unconditioned and conditioned responses (e.g., food-reinforced behaviors or learned avoidance behaviors) reveal effects of these substances at relatively low doses. In addition, these chemicals may have irreversible influences, especially with repeated use. Lead and mercury have known behavioral effects, especially in children. The June 2000 issue of *Environmental Health Perspectives* was dedicated to children's health and focused in part on the disturbingly high rate of developmental and behavioral disabilities that may be associated with toxic exposures of children to heavy metals and pesticides (May, 2000).

Ecosystems

Aquatic Toxicity

For ecotoxicology, the initial analyses involved taking water, air, and soil samples. The *Daphnia* species (especially *Daphnia magna*) were the original laboratory model for determining the impacts of water pollution in laboratory analysis of field samples (Organization for Economic Cooperation and Development [OECD], 1984). The LC_{50} and the EC_{50} mentioned for cells served as the toxicity indices. However, the static versus flow exposure method led to increased toxicity with higher flow rates and complicated the interpretation of results for algae (Schafer et al., 1994) and filter feeders such as *Daphnia* (Weltens et al., 2000). Subsequently, research moved from single species exposure to considerations of primary producers (algae) mixed with primary (zooplankton), secondary (fish that eat zooplankton), and tertiary (fish or other aquatic species that eat fish) consumers. This mixture could only be modeled in the wild or in microcosms (small aquaria) or stream or pond mesocosms (constructed small streams or lakes) (Mohr et al., 2005). This was and continues to be an expensive but useful method for investigating not only primary impacts on a species, but also the effect of other natural stresses and trophic levels on toxicity of chemicals such as herbicides that have a ripple effect through their trophic levels due to impacts on the primary producers. For example, the study of mesocosms identified further sensitivity of species such as algae to herbicides such as atrazine (Huggins et al., 1994). This is a controversial area, as some articles dispute the mesocosm analysis of atrazine.

As analyses became more sophisticated, a tiered approach was developed by the U.S. EPA for evaluating aquatic pollution. The tiered system for pesticide analysis was reviewed in 1994 (Baker et al., 1994). It required exposure of bluegill, rainbow trout, and *Daphnia* to determine the LC_{50}, the 95% confidence interval for that data, and the NOEC. A determination of the estimated **environmental concentration (EEC)** was then made. If the LC_{50} was less than 1 part per million (ppm), the EEC was greater than 0.1 LC_{50} or less than 0.01 LC_{50}, and the half-life of the chemical pesticide was more than 4 days (bioaccumulation potential), then it triggered early life stage testing in both a fish species and an invertebrate species. If the chemical was applied directly to water and the EEC was 0.1 NOEL or greater, then a full fish life cycle study was triggered.

The LC_{50} remains an essential tool in ecotoxicology, however, as lethality is more important than morbidity as long as it has no inference for human toxicity. In animal studies, morbidity is important, as these effects are usually used to predict human toxicity.

Synergy, Antagonism, and Endocrine Disruption

In the 1990s, a major change in the EPA's approaches to testing occurred due to the eruption of a phenomenon known as endocrine disruption. Although disturbances had been seen in earlier times, an article that appeared in *Science* (which was later withdrawn) indicated that low subthreshold concentrations of weak estrogens had a profound effect on the estrogen receptor when given in mixtures (McLachlan, 1997). Although these data were not reproduced, other evidence did support the hypothesis that extremely low concentrations of chemicals could cause higher than expected disruptions in endocrine function and development of organisms.

Toxicologists had already been aware of **synergisms** such as the increased toxicity of carbamate insecticides relative to acetylcholinesterase activity when xenobiotic metabolism was inhibited in *Drosophila* or other organisms by piperonyl butoxide. This combination is the basis for many commercially available insecticides. Synergisms are used to try to increase the effectiveness of the active toxic ingredient and fight resistance in insects (Wilson, 2001). The toxic antibiotic combination of sulfamethoxazole and trimethoprim synergizes to 100 times the effectiveness of either agent alone in the metabolic pathway in certain bacteria that make tetrahydrofolate from para-aminobenzoic acid. As mentioned earlier, antagonism at receptors serves the basis for toxicities and antidotes for overdosed medications or accidental exposure to toxins. The type of synergism reported for endocrine disruptors was new, however, as all the chemicals were supposed to be binding to the same receptor at concentrations that would not yield an effect alone.

In the 1990s, a report on Lake Apopka alligators' exposure to DDT shifted the focus in endocrine disruption research. In that study, females had two times the normal estrogen levels and abnormal ovarian morphology. Males had decreased testosterone, morphologically abnormal testes, and much reduced phallus size (Guilette et al., 1994). Since the publication of this study, a number of reports have verified endocrine disruption in the wild, with the new sensitive model being the amphibian, especially for malformations caused by estrogenic or thyroid-disrupting chemicals. Reports have also cited male fish that demonstrate such effects, and vitellogenin or egg yolk protein expression in the liver and other organs of these fish have become the new biochemical standard for evaluation of these effects in toxicology research.

Field Studies and Indices in Aquatic Ecotoxicology

Field studies appear to be the best indicator of how species are affected by environmental toxins. Unfortunately, they do not yield clean results because of the presence of confounding variables such as habitat destruction, introduction of non-native invasive species, and global climate change. Trying to parse the influence of a given toxin or mixture of toxins is difficult and requires a variety of consonant data. Given that *Daphnia magna* and EC_{50} data are well-researched values, sensitivities of other macroinvertebrate species may be ranked based on the **relative tolerance** $T_{rel} = \log (EC_i/EC_{D.\ magna})$ of species "i" to *D. magna* (Wogram and Liess, 2001). $T_{rel} > 0$ species are less sensitive than *D. magna*; $T_{rel} = 0$ are equally sensitive as *D. magna*.

Other units have also been developed for field work. Sometimes species are characterized as species at risk (**SPEARS**) versus species not at risk (SpEnotAR). This status can be determined from sensitivity to toxicants, generation time, migration ability, and the presence of aquatic stages during the time a chemical may appear at maximum concentrations in the aquatic environment (Liess and von der Ohe, 2005). The **toxic units (TU)** used in this type of analysis for a measured concentration of a pesticide "I" at concentration C (in µg/L) are represented by the expression $TU_{(D.\ magna)} = \log (C/LC_{50}i)$, where the LC_{50} expressed represents the 48-hour exposure of *D. magna* to that pesticide. When the final SPEARS units are calculated, species with a value of -0.36 or greater (median of the sensitivity based on all four factors) are regarded as sensitive. This makes ecological and toxicological sense.

Sometimes biotic indices and toxicological data need to be merged to determine the impact or risk posed by a chemical in an ecosystem. Clearly, various aquatic organisms, representing different trophic levels, can be use assess sensitivity and at-risk designations.

Terrestrial Ecotoxicology

The European Commission's Health and Consumer Protection Directorate-General, Directorate E—Food Safety: Plant Health, Animal Health and Welfare, International Questions (E1 Plant Health) produced a draft for determination of terrestrial ecotoxicology (http://ec.europa.eu/food/plant/protection/evaluation/guidance/wrkdoc09_en.pdf). In that document, the group indicated:

General adverse effects on the terrestrial environment include:

- Effects on soil functions, and particularly soil to act as a substrate for plants including effects on seed germination, and those on organisms (invertebrates, microorganisms) important for proper soil functions and nutrient cycle conservation.
- Effects on plant biomass production, related to contamination of soil or air including deposition on plant surfaces. Plants are the source of food for the whole system (including humans) and have additional roles in terms of land protection, nutrient cycles, equilibrium of gases in the atmosphere, etc.
- Effects on soil, above-ground and foliar invertebrates, which represent food for other organisms, and cover essential roles as pollinators, detrivores, saprophages, pest controllers, etc.
- Effects on terrestrial vertebrates exposed to contaminated food, soil, air, water, or surfaces, with obvious economic and/or social consequences. Poisoned birds and mammals probably constitute

the highest social concern, while reproductive effects, although less evident, represent a higher ecological hazard.

- Accumulation of toxic compounds in food items and through the food chain. Is a typical exposure route for animals within the contaminated ecosystems and represents an additional concern related to the consumption of this food by humans and domestic animals.

The no-observed-effect concentration (**NOEC**) may still be employed, but a regression-based parameter is preferred where determined on the EC curve approach. The **hazard quotient (HQ)** for every applied chemical, defined as $HQ = application\ rate/oral\ LD_{50}$, is determined in a given species that would have an oral route of ingestion of the chemical, such as a bee or a nontarget arthropod. A **toxicity to exposure ratio (TER)** (with a subscript used to denote "a" for acute exposure, "st" for short-term exposure, and "lt" for long-term exposure) is determined for all modeled terrestrial species of interest.

Notice that the TER and the HQ are inversely related. A high HQ or a low TER, therefore, would be problematic. The logarithmic nature of responses is still considered in determining the regulatory trigger ratio for either of these parameters. Triggers for both the TER and the HQ for testing have been identified.

In addition, the EC and the LD are still the curves of interest, along with the exposure concentration or dose. Endocrine effects (low-concentration or low-dose phenomena) and persistence of the agent in the environment (pulse or extended exposures) are also included in this analysis, as these results can determine which tests are really relevant when proceeding to **probabilistic risk assessment** (overlapping probits based on species and agent).

Air pollution fits under the terrestrial ecological assessment rubric, but LC_{50} curves in relevant sensitive animal species and EC_{50} curves looking at lung cancer, asthma, or other respiratory reactions to toxic gases, vapors, aerosols, and particles are important to note. Rats and mice are not as useful as human models of respiratory damage as they may be for the acute oral LD_{50}, because these animals lack well-developed respiratory bronchioles; by comparison, monkeys, dogs, pigs, and even ferrets (Sterner-Kock et al., 2000) experience toxic reactions similar to those demonstrated by humans. Note that the key commonality for all toxicology terms is they assess the concentration or amount at which sickness or death starts to occur and define how rapidly responses increase as a percentage of the population with increased levels of toxin.

Questions

1. For cells, which two factors are essential to know for exposure and toxicity characterization? Why?

2. Describe how an acute oral LD_{50} test is performed and explain the result's meaning.

3. What is the chronicity index and the therapeutic index? Why should the chronicity index be as low as possible and the therapeutic index be as high as possible?

4. Which routes of administration lead to the highest fastest peak concentration? Which routes would indicate toxicity if metabolites are more toxic than the original compound?

5. What are the EEC and LC_{50}, and how are they used to assess exposure and hazard to define a level of concern (LOC) in environmental toxicology?

References

Abramson SN, Radic Z, Manker D, Faulkner DJ, Taylor P. 1989. Onchidal: a naturally occurring irreversible inhibitor of acetylcholinesterase. *Mol Pharmacol.* 36:349–354.

Arthington JD, Corah LR, Blecha F. 1996. The effect of molybdenum-induced copper deficiency on acute-phase protein concentrations, superoxide dismutase activity, leukocyte numbers, and lymphocyte proliferation in beef heifers inoculated with bovine herpesvirus-1. *J Anim Sci.* 74:211–217.

Backe J. 2006. *Male breast cancer genetics.* 27. Deutscher Krebskongress. Berlin, 22.–26.03.2006. Düsseldorf, Köln: German Medical Science; Doc IS006.

Baker JL, Barefoot AC, Beasley LE, Burns L, Caulkins P, Clark J, Feulner RL, Giesey JP, Graney RL, Griggs R, Jacoby H, Laskowski D, Maciorowski A, Mihaich E, Nelson H, Parrish R, Siefert RE, Solomon KE, van der Schalie W. 1994. *Final report: aquatic risk assessment and mitigation dialogue group.* Pensacola, FL: SETAC Press.

Brown JG, Almond BD, Naglich JG, Eidels L. 1993. Hypersensitivity to diphtheria toxin by mouse cells expressing both diphtheria toxin receptor and CD9 antigen. *Proc Natl Acad Sci USA.* 90:8184–8188.

Buehler, EV. 1965. Delayed contact hypersensitivity in the guinea pig. *Arch Dermatol.* 91:171–177.

Burk RF, Lane JM. 1983. Modification of chemical toxicity by selenium deficiency. *Fundam Appl Toxicol.* 3:218–221.

Dubinsky JM. 1995. Excitotoxicity as a stochastic process. *Clin Exp Pharmacol Physiol.* 22:297– 298.

Epstein SS, Rohrborn G. 1981. Recommended procedures for testing genetic hazards from chemicals, based on the induction of dominant lethal mutations in mammals. *Nature.* 230:459–460.

Finney DJ. 1978. *Statistical methods in biological assay* (3rd ed.). London: Charles Griffin & Co.

Fischer LJ, Green MD, Harman AW. 1981. Levels of acetaminophen and its metabolites in mouse tissues after a toxic dose. *J Pharmacol Exp Ther.* 219:281–286.

Fukoto TR. 1990. Mechanism of action of organophosphorus and carbamate insecticides. *Environ Health Perspect.* 87:245–254.

Guilette LJ, Gross TS, Masson GR, Matter JM, Percival HF, Woodward AR. 1994. Developmental abnormalities of the gonad and abnormal sex hormone concentrations in juvenile alligators from contaminated and control lakes in Florida. *Environ Health Perspect.* 102:680–688.

Hayes WJ Jr. 1971. Insecticides, rodenticides and other economic poisons. In: Di Palma J, ed. *Drill's pharmacology in medicine* (4th ed.). New York: McGraw-Hill, pp. 1256–1276.

Heath DF. 1961. *Organophosphorous poisons.* New York: Pergamon Press, pp. 235–238.

Horio T. 1981. Evaluation of drug phototoxicity by photosensitization of *Trichophyton mentagrophytes.* *Br J Dermatol.* 105:365–370.

Huggins DG, Johnson ML, deNoyelles F Jr. 1994. The ecotoxic effects of atrazine on aquatic ecosystems: an assessment of direct and indirect effects using structural equation modeling. In: Graney RL, Kennedy JH, Rodgers JH Jr, eds. *Aquatic mesocosm studies in ecological risk assessment.* Boca Raton, FL: Lewis, pp. 653–697.

Kimber I, Basketter DA, Berthold K, Butler M, Garrigue J-L, Lea L, Newsome C, Roggeband R, Steiling W, Stropp G, Waterman S, Wiemann C. 2001. Skin sensitization testing in potency and risk assessment. *Toxicol Sci*. 59:198–208.

Liess M, von der Ohe PC. 2005. Analyzing the effects of pesticides on invertebrate communities in streams. *Environ Toxicol Chem*. 24:954–965.

Litchfield JT Jr, Wilcoxon F. 1949. A simplified method of evaluating dose-effect experiments. *J Pharmacol Exp Ther*. 96:99–113.

Magnusson B, Kligman AM. 1969. The identification of contact allergens by animal assay: the guinea pig maximization test. *J Invest Dermatol*. 52:268–276.

Matthews EJ, Kruhlak NL, Cimino MC, Benz RD, Contrera JF. 2006. An analysis of genetic toxicity, reproductive and developmental toxicity, and carcinogenicity data: I. identification of carcinogens using surrogate endpoints. *Regul Toxicol Pharmacol*. 44:83–96.

May M. 2000. Disturbing behavior: neurotoxic effects in children. *Environ Health Perspect*. 108:A262–A267.

McLachlan JA. 1997. Synergistic effect of environmental estrogens: report withdrawn. *Science*. 277:459–463.

Millard CB, Gertraud Koellner G, Ordentlich A, Shafferman A, Silman I, Sussman JL. 1999. Reaction products of acetylcholinesterase and VX reveal a mobile histidine in the catalytic triad. *J Am Chem Soc*. 121:9883–9884.

Miller L, Tainter M. 1944. Estimation of the ED-50 and error by means of logarithmic probit graph paper. *Proc Soc Exp Biol Med*. 57:261–264.

Mohr S, Feibicke M, Ottenströer T, Meinecke S, Berghahn R, Schmidt R. 2005. Enhanced experimental flexibility and control in ecotoxicological mesocosm experiments: a new outdoor and indoor pond and stream system. *Environ Sci Pollut Res Int*. 12:5–7.

Neubert D, Hopfenmüller W, Fuchs G. 1981. Manifestation of carcinogenesis as a stochastic process on the basis of an altered mitochondrial genome. *Arch Toxicol*. 48: 89–125.

Newell DR, Burtles SS, Fox BW, Jodrell DI, Connors TA. 1999. Evaluation of rodent-only toxicology for early clinical trials with novel cancer therapeutics. *Br J Cancer*. 81:760–768.

Organization for Economic Cooperation and Development (OECD). 1984. *Guidelines for testing chemicals. Daphnia sp. acute inmobilisation test and reproduction test*. Paris: OECD.

Prinsen MK. 2006. The Draize eye test and in vitro alternatives; a left-handed marriage? *Toxicol In Vitro*. 20:774–784.

Reifenrath WG, Chellquist EM, Shipwash, EA, Jederberg, WW. 1984. Evaluation of animal models for predicting skin penetration in man. *Fundam Appl Toxicol*. 4:S224–S230.

Sakaguchi H, Ashikaga T, Miyazawa M, Yoshida Y, Ito Y, Yoneyama K, Hirota M, Itagaki H, Toyoda H, Suzuki H. 2006. Development of an in vitro skin sensitization test using human cell lines; human Cell Line Activation Test (h-CLAT). II. An interlaboratory study of the h-CLAT. *Toxicol In Vitro*. 20:774–784.

Salles II, Tucker AE, Voth DE, Ballard JD. 2003. Toxin-induced resistance in *Bacillus anthracis* lethal toxin-treated macrophages. *Proc Natl Acad Sci USA*. 100:12426–12431.

Schafer H, Hettler H, Fritsche U, Pitzen G, Roderer G, Wenzel A. 1994. Biotests using unicellular algae and ciliates for predicting long-term effects of toxicants. *Ecotoxicol Environ Safety*. 27:64–81.

Schirmer K. 2006. Proposal to improve vertebrate cell cultures to establish them as substitutes for the regulatory testing of chemicals and effluents using fish. *Toxicology*. 224:163–183.

Sterner-Kock A, Kock M, Braun R, Hyde DM. 2000. Ozone-induced epithelial injury in the ferret is similar to nonhuman primates. *Am J Respir Crit Care Med*. 162:1152–1156.

Takenaka S, Heini A, Ritter B, Heyder J. 1998. The respiratory bronchiole of beagle dogs: structural characteristics. *Toxicol Lett*. 96–97:301–308.

Underwood EJ. 1959. Mineral metabolism. *Annu Rev Biochem*. 28:499–526.

Warkany J, Takacs E. 1959. Experimental production of congenital malformations in rats by salicylate poisoning. *Am J Pathol*. 35:315–331.

Weil CS. 1952. Tables for convenient calculation of median-effective dose (LD_{50} or ED_{50}) and instructions in their use. *Biometrics*. 9:249–263.

Weltens R, Goossens R, Van Puymbroeck S. 2000. Ecotoxicity of contaminated suspended solids for filter feeders (*Daphnia magna*). *Arch Environ Contam Toxicol*. 39:315–323.

Wilson TG. 2001. Resistance of *Drosophila* to toxins. *Annu Rev Entomol*. 46:545–571.

Wogram J, Liess M. 2001. Rank ordering of macroinvertebrate species sensitivity to toxic compounds by comparison with that of *Daphnia magna*. *Bull Environ Contam Toxicol*. 67:360–367.

CHAPTER 4

Hazard, Exposure, and Risk Modeling

This is a chapter outline intended to guide and familiarize you with the content to follow.

	Hazard	× Exposure	= Risk
Level of Organization			
Cellular	$LC_{50} \rightarrow$ NOEC $\rightarrow$ LOEC $\rightarrow$ Damage DNA? Cause cell proliferation (cancer)? MIC (bacterial) mechanism of action: receptor binding strength (K_D) QSAR— structurally similar to other known toxicants? Uncertainty factors (UF) For extrapolation to complex organism (possibly 3 log units) $\rightarrow$ Reference dose (RfD) = NOEC/UF $\times$ MF (modifying factors; e.g., cancer)	[Nominal] versus [Actual] $\rightarrow$ Does [outside] equilibrate with [Inside] or exclude, pump out, or metabolize (less)? Bioaccumulate (more)? Static (less) or flow-through (more) method of exposure?	RfD multiplied by factors better modeled by whole organism, such as body weight and route of administration
Whole organism	QSAR $\rightarrow$ Identify structural alerts LD_{50}, ED_{50}, TI, margin of safety $\rightarrow$ NOEL, LOEL, carcinogenesis (one-hit versus multi-hit sublingual, IV, IM, versus linearized multistage) $\rightarrow$ Mechanism of toxic action $\rightarrow$ RfD, ADI (NOEL/SF where SF = safety factor)	Routes of administration— dermal, inhalation, nasal spray, eye drops, PO, gavage, sublingual, IV, IM, IP, ICV, intrathecal, rectal $\rightarrow$ Toxicokinetics $\rightarrow C_{max}$, V_d (volume of distribution), AUC (area under the curve) $\rightarrow$ For industrial purposes, time-weighted average (TWZ), or environmental estimated exposure dose (EED) or therapeutic exposure = concentration $\times$ intake $\times$ duration $\times$ frequency/body weight; absorbed dose = exposure $\times$ absorption factor $\rightarrow$ AADD (average absorbed daily dose) $\rightarrow$ LADD (lifetime) $\rightarrow$ MDD (maximum daily dose); MRSD (maximum recommended starting dose)	Standards of exposure, permissible exposures based on ability to detect (LOD, LOQ) $\rightarrow$ [permissible] = RfD $\times$ body weight $\times$ duration $\times$ frequency or if MDD $>$ RfD and is within 2 orders of magnitude of NOEL = may be unsafe. Margin of exposure (MOE) = NOEL/EED (human dose) problem when NOEL $<$ EED. Regulatory dose (RgG) = NOEL/MOEi (i = regulated chemical). Carcinogenic risk (R) = $LADD_{POT \text{ or } INT} \times$ SF. Assign ADI or virtually safe dose (VSD).

CONCEPTUALIZING TOXICOLOGY 4-1

	Hazard	× Exposure	= Risk
Level of Organization			
Ecosystem	Predicted no effect concentration (PNEC) at population and community levels; select endpoints; select indicative species; field, lab, mesocosm, and microcosm tests; incorporate resilience and recovery factors of ecosystem. QSAR → toxic equivalency factor (TEF) from a myriad of databases → Benchmark dose (10% population affected) → Maximum allowable toxic concentration (MATC) → Toxic units, SPEARS, relative tolerance → Tiers of EPA (4 levels of analysis).	Predicted environmental concentration (PEC) from all emissions and fates derived from EPA models for groundwater, surface water, food chain, multimedia, air pollution from meteorological data, crop/agricultural practices, soil/sediment properties, pesticide properties, other factors (e.g., topography). Tiers of EPA exposure models (4 levels).	Risk characterization = PEC/PNEC ratio where <1 = low or no risk; for pesticides, if EEC < LC_5 for most sensitive species or EEC < NOEC for chronic data, then Tier 1 completed. If not, then if upper 10th percentile annual maximum EEC < lower 10th percentile LC_5 completes Tier 2. If not, soil and climate scenarios added to upper 10th percentile annual maximum EED and lower 10th percentile of LC_5 or NOEC. Only Tier 4 requires more realistic ecotoxicity analyses → Mitigation.

CONCEPTUALIZING TOXICOLOGY 4-1 (*continued*)

Framework

Toxicology is required to extrapolate beyond the LC_{50} or LD_{50} curves to a larger population than the data can adequately address. This is quite different from using standard calibration curves for protein determination or similar assay, in which case scientists must indicate only whether samples fell within the curve or were below detection limits. Statistics and safety factors are required in this extrapolation from the lethality or toxicity curve. **Risk assessment** assesses the hazard or toxic effect as well as the exposure and integrates those data into the determination of risk (**Conceptualizing Toxicology 4-1**). The problem with extrapolating the lethality or toxicity curve is that the shape of the curve may vary from a linear to nonlinear extrapolations.

For example, the effects of 2,3,7,8-tetrachlorodibenzo-*p*-dioxin (TCDD) on liver damage and cancer formation have generated controversy over the years; the relevant dose-response curves are seen in **Figure 4-1**. The U.S.

EPA has suggested that the chronic toxicity curve should be extended back linearly to provide a safety factor in TCDD risk assessment. When researchers noted that TCDD's biologic effects were mainly noted on binding of this chemical and chemicals of similar structure to the aryl hydrocarbon (Ah) receptor, it was suggested that a threshold might exist at a much higher dose than that indicated by a linear extrapolation. In contrast, industrial research scientists advocated for use of the nonlinear Ah receptor steep binding curve (Cook et al., 1987). However, cell proliferation data suggested that lower doses may, indeed, present some problems associated with tumor promotion.

In Figure 4-1, note that the liver effects of 0–100 ng/kg/day TCDD in diethylnitrosamine-initiated female rats fit a fairly linear curve. However, the induction of the isozyme of the drug-metabolizing enzyme that activates dioxin to a carcinogen, CYP1A2 (cytochrome P450 1A2), is a sigmoidal curve with no apparent threshold. Cell proliferation and development of preneoplastic

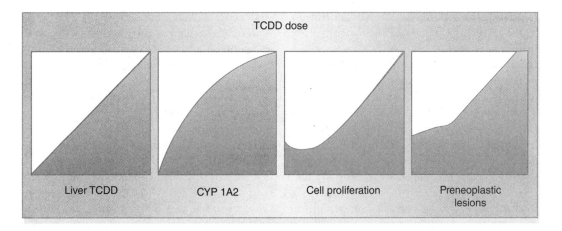

FIGURE 4-1 TCDD's Dose-Response Curves

Data from Tritscher AM, Goldstein JA, Portier CJ, McCoy Z, Clark GC, Lucier GW. 1992. Dose-response relationships for chronic exposure to 2,3,7,8-tetrachlorodibenzo-p-dioxin in a rat tumor promotion model: quantification and immunolocalization of CYP1A1 and CYP1A2 in the liver. *Cancer Res.* 52:3436–3442.; Vanden Heuvel JP, Lucier G. 1993. Environmental toxicology of polychlorinated dibenzo-p-dioxins and polychlorinated and polychlorinated dibenzofurans. *Environ Health Perspect.* 100:189–200.

lesions also show unusual curves, albeit at higher doses. If all of these data were used in the determination of the risk assessment for TCDD, then the EPA's extremely low standard of 0.006 pg/kg/day for an acceptable daily intake would be correct. However, the induction of cytochrome P450 occurs at doses lower than those that clearly cause carcinogenesis. Should the government follow the more mechanistic data, or should it mandate a conservative safety factor that might require an extremely high cost to achieve?

This is the fundamental problem in toxicological modeling and government regulation. The selection of biologic and statistical models, toxic endpoints, exposure assessments, safety factors, and finally risk models, and the determination of a government standard that is protective of nontarget species but not overly protective, are key factors to examine and discuss in risk assessment. The overriding priority should be to follow the Precautionary Principle that the United Nations Conference on Environment and Development adopted in 1992 or something akin to the Hippocratic Oath. The Precautionary Principle indicates that cost-effective steps should be taken to prevent the possibility of irreversible harm to the environment even when there is a lack of certainty about the effects of toxicants on the environment. Unfortunately, some very influential forces may seek to undermine this principle when it threatens to damage the short-term economic gain of a corporation or nation, or the possible ecological damage is superseded by the need of an overpopulated planet for food production (Adler, 2002).

Cells

Hazard

The hazard to a cell population still relies on the LC_{50} as a standard test for nontarget cells. The shape of the curve depends on the regression model selected, whether parametric or nonparametric. The most commonly used parametric models developed by Berkson and Bliss are probit and logit models, where the mechanism is less complex and better understood. The nonparametric models suggested by Spearman and Thompson were used early on in the development of the ED_{50} and should be used in complex phenomena where the mechanisms of action are not well understood (Muller and Schmitt, 1988). The proper selection of the exponential, probit, logit, or other model for analysis of linear or nonlinear data for the LC_{50} has been reviewed elsewhere (Hoekstra, 2006).

For cancer cells, the LC_{50} may be expressed as an LD_{50}, even though the units of dose (e.g., µg/mL) actually reflect concentration in the medium. The ratio of the toxicity of the medication to cancer cells versus normal cells is important in developing a therapeutic index (TI).

The development of an antibiotic relies on the **minimum inhibitory concentration (MIC)**. The effectiveness of the antibiotic is expressed as the time spent at greater than the MIC. The hazard posed to the infected cells by the antibiotic is a benefit to the host. The host would be tested under exposure to complex organisms—leading to therapeutic or human risk. The cells tested in that host would be assessed in terms of the EC_{50} for the development of that same antibiotic expressing the mortality of the microbial cells.

In cancer cells or microbial cells, the development of resistance to treatment or selection of a resistant population of cells by inadequate dose/concentration or time spent at the concentration lethal to those cells is important in determining hazard as well. For instance, important microbial pathogenic species such as certain strains of the gram-negative *Escherichia coli* or *Klebsiella pneumoniae* have a β-lactamase enzyme that cleaves penicillin and similar antibiotics into forms that no longer bind to the cell walls of those organisms. In this case, the MIC of a novel antibiotic from frog skin—that is, ascaphin-8 and its derivatives—would yield MICs in these resistant microbes. The LC_{50} in this case would refer to the toxicity of these compounds relative to the hemolytic activity of these agents in the host's cells (Eley et al., 2008).

Another form of resistance is the ability of bacteria to use an antibiotic/toxin as a nutrient source (Dantas et al., 2008). This adaptation turns a toxicity or lethality curve into a nutrient plot, which does not fit most toxicity analyses (with the exception of biphasic nutritional toxicity plots).

All tests should take into account possible additive, synergistic, or sensitizing effects, as well as tolerance, resistance, or antagonistic effects. The chemical should be given in a form that is likely to be used in industry or pharmaceuticals, including possible impurities. The teratogenicity/developmental toxicity of 2,4,5-trichlorophenoxyacetic acid, for example, was exploited following the discovery of a small contamination by an impurity of TCDD (Courtney et al., 1970). Metabolites need to

be determined, as they may be toxic chemical species; for example, the *N*-acetyl-*p*-benzoquinone imine metabolite of the over-the-counter analgesic acetaminophen is toxic to liver cells (Dahlin et al., 1984).

Extrapolation to the ends of the LC_{50} curve is used to ascertain where the no observed effect concentration (NOEC) or the **no observed adverse effect concentration (NOAEC)** is found at the intersection of the line with the *x*-axis. Statistically, the NOEC is the concentration on the extended LC_{50} curve where survival when the drug is taken is not significantly different from survival of controls. The lowest observed effect concentration (LOEC) is the lowest concentration at which survival with the drug is just significantly different from survival of controls. If these calculations are used to model larger organism, tissue, or ecosystem effects, then it is appropriate to use safety factors depending on how far removed this cell preparation is from the whole organism, species, route and time of exposure, flow conditions, or other relevant criteria. These factors are discussed further in this chapter where they are applied appropriately. Other factors would depend on measurements taken in cells depending on whether those cells are prokaryotic or eukaryotic. DNA damage and mutagenesis can be assessed in prokaryotes, while clastogenesis and sister chromatid exchanges are good measures of nuclear damage in mammalian cells (Kuroki and Matsushima, 1987). This information, along with the results of cell proliferation assays, is necessary to separate putative carcinogens from chemicals that carry little to no risk of carcinogenesis.

Risk assessment is subjected to different safety factors when a possible or likely carcinogen is encountered. These are important factors, especially given that regulatory toxicologists are encouraged or required by law to develop more in vitro or cellular models. Most toxicity tests that generate a LC_{50} may be considered **hazard identification**, not hazard characterization. The more mechanistically based tests that have human validation would be considered hazard characterization. For example, a **Scatchard plot** can be used to assess receptor **affinity**, which would determine the strength of action (potency or toxicity). For example, such findings have shown that cynomolgus monkey liver cells bind TCDD to the Ah receptor similarly to the beagle dog (Sandoz et al., 1999). **Figure 4-2** shows that high-affinity binding and high toxicity or potency results in a steep curve with a low dissociation constant (K_D or) at 50% receptor saturation (−1/slope of line) and B_{max} equal to the saturated receptor on the left side of the figure; by comparison, a low affinity or toxicity is evidenced by the line of low slope at the bottom of the figure. The reversibility of binding to the receptor and the toxicity to the cell should also be examined in hazard characterization.

Further analyses may involve modeling the **quantitative structure–activity relationships (QSAR)** to determine if the chemical of interest has a similar structure to chemicals that have been found to be problematic in a human population in a way not readily observable in a cellular assay. Once the MIC is determined for a microbe and the time required for sufficient

elimination of the microbe at the concentration is ascertained, the LC_{50} for host cells can be used to assess whether the risk to the host's cells justifies further development of this chemical as an antibiotic. Many **safety factors (SF)** and **uncertainty factors (UF)** have been suggested for adapting in vitro or cellular tests to human risk assessment for a variety of chemical exposures (**Figure 4-3**). Given that cells lack the integrity and interrelationships of complex organisms with intact systems for function (e.g., circulatory, immune, endocrine, nervous, and circulatory systems), they may indeed require more uncertainty factors. The 100-fold overall suggested uncertainty factor is equivalent to two logarithms. In toxicology, most uncertainty factors are 10-fold multiplied by another 10-fold uncertainty factor for being further removed from the species of interest, target organ, and route of administration, up to a possible 1000-fold ($10 \times 10 \times 10$) uncertainty factor for the data most removed from the true exposure route and time of exposure.

The dose at which human testing begins may be the **reference dose**, defined as **RfD = NOAEC/UF × MF**, where MF are modifying factors such as applying a carcinogenicity slope to the data for possible carcinogens. However, complete circumvention of animal testing is unwise, although these cellular tests may allow fewer animals to be used for hazard identification and characterization.

Exposure

The cellular toxicity assay assumes that at some time interval, the cell reaches equilibrium with environment, at which point the intracellular concentration may then equal that found in the environment. This is clearly a poor assumption for bacterial cells that use their cell wall to exclude certain antibiotics as part of their resistance mechanism (Hancock, 1997). Certain bacteria, the malarial parasite, and other cells have active extrusion mechanisms that keep intracellular concentrations lower than extracellular concentrations (Martin and Kirk, 2004). In the previous section, the metabolism of the toxin was included in resistance mechanisms that would limit exposure to the original chemical.

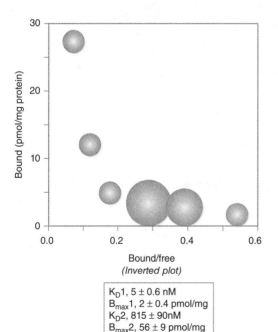

K_D1, 5 ± 0.6 nM
B_max1, 2 ± 0.4 pmol/mg
K_D2, 815 ± 90nM
B_max2, 56 ± 9 pmol/mg

FIGURE 4-2 The Binding of the Insecticide Avermectin B1a to Intact γ-Aminobutyric Acid A (GABAA) Receptors of Cultured Rat Cerebellar Neurons Showing High-Affinity and Low-Affinity Binding Sites

Data from Huang J, Casida JE. 1997. Avermectin B1a binds to high- and low-affinity sites with dual effects on the γ-aminobutyric acid-gated chloride channel of cultured cerebellar granule neurons. *J Pharmacol Exp Ther.* 281:261–266.

UNCERTAINTY FACTORS FOR IN VITRO DATA

From in vitro model system → complex living organism
$2.72^3 = 20.1$ (each factor being equally important)
(Metabolic factor differences × dosage discrepencies × differences between single cells or tissues and a complex multiorgan organism)

A

Uncertainties inherent in genetic and epigenetic differences within a species
$2.24^2 = 5.0$ (each factor being equally important)
(Polymorphisms in metabolism × toxicokinetic/toxicodynamic profiles)

B

Overall A × C = 100.5 multiplication for uncertaintes of moving from cells → complex organism but could be higher (150×) if using non-human cells and significant differences in receptors, etc. are taken into account

C

Similar to uncertainties for environmental assessments of inhaled toxicants going from rat oral LD_{50} → lifetime human inhalation: 10 (individual) × 10 (animal → human lifetime) × 40 (animal oral) × 500 (animal oral LD_{50}) at 95% confidence interval for each uncertainty. The closer to human epidemiology, the less the uncertainty (environmental uncertainty factors from Su and Wurzel, 1981).

D

FIGURE 4-3 Suggested Application of Uncertainty Factors to In Vitro Data

Data from Combes RD. 2005. Assessing risk to humans from chemical exposure by using non-animal test data. *Toxicol In Vitro.* 19:921–924.

Other cells actively bioaccumulate chemicals such as heavy metals (Sprocati et al., 2006). Equilibrium of some sort remains a good hypothesis over a period of time, but the time and method of exposure (e.g., static versus flow-through) must be specified. It would also be useful to assess the concentration of the chemical over time on an intracellular basis to help with interpretation of the data from the hazard analysis. For cellular models of human toxicity exposure characterization, the concentration range tested should model the concentration at the target organ for the dosage range anticipated.

Risk

Risk involves the combination (multiplication) of the reference dose with parameters better determined by the whole organism, such as body weight, and divided by exposure parameters. This topic will be discussed in more detail in conjunction with therapeutic or human risk assessment.

Complex Organisms—Tissues and Organs: Therapeutic or Human Risk

Medication Discovery and Development

An excellent summary of the events involved in risk assessment for therapeutic compounds can be found online (Fish, 2006). Before candidate selection takes place, several steps must be performed—namely, early safety prediction, candidate activity profiling, genetic toxicity and arrhythmia induction profiles, and acute (7-day) animal toxicity analysis. The period from candidate selection to first testing in humans is filled with definitive genetic toxicity tests, dose-range and 14- to 28-day toxicology studies, and safety pharmacology studies of the cardiovascular, central nervous system (CNS), and respiratory systems. The period from first testing in humans to proof-of-concept takes 3–12 months and is the time when reproductive toxicology testing takes place. The proof-of-concept to launch period additionally requires immunotoxicology data, juvenile or postnatal developmental studies, and 2-year rodent cancer tests.

Hazard

An excellent online summary of risk assessment is found at Extonet under the adverse health effects topic (http://extoxnet.orst.edu/faqs/risk/riskhome.htm). This process may start with a QSAR—QSARs are the predictive computational toxicology tools used in hazard identification and risk assessment (Ekins, 2007). Because QSARs only use data on similar structures and do not directly test animals, they may actually be considered risk prediction tools rather than true hazard identification in an experimental sense. However, the drive for pharmaceutical researchers to identify which of the thousands of synthesized structures warrant further testing in drug development requires this type of analysis, as it represents a less costly, preliminary method for hazard identification. QSARs identify **structural alerts**—that is, those molecular functionalities that are known to cause toxicity, such as mutagenic carcinogenic moieties of molecules (Ashby and Tennant, 1991). Computer programs allow these alerts to be quantified for original compounds or for impurities representing more than 0.1% of the medication or 1 mg/day, whichever is lower for a dose of 2.0 g/day or less (Kruhlak et al., 2007).

Qualitative SARs that are more rule based are also available. For example, the Organization for Economic Cooperation and Development (OECD) has developed a set of principles for QSAR known as the Setubal Principles. They involve defined endpoints of regulatory importance, unambiguous algorithm development, and defined applicability domain; include contain measures of goodness of fit, robustness, and predictability; and are based on the chemical's mechanism of action. The QSAR therefore tries to predict the adverse effects of a chemical, whether they involve biochemical, physiologic, anatomic, or behavioral alterations that impair the function of the impacted organism. It may also try to determine inherent toxicity associated with systemic or contact injury.

Along with the QSAR, additional hazard-related information on the chemical may emerge from epidemiological or case studies (relative risk = mortality or morbidity incidence in exposed versus unexposed populations), accident reports, cell culture studies, and animal studies (acute, subchronic and chronic exposures).

Dose–Response Relationship (Hazard Characterization)

The LD_{50}, ED_{50}, TI, and margin of safety describe the overall toxicity of the perspective medication and may be used to determine the no observed effect level (NOEL) or **no observed adverse effect level (NOAEL)**, and the lowest observed effect level (LOEL) or **lowest observed adverse effect level (LOAEL)**. Note that carcinogenicity as identified via a mutagenesis or promotion assay would prevent further consideration of the medication for human use, unless it will be administered to treat a terminal illness, especially cancer. Many genotoxic systemic cancer medications cause hair loss, emesis (nausea resulting in vomiting) and loss of cells of the mouth and gastrointestinal (GI) tract, lowered blood cell counts, and other overt signs of toxicity to fast-growing cell populations. In the best case, the cancer is forced into programmed cell death (**apoptosis**), while the normal cells do not suffer irreversible damage (Hickman and Dive, 1999). In this case, the susceptibility of the fast-growing cancer cells versus other cells is then considered, and quantified via the **therapeutic ratio**.

Other factors such as age, sex, pregnancy status, nutritional status, health status, immune status, genetics, **toxicokinetics** (toxin absorption, distribution, metabolism, and elimination [ADME]), and **toxicodynamics** (mechanistic actions) also play important roles in susceptibility to medications (Iyaniwura, 2004). These factors will be different in children with many fast-growing cell populations, high nutritional requirements, low fat content, less-developed xenobiotic metabolism, and poorly established blood–brain barriers. Elderly individuals may have decreased repair mechanisms, xenobiotic metabolism, kidney function (leading to higher half-lives of medications), and reserve functional capacity compared with young healthy adults. Sex-related body composition differences and variations in susceptibility to chemicals may occur as well. Chemical exposure during pregnancy may lead to risk for the mother and her embryo or fetus.

Since cancer appears to have an obesity component and treatment affects nutritional intake, this factor plays a role in effectiveness and toxicity of chemotherapy agents as well. Depending on the organ(s) affected by the cancer and other underlying health concerns, the toxicity of the chemotherapeutic agent may depend on both the remaining organ function and the need for more aggressive and toxic treatment of metastasized tumors. Immunity is affected by standard chemotherapeutic agents, and negative effects on the immune system may hinder recovery from the cancer or induce immune deficiencies that result in the development of infections. Genetics plays a role in the risk of acquiring certain cancers, such as through the lack of a repressor protein, and also causes increased or decreased metabolism of the cancer medications. Overall, these factors combine to ensure unique toxicokinetics and toxicodynamics in individual patients' responses to a combination of chemotherapy agents employed in treatment regimens.

The goal of the Food and Drug Administration's (FDA's) Center for Drug Evaluation and Research when approving new cancer agents is to identify effectiveness over existing agents versus adverse effects (disease-free survival). The National Cancer Institute (NCI) has joined with the FDA to speed the development and approval process for chemotherapy agents in the following ways (http://www.cancer.gov/newscenter/pressreleases/NciFdaCollab):

- Developing markers of clinical benefit (**biomarkers**) for evaluating new cancer medicines. The two agencies will work to develop a standard approach for evaluating biomarkers that demonstrate a drug's clinical effectiveness and that can potentially serve in clinical trials as surrogate endpoints, which are substitutes for more conventional measures, such as survival time or mortality. Better defined surrogate endpoints could help speed the development of new drugs.

- Creating a cancer **bioinformatics** infrastructure to improve data collection, integration, and analysis for preclinical, preapproval, and postapproval research across all of the sectors involved in the development and delivery of cancer therapies.

- Addressing joint technology development issues. NCI and FDA staff will continue their current collaboration on clinical **proteomics** (involving the discovery of protein markers in the blood that can be used to detect and monitor disease course and drug response) as a possible model for initiatives in areas such as diagnostic imaging and molecular targeting.

- Advancing the development and evaluation process for cancer chemoprevention agents, including the development of clinically meaningful endpoints.

- Conducting a systematic review of current policies to identify other ways in which FDA–NCI collaborations can enhance the development and regulatory process for cancer technologies.

- Improving consumer awareness of the consequences of their choices about diet and nutrition for cancer prevention.

- Enhancing staff capabilities through collaborative training, joint rotations, and joint appointments.

Once the mechanism of action of a chemical is better understood (i.e., noncarcinogen or carcinogen), calculations can be done to better assess the hazard. Since the NOEL and LOEL are established prior to this phase for the most sensitive endpoint (toxic damage to the organ or function affected at the lowest dose range, such as reproduction), the use of uncertainty factors and modifying factors becomes important. These factors are based on the quality and closeness of the animal model to the human situation and whether the compound is a carcinogen.

For example, an older model to assess possible human exposure to air pollution was applied in the state of Michigan (Su and Wurzel, 1993). This model indicated that if the human lifetime inhalation NOEL was known for a given toxic emission, an uncertainty factor of 10 for individual differences was necessary to divide into the NOEL to obtain an acceptable ambient concentration (AAC). This determination would be similar to the U.S. Environmental Protection Agency's (EPA's) calculation of an **acceptable daily intake** (**ADI**; ADI = NOAEL/SF), where SF is the safety factor or that of a reference dose (RfD = NOEL/ UF × MF), UF is the uncertainty factor, and MF is the modifying factor (EPA, 1993). Further uncertainty factors for the Michigan model would multiply the factor of 10 for individual differences × 10 if only animal lifetime inhalation were available (now two log units), × 40 if only animal lifetime oral data were available (95th percentile oral LD_{50}/inhalation LD_{50} or LC_{50} ratio), × 5 if only 90-day animal oral data were available (95th percentile extrapolating 90-day to lifetime exposure), and × 7 if only 7-day animal oral data were available (95th percentile extrapolating 7-day to 90-day exposure). If only a short-term animal LC_{50} was available, then AAC = LC_{50}/100 × 500. If only the acute LD_{50} was available, then AAC = 100 × 40 × 500.

The EPA takes a less conservative approach than the Michigan model for air pollution exposure. The federal agency has established a set of standard UFs. It still uses a 10-fold factor to account for variation in human sensitivity, known as 10H. An additional 10-fold factor is used to extrapolate from animal data to humans similar to the Michigan model, known as 10A. This is where the EPA model and the Michigan model diverge, however. The EPA employs an additional 10-fold factor when extrapolating from less than chronic NOAELs to chronic NOAELs, known as 10S. Another 10-fold factor is used when the RfD is determined from a LOAEL instead of a NOAEL, known as 10L. The MF is greater than 0 but less than 10, and is determined through the use of professional judgment of scientific uncertainties of toxicology studies. An MF = 1 is used as the default value in the EPA model.

If a chemical is determined to be carcinogenic or oncogenic based on epidemiological evidence or animal studies, short-term in vitro experiments, increasing tumor size, or type in tumor models, or if the mechanism of action is known and represents the type of chemical species that has been found to cause tumorigenesis, then the linear dose–response curve assumes no threshold and a multistage process is employed where increasing the concentration of the carcinogen yields increased cancer. A cancer risk slope factor is generated to assess the oncogenic potency of the new chemical. In the generation of the cancer slope, the uncertainty factor for species differences is considered irrelevant, because cancer mechanisms are considered to be conserved by individuals and do not change up the evolutionary tree. Certain genetic differences may increase the risk of cancer such as the *BRCA1* and *BRCA2* mutations, which are associated with greater breast cancer incidence.

The type of data derived in such cases can be seen by examining the data for DDT from the EPA's Integrated Risk Information System (IRIS). DDT has a NOEL of 1 ppm (diet) or 0.05 mg/kg body weight/day, with a UF of 100 and a MF of 1, giving a RfD of 5 × 10^{-4} mg/kg/day based on a 27-week rat feeding study (Laug et al., 1950). A 100-fold UF was employed due to the uncertainty of interspecies conversion (factor of 10) and to protect sensitive human subpopulations (second factor of 10). As another chronic animal study was already found in the EPA database, it was considered unnecessary to include another 10-fold uncertainty factor for conversion from subchronic to chronic data. The older studies on DDT were shorter than the EPA currently requires, so the confidence in the RfD is considered medium to low. DDT is classified as B2—a probable human carcinogen—based on sufficient rat and mice liver tumor development, but inadequately verified in human populations by three studies that indicated elevated DDT and DDE (a metabolic product of DDT) in cancer victims versus those who died of other causes. The carcinogenicity oral slope factor is 3.4×10^{-1} mg/kg/day using a linearized multistage procedure including extra risk. The drinking water risk is 9.7×10^{-6} µg/L. For drinking water, the 1/10,000, 1/100,000, and 1/1,000,000 risk factors are 1.0×10^{1}, 1.0, and 1.0×10^{-1} µg/L, respectively.

Exposure

There are a number of routes of exposure, including dermal or dermal patch, inhalation or nasal spray, eye drops or exposure, oral (PO) or oral gavage, sublingual, intravenous (IV), intramuscular (IM), intraperitoneal (IP), intracerebroventricular (ICV; injected into the cerebrospinal fluid [CSF] in the brain) and intrathecal (injected in the CSF of the spinal cord), and rectal or rectal suppository. Here, the toxicokinetics are important for assessing time to peak. Indeed, the route of administration is extremely important in the development of maximum concentration, C_{max} (**Figure 4-4**). With the IV route, 100% bioavailability is apparent instantaneously on administration. This outcome is similar for the sublingual, ICV, intrathecal, and inhalation routes. Lower doses give a rapid peak equal to that of administration of the same drug by the PO or similar routes at much higher doses. The peak also drops rapidly in a biphasic manner related to the apparent **volume of distribution**, V_d, followed by a sustained metabolism and elimination line.

If the original compound (e.g., cocaine, ethanol) produces a threshold toxic effect, then these rapid peak routes will indicate the acute toxicity more readily. If metabolism is required to activate the compound to a toxic form and then a threshold is reached, then those routes that must first pass through the liver may yield the highest peak toxicity (e.g., PO or IP). However, for other compounds, the development of cancer or other chronic toxicities such as liver cirrhosis is seen with an increased **area under the curve (AUC)**. In Figure 4-4, note that the oral route sustains the absorption and elimination and, therefore, the AUC is larger for this route, although the peak is lower for the same dosage. If toxicity is not significant by either of these routes, except that children may be more susceptible to apparent CNS effects, the ICV or intrathecal route should indicate whether the blood–brain barrier is effectively excluding the compound of interest due to its charge and size. The only routes necessary to consider for therapeutic risk assessment are oral, inhalation, and dermal.

In nontherapeutic tests to model environmental human exposures, the assessment of dose usually involves the concentration of the toxicant (e.g., lead in paint chips, mercury in fish, ozone in the air) multiplied by the amount ingested or the time spent inhaling the average concentration (**time-weighted average [TWA]**). The EPA calculates an **estimated exposure dose (EED)**. For therapeutic models, **exposure = concentration × intake × duration × frequency/body weight**. Intake is the amount organisms are actually exposed to by a given route, while uptake is the amount actually absorbed into the body. Thus **absorbed dose = exposure × absorption factor**. Hydrophobicity, charge, molecular weight, and size of the compound, along with tissue hydration, heart rate, plasma volume and protein binding, kidney function, and metabolic rate, are all factors that affect the absorption, distribution, metabolism, and elimination—that is, the toxicokinetics—of the compound. The absorbed doses from the oral, inhalation, and dermal routes are added to obtain an **average absorbed daily dose (AADD)**.

As aging changes the metabolic rates, growth, and organ functions, a **lifetime average daily dose (LADD)** is calculated as $(1/70 \times \text{AADD}_{infant}) + (5/70 \times \text{AADD}_{1-6}) + (6/70 \times \text{AADD}_{7-12}) + (6/70 \times \text{AADD}_{13-18}) \times (52/70 \times \text{AADD}_{19-70})$. Although the adult portion appears

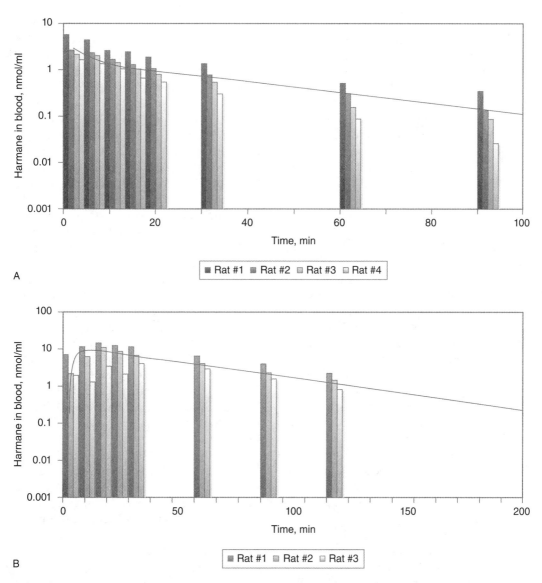

FIGURE 4-4 Toxicokinetic Blood Concentration Versus Time Curve for (A) 0.5 mg/kg IV Dosage and (B) 20 mg/kg Oral Carboline Tremorogenic Agent Harmane into Male Sprague-Dawley Gavage of the Rats

Data from Guan Y, Louis ED, Zheng W. 2001. Toxicokinetics of tremorogenic natural products, harmane and harmine, in male Sprague-Dawley rats. *J Toxicol Environ Health.* 64:645–660.

to dwarf the other stages of life, much of pesticide exposure that impacts a human may occur in the earliest stages of life due the lipophilicity of the compounds and breast milk concentrations. For many adult therapeutic compounds, this may not be as important a consideration (especially if age restrictions result from FDA analysis of human case reports of morbidity and mortality in children, such as occurred with cold medication use in children younger than 2 years of age).

The **maximum daily dose (MDD)** or **maximum recommended therapeutic dose (MRTD)** is also assessed in the target population by known use, as opposed to animal experiments that require safety factors. The FDA quotes an article indicating that the **maximum recommended starting dose (MRSD)** for Phase I clinical trials as well as the NOEL can be extrapolated from animal studies, while the NOAEL involves multiple species and a most sensitive species. While extrapolation to humans involves multiple uncertainty factors, the MRTD is determined from human studies at a dose above which no increased therapeutic advantage is gained and adverse effects do not exceed benefits (Contrera et al., 2004).

Risk

Risk characterization involves **standards of exposure** and **permissible exposures**. Risk managers may incorporate more than the scientific evidence mentioned previously; in particular, they may consider economic considerations, the **limit of detection (LOD)**, and the **limit of quantification (LOQ)**. The last two are analytical chemistry functions determined by the latest, most sensitive, reproducible technological means (Mocak et al., 1997). The limit of detection is the smallest amount or concentration that can be detected with reasonable certainty, but does not account well for the blank signal. The limit of quantification accounts for the blank versus the standard signals and represents the smallest concentration or mass that can be reasonably analyzed by a given procedure.

Permissible exposures use only the scientific data associated with published adverse health effects. The chemical must again be separated into carcinogen and noncarcinogens. The **permissible concentration = RfD × body weight/intake × duration × frequency** (referred as the **permissible exposure limit [PEL]** by EPA). This may be considered more easily by looking at the RfD and the MDD. If MDD < RfD, then the exposure is considered as safe as can be determined if proper safety factors are employed. If MDD > RfD and approaches two log units from the NOEL, then the exposure may be considered unsafe. Safety is a relative factor. For example, people with certain enzyme deficiencies, such as those with phenylketonuria who lack the phenylalanine hydroxylase enzyme, must avoid compounds

such as aspartame, which is safe to the general population; individuals with severe allergies, such as peanut allergy, must avoid all forms of peanut protein in foods and even inhalation of small concentrations of this substance.

The EPA sets a **margin of exposure (MOE)** as well, where the MOE = NOAEL (experimental dose) / EED (human dose). A problematic exposure is considered when the NOAEL < EED. MOE > 10 is considered relatively low risk if all extrapolations have been made properly. The EPA also considers the **regulatory dose, RgD(i) = NOAEL/MOE(i)**, where (i) is the chemical under regulatory scrutiny. Different RgDs are possible for a given chemical with a single RfD. Comparing the RfD to a particular RgD(i) is equivalent to comparing the MOE(i) with the UF × MF: RfD/RgD(i) = MOE(i) / (UF × MF). Risk managers at EPA are asked to look carefully at case-specific data from risk assessors whenever the RgD is > or < the RfD. "In assessing the significance of a case in which the RgD is greater (or less) than the RfD, the risk manager should carefully consider the case-specific data compiled by the risk assessors, as discussed in Section 1.3.4" (EPA, 1993).

Carcinogens carry a carcinogenicity slope that can be a modifying factor for an ingested substance. The EPA assesses the risk of carcinogens by using a methodology examined by the National Academy of Sciences (Committee on the Institutional Means for Assessment of Risks to Public Health, 1983). It calculates carcinogenic risk as $R = LADD_{POT \text{ or } INT} \times SF$, where POT represents dermal exposures, INT represents oral administrations, and SF is the carcinogenicity slope factor. The total should represent 1 in 1 million risk or $1 \times 10^{-6}/SF$.

As an example, for a study of uranium in Korean groundwater, the RfD for uranium as a chemical is 0.6 µg/kg/day. The LADD for the most contaminated site at Daejeon was 0.074 µg/kg/day, meaning that the RfD exceeded the LADD by a factor of 8.1 (Kim et al., 2004). Since a factor of 10 was not yet achieved, risk was determined. The carcinogenicity slope factor for the uranium isotope ^{238}U (isotope ^{238}U is 99.3% of the natural uranium concentration) is 2.1×10^{-10} risk/pCi for ingested uranium due to the low intestinal absorption of approximately 1–2% (picocuries [pCi] are radiation decomposition units). The Health Physics Society indicates that 1 pCi of ^{238}U represents 2.97 mg/L (http://www.hps.org/Publicinformation/ate/q6747.html). This corresponds to a slope factor in risk per milligram of 2.1 $\times$ 10^{-10} risk/pCi $\times$ 1 pCi/2.97 mg or 7.1 $\times$ 10^{-11} risk/mg. R = LADD $\times$ SF, so R = 0.074 $\times$ 7.1 $\times$ 10^{-11} risk/mg ^{238}U = 5.2 $\times$ 10^{-12} risk or 5.2 cancer risk per 1 trillion population. Actually, if other factors are included, the risk is still small and less than 1 in 10 million for the Korean study.

This example demonstrates that for some compounds, the model predicts low risk. Other reports, such as for the pesticide Aldrin at Extoxnet, predict a much higher cancer risk (1/29) than actually exists. For these chemicals, the human data should be examined rather than relying on the risk model. If the model is inverted (R/SF = LADD) setting the risk at 1 per 1 million, DDT would have a 0.000001/0.34 mg/kg/day slope factor or 0.00000294 mg/kg/day for a LADD. At this extremely low level, the data would suggest banning DDT and sequestering the remaining contamination in some safe hazardous waste facility. This result is even below the ADI set by the World Health Organization (WHO) for breastfeeding women. The developing countries of the world have problems with malaria that kill millions of people per year; the incidence of this infection may be greatly reduced by DDT applications in homes of the affected regions. During the period of highest DDT use in the United States, when children literally ran in the DDT spray of trucks as a game, the cancer rate was not at a level that would have been calculated from the risk equation. The human data were reexamined and found to be weak regarding this pesticide. DDT was, in fact, banned due to its adverse effects on condor egg shell strength, not based on its carcinogenicity (Hickey et al., 1968).

As the DDT example suggests, both the regulatory agency and the toxicologist must consider the calculation of a risk value in light of the strength of the empirical human evidence. Otherwise, unwise and expensive unnecessary regulations will cause mistrust in the science

of toxicology and other undesired societal outcomes. These risk factors can also be used to calculate when an area sprayed with pesticide is safe for workers to return to manage crops— that is, where the reentry dose level is equal to the toxicological endpoint/safety factor. Note that this relationship is similar in structure to other toxicological risk assessment calculations. Evidence indicates there are a "safe" level and a sensitive toxic endpoint for any chemical. Uncertainty about individual differences and the quality of the data used in assessing this endpoint may lead to identification of safety factors that should provide adequate protection if all assumptions or models have the most sensitive toxicity targeted and the human range of response well addressed. For carcinogens, ADIs have been disallowed, with a virtually safe dose (VSD) being assigned instead; ADIs are reserved for noncarcinogens.

Ecosystems

Overview

Some ecosystem analyses have used laboratory exposures of selected species as predictive of the whole. In such a case, looking retrospectively into the effects of certain compounds on species or metrics used to evaluate ecosystems needs to be combined with the generation of the predictive data by proper modeling and testing. Entire books have been developed that examine environmental risk assessment and ecological risk assessment (Suter, 2007). However, the EPA offices (e.g., Office of Pollution Prevention and Toxics or OPPT), the European Environmental Agency (EEA), and other agencies worldwide have not yet brought their analysis under one commonly accepted set of criteria. The chief problems appear to be the production of an integrated risk assessment that WHO can agree will serve all purposes of this assessment (Bridges, 2003). The EEA has produced a document that summarizes the techniques, which are similar to those described earlier. The hazard and dose-response relationship are classified together as an effects assessment based on physicochemical properties of the chemical, its ecotoxic effects, its intended use, and the predicted no effect concentration (PNEC) using all appropriate ecological impacts and assessment criteria. Exposure is determined by the predicted environmental concentration (PEC). Modeling should consider release, degradation, transport, and fate and include worst-case situations. Monitoring should also be a component when deriving real-world data. Risk characterization uses the PEC/PNEC ratio (less than 1 defines low or no risk to the environment). The scheme for an environmental risk analysis is presented in **Figure 4-5** (Fairman et al., 1998).

Note that all emissions and fates should be considered; that is, the air, various soil use areas (e.g., grassland and agricultural land), waters (surface and groundwater), and sediments should be considered. The EEC report also indicates that the following problems need to be addressed:

- Determining the effects at population and community level

- Selection of endpoints
- Selection of indicative species;
- Selection of field, laboratory, mesocosm, and microcosm tests
- Incorporation of resilience and recovery factors of the ecosystem

Hazard

The definition of the hazard may start with a QSAR and attention to a variety of databases. The QSAR may involve something akin to the **toxic equivalency factor (TEF)**, which assigns a value to chlorine positions of dioxins, furans, and polychlorinated biphenyls (PCBs), or a **total dioxin-toxic equivalent (TEQ)** (Van den Berg, 1998). The databases used include the following:

- Agency for Toxic Substances and Disease Registry HazDat: hazardous substance release/health effects database based on

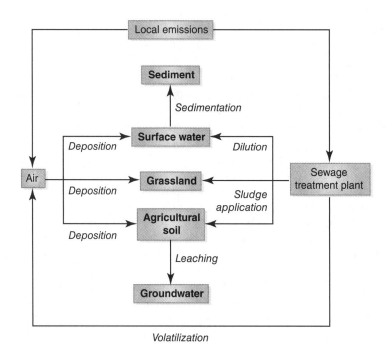

FIGURE 4-5 Local Relevant Emission and Distribution Routes

Data from Fairman R, Mead CD, Williams WP. 1998. Environmental risk assessment: approaches, experiences and information sources. EEA at http://reports.eea.europa.eu/GH-07-97-595-EN-C2/en/riskindex.html

U.S. data and exposure scenarios including toxicological profiles (http://atsdr1.atsdr.cdc.gov:8080/ hazdat.html#A3.1)

- Aquatic Information Retrieval or AQUIRE: aquatic toxicity studies
- Bielstein: information on all organic compounds including toxicity and environmental effects (http://www .beilstein.com/)
- BIG (Data Bank Brandweerinformatiecentrum Gevaarlijke Stoffen): names, physical properties, handling and response, health effects of chemicals
- Carcinogenic Potency Database (http://potency .berkeley.edu/cpdb.html)
- CHEMBANK: HSDB, OHMTADS, CHRIS, RTECS, and IRIS databases
- CHEMBASE Physical Properties Database: chemical names, physicochemical properties and structures
- CHEMDATA: physical properties, names and codes, handling information, health effects
- CHEMEST: physicochemical properties
- Chemical Abstracts: includes environmental fate and ecotoxicity
- Chemical Hazards Response Information System (CHRIS): physicochemical properties and biological/fire hazard potential use in spill situations
- Chemical Information System (CIS): chemical and physical properties, handling and response, health effects, environmental effects
- Chemical Safety Newsbase: bibliographic information, abstracts, and other data from all types of media on hazards of chemicals, including spillages, disposal, and accidental releases of chemicals
- CHEMTOX: physicochemical properties, toxicity, effects, spill data
- Dictionary of Substances and Their Effects (DOSE): occupational exposure limits, mammalian and avian toxicity, ecotoxicity and environmental fate, and physical properties
- ECETOC Aquatic Toxicity (EAT)
- EINECS Plus-CD: European Inventory of Existing Chemicals (EINECS) and European List of Notified Chemical Substances (ELINCS); names, CAS numbers and formulae

- Environmental Chemicals Data and Information Network (ECDIN): European databank on chemical names, chemical and physical properties, toxicity, health and environmental effects, environmental fate and transport (http://ulisse .ei.jrc.it/Ecdin/Ecdin.html)
- Environmental Chemistry, Health and Safety: information on chemicals deemed to cause actual or potential problems to humans or the environment
- Environmental Fate (ENVIROFATE): physicochemical properties and environmental transformation rates extracted from published literature
- Environmental Fate Databases: physicochemical properties and environmental transformation rates
- Environmental Fate/Exposure Databases (EFEDB): four interrelated files providing physicochemical properties and environmental transformation rates
- EXICHEM: details of areas of research conducted by OECD member countries on existing chemicals (http://oracle.bangor . ac.uk/exichem/)
- Extension TOXicology NETwork (Extoxnet): pesticide information briefs, related toxicity information and FAQs (http://ace.ace.orst.edu/info/extoxnet/ghindex.html)
- Hazardous Chemical Database (http://odin .chemistry.uakron.edu/erd/)
- HAZDATA: chemical risk assessment database
- IARC and NTP Carcinogen List (http://ntp .niehs.nih.gov/go/roc)
- INFOTOX: chemical and physical properties, handling and response, health effects
- Integrated Risk Information System (IRIS; http://www.epa.gov)
- International Register of Potentially Toxic Chemicals (IRPTC; http://www.unep.ch/irptc/databank.html)
- IUCLID (International Uniform Chemical Information Database): basic tool for priority setting and risk assessment within the EU-Risk Assessment Programme
- Material Safety Data Sheets (MSDS): many are available online by searching for MSDS

- Oceanic Abstracts (OA)
- OECD SIDS Profiles: Screening Information Data Set profiles of chemicals from the OECD High Production Volume Investigation (http://www .unep.ch/irptc/tcontent.html)
- OHS MSDS Database
- Oil and Hazardous Materials Technical Assistance Data System (OHM-TADS)
- PEST-BANK: information on registered pesticides in the United States
- PESTIS (Pesticide Information Service): an online database that contains pesticide reform-related material generated by nongovernmental organizations (NGOs), including articles, newsletters, reports, and action alerts, all of which can be full-text searched
- POLTOX I: citations of the world's pollution and toxicology literature from seven databases, including TOXLINE, Toxicology Abstracts and Ecology Abstracts
- Portfolio–Chemical Safety: Stanford University searchable database of hazard information on chemicals (http://www .portfolio.stanford.edu/ no-form/100369/5)
- Registry of Toxic Effects of Chemical Substances (RTECS)
- RISKLINE: bibliographic databank containing information on the toxic effects of chemical substances in the form of peer-reviewed documents
- SOLVE-DB: common names/synonyms, physicochemical properties, environmental fate of solvents
- CHEMTOX Database: chemical names, CAS numbers, synonyms, physicochemical properties, toxicological data, and transport hazard/emergency response data
- Toxfaqs: toxicity and human health effects of chemicals in fact sheet format (http://atsdr1.atsdr.cdc.gov:8080/toxfaqf .html)
- TOXLINE: adverse effects of chemicals, drugs, and physical agents on humans and animals
- U.S. EPA Chemicals Substance Factsheets and Material Safety Data Sheets: chemical safety data sheets providing information such as toxicological and ecotoxicological

information, effects endpoints, and exposure limits (http://www.epa.gov)

This list is not complete but gives the overwhelming amount of data in a variety of formats. It is clear that a single reliable source of data has not yet been developed in a commonly accepted format that is best for ecotoxicological hazard assessment.

Hazard Characterization/Dose–Response Relationship

Figure 4-6 gives a sense of which data might likely be provided by an environmental toxicity analysis. New to this analysis is the **maximum-allowable toxic concentration (MATC)**. Another measure suggested by regulatory researchers is the **benchmark dose**, meaning the dose that causes a 10% increase in population affected over the untreated background population (Gaylor and Aylward, 2004). The aquatic toxicity measures of toxic units, SPEARS, and relative tolerance would come into play here.

The EPA's analysis of aquatic toxicity of pesticides requires a tiered approach. In Tier 1 (deterministic), acute toxicity and slope data are required for three species of freshwater (and saltwater) aquatic animals and one species of aquatic plant and, only in some cases, chronic studies of four species of aquatic organisms. In Tier 2 (probabilistic), additional acute toxicity tests on four species are performed for the group of organisms (e.g., fish, algae) observed to be most sensitive in Tier 1 data. If triggered by other criteria such as persistence, chronic studies on four species of aquatic organisms would be required. Tier 3 requires no additional toxicity data. Tier 4 indicates that the regulator or registrant must require or furnish additional field-derived toxicity data that are more realistic, or special tests for pulse exposures or compounds with very short half-lives may be used to obtain a better estimate of the toxicity distribution. Moving up the tiers requires an EEC (exposure) determination and a risk assessment. Ecotoxicology researchers would like to include more ecologically relevant macrobiotic invertebrate, benthic fish species, and other metrics in

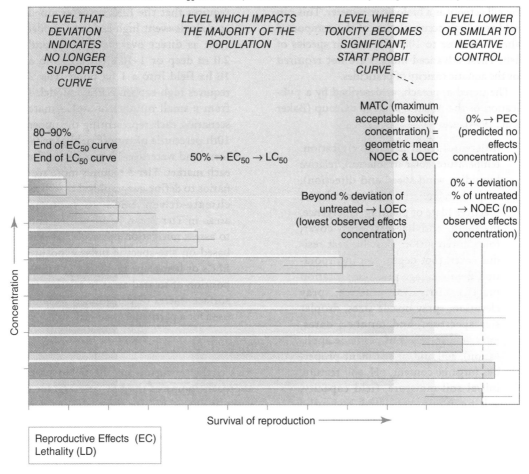

Environmental effluent toxicity testing
(Inverted plot)

Acute to chronic ratio = LC_{50}/MATC helps determine chronic toxicity using acute toxicity data

FIGURE 4-6 Environmental Effluent Toxicity Testing

Data from Stewart AJ. 1999. Insights from ambient toxicity testing. In *Measures of environmental performance and ecosystem condition*. Schulze PC, ed. Washington, DC: National Academy Press, pp. 199–216.

these analyses to assess impacts on an ecological scale rather than single-species laboratory tests, as well as limited-species microcosm or mesocosm analyses.

Exposure

For exposure, a true examination would not only use laboratory exposures, but also consider bioaccumulation up the food web, especially for persistent compounds, such as the halogenated hydrocarbons. The EPA's Center

for Exposure Assessment Modeling (CEAM) has a variety of models to assess exposure through groundwater, surface water, food chain, and multimedia. Air pollution models are handled by another laboratory.

One food chain program for fish that has been used is the Food and Gill Exchange of Toxic Substances (FGETS) program. Using physicochemical parameters of a compound such as the octanol–water partition coefficient (hydrophobicity of the compound), along with the molecular weight and molecular volume of

the chemical, the percent active gill of the fish, the concentration in the fish, and bioaccumulation may be modeled. Especially important is the gill activity as a biologic parameter. This can yield very high accumulation of the compound when it is close to 100% for certain species of fish. These advanced models are not required for the aquatic toxicity of pesticides.

The tiered approach, as described by a publication of the Aquatic Dialogue Group (Baker et al., 1994), uses

> [M]eteorological data (precipitation, temperature, solar irradiation, relative humidity, wind speed and direction), crop characteristics and agricultural practices (date of planting, emergence, maturity, and harvest; crop cover, foliar interception, post-harvest residue cover, root depth, soil incorporation depth, tillage practices, rotation practices, irrigation practice, spray elevation, spray nozzle sizes, droplet size spectrum; and number, dates, rates, and methods of pesticide application), soil and/or sediment properties (organic content, pH, soil texture, initial soil moisture, field capacity, wilting point, saturated hydraulic conductivity, slope, temperature, bulk density and porosity as a function of vertical and/or horizontal segmentation), pesticide properties (aqueous solubility, pK_as, Henry's constant, octanol/water partition coefficient, aqueous diffusivity, organic normalized soil/water and/or sediment/water partition coefficients, foliar washoff and degradation, overall and process-specific half-lives, and degradate formation rate constants), and surface water characteristics (pesticide loadings due to runoff, soil erosion, and spray drift; pH, temperature, suspended sediment concentrations, dissolved natural organic concentrations, redox potentials, base flows, depth, width, cross-sectional areas, and dispersion coefficients). Models employed involve categories or

dissolved runoff, soil erosion, and leaching models; spray drift models; and surface water models. Tier 1 requires that the EEC be determined as a single-event high-exposure model such as direct overspray of a pond 2.0 m deep or 1–10% runoff from a 10 ha field into a 1 ha pond. Tier 2 requires high-exposure EECs modeled from a small number of soil/climate scenarios, each representing the upper 10th percentile of runoff yield of sediment and water for 10-year return for each market. Tier 3 requires more scenarios to define geographical as well as climate-driven EECs so problem areas in Tier 2 can be identified and to assess mitigation options. Tier 4 is based on site-specific pulse exposure EECs or landscape modeling to assess position of treated areas in relation to surface waters or percentages of land used for a particular chemical.

Risk

Risk characterization for the tiered pesticide approach compares the EEC and LC_5 for most levels. If EEC $<$ LC_5 for the most sensitive species and (where chronic data are available) if EEC $<$ NOEC for the most sensitive species, then Tier 2 is employed. In such a case, the environmental assessment is completed and an ecotoxicological analysis is not required beyond this information. To move from Tier 2 to Tier 3, each market for which the upper 10th percentile annual maximum EEC for the duration of interest and its high-exposure soil/climate scenario is less than the lower 10th percentile of the distribution of the LC_5 estimates from acute tests or this EEC is less than the lower 10th percentile of the distribution of the NOEC from chronic test must be evaluated. To move from Tier 3 to Tier 4, the same analysis is done as occurred at the lower tier, but adding the soil/climate scenarios to compare the upper 10th percentile annual maximum EEC to the lower 10th percentile of the distribution of the LC_5 or NOEC. Only Tier 4 calls for "more realistic toxicity tests" that may really

ECOLOGICAL RISK ASSESSMENT PARADIGM

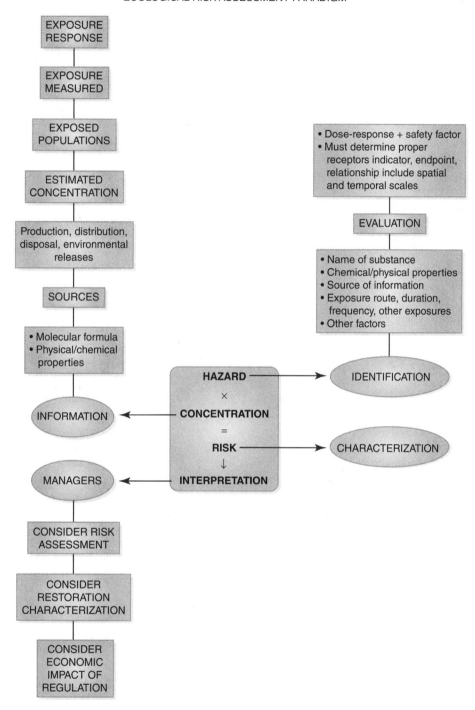

FIGURE 4-7 Ecological Risk Assessment Paradigm as Proposed by the National Research Council

Data from Burger J. 1997. The historical basis of ecological risk assessment. *NY Acad Sci.* 837:360–371.

start to broach an ecotoxicological analysis that either leads to mitigation or sparks studies by the research laboratories of EPA or academic institutions that are interested in species abundance, richness, habitat, food web effects, and other outcomes that may indicate the degraded condition of watersheds in agriculturally intensive areas or urban areas impacted by industrial emissions.

Some regional reestablishment of habitat and quality has occurred, as in the urban previously highly contaminated New Jersey Meadowlands (a research article list can be found at http://meri.njmeadowlands.gov/About_Meri/publications.php). At these sites, ecological and toxic substance monitoring is used to evaluate the recovery of an important aquatic ecosystem.

Current agricultural practices that have been allowed to degrade systems have led to the dead zone in the Gulf of Mexico that is a focus of the EPA at this time (Mississippi River/Gulf of Mexico Watershed Nutrient Task Force; http://www.epa.gov/msbasin/). As long as the former potential of an ecosystem or ecoregion is not considered, environmental assessments represent justifications based on economic decisions to accept the degraded current system as a control on which to base risk decisions employing species very tolerant to pollution, such as the fathead minnow, as a model EPA species. This point has been well made by Zhou and coworkers (2004), who note that most ecological risk assessments ignore the ecology framework of understanding community and ecosystem structure and function. They proposed a model that simulates "the structure and dynamics of complex ecological networks to generally estimate the risk under environmental stressors." In doing so, Zhou et al. employed a food-web structure model (Williams and Martinez, 2000) as well as a trophic predator–prey dynamics model (Yodzis and Innes, 1992). In summary, they "propose a generic framework for estimating and predicting community risks that may be extended to address many other risks such as those posed by toxics in the environment combined with global warming." This combination approach is necessary if single-species toxicity testing or multiple-species testing moves to

ecotoxicological testing for the interaction of species in a changing environment. **Figure 4-7** demonstrates this understanding, as expressed by Burger and Handel (n.d.).

The U.S. EPA also has developed a number of metrics that it recommends for stream evaluation, landscape evaluation, and other assessments and has provided grants to study and integrate metrics into its regulatory structure.

Questions

1. What is an RfD and how is it assembled for cells? For the whole organism?
2. How are the EEC and the LC_5 used to assess environmental toxicity?
3. What is a TEF and why is it necessary?

References

Adler JH. 2002. Dangerous precaution: the precautionary principle's challenge to progress. *Nat Rev.* http://www.nationalreview.com/adler/adler091302.asp.

Ashby J, Tennant RW. 1991. Definitive relationships among chemical structure, carcinogenicity and mutagenicity for 301 chemicals tested by the U.S. NTP [National Toxicology Program]. *Mutat Res.* 257:229–306.

Baker JL, Barefoot AC, Beasley LE, Burns L, Caulkins P, Clark J, Feulner RL, Giesey JP, Graney RL, Griggs R, Jacoby H, Laskowski D, Maciorowski A, Mihaich E, Nelson H, Parrish R, Siefert RE, Solomon KE, van der Schalie W. 1994. *Final report: aquatic risk assessment and mitigation dialogue group.* Pensacola, FL: SETAC Press.

Bridges J. 2003. Human health and environmental risk assessment: the need for a more harmonised and integrated approach. *Chemosphere.* 52:1347–1351.

Burger J. 1997. The historical basis of ecological risk assessment. *NY Acad Sci.* 837:360–371.

Burger J, Handel S. Using restoration ecology as a tool for risk assessment. *Risk Anal. CRESP.* Unpublished Report 20.

Committee on the Institutional Means for Assessment of Risks to Public Health, National Research Council. 1983. *Risk assessment in the federal government: managing the process.* Washington, DC: National Academies Press.

Contrera JF, Matthews EJ, Kruhlak NL, Benz, RD. 2004. Estimating the safe starting dose in Phase I clinical trials and no observed effect level based on QSAR modeling of the human maximum recommended daily dose. *Regul Toxicol Pharmacol.* 40:185–206.

Cook JC, Gaido KW, Greenlee WF. 1987. Ah receptor: relevance of mechanistic studies to human risk assessment. *Environ Health Perspect.* 76:71–77.

Courtney KD, Gaylor DW, Hogan MD, Falk HL, Bates RR, Mitchell I. 1970. Teratogenic evaluation of 2,4,5-T. *Science.* 168:864–866.

Dahlin DC, Miwa GT, Lu AY, Nelson SD. 1984. *N*-Acetyl-p-benzoquinone imine: a cytochrome P-450–mediated oxidation product of acetaminophen. *Proc Natl Acad Sci USA.* 81:1327–1331.

Dantas G, Sommer MOA, Oluwasegun RD, Church GM. 2008. Bacteria subsisting on antibiotics. *Science.* 320:100–103.

Ekins S, ed. 2007. *Computational toxicology: risk assessment for pharmaceutical and environmental chemicals.* Hoboken, NJ: John Wiley & Sons.

Eley A, Ibrahim M, Kurdi SE, Conlon JM. 2008. Activities of the frog skin peptide, ascaphin-8 and its lysine-substituted analogs against clinical isolates of extended-spectrum β-lactamase (ESBL) producing bacteria. *Peptides.* 29:25–30.

Fairman R, Mead CD, Williams WP. 1998. Environmental risk assessment: approaches, experiences and information sources. http://reports.eea.europa .eu/GH-07-97-595-EN-C2/en/riskindex.html.

Fish C. 2006. Risk assessment in drug development [or how much of compound X is safe?]. Glaxo-SmithKline. http://www.mmsconferencing.com/ pdf/eyp//c.fish.pdf.

Gaylor DW, Aylward LL. 2004. An evaluation of benchmark dose methodology for non-cancer continuous-data health effects in animals due to exposures to dioxin (TCDD). *Regul Toxicol Pharmacol.* 40:9–17.

Hancock REW. 1997. The bacterial outer membrane as a drug barrier. *Trends Microbiol.* 5:37–42.

Hickey JJ, Daniel W, Anderson DW. 1968. Chlorinated hydrocarbons and eggshell changes in raptorial and fish-eating birds. *Science.* 162:271–273.

Hickman JA, Dive C, eds. 1999. *Apoptosis and cancer chemotherapy: cancer drug discovery and development.* Totowa, NJ: Humana Press.

Hoekstra HA. 2006. Estimating the LC_{50}: a review. *Environmetrics.* 2:139–152.

Iyaniwura TT. 2004. Individual and subpopulation variations in response to toxic chemicals: factors of susceptibility. *Risk World.* http://www.riskworld .com/Nreports/2004/Iyaniwura.htm.

Kim Y-S, Park H-S, Kim J-Y, Park S-K, Cho B-W, Sung I-H, Shin D-C. 2004. Health risk assessment for uranium in Korean groundwater. *J Environ Radioact.* 77:77–85.

Kruhlak NL, Contrera JF, Benz RD, Matthews EJ. 2007. Progress in QSAR toxicity screening of pharmaceutical impurities and other FDA regulated product. *Adv Drug Deliv Rev.* 59:43–55.

Kuroki T, Matsushima T. 1987. Performance of short-term tests for detection of human carcinogens. *Mutagenesis.* 2:33–37.

Laug EP, Nelson AA, Fitzhugh OG, Kunze FM. 1950. Liver cell alteration and DDT storage in the fat of the rat induced by dietary levels of 1–50 ppm DDT. *J Pharmacol Exp Therap.* 98:268–273.

Martin RE, Kirk K. 2004. The malaria parasite's chloroquine resistance transporter is a member of the drug/metabolite transporter superfamily. *Mol Biol Evol.* 21:1938–1949.

Mocak J, Bond AM, Mitchell S, Scollary G. 1997. A statistical overview or standard (IUPAC and ACS) and new procedures for determining the limits of detection and quantification: application to voltammetric and stripping techniques. *Pure Appl Chem.* 69:297–328.

Muller H-G, Schmitt T. 1988. Kernel and probit estimates in quantal bioassay. *J Am Statist Assoc.* 83:750–759.

Sandoz C, Lesca P, Narbonne JF. 1999. Hepatic Ah receptor binding affinity for 2,3,7, 8-tetrachlorodibenzo-*p*-dioxin: similarity between beagle dog and cynomolgus monkey. *Toxicol Lett.* 109:115–121.

Sprocati AR, Alisi C, Segre L, Tasso F, Galletti M, Cremisini C. 2006. Investigating heavy metal resistance, bioaccumulation and metabolic profile of a metallophile microbial consortium native to an abandoned mine. *Sci Total Environ.* 366: 649–658.

Stewart AJ. 1999. Insights from ambient toxicity testing. In: Schulze PC, ed. *Measures of environmental performance and ecosystem condition.* Washington, DC: National Academy Press, pp. 199–216.

Su G, Wurzel KA. 1993. A regulatory framework for setting air emission limits for non-criteria pollutants. *J Air Pollut Control Assoc.* 1:160–162.

Suter GW II. 2007. *Ecological risk assessment* (2nd ed.). Boca Raton, FL: CRC Press.

U.S. Environmental Protection Agency (EPA). 1993. An ADI for fluoride use on human teeth would have a safety factor of one according to the EPA due to the known sensitive human population's response. Reference dose (RfD): description and use in health risk assessments. http://www.epa.gov/ iris/rfd.htm.

Van den Berg M, Birnbaum L, Bosveld BTC, Brunstrom B, Cook P, Feeley M, Giesy JP, Hanberg A, Hasegawa R, Kennedy SW, Kubiak T, Larsen JC, van Leeuwen FXR, Liem AKD, Nolt C, Peterson RE,

Poellinger L, Safe S, Schrenck D, Tillitt D, Tysklind M, Younes M, Waern F, Zacharewski T. 1998. Toxic equivalency factors (TEFs) for PCBs, PCDDs, PCDFs for humans and for wildlife. *Environ Health Perspect.* 106:775–792.

Williams RJ, Martinez ND. 2000. Simple rules yield complex food webs. *Nature.* 404:180–183.

Yodzis P, Innes S. 1992. Body-size and consumer-resource dynamics. *Am Nat.* 139:1151–1173.

Zhou Y, Brose U, Kastenberger W, Martinez ND. 2004. A new approach to ecological risk assessment: simulating effects of global warming on complex networks. necsi.org/events/iccs/openconf/author/papers/f422.pdf.

PART II

Toxic Reactions of Cells

Absorption and Transport of Toxicants Through Membranes: Toxic Damage to Membranes

This is a chapter outline intended to guide and familiarize you with the content to follow.

I. Absorption of Toxicants

   A. Examples

→ Large (Hg^0) or highly charged (acetylsalicylic acid) → Skin	X No/Low absorption
→ Hydrophobic (dimethylmercury) or + DMSO (dimethylsulfoxide) → Skin	→ High absorption
→ Hydrophobic + small (gases such as anesthetic gases) → Lung	→ High absorption
→ Very small (nanoparticles, nanofibers) → All routes	→ High absorption
→ Strong acids, bases, solvents → Damage membrane components	→ High absorption

High absorption follows Fick's first law of diffusion

   B. Mechanisms of transport

Certain metals such as arsenite → Specialized transport through water channels (see AQPs)

Other heavy metals → Through ion channel (Cd and Ca channels)

→ Bind to proteins and form diffusible complexes (Hg^{+1} or Hg^{+2})

→ ATP-binding cassette (ABC) transporter (molybdate/tungstate)

Organic compounds → ABC transporter (charged monosaccharides, antibiotics, peptides; may confer resistance to cancer chemotherapy agents and transport them out of the cell; can block this transport with biricodar)

→ Organic anion transporters (OATs), organic cation transporters (OCTs)

II. Membrane Barrier and Transport Affected by Toxicants

   A. Disrupts water movement through aquaporins (AQPs; protein water channels)

→ Decrease aquaporin + Na,K ATPase formation (Li) → Kidney cell × **Low water reabsorption**

→ Affect AQP4 (type D epsilon toxin of *Clostridium perfringens*) → Brain × **Cerebral edema**

→ LPS (lipopolysaccharide) → ↑ TNFα (cytokine) → ↓ APQ5 → Liver × **Sepsis-induced cholestasis**

   B. Disrupts osmotic flow by inhibiting facilitated diffusion of glucose

      Example: Cytochalasin B and similar agents

   C. Penetration agents such as organic solvents, cationic polymers, pore-forming bacterial toxins, heavy metals that bind to and disrupt the membrane

   D. Loss of membrane phospholipids by agents such as surfactants

   E. Surfactant action of lipid breakdown products

   F. Cytoskeletal changes by compounds such as cytochalasin B

   G. Oxygen free-radical generation

   H. Energy metabolism losses related to phospholipid synthesis

   I. Detection: leakage of ions and enzymes, conductivity changes, electron micrographs

Cellular Barriers

Mammalian Cell Membrane

The contents of a cell are bounded by a membrane that serves as a semi-permeable barrier. As a consequence, certain substances are essentially excluded from entry into or exit out of the cell without specialized transporters (**Conceptualizing Toxicology 5-1**). Nutrients that the cell requires for function either pass through the membrane due to their chemical nature or are given pores, channels, gates, or transporters to facilitate their entry. Other mechanisms transport wastes out of cells or ions that serve to transiently depolarized the cell or signal the cell. Toxicants that mimic these nutrients or have chemical or structural properties that take advantage of these mechanisms can gain access to the cell disproportionally to other xenobiotics or foreign substances. Also, those substances that block pores or channels, interfere with gate function, or disrupt transporters cause cellular toxicity. Even nutrients may become toxic at high concentrations or with increased time in a cell. Substances that form holes in the cellular membrane, alter the porosity of the membrane, or alter the membrane potentials also yield cellular damage.

Mechanisms that cause or prevent these disturbances in cellular homeostasis are important in understanding toxicity and pathology of cells. Cell membrane composition and function are different in specialized cells that promote absorption, such as the brush border cells of the intestinal tract and the proximal convoluted tubule cells of the kidney. Age, hormonal influences, diet, and other factors can change the composition and function of cell membranes. Some cells, because of their location, are highly hydrated; others, because of their location (outer epithelium of the skin of the hand or foot), are covered by a keratin layer and are rather dry on their surface. This dryness or thick protective layer increases the likelihood that the cell membrane will serve as a barrier. The infant child has a poor intestinal barrier and a poor blood–brain barrier whose effectiveness increases with age. Hair follicles offer a way that toxins may gain entry to a cell or a group of cells, so this route has to be considered as well. Thus, any mention of generalities of a mammalian cell membrane should be viewed in light of differences in structure and function of specialized cell membranes that increase or decrease the possibility of toxicant absorption through or damage to the membrane's integrity.

The mammalian cell membrane is shown in **Figure 5-1**. The integral structure of this

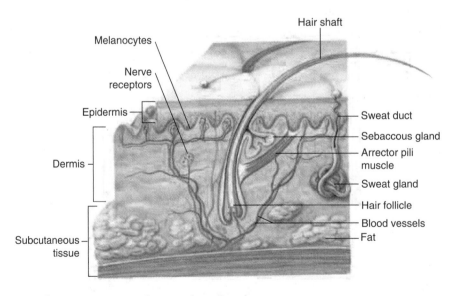

FIGURE 5-1 A Schematic Representation of a Mammalian Cell Membrane

membrane is a hydrophobic bilayer of lipids containing a polar phosphate moiety that interacts with the hydrophilic fluid outside and inside of the cell. This interaction creates a barrier against charged hydrophilic substances unless pores, channels, gates, or specialized active or passive transporters are available to aid them in crossing the membrane. Highly hydrophobic substances will cross a membrane with relative ease.

Carbohydrate groups attached to proteins (glycoproteins) provide a binding region for certain toxins (e.g., plant lectins). These proteins can be found at the surface of the membrane, or they may span the entire membrane (transmembrane proteins). Proteins serve as receptors, gates, channels, carriers, or enzymes. They are the main way that hydrophilic substances enter or leave the cell or become involved in signal transduction across the membrane. Proteins can support passive transport mechanisms such as a leak channel or facilitated diffusion of a gate or carrier (no cellular energy required), or they may require ATP (primary active transport) or use the diffusion of one substance down its concentration gradient to drive another up its concentration gradient (secondary active transport).

Bacterial, Fungal, and Plant Cell Walls

Bacteria have a cell wall that makes provides additional barriers to entrance of toxicants. Gram stain may be applied to highlight that the cell wall composition of gram-positive bacteria is significantly different from that of gram-negative bacteria. Gram-positive bacteria's cell walls contain peptidoglycans, proteins, and teichoic acids, but very few lipids or amino acids. This composition has made it easier for antibiotics to cause toxic reactions by binding to and preventing cell wall synthesis. In contrast, gram-negative bacteria's cell walls not only contain enzymes that may cleave certain types of antibiotics, but also are able to exclude toxins owing to the presence of a number of lipopolysaccharide layers cross-linked by proteins. In addition, these bacteria's cell walls contain a significant amount of lipids and amino acids linking structures, which decreases the diffusion

potential. Additionally, peptidoglycans account for a smaller portion of the cell wall in gram-negative bacteria compared to gram-positive bacteria (Aceret et al., 1998).

Fungi also have a well-developed cell wall and cell membrane that resist toxin entry. The outer wall consists of first mannoproteins, followed by glucans and chitin in polymers (Adams, 2004). The phospholipid bilayer of the inner cell membrane contains ergosterol instead of cholesterol—a difference that has been exploited as a site for toxic antifungal agents (Lewis, 2007).

The cellulose or other polysaccharide composition of the cell wall of a plant makes it hold more water molecules and renders it more vulnerable to hydrophilic toxicants. This can change, for example, in fruit ripening, where the pectin composition is affected by synthesis of the polysaccharide chains as well as the protein composition (Nunan et al., 1998). Plants also contain channels or ectodesmata in the cell walls, trichomes or leaf hairs, and other structures that are susceptible to herbicides or other toxicants.

As these differences in structure imply, certain toxins will have higher or lower toxicity in mammalian cells than in bacteria, fungi, or plants based simply on the cellular barrier composition.

Mechanisms of Cellular Transport

Water Movement

Since membranes have a lipid component and other barriers, the movement of hydrophobic substances was more easily deciphered. The movement of water through cell membranes was traditionally considered to be a passive process involving osmosis and pores in membranes. A set of proteins was discovered that changed that viewpoint, as water movement was faster than could be accounted for via passive channels.

Aquaporins (AQP) are a group of proteins found in the membranes of cells, in organisms ranging from bacteria to humans. Aquaporin Z from *Escherichia coli* conducts water at high rates, and its crystal structure has been analyzed for functional groups. The 28 Å long aquaporin channel is less than 4 Å in diameter and is lined with helices M1–M3 and M5–M7. This amphipathic channel allows water molecules to pass in only one at a time, due to the hydrophilic nature of the four adjacent carbonyls of G59 (GlpF number 64), G60(65), H61(66), and F62(67) from the amino-terminal domain and the quasi-2-fold related N182(199), T183(200), S184(201), and V185(202) from the carboxy-terminal domain. The hydrophobic portion of the channel results from the presence of many valines, phenylalanines, and isoleucines within the channel (Savage et al., 2003).

Certain toxicants exert at least a portion of their toxic effect through disruption of aquaporins. Lithium therapy in humans for manic depression, for example, was long known to induce polyuria, though scientists did not understand how this occurred. Laursen and coworkers (2004) demonstrated that decreased expression of mRNA for AQP2 and the $3Na^+,2K^+$-ATPase in the kidney appears to lead to the diabetes insipidus–like action of lithium. AQP4 appears to be involved in the acute cerebral edema caused by type D epsilon toxin of *Clostridium perfringens* (Finnie et al., 2008). Lipopolysaccharide induces a cytokine, TNFα, that down-regulates aquaporin-8 in sepsis-induced cholestasis (Lehman et al., 2008) and causes subcellular distribution alterations in AQP5 and plasma membrane water permeability changes in the lung (Ohinata et al., 2005). Necrosis induced through hemolysin causes accumulation of aquaporin-1 (Schweitzer et al., 2008). Certain high-profile toxic substances such as mercuric ion (Hg^{+2}) and other sulfhydryl-reactive mercurial compounds are nonspecific toxic blockers of AQP1. Gold (Au^{3+}) also inhibits AQP1. Some reports indicate that the solvent DMSO (which makes membranes more porous), acetazolamine, and quaternary ammonia compounds, such as the channel blocker tetraethylammonium, which cannot cross lipid membranes, affect AQP channels. However, compounds such as DMSO affect water movement via an "osmotic clamp" mechanism rather than affecting the AQP1, and tetraethylammonium and acetazolamide do not specifically inhibit AQP1, according to Yang and colleagues (2006). Nevertheless, it is clear that a number of mechanisms cause toxins to disrupt water movement in cells.

Certain gases, such as ammonia, but not the water-soluble charged ammonium ion, may have their own APQ transport channel, as has been demonstrated in wheat (Bertl and Kaldenhoff, 2007). Similar ideas have been considered in connection with lung tissue, but a controversy exists about how much gas transport occurs directly or rapidly through the lipid or via the AQPs.

AQPs appear to be involved in the transport of certain toxins, such as arsenite (Liu et al., 2002). As a consequence, caution should be used when assuming simple diffusion is the mechanism for transporting many toxicants, even if the absorption process is explained easily in that form. Protein mediators of toxicant and water movement may ultimately prove to account for a significant portion of the toxic action of a given compound.

Simple Diffusion of Hydrophobic and Non-ionized Small Molecules

The assumption of simple diffusion down a concentration gradient without a carrier molecule should be tempered with the understanding that protein mediators may play a role in this process. Competition for absorption would be the only mechanism that would decrease the absorption of substances that enter via simple diffusion, as contact with the lipid portion of the membrane (concentration), lipid solubility, temperature, viscosity, and size of the molecule would be important factors in limiting or increasing absorption.

Facilitated diffusion infers that the concentration gradient is still the driving force, but implies that proteins can act as mediating gates or carriers. The transport of glucose and amino acids into red blood cells (RBCs) is an example of facilitated diffusion. Inhibitors of glucose-facilitated diffusion also inhibit osmotic flow—such as cytochalasin B, diallyldiethylsilbesterol, a glucose analog (ethylidene-D-glucose), and phloretin (a known inhibitor of facilitated diffusion)—and yield toxicity partially by this effect (Fischbarg et al., 1987).

Pharmacologists have sought to increase the diffusion of charged substances, peptides, and proteins through the use of low-molecular-weight transmucosal penetration enhancers, albeit with mixed results (Junginger and Verhoef, 1998). Changing membrane permeability has yielded cellular toxicity. For single cells, toxicants can choose only whether to go through the membrane or around the cell. For highly hydrophobic and small toxicants (including gases), this may be accomplished through the lipid. This transcellular pathway or transport is illustrated in **Figure 5-2** as the paracellular and transcytotic pathway (with endocytosis reserved for macromolecules).

This kind of transport may follow **Fick's first law of diffusion**, which states that the flux across the membrane in number of moles per second ($\Delta n/\Delta t$) is equal to $-DA(\Delta C/\Delta x)$, where

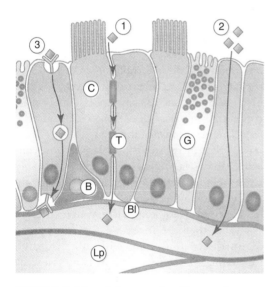

FIGURE 5-2 Schematic Representation of Transport Routes Across Nasal Respiration Mucosa: (1) Paracellular Across Tight Junctions, (2) Transcellular, and (3) Transcytotic. Mucus-Secreting Goblet Cells (G), Ciliated Columnar Cells (C), and Tight Junctions (Tj) are Represented. Basal Cells (B) are Located on the Basal Lamina (Bl) Adjacent to the Lamina Propria (Lp) with Blood Vessels

Data from Junginger HE, Verhoef JC. 1998. Macromolecules as safe penetration enhancers for hydrophilic drugs—a fiction? *Pharm Sci Technolo Today.* 1:370–376.

D is the diffusion coefficient in cm²/sec, A is the membrane barrier surface area in cm², and ΔC is the change in concentration in moles over the distance of Δx of the membrane. D can also be expressed as $kT/6\pi r\eta$, where k is Boltzmann's constant, or the average energy of a molecule in joules per degree kelvin (1.38×10^{-23} J/K); T is absolute temperature (K); r is the molecular radius, and η is the viscosity of a solution of the chemical.

When size is considered, the shape of a molecule is also a factor in the transport process. Long, thin molecules tend to find holes in membranes more easily and diffuse more rapidly (Goodman, 2002). However, for most purposes, the hydrophobicity is determined by the octanol–water partition coefficient or log P. This works well when considering the absorption of Hg^0 mercury versus methylmercury across the human skin. This factor can be overstated and misused to indicate that this is the key factor in bioaccumulation of hydrophobic versus hydrophilic toxins. Note that for phytoplankton, the hydrophobicity of inorganic versus methylmercury does not explain why methylmercury accumulates in phytoplankton and up the food chain. Rather, the binding of the inorganic form to the membrane and the cytoplasmic partitioning of the methylmercury accounts for its food web effects and high toxicity (Mason et al., 1995).

For tissues, there is a choice between the transcellular pathway and the **paracellular pathway**. The latter involves an entry through the "tight junctions" of cells, which for cells of the duodenum or proximal tubule of the kidney or epithelium would not be as tight as the name implies. This route allows water and associated small ions in a solvent drag mechanism to enter tissues between cells. It is a target for pharmacologists, who seek to enhance the penetration of medications such as proteins across membranes, as there are no proteases in this region (Fasano, 1998).

A determination of which substances are non-ionized must be accomplished by measuring the pH of the environment surrounding a cell for weak acids and weak bases. Strong acids and bases have an ability to penetrate that is based on their ability to damage components of the membrane. The rule of thumb is that acids in more acidic media become uncharged, such as the carboxylic moiety of amino acids —COO$^-$ (ionized) + H$^+$ ↔ —COOH (non-ionized), and bases in more basic media become more uncharged, such as the amine of amino acids —NH$_3^+$ (ionized) + OH$^+$ ↔ —NH$_2$ (non-ionized) + H$_2$O. Each reaction has an ionization constant. Thus, for the weak acid, the expression would be K$_a$ = [—COO$^-$][H$^+$]/[—COOH]. For the weak base, the corresponding expression is K$_b$ = [—NH$_3^+$][OH$^-$]/[—NH$_2$] in a dilute solution. Rearrangement of the expression for the weak acid leads to the equation 1/[H$^+$] = [—COO$^-$]/K$_a$ [—COOH]. Taking the logarithm of both sides yields log 1/[H$^+$] = log 1/K$_a$ + log [—COO$^-$]/[—COOH] or —log [H$^+$] = —log K$_a$ + log [—COO$^-$]/[—COOH]. The Henderson-Hasselbalch equation further defines this relationship as pH = pK$_a$ + log [—COO$^-$]/[—COOH] or pH = pK$_a$ + log [ionized]/[non-ionized]. Thus, as pH drops for the weak acid, the fraction of ionized to non-ionized must decrease as well, because the non-ionized portion predominates (acid in more acidic environment). Since the case for the base is just the opposite, the fraction is reversed: pH = pK$_a$ + log [non-ionized]/[ionized]. As the pH drops for the weak base, more of the compound is ionized (acid in base).

In humans, the pH of the GI tract is approximately 6 and the pH of the plasma is 7.4. That explains why a weak acid is less likely to be absorbed, while a weak base is more likely to be absorbed. For example, it explains why the herbicide 2,4-dichlorophenoxyacetic acid (2,4-D; pK$_a$ = 2.8), which is widely used for lawn applications, has a low skin absorption in humans—it stays a charged salt (Ross et al., 2005). Some of the increased absorption and toxicity to aquatic species of the widely used agricultural herbicide atrazine may be due to its chemistry as a weak base (pK$_a$ = 1.7).

Transport of Ions and Heavy Metals

The transport of ions across membranes involves specialized protein channels and carriers. For this process, pertinent factors include the concentration difference across the membrane, the electromotive force (like charges would repel an ion across a membrane), the size of the ion, the ability of the ion to associate nonspecifically with certain proteins or moieties, the transport mechanism (passive or active), and the presence of other ions that may compete for transport or absorption. Physiology is interested in metals like sodium and potassium for their effects on the action potential and the activity of Na and K channels and for the primary active transport accomplished by 3Na$^+$,2K$^+$-ATPase, which keeps a cell properly polarized. Calcium has been similarly studied for its role as a second messenger and in apoptosis (programmed cell death), necrosis (resulting in cell death and damage to surrounding tissues and cells), muscle contraction, heart potentials, and the primary active transport via Ca^{2+}-ATPase, which prevents the build-up of Ca in functional cells.

Foulkes (2000) has reviewed heavy metal transport, describing four categories of metals (classes A-D). Iron is the compound most representative of metals that are nutrients required at high concentrations (class A). Strontium is an example of those compounds that have low toxicity at low concentrations (class B). Trace metal nutrients such as zinc are essential at low concentrations (class C). Mercury is the quintessential representative of the group of toxic heavy metals that disrupt cells at relatively low concentrations (class D). Mercury binds strongly to proteins; likewise, other heavy metals are thought to move across cell membranes in diffusible complexes. Some metals enter through channels that are intended for the uptake of nutrients. Cadmium will enter through Ca channels in many cells, but is inhibited by Zn and other metals in human liver cells. The presence of a separate Zn transporter has been suggested by kinetics, but the complexity of the transport does not yield clear analysis by biochemical competition modeling (Lineweaver-Burk, Eadie–Hofstee, or Michaelis-Menton). Part of the complexity is the presence of more than one parallel mechanism for uptake of heavy metals, such as the two pathways for Cd that are distinguishable by their temperature dependence in human hepatocytes (Souza et al., 1997).

Some heavy metals may be assisted in their entry into cells by active transport, as indicated by the action of P-type ATPases (Solioz and Vulpe, 1996). A variety of protein transporters of heavy metals may function in that role due to their strong binding, such as the binding of mercury to sulfhydryl groups, which can transport methionine or other amino acids or ions. However, these transports can also be trans-inhibited by the heavy metals, or cause the transporter to be dysfunctional following translocation. Trans-inhibition has been described for transporters of ions, amino acids, and ATP-binding cassette (ABC) transporters. One such inhibition has been studied structurally with a molybdate/tungstate ABC transporter of *Methanosarcina acetivorans* (Gerber et al., 2008).

In other bacteria, resistance to heavy metals may be coded for by plasmids (Hassan et al., 2008). Alternatively, it may be associated with antibiotic-resistant bacteria, which synthesize increased amounts of outer membrane proteins but are not plasmid associated (Choudhury and Kumar, 1996).

Transport of Organic Compounds

ABC transporters not only transport ions, but can also transport charged organic compounds, such as small monosaccharides or amino acids, or larger antibiotics, other medications, lipids, and oligopeptides. This makes them a key primary active transporter for toxicants that are large or charged organic compounds. ABC transporters are found in many organisms, ranging from bacteria to humans. Bacteria express both prokaryotic- and eukaryotic-type ABC transporters (Moussatova et al., 2008).

All ABC transporters have two transmembrane domains composed of alpha-helices and two nucleotide binding domains containing the water-soluble proteins of the Walker A and B motifs that are part of all ATP-binding proteins on only one side of the membrane. If the organic compounds do not come from the lipid bilayer, then specialized binding proteins can deliver the substrate from the aqueous

phase to the transporter (usually in gram-negative bacteria). The binding of ATP to the nucleotide-binding domains causes a conformational change in both domains, which opens a conduit between the transmembrane domain and either the outside or the inside of the cell (Kerr, 2002). Subsequently, organic molecules that resemble nutrients can be pumped into the cell, while recognized toxic agents are pumped outside the cell. Fungi also have a pleiotropic drug resistance, such as is found in *Saccharomyces cerevisae*, which appears to involve the ABC and major facilitator superfamily (MFS) transporters.

One of the key ABC transporters important in the transport of organic toxicants out of the cell is the first identified P-glycoprotein (Matheney et al., 2001). It is especially important in chemotherapy of cancer, as many cytotoxic chemotherapy agents, such as paclitaxel (which induces microtubule formation and metaphase arrest), are removed by P-glycoprotein and confer resistance to the toxicants. Relatively weak inhibitors of this transporter include the calcium-channel blocker verapamil, the immunosuppressant agent cyclosporine, the antibacterial erythromycin, the antifungal ketoconazole, and the weak estrogenic/antiestrogen chemotherapeutic agent tamoxifen. Second-generation P-glycoprotein inhibitors, such as biricodar, increase the chemotherapeutic value and toxicokinetics of paclitaxel in human cancer patients (Rowinsky et al., 1998). This effect indicates that inhibition of ABC transporters may increase the toxicity of a wide variety of organic toxicants—a finding that may have therapeutic value in cancer patients.

Another group of organic compound transporters are the organic anion transporters (OATs). The first OAT was discovered in 1996 and originally named NKT; most of the research into this type of transport has supported its role in this mechanism. NKT is now known as OAT1 and is part of the *SLC22* gene family, which includes the organic cation transporters (OCTs), organic cation transporters of carnitine (OCTNs), and fly-like putative transporters (Flipts). This superfamily has been studied in the human kidney but is also present in species such as the fly and the worm (Nigam et al., 2007). These transporters in the human kidney, in combination with urea transporters in mammalian cells (Goodman, 2002), not only confer resistance of cells to toxic substances, but also are considered secretory pathways and a portion of the excretory route for waste products of catabolism and xenobiotics. Species-related differences in the cell's ability to remove these toxicants partially explain both individual and species differences in sensitivity to toxicants.

Mechanisms of Membrane Damage

The mechanisms of cell membrane or cell wall injury may be due to penetration agents, loss of membrane phospholipids or the surfactant action of lipid breakdown products that may accumulate in a damaged cell, cytoskeletal changes, oxygen free radical generation, and energy metabolism losses that relate to phospholipid synthesis. These will be discussed below in greater detail to understand the importance of the integrity of the cell barriers and how they may be breached.

Penetration Enhancers and Cytoskeleton Disruption Agents

Junginger and Verhoef (1998) describe three methods of breaching the membrane:

- By acting on the mucous layer
- By altering membrane components
- By changing the diffusion characteristics of tight junctions

Table 5-1 lists the mechanisms for increasing membrane absorption.

Membrane proteins and lipids are altered by lipid components (fatty acids, monoglycerides, fatty acid–bile salt micelles) and detergents to increase membrane permeability. The surfactant itself may solubilize or extract the

TABLE 5-1	Mechanisms for Increasing Membrace Permeability		
Class	**Examples**	**Mechanism**	**Transport Ways**
Surfactants	Na-laurylsulfate Polyoxyethyle ne-9-laurylether	Phospholipid acyl chain perturbation	Transcellular ↑
	Bile salts: Na-deoxycholate Na-glycocholate Na-taurocholate	Reduction mucus viscosity Peptidase inhibition	Paracellular ↑
Fatty acids	Oleic acid Short fatty acids	Phospholipid acyl chain perturbation	Transcellular ↑ Paracellular ↑
Cyclodextrins	α-, β- and γ-cyclodextrin Methylated β-cyclodextrins	Inclusion of membrane compounds	Transcellular ↑ Paracellular ↑
Chelators	EDTA	Complexation of Ca^2	Transcellular ↑ Paracellular ↑
	Polyacrylates	Opening of tight junctions	Paracellular ↑
Positively charged polymers	Chitosan salts Trimethyl chitosan	Ionic interactions with negatively charged groups of glycocalix	Paracellular ↑

Data from Junginger HE, Verhoef JC. 1998. Macromolecules as safe penetration enhancers for hydrophilic drugs—a fiction? *Pharm Sci Technolo Today.* 1:370–376.

phospholipids and membrane proteins and may enter the cell to damage the cell organelles. Organic solvents may act in similar fashion with cells. Cationic polymers are used to increase permeation by adhering to the mucous or lipid membrane through ion–ion interaction, thereby allowing water-soluble medications to penetrate the membrane. Some of these agents, such as chitosan, poly-L-arginine, animated gelatins, and sperminated pullulans, are being evaluated as means of pharmaceutical delivery (Seki et al., 2008).

Another method of penetrating the membrane is to interfere with the cytoskeletal structure. Cytochalasin B is a mycotoxin that inhibits actin polymerization. This action, in turn, prevents microtubule formation. Exploitation of this mechanism has allowed penetration of a variety of agents, such as peptides, into corneal cells without the epithelial disruption caused by other cell penetrators (Harris et al., 1992) and facilitated sperm penetration into an egg (Ohta et al., 1998).

Biological Toxins and Penetration of the Membrane

Exotoxins of bacteria are known to damage to cell membranes of the host cells. For example, *Clostridium perfringens* produces an alpha-toxin lecithinase, a kappa-toxin collagenase, and a mutoxin hyaluronidase. Some endotoxins, such as the delta-endotoxins of *Bacillus thuringiensis*, bind to the cell surface of water-soluble proteins, then transform the proteins and insert the complexes into the membranes, thereby forming pores. One gene family of these delta-endotoxins, known as *Cry*, has an N-terminal helical domain that forms the channel with two beta-sheet domains that bind to the membrane receptors. The other *Cyt* gene family forms toxins that have three layers—two outer layers plus an inner amphiphilic beta-sheet that acts as the pore-former (Li et al., 2001).

Note that these examples define a wide variety of permeation enhancement by bacteria. They can be divided into pore-forming toxins, which are not true translocators, and translocators that have pore-forming and enzymatic activity (Rádis-Baptista et al., 2008). The poreforming

toxins form channels by insertion of either amphipathic alpha-helices (*Staphylococcus* delta-hemolysins) or beta-hairpins (*Clostridium* perfrigolysin). The beta-hairpins bind to a receptor that is either cholesterol, a ganglioside, or a glycosylphosphatidylinositol (GPI)-anchored protein. Streptolysin is an especially notable pore-former: It was the first chemical to be recognized as an evolutionary adaptation to translocate a protein, the NAD:glycohydrolase complex (Geny and Popoff, 2006). Cytotoxic peptides that produce pores (cytolysins) also are found as melittin in the venom of *Apis mellifera* (honeybee), ectatomin in the venom of *Ectatomina tuberculatum* (ants), and equinatoxin of *Actina equina* (R. Tebben's flower anemone). The alkyl pyridinium sponge toxins poly-3-alkylpyridinium salt (APS) isolated from *Reniera sarai* and halitoxin isolated from the *Amphimedon* genus form transient pores in cell membranes that some researchers have used to perform transfection of mammalian cells (Tucker et al., 2003).

Bacterial binary toxins have one catalytic A moiety and one receptor-binding B moiety; they include some of the most toxic substances produced by pathogenic bacteria, such as the neurotoxins from *Clostridium botulinum*, and other toxins relevant to human disease, such as tetanus, diphtheria, pertussis, and cholera. These toxins bind to receptors such as heparin-binding epidermal growth factor (EGF)–like growth factor receptor (diphtheria toxin), α_2-macroglobulin receptor (pertussis exotoxin A), glycolipid $G\beta_3$ (Shiga toxin), and ganglioside GM1 (cholera toxin). The receptor mediates an endocytosis aided by the proteins clathrin and caveolin to the Golgi apparatus and endoplasmic reticulum. These toxins form a pore in the early endosome phase or, by retrograde transport, to the Golgi apparatus and endoplasmic reticulum.

Similarly, an extremely toxic plant lectin isolated as the protein ricin from *Ricinus communis* (castor bean plant) is a binary preformed protein. Ricin binds to galactose residues of glycoproteins and glycolipids of eukaryotic cells via binding to its B lectinic receptor domain and is subsequently translocated by receptor-mediated endocytosis. The catalytic A domain then proceeds to profoundly inhibit protein translation in the cytoplasm. The transport is accomplished via the endosome retrograde via the trans-Golgi network (TNG) to the Golgi apparatus and then to the endoplasmic reticulum.

Bacteria are also susceptible to pore-forming substances based on the negative charge on the outside of bacterial membranes caused by the peptidoglycan and lipoteichoic acid of gram-positive bacteria or the lipopolysaccharide of gram-negative bacteria.

Antimicrobial peptides (AMPs) are part of the innate immunity of invertebrates, plants, and animals. The AMPs from mammals and insects (defensins) as well as other organisms are pore-formers that cause extensive rupture of the membranes. Three models of peptide insertion have been proposed, known as the toroidal pore, carpet, and barrel stave models (Brogden, 2005). In the toroidal pore model, lipid monolayers from the alpha-helices bend through the pores. In the carpet model, the surfactant or micelle-forming property of the peptides produces the pores. Finally, in the barrel stave model, the hydrophobic portions of the alpha-helices associate with the lipid leaving the hydrophilic groups, thereby forming the pore. These AMPs also may translocate and have other toxic actions as well, but their major feature is the pore formation. They are agents of interest not only for microbial diseases, but also for their antitumor properties (magainin-induced apoptosis in leukemia KL-60 cells; Cruz-Chamorro et al., 2006).

Cell-penetrating peptides (CPPs) may be made by the virus HIV-1 (the Tat protein) and by *Drosophila* (fruit fly; Antennapedia). The characteristics of these agents that can aid in transport of protein, nucleic acids, medications, and nanometric biomaterials are their short length, cationic charge, amphipathicity, and structural arrangement. While AMPs make transient pores, the CPPs use receptor-mediated endocytosis to create pores. Crotamine—the cationic peptide from *Crotalus durissus* (South American rattlesnake)—enters mouse embryonic stem cells during the G_1/S phase in a time- and concentration-independent fashion (Kerkis et al., 2004). Other substances produced naturally, such as bilirubin in animals, which may be beneficial at low concentrations.

Bilirubin is a powerful antioxidant that protects cell membranes at normal or slightly elevated levels (Baranano et al., 2002), yet at high concentrations causes a loss of the inner-located phospholipids, phosphatidylethanolamine and phosphatidylserine, in the lipid membrane of RBCs, which may induce more hemolysis (Brito et al., 2002).

For a more complete review of bacterial and plant toxins' mechanisms of breaching the membrane of mammalian cells (penetration, endosomal entry, endoplasmic reticulum retrograde movement), refer to the review by Watson and Spooner (2006).

Chemical Agents That Bind to and Disrupt the Membrane

Heavy metals attach to portions of the lipid membrane. For example, arsenic attaches to the phosphate head and the choline moiety of 1-palmitoy-2-oleoyl-*sn*-glycero-3-phosphocholine liposomes or to algal cell membranes (Houng et al., 2006). This changes the membrane fluidity, apart from the damage that arsenic may cause via oxidative stress or binding to dithiols (van Iwaarden et al., 1992). Modification of the membrane can also cause the cell to be recognized by the immune system as foreign if the changes go beyond the individual cell or cells.

Organic metals are more lipophilic and can increase the toxicity to membranes. Triorganic tin compounds, for example, cause hemolysis of human erythrocytes, leading to transport of organic anions across lipid membranes by exchange diffusion with chloride (Ortiz et al., 2005).

Other toxins that are not known primarily for their membrane binding and damage are compounds similar to puromycin. This protein synthesis inhibitor causes internalization of the rabbit or human erythrocyte membrane, resulting in vacuolization of the cells. Because RBCs from these species do not synthesize protein, this effect must be due to direct binding and disruption of the membrane (Burka et al., 1975).

Many antibacterial agents bind to moieties outside of the membrane and disrupt cell-wall synthesis. For example, penicillin is a compound isolated from the fungus of the *Penicillium* genus, and other beta-lactam antibiotics appear structurally similar to D-alanyl-D-alanine. These antibiotics bind to the transpeptidase, thereby inhibiting cross-linking of the glycopeptide polymers. Penicillin-binding proteins that confer resistance have a structural similarity to the transpeptidase (Fan et al., 2007). Vancomycin is an antibacterial isolated from the bacterium *Staphylococcus orientalis* used to treat methicillin-resistant *Staphylococcus aureus* infections. It binds with high affinity to the D-alanyl-D-alanine terminus of cell-wall precursor units (Perkins, 1969). Polyene antifungal (macrolide antibiotic) agents such as amphotericin B bind to the ergosterol that is present in fungal membranes, depolarizing the membrane and forming pores (Gale et al., 1975). These toxicities due to membrane binding of various components essential for the integrity or synthesis of the membrane indicate that compounds can affect a cell in many ways. Additionally, these toxins can be turned into therapeutic agents to target specific membranes or organisms.

A particular chemical is not always required to disrupt membranes. Guinea pig macrophages, for example, show changes in cell membrane potential in response to small dust particles. The more a dust particle causes hemolysis of RBCs, the more the lasting influence on the membrane potential (Gormley et al., 1978).

Compounds that do not damage lipid membranes directly but are highly lipophilic, such as the polycyclic aromatic hydrocarbons (PAHs), may have limited rates of absorption at or above the saturation level. The PAHs, which come from incomplete combustion of organic material, show a first-order absorption rate into lung cells at low concentrations that goes to zero order at high concentrations (Ewing et al., 2006). Only those compounds that damage membrane components increase their own absorption.

Oxygen Radicals

The paradox of non-anaerobes is that they require oxygen as the terminal recipient of electrons in oxidative phosphorylation, yet suffer from the toxicity of oxygen radicals and the aging effects of oxidation. This phenomenon may be best understood in terms of how various food substances are sensitive to oxidation. Oils of various types have a limited shelf life based on the time it takes them to become rancid. In scientific terms, the oxidation or peroxidation of lipids leads to disruption of the membrane. It has been known for decades that vitamin E plays a key role as an antioxidant that prevents the chain reaction of lipid peroxidation in a membrane (Tinberg and Barber, 1970). Depending on the lipid composition of a membrane and its antioxidants, the membrane will be more or less responsive to oxidant damage. For example, brain cells contain a high proportion of polyunsaturated fatty acids that are prone to forming reactive oxygen species (ROS). ROS include superoxide radicals ($O_2^{\cdot-}$), hydrogen peroxide (H_2O_2) and hydroxyl radicals (OH^-), and reactive nitrogen species (RNS) such as nitric oxide (NO) and peroxynitrite. Hypertension in rats is associated with an increase in oxidative stress in brain cells (Hirooka, 2008) as indirectly measured by an increased concentration of thiobarbituric acid-reactive substances (TBARS).

The organism that produces Lyme disease, *Borrelia burgdorferi*, does not contain intracellular iron. As a consequence, the organism cannot generate oxygen radicals via Fenton's reaction, which produces hydroxyl radicals as follows: $Fe^{2+} + H_2O_2 \rightarrow Fe^{3+} + {}^-OH^{\cdot} + {}^-OH$ and $Fe^{3+} + H_2O_2 \rightarrow Fe^{2+} + {}^-OOH + H^+$ (Fenton, 1894; Haber and Weiss, 1934). Superoxide ($O_2^{\cdot-}$) generation and dismutation lead to the formation of the hydrogen peroxide. The lack of Fenton's reaction in the Lyme's disease bacterium eliminates any damage done by oxygen radicals to the cell wall, unlike the DNA damage that follows from exposure to hydrogen peroxide and similar agents. Since *Borrelia burgdorferi* has shown irregularities in electron micrographs in response to peroxides, damage to the large amounts of polyunsaturated lipids found in the membranes of these organisms might be expected (Boylan et al., 2008).

As shown in Fenton's reaction, iron can form ROS. Other metals that are chelated to biomolecules, such as ATP, ADP, and citrate, or are in acidic pH will also generate oxygen radicals in the favored oxidation state (Jacobs, 1977;

Weaver and Pollack, 1989). The favored state is +2 for Be, Cd, Co, Cu, Hg, Pb, and Ni, and +5 for As. Cr(IV-VI) can generate oxygen radicals, but is more damaging to DNA. For alveolar macrophages, silica asbestos fibers induce cellular membrane perturbations and generate significant oxygen radicals, especially in the presence of iron (Kamp et al., 1992). Similarly, coal and other fine dusts may generate oxygen radicals with similar cell types.

Ozone (O_3) is an oxidative molecule that can cause membrane damage (Pryor, 1994). Ionizing radiation (high frequency, low wavelength), such as X- and γ-rays and low-wavelength ultraviolet (UV) radiation, generates oxygen radicals via the following reactions: H_2O + radiation → HOH^+ + e^-; e^- + H_2O → HOH^-; HOH^+ → H^+ + $\cdot OH$; HOH^- → OH^- + $\cdot H$ (hydrogen radical). The net yield is two radicals (Tubiana et al., 1990). These radicals can then interact with the biomolecules found in membranes. Membrane lipids are especially sensitive to radiation-induced ROS damage (Pandey and Mishra, 2003). Compounds such as ellagic acid from fruit, tocopherol succinate (vitamin E analog), Triphala (herbal fruit extracts), and arachidonic acid additions (a polyunsaturated fatty acid) have been used to sensitize radiation-resistant cancer cells to the oxidative damage by radiation (Girdhani et al., 2005).

Certain antioxidants are also pro-oxidants under conditions of degradation in aqueous media. Polyphenols such as plant-derived flavonoids, catechols, and derivatives of gallic acid generate oxidized lipid degradation products, as measured by the development of malondialdehyde, on exposure of these compounds to human promyelocytic leukemia cells (Sergediene et al., 1999). One way this oxidation may be accomplished is through auto-oxidation, a condition that is known to occur with flavonoids, or through the generation of superoxide in the auto-oxidation of epinephrine (Brusov et al., 1976). The generation of superoxide and hydrogen peroxide during the auto-oxidation of 2,5-dihydroxyphenylacetic acid (homogentisic acid) may play an important role in the membrane and tissue damage associated with inflammatory arthritis (Martin and Batkoff, 1987). Ascorbic acid (vitamin C) also autooxidizes under physiological conditions.

Certain pro-oxidant medications, such as quinine, the antimalarial compound present in tonic water, cause lipid peroxidation and damage to the sperm and reproductive tract cells (Osinubi et al., 2007). Another antimalarial medication, chloroquine, increases lipid peroxidation; part of its therapeutic action entails increasing oxidative stress in the protozoan parasitic cell (Toler et al., 2006). A number of compounds, such as paraquat, diquat, and polycyclic aromatic hydrocarbons, require metabolism by enzymes found primarily in the endoplasmic reticulum to generate oxygen radicals. It would be more appropriate to view the damage done to membranes as occurring in the cytosol, such as in the endoplasmic reticulum, or to the mitochondrial membrane, even though some of the ROS would damage the cell membrane as well.

Not only is lipid peroxidation a toxic effect of ROS, but it also changes ion permeability across membranes. ROS affect the ion transport proteins involved in transmembrane signal transduction via oxidation of sulfhydryl groups, lipid peroxidation, inhibition of membrane-bound regulatory enzymes, and mitochondrial effects that inhibit oxidative phosphorylation. These species impact calcium, potassium, sodium, and chloride channels. ROS may damage ion pumps for calcium, sodium and potassium, and protons as well as ion exchangers for sodium-calcium and sodium–hydrogen ion antiport. Additionally, ion cotransporters are affected, such as potassium chloride, sodium potassium chloride, and sodium phosphate. The perturbations in calcium level signal the cell to further degrade (Kourie, 1998). Other actions on cell signaling are seen as well by reactive nitrogen species (RNS), such as the effects of peroxynitrite on tyrosine phosphorylation and phosphoinositide signaling in human neuroblastoma SH-SY5Y cells (Li et al., 1998).

Energy Metabolism/Mitochondrial Disruption

Anoxia (lack of oxygen) induces ischemic cell injury in a progressive fashion, with larger molecules gaining greater access to the damaged cell over time (Chen et al., 2001). In the first phase, propidium iodide (molecular weight = 668) crosses the membrane; this phase is reversible by oxygenation but cannot be prevented by glycine. In phase 2, 3-kDa dextrans are allowed into the cell; this phase is inhibited by glycine. In phase 3, 70-kDa dextrans or lactate dehydrogenase enter the cell; this phase is inhibited by homobifunctional cross-linkers, such as dimethyl-pimelimidate. In contrast, necrotic cell injury is more or less an "all-or-none" process in allowing molecules to cross the membrane. This difference is important, because the effect of anoxia would be expected to be similar to that of toxicants that disrupt mitochondrial (or chloroplasts in plants) energy pathways but do not cause extensive damage elsewhere that would lead to necrosis.

In 3T3 transformed mammalian cells, the cytoplasmic ATP concentrations are essential in maintaining a pore barrier to prevent escape of nucleotide pools and ions; externally added ATP or internal decreases in ATP due to inhibition of ATP synthesis result in similar release of these small molecules (Makan, 1979). The question of the relative importance of mitochondrial versus cytosolic-derived ATP synthesis in cell membrane integrity and damage arises because in fibroblasts, the inhibition of cytosolic energy production makes the insult by external exposure to lysophosphatidyl choline or phospholipase C much worse than the inhibition of oxidative phosphorylation alone (Kristensen, 1994).

In the mid-1960s, the finding that fatty acid synthesis dependent on the mitochondria stimulated other studies of inhibitors of mitochondrial energy generation (Youngs and Cornatzer, 1963) and lipid membrane synthesis (Bhaduri and Srere, 1964). Fats are synthesized from acetylCoA and glycerol—both products of glycolysis from cytosolic energy production. Lipid synthesis also involves citrate, which is derived from an intermediate in the Krebs cycle in mitochondria. Phospholipids start their synthesis pathway with phosphatidic acid. Each portion of energy metabolism plays an essential role in the synthesis of lipids. Thus it is not surprising that inhibitors of any stage of the electron transport that is essential for oxidative phosphorylation (complex I inhibitor, rotenone; complex II inhibitor, 2-thenoyltrifluoroacetone; complex III inhibitor, antimycin A1; and the most used or known inhibitors of complex IV, sodium azide, cyanide compounds, and carbon monoxide) and compounds that uncouple ATP synthesis from electron transport (2,4-dinitrophenol) will have some impact on the membrane by reducing lipid synthesis, and especially synthesis of phospholipids.

Conversely, it is interesting to see how membrane composition may play a role in resistance to these agents. *Bacillus subtilis* mutants that grew on carbonyl cyanide m-chlorophenyl-hydrazone, depending on the mutation, were resistant to 2,4-dinitrophenol (DNP) and/or tributyltin and neomycin. The membrane lipids of mutants resistant to the uncoupler, 2,4-DNP, had reduced amounts of monounsaturated C16 fatty acids and increased ratios of iso/anteiso branches on the C15 fatty acids. These resistant cells also were able to synthesize more ATP at low bulk transmembrane electrochemical gradients of protons (Guffanti et al., 1987). This makes the membrane–mitochondrial connection a more complex interaction involving ion transport and lipid synthesis, both of which are important to the function of the cellular membrane or wall and the mitochondrion.

Methods for Detecting Membrane Insults

The first methods for detecting a membrane breach relied on determination of the leakage of ions, other small molecules, and finally enzymes from heavily damaged cells. Also, electron micrographs can indicate when a membrane is severely altered. One assay focuses on the release of a radiolabeled nonmetabolized amino acid from fibroblasts as an indication of membrane damage from phospholipase C and theta-toxin from *Clostridium perfringens*; alpha-, beta-, delta-, and gamma-toxins from *Staphylococcus aureus*; and streptolysin S from *Streptococcus pyogenes* (Thelestam and Möllby, 1975).

More recently, sensitive electrical measurements have been developed as means to detect any ion leakage. A conductivity assay detected damage done to *Elodea canadensis* leaves by the benzalkonium chloride surfactant and examined other parameters such as photochemical efficiency, plasmolysis capacity, nitro blue tetrazolium reduction, and electron microscopy (Eich et al., 2000). This technique holds promise for sensitive detection of the effects of other detergents, organic solvents, radical formers, and biological toxins on cell membrane function.

Another group used a dielectrophoresis cross-over method for detecting dose- and time-related adverse effects of exposure of cells to the oxygen radical–forming paraquat; simultaneous membrane and nucleic acid attacks by styrene oxide; a nucleic acid alkylation agent, *N*-nitroso-*N*-methylurea; and a protein synthesis inhibitor, puromycin. As described earlier, puromycin may cause membrane damage as well as protein synthesis inhibition. This method showed effects that were correlated with and confirmed by electron micrographs. This method detected changes made by agents that directly affected the membrane (paraquat and styrene oxide) in half the time it took for those agents whose target was within the cell (puromycin and *N*-nitroso-*N*-methylurea). It appears that sensitive electrical measurements are good ways to identify membrane damage from fast-acting direct agents or compounds that alter membrane function indirectly via transcription, translation, or energy pathways.

Questions

1. Which factors lead to high absorption and toxicity? Give an example.
2. What are the heavy metal transporters?
3. How do toxicants disrupt the membrane barrier?
4. What are ways of detecting membrane damage?

References

Aceret TL, Coll JC, Uchio Y, Sammarco PW. 1998. Antimicrobial activity of the diterpenes fleibilide and sinulariolide derived from *Sinularia flexibilis* Quoy and Gaimard 1833 (Coelenterata: Alcyonacea, Octocorallia). *Comp Biochem Physiol Part C.* 120:121–126.

Adams DJ. 2004. Fungal cell wall chitinases and glucanases. *Microbiol.* 150:2029–2035.

Baranano DE, Rao M, Ferris CD, Snyder SH. 2002. Biliverdin reductase: a major physiologic cytoprotectant. *Proc Natl Acad Sci USA.* 99:16093–16098.

Bertl A, Kaldenhoff R. 2007. Function of a separate NH_3-pore in aquaporin TIP2;2 from wheat. *FEBS Lett.* 581:5413–5417.

Bhaduri AM, Srere PA. 1964. Mitochondrial stimulation of fatty acid biosynthesis. *J Biol Chem.* 239:1357–1363.

Boylan JA, Lawrence KA, Downey JS, Gherardini FC. 2008. *Borrelia burgdorferi* membranes are the primary targets of reactive oxygen species. *Mol Microbiol.* 68:786–799.

Brito MA, Silva RFM, Brites D. 2002. Bilirubin induces loss of membrane lipids and exposure of phosphatidylserine in human erythrocytes. *Cell Biol Toxicol.* 18:181–192.

Brogden KA. 2005. Antimicrobial peptides: pore formers or metabolic inhibitors in bacteria? *Nat Rev Microbiol.* 3:238–250.

Brusov OS, Gerasimov AM, Panchenko LF. 1976. [The influence of natural inhibitors of radical reactions on auto-oxidation of adrenaline.] *Biull Eksp Biol Med.* 81:33–35.

Burka EF, Ballas SK, Sabesin SM. 1975. Toxic effect of puromycin on erythrocyte membranes which is unrelated to inhibition of protein synthesis. *Blood.* 45:21–27.

Chen J, Liu X, Mandel LJ, Schnellmann RG. 2001. Progressive disruption of the plasma membrane during renal proximal tubule cellular injury. *Toxicol Appl Pharmacol.* 171:1–11.

Choudhury P, Kumar R. 1996. Association of metal tolerance with multiple antibiotic resistance of enteropathogenic organisms isolated from coastal region of deltaic Sunderbans. *Indian J Med Res.* 104:148–151.

Cruz-Chamorro L, Puertollano MA, Puertollano E, de Cienfuegos GA, de Pablo MA. 2006. *In vitro* biological activities of magainin alone or in combination with nisin. *Peptides.* 27:1201–1209.

Eich J, Dürholt H, Steger-Hartmann T, Wagner E. 2000. Specific detection of membrane-toxic substances with a conductivity assay. *Ecotoxicol Environ Saf.* 45:228–235.

Ewing P, Blogger B, Ryrfeldt A, Gerde P. 2006. Increasing exposure levels cause an abrupt change in the absorption and metabolism of acutely inhaled benzo(a)pyrene in the isolated, ventilated, and perfused lung of the rat. *Toxicol Sci.* 91:332–340.

Fan X, Liu Y, Smith D, Konermann L, Siu KW, Golemi-Kotra D. 2007. Diversity of penicillin-binding proteins: resistance factor FmtA of *Staphylococcus aureus. J Biol Chem.* 282:35143–35152.

Fasano A. 1998. Innovative strategies for the oral delivery of drugs and peptides. *Trends Biotechnol.* 16:152–157.

Fenton HJH. 1894. Oxidation of tartaric acid in the presence of iron. *J Chem Soc.* 65:899–910.

Finnie JW, Manavis J, Blumbergs PC. 2008. Aquaporin-4 in acute cerebral edema produced by *Clostridium perfringens* type D epsilon toxin. *Vet Pathol.* 45:307–309.

Fischbarg J, Liebovitch LS, Koniarek JP. 1987. Inhibition of transepithelial osmotic water flow by blockers of the glucose transporter. *Biochim Biophys Acta.* 898:266–274.

Foulkes EC. 2000. Transport of toxic heavy metals across cell membranes. *Proc Soc Exp Biol Med.* 223:234–240.

Gale EF, Johnson AM, Kerridge D, Koh TY. 1975. Factors affecting the changes in amphotericin sensitivity of *Candida albicans* during growth. *J Gen Microbiol.* 87:20–36.

Geny B, Popoff MR. 2006. Bacterial protein toxins and lipids: pore formation or toxin entry into cells. *Biol Cell.* 98:667–678.

Gerber S, Comellas-Bigler M, Goetz BA, Locher KP. 2008. Structural basis of trans-inhibition in a molybdate/tungstate ABC transporter. *Science.* 321:246–250.

Girdhani S, Bhosle SM, Thulsidas SA, Kumar A, Mishra KP. 2005. Potential of radiosensitizing agents in cancer chemo-radiotherapy. *J Cancer Res Ther.* 1:129–131.

Goodman BE. 2002. Transport of small molecules across cell membranes: water channels and urea transporters. *Adv Physiol Educ.* 26:146–157.

Gormley IP, Wright MO, Ottery J. 1978. The effect of toxic particles on the electrophysiology of macrophage membranes. *Ann Occup Hyg.* 21:141–149.

Guffanti AA, Clejan S, Falk LH, Hicks DB, Krulwich TA. 1987. Isolation and characterization of uncoupler-resistant mutants of *Bacillus subtilis. J Bacteriol.* 169:4469–4478.

Haber F, Weiss JJ. 1934. The catalytic decomposition of hydrogen peroxide by iron salts. *Proc R Soc Lond Sect A.* 147:332–352.

Harris D, Liaw J-H, Robinson JR. 1992. (D) Routes of delivery: case studies: (7) ocular delivery of peptide and protein drugs. *Adv Drug Deliv Rev.* 8:331–339.

Hassan SH, Abskharon RN, El-Rab SM, Shoreit AA. 2008. Isolation, characterization of heavy metal resistant strain of *Pseudomonas aeruginosa* isolated from polluted sites in Assiut city, Egypt. *J Basic Microbiol.* 48:168–176.

Hirooka Y. 2008, July 21. Role of reactive oxygen species in brainstem in neural mechanisms of hypertension. *Auton Neurosci.* [Epub ahead of print].

Houng TTT, Tuan LQ, Umakoshi H, Kuboi R. 2006. Toxic effect of arsenic (As) on biomembrane. Workshop on biotechnology in agriculture. Nong Lam University, Ho Chi Minh City, Vietnam, 20 October 2006. http://www.hcmuaf.edu.vn/cpb/phtqt/biotech2006/papers/thuysan/TTTHuong.pdf.

Jacobs A. 1977. Low molecular weight intracellular iron transport compounds. *Blood.* 50:433–439.

Junginger HE, Verhoef JC. 1998. Macromolecules as safe penetration enhancers for hydrophilic drugs—a fiction? *Pharm Sci Technol Today.* 1:370–376.

Kamp DW, Graceffa P, Pryor WA, Weitzman SA. 1992. The role of free radicals in asbestos-induced diseases. *Free Radic Biol Med.* 12:293–315.

Kerkis A, Kerkis I, Rádis-Baptista G, Oliveira EB, Vianna-Morgante AM, Pereira LV, Yamane T. 2004. Crotamine is a novel cell-penetrating protein from the venom of rattlesnake *Crotalus durissus terrificus. FASEB J.* 18:1407–1409.

Kerr ID. 2002. Structure and association of ATP-binding cassette transporter nucleotide-binding domains. *Biochim Biophys Acta.* 1561:47–64.

Kourie JI. 1998. Interaction of reactive oxygen species with ion transport mechanisms. *Am J Physiol.* 275:C1–C24.

Kristensen SR. 1994. Importance of various types of metabolic inhibition for cell damage caused by direct membrane damage. *Mol Cell Biochem.* 140:81–84.

Laursen UH, Pihakaski-Maunsbach K, Kwon TH, Østergaard Jensen E, Nielsen S, Maunsbach AB. 2004. Changes of rat kidney AQP2 and Na,K-ATPase mRNA expression in lithium-induced nephrogenic diabetes insipidus. *Nephron Exp Nephrol.* 97:e1–e16.

Lehman GL, Carreras FI, Soria LR, Gradilone SA, Marinelli RA. 2008. LPS induces the TNF-alpha-mediated downregulation of rat liver aquaporin-8: role in sepsis-associated cholestasis. *Am J Physiol Gastrointest Physiol.* 294:G567–G575.

Lewis RE. 2007. Antifungal pharmacology. http://www.doctorfungus.org/thedrugs/antif_pharm.htm.

Li J, Derbyshire DJ, Promdonkoy B, Ellar DJ. 2001. Structural implications for the transformation of the *Bacillus thuringiensis* d-endotoxins from water-soluble to membrane-inserted forms. *Biochem Soc Trans.* 29:571–578.

Li X, De Sarno P, Song L, Beckman JS, Jope RS. 1998. Peroxynitrite modulates tyrosine phosphorylation and phosphoinositide signalling in human neuroblastoma SH-SY5Y cells: attenuated effects in human 1321N1 astrocytoma cells. *Biochem J.* 331:599–606.

Liu Z, Shen J, Carbrey JM, Mukhopadhyay R, Agre P, Rosen BP. 2002. Arsenite transport by mammalian aquaglyceroporins AQP7 and AQP9. *Proc Natl Acad Sci USA*. 99:6053–6058.

Makan NR. 1979. Role of cytoplasmic ATP in the restoration and maintenance of a membrane permeability barrier in transformed mammalian cells. *J Cell Physiol*. 101:481–492.

Martin JP Jr, Batkoff B. 1987. Homogentisic acid autoxidation and oxygen radical generation: implications for the etiology of alkaptonuric arthritis. *Free Radic Biol Med*. 3:241–250.

Mason RP, Reinfelder JR, Morel FMM. 1995. Bioaccumulation of mercury and methylmercury. *Water Air Soil Pollut*. 80:915–921.

Matheney CJ, Lamb MW, Brouwer KLR, Pollack GM. 2001. Pharmacokinetic and pharmacodynamic implications of P-glycoprotein modulation. *Pharmacotherapy*. 21:778–796.

Moussatova A, Kandt C, O'Mara ML, Tieleman DP. 2008, June 18. ATP-binding cassette transporters in *Escherichia coli*. *Biochim Biophys Acta*. [Epub ahead of print].

Nigam SK, Bush KT, Bhatnagar V. 2007. Drug and toxicant handling by the OAT organic anion transporters in the kidney and other tissues. *Nat Clin Pract Nephrol*. 3:443–448.

Nunan KJ, Sims IM, Bacic A, Robinson SP, Fincher GB. 1998. Changes in cell wall composition during ripening of grape berries. *Plant Physiol*. 118:783–792.

Ohinata A, Nagai K, Nomura J, Hashiomoto K, Hisatsune A, Miyata T, Isohana Y. 2005. Lipopolysaccharide changes the subcellular distribution of aquaporin 5 and increases plasma membrane water permeability in mouse lung epithelial cells. *Biochem Biophys Res Commun*. 326:521–526.

Ohta T, Yoshida M, Kato S. 1998. Electron microscopic observations on sperm penetration in cytochalasin-treated eggs of the rose bitterling. *Cell Struct Funct*. 23:179–186.

Ortiz A, Teruel JA, Aranda FJ. 2005. Effect of triorganotin compounds on membrane permeability. *Biochim Biophys Acta*. 1720:137–142.

Osinubi AA, Daramola AO, Noronha CC, Okanlawon AO, Ashiru OA. 2007. The effect of quinine and ascorbic acid on rat testes. *West Afr J Med*. 26:217–221.

Pandey BN, Mishra KP. 2003. *In-vitro* studies on radiation induced membrane oxidative damage in apoptotic death thymocytes. *Int J Low Radiat*. 1:113–119.

Perkins HR. 1969. Specificity of combination between mucopeptide precursors and vancomycin or ristocetin. *Biochem J*. 111:195–205.

Pryor WA. 1994. Mechanisms of radical formation from reactions of ozone with target molecules in the lung. *Free Radic Biol Med*. 17:451–465.

Rádis-Baptista G, Kerkis A, Prieto-Silva AR, Hayashi MAF, Kerkis I, Yamane T. 2008. Membrane-translocating peptides and toxins: from nature to bedside. *J Braz Chem Soc*. 19:211–225.

Ross JH, Driver JH, Harris SA, Maibach HI. 2005. Dermal absorption of 2,4-D: a review of species differences. *Regul Toxicol Pharmacol*. 41:82–91.

Rowinsky EK, Smith L, Wang YM, Chaturvedi P, Villalona M, Campbell E, Aylesworth C, Eckhardt SG, Hammond L, Kraynak M, Drengler R, Stephenson J Jr, Harding MW, Von Hoff DD. 1998. Phase I and pharmacokinetic study of paclitaxel in combination with biricodar, a novel agent that reverses multidrug resistance conferred by overexpression of both MDR1 and MRP. *J Clin Oncol*. 16:2964–2976.

Savage DF, Egea PF, Robles-Colmenares Y, O'Connell JD 3rd, Stroud RM. 2003. Architecture and selectivity in aquaporins: 2.5 a X-ray structure of aquaporin Z. *PLoS Biol*. 1:E72.

Schweitzer K, Li E, Sidhaye V, Leitch V, Kuznetsov S, King LS. 2008. Accumulation of aquaporin-1 during hemolysin-induced necrotic cell death. *Cell Mol Biol Lett*. 13:195–211.

Seki T, Fukushi N, Chono S, Morimoto K. 2008. Effects of sperminated polymers on the pulmonary absorption of insulin. *J Control Release*. 125:246–251.

Sergediene E, Jönsson K, Szymusiak H, Tyrakowska B, Rietjens IM, Cenas N. 1999. Prooxidant toxicity of polyphenolic antioxidants to HL-60 cells: description of quantitative structure–activity relationships. *FEBS Lett*. 462:392–396.

Solioz M, Vulpe C. 1996. Cpx-type ATPases: a class of P-type ATPases that pump heavy metals. *Trends Biochem Sci*. 21:237–241.

Souza B, Bucio L, Guiterrez-Ruiz MC. 1997. Cadmium uptake by a human hepatic cell line. *Toxicology*. 120:215–220.

Thelestam M, Möllby R. 1975. Sensitive assay for detection of toxin-induced damage to the cytoplasmic membrane of human diploid fibroblasts. *Infect Immun*. 12:225–232.

Tinberg HM, Barber AA. 1970. Studies on vitamin E action: peroxidation inhibition in structural protein–lipid micelle complexes derived from rat liver microsomal membranes. *J Nutr*. 100:413–418.

Toler SM, Noe D, Sharma A. 2006. Selective enhancement of cellular oxidative stress by chloroquine: implications for the treatment of glioblastoma multiforme. *Neurosurg Focus.* 21:E10.

Tubiana M, Dutreix J, Wambersie A. 1990. *Introduction to radiobiology.* Bewley DR, trans. Bristol, PA: Taylor and Francis.

Tucker SJ, McClelland D, Jaspars M, Sepcic K, MacEwan DJ, Scott RH. 2003. The influence of alkyl pyridinium sponge toxins on membrane properties, cytotoxicity, transfection and protein expression in mammalian cells. *Biochim Biophys Acta.* 1614:171–181.

van Iwaarden PR, Driessen AJM, Konings WM. 1992. What we can learn from the effects of thiol reagents on transport proteins. *Biochim Biophys Acta.* 1113:161–170.

Watson P, Spooner RA. 2006. Toxin entry and trafficking in mammalian cells. *Adv Drug Deliv Rev.* 58:1581–1596.

Weaver J, Pollack S. 1989. Low-Mr iron isolated from guinea pig reticulocytes as AMP-Fe and ATP-Fe complexes. *Biochem J.* 261:787–792.

Yang B, Kim JK, Verkman AS. 2006. Comparative efficacy of $HgCl_2$ with candidate aquaporin-1 inhibitors DMSO, gold, TEA and acetazolamide. *FEBS Lett.* 580:6679–6684.

Youngs JN, Cornatzer WE. 1963. Effect of oxidative phosphorylation inhibitors on synthesis of liver mitochondria phospholipids. *Proc Soc Exp Biol Med.* 112:308–311.

CHAPTER 6

Receptor-Mediated Toxicities
on the Outside of Cells

This is a chapter outline intended to guide and familiarize you with the content to follow.

I. Receptor Function

Ligand → Binds to receptor (usually a protein) → High affinity → Potent → Increases normal function = potent agonist

Example: nicotine from tobacco binds more strongly to cholinergic receptors than to acetylcholine → Blocks normal function = potent antagonist

Example: atropine blocks the muscarinic subset of cholinergic receptors → Low affinity → Low potency

Scatchard plot revisited: K_D = dissociation (affinity) constant, B_{max} = receptor saturation (usually toxic at saturation)

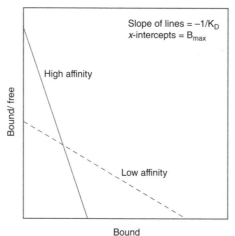

Slope of lines = $-1/K_D$
x-intercepts = B_{max}

High affinity

Low affinity

Bound/ free

Bound

Chronic toxicant binding → Down-regulation of receptor → Less sensitivity—tolerance → Take away toxicant stimulation abruptly → Withdrawal—dependence

Up-regulation of receptor for a variety of reasons/conditions → Sensitization

Downstream effects (signal transduction) → Actions in the cell cytoplasm affecting other organelles such as the nucleus (affects gene expression) or the mitochondrion (affects energy functions and can lead to effects ranging from cell death [apoptosis] to necrosis)

II. Receptor Inhibitors (for Enzymes) or Blockers (for Receptors)

A. Competitive (least toxic, as a normal substance may be increased to compete with agent). The full binding and receptor response is still available (V_{max}), where $1/V_{max}$ is the inverse of the maximum rate of enzyme product formation (and $-1/K_m$ is normally the x-intercept in enzyme kinetics, where K_m = concentration at ½ V_{max})

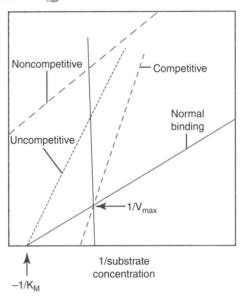

Emaduddin M, Takeuchi H. 1996. Lineweaver–Burk analysis for the blocking effects of mammalian dopamine receptor antagonists on dopamine-induced currents in *Achatina* giant neurones. *Gen Pharmacol.* 27:1209–1213. This article shows how an enzyme inhibition plot is transformed into a receptor antagonist analysis.

B. Uncompetitive: Maintains the affinity (represented in the plot as the inverse function $1/K_M$), but the blocker/inhibitor binds elsewhere (allosteric site) and affects the maximum binding and is more toxic than competitive

C. Noncompetitive: Affects binding and affinity, with parallel curves representing changes in both functions. This is the most toxic type of binding, except for binding of irreversible inhibitors that may destroy a receptor or an enzyme

III. Receptor-Mediated Toxicities

A. Target ion channels (superfamily of ligand-gated Cl^- channels, Na^+ channels, K^+ channels, Ca^{2+} channels)

1. Changes membrane potential
2. Produces neurotoxicity/cardiotoxicity or paralysis of metazoans
3. Leads to apoptosis and necrosis
4. Induces immune suppression

B. Target transmembrane enzyme receptors and downstream enzymes

1. Coupled to tyrosine kinase—proliferation, angiogenesis, survival, motility
   a. AhR (aryl hydrocarbon receptor) also linked to cell proliferation
   b. Transcriptional regulators such as NF-κB can be activated via cytokines such as TNFα or oxidative stress to yield cell proliferation
2. Coupled to guanylate cyclase

C. Target G protein–linked receptors and downstream signal transduction

1. Group of seven transmembrane receptors responding to neurochemicals and hormones—in cardiac myocyte, leads to inotropy, apoptosis, and hypertrophy, but is more universally linked in cells to cell proliferation and survival
2. VEGF (vascular endothelial growth factor) stimulates angiogenesis
3. Some linked to Ca^{2+} channels → Important second messenger signal in the cytosol → Will alter signal transduction pathways including in immune cells (e.g., interference with calcium signaling will cause immune suppression in T cells) and when combined with high Ca^{2+} levels will lead to cell death

CONCEPTUALIZING TOXICOLOGY 6-1 (*continued*)

Receptors and Signal Transduction Mechanisms

Cells respond rapidly to changes in their external environment through the use of receptors and signal transduction mechanisms (**Conceptualizing Toxicology 6-1**). On the outside of cells, the receptor is generally a protein that must be saturable and have specificity for a limited number of binding ligands; the ligand remains unchanged by interaction with the receptor. The concentration of the ligand and its affinity or binding strength for the receptor plus the number of receptors on the cell surface should determine the degree of resultant activity. This characteristic distinguishes the receptor from nonspecific binding sites such as proteins and lipids, which are not receptors. The affinity for a receptor is defined by a Scatchard plot. High-affinity ligands bind at low concentrations and are the most potent or toxic. Low-affinity ligands bind at high concentrations and have low potency or toxicity through that receptor.

The toxicant–receptor interaction works by mass action as follows: Toxicant + Receptor ↔ Toxicant–Receptor Complex. Although this relationship is depicted as a two-directional binding–unbinding reaction, some toxicants form covalent bonds that make their reactions more unidirectional as far as the cell's function is concerned. Two constants are derived from the forward and backward interactions, which will be referred to as k_{bind} and k_{unbind}, respectively. If an equilibrium is reached, then k_{bind}[Toxicant][Receptor] = k_{unbind} [Toxicant–Receptor Complex]. The dissociation constant $K_D = k_{unbind}/k_{bind}$ = [Toxicant][Receptor]/[Toxicant–Receptor Complex] or, rearranging the equation, [Receptor] = K_D[Toxicant–Receptor Complex]/[Toxicant]. The maximum amount of receptor sites that can be bound by the toxicant, B_{max}, is defined as follows: B_{max} = [Receptor] + [Toxicant–Receptor Complex] = K_D[Toxicant–Receptor Complex]/[Toxicant] + [Toxicant–Receptor Complex]. The [Toxicant] is free unbound toxicant, which in enzyme kinetics or Scatchard plots is referred to as free (F). The [Toxicant–Receptor Complex] is the bound (B) toxicant. Thus $B_{max} = K_D B/F + B$. If B is factored

out of the right side of the equation, B_{max} = $B(K_D/F + 1)$. Rearranging gives B = $B_{max}F/(F + K_D)$, which is in the same form as the enzyme kinetics equation v = $V_{max}S/(K_m + S)$, where v is velocity (instead of binding) and V_{max} is maximum velocity (instead of maximum binding). S is the [substrate] instead of the [bound ligand].

An inverse form of the equation makes it easier to see how competitive binding, noncompetitive binding, and uncompetitive binding may affect a receptor (Eadie–Hofstee relationship). If K_D appears to change but not B_{max}, the toxicant would be competitive with the natural ligand. If K_D is unaffected but B_{max} appears to change, then the toxicant is considered noncompetitive. If both appear to change and generate parallel lines with increased toxicant concentration, then uncompetitive binding is present.

To see if the toxicant binds to low-affinity or high-affinity binding sites (or both), the Scatchard arrangement of the equation is used: $B/F = B/K_D + B_{max}/K_D$. In a Scatchard plot, high-affinity binding yielding toxicity at low concentrations is observed by a high negative slope. Low-affinity binding yielding toxicity only at high concentrations is observed for a toxicant whose binding plot has a low negative slope. It is important that the toxicity matches the binding curve; otherwise, either the binding is nonspecific or its meaning is unclear.

Toxicants may cause damage by abusively stimulating a receptor, blocking a receptor, modifying a receptor, down- or up-regulating a receptor, or changing the response rate to that receptor. Receptor mechanisms for signaling across a membrane have been organized into at least three receptor superfamilies: ligand-regulated oligomeric ion channels, ligand-regulated enzymes, and GTP-dependent ligand-regulated or G protein–linked receptors (**Figure 6-1**) (Hollenberg, 1991).

Many other receptor definitions of superfamilies have been proposed, such as the one for interleukins (Viola and Luster, 2008) or, more specifically, that for receptors such as toll-like receptor superfamilies and scavenger receptors that comprise pattern recognition receptors whose functions link them to intracellular molecular chaperones such as heat

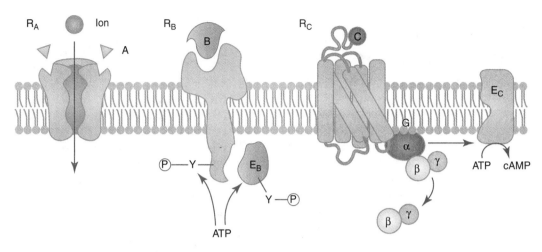

FIGURE 6-1 Receptor Types/Models for Toxicant Action

Note: R_A is a ligand-regulated channel that alters ion flux into the cell. This is modeled after the nicotinic cholinergic receptor. R_B is a ligand-regulated enzyme that starts a cascade of signaling through the cell. This is modeled after the tyrosine kinase receptor such as the single-chained epidermal growth factor-urogastrone or for platelet-derived growth factor. The receptor is autophosphorylated while phosphoylating E_B, the target substrate. R_C is a receptor that is linked to a G protein and then to an enzyme that forms a second messenger such as cAMP depicted as the most used pathway and model for cellular activation via G proteins.

Data from Hollenberg MD. 1991. Structure-activity relationships for transmembrane signaling: the receptor's turn. *FASEB J.* 5:178–186.

shock proteins (Calderwood et al., 2007). Signal transduction is the pathway that begins with the substance binding to its receptor, followed by transmembrane signaling, second messenger modulation, and finally the internal cascade of cellular events that lead to the cell's responses to the binding to a receptor or multiple receptors. Changes in the signal transduction pathway can result in both transcriptional and translational events (and nuclear activity for eukaryotes). Toxicants can disrupt signal transduction mechanisms in a variety of ways that modify the response to receptor binding.

Targeting Ion-Channel Receptors

Some key ion channels involve the entry of sodium, calcium, and chlorine into the cell or potassium leaving the cell. For example, kainic acid from the red algae *Digenea simplex* simulates specific stimulatory glutamate receptors of mammalian neuronal cells, thereby increasing Na^+ movement into the cells (Kirischuk et al., 2007), but also alters the $GABA_A$ subunit for the inhibitory neurotransmitter γ-aminobutyric acid (GABA) so as to alter the influx of Cl^- (Laurén et al., 2005). Glutamate receptors can

also be abusively stimulated in neuronal cells subjected to high concentrations of glutamate (or high concentrations of the flavor enhancer monosodium glutamate) during ischemic episodes (Manev et al., 1990).

Glutamate receptor–gated Cl^- channels occur in nematodes such as *Caenorhabditis elegans* as well. Avermectins such as ivermectin (22,23-dihydroavermectin-B_1), a semisynthetic analog of avermectin B_{1a} from *Streptomyces avermitilis*, produce a tonic paralysis in these organisms. Avermectins bind with 100 times the affinity for nonresistant nematode receptors as for rat brain receptors (Schaeffer and Haines, 1989). Sleep medications such as barbiturates and benzodiazepines target subunits of the $GABA_A$ receptor as agonists, while the $GABA_A$ selective antagonists bicuculline and picrotoxin produce excitation of mammalian neuronal cells or inhibit the whirling and forward swimming behavior in *Paramecium primaurelia* induced by the $GABA_A$ receptor agonist muscimol (Bucci et al., 2005).

$GABA_A$ receptors are part of a larger superfamily of ligand-gated chloride channels, which include nicotinic acetylcholine receptors, strychnine-sensitive glycine receptors, and 5-HT$_3$

serotonin receptors. Other effectors at the GABA$_A$ site are steroids and ethanol (Bormann, 2000).

Cholinergic receptors for mammalian systems have been demonstrated in the Pacific electric ray (*Torpedo californica*). Subsets of receptors have been mapped in human cerebral cortical cells for high-affinity agonists that are strong stimulants, such as the plant-derived toxin nicotine, cytisine, and epibatidine (Sihver et al., 1998). High-affinity and low-affinity sites for binding of alpha-bungarotoxin, which is a potent nicotinic antagonist, have been described (Dunn et al., 1983). The cone snail *Conus leopardus* produces an alpha-conotoxin that is an antagonist to the nicotinic receptor of neuronal and neuromuscular cells; this toxin can induce seizures and paralysis of freshwater goldfish (Peng et al., 2008). Among the most famous nicotinic antagonists is D-tubocurarine, derived from a South American vine. Modulation of the action of nicotinic receptors can occur via a number of substances, including botulinum toxin. Botulinum toxin not only destroys nerve endings and acetylcholine release, but also makes adult nicotinic receptors in muscle cells act as their embryonic counterparts (Költgen et al., 1994).

High concentrations of glycine abusively stimulate glycine receptors and NMDA (*N*-methyl-D-aspartate) subset of glutamate receptors (Barth et al., 2005). Strychnine poisons spinal cord cells via antagonistic binding to glycinergic receptors (Young and Snyder, 1973). The 5-HT$_3$ receptor depresses spinal reflex potentials in rat spinal cord cells, as indicated by the agonistic action of the *Ptychodiscus brevis* toxin and its antagonism by ondansetron (Singh et al., 2006).

Certain receptors are better known for transporting organic toxins out of cells, such as the ABC receptors, but have ion transport activities as well. The cystic fibrosis transmembrane receptor and the sulfonylurea receptor are such atypical ABC proteins. The sulfonylurea receptor regulates the potassium (ATP) channel (Burke et al., 2008).

Receptors linked to ion channels may not only cause abusive stimulation or depression of cells, but also lead to pain pathways such as the NMDA portion of the spinal extracellular signal-regulated kinase signaling pathway produced by polypeptides of the scorpion *Buthus martensi's* Karch venom (Pang et al., 2008). Stimulation and depression of receptors controlling Na$^+$, K$^+$, and Cl$^-$ affect the potentials of cells, however; those that also influence Ca^{2+} can alter apoptosis and necrosis if not pumped out by Ca^{2+} ATPases (Orrenius et al., 1992). Normally cells regulate Ca^{2+} concentrations within a 100-nM range and expend a great deal of cellular energy to keep a large gradient between extracellular and intracellular Ca^{2+}. As a result, increases in Ca^{2+} can serve as a second messenger for a number of pathways, including the calmodulin-dependent kinase II, mitogen-activated protein kinase, protein kinase C, and calcium-dependent protease pathways. Interference in this mechanism in T cells produces the immunosuppressive action of cyclosporine A, which also inhibits other Ca-mediated events in these cells, such as Na$^+$/H$^+$ antiport (Rosoff and Terres, 1986). The NMDA receptor not only regulates Na and K conductance, but also supports an extremely high Ca^{2+} conductance (Contestabile, 2000). The ryanodine receptor is located in the endoplasmic reticulum and the sarcoplasmic reticulum of muscle cells (rather than on the plasma membrane), but it is regulated by Ca^{2+}, Mg^{2+}, ATP, and voltage-dependent channels. The IP$_3$ (inositol 1,4,5,-triphosphate) receptor is a tetrameric calcium channel affected by reactive oxygen or nitrogen species. L-, N-, and R-type Ca^{2+} channels are affected by heavy metals. Transient receptor potential channels are also considered a superfamily of non-voltage-gated calcium channels (Waring, 2005).

General anesthetic agents are known for their inhibition of central nervous system cell functions; however, they can also increase inflammation in peripheral neuronal cells, excite these nerve cells directly via the transient receptor potential A$_1$ channel (mustard oil or allyl-isothiocyanate receptor), and increase pain or nociception in these same neuronal cells via stimulation of the transient potential receptor V$_1$ (capsaicin receptor) in HEK 293F cells (Cornett et al., 2008). Cigarette smoke–derived α,β-unsaturated aldehydes also increase neuronal cell inflammation via the mustard oil receptor (Andrè et al., 2008).

GABA$_B$ receptors control the Ca^{2+} and K$^+$ channels. The GABA$_B$ receptor agonist baclofen suppresses the membrane Ca^{2+} current via a pertussis toxin-sensitive G protein (Tatebayashi and Ogata, 1992). The GABA$_B$ receptor antagonists appear to suppress absence seizures in thalamic cells while increasing tonic or clonic seizures in rats, depending on the model system used (Vergnes et al., 1997). Although antagonism of receptors usually has the opposite effect to agonism, effects related to changes in sensitivity of the receptors can occur as a result of excessive stimulation by an agonist or an antagonist. For example, blocking receptors can increase the number of receptors, thereby making the cells more sensitive to future stimulation, such as occurs with hippocampal neuronal cells containing the NMDA receptors (Rao and Craig, 1997).

Targeting Transmembrane Enzyme Receptors and Downstream Enzymes

Interaction with transmembrane enzyme receptors becomes more complex when multiple signal transduction factors are present downstream or in the cytoplasm of the cell. Examples of this receptor class include insulin, epidermal growth factor–urogastrone, platelet-derived growth factor that is coupled to a tyrosine kinase, and platelet-derived growth factor coupled to atrial natriuretic factor coupled to a guanylate cyclase. A variety of other internal kinases and cascades are triggered by these receptors. The activation or inhibition of tyrosine kinase receptors and the resulting signal transduction mechanisms are illustrated in **Figure 6-2**.

For example, the appetite suppressing peptide obestatin activates cell proliferation of a gastric cancer cell line, KATOIII, through mitogen-activated kinase/extracellular signal–regulated kinases-1/2 phosphorylation. This effect can be blocked partially by pertussis toxin, an inhibitor of phosphoinositide 3-kinase (wortmannin), an inhibitor of protein kinase C (staurosporine), and an inhibitor of the nonreceptor tyrosine kinase Src (4-amino-5-(4-chlorophenyl)-7-(t-butyl) pyrazolo[3,4-D]pyrimidine) (Pazos et al., 2007).

The snake venom toxin rhodocytin triggers powerful platelet aggregation via the C-type lectin-like receptor. Cross-linkage of the C-type lectin receptor leads to Src kinase–dependent tyrosine phosphorylation of the Tyr-Xaa-Xaa-Leu domain sequence, inducing activation of the tyrosine kinase Syk and initiation of a signaling pathway that culminates in activation of phospholipase Cg (Fuller et al., 2007). The mycotoxin ochratoxin A causes increased phosphorylation of atypical protein kinase C and downstream activation of mitogen-activated protein (MAP) kinase isoforms 1 and 2 in rat kidney cells. MAP kinases are serine/threonine kinases that are activated by multiple toxicants and physiological ligands; they mediate signal transduction from the cell surface to membrane targets and cytoplasmic pathways, and may translocate to the nucleus. For example, copper concentrations that were toxic to trout hepatocytes caused an increase in phosphorylated extracellular signal–regulated protein kinase (pERK), but did not translocate this messenger into the nucleus. This mechanism may serve to protect hepatocyte cells, as nuclear accumulation of pERK might otherwise induce damage, as has occurred in mouse hippocampal cells (Ebner et al., 2007). Thus not only are the precise receptor and signaling pathway that are activated or inhibited by a toxicant important, but also the extent that the signals translocate in the cell.

The strength of binding to receptors appears also to play a role. Diethylstilbestrol, a strong synthetic estrogen linked to cancer of the vagina and cervix of daughters of women who were treated with this medication (which has since been withdrawn from the market), reduces the androgen receptor protein concentration in Sertoli cells, thereby increasing the expression of epidermal growth factor and downstream ERK1/2 in spermatogonia and spermatocytes. This effect has been linked to increased cell proliferation and impaired testicular development, but not to apoptosis. By comparison, genistein, a weak estrogen found in soy, neither altered these activities nor affected testicular development (Fritz et al., 2003).

Another famously potent cell-proliferative toxicant is 2,3,7,8-tetrachlorodibenzodioxin (TCDD). It activates the aryl hydrocarbon

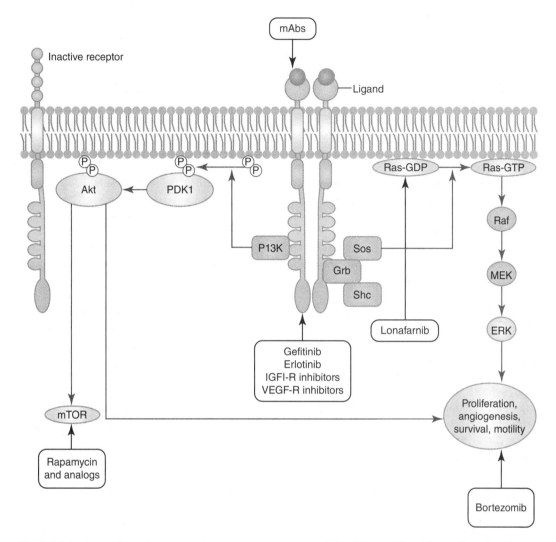

FIGURE 6-2 The Signal Transduction Through Tyrosine Kinase Receptors and the Inhibitors of that Pathway Indicated in Color

Note: mAbs = monoclonal antibodies, Sos = nucleotide exchange factor son of sevenless, Grb = growth factor receptor bound protein, Shc = Src 2 homology 2 domain containing, Ras = GTPase, Raf = Ser/Thr protein kinase, MEK = mitogen-activated protein kinase / Ser/Thr kinase kinase (MAPK/ERK kinase), ERK = a MAP kinese ERK that is a Ser/Thr kinase. This left side represents the ERK signaling pathway involved in growth and cancer. PI3K = 1-phosphatidylinositol 3-kinase, PDK1 = 3-phosphoinositide-dependent protein kinase 1, Ak1 = adenylate kinase 1 and is a key mediator in control of cell proliferation and survival , mTOR = mammalian target of rapamycin is a protein kinase that is hyperactive in cancer cells.

Data from Cruz JJ, Ocaña A, Del Barco E, Pandiella A. 2007. Targeting receptor tyrosine kinases and their signal transduction routes in head and neck cancer. *Ann Oncol*. 18:421–430.

receptor (AhR), which induces isoforms of the xenobiotic metabolizing enzyme cytochrome P450 that activate aryl hydrocarbons and cause them to become cell-proliferative or toxic-carcinogen metabolites. TCDD also induces cleft palate and hydronephrosis in mice through

cell-proliferative events mediated by epidermal growth factor receptor, epidermal growth factor, and transforming growth factor-α. The degree to which each of these pathways is involved in the proliferative action leading to developmental abnormalities has been demonstrated by knockout mice that are deficient in these factors (Abbott et al., 2003). As these various cellular effects demonstrate, such transmembrane receptor pathway activations are significant—they play roles in cell proliferation, cell survival, anti-apoptotic activity, developmental defects, and cancer development (Marin-Kuan et al., 2007).

Other signals may indirectly act at these sites. For example, oxidative stress induced in lymphocytes during the inflammatory response activates tumor necrosis factor-alpha (TNFα) and reperfusion injury appears to deplete cells of the antioxidant glutathione and cause the transloca-tion of transcriptional regulators such as nuclear factor-kappa B (NF-κB). The result is inhibition of interleukin-2 (IL-2) production by mitogen-activated T cells. Ultimately, it is thought to be the activation of the protein tyrosine kinase (PTK)-dependent signals that leads to the down-stream responses by activation of phospholipase C_{gamma1} (PLC$_{g1}$) and uncoupling of PLC$_{g1}$. This relationship has been confirmed by blocking the response by a PTK inhibitor, herbimycin A. Although this activation of PLC$_{g1}$ was considered a problematic outcome (Holsapple et al., 1996), later research with a knockout mouse cell line showed that this mechanism actually protects fibroblasts from oxidative stress (Bai et al., 2002). It is this kind of result that changes the inter-pretation of cellular responses to toxic insult. The Ca^{2+} disruption that occurs during oxidative stress, however, is still viewed as a negative event for certain cellular functions, as it triggers apop-tosis. Protein tyrosine phosphatases are inhib-ited by oxidative stress, because they are sensitive to thiol-reactive substances. These responses are linked to activation of the ZAP70 and Syk tyrosine kinases, which have been implicated in the signaling of the Src-family kinases associated with antigen signaling.

Targeting G Protein–Linked Receptors and Downstream Signal Transduction

Changes involving GTP-dependent or guanine nucleotide binding protein (G protein)-linked receptors can also affect both proliferative and destructive pathways. These G protein-linked receptors are the ones most often referred to in signal transduction research as linked to a group of seven transmembrane receptors that respond to neurochemicals and hormones (Gutman, 1997). Binding to a receptor that is coupled to a G protein activates pathways downstream that regulate the cell, but can also activate other powerful pathways (**Figure 6-3**).

Toxicants that affect vascular endothelial growth factor (VEGF) alter the development of new blood vessels or angiogenesis. This process is important in cancer development, but can also remodel capillaries. As(III) is a form of arse-nic known to cause cancer, noncirrhotic fibrosis, portal hypertension, and vascular remodeling. In sinusoidal endothelial cells, the signaling that maintains fenestrations and suppresses cell spreading is accomplished via a nitric oxide (NO)-mediated pathway. As(III) stimulates a NADPH oxidase generation of superoxide that consumes NO or decreases the availability of tetrahydrobipterin, which is required for NO synthase. This effect is evident as an increase in ras-related C3 botulinum toxin substrate 1 (rho family, small GTP binding protein Rac1), which is part of the NADPH oxidase. The result is a disruption of the vessel's porosity. VEGF signaling is disrupted as well, and caveolin-1 levels increase. Caveolin-1 helps maintain the caveolae—that is, the small invaginations of the cell surface that play an important role in cell signaling. As a consequence, vascular remodel-ing occurs (Straub et al., 2007).

Changes involving a GTP- or G protein-linked receptor can have far-reaching effects that change the cell surface, cell signaling, and ultimately cell proliferation and survival. For example, disrupting these G protein-linked mechanisms via exposure to pertussis toxin or cholera toxin can decrease the metallothionein-linked chemotaxis and, therefore, function of leukocytes (Yin et al., 2005). The plant from which marijuana is derived, *Cannabis sativa*, has receptors to its active ingredient, Δ^9-tetrahydrocannabinol, referred to as canna-binoid brain receptor 1 (CB$_1$) centrally and 2 (CB$_2$) peripherally. This substance not only pro-duces psychoactive effects, but also is a known immunosuppressive toxicant. CB$_1$ receptors

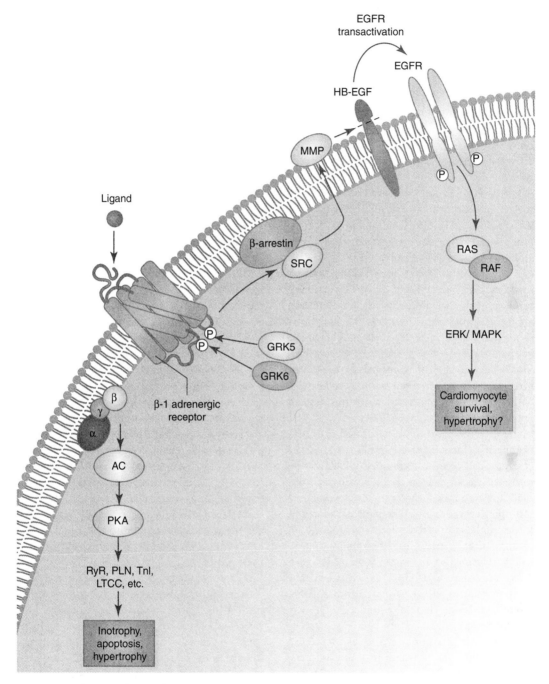

FIGURE 6-3 Classic β_1 Adrenergic Receptor (β_1AR) Activation Pathway via a G_s Protein for a Cardiomyocyte (Left-Hand Pathway) and an Antiapoptotic Pathway Through β-Arrestin

Note: The a_s, g, and b subunits of the G protein are indicated in the figure and how they relate to the activation of the adenylyl cyclase (AC), a cAMP-dependent protein kinase (PKA), and phosphorylation of target proteins such as the ryanodine receptor (RyR), phospholamban (PLN), troponin I (TnI), and the L-type Ca^{2+} channel (LTCC). GRK5 and GRK6 = G protein-coupled receptor kinases, SRC = tyrosine kinase first isolated as a gene product of a transforming rous sarcoma virus, MMP = membrane-type matrix metalloproteinases, HB-EGF = heparin-binding epidermal growth factor, EGFR = epidermal growth factor receptor, Ras = an oncogene whose name was derived from a rat sarcoma, Raf = serine/threonine protein kinase involved in tyrosine kinase signal transduction pathways, ERK/MAPK = extracellular signal-regulated kinase/mitogen-activated protein kinase.

Data from Engelhardt S. 2007. Alternative signaling: cardiomyocyte b1 adrenergic receptors signal through EGFRs. *J Clin Invest*. 117:2396–2398.

couple to $G_{i/o}$ to inhibit cAMP production, decrease Ca^{2+} conductance, increase K conductance, and increase mitogen-activated protein kinase activity centrally (Howlett et al., 2004). CB_2 is a receptor on immune cells that similarly decreases cAMP. However, cAMP has been viewed as an immunosuppressant rather than a stimulant. This apparent contradiction is based on a misunderstanding of the concentration-response relationship that toxicologists emphasize. At physiologically relevant concentrations (less than 100 μM), cAMP has immunostimulatory effects. Studies that have increased cAMP with analogs have approached immunosuppressive toxic concentrations of between 250 and 500 μM (Holsapple et al., 1996).

A ubiquitous plasticizer found in the environment, diethyl-(2-ethylhexyl) phthalate (DEHP), forms a metabolite mono-(2-ethylhexyl) phthalate (MEHP) toxic to Sertoli cells, which appears to mediate its effects first via a G protein-coupled receptor family that may be involved in cell–cell adhesion (flamingo1). MEHP then proceeds to cell-death receptors such as DR4,5,6 and FAS-signaling pathways to start germ cell apoptosis (Richburg et al., 2002).

Certain G proteins are linked to Ca^{2+} channels. For example, the inhibitory effect of ethanol on L-type Ca^{2+} channels appears to be mediated via a pertussis toxin–sensitive G protein. However, it is likely that toxicants work via multiple receptors and mechanisms. Mercury, for example, is a well-known neurotoxin with multiple sites of action based on its binding to sulfhydryl moieties. Interactions with both protein kinase A and the G_i/G_o proteins underlie the potentiating effect of mercury on $GABA_A$ receptor–chloride channel complexes. The second messenger cAMP and its signaling pathway play a role in this potentiation, as increasing cAMP in the cells decreases mercury's effects. Protein kinase A is also involved, as indicated by the fact that potentiation decreases when levels of this enzyme increase in the cells affected by mercury. Addition of GTP-γ-S decreases mercury's potentiation, indicating a role for G proteins in this phenomenon. In the presence of the cholera toxin, which is a G_s stimulator, mercury does not potentiate the action of GABA. Application of the inhibitors of G_i/G_o

protein function, GDP-β-S and pertussis toxin, also blocked the potentiating action of mercury. Likewise, methylmercury can redistribute the cell's intracellular Ca^{2+} stores, as does polycyclic aromatic hydrocarbons and TCDD.

Lead works similarly to other heavy metals—that is, a number of mechanisms may induce its neurotoxic or other cytotoxic actions. Its ability to decrease the exocytosis of secretory cells at low concentrations appears to be mediated via lead's extracellular block of voltage-gated Ca^{2+} channels. Once lead enters the cell via those same Ca channels, it affects L-type Ca channels and activation of protein kinase C (Narahashi et al., 1998). Lead (Pb^{2+}), along with other divalent ions such as Ca^{2+}, Ba^{2+}, Cd^{2+}, Co^{2+}, Fe^{2+}, Gd^{3+}, and Ni^{2+} and the antibiotic neomycin (but not Hg^{2+}), also affects the calcium-sensing receptor (CaR), which is a G protein–coupled receptor family. This receptor's action is mediated through the activity of phospholipase A_2 (PLA_2) and the mitogen-activated protein kinase p42ERK (Handlogten et al., 2000).

Some toxins alter the G protein content of cells. The herbicide dichlobenil causes olfactory toxicity in *Ictalurus punctatus*, the channel catfish, via reduction of G alpha q and G alpha 11 (Andreini et al., 1997). The importance of G proteins is that they can dissociate into subunits (α and β/γ), that regulate (Ca^{2+}) ion channels or enzymes that generate second messengers such as cAMP, cGMP, inositol phosphate, and diacylglycerol. This serves to amplify the signal significantly and is involved in the feedback control of these receptors (Hollenberg, 1991).

As complex as the interaction of toxic ligands with receptors appears to be, the importance of finding the pathways that are associated with toxicities has led to better understanding of the toxic versus protective pathways that cells use to cope with toxic insults and the development of pharmacologic agents, antidotes, and model agonists and antagonists of specific receptors for use in research. The goal of the toxicologist is to understand which mechanism(s) initiate a toxic action and which represent a true "tipping point" that irrevocably moves a cell toward oncogenic transformation or other dysfunctions such as fibrosis, apoptosis, and necrosis. The method used in this chapter for characterizing groups of receptors that react with toxicants is not the only way of ordering receptors and signal transduction mechanisms. Gutman (1997) indicates that there are seven transmembrane receptors for neurotransmitters and hormones, guanylyl cyclase receptors, tyrosine kinase receptors, T-cell and immunologic-stimulated hormone receptors, and growth hormone receptors.

Questions

1. Describe how a receptor agonist or antagonist may be toxic.
2. Why does down-regulation of receptors prevent toxicity, yet can generate toxicity when the toxicant is abruptly removed?
3. What are classes of receptor-mediated toxicities?

References

Abbott BD, Buckalew AR, DeVito MJ, Ross D, Bryant PL, Schmid JE. 2003. EGF and TGF-alpha expression influence the developmental toxicity of TCDD: dose response and AhR phenotype in EGF, TGF-alpha, and EGF + TGF-alpha knockout mice. *Toxicol Sci.* 71:84–95.

Andrè E, Campi B, Materazzi S, Trevisani M, Amadesi S, Massi D, Creminon C, Vaksman N, Nassini R, Civelli M, Baraldi PG, Poole DP, Bunnett NW, Geppetti P, Patacchini R. 2008. Cigarette smoke–induced neurogenic inflammation is mediated by alpha,beta-unsaturated aldehydes and the TRPA1 receptor in rodents. *J Clin Invest.* 118:2574–2582.

Andreini I, DellaCorte C, Johnson LC, Hughes S, Kalinoski DL. 1997. G-protein(S), G alpha q/G alpha 11, in the olfactory neuroepithelium of the channel catfish (*Ictalurus punctatus*) is altered by the herbicide, dichlobenil. *Toxicology.* 117:111–122.

Bai XC, Deng F, Liu AL, Zou ZP, Wang Y, Ke ZY, Ji QS, Luo SQ. 2002. Phospholipase C-gamma$_1$ is required for cell survival in oxidative stress by protein kinase C. *Biochem J.* 363:395–401.

Barth A, Nguyen LB, Barth L, Newell DW. 2005. Glycine-induced neurotoxicity in organotypic hippocampal slice cultures. *Exp Brain Res.* 161:351–357.

Bormann J. 2000. The "ABC" of GABA receptors. *Trends Pharmacol Sci.* 21:16–19.

Bucci G, Ramoino P, Diaspro A, Usai C. 2005. A role for GABA$_A$ receptors in the modulation of paramecium swimming behavior. *Neurosci Lett.* 386: 179–183.

Burke MA, Mutharasan RK, Ardehali H. 2008. The sulfonylurea receptor, an atypical ATP-binding cassette protein, and its regulation of the KATP channel. *Circ Res.* 102:164–176.

Calderwood SK, Jimmy Theriault J, Gray PJ, Jianlin Gong J. 2007. Cell surface receptors for molecular chaperones. *Methods.* 43:199–206.

Contestabile A. 2000. Roles of NMDA receptor activity and nitric oxide production in brain development, *Brain Res Rev.* 32:476–509.

Cornett P, Matta J, Ahern G. 2008, August 8. General anesthetics sensitize the capsaicin receptor TRPV1. *Mol Pharmacol.* [Epub ahead of print].

Dunn SM, Conti-Tronconi BM, Raftery MA. 1983. Separate sites of low and high affinity for agonists on *Torpedo californica* acetylcholine receptor. *Biochemistry.* 22:2512–2518.

Ebner HL, Blatzer M, Nawaz M, Krumschnabel G. 2007. Activation and nuclear translocation of ERK in response to ligand-dependent and -independent stimuli in liver and gill cells from rainbow trout. *J Exp Biol.* 210:1036–1045.

Fritz WA, Cotroneo MS, Wang J, Eltoum IE, Lamartiniere CA. 2003. Dietary diethylstilbestrol but not genistein adversely affects rat testicular development. *J Nutr.* 133:2287–2293.

Fuller GL, Williams JA, Tomlinson MG, Eble JA, Hanna SL, Pohlmann S, Suzuki-Inoue K, Ozaki Y, Watson SP, Pearce AC. 2007. The C-type lectin receptors CLEC-2 and dectin-1, but not DC-SIGN, signal via a novel YXXL-dependent signaling cascade. *J Biol Chem.* 282:12397–12409.

Gutman Y. 1997. Overview of signal transduction. In: Gutman Y, Lazarovici P, eds. *Toxins and signal transduction.* Amsterdam: Harwood Academic, pp. 1–14.

Handlogten ME, Shiraishi N, Awata H, Huang C, Miller RT. 2000. Extracellular Ca(2+)-sensing receptor is a promiscuous divalent cation sensor that responds to lead. *Am J Physiol Renal Physiol.* 279:F1083–F1091

Hollenberg MD. 1991. Structure–activity relationships for transmembrane signaling: the receptor's turn. *FASEB J.* 5:178–186.

Holsapple MP, Karras JG, Ledbetter JA, Schieven GL, Burchiel SW, Davila DR, Schatz AR, Kaminski NE. 1996. Molecular mechanisms of toxicant-induced immunosuppression: role of second messengers. *Annu Rev Pharmacol Toxicol.* 36:131–159.

Howlett AC, Breivogel CS, Childers SR, Deadwyler SA, Hampson RE, Porrino LJ. 2004. Cannabinoid physiology and pharmacology: 30 years of progress. *Neuropharmacology.* 47(suppl 1):345–358.

Kirischuk S, Kettenmann H, Verkhratsky A. 2007. Membrane currents and cytoplasmic sodium transients generated by glutamate transport in Bergmann glial cells. *Pflugers Arch.* 454:245–252.

Költgen D, Ceballos-Baumann AO, Franke C. 1994. Botulinum toxin converts muscle acetylcholine receptors from adult to embryonic type. *Muscle Nerve.* 17:779–784.

Laurén HB, Lopez-Picon FR, Korpi ER, Holopainen IE. 2005. Kainic acid–induced status epilepticus alters GABA receptor subunit mRNA and protein expression in the developing rat hippocampus. *J Neurochem.* 94:1384–1394.

Manev H, Costa E, Wroblewski JT, Guidotti A. 1990. Abusive stimulation of excitatory amino acid receptors: a strategy to limit neurotoxicity. *FASEB J.* 4:2789–2797.

Marin-Kuan M, Nestler S, Verguet C, Bezençon C, Piguet D, Delatour T, Mantle P, Cavin C, Schilter B. 2007. MAPK-ERK activation in kidney of male rats chronically fed ochratoxin A at a dose causing a significant incidence of renal carcinoma. *Toxicol Appl Pharmacol.* 224:174–181.

Narahashi T, Treistman SN, Suszkiw JB, Miletic V, Atchison WD. 1998. Symposium overview: chemical modulation of neuroreceptors and channels via intracellular components. *Toxicol Sci.* 45:9–25.

Orrenius S, McCabe MJ Jr, Nicotera P. 1992. Ca(2+)-dependent mechanisms of cytotoxicity and programmed cell death. *Toxicol Lett.* 64–65:357–364.

Pang XY, Liu T, Jiang F, Ji YH. 2008. Activation of spinal ERK signaling pathway contributes to pain-related responses induced by scorpion *Buthus martensi* Karch venom. Toxicon. 51:994–1007.

Pazos Y, Alvarez CJ, Camiña JP, Casanueva FF. 2007. Stimulation of extracellular signal–regulated kinases and proliferation in the human gastric cancer cells KATO-III by obestatin. *Growth Factors.* 25:373–381.

Peng C, Han Y, Sanders T, Chew G, Liu J, Hawrot E, Chi C, Wang C. 2008. Alpha4/7-conotoxin Lp1.1 is a novel antagonist of neuronal nicotinic acetylcholine receptors. *Peptides.* 29:1700-1707.

Rao A, Craig AM. 1997. Activity regulates the synaptic localization of the NMDA receptor in hippocampal neurons. *Neuron.* 19:801–812.

Richburg JH, Johnson KJ, Schoenfeld HA, Meistrich ML, Dix DJ. 2002. Defining the cellular and molecular mechanisms of toxicant action in the testis. *Toxicol Lett.* 135:167–183.

Rosoff PM, Terres G. 1986. Cyclosporine A inhibits Ca^{2+}-dependent stimulation of the Na^{+}/H^{+} antiport in human T cells. *J Cell Biol.* 103:457–463.

Schaeffer JM, Haines HW. 1989. Avermectin binding in *Caenorhabditis elegans*: a two-state model for the avermectin binding site. *Biochem Pharmacol.* 38:2329–2338.

Sihver W, Gillberg PG, Nordberg A. 1998. Laminar distribution of nicotinic receptor subtypes in human cerebral cortex as determined by [3H](–) nicotine, [3H]cytisine and [3H]epibatidine in vitro autoradiography. *Neuroscience.* 85:1121–1133.

Singh JN, Gupta R, Deshpande SB. 2006. *Ptychodiscus brevis* toxin-induced depression of spinal reflexes involves 5-HT via 5-HT$_3$ receptors modulated by NMDA receptor. *Neurosci Lett.* 409:70–74.

Straub AC, Stolz DB, Ross MA, Hernández-Zavala A, Soucy NV, Klei LR, Barchowsky A. 2007. Arsenic stimulates sinusoidal endothelial cell capillarization and vessel remodeling in mouse liver. *Hepatology.* 45:205–212.

Tatebayashi H, Ogata N. 1992. GABA$_B$-mediated modulation of the voltage-gated Ca^{2+} channels. *Gen Pharmacol.* 23:309–316.

Vergnes M, Boehrer A, Simler S, Bernasconi R, Marescaux C. 1997. Opposite effects of GABA$_B$ receptor antagonists on absences and convulsive seizures. *Eur J Pharmacol.* 332:245–255.

Viola A, Luster AD. 2008. Chemokines and their receptors: drug targets in immunity and inflammation. *Annu Rev Pharmacol Toxicol.* 48:171–197.

Waring P. 2005. Redox active calcium ion channels and cell death. *Arch Biochem Biophys.* 434:33–42.

Yin X, Knecht DA, Lynes MA. 2005. Metallothionein mediates leukocyte chemotaxis. *BMC Immunol.* 6:21.

Young AB, Snyder SH. 1973. Strychnine binding associated with glycine receptors of the central nervous system. *Proc Natl Acad Sci* USA. 70:2832–2836.

CHAPTER 7

Detoxication and Activation by Cells: Metabolism of the Original Toxicant

This is a chapter outline intended to guide and familiarize you with the content to follow.

I. Biotransformation: Detoxicating/activating foreign compounds and in the process trying to make them suitable for excretion (water soluble)

   A. Anaerobic biotransformation

   1. Polycyclic aromatic hydrocarbons (from Karthikeyan and Bhandari, 2001)

Hydrogenation	Hydration	Dehydrogenation	Ring cleaving	Mineralization	Carboxylation
PAH	Reduced PAH	Oxidized PAH	Further oxidized PAH	Hydrolyzed PAH	PAH
H_2	H_2O	H_2	H_2O	H_2O	CO_2 H_2O
Reduced PAH	Hydrated/ oxidized PAH	Further oxidized PAH	Hydrolyzed PAH	Mineralized ($CO_2 + H_2O$)	Oxidized/ carboxylated PAH

   2. Metals: methylation Hg + SAM (S-adenosylmethionine) → CH^3-Hg; (see Challenger mechanism in Figure 7-1)

   B. Facultative anaerobes' biotransformation

   1. Formation of CoA esters starts the hybrid pathway in Figure 7-2

   C. Aerobes' biotransformation

   1. Phase 1 monooxygenases and dioxygenases (Figure 7-3)

      a. Cytochrome P450 monooxygenase catalytic cycle (Figure 7-4 and reactions (Figure 7-5)

         (1) Activation of benzo[a]pyrene by CYPs (Figure 7-6), especially CYP1 (Figure 7-7)

         (2) Drug metabolism by CYP3A4 (most abundant) + CYPs 1A2, 2B6, 2C9, 2C19, and 2D6

CONCEPTUALIZING TOXICOLOGY 7-1

Data from Karthikeyan R, Bhandari A. 2001. Anaerobic Biotransformation of Aromatic and Polycyclic Aromatic Hydrocarbons in Soil Microcosms: A Review. *J Hazard Substance Res* Volume III-3:3-1–3-19.

(3) Different CYPs are inducible based on their activity to metabolizing that toxicant (aryl hydrocarbons by AhR versus phenobarbital versus glucocorticoids versus ethanol versus peroxisome proliferators)

(4) Inhibitors of CYPs: reversible and irreversible

b. Flavin-containing monooxygenases

(1) Similar to CYPs: catalyze N- and S-oxidations; FMO1 works primarily with tertiary amines; FMO3 metabolizes primary, secondary, and tertiary amines

(2) Catalytic cycle (Figure 7-8)

c. Monoamine oxidases (MAOs)

(1) MAO-A metabolizers: epinephrine, norepinephrine, metanephrine, and serotonin (inactivate neurotransmitters and structurally related pharmaceutical amines)

(2) MAO-B oxidizes amines on β-phenylephrine, phenylethanolamine, o-tyramine, and benzylamine

(3) MAO inhibitors (MAOIs) were first used as pharmaceutical agents to treat depression but patients are now mostly warned about simultaneously taking agents that inhibit MAO and increase neurotransmitter levels (such as SSRIs + MAO-A inhibitors = serotonin syndrome = seizures or MAOIs and tyramines in cheese = hypertension)

d. Cyclooxygenases

(1) Important in formation of pro-inflammatory prostaglandins

(2) Inhibition (COX inhibitors) used to reduce inflammation (NSAIDs) by increasing bleeding via reduction of thromboxane A_2 formation

(3) Reaction sequence(s) shown in Figure 7-9

(4) COX-2 is induced by cigarette smoke and appears to form mutagenic/genotoxic products

e. Mammalian heme peroxidases

(1) Oxidize the MPTP neurotoxin that forms in Parkinson's disease, which MAOs and CYPs cannot

(2) Thyroid peroxidase disrupted by goitrogens

f. Molybdoenzyme oxidases/hydrolases

(1) Cytosolic aldehyde oxidase and xanthine oxidase (lactating mammary gland) oxidize N-heterocyclic compounds and aldehydes → ROS and involved in liver damage from CCl_4, $HCCl_3$, and thioacetamide

(2) Inhibited by sodium tungstate

2. Phase I dehydrogenases/oxidases

a. Alcohol dehydrogenase

(1) Generates the toxic aldehyde, which may be further metabolized

b. Aldehyde dehydrogenase

(1) Generates the toxic formic acid product from formaldehyde (a product of methanol via alcohol dehydrogenase) and the glycolic acid product from glycoaldehyde (a product of the ethylene glycol portion of antifreeze via alcohol dehydrogenase)

3. Phase 1 carbonyl reductases (cytosol) and hydroxysteroid dehydrogenases (endoplasmic reticulum)

a. Aldo-keto reductases: aldehyde reductase and aldose reductase

b. Short-chain dehydrogenases: carbonyl reductase

c. Both types are considered detoxication steps in reducing reactive moieties of compounds (except for daunorubicin and doxorubicin, which are activated by reduction)

CONCEPTUALIZING TOXICOLOGY 7-1 (*continued*)

4. Phase 1 NADPH cytochrome P450 reductase and redox cycling

   a. Generates $O_2^{\cdot-}$ radicals by reducing oxidation–reduction indicators such as paraquat, which then donates its electron to oxygen without any need for enzymes

5. Phase 1 carboxyesterases

   a. Hydrolysis of pyrethroid insecticides, plasticizers, and narcotics

   b. Target of insecticides and chemical warfare nerve gas agents

6. Phase 1 amidases and esterases

   a. Hydrolyze aryl esters (A), carboyl esters (B), acetyl esters (C), and S-formylglutathione (D)

   b. A-type esterases confer protection to mammals via hydrolysis of the "oxon" metabolite of parathion or malathion by CYP = basis of selective toxicity of these insecticides

7. Phase 1 alkaline phosphatases

   a. Hydrolyze esters of phosphoric acid

8. Phase 1 peptidases/proteinases

   a. Limit availability of peptides injected into the bloodstream to cells

9. Antioxidant enzymes

   a. Catalase

      (1) Remove oxygen from hydrogen peroxides (peroxisomes of mammals, but cytosol of guinea pig liver cells)

   b. Selenium-dependent glutathione peroxidase (Se GSHpx)

      (1) Uses glutathione to reduce peroxides in the cytosol, plasma, and the GI tract

   c. Superoxide dismutases (SODs)

      (1) $O_2^{\cdot-}$ in the presence of water $\rightarrow H_2O_2 + O_2$

   d. Peroxiredoxins

      (1) Thioredoxin in mammalian mitochondria reduces hydrogen peroxides, lipid peroxides, alloxan, and a number of other thiols

         (a) Inhibited irreversibly by dinitrobenzene

   e. GSH reductase (also could be included in the reductase category): reduces GSSG and provides reduced glutathione for maintenance of cell oxidation/reduction state and a substrate for glutathione transferase of phase 2 biotransformation

   f. Epoxide hydrolase (also could be included in the hydrolase category)

      (1) Converts reactive epoxides from an oxirane ring to a dihydrodiol

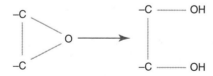

10. Phase 2 conjugation enzymes

    a. Acetylation of hydrazines and arylamine

    b. Acyl-CoA amino acid N-acyl and methyl transferases; acyltransferases involved in synthesis of glycerophospholipids; glycine conjugate represents mitochondria detoxication pathway

    c. Cytosolic N-methylatoins of azaheterocyclics part of toxic product

CONCEPTUALIZING TOXICOLOGY 7-1 (*continued*)

d. Parkinson's disease: neurotoxic 2,9-di-[N, N']-methylated beta-carbolinium cations

e. Rhodanese (thiosulfate sulfurtransferase)

(1) CN → Less toxic thiocyanate

f. Acetaminophen detoxication as exemplified by glucuronidation or sulfation (primary conjugation pathways for chemicals with a hydroxyl /phenol moiety) versus glutathione conjugation (conjugation to a reactive moiety as is formed in acetaminophen metabolism by CYPs) (Figure 7-10)

g. Phosphorylation

CONCEPTUALIZING TOXICOLOGY 7-1 (*continued*)

Biotransformation

The cell cannot withstand the accumulation of a lipophilic toxicant in its membranes until a lethal concentration is reached. It also cannot allow signals to remain intact and abusively stimulate receptors. Metabolism of nutrients by catabolic means for energy production or anabolism to build new cellular components is clearly understood as necessary for survival. The cell transporters that may allow certain substances to be pumped out of a cell, however, are insufficient to remove xenobiotics or inactivate extracellular or intracellular signals. Biotransformation allows signals to be metabolized into inactive smaller molecules, waste products to be altered into excretable forms, or unneeded molecules to be conjugated to groups that favor transport out of a cell or a more complex organism (**Conceptualizing Technology 7-1**).

Removal of hydrophobic substances is of most concern. These molecules need to be made more water soluble for easier sequestration and transport out of the cell, which requires covalent bonds to be attacked by highly reactive molecules produced by the cell's enzymes that will yield more hydrophilic moieties on the toxicant. Otherwise, bioaccumulation occurs. Certain cells live in more aerobic environments and can utilize oxidation and reduction. Others are found in more hypoxic or anaerobic environments and are more reductive. All cells contain

water, so use of water in the reaction or hydrolysis is always a possibility. This process is characteristic of phase 1 metabolism and adds a functional group that may be conjugated with a larger compound in phase 2 via any of the following means:

- Oxidation reactions including epoxidation, hydroxylation, dealkylation of specific heteroatoms (O-, N-, or S-; the heteroatom is any atom bound to a carbon atom that is not carbon or hydrogen), substitution of oxygen for heteroatoms, and dehydrogenation
- Reduction of azo, carbonyl, and nitro moieties of larger chemical structures
- Hydrolysis of amides, epoxides, and esters

Phase 2 metabolism entails conjugation by acetylation, amino acids, glucuronidation, glutathione, methylation, or sulfonation.

As far as a toxicologist is concerned, the metabolism and excretion of a compound determines the toxicokinetics or the concentration and distribution of the toxicant over a period of time, such as the half-life of a compound in a cell or organism (i.e., the amount of time it takes to halve the absorbed concentration). The formation of a metabolite may yield a less toxic compound, a process known as detoxication. The formation of a highly reactive more toxic metabolite is termed activation; it occurs with those compounds containing benzene rings or other structures that yield to unstable intermediates and attach themselves to macromolecules in the cell.

Anaerobic Bacteria

Anaerobic bacteria have a wide variety of species and activities. Strict anaerobes lack catalase, so they have no ability to handle reactive oxygen species. They also do not contain the cytochromes that are so important for aerobic xenobiotic biotransformation. Interest in these organisms ranges from the anaerobic environment of the mammalian gastrointestinal tract to wastewater treatment. Anaerobic bacteria are also involved in the environmental fates of dense substances that are metabolized at the bottom of lakes or streams or deep within the soil. In addition, they are found at volcanic vents and other places where high temperatures and high concentrations of heavy metals are found naturally. Anaerobic bacteria have been implicated in metabolism that leads to bioaccumulation of heavy metals or the biodegradation of organic compounds. Given that evolution started under what is assumed to be anoxic conditions, the anaerobic bacteria were likely some of the earliest organisms that metabolized toxic compounds under conditions viewed by humans as being extreme, such as high or low temperatures, low or high pH, and the high pressures found at the bottom of the oceans (Mesbah and Juergen Wiegel, 2008). For those organisms, the oxygen and other conditions considered normal for human function would be considered an extreme environment.

Anaerobic Metabolism of Aromatic Compounds

Many organic aromatic compounds are synthetic compounds of petroleum origin or natural compounds that arise from burn products, aromatic amino acids (tyrosine and tryptophan), lignin, flavonoids, phenolics, tannins, quinones, and lignans. These extremely hydrophobic compounds require some method of adding moieties to the ring structures to eliminate them; otherwise, some method is needed to open the ring structure for catabolism. Strict

anaerobes cannot utilize toxic oxygen, so they must employ other methods (Fuchs, 2008).

Even phototrophic bacteria and denitrifying bacteria employ anaerobic pathways to metabolize aromatic compounds. These bacteria use coenzyme A (CoA) esters to convert aromatic substrates to compounds such as benzoyl-CoA, resorcinol (1,3 hydroxybenzene), and phloroglucinol (1,3,5-trihydroxybenzene). Any phenolic compounds clearly are not formed by oxidative processes in phototrophic and denitrifying bacteria, but rather are reduced by these organisms, thereby forming alicyclic compounds (aliphatic and cyclic). Pyridine nucleotides are the source of electrons for reduction of phloroglucinol, while ferredoxin is required for reductive removal of the phenolic hydroxyl groups in resorcinol. The reduction of benzoyl-CoA requires the hydrolysis of one high-energy ATP molecule for each electron transferred. Hydrolysis also opens the nonaromatic ring. The final product is acetyl-CoA, as catalyzed by beta-oxidation.

Some anaerobes, such as clostridia, use a carboxylation step to metabolize phenolics. Others use a decarboxylase to deal with benzoic acid. Nevertheless, all of these organisms must still obtain access to the CoA ester intermediate and avoid using too much ATP in the process for energetically disfavored reactions. This requires the activation of benzoate to benzoyl-CoA by an ATP-dependent benzoate-CoA ligase (AMP plus PPi forming EC 6.2.1.25).

Sulfate-reducing bacteria can oxidize sn-alkanes or alkylbenzenes in oil to produce electrons for the reduction of sulfate to sulfide (Rueter et al., 1994). For chlorinated benzenes, dehalorespiration is a process by which certain anaerobic organisms, such as *Dehalococcoides ethenogene*, use an electron from hydrogen to initiate reductive dechlorination, thereby meeting their respiratory needs (Adrian et al., 2000).

Anaerobic Metabolism of Heavy Metals

Sulfate-reducing bacteria generate hydrogen sulfide; sulfide, an insoluble metal, causes heavy metals to precipitate out of water (Webb et al., 1998). These bacteria are also responsible for the

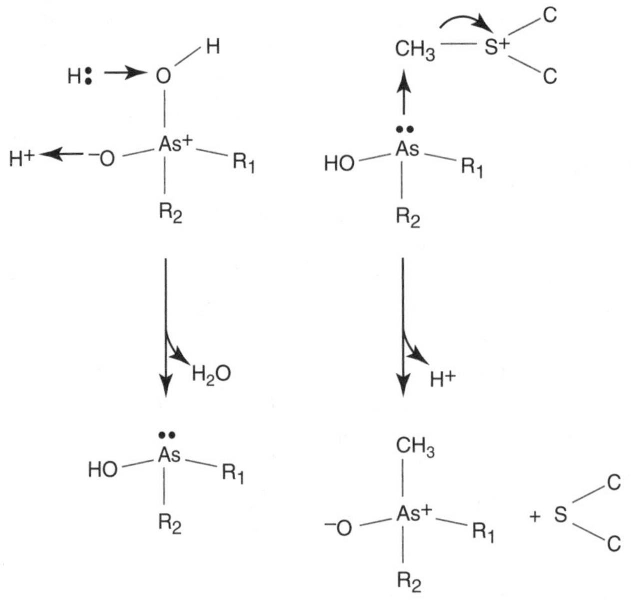

FIGURE 7-1 Typical Reactions of the Challenger Mechanism

Note: The top line indicates a mechanism for the reduction, As(V) → As(III), resulting in an unshared pair of electrons on As. Structures are as follows: $R_1 = R_2 = OH$, arsenate; $R_1 = CH_3$, $R_2 = OH$, methylarsonate; $R_1 = R_2 = CH_3$, dimethylarsinate. For reduction of trimethylarsine oxide to trimethylarsine, the process is a little different. Following proton addition, the structure $H-O-As^+-(CH_3)_3$ reacts with hydride ion leading to elimination of H_2O. The bottom line indicates the methylation of an As(III) structure with SAM [shown in abbreviated form as $CH_3-S^+-(C)_2$]. A proton is released and SAM is converted to S-adenosylhomocysteine [abbreviated form, $S-(C)_2$].

methylation of mercury, as inhibition of sulfate reduction by molybdenum almost totally eliminates the formation of methylmercury species (Compeau and Bartha, 1985). Methylation of arsenic and similar metalloids appears to use S-adenosylmethionine (SAM) as the universal donor of methyl groups in most biological systems (Bentley and Chasteen, 2002). The challenger mechanism by which As(V) is first reduced by two electrons and then methylated by SAM is depicted in **Figure 7-1**.

Hybrid Reactions of Facultative Anaerobes: Metabolism of Aromatic Compounds

The hybrid pathway for metabolism of benzoic acid is shown in **Figure 7-2**. As shown in this figure, bacteria may employ both reductive and oxidative approaches; both of these pathways are initiated by formation of the CoA esters. The second step differs in an important way from a benzoyl-CoA reductase (EC 1.3.99.15), which is inhibited/poisoned by oxygen. In contrast, in the facultative anaerobe, this step involves an oxidase, which under oxidative conditions can still yield the nonaromatic *cis*-dihydrodiols. This prevents a lethal accumulation of the CoA intermediate. The ring opens at this step by CoA thioesterification of the carboxyl group. Hydrolysis reactions are mostly featured in the remaining steps (Fuchs, 2008).

Aerobic Organisms' Phase 1 Metabolism

Bacterial and Fungal Metabolism of Aromatic Compounds

The key reaction in bacterial and fungal metabolism of aromatic compounds is the transfer of both atoms of molecular oxygen to these compounds via a dioxygenase reaction using Rieske-type non-heme iron oxygenases (EC 1.14.12.3–18

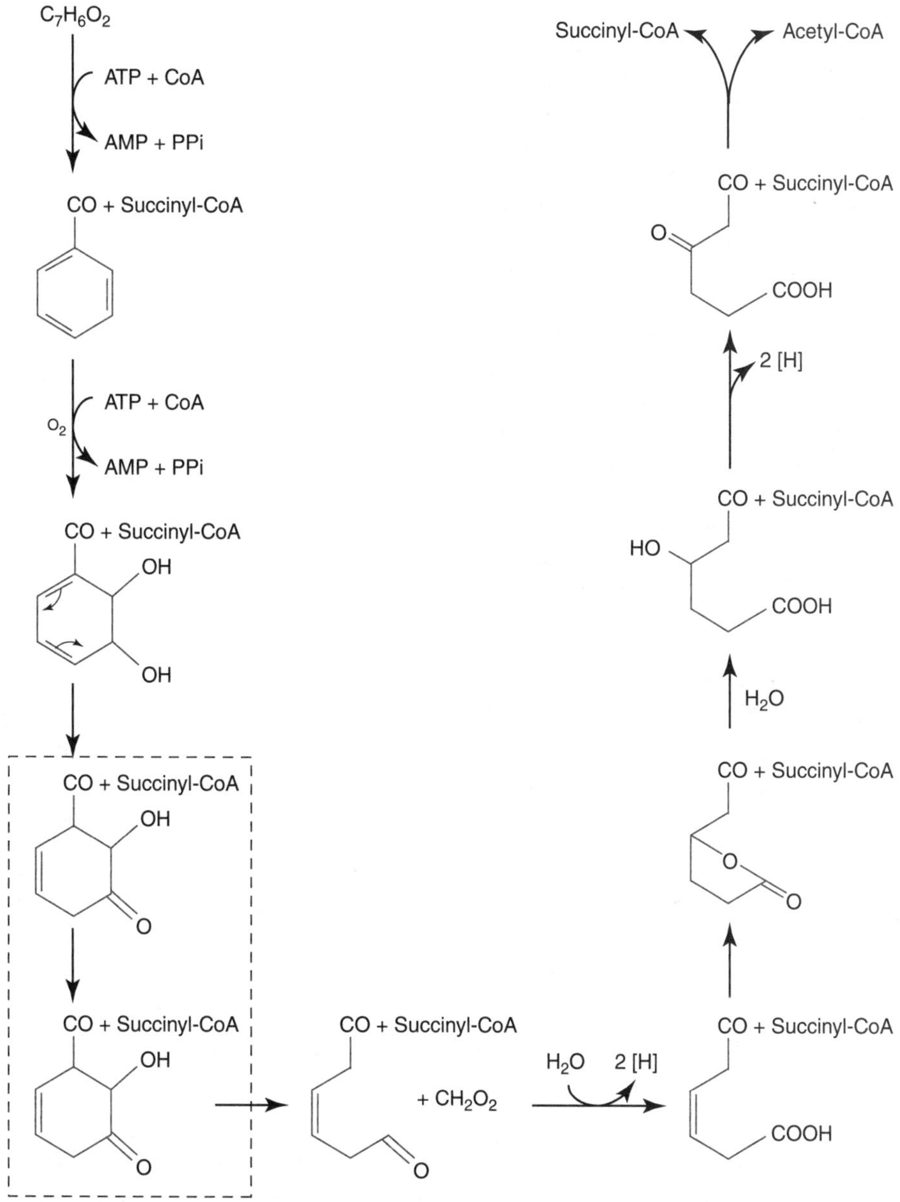

FIGURE 7-2 The Pathway for Conversion of Benzoic Acid to acetyl-CoA or succinyl-CoA Utilizing Either Anaerobic or Aerobic Pathways in a Facultative Anaerobe

depending on the substrate; Pieper et al., 2004). Highly chlorinated dioxins are metabolized via reductive dechlorination by the anaerobic bacteria, but have multiple enzyme systems for oxidative degradation. Dioxygenases of aerobic bacteria, bacterial and fungal cytochrome P450 monooxygenases, fungal lignolytic enzymes, and direct ether-ring cleavage by fungi containing

etherase-like enzymes allow for degradation of these compounds prior to plant uptake or animal consumption (Chang, 2008). As oxidation leads to a number of faster and alternative pathways to metabolism of xenobiotics, this principle has been utilized in bioremediation efforts, sewage treatment, and development of chemical agents ranging from pesticides to pharmaceuticals. Plants also benefit from mineralization/degradation of xenobiotics via oxidative pathways.

Although the phase 1 biotransformation involves oxidation, reduction, and hydrolysis reactions, the most important of these for plants is done by monooxygenases, also known as mixed function oxidases of the cytochrome P450 system (Komives and Gullner, 2005). In this reaction, half of the oxygen molecule oxidizes the substrate, while the other half becomes part of a water molecule (**Figure 7-3**).

This system is essential for metabolism in all higher-level cells, including human cells. Phase 2 biotransformation, in contrast, involves conjugation reactions. Next, these reactions are examined more closely in mammalian cells, where the functions of many of the enzymes in these two phases of metabolism were first discovered.

Cytochrome P450 Monooxygenase System Metabolism: Oxidation and Reduction

Omura and Sato (1964) described a carbon monoxide–binding pigment of liver microsomes that had a peak of 450 nm as analyzed with a dual beam spectrophotometer. Its initial function in bovine adrenocortical microsomal preparations was a very specific 21-hydroxylation of corticosteroids that was inhibited by carbon monoxide and reversed by an intense light beam of 450 nm (Cooper et al., 1965).

The discovery of cytochrome P450 was the basis for much of the present understanding of xenobiotic metabolism. Cytochrome P450 is a heme-containing enzyme that requires two electrons to reduce the heme iron from Fe^{3+} to Fe^{2+} and then transfer electrons from the reduced ferrous iron to oxygen; thus it is considered part of a monooxygenase system. Cytochrome P450 produces a very reactive oxygen molecule, O_2^{2-}. Its formation splits the oxygen molecule and can produce reactive oxygen species as well as an oxidized substrate and water. Potential sources of electrons include flavoproteins from the FAD or FMN domain, iron–sulfur proteins, and cytochrome b_s.

Ten classes of P450 systems are distinguished based on the topology of the protein components that transfer electrons to the

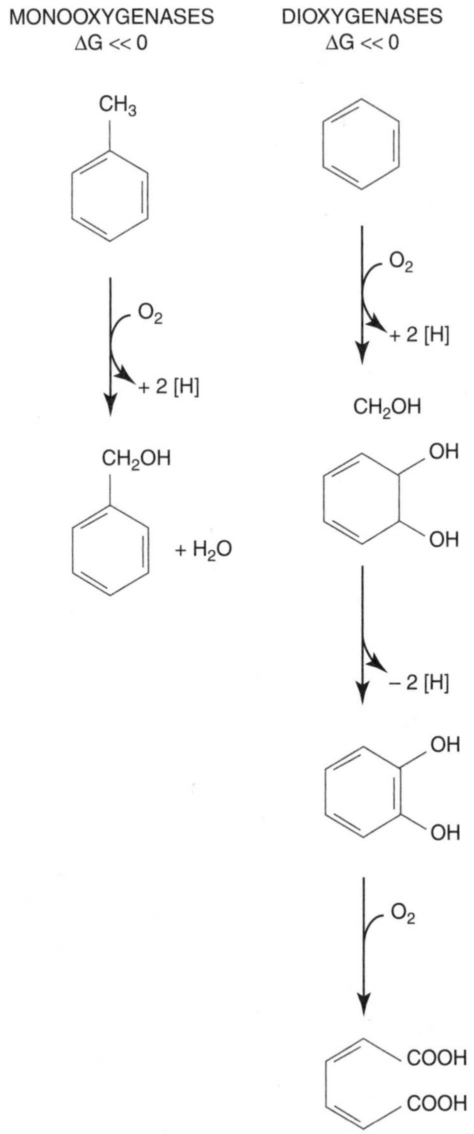

FIGURE 7-3 The Monooxygenases and Dioxygenases that are Found in Aerobes and Their Reactions with Toluene and Benzene Respectively

P450 enzyme (Hannemann et al., 2007). *Bacillus megaterium* contains a single polypeptide chain with a flavin and a heme that is a unique cytochrome P450 system. The type I cytochrome P450 systems are found in bacteria and mitochondria; they contain a three-protein system consisting of a flavin adenine dinucleotide (FAD)-containing NADPH or NADH-dependent reductase, an iron–sulfur protein, and cytochrome P450. Eukaryotic cells

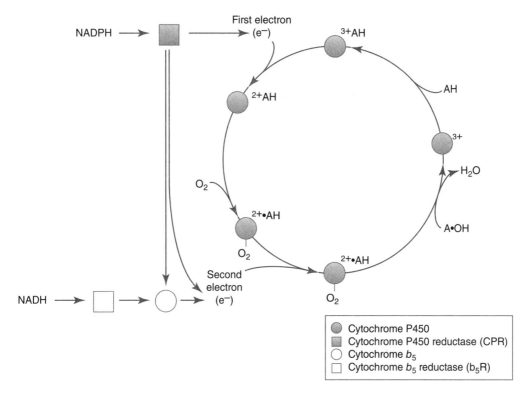

FIGURE 7-4 Catalytic Cycle of Cytochrome P450 in Microsomes of Eukaryotes

Note: The cycle starts with binding of the substrate (AH) to the ferric iron of cytochrome P450 at the top left of the circle. A first electron from NADPH in the cytosol to the cytochrome P450 reductase (CPR) reduces iron from the ferric to ferrous form. This is followed by the binding of a molecule of oxygen. The second electron also prefers to come from NADPH and CPR, but the electron may also in some systems (*Candida albicans*) be provided by cytochrome b5 (b5) and its reductase (b5R) which uses NADH as its electron source. In either case the oxygen becomes doubly reduced at the bottom of the circle leading to an oxidized (hydroxyl in this example) product and a molecule of water, regenerating the original oxidized ferric heme enzyme.

have a FAD and flavin mononucleotide (FMN)–containing NADPH:P450 reductase (EC 1.6.2.4) that transfers electrons to cytochrome P450 in the endoplasmic reticulum of cells. The reducing systems derive from the adrenodoxins and the adrenodoxin reductases (EC 1.18.1.2), cytochrome b_5 and cytochrome b_5 reductases (EC 1.6.2.2), Fe_3S_4 ferredoxins and NADH-ferredoxin reductases (EC 1.18.1.3), and NADPH:P450 reductases. Homologues of these systems are alkyl hydroperoxide reductases (EC 1.11.1.15), cytochrome b_5 domain-containing proteins, dihydrolipoamide dehydrogenases (EC 1.8.1.4), ferredoxin:NADP$^+$-reductases (EC 1.18.1.2), flavodoxins, glutathione reductases (EC 1.6.4.2), mercuric reductases (EC 1.16.1.1), NADPH:sulfite reductases flavoprotein, nitric oxide synthetases (EC 1.14.13.39), plant and fungal nitrate reductases (EC 1.6.6.2), thiodoxin reductases (EC 1.8.1.9), and trypanothione reductases (EC 1.8.1.12) (Degtyarenko, 2007). Cytochrome P450 accepts the electrons, reduces oxygen, and generates oxidized substrate in the manner depicted in **Figure 7-4**.

A more modern scheme proposes that a short-lived perferryl oxygen (FeO^{3+}) intermediate exists, which may be represented as a Fe^{IV} = O/porphyrin radical species (Guengerich, 2007). This species will remove a hydrogen atom from the molecule and form a FeOH^{3+} ion, which collapses and recombines rapidly into the alcohol or similar oxidized product. The reactions associated with this scheme are summarized in **Figure 7-5**.

Attack of the carbon atom in an alkane or the lone non-ring carbon on toluene (methyl

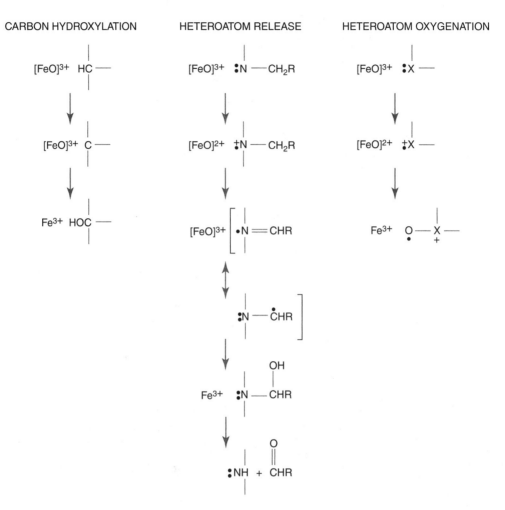

FIGURE 7-5 Reactions of Cytochrome P450 as Peformed by the Perferryl Oxygen Species

benzene) will yield the alcohol—a process referred to as aliphatic hydroxylation. Further attack would lead to the carboxylic acid (or benzoic acid, in the case of toluene oxidized twice). These compounds are generally more water soluble and less toxic than their original lipophilic structures. Oxidation of the second carbon may yield exceptions to this rule. For example, alcohols and ketones with structures such as ethanol, isopropanol, acetone, 2-butanol, and 2-hexanone, as well as the ketones that form in persons with uncontrolled diabetes mellitus, can potentiate chloroform toxicity and increase toxicity based on the increased aliphatic chain length. The modification of cytochrome P450 parameters to increase reactive metabolites during CCl_3 biotransformation appears to correlate well with the potentiating ability of these chemicals (Hewitt et al., 1987). Another exception would be the hydroxylation of cyclophosphamide, a genotoxic alkylating medication used in the treatment of cancer. The hydroxylation on the carbon at position 4 leads to opening of the ring and formation of the highly reactive metabolites phosphoramide mustard and acrolein (Sladek, 1988).

The next reaction scheme in Figure 7-5 involves the dealkylation at the heteroatom. This more reactive heteroatom is represented in the figure by nitrogen being released from an alkyl group. This dealkylation reaction forms the aldehyde and a heteroatom with a hydrogen moiety now attached. The aldehydes generated by this reaction tend to be more reactive or toxic than the corresponding alcohols (i.e., formaldehyde's genotoxicity and neurotoxicity compared to that of unmetabolized methanol, or acetaldehyde's hepatoxicity compared to that of unmetabolized ethanol).

The next scheme in Figure 7-5 focuses on oxidation of the heteroatom. The oxidation of the heteroatom in the case of nitrogen would yield a toxic nitrogen oxide (nitroso) group or hydroxylamine and further oxidation of the nitrogen group. These groups are highly reactive nitrogen species.

The epoxide formed in the last step in Figure 7-5 is always a very toxic product that yields short-lived highly reactive radicals, which themselves can damage macromolecules by forming adducts to proteins and nucleic acids. The compounds that form these epoxides contain either an aromatic ring, such as benzene, or a double bond close to an electron-withdrawing group such as halide (e.g., F, Cl, Br). Such is the case for vinyl chloride monomer, which causes mutations and cancer at a very high rate compared with the much less reactive polymer found in polyvinyl chloride (PVC) pipe.

The most dangerous substrates for cytochrome P450 involve aromatic compounds, many of which are formed during long organic synthesis procedures under higher temperatures or come from burn products of wood (polycyclic aromatic hydrocarbons) or plastics (dibenzodioxins and dibenzofurans). In essence, the monster of Dr. Frankenstein in the old horror movies was correct: The alcohol he drank was "good" at concentrations that would not be tolerated for most pharmaceuticals or toxicants, and the burning match and cigar were to be feared as chronically dangerous.

The compound 2-acetylaminofluorene is a case in point. This aromatic structure forms some metabolites that cause profound changes to mitochondrial integrity and disrupt apoptosis, while other metabolites are genotoxic or cell proliferative in nature. The adaptations the cell tries to make after injury by these toxic metabolites are well illustrated by liver cells and their transformation into cancer cells. The liver experiences carcinogenesis with no apparent threshold, while the bladder shows such a threshold at much higher concentrations associated with 2-acetylaminofluorene metabolites that promote cell growth (Bitsch et al., 1999). The lack of threshold for this carcinogen is reminiscent of the effects of radiation, which include cumulative, no-threshold toxic injury by radicals formed from ionization of water.

For polycyclic aromatic hydrocarbons (PAHs), the site at which the oxides form is an important determinant of their carcinogenic potency. The bay region is so named because the aromatic rings appear to form a "bay" in the "ocean" of fluid and enzymes and, unfortunately, are protected from further detoxication by other enzymes such as epoxide hydrolases that have difficulty accessing this region. Within the bay region, oxides (7,8-diol and 9,10-epoxides) of benzo[a]pyrene or B[*a*]P are the ultimate carcinogenic metabolites; they can be seen in the metabolic biotransformation of B[*a*]P in **Figure 7-6**.

Liver CYPs located close to the central hepatic vein function in a hypoxic environment. Whereas most aerobic transformations of chlorinated compounds by cytochrome P450 involve the generation of an unstable halohydrin, which can then form adducts to macromolecules, under anaerobic conditions the electrons proceed directly to reductive dehalogenation and formation of a carbon-centered radical and the inorganic form of the halide atom. P450 can also reduce azo- and nitro-compounds along with NAD(P)H-quinone oxidoreductase in an hypoxic environment, albeit less efficiently than anaerobic bacteria (Guengerich, 1991). In this way, this enzyme is a good example of oxidoreductases, which all oxidases and reductases really represent.

Cytochrome P450 Superfamily

Not only is the cytochrome P450 system composed of more than one enzyme, but cytochrome P450 also has many isozymes with optimal activities for groups of compounds. These isozymes are designated as CYPs. The letter following the "CYP" designation indicates the family, followed by a letter for the subfamily, followed by a number for the individual gene. For example, the isozymes responsible for bay- or fjord-region epoxides or diol-epoxides are the human CYP1 enzymes known as CYP1A1, CYP1A2, and CYP1B1 (Shimada, 2006). Numerous isozymes from *CYP1A1* genes have been identified in humans, long-tailed and Rhesus macaques, sheep, dogs, wildcats, European rabbits, guinea pigs, Syrian hamsters, and fish (four-eye butterfly fish, European seabass, dab, golden grey mullet, leaping mullet, Atlantic tomcod, rainbow trout, oyster toadfish, Japanese medaka, red seabream, gilthead seabream, right-eye flounders, European plaice, scup). CYP725A2 has been identified in the Japanese yew shrub.

It is not possible in this limited review of biotransformation to do justice to all of the CYP isozymes, except to note that all isozymes are not present in equal concentrations in each cell or organ of a species and do not have equal activity toward producing or detoxifying a toxic chemical species. Clearly, the presence

of CYP1 in many animal species indicates that these organisms are susceptible to carcinogenic transformations and may have a long history with PAHs arising from natural sources. As seen in **Figure 7-7**, CYP1 does, indeed, cause most of the known genotoxic/carcinogenic metabolites.

Although other CYPs (e.g., CYP2C9, CYP2W1, CYP3A4) demonstrate the ability to create some of these metabolites, their rate of formation is much slower than those more specific for aryl hydrocarbons. Some CYPs have no ability to transform PAHs into genotoxic metabolites (e.g., human CYP2A6, CYP2C8, CYP2D6, CYP2E1, and CYP4A11). This description does not give the complete picture regarding the susceptible cells, however, because each CYP may have different organ distributions. For example, CYP1A2 is mainly expressed in liver cells, where the first-pass metabolism of orally administered medications and toxins occurs. CYP1A1 messenger RNA expression is greater than expression of CYP1B1 in the digestive structures of the pancreas, small intestine, and the colon and catalyzes the activation of many aryl hydrocarbons and oxidation of 7-ethoxyresorufin (O-deethylase), 7-ethoxycoumarin, caffeine, theophylline, chlorzoxazone, and the endogenous hormones 17β-estradiol and estrone. CYP1B1 expression exceeds expression of CYP1A1 in the excretory organ cells of the kidney, the gonadal structures (mammary gland, uterus, ovary, prostate, and testis), the neuroendocrine pituitary gland, peripheral leukocytes, fetal tissues, and human cancer cells (breast, uterine myoma, and renal and adrenal carcinoma); this CYP catalyzes the activation of aromatic amines, nitroarenes, and estrogen to a metabolite that may initiate breast cancer as well as the oxidation of ethoxyresorufin, theophylline, caffeine, ethoxycoumarin, and bufaralol. No CYP1B1 expression is found in the pancreas.

These isozymes with the most activity for aryl hydrocarbons are inducible by the aryl hydrocarbon receptor (AhR)—for example, PAHs, TCDD, and 3,4,3′,4′-tetrachlorobiphenyl (3,4,3′,4′-TCB). Otherwise, the expression of CYP1A1 is low in naïve (untreated) animals, while the expression of CYP1B1 is low in male liver cells and female lung cells. Constitutive expression of CYP1B1 is biologically relevant in the other organs mentioned previously. Induction of CYP1A1 is very

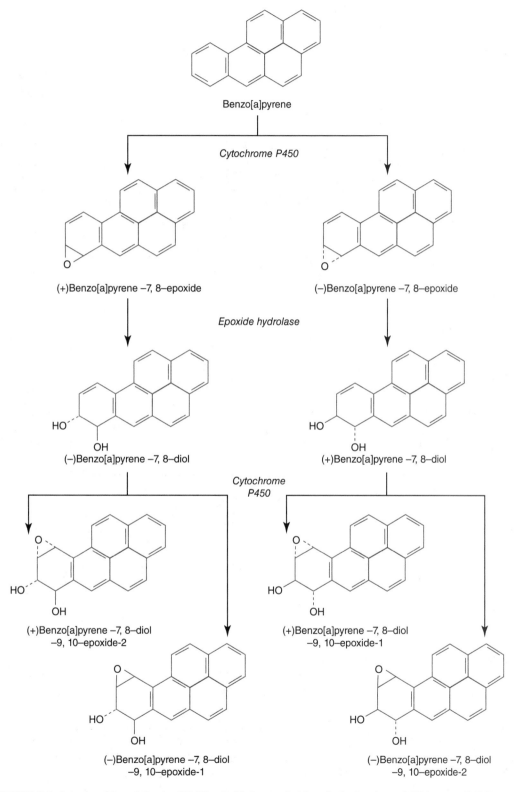

FIGURE 7-6 Activation of Benzo[*a*]pyrene (B[*a*]P) to Highly Reactive Diol-Epoxides by Cytochrome P450 Isozymes (P450) and Epoxide Hydrolase (EH)

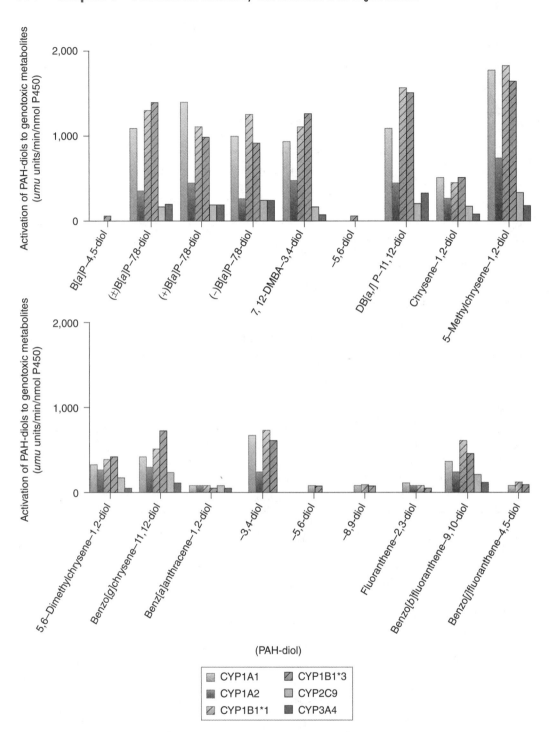

FIGURE 7-7 Activation of the Polycyclic Aromatic Hydrocarbons Benzo[*a*]pyrene (B[*a*]P), 7,12-Dimethylbenz[*a*]anthracene (7,12-DMBA), Dibenzo[*a,l*]pyrene (DB[*a,l*]P, Chrysene, 5-Methylchrysene, 5,6-Diemthylchrysene, Benzo[*g*]chrysene, Benz[*a*] anthracene, Fluoranthene, Benzo[*b*] Fluoranthene, and Benzo[*j*] Fluoranthene to Genotoxic Metabolites by Recombinant (*Escechrichia coli*) Human Cytochrome P450 Enzymes in a Tester Strain *Salmonella typhimurium* NM2009

Data from Shimada T. 2006. Xenobiotic-metabolizing enzymes in activation and detoxification of carcinogenic polycyclic aromatic hydrocarbons. *Drug Metab Pharmacokinet.* 21: 257–277.

high (e.g., 30- to 60-fold in female mouse lung cells induced with 3-methylcholanthrene and 3,4,3′,4′-TCB, respectively) and greater than that for CYP1B1, which has more constitutive expression. The importance of these isozymes and their induction cannot be overestimated, as genetic polymorphisms as the *CYP1A1* gene (*MspI* or *CYP1A1*2A*; *Ile-Val* or *CYP1A1*2B*) are linked to cigarette smoking–associated squamous cell carcinomas. The *CYP1A1*5* polymorphism is associated with lung cancer risk as well (Shimada, 2006).

CYP1A2 accounts for approximately 10–15% of adult human liver cell's expression of P450 protein, though this rate varies 40-fold among individuals (i.e., induced by cigarette smoke condensates and consumption of broiled food). CYP1A2 catalyzes the activation of aromatic amines as well as oxidation of acetaminophen, antipyrene, caffeine, 7-ethoxyresorufin, lidocaine, phenacetin, theophylline, and *R*-warfarin.

Polymorphisms of the *CYP1B1* gene have been associated with susceptibility to breast or squamous cell carcinoma of the lung (*2) in a Japanese population and breast cancer in a Chinese population (codon 432). Ethnic differences may be important here, as polymorphisms of these types are not necessarily associated with increased cancer risk in other human populations.

CYP2C9 represents approximately 20% of the P450 protein expression in human liver cells. This CYP slowly activates aryl hydrocarbons and oxidizes flubiprofen, losartan, phenytoin, tolubutamide, and warfarin.

CYP3A4 is the most abundant form (approximately 30%) of hepatic and intestinal cells expression of P450 and metabolizes approximately 50% of all medications currently in use (Zhou, 2008). This isozyme is also involved in the activation of the mycotoxins aflatoxin B_1 and G_1 and sterigmatocystin, turning them into active metabolites that can cause irreversible liver damage (when the metabolites are present in high concentrations in moldy feed) or cancer of the liver, especially in concert with hepatitis B and alterations to the *p53* gene (*Arg249Ser* mutation for aflatoxin B_1; Pineau et al., 2008).

In short, it appears as if CYP1A and CYP2E induction is associated with metabolic activation

of chemicals to carcinogenic intermediates. CYP1A1 is associated with lung cancer, but not liver cancer, because it is inducible by PAHs from burn products. CYP1A2 is more closely associated with metabolic activation of the polyaromatic and heterocyclic amines and amides formed during broiling of meat. CYP2E's induction by benzene, ethanol, acetone, carbon tetrachloride, and dichloromethane generates reactive oxygen species (ROS). However, cytochrome P450s must also be viewed in light of the detoxication pathways, which are especially significant for healthy subjects exposed to low concentrations of procarcinogens (Lewis et al., 1998). High doses of carcinogens that approach the maximum tolerated dose or chronic exposure of the type that occurs in cigarette smokers or those people or animals that consume mycotoxins or similar agents in their daily diets raise concerns about effects produced through the activation pathways. This is especially true in populations that already show genetic susceptibility to carcinogens, whether this represents a P450 gene polymorphism or some other genetic susceptibility factor (e.g., expression of a cancer susceptibility protein such as BRCA2).

Complicating this picture is the finding that cells in organ systems do not contain equal concentrations of cytochrome P450s or equal amounts of substances such as glutathione that can be used subsequent to activation in phase 2 metabolism. For example, greater activation of 1,1,-dichloroethylene is observed in lung bronchiolar Clara cells and liver centrilobular cells, along with greater damage due to higher cytochrome P450 concentrations and lower glutathione concentrations (Forkert, 1997). Similar results have been found in relation to acetaminophen hepatotoxicity.

CYP3A4 is the most abundant hepatic and intestinal phase 1 enzyme of the 57 genes that code for isozymes of human CYPs. The other enzymes that participate in drug metabolism are the CYPs designated as 1A2, 2B6, 2C9, 2C19, and 2D6. Taken together, CYP families 1, 2, and 3 account for 70% of the total liver content of cytochrome P450s and 94% of hepatic drug metabolism (Chang and Kam, 1999).

The isoforms of the CYP3A family numbered 4, 5, 7, and 43 are found on chromosome 7 of

Homo sapiens. The promoter region contains a basal transcription element, a mammalian heterotetrameric adapter protein 3 (AP-3) element that binds preferentially in vitro to dileucine- and tyrosine-based sorting signals of lysosomal transmembrane proteins, a p53 tumor-suppressing protein-binding motif, a hepatocyte nuclear factor 4 (HNF-4) region, two HNF-5 elements, a pregnane X receptor region, and an estrogen response motif. Model medication substrates for this isoform are clarithromycin, cyclosporine, and erythromycin for *N*-demethylation alone. *N*-Dealkylation occurs with alfentanil. *N*-Demethylation with 3-hydroxylation is represented by diazepam, flunitrazepam, and lidocaine (*N*-deethylation instead of *N*-demethylation). 1′-Hydroxylation is the product of alprazolam, atorvastatin, mexazolam, midazolam, and triazolam (with 4-hydroxylation occurring as well) metabolism. Hydroxylation at the 2 and 4 positions occurs with ethynyl estradiol. 3′-Hydroxylation results from this isoform's reactions with paclitaxel and simvastatin (with 3′,5′-dihydroxylation). 5-Hydroxylation occurs with diclofenac. 6β- or 6′β-hydroxylation is the product of cortisol and testosterone or lovastatin metabolism, respectively. Dehydrogenation alone occurs with felodipine, nifedipine, and nisoldipine.

Most of the medications that inhibit CYP3A4 are reversible and inhibit a series of reactions in a certain number of medications, but not all reactions with all medications. For instance, troleandomycin, fluoxetine, and erythromycin inhibit the 1′-hydroxylation of alprazolam, whereas ketoconazole, itraconazole, and fluconazole inhibit the 1′-hydroxylation of atorvastatin. Another example is the broad action of troleandomycin, which inhibits the *N*-dealkylation of alfentanil, the *N*-demethylation of clarithromycin and erythromycin, the 1′-hydroxylation of alprazolam, the 3′-hydroxylation of paclitaxel, the 6′β-hydroxylation of lovastatin, the *N*-hydroxylation of dapsone, the demethylation of tacrolimus, the *N*-demethylation and 3-hydroxylation of diazepam, the *N*-deethylation and 3-hydroxylation of lidocaine, the demethylation and deacetylation of rifabutin, and the dehydrogenation of nisoldipine. Most of the drug inhibitors are reversible except for

the macrolide antibiotics (e.g., azithromycin, clarithromycin derivatives, erythromycin derivatives, oleandomycin, roxithromycin, and troleandomycin) and cancer chemotherapeutic medications such as irinotecan and its active metabolites.

For induction of CYP3A4, production of the enzyme may be increased in three ways:

- Up-regulation of gene expression to increase enzyme synthesis (e.g., rifampicin)
- Stabilization of mRNA transcripts (e.g., erythromycin)
- Decreased degradation of the CYP protein

Whereas enzyme inhibition is immediate, increased enzyme production takes days to develop. The antibiotics rifampin and fibabutin are the most potent inducers (20- to 40-fold reduction of unmetabolized drug in plasma), followed by anticonvulsants such as carbazepine, and then by phenytoin, primidone, and the classical inducer phenobarbital. The antimycotic agent clotrimazole, cholesterol-synthesis–inhibiting statins (HMG-CoA reductase inhibitors), and the chemotherapeutic medications paclitaxel, cyclophosphamide, and ifosfamide are inducers as well. All inducers share a high lipophilicity. Medications that induce their own metabolism (i.e., autoinducers) are found in many drug classes, such as analgesics, antibiotics, anticonvulsants, antimalarial compounds, cancer chemotheraeutic agents, diuretics, and sedative-hypnotics.

The induction of CYP3A4 occurs by binding to the pregnane receptor, the constitutive androstane receptor, HNF4α, glucocorticoid receptor, or vitamin D receptor (Zhou, 2008). The binding to the first two receptors yields xenobiotic nuclear receptors that coordinate the protective responses of the liver to potentially toxic insults, including the accumulation of bile acids (Stedman et al., 2005). The binding to the pregnane X receptor produces an activated complex that forms a heterodimer with the retinoid X receptor; this heterodimer then binds to the pregnane X receptor response element region or the so-called xenobiotic responsive enhancer module. The final increased expression of CYP3A4 is accompanied by increased amounts of the important ABC organic toxin transporter

P-glycoprotein and phase 2 conjugation enzymes such as glutathione *S*-transferases (Liu et al., 2007). This combination will transport out unmetabolized toxic xenobiotics, increase metabolism of more water-soluble products, and detoxify via conjugation and transport toxic metabolites. In this way, the induction of CYP3A4 creates an integrated xenobiotic defense system, rather than just ensuring specific metabolism of selected compounds useful as medications at prescribed doses.

Not only do the isoforms of cytochrome P450 differ within cells of the same species, but some major differences in these isoforms are observed between species. This factor is important when toxicologists use a rodent model of carcinogenesis. For example, coumarin is activated via 3,4-epoxidation in the rat and detoxified by 7-hydroxylation in the mouse. Conversely, butadiene produces a monoepoxide and a diepoxide in the mouse, but does not form any epoxides in the rat. Human differences also exist. For example, tamoxifen is a weak agonist of estrogen and is used as an estrogen antagonist and breast cancer treatment chemotherapy agent. It is metabolized to nontoxic metabolites by CYP2C9 and CYP3A4 in humans, but is activated in rodents to an epoxide or undergoes hydroxylation of an ethyl group that yields a reactive and genotoxic carbonyl ion intermediate (Lewis et al., 1998).

P450 Inducers and Inhibitors

The inducers of cytochrome P450 were covered in the discussion of the CYP superfamilies. There, the CYP1 and CYP2 families were described as being linked to the Ah receptor, and the CYP3 drug metabolism and P-glycoprotein transporter of xenobiotics as being linked to ligand-activated nuclear receptors, constitutively active receptors, and the pregnane receptor. The inducer categories for all CYPs are as follows:

- Phenobarbital and phenytoin
- PAHs
- Pregnalone 16α-caronitrile and glucocorticoids
- Ethanol and isoniazid
- Peroxisome proliferators such as clofibrate and phthalates

Cytochrome P450 activity is also affected by reversible competitive or noncompetitive inhibitors, quasi-irreversible inhibitors, and irreversible inhibitors. The quasi-irreversible and irreversible inhibitors usually involve bioactivation to a reactive intermediate, which then covalently alters an amino acid residue of the apoprotein (not the heme group), alkylates the heme prosthetic group, and/or coordinates with the heme iron. The formation of a metabolite-inhibitor complex is determined by three factors:

- The appearance of a ferrous (reduced) iron form of P450 that absorbs light with a wavelength of 448–456 nm
- The lack of catalytic activity
- The inability to bind carbon monoxide

If the reactant group is an amine, ferricyanide dissociates the inhibitor from P450. If the complex is not formed with an amine, however, this process will not work.

Quasi-irreversible inhibitors have more profound effects after multiple doses than do reversible inhibitors. Aliphatic and aromatic amines form a nitrosoalkane that coordinates tightly to the ferrous iron form of cytochrome P450. Certain macrolide antibiotics with high C log P and a nonhindered, readily accessible *N,N*-dimethyl-amino group, such as erythromycin and clarithromycin, work via this mechanism. Other macrolide antibiotics rarely or never form these inhibitor complexes.

Cyclopropylamines either modify the enzyme via a one-electron reduction of the nitrogen and subsequent ring opening to a reactive intermediate or act via a nitroso metabolite. Calcium-channel blockers that have a tertiary amine are *N*-dealkylated to the primary amine prior to formation of an inhibitor complex with P450. *N*-Demethylation does not always yield a group that interacts with the heme; for example, tamoxifen metabolites that bind to the apoprotein and inhibit cytochrome P450 function do not interfere with carbon monoxide binding. Chemicals that have a 1,3-benzdioxole group, such as the selective serotonin reuptake inhibitor paroxetine (a widely used antidepressant) or the phosphodiesterase-5 inhibitor tadalafil, form a carbene intermediate by either abstraction of a hydrogen atom from the methylene carbon or removal of a water molecule (H_2O) from a hydroxymethylene intermediate.

HIV protease inhibitors are known inhibitors of cytochrome P450, whose activity involves reactive intermediates or ROS. Some covalent linkages that occur via reactive metabolites will occasionally lead to development of immunoallergic hepatitis by generating anti-P4501A2 antibodies; this effect has been demonstrated with dihydralazine. Although acetaminophen's reactive metabolites do not appear to inhibit P450, an isomer of acetaminophen, 3-hydroxyacetanilide, is metabolized by the same CYP2E1 isoform to a dihydroxy species, which is then further oxidized to benzoquinone reactive metabolites; these metabolites irreversibly inactivate the 3-hydroxyacetanilide isozyme.

Furans inactivate cytochrome P450 and lead to liver and kidney toxicity and hepatic cancer via an epoxide opening of the ring to a *cis*-2-butene-1,4-dial reactive metabolite. A dihydrofuranone moiety in the cyclooxygenase-2 (COX2) inhibitor rofecoxib appears to be involved in this compound's inactivation of CYP1A2. This is consistent with the interaction of theophylline and tizanidine with this isozyme.

Thiophenes, such as sudoxicam and ticlopidine, are activated via CYP2C19 and 2B6 to hydroxythiophenes and then undergo sulfur oxidation to unstable, reactive sulfoxides or form an epoxide that opens the ring to a reactive intermediate.

Alkenes, such as the sedative-hypnotic medication 2-isopropyl-4-pentenamide, irreversibly inhibit P450 via an epoxidation of the π-bond, which covalently binds to the nitrogen in the porphyrin ring and undergoes cyclization to a lactone. Alkynes may form a reactive species via oxygenation of the terminal carbon in terminal alkynes and formation of a ketene for acylation of the heme (oral contraceptive 17α-ethynylestradiol mechanism). Alternatively, for internal alkynes, oxidation and subsequent rearrangement yield an alkylating oxirene (antiprogestin medication mifepristone mechanism). 4-Alkyl-1,4-dihydroxypyridines are subject to dehydrogenation of the ring and aromatization by cytochrome P450. In this process, the 4-alkyl or 4-alkylaryl group is removed as a radical. 2-Alkylimidazoles, such as

furafylline, inhibit CYP1A2, but not through the furan ring activation as might be anticipated. Rather, an intermediate formed in the oxidation of the methyl group at position 8 appears to be involved; otherwise, the formation of a reactive imine-methide metabolite appears to occur with the benzodiazepine derivative midazolam. Dihaloalkanes, such as the antibiotic chloramphenicol, inactivate P450 via an acyl chloride formed following oxidative dechlorination of the dichloromethyl group.

Cyclopropylamines inhibit monoamine oxidase (MAO) B as well as cytochrome P450. This mechanism involves either oxidation—that is, transfer of a single electron on the amine nitrogen to a cation radical—or direct hydroxylation via hydrogen atom transfer to the α-carbon of the cyclopropyl moiety. Hydrazines, such as the antidepressant phenelzine, also inhibit MAO as well as P450 via oxidation of a phenyldiazene intermediate and degradation to a phenethyl radical (MAO inhibitor) or oxidative formation of the 2-phenylethyl radical (human CYP3A4 and rat CYP2C11), raloxifine (CYP3A4), troglitazone (CYP2C and CYP3A), N-phenylmorpholino potassium-channel opener (CYP3A4), tacrine (CYP1A2), delavirdine (CYP3A4), mibefradil (CYP3A4), imipramine (rat CYP3A2, CYP2D, and CYPC11), propranolol (rat CYP2D), N,N′,N″-triethylenethiophosphoramide (rat and human CYP2B), phencyclidine (CYP2B, CYP2C, and CYP2D), and gemfibrozil (clinical human CYP2C8 > CYP2C9).

Natural products that inhibit cytochrome P450 include methysticin and 7,8-dihydromethysticin (kava), gomisin C (schisandra fruit extract), rutaecarpine (evodia fruit), glabridin and 2,4-dimethylglabridin (licorice root), diallylsulfide (garlic), benzyl and phenethylisocyanate (cruciferous vegetables), menthofuran (pennyroyal oil), resveratrol (red wine and peanuts), silybin (milk thistle), ipomeanol (sweet potatoes), oleuropein (olive oil), capsaicin (capsaicin fruit), limonin (evodia fruit and citrus), 8-methoxypsoralen (parsley, parsnips, figs, celery, and grapefruit juice), and bergamottin and 6′,7′-dihydroxy bergamottin (grapefruit juice) (Kalgutkar et al., 2007). The inhibitory influence of furanocoumarins in grapefruit juice on both CYP3A4 and organic transporters such as P-glycoprotein and organic anion-transporting polypeptides cannot be overstated (Uno and Yasui-Furukori, 2006). In one study, 240 mL of grapefruit juice given to human subjects increased the area under the curve (concentration versus time curve) for felodipine only when the natural furanocoumarins were present in the juice (Paine et al., 2006).

Flavin-Containing Monooxygenases: Oxidation

The flavin-containing monooxygenases (FMOs; EC 1.14.13.8) are similar to the cytochrome P450 family of microsomal enzymes that metabolize medications, toxicants, and nutrients. The FMOs catalyze the nitrogen and sulfur oxidation of these compounds. Researchers have identified a five-gene cluster consisting of *FMO1–4* and *FMO6p*, another five-gene cluster that transcribes into *FMO7p–11p*, and a single gene *FMO5* that encodes for a total of five active proteins in *Homo sapiens*. FMO1 is the most abundant enzyme in the human fetal liver, whereas FMO3 appears to be absent at this site (Hines, 2006). In the adult, FMO3 is the enzyme that is present in highest concentration and activity and compares favorably with the activity of the abundant CYP3A4 and CYP2C9 isoforms. In other animals, FMO1 appears to be the predominant form of the enzyme. Significant polymorphisms of FMO3 are observed in various ethnic and racial populations, with FMO3 N61K being devoid of activity to the FMO3 substrates of methimazole, trimethylamine, sulindac, and ethylenethiourea. A total of 27 FMO3 missense, nonsense, or deletion mutants confer a complete loss of activity and lead to a build-up of trimethylamine in the urine, which creates a characteristic "fish-odor syndrome."

Induction of FMOs is not well established as a link to individual differences that differentiate these monooxygenases from the members of the cytochrome P450 family. An 80-fold induction of FMO3 mRNA expression in male mice exposed to 2,3,7,8-TCDD was found to be dependent on the presence of the AhR; it may indicate that suppression of testosterone is overcome by transcription of the FMO3 gene in this species (Koukouritaki et al., 2007). The FMOs also differentiate themselves from the P450 isozymes based on their catalytic cycle, which proceeds as follows:

1. The FMOs are first subject to a two electron reduction by NADPH to form $FADH_2$; the NADPH remains bound until it dissociates at the last step prior to being reduced and binding a subsequently FMO.
2. They bind molecular oxygen prior to binding with the substrate, thereby forming FADH-4α-hydroperoxide (peroxyflavin).
3. One atom of oxygen oxidizes the substrate (nucleophile).
4. A water molecule is released, leaving the oxidized FAD prior to release of the $NADP^+$ (**Figure 7-8**).

The most important role of the FMOs is the conversion of nucleophilic chemicals containing heteroatoms into more water-soluble and excretable forms. Human FMO3 metabolizes primary, secondary, and tertiary amines, while FMO1 works primarily with tertiary amines. Both forms oxidize sulfur-containing compounds, with some selectivity for specific stereoisomers. FMO3 in the human prefers a nitrogen atom bound to a large aromatic group (more than five carbons) rather than a nitrogen atom bound to a two- to three-carbon structure. Efficient metabolites include the phenothiazines and the phenylethylamines. Trimethylamine conversion to trimethylamine N-oxide, cimetidine S-oxygenation, or ranitidine N-oxidation offers a way to probe for human conversion by FMO3, while a stereoselective probe comprises the formation of (*S*)-nicotine *N*-1'-oxide from exposure to the nicotine tobacco plant alkaloid. The importance of FMOs in clinical practice is that certain medications undergo adverse reactions in some individuals, especially those persons with poor metabolism phenotypes (Cashman, 2000).

Amine Oxidases

Monoamine oxidase (MAO; EC 1.4.3.4) is another flavin-containing enzyme localized primarily on the outer mitochondrial membrane of cells. There are two distinct isozymes: MAO-A and MAO-B. MAOs have distinct substrate

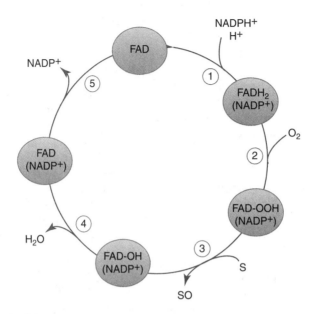

FIGURE 7-8 Catalytic Cycle of Flavin-Containing Monooxygenase

Note: 1) Fast reduction of FAD by NADPH. 2) Fast reaction of molecular oxygen with $FADH_2$ forming the stable flavin-hydroperoxide (FAD-OOH). 3) The FAD-OOH reacts with any suitable nucleophile at the active site. No substrate is necessary at this step. 4) One atom of O_2 reacts with the substrate, while the other atom goes to water similar to CYP monooxygenases. 5) FAD-OH regenerates as FAD via release of water in the rate-limiting step and the $NADP^+$ is also released in this slow step.

specificities when chemicals are at low concentrations. MAO-A is specific for epinephrine, norepinephrine, metanephrine, and serotonin (5-hydroxytryptamine [5-HT]). MAO-B selectively metabolizes β-phenylephrine, phenylethanolamine, o-tyramine, and benzylamine. Both isozymes metabolize *m,p*-tyramine, dopamine, octopamine, synephrine, tryptamine, *N*-methyltryptamine, and *N,N*-methyltryptamine. Inhibitors of MAO-A are reversible, such as harmaline, amiflamine, cimoxatone, moclobemide, and brofaramine; an irreversible inhibitor of this form of MAO is clorgyline. An irreversible inhibitor for MAO-B is (–)deprenyl, while irreversible inhibition of all MAOs occurs with phenelzine, tranylcypromine, isocarboxide, and pargyline.

In humans, MAO-A predominates in monoaminergic neurons, the placenta, liver (slightly), and brain, while MAO-B is exclusively found in platelets and is favored in serotonergic neurons, intestine, and extraneural cells. The human liver has the highest MAO-A activity of any species studied, with the rat liver having comparable kinetic activities and MAO-A/MAO-B ratios. Subhuman primates have little MAO-A activity. MAO-B is the principal enzyme of most tissues in most species. The rabbit brain and liver have very low MAO activities (Inoue et al., 1999).

MAOs mainly control the concentrations of catecholamines and indolamines following their release from nerve endings. They are also capable of oxidizing from primary to tertiary amines, generating ammonia (an amine) and possibly toxic concentrations of hydrogen peroxide (an aldehyde). Inhibition of these activities breaks down the defense against monoamines in herbs such as *Cytisus scoparius* (Scotch broom) and foods such as tyramine and β-phenylethanolamine, leading to an increase in blood pressure known as the "cheese effect" (Wells and Bjorksten, 1989). Given that tryptophan may also be influenced by MAO inhibition, this food substance's effect may be amplified as it is transported to the brain. Certain herbs may be either mild MAO inhibitors or increase sympathetic activity, such as occurs with the harmane alkaloids in *Passiflora incarnata* (passion flower), *Peganum harmala* (Syrian rue), hypericin in *Hypericum perforatum* (St. John's wort), isoliquiritigenin and glycyrrhizins in *Glycyrrhiza glabra* (licorice root), mescaline in *Lophophora williamsii* (peyote), myristicin in *Myristica fragrans* (nutmeg), and yohimbine in *Pausinistalia yohimbe* (http://home.caregroup.org/clinical/altmed/interactions/Drug_Classes/Monoamine_Oxida.htm).

A catecholamine neuron toxicant, 1-methyl-4-phenyl-1,2,3,6-tetrahydropyridine (MPTP), is prevented from causing damage if an inhibitor of MAO-B (Ro 19-6327), but not MAO-A (clorgyline), is given to cultured bovine adrenomedullary chromaffin cells. The toxic product 1-methyl-4-phenylpyridinium (MPP$^+$) is taken up by nigrostriatal dopaminergic neurons and blocks mitochondrial metabolism leading to Parkinson's disease. MAO inhibitors will not prevented MPP$^+$ from depleting catecholamines or reducing the activities of tyrosine kinase and lactate dehydrogenase activity. However, the inclusion of an inhibitor of cellular catecholamine uptake, desmethylimipramine, antagonized the cytotoxic action of MPP$^+$. MPP$^+$ is formed by MAO through a 1-methyl-4-phenyl-2,3-dihydropyridinium intermediate (Reinhard et al., 1990).

The intracellular form of polyamine oxidase (EC 1.5.3.3) may be grouped with the MAOs since it also uses flavin adenine nucleo-tide (FAD) and its cofactor. It is constitutively expressed in all vertebrates. Lysyl oxidase (EC 1.4.3.13), which is found in connective tissue, and semicarbazide-sensitive copper-containing amine oxidase (SSAO), which is found in endothelial cells, smooth muscle cells, and blood, use compounds containing carbonyl moieties as their cofactor, making them sensitive to inhibition by these same groups as occurs with semicarbazide (Gong and Boor, 2006). Diamine oxidase (EC 1.4.3.6) is an SSAO that catalyzes the rate-limiting step in polyamine metabolism. This enzyme prevents the inflammatory substance histamine and the toxic odiferous substances that are formed following degradation of dead organisms, putrescine and cadaverine, from having profound effects on cells. Polyamine oxidase has protective functions due its

catalysis of substrates that are not common to diamine oxidase, such as spermidine and spermine (Tunici et al., 1999). Aldehydes, ammonia, and superoxide produced by SSAOs cause vascular cell damage and low-density lipoprotein (LDL) oxidation due to the presence of copper in the enzyme (Exner et al., 2001).

Cyclooxygenases/Prostaglandin Synthases, Peroxidases, and Antioxidant Enzymes: Oxidation, Reduction, and Dismutation

The arachidonic acid cascade is an important biochemical pathway in the development of eicosanoids from membrane lipids. The enzymes of this cascade have been targeted for inhibition due the role of the products of their activities—namely, the prostaglandins (PGs; EC 1.14.99.1), prostacyclin, and thromboxane A$_2$ (TXA$_2$). These potent substances mediate effects on the cardiovascular system, inflammation and immunity, bronchial and tracheal smooth muscle, uterine smooth muscle, gastric and intestinal secretions, kidney function, central nervous system function, endocrine organs, and bone metabolism. They are formed by the microsomal cyclooxygenases (and phospholipase).

Cyclooxygenases (COX) represent the rate-limiting step in the formation of the prostaglandins due in part to the reversible self-inactivating property of these enzymes following a short catalytic period. Growth factors and cytokines both regulate COX enzymes. Cytokine interleukin-1 (IL-1), which starts the immune and inflammatory cascades, inhibits endothelial growth in vitro and stimulates prostacyclin synthesis, while the endothelial growth mitogen heparin-binding growth factor 1 inhibits prostacyclin synthesis in human umbilical vein endothelial cells (Hla and Maciag, 1991). Two COX isoforms (1 and 2) have important functions, while a third (COX-3) found in mouse neural cells is almost identical to COX-1, with the exception of its in-frame retention of intron 1 (Shaftel et al., 2003).

The COX enzymes convert arachidonic acid to prostaglandin H$_2$ first by using two molecules of oxygen to form a cyclic peroxide and the hydroperoxide portion of the first prostaglandin in the cascade (PGG$_2$). Next, a lipophilic organic compound (e.g., a phenol or aromatic amine) is oxidized and used as the source of electrons to reduce the hydroperoxide to a hydroxyl in the formation of PGH$_2$ (**Figure 7-9**).

In the formation of the oxidized organic compound, a radical is created that has toxic implications. The COX-1 and COX-2 enzyme inhibitors are known as nonsteroidal anti-inflammatory drugs (NSAIDs). A newer group of NSAIDs have only COX-2 inhibitory activity; that is, they mainly reduce inflammation. COX-1 acetylation in platelets and irreversible inhibition by compounds such as acetylsalicylic acid (aspirin) decreases TXA$_2$, which increases clotting times. Because COX-1 is also the source of cytoprotective prostaglandins in the gastrointestinal (GI) tract, such as PGE$_2$ and PGI$_2$, COX-1 inhibitors cause GI disturbances and increase bleeding. The COX-2 inhibitors, in contrast, promote clot formation, which increases the risk of myocardial infarction. Weak inhibitors of COX-1 and COX-2, such as paracetamol (acetaminophen), have neither problem, but acetaminophen forms toxic metabolites with CYPs.

COX-1 is the constitutively expressed enzyme that maintains function of the cells of the GI tract, platelets, and kidney. COX-2 is inducible by inflammatory mediators and has implications for conditions such as rheumatoid arthritis (Spangler, 1996) and cancer via regulation of cell growth. A newer hypothesis suggests that inflammation may produce a disrupting environment that promotes the development of certain cancers. For example, cigarette smoke induces COX-2 mRNA production, prostaglandin E synthase and PGE$_2$ production, phosphorylation of ERK1/2, and nuclear translocation of p50 and p65 subunits for NF-κB in human lung fibroblasts. Acrolein and acetaldehyde in smoke induce COX-2 and increase release of PGE$_2$. Increased PGE$_2$ levels abolish activating tumor suppressors such as p53 and Rb, and increase the activity of oncogenic proteins such as K-ras. It has been hypothesized that aryl hydrocarbons such as the benzanthracenes and benzopyrenes found in cigarette smoke also may undergo significant metabolism by COX-2, which then leads to mutagenic/genotoxic products. The carcinogen benzo[a]pyrene (B[a]P) is converted

to the reactive B[a]P-7,8-dihydrodiolepoxide by the second step of COX-2 enzyme conversion of PGG$_2$ to PGH$_2$; this compound increases the cellular content of COX-2 and the rate of PGE$_2$ synthesis in epithelial cells and vascular smooth muscle cells. The lipid peroxidation product that results from arachidonic acid metabolism by COX enzymes, malondialdehyde, can alkylate DNA (Martey et al., 2004). COX-2 has also been found to be a useful marker for kidney tumors (Sakurai et al., 2005). In total, it appears that the induction of COX-2, its metabolic products, and tumorigenesis are linked via multiple mechanisms.

Mammalian heme peroxidases (EC 1.11.1.7) include myeloperoxidase (MPO) of neutrophils, eosinophil peroxidase (EC 1.11.1.7), and lactoperoxidase (EC 1.11.1.7) of secretory cells of exocrine glands with anti-inflammatory and antimicrobial activities. They and the plant-derived horseradish peroxidase are able to oxidize analogs of the MPTP neurotoxin that are prevalent in Parkinson's disease, such as 2-methyl-1,2,3,4-tetrahydro-β-carboline, to the pyridinium-like (β-carbolinium) cations. In contrast, MAOs and CYPs cannot stimulate this transformation. They do not perform the toxic conversion of MPTP to MPP+, but are able to convert a metabolite 1-methyl-4-phenyl-2, 3-dihydropyridinium cation (MPDP$^+$) to MPP$^+$ (Herraiz et al., 2007). The heme peroxidases form hypohalous acid from halides, and oxidant products from their substrates such as hypothiocyanous acid, RNS, singlet oxygen, ozone, and phenoxy (from benzene and etoposide catalyzed by MPO in bone marrow cells) and hydroxyl radicals (Davies et al., 2008). Other mammalian heme-containing peroxidases include uterine peroxidase, salivary peroxidase, and prostaglandin H$_1$/H$_2$ synthases. Peroxidases can activate the 4-hydroyx metabolite of the breast cancer medication tamoxifen via a phenoxy radical. Thyroid peroxidase (TPO; EC 1.11.1.8) is a glycoprotein with a heme prosthetic group that is disrupted by goitrogens. A clinically important interaction is the suicidal inactivation of TPO by resourcinol and flavonoids (i.e., isoflavones genistein and daidzein in soy products) in food via formation of phenoxy radicals (O'Brien, 2000).

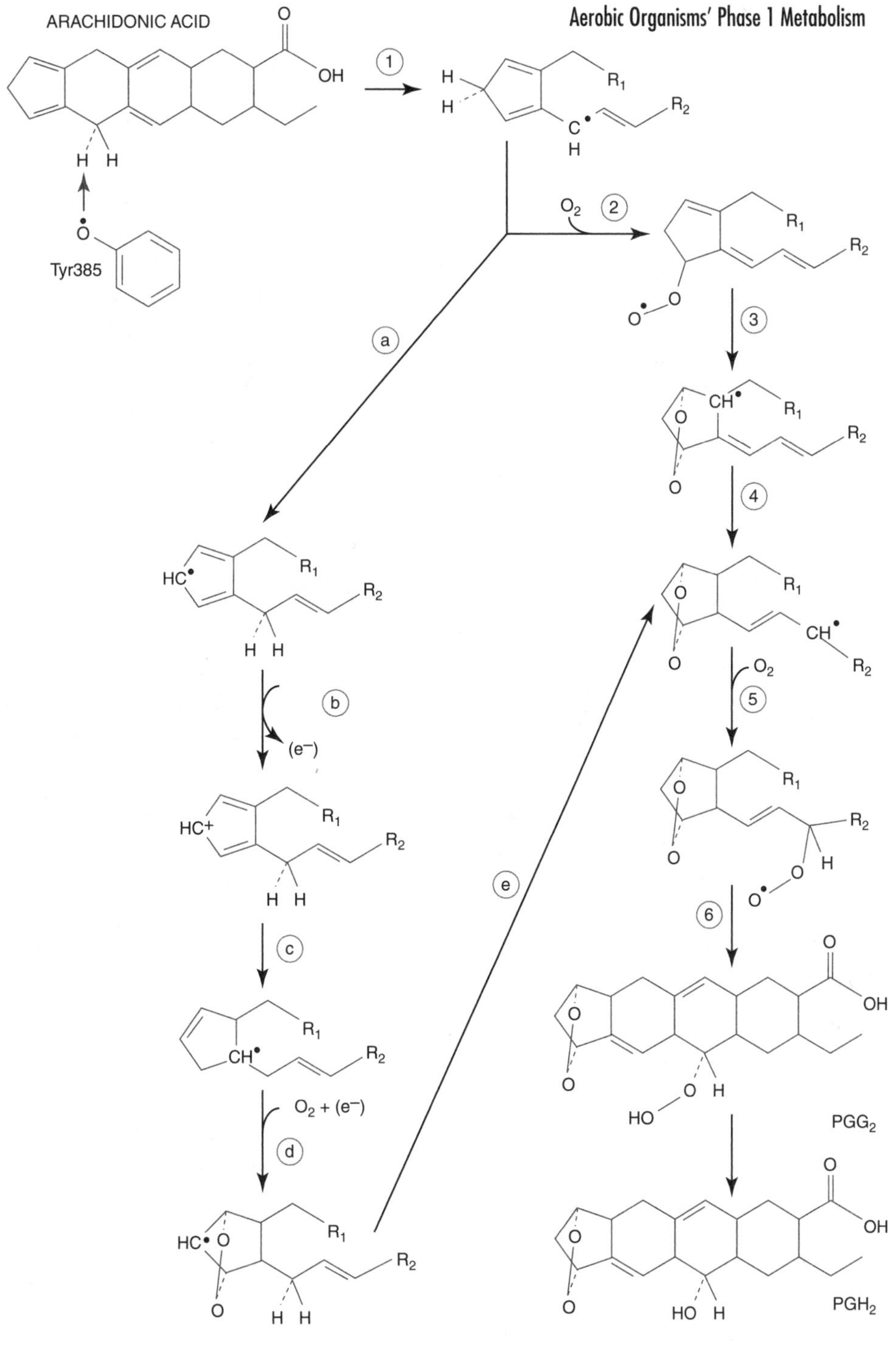

FIGURE 7-9 The Cyclooxygenase Reaction Mechanism

1) A protein-based radical removes the 13-pro-S hydrogen from bound arachidonic acidà C11-C15 delocalized pentadienyl radical. In steps 2-5 this structure reacts with two molecular oxygens to form the bicyclic hydroperoxide, PGG$_2$. This sequence is supported the identification of a tyrosyl radical as catalytic initiator, the X-ray structures of arachidonic acid bound at active site of the protein, EPR spectroscopy detection of a substrate-based pentadienyl radical, and the postulation of a carbocation at C10 to explain the stereospecificity of the cyclooxygenase reaction (introduction of 5 five chiral centers in an achiral molecule). The dashed arrows indicate a sigmatropic H-shift from C10 to the radical present in C13, which yields a C8-C12 delocalized pentadienyl radical . This radical loses an e-àcarbocation that forms a cyclic structure with the proper stereochemistry. After cyclization reduction produces the radical and the reaction continues through the radical-only pathway. The observed pentadienyl radical which includes the C11-C15 carbons instead of C8-C12 does not support the combined radical/carbocation mechanism. However, the observed radical might be a thermodynamically but not kinetically favored artifact. It is postulated that cyclooxygenation is favoed via the radical/carbocation mechanism rather than through the radical-only mechanism. A density-functional (DFT B3LYP/6-311+G(3df,2p)//B3LYP/6-31G*) study on both mechanisms, indicates the correct one.

Antioxidant Enzymes

Catalase

It may seem unusual to discuss antioxidant enzymes among the peroxidases unless the point is to indicate the high rate of ROS or NOS produced by these enzymes. However, catalase (EC 1.11.1.6) is an unusual enzyme in this regard. The typical heme-containing catalases protect Eubacteria, Archaeabacteria, Protista, Fungi, Plantae, and Animalia from the toxic effects of hydrogen peroxide via the reaction $2 H_2O_2 \rightarrow 2H_2O + O_2$. However, a second group of heme-containing catalases has the combined activity of catalases and peroxidases and is not found in plant and animal cells.

Another bacterial enzyme is the (di)manganese catalase (Zamocky et al., 2008). The mammalian enzyme is localized in the matrix of peroxisomes in cells, such as the human liver or neutrophils or rat kidney and neuronal cells. It is also found in the cytosol of liver cells from guinea pigs, Rhesus monkeys, and sheep. In the hearts of transgenic mice that overexpress catalase, the increased injury was found to be due to elevated catalase activity in the cardiomyocytes—more specifically, in the nucleus, peroxisomes, and the sarcoplasm, but not in the mitochondria (Zhou and Kang, 2000).

Se-GSHpx

Because catalase is expressed normally mainly in the peroxisomes, the protection of the cytoplasm falls to another peroxidase, the selenium-dependent glutathione peroxidase (GPx; EC 1.11.1.9). The reaction of these enzymes proceeds as follows: $ROOH + 2GSH \rightarrow ROH + GSSG + H_2O$, where GSH represents the most abundant thiol antioxidant glutathione. Four members of this family of enzymes are found in mammals: the cytosolic (cGPx), plasma (pGPx), GI tract, and phospholipidihydroperoxide forms (PHGPx) (Gross et al., 1995).

GPx was the first identified and is the most abundant form of the 18 mammalian selenoproteins. It is mainly known for its protection against the formation of ROS and resultant apoptosis of injured cells, but actually increases apoptosis in conjunction with peroxynitrite, a potent RNS (Fu et al., 2001). The hydrogen peroxide ROS usually is generated by superoxide first. The enzymes involved in production of ROS vary from reductases for redox cycling compounds like paraquat (methyl viologen) or diquat, to oxidases (e.g., NADPH oxidase; EC 1.6.3.1) that serve as a target for prevention of ROS and cancer (Ushio-Fukai and Nakamura, 2008), to synthase of cell signals (e.g., NO synthase; EC 1.14.13.39).

Superoxide Dismutases

Superoxide dismutases (SOD; EC 1.15.1.1) catalyze the dismutation of superoxide ion to hydrogen peroxide and molecular oxygen. Three isoforms of SOD exist: the copper/zinc SOD1, the manganese SOD2, and the extracellular SOD3.

- SOD1 is an enzyme found in abundance in the cytosol, inner membrane of the mitochondria, nucleus, and peroxisomes of mammalian cells. Its role is to maintain low steady-state concentrations of $O_2^{-\cdot}$. SOD1 deficiency phenotypes lead to amyotrophic lateral sclerosis in humans and can be used as targets of an in vivo assay for determining the role of superoxide in yeast cells (Wallace et al., 2005).
- SOD2 is a mitochondrial enzyme that is inducible by pro-oxidant conditions. It keeps superoxide generated from oxidative phosphorylation in check.
- SOD3 is a secreted enzyme found in organs (blood vessels, heart, lung, kidney, placenta, and extracellular fluids). It is responsible for regulation of blood pressure via controlling superoxide and NO concentrations that alter vascular contraction (Qin et al., 2008).

Iron-containing superoxide reductases (also known as desulfoferrodoxin; EC 1.18.96.1, transferred to EC 1.15.1.2) are not found in humans but provide antioxidant protection in sulfate-reducing anaerobic bacteria.

Peroxiredoxins

Peroxiredoxins (Prx, thioredoxin peroxidases; EC 1.11.1.15) directly reduce hydrogen peroxide and alkyl hydroperoxides. The AhpF component of the alkyl hydroperoxide reductase system of *Salmonella typhimurium*, the mammalian mitochondrial thioredoxin system, and the trypanothione in trypanosomatids have this activity. The thioredoxin system is composed of two oxidoreductases: thioredoxin reductase (TrxR, a FAD-containing NADPH-dependent homodimer protein) and thioredoxin (Trx). The mammalian TrxR can reduce mammalian and bacterial Trx, while the E. *coli* enzymes reduce only bacterial Trx. TrxR also reduces hydrogen peroxides, lipid peroxides, the disulfide moiety of Ellman's thiol reagent (used to determine free thiols) 5,5'-dithio-*bis*(2-nitrobenzoic acid), nitro-blue tetrazolium (used to detect NADPH diaphorase activity), alloxan, L-cystine, vitamin K, antibacterial polypeptide NK-lysin, and protein disulfide isomerases (post-translational folding enzymes of the endoplasmic reticulum). Inhibitors of TrxR include arsenic-containing compounds, gold-containing medications for rheumatoid arthritis, cancer chemotherapeutic agents such as cisplatin, iodo-acetic acid, and 4-vinyl pyridine.

The delayed-type hypersensitivity-provoking chemical known as 1-chloro-2,4-dinitrobenzene (DCNB) is an unusual irreversible inhibitor of TrxR. DCNB turns the enzyme into a superoxide-producing NADPH oxidase via derivatization of the C-terminal selenocysteine and FAD-catalyzed generation of nitro anion radicals. The other portion of the thioredoxin system—that is, reduced thioredoxin—is extremely efficient in the reduction of oxidized disulfides of proteins and peptides and oxidized glutathione.

Three Trx isozymes have been identified:

- Trx-1 is a 12,000-Da enzyme.
- Trx-2 is a mitochondrial enzyme with a 60-amino-acid mitochondrial translocation signal.
- SpTrx, the third variant, is found in spermatozoa.

All three isozymes have the -Cys-Gly-Pro-Cys-active site essential for protein disulfide oxidoreductases, which targets the reduction of ribonucleotide reductase, as well as important transcription factors p53, NF-κB, and AP-1.

The transcription factors appear to be important in induction of Trx by oxidative stress.

Ionizing radiation- and ferric nitrilotriacetate-induced oxidative damage stimulates Trx translocation to the nucleus, where Trx enhances the binding of NF-κB by reduction of an essential cysteine residue. It also enhances binding of AP-1 via Ref-1 in the nucleus. Trx prevents apoptosis by an inhibitory binding to apoptosis signal-regulating kinase 1 (ASK-1) as well as protects against the actions of peroxides. By these mechanisms, Trx is able to prevent oxidative stress–induced cataracts in lens cells and reperfusion-induced arrhythmias in rat heart. It is also found to at elevated levels in the plasma of human patients with AIDS, hepatocellular carcinoma, rheumatoid arthritis, and Sjögren's syndrome (Nordberg and Arnér, 2001).

The regulation of cytoprotective enzymes against environmental toxicants and their reactive metabolites is performed by NF-E$_2$-related factor (Nrf2). Nrf2 induces expression of a number of enzymes responsible for the synthesis of the antioxidant peptide GSH, direct-acting antioxidants, and reducing equivalents. Agents that increase Nrf2 induce cysteine ligase, glucose-6-phosphate dehydrogenase, heme oxygenase-1, malic enzyme, and UDP-glucose dehydrogenase. Nrf2 also regulates the basal expression of aldehyde dehydrogenase 1A1, carbonyl reductase, epoxide hydrolase, ferritin light chain subunit 1, glutathione peroxidase, glutathione-S-transferases (α4, μ1, and μ5), NADPH-quinone oxidoreductase, and UDP gluronosyltransferases 2B5 and 1A6 (Osburn and Kensler, 2008).

Molybdoenzyme Oxidases/Hydrolases

Cytosolic aldehyde oxidase (EC 1.2.3.1) and xanthine oxidase (EC 1.1.3.22) are non-CYP enzymes that oxidize substrates such as *N*-heterocyclic compounds and aldehydes and generate ROS via the reaction $RH + H_2O \rightarrow ROH + 2e^- + 2H^+$. Aldehyde oxidase (AO) is primarily found in liver cells, while xanthine oxidase (XO) predominates in the lactating mammary gland and is found in cow's milk.

These enzymes can have either positive or negative consequences, depending on the substrate and the cell. Both are known for the detoxication of nitrogen-containing heterocyclic chemicals. AO works most effectively on aromatic chemicals with two fused six-member rings, such as in the catalysis of phthalazine to 1-hydroxyphthalazine. XO performs this reaction less well, but is able to oxidize an inhibitor of AO, 3-hydroxy4-methoxybenzaldehyde (isovanillin; Panoutsopoulos and Beedham, 2004). Conversely, AO's conversion of 1-methyl-4-phenyl-1,2,3,6-tetrahydropyridine (MPTP) to the MPTP lactam (1-methyl-4-phenyl-5, 6-dihydro-2-pyridone) avoids the formation of the toxic 1-methyl-4-phenylpyridinium (MPP⁺) metabolite of mitochondrial MAO-B in liver cells (Yoshihara and Shigeru Ohta, 1998). The metabolism of ethanol also yields NADH and acetaldehyde, both of which are substrates for aldehyde oxidase. The generation of $O_2{}^{\cdot-}$ occurs via both reactions, as does peroxidation of membrane lipids (Mira et al., 1995). These enzymes are also involved in damage done to liver cells by activation of compounds such as $CHCl_3$, CCl_4, and thioacetamide; their conversion to free radicals is performed by these molybdenum iron–sulfur flavin hydroxylases, as indicated by decreased biochemical and oxidant stress markers in the presence of their common inhibitor, sodium tungstate (Ali et al., 2008).

Metabolism of Alcohols: Dehydrogenases and Oxidases

Alcohols appear to be some of the best-tolerated substances in the body, although the same is not true of some of their metabolites. Ethyl alcohol has an extremely high metabolism rate for a xenobiotic, averaging 20–25 mg in a nonalcoholic individual and even higher in an alcoholic individual. During its metabolism, ethanol is converted by microsomal CYP2E1, cytosolic alcohol dehydrogenase (EC 1.1.1.1), and the peroxisome catalase (EC 1.11.1.6) system to acetaldehyde. Alcohol dehydrogenase (ADH) is the major enzyme in the conversion of ethanol and is a NAD-dependent enzyme:

$$CH_3CH_2OH + NAD^+ \rightarrow$$
$$CH_3CHO + NADH + H^+$$

This reaction generates the more toxic and aversive aldehyde product in humans, who consume ethanol for its solvent euphoric effects on the CNS.

Polymorphisms of this enzyme have been noted. Persons who have the *ADH2*2* and *ADH3*1* alleles encode for the high-activity ADH isoform. The cytosolic and mitochondrial aldehyde dehydrogenase forms (EC 1.2.1.3), ALDH1 and ALDH2, respectively, convert acetaldehyde to the nutrient acetic acid, which can enter the Krebs cycle via acetylCoA:

$$RCHO + NAD(P)^+ + H_2O \leftrightarrow$$
$$RCOOH + NAD(P)H + H^+$$

The *ALDH2*2* allele encodes for a low-activity isoform that leaves more acetaldehyde unconverted over time. Both enzymes are inducible by drinking ethanol. Collectively, East Asians are more likely to have the *ADH2*2* and *ALDH2*2* alleles, which lead to more acetaldehyde or increased toxicity (Chen et al., 1999); as a consequence, these individuals are less likely to become alcoholic due to the more aversive reactions they experience after consuming alcohol.

For other alcohols, the aldehyde product created during metabolism is the problem. Methanol is converted to a formaldehyde product, which causes crystallization in brain cells and death at high concentrations. Aldehyde dehydrogenase leads to a formic acid product, which is metabolized to folic acid, then to folinic acid, and ultimately to carbon dioxide and water. Ethanol is the known antidote to methanol poisoning, as it would compete for alcohol dehydrogenase with methanol.

Isopropyl alcohol is converted to acetone by ADH. Ethylene glycol (antifreeze additive) is metabolized by ADH into glycoaldehyde and rapidly transformed into glycolic acid (which causes severe acidosis when present at high concentrations) by ALDH. The conversion to glyoxylic acid is the rate-limiting step in this pathway. Glycolic acid is converted to either oxalic acid, glycine (pyridoxine as cofactor), or α-hydroxy-β-keoadipate (thiamine as cofactor) (Levine, 2008). The oxalic acid chelates with calcium to form calcium oxalate monohydrate crystals, which at high concentrations can be lethal to renal proximal tubule cells due to their inhibition of mitochondrial respiration (Pomara et al., 2008).

Another important difference in ADH is its species specificity. The medium-chain zinc enzymes constitute one family; they are the versions usually found in prokaryotes and eukaryotes, including liver or yeast enzymes, whereas the short-chain enzymes are found mainly in insects. *Drosophila* has been found to contain a medium-chain enzyme similar to the evolutionarily conserved class III form found in humans. The familiar liver enzyme for ADH is a class I form and has α, β, and γ subunits, while class III includes the glutathione-dependent formaldehyde dehydrogenase with the χ subunit. Class IV includes the stomach enzyme, which has a σ subunit. Classes II (liver π subunit), V, and VI are less studied but distinct from one another. Gene duplications in vertebrate evolution led to I/III (early) and IV/I duplications. Class I is considered the most variable, whereas class III appears to be most constant (Danielsson et al., 1994).

Carbonyl Reductases and Hydroxysteroid Dehydrogenases: Reduction

Carbonyl reduction of aldehydes, ketones, and quinones to their hydroxy metabolites involve two superfamilies: the aldo-keto reductases (AKR) and the short-chain dehydrogenases/reductases (SDR).

Aldehyde reductase (EC 1.1.1.2) and aldose reductase (EC 1.1.1.21) belong to the AKR superfamily, while carbonyl reductase (EC 1.1.1.184) belongs to the SDR protein superfamily. The members of the aldehyde reductase AKR family are alcohols: NADP$^+$-oxidoreductase, high-K_m aldehyde reductase, mevaldate reductase, daunorubicin (pH 8.5) reductase, hexonate dehydrogenase, lactaldehyde reductase, glucuronate reductase, and aluminum resistance gene protein 1 (ALR 1). Aldose reductase AKR family members form alditols: NADP$^+$-oxidoreductase, low-K_m aldehyde reductase, and ALR 2. Carbonyl reductase SDR family members are NADPH: secondary-alcohol oxidoreductase, prostaglandin 9-ketoreductase, daunorubicin (pH 6.0) reductase, and ALR 3. The pluripotent hydroxysteroid dehydrogenases (HSDs) are either AKR1C or SDR (several forms of dihydrodiol dehydrogenases and several HSDs are distinguished

based on the carbon atom involved in catalysis). The AKR 1–14 superfamily of enzymes (AKR 1–7 are mammalian, while AKR 2–5 and 8–14 are found in bacteria, plants, and yeast) are monomeric (α/β)8-barrel proteins that are approximately 320 amino acids in length and lack a Rossmann fold motif. The active sites of AKRs contain the amino acids tyrosine, histidine, aspartic acid, and lysine.

The SDR superfamily consists of enzymes that are 250–350 amino acids in length. The length is used to subdivide this superfamily in two large subfamilies, which are then further subdivided into seven classical SDRs and three extended SDRs. SDRs are soluble or membrane-bound homodimeric or homotetrameric proteins that function independently of metal cofactors. NAD(H) or NADP(H) binds to SDRs at a βαβ motif of a Rossmann fold, similar to other dehydrogenases.

The reactions catalyzed by AKR and SDR enzymes are considered mainly detoxication steps, as the groups reduced are reactive moieties. HSDs are pyridine nucleotide-dependent oxidoreductases that catalyze the interconversion of secondary alcohols and ketones. Biogenic amines, steroids and other hormones, prostaglandins, lipid peroxidation products (acrolein, 4-hydroxynonenal, 4-oxononenal, and malondialdehyde), aldehydes from fruits, ethanol and its acetaldehyde metabolite, and a variety of medications are reduced by these enzymes to less toxic substances. Conversely, daunorubicin and doxorubicin are activated by this reaction. It appears as if the physiological role of HSDs is steroid metabolism, as might be expected from this group's name.

Carbonyl reductases appear to have an important protective effect by detoxifying quinones (two-electron reduction to hydroquinone, which can be conjugated to glucuronide or sulfate) , aflatoxin B$_1$, aldophosphamide, tripeptidyl aldehydes, chordecone, and tobacco-specific nitrosamine 4-(methylnitrosamino)-1-(3-pyridyl)-1-butanone (NNK). NNK is considered to be the major carcinogen in tobacco smoke; it is activated by CYPs via hydroxylation of the carbons adjacent to the *N*-nitroso group or detoxication via reduction of the ketone by 11β-HSD1,

CBR1, AKR 1C1, AKR 1C2, and AKR 1C4 to the alcohol. These reductases also appear to protect brain cells against ROS, especially regarding the formation of active aldehydes during lipid peroxidation including 4-oxonon-2-enal. The reduction of 1,4-naphquinones and their glutathione conjugates has the opposite effect—that is, it induces redox cycling and generation of ROS via auto-oxidation. Additionally, generation of the hydroxy compound is not always a less toxic outcome, as indicated by the formation of cataracts from the conversion of naphthalene dihydrodiol to 1,2-dihydroxynaphthalene (Lou et al., 1996).

Carbonyl-reducing enzymes have been described in plants, bacteria, yeast, fish, insects, and mammals. Human cells that contain these reductases are found in liver, lung, heart, kidney, brain, ovary, and adrenal cells.

While carbonyl reductase and NAD(P)H: quinone oxidoreductase (formerly DT-diaphorase) offer protection to cells in the cytosol, 11β-HSD1 prevents the endoplasmic reticulum from semi-quinone oxygen radical formation via hydroquinone generation. Carbonyl reduction by CBR1, AKR 1A1, AKR 1B1, and AKR 1C2 also appears to play a role in the development of cancer cells' resistance to anthracyclines, such as through the conversion of duanorubicin to daunorubicinol (Hoffmann and Maser, 2007). However, NAD(P)H: quinone oxidoreductase can also become bioactivated by two-electron reduction of quinodal medications and other aromatic nitro compounds to aromatic hydroxyl amines (Anusevicius et al., 2002).

Glutathione Reductases

Earlier in this chapter, GPx was identified as an important antioxidant reductase. The oxidized glutathione (GSSG) formed from this reaction or other glutathione-dependent reactions, such as the conjugation by glutathione (to be discussed later in terms of phase 2 metabolism), is reduced to 2GSH by glutathione reductase (GR; EC 1.6.4.2). *Escherichia coli*, *Drosophila melanogaster* (has no GR), *Homo sapiens*, and *Plasmodium falciparum* reduce GSSG by thioredoxins as well. Glutaredoxins (Grx) are similar to thioredoxins, with the notable difference that Grx can be reduced by GSH and, in turn, reduce GSH mixed-protein disulfides created by oxidative stress (Nordberg and Arnér, 2001).

NADPH Cytochrome P450 Reductase and Redox Cycling

The NADPH cytochrome P450 reductase (CYPOR) transfers electrons not only to CYPs, but also to heme oxygenase, cytochrome b_5, squalene monooxygenase, 7-dehydrocholesterol reductase, and the fatty acid elongase. It has been characterized in organisms ranging from mammals to mosquitos to *E. coli*, where it is known by its classical designation of NADPH-cytochrome *c* oxidoreductase (Sarapusit et al., 2008). This enzyme appears to be primarily responsible for the generation of ROS, especially superoxide, from the reduction of redox cycling compounds, such as the bipyridylium herbicides paraquat (1,1'-dimethyl-4,4'-bipyridyl) and diquat (N,N'-ethylene,1,1'-bipyridyl), the antibiotic nitrofurantoin (*N*-[5-amino-2-furfurylidene)-1-amino hydantoin; used to treat urinary tract infections), and a toxicological probe to induce oxidative stress menadione (2-methyl-1,4-naphthquinone). Diquat and menadione have higher affinities for CYPOR, as indicated by the K_m for CYPOR from rat lung and liver cells, than do paraquat and nitrofurantoin; they also have an order of magnitude higher consumption of oxygen and NADPH. Only the uptake differences account for the increased pulmonary cell toxicity of paraquat compared with the other compounds (Adam et al., 1990). Other oxidoreductases generate redox cycling (as indicated by other examples in this chapter), but CYPOR is given special consideration in this section because it has been clearly linked to numerous accounts of human clinical and animal toxicity in published studies.

Epoxide Hydrolases

It is fitting to end the discussion of the oxidoreductases with the beginning of the hydrolases, especially epoxide hydrolases (EC 3.3.2.3). Every aerobic organism has to live with the paradox of coordinating oxygen as its terminal electron acceptor for energy functions and metabolism, while being prepared to handle the inevitable production of reactive oxygen species. Epoxides are short-lived, very unstable, reactive intermediates that may proceed to an oxygen radical that will form adducts, as occurs via P450 metabolism of benzene or vinyl chloride. Forming the phenol in the case of benzene or a diol is preferred for oxidant protection and provides for greater water solubility. Epoxide hydrolases are a group of α/β hydrolases that catalyze the formation of a dihydrodiol from oxides (oxirane rings) of physiological substrates such epoxyeicosatrienoic acids (Inceoglu et al., 2007) or from xenobiotics. The aspartate group of the active site of these hydrolases performs a nucleophilic attack on the ring forming an ester, which is hydrolyzed to the diol product.

Microsomal epoxide hydrolases (mEH) and soluble or cytosolic forms (sEH) of the enzyme play a role in toxicity, although the microsomal form of the enzyme has been studied more intensively owing to its role in the bioactivation of compounds such as PAHs to the highly reactive diol-epoxides in conjunction with the oxidation by CYPs. Mice lacking the mEH gene (created by genetic engineering) produce smaller quantities of the 3,4-diol metabolite of 7,12-dimethylbenzanthracene (DMBA) and, therefore, succumb less to its toxicity or its carcinogenicity. Human colon cells appear to have less of a risk of developing adenomas with exon 3 (Tyr113His substitution) or exon 4 (His139Arg substitution) polymorphisms, while lung cancers are less likely to occur when exon3 polymorphism is present (Shimada, 2006).

Based on these two genotypes, four phenotypes for epoxide hydrolase activity have been identified: fast, normal, slow, and very slow. In chronic obstructive pulmonary disease (COPD), the polymorphisms have been found to lead to increased disease incidence associated with the 113 mutant homozygote in Asians but not in Caucasian populations. The slow activity phenotype increased COPD incidence, whereas the very slow activity phenotype increased the disease incidence only in Caucasians. The fast activity phenotype protected only the Asian population, so the relationship is a complex one (Hu et al., 2008).

The sEH enzymes are primarily responsible for converting epoxyeicosatrienoic acids (EETs) formed from arachidonic acid by P450 epoxygenase. The EETs are antihypertensive eicosanoids, whereas the diol metabolites are not. Disruption of the sEH gene in male mice or inhibition of this enzyme decreases blood pressure (Fang, 2006). The sEHs also exhibit polymorphisms. For example, increased risk of cerebral vascular accident (ischemic stroke) and coronary artery disease are noted with single nucleotide differences, while kidney grafts are protected by a variant allele (Lee et al., 2008).

Carboxylesterases: Hydrolysis

As the examination of the esterases moves further toward carboxylesterases (CEs; EC 3.1.1.1) and the A (mammalian paraoxonase or aryl esterase; EC 3.1.8.1 [Sorenson et al., 1995]), B (includes acetylcholinesterase and butyrylcholinesterase), and C esterases (acetyl esterases), the catalytic speed of these enzymes becomes important, because neurotoxic neurotransmitters and toxicants may reversibly or irreversibly inhibit these enzymes. The carboxylesterases are important in the hydrolysis of pyrethroid insecticides, plasticizers such as the phthalate esters, chemotherapeutic prodrugs such as irinotecan, angiotensin-converting enzyme inhibitors, and narcotics such as the esterified "caines" and opioids in human cells. CEs are part of the α,β-serine hydrolase multigene family, which act inefficiently on esters, amides, and thioesters.

Two CE isoforms predominate in high amounts in the human liver: hCE1 (CES1) and hCE2 (CES2). The hCE2 form appears to be the only isoform found in the small intestinal enterocytes, and may represent a metabolic barrier to xenobiotic exposure. The hCE1 form appears to be the only form that catalyzes the hydrolysis of the 2S, αS-isomer of the active ingredient in the insecticide esfenvalerate. In contrast, hCE2 appears to have a strong preference for activity with the (R)-configuration at the second carbon position of fenvalerate regardless of the α-carbon configuration. hCE1 hydrolyzes (αS)-enantiomers of the same compound three times faster than the (αR)-enantiomers, independent of the configuration at position 2. This difference highlights the different roles of both enzymes in structure–activity relationships and the possibilities for toxicity from a given compound or sets of compounds with related structures if either isozyme is deficient (Nishi et al., 2006).

Species differences are extremely important with CEs. For example, rat and mice models of human exposure express high levels of CEs in their plasma, whereas no detectable level of the enzyme is found in human plasma (Crow et al., 2007). The rat has many isoforms of CEs, three of which (ES10, ES4, and ES3) appear to account for 95% of the hydrolysis activity of these enzymes (Sanghani et al., 2002). Rat CEs are inducible by chemicals that also induce the CYPs, such as phenobarbital, aminopyrine, and peroxisome proliferators such as clofibrate. CES1 is inhibited by oxons formed by oxidation of organophosphate pesticides such as parathion and the macrophage reverse cholesterol transport (Crow et al., 2008). The mouse CES2 is similarly subject to inhibition and appears to play a larger role in the metabolism of lipids (Furihata et al., 2006).

Amidases and Esterases: Hydrolysis

The enzymes of these pathways became of interest as neurotoxic insecticides and biological warfare agents were developed. Many serine hydroxylases are affected by organophosphorus compounds, partially explaining the lethality of these compounds or their metabolism and resistance by selected organisms. Lysis of the ester linkage is usually reversible, so these enzymes can also function to synthesize esters. At least three classical categories of esterases exist that cleave esters of alcohols—namely, mineral acids, organic acids, and phenols. Those compounds that cleave aryl esters have been labeled as A-type esterases. Cleavage by carboxylesterases is performed by B-type esterases. As it is often desirable to separate the cholinesterases from the "true" carboxylesterases, this section reviews the cholinesterases. The C-type esterases are acetyl esterases (Barbier et al., 2000). Most of the work on insecticides has focused on types A and B.

A human esterase D has also been isolated. This S-formylglutathione hydrolase is found in most human tissues has major carboxylesterase activity in the human liver cytosol. It catalyzes the hydrolysis of p-nitrophenyl acetate and 4-methylumbelliferyl acetate, is inducible by methylmethane sulfonate or phenobarbital, and is overexpressed in at least one breast cancer cell line (Legler et al., 2008).

Esterases have bound and soluble forms in rat brain. The A-type esterases are localized in droplets associated with lysosomal structures. The B-type esterases are located primarily in the neuron's cytoplasm (Bernsohn et al., 1966).

Another way of categorizing the effects of hydrolases is to differentiate between lipases (triacylglycerol hydrolases; EC 3.1.1.1) and the "true" esterases (carboxyl ester hydrolases; EC 3.1.1.3). Lipases require a minimum substrate concentration before high activity is achieved, while esterases conform strictly to Michaelis–Menten kinetics (Aurilia et al., 2008). Their ability to metabolize organophosphates serves as a good way to differentiate them toxicologically. Organophosphates (OPs) inhibit a variety of esterases with different functions such as cholinesterases, including both acetylcholinesterase (AChE; EC 3.1.1.7), which is involved in neurotransmission and neurotoxicity, and butyrylcholinesterase (BChE; EC. 3.1.1.8), which is involved in detoxication, lipid metabolism, peptidases, blood clotting enzymes, digestive proteases, and a variety of enzymes that play roles in nicotinamide synthesis, blood pressure regulation, immunity, cancer cell function or dysfunction, and cell surface recognition. OPs also inhibit the detoxifying carboxylesterases and interact with anandamide (cannabinoid) and muscarinic (cholinergic) neurotransmitter receptors (Casida and Quistad, 2005). Resistance to these substances occurs either via induction of these enzymes or through species differences in the ability of esterases to hydrolyze the compound to a less neurotoxic metabolite, as in the case of a malathion- and permethrin-resistant strain of *Pediculus capitis*, the head louse (Gao et al., 2006).

The A-type esterases (EC 3.1.1.2) have been renamed paraoxonases, as they confer to mammals a distinctly lower toxicity to the P450 metabolite of parathion, paraoxon, through hydrolysis of paraoxon. Human paraoxonase-1

(PON1; EC 3.1.8.1) is a versatile enzyme that functions primarily as a lactonase but also has activities of a phosphotriesterase, arylesterase, and lactonase, as well as antioxidative, phospholipid-binding, and anti-atherogenic properties. Human PON1 associates with and is provided with increased heat stability via human phosphate-binding protein. It is usually found on high-density lipoprotein (HDL) particles (Rochu et al., 2007), but is also found in liver microsomes. A single enzyme in human serum has both paraoxonase and arylesterase activity (Gan et al., 1991). Although PON enzymes protect best against paraoxon, the parent compound paraoxon is first—and best—protected by direct hydrolysis by carboxylesterases, followed by paraoxonases. This relationship is indicated by the increased sensitivity of neonatal and juvenile rats, which have low activities of these enzymes compared with adults (Karanth and Pope, 2000).

Other isozymes of PON in the human are PON2 (distributed in multiple tissues) and PON 3 (found in liver and kidney microsomes and serum). Serum PON1 is also polymorphic in humans, as its Arg192 isoform (PON1R192) has a high activity to paraoxon hydrolysis, while the Gln192 isozyme (PON1Q192) has low activity for this toxic metabolite. The activity to diazonon, soman, and particularly sarin is reversed, with the PON1Q192 form having the highest activity (Furlong et al., 2000).

Type B esterases are the focus of the toxic action of organophosphates. In humans, acetylcholinesterase is found both centrally (where it is the predominate cholinesterase) and peripherally in the nervous system, including in autonomic and motor nerves. In contrast, in fish it is found primarily in the brain and muscle (Huang et al., 1997), and in insects it is an enzyme of the central nervous system with some peripheral nerve activity, as is the case in the tick (Carson et al., 1987). In fish and humans, butyrylcholinesterase is a nonspecific choline esterase sometimes considered to be plasma cholinesterase or pseudocholinesterase and is a detoxifying enzyme found in the blood serum, pancreas, liver, and central nervous system. It has activity toward acetylcholine, but is named for its activity in hydrolyzing the larger butyrylcholine.

AChE's activity is clearer, but its localization leads to some interesting problems. Pyridostigmine bromide, a drug used to protect Gulf War soldiers against the irreversible AChE inhibition by soman, inhibits both AChE and BChE peripherally. It prevents soman from binding to the peripheral AChE by carbamylation, but does not pass through the blood–brain barrier and thereby protect the central nervous system. Also, its binding to both enzymes presents a problem, as it keeps lipophilic compounds from being metabolized and becoming more available for binding to acetylcholinesterases in the brain. Huperzine A provides an alternative mechanism for protecting AChE: It provides for specific inhibition of red blood cell AChE without affecting serum BChE (Haigh et al., 2008). The BChE gene has 65 identified variants and is responsible for metabolism of the muscle relaxants succinylcholine and mivacurium, as well as the narcotic cocaine (Mikami et al., 2008). AChE inhibitors that are milder than those used for warfare purposes are used in the treatment of Alzheimer's disease or an antidote to overdose with the cholinergic muscarinic antagonist atropine, which is used in war as an antidote to nerve agent exposure.

Species differences are noted in AChE inhibition. For example, rivastigmine, which is used to treat Alzheimer's disease, inhibits human AChE 1000-fold faster than the first AChE isolated, the AChE of *Torpedo californica*. A serine protease inhibitor phenylmethylsulfonyl fluoride (PMSF) inhibits mammalian AChE, but not electric eel or goldfish AChE. However, if just one methylene group is removed from PMSF to form benzenesulfonyl fluoride, then inhibition of *Torpedo* and mouse enzymes occurs (Silman and Sussman, 2008). Cholinesterase genes have three types of exons encoding for C-terminal domains, referred to as H (AChE$_H$) or hydrophobic, T (AChE$_T$) or tailed, and S (AChE$_S$) or soluble or snake. There is also a read-through (R) transcript from *Torpedo* and mammals, known as AChE$_R$. Invertebrates like *Drosophila* may contain one cholinesterase gene, whereas *Culex* has two genes. *Caenorhabditis* has four genes, but each codes for just one C-terminal domain. Insects and prochordate amphioxus produce only type H cholinesterases, while *Caenorhabditis* produces type T from the major *ace-1* gene and type H from the less expressed *ace-2* gene, with minor *ace-3* and *ace-4* gene production also occurring.

Tissue distributions of AChEs also vary based on species. AChE$_H$ is used by *Drosophila* in its nervous system and by *Torpedo* in its muscles. AChE$_T$ appears to be the only type used by mammals in these tissues.

The cholinesterases can be further grouped based on whether they stay as monomers or group up through triple tetramers, and how that behavior changes their solubility. Both forms are found in human muscle, the brain contains the G4 tetramer, and the red blood cells contain the dimer. As variants in AChE may lead to a nonfunctional organism based on this cholinesterase's key role in neurotransmission in the central nervous system, the importance of these forms may simply reflect whether they are membrane associated (Massoulié et al., 1998).

Strangely, acetylcholinesterase and butyrylcholinesterase are both mediators of inflammatory reactions. Acetylcholine is an anti-inflammatory compound that works via nicotinic receptors. Nicotine is the model agonist for this receptor and has anti-inflammatory action. It appears as if the anti-inflammatory action of nicotinic receptors signals the efferent vagus nerve to release acetylcholine peripherally onto nicotinic receptors of macrophages. This initiates NF-κB activation in the macrophages, leading to preservation of high mobility group box 1 (HMGB1) nuclear localization and reduced production of inflammatory cytokines (Das, 2007). Thus these enzymes mediate one form of toxicity, which is more chronic in nature, while preventing acute neurotoxicity.

Alkaline Phosphatases: Hydrolysis

Alkaline phosphatases (APs or ALPs or ALKPs or AKPs; EC 3.1.3.1) are part of large superfamily of enzymes that include nucleotide pyrophosphatase/phosphodiesterase and are present in cells from organisms ranging from bacteria to humans. APs are homodimeric proteins with serine and three metal ions (two Zn^{2+} ions and one Mg^{2+} ion) in their active sites. They hydrolyze esters of phosphoric acid and, in the

presence of a high concentration of phosphate acceptors, catalyze transphosphorylation. Mammalian APs have higher specific activities, K_m, more alkaline pH, and lower heat stability than their bacterial counterparts. The mammalian enzymes are also membrane bound and uncompetitively inhibited by peptides and amino acids.

Bone mineralization is accomplished by the tissue nonspecific human *ALPL* and the mouse *Akp2* isozymes. Intestinal/fat absorption appears to be the role of the human *ALPI* and murine *Akp3*. Human placental and mouse embryonic ALP isoforms are *ALPP* and *Akp5*, respectively. *ALPP* appears to be associated with tumors as well. Human *ALPP2* is found in testes and testicular cancer, as well as malignant trophoblasts. Based on the homology, the AP superfamily also contains the cofactor-independent phosphoglycerate mutase (iPGM; EC 5.4.2.1) and phosphopentomutases (EC 5.4.2.7; Millán, 2006).

ALPs appear to be sensitive to heavy metal poisoning, which may inhibit the enzyme and change the pattern of isozymes. For example, this effect has been demonstrated with cadmium in gypsy moth larvae and copper in gastropod hemolymph phosphatase (Vlahović et al., 2009). ALPs appear to be decreased by toxic herbicide concentrations of heptachlor in amphibians exposed at stages of development ranging from tadpole to complete metamorphosis, indicating a decrease in skin transport vital to the function of these organisms (Fenoglio et al., 2009). Elevations in serum alkaline phosphatase have also been used extensively as a measure of liver cell damage by compounds such as carbon tetrachloride.

The field of prodrugs tries to use ALPs to advantage, based on the fact that the phosphate form of the prodrug is more water soluble. Thus such compounds are extensively used as IV promedications. ALPs then cleave the drug free from the phosphate. However, there is usually the need for a spacer molecule to aid the enzymes in navigating around the bond, such as an oxymethyl or ethyldioxy group. The oxymethyl is liberated as the genotoxic formaldehyde, while the ethyldioxy is cleaved off as acetaldehyde, the less toxic product that appears to be the metabolite of ethanol responsible for liver cirrhosis. The design of the prodrug is important as to limit toxicity of undesirable metabolites (Kumpulainen et al., 2008).

Peptidases

Peptidases (serine proteases; EC 3.1.14.x) may limit the ability of peptides to be injected into the bloodstream and become available to cells. They also regulate other molecules that have important physiological functions. For example, amino boronic dipeptides inhibit dipeptidyl peptidases and accelerate neutrophil and erythrocyte regeneration in mouse models of neutropenia and acute anemia (Jones et al., 2003). Targeting of these enzymes, cell adhesion molecules, and receptors involved in endocytosis of endothelial cells can also aid in the delivery of medications to treat acute vascular cell disorders such as ischemia, oxidative stress, inflammation, and clot formation (Simone et al., 2009).

Aerobic Organisms' Phase 2 Metabolism: Conjugation

Acetylation of Hydrazines and Arylamines

A key mechanism for detoxication of hydrazines and arylamines is acetylation. This is accomplished by cytosolic isozymes of N-acetyltransferase (NAT; EC 2.3.1.x), which have a dramatically different and clinically relevant toxicity profile. Both a slow acetylator gene and a rapid acetylator gene have been identified.

Those organisms with two copies (homozygous) for the slow acetylator gene show peripheral neurotoxicity and hepatotoxicity to pyridine-4-carboxy hydrazide, which also known as the antituberculosis medication isoniazid (Preziosi, 2007). The N-acetylated compound is less toxic for arylamines. However, O-acetylation following oxidation of the arylamine to N-hydroxyarylamine by cytochrome P450 leads to an acetoxy arylamine that spontaneously converts to an arylnitrenium ion, a highly reactive species that is mutagenic/carcinogenic (Hein et al., 1992).

Intermediate and rapid acetylators are combined into a rapid acetylator group whose members are heterozygous or homozygous for the rapid N-acetyltransferase gene. This pattern has been discovered in both humans and mice. In the mouse, the gene for N-acetyltransferase is closely linked to esterase-1 on chromosome 8 (Weber, 1990). The rat has three NATs (1–3); rat NAT1 and NAT2 are expressed mainly in the colon, while NAT3 is a minor contributor to acetylation. The rat liver shows a developmental increase in NAT1, but not NAT2. NAT2 in the colon increases dramatically following birth, although the same is not true for NAT1. Polymorphisms of NAT2 are used to model similar changes in the human (Barker et al., 2008).

Acyl-CoA Amino Acid N-Acyl and Methyl Transferases

The acyltransferases cover a broad group of enzymes, including 1-acylglycerophosphocholine O-acyltransferase, choline O-acetyltransferase, 3-oxoacyl-(acyl-carrier protein) synthase, diacylglycerol O-acyltransferase, 5-aminolevulinic acid synthase, dihydrolipoamide S-acetyltransferase, acetyl-CoA C-acetyltransferase, dihydrolipoamide S-succinyltransferase, acetyl-CoA C-acyltransferase, glycerol-3-phosphate O-acyltransferase, arylamine N-acetyltransferase, histone acetyltransferase, carnitine O-acetyltransferase, phosphate acetyltransferase, carnitine O-palmitoyltransferase, phosphatidylcholine-sterol O-acyltransferase, chloramphenicol O-acetyltransferase, and sterol O-acyltransferase. Many of the acyltransferases are involved in the synthesis of glycerophospholipids (Shindou, 2009). Since the acetyltransferases important to detoxication and activation have already been covered in this chapter, the conjugation to amino acids will be described in this section, along with the conjugation of a compound to a methyl group.

The amino acid conjugation in humans is mainly a function of the mitochondria, so its functions are limited. Prior to formation of the conjugate, which is usually glycine, a carboxylic acid group of the xenobiotic must first form an acyl-CoA thioester. However, this does not always mean that the resulting compound is a conjugate to an amino acid. The formation of an acyl-CoA thioester does interfere with mitochondrial function if the glycine conjugate is not made. In this respect, this process represents a mitochondrial detoxication pathway (Knights et al., 2007). Interestingly, the bile acids form glycine conjugates only due to bacterial enzymes, but conjugate to the amino acid taurine in mammals. As indicated in the earlier discussion of the N-acetyltransferases, the conjugation of an N-hydroxy aromatic amine will result in a nitrenium (or carbonium) ion, no matter what the form of the acyl group (acetyl or amino acid). This transfer is accomplished by cytosolic tRNA synthetases (EC 6.1.1.x; Kato et al., 1983).

The S-adenosylmethionine (SAM)-dependent methyl transferases (EC 2.1.1.x) are important bacterial enzymes that confer resistance to a number of substances, ranging from heavy metals to aminoglycoside antibiotics (Savic et al., 2008). Methylation of DNA is disrupted by arsenic, which interferes with SAM formation, so there are toxic factors that change the ability of the cell to utilize or synthesize the cofactor needed for conjugation (Coppin et al., 2008). Enzymes catalyze the N-methylation, O-methylation, and S-methylation reactions. Cytosolic N-methylations are performed on azaheterocyclics. This methylation in the brain for beta-carbolines may be responsible for some of the toxic products that produce Parkinson's disease, such as the neurotoxic 2,9-di-[N, N']-methylated beta-carbolinium cations (Matsubara, 1998). Catechol-O-methyltransferase found in the cytosol and microsomes deactivates genotoxic estrogens into easily excreted methyl ethers, but the link between polymorphisms in this gene and breast cancer has not been clearly demonstrated (Wedrén et al., 2003). Pheno-O-methyltransferase is a microsomal enzyme that methylates phenols, but is important in fungi for its ability to detoxify chlorinated phenols and in the use of a chlorinated compound such as methyl chloride to form veratryl alcohol and methyl benzoate (Coulter et al., 1993).

Thiopurine methyltransferse (TMPT; EC 2.1.1.67) detoxifies 6-mercaptopurine and 6-thioguanine. Polymorphisms in this gene have led to near-fatal hematological reactions to clinically relevant doses and concentrations of these compounds (McLeod et al., 2000). Other S-methylation reactions through TMPT involve other aromatic and heterocyclic sulfhydryl compounds. Inhibitors of TMPT include the metabolite salicylic acid, which is produced after a therapeutic dose of aspirin, and sulfasalazine, an anti-inflammatory medication that is metabolized to 5-aminosalicylic acid (5ASA) and sulfapyridine by bacteria in the colon. Furosemide, a loop diuretic, when given with sulfasalazine, could influence the S-methylation of thiopurines. Disulfiram is a medication that is used to make alcoholics ill by increasing the acetaldehyde formed from ethanol. TMPT S-methylates the diethylthiocarbamate active metabolite of this medication, making it less effective (Lennard, 1998).

Thiosulfate Sulfurtransferase and Rhodanese

In a television series that ran from 1985 to 1992, a photographic fixing chemical, sodium thiosulfate, was used by MacGyver, the hero, to treat cyanide poisoning in his boss. Except for the instant and complete recovery by the boss, the science was essentially sound: $CN^- + S_2O_3 \rightarrow SCN^- + SO_3$. CN is a naturally occurring compound, so it is not surprising that a mitochondrial enzyme present in prokaryotes and eukaryotes tries to prevent its unmetabolized inhibition of cytochrome oxidase and poisoning of oxidative phosphorylation by catalyzing the transfer of a sulfur atom from thiosulfate to sulfur acceptors like cyanide and thiol compounds. Thiocyanate is less toxic than cyanide, but still quite toxic. Thiosulfate sulfurtransferase (TST) not only detoxifies cyanide, but also regenerates iron–sulfur clusters and metabolizes organo-sulfane sulfur compounds. TST is expressed at high concentrations in the human colon and the rectum as well, which helps detoxify the hydrogen sulfide gas produced by the active anaerobic bacteria of the intestinal flora. Human polymorphisms have been discovered that may explain why patients with ulcerative colitis have three times the H_2S release as unaffected humans (Billaut-Laden et al., 2006). In the rat, high TST activity is found in the liver and the kidney.

It is also not surprising that the central nervous system has high expression of this enzyme, as cyanide toxicity appears to manifest its toxicity there. An inhibitor of TST, sodium 2-propenyl inhibits the sulfur-free form of rhodanese (EC 2.8.1.1) by thiolation of the cysteine at the active site. Thioredoxin is capable of restoring activity following this inhibitory thiolation reaction. This last finding appears to explain the cancer cell cytotoxicity of organosulfane sulfur compounds and links the apoptosis induced by these compounds to the damage to mitochondrial enzymes engaged in Fe-S cluster repair and the detoxication system of this organelle (Sabelli et al., 2008).

Acetaminophen Detoxication as an Example of Sulfonation, Glucuronidation, and Glutathione Conjugation

Conjugation reactions are generally viewed as detoxication mechanisms of the cell. Occasionally, they can activate specific chemical species. However, acetaminophen is a good case study of detoxication reactions. The term "phase 2 metabolism" appears to imply that this process follows phase 1, but that is not always the case. Moieties that are readily amenable to conjugation, such as phenols, may be immediately conjugated by sulfate, a methyl group, or may become a glucuronide, depending on the availability of the enzyme (biological species, stage of development, and cellular compartment) and the conjugate donor. Similarly, thiols may be conjugated by a glucuronide group or a sulfate. Amines may be subject to sulfonation, glucuronidation, methylation, or acetylation. Carboxylic moieties are subject to conjugation by amino acids and glucuronic acid. Glutathione conjugation is reserved for the reactive electrophiles usually generated by phase 1 metabolism. Acetaminophen is a good case in point (**Figure 7-10**).

The pathway of acetaminophen metabolism in adult mammalian liver cells is shown in the figure with the formation of an N-acetyl-p-quinoneimine as the reactive metabolite from oxidation by CYPs, which binds to liver proteins and causes centrilobular necrosis. The kidney cell metabolite of CYPs, the free radical N-acetyl-benzosemiquinoneimine, which damages medullary renal cell proteins, is not indicated in Figure 7-10. Note that prior to phase 1 metabolism, the presence of a hydroxyl group (phenol) allows for detoxication via a sulfate or glucouronide conjugate. In general, the formation of these conjugates indicates that the compound has not been through activation by a phase 1 enzyme and is a less toxic product. The glutathione conjugate is formed and saves the liver cells from assured damage as long as the glutathione concentration is approximately an astounding 10 mM in liver cells. Depletion of glutathione increases the likelihood of damage while increasing levels of glutathione—for example, in selenium-deficient cells that have less glutathione utilization through the glutathione peroxidase—and decreases necrotic cell formation. The formation of a glutathione conjugate indicates the activation of a compound to a reactive metabolite. This example is a rule of thumb that is worth considering, with specific exceptions to it indicated in the following sections on sulfonation, glucuronidation, and glutathione conjugate formation.

Sulfonation

The sulfotransferases (STs; EC 2.8.2.x) are responsible for the transfer of a SO_3^{-1} sulfonate group that uses 3'-phosphoadenosine-5'-phosphosulfate (PAPS) as its donor. In the process, the conjugate compound (sulfate ester or sulfamate) becomes more water soluble. The donor group is synthesized from ATP and inorganic sulfate via a two-step process.

Two families of sulfotransferases are distinguished: the cytosolic STs and the Golgi membrane-bound STs. The membrane-bound STs catalyze the sulfonation of glycosaminoglycans, glycoproteins, and proteins for subsequent secretion by the Golgi apparatus. The human cytosolic enzymes conjugate xenobiotics and are represented by four different isozymes: the liver and adrenal hydroxysteroid or dehydroepiandrosterone (DHEA) ST; the liver, platelets, intestines, adrenal, brain, and lung phenol-sulfating (P-PST) and monoamine-sulfating (M-PST) forms of the phenol ST; and the estrogen ST (EST). The hydroxysteroid STs

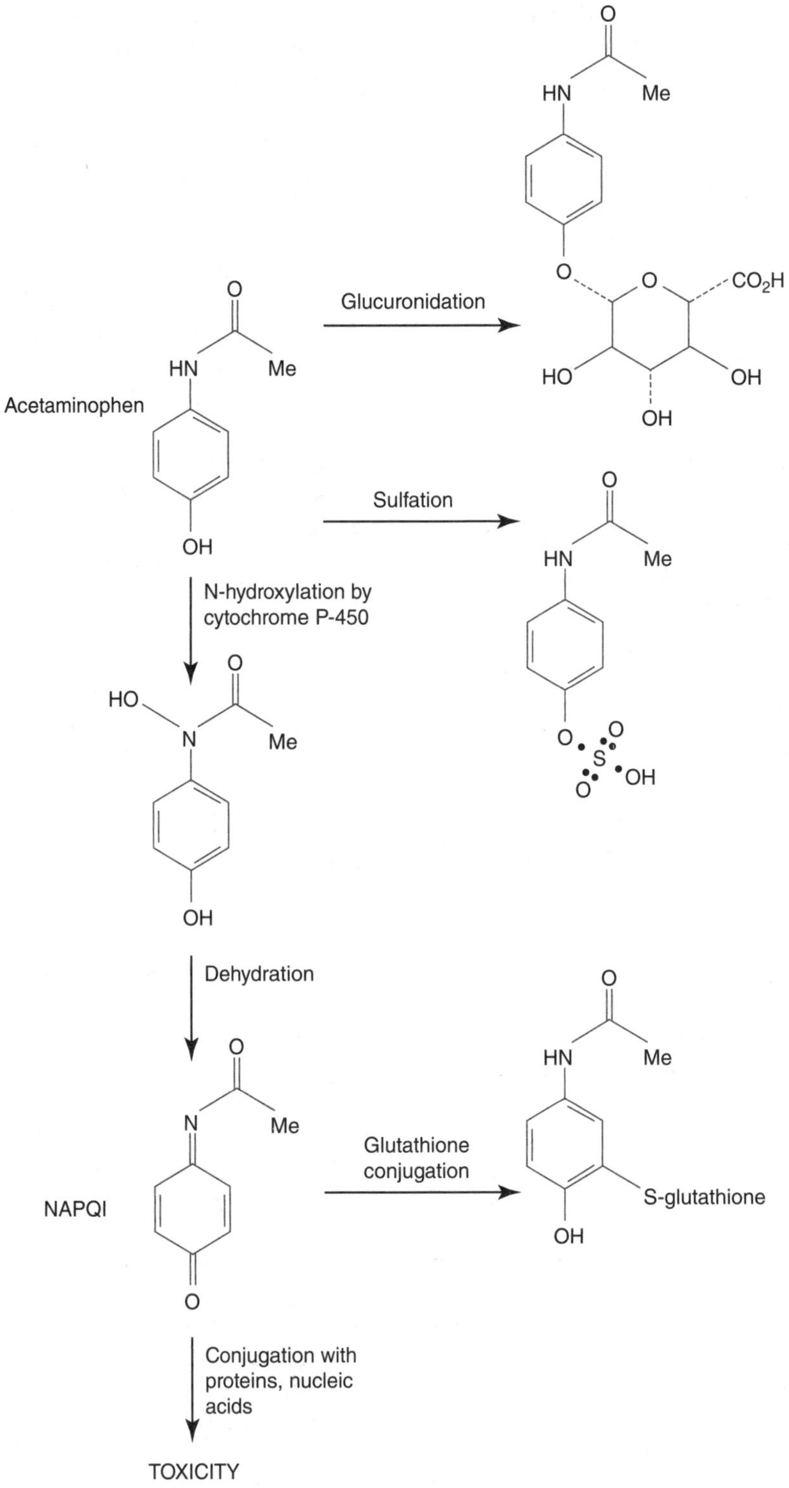

FIGURE 7-10 Acetaminophen Metabolism and Toxicity

Data from James LP, Mayeux PR, Hinson JA. 2003. Acetaminophen-induced hepatotoxicity. *Drug Metab Dispos.* 31:1499–1506.

have been found in bacterial and mammalian cells, and six isoforms of the enzyme are present in the rat. P-PST conjugates amino-terminal and internal tyrosine residues of peptides, aromatic amines, estrogenic steroids (similar to EST), the nitrogen oxide of minoxidil, and thyroid hormones. The K_m for neutral phenolic compounds is lower for P-PST than for M-PST, which makes P-PST catalytically more active toward acetaminophen at lower concentrations. However, M-PST has high affinity for catecholamines (adrenergic neurotransmitters). M-PST also shows a stereoselectivity that P-PST does not, by favoring the (+)-enantiomer of 4′-hydroxypropanolol, terbutaline, and isoproteranol and the (−)-enantiomer of albuterol. M-PST has no activity toward estrogens, hydroxysteroids, genistein, or diethylstilbestrol. M-PST and P-PST conjugate thyroid hormones. M-PST activity is higher in platelets, while P-PST predominates in the cytosol. PSTs are higher in male rats, but no sex difference is observed in the human. P-PST is found to predominate in the periportal region of the liver, where it represents a first-pass enzyme for ingested xenobiotics. PSTs in the lung and kidney provide further metabolic inactivation pathways, while PSTs in the brain represent catecholamine inactivation. Activation by sulfonation has been studied extensively for the carcinogenic N-hydroxyacetylaminofluorene, and also occurs for PSTs for other N-hydroxylated aromatic amines and heterocyclic amines. The hydroxysteriod STs activate hydroxymethyl polyaromatic hydrocarbons (Falany, 1997).

A more modern approach to categorizing the bioactivating and inactivating STs identifies six families. The most studied cytosolic enzyme is SULT1, which is involved in xenobiotic and steroid sulfonation. SULT1 may be subdivided further into five families. SULT1A has been characterized in the cow, dog, guinea pig, monkey, mouse, platypus, and rat; three similar forms, SULT1A1–3, in the human. The human SULT1A1 conjugates a variety of small phenolic compounds, including the model substrate of p-nitrophenol ($K_m \approx 1$ μM). It is referred to as P-PST, is inhibited by 2,6-dichloro-4-nitrophenol (DCNP), and is thermostable at 45°C. SULT1A1 is the major sulfonation enzyme, including

the conjugation of estrogens. This enzyme is responsible for DNA adduct formation from reactive intermediates of sulfonated forms of hydroxymethyl polycyclic aromatic hydrocarbons. Polymorphisms of SULT1A1 have been studied with regard to the etiologies of a variety of cancers (Hempel et al., 2007). The human fetus has substantial sulfation capability, which is not true for glucuronidation until the perinatal period (Richard et al., 2001).

Glucuronidation

Glucuronidation does not play a major conjugation role until the neonatal period (Lucier et al., 1979). Microsomal UDP-glucuronosyltransferase (UGT; EC 2.4.1.17) becomes important for the adult detoxication of xenobiotics, bilirubin, bile acids, and steroid hormones. Two major families of UGTs exist: UGT1A and UGT2. Since UGT2 is mainly involved in the conjugation of endogenous substrates, it will not be discussed further here, other than to mention that the UGT2B isoform is inducible by phenobarbital in the rat and that the UGT2B7 and UGT2B15 isoforms have substantial liver activity.

Polymorphisms of UGTs have clinical implications, as Caucasian populations that are homozygous for UGT1A1*28 tend to have a mild hyperbilirubinemia referred to as Gilbert's syndrome. That same polymorphism appears to cause a severe hematologic toxicity known as neutropenia upon use of the cancer chemotherapy medication irinotecan (Biason et al., 2008). The liver transformation results in detoxified metabolites, but the distribution following liver cell conjugation may involve the bile or the kidney. Since the bile goes into the gastrointestinal tract, the β-glucuronide formed from exogenous compounds may be cleaved and subject to enterohepatic recirculation, which increases the half-life of the compound and complicates simple toxicokinetic modeling. Moreover, inducers of liver cytochrome P450 also induce UGT1 isoforms, such as clofibrate, 3-methylcholanthrene, and phenobarbital.

The isoforms most responsible for liver glucuronidation are UGT1A1, UGT1A4, and UGT1A9. The rate of glucuronidation of aromatic amines has been established as

UGT1A9 > UGT1A4 >> UGT2B7 > UGT1A6 = UGT1A1. The glucuronidation of aromatic amines is unusual in that the *O*-glucuronides represent the usual detoxication mechanism of these enzymes, while the *N*-glucuronides of the *N*-hydroxyl metabolites proceed to activation in the cells of the urinary bladder (Ciotti et al., 1999). Although most of the metabolism is usually concentrated on liver cells, colon cell cancer following from UGT1 metabolism has arisen as a concern. Most UGT1A enzymes are expressed at low levels in the colon, but UGT1A7, UGT1A8, and UGT1A10 are expressed exclusively extrahepatically. However, individuals with variants of the *UGT1A6*2* allele show decreased rates of phenol and planar heterocyclic amine conjugation and increased risk of tumors of proximal colon cells, which is reversed in the case of the presence of acetylsalicylic acid (aspirin). The planar heterocyclic amines are of interest to researchers studying the link between pan-fried or well-done red meat and colorectal cancer risk. UGT1A7, which conjugates benzo[*a*]pyrene (low in *2 or *3 polymorphisms), which is found in cigarette smoke and dietary heterocyclic amines, also has variants associated with this cancer (van der Logt et al., 2004).

Other UGTs isolated is various species can be found at http://som.flinders.edu.au/FUSA/ClinPharm/UGT/udgpa.html.

Glutathione *S*-Transferases

Cytosolic glutathione *S*-transferases (GSTs; EC 2.5.1.18) are important in the detoxication of the reactive electrophiles produced mainly by phase 1 enzymes via nucleophilic conjugation to glutathione (GSH). Tumor resistance to chemotherapeutic medications, cellular aging, Alzheimer's disease, atherosclerosis, cataract formation, cirrhosis of the liver, and Parkinson's disease are all, in some fashion, linked to alterations in GST activity (Dourado et al., 2008). Research into the cytosolic enzymes has mainly focused on the alpha, mu, pi, and theta enzymes, which are mapped on different chromosomes. However, zeta, sigma, and omega forms also exist. Likewise, a mitochondrial form (kappa) and multiple microsomal forms (gp I, II, and IV) have been identified.

The GSTs must dimerize to become catalytically active. The active site binds GSH (G site) and the hydrophobic substrate (H site). GST subunits that contribute fully to the dimerization have a small N-terminal α/β domain reminiscent of GPx or thioredoxin of bacterial cells, plus a larger domain consisting of five α-helices. The tyr residue near the N-terminus stabilizes the thiolate anion's reactive state. Human polymorphism at nucleotide 69 in the 5′-regulatory region of the *GSTA1* gene known as *GSTA1*B* has homozygotes that have reduced GST activity compared with homozygotes of *GSTA1*A*. GSTP1 (pi class) appears to be the most widely present isoform in various cells. Of the five major genes for the mu class (*M1–M5*), *GSTM1* seems most important for intestinal cell conjugation of electrophilic species (van der Logt et al., 2004), increasing the hepatocellular cancer risk. Approximately 10–20% of Caucasians express the *GSTT1* (theta) null genotype and 40–60% of Caucasians have the *GSTM1* null genotype, which suggests that these isoforms are essential protective conjugation liver enzymes in humans (White et al., 2008).

It is interesting how these null isoforms can work for or against a cell or organism, depending on the substrate. For instance, most carcinogens that are already electrophiles (e.g., compounds with an electron-withdrawing group that allows displacement of another electron-withdrawing group, such as a halogen/halide or nitro group) or that become activated electrophiles (e.g., epoxides) on metabolism will be more toxic with a null gene such as *GSTT1* or *GSTM1*. The nucleophilic substitution and nucleophilic addition reactions of GSTs there represent important protection functions, as does the reduction of hydroperoxides. The isomerization of organic compounds is not clearly a detoxication pathway, but represents a fourth reaction. However, *GSTM1* disposes of isothiocyanates, which are derived from metabolites of glucosinates (present in high concentrations in cruciferous vegetables). The glucosinates are strong inducers of GSTs and other detoxication enzymes. This indicates that the null enzyme will keep these metabolites in the cells longer and have chemopreventive effects. Men who have the *GSTT1* and *GSTM1* null variants have less lung cancer.

GSTs can also increase toxicity via reaction with halogenated hydrocarbons, generating a halide anion and a thiiranium ion (mutagenic and nephrotoxic metabolites from S-[2-haloethyl] glutathione conjugates; Dekant, 2001) from a vicinal dihaloalkane or the nephrotoxic thioketene product of a perchloroethylene (from the formation of S-[trichlorovinyl]glutathione; Völkel and Dekant, 1998). As usual, it appears that the nature of the chemical determines whether a reaction that is meant to provide a more soluble and less reactive product leads to detoxication, activation, or removal of antioxidants or other protective agents from the cell.

Phosphorylation

Phosphorylation of nucleoside/nucleotide antiretroviral medications is an exception to the rule that it is not smart to make a compound less able to leave a cell and use a vital cellular energy and signaling group in the process of conjugation (Lai et al., 2008). However, phosphorylation is a very useful signal to activate biotransformation enzymes such as cytochrome P450s (Oesch-Bartlomowicz and Oesch, 2008) or UDP-glucuronosyltransferases (Basu et al., 2003).

Questions

1. What are the anaerobic reactions available to convert polycyclic aromatic hydrocarbons for removal from cells? From metals?
2. Indicate the key steps in the CYP catalytic cycle. What does the cycle yield?
3. How is acetaminophen metabolized? What does the formation of phase 2 conjugates mean in terms of decreased and increased toxicity of the reactive intermediates produced in phase 1?

References

Adam A, Smith LL, Cohen GM. 1990. An assessment of the role of redox cycling in mediating the toxicity of paraquat and nitrofurantoin. *Environ Health Perspect*. 85:113–117.

Adrian L, Szewzyk U, Wecke J, Görisch H. 2000. Bacterial dehalorespiration with chlorinated benzenes. *Nature*. 408:580–583.

Ali S, Pawa S, Naime M, Prasad R, Ahmad T, Farooqui H, Zafar H. 2008. Role of mammalian cytosolic molybdenum Fe-S flavin hydroxylases in hepatic injury. *Life Sci*. 82:780–788.

Anusevicius Z, Sarlauskas J, Cenas N. 2002. Two-electron reduction of quinones by rat liver NAD(P)H:quinone oxidoreductase: quantitative structure-activity relationships. *Arch Biochem Biophys*. 404:254–262.

Aurilia V, Parracino A, D'Auria S. 2008. Microbial carbohydrate esterases in cold adapted environments. *Gene*. 410:234–240.

Barbier M, Prevot P, Soyer-Gobillard M-O. 2000. Esterases in marine dinoflagellates and resistance to the organophosphate insecticide parathion. *Int Microbiol*. 3:117–123.

Barker DF, Walraven JM, Ristagno EH, Doll MA, States JC, Hein DW. 2008. Quantitative tissue and gene specific differences and developmental changes in Nat1, Nat2 and Nat3 mRNA expression in the rat. *Drug Metab Dispos*. 36:2445–2451.

Basu NK, Kole L, Owens IS. 2003. Evidence for phosphorylation requirement for human bilirubin UDP-glucuronosyltransferase (UGT1A1) activity. *Biochem Biophys Res Commun*. 303:98–104.

Bentley R, Chasteen TG. 2002. Microbial methylation of metalloids: arsenic, antimony, and bismuth. *Microbiol Mol Biol Rev*. 66:250–271.

Bernsohn J, Barron KD, Doolin PF, Hess AR, Hedrick MT. 1966. Subcellular localization of rat brain esterases. *J Histochem Cytochem*. 14:455–472.

Biason P, Masier S, Toffoli G. 2008. UGT1A1*28 and other UGT1A polymorphisms as determinants of irinotecan toxicity. *J Chemother*. 20:158–165.

Billaut-Laden I, Allorge D, Crunelle-Thibaut A, Rat E, Cauffiez C, Chevalier D, Houdret N, Lo-Guidice JM, Broly F. 2006. Evidence for a functional genetic polymorphism of the human thiosulfate sulfurtransferase (Rhodanese), a cyanide and H_2S detoxification enzyme. *Toxicology*. 225:1–11.

Bitsch A, Klöhn PC, Hadjiolov N, Bergmann O, Neumann HG. 1999. New insights into carcinogenesis of the classical model arylamine 2-acetylaminofluorene. *Cancer Lett*. 143:223–227.

Carson KA, Sonenshine DS, Boland LM, Taylor D. 1987. Ultrastructural localization of acetylcholinesterase in the synganglion of the tick, *Dermacentor variabilis* (Say). *Cell Tissue Res*. 249:615–623.

Cashman JR. 2000. Human flavin-containing monooxygenase: substrate specificity and role in drug metabolism. *Curr Drug Metab*. 1:181–191.

Casida JE, Quistad GB. 2005. Serine hydrolase targets of organophosphorus toxicants. *Chem Biol Interact*. 157–158:277–283.

Chang GW, Kam PC. 1999. The physiological and pharmacological role of CYP450 isoenzymes. *Anesthesia.* 54:42–50.

Chang YS. 2008. Recent developments in microbial biotransformation and biodegradation of dioxins. *J Mol Microbiol Biotechnol.* 15:152–171.

Chen C-C, Lu R-B, Chen Y-C, Wang M-F, Chang Y-C, Li T-K, Yin S-J. 1999. Interaction between the functional polymorphisms of the alcohol-metabolism genes in protection against alcoholism. *Am J Hum Genet.* 65:795–807.

Ciotti M, Lakshmi VM, Basu N, Davis BB, Owens IS, Zenser TV. 1999. Glucuronidation of benzidine and its metabolites by cDNA-expressed human UDP-glucuronosyltransferases and pH stability of glucuronides. *Carcinogenesis.* 20:1963–1969.

Compeau G, Bartha R. 1985. Sulfate reducing bacteria: principal methylators of Hg in anoxic estuarine sediments. *Appl Environ Microbiol.* 50:498–502.

Cooper DY, Levin S, Narasimhulu S, Rosenthal O. 1965. Photochemical action spectrum of the terminal oxidase of mixed function oxidase systems. *Science.* 147:400–402.

Coppin JF, Qu W, Waalkes MP. 2008. Interplay between cellular methyl metabolism and adaptive efflux during oncogenic transformation from chronic arsenic exposure in human cells. *J Biol Chem.* 283:19342–19350.

Coulter C, Kennedy JT, McRoberts WC, Harper DB. 1993. Purification and properties of an S-adenosylmethionine: 2,4-disubstituted phenol O-methyltransferase from *Phanerochaete chrysosporium. Appl Environ Microbiol.* 59:706–711.

Crow JA, Borazjani A, Potter PM, Ross MK. 2007. Hydrolysis of pyrethroids by human and rat tissues: examination of intestinal, liver and serum carboxylesterases. *Toxicol Appl Pharmacol.* 221:1–12.

Crow JA, Middleton BL, Borazjani A, Hatfield MJ, Potter PM, Ross MK. 2008. Inhibition of carboxylesterase 1 is associated with cholesteryl ester retention in human THP-1 monocyte/macrophages. *Biochim Biophys Acta.* 1781:643–654.

Danielsson O, Atrian S, Luque T, Hjelmqvist L, Gonzàlez-Duarte R, Jörnvall H. 1994. Fundamental molecular differences between alcohol dehydrogenase classes. *Proc Natl Acad Sci USA.* 91:4980–4984.

Das UN. 2007. Acetylcholinesterase and butyrylcholinesterase as possible markers of low-grade systemic inflammation. *Med Sci Monit.* 13:RA214–RA221.

Davies MJ, Hawkins CL, Pattison DI, Rees MD. 2008. Mammalian heme peroxidases: from molecular mechanisms to health implications. *Antioxid Redox Signal.* 10:1199–1234.

Degtyarenko K. 2007. Directory of P450-containing systems. http://www.icgeb.org/~p450srv/.

Dekant W. 2001. Chemical-induced nephrotoxicity mediated by glutathione S-conjugate formation. *Toxicol Lett.* 124:21–36.

Dourado DF, Fernandes PA, Ramos MJ. 2008. Mammalian cytosolic glutathione transferases. *Curr Protein Pept Sci.* 9:325–337.

Exner M, Hermann M, Hofbauer R, Kapiotis S, Quehenberger P, Speiser W, Held I, Gmeiner BMK. 2001. Semicarbazide-sensitive amine oxidase catalyzes endothelial cell-mediated low density lipoprotein oxidation. *Cardiovasc Res.* 50:583–588.

Falany CN. 1997. Enzymology of human cytosolic sulfotransferases. *FASEB J.* 11:206–216.

Fang X. 2006. Soluble epoxide hydrolase: a novel target for the treatment of hypertension. *Recent Patents Cardiovasc Drug Discov.* 1:67–72.

Fenoglio C, Grosso A, Boncompagni E, Gandini C, Milanesi G, Barni S. 2009. Exposure to heptachlor: evaluation of the effects on the larval and adult epidermis of *Rana* kl. *esculenta. Aquat Toxicol.* 91:151–160.

Forkert PG. 1997. Conjugation of glutathione with the reactive metabolites of 1, 1-dichloroethylene in murine lung and liver. *Microsc Res Tech.* 36:234–242.

Fu Y, Sies H, Lei XG. 2001. Opposite roles of selenium-dependent glutathione peroxidase-1 in superoxide generator diquat- and peroxynitrite-induced apoptosis and signaling. *J Biol Chem.* 276:43004–43009.

Fuchs G. 2008. Anaerobic metabolism of aromatic compounds. *NY Acad Sci.* 1125:82–99.

Furihata T, Hosokawa M, Masuda M, Satoh T, Chiba K. 2006. Hepatocyte nuclear factor-4alpha plays pivotal roles in the regulation of mouse carboxylesterase 2 gene transcription in mouse liver. *Arch Biochem Biophys.* 447:107–117.

Furlong CE, Li WF, Richter RJ, Shih DM, Lusis AJ, Alleva E, Costa LG. 2000. Genetic and temporal determinants of pesticide sensitivity: role of paraoxonase (PON1). *Neurotoxicology.* 21:91–100.

Gan KN, Smolen A, Eckerson HW, La Du BN. 1991. Purification of human serum paraoxonase/arylesterase: evidence for one esterase catalyzing both activities. *Drug Metab Dispos.* 19:100–106.

Gao J-R, Yoon KS, Frisbie RK, Coles GC, Clark JM. 2006. Esterase-mediated malathion resistance in the human head louse, *Pediculus capitis* (Anoplura: Pediculidae). *Pestic Biochem Physiol.* 85:28–37.

Gong B, Boor PJ. 2006. The role of amine oxidases in xenobiotic metabolism. *Expert Opin Drug Metab Toxicol.* 2:559–571.

Gross M, Oertel M, Köhrle J. 1995. Differential selenium-dependent expression of type I 5′-deiodinase and glutathione peroxidase in the porcine epithelial kidney cell line LLC-PK1. *Biochem J.* 306(Pt 3):851–856.

Guengerich FP. 1991. Reactions and significance of cytochrome P-450 enzymes. *J Biol Chem*. 266:10019–10022.

Guengerich FP. 2007. Mechanisms of cytochrome P450 substrate oxidation: minireview. *J Biochem Mol Toxicol*. 21:163–168.

Haigh JR, Johnston SR, Peppernay A, Mattern PJ, Garcia GE, Doctor BP, Gordon RK, Aisen PS. 2008. Protection of red blood cell acetylcholinesterase by oral huperzine A against ex vivo soman exposure: next generation prophylaxis and sequestering of acetylcholinesterase over butyrylcholinesterase. *Chem Biol Interact*. 175:380–386.

Hannemann F, Bichet A, Ewen KM, Bernhardt R. 2007. Cytochrome P450 systems: biological variations of electron transport chains. *Biochim Biophys Acta*. 1770:330–344.

Hein DW, Rustan TD, Doll MA, Bucher KD, Ferguson RJ, Feng Y, Furman EJ, Gray K. 1992. Acetyltransferases and susceptibility to chemicals. *Toxicol Lett*. 64–65:123–130.

Hempel N, Gamage N, Martin JL, McManus ME. 2007. Human cytosolic sulfotransferase SULT1A1. *Int J Biochem Cell Biol*. 39:685–689.

Herraiz T, Guillén H, Galisteo J. 2007. *N*-Methyltetrahydro-beta-carboline analogs of 1-methyl-4-phenyl-1,2,3,6-tetrahydropyridine (MPTP) neurotoxin are oxidized to neurotoxic beta-carbolinium cations by heme peroxidases. *Biochem Biophys Res Commun*. 356:118–123.

Hewitt LA, Valiquette C, Plaa GL. 1987. The role of biotransformation–detoxication in acetone-, 2-butanone-, and 2-hexanone-potentiated chloroform-induced hepatotoxicity. *Can J Physiol Pharmacol*. 65:2313–2318.

Hines RN. 2006. Developmental and tissue-specific expression of human flavin-containing monooxygenases 1 and 3. *Expert Opin Drug Metab Toxicol*. 2:41–9.

Hla T, Maciag T. 1991. Cyclooxygenase gene expression is down-regulated by heparin-binding (acidic fibroblast) growth factor-1 in human endothelial cells. *J Biol Chem*. 266:24059–24063.

Hoffmann F, Maser E. 2007. Carbonyl reductases and pluripotent hydroxysteroid dehydrogenases of the short-chain dehydrogenase/reductase superfamily. *Drug Metab Rev*. 39:87–144.

Hu G, Shi Z, Hu J, Zou G, Peng G, Ran P. 2008. Association between polymorphisms of microsomal epoxide hydrolase and COPD: results from meta-analyses. *Respirology*. 13:837–850.

Huang TL, Obih PO, Jaiswal R, Hartley WR, Thiyagarajah A. 1997. Evaluation of liver and brain esterases in the spotted gar fish (*Lepisosteus oculatus*) as biomarkers of effect in the lower Mississippi River Basin. *Bull Environ Contam Toxicol*. 58:688–695.

Inceoglu B, Schmelzer KR, Morisseau C, Jinks SL, Hammock BD. 2007. Soluble epoxide hydrolase inhibition reveals novel biological functions of epoxyeicosatrienoic acids (EETs). *Prostaglandins Other Lipid Mediat*. 82:42–49.

Inoue H, Castagnoli K, Van Der Schyf C, Mabic S, Igarashi K, Castagnoli N Jr. 1999. Species-dependent differences in monoamine oxidase A and B-catalyzed oxidation of various C4 substituted 1-methyl-4-phenyl-1,2,3,6-tetrahydropyridinyl derivatives. *J Pharmacol Exp Ther*. 291:856–864.

Jones B, Adams S, Miller GT, Jesson MI, Watanabe T, Wallner BP. 2003. Hematopoietic stimulation by a dipeptidyl peptidase inhibitor reveals a novel regulatory mechanism and therapeutic treatment for blood cell deficiencies. *Blood*. 102:1641–1648.

Kalgutkar AS, Obach RS, Maurer TS. 2007. Mechanism-based inactivation of cytochrome P450 enzymes: chemical mechanisms, structure-activity relationships and relationship to clinical drug–drug interactions and idiosyncratic adverse drug reactions. *Curr Drug Metab*. 8:407–447.

Karanth S, Pope C. 2000. Carboxylesterase and A-esterase activities during maturation and aging: relationship to the toxicity of chlorpyrifos and parathion in rats. *Toxicol Sci*. 58:282–289.

Karthikeyan R, Bhandari A. 2001. Anaerobic biotransformation of aromatic and polycyclic aromatic hydrocarbons in soil microcosms: a review. *J Hazard Substance Res*. III-3:3-1–3-19.

Kato R, Kamataki T, Yamazoe Y. 1983. *N*-Hydroxylation of carcinogenic and mutagenic aromatic amines. *Environ Health Perspect*. 49:21–25.

Knights KM, Sykes MJ, Miners JO. 2007. Amino acid conjugation: contribution to the metabolism and toxicity of xenobiotic carboxylic acids. *Expert Opin Drug Metab Toxicol*. 3:159–168.

Komives T, Gullner G. 2005. Phase I xenobiotic metabolic systems in plants. *Z Naturforsch [C]*. 60:179–185.

Koukouritaki SB, Poch MT, Henderson MC, Siddens LK, Krueger SK, VanDyke JE, Williams DE, Pajewski NM, Wang T, Hines RN. 2007. Identification and functional analysis of common human flavin-containing monooxygenase 3 genetic variants. *J Pharmacol Exp Ther*. 320:266–273.

Kumpulainen H, Järvinen T, Mannila A, Leppänen J, Nevalainen T, Mäntylä A, Vepsäläinen J, Rautio J. 2008. Synthesis, in vitro and in vivo characterization of novel ethyl dioxy phosphate prodrug of propofol. *Eur J Pharm Sci*. 34:110–117.

Lai J, Wang J, Cai Z. 2008. Nucleoside reverse transcriptase inhibitors and their phosphorylated metabolites in human immunodeficiency virus-infected human matrices. *J Chromatogr B Analyt Technol Biomed Life Sci*. 868:1–12.

Lee SH, Lee J, Cha R, Park MH, Ha JW, Kim S, Kim YS. 2008. Genetic variations in soluble epoxide hydrolase and graft function in kidney transplantation. *Transplant Proc.* 40:1353–1356.

Legler PM, Kumaran D, Swaminathan S, Studier FW, Millard CB. 2008. Structural characterization and reversal of the natural organophosphate resistance of a D-type esterase, *Saccharomyces cerevisiae* S-formylglutathione hydrolase. *Biochemistry.* 47:9592–9601.

Lennard L. 1998. Clinical implications of thiopurine methyltransferase: optimization of drug dosage and potential drug interactions. *Ther Drug Monit.* 20:527–531.

Levine MD. 2008. Toxicity, alcohols. http://www.emedicine.com/EMERG/topic19.htm.

Lewis DFV, Ioannides C, Parke DV. 1998. Cytochromes P450 and species differences in xenobiotic metabolism and activation of carcinogen. *Environ Health Perspect.* 106:633–641.

Liu YT, Hao HP, Liu CX, Wang GJ, Xie HG. 2007. Drugs as CYP3A probes, inducers, and inhibitors. *Drug Metab Rev.* 39:699–721.

Lou MF, Xu GT, Zigler S Jr, York B Jr. 1996. Inhibition of naphthalene cataract in rats by aldose reductase inhibitors. *Curr Eye Res.* 15:423–432.

Lucier GW, Lui EM, Lamartiniere CA. 1979. Metabolic activation/deactivation reactions during perinatal development. *Environ Health Perspect.* 29:7–16.

Martey CA, Pollock SJ, Turner CK, O'Reilly KM, Baglole CJ, Phipps RP, Sime PJ. 2004. Cigarette smoke induces cyclooxygenase-2 and microsomal prostaglandin E$_2$ synthase in human lung fibroblasts: implications for lung inflammation and cancer. *Am J Physiol Lung Cell Mol Physiol.* 287:L981–L991.

Massoulié J, Anselmet A, Bon S, Krejci E, Legay C, Morel N, Simon S. 1998. Acetylcholinesterase: C-terminal domains, molecular forms and functional localization. *J Physiol Paris.* 92:183–190.

Matsubara K. 1998. [Metabolic activation of azaheterocyclics induced dopaminergic toxicity: possible candidate neurotoxins underlying idiopathic Parkinson's disease.] *Nihon Hoigaku Zasshi.* 52:301–305.

McLeod HL, Krynetski EY, Relling MV, Evans WE. 2000. Genetic polymorphism of thiopurine methyltransferase and its clinical relevance for childhood acute lymphoblastic leukemia. *Leukemia.* 14:567–572.

Mesbah NM, Juergen Wiegel J. 2008. Life at extreme limits: the anaerobic halophilic alkali thermophiles. *NY Acad Sci.* 1125:44–57.

Mikami LR, Wieseler S, Souza RL, Schopfer LM, Nachon F, Lockridge O, Chautard-Freire-Maia EA. 2008. Five new naturally occurring mutations of the *BCHE* gene and frequencies of 12 butyrylcholinesterase alleles in a Brazilian population. *Pharmacogenet Genomics.* 18:213–218.

Millán JL. 2006. Alkaline phosphatases: structure, substrate specificity and functional relatedness to other members of a large superfamily of enzymes. *Purinergic Signal.* 2:335–341.

Mira L, Maia L, Barreira L, Manso CF. 1995. Evidence for free radical generation due to NADH oxidation by aldehyde oxidase during ethanol metabolism. *Arch Biochem Biophys.* 318:53–58.

Nishi K, Huang H, Kamita SG, Kim IH, Morisseau C, Hammock BD. 2006. Characterization of pyrethroid hydrolysis by the human liver carboxylesterases hCE-1 and hCE-2. *Arch Biochem Biophys.* 445:115–123.

Nordberg J, Arnér ES. 2001. Reactive oxygen species, antioxidants, and the mammalian thioredoxin system. *Free Radic Biol Med.* 31:1287–1312.

O'Brien PJ. 2000. Peroxidases. *Chem Biol Interact.* 129:113–139.

Oesch-Bartlomowicz B, Oesch F. 2008. Phosphorylation of xenobiotic-metabolizing cytochromes P450. *Anal Bioanal Chem.* 392:1085–1092

Omura T, Sato R. 1964. The carbon monoxide-binding pigment of liver microsomes. I. Evidence for its hemoprotein nature. *J Biol Chem.* 239: 2370–2378.

Osburn WO, Kensler TW. 2008. Nrf2 signaling: an adaptive response pathway for protection against environmental toxic insults. *Mutat Res.* 659:31–39.

Paine MF, Widmer WW, Hart HL, Pusek SN, Beavers KL, Criss AB, Brown SS, Thomas BF, Watkins PB. 2006. A furanocoumarin-free grapefruit juice establishes furanocoumarins as the mediators of the grapefruit juice–felodipine interaction. *Am J Clin Nutr.* 83:1097–1105.

Panoutsopoulos GI, Beedham C. 2004. Enzymatic oxidation of phthalazine with guinea pig liver aldehyde oxidase and liver slices: inhibition by isovanillin. *Acta Biochim Pol.* 51:943–951.

Pieper DH, Martins dos Santos VA, Golyshin PN. 2004. Genomic and mechanistic insights into the biodegradation of organic pollutants *Curr Opin Biotechnol.* 15:215–224.

Pineau P, Marchio A, Battiston C, Cordina E, Russo A, Terris B, Qin LX, Turlin B, Tang ZY, Mazzaferro V, Dejean A. 2008. Chromosome instability in human hepatocellular carcinoma depends on p53 status and aflatoxin exposure. *Mutat Res.* 653:6–13.

Pomara C, Fiore C, D'Errico S, Riezzo I, Fineschi V. 2008. Calcium oxalate crystals in acute ethylene glycol poisoning: a confocal laser scanning microscope study in a fatal case. *Clin Toxicol (Phila).* 46:322–324.

Preziosi P. 2007. Isoniazid: metabolic aspects and toxicological correlates. *Curr Drug Metab.* 8:839–851.

Qin Z, Reszka KJ, Fukai T, Weintraub NL. 2008. Extracellular superoxide dismutase (ecSOD) in vascular biology: an update on exogenous gene transfer and endogenous regulators of ecSOD. *Transl Res*. 151:68–78.

Reinhard JF Jr, Carmichael SW, Daniels AJ. 1990. Mechanisms of toxicity and cellular resistance to 1-methyl-4-phenyl-1,2,3,6-tetrahydropyridine and 1-methyl-4-phenylpyridinium in adrenomedullary chromaffin cell cultures. *J Neurochem*. 55:311–320.

Richard K, Hume R, Kaptein E, Stanley EL, Visser TJ, Coughtrie MW. 2001. Sulfation of thyroid hormone and dopamine during human development: ontogeny of phenol sulfotransferases and arylsulfatase in liver, lung, and brain. *J Clin Endocrinol Metab*. 86:2734–2742.

Rochu D, Chabrière E, Renault F, Elias M, Cléry-Barraud C, Masson P. 2007. Stabilization of the active form(s) of human paraoxonase by human phosphate-binding protein. *Biochem Soc Trans*. 35:1616–1620.

Rueter P, Rabus R, Wilkes H, Aeckersberg F, Rainey FA, Jannasch HW, Widdel F. 1994. Anaerobic oxidation of hydrocarbons in crude oil by new types of sulphate-reducing bacteria. *Nature*. 372:455–458.

Sabelli R, Iorio E, De Martino A, Podo F, Ricci A, Viticchiè G, Rotilio G, Paci M, Melino S. 2008. Rhodanese-thioredoxin system and allyl sulfur compounds. *FEBS J*. 275:3884–3899.

Sakurai M, Oishi K, Watanabe K. 2005. Localization of cyclooxygenases-1 and -2, and prostaglandin F synthase in human kidney and renal cell carcinoma. *Biochem Biophys Res Commun*. 338:82–86.

Sanghani SP, Davis WI, Dumaual NG, Mahrenholz A, Bosron WF. 2002. Identification of microsomal rat liver carboxylesterases and their activity with retinyl palmitate. *Eur J Biochem*. 269:4387–4398.

Sarapusit S, Xia C, Misra I, Rongnoparut P, Kim JJ. 2008. NADPH-cytochrome P450 oxidoreductase from the mosquito *Anopheles minimus*: kinetic studies and the influence of Leu86 and Leu219 on cofactor binding and protein stability. *Arch Biochem Biophys*. 477:53–59.

Savic M, Ilic-Tomic T, Macmaster R, Vasiljevic B, Conn GL. 2008. Critical residues for cofactor binding and catalytic activity in the aminoglycoside resistance methyltransferase Sgm. *J Bacteriol*. 190:5855–5861.

Shaftel SS, Olschowka JA, Hurley SD, Moore AH, O'Banion MK. 2003. COX-3: a splice variant of cyclooxygenase-1 in mouse neural tissue and cells. *Brain Res Mol Brain Res*. 119:213–215.

Shimada T. 2006. Xenobiotic-metabolizing enzymes in activation and detoxification of carcinogenic polycyclic aromatic hydrocarbons. *Drug Metab Pharmacokinet*. 21:257–276.

Shindou H, Shimizu T. 2009. Acyl-CoA: lysophospholipid acyltransferases. *J Biol Chem*. 284:1–5.

Silman I, Sussman JL. 2008. Acetylcholinesterase: how is structure related to function? *Chem Biol Interact*. 175:3–10.

Simone E, Ding BS, Muzykantov V. 2009. Targeted delivery of therapeutics to endothelium. *Cell Tissue Res*. 335:283–300.

Sladek NE. 1988. Metabolism of oxazaphosphorines. *Pharmacol Ther*. 37:301–355.

Sorenson RC, Primo-Parmo SL, Kuo CL, Adkins S, Lockridge O, La Du BN. 1995. Reconsideration of the catalytic center and mechanism of mammalian paraoxonase/arylesterase. *Proc Natl Acad Sci USA*. 92:7187–7191.

Spangler RS. 1996. Cyclooxygenase 1 and 2 in rheumatic disease: implications for nonsteroidal anti-inflammatory drug therapy. *Semin Arthritis Rheum*. 26:435–446

Stedman CA, Liddle C, Coulter SA, Sonoda J, Alvarez JG, Moore DD, Evans RM, Downes M. 2005. Nuclear receptors constitutive androstane receptor and pregnane X receptor ameliorate cholestatic liver injury. *Proc Natl Acad Sci USA*. 102:2063–2068.

Tunici P, Sessa A, Rabellotti E, Grant G, Bardocz S, Perin A. 1999. Polyamine oxidase and tissue transglutaminase activation in rat small intestine by polyamines. *Biochim Biophys Acta*. 1428:219–224.

Uno T, Yasui-Furukori N. 2006. Effect of grapefruit juice in relation to human pharmacokinetic study. *Curr Clin Pharmacol*. 1:157–161.

Ushio-Fukai M, Nakamura Y. 2008. Reactive oxygen species and angiogenesis: NADPH oxidase as target for cancer therapy. *Cancer Lett*. 266:37–52.

van der Logt EM, Bergevoet SM, Roelofs HM, van Hooijdonk Z, te Morsche RH, Wobbes T, de Kok JB, Nagengast FM, Peters WH. 2004. Genetic poly-morphisms in UDP-glucuronosyltransferases and glutathione S-transferases and colorectal cancer risk. *Carcinogenesis*. 25:2407–2415.

Vlahović M, Lazarević J, Perić-Mataruga V, Ilijin L, Mrdaković M. 2009. Plastic responses of larval mass and alkaline phosphatase to cadmium in the gypsy moth larvae. *Ecotoxicol Environ Saf*. 72:1148–1155.

Völkel W, Dekant W. 1998. Chlorothioketene, the ultimate reactive intermediate formed by cysteine conjugate beta-lyase–mediated cleavage of the trichloroethene metabolite S-(1,2-dichlorovinyl)-L-cysteine, forms cytosine adducts in organic solvents, but not in aqueous solution. *Chem Res Toxicol*. 11:1082–1088.

Wallace MA, Bailey S, Fukuto JM, Valentine JS, Gralla EB. 2005. Induction of phenotypes resembling CuZn-superoxide dismutase deletion in wild-type yeast cells: an in vivo assay for the role of superoxide in the toxicity of redox-cycling compounds. *Chem Res Toxicol*. 18:1279–1286.

Webb JS, McGinnes S, Lappin-Scott HM. 1998. Metal removal by sulphate-reducing bacteria from natural and constructed wetlands. *J Appl Microbiol.* 84:240–248.

Weber WW. 1990. Acetylation. *Birth Defects Orig Artic Ser.* 26:43–65.

Wedrén S, Rudqvist TR, Granath F, Weiderpass E, Ingelman-Sundberg M, Persson I, Magnusson C. 2003. Catechol-*O*-methyltransferase gene polymorphism and post-menopausal breast cancer risk. *Carcinogenesis.* 24:681–687.

Wells DG, Bjorksten AR. 1989. Monoamine oxidase inhibitors revisited. *Can J Anaesth.* 36:64–74.

White DL, Li D, Nurgalieva Z, El-Serag HB. 2008. Genetic variants of glutathione S-transferase as possible risk factors for hepatocellular carcinoma: a HuGE systematic review and meta-analysis. *Am J Epidemiol.* 167:377–389.

Yoshihara S, Shigeru Ohta S. 1998. Involvement of hepatic aldehyde oxidase in conversion of 1-methyl-4-phenyl-2,3-dihydropyridinium (MPDP$^+$) to 1-methyl-4-phenyl-5,6-dihydro-2-pyridone. *Arch Biochem Biophys.* 360:93–98.

Zamocky M, Furtmüller PG, Obinger C. 2008. Evolution of catalases from bacteria to humans. *Antioxid Redox Signal.* 10:1527–1548.

Zhou SF. 2008. Drugs behave as substrates, inhibitors, and inducers of human cytochrome P450 3A4. *Curr Drug Metab.* 9:310–322.

Zhou Z, Kang YJ. 2000. Cellular and subcellular localization of catalase in the hearts of transgenic mice. *J Histochem Cytochem.* 48:585–594.

CHAPTER 8

Damage to Cytosolic and Endoplasmic Reticulum Activities

This is a chapter outline intended to guide and familiarize you with the content to follow.

I. Moving through the outer membrane into the cytosol (second messenger; signal transduction) and endoplasmic reticulum (protein synthesis and xenobiotic metabolism plus other functions) shows how compounds or their metabolites can confer damage

  A. Types of reactants based on their chemical nature

    1. Nonionic electrophiles—compounds deficient in electrons, such as:

      Aldehydes and ketones:

Allyl alcohol

Alcohol dehyrogenase

Acrolein (toxic electrophile)

Neurotoxic acrylamide monomer =

      a. (Thiono)acyl halides and thioketenes ($R_2C = C = S$)

      b. Quinones (cyclic dione) or quinone imines—can form DNA adducts

      c. Oxiranes = oxygen in a highly unstable three-member ring with two carbons

      d. N-nitroso (nitrosamines $R_2N-N=O$) compounds

      e. Oxon (P-S bond becomes a P-O bond; malathion → malaoxon, which inhibits cholinesterases)

      f. Sulfoxide (R-S(O)-R′ where R and R′ = organic moieties)

CONCEPTUALIZING TOXICOLOGY 8-1

2. Cationic electrophiles

   a. Protonation of the nonionic electrophiles aziridinyl quinones → "hard" electrophile, which alkylates DNA of the quinones phosphate group

   b. Triphenylmethane dyes—some carcinogenic

   c. Triphenylphosphonium cation—mitochondrial damage

   d. Benzyl carbonium cation = mutagen vs. benzyl alcohol (not mutagenic)

   e. Aristolochic acids → nitrenium ions (via CYPs)—react with DNA and protein

   f. Glutathione conjugates form episulfonium ion intermediates with a nematocide, 1,2-dibromo-3-chloropropane via glutathione transferases (located in cytosol and mitochondria)

   g. Metals in charged states

3. Oxidation to a free radical—reactive oxygen species (ROS)

   a. Formation of superoxide, hydrogen peroxide, hydroxyl radical (Figure 8-1, Figure 8-2)

4. Oxidation to a free radical—reactive nitrogen species (RNS)

   a. Overproduction of NO (cell signaling molecule) → genotoxic lesions (during infection, NO increases endogenous nitrates, nitrites, and nitrosamines—similar to cooking food)

5. Other free radical species

   a. Sulfur-centered (–S˙), halogen (–Cl˙), and carbon free radical species (–HC˙–)

6. Nucleophiles—donate electron pair to an electrophile

   a. Phenols (nucleophile) → phenoxy radical (after donation)

phenol → phenoxy radicals

   b. Aromatic amines → amine radical cations + aminyl radicals (R—N⁺—R) and similar reactions possible for hydrazines, hydroquinones, phenothiazines, and thiols

   c. Amygdalin (structure below) releasing the cyanide (CN)nucleophile

Structure from http://upload.wikimedia.org/wikipedia/commons/4/4a/Amygdalin_skeletal.png.

   d. Carbon monoxide (CO)

   e. Selenomercaptans (selenol)

7. Changes in redox state of cell

   a. Methylmercury, Pb, and Paraquat increase oxidative state via redox/Fyn/c-Cbl pathway; cause activation of Fyn kinase = nonreceptor tyrosine kinase Src family; the c-Cbl enzyme modifies receptors responsible for mitosis and cell survival; disruption leads to degraded receptors/downstream signaling (Figure 8-3)

   b. Redox cycling (continuously form oxygen radicals; As + thiol binding + generation of H_2O_2) (Figure 8-4)

CONCEPTUALIZING TOXICOLOGY 8-1 (*continued*)

B. Types of cellular damage

1. Covalent binding to macromolecules

   a. Acetaminophen → quinone imine metabolite → damages liver → semiquinone imine metabolite → damages kidney

   b. Targets endoplasmic reticulum (ER stress) and associated metabolic enzymes (e.g., CYPs, glutathione S-transferase) > cytoplasm > mitochondria >> nuclear, peroxisomal, lysosomal, plasma membrane, Golgi

2. Depletion of glutathione

   a. Acetaminophen, diethylmaleate, phorone.

   b. Activation of JNK pathway appears to lead to damage and cell death by oxygen radicals, and this pathway is not attenuated by other signaling molecules such as NF-κB in severe GSH depletion. Damage is increased by TNFα signal

   c. Extrahepatic cells can have apoptosis initiate in cytosol via caspase 8 cleavage of procaspase 3 (mitochondrial in hepatocytes)

3. Lipid peroxidation and redox cycling

   a. Figure 8-4 illustrates redox cycling to generate ROS

   b. Lipid peroxidation is shown in Figure 8-5

   c. Lipid peroxidation products first stimulate cell survival mechanisms via heme-oxygenase and thioredoxine-1 gene expression → inhibit growth factor receptors EGFR and PDGFR at high concentrations → inhibit CREB-responsive promoters while increasing c-jun responsive promoter leading to cell degeneration and apoptosis

   d. Lipid peroxidation products damage DNA via mechanisms presented in Figure 8-6 (HO• radical damage, single-stranded breaks, and adduct formation); cytosolic damage important in prokaryotic cells as they have no nuclear compartment

4. Cell rupture and repair

   a. Wound healing → initiated by sphingosine-1-phosphate and mediated by the nuclear translocation of FHL2 → disruption lays down less elastic forms of collagen and may cause cell proliferation via factors such as TGF-β, platelet-derived growth factor, fibroblast growth factor, hepatocyte growth factor as mediated by members of the epidermal growth factor families and metalloproteinases

5. Cell death from apoptosis through necrosis

   a. Ca^{2+} depletion of ER stores by cholesterol → apoptosis

   b. Release of intracellular Ca^{2+} stores mediated by IP_3 and ryanodine receptors and cytosolic free Ca^{2+} concentrations—up to 500 nM opens channel synergistically with IP_3 and higher cytosolic Ca^{2+} concentrations are inhibitory to channel opening

   c. Necrosis is initiated by cytoplasmic and mitochondrial swelling → loss of membrane integrity, no vesicle formation, organelle disintegration, and cell lysis

6. Protein synthesis inhibition

   a. Ribosome binding of aminoglycoside antibiotics (on rough endoplasmic reticulum), puromycin, etc.

C. Antidotes

1. Limiting absorption–nonspecific = albumin binding of toxicant; specific = metal chelator, binding agent, or alternate target

2. Increasing excretion–nonspecific = hemodialysis or hemoperfusion; specific = metal chelator, antibody to toxin, or drug

3. Raising threshold–nonspecific = artificial respiration, renal dialysis, heart-lung machine, etc. for higher organism and electrolyte balance for cells; specific is antagonist to receptor (naloxone for heroin) or alternative pathway as folinic acid for overdose of cancer chemotherapy agent methotrexate that prevents the formation of tetrahydrofolate from folic acid

CONCEPTUALIZING TOXICOLOGY 8-1 (*continued*)

Moving into the cytosol and the endoplasmic reticulum really engages the modification of macromolecules and the metabolites that develop as a result of activation by enzymes in the cytosol or the endoplasmic reticulum. First, this chapter examines the reactive chemical species that are generated in the cytosol and the endoplasmic reticulum and their effects. This is followed by a discussion of cellular damage and adaptation mechanisms. Finally, antidotes are considered.

Reactive Chemical Species

Electrophiles — Nonionic

Electrophile means "electron loving"; chemically, it refers to a compound deficient in an electron that can attract electrons to that deficient center of the compound. If the compound is truly positively charged, it is a cationic electrophile; otherwise, it is a nonionic electrophile. Aldehydes and ketones start the list of nonionic electrophiles. Alcohol dehydrogenase (liver cytoplasmic enzyme) converts allyl alcohol to the potent electrophile acrolein (Glascott et al., 1996). Acrolein (type-2 alkene) can be found as an oxidation product in oils or by heating the triglycerides in oil. In a reaction by the methylglyoxal synthase in *Escherichia coli*, a similarly toxic endogenous aldehyde electrophile is formed (Benov et al., 2004). The neurotoxic electrophile acrylamide is formed from amino acids heated in oils as occurs in fried food (Ehling et al., 2005) or by microbial nitrile hydratase (Kobayashi et al., 1992). Other neurotoxic soft electrophiles are methyl acrylate or acrylamine, *N*-ethylmaleimide, acrolein, and methyl vinyl ketone (LoPachin et al., 2007). Alcohol dehydrogenase is involved in the formation of other aldehydes, such as the formation of acetaldehyde from ethanol and the ability of this electrophile to cause liver fibrosis through transforming growth factor beta 1 (TGF-β1) that is inhibited by interferon-gamma (IFNγ) (Ha et al., 2008). Oxidation to an aldehyde or ketone is also possible via cytochromes P450 (CYPs—liver enzymes in the endoplasmic reticulum) and monoamine oxidases (MAOs—outer mitochondrial membrane enzymes, but small

amount in endoplasmic reticulum). The CYP-conversion of n-hexane or n-butyl ketone to 2,5-hexanedione leads to a progressive decline of cytoskeletal protein contents of nerve cells, with neurofilament-H as the most sensitive index of neurotoxicity (Wang et al., 2008). Compounds that are activated by MAO to electrophiles tend to inhibit the enzyme directly, as does the conversion of allylamine to acrolein and at least in part the metabolites of benzylamines (Lu et al., 2003). Even acyl glucuronides form nonionic electrophiles of the aldehyde/ketone class due to the migration of the aglycone resulting in positional and stereoisomers under conditions normally found in the cell (Walker et al., 2007). Ketosis is also observed under low carbohydrate conditions such a low dietary intake and diabetes mellitus, as well as from extensive lipid peroxidation. Although the dietary restriction of carbohydrates on its own is not problematic, ketosis plays a role in the potentiation of the toxicity of haloalkanes (Hewitt et al., 1980).

Because acyl compounds were just mentioned along with haloalkanes, it is worth noting that (thiono)acyl halides and thioketenes represent the next class of nonionic electrophiles. Chloroform is oxidized by CYP2E1 to phosgene, which is inhibited by 4-methylpyrazole and increased 10- to 15-fold by acetone and pyrazole treatment (Testai et al., 1996). Glutathione S-transferases save liver cells from the toxicity of many haloalkanes and haloalkenes. Of special interest here are the glutathione conjugates of the haloalkenes, such as chlorotrifluoroethylene, hexachlorobutadiene, trichloroethylene, and tetrafluoroethylene. The conjugates leave the liver cells and are subject to kidney cell beta-lyase-dependent bioactivation to thioacylating reactive intermediates such as thioacyl halides, 2,2,3-trihalothiiranes, and thioketenes that result in renal cell necrosis (Anders, 2004). Acetaminophen, through CYP2E1 and CYP1A2, produces the N-acetyl-p-quinoneimine in liver cells (Zaher et al., 1998), but this reactive quinone electrophile may be produced through mammalian or plant peroxidases (Fischer et al., 1985). 2-Methoxyaniline (*o*-anisidine) is a compound similarly activated by horseradish peroxidase or mammalian peroxidases (e.g., prostaglandin H synthase or lactoperoxidase) to a carcinogenic quinone imine that forms DNA adducts (Stiborová et al., 2002). Stilbene estrogen (diethylstilbestrol, or DES) through microsomal, mitochondrial, and nuclear enzymes can convert DES to a reactive semiquinone or quinone that covalently binds to DNA and causes breast cancer. Chemopreventive diallyl sulfide from garlic inhibits this conversion of stilbene estrogens to nonionic electrophiles (Thomas et al., 2004).Oxiranes formed from aromatic hydrocarbons such as benzene show increased mutagenicity with the presence of a double bond in formal conjunction with the epoxide ring. The presence of a bromide or hydroxyl group would be expected to increase the electrophilicity; however, the presence of a 4-hydroxyl group in *syn* position to a 1,2-epoxide ring creates a dihydrodiol epoxide with little mutagenic activity. Additionally, other epoxide groups do not appear to increase the mutagenic activity of the first group on the same molecule (Jung et al., 1981).

Other epoxides, such as those formed from aflatoxin, benzo[*a*]pyrene, or vinyl chloride are known potent carcinogens, while N-nitroso compounds similarly have nonionic electrophilic properties that lead to mutations and cancer (Preussmann, 1978). One important neurotoxic mechanism of conversion of chemicals via CYPs to nonionic electrophiles is the desulfuration of the phosphonates (e.g., parathion, malathion) to their oxons, which inhibits cholinesterases. The relative toxicity of *O,O*-diisopropyl *O-p*-nitrophenol phosphorothioate (isopropyl parathion) to houseflies was higher than for honeybees given the same 4.7 µg per gram dosage, due to the high conversion to the paraoxon in houseflies (0.67 µg per gram) compared to the bees (0.29 µg per gram) 4 hours following external application. Additionally, the houseflies' cholinesterase is 36 times more sensitive ($I_{50} = 2.8 \times 10^{-7}$ M) than that of the bees ($I_{50} = 1.0 \times 10^{-5}$ M; Camp et al., 1969).

The last nonionic electrophile to be examined is the sulfoxide. The generation of liver cell fibrosis and cirrhosis is linked to the oxidation of thioacetamide to thioacetamide S-oxide and subsequent oxidative stress via flavin adenine dinucleotide (FAD)–containing monooxygenase (FMO) and CYPs. The downregulation of fatty acid beta-oxidation, branched chain amino acids, and methionine breakdown reduction is thought to implicate a depletion of succinyl-CoA, while the upregulation of proteins engaged in mediating the effects of oxidative stress and lipid peroxidation appears to complete a snapshot of events preceding the induction of cirrhosis (Low et al., 2004).

Electrophiles — Cationic

The antitumor compound 2,5-diaziridinyl-1,4-benzoquinone (DZQ), $pK_a = 3.8$, is an aziridinyl quinone, which links to the nonionic electrophiles describe in the previous section. However, when protonated, DZQ becomes a hard electrophile that alkylates ~35% of bulk DNA by attaching to the phosphate groups (Skibo and Xing, 1998). Triphenylmethane (trityl) dyes are commercially useful and the trityl groups form stable cations useful as labile protective groups in organic synthesis. These trityl cationic electrophiles are generated from alcohols under acidic conditions (Denekamp and Yaniv, 2006). Some of these dyes are carcinogenic (Vachálková et al., 1996), while others are not (Lin and Brusick, 1992). Triphenylmethane alone appears to be a chemopreventive agent with respect to 3-methylcholanthrene (Cooney et al., 1992), so the specific chemical structure of the electrophile is vitally important in the toxicity produced. Triphenylphosphonium cation is a similar electrophile that does more mitochondrial damage as lipophilic cations are accumulated in mitochondria by the $\Delta\psi_m$, the mitochondrial membrane potential (Ross et al., 2008). N-nitroso-N-benzyl-methylamine (NBzMA) is converted by CYPs to benzyl alcohol, which is not mutagenic, and benzyl carbonium cation (through hydroxylation of the methyl group), which is mutagenic. This indicates the cationic carbonium ion is the electrophile responsible for the benzylation of DNA and carcinogenesis associated with these compounds (Lin et al., 1990). The *Aristolochia* species (birthwort plants) contain aristolochic acids that are reduced by CYP1A1/2 or peroxidases in extrahepatic cells that have cyclic nitrenium ions as a highly reactive intermediate. These cationic electrophiles react with DNA and protein, activate the H-ras oncogene, cause gene mutation in kidney cells, and finally result in renal cancer (Zhou et al., 2007). As usual, CYPs and peroxidases appear to generate most of these reactive species, but glutathione transferases (GSTs—located in the cytosol and mitochondria; Raza, 2011) generate cationic electrophiles. The nematocide and soil fumigant 1,2-dibromo-3-chloropropane (DBCP) is also a mutagenic carcinogen in kidney and testes cells. Five metabolites that were products of glutathione conjugation by glutathione S-transferase were identified as S-(2,3-dihydroxy-propyl) glutathione, S-(2-hydroxypropyl)glutathione, S-(3-chloro-2-hydroxypropyl)glutathione, 1,3-di(S-glutathionyl)propan-2-ol, and 1-(glycyl-S-cysteinyl)-3-(S-glutathionyl)propan-2-ol.S-(2,3-dihydroxy-propyl)glutathione, S-(3-chloro-2-hydroxypropyl)glutathione, and 1-(glycyl-S-cysteinyl)-3-(S-glutathionyl)propan-2-ol were found to involve a cationic episulfonium ion intermediate (Pearson et al., 1990).

Metals are the most obvious cationic species, with the exception of the elemental forms of these compounds. The heavy metals are known to damage most cells, but especially where they are accumulated or biotransformed to more toxic electrophilic species. Because they may be bound to metallothionein in liver cells, hepatic damage may be avoided at lower concentrations and be concentrated instead in kidney cells. Mercury is an ever-present example of a ubiquitous heavy metal toxicant that damages kidney cells in the form of mercuric chloride. Unlike other toxicants that may synergize, the presence of the prooxidant metal selenium reduces the toxicity of the other heavy metal while at the same time increasing its concentration in liver, kidney, and brain cells. Mercury alone decreases superoxide dismutase (SOD) in liver and kidney cells and glutathione peroxidase (GPx) activity in hepatic cells, while increasing catalase activity in the liver and brain. Selenium causes a similar elevation of catalase activity (Agarwal and Behari, 2007). This is important, because the activity of catalase not only reflects the generation of reactive oxygen species (ROS), but also converts Hg(0) to Hg(II) and increases the uptake of mercury into the brain. Aminotriazole, an inhibitor of catalase, only reduced mercury uptake when injected directly by brain

cells. In an interesting counterpoint, liver cell accumulation of mercury increased with catalase inhibition, possibly reflecting its availability when not taken up into the brain (Eide and Syversen, 1983a). Of interest is the role of glutathione (GSH) and GPx in the uptake of Hg into brain cells. GSH depletion by diethyl maleate only marginally increases Hg uptake, while GPx inhibition by iodoacetate causes a much larger increase in mercury uptake (Eide and Syversen, 1983b).

Oxidation to a Free Radical—ROS

A simplified scheme for generation of ROS is indicated by the following:

O_2 (molecular oxygen) + e^- (one electron) → $O_2^{\bullet-}$ (superoxide anion radical)

$O_2^{\bullet-}$ + e^- + $2H^+$ (protons) → H_2O_2 (hydrogen peroxide)

H_2O_2 + e^- → $^{\bullet}OH$ (hydroxyl radical) + OH^- (hydroxide anion)

$OH + OH^- + e^- + 2H^+ → 2H_2O$

Note the overall picture of the development of these radicals in the cytosol and the mitochondria of the cell in **Figure 8-1**.

Each step that appears in the figure is examined more thoroughly here. The first step in this process is the generation of superoxide. Herbicides such as Paraquat (N,N′-dimethyl-4,4′-bipyridinium dichloride) and diquat, the antibiotic nitrofurantoin, and the cancer chemotherapy agent doxorubicin all generate superoxide following reductase action. This can happen spontaneously as is the case for Paraquat, which is known as methyl viologen. If this oxidation-reduction indicator is reduced by sodium hydrosulfite under alkaline conditions, it turns purple in a test tube. If the tube is shaken too vigorously in the analysis, the color disappears as superoxide is formed to the detriment of the Paraquat calibration curve. However, Paraquat and diquat do not damage the same cells. Paraquat is selectively taken up as if it were an endogenous diamine or polyamine by the lung cells and causes damage there irrespective of its administration, even though it is extremely hydrophilic (Smith, 1985). Diquat is more damaging to kidney cells despite its lower

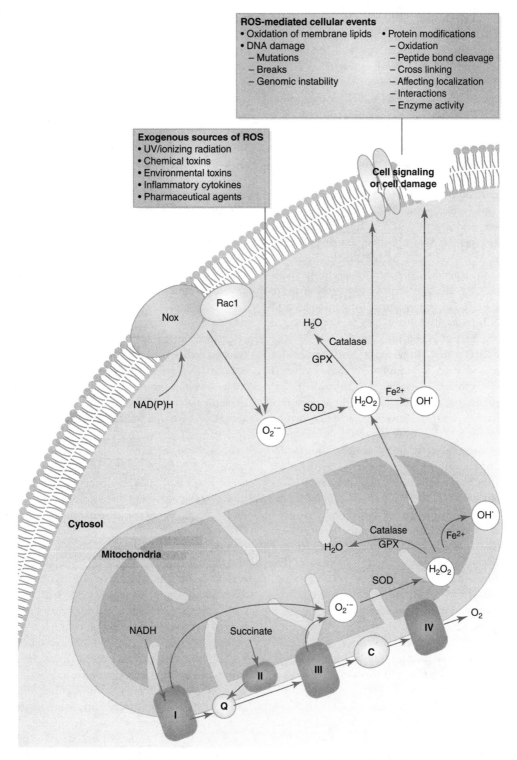

FIGURE 8-1 The Generation of ROS in the Cytosol and the Mitochondria and the Damage They Produce

Note: Nox = NADPH oxidase; Rac1 = Ras-related C3 botulinum toxin substrate 1 (rho family, small GTP binding protein Rac1); SOD = superoxide dismutase; GPx = selenium-dependent glutathione peroxidase.

K_m for one electron reduction by microsomes or mitochondria of lung, liver, or kidney cells, because it has a much shorter half-life in lung cells (Tomita, 1991). Note in Figure 8-1 that Rac1 can also stimulate nicotinamide adenine dinucleotide phosphate (NADPH) oxidase (Nox) activity that increases the redox cycling by Paraquat and similar agents. By itself, the superoxide radical is not as reactive as it appears, and it is trapped in the compartment where it was produced because its charge excludes it from crossing lipid membranes. It is produced during ischemia-reperfusion via the xanthine oxidase system and is also made by lipoxygenase and cyclooxygenase. Hydrogen peroxide is produced from superoxide as indicated in the figure by SOD and penetrates membranes more readily, serving as an intermediate for other more toxic ROS. The generation of hypochlorous acid (HOCl) from myeloperoxidase is not shown in the figure, but is generated in the peroxisomes of neutrophils. Superoxide and hypochlorous acid react spontaneously into hydroxyl radical, molecular oxygen, and chloride anion. Together, hydroxyl radical and hypochlorous acid are toxicants to invading bacteria. Further, in Figure 8-1, the Fenton reaction is shown in the generation of hydroxyl radical from oxidation of transition metals—Fe(II) → Fe(III) most likely reaction or Cu(I) → Cu(III) or Cr(V) → Cu(VI) or Ni(II) → Ni(III)—by hydrogen peroxide. The transition metals can then be reduced back by superoxide to finish the Haber-Weiss reaction cycle. If transition metals are stripped from the metalloproteins by superoxide, this is known as the *in vivo* Haber-Weiss reaction. Hydroxyl radical is the most reactive of the ROS with regard to macromolecules it contacts (Nordberg and Arnér, 2001). The generation of ROS leads to protective cell survival mechanisms in the cytoplasm at low levels, but high levels or production of ROS in the mitochondria lead to tumor necrosis factor-alpha (TNFα)-induced apoptosis.

As shown in **Figure 8-2**, the damage resulting in cell death is due to a number of factors. The damage is mediated in the cytosol by Nox and in the mitochondria by the electron transport chain (mETC). There is damage by Ca^{+2}-induced opening of the mitochondrial permeability transition (PT) pore, which is partially prevented by the 1,4-dihydropyridine derivative cerebrocrast, but not by diethone, gamma-pyrone, and glutapyrone (Fernandes et al., 2003). The outer mitochondrial membrane voltage–dependent anion channel (VDAC) and the inner membrane adenine nucleotide translocator (ANT) are part of the PT pore and, more importantly, are involved in the mitochondrial apoptosis pathway (Veenman et al., 2008). This transition to induced cell suicide is shown in part A of Figure 8-2 on the far right side.

Nanoparticles are new concerns for toxicology as nanotechnologies develop smaller, stronger fibers from materials such as titanium dioxide, which lead to ROS. These ROS cause, among other things, the activation of cytosolic caspase-3 and chromatin condensation that leads to apoptosis (Park et al., 2008). Greater damage to macromolecules in the cytosol, mitochondrial energy functions, and DNA in the nucleus results in necrosis.

Survival mechanisms utilizing ROS include the neutrophil protection against bacteria mentioned earlier or macrophage oxidative burst activation of nuclear factor kappa beta (NF-κB), activating protein-1 (AP-1), mitogen-activating protein kinase (MAPK), and phosphatidyl inositol-3 kinase (PI3K) pathways (Gwinn and Vallyathan, 2006). Another survival function is sensing oxygen, for example, via the stabilization of hypoxia-inducible factor-1 alpha (HIF-1α) that responds to hypoxia by induction of genes involved in anaerobic glycolysis and factors that increase blood vessel formation (vascular endothelial growth factor, or VEGF), vasodilation (inducible nitric oxide synthase, or iNOS), hemoglobin and red blood cell (RBC) formation, and tissue oxygenation (erythropoietin, or EPO; Taylor, 2008). The activation of hepatic heat shock transcription factor (HSF-1) is induced by ROS as a protective factor, but is also associated with the ethanol enhancement of hyperthermia associated with 3,4-methylenedioxymethamphetamine (MDMA; ecstasy). This interaction of ethanol and ecstasy also interferes with antioxidant enzyme function and induces NF-κB, indicating a pro-inflammatory effect (Pontes et al., 2008). This indicates that these signals may have survival functions or

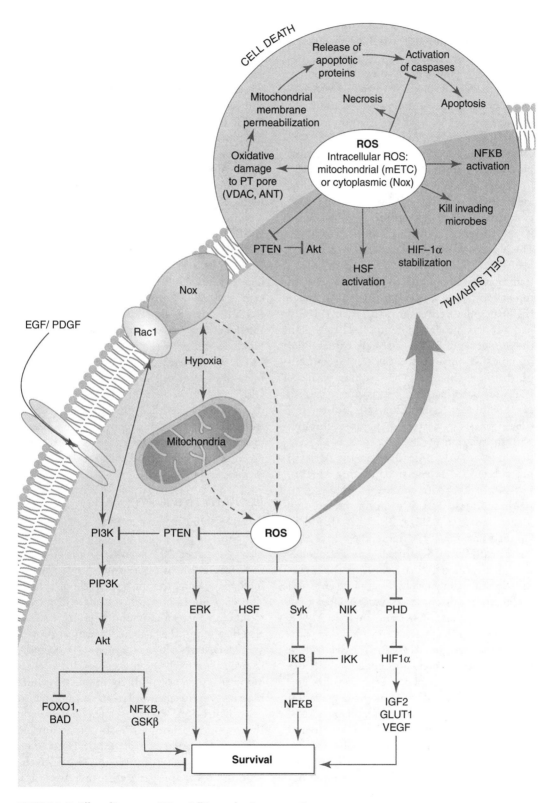

FIGURE 8-2 Effect of Increasing ROS on Cell Survival to Apoptosis to Necrosis

may indicate toxic damage that could lead to cell dysfunction and death. ROS or phosphorylation can lead to the downregulation of the activity of the phosphatase and tensin homolog (PTEN) protein. PTEN is the main negative regulator of the PI3K/Akt pathway. Because PI3K, as increased by the serine/threonine kinase Akt (also known as protein kinase B or PKB), catalyzes the formation of the second messenger phosphatidylinositol 3,4,5-trisphosphate (PIP3), it induces mechanisms involved in cell viability, metabolism, motility, and proliferation. However, this also has a downside as indicated by its role in cancer formation (Silva et al., 2008). These pathways are further delineated in part B of Figure 8-2. These are the pathways that lead to survival, but also to inflammation and tumor formation. The epidermal growth factor (EGF)/platelet-derived growth factor (PDGF) pathway acts through PI3K and Rac1 to Nox in the generation of ROS as discussed earlier. PIP3 as indicated previously is the second messenger that links the EGF/PDGF pathway with the PTEN regulated pathway. Akt is another a protein kinase that leads to survival, growth, and tumorigenesis by decreased apoptosis through phosphorylation of proteins such as FOXO1 (forkhead box O1), BAD (Bcl-2-associated death promoter), ASK1 (signal regulating kinase), FoxO4 (forkhead factor O4), and glycogen synthase kinase 3beta shown on the left side of the figure (GSK3beta; Zhong et al., 2008). On the right side of the figure, the role of HSF has already been described. The extracellular signal-regulated kinase (ERK) pathway is a MAP kinase mainly involved in cell survival and proliferation as opposed to stress-related c-*jun* N-terminal kinase (JNK) and the p38 MAPK that mediate inflammatory and apoptotic pathways (Kim, Jeong, et al., 2008). The Syk (spleen tyrosine kinase) protein is essential in the H_2O_2-induction of tyrosine phosphorylation of inhibitor kappa B (IκB), which leads the degradation of this inhibitory protein regulator of NF-κB. The NF-κB pathway, which is also stimulated by cytokines IL-1 and TNFα, lipopolysaccharides, and the human T-cell transactivator protein Tax, prevents apoptosis and immune/inflammatory cellular responses (Takaesu et al., 2003). Hydrogen peroxide appears to mediate

some of its influence via the NF-κB–inducing kinase (NIK) and lipopolysaccharide (LPS)-induced IκB kinase (IKK) activation. The antioxidant carotenoid, lutein, reduces H_2O_2 and NF-κB activation apparently at least partially through its inhibitory effect on LPS-induced IKK activation, IκB degradation, nuclear translocation of NF-κB, and binding of NF-κB to the κB motif of the iNOS promoter (Kim, Na, et al., 2008). Although the stabilization of HIF-1α has been linked to cell survival (as indicated earlier), its regulation through oxygen-dependent *trans*-4-hydroxylation of prolines by prolyl hydroxylase domain–containing proteins (PHD1, PHD2, and PHD3) has not been described earlier. Hypoxia or ROS (sometimes generated during hypoxia) inhibits PHD, which stabilizes HIF-1α (Yin et al., 2007). Insulin-like growth factor-2 (IGF2), glucose transporter-1 (GLUT1), and VEGF not only are survival mechanisms, but are highly expressed in tumors. HIF-1α's action on VEGF stimulates tumor angiogenesis; on IGF2 increases tumor cell survival; and on GLUT1, GLUT3, aldolase A and C, enolase 1, hexokinase 1 and 3, lactate dehydrogenase A, phosphofructokinase L, and phosphoglycerate kinase 1 promotes glucose transport and glycolysis that provides energy for rapidly dividing cancer cells (Semenza, 2002).

Oxidation to a Free Radical — RNS

Because ROS can serve to induce positive cell signaling or protection mechanisms, reactive nitrogen species (RNS) can act similarly at low concentrations. Nitrogen oxides play a key role in cell signaling; the nitrogen cycle of conversion of oxidized nitrogen (nitrate and nitrite) to ammonia gas or ammonium ion in water is also involved in the anabolic process or protein synthesis. Physiologically, nitric oxide (NO) is produced by NO synthase and decreases blood pressure, cell proliferation, extracellular matrix protein accumulation, mononuclear cell infiltration, and platelet degranulation through activation of the soluble guanylate cyclase and generation of cGMP. High levels of NO generated through iNOS affect the immune response, generate other free radicals or free radical damage, and other toxic nitrogen species (Wang-Rosenke et al., 2008).

To complicate the picture, high levels of NO can generate genotoxic lesions resulting in cancer initiation, promotion, and progression via stimulating angiogenesis, tumor cell growth, and invasion. Conversely, it can prevent colon cancer in mice via iNOS activation and its effect on immune function. This same dichotomy is observed in the function of macrophages and cancer. The generation of NO was observed to be an arginine-dependent function that disrupted mitochondrial respiration and iron metabolism, causing the mortality of neoplastic cells and bacteria. However, this generation of NO during infection increases endogenous nitrates, nitrites, and nitrosamines similar to that which occurs during cooking and metabolism of foods preserved with antimicrobial concentrations of nitrates and nitrites. This will generate more genotoxicity and cancer formation. Smog formation from air pollution is rich in intermediates such as NO, NO_2, and N_2O_3. These compounds deaminate nucleic acids and cause transitions similar to those found in p53 mutations in colon cancer, rather than the transversions caused by ROS and peroxynitrite. Lung cancers generated by smoking cigarettes generate both transitions and transversions in p53, indicating that oxidants in tar and RNS in smoke may be responsible for these mutations. However, RNS generate ROS that could also be responsible for the transversions. There appears to be an important interaction of iNOS and p53 in the generation/mortality of tumors. NO generation induces p53 and causes cell cycle arrest in normal cells but increased VEGF and tumor formation in the p53 mutants. The stabilization of HIF-1α mediated through PHD with reactive oxygen species may also be achieved through NO generation, leading to stimulation of VEGF expression and the induction of endothelial NOS (eNOS). This will generate low levels of NO, which stimulates angiogenesis and endothelial function. If NO is high, this may also kill tumor cells via DNA mutation/adduct formation and DNA repair disruption. NO or molecular oxygen sensitizes hypoxic mammalian solid tumors to ionizing radiation, as does iNOS gene therapy. However, eNOS knockout animals show decreased sensitivity to radiation. NO also sensitizes tumor cells to chemotherapeutic alkylating agents, partly due to nitrosation of critical thiols in DNA repair enzymes such as alkyltransferase (Wink et al., 2008).

Other Free Radical Species

Oxygen and nitrogen are not the only free radical species that yield toxicity and disease. Sulfur-centered free radicals (Løvaas, 1992), halogen free radicals, and carbon-free radical species (Lin et al., 2008) are examples of intermediates that further become cationic electrophiles or negatively charged nucleophiles. They also are used in chemical synthesis for polymerization reactions. It is this reactive property that makes these monomers very toxic and attach easily to macromolecules. Because many of these compounds are generated under oxidative conditions or as part of oxidation/reduction reactions, they are often lumped into the category of the oxygen radicals or oxygen radical reactions.

Nucleophiles

As a link to the previous section, certain nucleophiles such as phenols (or aminophenols) generate phenoxy radicals that are short-lived reactive intermediates that irreversibly yield the parent phenol and the reactive quinone methide (Omura, 2008). Aromatic amines also have a relatively weak N-H bond, so that aniline or secondary aromatic amines act as H donors in radical reactions, forming amine radical cations and aminyl radicals (Maroz et al., 2005). Similar reactions are possible for hydrazines, hydroquinones, phenothiazines, and thiols. The creation of a nucleophile is best represented by the formation of cyanide from amygdalin. D-amygdalin (D-mandelonitrile-β-D-gentiobioside) is treated from extracts of plant seeds (prunasin family) to detoxify foods or to create a cancer chemotherapy compound (formerly known as laetrile). *Armeniacae semen* has been used in the treatment of asthma, bronchitis, colorectal cancer, emphysema, leprosy, leucoderma, and pain. Amygdalin is found to induce apoptosis in prostate cancer cells via activation of caspace-3 activation through downregulation of Bcl-2 and upregulation of Bax. Bcl-2 is a suppressor of programmed cell death that homodimerizes with itself and forms heterodimers with a homologous protein Bax, which promotes cell death (Chang et al., 2006). The cleavage of amygdalin occurs via beta-glucosidase (EC 3.2.1.117 used to increase toxicity of amygdalin to cancer cells; Syrigos et al., 1998) of bacteria, fungi, termites, or plants and is enhanced by the presence of pharmacological doses of ascorbic acid (vitamin C, which also depletes cysteine stores that detoxify cyanide; Bromley et al., 2005).

Carbon monoxide (CO) is a nucleophilic species that is very important to toxicity of aerobic organisms and is a well-known toxicant to humans in confined spaces when using incomplete combustion for heating, cooking, and so forth. It is generated by heme oxygenase in metabolic syndrome experienced by obese Zucker rats and subsequently inhibits NO synthase, increases hypertension, and causes endothelial dysfunction (Johnson et al., 2006). However, carboxidotrophic bacteria such as *Oligotropha carboxidovorans* have adapted to live on "coal gas" via oxidation and fixation utilizing the Wood-Ljungdahl pathway with the molybdenum-containing iron-sulfur flavoprotein CO dehydrogenase (EC 1.2.99.2; $CO + H_2O \rightarrow CO_2 + 2e^- + 2H^+$; Dobbek et al., 1999) and acetyl-CoA synthase (EC 6.2.1.13) as the key enzymes (Ragsdale, 2004).

A nutritional example of a nucleophile is the formation of selenomercaptans (selenol) from selenium. Selenols are stronger acids than other mercaptans that exist at physiological pH as the anionic nucleophile—as opposed to sulfhydryls, which predominate as the protonated form (Reddy and Massaro, 1983).

Active Redox States

Most discussions of redox states focus on the compounds rather than the cell. A different and more toxicological approach is found in the response of central nervous system progenitor cells to small changes in redox state/oxidation. Environmentally relevant concentrations of methylmercury, lead, and Paraquat show that the redox/Fyn/c-Cbl pathway is a good model for the impact of an increased oxidative state on cellular functions. Relatively small changes

in the redox state of the cell (oxidation) result in activation of Fyn kinase (nonreceptor tyrosine kinase Src family located on the growth cones and postsynaptic membranes of neurons that may phosphorylate nicotinic acetylcholine receptors). This causes a secondary activation of the c-Cbl ubiquitin ligase, which leads to reductions in c-Cbl target platelet-derived growth factor receptor-α and other c-Cbl targets. This does not affect the TrkC receptor tyrosine kinase, which is not a c-Cbl target. This is important, because c-Cbl enzyme targets modify specific receptor proteins that are necessary to promote mitosis and cell survival. If these are degraded during this oxidative change in the redox state of the cell, this initiates the degradation of the receptors, disrupting their downstream signaling functions (Zaibo et al., 2007). The use of quantitative, real-time polymerase chain reaction (qRT PCR) has shown that those changing the redox state via oxidant stress unregulate 28 genes in common in DNA microarrays of the isogenic (cloned) rainbow trout *Oncorhynchus mykiss* for diquat and benzo[a]pyrene. Each compound tested—ethynylestradiol (xeno-estrogen), 2,2,4,4′-tetrabromodiphenyl ether (BDE-47, thyroid active), chromium(VI), and trenbolone (anabolic steroid/model androgen)—had its own fingerprint, sharing genes in common to their toxicity such as CYPs, steroid synthesis pathways, and estrogen-responsive genes (Hook et al., 2006). This means that the effects of compounds on various states of the cell may be quantifiable and categorized in a more precise manner in the future.

The discussion of electrophiles has a caveat, however. Whether the electrophile is neurotoxic or neuroprotective is determined by the cell's response. Neurotoxicity results from a decrease in the total reductive capacity/redox state of the cell by compounds such as doxorubicin and menadione. Neuroprotective actions occur via launching a counterattack by increasing essential cellular redox factors such as reduced glutathione and inducing the expression of phase-2 enzymes, such as NAD(P)H:quinone oxidoreductase and heme oxygenase-1, often through the Keap1–Nrf2 transcription factor pathway against weak electrophiles such as *tert*-butyl hydroquinone and neurite outgrowth-promoting prostaglandin compounds (Satoh and Lipton, 2007).

Currently, knowing the chemistry of redox states is valuable information in predicting toxicant action. The preceding discussions of electron-deficient electrophiles to free radicals and the important nucleophiles have made it clear that the most destructive molecules are unstable molecular fragments such as free radicals, followed by electrophiles, and some nucleophiles. A quantitative structure–activity relationship between metals and their toxicity in rodents became apparent primarily based on their electrode potential, when factors such as energy levels, redox potentials, free energies of formation, and ionic and covalent radii were collated for more than 30 metals as shown in **Figure 8-3** (Lewis et al., 1999). However, the mechanism of toxicity of those compounds and organic compounds in their various redox states is not so clearly defined as just the electrode potential. For example, redox cycling appears to be the major route through which chromium, cobalt, copper, iron, and vanadium achieve their

toxic endpoint, while cadmium, mercury, and nickel deplete cellular glutathione levels and bind to sulfhydryl moieties of proteins. Arsenic appears to bind to thiols and generate oxidative damage via H_2O_2 formation (Valko et al., 2005). More specifically, As(III) versus As(V) shows that the As(V) metalloid has the identical structure and acid dissociation constants as phosphate and is able to substitute for this molecule. Although both forms will substitute for nitrogen or phosphorus groups and perform oxidationreduction reactions, only the As(III) form with electron-rich groups binds to proteins (Carter et al., 2003). So, as useful as the quantitative structure–activity model is to determine overall toxicity risk, specific mechanisms of damage still rely on the study of the response of organisms to increasing doses of a variety of formulations and oxidation states of that compound.

Cellular Damage and Adaptation Mechanisms

Covalent Binding to Macromolecules

The binding of chemicals to macromolecules can result in necrotic injury or cancer initiation if covalent bonds form with DNA. For example, the administration of benzoquinol-glutathione conjugate to rats causes necrosis of the S_3 segment of renal proximal tubule cells. This is suspected to be a result of the oxidation of the quinol to the quinone and covalent binding to macromolecules in the cells. Administration of the 2-methyl-3-(*N*-acetylcystein-*S*-yl)-1,4-naphthoquinone caused necrosis, while 2-methyl-3-(glutathion-*S*-yl)-1,4-naphthoquinone did not. 2-(Glutathion-*S*-yl)-1,4-naphthoquinone and 2,3-(diglutathion-*S*-yl)-1,4-naphthoquinone had weak toxicity to these cells, implicating the *N*-acetylcysteine conjugate as the toxic species. Similarly, acetaminophen, carbamazepine, diclofenac, indomethacin, nefazodone, sudoxicam, and tienilic acid demonstrated covalent binding *in vitro* with hepatic cells consonant with their hepatotoxicity. However, buspirone, diphenhydramine, meloxicam, paroxetine, propranolol, raloxifene, and simvastatin

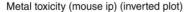

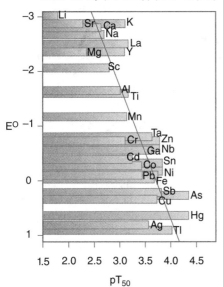

FIGURE 8-3 Correlation between Acute (Ip) Toxicity (pT_{50}) in the Mouse and Metal or Ion Redox Potential (E°) for 30 Metals Based on the Equation: Mouse $pT_{50} = 0.41$ (+ 0.05)E° + 3.72

indicated covalent binding, but are not viewed as hepatotoxins. Benoxaprofen and felbamate are hepatotoxic, but do not result in covalent binding, while ibuprofen and theophylline do not show covalent binding and are not hepatotoxic. Covalent binding intrinsic clearance offers no better solution, as paroxetine has the highest covalent binding to microsomes yet is not hepatotoxic.

A better but not perfect model predicting hepatotoxic compounds results when the total fraction of metabolism causing covalent binding and the daily dose of the compound are considered (Obach et al., 2008). Not only is it important to know the chemical species that causes the formation of a covalent link, but also the protein it adducts. This can be tested by highly reactive electrophilic (biotin) tagged species such as 1-biotinamido-4-(4'-[maleimidoethylcyclohexane]-carboxamido) butane (BMCC) and N-iodoacetyl-N-biotinyl-hexylenediamine (IAB). When adducts are identified by liquid chromatography-tandem mass spectrometry, BMCC and IAB identified 376 microsomal cysteine thiol targets in 263 proteins. BMCC formed adducts with 223 proteins, while IAB covalently bound to 243 proteins. Both formed the most adducts with the endoplasmic reticulum ($\geq$ 31%), followed by the cytoplasm ($\geq$ 25%), and the mitochondria ($\geq$ 20%), with the remainder associated with the nuclear, peroxisomal, lysosomal, or plasma membrane or Golgi apparatus. Only approximately 25% of these targets/proteins were in common to both electrophiles. One of those shared targets is the microsomal glutathione-S-transferase cysteine 50 that is adducted by the toxic acetaminophen metabolite N-acetyl-p-benzoquinoneimine. Targets shared in common to the two electrophiles are functions of the endoplasmic reticulum (ER), such as drug metabolism (CYP, GST, and UGT enzymes), ion transport (SERCA2), and protein folding (calreticulin). However, the interesting part is that the iodoacetamide-like electrophile IAB alone induced stress of the ER as indicated by activation of BiP, a prosurvival ER member of the Hsp 70 family of protein chaperones. The binding of the ER resident chaperone Bip/GRP78 to unfolded or misfolded proteins in the ER lumen dissociates BiP from and activates the proteins PERK, ATF6, and IRE1, and initiates the ER stress response. This results in a downregulation of protein translation and upregulation of transcription of ER stress response genes. Other stress pathways are also activated. Reactive electrophiles, such as IAB, activate this ER stress pathway, which appears to determine whether necrotic reactions will occur versus adaptive survival mechanisms. In neurodegenerative diseases, the S-nitrosylation of ER proteins is thought to induce ER stress that mediates the toxic response (Shin et al., 2007).

Depletion of Glutathione (GSH)

Glutathione is a tripeptide composed of cysteine, glutamate, and glycine that plays a prominent role in protection against cellular oxidation, maintains the redox state of cells, and participates in cellular signaling pathways. GSH is synthesized in the cytosol via the first rate-limiting step of γ-glutamylcysteine synthetase, followed by addition of the glycine via GSH synthetase, and in the process utilizing the energy of two adenosine triphosphates (ATPs). γ-Glutamylcysteine synthetase is negative feedback regulated by GSH concentrations, which turn over based on its efflux, utilization, and transport within the cell. Hepatocytes export GSH into the plasma, which is stimulated by uncharged thiols such as dithiothreitol and inhibited intracellular by disulfides such as cystine, oxidized glutathione (GSSG), or extracellular methionine. Rat hepatocytes use the organic transporter, OAT1, to exchange organic anions for GSH in a disulfide-sensitive, electrically neutral but thiol-insensitive fashion. Multidrug-resistant proteins, particularly Mrp2, appear to mediate the efflux of half of the GSH into the bile though glutathione S-conjugates of xenobiotics. When approximately 75% of GSH is rapidly exported from human Jurkat T lymphocytes, HepG2 cells, or rat hepatocytes, this stimulates the Fas-induced apoptosis pathway through increasing oxidative stress. The small mitochondrial pool of GSH anion occurs due to the exchange for P_i^{2-} and matrix 2-oxoglutarate via the dicarboxylate carrier and 2-oxoglutarate carrier, respectively. This transport is reduced by changing the fluidity of the mitochondrial membrane through chronic excess cholesterol or ethanol administration. The GSH/GSSG reducing couple is at 100- to ~10,000-fold more than $NADP^+$/NADPH and thioredoxin ($TrxSS$/$Trx(SH)_2$), which keep the cell sufficiently (not oxidized) but not excessively (as in hypoxia) reduced. The Nernst equation, $\Delta E = E_0 - (RT/nF)\ln Q$ at 25°C and pH 7 where $Q = \log([GSH][GSH])/[GSSG]$, indicates that the redox potential of the cell generated from the reaction $GSH + GSH \leftrightarrow GSSG + 2H^+$ is a function both of the reduced GSH concentration of ~10.0 mM hepatic or ~1.0 mM neuronal and the ratio of reduced to oxidized glutathione. This indicates that the redox state of the cell could be altered by consuming GSH without altering the GSH/GSSG ratio. Not only does GSH help protect against ROS and reactive chemical species through conjugation in the cytosol, it also reduces hydrogen peroxide in the mitochondria of hepatic cells as aided by peroxiredoxins-thioredoxin2 (no catalase present in these mitochondria). GSH keeps protein sulfhydrils reduced, which affects their function and signaling pathways. GSH reacts rapidly with sulfenic acids (S—OH), which forms reversibly as a cysteine oxidation product, along with disulfides (—S—S—). This prevents the irreversible oxidation to sulfinic acids ($S—O_2H$) and sulfonic acids ($S—O_3H$).

Following oxidation or other radical-induced injury, will the death state of the cell yield apoptosis or necrosis? High concentrations of compounds that deplete cellular GSH, such as acetaminophen, diethyl maleate, or phorone have induced necrosis of hepatic cells. Lower doses of the same compounds or addition of TNFα have produced apoptosis instead. What is the role of TNFα in this process? Macrophages make substantial TNFα in response to inflammatory reactions or infection, hypoxic injury resulting in ischemia, oxidative stress, and exposure to toxic substances. There is a receptor to this cytokine on the hepatocyte surface, TNFR1, which triggers the TNFR1-DD (death domain) to form complex I with mediators TNFR-associated death domain (TRADD), receptor-interacting protein 1 (RIP1) and TNFR-associated factor 2 (TRAF2). NF-κB, c-jun

N-terminal kinase (JNK), and P38 cascades are activated by complex I to induce inflammation but promote survival. TRADD, RIP, and TRAF2 dissociate from TNFR1-DD and associate with Fas-associated death domain-containing protein (FADD), whose death-effector domain recruits procaspase 8 to be cleaved into caspase 8. FADD can also be activated by the binding of FasL on T lymphocytes to Fas, causing trimerization of Fas. Fas forms death-induced signal complex (DISC) with FADD and procaspase 8. In some extrahepatic cells, apoptosis originates in the cytosol from caspase 8 cleavage of procaspase 3. In hepatocytes, the mitochondria must be signaled via the lysis of Bid to tBid. Mitochondrial membrane permeability is increased by pro-apoptotic members of the Bcl-2 homology, Bax, and Bak, activated by tBid. Cytochrome c is then released from the mitochondrial intermembrane space, where it forms apoptosome with Apaf-1 and procaspase 9. The self-cleavage of procaspase 9 to caspase 9 helps form the true apoptosis executioner by cleaving procaspase 3 into caspase 3. It appears that TNFα and cytochrome c play the key role in inducing apoptosis rather than the more damaging effects of necrosis that occur when the cell is not given to chance to activate these pathways in time to mediate the toxic impact. The reason the cell may not have the machinery left to induce apoptosis is that ROS and RNS may oxidize the caspases as may other inhibitors of these essential enzymes, or ATP may be depleted too far to provide energy for the intensive process of apoptosis.

When does glutathione depletion yield less severe results? This requires a further inspection of the earlier formation of complex I via NF-κB, JNK, and P38 activation. Survival gene expression is induced by activation of NF-κB. When 50% of GSH is depleted by diethyl maleate in hepatocytes, the mitochondria are usually fine and the generation of ROS is not a particular problem. NF-κB is no longer activated by TNF with moderate GSH depletion as indicated by the lack of expression of downstream anti-apoptotic genes such as iNOS, cIAP1, and $cFLIP_L$, but activation of IKK, NF-κB nuclear translocation, and p50/p65 DNA binding remain unchanged. At 80% GSH depletion, IKK activation is inhibited due to the prevention of the polyubiquitination of RIP1, but can be restored with an antioxidant such as Trolox.

However, this severe GSH depletion and ROS generation will not allow restoration of NF-κB transcriptional activity. Regarding JNK, NF-κB can attenuate its response until sustained pressure by more severe damage and release of TNF activates JNK leading to cell death. JNK activates upstream mitochondrial apoptotic/death pathways via the ubiquitin ligase Itch and cleavage of Bid. Itch releases the inhibition of caspase 8 by ubiquitination of cFLIP_L. Similarly, the inhibition of caspase 8 can also be relieved by cleavage of Bid to jBid, which releases Smac to inhibit IAP. IAP inhibition prevents the deactivation of caspase 8. Sustained action on JNK by concanavalin A induction of TNFα release from T cells results in severe hepatic cell death. Formation of ROS appears extremely important in the sustained stimulation of JNK, as the antioxidant butylated hydroxyanisole (BHA) appears to prevent its activation. This sustained action of ROS may be mediated through the ASK1/Trx pathway or just by direct inactivation of JNK phosphatases, which will then leave JNK in its activated phosphorylated state. On the other hand, a transient stimulatory phosphorylation of JNK results in hepatic cell proliferation as occurs following partial liver removal through activation of cyclin D1 and the stimulation of DNA synthesis through a G0 to G1 transition (Yuan and Kaplowitz, 2008).

GSH depletion is also important in cells other than hepatocytes, as demonstrated by the human neurodegenerative diseases of Parkinson's disease and incidental Lewy body disease, which have close to half of the GSH depleted compared with healthy subjects (Zeevalk et al., 2008).

Lipid Peroxidation and Redox Cycling

Because the formation of ROS, RNS, and other free radical species has already been covered, it is unnecessary to reiterate that information. Note in **Figure 8-4** how a redox cycling reaction occurs that generates superoxide. The radical species is created in this example by superoxide, which generates hydrogen peroxide and the anion radical. Another superoxide species

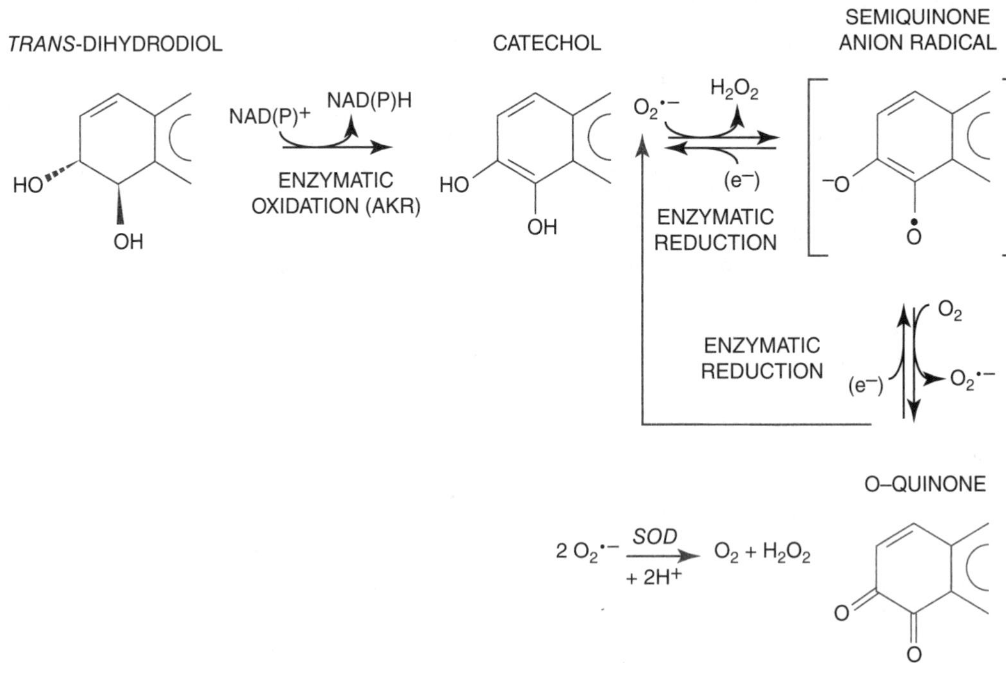

FIGURE 8-4 Catechol-Quinone Redox-Cycling and Dismutation of Superoxide to Hydrogen Peroxide toward the Formation of Hydroxyl Radical

is generated and so on unless an antioxidant such as d-α-tocopherol (vitamin E) or superoxide dismutase converts the superoxide to peroxide. Unfortunately, hydrogen peroxide plus superoxide generates a hydroxyl radical in the presence of a transition metal (Fenton reaction). The free radicals can form covalent bonds with each other and other molecules (e.g., protein [Negre-Salvayre et al., 2008] and DNA [Goetz and Luch, 2008]).

Another revolving chain of reactions occurs when oxygen radical species encounter lipid present in the membranes of the cell such as the ER. This process, known as lipid peroxidation, generates a chain reaction of reactive species—especially in conjunction with polyunsaturated fatty acids (PUFA). As shown in **Figure 8-5**, the generation of hydroperoxides and endoperoxides from PUFA may fragment into reactive intermediates such as alkanals, alkenals, hydroxyalkenals, hydroxynonenal, and malondialdehyde. These products have been used to assess lipid peroxidation by visible spectroscopy as thiobarbituric acid reactive substances (TBARS; not a specific indicator without other measures), UV spectroscopy as conjugated dienes, chemiluminescence and iodometric analysis as lipid hydroperoxides, and gas chromatography (GC) or high pressure liquid chromatography (HPLC) or immunoassay of aldehydes, alkanes, and isoprostanes. Approximately 2–3% of cellular oxygen consumption results in free radicals that can cause lipid peroxidation that may be part of normal aging processes (Praticò, 2002). Oxidation of *n*-6 PUFAs (omega-6 fatty acids such as linoleic and arachidonic acid components of many animal-derived food sources) leads to degradation products such as 4-hydroxynonenal, whereas oxidation of *n*-3 PUFAs (omega-3 fatty acids such as docosahexaenoic acid, eicosapentaenoic acid, and linolenic acid that may originate from salmon, tuna, halibut, algae, krill, and certain plants and nut oils) leads to 4-hydroxyhexenal formation (Negre-Salvayre et al., 2008). Lipid peroxidation products' reactivity lead to protein and DNA adducts as well, which increase on lower antioxidant protection as occurs during glutathione depletion (4-hydroxy-2[*E*]-nonenal and DNA damage; Falletti and Douki, 2008).

Amino acid residues that are susceptible to electrophilic attack by 4-hydroxynonenal are histidine, cysteine, and lysine, forming a stable Michael adduct with a hemiacetal structure. A Schiff base adduct may be formed with the primary amine of a lysine residue, or Michael addition may occur with the amino groups of

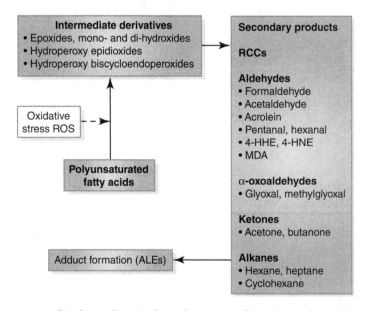

FIGURE 8-5 Schematic Steps of Lipid Peroxidation Leading to the Formation of Secondary Products and ALEs

lysine or histidine or the thiol group of a cysteine (or glutathione) by 4-hydroxyhexenal. Some of the proteins modified have a critical role to play in disease. The formation of foam cells and atherosclerotic lesions result from the oxidation of low density lipoprotein (LDL) and the subsequent modification of the receptor for LDL, apoB/E. Modification of tyrosine kinase receptors leads at low concentrations of lipid peroxidation products to growth enhancement of cells and at high concentrations to growth inhibition. Growth enhancement appears to occur due to modification of the tyrosine kinase receptor, which leads to enhanced autophosphorylation and the stimulation of the downstream ERK1/2 phosphorylation and cell cycle progression pathway. High concentrations of reactive lipid peroxidation products such as 4-hydroxynonenal appear to inhibit growth factor receptors EGFR and PDGFR. Following concentrations exceeding 10 µM, oxidized LDL or 4-hydroxynonenal caused a progressive desensitization of PDGFRβ to its own ligand PDGF-BB in smooth muscle cells. These toxic lipid peroxidation products at lower concentrations may stimulate cell survival mechanisms as appears to occur via induction of the expression of antioxidant genes (e.g., heme oxygenase, thioredoxine-1) through stimulation of the mitogen-activated protein kinase pathway and transcription factor Nrf2. The NF-κB signaling pathway for regulation of inflammatory reactions, cell survival, and proliferation appears to be inhibited by acrolein or 4-hydroxynonenal (4-HNE) or conversely activated by aldehydes produced by lipid peroxidation leading to inflammation. Acrolein and 4-HNE activate the phosphorylation of transcription factors c-jun involved in apoptosis and CRE-binding protein that mediates survival. Conversely, they inhibit the activity of the CREB-responsive promoters while augmenting c-jun responsive promoter. This series of events lead to neuronal cell degeneration and apoptosis.

Because lipid peroxidation products appear to play a role in cancer and cardiovascular, inflammatory, and neurodegenerative diseases, inhibitors have been developed to deal with some of these products. These include amino acid derivatives (especially histidine, cysteine, and methionine), angiotensin-converting enzyme inhibitors, AT1 angiotensin receptor inhibitor, antioxidants, hydrazines, and pyridoxal (vitamin B6) derivatives (Negre-Salvayre et al., 2008). As shown in **Figure 8-6**, DNA damage is possible by ROS themselves, which foreshadows damage to nuclear material. This is important for the cytosolic damage done to prokaryotic organisms as they have no nucleus. The toxic α,β-unsaturated aldehydes lipid peroxidation products mentioned earlier (i.e., 4-HNE) are seen to cause the formation of low amounts of cyclic adducts of DNA, such as (1-hydroxyhexyl)-8-hydroxy-1, N^2-propano-2'-deoxyguanosine (HNE-dGuo) without the addition of any pro-oxidant compound. Usually, GSH concentrations are high enough to result in ~80% of the 4-HNE metabolism, with the rest oxidized to the primary alcohol or carboxylic acid. As lipid peroxidation increases, the cellular survival rate of cells such as monocytes decreases as HNE-dGuo adducts increase. This is not just a function of the cell content of GSH, as the addition of the GSH synthesis inhibitor buthionine sulfoximine results in a 75% drop in GSH without a statistically significant fall in viability (Falletti and Douki, 2008).

Cell Rupturing and Repair

The process of rupture and repair is part of a process called wound healing. A number of cell signaling functions are involved in the process, but it may be disrupted by toxicants. Intestinal cells must lay down collagen III to repair physical damage. The signaling cascade is initiated by sphingosine-1-phosphate and mediated by the nuclear translocation of FHL2, which is a four-and-a-half LIM domain protein involved in tissue repair function regulation such as cell adhesion, cytoarchitecture, gene expression, migration, and signal transduction (Kirfel et al. 2008). Toxicants that cause fibrosis may cause different less elastic forms of collagen to be laid down and may also cause excess cell proliferation and increased damage, leading to cancer formation. For example, injured mesothelial cells also release growth factors that mediate cell proliferation,

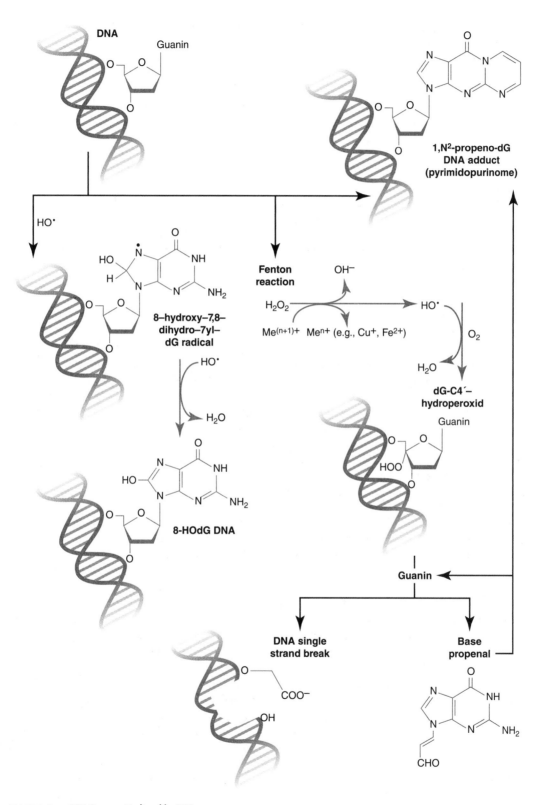

FIGURE 8-6 DNA Damage Mediated by ROS

migration, and extracellular matrix synthesis, including TGF-β, platelet-derived growth factor, fibroblast growth factor, and hepatocyte growth factor as mediated by members of the epidermal growth factor families (Mutsaers et al., 1997). These cells synthesize collagen types I, III, and potentially IV; elastin; fibronectin; and laminin and organize these components into extracellular matrix. Mesothelial cells secrete matrix metalloproteinases and tissue inhibitors of metalloproteinases to regulate turnover of the extracellular matrix (Mutsaers, 2004). Mutagenic/carcinogenic cigarette smoke stimulates formation of matrix metalloproteinase-1 and tissue inhibitors of metalloproteinase-1 mRNA, while reducing tissue inhibitors of metalloproteinase-2 and type I collagen mRNA expression in rat lungs. Chrysotile asbestos or alumina silicate ceramic fibers increased the expression of matrix metalloproteinase-1 mRNA expression. The asbestos fiber plus cigarette smoke generated the highest expression of matrix metalloproteinase-1 mRNA (Morimoto et al., 1997). Arsenic interferes with wound healing in lung cells via induction of metalloproteinase-9, whose inhibitor GM6001 improves healing (Olsen et al., 2008). Asbestos also damages via ROS that induce various clastogenic activities. ROS play a role in abnormal wound healing (Schäfer and Werner, 2008) and stimulate tumorigenic conversion and progression in asbestos and related foreign body–stimulated toxicities (Okada, 2007). Asbestos also stimulates the ERK cascade to proliferate mesothelial cells (Zanella et al., 1996). In a syngenic mouse breast cancer model of enhanced tumor growth, T cells secrete cytokines and/or growth factors in response to acute wounding that increase tissue repair and stimulate residual tumor enlargement (Stuelten et al., 2008). Thus, it appears that both toxicants and wound repair mechanisms lead to untoward outcomes in cells.

Starting Apoptosis or Necrosis by Calcium — Cell Signaling following Damage

Ca^{2+} is an important second messenger for many cells. Calcium concentrations are stochastic or pulse events that increase via external entry through voltage- and ligand-gated Ca^{2+} channels in the plasma membrane and from internal stores from the endoplasmic reticulum. Significant Ca^{2+} concentrations are not found in the mitochondria, as this would stimulate apoptosis. Depletion of Ca^{2+} stores from the endoplasmic reticulum by cholesterol has been shown to be a mediator of cell death through apoptosis. Ca^{2+} is the primary stimulant for opening the mitochondrial permeability transition pore. As the mitochondrial membrane potential ($\Delta\Psi_m$) collapses due to pore opening and rupture of the outer mitochondrial membrane, the role of Ca^{2+} in inducing a perturbation cannot be underestimated. It is by these means that oxidized LDL appears to induce apoptosis in macrophages (Deng et al., 2008). The mechanism for the release of intracellular stores of Ca^{2+} appears to involve the inositol 1,4,5-triphosphate (IP_3) receptors and the ryanodine receptors. IP_3 receptors are large tetramers that are dependent both on the presence of IP_3 and the free cytosolic Ca^{2+} concentrations, with up to 500 nM calcium leading to opening of the channel synergistically with IP_3 and higher concentrations being inhibitory. The construction and biphasic response to Ca^{2+} concentrations of ryanodine receptors is similar to that of the IP_3 receptors. Both have the calcium-activated calcium release and the negative feedback at high concentrations that prevent calcium toxicity and cause a rapid oscillation in conjunction with Ca^{2+}-ATPase pumps, unless extended by cholecystokinin. The IP_3 receptors have three isoforms with functional redundancy, while the ryanodine receptors are expressed in distinct patterns and exhibit differing gating mechanisms. Type 2 cardiac ryanodine receptors are distinctly activated by external calcium concentrations, as opposed to Type 1 skeletal muscle ryanodine receptors that function in the intact muscle based on protein–protein interactions. The complex regulation of these channels by a large number of accessory proteins is important in understanding cell physiology and toxicology. Multiple signal transduction pathways appear to intersect at these receptors, with factors such as Brc-2 and phosphorylation of the channels by protein kinase A altering their functional state. Because apoptosis appears to be mainly a mitochondria-mediated event, the calcium transporters there must be considered: a Ca^{2+} uniporter and a Na^+/Ca^{2+} exchanger (Thul et al., 2008). The application of this information to cellular toxicity is dependent on the toxic species formed, the type of cell, and the degree of damage induced. For example, the trichloromethyl radical, CCl_3, is formed from dechlorination of carbon tetrachloride by CYPs. This toxic chemical species in hepatic cells is more likely to bind to nucleic acids, proteins, and lipids, causing disruptions in lipid metabolism or steatosis and adduct formation leading to hepatocarcinomas. When CCl_3 reacts with oxygen, it forms the trichloromethylperoxy radical CCl_3OO. This reactive oxidative species forms lipid peroxides that increase the permeability of plasma, endoplasmic reticulum, and mitochondrial membranes, resulting in a loss of cellular calcium sequestration and homeostasis. This is one event that has a direct bearing on apoptotic or necrotic events. Reactive lipid peroxidation products such as aldehydes inhibit critical enzyme activities. The toxicity of carbon tetrachloride leads to inhibition of both protein synthesis and lipoprotein secretion by inducing hypomethylation. CCl_4 also stimulates the activation of TNFα (an apoptosis promoter), nitric oxide, and transforming growth factors alpha and beta (fibrosis promotion) in the cell. Cytokines IL-6 induced by TNFα and IL-10 appear to reverse the action of TNFα as antiapoptotic factors (Weber et al., 2003).

Despite the presence of apoptotic and survival mechanisms present in hepatic cells, most hepatotoxins induce necrosis. The alkylation of vital macromolecules and/or generation of oxidative stress disrupt calcium homeostasis before lysis of the plasma membrane. Compromised mitochondria produce less ATP, leading to less activity of the plasma membrane Ca^{2+}-ATPase. Calcium-dependent endonucleases catalyze double-stranded breaks in DNA prior to cell lysis. Because these biochemical pathways are similar between necrosis and apoptosis, it is the extracellular and intracellular control points that mark the difference between an orderly cell death of apoptosis mediated by newly synthesized proteins in an energy-intensive fashion

or the random wholesale destruction of necrosis leading to damage of surrounding cells and inflammation (Kedderis, 1996). Apoptosis is marked at the start by shrinkage of the cytoplasm and nuclear condensation followed by aggregation of chromatin, membrane blebbing, formation of membrane-bound vesicles, and leaky mitochondria induced by Bcl-2 pore formation, and it ends with cell fragmentation into smaller bodies. Necrosis is initiated by swelling of the cytoplasm and mitochondria and subsequently exhibits loss of membrane integrity, no vesicle formation, and disintegration of organelles, and it ends with total cell lysis.

Protein Synthesis Inhibition

If the rough endoplasmic reticulum is considered in this section, then protein synthesis inhibitors' mechanisms should be considered. The target of many antibacterials is the bacterial ribosome, composed of 30S and 50S subunits composed of rRNA and protein. Aminoglycoside antibiotics bind to the 30S subunit at the A site as do the tetracyclines. The antibacterial effect of aminoglycosides appears to allow noncognate tRNAs to incorporate their amino acids into the growing polypeptide chain thus "misreading" the mRNA. The oxazolidinone antibiotics bind to the 23S rRNA present within the 50S subunit, preventing the binding of initiator tRNA from binding to the P site. Chloramphenicol also prevents protein synthesis in bacteria by binding to the 50S subunit as well and has less influence on eukaryotic protein synthesis. Clindamycin binds in very close proximity to chloramphenicol and erythromycin. Macrolide and ketolide antibiotics similarly affect protein synthesis by 50S binding. Inhibition of aminoacyl-tRNA synthetases also provides a way of stopping protein synthesis. Alternatively, inhibiting the aminoacylation reaction is one mechanism utilized by the aminoglycosides for preventing bacterial protein synthesis. Aminoglycosides also bind to the T box region that is a 14-nucleotide conserved sequence that is involved in the binding of specific noncharged tRNAs in gram-positive bacteria (Thomas and Hergenrother, 2008).

Eukaryotic protein synthesis inhibitors focus on the treatment of cancer. Most were developed prior to the late 1970s and represent the translation inhibitors used in research labs such as didemnin B, cephaeline, bouvardin, baccharinol, bruceantin, verrucarin, anisomycin, homoharringtonine, emetine, sparsomycin, and especially puromycin. Phyllanthoside and nagilactone C inhibit protein synthesis exclusively in eukaryotic cells, with an IC_{50} of ~0.4 µM and 3 µM for phyllanthoside and nagilactone C, respectively, for incorporation of ^{35}S-methionine into HeLa cells. *E. coli* were unaffected by these two agents. Cycloheximide, phyllanthoside, and nagilactone C appear to inhibit chain elongation. A nonhydrolyzable GTP analogue, GMP-PNP, inhibits initiation by preventing the joining of the 60S ribosome subunit as well as release of eIF2. This prevents protein synthesis by halting the formation of 80S initiation complexes and traps a 40S ribosome on the mRNA template. Homoharringtonine alternatively prevents reinitiating of ribosomes. Anisomycin interferes with protein synthesis by stalling ribosomes on mRNA templates. Other protein synthesis inhibitors may be classified by their ability to bind to nucleic acids (e.g., doxorubicin, etoposide), poison cytoskeletal formation (e.g., vinca alkaloids, paclitaxel), or by various other mechanisms or unknown (of which phyllanthoside and nagilactone C were members prior to more intensive study; Chan et al., 2004). More disruptions in protein synthesis can occur via nuclear events.

Antidotes

Antidotal therapy should involve three possible mechanisms—limiting absorption, increasing excretion, and raising the threshold for toxicity. This relates well to the concentration-versustime curve generated to follow the toxicokinetics of the chemical and the response of the organism during that time curve. Cells already provide much of their own antidotal protection through absorption barriers, pumps that confer resistance to toxic substances, cellular synthesized antioxidants, and signaling pathways that increase the chances of cellular survival. There are two types of antidotes in each category. A nonspecific antidote will not depend on the specific toxicant, while a specific antidote is related to the structure and effects of the toxicant. Both are discussed in each of the following sections.

Decreasing Absorption

At the cellular level, there is no way of using activated charcoal, vomiting, or other gastrointestinal responses to prevent absorption. Providing other targets to bind or inactivate toxicants may reduce the absorption of the compound in a nonspecific or specific manner. A nonspecific method may be the use of a protein such as albumin to bind up the toxicant and make it too large to transport into the cell or acid–base neutralization. Also eliminated are the more extreme gastrointestinal-specific treatments with oxidizing agents such as potassium permanganate to treat ingested strychnine or nicotine. The key nonspecific treatments available would be changing the pH of the extracellular fluid within parameters that do not cause more injury and infusion of a fatty acid emulsion for toxicity due to anesthetic agents and other hydrophobic chemicals (Turner-Lawrence and Kerns 2008).

Some of the newest specific antidotes to prevent absorption were begun with development of antibodies to toxic components of snake venom and cardiac glycosides, such as digitalis (digoxin immune Fab; Scherrmann et al., 1989), and have since been developed for low-molecular-weight toxicants (Baud et al., 1997). Another specific approach is to provide a biological scavenger for the toxicant externally to the cell, such as the use of human serum butyrylcholinesterase for the protection against organophosphorus compounds (Saxena et al., 2006). Other more traditional approaches to preventing absorption include producing a less toxic complex such as excess iron from vitamins with mineral overdose that may be treated with sodium bicarbonate–producing ferrous carbonate or the iron chelator desferrioxamine. Another example is treading the photograph-developing agent silver nitrate with sodium chloride to become silver chloride, and so on. However, this is not the only way of preventing the increase in the toxic product in the cell. Binding up the toxic agent, enzyme inhibitors, or competition may serve the purpose in these cases. For example, cyanide will not bind to hemoglobin, but it does bind to oxidized hemoglobin known as methemoglobin. Some sodium nitrite will produce the correct amount of methemoglobin to bind up the cyanide without a major reduction in pO_2 that is required for aerobic mitochondrial energy production through oxidative phosphorylation. This is an interesting example, because cyanide would also prevent oxidative phosphorylation via binding to cytochrome a_3, part of the terminal cytochrome c oxidase (Hill et al., 1983). Thiosulfate can also be used as an antidote to cyanide by producing the thiocyanate complex. Examples of competition include ethanol, which can be used to compete for alcohol dehydrogenase with methanol to prevent the formation of formic acid and instead make the less toxic acetaldehyde. The use of acetate, Monoacetin or acetamide competes with fluoroacetate (used to control the feral fox population) for mitochondrial transport and reduced toxicity in other domestic animals such as the dog or the cat (Goh et al., 2005). However, it is not as easy as it sounds to give these antidotes, because there are concerns regarding calcium depletion and severe acidosis that is exacerbated by Monoacetin antidotal therapy for fluoroacetate poisoning (Taitelman et al., 1983).

Increasing Elimination

In this case, the nonspecific methods involve hemodialysis or hemoperfusion, exchange transfusion, adjusting the pH and diuresis, or peritoneal dialysis in intact higher organisms (Goldberg et al., 1986). However, in cellular environments adjusting the pH or a fluid treatment system might work, but other specific methods make more sense here. Clearly, anything that enhances renal excretion— such as chloride or bromide or calcium for strontium or radium poisoning—is for higher organisms. Chelators, on the other hand, are very likely good agents for use in organisms and environments. Ethylenediamine tetra-acetic acid with the structure, $(HOOCH_2C)_2\text{-}NCH_2$ $CH_2N\text{-}(CH_2COOH)$, is a strong chelating agent, especially for Cu(II), Co(III), and

Fe(III), but it has an affinity for calcium, lead, mercury, and nickel. British antilewisite (BAL), known also as dimercaprol, is a chelator for arsenic, mercury, and gold, especially, but also serves to complex antimony, bismuth, chromium, and nickel. Dimethylmercury is better served by chelation by N-acetyl cysteine or D-penicillamine. The combination of nutritional supplementation with Se worked better against the organic form of mercury in combination with N-acetyl cysteine, as did Mg with D-penicillamine (Singh et al., 2007). Again, this is not as easy as it sounds, because delayed treatment for organic mercury poisoning still results in neural cell death as occurred with an accidental tragic exposure of a human (Nierenberg et al., 1998). D-penicillamine has also been used in Wilson's disease as a copper chelator, where an abnormality in ATP-linked Cu transport, incorporation into ceruloplasmin, and excretion from the liver cells into the bile does not occur, and copper accumulation results in liver cirrhosis and extrahepatic accumulation of copper that causes neural cell degeneration (Aoki, 2005). Emergency rooms also have an antibody to botulinum toxin due to problems with contaminated food, misinjected doses of the toxin for medical treatments, and concerns about bioterrorism (Betten et al., 2006).

Increasing Cellular/Organism Threshold

In the intact higher organism, artificial respiration, renal dialysis to maintain filtering during acute renal failure, and other life-saving equipment make possible the raising of the threshold for toxicity in ways not directly specific to the toxin and its effects. Electrolyte balance is another way of increasing the threshold that also works for cells. Antagonism of receptors/binding sites is the most prevalent way of raising the threshold followed by alternative pathways. *The Wizard of Oz* provides an excellent example of this, where the little girl Dorothy, her dog Toto, and the cowardly lion all succumbed to the toxicant in the opium poppy because they had opioid receptors, and the tin man and scarecrow of course did not. Naloxone is the preferred antidote to opioid overdose, because it binds to all the receptors and antagonizes the action of opium and its derivatives. Similarly, people in cold climates use incomplete combustion to heat their houses and run their automobiles, which often causes carbon monoxide poisoning. As carbon monoxide binds > 200 (reported from 200–245) times stronger than oxygen to hemoglobin, hyperbaric oxygen is used to compete for hemoglobin in severely poisoned individuals (Prockop and Chichkova, 2007). Unless the carboxyhemoglobin concentrations are assessed immediately, the COHb level in the blood is not the best assessment of clinical outcome by the time the patient is brought to a treatment center (Hampson and Hauff, 2008). This is also true of a cell, because how fast and long a cell has spent time with the toxicant may best determine its viability. Similarly, organophosphate poisonings are treated with the muscarinic cholinergic receptor antagonist atropine and oximes to reactivate acetylcholinesterase. However, the central nervous system activation by these poisons may also require prevention of sympathetic outflow through use of alpha-2 presynaptic adrenergic agonist (negative feedback mechanism) as well as a GABAergic (inhibitory neurotransmitter) central nervous system (CNS) agonist such as diazepam that inhibits other CNS functions (Peter et al., 2008). Atropine may also be given for excess nicotine ingestion or patch use and help overstimulated neural and muscle cells (Rogers et al., 2004). Conversely, d-tubocurarine acts as an inhibitor of nicotinic receptors in neuromuscular transmission and must be antagonized by inhibitors of acetylcholinesterase, such as neostigmine or edrophonium (Narimatsu et al., 1999). Antagonists are excellent ways of combating receptor-mediated toxic effects on cells, but alternative pathways may also be necessary to reverse untoward effects. Methotrexate is used to treat leukemias, other cancer cells, and rheumatoid arthritis via inhibition of dihydrofolate reductase, but may require reduced folate known as leucovorin or folinic acid to come to the aid of normal cells (Comandone et al., 2005). Other compounds that treat cancer cells also require similar "rescues" of normal cells, such as the use of thymidine to alter the effects of inhibition of thymidine monophosphate synthesis

by 5-fluorouracil (its metabolite fluorodeoxyuridine monophosphate inhibits thymidylate synthase; Thomas and Zalcberg, 1998) or the use of purine for substitution when 6-mercaptopurine inhibits the first step in the *de novo* synthesis of the purine base (through accumulation of its metabolite 6-thioinosine-5′-monophosphate; Worthley, 2002). In clinical toxicology settings, the use of nonspecific ventilation to keep proper oxygenation of tissues and cells is vital for most poisonings, with the exceptions being those that generate oxygen radicals in the lung cells such as Paraquat.

Specific antidotes or alternative pathways are important, but not many of the intensive care units of hospitals stock more than the following remedies: N-acetylcysteine, atropine, botulism antitoxin, calcium gluconate and chloride, Crotaline snake antivenom, cyanide antidote kit, deferoxamine, digoxin immune Fab, ethanol, flumazenil, fomepizole, glucagon, methylene blue, naloxone, octreotide, physostigmine, phytonadione, pralidoxime, pyridoxine, and sodium bicarbonate (Betten et al., 2006). Because this text has covered many of these agents, try to figure out what they treat, what cells would benefit the most, and whether they represent mainly nonspecific or specific remedies for absorption, excretion, and raising the threshold. Also, it is informative to consider how many other mechanisms of toxic action may be missed by this limited group of compounds. Poison control centers provide information that usually assumes ingestion rather than cellular protective mechanisms that toxicologists must be able to provide through research.

Questions

1. What is an electrophile, and which nucleophile is most reactive? How are these most reactive electrophiles formed from an enzyme that usually protects against reactive intermediates? Conversely, what is a nucleophile?

2. Indicate how the generation of superoxide leads to the generation of other oxygen radicals.

3. If NO is a normal signaling molecule for immune function, why might an infection yield cancer?

4. How is the Fyn kinase signaling pathway involved in the effect of changes in redox state of certain cells?

5. What are the main targets of covalent binding that occurs from metabolic activation?

6. How does GSH depletion lead to cell death?

7. How do lipid peroxidation products lead to cell degeneration and apoptosis? What are three mechanisms of DNA damage done by ROS/lipid peroxidation products?

8. How do wound healing mechanisms lead to fibrosis and/or cell proliferation?

9. Why does disruption of calcium storage in the cell, such as in the ER, lead to cell death?

10. Give examples of specific and nonspecific antidotes for the three methods of preventing toxicity.

References

Aoki T. 2005. Genetic disorders of copper transport—diagnosis and new treatment for the patients of Wilson's disease [in Japanese]. *No To Hattatsu*. 37:99–109.

Agarwal R, Behari JR. 2007. Role of selenium in mercury intoxication in mice. *Ind Health*. 45:388–395.

Anders MW. 2004. Glutathione-dependent bioactivation of haloalkanes and haloalkenes. *Drug Metab Rev*. 36:583–594.

Azad MB, Chen Y, Gibson SB. 2008. Regulation of autophagy by reactive oxygen species (ROS): implications for cancer progression and treatment. *Antioxid Redox Signal*. 11(4):777–790.

Baud FJ, Borron SW, Scherrmann JM, Bismuth C. 1997. A critical review of antidotal immunotherapy for low molecular weight toxins. Current antidotes and perspectives. *Arch Toxicol Suppl*. 19:271–287.

Benov L, Sequeira F, Beema AF. 2004. Role of rpoS in the regulation of glyoxalase III in Escherichia coli. *Acta Biochim Pol*. 51:857–860.

Betten DP, Vohra RB, Cook MD, Matteucci MJ, Clark RF. 2006. Antidote use in the critically ill poisoned patient. *J Intensive Care Med*. 21:255–277.

Bromley J, Hughes BG, Leong DC, Buckley NA. 2005. Life-threatening interaction between complementary medicines: cyanide toxicity following ingestion of amygdalin and vitamin C. *Ann Pharmacother*. 39:1566–1569.

Camp HB, Fukuto TR, Metcalf RL. 1969. Toxicity of isopropyl parathion. Metabolism in the housefly, honey bee, and white mouse. *J Agric Food Chem*. 17:249–254.

Carter DE, Aposhian HV, Gandolfi AJ. 2003. The metabolism of inorganic arsenic oxides, gallium arsenide, and arsine: a toxicochemical review. *Toxicol Appl Pharmacol*. 193:309–334.

Chan J, Khan SN, Harvey I, Merrick W, Pelletier J. 2004. Eukaryotic protein synthesis inhibitors identified by comparison of cytotoxicity profiles. *RNA*. 10:528–543.

Chang HK, Shin MS, Yang HY, Lee JW, Kim YS, Lee MH, Kim J, Kim KH, Kim CJ. 2006. Amygdalin induces apoptosis through regulation of Bax and Bcl-2 expressions in human DU145 and LNCaP prostate cancer cells. *Biol Pharm Bull*. 29:1597–1602.

Comandone A, Passera R, Boglione A, Tagini V, Ferrari S, Cattel L. 2005. High dose methotrexate in adult patients with osteosarcoma: clinical and pharmacokinetic results. *Acta Oncol*. 44:406–411.

Cooney RV, Pung A, Harwood PJ, Boynton AL, Zhang LX, Hossain MZ, Bertram JS. 1992. Inhibition of cellular transformation by triphenylmethane: a novel chemopreventive agent. *Carcinogenesis*. 13(7):1107–12.

Denekamp C, Yaniv M. 2006. Benzene loss from trityl cations—a mechanistic study. *J Am Soc Mass Spectrom*. 17:730–736.

Deng T, Zhang L, Ge Y, Lu M, Zheng X. 2008. Redistribution of intracellular calcium and its effect on apoptosis in macrophages: induction by oxidized LDL. *Biomed Pharmacother*. 63(4):267–274.

Dobbek H, Gremer L, Meyer O, Huber R. 1999. Crystal structure and mechanism of CO dehydrogenase, a molybdo iron-sulfur flavoprotein containing S-selanylcysteine. *Proc Natl Acad Sci USA*. 96: 8884–8889.

Eide I, Syversen TL. 1983a. Relationship between catalase activity and uptake of elemental mercury by rat brain. *Acta Pharmacol Toxicol (Copenh)*. 52:217–223.

Eide I, Syversen TL. 1983b. Uptake of elemental mercury by brain in relation to concentration of glutathione and activity of glutathione peroxidase. *Toxicol Lett*. 17:209–213.

Ehling S, Hengel M, Shibamoto T. 2005. Formation of acrylamide from lipids. *Adv Exp Med Biol*. 561:223–233.

Falletti O, Douki T. 2008. Low glutathione level favors formation of DNA adducts to 4-hydroxy-2 (E)-nonenal, a major lipid peroxidation product. *Chem Res Toxicol*. 21(11):2097–2105.

Fernandes MA, Santos MS, Vicente JA, Moreno AJ, Velena A, Duburs G, Oliveira CR. 2003. Effects of 1,4-dihydropyridine derivatives (cerebrocrast, gammapyrone, glutapyrone, and diethone) on mitochondrial bioenergetics and oxidative stress: acomparative study. *Mitochondrion*. 3:47–59.

Fischer V, West PR, Harman LS, Mason RP. 1985. Free-radical metabolites of acetaminophen and a dimethylated derivative. *Environ Health Perspect*. 64:127–137.

Glascott PA Jr, Gilfor E, Serroni A, Farber JL. 1996. Independent antioxidant action of vitamins E and C in cultured rat hepatocytes intoxicated with allyl alcohol. *Biochem Pharmacol*. 52:1245–1252.

Goetz ME, Luch A. 2008. Reactive species: a cell damaging rout assisting to chemical carcinogens. *Cancer Lett*. 266:73–83.

Goh CS, Hodgson DR, Fearnside SM, Heller J, Malikides N. 2005. Sodium monofluoroacetate (Compound 1080) poisoning in dogs. *Aust Vet J*. 83:474–479.

Goldberg MJ, Spector R, Park GD, Roberts RJ. 1986. An approach to the management of the poisoned patient. *Arch Intern Med*. 146:1381–1385.

Gwinn MR, Vallyathan V. 2006. Respiratory burst: role in signal transduction in alveolar macrophages. *J Toxicol Environ Health B Crit Rev*. 9:27–39.

Ha MH, Wei L, Rao HY, Liu F, Wang XY, Feng B, Fei R, Chen HS, Cong X. 2008. Effect of interferon-gamma on hepatic stellate cells stimulated by acetaldehyde. *Hepatogastroenterology*. 55:1059–1065.

Hampson NB, Hauff NM. 2008. Carboxyhemoglobin levels in carbon monoxide poisoning: do they correlate with the clinical picture? *Am J Emerg Med*. 26:665–669.

Hewitt WR, Miyajima H, Côté MG, Plaa GL. 1980. Modification of haloalkane-induced hepatotoxicity by exogenous ketones and metabolic ketosis. *Fed Proc*. 39:3118–3123.

Hill BC, Brittain T, Eglinton DG, Gadsby PM, Greenwood C, Nicholls P, Peterson J, Thomson AJ, Woon TC. 1983. Low-spin ferric forms of cytochrome a3 in mixed-ligand and partially reduced cyanide-bound derivatives of cytochrome c oxidase. *Biochem J*. 215:57–66.

Hook SE, Skillman AD, Small JA, Schultz IR. 2006. Gene expression patterns in rainbow trout, *Oncorhynchus mykiss*, exposed to a suite of model toxicants. *Aquat Toxicol*. 77:372–385.

Johnson FK, Johnson RA, Durante W, Jackson KE, Stevenson BK, Peyton KJ. 2006. Metabolic syndrome increases endogenous carbon monoxide production to promote hypertension and endothelial dysfunction in obese Zucker rats. *Am J Physiol Regul Integr Comp Physiol*. 290:R601–R608.

Jung R, Beermann D, Glatt HR, Oesch F. 1981. Mutagenicity of structurally related oxiranes: derivatives of benzene and its hydrogenated congeners. *Mutat Res*. 81:11–19.

Kedderis GL. 1996. Biochemical basis of hepatocellular injury. *Toxicol Pathol*. 24:77–83.

Kim JH, Na HJ, Kim CK, Kim JY, Ha KS, Lee H, Chung HT, Kwon HJ, Kwon YG, Kim YM. 2008. The non-provitamin A carotenoid, lutein, inhibits NF-kappaB-dependent gene expression through redox-based regulation of the phosphatidylinositol 3-kinase/PTEN/Akt and NF-kappaB-inducing kinase pathways: role of H(2)O(2) in NF-kappaB activation. *Free Radic Biol Med*. 45:885–896.

Kim SJ, Jeong HJ, Myung NY, Kim MC, Lee JH, So HS, Park RK, Kim HM, Um JY, Hong SH. 2008. The protective mechanism of antioxidants in cadmium-induced ototoxicity in vitro and in vivo. *Environ Health Perspect*. 116:854–862.

Kirfel J, Pantelis D, Kabba M, Kahl P, Röper A, Kalff JC, Buettner R. 2008. Impaired intestinal wound healing in Fhl2-deficient mice is due to disturbed collagen metabolism. *Exp Cell Res*. 314(20):3684–3691.

Kobayashi M, Nagasawa T, Yamada H. 1992. Enzymatic synthesis of acrylamide: a success story not yet over. *Trends Biotechnol*. 10:402–408.

Lewis DFV, Dobrota M, Taylor MG, Parke DV. 1999. Metal toxicity in two rodent species and redox potential: evaluation of quantitative structu-reactivity relationships. *Environ Toxicol Chem*. 18:2199–2204.

Lin CY, Coote ML, Gennaro A, Matyjaszewski K. 2008. Ab initio evaluation of the thermodynamic and electrochemical properties of alkyl halides and radicals and their mechanistic implications for atom transfer radical polymerization. *J Am Chem Soc*. 130:12762–12774.

Lin DX, Malaveille C, Park SS, Gelboin HV, Bartsch H. 1990. Contribution of DNA methylation and benzylation to N-nitroso-N-benzyl-methylamine-induced mutagenesis in bacteria: effects of rat liver cytochrome P450 isozymes and glutathione transferases. *Carcinogenesis*. 11:1653–1658.

Lin GH, Brusick DJ. 1992. Mutagenicity studies on two triphenylmethane dyes, bromophenol blue and tetrabromophenol blue. *J Appl Toxicol*. 12:267–274.

Low TY, Leow CK, Salto-Tellez M, Chung MC. 2004. A proteomic analysis of thioacetamide-induced hepatotoxicity and cirrhosis in rat livers. *Proteomics*. 4:3960–3974.

Løvaas E. 1992. Free radical generation and coupled thiol oxidation by lactoperoxidase/SCN-/H_2O_2. *Free Radic Biol Med*. 13:187–195.

Lu X, Rodríguez M, Gu W, Silverman RB. 2003. Inactivation of mitochondrial monoamine oxidase B by methylthio-substituted benzylamines. *Bioorg Med Chem*. 11:4423–4430.

LoPachin RM, Gavin T, Geohagen BC, Das S. 2007. Neurotoxic mechanisms of electrophilic type-2 alkenes: soft soft interactions described by quantum mechanical parameters. *Toxicol Sci.* 98:561–570.

Maroz A, Hermann R, Naumov S, Brede O. 2005. Ionization of aniline and its N-methyl and N-phenyl substituted derivatives by (free) electron transfer to n-butyl chloride parent radical cations. *J Phys Chem A.* 109:4690–4696.

Morimoto Y, Tsuda T, Nakamura H, Hori H, Yamato H, Nagata N, Higashi T, Kido M, Tanaka I. 1997. Expression of matrix metalloproteinases, tissue inhibitors of metalloproteinases, and extracellular matrix mRNA following exposure to mineral fibers and cigarette smoke in vivo. *Environ Health Perspect.* 105(Suppl 5):1247–1251.

Mutsaers SE. 2004. The mesothelial cell. *Int J Biochem Cell Biol.* 36:9–16.

Mutsaers SE, McAnulty RJ, Laurent GJ, Versnel MA, Whitaker D, Papadimitriou JM. 1997. Cytokine regulation of mesothelial cell proliferation in vitro and in vivo. *Eur J Cell Biol.* 72:24–29.

Mutsaers SE, Bishop JE, McGrouther G, Laurent GL. 1997. Mechanisms of tissue repair: from wound healing to fibrosis. *Int J Biochem Cell Biol.* 29:5–17.

Negre-Salvayre A, Coatrieux C, Ingueneau C, Salvayre R. 2008. Advanced lipid peroxidation end products in oxidative damage to proteins. Potential role in diseases and therapeutic prospects for the inhibitors. *Br J Pharmacol.* 153:6–20.

Narimatsu E, Nakayama Y, Sumita S, Iwasaki H, Fujimura N, Satoh K, Namiki A. 1999. Sepsis attenuates the intensity of the neuromuscular blocking effect of d-tubocurarine and the antagonistic actions of neostigmine and edrophonium accompanying depression of muscle contractility of the diaphragm. *Acta Anaesthesiol Scand.* 43:196–201.

Nierenberg DW, Nordgren RE, Chang MB, Siegler RW, Blayney MB, Hochberg F, Toribara TY, Cernichiari E, Clarkson T. 1998. Delayed cerebellar disease and death after accidental exposure to dimethylmercury. *N Engl J Med.* 338:1672–1676.

Nordberg J, Arnér ES. 2001. Reactive oxygen species, antioxidants, and the mammalian thioredoxin system. *Free Radic Biol Med.* 31:1287–1312.

Obach RS, Kalgutkar AS, Soglia JR, Zhao SX. 2008. Can in vitro metabolism-dependent covalent binding data in liver microsomes distinguish hepatotoxic from nonhepatotoxic drugs? An analysis of 18 drugs with consideration of intrinsic clearance and daily dose. *Chem Res Toxicol.* 21:1814–1822.

Okada F. 2007. Beyond foreign-body-induced carcinogenesis: impact of reactive oxygen species derived from inflammatory cells in tumorigenic conversion and tumor progression. *Int J Cancer.* 121:2364–2372.

Olsen CE, Liguori AE, Zong Y, Lantz RC, Burgess JL, Boitano S. 2008. Arsenic upregulates MMP-9 and inhibits wound repair in human airway epithelial cells. *Am J Physiol Lung Cell Mol Physiol.* 295:L293–L302.

Omura K. 2008. Electron transfer between protonated and unprotonated phenoxyl radicals. *J Org Chem.* 73:858–867.

Park EJ, Yi J, Chung KH, Ryu DY, Choi J, Park K. 2008. Oxidative stress and apoptosis induced by titanium dioxide nanoparticles in cultured BEAS-2B cells. *Toxicol Lett.* 180:222–229.

Praticò D. 2002. Lipid peroxidation and the aging process. *Sci Aging Knowledge Environ.* 2002:re5.

Pearson PG, Soderlund EJ, Dybing E, Nelson SD. 1990. Metabolic activation of 1,2-dibromo-3-chloropropane: evidence for the formation of reactive episulfonium ion intermediates. *Biochemistry.* 29:4971–4981.

Peter JV, Moran JL, Pichamuthu K, Chacko B. 2008. Adjuncts and alternatives to oxime therapy in organophosphate poisoning—is there evidence of benefit in human poisoning? A review. *Anaesth Intensive Care.* 36:339–350.

Pontes H, Duarte JA, de Pinho PG, Soares ME, Fernandes E, Dinis-Oliveira RJ, Sousa C, Silva R, Carmo H, Casal S, Remião F, Carvalho F, Bastos ML. 2008. Chronic exposure to ethanol exacerbates MDMA-induced hyperthermia and exposes liver to severe MDMA-induced toxicity in CD1 mice. *Toxicology.* 252:64–71.

Preussmann R. 1978. [Environmental carcinogens: mechanisms of action and occurrence. Some aspects (author's transl)]. *Zentralbl Bakteriol* [Orig B]. 166:144–158.

Prockop LD, Chichkova RI. 2007. Carbon monoxide intoxication: an updated review. *J Neurol Sci.* 262:122–130.

Ragsdale SW. 2004. Life with carbon monoxide. *Crit Rev Biochem Mol Biol.* 39:165–195.

Raza H. 2011. Dual localization of glutathione S-transferase in the cytosol and mitochondria: implications in oxidative stress, toxicity and disease. *FEBS J.* 278:4243–4251.

Reddy CC, Massaro EJ. 1983. Biochemistry of selenium: a brief overview. *Fundam Appl Toxicol.* 3:431–436.

Rogers AJ, Denk LD, Wax PM. 2004. Catastrophic brain injury after nicotine insecticide ingestion. *J Emerg Med.* 26:169–172.

Ross MF, Prime TA, Abakumova I, James AM, Porteous CM, Smith RA, Murphy MP. 2008. Rapid and extensive uptake and activation of hydrophobic triphenylphosphonium cations within cells. *Biochem J.* 411:633–645.

Satoh T, Lipton SA. 2007. Redox regulation of neuronal survival mediated by electrophilic compounds. *Trends Neurosci.* 30:37–45.

Saxena A, Sun W, Luo C, Myers TM, Koplovitz I, Lenz DE, Doctor BP. 2006. Bioscavenger for protection from toxicity of organophosphorus compounds. *J Mol Neurosci.* 30:145–148.

Schäfer M, Werner S. 2008. Oxidative stress in normal and impaired wound repair. *Pharmacol Res.* 58:165–171.

Scherrmann JM, Terrien N, Urtizberea M, Pierson P, Denis H, Bourre JM. 1989. Immunotoxicotherapy: present status and future trends. *J Toxicol Clin Toxicol.* 27:1–35.

Semenza GL. 2002. HIF-1 and tumor progression: pathophysiology and therapeutics. *Trends Mol Med.* 8(4 Suppl):S62–S67.

Shin NY, Liu Q, Stamer SL, Liebler DC. 2007. Protein targets of reactive electrophiles in human liver microsomes. *Chem Res Toxicol.* 20:859–867.

Silva A, Yunes JA, Cardoso BA, Martins LR, Jotta PY, Abecasis M, Nowill AE, Leslie NR, Cardoso AA, Barata JT. 2008. PTEN posttranslational inactivation and hyperactivation of the PI3K/Akt pathway sustain primary T cell leukemia viability. *J Clin Invest.* 118(11):3762–3774.

Singh V, Joshi D, Shrivastava S, Shukla S. 2007. Effect of monothiol along with antioxidant against mercury-induced oxidative stress in rat. *Indian J Exp Biol.* 45:1037–1044.

Skibo EB, Xing C. 1998. Chemistry and DNA alkylation reactions of aziridinyl quinones: development of an efficient alkylating agent of the phosphate backbone. *Biochemistry.* 37:15199–151213.

Smith LL. 1985. Paraquat toxicity. *Philos Trans R Soc Lond B Biol Sci.* 311:647–657.

Stuelten CH, Barbul A, Busch JI, Sutton E, Katz R, Sato M, Wakefield LM, Roberts AB, Niederhuber JE. 2008. Acute wounds accelerate tumorigenesis by a T cell-dependent mechanism. *Cancer Res.* 68:7278–7282.

Stiborová M, Miksanová M, Havlícek V, Schmeiser HH, Frei E. 2002. Mechanism of peroxidase-mediated oxidation of carcinogenic o-anisidine and its binding to DNA. *Mutat Res.* 500:49–66.

Syrigos KN, Rowlinson-Busza G, Epenetos AA. 1998. In vitro cytotoxicity following specific activation of amygdalin by beta-glucosidase conjugated to a bladder cancer-associated monoclonal antibody. *Int J Cancer.* 78:712–719.

Taitelman U, Roy A, Raikhlin-Eisenkraft B, Hoffer E. 1983. The effect of monoacetin and calcium chloride on acid-base balance and survival in experimental sodium fluoroacetate poisoning. *Arch Toxicol Suppl.* 6:222–227.

Takaesu G, Surabhi RM, Park KJ, Ninomiya-Tsuji J, Matsumoto K, Gaynor RB. 2003. TAK1 is critical for IkappaB kinase-mediated activation of the NF-kappaB pathway. *J Mol Biol.* 326:105–115.

Taylor CT. 2008. Mitochondria and cellular oxygen sensing in the HIF pathway. *Biochem J.* 409:19–26.

Testai E, De Curtis V, Gemma S, Fabrizi L, Gervasi P, Vittozzi L. 1996. The role of different cytochrome P450 isoforms in in vitro chloroform metabolism. *J Biochem Toxicol.* 11:305–312.

Thomas DM, Zalcberg JR. 1998. 5-fluorouracil: a pharmacological paradigm in the use of cytotoxics. *Clin Exp Pharmacol Physiol.* 25:887–895.

Thomas JR, Hergenrother PJ. 2008. Targeting RNA with small molecules. *Chem Rev.* 108:1171–1224.

Thomas RD, Green MR, Wilson C, Sadrud-Din S. 2004. Diallyl sulfide inhibits the oxidation and reduction reactions of stilbene estrogens catalyzed by microsomes, mitochondria and nuclei isolated from breast tissue of female ACI rats. *Carcinogenesis.* 25:787–791.

Thul R, Bellamy TC, Roderick HL, Bootman MD, Coombes S. 2008. Calcium oscillations. *Adv Exp Med Biol.* 641:1–27.

Tomita M. 1991. Comparison of one-electron reduction activity against the bipyridylium herbicides, paraquat and diquat, in microsomal and mitochondrial fractions of liver, lung and kidney (*in vitro*). *Biochem Pharmacol.* 42:303–309.

Turner-Lawrence DE, Kerns W II. 2008. Intravenous fat emulsion: a potential novel antidote. *J Med Toxicol.* 4:109–114.

Vachálková A, Novotný L, Blesová M. 1996. Polarographic reduction of some triphenylmethane dyes and their potential carcinogenic activity. *Neoplasma.* 43:113–117.

Valko M, Morris H, Cronin MT. 2005. Metals, toxicity and oxidative stress. *Curr Med Chem.* 12:1161–1208.

Veenman L, Shandalov Y, Gavish M. 2008. VDAC activation by the 18 kDa translocator protein (TSPO), implications for apoptosis. *J Bioenerg Biomembr.* 40:199–205.

Walker GS, Atherton J, Bauman J, Kohl C, Lam W, Reily M, Lou Z, Mutlib A. 2007. Determination of degradation pathways and kinetics of acyl glucuronides by NMR spectroscopy. *Chem Res Toxicol.* 20:876–886.

Wang QS, Hou LY, Zhang CL, Song FY, Xie KQ. 2008. Changes of cytoskeletal proteins in nerve tissues and serum of rats treated with 2,5-hexanedione. *Toxicology.* 244:166–178.

Wang-Rosenke Y, Neumayer HH, Peters H. 2008. NO signaling through cGMP in renal tissue fibrosis and beyond: key pathway and novel therapeutic target. *Curr Med Chem.* 15:1396–1406.

Weber LW, Boll M, Stampfl A. 2003. Hepatotoxicity and mechanism of action of haloalkanes: carbon tetrachloride as a toxicological model. *Crit Rev Toxicol.* 33:105–136.

Wink DA, Ridnour LA, Hussain SP, Harris CC. 2008. The reemergence of nitric oxide and cancer. *Nitric Oxide*. 19:65–67.

Worthley LI. 2002. Clinical toxicology: part II. Diagnosis and management of uncommon poisonings. *Crit Care Resusc*. 4:216–230.

Yin L, Kharbanda S, Kufe D. 2007. Mucin 1 oncoprotein blocks hypoxia-inducible factor 1alpha activation in a survival response to hypoxia. *J Biol Chem*. 282:257–266.

Yuan L, Kaplowitz N. 2008. Glutathione in liver diseases and hepatotoxicity. *Mol Aspects Med*. 30(1–2):29–41.

Zaher H, Buters JT, Ward JM, Bruno MK, Lucas AM, Stern ST, Cohen SD, Gonzalez FJ. 1998. Protection against acetaminophen toxicity in CYP1A2 and CYP2E1 double-null mice. *Toxicol Appl Pharmacol*. 152:193–199.

Zaibo L, Tiefei D, Pröschel C, Noble M. 2007. Chemically diverse toxicants converge on fyn and c-Cbl to disrupt precursor cell function. *PLoS Biol*. 5:e35.

Zanella CL, Posada J, Tritton TR, Mossman BT. 1996. Asbestos causes stimulation of the extracellular signal-regulated kinase 1 mitogen-activated protein kinase cascade after phosphorylation of the epider-mal growth factor receptor. *Cancer Res*. 56:5334–5338.

Zeevalk GD, Razmpour R, Bernard LP. 2008. Glutathione and Parkinson's disease: is this the elephant in the room? *Biomed Pharmacother*. 62:236–249.

Zhong D, Liu X, Kure FR, Sun SY, Vertino PM, Zhou W. 2008. LKB1 is necessary for Akt-mediated phosphorylation of proapoptotic proteins. *Cancer Res*. 68:7270–7277.

Zhou SF, Xue CC, Yu XQ, Wang G. 2007. Metabolic activation of herbal and dietary constituents and its clinical and toxicological implications: an update. *Curr Drug Metab*. 8:526–553.

CHAPTER 9

Damage to Mitochondrial and Chloroplast Activities

This is a chapter outline intended to guide and familiarize you with the content to follow.

I. Mitochondrial damage (energy organelle in plants in dark and non-photosynthetic cells at all times)

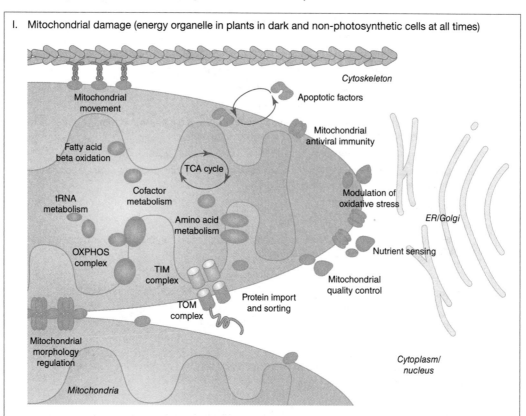

A. Overview—See Figure 9-1 including protonophoretic activity (uncoupling), inhibition of citric acid cycle, inhibition of fatty acid uptake or oxidation, binding of xenobiotics to cardiolipin, ROS damage that may lead to apoptosis or affect membrane lipid, opening of the mitochondrial permeability transition pore (PT), inhibition of adenine nucleotide translocase (ANT), inhibition of ATPase, mitochondrial DNA (mtDNA) depletion and inhibition of protein synthesis, and inhibition of electron transport

   1. Outer membrane

      a. point mutations of mtDNA that alter the voltage-dependent anion channel (eukaryotic porin)
         ↓ passage of charged biomolecules and cell viability; this porin plays a critical role in damage

and apoptosis produced by $O_2^{-\cdot}$ as inhibitors of this channel such as Konig's polyanion inhibit cyt c release and apoptosis caused by superoxide generated by xanthine/xanthine oxidase; cardiolipin oxidation in the outer membrane also generates cyt c release → apoptosis

2. Inner membrane

   a. Disruption of the transmembrane potential, $\Delta\psi$, can be disturbed by organophosphate poisoning (parathion → paraoxon), organochlorines (endosulfan, 3,4-dichloroanaline), and heavy metals (organotin, Cd)

   b. Opening of the PT is cyclosporine-sensitive and generated by oxidative stress (ROS and NO), TNFα exposure, Fas ligation, ganglioside GD3, and excessive Ca^{2+}

   c. ANT inhibition by dimaleimides—antiport reversed = pump protons out of mitochondria matrix

   d. Signal transduction through JNK and subsequent inactivation of BCL-2 and Bcl-xL

3. Oxidative phosphorylation—see Figure 9-2

   a. NADH uses complexes I, III, and IV to produce ATP and then moves on to reduce O_2

   b. Succinate uses complexes, II, III, and IV and then reduces O_2

   c. $FADH_2$ only uses complexes III and IV to generate 2 ATP

   d. Fluoroacetate reduces the substrates needed to fuel the electron transport chain

   e. Rotenone = classic complex I inhibitor (also oximes and pyrrolines)

   f. Thenoyl trifluoroacetone = complex II inhibitor

   g. Antimycin A = classic complex III inhibitor

   h. Classic poisons CN^-, CO, and NO inhibit complex IV (cyt c oxidase), with only cyanide and carbon monoxide being additive (NO antagonistic to other 2)

   i. Oligomycin inhibits complex V

   j. Uncouplers (protonophoric)—weak acids such as phenols that are able to transfer protons through a proton-impermeable membrane

4. Mitochondrial DNA

   a. Mutates 10× faster than nuclear DNA

   b. Inhibitors of mitochondrial protein synthesis (aminoglycoside antibiotics) lead to mitochondrial dysfunction, ototoxicity, and nephrotoxicity

II. Chloroplast damage (energy organelle in photosynthesizing cells in light)

   A. Mitochondria linked to chloroplast energy generation (complex I + additional dehydrogenase + alternate oxidase[s])—see Figure 9-3

   B. Photosystems I (PSI) + II (PSII) in chloroplast—see Figure 9-4 for light reactions in thylakoid membrane of chloroplast

      1. 3-(3,4-dichloro-phenyl)-1,1-dimethylurea ↑ rate of charge recombination between PSII acceptor and donor measured in thylakoids with the membrane potential and transmembrane electrochemical proton gradient ($\Delta\mu_H+$)

      2. Tributyltin inhibits ATP synthase

      3. Uncouplers nigericin and nonactin fully collapse $\Delta\mu_H+$ preexisting in the dark

      4. Because much ATP for dark reactions comes from mitochondria, antimycin A collapses $\Delta\mu_H+$

      5. Paraquat and diquat inhibit PS1 as they act as electron receptors

      6. Iodoacetamide inhibits NADP(H)-glyceraldehyde-3-phosphate dehydrogenase and prevents photooxidation of P700 in PSI

      7. Diphenyl ether herbicides generate a light-dependent free radical chain reaction through activation of carotenoid cofactors by binding to coupling factor CF1 associated with PSI in thylakoid membrane of chloroplasts occupied by Fd-NADP and Fd-thioredoxin reductases; $O_2^{-\cdot}$ generation may be responsible for chlorosis and desiccation

CONCEPTUALIZING TOXICOLOGY 9-1 (*continued*)

8. Cyanide inhibits all terminal oxidases under aerobic conditions as well as carbon dioxide assimilation

9. Hill reaction = one of first steps of photosynthesis going into PSII—inhibited by nitrofluorfen

10. Triazine herbicides such as atrazine are classic inhibitors of PSII at Q_B interrupting the electron transfer from Q_A to Q_B and have a long history of use in agriculture. Triazines/urea herbicides do not degrade D1 protein in the process, but phenol-type inhibitors degrade D1 and inhibit the electron transfer. However, the urea-type and phenol-type inhibitors do not bind to a bacterial reaction center of *Rhodobacter sphaeroides*, despite the homology with the plant Q_B binding site

11. Pb affects PSII electron transfer (but not PSI) between primary donor of PSII and site of water oxidation

12. Other herbicides work via interference with amino acid biosynthesis (glyphosate), cause porphyrin accumulation (*p*-nitrodiphenylethers and *N*-phenyl imides), use oxygen radicals to disrupt PSI and cause photobleaching by producing ROS (Paraquat), disrupt lipid synthesis (aryloxyphenoxy propionates and cyclohexane diones), result in mitotic arrest (dinitroanilines and phosphoric amides), inhibit folate synthesis (asulam), and block cellulose synthesis (dichlobenil)

CONCEPTUALIZING TOXICOLOGY 9-1 (*continued*)

This chapter builds on the concepts of energy functions and apoptotic activities. This discussion will proceed from the outside of the energy organelle into the generation of ATP. Clearly, significant damage to these organelles signals problems for the viability of the cell. Absence of adenosine triphosphate (ATP) guarantees necrosis, while significant ATP stores are required for apoptosis and less destructive survival pathways. Note the location and variety of functions in the mitochondrial schematic in the **Conceptualizing Toxicology** feature.

Mitochondria

Mitochondria are the energy-producing organelles that are mostly associated with aerobic ATP synthesis, while anaerobic energy functions can occur in the cytosol. This is also the energy-producing portion of plant cells; the ATP and nicotinamide adenine dinucleotide phosphate-oxidase (NADPH) generated during photosynthesis in chloroplasts in the light period are used in the biosynthesis of glucose from carbon dioxide. Mitochondrial numbers vary widely by cell type within a species and between species depending on the metabolic needs of those cells. The highest mitochondrial content appears to exist in mammalian muscle and cardiac cells,

with high numbers in liver cells (Allard et al., 1952) and fish gills (rainbow trout; Galvez et al., 2002), low numbers in plants (Avers and King, 1960), and even lower amounts in unicellular protists. The exact numbers are not reported here, because the number of mitochondria from histological analyses may be contrasted with virtual mitochondrial number per cell. This is based on the evidence that the amount of mitochondrial DNA does not vary per mitochondria in mammals but the mitochondrial DNA per cell and mitochondria per cell vary eight-fold among various cell types (Robin and Wong, 1988).

An overview of the toxic insults that can disrupt mitochondrial functions is shown in **Figure 9-1**. The figure is not an accurate morphological schematic of a mitochondrion, but it is an excellent concept map. Note that the outer cell membrane is indicated by the dotted line. The critical inner cell membrane is the solid line, and the functions associated with the cristae and more internally to the (maternal) DNA of the mitochondrion are indicated as well. When considering mitochondrial function and toxicity, bacteria are the best models. The reasons are that mitochondria likely came into being by invasion of symbiotic bacteria. Mitochondria arise clonally only from other mitochondria. Mitochondrial membranes remain distinct from

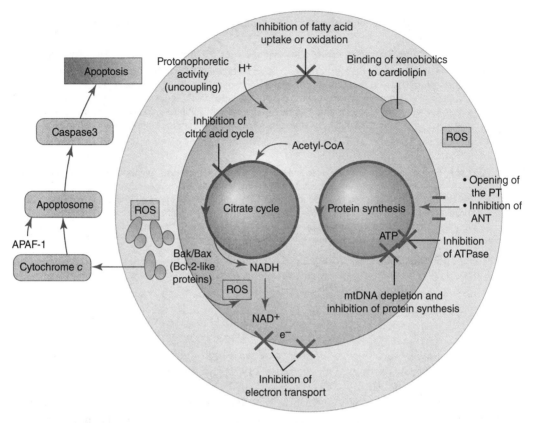

FIGURE 9-1 Mitochondrial Function Can Be Inhibited in Many Ways in Addition to Inhibition of Electron Transport and Uncoupling of It from the Membrane Potential

Note: For example, impairment of exchange of requisite substrates via membrane transporters, inhibition of metabolic pathways that fuel respiration, and direct effects of drugs on cardiolipin can acutely undermine mitochondrial function. Such acute effects frequently accelerate autoxidation of electron transport components that yields oxygen-centered and nitrogen-centered free radicals. By contrast, drugs that impair DNA replication or protein synthesis will diminish mitochondrial and hence bioenergetic capacity over a longer time period. In addition, many drugs can precipitate irreversible mitochondrial collapse via formation of the permeability transition pore leading to release of pro-apoptotic factors such as cytochrome c. Drugs that alter the normal equilibrium between pro-apoptotic and anti-apoptotic proteins, such as Bak/Bax and Bcl-2, among many others, can also induce mitochondrial failure.

cytoplasmic membranes and do not fuse with cytoplasmic structures. Mitochondrial DNA and protein synthesis are separate and resemble structures and mechanisms of the α-Proteobacteria, including protein and rRNA sequences. Even genes for mitochondrial proteins located in the nucleus of eukaryotic cells resemble those of α-Proteobacteria (Searcy, 2003).

Outer Membrane

The outer membrane of mitochondria appears to be freely permeable to many chemicals including charged substances, while the inner

membrane's lack of permeability is vital to the functional integrity of this organelle. This would indicate that toxicity to this structure is unlikely or would have little effect. One of the reasons for the permeability of the outer membrane is the voltage-dependent anion channel (VDAC) or eukaryotic porin that allows passage of charged biomolecules that are substrates for oxidative phosphorylation and other mitochondrial reactions. Point mutations of mitochondrial DNA that alter this channel protein can greatly diminish cell viability, or in the case of yeast seriously impair growth (Angeles et al., 1999). This channel also appears to play a critical role in the damage and subsequent apoptosis produced by superoxide. It was thought that only inner cell membrane cardio-lipid damage as produced by reactive oxygen species (ROS) generated by compounds such as dexamethasone led to apoptosis. The involvement of the mitochondrial permeability transition pore (PTP) opening and resultant swelling of the mitochondrial matrix space created a possible route for causing rupture of the outer mitochondrial membrane.

Other possibilities for mitochondrial damage by ROS involved the release of cytochrome c and the Brcl-2 family proteins. However, exposure of permeabilized HepG2 cells to superoxide but not hydrogen peroxide stimulated cytochrome c release. The PTP opening inhibitor cyclosporin A or bongkrekic acid failed to prevent the massive cytochrome c release. An inhibitor of the F_0F_1-ATPase, oligomycin, also did not prevent the release caused by superoxide. Inhibitors of the VDAC, 4,4′-diisothiocyanatostilbene-2,2′-disulfonic acid (DIDS) and Konig's polyanion, completely inhibited the release of cytochrome c produced by xanthine/xanthine oxidase-generated superoxide (Madesh and Hajnóczky, 2001). From this, a whole new model of ischemia-generated superoxide damage to mitochondria has been generated.

There is additionally an exclusively outer membrane free radical–producing mitochondrial NADH–quinone oxidoreductase that appears to participate in redox-cycling Paraquat toxicity. It is inhibited by higher concentrations of dicoumarol than those required to inhibit the NAD(P)H-quinone oxidoreductase. It is also insensitive to the antibody to cytochrome b_5 reductase or the cytochrome b_5 inhibitor, p-hydroxymercuribenzoate. The activity of this novel quinone oxidoreductase is also rotenone-insensitive, ruling out the participation of oxidative phosphorylation in this process (Shimada et al., 1998).

It appears that the outer mitochondrial membrane may mediate damage further into the mitochondria as well. The apoptosis signaling phospholipid cardiolipin will be translocated in high quantities to the outer cell membrane during damage-induced apoptosis. There, the cardiolipin complexes with cytochrome c and functions as a peroxidase. This oxidizes cardiolipin in the outer membrane and subsequent release of pro-apoptotic molecules from the mitochondria (O'Brien, 2006).

Inner Membrane and the Mitochondrial Transmembrane Electric Potential ($\Delta\Psi$)

The inner membrane is critical for mitochondrial function and its perturbation to make it more permeable. Changes in energy functions, protein synthesis inhibition, or mitochondrial DNA damage that undermine support of the transmembrane electric potential cause cell dysfunction to cell death as mediated by apoptosis or necrosis, depending on the severity of the damage. The use of the mitochondria as a subcellular toxicity model (or taken from an evolutionary perspective of as a bacterial sensor of cell damage) has been utilized in ecotoxicology. This was tested through the use of rat liver mitochondria exposed to concentrations of an organophosphate parathion (O,O-diethyl O-p-nitrophenol phosphorothioate); two organochlorine compounds, endosulfan (6,7,8,9,10,10-hexachloro-1,5,5a,6,9,9a-hexahydro-6,9-methano-2,4,3-benzo(e)-dioxathiepin-3-oxide) and 3,4-dichloroanaline (3,4-dichlorobenzeneamine); an organotin toxicant tributyltin; a heavy metal Cd called a "substance of reference" by the researchers; and treated and untreated domestic wastewater from the city of Coimbra, Portugal (da Silva et al., 1998). The transmembrane potential was assessed using the transmembrane distribution of the tetraphenylphosphonium ion (TPP$^+$) and a TPP$^+$-selective electrode. The fluctuations in $\Delta\Psi$ (mV) associated with succinate energization and phosphorylative cycle at 25°C upon addition of adenosine diphosphate (ADP) was calculated by the equation: $\Delta\Psi = 59*\log(v/V) - 59*\log(10^{\Delta E/59} - 1)$, where v, V, and ΔE are the volume of mitochondria, volume of incubation medium, and the deflection of the electrode potential from baseline, respectively. Parathion, 3,4-dichloroanaline, endosulfan, and cadmium affected succinate polarization with EC$_{50}$s of 1.96 mM, 2.02 mM, 24.66 μM, and 3.82 μM, respectively. Wastewater influent and tributyltin affected ADP phosphorylation with EC$_{50}$s of 2.53% and 0.28 μM, respectively, while primary clarifier and effluent had no apparent effects. Unfortunately, these effects were diminished from an order of magnitude to several orders of magnitude when compared to those observed by exposing intact *Daphnia magna* to parathion, 3,4-dichloroaniline, endosulfan, cadmium, and tributyltin with EC_{50}s 7.55 nM, 0.86 µM, 1.81 µM, 0.087 µM, and 0.030 µM, respectively (da Silva et al., 1998). This indicates that a cellular organelle or possibly a single cell is not necessarily as sensitive or has only mitochondrial damage as the basis for toxic responses.

Another classic example of how mitochondrial toxicity has been monitored, oxygen utilization or uptake, was measured by oxygen-detecting polarographic electrodes. This technique will determine only how oxidative phosphorylation is proceeding apart from direct toxicity to the membrane structures. It uses fluorescent dyes that register changes in $\Delta\psi$, but cannot tell the difference between inhibition, uncoupling, or mitochondrial permeability transition. Although whole organ models and whole animal models may better match the clinical outcome, they fail to discern specific mitochondrial events. This may be changing as mice have been developed with deficiencies in uncoupling protein, mitochondrial transcription factor A (*tfam*), glutathione peroxidase-1, γ-glutamyl transpeptidase, and adenine nucleotide translocase. A model for ROS-generating medications and toxicants is the heterozygous knockout mouse that expresses only half of the Mn-SOD activity.

Although biopsy for histopathological analysis of mitochondrial damage remains an important standard for detecting toxicities, there is also a less invasive method of using the ^{13}C (heavy)-labeled compounds such as methionine and following the evolution of $^{13}CO_2$ using isotope ratio mass spectrometry (Dykens and Will, 2007). These different methods are important for they combine the sensitivity of the intact organism with the specific toxicity assays needed to determine the focus of the toxic action. Others are using the yellow compound MTT (3-(4,5-dimethylthiazol-2-yl)-2,5-diphenyltetrazolium bromide) that is reduced to a purple formazan in the mitochondria of living cells to assess cell viability in preparations such

as retinal pigmented epithelial cells. Retinal cells exposed to acrolein show > 79% loss in this function by exposure for 24 hours to > 50 µM of acrolein, a cytotoxic and genotoxic compound found in cigarette smoke. Acrolein reduced mitochondrial function as assessed by decreases in $\Delta\psi$, glutathione, antioxidant capacity, Nrf2 expression, activities of mitochondrial complexes I/II/III, antioxidant enzyme activities of superoxide dismutase (SOD), and glutathione peroxidase. Increases were observed in oxidant levels, protein carbonyls, and calcium. R-α-lipoic acid pretreatment prevented these effects (Jia et al., 2007).

How can scientists parcel out the individual effects that led to this multitude of effects in the mitochondria? A correct assumption could be made that part of acrolein's effects are mediated by ROS, but that assumption would lead to the actions of Paraquat, which starts with damage to the outer membrane. The genotoxicity and reactivity of acrolein to other macromolecules is too broad to decipher one definitive cause for the decrease in cell viability. Other toxicants are better models of specific and selective damage to mitochondrial structures and functions. One relatively clear event is the permeabilization of the inner membrane. The cyclosporine A–sensitive (cyclophilin D binding site) opening of the permeability transition pore to small solutes is stimulated by a variety of toxicants that generate oxidative stress (ROS and nitric oxide) or ischemia/reperfusion injury, TNFα exposure, Fas ligation, ganglioside GD3, and excessive Ca^{2+}. This event can be followed by the translocation of permeable fluorophores such as calcein (Lemasters et al., 2002). The involvement of the outer membrane in this process appears to be controversial, because the permeabilization of these membranes is perceived as independent processes.

A key player to focus attention on in the process of initiating permeabilization of the inner cell membrane is adenine nucleotide translocator (ANT), which is a member of a family of inner membrane carriers involved in the exchange of ADP into the mitochondria and ATP export. This transport is driven by the $\Delta\psi$ resulting in the import of one positive charge per antiport (ATP^{4-} for ADP^{3-}).

When the electron transport that generates ATP is inhibited, the antiport may occur in the opposite direction. In that case, the $F_{0/1}$ ATP synthase would then function as an ATPase and pump protons out of the mitochondrial matrix. The adenine nucleotide translocator has two forms in the human, ANT1 and ANT2. ANT2 is expressed during cell growth as negatively regulated by general transcription factor Sp1 and a hexanucleotide silencer element in the ANT2 promoter region. ANT isoforms are comprised of three repeating segments of approximately 100 amino acids each. Each segment has two hydrophobic transmembrane helices separated by a stretch of amino acids that bulges into the matrix. ANT is a basic protein with excess cationic charges that interact closely with the acidic cardiolipin mentioned earlier. Two inhibitors force the molecule into an m-state conformation (bongkrekic acid binding to the matrix face of ANT) or c-state conformation (carboxyatractyloside or atractyloside binds to the intermembrane side of ANT). ANT's function depends on changing from the m- to the c-state during ADP/ATP exchange. Methyl methanethiosulfonate derivatizes the thiol on Cys56, which also freezes ANT in its m-state conformation by irreversible extrusion of the first loop facing the matrix. Dimaleimides also freeze ANT in the same m-state by cross-linking the Cys56 residues. ADP can be displaced from its binding site by 7-azido-5-isopropyl-acridone, which reacts with Cys159 of ANT. t-Butyl hydroperoxide or cross-linking Cys56 by diamide decreases ADP binding to ANT. When ANT proteoliposomes are prepared, they are shown to be permeabilized by atractyloside, Ca^{2+}, diamide, t-butyl hydroperoxide, Bax, and viral protein R encoded by human immunodeficiency virus-1 (HIV-1). Nonspecific pore formation has also been observed for other carriers such as the aspartate/glutamate antiporter transformed to a channel-like uniporter by thiol-specific chemicals. As discussed in apoptotic mechanisms, ANT interacts with Bcl-2, Bcl-XL, Bax, and Bak in the inner membrane and binds to VDAC of the outer cell membrane. Bax and Bcl-2 target VDAC to form a cytochrome c conduit in the activation of apoptotic mechanisms. The VDAC1

gene is upregulated by γ-irradiation-induced apoptosis, which may aid this process. The peripheral benzodiazepine receptor is located on the outer membrane, but copurifies with VDAC and ANT. Cytotoxic medications such as PK111195 (1-(2-chlorophenyl)-N-methyl-N-(1-methylpropyl)-isoquinolinecarboxamide), FGIN-I-27 (N,B-di-n-hexyl 2-(4-fluorophenyl)indole-3-acetamide), and chlorodiazepam overwhelm the protective influence of BCl-2 and increase apoptosis in response to arsenite, ceramide, doxorubicin, etoposide, lonidamine, and TNF. Creatine kinase, which also copurifies with ANT, has the opposite effect as creatine and creatine phosphate appear to have protective influences. Viral products may be pro-apoptotic in combination with ANT (viral protein R from HIV1) or anti-apoptotic (a product of the cytomegalovirus UL37 gene vMIA). Because ANT facilitates the electrophoretic transition between the inner and outer leaves of the inner membrane, fatty acid anions such as palmitate or stearate uncouple mitochondria through their interactions with ANT. Some nonsteroidal anti-inflammatory drugs (NSAIDs) such as diclofenac inhibit ANT activity and induce pore opening. Lipid peroxidation toxic unsaturated aldehydes 4-hydroxynonenal and 4-hydroxyhexenal inhibit ANT's antiport functions and induce permeabilization. The critical region for ANT inducing apoptosis appears to involve amino acid residues 102–141, which is also the binding region of Bcl-2/Bax and contains a Vpr-binding peptide motif. A universal apoptosis inducer, staurosporin, demonstrates that overexpression of Bax induces alkalinization of the mitochondrial matrix and cytosolic acidification leading to an increase in $\Delta\psi$ prior to the collapse of $\Delta\psi$ (Vieira et al., 2000).

The sequence of these events is important in understanding toxicant action and prevention of mitochondrial collapse and apoptosis. Although the disruption of $\Delta\psi$ might just be a function of inhibition of the process of oxidative phosphorylation as occurs via fibrates and thiazolidinediones or uncoupling electron transport from ATP synthesis as induced by NSAIDs, other medications may cause multiple problems. Acetaminophen, doxorubicin, and ethanol induce oxidative stress, which not only affects electron transport, but depletes glutathione as well. The delayed toxicity of acetaminophen by leflunomide points to the c-jun NH_2-terminal protein kinase (JNK) activation and subsequent Bcl-2 and Bcl-xL inactivation in mitochondrial toxicity. Induction of the mitochondrial permeability transition and subsequent collapse of $\Delta\psi$ and apoptosis can be induced by some statins and thiazolidinediones. These events can be prevented by overexpression of Bcl-xL. Inhibition of fatty acid p-oxidation pathways and the Krebs cycle also affect the $\Delta\psi$ through prevention of formation of substrates for oxidative phosphorylation, as does the blockade or destruction of inner membrane carriers such as the crucial one that transports the acetylCoA into the cell (Dykens and Will, 2007).

Oxidative Phosphorylation

Mitochondria account for more than 90% of the ATP synthesized and O_2 consumed by cells as part of cellular respiration. The classic mitochondrial inhibitors affect oxidative phosphorylation. The electron transport chain is shown in **Figure 9-2**. The order inhibitors of the chain are normally given to evaluate cellular respiratory function; the substrates used at various points that donate electrons to the electron transport chain are also shown in the oxygen electrode tracing. Electrons are transferred to oxygen via the energy-transducing complexes of the electron transport or respiratory chain. NADH-producing reactions use complexes I, III, and IV to reduce oxygen and generate three ATP for each electron from NADH. Succinate reduces oxygen through complexes II, III, and IV. Reactions that generate $FADH_2$ (i.e., Krebs cycle) reduce oxygen by utilizing complexes III and IV and only generating two ATP for each electron from $FADH_2$. The extremely hydrophobic quinone CoQ and cytochrome c "shuttle" between complexes. Complexes I, III, and IV pump protons from the inner (matrix) side of the mitochondrial membrane into the space between the inner and outer membrane, creating a temporary localized acidic environment and a transmembrane proton gradient. ATP is synthesized from the energy generated when complex V (ATP synthase) allows protons to flow back into

the mitochondrial matrix (Rötig and Munnich, 2003). The first step in the process is the arrival of an NADH molecule or an $FADH_2$ molecule. These and other substrates that donate electrons come primarily from the Krebs cycle. Fluoroacetate or similar toxic substrates for that cycle reduce the amount of true substrates and products necessary to fuel the electron transport chain, but are not considered true toxicants of oxidative phosphorylation (Proudfoot et al., 2006). The true toxicants affect the electron transport chain by inhibiting reactions or uncoupling the chain from the synthesis of ATP, although both types of inhibitors will exert their toxicity similarly, such as in the development of mouse ovarian follicles (Wycherley et al., 2005). Rotenone is the classic respiratory chain complex I inhibitor that blocks the flow of electrons from NADH to coenzyme Q, but doesn't prevent the flow of electrons from complex II on down the chain.

Other inhibitors of NADH oxidase activity (complex I) are a variety of natural and synthetic insecticides, including certain oximes and pyrrolines (Cantín et al., 2005). Amobarbital (amytal) is another classic mitochondrial energy inhibitor that prevents NADH oxidation (Peng and Hertz, 2002). Complex II (succinate: ubiquinone oxidoreductase) can feed in electrons from succinate even if complex I is blocked. Complex II is blocked by thenoyltrifluoroacetone as it was used to evaluate the function of complex III in embryoid bodies toward the differentiation into cardiomyocytes (Spitkovsky et al., 2004). The competitive succinate dehydrogenase inhibitor malonate may serve a somewhat similar function in the direction of electrons to complex II, although technically succinate dehydrogenase is an enzyme of the Krebs cycle. Antimycin A was shown to be the classic inhibitor of complex III (ubiquinol: cytochrome c oxidoreductase) at center i and by myxothiazol at center o in an evaluation of mitochondrial function in chickens (Ojano-Dirain et al., 2004).

The classic poison gases cyanide (CN^-), carbon monoxide (CO), and nitric oxide (NO) block the entire respiratory chain by binding to cytochrome c oxidase (complex IV). However, only CN^- plus CO show additive effects, while NO antagonizes the action of the other

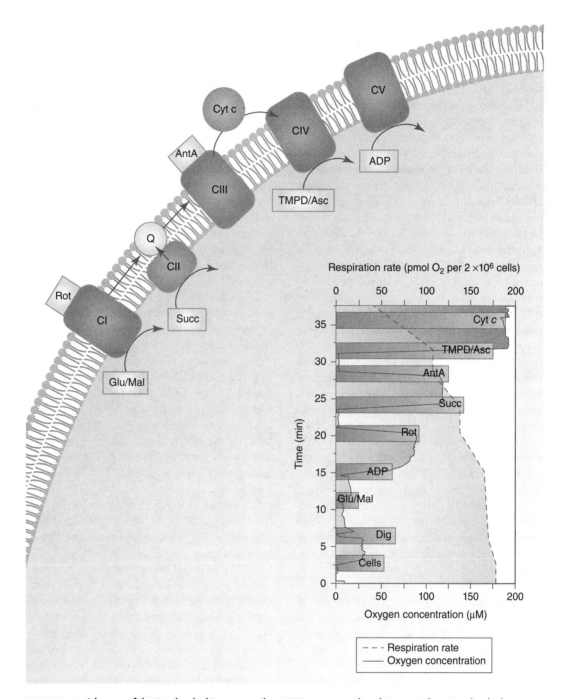

FIGURE 9-2 Schematic of the Mitochondrial Respiratory Chain (MRC - upper panel) and How to Evaluate Mitochondrial Respiratory Function Using Inhibitors and Substrates (lower panel)

Note: MRC complexes I (CI, NADH/CoQ oxidoreductase), II (CII, succinate/CoQ oxidoreductase), III (CIII, CoQH2/cytochrome *c* oxidoreductase), IV (CIV, cytochrome *c* oxidase) and V (CV, ATP synthase). Inhibitors of CI = Rot (rotenone) and of CIII = AntA (antimycin A). Electron-donating substrates = Glu/Mal (glutamate + malate); Succ (succinate); TMPD/ascorbate (trimethylpentane-1,3-diol/cytochrome *c* + ascorbate). The lower panel shows a trace of mitochondria evaluated using permeabilized cells and an oxygen electrode with maximal respiration capacity achieved by stimulating with ADP at its saturating concentration (2 mM) and cell density at 2 10^6 cells/ml. Additions: Dig, digitonin 15 mg ml^{-1}; Glu/Mal, 10 mM glutamate + 5 mM malate; ADP, 1 mM ADP; Rot, 0.5 mM rotenone; Succ, 10 mM succinate; AntA, 5 mM antimycin A; TMPD/Asc, 0.5 mM TMPD + 2 mM ascorbate; Cyt *c*, 10 mM cytochrome *c*.

two gases. NO displaces CN^- from ferric hemoproteins as regulated by heme reduction, which is facilitated by nonligand-binding electron-transfer centers (Pearce et al., 2008). Hydrogen sulfide poisoning was also formerly considered to be a function of the inhibition of complex IV, but now appears to be more related to a reactive sulfur species that depletes reduced glutathione and generates ROS (Truong et al., 2006). Complex V or F_0F_1-ATPase (ATP synthase) is inhibited severely in a time-dependent, high-affinity manner by the mixed inhibitor oligomycin and depletes ATP from the cell (more likely to head toward necrosis). However, Bz-423, a 1,4-benzodiazepine binds to the oligomycin sensitivity-conferring protein subunit of the mitochondrial F_0F_1-ATPase, only producing moderate inhibition. This milder inhibition of ATP synthesis increases superoxide, resulting in redox-regulated apoptosis (Johnson et al., 2006).

Another important class of toxicants in cellular respiration is the uncouplers. The uncoupling reagents separate the electron transport chain from phosphorylation. Most uncouplers are hydrophobic weak acids, such as acyldithiocarbazates, aromatic amines, benzimidazoles, cumarines, phenols, N-phenylanthranilates, phenylhydrazones, and salicylic acids, which are able to transfer protons through a proton-impermeable membrane (protonophoric). Because Mitchell's chemiosmotic theory postulates that the energy for ATP synthesis comes from redox reactions that set up an H^+ gradient across an impermeable inner membrane, it is clear to see how these protonophores disrupt the proton motive forces provided from electron transport and thereby prevent ATP synthesis. Because this proton motive force is both a pH difference and a membrane potential difference, anything that disrupts either pH or $\Delta\psi$ will be an uncoupler, including aging or osmotic shock. Some weaker uncouplers, such as the cationic cyanide dyes, require inorganic phosphate to be effective. They are thought to inhibit the ADP/ATP transporter, as do the compounds bongkrekic acid and atractyloside mentioned earlier in regard to the disruption of the inner membrane and $\Delta\psi$ (Terada, 1990). One of the most classic and utilized uncoupling agents is a dinitrophenol, while others prefer to use carbonyl cyanide phenylhydrazones.

Mitochondrial DNA and Protein Synthesis

Much of the damage that occurs to mitochondria that does not directly come from toxicant-induced dysfunction results from reactive oxygen species damage—not only to oxidative phosphorylation but also to mitochondrial DNA. Mitochondrial DNA mutates at one log unit faster than nuclear DNA. This is important in considering the aging or toxic sensitivity of various organelles. In a 65-year-old human, approximately half of the mitochondrial DNA is damaged, with an accompanying loss in capacity for oxidative phosphorylation. Nerve cells are very sensitive as they have high metabolic requirements and little space for energy organelles. Because nerve cells don't generate much excess respiratory capacity, the loss of mitochondrial function during aging appears to play a role in Alzheimer's disease, Parkinson's disease, and late-onset Type 2 diabetes mellitus. A dozen known mutations of mitochondrial DNA are related to mitochondrial dysfunction leading to retinal cell death by age 30 in humans—known as Leber's hereditary optic neuropathy (Searcy, 2003). The nucleoside reverse transcriptase inhibitors used in the treatment of HIV also inhibit the mitochondrial polymerase, inducing toxicity to muscle and liver cells and lipodystrophy and lipoatrophy. Mitochondrial protein synthesis inhibition by aminoglycoside antibiotics such as streptomycin or neomycin also lead to mitochondrial dysfunction, ototoxicity (vestibulocochlear nerve damage), and nephrotoxicity (kidney cell damage; Dykens and Will, 2007). Other compounds not related to antiretroviral medications also deplete mtDNA in mammalian cells. These agents include intercalating (e.g., ethidium bromide) and non-intercalating (e.g., polyamine analogues) DNA-binding compounds, the bacterial type II topoisomerase inhibitors ciprofloxacin and nalidixic acid, and lipophilic cationic compounds such as dequalinium, MKT-077, and 1-methyl-4-phenylpyridinium ion (MPP^+; Rowe et al., 2001). This is not surprising, because mitochondrial DNA is like the bacterial version of viral DNA that are the targets of medications or are very sensitive to other clastogenic agents.

Chloroplasts and Plant Mitochondria

Plant mitochondria have a number of unique features that other eukaryotic organisms do not have. For example, the light/dark cycle of the plant cell requires this photoautotrophic organism to adjust to changes in cellular energy, organelle function, and redox status throughout the day. The interactions of the mitochondria with the chloroplasts have revealed that complex I is essential for optimal photosynthetic performance in photorespiratory conditions and during transients in tobacco leaves, for example, and that a plant mitochondrial uncoupling protein is similarly necessary for photosynthesis. Additionally, the plant mitochondrial chain has a l-galactono-1,4-lactone dehydrogenase and several homologues of type II NAD(P)H dehydrogenases and alternative oxidases that bypass energy conservation in addition to the complexes found in other eukaryotic mitochondria. The functional diversity and flexibility of plant mitochondria are due to the 12 functionally distinct dehydrogenases in the electron transport chain. Additionally, certain components counter metabolic imbalances produced by altered stimulation of the chloroplast. For instance, the alternative oxidase is found to upregulate when the chloroplast over-reduces in excess light.

Plant DNA, RNA, and protein expression are different in plants as compared to animal mitochondria. The evolution of plant mitochondrial DNA has been to larger rather than smaller genomes. Part of that increase is the encoding for biosynthesis of proteins of the electron transport chain. As part of that encoding is a four-gene unit utilized for synthesis of proteins involved in cytochrome c maturation, which is similar to bacteria but not mammalian or fungal mitochondria. Self-splicing introns of types I and II are present in plants, but with notable exceptions not in animals. Type II introns

appear essential for plant gene expression as does a peculiar type of RNA editing, in which C DNA residues are encoded into U in mRNA post-transcriptionally. Another unusual feature is that the nucleus not only controls some functions of the mitochondria, but the mitochondrial DNA also involves retrograde regulation of the nucleus, such as in flower development (Rasmusson et al., 2008).

This discussion now focuses on the role of energy transfer between plant mitochondria and chloroplasts and ATP synthesis in the chloroplast. Note the ATP synthesis schematic and energy transfer in **Figure 9-3**. The active ATP transporter is similar to that of mammals in that the mitochondria are the major sources of ATP for the cytosol. The ATP transporter of the chloroplasts is low activity and only active in younger chloroplasts. The dihydroxyacetone 3-phosphate (DHAP)/3-phosphoglycerate (3-PGA) shuttle using the phosphate translocator of the chloroplast membrane is capable of exporting some ATP as well as NADPH, but under physiological conditions the export of reducing equivalents as the nonphosphorylating system predominates via the DHAP/3-PGA translocator shuttle or via the malate/oxaloacetate (Mal/OAA) shuttle. The mitochondria also export reducing equivalents via a Mal/OAA shuttle, but in the case of the chloroplast the malate dehydrogenase (MDH) is $NADP^+$-dependent and light-activated, whereas an NAD^+-MDH operates in the cytosol and the mitochondria. Light-activated photosystems I and II (PSI and PSII) are shown in **Figure 9-4**.

The Calvin cycle that fixes CO_2 is not shown in the figure, because the focus is on energy production by the cell for survival. Even though the chloroplast provides ATP for the Calvin cycle, it is not always enough for all the functions of the chloroplast. The degree to which mitochondria supplement ATP to the chloroplast depends on the amount generated from cyclic and pseudocyclic phosphorylation. Cyclic phosphorylation yields ATP as the sole product via PSI's transfer of electrons via its Fd or NADPH acceptors to plastoquinone, which serves as a donor to PSI. This occurs in pea leaves, for example, only under conditions of high irradiances in combination with very low CO_2 concentrations. Oxidation of the PSI acceptor produces the ROS H_2O_2 in the process of pseudocyclic phosphorylation, which utilizes both PSI and PSII. The reason H_2O_2 generation does not yield toxicity physiologically is due to the activity of catalase, which is rapidly converted to hydrogen peroxide then to water and oxygen.

Noncyclic photosynthetic electron transport produces ATP and NADPH in a ratio of 2.6:2, which does not satisfy the requirements of a ratio of $\geq$ 3:2 for CO_2 fixation to yield DHAP.

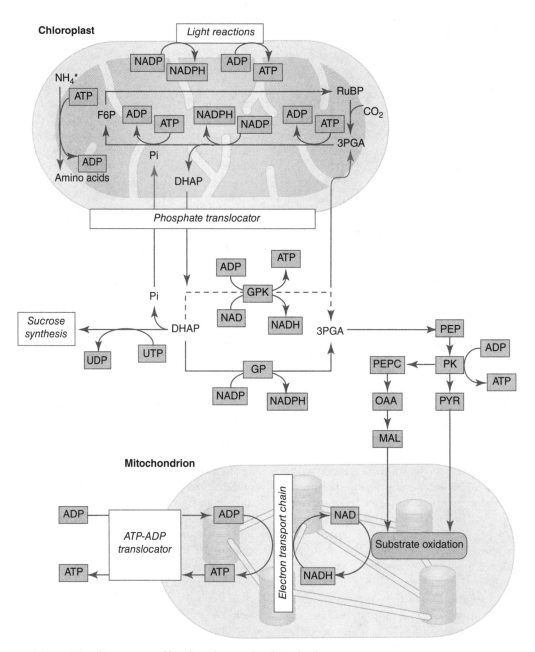

FIGURE 9-3 ATP Exchanges among Chloroplasts, the Cytosol, and Mitochondria

Note: ETC, Electron Transport Chain; GP, NADP+-GAPDH (glyceraldehyde-3-P dehydrogenase); GPK, PGK (phosphoglycerate kinase) and NAD+GAPDH (glyceraldehyde-3-P dehydrogenase); PEPC, PEP (phosphoenol pyruvate) Carboxylase; PK, Pyruvate Kinase; DHAP, dihydroxyacetone phosphate; MAL, malate; OAA, oxaloacetate; PEP, phosphoenol pyruvate; 3-PGA, 3-phosphoglycerate; RuBP, ribulose 1,5-bisphosphate.

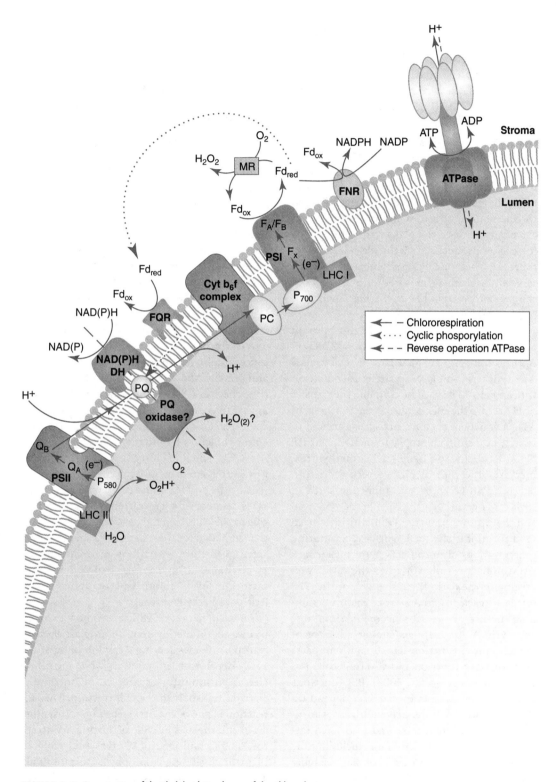

FIGURE 9-4   Organization of the Thylakoid Membrane of the Chloroplast

Note: FNR, ferredoxin-NADP+ oxidoreductase; FQR, ferredoxin-plastoquinone reductase; LHC, light harvesting complex; MR, Mehler reaction; PC, plastocyanin; NAD(P)HDH, NAD(P)H dehydrogenase; PQ, plastoquinone; PS, photosystem. The elements of the suggested chlororespiratory pathway are indicated by dark-shaded rectangles.

Additional ATP molecules must be provided for sucrose synthesis, protein synthesis, NH_4^+ assimilation, metabolite transport, and maintenance. The plant mitochondria provide additional ATP as necessary, as they produce up to 3 ATP per NAD(P)H compared to the 1.5–2 ATP per NAD(P)H in the chloroplast (Hoefnagel et al., 1998).

Note that because ATP can be generated both in the mitochondria and in the chloroplast, the usual mitochondrial toxicants may or may not affect the plant cell as effectively depending on the mechanism of action and concentration in the organelle since the plant has more options for energy production. Herbicides clearly have overcome these mechanism in specific plants targeted by these agent based on the ability of the plant to metabolize them (e.g., maize) or respond to their action.

The transmembrane electrochemical proton gradient or difference, $\Delta\mu H^+ = \Delta\psi - (2.3RT/F)$ ΔpH (Rottenberg, 1975), drives the chloroplast ATP synthesis similarly to the mitochondrion with an F_0F_1 ATP synthase coupling the transfer of H^+ across the membrane to the synthesis of ATP. A variety of chemicals has been utilized to analyze or disturb chloroplast function. DCMU, or 3-(3,4-dichloro-phenyl)-1,1-dimethylurea, increases the rate of charge recombination between PSII acceptor and donor measured in thylakoids with both the membrane potential and the proton gradient. Tributyltin has been used to inhibit the ATP synthase. Saturating concentrations of uncouplers 2 μM nigericin + 2-μM nonactin fully collapses the $\Delta\mu H^+$ preexisting in the dark. Because much of the ATP for dark reactions comes from the mitochondria, the use of the cytochrome b/c inhibitor antimycin A (40 μM) or a similar inhibitor of mitochondrial function has dramatic impacts on chloroplast function and also fully collapses $\Delta\mu H^+$ (Joliot and Joliot, 2008). PSI functions of chloroplasts and cyanobacteria depend on the function of light-driven plastocyanin-ferre-doxin oxidoreductase and associated factors in the thylakoid membrane, including the essential cofactor and measure of plant viability in ecotoxicology, chlorophyll a (Chitnis, 2001).

Chlorophyll a plays a much more central role in PSII. The bipyridylium herbicides Paraquat and diquat famously inhibit PSI if allowed access to the chloroplast; otherwise, the plant would be resistant to its action. These redox cycling herbicides act as electron acceptors from one of the iron-sulfur proteins, generating a radical that is not toxic to the plant. However, this alone prevents PSI from transferring electrons to PSII. Additionally, the creation of ROS superoxide, hydrogen peroxide, followed by hydroxyl radical from oxidation of the bipyridylium radical species does cause lipid damage and observed loss of membrane integrity (Fuerst et al., 1985). PSI can be studied by use of 730 nm light and DCMU to inhibit PSII electron transfer. Potassium cyanide acts both as an inhibitor of terminal oxidases under aerobic conditions and as and assimilator of carbon dioxide under anaerobic conditions. Pentachlorophenol similarly acts as an inhibitor of terminal oxidases under aerobic conditions and as an uncoupling agent. Iodoacetamide inhibits NADP(H)-glyceraldehyde-3-phosphate dehydrogenase and prevents the photooxidation of P700 in PSI (Bolychevtseva, 2007). Diphenyl ether herbicides appear to generate a light-dependent free radical chain reaction through activation of the carotenoid cofactors by binding to a coupling factor, CF1, which is closely associated with PSI in the thylakoid membrane in the area occupied by the Fd-NADP and Fd-thioredoxin reductases. Superoxide generation may still play a role in the chlorosis and desiccation observed in treated plants for these herbicides such as fomesafen (5-[2-chloro-4-trifluoromethylphenoxy]-N-methanesulfonyl-2-nitrobenzamide) and nitrofluorfen (2-chloro-1-[4-nitrophenoxy]-4-[trifluoromethyllbenzene]).

An examination of PSII reveals how two herbicides act differently upon chloroplast electron transport. Fomesafen is a weak inhibitor of the FeCN-dependent Hill reaction, while nitrofluorfen is an inhibitor of coupled or uncoupled electron transport in the Hill reaction. The Hill reaction is one of the first steps in photosynthesis in chloroplasts in PSII, as the primary acceptor P680 (a multimer of several weakly colored pigments including chlorophyll; Durrant et al., 1995) has two electrons donated to it from the splitting of water as follows: $H_2O + NADP +$ light + chloroplasts $\rightarrow$ NADPH + ½ $O_2 + H^+$.

The electrons move to P700 (PSI) and on to NADP to produce NADPH (refer back to Figure 9-4). Photosystem II's part of this reaction can be monitored by substituting the blue dye 2,6 dichlorophenolindophenol (DCIP) as the acceptor instead of going to P700 and PSI: H_2O + DCIP (blue) + light + PSII $\rightarrow$ DCIP (clear reduced form) + ½ O_2. Then the action of the PSII-inhibiting herbicides can be followed with less DCIP formation. The herbicide diuron (DCMU; 3-[3,4-dichlorophenyl]-1, 1-dimethylurea]) appears to work prior to the site where Paraquat or diquat is active, and nitrofluorfen works after that site (Ridley, 1983). Diuron moves the focus onto subgroups of PSII inhibitors, as most PSII inhibitors that are used as herbicides are usually grouped in diuron/triazine-types (serine 264) and phenol-types (histidine 215) as the commercially available photosynthesis-inhibiting herbicides bind to D-1 quinone-binding protein (Duke, 1990). Triazines such as atrazine are heavily used herbicides that inhibit PSII. The reason that these classifications of PSII inhibitors exist is clarified by the mechanisms of action, even though both types appear to bind at the Q_B site, interrupting the electron transfer from Q_A^- to Q_B^-.

This section concludes with a discussion of what happens during photoinhibitory illumination to the D1 protein and PSII activity. D1 protein is degraded under these conditions even in the presence of phenol-type inhibitors but not in the presence of urea/triazine-type inhibitors. Both lead to formation of a 41 kDa adduct to the D1 protein, but only the urea/triazine-type inhibitors also causes an adduct of the α-subunit of Cyt b_m. The lack of D1 protein degradation leads to suppression of the inactivation of PSII by urea/triazine-type inhibitors. Trypsin modification of the D1 binding site for DCMU or similar inhibitors eliminates their protective influences in this study (Nakajima et al., 1996). This indicates very specific binding regions and functional differences between these PSII disruptors despite the fact that both have potent herbicidal action due the disruption of this system. Lead is a toxic heavy metal that does not appears to affect PSI, but inhibits the oxidizing side of PSII electron transfer between the primary electron donor of PSII and

site of water oxidation as demonstrated by the restoration of normal chlorophyll fluorescence in the presence of hydroxylamine (Miles et al., 1972). The reducing side of PSII or at the bacterial reaction center from *Rhodobacter sphaeroides* at Q_B is weakly inhibited by the natural quinone analog capsaicin from the red pepper species as opposed to strong inhibition by certain herbicides, such as the atrazines and 2-iodo-4-nitro-6-isobutyl-phenol. However, other urea-type and phenol-type inhibitors do work on PSII but do not act on Q_B of the bacterial reaction center (Spyridaki et al., 2000). Other herbicides interfere with the biosynthesis of amino acids (e.g., 5-enolpyruval-shikimate-3-phosphate synthase inhibition by glyphosate); cause accumulation of photodynamic porphyrins by inhibiting protoporphyrinogen oxidase (*p*-nitrodiphenylethers and *N*-phenyl imides); use oxygen radicals not only to disrupt PSI, but also to generate photobleaching by the production of ROS (Paraquat); disrupt lipid synthesis (acetyl CoA carboxylase inhibition by aryloxyphenoxy propionates and cyclohexanediones); cause mitotic arrest by interaction with tubulin (dinitroanilines and phosphoric amides); inhibit folate synthesis (asulam inhibition of dihydropteroate synthase); and block cellulose synthesis (dichlobenil; Duke, 1990). Clearly these actions would have dramatic but indirect effects on energy production in photosynthetic organism.

Questions

1. What is the most important transporter of the outer membrane of mitochondria that mediates superoxide toxicity?
2. What are the measures of inner membrane disturbance?
3. Give examples of inhibitors of oxidative phosphorylation/electron transport chain and indicate where they block the transfer of electrons.
4. Why are mitochondrial DNA and mitochondrial protein synthesis key features in mitochondrial dysfunction?
5. How are plant mitochondria different from mammalian mitochondria? How does this affect toxicity to mitochondrial toxicants?

6. What are the classic inhibitors of PSI → PSII electron transport?
7. What inhibits the Hill reaction, and what is the importance of this reaction to PSII?
8. Triazine herbicides used classically in corn agriculture affect what transfer in PSII?

References

Allard C, de Lamirande G, Cantero A. 1952. Mitochondrial population of mammalian cells. II. Variation in the mitochondrial population of the average rat liver cell during regeneration; use of the mitochondrion as a unit of measurement. *Cancer Res.* 12:580–583.

Angeles R, Devine J, Barret R, Goebel D, Blachyl-Dyson E, Forte M, McCauley R. 1999. Mutations in the voltage-dependent anion channel of the mitochondrial outer membrane cause a dominant nonlethal growth impairment. *J Bioenerg Biomembr.* 31:143–151.

Avers CJ, King EE. 1960. Histochemical evidence of intracellular enzymatic heterogeneity of plant mitochondria. *Am J Bot.* 47:220–225.

Bolychevtseva YV, Terekhova IV, Roegner M, Karapetyan NV. 2007. Effects of oxygen and photosynthesis carbon cycle reactions on kinetics of P700 redox transients in cyanobacterium *Arthrospira platensis* cells. *Biochemistry (Mosc).* 72:275–281.

Cantín C, López-Gresa MP, González MC, Moya P, Miranda MÁ, Primo J, Romero V, Peris E, Estornell E. 2005. Novel inhibitors of the mitochondrial respiratory chain: oximes and pyrrolines isolated from *Penicillium brevicompactum* and synthetic analogues. *J Agric Food Chem.* 53:8296–8301.

Chitnis PR. 2001. Photosystem I: function and physiology. *Annu Rev Plant Physiol Plant Mol Biol.* 52:593–626.

da Silva EM, Soares AM, Moreno AJ. 1998. The use of the mitochondrial transmembrane electric potential as an effective biosensor in ecotoxicological research. *Chemosphere.* 36:2375–2390.

Duke SO. 1990. Overview of herbicide mechanisms of action. *Environ Health Perspect.* 87:263–271.

Durrant JR, Klug DR, Kwa SL, van Grondelle R, Porter G, Dekker JP. 1995. A multimer model for P680, the primary electron donor of photosystem II. *Proc Natl Acad Sci USA.* 92:4798–4802.

Dykens JA, Will Y. 2007. The significance of mitochondrial toxicity testing in drug development. *Drug Discov Today.* 12:777–785.

Fuerst EP, Nakatani HY, Dodge AD, Penner D, Arntzen CJ. 1985. Paraquat resistance in *Conyza. Plant Physiol.* 77:984–989.

Galvez F, Reid SD, Hawkings G, Goss GG. 2002. Isolation and characterization of mitochondria-rich cell types from the gill of freshwater rainbow trout. *Am J Physiol Regul Integr Comp Physiol.* 282:R658–R668.

Hoefnagel MHN, Atkin OK, Wiskich JT. 1998. Interdependence between chloroplasts and mitochondria in the light and the dark. *Biochim Biophys Acta.* 1366:235–255.

Jia L, Liu Z, Sun L, Miller SS, Ames BN, Cotman CW, Liu J. 2007. Acrolein, a toxicant in cigarette smoke, causes oxidative damage and mitochondrial dysfunction in RPE cells: protection by (R)-alpha-lipoic acid. *Invest Ophthalmol Vis Sci.* 48:339–348.

Johnson KM, Cleary J, Fierke CA, Opipari AW Jr, Glick GD. 2006. Mechanistic basis for therapeutic targeting of the mitochondrial F1F0-ATPase. *ACS Chem Biol.* 1:304–308.

Joliot P, Joliot A. 2008. Quantification of the electrochemical proton gradient and activation of ATP synthase in leaves. *Biochim Biophys Acta.* 1777:676–683.

Kuznetsov AV, Veksler V, Gellerich FN, Saks V, Margreiter R, Kunz WS. 2008. Analysis of mitochondrial function *in situ* in permeabilized muscle fibers, tissues and cells. *Nat Protoc.* 3:965–976.

Lemasters JJ, Qian T, He L, Kim JS, Elmore SP, Cascio WE, Brenner DA. 2002. Role of mitochondrial inner membrane permeabilization in necrotic cell death, apoptosis, and autophagy. *Antioxid Redox Signal.* 4:769–781.

Madesh M, Hajnóczky G. 2001. VDAC-dependent permeabilization of the outer mitochondrial membrane by superoxide induces rapid and massive cytochrome *c* release. *J Cell Biol.* 155:1003–1015.

Miles CD, Brandle JR, Daniel DJ, Chu-Der O, Schnare PD, Uhlik DJ. 1972. Inhibition of photosystem II in isolated chloroplasts by lead. *Plant Physiol.* 49:820–825.

Nakajima Y, Yoshida S, Ono T. 1996. Differential effects of urea/triazine-type and phenol-type photosystem II inhibitors on inactivation of the electron transport and degradation of the D1 protein during photoinhibition. *Plant Cell Physiol.* 37(5):673–680.

O'Brien PJ. 2006. Mitochondrial toxicity. *Chem Biol Interact.* 163:1–3.

Peng L, Hertz L. 2002. Amobarbital inhibits K(+)-stimulated glucose oxidation in cerebellar granule neurons by two mechanisms. *Eur J Pharmacol.* 446:53–61.

Proudfoot AT, Bradberry SM, Vale JA. 2006. Sodium fluoroacetate poisoning. *Toxicol Rev.* 25:213–219.

Ojano-Dirain CP, Iqbal M, Cawthon D, Swonger S, Wing T, Cooper M, Bottje W. 2004. Determination of mitochondrial function and site-specific defects in electron transport in duodenal mitochondria in broilers with low and high feed efficiency. *Poult Sci.* 83:1394–1403.

Pearce LL, Lopez Manzano E, Martinez-Bosch S, Peterson J. 2008. Antagonism of nitric oxide toward the inhibition of cytochrome *c* oxidase by carbon monoxide and cyanide. *Chem Res Toxicol.* 21(11):2073–2781.

Rasmusson AG, Handa H, Mølle IM. 2008. Plant mitochondria, more unique than ever. *Mitochondrion.* 8:1–4.

Ridley SM. 1983. Interaction of chloroplasts with inhibitors: effects of two diphenylether herbicides, fomesafen and nitrofluorfen, on electron transport, and some comparisons with dibromothymoquinone, diuron, and paraquat. *Plant Physiol.* 72:461–468.

Robin ED, Wong R. 1988. Mitochondrial DNA molecules and virtual number of mitochondria per cell in mammalian cells. *J Cell Physiol.* 136:507–513.

Rötig A, Munnich A. 2003. Genetic features of mitochondrial respiratory chain disorders. *J Am Soc Nephrol.* 14:2995–3007.

Rottenberg H. 1975. The measurement of transmembrane electrochemical proton gradients. *J Bioenerg.* 7:61–74.

Rowe TC, Weissig V, Lawrence JW. 2001. Mitochondrial DNA metabolism targeting drugs. *Adv Drug Deliv Rev.* 49:175–187.

Searcy DG. 2003. Metabolic integration during the evolutionary origin of mitochondria. *Cell Res.* 13:229–238.

Shimada H, Hirai K, Simamura E, Pan J. 1998. Mitochondrial NADH-quinone oxidoreductase of the outer membrane is responsible for paraquat cytotoxicity in rat livers. *Arch Biochem Biophys.* 351:75–81.

Spitkovsky D, Sasse P, Kolossov E, Böttinger C, Fleischmann BK, Hescheler J, Wiesner RJ. 2004. Activity of complex III of the mitochondrial electron transport chain is essential for early heart muscle cell differentiation. *FASEB J.* 18:1300–1302.

Spyridaki A, Fritzsch G, Kouimtzoglou E, Baciou L, Ghanotakis D. 2000. The natural product capsaicin inhibits photosynthetic electron transport at the reducing side of photosystem II and purple bacterial reaction center: structural details of capsaicin binding. *Biochim Biophys Acta.* 1459:69–76.

Terada H. 1990. Uncouplers of oxidative phosphorylation. *Environ Health Perspect.* 87:213–218.

Truong DH, Eghbal MA, Hindmarsh W, Roth SH, O'Brien PJ. 2006. Molecular mechanisms of hydrogen sulfide toxicity. *Drug Metab Rev.* 38:733–744.

Vieira HLA, Haouzi D, El Hamel C, Jacotot E, Belzacq A-S, Brenner C, Kroemer G. 2000. Permeabilization of the mitochondrial inner membrane during apoptosis: impact of the adenine nucleotide translocator. *Cell Death Differ.* 7:1146–1154.

Wycherley G, Kane MT, Hynes AC. 2005. Oxidative phosphorylation and the tricarboxylic acid cycle are essential for normal development of mouse ovarian follicles. *Hum Reprod.* 20:2757–2763.

CHAPTER 10

Damage to Nuclear Structures/DNA: Mutagenesis and Carcinogenesis

This is a chapter outline intended to guide and familiarize you with the content to follow.

I. Damage to nuclear structures/DNA

   A. Tests

      1. 4,6′-diaminodino-2-phenylindole dihydrochloride (nonintercalating DNA-specific) dye exclusion test

      2. DNA staining and ultrastructural biological analysis

      3. Mass spectrometry (or accelerator MS for isotope ratios), fluorescence microscopy, electrochemical detection, immunochemical, or radiolabel analysis of adducts formed on DNA bases

      4. Bacterial reversion assays (Ames test)

      5. Flow cytometry followed by DNA sequencing

      6. Ethidium bromide staining and densitometry (interstrand cross-links or ICLs)

      7. Create a mutagenesis reporter construct into the DNA (using a pSP189 or similar vector)

      8. Solid-phase oligodeoxyribonucleotide synthesis and restriction endonucleases indicate target bases or sequences for cross-linking

      9. Sister chromatid exchanges (SCEs = cross-over/repair)—see Figure 10-2

     10. Micronuclei formation frequency (clastogenesis)

     11. Comet assay (clastogenesis)—see Figure 10-3

     12. Sperm chromatin structure (denatures DNA at strand breaks with acid + flow cytometry)

     13. TUNEL assay—uses terminal deoxynucleotidyl transferase dUTP to label nick ends due to apoptotic signal cascades or severe DNA damage

     14. Mutagenicity of mixtures determined with Ames test ± strains that overexpress nitroreductase to be sensitive to nitroarenes and aromatic amines, SOS Chromotest and *umu*-test system, Mutatox test, Microscreen phage-induction assay, DNA repair assay, DNA adduct quantitation, DNA strand break assay, micronuclei formation, SCEs, chromosome aberration tests, and *Tradescantia* clone 4430 stamen hair mutation assay

   B. Nuclear membrane damage

      1. Ethylmercury → inorganic Hg → membrane damage and DNA damage (mutagenic and breaks)

      2. Nuclear pyknosis (apoptosis or necrosis-related irreversible chromatin condensation) as caused by Cd and thymic cells irradiation → ↑ ^{3}H-conconavalin A binding, ↓ autologous rosette-forming cell receptors, ↑ nuclear pyknosis, and post-irradiation relaxation of supercoiled DNA

      3. Progerin bound by farnesylation to nuclear membrane (farnesyltransferase causes a 15-carbon isoprenoid or farnesyl group to be added to proteins) → causes membrane blebbing

CONCEPTUALIZING TOXICOLOGY 10-1

C. Mutagenesis

1. Strong mutagens = carcinogens, but not weak mutagens. Some strong carcinogens such as 2,3,7,8-TCDD are not mutagens but cell proliferation agents (mitogens). Increased mitogenesis also leads to more mutagenesis

2. Single nucleoside point mutations (single base alterations + adducts)

Point mutations

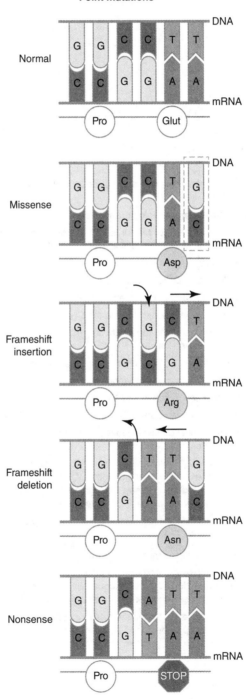

a. Test *in vivo* by examining hemoglobin or glycophorin-A for somatic cell mutations of bone marrow cells of abnormal forms of hypoxanthine-guanine phosphoribosyltransferase and HLA genes in T-lymphocytes

b. Nitrous acid: C → U and A → G in RNA of tobacco mosaic virus

c. N-ethyl N-nitrosourea: AT → TA transversions or AT → GC transitions

d. N-alkyl groups of alkylating agents add the alkyl to the DNA base (7N-guanine residues as mono-alkylating or di-alkylating agents)—classic agents = nitrogen mustards (cyclophosphamide), nitrosoureas, alkyl sulfonates

Mechanism for nitrogen mustards' alkylation:

$$ClCH_2\ CH_2\text{-}N(CH_3)\text{-}\ CH_2\ CH_2Cl \rightarrow ClCH_2\ CH_2\text{-}N^+(CH_3)\text{-}(CH_2)_2 + Cl^-$$
$$+\ RNH_2\ \text{from guanine} \rightarrow ClCH_2\ CH_2\text{-}N(CH_3)\text{-}\ CH_2\ CH_2\text{-}NR(H) + HCl$$

e. ROS alter DNA bases and sugars, cross-link DNA-protein, induce tandem and cluster lesions, + strand breaks—see Figure 10-1. The formation of an 8-hydroxypurine is a precursor to formamidopyrimidines. The formation of 8-OH-G is a premutagenic lesion associated with the process of carcinogenesis. Hydroxyl radical, UV irradiation, or photosensitization → 4,6-diamino-5-formamidopyrimidine and 2,6-diamine-4-hydroxy-5-formamidopyrimidine, which are bypassed by DNA polymerase → wrong DNA base inserted opposite adducted bases

f. Aflatoxin B$_1$ + CYP3A4 → epoxide → unstable N-7 adduct of guanine → AFB$_1$-guanine in urine (depurination) → hepatocarcinoma

g. Aristolochic acid activated by nitro reduction → guanine and more stable adenine adducts; pyrrolizidine alkaloids → DNA adducts → cancer; propenylbenzene safrole → reactive sulfate ester generates DNA adducts; agaritine → hydrazine derivative → DNA adducts

h. PAHs + CYPs → epoxides especially problematic in bay region → bulky DNA adducts

i. Acrylamide → glycidamide metabolite → N7-(2-carbamoyl-2-hydroxyethyl)guanine and N3-(2-carbamoyl-2-hydroxyethyl)adenine adducts

3. Intercalating frameshift mutagens (get between strands and mispair)

a. Pure intercalating agents = 9-aminoacridine dyes

b. Planar PAHs intercalate in space between base pairs → unwinding of double helix, lengthening of strand, mutagenesis

(1) Increases genotoxicity with addition of alkylation (acridine mustards), topoisomerase inhibition (anthracyclines), and DNA adducts (epoxides, etc.)

(2) Only (+)-antiBPDE dG isomer adduct results in mutagenic events leading to carcinogenesis and inhibition of RNA and DNA polymerases

(3) Oxiranes formed by these compounds as metabolized by CYP can also cross-link with preferred sequence of 5′-GNC-3′

c. Mono- and bis-intercalators (strong DNA binding) depends upon alkyl chain length separating the chromophores

4. Cross-linking DNA bases (between adjacent bases or interstrand although bases do not have to be directly paired such as a cytosine-adenine crosslink by UV irradiation) DNA bases labeled by position to visualize adduct/cross-link attack:

Purines

Adenine   Thymine

Pyrimidines

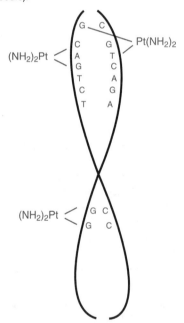

Cytosine   Guanine

a. Cross-links from hydroxyl radical can be initiated by abstracting a hydrogen atom from the C5 or C6 position of cytosine, thymine, or 5-methylcytosine, yielding the pyrimidine radical. This radical may attack neighboring purine base or aerobically yields a cation radical of cytosine (deprotonate exocyclic amino group) → nitrogen-centered radical which couples to neighboring 5'-cytosine (yields 2 types of cross-links)

b. Cross-linking with cisplatin (a chlorinated platinum compound activated by CYP dechlorination and addition of a water molecule):

In the above figure, cisplatin attacks the N-7 position of guanine linked to adjacent guanines or guanine-adenine pairs on the same strand or guanine-guanine pairs between strands.

c. Bidirectional alkylating agents can produce intrastrand/interhelical and interstrand cross-links. Nitrogen mustards form aziridinium followed by alkylation and repeat the cycle to form bisalkylated cross-links. Nitrosoureas, especially chloronitrosourea, target the N-1 of deoxy-guanosine and N-3 of base pairing deoxycytosine + use an ethane linkage to form intrastrand cross-links. Chlorinated α-acetoxy nitrosamines also were more mutagenic (form ICLs) than unchlorinated counterparts. 1,3-Dialkyl-3-acyltriazines transfer N-1 and N-3 alkyl groups to N-7 and O-6 positions of deoxyguanosine

d. Busulfan and congeners = only di-sulfonyls to form ICLs

e. Reduction of Cr(VI) → Cr(III) by ascorbate caused adducts (cross-links) so metals can be involved in cross-linking as well

CONCEPTUALIZING TOXICOLOGY 10-1 (*continued*)

f. 2-chlorothethyl (methylsulfonyl)methanesulfonate chloroethylates at N-1 of dG forming a dC-dG ICL (plus formation of an N-7-chloroethylguanosine) is more selective in action than triazines and nitrosoureas

g. Cross-linking by large oxiranes such as metabolites of PAHs distort DNA structure. However, covalent and noncovalent dimer formation by proteins that interact with DNA indicate that there are high affinity dimer domains on genes that favor binding of larger cross-linking agents despite the structural distortion of DNA. Natural dimeric products (sandramycin, luzopeptins) that have a peptide backbone and aromatic moieties lead to π-stacking and intercalate their aromatic groups with extensive hydrogen bonding in minor groove of DNA. Isochrysohermidin is a natural dimeric N-methylcarbinolamide that proceeds through ring opening and an electrophilic carbonyl that reacts with accessible nucleophiles within minor groove of DNA

h. Bizelesin is a dimeric antitumor medication that alkylates N-3 of adenines in 5′-TAATTA-3′ sequence, cross-linking the first and last base of this sequence. Bizelesin increases cytotoxicity via forming furans or pyrroles

i. Anthramycin, tomaymycin, and sibiromycin are natural pyrrolo[2,1-c][1,4]benzodiazepines that reversibly alkylate in minor groove of exocyclic N-2 amine of dG (carbinolamine at C-11 becoming an imine). The twist in their chemical structures allows hydrogen bonding to O-2 group of paired cytosine as well

j. Psoralens = aromatic compounds with a furan fused to a coumarin. ICL proceeds via intercalation into duplex with 5′-AT or 5′-TA → quantum of light absorbed by compounds 3,4-pyrone or 4′,5′-furan double bond → photocycloaddition to the dT 5,6-double bond → (if pyrone reacts, no ICLs due to destruction of coumarin nucleus) if furan reacts, the coumarin absorbs another quantum of energy → excites 3,4-double bond to a triplet state → cyclizing 5,6-double bond of neighboring pyrimidine forming ICL

k. CYP activation is responsible for oxidatively activated cross-linkers such as cyclophosphamide (nitrogen mustard), N,N,N',N',N',N'-hexamethylmelamine (trimelamol product = cross-linker), pyrrolizidine alkaloids

l. Reductive active agents are created in hypoxic conditions such as nitroaromatic alkylating agents, transition metal complexes, anthracyclines (doxorubicin + e^- → $O_2^{-\cdot}$ + H_2O_2 (Fenton in presence of Fe) → HCO + 3′amino group of doxorubicin → aminal linkage to 2-amino group of proximal dG), aziridinylquinones (form semiquinone on 1 e^- and hydroquinone on 2 e^- reduction alkylate the N-7 of dG in major groove of DNA with strong preference fo 5′-TGC-3′), mitomycin C (quinone moiety cross-links at dG to halt DNA synthesis and promotes phosphodiester strand cuts, alkylates, and produces ROS)

5. Clastogenic mutagens (break DNA into fragments)

a. Crossover in ct-f region close to the centromere of y ct f/+ + + $Drosophila$ $melanogaster$ females exposed to intercalating agents acridine orange, acriflavine, and ethidium bromide.

b. Inhibition of topoisomerase II (topo II) by coumestrol and genistein ↑ micronuclei formation, strand breaks, and hypoxanthine (guanine) phosphoribosyltransferase (hprt) locus mutations in Chinese hamster V79 ovary cells. Certain agents catalytically inhibit topo II (9-aminoacridine, chloroquine, ethidium bromide, tacrine) or poison topo II (auramine, curcumin, proflavine) or have no known direct influence on topo II (2-aminoanthracene, iminostilbene, imipramine, promethazine, quinacrine)

c. SCEs generated by streptonigrin (contains a ROS-generating quinone)

II. Carcinogenesis—see Figure 10-4

A. Activation of oncogenes (embryonic genes for cell proliferation)

1. Viral oncogenes

2. Cellular or proto-oncogenes

a. Growth factors (platelet-derived growth factor)

b. Growth factor receptors—invasive breast cancers and leukemia (ErbB2)

c. Signal transducers—Bcr-Abl construct for acute leukoblastic leukemia

d. Transcription factors (Myc)

e. Apoptosis regulators (bcl-2 prevents apoptosis)

CONCEPTUALIZING TOXICOLOGY 10-1 (*continued*)

B. Inactivate tumor suppressor genes (BRCA2 = region of famous inherited breast cancer abnormalities)

C. Gene abnormalities that predispose cells to becoming cancerous—Table 10-1

D. Mutations around oncogenes or tumor suppressor genes (strong mutagens)

   1. Chromosome rearrangements—new chimeric fusion protein with new or affected function → cancer; reciprocal rearrangement does not; see Figure 10-5

   2. Unbalanced deletions by alkylating agents → acute myeloid leukemia

   3. DNA topoisomerase II inhibitors → leukemias

   4. Tyrosine kinases (abnormal) = key enzyme sequences for cancer formation

   5. Transcription factors can be produced that enhance or produce abnormal transcriptional activity (Ewing's sarcoma) or repress transcription (repression of genes for normal myeloid differentiation → ↑ immature myeloid ells → acute myeloid leukemia).

   6. Toxicogenomics

      a. Covers alkylating agents/ cross-linking agents, oxidative agents, radiation, certain metals (Cd, Cr), certain highly chlorinated pesticides, aryl amines, PAHs, TCDD, diethyl-stilbestrol (DES)

      b. Assay uses a stable transfected human hepatocellular liver carcinoma cell line HepG2 + a luciferase reporter gene and compared with comet assay—see Table 10-2

         (1) All carcinogenic materials ↑ DNA fragmentation (= ↑ olive tail moments in comet assay; luciferase assay = several orders of magnitude more sensitive for PAH benzo[a]pyrene)

E. Multistep process of cancer from gene mutation and chromosome damage → malignancy

   1. Initiation = genotoxicity/mutagenicity—see Figure 10-6

      a. Best measured at early times following treatment (first 8 weeks)

      b. Genotoxic hepatocarcinogens → upregulation of p53 gene (survival and proliferative pathways)

      c. Represented by aflatoxin B_1

   2. Nongenotoxic mechanisms (discriminated from genotoxic agents by apoptotic pathways = weak action on p53, while overexpress transcription factor c-myc)

      a. Proliferation—regenerative hyperplasia and hormone alterations

      b. Nuclear hormone receptor activation

      c. Epigenetics—miRNA and methylation (especially hypomethylation and ↑ gene expression)

      d. Represented by DES

   3. Progression to organ cancer to multi-organ metastasis

      a. Example—Friend leukemia virus → infects cells → 2 weeks later proerythroblasts preventing from maturation first in spleen and then as invading population (glycosylated gp55 glycoprotein interacts with erythropoietin hormone receptor to promote formation of erythroid progenitor cells) → recruits member of tyrosine kinase family in cells → causes dysfunction in cell signaling through a variety of signal transduction and transcription pathways (mostly kinases as indicated by STATs, PI3-kinase/AKT, Grb2/Gab2 molecular adaptors, Lyn kinase, p38MAP kinase, and ERK1/2 MAP kinases) → virus also causes insertional mutagenesis at *spi-1* locus (overexpression) causing arrest of differentiation and turns abnormal cells malignant

      b. Dysregulation of signaling pathway occurs via overactivation, sequence insertion, or mutation of a particular region—allelic deletions or missense mutation by tumor suppressor *p53* gene ↑ susceptibility to cancers such as Friend leukemia virus (increase survival of proerythroblasts rather than affecting differentiation) late in the development of the cancer

      c. Dysregulation can also involve activation of proto-oncogenes and decreasing expression of tumor suppressor genes and apoptotic signaling (mutagens such as aflatoxin B_1 at levels that don't cause liver failure and death)

      d. Another signaling pathway example of carcinogen: 2,3,7,8-TCCD → CYP1A1 and CYP1B1 → activated to toxic metabolites → bind to AhR (aryl hydrocarbon receptor) and AhR nuclear translocator

CONCEPTUALIZING TOXICOLOGY 10-1 (*continued*)

     e. Angiogenesis promotes growth of tumor by providing nutrients and tumor cell movement via new blood supply

F. Cancer risk models

  1. One-hit

     a. Better for As because it has more moderate dependence on time of exposure

     b. Worse for ethylene dibromide, which is strongly dependent on time of exposure

     c. Using high doses to extrapolate to low doses

  2. Multi-hit

  3. Multistage (initiation → promotion → progression)

     a. Clonal two-stage/intermediate stage clonal growth advantage

     b. True multistage models

     c. Short exposure times for these models have high error (3.4-fold error for As, 8-fold for ethylene dibromide)

     d. Using rat lifetime to assume human lifetime

     e. PAHs with only 3–4 rings are better models than those of genotoxic agents

     f. Confounding additional variables include multiple mechanisms of cancer development, species differences at any stage of carcinogenesis, and developmental, dietary, environmental, genetic, and lifestyle factors

     g. Hierarchical organization of multiple cells in a tissue or complex organism not well modeled by cell-free molecular targets or 2-dimensional cell cultures

     h. Certain chemicals require a preexisting condition (*N*-nitroso-*N*-methylurea-induced rat mammary tumors require rats to first have an Hras1 gene mutation)

     i. Extracellular (changes in hormone levels, interleukins, etc.), intracellular (epigenetic effects of compounds like DDT and TCDD on AhR, MAPK, and NF-κB), and intercellular (gap junctions affected by small PAHs affecting the toxicity of ROS) signals should be considered in cancer models

     j. Best model is a 3-dimensional (3D) dynamic culture system using stem cells, several cell types, organotypic cultures, and 3D organoids—see Figure 10-7

  4. Agencies that model cancer—see Table 10-3

     a. ATSDR—high-dose, short-exposure accounting for exposure routes, direct and indirect exposures, and nutritional and lifestyle variables. The history of exposures is also considered. Qualitative = weight of evidence from epidemiology, long-term animal bioassays, short-term tests, and SARs. Modeling assumes multistage process with both genotoxic and epigenetic mechanisms included. Quantitative = dose scaling based on metabolic rate, assumes no threshold, linear, multistage model in absence of plausible mechanism of action. Also relies on judgment of entire toxicology field including the U.S. National Toxicology Program, EPA, OSHA, NIOSH, FDA, and International Agency for Research on Cancer

CONCEPTUALIZING TOXICOLOGY 10-1 (*continued*)

Nuclear Membrane

Because a prokaryote does not have a nucleus, this section is not relevant to effects on eukaryotic cells. The substances that cause other membrane damage may also inflict damage to the nuclear membrane. How can a scientist determine the difference between plasma membrane damage and damage done to the nuclear membrane in particular? DNA staining and ultrastructural histological analyses are two ways of determining that breaches in the nuclear envelope have occurred. An excellent example of this type of testing is a study of the nuclear membrane damage caused by the controversial use of thimerosal (sodium ethylmercurythiosalicylate) as an antibacterial and antifungal preservative in biological products and vaccines in concentrations ranging from 0.003–0.01% (30–100 µg/mL). The mercury content by weight of thimerosal is 49.6% and forms ethylmercury as a metabolite. Ethylmercury can be converted to inorganic mercury, which preferentially accumulates in the cells of the kidneys and brain. Inorganic mercury causes membrane and DNA damage resulting in mutagenic alterations and generating DNA breaks at concentrations below 500 nM. The way the researchers in this study looked for nuclear membrane damage was to utilize the 4′,6-diamidino-2- phenylindole dihydrochloride (DAPI) dye exclusion test. In this assay, the viability of the cells and the presence of nuclear membrane damage were determined by incubating the cells with this nonintercalating DNA-specific dye with an emission maximum in the blue spectrum, with a final concentration of 100 ng/mL DAPI. The method required monitoring of a fluorescent signal, and representative images were taken using a fluorescent scope at 45 minutes and 2, 4, 6, and 24 hours after the addition of thimerosal, with the final for 30 minutes at 20°C in the presence of the dye. Micrographs were analyzed in the center of the wells, where the HCN-1A human cerebral cortical neuron or neonatal human foreskin HCA 2 fibroblast cultures were most uniform (Baskin et al., 2003). This damage is different from nuclear pyknosis, which is a thickening or a condensation and reduction in size of the nucleus as a stage of necrosis.

It is interesting to note that if another approach is taken with heavy metals with another assay, a different result emerges. For example, Cd is an extremely toxic metal. However, if thymic cells are irradiated, the changes toward necrosis usually include an increase in ^{3}H-conconavalin A binding, a reduction in autologous rosette-forming cell receptors, an increase in nuclear pyknosis, and a postradiation relaxation of nuclear supercoiled DNA. These effects have been shown to be reduced by Cd by binding to sites similar to other heavy metals (Zherbin et al., 1986). Thus, it appears that the model of damage and its interpretation indicate the nuclear toxicity directly by assessing damage or infer a toxic action by prevention of damage by alternative mechanisms. It is not surprising that heavy metals cause

nuclear membrane problems. Another interesting toxic product is progerin. This compound is persistently bound by farnesylation to the nuclear membrane. This compound appears to be responsible for nuclear membrane blebbing caused by mutations that disrupt proper nuclear lamina formation on the inside of the nuclear membrane. This makes the nuclear membrane more subject to damage and loss of cell viability. This occurs in premature aging syndromes, such as Hutchinson-Gilford progeria syndrome, and may be prevented by production of the farnesyl group, which is synthesized through the cholesterol biosynthetic pathway. Statin medications that inhibit HMG-CoA reductase and prevent cholesterol synthesis may have an important role in decreasing the toxicity of aging or premature aging on nuclear events. The fight against cancer has also led to farnesyl transferase inhibitors due to the participation of the farnesylation in the function of the oncoprotein ras (Korf, 2008).

Mutagenesis

Much of what was once considered mutagenic or clastogenic injury is now described as genetic toxicology or rolled into the genotoxic agents that cause carcinogenesis. The first and simple idea is that not all agents that modify DNA lead to cancer, unless they are strongly mutagenic. Some adduct formation of nucleic acids leads to apoptosis or necrosis such as damage from acetaminophen or amphetamine. Additionally, compounds that increase growth without modifying DNA are known as mitogens. They increase cancer formation as exemplified by 2,3,7,8-TCDD. However, it is not as clear as stated, because mitogenesis also increases the rate of mutation. Also, all DNA is subject to mutations or genetic damage, but not all cells can become cancer cells, such as prokaryotic cells. These cells may be able to indicate mutagenesis but require confirmation for ability to transform mammalian, avian, fish, or similar cells in complex organisms into cancer cells. This section considers all mutagenic events— from simple point mutations to large-scale DNA fragmentation or chromosomal breaks, which are true clastogenesis. Assays in somatic or germ cells are discussed as these represent noninheritable possible oncogenic events and inheritable mutational alterations. A discussion of cancer transformation mechanisms follows.

Single Nucleotide Point Mutations

Some of the earliest terminology in mutagenesis involved missense mutations where single amino acid replacements were noted in the triplet codon misreading due to alterations of a single nucleotide base. Nonsense mutations would cause early termination of a protein sequence. Hemoglobin and glycophorin-A have been used to look for somatic cell mutations in human red blood cells (RBCs) as a result of mutagen exposure to bone marrow cells. Similarly, T-lymphocytes may be examined for abnormal forms of hypoxanthine-guanine phosphoribosyltransferase and human leukocyte antigen (HLA) genes (Albertini et al., 1993). Early attempts at looking at the triplet codon results of point mutations involved the use of nitrous acid, which causes the transitions of $C \rightarrow U$ and $A \rightarrow G$ in the RNA tobacco mosaic virus (Sengbusch, 1967). The alkylating agent N-ethyl N-nitrosourea (ENU) is considered

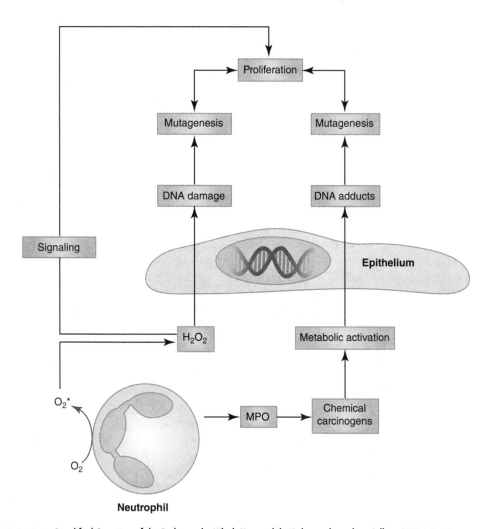

FIGURE 10-1 Simplified Overview of the Pathways by Which Neutrophils (Polymorphonuclear Cells or PMNs) May Impact on Pulmonary Genotoxicity

one of the most potent mutagens in mice and is estimated to induce a point mutation, most often with AT to TA transversions or AT to GC transitions. This agent is now used to elucidate the mouse genome and by inference human genome disease states by a forward genetics- or phenotype-driven approach—as differentiated from the reverse genetics approach of utilizing knockout mice (Acevedo-Arozena et al., 2008). Other alkylating agents such as nitrogen mustards (e.g., cyclophosphamide) were used in World War I as chemical weapons and are currently used in high doses to treat cancers via damaging the DNA of cells in any phase of the cell cycle. Four other classes of alkylating agents are used medically, including alkyl sulfonates, ethyleneimines, nitrosoureas, and triazenes.

It is important not to go too far into this topic without mentioning the effect of oxygen radicals that has been stressed heavily in former sections on DNA. **Figure 10-1** provides a simple illustration how an ROS-generating cell such as a neutrophil or metabolic activation and adduct formation can yield a mutagenic event or result in stimulation of cell signaling pathways that result in cell proliferation. Reactive oxygen species (ROS) modify DNA bases and sugars, cause DNA–protein cross-links, induce tandem and clustered lesions, and even result in strand breaks. Formamidopyrimidines resulting from the one-electron reduction of C8–OH-adduct radicals of purines have 8-hydroxypurines as their common precursor, which is generated by a one-electron oxidation. The generation of 8-hydroxyguandeoxyguanosine is a premutagenic lesion thought to be associated with the process of carcinogenesis (Knaapen et al., 2006). Hydroxyl radical attack, UV radiation, or photosensitization mainly generates 4,6-diamino-5-formamidopyrimidine and 2,6-diamino-4-hydroxy-5-formamidopyrimidine, which can be detected by mass spectrometry. These altered bases are bypassed by DNA polymerase. This process results in the wrong DNA base being inserted opposite of these adducted bases resulting in mutagenesis, which can be repaired by base excision utilizing prokaryotic or eukaryotic DNA glycosylases in the first step of this process (Dizdaroglu et al., 2008).

Other DNA-reactive products come from foods and have been associated with cancer formation. One of the most potent of these is aflatoxin B_1 (AFB$_1$), which is a product of *Aspergillus flavus*. After activation by CYP3A4 to an epoxide, the reactive intermediate of AFB$_1$ forms an unstable N-7 adduct of guanine residues. Depurination occurs (AFB$_1$-guanine in urine) or a ring-opening formamidopyrimidine derivative forms. These changes result in hepatocarcinomas, especially when in concert with hepatitis B exposure. Herbal teas and medicines contain aristolochic acid, which is activated by nitro reduction and yields guanine and adenine adducts. The adenine adducts tend to be more stable. Borage from *Borago officinalis* is used as a blood "purifier" and as a diuretic, but contains pyrrolizidines alkaloids that form DNA adducts inducing cancer formation. DNA adducts also are produced from the reactive sulfate ester (produced by hydroxylation and sulfonation) of the propenylbenzene safrole, which is found in natural root beer made from *Sassafras cortex*. Certain compounds from mushrooms such as agaritine are converted by the γ-glutamyl transpeptidase and possibly cytochrome P450 (CYP) to a hydrazine derivative that also forms DNA adducts (Jeffrey and Williams, 2005). Polycyclic aromatic hydrocarbons (PAHs) arise from broiling protein-rich foods. Their activation by CYP and formation of bulky-aromatic DNA adducts has been determined in human leukocytes (Peluso et al., 2008). Heating of food also cause acrylamide formation which can cause DNA damage as monitored by the DNA fragmentation comet assay or from the formation of DNA adducts such as N7-(2-carbamoyl-2-hydroxyethyl)guanine (N7-GA-Gua) and N3-(2-carbamoyl-2-hydroxyethyl)adenine (N3-GA-Ade). These adducts arise from the reactive glycidamide metabolite. The N7-GA-Gua is removed more slowly by DNA repair (Manière et al., 2005). It is apparent that the DNA bases modified by reactive intermediates, the extent of the adduct formation, the half-life of adducts in the cells or tissues, their likelihood of misreading or causing DNA breaks, and the genes they activate or inactivate by their presence must be considered in determining the risk of exposure and the probabilities of carcinogenesis versus apoptosis/necrosis.

Intercalating Frameshift Mutagens

Planar polycyclic aromatic hydrocarbons have the ability to intercalate in the space between two adjacent base pairs, leading to unwinding of the double helix, lengthening of the DNA strand, and mutagenesis. There is bulging of the unpair base of bases out of the helix, which can lead to a deletion or an addition depending on how the polymerase deals with the growing strand. Topoisomerase II can be involved in this process as well, because the effect of proflavine and analogues in bacteriophage T4 indicate a nick-processing model. In this model for chemicals that both intercalate and effect topoisomerase II, the DNA nicks of T4 topoisomerase II enzymes are subsequently processed in an error-prone fashion through the polymerase and exonuclease activities of T4 DNA polymerase. The model compounds that are pure intercalating agents are the dye 9-aminoacridine and its derivatives. These agents bind noncovalently and reversibly to DNA. The frameshift mutagenesis that occurs as a result of this binding is demonstrated most easily in bacteriophage and bacterial assays, especially in areas with repetitive sequences, but is less clastogenic in mammalian cells. Only in cases where acridines tether other chemicals to DNA do base substitutions and frameshifts occur at higher frequencies. 9-Aminoacridine is a monointercalator, as is quinoline. They rarely cause cancer on their own as indicated by the weak intercalation caused by the flavonoids. A monointercalator becomes more genotoxic as it does other functions as well such as alkylation (acridine mustard or nitroacridines), topoisomerase II inhibition (anthracyclines), or forming DNA adducts (aflatoxin B_1, aminofluorene, diol epoxides, tamoxifen). Di-acridines or diquinolines can be mono- or bisintercalators dependent upon the alkyl chain length separating the chromophores. The bisintercalators show strong DNA binding and may induce "petite" mutagenesis, which is the term given to mutations of small DNA found in the more susceptible mitochondria rather than the larger genome

of the nucleus. The Ames test is a simple way of picking up point mutations or frameshift mutations, as the *Salmonella*-mammalian microsome mutagenicity test indicates a mutation via the number of reversions to His$^+$ colonies that will grow under low histidine concentrations in the growth medium. This has been used as the premier assay for activation via P450 and subsequent mutagenic action. Because the His$^+$ reversion requires a frameshift in the GC repeat sequence, acridines and similar agents' action is also detected easily by this assay. Similarly, a reversion assay of mutagenicity of acridines can be detected in a reversion assay based on tetracycline resistance in plasmid pBR322 in *Escherichia coli*. The compounds 9-aminoacridine and quinacrine effectively induce −1 frameshifts and weakly induce +1 frameshifts, while acridine mustards induce both −1 and +1 frameshifts as well as other events. If an *E. coli* lacZ reversion assay is employed, simple acridines have −1 frameshifts for poly G residues and weaker +1 frameshifts for poly A residues. Nitroacridines induce a wide range of responses as expected. Similar work can be done in eukaryotic cells employing enhanced green fluorescence protein (EGFP) reporter plasmids. The EGFP is inserted out of frame so that initially it does not report in mouse cell lines C3H10T1/2 and mismatch repair-deficient MC2a. EGFP reversions could be detected by a variety of mutagens, including the frameshift type acridines. This is then measured by flow cytometry and confirmed by DNA sequencing. An *in vitro* bleomycin amplification method employing V79 Chinese hamster cells can quantify the potential strength of DNA intercalative binding through a three- dimensional DNA computational docking model. This method indicates that DNA intercalation is necessary but insufficient for genotoxicity for many classes of chemical agents (Ferguson and Denny, 2007).

Cross-Linking Mutagens

Cross-linking between adjacent DNA strands in a double helix prevents replication by inhibiting separation of the strands into a fork that allows replication. That these interstrand crosslinks (ICLs) completely halt replication was one early way of detecting the dramatic inhibitory effects of a cross-linking sulfur mustard di-2-chloroethyl sulfide on T7 phage's ability to infect *E. coli* in the late 1960s (Rajski and Williams, 1998). Cross-links from ultraviolet (UV) irradiation can usually start from an oxygen (hydroxyl) radical that will abstract a hydrogen from C5 or C6 on cytosine, thymine, or 5-methylcytosine, generating a pyrimidine radical. Either this radical attacks the neighboring purine base or yields a cation radical of cytosine (nitrogen-center radical) that couples to the neighboring 5′-cytosine (Hong and Wang, 2005). Cross-links can also be detected by heat-denaturing, double-stranded plasmid DNA in a strand-separating buffer followed by chilling and loading onto an agarose gel for electrophoretic analysis. Ethidium bromide staining and densitometry allow quantitation for the presence of double-stranded DNA as ICLs. There are other types of DNA modifications possible with cross-linking reagents including adducts of single bases or hydrolyzed single bases detectable by the usual reversion assays and nucleotide sequencing using mass spectrometry. DNA-protein cross-links are also possible as are intrastrand or interhelical cross-links. Bidirectional alkylating agents are in theory capable of all these types of interactions. When three α-acetoxy nitrosamines were evaluated versus those that contained chloroethyl, chloropropyl and chlorobutyl groups, it was discovered that the chlorinated nitrosamines were more mutagenic than their unchlorinated counterparts. They were more mutagenic in *Salmonella typhimurium* strains deficient in the *ogt* gene (YG7108 and YG7104) compared to those not deficient in that gene (TA1535), which appears to identify the O^6- alkylguanine adducts as the cause of the mutations. Loss of excision repair increased mutagenicity manifold for all nitrosamines when comparing TA1975 (*uvrB+*) versus TA1535 ($\Delta uvrB$) strains. However, *N*-nitroso-*N*-(acetoxymethyl)-2-chloroethylamine caused the most ICLs, followed by the *N*-nitroso-*N*-(acetoxymethyl)-4-chlorobutylamine derivative. The weaker cross-linking capability of the chlorobutyl derivative appears to be due to the lack of appropriate bond length between the two DNA strands. *N*-(acetoxymethyl)-3-chloropropylamine and the other nonchlorinated nitrosamines caused no observable cross-links in the plasmid DNA assay.

The cross-linking ability of the chlorinated forms appears similar in action to the antitumor chloroethylnitrosoureas (Ishikawa and Mochizuki, 2003). Cisplatin (cis-diaminodichloroplatinum) is a good example of a chlorinated metal species that causes cross-linking, which appears to be important in its chemotherapeutic action against cancer cells. The chloride atoms are displaced in the cell and replaced by water to produce the species that creates intrastrand and interstrand cross-links of DNA. Cisplatin especially attacks at the N-7 position of guanine, linking adjacent guanines on the same strand or guanine-adenine pairs between strands. As with other cross-linking agents, other mutations are much more favored reactions. The repair of this damage appears to be linked to a trimeric protein phosphatase complex (Vázquez-Martin, 2008). Another group used a pSP189 vector to create a mutagenesis reporter construct in flies based on the *supF* gene and a second assay employing the *lats* tumor suppressor gene. They found that a gene sequence discovered in a disorder known as Fanconi anemia used in DNA repair. In the human autosomal recessive cancer susceptibility that characterizes Fanconi anemia, there is both a sensitivity to mitomycin C and ionizing radiation. A nuclear complex containing FANCA, FANCC, FANCFm, and FANCG proteins is required for activation of the FANCD2 protein to a monoubiquitinated isoform. In normal cells, FANCD2 is monoubiquitinated in response to DNA damage and is co-localized to the breast cancer susceptibility protein BRCA1. This pathway is indicated by the mutagenesis reporter system as being involved in cross-link repair. Additionally, the multiple endocrine neoplasia type I (MEN1) gene appears to be involved in cross-link repair, transcriptional regulation, control of cell proliferation, apoptosis regulation, and bone development. The *supF* gene reporter model showed that cross-linked DNA was more subject to single base deletions in a homopolymeric tract in MEN1 mutants, while FANCD2 mutants had a mutation spectrum and frequency similar to wild-type cells. The *lats* assay demonstrated the high frequency or large deletions in cross-linked DNA of FANCD2 mutants but rarely in MEN1 mutants not detected by the other assay. So, to detect cross-linking and its repair mechanisms, more than one assay is appropriate in deciphering differing mechanisms of action and repair (Marek et al., 2008).

In addition to chlorinated species, certain metals, such as the ascorbate reduction of Cr(VI) to between 5 and 60 μM Cr(III), cause from 2–40 adducted sites per 1000 nucleotide bases, with 18.5% resulting in polymerase arrest (cross-linking). Chromium also binds to the phosphate backbone resulting in interhelical binding, but only the base cross-linking leads to polymerase arrest. A method has been developed for truly evaluating where these cross-links form in regard to target bases or sequences through the use of solid-phase oligodeoxyribonucleotide synthesis and restriction endonucleases. Through the use of these and other technologies, the following categories of cross-linking agents have emerged: inherently labile compounds (nitrogen mustards, chlorethylating agents, nitrosoureas, triazines, alkyl sulfonates, oxiranes, diepoxybutane, carzinophilin/azinomycin B, *cis*-diamminedichloroplatinum[II; cis-DDP], dimeric DNA-binding and cross-linking agents, sandramycin, luzopeptins, isochrysohermidin, bizelesin and related structures, pyrrolobenzodiazepine dimers, dinuclear *cis*-DDP analogues), photoactivated agents (psoralens), oxidatively activated cross-linkers (cyclophosphamide, N,N,N',N',N',N'-hexamethylmelamine and related structures, pyrrolizidine alkaloids), and hypoxia-selective or reductively activated agents (masked nitrogen mustards, transition metal complexes, anthracyclines, aziridinylbenzoquinones, mitomycin C and related structures, FR-900482 and related structures, and interstrand DNA cross-linking DNA–protein cross-linking by FR-66979). Some of these agents have been discussed earlier, but the mechanisms of others are examined in the paragraphs that follow.

The nitrogen mustards represent the earliest and most widely evaluated inherently labile compounds. The nitrogen mustards covalently cause aziridinium formation followed by alkylation and repeat the cycle to form the bisalkylated cross-link. The nitrosoureas, especially the chloronitrosoureas, are also inherent cross-linking agents targeting the N-1 of deoxyguanosine and the N-3 of its base pairing partner deoxycytosine. An ethane linkage forms the interstrand cross-link. The 1,3-dialkyl-3-acyltriazenes transfer the N-1 and N-3 alkyl groups to deoxyguanosine N-7 and O-6 positions. This may be achieved by two different degradative routes. The major route generates the alkane diazonium preceded by heterolytic scission of the N-2-to-N-3 bond. This is completed by generation of the alkane diazonium, DNA alkylation, or hydrolysis giving rise to dG adducts. The minor pathway transfers the N-3 alkyl group via deacylation and tautomerization. If the N-1 alkyl group is a chloroethyl moiety, quenching of the diazonium yields chloroethylation at either dG N-7 or O-6. Similar to nitrosoureas, O-6 and N-7 chloroethylation yield dG-dC interstrand cross-links and dG-dG intrastrand lesions (if there is a deoxyguanosine proximal to the initial N-7 lesion), respectively. Busulfan and its congeners are the only disulfonyls to form ICLs. They form 1,4-bis(7-guanyl)butane and 7-(4-hydroxybutyl)guanosine. Introduction of a 2-chloroethyl group alone to these compounds does not generate the expected higher level of ICL formation. However, 2-chloroethyl (methylsulfonyl)methanesulfonate (clomesone) chloroethylates at the N-1 position of dG, forming a dC-dG ICL. The adduct formation of this compound to an N-7-chloroethylguanosine is much more selective than those of the triazenes and nitrosoureas, which form a variety of covalent links to DNA. Additionally, clomesone does not perform carbamoylation, which is a reaction common to proteins treated with chloronitrosourea. Oxiranes are toxic products, especially for compounds such as benzo[*a*]pyrene (B[*a*]P). Four carcinogenic stereoisomers of 7,8-dihydroxy-9,10-epoxy-7,8,9,10-tetrahydrobenzo[a]pyrene (BPDE) form from oxidative metabolism of B[*a*]P. The benzylic epoxides form adducts mainly by ring-opening and forming the bulky BPDE C-10 covalent linkage to an exocyclic amine N-2 of dG. Only the (+)-antiBPDE dG isomer adduct results in mutagenic events that lead to carcinogenesis and inhibits RNA and DNA polymerases.

Diepoxybutane was the first oxirane demonstrated to cause cancer and the simplest oxirane with cross-linking ability. Its preferred cross-linking DNA sequence is 5'-GNC-3', predominating four-fold over the sequences from 5' to 3' of TGCA or TCGA, which are preferred over CCGG and the least attacked TATA. It is unusual that a cross-linking reagent could be this small, as the 6.8 Å distance between the N-7 and N-7 bases in the preferred GNC sequence is larger than the diepoxybutane of 5.1 Å. It is expected that there is a large distortion in the bases to accommodate such a linkage. The complex oxirane carzinophilin from *Streptomyces sahachiroi* (azinomycin B from *Streptomyces griseofuscus* S42227) contains both a labile epoxide and a bicyclic aziridinopyrolidine along with the C-6 amide. Piperidine labile site cleavage and solid-phase oligodeoxyribonucleotide containing deoxyinosine and 7- deazaguanosine to probe the effects of functional group deletions on cross-linking efficiency indicated akylations occur with 5'-GNC-3' and 5'-GNT-3' sequences between the N-7 groups of two deoxyguanosines or dG and an adjacent dA. The assignments made by piperidine reactions were confirmed by employing bis(1,10-phenanthroline)copper, a chemical nuclease reagent. Covalent and noncovalent dimer formation by proteins that interact with DNA indicate that there are high affinity dimer domains on genes that would favor binding with larger cross-linking agents rather than small ones that also require substantial distortion of the DNA structure. There are some natural dimeric products that have a peptide backbone and aromatic moieties leading to π-stacking. These compounds intercalate via their aromatic groups and have extensive hydrogen bonding with the minor groove. Whether these compounds have the decadepsipeptide backbone of sandramycin and the luzopeptins or the bicyclic octadepsipeptides of echinomycin and triostin A, they all can bisintercalate in DNA in a syn fashion due to their dimer structure (Rajski and Williams, 1998). The natural cross-linking product isochrysohermidin from *Mercurialis perennis* is a dimeric N-methylcarbinolamide that proceeds via slow ring-opening to a *d,l-* and *meso-*isochrysohermidin.

An electrophilic carbonyl is exposed, which reacts with accessible nucleophiles within the minor groove of duplex DNA (C-2 amine of dG; Yeung and Boger, 2003). Cyclopropylpyrroloindoles induce alkylation at the N-3 group of adenines. The synthesis of dimers of these compounds has yielded a crosslinking antitumor medication bizelesin, whose cytotoxicity increases by forming furans or pyrroles from the parent compound. As a cyclopropylpyrroloindole, bizelesin selectively alkylates the N-3 of adenine in the 5'-TTA-3' sequence. Based on its size, it prefers to cross-link the first and last bases of a 5'-TAATTA-3' sequence. The inherent instability of the central AT step of this short sequence leads to base opening, which hydrogen bonds with the ureylene amido protons of bizelesin. This stabilizes the transient Hoogsteen and open base pair conformations. These steps increase the specificity and the probability of cross-link formation. Anthramycin, tomaymycin, and sibiromycin are natural pyrrolo[2,1-*c*][1,4]benzodiazepines. Reversible alkylation in the minor groove of the exocyclic N-2 amine of dG occurs from these compounds by the carbinolamine at C-11 becoming an imine. The binding of these compounds to the minor groove binding is facilitated by the twist in their chemical structure (S configuration at the bicyclic C-11a position) and hydrogen bonding between the O-2 group of the cytosine across from its alkylated guanine pair and the phenolic 9-OH of the alkylating agent. The pyrrolo[2,1-*c*] [1,4] benzodiazepines dimerized via a propane–diyldioxy ether linkage are excellent irreversible ICL formers.

As indicated earlier, cisplatin is a cross-linking medication used to treat aggressive forms of cancer. However, its usefulness in forming ICLs may be limited by its size. Dinuclear Pt complexes containing one chloride group per platinum allows for excellent cross-linking, as only one adduct formation per platinum group. The use of pyridyl moieties in these compounds aids in the unwinding of DNA. The *trans-* isomer of these compounds is the only one capable of both ICLs and intrastrand cross-links in 5'-GGCC-3' sequences. *Cis* chloride placements do not allow the butanediamine chain the correct orientation for intrastrand linkages. This finishes the discussion on the inherently labile cross-linking compounds.

There is only one group of compounds that activate by photolysis as isolated from the *Umbelliferae, Rutaceae,* and *Leguminosae* plant families and from fungi: the psoralens— aromatic chemicals with a furan fused to a coumarin. These agents induce ICLs and also generate A to C mutations. The ICL process is done in three steps. The planar tricyclic psoralen first intercalates into the duplex between two bases of either 5′-AT or 5′-TA. A quantum of light absorbed into the 3,4-pyrone double bond or the 4′,5′-furan double bond causes a photocycloaddition to the dT 5,6-double bond. If the pyrone reacts, this destroys the coumarin nucleus and prevents ICL formation. If the furan reacts, the coumarin can absorb a second quantum of light energy. This excites the 3,4-double bond to a triplet state ($\pi \rightarrow \pi^*$), cyclizing the 5,6-double bond of the neighboring pyrimidine forming the ICL.

CYPs are responsible for the oxidatively activated cross-linkers. Cyclophosphamide has been mentioned earlier as a chemical warfare and a tumor treatment agent. Oxazaphosphorines such as cyclophosphamide are oxidized at the C-4 position next to the ring nitrogen to a 4-hydroxy metabolite that spontaneously and reversibly opens the ring to an aldophosphamide. ICLs will not form if the C-4 hydroxyl is oxidized by alcohol dehydrogenase or the aldophosphamide is oxidized by aldehyde dehydrogenase ALDH1. However, the active products of phosphoramide mustard (actual ICL former) and acrolein are yielded from removal of the phosphoryl group from the aldehyde. The phosphoramide mustard may be hydrolyzed into nor-HN2, which is the secondary amine form of mechlorethamine. N,N,N',N',N',N'-hexamethylmelamine is a cancer chemotherapy agent that is demethylated to form a potent electrophile with cross-linking activity. This compound as well as trimelamol may not always in fact be the cross-linking agent, because a formaldehyde product can form a methylene bridge between the two N-6 exocyclic amines of dA from a 5′-ApT-3′ sequence. However, the lack of deformation ICLs, exclusive formation of the trisubstituted

thioether adducts, and no ICLs formed with a concentration of formaldehyde that might occur in these reactions implicate the trimelamol as the cross-linking agent. The pyrrolizidine alkyloids mentioned earlier from borage and other similar herbal products are oxidized to a highly toxic pyrrole and a less toxic *N*-oxide. The most potent ICL formers of this group have an α,β-unsaturated, 12-member macrocyclic necine diester moiety. These compounds attack a 5′-CpG-3′ sequence similarly to mitomycin C. However, certain of the pyrrolizidine alkaloids also show abilities to attack 5′-GpC-3′, 5′-TCGA-3′, and 5′-GCGC-3′ sequences. This indicates that mitomycin C is much more selective than the pyrrolizidines.

Reductively active agents generated during hypoxic conditions existent in solid tumors are important cross-linking chemotherapy agents, because ionizing radiation does not work in tumor cells of this type. Nitroaromatic alkylating agents are activated by reduction to a more reactive form. Nitrobenzyl chemicals are reduced to form iminoquinone methide. The conversion of the electron-withdrawing nitro moiety to an intermediate hydroxylamine or an electron-donating amine is the mechanism for activation for the nitroimidazoles to form adducts or ICLs. Transition metal complexes can also facilitate activation of cross-linking reagents via one-electron reduction activation by enzymes such as such as cytochrome P-450 reductase. Two-electron reductions of quinones and nitroheterocycles may be catalyzed by NAD(P)H:quinone oxidoreductases (DT diaphorase) and xanthine dehydrogenase under aerobic conditions. The advantage of one-electron reductions is their specificity, as irreversible two-electron reductions bypass the possible selectivity generated by the oxidation of the one-electron reduced agent and production of superoxide. Co(III) complexes serve well as one-electron reduction substrates depending on the attached ligands. $Co^{3+}(NH_3)_6$ is a very stable compound in water, but the reduction to Co(II) results in rapid, irreversible exchange to an extremely stable $[Co(H_2O)_6]^{2+}$ species. If polydendate ligands are used, then the stabilization of the Co(II) species allows the oxygen reversibility required for selectivity of action in a hypoxic state. Anthracyclines are compounds having a tetracyclic quinophenolic ring system with associated carbohydrate groups that are reducible. The effectiveness of doxorubicin on cancer cells is its ability to intercalate in a distorted B-DNA duplex between the 5′-CpG-3′ sequences at both ends. The D-ring of the anthracyclines protrudes into the major groove and the amino sugar in the minor groove of the DNA helix. Anthracyclines without a C-9 hydroxyl group to coordinate with the N-3 and N-2 nitrogens of dG are not ICL reagents. These agents also inhibit topoisomerase II, causing DNA double-stranded breaks. These compounds additionally bind to negatively charged phospholipids increasing cell growth at low subcytoxic concentrations and inhibiting growth with increased cytotoxicity. One severe limitation of the use of doxorubicin in the treatment of cancer is its ability to generate superoxide and prevent the repair mechanisms in cardiac cells, resulting in cardiomyopathy. ICL formation may occur from dimers that result from condensation of two quinone methides following reduction of the original compound. However, the formation of quinone methides is not an obligatory step in the formation of crosslinks. Research with doxorubicin showed that reduction was an obligatory step in its activity as an ICL agent. The involvement of Fe(II)-Fe(III) redox in this process appears to the other essential ingredient in ICL formation for this and structurally similar compounds. The ICL is then formed from doxorubicin as follows. The reductive activation results in superoxide formation and hydrogen peroxide, which combine in a Fenton- type reaction scheme to produce formaldehyde. This formaldehyde condenses with the 3′-amino group of doxorubicin and forms an aminal linkage to the 2-amino group of the proximal dG. Anthracyclines are grouped into those that inhibit DNA and nucleolar precursor RNA synthesis at similar concentrations (class I) and those that affect nucleolar synthesis at 200–1300-fold lower concentrations than those that alter DNA synthesis (class II). Aziridinylquinones are nonaromatic quinones that upon reduction become an aromatic semiquinone on one-electron transfer or hydroquinone with a two-electron reduction. Because these structures no longer have the nitrogen's lone pair of

electrons tied to the carbonyl group, this allows protonation of the now alkaline tertiary amines and the electrophilic strength of the aziridine. Alkylation of the DNA base is followed by regenerating the quinone via autoxidation. These compounds appear to alkylate the N-7 position of dG in the major groove of DNA with strong preference for the 5′-TGC-3′ motif forming the ICL. However, some dA alkylation occurs, especially for the 5′-(A/T)AA-3′ sequences.

As indicated earlier, mitomycin C has a very constrained specificity for adduct and ICL formation. It is an intercalating agent with a quinone moiety that is similar to other crosslinking agents of this type. However, it can both alkylate DNA and produce DNA-damaging superoxide and subsequent other ROS. It is the aziridinomitosene moiety that reacts with dG to halt DNA synthesis and promote phosphodiester strand cuts. Cell death results from ICL formation and not from strand scissions caused by mitomycins. The antitumor agents FR-900482 (4-formyl-6,9-dihydroxy-14-oxa-1, 11-diazatetracyclo[7.4.1.0.0]tetradeca-2,4, 6-triene-8-yl methyl carbamate) and its dihydro congener, FR-66979 are fermentation products of *Streptomyces sandaensis* 6897. They are structurally similar to mitomycin C. The interesting portion of these cross-linking agents is that FR-900482 is effective in multidrug-resistant P388 cells, where mitomycin C has little activity. They are still activated by reduction, but do not produce the superoxide-generated, single-strand DNA break due to their lack of participation in Fenton or Haber-Weiss reactions. This makes them more potent than mitomycin C with less toxicity against neoplastic cells. Their lack of oxidative damage is due to the structural absence of the quinone. It appears instead that the hydroxylamine hemiketal's N-O bond is its important reactive moiety. Upon reduction, these compounds form mitocenes that would be expected to attack the same 5′-CpG-3′ as do the mitocenes formed from the mitomycin C. Iron(II) salts are extremely important in the reductive and cross-linking process, because the FR compounds only cross-link DNA at approximately 5% efficiency in the presence of only a thiol reductive reagent. The addition of Fe(II) increases the ICL efficiency to 55–62%. The phenolic moiety of these FR compounds appears to play a large role in their ability to form DNA adducts, ICLs, and cross-links to proteins. The formation of the DNA-FR-66979-peptide adduct shows that the dG-FR-66979 adduct coordinates with two arginine groups of the binding domain (BD) of the High Mobility Group I/Y (HMG I/Y) peptide substrate as indicated by 1H NMR studies. This indicates a likely reaction between the C-10 position of the mitocene metabolite and an essential arginine moiety. Ligand-DNA exchange reactions and negative ion spray mass spectrometry of the gel-purified DNA-mitocene-peptide conjugate indicated that this cross-linked combination was indeed covalent. Reduced bioxalomycin α_2 of *Streptomyces viridostaticus litoralis* also cross-links in the 5′-CpG-3′ motif. It is the exocyclic amine (N-2) of the minor groove dG that participates in the cross-link as indicated by piperidine digestion. The structure of bioxalomycin again contains a quinone capable of producing ROS and also resultant DNA and protein damage (Rajski and Williams, 1998).

Clastogenic Mutagens

A number of mutagens discussed earlier cause fragmentation of DNA, induce problems that require DNA repair and can cause exchange of genetic material, form micronuclei, and lead to chromosomal abnormalities. It appears that this may be a dose-dependent phenomenon, with smaller changes such as point mutations or adduct formation preceding larger DNA fragmentation at higher doses. This section examines the various agents that cause clastogenic actions and how they are measured. One early measure for clastogenesis was crossingover. There is some mutual exchange of parts of chromatids of homologous chromosomes during meiosis and in some species during mitosis that is known as crossing-over. Because DNA sequences are altered, this is considered mutagenic. Additionally, this is a clastogenic event as DNA pieces are cleaved off their original chromosomes. The increased frequencies of recombination events increase with mutagens. In one study, intercalating agents increased the crossing-over events in the ct-f region close to the centromere of y *ct f*/+ + + *Drosophila melanogaster*

females exposed to intercalating agents acridine orange, acriflavine, and ethidium bromide. The changes were followed by a classic genetics technique of phenotypic expression following larval stage exposure (Xamena et al., 1985). Further investigation reveals that the DNA intercalating agent 8-methoxy pyrimido[4′,5′:4,5]thieno (2,3-b)quinoline-4(3H)-one causes clastogenesis in mouse bone marrow cells and induces sperm abnormalities. More modern research tools have determined that these events originate from protein-associated DNA strand breaks that are facilitated by inhibition of the topoisomerase enzymes. The use of three phytoestrogens confirms this finding. Two of them (coumestrol and genistein but not daidzein) inhibit topoisomerase II and therefore increase the formation of micronuclei, strand breaks, and hypoxanthine (guanine) phosphoribosyltransferase (hprt) locus mutations in cultured Chinese hamster V79 cells. This indicates that for certain agents that are less disruptive such as the intercalators, the inhibition of topoisomerase enzymes may be necessary for larger disruptive effects. When the micronucleus assay detectable by microscopy is modified, it can detect those intercalating compounds that catalytically inhibit type II topoisomerase (9-aminoacridine, chloroquine, ethidium bromide, tacrine), are topo II poisons (auramine, curcumin, proflavine), or have no detectable influence on that key DNA-interacting enzyme (2-aminoanthracene, iminostilbene, imipramine, promethazine, quinacrine; Ferguson and Denny, 2007).

Micronuclei appearance is also indicative of cancer risk or cancer treatment, because it marks chromosomal damage and genome instability. A meta-analysis of cancer patients, thyroid cancer patients treated with radioactive iodine, and the radiosensitivity of lymphocytes from untreated cancer patients found increased micronuclei in untreated cancer patients and thyroid cancer patients following radioiodine therapy. However, a reduction in micronuclei in assessing radiosensitivity of untreated cancer patients' lymphocytes indicated a high rate of apoptosis following irradiation (Iarmarcovai et al., 2008). These studies indicate care must be taken in interpreting the damage from these tests, because other mechanisms such as apoptosis may confound the data.

A researcher can look for clastogenesis by other light microscopic methods. For example, if micronuclei do not form, then chromosome abnormalities may be picked up by staining the chromosomes and doing a classical karyotype. If more subtle DNA damage and repair has occurred, then that can be detected by a fairly old technique known as sister chromatid exchange. In that technique, the recombinations indicated by crossing-over are visualized by light microscopy as shown in **Figure 10-2**. The experimental metal-dependent quinone-containing antitumor agent streptonigrin induces ROS via the Fenton reaction and causes dose-dependent chromosomal abnormalities and sister chromatid exchanges. The metal chelating agent 1, 10-phenanthroline severely inhibits but does not totally eliminate these reactions (Bolzán et al., 2001). These tests clearly can point to reactions that lead to wholesale DNA damage and to what degree they are dependent on oxidative mechanisms or those from adduct formation, and so forth.

A more recent technique developed for light microscopy is the comet assay. By multiple staining not only can DNA fragmentation be detected, but also the development of apoptosis or necrosis can be parceled out as indicated in **Figure 10-3**. Deeper examination reveals the interpretations possible from utilization of the comet assay or single-cell gel electrophoresis assay. The comet assay is capable of detecting alkali labile sites, cross-linking, and single-strand breaks. The assay developed from a neutral lysis and electrophoresis with acridine orange stain that showed an intact DNA "head" and a "comet tail" of broken DNA strands to an alkaline method that increased the sensitivity for strand breaks. When used in combination with fluorescence *in situ* hybridization (FISH), the comet-FISH assay can determine sequence damage and repair. Isolating the comet assay, is this assay alone capable of resolving the difference between genotoxic agents, epigenetic chemicals that affect DNA expression but not sequence (not mutagenic), and cytotoxic chemicals that do not directly alter DNA? In one study, three dose levels were given to male rats after determining the maximum tolerated dose (MTD) used for cancer analyses: a maximum

recommended dose of 2000 mg/kg for nontoxic products, 50% of that dose, and 25% of that dose. The kidney was chosen as the target organ for the genotoxic agents aristolochic acids (forms deoxyadenosine adduct of AA-I [7-(deoxyadenosin- N^6-yl)-aristolactam I]; Schmeiser, 1996), cisplatin (cross-linking agent mentioned earlier), 2-nitroanisole (forms dG adducts derived from the reductive metabolite N-(2-methoxyphenyl) hydroxylamine; Stiborová et al., 2004), potassium bromate (causes oxidative DNA damage with double-stranded DNA breaks and large deletions; Luan et al., 2007), and streptozotocin (forms free radical DNA damage and alkylates DNA bases; Błasiak et al., 2004). All these genotoxic compounds were determined directly or indirectly via the comet assay using 20 mg/kg streptozotocin increase of mean Olive Tail Moment (OTM) median value as a positive control in all assays. Cisplatin decreased the DNA migration as would be expected for a cross-linking reagent. This effect was amplified by increasing the time of electrophoresis. Epigenetic carcinogens D-limonene and cyclosporine or nephrotoxic agents streptomycin and indomethacin did not cause any significant increases in DNA migration (Nesslany et al., 2007).

Returning to the FISH assay used in combination with the comet assay, this technique can indicate what sequences of DNA are most sensitive to certain genotoxic agents. For example, it is known that ionizing radiation produces a variety of cancers including leukemia and thyroid cancer. The high degree of RET (rearranged during transfection) proto-oncogene (multiple endocrine neoplasia MEN2A, MEN2B and medullary thyroid carcinoma 1, Hirschsprung disease)/papillary thyroid carcinoma (PTC) rearrangements for patients treated with external radiation indicate that perhaps this genomic region is more sensitive than others to the effects of ionizing radiation. The comet-FISH assay showed indeed that RET fractionation was significantly higher than the SDF1/ CXCL12 (chemokine stroma-derived factor pathway mediates tumor pathogenesis; CXCL12 increases tumor growth/malignancy, induces angiogenesis, facilitates tumor metastasis, and promotes immunosuppressive networks; Kryczek

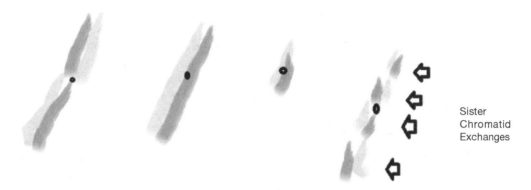

FIGURE 10-2 Sister Chromatid Exchanges (SCEs) Noted in Giemsa Stain Normal DNA (Dark Stain) and Those Labeled for Two Cell Cycles with Bromodeoxyuridine (BrdU), Which Stain More Lightly. SCEs Are Indicated by Chromatids on Either Side of the Centromere with Sections Staining Intermittently Dark and Bright (Not Uniform for the Chromatid)

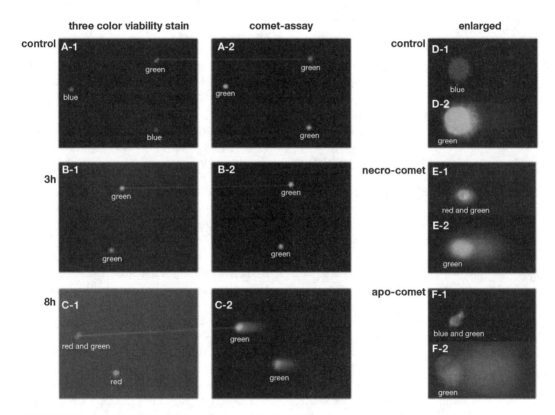

FIGURE 10-3 Apoptosis Induction by Etoposide Treatment in HaCaT Cells

Note: Images marked **(A)** show typical control cells with high cytosolic esterase activity (blue: A-1) and no detectable DNA fragmentation (A-2). After 3 h post-etoposide incubation **(B)** apoptosis is visible indicated by an Annexin V green fluorescence (B-1), no DNA fragmentation is detectable (B-2). At 8 h postincubation **(C)** the cells show a strong apoptotic/necrotic signal (C-1) indicated by annexin V and Ethidium-HD (green and red) positive cells. The comets of these cells also show a high level of DNA fragmentation (C-2). Images D-1 and D-2 show an enlarged healthy cell and the resulting comet, E and F for necro-comets and apo-comets, respectively. The white lines indicate the cell from which the comet originates in the merge images.

Reproduced from Morley N, Rapp A, Dittmar H, Salter L, Gould D, Greulich KO, Curnow A. 2006. UVA-induced apoptosis studied by the new apo/necro-Comet-assay which distinguishes viable, apoptotic and necrotic cells. *Mutagenesis*. 21:105–114.

et al., 2007), Abl (Abelson murine leukemia viral oncogene homolog 1 whose protein translation product has an ATP-binding region on a tyrosine kinase for which the leukemia chemotherapy agent imatinib [Gleevec] binds unless mutations are present on the Abl gene; Iqbal et al., 2004), MYC (proto-oncogene prevents cell cycle arrest in response to growth-inhibitory signals; Amati et al., 1998), PLA2G2A (phospholipase A2, group IIA of platelets and synovial fluid is elevated in early gastrointestinal tumors but appears to inhibit invasive metastasis; Ganesan et al., 2008), p53 (tumor suppressor gene promotes apoptosis unless TNFα inhibits this action through the activation of nuclear factor (NF)-κB, unless an NF-κB inhibitor such as parthenolide is given; Szołtysek et al., 2008), and JAK2 (janus kinase 2 gene is responsible for the production of a signaling protein for cytokine-induced activation of transcription and abnormal growth of hematopoietic cells; Kralovics et al., 2005) genomic regions in a lymphoblastoid and a fetal thyroid cell line (Volpato et al., 2008). This indicates that the agent that causes clastogenesis is not uniformly causing DNA damage in all cells in all regions at doses that are not immediately lethal. The molecular technology presently available can now discern those differences and indicate why mutations and cancer may be caused by certain agents but not others.

Although somatic cells serve well for these clastogenic or other mutagenic analyses, so do germ cells such as sperm. Four clastogenic assays for sperm are the Comet assay described earlier, the acridine orange test, and the sperm chromatin structure and TUNEL assays (uses terminal deoxynucleotidyl transferase dUTP to label nick ends due to apoptotic signal cascades or severe DNA damage). The comet assay is modified for sperm by mixing sperm cells with melted agarose on a glass slide. The cells are then lysed and DNA fragments separated by horizontal electrophoresis. The results from this assay are limited, because a clinical threshold has not been established and it uses only a few hundred sperm in its analysis. The results are also complicated by differing methodologies employed by different researchers. The positive side is that through the use of positive and negative controls, some studies have

shown an ability to diagnose or offer a disease prognosis. The acridine orange is a simple light microscopy technique that employs the metachromatic properties of the dye to stain sperm cells in various states of fragmentation. The dye stains intact DNA as green and single-stranded break segments as red. This is not a very reliable assay as a strict ratio of two molecules of dye per DNA phosphate is necessary for proper staining, which is not achievable on a simple slide with a cover slip. The sperm chromatin structure assay first employs acidic pH to denature the DNA at the strain breaks. Acridine orange stains the intact DNA as red, while fragments are deciphered and quantified by their red signal by flow cytometry. The TUNEL assay uses a terminal deoxynucleotidyl transferase to label broken 3′OH groups of broken DNA strands. Flow cytometry can separate sperm and determine fluorescence intensity for fragmentation quantitation or use a light microscope to do a fluorescence intensity to score for those affected sperm. Unfortunately, the results of this assay appear to vary depending on the researcher and require greater standardization prior to adoption as a clinical test (Evenson and Wixon, 2006).

Another relatively new avenue for mutagenic testing and developmental toxicity is available through the use of stem cells (Cho and Li, 2007). How does the environmental toxicologist determine the mutagenicity of mixtures, such as may be found in surface water samples, while retaining the ability to decipher the genotoxic mechanisms? The Ames test with two different strains of *Salmonella typhimurium* (TA98 and TA 100), the same test done with strains of *S. typhimurium* YG1021 and YG1026 that overexpress nitroreductase or *S. typhimurium* YG1041 and YG1042 sensitive to nitroarenes and aromatic amines due to increased nitroreductase and O-acetyltransferase, the SOS Chromotest and *umu*-test system that uses a bacteria strain of E. coli or *S. typhimurium* with a galactosidase gene linked to an SOS response gene to provide photometric quantitation of genotoxic events, the Mutatox test using a dark mutant strain of luminescent *Photobacterium phosphoreum*, the microscreen phage-induction assay with an *E. coli* strain, the DNA repair assay with E. coli strain, the

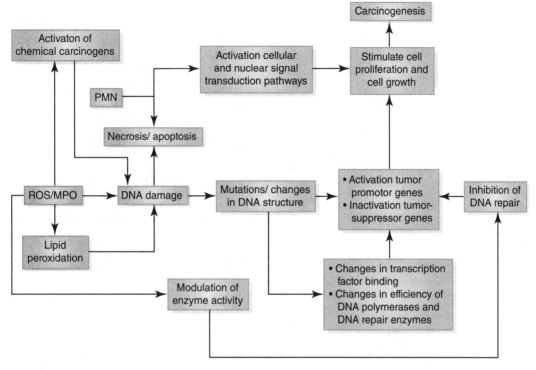

FIGURE 10-4 Overview of a Variety of Processes by Which Neutrophil-Derived ROS May Promote Tumor Development

Ara-test (L-arabinose resistance mutagenesis test) with *S. typhimurium*, DNA adduct quantitation, DNA strand break assay, micronuclei formation, sister chromatid exchange assays, chromosome aberration tests, and *Tradescantia* clone 4430 stamen hair mutation assay (phenotypic color change) reveal a number of known and unknown chemicals in surface waters that are mutagenic and possibly carcinogenic. The use of more than one assay makes for a more reliable detector. It is clear that except for the use of *Salmonella* strains, a standard system that scores both degree and type of mutagens is not currently used by all researchers. However, some useful information has come from these analyses regarding what are likely newly discovered mutagenic species of chemicals found in surface waters, such as heterocyclic aromatic amines (HCAs) arising from human feces, 2-phenylbenzotriazole- type chemicals emitted by textile dyeing factories, and 4-amino-3,3′-dichloro-5, 4′-dinitrobiphenyl released from chemical plants manufacturing polymers or as dye intermediates (Ohe et al., 2004).

Carcinogenesis

Clearly the pervious section involves genotoxic carcinogens, but the question to explore now is: What is cancer and why do toxic insults to DNA, cell signaling, and/or expression of DNA in proteins lead to tumor formation? **Figure 10-4** provides an overview of the answers to this question. The figure displays the oxidation that can occur from the activity of the most abundant phagocytic white blood cell, the polymorphonuclear (PMN) neutrophil. Oxidation events are known to be involved in aging, and cancer is mostly a disease of aging. Additionally, it is a disease that some people, sexes, and species are more susceptible to than others due to genetic differences. Why does cancer form and what types of genes would cause the development of uncontrolled growth that is a function of metastatic cancer cells? An organism starts at the embryonic stage, and throughout its development its genes are controlled during differentiation of tissues and organs. If they turn on unexpectedly to the detriment of the organism, clinicians view them no longer as embryonic genes but as oncogenes. So, the figure shows what happens if toxicants turn on these oncogenes by initiating a cancer cell via DNA damage that may activate tumor promoter sequences and/or inactivate tumor suppressor genes or modify tumor suppressor proteins directly. DNA damage or protein adduction may also affect DNA repair enzymes, affect the faithful transcription or efficiency of DNA polymerases, or may alter the binding of DNA transcription factors. Higher levels of damage may not yield cancer or lead to the death of tumor cells if apoptosis or necrosis is engaged, as is likely from chemotherapeutic medications. The right side of the figure indicates growth signaling pathways that are also considered tumorpromotion or -proliferation pathways.

Oncogenes have been studied extensively, yielding more than 100 types of oncogenes. There are viral oncogenes such as Rous sarcoma virus isolated in 1910. There are cellular oncogenes or proto-oncogenes (Hall, 1984). These proto-oncogenes may be classified into five categories. One is growth factors such as the platelet-derived growth factor (PDGF) and v-sis. PDGF not only stimulates the formation of tumors and promotes tumor growth, it also has inflammatory and atherosclerotic functions. The PDGF-B chain gene is related to the v-sis oncogene from simian sarcoma virus by a 92% homology, so it is also known as the c-sis proto-oncogene. This gene's transcription can be blocked by triplex-forming oligonucleotides (Liu et al., 2001).

Another class of oncogenes is the growth factor receptors. These may amplify the gene by causing more than two copies to be available for transcription. These amplifications appear to be important in diagnosis, as in the case of v-erb-bs (erythroblastic leukemia viral oncogene homolog 2, or ErbB2 [human epidermal growth factor receptor-2, or HER2/neu]) and invasive breast cancers (Ni et al., 2007). Note that these factors may have multiple names, because they have been described for various functions.

Another class of oncogenes is signal transducers. These intermediate pathways between the growth factor receptor and the nucleus may be turned on or off. In cancer cells they are activated. The Abl gene mentioned twice earlier in the chapter is a target of the chemotherapy agent imatinib (Gleevec). The expression of the Bcr-Abl construct codes for a p185 protein associated with acute lymphoblastic leukemia. Mutations can keep these genes activated and/or make them insensitive to certain chemotherapy agents. Such is the case with the T315I mutated form of Abl and the insensitivity of the tyrosine kinase produced by the gene to imatinib mesylate but its sensitivity to C6-unsubstituted and substituted pyrazolo[3,4-d]pyrimidines that are dual Src/Abl inhibitors (Santucci et al., 2008). Although changes in the Ras gene appear to signal cancer formation, there are many times other signaling pathways are required for the transformation of the cell. For example, oncogenic K-Ras is insufficient to transform lung epithelial cells, although its expression is found in non-small cell lung cancer. Expression of K-Ras activates ERK signaling, which induces COX-2 synthesis, which then generates the production of prostaglandin E_2. ERK also induces metalloproteinase-9 and cleavage of E-cadherin at two specific sites. By performing these functions, K-Ras increases cell proliferation and decreases cell–cell contacts that are indicative of normal epithelial cell function (Wang et al., 2008). This shows that some functions that are not directly linked to a transformation into a cancer cell may lead to phenotypic changes that produce fast growth or hyperplasias.

A fourth class of oncogenes is transcription factors. These factors control which genes are transcribed to produce mRNA and subsequently translated into protein. Changes in Myc play a large role in cancer formation and how aggressive or treatable the cancer is. Diffuse large cell B-cell lymphoma patients (non-Hodgkin's lymphoma) with the 8q24/c-Myc translocation appeared to have had a poor prognosis. Addition of the t(14;18) translocation resulted in further degradation of their prognosis (Niitsu et al., 2008). Thus, it appears that the type of mutations or translocations plays a role in the cancers developed and the ability of the abnormal cells to yield to current chemotherapy.

The last class of oncogenes is the apoptosis regulators. One of the most important of these

TABLE 10-1   Genes Involved in Inherited Cancer (A) or Oncogenes or Tumor Suppressor Genes That May Form Cancer as a Result of Toxic Insult (B) Taken from the American Cancer Society

Inherited Cancer	Abnormal Gene	Other Non-Inherited Cancers Seen with This Gene
Retinoblastoma	*RBI*	Many different cancers
Li-Fraumeni syndrome (sarcomas, brain tumors, leukemia)	*P53*	Many different cancers
Melanoma	*INK4a*	Many different cancers
Colorectal cancer (due to familial polyposis)	*APC*	Most colorectal cancers
Colorectal cancer (without polyposis)	*MLH1, MSH2,* or *MSH6*	Colorectal, gastric, endometrial cancers
Breast and/or ovarian	*BRCA1, BRCA2*	Only rare ovarian cancers
Wilms tumor	*WTI*	Wilms tumors
Nerve tumors, including brain	*NF1, NF2*	Small numbers of colon cancers, melanomas, neuroblastoma
Kidney cancer	*VHL*	Certain types of kidney cancers

Oncogene/Tumor Suppressor Gene	Related Cancers
BRCA1, BRCA2	Breast and ovarian cancer
bcr-abl	Chronic myelogenous leukemia
bcl-2	B-cell lymphoma
HER2/neu (erbB-2)	Breast cancer, ovarian cancer, others
N-myc	Neuroblastoma
EWS	Ewing tumor
C-myc	Burkitt lymphoma, others
p53	Brain tumors, skin cancers, lung cancer, head and neck cancers, others
MLH1, MSH2	Colorectal cancers
APC	Colorectal cancers

Table includes oncogenes or tumor suppressor genes that may form cancer as a result of toxic insult.

genes that prevent apoptosis is Bcl-2. These pathways are also important in successful chemotherapy agents. Diallyl disulfide (extract of garlic *Allium sativum*) treatment of a human colon cancer cell line COLO 205 results in G2/M phase arrest and mitochondrial pathway–induced apoptosis through downregulation of Bcl-2 and Bcl-xL anti-apoptosis genes and upregulation of Bak and Bax apoptosis genes. Ultimately, the induction of caspase-3 results in apoptosis from these events, unless inhibitors of caspase-3 are administered (broad spectrum caspases inhibitor Z-VAD-FMK; Yang et al., 2008).

Chromosomal Abnormalities Leading to Cancer

Table 10-1 indicates that there are certain gene abnormalities that predispose cells to become cancerous, especially certain fast-growing or susceptible cell populations. Additionally, certain mutations around oncogenes or tumor

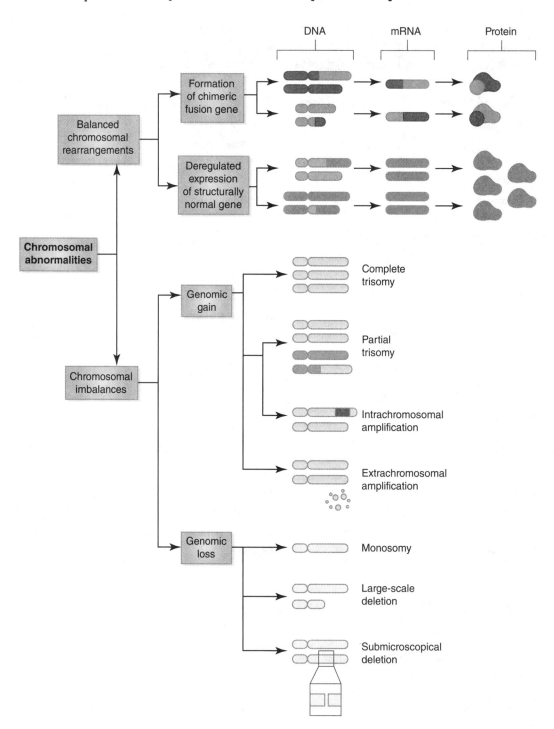

FIGURE 10-5 Generation of Chromosomal Abnormalities

suppressor genes caused by toxicants can lead to cancer transformations or lead to the treatment of those cancers. Clonal chromosomal abnormalities have been found in all cancer patients (> 54,000) studied and classified by the World Health Organization. Chromosomes are divided by the centromere into the short p arms and the long q arms that are essential for chromosome segregation during mitosis. The telomeres cap the arms leading to the structural integrity and replication of the chromosome and the threedimensional shape of the nucleus. Just prior to or during metaphase, chromosomes are dyed and identified by shape and dark and light banding. This banding pattern can be part of the identification process for abnormal chromosomes that are found in cancer cells.

Note in **Figure 10-5** that chromosomal abnormalities arise from two different events. Balanced chromosome rearrangements indicated on the left side of the figure either yield a chimeric fusion gene or the insertion of gene regulatory elements next to a structurally intact gene. In the first case, a new chimeric fusion protein with a new or affected function is synthesized that may influence the cancer process, while the protein produced by the reciprocal rearrangement does not yield a cancer pathway. The second abnormal combination of gene regulatory elements from one gene to that of an intact gene leads to deregulation of that gene and the unregulated expression of a normal protein.

The right side of the figure deals with chromosomal gains or losses. The gains can be observed as homogeneously staining regions and double-minute chromosomes for partial or complete trisomies and intrachromosomal or extrachromosomal amplifications, respectively. Losses can be detected as monosomies or deletions of various sizes. Alkylating agents can cause the unbalanced deletions of chromosomes 5 and/or 7 that may lead to myelodysplastic syndrome or acute myeloid leukemia (Frohling and Dohner, 2008). Epipodophyllotoxins and other DNA topoisomerase II inhibitors cause leukemias with balanced translocations of the MLL gene at chromosome band 11q23 or, less often, t(8;21), t(3;21), inv(16), t(8;16), t(15;17), or t(9;22) (Felix, 1998).

Most cancer etiologies from chromosomal abnormalities have unknown causal agents. For the chimeric fusion proteins, for example, the tyrosine kinases are the key enzyme sequences involved in cancer formation. The Philadelphia truncated chromosome 22 results from a balanced translocation t(9;22)(q34.1;q11.23). This designation indicates that sequences of band 22q11.23 of the BCR gene join to the cytoplasmic ABL1 tyrosine kinase on band 9q34.1 yielding chronic myeloid leukemia, one-fifth of the cases of acute lymphoblastic leukemia, and a small group of acute myeloid leukemia patients from BCR-ABL1. As mentioned earlier, this led to the development of imatinib mesylate chemotherapy directed against abnormal tyrosine kinases and further therapies for those kinases resistant to this medication. Other abnormal tyrosine kinases from translocations can be found in acute lymphoblastic leukemia (NUP214-ABL1 fusion), anaplastic large-cell lymphoma (ALK-NPM1 fusion), multiple myeloma (WHSC1-IGHG1 fusion), myeloid cancer with eosinophilia (FIP1L1- PDGFRA or PDGFRB-ETV6 fusion), non-small cell lung cancer (EML4-ALK fusion), papillary thyroid cancer (RET-CCDC6 or RET-NCOA4 fusion), and various cancers that are started by the ETV6-NTRK3 fusion.

Disruption of transcription factors is the other chimeric fusion gene consequence that leads to many cancers. Two possible outcomes are possible: the production of transcription factors with enhanced or abnormal transcriptional activity or fusion proteins that repress transcription. For example, Ewing's sarcoma features an enhanced or abnormal transcriptional activity in a fusion protein FLI1-EWSR1 from t(11;22)(q24.1-q24.3;q12.2) and t(21;22)(q22.3;q12.2) translocations. This indicates that the EWSR1 gene on band 22q12.2 fuses most frequently (85% of patients) to FLI1 on band 11q24.1-q24.3 (ETS family of transcription factors) and ERG on band 21q22.3 (~10% of patients). This still leads to DNA binding through the ETS family of transcription factors, but the EWSR portion of the fusion protein is a potent transactivation domain that causes abnormal expression required for cancer cell growth. Conversely, acute myeloid leukemia features the fusion of genes such as PML-RARA, RUNX1-RUNX1T1, and CBFB-MYH11. These fusions still retain the DNA-binding motif of the other abnormal transcription fusion proteins, but also have an unrelated protein that interacts with inhibitors of gene transcription. The abnormal inhibition caused by these fusion proteins targets genes required for normal myeloid differentiation. As a result, immature myeloid cells accumulate in acute myeloid leukemia. These fusion proteins can be inhibited by all-trans retinoic acid and arsenic trioxide in the treatment of acute promyelocytic leukemia. These compounds reverse the repression of the PML-RARA fusion protein by forcing the release of transcription inhibitors from the fusion protein or stimulating degradation of PML-RARA or both. The deregulated expression of structurally normal genes puts enhancer or promoter sequences next to proto-oncogenes as occurs with Burkitt's lymphoma. In these cancer cells, IGHG1, band 14q32.33; IGKC, 2p12; and IGLC1, 22q11.2 (enhancer of the immunoglobulin gene) increase the expression of MYC transcription factor on band 8q24.21. Another fusion of interest is that for prostate cancer, which fuses ERG's coding exons to androgen-regulated sequences in the promoter of the prostate-specific TMPRSS2 gene. This leads to abnormal expression of ERG in prostate tissue. Other cancers of this type are acute myeloid leukemia mentioned earlier (this fusion is ETV6-CDX2), follicular lymphoma (IGHG1-BCL2 fusion), and mantle-cell lymphoma (CCND1-IGHG1 fusion).

Chromosomal gains are seen in a variety of cancers and proliferative disorders. Of these, the gene targets are known for BIRC2 (hepatocellular carcinoma), CCND1 (various cancers), CDX2 (acute myeloid leukemia), EGFR (various cancers treatable by cetuximab and similar agents), ERBB2 (various cancers treatable by trastuzumab), ERG (acute myeloid leukemia), ESR1 (breast cancer treatable by tamoxifen), IKBKE (breast cancer), IKCF1 (BCR-ABL1- positive acute lymphoblastic leukemia or lymphoid blast crisis of chronic myeloid leukemia), JAK2 (polycythemia vera), KRAS (various cancers), MET (various cancers), MITF (malignant melanoma), MYB (acute lymphoblastic leukemia), MYC (various cancers), MYCN (neuroblastoma), NKX2-1 (non-small cell lung cancer), and YAP1 (hepatocellular carcinoma). Genomic losses are known for APC (colon cancer), ATM (various cancers), CDKN2A/B (various cancers), ETV6 (acute myeloid leukemia, acute lymphoblastic leukemia), FAM123B (Wilms' tumor), NF1

(various cancers), PAX5 (acute lymphoblastic leukemia), PTEN (various cancers treatable by sirolimus), RB1 (retinoblastoma), REST (colon cancer), RPS14 (myelodysplastic syndrome or 5 q minus syndrome treatable by lenalidomide), TP53 (various cancers), and VHL (renal cell cancer; Frohling and Dohner, 2008).

One of the most studied cancer susceptibility genes is the BRCA2 tumor suppressor gene. From the investigation of this gene and the use of bioinformatics, it was found that a protein structure model was able to correctly ascertain the risk of 229 unclassified missense variants found in cells of families at high risk for breast and ovarian cancers. The model indicated that the most untoward changes were found in the BRCA2 OB1 domain, which would destabilize the formed protein and its small acidic binding partner DSS1 (Karchin et al., 2008). This kind of data are useful in determining the likelihood of cancer type from a variety of agents once the mechanisms of action are known, the most susceptible sequences of DNA affected are identified, and the degree of damage is assessed in cells and whole organisms.

Genotoxic Carcinogens and Toxicogenomics

Because most of the genotoxic carcinogens were covered under mutagens, how do toxicological researchers screen toxicants for genotoxicity? This question is answered in this section and is followed by a discussion of the modern field of toxicogenomics and how toxicogenomics is used to evaluate mechanisms of genotoxicity and carcinogenicity. One study of genotoxicity (Zhang et al., 2008) employed a series of agents including alkylating agents; cross-linking agents; oxidative agents; radiation; nongenotoxic carcinogens; precarcinogenic agents, which included metals (cadmium chloride, chromium trichloride, mercuric chloride, and lead nitrate), pesticides (dichloro-diphenyl-trichloroethane [DDT] and deltamethrin), arylamines (biphenylamine and 2-aminofluorene), polycyclic aromatic hydrocarbons (benzo[a]pyrene, 2,3,7,8,-tetrachlorodibenzo-p-dioxin [TCDD], and diethyl-stilbestrol; a chlorinated hydrocarbon (carbon tetrachloride); antineoplastic agents mitomycin C and hydroxycamptothecin;

TABLE 10-2   Summary of the gadd153-Luc Test and Comparison with Comet Assay (the Threshold Concentration)

Agents	Luciferase Activity		Comet Assay	
	Concentration	RLU	Concentration	OTM
Control	0 μmol/L	1.0 ± 0.12		0.53 ± 0.08
Metals				
CdCl$_2$	1 μmol/L	1.35 ± 0.18	0.3 mmol/L	1.10 ± 0.12
CrCl$_3$	1 μmol/L	2.12 ± 0.25	17 μmol/L	0.92 ± 0.11
HgCl$_2$	0.1 μmol/L	1.67 ± 0.25	6 μmol/L	1.33 ± 0.18
Pb(NO$_3$)$_3$	30 μmol/L	1.61 ± 0.28	51 μmol/L	1.95 ± 0.21
Pesticide				
DDT	0.1 nmol/L	1.50 ± 0.24	70 nmol/L	0.99 ± 0.15
Deltamethrin	1 μmol/L	3.48 ± 0.20	10 μmol/L	1.89 ± 0.06
Arylamine				
Biphenylamine	5 μmol/L	1.49 ± 0.20	45 μmol/L	1.82 ± 0.21
2-Aminofluorene	0.5 μmol/L	1.44 ± 0.16	55 μmol/L	1.22 ± 0.08
Polycyclic aromatic hydrocarbon				
Benzopyrene	10 nmol/L	2.20 ± 0.39	10 μmol/L	1.94 ± 0.17
TCDD	1 nmol/L	2.63 ± 0.41	5 nmol/L	0.98 ± 0.11
Diethylstilbestrol	0.37 μmol/L	1.58 ± 0.19	3.7 μmol/L	1.53 ± 0.14
Chlorinated hydrocarbon				
Carbon tetrachloride	65 μmol/L	1.48 ± 0.22	2.6 mmol/L	2.02 ± 0.23
Antineoplastic agent				
Mitomycin C	0.01 μmol/L	1.44 ± 0.18	0.04 μmol/L	1.76 ± 0.10
Hydroxycamptothecin	10 μmol/L	2.95 ± 0.40	5 μmol/L	1.02 ± 0.19
Physical agent				
UV	30 J/m^2	3.25 ± 0.72	10 J/m^2	1.12 ± 0.08
Others				
NaF	24 μmol/L	1.37 ± 0.17	0.12 mmol/L	1.66 ± 0.14
Acrylamide	1.4 mmol/L	1.75 ± 0.60	0.14 mmol/L	1.01 ± 0.13
Pollutants in environment				
Raw water	1 mL/mL	1.69 ± 0.21	10 mL/mL	1.53 ± 0.46
Chlorinated drinking water	0.5 mL/mL	1.32 ± 0.13	10 mL/mL	2.84 ± 0.88
Noncarcinogen				
Benzylpenicillin sodium	—		—	
Vitamin C	—		—	
4-Acetylaminofluorene	—		—	
Pyrene	—		—	

Data were expressed as means ± SD (standard deviation). Each data point was an average of three independent experiments. RLU = relative luciferase unit where the control is set to 1.0 and samples are done in ratio to the control; OTM = olive tail moment.

a physical agent UV, which is ionizing at low wavelengths; two listed as "others" (sodium fluoride and acrylamide); and the oxidant hydrogen peroxide. In addition, two complex genotoxic agents were given as raw water and chlorinated drinking water originating from the Han River in China and more specifically from the Zongguan Water Treatment Plants, Wuhan, China. The four noncarcinogens tested included a derivative of aminofluorene (4-acetylaminofluorene), a compound similar in structure to benzo[a]pyrene (pyrene), benzylpenicillin sodium, and vitamin C (ascorbic acid). The study proceeded with three different tests. First, the novel assay employed a stable transfected human hepatocellular liver carcinoma cell line HepG2. A pGadd153-EGFP (enhanced green fluorescent protein) containing hamster gadd153 promoter sequences had the promoter excised using KpnI and HindIII. T4 DNA polymerase ligated the promoter fragment into a KpnI/HindIII double-digested pGL3-Basic vector and received the plasmid gadd153-Luc. The Luc refers to a luciferase reporter gene whose activation can be determined colorimetrically using 3-(4,5-dimethylthiazol-2-yl)2,5-diphenyltetrazolium bromide (MTT). The comet assay was used as a comparison. A third test was done specifically with cadmium chloride to test for its effect on the expression of endogenous gadd153 mRNA by reverse transcriptase-polymerase chain reaction (RT-PCR). The doses selected in this study were based on firm toxicology, with a 50% reduction in viability 24 hours following treatment was set as the highest dose level. Results were reported for effects on genotoxic assays at a sublethal dose.

The first aspect of this study to examine is the comet assay, which is summarized in **Table 10-2**. Note the OTM is low for the controls; however, all carcinogenic chemicals increased the fragmentation as noted by increase in the OTMs at a concentration varying from 5 nM for TCDD to 10 mL/mL for water samples. The luciferase reporter gene gave much more sensitive results by a smaller amount for lead to several orders of magnitude for benzo[a]pyrene. This system is not only sensitive, but also is able to generate toxic metabolites that are the basis for the carcinogenicity

for a number of these agents. The third assay looked for the induction of the reporter gene by cadmium. A suitable reporter would respond to a low level of damage and have a high level of induction. When gadd153, gadd45, and gadd34 responses to cadmium chloride were compared, all were inducible. However, the gadd153 was the most sensitive as indicated by the most mRNA produced per gadd gene that was threefold higher than the highest response for the gadd45 reporter at the lowest concentration of $CdCl_2$ (1.25 μM). When gadd153 was compared with a SV40 promoter, the results indicated a 2.9-fold induction by $CdCl_2$ by the gadd153 promoter and no significant effects noted by the SV40 promoter 24 hours following treatment. It appears that this promoter assay has the sensitivity and the versatility to determine a number of toxic substances that are also carcinogens (Zhang et al., 2008).

The field of toxicogenomics has a major focus on predicting cancer formation and determining the mechanism of action of genotoxic agents. The formation of cancer is a multistep process. Gene mutation and chromosomal damage are followed by transformation to malignancy and ultimately disease characteristics of cancer in an organ or multiple organ systems. The importance of the first step in initiating this process has led to the testing for genotoxicity of chemicals, especially in the development of medicines. Note how normal cancer testing proceeds in the case of drug development in **Figure 10-6**.

Both genotoxic and nongenotoxic mechanisms must be sought, and whole animal cancer models must then be tested. The assays that are standard to a drug study must currently involve the primary bacterial gene mutation assay such as the Ames test, a second *in vitro* mammalian mutation and/or chromosome damage assay to insure that mammalian DNA is not uniquely sensitive to damage, and a third *in vivo* chromosome damage assay that includes physiological mechanisms not present in the other tests. Because these assays may not discover those chemicals that are mainly epigenetic in nature, a chronic 2-year bioassay in rats and mice (effectively one lifespan) that was developed at the National Cancer Institute in the early 1960s

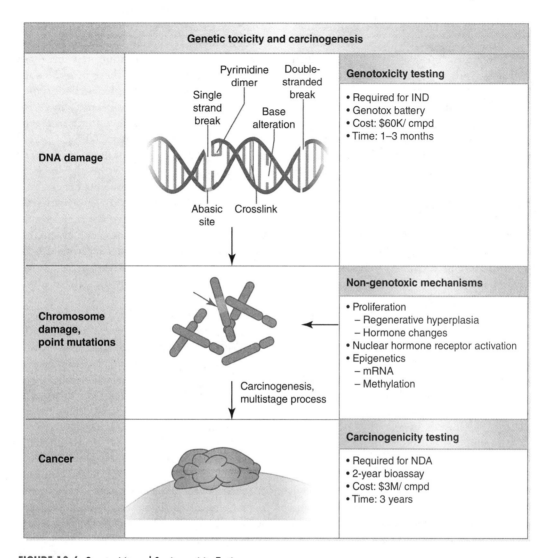

FIGURE 10-6 Genotoxicity and Carcinogenicity Testing

is also required using three concentrations of tested agent, plus controls. Cancer-susceptible transgenic mice models such as p53+/−, Hras2, and Tg.AC have drawn attention and may represent future alternative approaches to the current model systems such as the Sprague-Dawley female rat breast cancer assay. Although the standard genotoxicity tests successfully screen for 93% of carcinogens, they also yield false positives for 50% of the noncarcinogenic compounds by identifying some minor genotoxicity. The genotoxic substances' risk is determined by a linear extrapolation to low doses, because a single

mutation has the possibility of yielding a cancer transformation. Nongenotoxic carcinogens' risk may involve threshold models, because they affect growth and tissue regeneration, prevent apoptosis, promote endocrine disruption, and/or suppress the immune response indicative of DNA expression or cellular function alterations, but do not directly alter DNA sequences (Ellinger-Ziegelbauer, Aubrecht, et al., 2008).

Some non-DNA-reactive toxicants are still genotoxic: They interfere with the enzymes of DNA and protein synthesis, prevent Na/K transport in cells, inhibit topoisomerases, produce an imbalance of DNA precursor molecules, interfere with energy functions by producing mitochondrial failure (Fosslien, 2008), generate ROS and lipid peroxidation products, and release nuclease from lysosomes. However, because only one-third of medications that cause cancer also are genotoxic, it is important to quantitate and evaluate the genotoxic and the nongenotoxic carcinogens through mechanisms of action. One method for assessment of damage is the gene reporter model examined earlier. Reporters could look for alterations in critical functions such as DNA repair, cell growth arrest, signal transduction mechanisms, and apoptosis. cDNA or oligonucleotide microarray analyses bring toxicologists into the genome age and can be standardized as indicated by inter- and intra-platform reproducibility of gene expression measurements in the MicroArray Quality Control project. It is easiest to visualize the damage done to DNA and signaling pathways via a known carcinogen that affects all systems, specifically ionizing radiation. Treatment of cancer requires higher doses of radiation that causes necrosis or halts the cell cycle and starts apoptosis via the activation of MAPK cascades, NF-κB, and the AP-1 transcription complex.

How to monitor effects of carcinogens or antitumor agents involves monitoring signaling pathways affected by ionizing radiation through mRNA expression. CDKN1A, GADD45, and Cyclin E gene products monitor changes in the cell cycle. As described earlier, BAX and BCL-XL expression indicates apoptosis. XPC, DDB2, and GADD45 (or GADD153 mentioned earlier) would report DNA repair alterations (Ellinger-Ziegelbauer, Aubrecht, et al., 2008). Mitogenic stimulation may be monitored through the activation of proto-oncogenes c-fos and c-jun that form a heterodimer as part of AP-1 and modulate a wide variety of genes that facilitate cancer development (O'Shea et al., 1992). FRA-1 is a critical promoter of AP-1 (fos/jun) whose expression may be monitored separately to determine stimulation of tumor cell motility and metastasis (Adiseshaiah et al., 2008). Changes in tumor suppression can be monitored via the ubiquitin ligase MDM2, which is a negative regulator of the tumor suppressor p53 mentioned in an earlier section (Chan et al., 2006). Pancreatic cancer

cells' expression of CYCL8/IL8 and fibroblasts' expression of CYC12/SDF-1α indicate that they are factors that may be monitored in cancer development. Specifically, these factors cooperatively induce angiogenesis required for tumor growth and promote the proliferation, invasion, and tube formation of human umbilical vein endothelial cells (Matsuo et al., 2008).

Another factor important in maintaining the cancer cell is the expression of heat shock protein 70, which protects cancer cells from an apoptotic reaction to various stresses. This protein may be targeted for downregulation by chemotherapy agents such as quercetin. However, the pro-survival chaperone GRP78 induction may lead to quercetin resistance. Green tea (-)-epigallocatechin gallate binds to the ATP-binding domain of the chaperone and increases cancer susceptibility to quercetin (Li et al., 2008). This indicates that the factors to be measured should fit the cancer and mechanism that fits the organ-specific carcinogenesis caused by specific classes of chemicals or targeted tumor therapies by toxic chemicals. For example, the cross-linking chemotherapy agent cisplatin and the noncarcinogenic nonsteroidal anti-inflammatory drugs have clearly different gene expression patterns.

Even more important is the ability to discern the difference in gene expression between genotoxic agents as has been accomplished for equitoxic doses of two differing radiation treatments (ionizing and UV), and an oxidant (t-butyl hydroperoxide). In this analysis it is apparent that ionizing radiation has a mechanism that is more like that of oxidants than UV irradiation. The human lymphoblast TK6 line has tested genotoxic versus cytotoxic chemicals in p53-proficient and -deficient cell lines employing 1451 responsive genes. As expected, those causing damage to DNA elicited the p53-dependent pathway, but the cytotoxic agents did not show any indication of a p53 response. For example, genotoxic agents such as cisplatin show a linear dose-response pattern with no threshold for p53-regulated genes (e.g., CDKN1A [p21], GADD45A, FOS) and adduct formation. However, adduct formation is still a more sensitive tool for assessing DNA damage as indicated by exposure of TK6 p53–proficient cells to benzo[*a*]pyrene diol epoxide. Although it might be expected that the damage to DNA repair enzymes would be critical in developing cancer, it appears that only relatively small changes in the expression of a relatively minor group of repair enzyme genes was caused by DNA-reactive genotoxic agents, but major inductions were reserved for genes involving apoptosis, cell cycle, inflammation, and senescence control. If time-dependence of reactions is considered, the AH receptor–responsive elements (CYP 1A1/1B1) respond first followed by alterations in cell cycle–controlling genes when HepG2 cells are exposed to benzo[*a*]pyrene. When comparing genotoxic agents of this type to nongenotoxic carcinogens, apoptotic pathways discriminate well. However, the cancer-causing nature of PAHs appears to be manifested through their influence on cholesterol and fatty acid biosynthetic pathways.

Even though cancer is a multistage process involving initiation, promotion, and progression, gene expression effects of genotoxic carcinogens are best measured at early times following treatment. In one study, the hepatocarcinogen *N*-nitroso-morpholine showed that the gene expression in the first 8 weeks was representative of genotoxicity. Later times had few genes exhibiting deregulation in the nondissected liver. Because toxicology emphasizes dose-response, these toxicogenomic analyses should indicate that these properties are followed and how they develop with dose. The development of a mean benchmark dose for deregulation of the expression of key genes should be used to normalize toxicogenomic analyses. However, most of the studies use an equitoxic amount of different cancer-causing agents to look for mechanistic differences. These mechanistic studies look for the difference in genotoxic carcinogens versus noncarcinogenic isomers, genotoxic verus nongenotoxic carcinogens, and nongenotoxic carcinogens versus noncarcinogenic chemicals. The genotoxic carcinogens cause distinct changes in gene expression compared with noncarcinogens. Genotoxic hepatocarcinogens show an upregulation of the p53 gene characteristic of survival and proliferation pathways, while nongenotoxic carcinogens have a weak action against these genes reflecting

oxidative damage to DNA, proteins, or other oxidative damage that leads to regeneration and cell cycle progression pathway induction. DNA damage caused by ROS formation from nongenotoxic carcinogens may be monitored by induced expression of apurinic/apyrimidinic endonuclease 1 (APEX1). The nongenotoxic carcinogens also cause overexpression of pathways linked to the proto-oncogene c-myc. However, it is not that simple to discriminate between genotoxic and nongenotoxic carcinogens. A systems biology approach would indicate a pattern of gene expression that would definitively identify one carcinogen class from another (Ellinger-Ziegelbauer, Aubrecht, et al., 2008).

How might a proper toxicogenomic analysis be performed? First, the selection of compounds must train the toxicogenomic model. Compounds were selected based on their ability to be genotoxic hepatocarcinogens (aflatoxin B_1, the azo compound C.I. Direct Black, dimethylnitrosamine, 2-nitrofluorene, and N-nitrosomorpholine), nongenotoxic hepatocarcinogens (diethylstilbestrol, methapyrilene HCl, piperonyl butoxide, thioacetamide, and the peroxisome proliferator-activated receptor activator WY-14643 or 4-chloro-6-[2,3-xylidino]-2-pyrimidinylthioacetic acid), and non-hepatocarcinogens (cefuroxime, nifedipine, and propanolol). There were also validation compounds to be evaluated by the generated model, including more genotoxic hepatocarcinogens (2-acetylaminofluorene, methylenedianiline, 4-[methylnitrosamino]-1-[3-pyridyl]-1-butanone, and N-nitrosopiperidine), nongenotoxic hepatocarcinogens (acetamide, acetaminophen, cyproterone acetate, dehydroepiandrosterone, ethionine, and methylcarbamate), and non-hepatocarcinogens (allyl alcohol, clonidine, 1,4-dichlorobenzene, ibuprofen, 3-methylcholanthrene, and prazosin). It is odd that this group picked 3-methylcholanthrene as a non-hepatocarcinogen as it is a strong mutagen following CYP activation. The dose varied based on compound and published effects (development of a hepatic cancer in a long-term rodent assay), and the time of exposure varied from 1, 3, 7, and/or 14 days depending on the compound. This short-term text was meant to be an alternative to the 2-year assay and consistent with the finding that gene expression disruptions were most easily discernable at short times following exposure. The microarray contained 5,399 annotated rat genes and 10,467 expressed sequence tags. The microarray results were validated through the use of quantitative real-time polymerase chain reactions. Gene ranking was performed using the training chemical exposure results to optimize the marker genes with cross-validation to determine the best prediction model. Gene ranking used three statistical measures. The first one was the analysis of variance (ANOVA), which determined variance within a carcinogen class and between classes. The second was support vector machine (SVM) weight, which determines the important of a gene in a classifier system. The third was recursive feature elimination (RFE), which refined the SVM by doing the SVM ranking and eliminating the worst 10% of the scores. Three algorithms were used to cross-validate the best prediction models for the training compound profiles. The first was SVM. The second was sparse linear discriminant analysis. The third was k-nearest neighbors, which determines for a given test point the k nearest neighbors. This is then used to assign the test point to a class with the largest number of nearest neighbors. Microarray results algorithms worked best with $k = 1$. Misclassifications were avoided by eliminating the worst gene and then rerunning the analysis. This was repeated 100 times to obtain the minimal number of critical genes to classify carcinogens. Gene groups were then selected mechanistically based on the lowest misclassifications rates. The four genotoxic and four nongenotoxic carcinogens were represented by toxicological categories of cell cycle progression, cell survival/proliferation, DNA damage response, oxidative protein damage response, oxidative stress response in general, and regeneration. The probe sets that matched these categories were then mapped using a best match mapping table. Finally, there were 186 ratio profiles that were put into the three mechanistic classes using an affinity value assigned to each of the three classes. Affinity values below zero were considered unclassified. Using up to 12 predictions per compound, the compound

was assigned as true positive if at least one profile was as expected for that group, while the rest were unclassified. It was a false negative if all the profiles were unclassified for a known class of compound. A false positive was assigned if one or more profiles fit another class of carcinogen. A Fisher's exact test was run at the end to ensure that there were no over- or underrepresented biochemical categories in each gene group. Weak apoptosis, necrosis, and inflammation were noted for the genotoxic agents, and early or regenerative hyperplasia marked the nongenotoxic carcinogens. The exception was ethionine, which did not show any hyperplasia, but did cause short-term apoptosis and inflammation. Venn diagrams were constructed to look for overlap of gene groups. Very little overlap was found, with the exception of the RFE-SVM pairing. This was expected as RFE is just a refinement of the SVM data. The overrepresented expressions in all groups are the oxidative stress response, regulation of proliferation and apoptosis characteristic of the genotoxic chemicals and the cell cycle, and proliferation category characteristic of the nongenotoxic hepatocarcinogens. Once the training was complete, it was clear that all genotoxic compounds were categorized as genotoxic, with the exception of the false negative for the test compound methylenedianiline. The 1,4-dichlorobenzene was a false positive for a nongenotoxic hepatocarcinogen in the ANOVA analysis, while 3-methylcholanthrene was a false positive for a nongenotoxic carcinogen in mechanistic or ANOVA analyses (Ellinger-Ziegelbauer, Gmuender, et al., 2008). As stated earlier, 3-methylcholanthrene's mutagenic potential should at higher doses yield cancer at high rates, so toxicologists should question the selection of this agent as a negative test substance. Because these tests should be 100% accurate, the whole animal remains a better predictor, although these expensive and statistically intensive analyses offer some hope for short-term probes for cancer mechanisms.

Epigenetic Carcinogens

As indicated earlier, the genotoxic and the nongenotoxic carcinogens appear to stimulate the expression of different pathways.

The nongenotoxic agents appear to promote cell proliferation over other pathways. Is that the sole difference around the epigenetic carcinogens that do not affect the DNA sequence directly? Apparently, alteration of DNA methylation rates is viewed as a possible reason for how epigenetic carcinogens may act. Hypomethylation or hypermethylation of DNA CpG islands found at the 5′ end of genes may play a role in cancer, as increased methylation of cytosines appears to silence the adjacent gene. Phenobarbital, for example, is a nongenotoxic medication that induces hepatic tumors in a sensitive B6C3F1 mouse strain at a dose that reduces DNA methylation. In a tumor-resistant C57BL/6 mouse strain, the same dose of phenobarbital increases cell proliferation but does not change DNA methylation rates. Conversely, another group used phenobarbital and found increased methylation rates in GC-rich regions using PCR-based technology to detect the methylations, especially in tumorprone mice. In either case, a disruption of gene expression would be observed (overexpression in the first study and underexpression in the latter study).

In another study, cigarette smoke condensate used as a promoter of dimethylbenz[a]anthracene-initiated tumors altered DNA methylation rates, especially in the GC regions of the tumor versus healthy cells. These changes may reverse during a recovery period depending on the degree of damage and the transformation to a cancer cell. Trichloroethylene, dichloroacetic acid, and trichloroacetic acid induce liver cancers as might be indicated by their metabolism as organochlorines. Within the first 100 minutes of exposure, these compounds increase expression of proto-oncogenes *c-jun* and *c-myc* as indicated by hepatic mRNA and protein synthesis. Demethylation of CpG dinucleotides in the regulatory regions of both genes is noted in liver cells following 5 days of exposure to these organochlorines.

Metals have been identified for a while as epigenetic carcinogens. Cd alters methylation rates dependent on the time of exposure, with shorter exposures (1 week) causing hypomethylation and a logarithm longer (10 weeks) resulting in hypermethylation. Arsenic is more consistent in that it yields hypomethylation dependent on time and concentration/dose. Nickel is a carcinogenic metal that induces hypermethylation This hypermethylation of the coding and flanking regions of a gene, such as a transgene, induces silencing of genes associated with the transgene. This was noted for a bacterial gene inserted by the transgene. This DNA hypermethylation induces a highly compacted state of chromatin associated with the DNA known as heterochromatin.

It is important to investigate in detail how changes in methylation rates affect the formation of cancer by epigenetic mechanisms. The DNA methyltransferases, especially DNMT1, DNMT3A, and DNMT3B in mammals, are responsible for DNA methylation. The first one (DNMT1) maintains the DNA methylation rates and patterns in a cell following replication to insure consistent regulation following cell growth and division. The *de novo* methylators are represented by the other two enzymes. The greater the methylation, the more chromatin is compacted. This compaction excludes the cellular transcription enzymes and therefore silences gene expression. Four proteins lead to this silencing through compaction: ATP-dependent chromatin DNA remodeling enzymes, two sets of enzymes which acetylate (histone acetyltransferases) and deacetylate (histone deacetylases) lysine residues of the histone protein moieties of chromatin, and enzymes that methylate arginine or lysine residues of histone proteins (histone methyltransferases). Metals interact with these enzymes by interfering with the binding domain of the methyltransferases (Cd) or inhibit acetylation enzymes (Ni). Other chemicals such as 5-aza-cytidine and suberoylanilide hydroxamic acid have been found to alter methylation rates and gene expression via inhibition of key methylation enzymes that may cause carcinogenesis or reverse the alterations in these parameters and also serve as chemotherapeutic agents. Certain other chemicals such as the chlorinated hydrocarbons mentioned earlier lower methylation rates by interfering with the synthesis of the methyl donor S-adenosylmethionine (SAM). Similarly, dietary undernutrition of methyl donor substances and those used as cofactors in transferring the methyl group such as choline, folic acid, methionine, and vitamin B_{12}

lead to hypomethylation. In fact, a choline deficiency induces hepatocarcinogenesis in rats. Also, a transgenic mouse that does not synthesize the specific liver methionine adenosyltransferase (MAT1A) is deficient in SAM and is sensitive to liver damage.

Synthetic estrogens such as diethylstilbestrol have been associated with vaginal cancers, especially in the female children of women who took this compound. The phytoestrogen genistein from soy products also causes uterine epithelial cell cancers in mice. It would make sense that the epigenetic cause of cancer could be caused by estrogen-receptive reproductive cell proliferation due to effects of developmental receptors encoded by homeobox genes *Hoxa-10* and *Hoxa-11* and alterations of regulation of genes such as *c-fos*, *c-jun*, *c-myc*, EGF, or lactoferrin. Neonatal mice exposed to diethylstilbestrol (DES) show upregulation of lactoferrin and *c-fos* and changes in methylation not observed in adult mice with the same dose of DES. The cancer found in the offspring of women who took DES usually appears following puberty, and DNA methylation perturbations also require both estrogenic signals neonatally and also around puberty. It is also pertinent that the CpG methylations occur within or close to the estrogen receptor–regulated genes. Although genetic theory indicates that these epigenetic changes should not be transmitted to the next generation, it appears that some methylation rates persist between a treated mother and her offspring. Pups born to mice fed a diet rich in choline, methionine, betaine, folic acid, and vitamin B_{12} for 2 weeks prior to mating were lean and brown, which is consistent with hypermethylation of the locus and less expression of the *agouti* protein (expression leads to obese, yellow pups). Mothers fed a control diet prior to mating had obese, yellow pups (Bombail et al., 2004). Thus, epigenetic origins of cancer may not only be due to signals that occur in the organism, but also in the parent prior to mating or birth.

Multistage Carcinogenesis

Cancer is a multistage process, so a normal cell is initiated via chemicals, irradiation, or viruses into a focus that may be clonally expressed into a preneoplastic lesion. From there it is promoted into a malignant tumor. It may then become clinical cancer in a whole organism and then further progress into a metastatic cancer. This section examines multistage cancer development through a viral infection. It may not immediately be apparent why this might lead to an understanding of how toxicants interact with the genome or epigenetically to initiate a cancer focus or promote or cause progression to metastatic disease. The link between viral hepatitis, toxins such as alcohol and aflatoxin, insulin resistance, and hepatocarcinomas has clearly been established (Gomaa et al., 2008). Because multiple factors appear to work together to produce advanced cancer, it is important to examine how these factors transform normal cells over the course of the disease.

Because fast-growing cell populations appear to be more sensitive to cancer formation, a good place to start is with the examination of cells of the bone marrow with regard to the formation of leukemia using the Friend spleen focus-forming virus (SFFV) multistep model of erythroleukemia in certain susceptible strains of mice. The Friend retroviruses are resisted by murine cells containing the retroviral restriction factor Fv1 (Friend virus susceptibility factor 1) or the Ref1/Lv1/TRIM5 factor that mediates resistance to a variety or retroviruses in primates. Other factors important in retroviral resistance are the murine gene *Rfv3* (Recovery from Friend virus 3) and retroviral-neutralizing antibody responses encoding an antiretroviral factor APOBEC3. The Friend leukemia viruses are categorized by their ability to form anemia due to hemodilution (FLV-A) or induction of polycythemia (FLV-P). These strains are also differentiated by the formation of abnormal erythrocytes in the absence of kidney hormone erythropoietin (FLV-P) or hypersensitive to erythropoietin (FLV-A). The target cell for these viruses is the erythropoietin-responsive progenitor cell (late BFU-E or CFU-E). Two weeks after inoculation with the virus, the proerythroblasts are found to be blocked in their differentiation into mature erythrocytes first in the spleen and then as an invading population. These cells are not permanently prevented from differentiation, as indicated by treatment by butyric acid, dimethyl sulfoxide, hemin, or hexamethylene bisacetamide. This differentiates the murine viral mechanism from the irreversible leukemia viruses in cattle (bovine leukemia virus) or humans (human T-cell leukemia virus). The FLVs contain a replication-competent Friend murine leukemia virus (F-MuLV) and a replication-defective SFFV, which is the basis of the examined model. SFFV is responsible for the acute erythroblastosis and differs from other retroviruses, because it does not contain a sequence that may originate from a proto-oncogene. The gp55 or a glycoprotein of 55 kDa encoded by the *env* gene determines the pathogenicity of SFFV and must be glycosylated for its leukemic activity. This gp55 interacts with the erythropoietin receptor and promotes the erythropoietin-independent differentiation and proliferation of erythroid progenitor cells. Gp55 also recruits the short form of the stem-cell-kinase receptor for cell signaling. This additional receptor is a member of the transmembrane tyrosine kinase family of receptors, lacking only the extracellular binding domain of the stem-cell-kinase receptor. This larger stem-cell-kinase receptor is encoded by the *Fv2* gene (Friend virus susceptibility gene 2) that mediates the susceptibility of sensitive strains of mice to the leukemia virus (Fv2$^{s/s}$). This is important, because genetic susceptibilities to cancer appear to involve dysfunctions in cell signaling.

Mice resistant to the leukemia virus have deleted the internal promoter within the stem-cell-kinase receptor gene. For those infected mice that encode gp55, erythropoietin receptor, and the short form of the stem-cell-kinase receptor, this also leads to dysregulation of proliferation, survival, and differentiation via affecting signal transduction and transcription activation pathways involving STATs, PI3-kinase/AKT, Grb2/Gab2 molecular adaptors, Lyn kinase, p38MAP kinase, and ERK1/2 MAP kinases. SFFV causes insertional mutagenesis by preferential integration into the *spi-1* locus. Dimethyl sulfoxide's influence on continuing differentiation rather than carcinogenesis was noted by decreased Spi-1 expression. The arrest of differentiation and increased proliferation appear to require coexpression of Spi-1 with

gp55 activation of the erythropoietin receptor or by a mutation of the R129C residue, which mimics this activation. From this example, it becomes clearer how dysregulation of signaling pathways can occur via over-activation, sequence insertion, or by mutation in a particular region. Allelic deletions or missense mutations in the tumor suppressor gene *p53* made mice more susceptible to the development of Friend disease due to increased survival of leukemic proerythroblasts rather than affecting differentiation. This happens late in the leukemic process, as do point mutations in the *Kit* gene. The *Kit* gene controls ERK1/2 MAP kinases, PI3Kinase, and Src kinases, thereby in combination with Spi-1 overexpression causing the abnormal cells to become malignant.

Human leukemias confirm that a single mutation alone may lead only to a myeloproliferative disorder. Leukemic progression has too long a latency period to be caused by that single event. Instead, there may be a second mutational event or leukemia may then be induced through the use of genotoxic compounds in addition to the initiating damage. Mechanistically, consider the first event to involve a mutation in a gene involving a transcription factor, such as promyelocytic leukemia-retinoic acid receptor α (PML/RARα). PML/RARα is linked to 99% of acute promyelocytic leukemia and acts as a transcriptional repressor for the hormonal receptor RARα. So modification of this or similar factors will arrest the differentiation of stem cells that are more prone to cancer development. The second mutation would likely involve tyrosine kinase genes signaling an increase in proliferation of those abnormal undifferentiated cells (Moreau-Gachelin, 2008). Another cell signaling theory involves the mechanisms that lead to dysregulation, such as decreasing the action of tumor suppressors and activating proto-oncogenes, also influence metabolism and decrease apoptotic signaling. Scientists can then describe a "metabolic phenotype" that unifies metabolic and genetic models of cancer (DeBerardinis, 2008).

Another way that signaling pathways may influence development of cancer is indicated by the malignant transformation induced by 2,3,7,8-tetrachlorodibenzo-p-dioxin (TCDD) and its prevention by the oxidative stress-inducing agent curcumin. TCDD increased the formation of CYP 1A1 and 1B1 through which genotoxic metabolites are generated. TCDD mediates its action via the aryl hydrocarbon receptor (AhR) and AhR nuclear translocator (ARNT). Curcumin prevents TCDD's carcinogenic action by creating ROS that degrade AhR and ARNT in the nucleus but not in the cytoplasm (Choi et al., 2008). Another multiphase model has also been developed to look at angiogenesis which supplies the growing tumor with the blood flow necessary to sustain the growth and provide the necessary tumor cell movement to relieve mechanical stress caused by the increased mass of the tumor (Breward et al., 2003).

The cancer risk models try to assess time of exposure and target tissue concentrations of toxicants to account for various mechanisms that cancer can initiate, promote, or progress. The time-averaged tissue concentrations of the toxicants serve the one-hit high dose or multi-hit models well. Detailed concentration histories are required for the clonal two-stage (intermediate-stage clonal growth advantage) model or multistage models. However, these assume long or lifetime exposures. Certain substances such as arsenic show more moderate dependence on time of exposure while ethylene dibromide is strongly dependent on exposure time. Short exposures show the most problems when these two or more stage models are employed resulting in errors of several orders of magnitude. This is unacceptable when dose–response is a logarithmic function. Even when the exposure may be two-thirds of a lifetime, these models average those exposures over a full lifetime and lead to a 3.4-fold error for arsenic and 8-fold error for ethylene dibromide (Morrison, 1987). This indicates that the models alone will not bail researchers out of assessing cancer risk from a variety of exposures. Researchers use high doses extrapolated to low doses, and assume rat lifetime is applicable to human lifetime. Many of the assumptions are not based on mechanistic realities of how cell populations respond to a variety of insults.

Is toxicogenomics the answer, or must other models be used to account for a variety of exposure patterns? A scathing analysis of toxicogenomics and the model of the carcinogen as only a mutagen indicates that much of the focus on gene alterations appears to miss the major roles epigenetic alterations play in carcinogenesis (Trosko and Upham, 2005). This includes changes in cell signaling and the important role that stem and progenitor cells play in the process of tumor development. This analysis indicates that low-molecular-weight (three to four rings) polycyclic aromatic hydrocarbons are better models of cancer development than those of genotoxic agents. The complexity of cancer development indicates that a two-dimensional analysis of *in vitro* assays employing normal, primary rodent or human cells, or immortalized normal or cancer cell lines, can never truly represent the *in situ* living complex human organism with intricate interactions between stem cells, proliferating progenitor cells, and the terminally differentiated cells with a given tissue or between tissues, including physiological responses.

Further confounding a cellular or animal model of cancer is the multistage, multiple mechanisms of cancer development, the species differences that may affect any of these stages, the variety of developmental, dietary, environmental, genetic, and even lifestyle factors that influence cancer risk and stages of cancer, and the hierarchical/cybernetic organization of multiple cells within a tissue or organism that is not adequately mimicked by cell-free molecular targets or two-dimensional cell cultures. Only the use of human stem cells may provide the additional information necessary to inform both genotoxicity assays and epigenetic models of cancer development in animals. The high-dose model of animal carcinogenesis has assumptions that either the high dose of the chemical is fully capable of accomplishing all phases of cancer development by multiple mechanisms that can be found in mixtures such as cigarette smoke or that the high dose has a large impact on the physiology of the animal that mainly influences one stage of cancer initiation, promotion, or progression. Even mutation assays generate mainly phenotypic changes that identify many false positives that may not lead to cancer in a whole organism at the given dose/concentration used in the tests. Rodent models have their shortcomings as well, because an agent may select a spontaneously generated mutation in an oncogene or tumor suppressor gene and be considered a carcinogen based on the false interpretation of that test alone.

It would be a mistake to see promotion by epigenetic mechanisms as only involving toxic chemical action rather than inclusion other processes such as tissue irritation, cell death, and removal of cells by surgery. The best model should incorporate aspects of initiation, promotion, and progression and should not rely on genotoxic indices that do not account mechanistically for epigenetic mechanisms. Additionally, tumor-promotion agents represent many of the chemicals labeled as epigenetic carcinogens. Many of the chemicals labeled as carcinogenic mutagens with one cell type would likely cause tissue necrosis for other cell populations or death of the whole animal and are probably more reasonably assessed as epigenetic but not mutagenic or genotoxic. For example, a report has indicated that N-nitroso-N-methylureainduced rat mammary tumors appear to result from cells with preexisting oncogenic Hras1 gene mutations (Cha et al., 1994). This is not an easy regulatory endpoint that defines a carcinogen based on its outcome rather than its mechanism and sensitivity of the organism. Additionally, two reports indicated that a model mutagenic carcinogen 7,12-dimethylbenz[a] anthracene (DMBA) did not cause any mutations of the Ki-ras and Ha-ras oncogene of the DMBA-transformed cells (Brookes et al., 1988; Mass and Austin, 1989).

The focus of toxicologists has been on the high-molecular-weight PAHs such as benzo[a] pyrene and benzo[e]pyrene that have mutagenic activity when biotransformed. However, the low-molecular-weight epigenetic PAHs are at 62 times the concentration of these higher molecular weight mutagenic components of cigarette smoke and are the powerful co-carcinogens that account for the total response to the smoke PAHs. This also explains the reversal of effects after smoking cessation due to the low mutagenicity of the smoke mixture. These low-molecular-weight PAHs that have bay regions, but have not been converted to electrophiles via metabolism, also inhibit gap junctional intercellular communications, which is important in ROS toxicity. Similarly, carcinogenic substances such as DDT, TCDD, the pesticide tetrachloroterephthalic acid (TPA), the medication phenobarbital, pentachlorophenol, and peroxisome proliferators do not damage DNA, but rather promote tumor growth. For example, treatment of rodents with organic and hydrogen peroxides was found to promote but not initiate cancer formation. ROS are known to affect the expression of 127 genes and signal transducing proteins at doses that are not cytotoxic. This indicates a shift from DNA damage to a more complex epigenetic toxic action of oxidative chemicals. Two of those pathways are the mitogen-activated protein kinases (MAPK) and NF-κB. The activation of MAPK requires both ROS and internally produced hydrogen peroxide. Solid tissue cell types depend on both extracellular signals and intercellular signals through gap junctions. ROS inhibit gap junctional intercellular communications, thereby preventing the escape of the H_2O_2 necessary to assist the induction of MAPK-dependent activation of transcription factors. Additionally, it would be expected that this effect would be exacerbated by the absence of antioxidants in cells. However, depletion of GSH reverses the inhibition of gap junctional intercellular communications, induction of c-jun, and activation of NF-κB. This indicates that extracellular, intracellular, and intercellular signals should be considered in cancer models and how other cellular factors are required for activation of or block expression of key genes (Trosko and Upham, 2005).

An example of how whole animal models may be misinterpreted is the effect of atrazine on mammary tumors in Sprague-Dawley rats. It appears that the maximum tolerated dose of atrazine lengthens the estrous cycle and should have been classified as an endocrine disruptor rather than a carcinogen, because it only makes the spontaneous formation of mammary and pituitary tumors occur at an earlier age (Wetzel et al., 1994). This result caused a regulatory challenge to the carcinogen risk assessment process when these data were submitted to the Office of Prevention, Pesticides, and Toxic Substances (now called the Office of Chemical Safety and Pollution Prevention) at the U.S. Environmental Protection Agency (EPA).

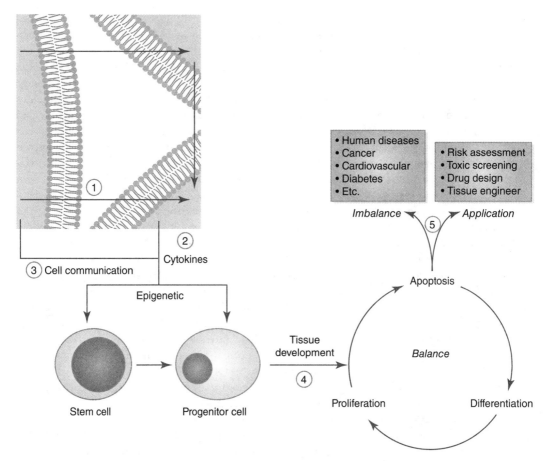

FIGURE 10-7 Summary Statement: In Response to Environmental and Foodborne Toxicants and Toxins That May Induce Oxidative Stress, the Stem and Progenitor Cells Can Be Affected at the (1) Genotoxic Level, Leading to Somatic Mutations. However, the significance of genotoxicity has been questioned and genotoxic level also leads to cytotoxicity. (2) Cytotoxic (necrotic) levels, acute death of cells in a tissue by toxic compounds often results in the compensatory release of cytokines that affect distal cells. (3) Epigenetic level, toxic agents can directly affect the expression of genes at the transcriptional, translational and post-translational levels by altering the integrated cell signaling systems controlling gene expression resulting in (4), the interruption of the homeostatic balance of a tissue by disturbing the equilibrium between apoptosis, proliferation and differentiation. Such imbalances lead to (5), chronic disease such as cancer. Assessment of epigenetic events and the use of stem cells have numerous applications in human health.

So, what is the best model? A three-dimensional dynamic culture system has been developed through the use of stem cells (embryonic and adult), culturing several cell types together, organotypic cultures, creation of three-dimensional organoids, and through the use of insert wells to measure soluble factors that indicate stromal–epithelial. It is important to represent the three basic cell types with a few adult stem cells, many committed progenitor or transit cells

that are not immortal, and terminally differentiated cells. These tests should not involve high pO_2, high Ca^{2+}, or other growth factors such as serum that do not replicate the true physiological state of a tissue in an intact organism. The closest that human testing can be done ethically is to use a tissue-appropriate mixture of human stem cells, their differentiated progenitor daughter cells, and terminally differentiated progeny. This approach is modeled in **Figure10-7**. Note that the cellular distribution and the epigenetic effects are more central to this analysis. Cancer is just one possibility in proliferative diseases. Note that the toxicologist also becomes the key to medication development, because the toxicologist must consider proliferation versus differentiation pathways for treatment options in addition to a straightforward cancer risk assessment by traditional approaches (Trosko and Upham, 2005).

Regulatory Agencies' Assessment of Cancer Risk from Toxic Substances

This chapter concludes with an examination of how regulatory agencies assess cancer risk from toxic substances and attempt to keep in consideration the multitude of parameters that lead to metastatic disease. The Agency for Toxic Substances and Disease Registry (ATSDR) has a process that accounts from high-dose short exposures to low-dose chronic exposure (http://www.atsdr.cdc.gov/cancer.html). It accounts for all exposure routes and direct and indirect exposures with the intention of estimating the dose at the biologic target cells/tissue(s). It substitutes mathematical modeling where complete monitoring information is unavailable. If inhalation rates, water consumption, lifespan, body weight, or other factors that influence the exposure are not known, default values with uncertainty factors are employed to assess risk. Nutritional and lifestyle variables are considered in the behavioral factors that determine exposure and risk. The history of past and current exposures as well as potential future exposures is taken into account. The qualitative issues for cancer risk include a weight-of-evidence approach that includes studies, epidemiologic studies, long-term animal bioassays, short-term tests, and structure–activity relationships (SARs). The peer-reviewed studies are analyzed for use of proper controls, number of animals per group to make the correct statistical analyses and the correct animal model for extrapolation to humans, administration route(s), selection of doses, and tumor types confirmed by accepted techniques. Under mechanistic inference and species concordance, the agency states that "carcinogenesis is generally viewed

as a multistage process, proceeding from initiation, through promotion and progression." The statement then goes on to indicate that both genotoxic and epigenetic mechanisms are important. ATSDR assumes that most cancer-causing chemicals have no threshold for tumor formation. It will not rule out that a threshold may exist for any step in the multistage process and evaluates studies on a case-by-case basis for relevance to the human population. The agency is aware that a route of administration in an animal that causes cancer may not do so in a human and vice versa, so relevant routes are indicated for the assessment of risk. Finally, the qualitative analysis indicates that epidemiological studies really provide direct data for human risk and must be given a higher weight, especially if they are intelligently designed and implemented. This means that, as with any good toxicological analyses, a dose–response relationship is established and a temporal sequence of exposure and then response is determined. The study should have no confounding bias, should be consistent with other scientific evidence, is biologically plausible, and shows a strong association with the toxicant and cancer in the population (e.g., cigarette smoke components). The analysis then takes into account susceptible populations who may have genetic, nutritional, age, physiological factors, and/or an unusually high exposure profile compared to the general population. SARs may provide confirming evidence, but are considered inadequate alone as refinements and validation have not reached the level of certainty with regard to animal or human disease. Although ATSDR is aware that the real world has exposure to mixtures, there is inadequate modeling that currently can substitute for animal or human exposure in this arena. Based on these qualitative factors, it does appear that regulators view the entire carcinogenic process rather than focusing on any one aspect as having more value.

The quantitative issues for the ATSDR include dose scaling that accounts for metabolic rate through the use of $mg/kg^{3/4}/day$ as the scaling factor. It prefers that more accurate information be developed through the use of physiologically based toxicokinetic modeling to determine both the degree and the time course

TABLE 10-3 Classification of Carcinogens			
EPA	**IARC**	**NTP**	**OSHA**
(Group A) Human Carcinogen	(Group 1) Carcinogenic to Humans	Human Carcinogen	Category I
(Group B1, B2) Probable Human Carcinogen	(Group 2A) Probably Carcinogenic to Humans	Reasonably Anticipated to be a Carcinogen	Category II
(Group C) Possible Human Carcinogen	(Group 2B) Possibly Carcinogenic to Humans		
(Group D) Not Classifiable as to Human Carcinogenicity	(Group3) Not Classifiable as to Human Carcinogenicity		
(Group E) Evidence of Non-carcinogenicity for Humans			

EPA, Environmental Protection Agency; IARC, International Agency for Research on Cancer; NTP, National Toxicology Program; OSHA, Occupational Safety and Health Administration.

Reproduced from ATSDR - Cancer Policy Framework, January 1993. Available at http://www.atsdr.cdc.gov/cancer.html.

of the exposure at the target site on or within cells or tissues. Without a plausible mechanism of action, the agency selects the conservative no-threshold, linear, multistage model of lowdose exposure to genotoxins, because high doses for shorter period exposures have historically predominated in the animal exposure literature and are not necessary easily converted into relevant human cancer risk without uncertainties. ATSDR realizes that this modeling may be inappropriate for epigenetic agents and thresholds must be demonstrated along with the "plausible potency" estimates for reaching conclusions that are quantifiable. Biomarkers of molecular epidemiology are acceptable for assessing increased risk such as DNA adducts, activated oncogenes and their protein products, and/or loss of suppressor gene activity. Prior exposure that may also increase risk may be properly indicated by the activity of certain aryl hydroxylase isozymes. However, these factors must be combined with experimental models and epidemiology to provide confirming evidence of their usefulness in determination of individual cancer risk.

ATSDR also relies on the judgment and experience of the whole toxicological field through peer review and other agencies such as the National Toxicology Program, the EPA, the Occupational Safety and Health Administration (OSHA), the National Institute for Occupational Safety and Health (NIOSH), the Food and Drug Administration (FDA), and other prominent government scientific programs in this arena such as the International Agency for Research on Cancer (IARC).

The categories of carcinogenic substances are indicated in **Table 10-3**. This is placed as a higher value than that of computer programs that assess risk in ways that may not agree with currently held conclusions based on previous animal or especially human epidemiological evidence. As new studies challenge the view of cancer mechanisms, the policy is dynamic in that it recognizes the importance of insights that change our understanding and therefore determination of cancer risk. Accordingly, the challenge to future toxicologists is to do the rigorous mechanistic studies with cell preparations, the intact animal, and finally epidemiologists to evaluate how genotoxic and epigenetic pathways lead to advanced cancer and to gauge the weight of other factors in decreasing or increasing the risk of oncogenesis.

Questions

1. What happens during apoptosis or necrosis that leads to nuclear membrane changes?

2. Why aren't all mutagens carcinogens or carcinogens mutagenic?

3. Based on the point mutagens, which DNA base seems most prone to adduct formation by alkylation and formation by ROS of formamidopyrimidines?

4. Why can PAHs be both point mutagens and frameshift mutagens?

5. Which are the most toxic cross-links?

6. Which is more toxic: agents that cross-link and produce ROS or those that just cross-link? Explain.

7. Three good assays for clastogenesis are the micronucleus assay, sister chromatid exchanges, and the comet assay. How are they done and interpreted?

8. How can strong mutagens inactivate certain genes and activate others, and how can both initiate cancer?

9. Which signaling pathways differentiate between genotoxic agent action versus nongenotoxic action?

10. Why is the single-hit model good for highdose, short-term exposures and the multistage better for long-term exposure? Which would be the best model toxicant for cancer: a small PAH or a large one?

References

Acevedo-Arozena A, Wells S, Potter P, Kelly M, Cox RD, Brown SD. 2008. ENU mutagenesis, a way forward to understand gene function. *Annu Rev Genomics Hum Genet.* 9:49–69.

Adiseshaiah P, Li J, Vaz M, Kalvakolanu DV, Reddy SP. 2008. ERK signaling regulates tumor promoter induced c-Jun recruitment at the Fra-1 promoter. *Biochem Biophys Res Commun.* 371:304–308.

Albertini RJ, Nicklas JA, O'Neill JP. 1993. Somatic cell gene mutations in humans: biomarkers for genotoxicity. *Environ Health Perspect.* 101(Suppl 3): 193–201.

Amati B, Alevizopoulos K, Vlach J. 1998. Myc and the cell cycle. *Front Biosci.* 3:d250–d268.

Baskin DS, Ngo H, Didenko VV. 2003. Thimerosal induces DNA breaks, caspase-3 activation, membrane damage, and cell death in cultured human neurons and fibroblasts. *Toxicol Sci.* 74:361–368.

Błasiak J, Sikora A, Wozniak K, Drzewoski J. 2004. Genotoxicity of streptozotocin in normal and cancer cells and its modulation by free radical scavengers. *Cell Biol Toxicol.* 20:83–96.

Bolzán AD, Bianchi MS, Correa MV. 2001. Modulation of streptonigrin's clastogenic effects in CHO cells by the metal-chelating agent 1,10-phenanthroline. *Environ Mol Mutagen.* 38:306–310.

Bombail V, Moggs JG, Orphanides G. 2004. Perturbation of epigenetic status by toxicants. *Toxicol Lett.* 149:51–58.

Breward CJ, Byrne HM, Lewis CE. 2003. A multiphase model describing vascular tumour growth. *Bull Math Biol.* 65:609–640.

Brookes P, Cooper CS, Ellis MV, Warren W, Gardner E, Summerhayes IC. 1988. Activated Ki-ras genes in bladder epithelial cell lines transformed by treatment of primary mouse bladder explant cultures with 7,12-dimethylbenz[a]anthracene. *Mol Carcinog.* 1:82–88.

Cha RS, Thilly WG, Zarbl H. 1994. N-Nitroso-N-methylurea-induced rat mammary tumors arise from cells with preexisting oncogenic Hras1 gene mutations. Proc. *Natl Acad Sci USA.* 91:3749–3753.

Chan WM, Mak MC, Fung TK, Lau A, Siu WY, Poon RY. 2006. Ubiquitination of p53 at multiple sites in the DNA-binding domain. *Mol Cancer Res.* 4:15–25.

Cho E, Li WJ. 2007. Human stem cells, chromatin, and tissue engineering: boosting relevancy in developmental toxicity testing. *Birth Defects Res C Embryo Today.* 81:20–40.

Choi H, Chun YS, Shin YJ, Ye SK, Kim MS, Park JW. 2008. Curcumin attenuates cytochrome P450 induction in response to 2,3,7,8-tetrachlorodibenzo-p-dioxin by ROS-dependently degrading AhR and ARNT. *Cancer Sci.* 99(12):2518–2524.

DeBerardinis RJ. 2008. Is cancer a disease of abnormal cellular metabolism? New angles on an old idea. *Genet Med.* 10(11):767–777.

Dizdaroglu M, Kirkali G, Jaruga P. 2008. Formamidopyrimidines in DNA: mechanisms of formation, repair, and biological effects. *Free Radic Biol Med.* 45(12):1610–1621.

Ellinger-Ziegelbauer H, Aubrecht J, Kleinjans JC, Ahr HJ. 2008. Application of toxicogenomics to study mechanisms of genotoxicity and carcinogenicity. *Toxicol Lett.* 186(1):36–44.

Ellinger-Ziegelbauer H, Gmuender H, Bandenburg A, Ahr HJ. 2008. Prediction of a carcinogenic potential of rat hepatocarcinogens using toxicogenomics analysis of short-term *in vivo* studies. *Mutat Res.* 637:23–39.

Evenson DP, Wixon R. 2006. Clinical aspects of sperm DNA fragmentation detection and male infertility. *Theriogenology.* 65:979–991.

Felix CA. 1998. Secondary leukemias induced by topoisomerase-targeted drugs. *Biochim Biophys Acta.* 1400:233–255.

Ferguson LR, Denny WA. 2007. Genotoxicity of noncovalent interactions: DNA intercalators. *Mutat Res.* 623:14–23.

Fosslien E. 2008. Cancer morphogenesis: role of mitochondrial failure. *Ann Clin Lab Sci.* 38:307–329.

Frohling S, Dohner H. 2008. Molecular origins of cancer: chromosomal abnormalities in cancer. *N Engl J Med.* 359:722–734.

Ganesan K, Ivanova T, Wu Y, Rajasegaran V, Wu J, Lee MH, Yu K, Rha SY, Chung HC, Ylstra B, Meijer G, Lian KO, Grabsch H, Tan P. 2008. Inhibition of gastric cancer invasion and metastasis by PLA2G2A, a novel beta-catenin/TCF target gene. *Cancer Res.* 68:4277–4286.

Gomaa AI, Khan SA, Toledano MB, Waked I, Taylor-Robinson SD. 2008. Hepatocellular carcinoma: epidemiology, risk factors and pathogenesis. *World J Gastroenterol.* 14:4300–4308.

Hall A. 1984. Oncogenes—implications for human cancer: a review. *J R Soc Med.* 77:410–416.

Iarmarcovai G, Ceppi M, Botta A, Orsière T, Bonassi S. 2008. Micronuclei frequency in peripheral blood lymphocytes of cancer patients: a meta-analysis. *Mutat Res.* 659:274–283.

Hong H, Wang Y. 2005. Formation of intrastrand cross-link products between cytosine and adenine from UV irradiation of d((Br)CA) and duplex DNA containing a 5-bromocytosine. *J Am Chem Soc.* 127:13969–13977.

Iqbal Z, Siddiqui RT, Qureshi JA. 2004. Two different point mutations in Abl gene ATP-binding domain conferring primary imatinib resistance in a chronic myeloid leukemia (CML) patient: a case report. *Biol Proced Online.* 6:144–148.

Ishikawa S, Mochizuki M. 2003. Mutagenicity and cross-linking activity of chloroalkylnitrosamines, possible new antitumor lead compounds. *Mutagenesis.* 18:331–335.

Jeffrey AM, Williams GM. 2005. Risk assessment of DNA-reactive carcinogens in food. *Toxicol Appl Pharmacol.* 207(2 Suppl):628–635.

Karchin R, Agarwal M, Sali A, Couch F, Beattie MS. 2008. Classifying variants of undetermined significance in BRCA2 with protein likelihood ratios. *Cancer Inform.* 6:203–216.

Knaapen AM, Güngör N, Schins RP, Borm PJ, Van Schooten FJ. 2006. Neutrophils and respiratory tract DNA damage and mutagenesis: a review. *Mutagenesis.* 21:225–236.

Korf B. 2008. Hutchinson-Gilford progeria syndrome, aging, and the nuclear lamina. *N Engl J Med.* 358:552–555.

Kralovics R, Passamonti F, Buser AS, Teo SS, Tiedt R, Passweg JR, Tichelli A, Cazzola M, Skoda RC. 2005. A gain-of-function mutation of JAK2 in myeloproliferative disorders. *N Engl J Med.* 352:1779–1790.

Kryczek I, Wei S, Keller E, Liu R, Zou W. 2007. Stroma-derived factor (SDF-1/CXCL12) and human tumor pathogenesis. *Am J Physiol Cell Physiol.* 292:C987–C995.

Li M, Wang J, Jin J, Hua H, Luo T, Xu L, Wang R, Liu D, Jiang Y. 2008. Synergistic promotion of breast cancer cells death by targeting molecular chaperone GRP78 and heat shock protein 70. *J Cell Mol Med.* 13(11–12):4540–4550.

Liu J, Xu R, Jin Y, Wang D. 2001. *In vitro* triplex formation and functional analysis of TFOs designed against human c-sis/PDGF-B proto-oncogene. *Sci China C Life Sci.* 44:83–91.

Luan Y, Suzuki T, Palanisamy R, Takashima Y, Sakamoto H, Sakuraba M, Koizumi T, Saito M, Matsufuji H, Yamagata K, Yamaguchi T, Hayashi M, Honma M. 2007. Potassium bromate treatment predominantly causes large deletions, but not GC>TA transversion in human cells. *Mutat Res.* 619:113–123.

Manière I, Godard T, Doerge DR, Churchwell MI, Guffroy M, Laurentie M, Poul JM. 2005. DNA damage and DNA adduct formation in rat tissues following oral administration of acrylamide. *Mutat Res.* 580:119–129.

Marek LR, Kottemann MC, Glazer PM, Bale AE. 2008. MEN1 and FANCD2 mediate distinct mechanisms of DNA crosslink repair. *DNA Repair (Amst).* 7:476–486.

Mass MJ, Austin SJ. 1989. Absence of mutations in codon 61 of the Ha-ras oncogene in epithelial cells transformed *in vitro* by 7,12-dimethylbenz(a)anthracene. *Biochem Biophys Res Commun.* 165:1319–1323.

Matsuo Y, Ochi N, Sawai H, Yasuda A, Takahashi H, Funahashi H, Takeyama H, Tong Z, Guha S. 2008. CXCL8/IL-8 and CXCL12/SDF-1alpha cooperatively promote invasiveness and angiogenesis in pancreatic cancer. *Int J Cancer.* 124(4):853–861.

Moreau-Gachelin F. 2008. Multi-stage Friend murine erythroleukemia: molecular insights into oncogenic cooperation. *Retrovirology.* 5:99.

Morrison PF. 1987. Effects of time-variant exposure on toxic substance response. *Environ Health Perspect.* 76:133–139.

Nesslany F, Zennouche N, Simar-Meintières S, Talahari I, Nkili-Mboui EN, Marzin D. 2007. *In vivo* Comet assay on isolated kidney cells to distinguish genotoxic carcinogens from epigenetic carcinogens or cytotoxic compounds. *Mutat Res.* 630:28–41.

Ni R, Mulligan AM, Have C, O'Malley FP. 2007. PGDS, a novel technique combining chromogenic in situ hybridization and immunohistochemistry for the assessment of ErbB2 (HER2/neu) status in breast cancer. *Appl Immunohistochem Mol Morphol.* 15:316–324.

Niitsu N, Okamoto M, Miura I, Hirano M. 2008. Clinical significance of 8q24/c-MYC translocation in diffuse large B-cell lymphoma. *Cancer Sci.* 100(2):233–237.

Ohe T, Watanabe T, Wakabayashi K. 2004. Mutagens in surface waters: a review. *Mutat Res.* 567:109–149.

O'Shea EK, Rutkowski R, Kim PS. 1992. Mechanism of specificity in the Fos-Jun oncoprotein heterodimer. *Cell.* 68:699–708.

Peluso M, Airoldi L, Munnia A, Colombi A, Veglia F, Autrup H, Dunning A, Garte S, Gormally E, Malaveille C, Matullo G, Overvad K, Raaschou-Nielsen O, Clavel-Chapelon F, Linseisen J, Boeing H, Trichopoulou A, Palli D, Krogh V, Tumino R, Panico S, Bueno-De-Mesquita BH, Peeters PH, Kumle M, Agudo A, Martinez C, Dorronsoro M, Barricarte A, Tormo MJ, Quiros JR, Berglund G, Jarvholm B, Day NE, Key TJ, Saracci R, Kaaks R, Riboli E, Bingham S, Vineis P. 2008. Bulky DNA adducts, 4-aminobiphenyl-haemoglobin adducts and diet in the European Prospective Investigation into Cancer and Nutrition (EPIC) prospective study. *Br J Nutr.* 100:489–495.

Rajski SR, Williams RM. 1998. DNA cross-linking agents as antitumor drugs. *Chem Rev.* 98:2723–2796.

Santucci MA, Corradi V, Mancini M, Manetti F, Radi M, Schenone S, Botta M. 2008. C6-unsubstituted pyrazolo[3,4-d]pyrimidines are dual Src/Abl inhibitors effective against imatinib mesylate resistant chronic myeloid leukemia cell lines. *Chem Med Chem.* 4(1):118–126.

Schmeiser HH, Bieler CA, Wiessler M, van Ypersele de Strihou C, Cosyns JP. 1996. Detection of DNA adducts formed by aristolochic acid in renal tissue from patients with Chinese herbs nephropathy. *Cancer Res.* 56:2025–2028.

Sengbusch PV. 1967. Influence of protein structure on selection of nitrous acid induced mutants of TMV. *Mol Gen Genet.* 99(2):171–180.

Stiborová M, Miksanová M, Smrcek S, Bieler CA, Breuer A, Klokow KA, Schmeiser HH, Frei E. 2004. Identification of a genotoxic mechanism for 2-nitroanisole carcinogenicity and of its carcinogenic potential for humans. *Carcinogenesis.* 25:833–840.

Szołtysek K, Pietranek K, Kalinowska-Herok M, Pietrowska M, Kimmel M, Widłak P. 2008. TNFalpha-induced activation of NFkappaB protects against UV-induced apoptosis specifically in p53-proficient cells. *Acta Biochim Pol.* 55(4):741–748.

Trosko JE, Upham BL. 2005. The emperor wears no clothes in the field of carcinogen risk assessment: ignored concepts in cancer risk assessment. *Mutagenesis.* 20:81–92.

Vázquez-Martin C, Rouse J, Cohen PT. 2008. Characterization of the role of a trimeric protein phosphatase complex in recovery from cisplatin-induced versus noncrosslinking DNA damage. *FEBS J.* 275:4211–4221.

Volpato CB, Martínez-Alfaro M, Corvi R, Gabus C, Sauvaigo S, Ferrari P, Bonora E, De Grandi A, Romeo G. 2008. Enhanced sensitivity of the RET proto-oncogene to ionizing radiation *in vitro*. *Cancer Res.* 68:8986–8992.

Wang XQ, Li H, Van Putten V, Winn RA, Heasley LE, Nemenoff RA. 2008. Oncogenic K-Ras regulates proliferation and cell junctions in lung epithelial cells through induction of COX-2 and activation of MMP-9. *Mol Biol Cell.* 20(3):791–800.

Wetzel LT, Luempert LG III, Breckenridge CB, Tisdel MO, Stevens JT, Thakur AK, Extrom PJ, Eldridge JC. 1994. Chronic effects of atrazine on estrus and mammary tumor formation in female Sprague-Dawley and Fischer 344 rats. *J Toxicol Environ Health.* 43:169–182.

Xamena N, Creus A, Marcos R. 1985. Effect of intercalating mutagens on crossing-over in *Drosophila melanogaster* females. *Experientia.* 41:1078–1079.

Yang JS, Chen GW, Hsia TC, Ho HC, Ho CC, Lin MW, Lin SS, Yeh RD, Ip SW, Lu HF, Chung JG. 2008. Diallyl disulfide induces apoptosis in human colon cancer cell line (COLO 205) through the induction of reactive oxygen species, endoplasmic reticulum stress, caspases casade and mitochondrial-dependent pathways. *Food Chem Toxicol.* 47(1):171–179.

Yeung BKS, Boger DL. 2003. Synthesis of isochrysohermidin-distamycin hybrids. *J Org Chem.* 68:5249–5253.

Zhang R, Niu Y, Du H, Cao X, Shi D, Hao Q, Zhou Y. 2008. A stable and sensitive testing system for potential carcinogens based on DNA damage-induced gene expression in human HepG2 cell. *Toxicol In Vitro.* 23(1):158–165.

Zherbin EA, Chukhlovin AB, Köteles GJ, Kubasova TA, Vashchenko VI, Hanson KP. 1986. Effects *in vitro* of cadmium ions on some membrane and nuclear parameters of normal and irradiated thymic lymphoid cells. *Arch Toxicol.* 59:21–25.

CHAPTER 11

Selective Genetic Sensitivity of Cells to Toxicants

This is a chapter outline intended to guide and familiarize you with the content to follow.

I. Selective toxicity

  A. ↑ Dosage → hypersensitive responders → normal bell-shaped distribution of responding majority of population or species or cells → hyposensitive/resistant to toxicity

  B. Absorption and elimination (in vs. out)

   1. Chemosensitizers—inhibit ABC transporters of cancer cells and increase chemotherapy effects to those cells while having low toxicity to normal cells

   2. Q141K polymorphism = ↑ diarrhea from antitumor medication gefitinib

   3. OATP1B1 transporter important in limiting toxicity to statins in the liver → the polymorphism of the SLCO1B1 gene (c.521CC) had higher plasma levels, and others (c.521CC and c.521TC) had earlier peak time than normal = threshold toxicity; and c.521CC genotype had higher AUC (higher concentrations over time). Conversely, a multidrug-resistance-associated protein 2 (MRP2) confers resistance to a statin (pravastatin)

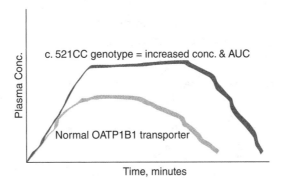

   4. Affecting Na- and Cl-dependent GABA transporter causes neurotoxicity by certain medications, which is reduced by a resistant polymorphism of the SLC6A1 gene in certain Tanzanians. Similarly, humans must have the LA/LA genotype of serotonin transporter 5-HTTLPR to be responsive to selective serotonin reuptake inhibitors (SSRIs) that treat depression and psychosis

   5. Polymorphisms in acid-sensing ion channel 3 (ASIC3) → hypertension in Taiwanese

   6. Secretion of organic acids by the kidney appears to be the reason for ↑ toxicity of phenoxyacetic acids (2,4-dichlorophenoxyacetic acid herbicide) in the dog

CONCEPTUALIZING TOXICOLOGY 11-1

C. Metabolism/CYP polymorphisms

1. CYP*2C I462 allele associated with cancers of the aerodigestive tract; more prominent when glutathione transferase (GSTM) gene is not expressed (null)

2. CYP1B1*3 allele = head and neck squamous cell cancers in smokers but also includes GSTMs, tumor suppressor mutation, DNA repair gene polymorphisms, and mitochondrial DNA mutations

3. CYP2E1 polymorphisms are related to environmental or industrial toxicant exposures

4. Acetylation status alterations via NAT2 are associated with bladder cancers of aromatic amines; bladder cancers due to PAHs appear in polymorphisms of GSTM1

5. Those with increased CYP1A1, CYP1A2, CYP1B1, CYP2A6, CYP2E1, and CYP3A4 have increased carcinogen activation

6. Medication metabolism related to fast (more resistant to action of medication) or slow metabolizing (longer or increased action of medication) by CYP1A2, CYP2A6, CYP2B6, CYP2C8, CYP2C9, CYP2C19, CYP2D6, CYP2E1, CYP3A4, and CYP3A5; CYP2C19 slow metabolizers 5 more effective treatment by proton pump inhibitors for ulcers

   a. CYP2A6*4 genotype 5 inactive toward metabolism of steroids, fatty acids, aflatoxin B$_1$, coumarins, cyclophosphamide, nicotine, nitrosamines

   b. CYP2B6*5 genotype 5 lower than normal activity toward steroids, fatty acids, bupropion, cyclophosphamide, methadone

   c. CYP2C9*2 and *3 genotypes have reduced activity toward limonene, amitriptyline, celecoxib, dapsone, diclofenac, ibuprofen, lornoxicam, meloxicam, (S)-naproxen, piroxicam, suprofen, warfarin, SSRIs, fluvastatin, glibenclamide, irbesartan and losartan, mephenytoin, phenobarbital, rosiglitazone, tamoxifen, torsemide, and zidovudine; CYP2C19*2A is inactive for limonene, amitriptyline, carisoprodol, citalopram, cyclophosphamide, indomethacin, omeprazole, certain anticonvulsants, benzodiazepines, barbiturates, and tricyclic antidepressants, among other medications that treat cancer, malaria, and HIV infection

   d. CYP2D6*4x, where x 5 a variety of alleles, produces inactivity toward beta-blockers, adrenergic stimulants, antipsychotics, atomoxetine, certain antihistamines, opiates, debrisoquine, dexfenfluramine, dextromethorphan, certain SSRIs, antiarrhythmic medications, halothane, lidocaine, among a variety of other agent used in cancer, treatment of emesis and digestive functions, and a variety of neuroactive and cardiovascular medicines

   e. Estrogens are metabolized by CYP1B

   f. Metabolism by CYP2D6 isoenzymes of tamoxifen (weak estrogenic breast cancer medication— slow metabolizers (*3/*4/*6 or absent in allele *5) show less endoxifen metabolite but increase effectiveness of medication; intermediate metabolizers lead to increased recurrences of breast cancer following treatment; ultra-rapid metabolizers have ↓ 5-year survival times

   g. Ultra-rapid ESR-Xbal/ESR2-02 metabolizers = change cholesterol/triglyceride levels rather than affect cancer outcome

   h. CYP2C8 and CYP2J2 responsible for arachidonic acid → epoxyeicosatrienoic acids; immunosuppressant calcineurin inhibitors increase kidney toxicity via prevention of vasodilation associated with epoxyeicosatrienoic acids

7. Aldehyde dehydrogenase

   a. ALDH2 polymorphisms lead to people who have increased illness due to drinking alcohol (increased acetaldehyde from conversion from alcohol dehydrogenase, ADH1/3, which is not converted at a proper rate to a less toxic metabolite, acetic acid, which can then be utilized as energy by transport into mitochondria by CoA)

   b. Aliphatic aldehydes metabolized by ALDH1B1

   c. ALDH3A1/2 (normal) versus ALDH3A2 (Sjögren-Larsson syndrome)

CONCEPTUALIZING TOXICOLOGY 11-1 (*continued*)

8. Alcohol dehydrogenase

   a. ADH3 metabolizes formaldehyde to a less toxic form

   b. ADH1/2 are known for their ability to convert ethanol and methanol to more toxic forms, while aldehyde dehydrogenase only detoxifies acetaldehyde:

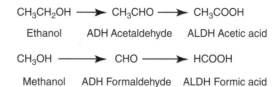

9. DT diaphorase (NQO2) activates antitumor quinones, and polymorphisms make these medications less effective

10. Dihydropyridine dehydrogenase metabolizes the chemotherapy agent 5-fluorouracil, and polymorphisms increase toxicity via lack of metabolism of this toxic agent

11. Uridine-glucuronosyltransferase polymorphisms are responsible for toxicity of mycophenolate mofetil, a solid organ transplantation immunosuppression agent

12. Decreased carbonyl reductase CBR3 11G > A = increased effectiveness and hematologic toxicity of doxorubicin (anthracycline cancer chemotherapeutic agent) and similar effects found with reduction of ABC transporter responsible for doxorubicin efflux. GST-null genotype reduced removal of chemotherapy-induced secondary oxidation products = decreased mortality with doxorubicin, as did gene polymorphism of MnSOD and MPO (increased oxidative stress in cancer cells)

13. Decreased cytidine deaminase = decreased clearance of gemcitabine chemotherapy agent in Japanese patients and increased neutropenia in combination therapy with Pt compounds or fluorouracil. Dihydropyrimidine dehydrogenase deficiencies (DPY*2A) increase fluorouracil toxicity without increasing the efficacy of this cancer chemotherapy agent

14. Steroid 5-α reductase type II (SRDA5A2): testosterone → dihydrotestosterone so SRD5A2 leucine isoform ↑ prostate cancer (including prostate-specific antigen, PSA)

15. Neuroactive metabolizing enzyme polymorphisms

    a. Catechol-O-methyltransferase Met/Val polymorphism associated with smoking cessation

16. Chemical effects on receptors controlling metabolic enzymes

    a. Paraquat and organophosphates affect human applicators' (δ)-aminolevulinic acid dehydratase (ALAD)

    b. Pesticide exposures to people with GSTT1 allele have increased ALA-D and AChE (less affected)

    c. Pesticide exposures to people with paraoxonase (PON1) R allele had lower AChE (opposite to effects noted in 16b)

    d. Pesticide exposures also increased variants of benzoylcholinesterase (BChE) gene

D. Receptor alterations

  1. AH receptor

     a. Rs2158041 and rs781198 associated with lung cancer risk; rs2066853 associated with smoking

     b. 2,3,7,8-TCDD equivalents (TEFs) and AH polymorphisms—see Figure 11-1

  2. Human epidermal growth factor 2 (HER2)—high levels of expression increase breast cancer risk

     a. E2F transcription factor 2 (E2F2), and cyclin D1 and D3 (CCND1 and CCND3) regulate HER2 expression and polymorphisms of these genes result in low expression and less downregulation of HER2

CONCEPTUALIZING TOXICOLOGY 11-1 (*continued*)

3. Estrogen receptor

   a. Polymorphisms rs2234670, rs2234693, rs9340799 associated with endometrial cancer

   b. ER$^+$/PR$^+$ (estrogen/progesterone receptors) stronger link to breast cancer than ER$^-$/PR$^-$

   c. Alpha estrogen receptor (ESR1) 4/5, 5/6, and 6/6 genotypes of GGGA repeat of first intron associated with late onset prostate cancer

4. Androgen receptor

   a. < 17 CAG repeats associated with late-onset prostate cancer

5. Vitamin cofactor receptors

   a. Retinoic acid (vitamin A acid) receptor α (RARA) gene responsible for myeloid cell differentiation associated with acute myeloid leukemia

   b. Vitamin D receptor (VDr) gene *BsmI* polymorphism associated with prostate cancer risk

6. Toll-like receptors (TLRs and immune response) and cytokine receptors

   a. Stevens-Johnson syndrome and toxic epidermal necrosis associated with TLR3 and 2999698T/G, 293248A/A, and 299698T/T genotypes

   b. Type I autoimmune diabetes mellitus and allergic asthma associated with TLR2 rs3804100 T polymorphism

   c. High-affinity IgE receptor associated with asthma

   d. TNF-308 GA/AA genotypes associated with childhood allergic diseases and coupled to pollution by nitrogen oxides and associated genotypes of glutathione-S-transferase P1 gene

7. Neurochemical receptors

   a. β,Gly49 polymorphism associated with norepinephrine and lower heart rate on standing (orthostatic hypotension)

   b. Heart arrhythmias associated with Ca^{2+} and cardiac ryanodine receptor channel (RyR2): autosomal-dominant catecholaminergic polymorphic ventricular tachycardia (CPVT1) or autosomal-recessive form involving calsequestrin gene (CASQ2)

   c. Serotonin (5-HT) and dopamine receptor and effectiveness of antipsychotic clozapine—less effective with 5HT$_{2A}$ gene with tyrosine instead of histidine at position 452, while a cytosine to serine substitution = increased clozapine effectiveness; as dopamine causes psychosis (schizophrenia), clozapine more effective when dopamine D2 receptor has one or two A1 alleles; D4 receptor with the 48-bp variant number tandem repeat polymorphism = effective of many neuroleptic agents such as Thorazine (chlorpromazine)

   d. Behavior

      (1) Adenosine A$_3$ knockout mice = ↑ locomotor activity, less stimulation by caffeine and amphetamine, and perinatal effects of MeHg on movement not found in wild-type mice

   e. Nicotinic cholinergic receptor A subunits (CHRNA) 3 and 5 genes at locus 15q24/15q25.1 associated with lung cancer risk. Those same genes with SNPs for CHRNA 3 (rs1051730) and CHRNA5 (rs16969968) associated with people who extract more nicotine from cigarette smoke and have higher dependence rates. They also have higher internal doses of the carcinogen 4-(methylnitrosamino)-1-(3-pyridyl)-1-butanone that may explain their increased lung cancer risk

8. Target enzymes

   a. Pb inhibits ALAD. People with *ALAD2* allele have increased Pb in blood but less impact on hemoglobin synthesis.

   b. Ethanol-induced cirrhosis of liver more likely in people with blood type A than blood type O. Transferrin C2 (*TF*C2* allele) frequency twice as high in cirrhosis than controls. Lower concentrations of proteinase inhibitors were also associated with cirrhotic liver cells. *GST1*0* and *2* associated with cirrhosis. Acid phosphatase locus *ACP1*C*, phosphoglucomutase locus 1 alleles *PGM1*1+*, *PGM1*1−*, *PGM1*2−* also had different frequencies associated with toxic cirrhosis

CONCEPTUALIZING TOXICOLOGY 11-1 (*continued*)

Selective Toxicity

In any biologically diverse population of animals, responses of certain animals or cells that express the genetic information differently show hypersensitivity or hyposensitivity that are significantly different from the median. Differences in the absorption of toxicants, their metabolism, and their receptor binding properties and activities that all have genetic links. As of May 12, 2015, the consensus coding sequence (CCDS) project of the GRCh38 reference genome has identified 31,371 CCDS IDs corresponding to 18,826 GeneIDs (National Center for Biotechnology Information, 2015a). Single gene polymorphisms in build 144 of the National Center for Biotechnology Information (2015b) show 9 organisms representing 537,677,189 submissions that have been reduced to 299,442,638 reference single nucleotide polymorphisms (SNPs) of which 102,899,581 have been validated. This might appear to be an overwhelming number of possible genetic variations that could lead to changes in the sensitivity to toxicants, but recognize that many of the polymorphisms are located between genes and appear to have little or no functional significance (Ingelman-Sundberg, 2001). The changes in toxicant transporters and metabolic enzymes that lead to changes in either the pharmacokinetics/toxicokinetics or pharmacodynamics/toxicodynamics may be termed *pharmacogenetics* or alternatively *toxicogenetics*. This is especially of interest to those researchers interested in cancer chemotherapy (Tan et al., 2008). There is an entire journal dedicated to this area titled *Pharmacogenetics and Genomics*.

Absorption and Elimination Differences

Absorption and elimination alterations due to genetic variability combined with metabolism represent the toxicokinetics portion of toxicogenetics. One example of the cellular absorption/elimination profile of chemical translocation is the expression of ABC transporters and multidrug resistance of cancer cells. In this example, the use of chemosensitizers that inhibit these transport proteins are sought to selectively treat cancer cells with chemotherapeutic toxicants while having low intrinsic toxicity to normal cells (Wu et al., 2008). A family of ABC transporters is the ABCG2, including ABCP, BCRP, and MXR. These transporters affect the absorption, distribution, and excretion of a number of medications and toxicants as this subfamily is highly expressed in the cells of the gastrointestinal tract and hepatocytes. The Q141K polymorphism increases the likelihood that the antitumor medication gefitinib will lead to diarrhea and changes the pharmacokinetics of other medications such as 9-aminocamptothecin, diflomotecan, irinotecan, rosuvastatin, sulfasalazine, and topotecan. This transporter does not always yield clear results as indicated by the data for important medications that have defined toxicity such as the anthracycline doxorubicin and a number of others including imatinib, nelfinavir, and pitavastatin (Cusatis and Sparreboom, 2008). Similarly, the organic anion transporting polypeptide 1B1 (OATP1B1) located on the sinusoidal membrane of human liver cells has polymorphisms on the solute carrier organic anion transporter family member 1B1 (SLCO1B1) gene that encodes for OATP1B1. This transporter is of importance to hepatic cells for compounds such as the statins, which are medications that are used to treat elevated cholesterol in humans via inhibition of HMGCoA reductase. These medications are known to cause liver damage and are monitored for toxicity through the increase in liver enzymes in the plasma. People with the normal homozygous genotype of the SLCO1B1 gene (c.521TT) had lower maximum plasma concentrations (C_{max}) of the metabolite (simvastatin acid) of a statin medication than those people possessing the c.521CC genotype and a later peak time than those having the c.521CC and c.521TC genotypes. This is important for threshold toxicity. Additionally, the area under the curve ($AUC_{0-\infty}$), which represents the toxicity of compounds that have not passed through a toxic threshold concentration, is lower in controls than c.521CC genotype individuals (Pasanen et al., 2006). Conversely, an SNP of the ABCC2 encoding for the multidrug resistance–associated protein 2 (MRP2) known as c.1446C>G leads to reduced systemic exposure to another statin (pravastatin). These findings would predict hypersensitivity for liver cell toxicity for those individuals expressing variants of the OATP1B1 protein and hyposensitivity and reduced efficacy for humans expressing specific alterations in the MRP2 protein (Niemi et al., 2006). An important relevant example of differences between species in kidney cell secretion of organic acids is the dog's increased toxicity response to the widely employed phenoxyacetic acid herbicide 2,4-dichlorophenoxyacetic acid (2,4-D) (Timchalk, 2004).

Other transporters may not directly affect the concentration of a toxicant in the cell, but instead predict the effect of toxicants on neurochemicals in synaptic neurotransmission. One such report is the polymorphisms expressed by Tanzanians expressing multiple copies of the SLC6A1 gene responsible for expressing the sodium-dependent and chloride-dependent [gamma]-aminobutyric acid (GABA) transporter. This insertion of promoter activity yields less to medications that inhibit this transporter and the toxicity that can result from excessive inhibition (Hirunsatit et al., 2009). In a similar manner, humans with the LA/LA genotype of 5-hydroxytryptamine (serotonin) transporters (5-HTTLPR) are the only ones that respond clinically to occupancy of these transporters by selective serotonin reuptake inhibitors (SSRIs) with clinical improvement for major depression (Ruhé et al., 2009). Certain channels may also predispose certain organisms to damage cells and organs via changes in blood pressure. The acid-sensing ion channel 3 (ASIC3) is a ligand-gated ion channel that is activated by extracellular protons. Polymorphisms in this channel in Taiwanese are related to hypertension (Ko et al., 2008). From this analysis it can be observed that changes in transport of toxicants can not only be altered by genetic differences in proteins that transport those toxicants, but they can also alter the electrical and/or neurochemical milieu of the cell, tissue, and whole organism.

Metabolism/CYP Polymorphisms

Genetic variations in metabolism are the major factors underlying the ethnic variations in responses to medications and toxicants. This is

also the reason certain mutated cell populations respond differently or selectively to medications and toxicants. This arena is especially important in cancer chemotherapy. Both metabolic enzymes and transporters may be different and therefore enhance the resistance or sensitivity of a cell population to a given toxicant. There are more metabolic polymorphisms that affect human populations than those that modify the expression of oncogenes. Health problems associated with expression of these genes stress the importance of this area of toxicogenetics. The cytochrome P450 CYP1A1 alleles and, more importantly, the *2C I462 allele have been associated with cancers of the aerodigestive tract. This is more prominent when the conjugation enzyme encoded by the glutathione transferase GSTM gene is not expressed, as is the case for the null allele. Smoking-related head-and-neck squamous cell cancer appears to be related to the CYP1B1 codon 432 polymorphism (CYP1B1*3). This is an oversimplification, because head-and-neck cancers are also related to tobacco smoke, lifestyle, oncogenous viral infections, and other genetic factors including glutathione transferases (GSTM1, GSTT1, GSTP1), tumor suppressor mutations (ATM, BRCA1, RB1, TP53), DNA repair genes polymorphisms (OGG1, RAD51, XPD, XRCC1), and mitochondrial DNA mutations (Rusin et al., 2008). CYP2E1 polymorphisms appear to be related to environmental or industrial toxicant exposures. Changes in acetylation status via NAT2 appear to be associated with bladder cancers of workers exposed to aromatic amines such as 4-aminodiphenyl, benzidine, or 1-naphthylamine. Polymorphisms of GSTM1 have also been associated with bladder cancers and may point to the polycyclic aromatic hydrocarbons as the source of the cancer (Thier et al., 2003). Increased carcinogen activation appears to occur primarily through polymorphisms of the cytochrome P450 isozymes CYP1A1, CYP1A2, CYP1B1, CYP2A6, CYP2E1, and CYP3A4. Medications are inactivated and rapid versus slow metabolizers that are characterized through cytochrome P450 isozymes CYP1A2, CYP2A6, CYP2B6, CYP2C8, CYP2C9, CYP2C19, CYP2D6, CYP2E1, CYP3A4, and CYP3A5. CYP2C19 slow metabolizers are more prone to have effective treatment by proton pump inhibitors (PPIs) used for ulcers caused by *Helicobacter pylori* and also affect the treatment of gastroesophageal reflux disease (GERD), reflux esophagitis, and duodenal ulcers (Chaudhry et al., 2008). For the Caucasian population, the poor metabolizers include a number of likely CYP polymorphisms. The CYP2A6 isozyme that metabolizes endogenous steroids and fatty acids, the hepatocarcinogen aflatoxin B1, anticoagulant coumarins, chemotherapeutic alkylating agents cyclophosphamide and ifosfamide, nicotine, and carcinogenic nitrosamines has a homozygous *CYP2A6*4* genotype that has a deletion in the gene sequence that causes a truncation in the polypeptide chain and an inactive protein. The CYP2B6 isozyme that metabolizes endogenous steroids and fatty acids, the antidepressant seizure-producing bupropion, cyclophosphamide, ifosfamide, and an opioid methadone has a homozygous genotype *CYP2B6*5* that forms the CYP2B6.5 isoform with much lower activity for these substrates. The CYP2C9 isoform that metabolizes endogenous (R)/(S) limonene; the antidepressant amitriptyline; the anti-inflammatory COX2 inhibitor celecoxib; the anti-leprosy topical antibacterial dapsone; the nonsteroidal anti-inflammatory drugs (NSAIDs) diclofenac, ibuprofen, lornoxicam, meloxicam, (S)-naproxen, piroxicam, and suprofen (topical); the anticoagulants dicoumarol and (S)-warfarin; the antidepressant SSRIs and CYP2C19 inhibitors fluoxetine and paroxetine; the cholesterol-lowering fluvastatin and pitavastatin; the anti-diabetic sulfonylureas glibenclamide, glimepiride, glipizide, and tolbutamide; the antihypertensive angiotensin II receptor blockers irbesartan and losartan; the anticonvulsant mephenytoin; the barbiturate and CYP2A6, CYP2B6, CYP2C8, CYP2C9, CYP2C19, CYP3A4, CYP3A5, CYP3A7, and CYP3A43 inducer phenobarbital; the thiazolidinedione antidiabetic rosiglitazone (increases congestive heart failure); the breast cancer medication tamoxifen; the loop diuretic torsemide; and the antiretroviral zidovudine has homozygous or heterozygous genotypes *CYP2C9*2* and *CYP2C9*3* that have much reduced activity. A splicing error causes the formation of the homozygous *CYP2C19*2A* genotype that is expressed as an inactive protein toward the normal CYP2C19 substrates that include

endogenous (R)/(S) limonene; amitriptyline; the centrally activating muscle relaxant carisoprodol; the antidepressant SSRIs citalopram, cyclophosphamide, benzodiazepine diazepam, and temazepam; the barbiturates hexobarbital, mephobarbital, and phenobarbital; the tricyclic antidepressants clomipramine and imipramine; the NSAID indomethacin; the proton-pump inhibitors anti-ulcer lansoprazole, omeprazole, pantoprazole, and rabeprazole; the anticonvulsants mephenytoin, phenytoin, primidone, and valproic acid; the MAO-inhibiting antidepressant moclobemide; the antiretroviral nelfinavir; the antiandrogen prostate cancer medication nilutamide; progesterone; antimalarial proguanil; beta-blocking anti-hypertensive propanolol; cytotoxic anticancer teniposide; (R)-warfarin; and zidovudine. Homozygous and heterozygous genotypes of alleles *CYP2D6*4A*, *CYP2D6*4B*, *CYP2D6*4C*, *CYP2D6*4D*, *CYP2D6*4E*, *CYP2D6*4F*, *CYP2D6*4G*, *CYP2D6*4H*, *CYP2D6*4J*, *CYP2D6*4K*, *CYP2D6*4L*, *CYP2D6*4M*, *CYP2D6*4N*, and *CYP2D6*4X2* lead to inactive proteins toward CYP2D6 substrates such as endogenous steroids; the beta-blockers alprenolol, bufuralol, carvedilol, (S)-metoprolol, nebivolol, propranolol, and timolol; adrenergic stimulants amphetamine, methoxyamphetamine, and 3,4 methylenedioxymethamphetamine (MDMA or ecstasy); amitriptyline; antipsychotics aripiprazole, chlorpromazine, haloperidol, perphenazine, promazine, risperidone, thioridazine, and zuclopenthixol; presynaptic norepinephrine transport inhibitor for attention-deficit disorder atomoxetine; antihistamines chlorpheniramine, doxylamine, and promethazine; tricyclic antidepressants clomipramine, desipramine, imipramine, and nortriptyline; opiates codeine, hydrocodone, oxycodone, and tramadol; metabolic marker for bladder (Benítez et al., 1990) and lung (Speirs et al., 1990) cancer debrisoquine; serotonin reuptake inhibitor, releasing agent, anti-obesity agent that caused pulmonary hypertension due to a nitric oxide deficiency (Archer et al., 1998) dexfenfluramine; anti-tussive dextromethorphan; selective serotonin and norepinephrine reuptake inhibitors duloxetine and venlafaxine; antiarrhythmics encainide, flecainide, mexiletine, and propafenone; SSRIs fluvoxamine and paroxetine; general anesthetic halothane; local anesthetic lidocaine; prokinetic antiemetics metoclopramide and ondansetron; tetracyclic antidepressant mianserin; antidepressant minaprine; PPI omeprazole; tricyclic anxiolytic opipramol; anti-anginal with neurotoxicity and hepatotoxicity perhexiline; analgesic phenacetin; antidiabetic causing fatal lactic acidosis phenformin; MAO-B inhibiting anti-Parkinson selegiline; oxytocic sparteine; tamoxifen; vinca alkaloid anti-tumor vincristine; and classic substrate for various CYPs 7-ethoxycoumarin (Waxman and Chang, 1998). Ultra-rapid metabolizers in Caucasians primarily have the phenotype *CYP2D6*2XN* whose substrates have just been described (Tomaszewski et al., 2008a, 2008b). Estrogens that feature prominently in breast and ovarian cancers are associated with metabolism via CYP1B1. Nicotine from cigarette smoke has varied metabolic rates determined by polymorphisms of the gene that encodes for the CYP2A6 isozyme.

Alcoholism and the ability to drink without illness are altered by polymorphisms of the aldehyde dehydrogenase ALDH1 gene, which produces the protein that metabolizes acetaldehyde. ALDH1A1 also plays a role in acetaldehyde and retinal metabolism. Aliphatic aldehydes are altered by ALDH1B1. Fatty and aromatic aldehydes depend on the normal expression of ALDH3A1/2 with the ALDH3A2 polymorphism leading to Sjögren-Larsson syndrome. Ethanol metabolism to acetaldehyde depends on two alcohol dehydrogenases (ADH1 and ADH3). ADH3 also metabolizes formaldehyde. DT-diaphorase (NQO2) activates the antitumor quinones, and, conversely, the enzyme dihydropyridine dehydrogenase polymorphism can lead to toxicity of unmetabolized 5-fluorouracil (Ingelman-Sundberg, 2001). Conjugation enzymes such as the uridine-glucuronosyltransferase (UGT) family have been found to be responsible for bioavailability of mycophenolic acid, the active metabolite of mycophenolate mofetil (MMF). MMF is used as an immunosuppressant in solid organ transplantation and its toxic side effects may be related to polymorphisms of the gene expressing this enzyme (Betonico et al., 2008).

What follows is a more thorough examination of the cancer chemotherapy agents and more specifically those used in the treatment of breast cancer cells. A medication that showed great promise in treating primary breast tumors was an intercalating chemical that inhibited topoisomerase II, amonafide. NAT2 polymorphisms caused varied acetylation rates. This was coupled to ethnic clearance differences and unpredictable toxicities that have prevented this from developing into a major antitumor medication. Tamoxifen is a weak estrogen that is used to shrink breast tumors. Cytochrome P450 isozymes metabolize approximately 90% of tamoxifen to *N*-desmethyl-tamoxifen (CYP3A4/5), and a much smaller portion to 4-hydroxy-tamoxifen (CYP2D6). Both metabolites are converted by CYP3A4/5 to endoxifen (4-hydroxy-*N*-desmethyl-tamoxifen). The 4-hydroxy metabolites of tamoxifen are all active. Sulfotransferases and UDP-glucuronosyl transferases conjugate and inactivate the metabolites of tamoxifen. Poor metabolizers show nonfunctional CYP2D6*3/*4/*6 or absent enzyme in *5 alleles that decrease the endoxifen metabolite. In this study, intermediate metabolizers had reduced CYP2D6*10/*17/*41 isozymes that many times lead to increased recurrences after tamoxifen treatment (Brauch et al., 2008). Ultra-rapid metabolizers had either increased WYP2D6*2xn or reduced CYP3A4*1B and CYP3A5*3, reduced conjugation enzymes of the sulfotransferase SULT1A1*2 or UDP glucuronosyltransferase UDT1A4 Leu[48]Val, or increased UGT2B15*2. Many of these variants had decreased 5-year survival times compared with normal metabolizers.

Another ultrametabolizer polymorphism is represented by the ESR-XbaI/ESR2-02 genotypes. These change cholesterol/triglyceride levels respectively in women with these genotypes, rather than alter the cancer outcome. The effectiveness of aromatase inhibitors is altered by polymorphisms of the CYP19A1 gene, because this is the gene that encodes for the aromatase isozyme of cytochrome P450. The anthracyclines as represented by doxorubicin can have decreased metabolism and increased effectiveness with hematologic toxicity with carbonyl reductase CBR3 11G>A or increased metabolism with CBR3 730G>A. This is the first step in reducing these chemotherapeutic agents, which can also be performed by aldo-keto reductases. Interestingly, the reduction of the

ABC cassette transporter ABCa 3435C>T, which decreases expression and function of P-glycoprotein (elimination category), made the anthracyclines more effective agents against breast tumors as these proteins mediate the efflux of doxorubicin. Anthracyclines are inactivated by CYPs. In this case, the lack of conjugation by GST null genotype, which causes reduced removal of chemotherapy-induced secondary oxidation products, showed decreased mortality with chemotherapy. This would be expected if cancer cells resulted in more rapid mortality than heart damage from the oxidative products. Alterations in enzymes that are involved in oxidative stress such as manganese superoxide dismutase (MnSOD CC) and myeloperoxidase (MPO GG) due to gene polymorphisms similarly decreased mortalities in anthracycline-treated patients. Oxidative stress may generate mitochondrial damage that can cause most of the idiosyncratic hepatotoxicity, as opposed to the predictable liver injury caused by compounds similar to acetaminophen. A heterozygous superoxide dismutase–deficient mouse model (SOD2$^{+/-}$) screens for these type of agents, which depend on the genetics polymorphisms of the person. This mouse model shows no apparent toxicity of the NSAID nimesulide given for 4 weeks to a wild-type mouse but yields unmistakable mitochondrial liver damage in the SOD-deficient mouse. Conclusive liver necrotic damage resulted from giving the insulin sensitizer and antidiabetic drug troglitazone to SOD-deficient but not wild-type mice. This was a two-phase toxicity with an adaptive response for 2 weeks followed by overt toxicity. Pharmacokinetics was not responsible, as both wild-type and SOD-deficient mice had the same toxic concentration profile over time in the target cells (Boelsterli and Hsiao, 2008). Thus, cellular or animal models may predict genetic predispositions to toxicity.

Another chemotherapy agent against breast cancer, gemcitabine, is transported into the cells via nucleoside transporters SLC28/29. The compound is then phosphorylated/activated by deoxycytidine kinase. It is incorporated into DNA following phosphorylation to its triphosphate form by nucleoside triphosphate where gemcitabine inhibits repair enzymes thymidylate synthase and ribonucleoside reductases.

Ribonucleotide reductases RRM1 −37/−524T polymorphisms showed better tumor lethality with a combination of gemcitabine and carboplatin. A decrease in the inactivating enzyme cytidine deaminase CDA*3 (208G>A) polymorphism in Japanese cancer patients decreased clearance of gemcitabine and increased neutropenia when administered together with platinum compounds or 5-fluorouracil. Dihydropyrimidine dehydrogenase deficiencies caused by DPY*2A are found to increase the toxicity of 5-fluorouracil alone or in combination with other agents, but do not increase the efficacy toward killing the cancer cells (Tan et al., 2008). A secondary way that metabolism can play a role in toxicity is the neurochemical changes it can cause externally or in neural cells, especially those associated with mechanisms involved in dependence and addictive behavior. A catechol-O-methyltransferase Met/Val functional polymorphism appears to be associated with smoking cessation (Omidvar et al., 2009) but not with schizophrenia (Fan et al., 2005). Another way of increasing the toxicity of a substance is the prevention of formation of protective cellular factors. CYP 2C8 and CYP 2J2 isozymes convert arachidonic acid to epoxyeicosatrienoic acids that promote kidney function. Calcineurin inhibitors cyclosporine A and tacrolimus block transplanted organ rejection by prevention of activation of the T cell, but cause significant kidney toxicity. This toxicity is augmented by kidney cells containing at least one CYP2C8*3 allele, which does not allow formation of the vasodilatory epoxyeicosatrienoic acids (Smith, Jones et al., 2008). It is apparent that genes involved in xenobiotic metabolism are the focus of most pharmacogenetic investigation, but it is clear to some researchers that multi-candidate gene-association and genome-wide analyses are possible. However, the pharmaceutical industry would need to partner with academia due to the lack of published pharmacogenetic data used in the development of medications that also bear on toxicant responses (Roses, 2008).

Receptor Interaction Alterations

Because the AH receptor plays such a large role in CYPs and cancer risk from exposure to cigarette smoke, it is important to examine polymorphisms of this receptor first. In a Chinese population sampling 500 lung cancer patients and 517 cancer-free controls, eight SNPs were examined with regard to lung cancer risk. Heterozygous genotypes rs2158041 and rs7811989 were associated with lung cancer risk and were in linkage disequilibrium. Haplotype analysis revealed a statistically significant interaction between smoking and the polymorphism rs2066853 (p.Arg554Lys). Heavy smoking was necessary to show a statistically significant association between the Lys/Lys genotype and lung cancer risk (Chen et al., 2009). It appears that the degree of risk depends on the specific

polymorphism and how that difference causes the expression of a protein receptor that is more sensitive to the effects of polycyclic aromatic hydrocarbons, dioxins, polychlorinated biphenyls, and similar agents (TEFs, or toxic equivalency factors—evaluation based on potency compared to 2,3,7,8-tetrachlorodibenzodioxin; Van den Berg et al., 1998). The interaction of the AH receptor along with polymorphisms in other associated gene products is shown in **Figure 11-1**. Note that the entire signaling pathway depends on the AH receptor and the complex it forms. Polymorphisms in receptors for other signaling proteins downstream from

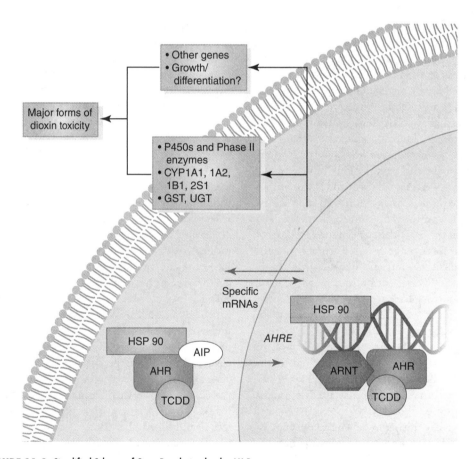

FIGURE 11-1 Simplified Scheme of Gene Regulation by the AH Receptor

Note: Ligands (exemplified by TCDD) bind to the AHR in cytoplasm where the receptor resides chaperoned by hsp90 and other receptor-interacting proteins (AIP). Ligand binding triggers translocation of the AHR into the cell nucleus, dissociation from chaperone proteins and dimerization with the ARNT protein. The ligand•AHR•ARNT complex binds to specific regulatory elements (AHREs) found in the 5'-flanking region of numerous genes. When occupied by the liganded AHR complex, AHREs act as transcriptional enhancers to increase the rate of production of mRNA. The AHR also can suppress transcription of some genes. Induction of Phase I and Phase II drug-metabolizing enzymes has its own consequences for the cell and organism, but induction of these enzymes is not required to produce the major classical manifestations of dioxin toxicity in rats.

the initial signal can also lead to different toxic outcomes. Breast cancer prognosis appears poor for those people expressing high levels of human epidermal growth factor receptor 2 (HER2). Regulators of HER2 expression E2F transcription factor 2 (E2F2), cyclin D1 (CCND1), and cyclin D3 (CCND3) have polymorphisms that result in low expression. This low expression of these regulators results in less downregulation of HER2 (Justenhoven et al., 2008). The estrogen receptor is also an important factor in endometrial cancers. Polymorphisms of the estrogen receptor alpha gene that are markers in strong linkage disequilibrium and associated with endometrial cancer are rs2234670, rs2234693, and rs9340799 (Wedrén et al., 2008). Estrogen (ER) and progesterone (PR) receptor status is linked to breast cancer through circulating levels of these hormones, where ER^+/PR^+ has a stronger association than ER^-/PR^- (Chen, 2008). The androgen and estrogen receptors are both linked to prostate cancer. The alpha estrogen receptor (ESR1) has 4/5, 5/6, and 6/6 genotypes of the GGGA repeat in the first intron that are associated with late onset prostate cancer. The androgen receptor gene (AR) with less than 17 CAG repeats is also associated with late-onset prostate cancer (Nicolaiew et al., 2009). Another factor is the irreversible metabolism of testosterone to dihydrotestosterone by the steroid 5-alpha reductase type II (SRD5A2) in male reproductive organ cells. Because testosterone is the relevant hormone associated with prostate cancer risk, polymorphisms of the converting enzyme play an important role in risk assessment. The SRD5A2 leucine isoform acts in a dose-dependent manner to predict a more severe case of prostate cancer as indicated by prostate-specific antigen (PSA) protease expression, clinical staging, and Gleason score (low differentiation indicates more malignant cells) when compared with men having the more common SRD5A2 valine variant (Scariano et al., 2008). However, the PSA gene polymorphism as determined by androgen response elements in the promoter region of PSA gene (PSA-158 G/A, rs266882) does not lead to total or free PSA level differences. There is also no interaction between the PSA SNP, AR CAG repeats, and prostate cancer (Jesser et al., 2008).

Other receptors more associated with the immune response, such as the Toll-like receptors, can mediate reactions both to infectious agents and to toxic responses to medications. SNPs of a Japanese population 299698T/G and the genotype patterns of 293248A/A and 299698T/T in Toll-like receptor (TLR) 3 exhibit a strong association with Stevens-Johnson syndrome and toxic epidermal necrolysis (Ueta et al., 2007). These represent a specific type of allergic reactions that indicate a sensitivity that can lead to the death of dermal cells. Similarly, type I diabetes mellitus and allergic asthma appear to be related to a TLR2 rs3804100 T polymorphism (Bjørnvold et al., 2009). In earlier studies, linkage of asthma to a number of other physiological receptors such as the beta-2 adrenergic receptor and its G protein that mediate bronchiole dilation (Wang et al., 2008) and the high affinity receptor for IgE have been associated with asthmatic response (Sanak et al., 2007). A class of toxicants in air pollution, the nitrogen oxides (NOx), appears to interact with the Ile105Val/Val105Val genotypes, which are SNPs of the glutathione S-transferase P1 gene. They result in childhood allergic diseases that are enhanced if the children also have the cytokine tumor necrosis factor (TNF)-308 GA/AA genotypes (Melén et al., 2008). Other cytokines, their functions, and their polymorphisms have been discussed in detail (Smith and Humphries, 2008).

Changes in neurochemical receptors also influence the neurotoxicity or other physiological responses. For example, idiopathic orthostatic intolerance, which results in extended low blood pressure on standing with increased heart rate and plasma norepinephrine concentrations, is protected by a β_1Gly49 polymorphism that is associated with a lower heart rate in the standing position (Winker et al., 2005). Some important cardiac arrhythmias involve factors that affect Ca homeostasis. The cardiac ryanodine receptor channel (RyR2) gene has an autosomal-dominant catecholaminergic polymorphic ventricular tachycardia form (CPVT1), while an autosomal-recessive form (CPVT2) appears to be associated with a polymorphism of the cardiac calsequestrin gene (CASQ2; Katz et al., 2009). Brain cells and regions have neurochemical receptor densities that may be associated with mental illness and treatment by psychoactive agents. Schizophrenia may be treated with agents that affect dopamine (decrease) or serotonin (increase) concentrations. One agent that works to treat the disease at these levels is the antipsychotic clozapine. Clozapine is less effective when the serotonin 5-HT$_{2A}$ receptor gene has expressed tyrosine instead of histidine at position 452 and has a homozygous cytosine allele at position 102. Conversely, a cysteine to serine substitution at position 23 expressed by the 5-HT(2C) gene improves clozapine effectiveness. One or two A1 alleles for the dopamine D2 receptor that is most associated with the development of schizophrenic symptoms results in better treatment results when antagonized by clozapine compared with those with no A1 allele (Taq1A genotype). Alternatively, a Del allele at position 141 of D2 resulted in a worse response to the antipsychotic medication. A homozygous serine/serine at position 9 of the expressed D3 receptor was associated with patients who did not respond to clozapine treatment. For the D4 receptor, the 48-bp variant number tandem repeat polymorphism appears to be associated with effectiveness of neuroleptics. Certain receptors are not generally considered neurochemical but have influences on behavior. The adenosine A$_3$ knockout mice show higher locomotor activity than that of control mice. They show less stimulation by caffeine and amphetamine. They also show perinatal effects of methylmercury on movement, which was not found in wild-type mice with an intact A$_3$ receptor (Björklund et al., 2008). This indicates interactions of receptor polymorphisms with toxicants on behavioral responses. Sprayers of the pro-oxidant herbicide Paraquat and insecticide acetylcholinesterase (AChE)-inhibiting organophosphates show effects on the erythrocyte delta (δ)-aminolevulinic acid dehydratase (ALA-D). Polymorphisms of the metabolic enzyme glutathione S-transferase GSTT1 null allele were associated with higher (less affected) ALA-D and AChE at periods of high exposure to pesticides. Conversely, the paraoxonase (PON1) R allele indicated increased impact (lower AChE) at low exposure to pesticides. Sprayers were less likely to have higher impact variants of the benzoylcholinesterase (BChE)

gene that expresses the enzyme that metabolizes acetylcholinesterase-inhibiting compounds than the general population (Hernández et al., 2005). Certain neurochemical receptor polymorphisms not only indicate susceptibility to toxicants at the behavioral level, but also predict cancer risk. The nicotinic (mainly CNS and peripheral motor) acetylcholine receptor A subunits 3 and 5 (CHRNA3 and CHRNA5) genes located at locus 15q24/15q25.1 are associated with lung cancer risk. It was discovered that CHRNA3 (rs1051730) and CHRNA5 (rs16969968) polymorphisms result in people who extract a higher amount of nicotine from cigarette smoke and have higher dependence rates. These polymorphisms also yield a higher internal dose of the carcinogen 4-(methylnitrosamino)-1-(3-pyridyl)-1-butanone that likely causes the increased risk of lung cancer (Le Marchand et al., 2008).

One form of receptor can be a target enzyme. Lead is known to be another toxicant that inhibits its δ-aminolevulinic acid dehydratase (ALAD), an enzyme with two co-dominantly expressed alleles, ALAD1 and ALAD2. People with the ALAD2 allele exhibited higher concentrations of lead in their blood and less impact on hemoglobin synthesis as indicated by higher hemoglobin concentrations and lower levels of zinc protoporphyrin, a factor inversely related to lead concentrations in the blood (Scinicariello et al., 2007). In this case, heavy metal poisoning is decreased by a polymorphism in the target gene product. In alcoholic toxic cirrhosis, a number of polymorphisms appear to be associated with this hepatic damage. People expressing the A type blood type (ABO*A allele) were more likely to have cirrhosis than the O type blood type (ABO*0 allele) were. Transferrin C2 (TF*C2 allele) frequency was twice as high in cirrhosis patients as controls. Lower concentrations of proteinase inhibitors as expressed by people with the PI*Z and PI*S alleles were more common in people with cirrhotic liver cells. Glutathione-S-transferase GST1*0 and GST1*2 alleles were more associated with cirrhosis. The acid phosphatase locus ACP1*C, phosphoglucomutase locus 1 alleles PGM1*1+, PGM1*1−, and PGM1*2− are also expressed at different frequencies in those people exhibiting the signs of toxic cirrhosis (Spitsyn et al., 2001). It may be easier to see how changes in alcohol dehydrogenase or aldehyde dehydrogenase may be important in the metabolism and therefore toxicity of ethanol. It is not always obvious how certain genetic associations may lead to the response to the toxic species of the chemical agent.

Alterations in the retinoic acid receptor alpha (RARA) are associated with the development of acute myeloid leukemia. This receptor protein plays a key role in myeloid differentiation (Parrado et al., 1999). There is a linkage between the vitamin D receptor (VDR) gene *Bsm*I polymorphism and the risk of prostate cancer, where the homozygous "bb" genotype carried a twofold higher risk of developing cancer for men under 72 years of age than the "BB" and heterozygous "Bb" genotypes (Huang et al., 2004). This indicates a linkage between nutrition, genetics, and toxicity.

Questions

1. Why is transport out of the cell as important as into the cell for toxicity? Give an example.
2. Why are the polymorphisms of certain CYPs related to carcinogen activation, while others are related to medication inactivation?
3. For which compound—acetaldehyde (metabolite of ethanol via alcohol dehydrogenase) or formaldehyde (metabolite of methanol via alcohol dehydrogenase)— is aldehyde dehydrogenase lowered activity more problematic in people with that polymorphism?
4. Why would CYP2D6 allele polymorphisms affect tamoxifen effectiveness in breast cancer patients?
5. Is the AH receptor's toxicity due to dioxin binding necessarily associated in rodents with the induction of CYPs (see Figure 11-1)?
6. It is easy to see how increased receptor action as with hormone receptors can lead to cancer, but how can the lack of a receptor sensitize animals to a toxicant? Give an example.
7. Explain Pb and ethanol toxicity in relationship to selective toxicity by genetic predisposition.

References

Archer SL, Djaballah K, Humbert M, Weir KE, Fartoukh M, Dall'ava-Santucci J, Mercier JC, Simonneau G, Dinh-Xuan AT. 1998. Nitric oxide deficiency in fenfluramine- and dexfenfluramine-induced pulmonary hypertension. *Am J Respir Crit Care Med*. 158:1061–1067.

Benítez J, Ladero JM, Fernández-Gundín MJ, Llerena A, Cobaleda J, Martínez C, Muñoz JJ, Vargas E, Prados J, González-Rozas F. 1990. Polymorphic oxidation of debrisoquine in bladder cancer. *Ann Med*. 22:157–160.

Betonico GN, Abudd-Filho M, Goloni-Bertollo EM, Pavarino-Bertelli E. 2008. Pharmacogenetics of mycophenolate mofetil: a promising different approach to tailoring immunosuppression? *J Nephrol*. 21:503–509.

Björklund O, Halldner-Henriksson L, Yang J, Eriksson TM, Jacobson MA, Daré E, Fredholm BB. 2008. Decreased behavioral activation following caffeine, amphetamine and darkness in A(3) adenosine receptor knock-out mice. *Physiol Behav*. 95:668–676.

Bjørnvold M, Munthe-Kaas MC, Egeland T, Joner G, Dahl-Jørgensen K, Njølstad PR, Akselsen HE, Gervin K, Carlsen KC, Carlsen KH, Undlien DE. 2009. A TLR2 polymorphism is associated with type 1 diabetes and allergic asthma. *Genes Immun*. 10(2):181–187.

Boelsterli UA, Hsiao CJ. 2008. The heterozygous Sod2(+/−) mouse: modeling the mitochondrial role in drug toxicity. *Drug Discov Today*. 13:982–988.

Brauch H, Schroth W, Eichelbaum M, Schwab M, Harbeck N; in cooperation with the AGO TRAFO Comission. 2008. Clinical relevance of CYP2D6 genetics for tamoxifen response in breast cancer. *Breast Care (Basel)*. 3:43–50.

Chaudhry AS, Kochhar R, Kohli KK. 2008. Genetic polymorphism of CYP2C19 and therapeutic response to proton pump inhibitors. *Indian J Med Res*. 127:521–530.

Chen D, Tian T, Wang H, Liu H, Hu Z, Wang Y, Liu Y, Ma H, Fan W, Miao R, Sun W, Wang Y, Qian J, Jin L, Wei Q, Shen H, Huang W, Lu D. 2009. Association of human aryl hydrocarbon receptor gene polymorphisms with risk of lung cancer among cigarette smokers in a Chinese population. *Pharmacogenet Genomics*. 19:25–34.

Chen WY. 2008. Exogenous and endogenous hormones and breast cancer. *Best Pract Res Clin Endocrinol Metab*. 22:573–585.

Cusatis G, Sparreboom A. 2008. Pharmacogenomic importance of ABCG2. *Pharmacogenomics*. 9:1005–1009.

Fan JB, Zhang CS, Gu NF, Li XW, Sun WW, Wang HY, Feng GY, St Clair D, He L. 2005. Catechol-O-methyltransferase gene Val/Met functional polymorphism and risk of schizophrenia: a largescale association study plus meta-analysis. *Biol Psychiatry.* 57:139–144.

Hirunsatit R, George ED, Lipska BK, Elwafi HM, Sander L, Yrigollen CM, Gelernter J, Grigorenko EL, Lappalainen J, Mane S, Nairn AC, Kleinman JE, Simen AA. 2009. Twenty-one-base-pair insertion polymorphism creates an enhancer element and potentiates SLC6A1 GABA transporter promoter activity. *Pharmacogenet Genomics.* 19:53–65.

Hernández AF, López O, Rodrigo L, Gil F, Pena G, Serrano JL, Parrón T, Alvarez JC, Lorente JA, Pla A. 2005. Changes in erythrocyte enzymes in humans long-term exposed to pesticides: influence of several markers of individual susceptibility. *Toxicol Lett.* 159:13–21.

Huang SP, Chou YH, Wayne Chang WS, Wu MT, Chen YY, Yu CC, Wu TT, Lee YH, Huang JK, Wu WJ, Huang CH. 2004. Association between vitamin D receptor polymorphisms and prostate cancer risk in a Taiwanese population. *Cancer Lett.* 207:69–77.

Ingelman-Sundberg M. 2001. Genetic variability in susceptibility and response to toxicants. *Toxicol Lett.* 120:259–268.

Jesser C, Mucci L, Farmer D, Moon C, Li H, Gaziano JM, Stampfer M, Ma J, Kantoff P. 2008. Effects of G/A polymorphism, rs266882, in the androgen response element 1 of the PSA gene on prostate cancer risk, survival and circulating PSA levels. *Br J Cancer.* 99:1743–1747.

Justenhoven C, Pierl CB, Haas S, Fischer HP, Hamann U, Baisch C, Harth V, Spickenheuer A, Rabstein S, Vollmert C, Illig T, Pesch B, Brüning T, Dippon J, Ko YD, Brauch H. 2008. Polymorphic loci of E2F2, CCND1 and CCND3 are associated with HER2 status of breast tumors. *Int J Cancer.* 124(9):2077–2081.

Katz G, Arad M, Eldar M. 2009. Catecholaminergic polymorphic ventricular tachycardia from bedside to bench and beyond. *Curr Probl Cardiol.* 34:9–43.

Ko YL, Hsu LA, Wu S, Teng MS, Chang HH, Chen CC, Cheng CF. 2008. Genetic variation in the ASIC3 gene influences blood pressure levels in Taiwanese. *J Hypertens.* 26:2154–2160.

Le Marchand L, Derby KS, Murphy SE, Hecht SS, Hatsukami D, Carmella SG, Tiirikainen M, Wang H. 2008. Smokers with the CHRNA lung cancer-associated variants are exposed to higher levels of nicotine equivalents and a carcinogenic tobacco-specific nitrosamine. *Cancer Res.* 68:9137–9140.

Melén E, Nyberg F, Lindgren CM, Berglind N, Zucchelli M, Nordling E, Hallberg J, Svartengren M,

Morgenstern R, Kere J, Bellander T, Wickman M, Pershagen G. 2008. Interactions between glutathione S-transferase P1, tumor necrosis factor, and traffic-related air pollution for development of childhood allergic disease. *Environ Health Perspect.* 116:1077–1084.

National Center for Biotechnology Information. (2015a). Consensus CDS protein set. http://www.ncbi.nlm.nih.gov/CCDS/CcdsBrowse.cgi

National Center for Biotechnology Information. (2015b). dbSNP short genetic variations. http://www.ncbi.nlm.nih.gov/projects/SNP/snp_summary.cgi

Nicolaiew N, Cancel-Tassin G, Azzouzi AR, Grand BL, Mangin P, Cormier L, Fournier G, Giordanella JP, Pouchard M, Escary JL, Valeri A, Cussenot O. 2009. Association between estrogen and androgen receptor genes and prostate cancer risk. *Eur J Endocrinol.* 160:101–106.

Niemi M, Arnold KA, Backman JT, Pasanen MK, Gödtel-Armbrust U, Wojnowski L, Zanger UM, Neuvonen PJ, Eichelbaum M, Kivistö KT, Lang T. 2006. Association of genetic polymorphism in ABCC2 with hepatic multidrug resistance-associated protein 2 expression and pravastatin pharmacokinetics. *Pharmacogenet Genomics.* 16:801–808.

Okey AB, Franc MA, Moffat ID, Tijet N, Boutros PC, Korkalainen M, Tuomisto J, Pohjanvirta R. 2005. Toxicological implications of polymorphisms in receptors for xenobiotic chemicals: the case of the aryl hydrocarbon receptor. *Toxicol Appl Pharmacol.* 207(2 Suppl):43–51.

Omidvar M, Stolk L, Uitterlinden AG, Hofman A, Van Duijn CM, Tiemeier H. 2009. The effect of catechol-O-methyltransferase Met/Val functional polymorphism on smoking cessation: retrospective and prospective analyses in a cohort study. *Pharmacogenet Genomics.* 19:45–51.

Parrado A, West R, Jordan D, Bastard C, McKenna S, Whittaker JA, Bentley P, White D, Chomienne C, Padua RA. 1999. Alterations of the retinoic acid receptor alpha (RAR alpha) gene in myeloid and lymphoid malignancies. *Br J Haematol.* 104:738–741.

Pasanen MK, Neuvonen M, Neuvonen PJ, Niemi M. 2006. SLCO1B1 polymorphism markedly affects the pharmacokinetics of simvastatin acid. *Pharmacogenet Genomics.* 16:873–879.

Roses AD. 2008. Pharmacogenetics in drug discovery and development: a translational perspective. *Nat Rev Drug Discov.* 7:807–817.

Ruhé HG, Ooteman W, Booij J, Michel MC, Moeton M, Baas F, Schene AH. 2009. Serotonin transporter gene promoter polymorphisms modify the association between paroxetine serotonin transporter occupancy and clinical response in major depressive disorder. *Pharmacogenet Genomics.* 19:67–76.

Rusin P, Markiewicz L, Majsterek I. 2008. Genetic pre-determinations of head and neck cancer. *Postepy Hig Med Dosw* [Online]. 62:490–501.

Sanak M, Potaczek DP, Nizankowska-Mogilnicka E, Szczeklik A. 2007. Genetic variability of the high-affinity IgE receptor alpha subunit (Fc epsilon RI alpha) is related to total serum IgE levels in allergic subjects. *Allergol Int.* 56:397–401.

Scariano JK, Treat E, Alba F, Nelson H, Ness SA, Smith AY. 2008. The SRD5A2 V89L polymorphism is associated with severity of disease in men with early onset prostate cancer. *Prostate.* 68:1798–1805.

Scinicariello F, Murray HE, Moffett DB, Abadin HG, Sexton MJ, Fowler BA. 2007. Lead and delta-aminolevulinic acid dehydratase polymorphism: where does it lead? A meta-analysis. *Environ Health Perspect.* 115:35–41.

Smith AJ, Humphries SE. 2008. Cytokine and cytokine receptor gene polymorphisms and their functionality. *Cytokine Growth Factor Rev.* 20(1):43–59.

Smith HE, Jones JP 3rd, Kalhorn TF, Farin FM, Stapleton PL, Davis CL, Perkins JD, Blough DK, Hebert MF, Thummel KE, Totah RA. 2008. Role of cytochrome P450 2C8 and 2J2 genotypes in calcineurin inhibitor-induced chronic kidney disease. *Pharmacogenet Genomics.* 18:943–953.

Speirs CJ, Murray S, Davies DS, Biola Mabadeje AF, Boobis AR. 1990. Debrisoquine oxidation phenotype and susceptibility to lung cancer. *Br J Clin Pharmacol.* 29:101–109.

Spitsyn VA, Nafikova AK, Spitsyna NK, Afanas'eva IS. 2001. Genetic predisposition to alcoholic toxic cirrhosis. *Russ J Genet.* 37:573–580.

Tan SH, Lee SC, Goh BC, Wong J. 2008. Pharmaco-genetics in breast cancer therapy. *Clin Cancer Res.* 14:8027–8041.

Thier R, Brüning T, Roos PH, Rihs HP, Golka K, Ko Y, Bolt HM. 2003. Markers of genetic susceptibility in human environmental hygiene and toxicology: the role of selected CYP, NAT and GST genes. *Int J Hyg Environ Health.* 206:149–171.

Timchalk C. 2004. Comparative inter-species phar-macokinetics of phenoxyacetic acid herbicides and related organic acids. evidence that the dog is not a relevant species for evaluation of human health risk. *Toxicology.* 200:1–19.

Tomaszewski P, Kubiak-Tomaszewska G, Łukaszkiewicz J, Pachecka J. 2008a. Cytochrome

P450 polymorphism—molecular, metabolic, and pharmacogenetic aspects. III. Influence of CYP genetic polymorphism on population differen-tiation of drug metabolism phenotype. *Acta Pol Pharm.* 65:319–329.

Tomaszewski P, Kubiak-Tomaszewska G, Pachecka J. 2008b. Cytochrome P450 polymorphism—molecular, metabolic, and pharmacogenetic aspects. II. Participation of CYP isoenzymes in the metabolism of endogenous substances and drugs. *Acta Pol Pharm.* 65:307–318.

Ueta M, Sotozono C, Inatomi T, Kojima K, Tashiro K, Hamuro J, Kinoshita S. 2007. Toll-like recep-tor 3 gene polymorphisms in Japanese patients with Stevens-Johnson syndrome. *Br J Ophthalmol.* 91:962–965.

Van den Berg M, Birnbaum L, Bosveld AT, Brunström B, Cook P, Feeley M, Giesy JP, Hanberg A, Hasegawa R, Kennedy SW, Kubiak T, Larsen JC, van Leeuwen FX, Liem AK, Nolt C, Peterson RE, Poellinger L, Safe S, Schrenk D, Tillitt D, Tysklind M, Younes M, Waern F, Zacharewski T. 1998. Toxic equivalency factors (TEFs) for PCBs, PCDDs, PCDFs for humans and wildlife. *Environ Health Perspect.* 106:775–792.

Wang WC, Mihlbachler KA, Bleecker ER, Weiss ST, Liggett SB. 2008. A polymorphism of G-protein coupled receptor kinase5 alters agonist-promoted desensitization of beta2-adrenergic receptors. *Pharmacogenet Genomics.* 18:729–732.

Waxman DJ, Chang TKH. 1998. Use of 7-ethoxycou-marin to monitor multiple enzymes in the human CYP1, CYP2 and CYP3 families. *Methods Mol Biol.* 107:175–179.

Wedrén S, Lovmar L, Humphreys K, Magnus-son C, Melhus H, Syvänen AC, Kindmark A, Landegren U, Fermér ML, Stiger F, Persson I, Baron JA, Weiderpass E. 2008. Estrogen recep-tor alpha gene polymorphism and endometrial cancer risk—a case-control study. *BMC Cancer.* 8:322.

Winker R, Barth A, Valic E, Maier R, Osterode W, Pilger A, Rüdiger HW. 2005. Functional adrener-gic receptor polymorphisms and idiopathic ortho-static intolerance. *Int Arch Occup Environ Health.* 78:171–177.

Wu CP, Calcagno AM, Ambudkar SV. 2008. Reversal of ABC drug transporter-mediated multidrug resistance in cancer cells: evaluation of current strategies. *Curr Mol Pharmacol.* 1:93–105.

CHAPTER 12

Nutritional Toxicity and Sensitivity

This is a chapter outline intended to guide and familiarize you with the content to follow.

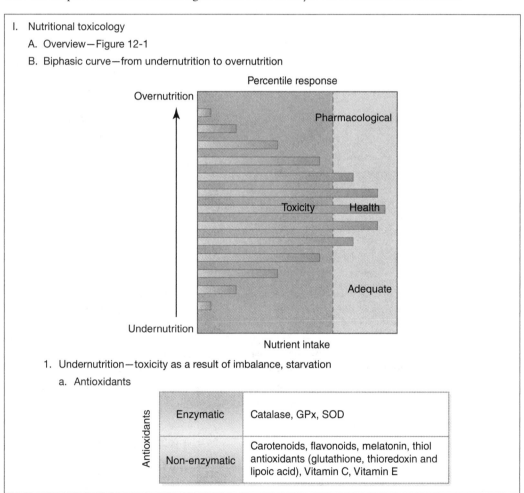

I. Nutritional toxicology
   A. Overview—Figure 12-1
   B. Biphasic curve—from undernutrition to overnutrition

   1. Undernutrition—toxicity as a result of imbalance, starvation
      a. Antioxidants

Antioxidants	Enzymatic	Catalase, GPx, SOD
	Non-enzymatic	Carotenoids, flavonoids, melatonin, thiol antioxidants (glutathione, thioredoxin and lipoic acid), Vitamin C, Vitamin E

CONCEPTUALIZING TOXICOLOGY 12-1

Reproduced from Flora SJS. 2009. Structural, chemical and biological aspects of antioxidants for strategies against metal and metalloid exposure. *Oxid Med Cell Longev.* 2:191–206.; Penniston KL, Tanumihardjo SA. 2006. The acute and chronic toxic effects of vitamin A. *Am J Clin Nutr.* 83:191–201.

(1) Ascorbic acid—increase in scurvy, Pb poisoning, quinine's toxic effects on testes, renal tubule damage by 3,4-dichloroaniline metabolite of 2-amino-2,4-dichlorophenol, plasma membrane damage by Cr, aldehyde toxicity, nitrosation, oxidative downregulation of pregnane X receptor and CYP3A11 mRNA expression (similar results for reduced CYP activity from protein, vitamin E, Mg, Zn, lipid, and riboflavin deficiencies), PCB toxicity

(2) Vitamin E and Se (glutathione peroxidase) deficiencies = prooxidant (Paraquat, nitrofurantoin); neurodegeneration prevented by α-tocotrienol, but not α-tocopherol; γ-tocotrienol, but not α-tocopherol inhibits inflammation by inhibiting COX2 formation of PGE_2 (see Figure 12-2)

(3) Vitamin A (retinoids from β-carotene) deficiency increases the toxicity of particle air pollutants on birth weight of children

(4) Mn (essential part of Mn-SOD) deficiency =↑ ROS damage; Mn also in oxidoreductases, transferases, hydrolases, lyases, isomerases, ligases, glutamine synthetase

b. Minerals and other vitamins

(1) Fe, thiamine, energy deficiencies induce CYPs; Fe deficiency increases Pb blood concentrations

(2) Calcium-related functions

(a) Pb retention increased by ↓ Ca^{2+}

(b) Blood clotting deficiency in absence of Ca^{2+} augmented by warfarin (anticoagulant that interferes with action of vitamin K)

CONCEPTUALIZING TOXICOLOGY 12-1 (*continued*)

(3) Vitamin D related to respiratory infections as aids in producing antimicrobial peptides

(4) Thiamine deficiency increases Pb toxicity; thiamine deficiency leads to neuropathies that are similar to poisoning by As

(5) Folate (radical scavenger on its own and precursor to tetrahydrofolate) deficiency = megaloblastic anemia, neural tube defects, pediatric leukemia and neuroblastoma, colon cancer, cardiovascular disease

(6) Choline deficiency = fatty liver; cancers of liver, breast, and colon; and mammalian cells in culture will not grow

(7) Glutathione deficiency—liver damage due to altered redox state and lack of conjugation of reactive groups on toxicants (e.g., acetaminophen metabolite)

(8) Vitamin B_{12} (cobalamin) deficiency = pernicious anemia → promote cancer, stroke, cardiovascular disease, impaired cognitive function, osteoporosis, neural tube defects, multiple sclerosis

(9) Vitamin B_6 (pyridoxine) deficiency = anemia, epileptic seizures, dermatitis, kidney failure, and promoting Alzheimer's disease, cardiovascular disease, colon cancer, and reduced cognition and/or depression

(10) Pantothenic acid (vitamin B_5 component of coenzyme A) deficiency increases cytotoxic action of decongestants, preservative benzalkonium chloride, and ototoxicity of chemotherapy agent cisplatin or antibiotic kanamycin

(11) Biotin deficiency—dry, scaly dermatitis, anorexia, nausea, and vomiting as caused by avidin in uncooked egg whites

(12) Cu and Se deficiency both ↓ plasma homocysteine and ↑ plasma GSH; Cu deficiency = early-onset Alzheimer's disease, anemia, neutropenia, reversible myelodysplasia + altered amyloid, ceruloplasmin, copper transport, cytochrome oxidase, myelination, organ analysis, and oxidative defense

(13) Mo (part of oxidases—xanthine, aldehyde and sulfite) deficiency = sulfite toxicity → mental retardation, neurological problems, ocular lens dislocation

(14) Zn (induces metallothionein for heavy metal chelation and activates genes involved in oxidant defense and immune response) deficiency = decreased wound healing/immune response, increased heavy metal toxicity

(15) Sulfur amino acids: methionine deficiency → ↓ protein synthesis and DNA hypomethylation; cysteine deficiency → ↓ GSH; taurine deficiency → neuronal and retinal dysfunctions

2. Overnutrition—toxicity as a result of too much nutrition (still an imbalance) as appears to be the key factors in cancer, heart disease, diabetes mellitus, dementia (most of the preventable diseases of aging as affected by calories in versus those utilized in exercise and other physical activity)

   a. Water soluble vitamins

(1) Vitamin C increases Fe absorption, so exacerbates hemochromatosis. Ascorbate's reducing power ↓ high-altitude resistance. ↑ Hemolysis associated with glucose-6-phosphate dehydrogenase deficiency. Critical problem of oxalate crystal deposition and kidney failure with excess ascorbate.

(2) Vitamin B_1 toxicity only occurs in people who are hypersensitive to B_1

(3) Vitamin B_2 not considered a problem in humans, but light-irradiated cultured rat lens cells generate H_2O_2 in presence of excess riboflavin

(4) Vitamin B_6 toxicity → sensory neuropathy (necrosis of dorsal root ganglion sensory neurons and degeneration of peripheral and central sensory projections) + degeneration of rat testes germinal epithelial cells + interferes with medications levodopa, penicillamine, and quinidine

CONCEPTUALIZING TOXICOLOGY 12-1 (*continued*)

(5) Vitamin B$_{12}$ + ascorbic acid or dithiothreitol → H$_2$O$_2$; in combination with folic acid may ↑ prostate cancer risk but ↓ hepatic fibrosis from dimethylnitrosamine

(6) Folic acid neurotoxicity similar to thiamine (B$_1$) if injected into CSF; a metabolite (folinic acid) ↑ 5-FU (cancer treatment) cytotoxicity due to locking thymidylate synthase in inhibited state; methyltetrahydrofolate may be a neurotoxic form of this vitamin

(7) Biotin injection into pregnant rats → estrogen deficiency signs

(8) "Conditional vitamins"—choline excess → ↓ male rat pachytene spermatocytes and lung lesions in guinea pigs; inositol interferes with intestinal absorption of Zn and Fe and role in IP3 is an inositol signaling molecule involved in calcium toxicity (apoptosis → necrosis); PABA and endocrine toxicity or allergic dermatitis of old formulations of sunscreens

b. Minerals: Ca^{2+}, Fe^{3+}, Fe^{2+}, Al^{3+}, and Mg^{2+} ↓ antibiotic tetracycline absorption; Ca^{2+} and calcification, apoptosis/necrosis, ventricular arrhythmias; PO$_4{}^{3-}$ excess unbalances Ca^{2+} homeostasis; Fe overload → hemosiderin hepatotoxicity; Mn excess = neurotoxicity (basal ganglia and ↓ dopamine → ↓ TSH); excess Na → dehydration, hypertension, oxidative stress, gastric cancer, acidosis/bone resorption; hyperkalemia → abnormal ECGs, acidosis, muscle weakness, ascending paralysis and exacerbated by certain medications (e.g., cardiac glycosides); sulfur excess; hypermagnesemia (due to kidney damage) → lethargy, confusion, arrhythmias, muscle weakness, hypotension; Mn excess → brain abscesses, Parkinsonian-like symptoms up to seizures; Cu → liver damage and neurotoxicity due to formation of a copper-dopamine complex and dopamine oxidation to aminochrome; Zn has opposite effects of Cu as it ↓ Cu status + causes developmental effects; Se → liver damage (toxic selenodiglutathione), skin and hair alterations, brittle fingernails, "garlic" breath (dimethylselenide exhaled) and neurological lesions in swine; Cr → anemia, thrombocytopenia, hemolysis, hepatotoxicity, kidney failure, apoptosis, and for Cr(III) deletion mutations and strand breaks (HO·) + skeletal disorders and neurotoxicity; Mo → ruminant kidney damage, reproductive failure, growth depression, decreased Hb and Hct; Vanadium → inhibit protein phosphatases; Boron → reproductive and developmental toxicity, rat kidney proximal tubule cell degeneration (see Figure 12-3); iodine → excess contributes to Hashimoto's thyroiditis and Graves' disease, is genotoxic to mammalian cells in drinking water

c. Excess sugar/fat intake (calories with lack of compensating activity = obesity → cardiovascular disease, diabetes mellitus II, cancer, dementia, fatty liver (steatosis requiring TNFα activation that is prevented by antioxidant-stimulating compound resveratrol) and hepatic cancer

(1) High fat intake (10% lipid)—turns vitamin C into a compound that prevents nitrosamine from forming into a compound that promotes its formation

(2) Specific fats

(a) O− cif3 fatty acids (lack clotting due to lower active TXA2), omega-6 fatty acids (high-fat diet effects on cardiovascular function, fatty liver [similar to goose liver pate] due to increased inflammatory prostaglandins

(b) Cholesterol → atherosclerotic plaques and VEGF signaling

(c) Fat-soluble vitamins

(i) Hypervitaminosis A and ↓ renal and immune function, skin toxicity, embryonic/fetal cell toxicity, liver fibrosis/portal hypertension + hyperplasia of Ito cells (liver storage site), eye alterations via ligand-dependent transcription-regulating retinoic acid receptors (RARs); humans eating bear liver (hibernating animal with high vitamin A storage); retinol plasma concentrations ↑ with DDE in frogs, TCDD or certain PCB congeners in rats and mice, and estradiol in sturgeon; toxic metabolites occur in people with too much vitamin A that overwhelms the liver storage capacity

CONCEPTUALIZING TOXICOLOGY 12-1 (*continued*)

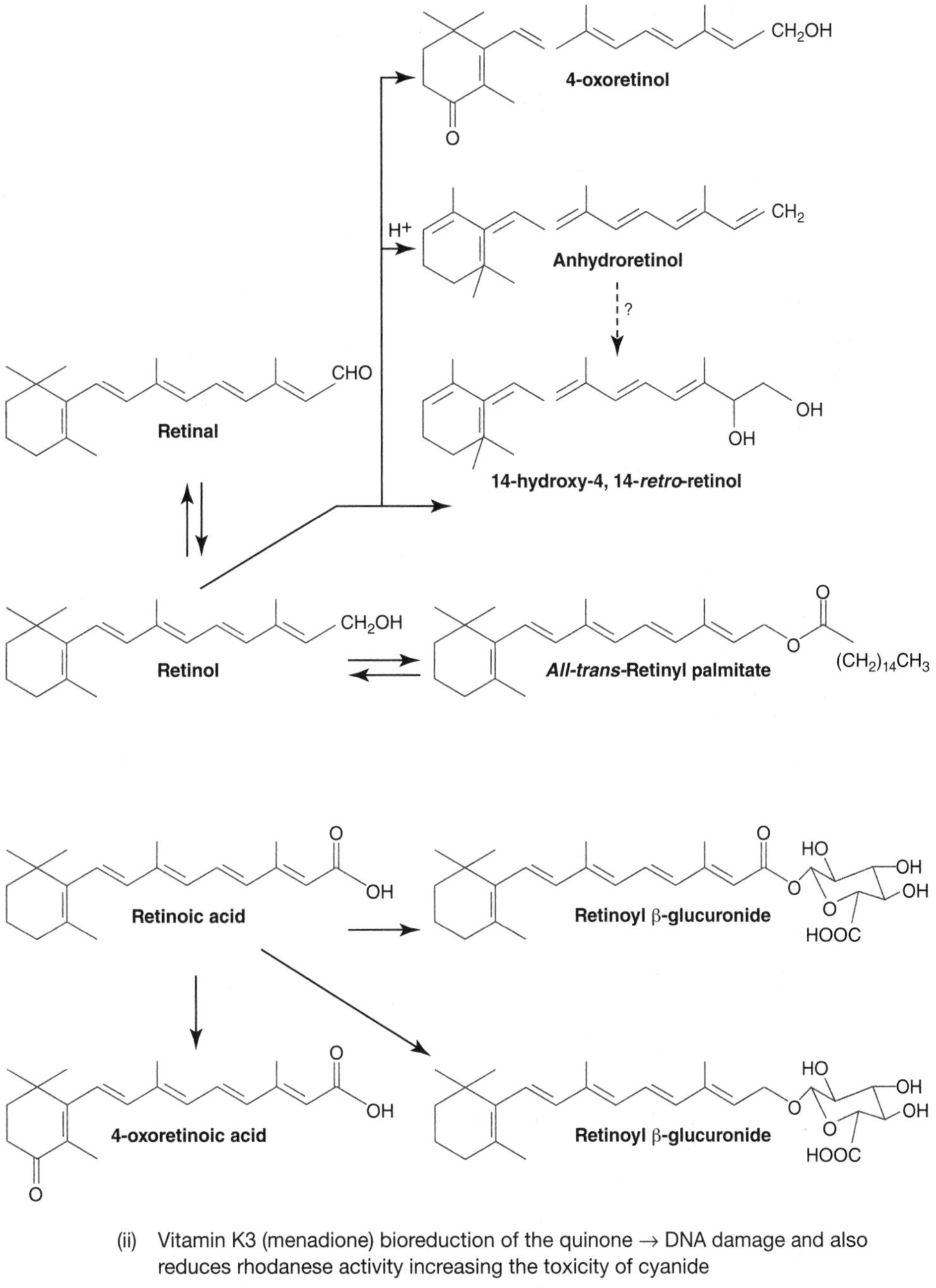

CH2OH
4-oxoretinol
O
H+
CH2
Anhydroretinol
?
CHO
Retinal
OH
OH
14-hydroxy-4, 14-retro-retinol
CH2OH
Retinol
O
O
All-trans-Retinyl palmitate
(CH2)14CH3
O
OH
Retinoic acid
O
HO
OH
O
OH
O
Retinoyl β-glucuronide
HOOC
O
OH
4-oxoretinoic acid
O
HO
OH
O
OH
O
Retinoyl β-glucuronide
HOOC

(ii) Vitamin K3 (menadione) bioreduction of the quinone → DNA damage and also reduces rhodanese activity increasing the toxicity of cyanide

(iii) Excess vitamin D (cholecalciferol) used as a rodenticide as it causes hypercalcemia → heart problems, bleeding as a result of the vessel mineralization (cardiovascular collapse) from the stomach wall, lungs, and kidneys (azotemia as a result of kidney failure)

(iv) Vitamin E excess via α-tocopherol supplementation ↓ γ-tocopherol which increases cardiovascular disease (less COX2 inhibition), other inflammatory damage, and premature membrane rupture during pregnancy

CONCEPTUALIZING TOXICOLOGY 12-1 *(continued)*

(3) Excess carbohydrates (high glycemic index) → hyperinsulinemia and insulin resistance; cardiovascular, eye, and brain alterations

d. Proteins and amino acids

(1) Excess protein → hyperaminoacidemia, hyperammonemia, hyperinsulinemia

(2) Amino acids → catabolism of enzymes, affect food consumption/eating patterns, neurotransmitter alterations; supplementing one amino acid alone may make other amino acids limit growth; sulfur amino acids → excess methionine (due to polymorphisms of transmethylation and transsulfuration pathways → brain edema; high doses of *N*-acCys → epileptic seizures/death; homocysteine → cardiovascular diseases and renal failure

e. Nucleic acids → constipation, uric acid formation from purines (gout)

3. Affected by toxicants (affect appetite, digestion, and absorption)

a. Vitamin A depleted by ROS (Cu), benzo[*a*]pyrene induction of CYP (metabolism of retinoids), also by PCBs in trout; opposite response = isotretinoin (retinoid used as anti-acne medication) yields birth defects + psychiatric symptoms + musculoskeletal alterations (enthesopathy)

b. Methylmercury interferes with the signaling (kinases) of all-trans-retinoic acid on differentiation of neuroblastoma cells

c. UV irradiation decreases vitamin A concentration in humans

d. PCB and mercury mixture overwhelms ability of vitamin C or Se to be protective

e. Pb exposure up-regulation of AH receptor → affects bone development; Cd ↑Ca^{2+} loss from bone (Itae-Itae disease)

f. Antilipemics and cephalosporins induce vitamin K deficiency

g. Thallium interaction with riboflavin may be responsible for a chronic energy deprivation neuropathy

h. Pyridoxine (vitamin B_6) and nicotinamide (niacin) interfered with by carbamazepine → cutaneous cell macular lesions

i. Dihydrofolate reductase inhibitors trimethoprim (antibiotic) and methotrexate (anticancer, rheumatoid arthritis medication) interfere with utilization of folic acid to become the methyl donation cofactor in thymidine synthesis

j. Heavy metals or glyphosate herbicide → Parkinson's disease, but also promoted by Mg deficiency, Mn toxicity, and CO poisoning

k. Chronic ethanol use → K and Mg wasting and transport of thiamine and folacin and promoted by heart disorders, diabetes mellitus II (obesity + aging), Gitelman and Bartter syndromes (kidney); cetuximab medication ↑ urinary excretion of Mg

l. Antacids (Na or Al) → Ca (this first one yields osteoporosis), Cu, folate, phosphate deficiencies (this last one yields osteomalacia; also promoted by high Cd)

m. Anticonvulsants phenobarbital, phenytoin, primidone → vitamin D and K deficiencies; valproic acid → carnitine deficiency

n. Tetracycline antibiotic or cisplatin chemotherapy agent → Ca deficiency

o. Gentamycin → altered K and Mg balance

p. Neomycin → lipid/cholesterol absorption impeded augmenting effect of statins

q. Boric acid or antipsychotic agent chlorpromazine → depletes riboflavin

r. Antimalarial isoniazid → pyridoxine, vitamin D, and niacin deficiencies; antimalarial pyrimethamine → depletes folate; antihypertensive hydralazine → ↓vitamin B_6

s. Asprin (acetylsalicylic acid) → depletes ascorbate, folate, Fe; estrogen depletes ascorbate, pyridoxine and folate

t. Anti-inflammatory sulfasalazine → depletes folate; steroid prednisone ↓ Ca

u. Microtubule agent colchicine → affects lipid and vitamin B_{12} concentrations; proton pump inhibitors and H_2 antagonists → ↓ acid → ↓ vitamin B_{12}

CONCEPTUALIZING TOXICOLOGY 12-1 (*continued*)

v. Diuretics deplete ions (e.g., HCTZ and hypokalemia); phytic acid from seeds chelates metal ions Ca, Fe, K, Mg, Mn, and Zn making them insoluble = ↓ absorption

w. Laxatives deplete vitamins (and promote dehydration)

x. Trypsin inhibitor in raw soybeans → pancreatic damage

4. Nutrient as pharmacological agent/chemoprevention

a. Ascorbic acid and recovering mitochondrial function of nephrotoxic dichlorovinyl-L-cysteine

b. Se decreases Hg toxicity (metal competition for absorption/utilization)

c. Gemini vitamin D analogues inhibit mammary tumors; vitamin D_3 increases sensitivity of squamous cell cancers to cisplatin (by ↑ Ca-induced apoptosis in those cells not resistant to this effect).

d. Thiamine supplementation treats Wernicke's encephalopathy related to ethanol-induced brain stem and cerebellar lesions

e. Pyridoxine treats a form of epilepsy caused by abnormality of α-amino adipic semialdehyde dehydrogenase leading to an accumulation of piperideine-6-carboxylic acid that inactivates pyridoxal phosphate via a condensation reaction and protects against isoniazid-induced convulsions, MSG reactions, monomethylhydrazine-containing mushrooms, and ethylene glycol poisoning

f. Cr^{3+} genotoxic, but chromium is a pharmacological agent/nutrient playing a role in insulin function and resistance in obesity and interferes with Fe absorption reducing diabetes mellitus heart disease in people consuming excess Fe

g. Hypermagnesemia as a chelation for excess ammonia resulting from liver cirrhosis

C. Naturally occurring toxicants in food

1. Mycotoxins—see Figure 12-4

a. Aflatoxins (infamous for contamination of corn and liver damage/cancer in humans) and ochratoxins (nephrotoxin, hepatotoxic, immunotoxic, teratogenic, carcinogenic)

b. Patulin genotoxicity on fruit

c. Zearalenone on corn (high affinity for estrogen receptors)

d. Alternariol → DNA strand breaks

e. Trichothecenes (grains) affect cell signaling from inflammation to apoptosis

f. Fumonisins → fatal leukoencephalomalacia in horses (interfere with sphingolipid metabolism)

g. Moniliformin → pyruvate dehydrogenase, glutathione peroxidase, and GSH reductase inhibition

h. Ergot alkaloids and sleepy grass toxicosis

i. Tremogens → shaking neurotoxicity

2. Cyanide

a. Inhibits cyt a_3 as oxygen-transferring step of oxidative phosphorylation

b. Cyanogenic glucosides found in 2500 plant species (phytoanticipins defense against herbivores) and in six spot moth

D. Nutritional genomics

1. Polyunsaturated fatty acids (PUFA) upregulate peroxisome proliferator activated receptor (PPAR) α

2. Amino acid nutrition influences mRNA expression

3. Zn regulates the metal response element transcription factor (promoter for metallothionein)

4. Grilling meat → heterocyclic amines → induces CYP1A2 and N-hydroxylation reactions on consumption of those amines

5. Grapefruit juice's furanocoumarins inhibit CYP3A4 → 10-fold increase in certain medications' AUC; St. John's wort has the opposite effect on CYP3A4

6. Antioxidants from fruit, onions, and soya milk reduce DNA damage from H_2O_2

7. Sucrose-rich diet augments mutations in mitochondrial genome by decreasing ATP synthesis efficiency, while vitamin A has opposite effect

CONCEPTUALIZING TOXICOLOGY 12-1 (*continued*)

Nutritional Toxicology

Nutritional toxicology is an important but often relatively minor portion of the coverage of toxicant action. This area is extremely important in disease, toxicant sensitivity, and aging. Malnutrition is defined as any state that increases disease processes, such as deficiency states caused by undernutrition or cardiovascular diseases, diabetes mellitus, increased aging, cancers, arthritis, and other diseases of excess consumption or overnutrition. Nutrients can cause direct toxicity by their absence, such as lack of antioxidants and blindness caused by 100% oxygen in neonatal humans. Excess nutrients such as excess trace minerals can cause death by metal poisonings. The lack of nutrients may directly increase the toxicity of a variety of chemicals or have an indirect action and decrease toxicity via lack of use of a cofactor (e.g., decreased acetaminophen toxicity due to selenium deficiency, which causes increased glutathione concentrations via less selenium-dependent glutathione peroxidase). Increased levels of nutrients may act pharmacologically or toxicologically on their own or may increase or decrease the disease process resulting from other chemicals. Consider again selenium. Excess selenium can cause selenosis and liver damage via selenodiglutathione. Excess selenium can also reduce dimethylbenzanthracene-induced tumors (Medina et al.,

1983). This action may be the basis for chemoprevention of cancer or aging that are current areas of intense investigation. For example, a new medication isolated from red wine resveratrol (3,5,4′-trihydroxy-trans-stilbene), a phytoalexin, would not be considered an essential nutrient or have a recommended daily allowance (RDA). However, as a pharmaceutical it has been effective in animals in preventing diseases of aging such as diabetes mellitus. It also reduces the carcinogenicity of a colon cell–specific carcinogen 1,2-dimethylhydrazine (adenoma and adenocarcinoma) and the glycoconjugates caused by this compound (Sengottuvelan et al., 2009). Because nutritional toxicity can yield hypersensitivities and hyposensitivities, affect the expression of genes, and alter signaling pathways, it should be viewed an important factor in selective toxicity. The way nutrition and toxicants interact is presented in **Figure 12-1**. Note that toxicants can alter nutrient intake. They can modify appetite, digestion, and absorption. Toxicants can alter functions of nutrients or modify signaling by nutrients. Xenobiotic and nutrient metabolism can be altered. The excretion of nutrients can be affected. Nutrients can also modify absorption of toxicants, serve as a binding competitor to serum albumin, which makes the toxicant more available, alter xenobiotic metabolism, and affect renal excretion of toxicants. Undernutrition and deficiency states

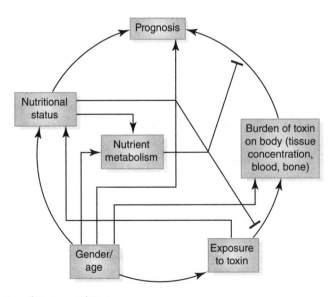

FIGURE 12-1 Interactions of Nutrients with Toxicants

are examined first in this chapter. Following that discussion, excess nutrient toxicities are noted. Next, naturally occurring toxicants in food are covered. Last, the investigation of this topic concludes with the interaction of genetics and nutrition, or nutritional genomics.

Undernutrition

Antioxidants

One of the easiest and earliest findings of undernutrition was the discovery of scurvy as a result of vitamin C or ascorbic acid deficiency. British sailors would use the juice of lemons or limes to avoid this dreaded dietary deficiency during long sea voyages. During the exploration for a Northwest Passage across the northern portion of Canada, the Franklin expedition had meat canned in tin with lead solder. They also used lemon juice to avoid scurvy, but were unaware that the ascorbic acid degraded as their ship was trapped in the ice. The combination of lead poisoning and scurvy caused them to be susceptible to disease and the cold of the arctic, and they all died in an historic tragedy (Beattie and Geiger, 2005). Quinine is a toxic medication used to prevent malaria that has deleterious effects on the testes. Ascorbic acid deficiency increases its toxic action, and supplementation decreases its toxicity (Osinubi et al., 2007). Kidney slices exposed to the toxic 2-amino-4,5-dichlorophenol metabolite of the renal proximal tubule toxicant 3,4-dichloroaniline show leakage of the enzyme lactate dehydrogenase and increased lipid peroxidation as measured by the formation of malondialdehyde. Ascorbic acid pretreatment reduced the toxicity to these cells (Valentovic et al., 2002). Vitamin C supplementation can prevent some of the plasma membrane oxidant damage induced by chromium, but not the functional toxicity (Dey et al., 2001). Certain functions such as renal proximal tubule injury and death caused by the nephrotoxic cysteine conjugate dichlorovinyl-L-cysteine are independent of ascorbic acid concentration as long as no deficiency exists, but pharmacological concentrations of vitamin C (500 µM) can aid in the recovery of mitochondrial function, active Na^+ transport, and proliferation following the toxic injury (Nowak et al.,

2000). Ascorbic acid can protect against toxic aldehydes (acetaldehyde, acrolein, and formaldehyde), while quercetin only protects against acetaldehyde and another important dietary antioxidant alph-atocopherol was not protective (Manzardo and Coppi, 1991). Ascorbic acid will prevent nitrosation of morpholine in the presence of nitrite (Archer et al., 1975). This will make the cells more deficient in vitamin C. Ascorbate will also cause increased nitrosation that will lead to metaplasia and adenocarcinoma in the presence of 10% lipid in the stomach, so the nutritional chemistry is altered by the presence of other nutrients in the diet (Combet et al., 2007). Lipopolysaccharide induces downregulation of pregnane X receptor and CYP3A11 mRNA expression. Ascorbic acid prevents this oxidative downregulation as well as the repressive effects of dexamethasone-, rifampicin-, mifepristone-, and phenobarbital-inducible CYP3A11 mRNA expression and erythromycin N-demethylase catalytic activity in mouse liver (Xu et al., 2004). Not only can ascorbic acid deficiency decrease CYP activity, but deficiencies in the antioxidant tocopherol (vitamin E), protein, magnesium, zinc, lipid, and riboflavin yield similar results. However, energy, iron, or thiamine (vitamin B_1) deficiencies have the opposite (inducing) effect (Hathcock, 1982). Combined deficiencies of vitamin E and selenium induce toxicity of a number of pro-oxidant redox-cycling compounds including the herbicide Paraquat (Combs and Peterson, 1983) and the antibiotic nitrofurantoin (Peterson et al., 1982). The nitric acid formation by ascorbic acid and nitrite can also increase forestomach and esophageal cancer as indicated by the enhancing action of sodium nitrite and ascorbic acid on the rat N-bis(2-hydroxypropyl)nitrosamine-initiated esophageal tumorigenesis model (Kuroiwa et al., 2008). Vitamin A is another antioxidant also known as part of the retinoids. Reactive oxygen species (ROS) deplete retinoids. Induction of CYPs also increases metabolism of and depletion of retinoids. Cu and benzo[a] pyrene deplete retinoids in zebrafish, but not sufficiently to affect reproduction (Alsop et al., 2007). Poland has very polluted air in its cities. There was a negative effect of fine particles ≤ 2.5 µm in diameter ($PM_{2.5}$) and birth weight of children from women on the third tertile of vitamin A intake

(Jedrychowski et al., 2007). Alltrans-retinoic acid mediates the differentiation of neuroblastoma cells (human SH-SY5Y line) and cell-cycle progression through extracellular signal-regulated kinase 1/2 (ERK1/2) and protein kinase C (PKC). Methylmercury disrupts these signaling pathways to induce neurotoxicity and interferes with vitamin A–induced differentiation (Kim et al., 2007). Ultraviolet irradiation also decreases vitamin A concentrations in the human (White et al., 1988).

Circling back to the antioxidants Se and ascorbic acid, it is interesting to note that they decrease the toxicity of each other. Polychlorinated biphenyl (PCB) toxicity is decreased by vitamin C. However, in mixtures of pollutants with PCBs and mercury, there is a decrease in the antioxidant enzyme superoxide dismutase and an increase in nitric oxide and neurotoxicity, which indicates oxidative stress and augmented neurotoxicity of the mixture that have limited protection offered by either Se prevention of Hg absorption or antioxidant protection by the selenium-dependent glutathione peroxidase or ascorbic acid (Cheng et al., 2009). This indicates that toxicants can overwhelm nutritional protection. A more thorough examination of antioxidants (and other nutrients) and toxicant action can be found elsewhere (Katsonis and Mackey, 2002).

Ca-Related Functions

Vitamin D and Ca maintain Ca homeostasis. Vitamin D analogs are now being considered for use in prevention and treatment of cancer. The reason vitamin D or its active 1α, 25-dihydroxyvitamin D_3 form cannot be used is the hypercalcemia that would result. Gemini vitamin D analogs show an inhibitory effect in the N-methyl-N-nitrosourea-induced estrogen receptor (ER)-positive mammary tumor model or a xenograft model of ER-negative mammary tumors (Lee, Paul et al., 2008). Because Ca is involved in apoptosis, the role of vitamin D in eliciting apoptosis in cancer cells is important for treatment options. 1α,25-dihydroxyvitamin D_3 increases the sensitivity of squamous cell carcinoma cells to the apoptotic effects of cisplatin, but does not occur in 1α,25-dihydroxyvitamin D_3–resistant cancer

cells (Ma et al., 2008). Because vitamin D is also responsible for the production of antimicrobial peptides, vitamin D deficiencies may be linked to frequent respiratory infections. Because an excess of one fat-soluble vitamin may also make another deficient, high levels of vitamin A intake through cod liver oil or vitamin supplementation may lead to vitamin D deficiency and increased respiratory infections (Cannell et al., 2008). Calcium alone is known to interact with xenobiotics. Ca^{2+} binds to the antibiotic tetracycline and prevents both from being absorbed, as do other polyvalent metal cations such as Fe^{3+}, Fe^{2+}, Al^{3+}, and Mg^{2+} (Neuvonen, 1976). Aromatic hydrocarbons may affect bone development through the AH receptor. Lead exposure sensitizes bone to toxicant exposure via upregulation of expression of the AH receptor (Ryan et al., 2007). Cadmium increases the Ca loss from bone in pregnant mice, simulating an Itae-Itae (ouch-ouch)–like syndrome with high cadmium exposure in humans (Wang et al., 1994). Ca deficiency appears to increase the retention of lead in animals (Mahaffey et al., 1973). Similarly, iron deficiency increases blood lead concentrations in humans (Bradman et al., 2001). Conversely, vitamin C decreases lead level in rats (Flora and Tandon, 1986) or humans (Dawson et al., 1999). Calcium also plays a key role in blood clotting along with vitamin K. Warfarin, which has been used as a rat poison, interferes with vitamin K action and increases clotting time as a medication. This is augmented by other toxicants or medications such as by the immunosuppressant chemotherapeutic medication 6-mercaptopurine (Buu-Hoï and Hien, 1968). Vitamin K, especially the synthetic vitamin K_3 (menadione), appears to play a role in cancer as well via a bioreductive activation of the quinone (Simamura et al., 2008). Antilipemics, cephalosporins, and other medications can induce vitamin K deficiencies (Roe, 1988).

Thiamine, Riboflavin, Niacin, Pyridoxine, Folate, Cyanocobalamin, Pantothenic Acid, Biotin, and Choline

As indicated earlier, lead toxicity is prevented by ascorbic acid and also by thiamine (Flora and Tandon, 1986). Thiaminase activity in alewives have caused large-scale salmonine deaths in the Laurentian Great Lakes (Lepak et al., 2008). There is also a suggestion of riboflavin deficiency leading to neuropathies that develop as a result of thiamine deficiency or arsenical poisoning. Thallium poisoning is also classified under the chronic energy deprivation neuropathies and may involve interactions of the thallium ion with riboflavin in the production of flavoproteins (Cavanagh, 1991). Alcoholics have lesions of the brain stem and cerebellum that cause Wernicke's encephalopathy characterized by progressive development of disorders of consciousness, oculomotor palsies, and ataxia. This is best treated by thiamine supplementation (Séréni and Degos, 1990). Human cutaneous cells show "sharply limited, sunburn-like brown reddish macular lesions with central scaling and partly hyperkeratotic areas on the hands, feet, face, knees, gluteal and axillar regions" associated with interference in the activities of vitamin B_6 (pyridoxine) and nicotinamide (niacin) by the anti-epileptic mediation carbamazepine (Heyer et al., 1998). Pyridoxine prevents a specific type of epilepsy on its own due to an abnormality of the alpha-amino adipic semialdehyde (AASA) dehydrogenase (antiquitin) in the cerebral lysine degradation pathway. As a result, piperideine-6-carboxylic acid (P6C) accumulates as a toxicant that inactivates pyridoxal phosphate (PLP) by a Knoevenagel condensation (Plecko et al., 2007).

The vitamins discussed in this section are mainly involved in mitochondrial energy functions considered to be one-carbon transfer cycles. Folate and choline promote methyl donation essential for nucleic acid and protein synthesis. Interference with folate to the 5-methyltetrahydrofolate pathway has been the basis for the action of an antibiotic (trimethoprim) and a chemotherapeutic medication (methotrexate). Folic acid on its own is a radical scavenger, repairing hydroxyl, peroxyl, and thiol radicals through oxidation of the purine hydroxyl groups. Folate deficiency is also associated with megaloblastic anemia, neural tube defects, pediatric leukemia or neuroblastoma, colon cancer, and cardiovascular disease. Choline prevents fatty liver, prevents certain cancers (e.g., liver, breast, colon), and is essential

for growth of mammalian cells in culture. Glutathione, which is an essential biochemical compound in maintaining the redox state of the mitochondria in the presence of oxidative toxicants, is synthesized from a cysteine source such a methionine. Cobalamin (vitamin B_{12}) may aid methyltetrahydrofolate in the synthesis of methionine. Deficiencies of vitamin B_{12} are associated with pernicious anemia, which is characterized by macrocytic anemia and subacute combined degeneration of the spinal tracts with polyneuritis. Vitamin B_{12} deficiency can also promote cancer, stroke, cardiovascular disease, impaired cognitive function, osteoporosis, neural tube defects, and multiple sclerosis. Vitamin B_6 appears to regenerate the methyl-bearing form of tetrahydrofolate and the conversion of homocysteine to glutathione. B_6 deficiencies result in anemia, epileptic seizures, dermatitis, and kidney failure. Additional associations have been made between B_6 and Alzheimer's disease, cardiovascular disease, colon cancer, and reduced cognition and/or depression (Depeint et al., 2006). Pantothenic acid also aids mitochondrial function and is a component of coenzyme A. The alcohol of pantothenic acid, dexpanthenol, serves a protective influence by promoting cell growth against the cytotoxic action of decongestants and the preservative benzalkonium chloride found in many nasal sprays (Klöcker et al., 2004). Biotin assists the B vitamins mentioned in this section, aids in the utilization of protein, and participates in the oxidation and synthesis of fatty acids. Biotin deficiency as noted by dry scaly dermatitis, anorexia, nausea, and vomiting can be caused by consumption of uncooked egg whites, which has been noted as early as 1936. The presence of avidin in egg whites is a strong binding agent for biotin as can be determined by single-molecule imaging (Wayment and Harris, 2009).

Chromium, Copper, Magnesium, Manganese, Molybdenum, and Zinc

Selenium has already been examined as related to antioxidant defense. The implications of iron deficiency have also been examined. As for other nutrient metals, chromium plays a key role in insulin function or insulin resistance in obesity (Roussel et al., 2007). However, some researchers argue that chromium is a pharmacological agent rather than a nutrient as its interference with iron absorption may reduce high iron concentrations and their linkage to diabetes mellitus and heart disease. The genotoxicity of Cr^{3+} also indicates its role as a toxic agent (Stearns, 2000). Copper and selenium deficiency both decrease plasma homocysteine and increase plasma glutathione (Uthus and Ross, 2008). This is important in conjugation reactions of xenobiotics and in cardiovascular disease. Copper deficiency is also associated with early onset of Alzheimer's disease and alterations in amyloid, ceruloplasmin, copper transport, cytochrome oxidase, myelination, organ analysis, and oxidative defense (Klevay, 2008). Low copper concentrations are also linked to anemia, neutropenia, and reversible myelodysplasia (Huff et al., 2007). Heavy metals and other environmental factors may be partially responsible for the development of Parkinson's disease. Among the mechanisms that appear to be associated with the damage that results in Parkinsonian syndrome are magnesium deficiency, manganese toxicity, and carbon monoxide poisonings (Guzeva et al., 2008). Potassium concentrations in cells are also tightly linked to magnesium concentrations but not vice versa. Possible reasons that high intracellular K^+ concentrations may not be maintained in a magnesium deficiency state are increased membrane permeability to K^+ and/or inhibition of the $3Na^+,2K^+$-ATPase. Chronic alcoholism, heart disorders, type 2 diabetes mellitus (linked to obesity and age), Gitelman syndrome and Bartter syndrome involving kidney potassium and magnesium wasting, severe diarrhea and vomiting, improper nutrition such as excess sodium, and certain medications lead to these deficiencies (Iezhitsa and Spasov, 2008). One medication that causes Mg deficiency is cetuximab, a monoclonal antibody against the epithelial growth factor receptor (EGFR), which increases urinary excretion of magnesium (Schrag et al., 2005). Manganese is part of a number of essential enzymes such as manganese superoxide dismutase (Mn-SOD). Because Mn-SOD is the principal antioxidant enzyme that protects against ROS, the damage by oxidants can be exacerbated by its absence. Mn is also important

in the activities of oxidoreductases, transferases, hydrolases, lyases, isomerases, ligases, and glutamine synthetase. Excess manganese (manganism) can cause neurotoxicity by damage to the nuclei of basal ganglia. The resulting reduction in dopamine may also affect the inhibitory effect of this hormone on the anterior pituitary cells' secretion of thyroid-stimulating hormone (Soldin and Aschner, 2007). Molybdenum is part of the enzymes that process purines (xanthine oxidase, XO), convert toxic aldehydes to acids (aldehyde oxidase, AO), and metabolize sulfur-containing amino acids (sulfite oxidase, SO). Sulfite is more toxic in molybdenum-deficient brain cells or in cells that have a deficiency of the molybdenum cofactor. This leads to mental retardation, neurologic problems, and ocular lens dislocation (Sardesai, 1993). Zinc binds to metallothioneins, which also bind heavy metals and prevent more hepatic cell damage than would be expected from their consumption. Zinc is also released and affects zinc-dependent genes that activate antioxidant enzymes in oxidative/nitrosative stress and affect the immune response (Mocchegiani et al., 2006).

Drug-Caused Nutritional Deficiencies

There is an extensive literature on the interactions of medications with nutrients. One compilation is fairly extensive by Roe (1989). Some medications and toxicants may lead to deficiency states depending on the individual and the dosage regimen. Antacids containing sodium bicarbonate and aluminum hydroxide can cause deficiencies in calcium, copper, folate, and phosphate. Anticonvulsants represented by phenobarbital, phenytoin, and primidone may yield deficiencies in vitamins D and K. Valproic acid can lead to a carnitine deficiency. Antibiotics such as tetracycline have already been mentioned as agents that cause Ca deficiency. Gentamycin may affect the K and Mg balance. Neomycin affects lipid/cholesterol absorption and appears to augment the effects of the statins (Vanhanen, 1994). Boric acid, which prevents bacterial growth in medications, can deplete riboflavin. The antibiotic trimethoprim (as mentioned earlier) causes a folate deficiency state. Isoniazid, used in the treatment of malaria, causes vitamins B_6 and D and niacin deficiencies. Pyrimethamine is another antimalarial agent that depletes folate. Acetylsalicylic acid (aspirin) depletes ascorbic acid, folate, and iron. Sulfasalazine is another anti-inflammatory agent that depletes folate. Because aspirin is also an anti-coagulant, it is important to emphasize that warfarin (Coumadin) works as an anticoagulant by a different mechanism that interferes with vitamin K function. The mitotic arrest agent colchicine affects lipid and vitamin B_{12} levels. The steroid anti-inflammatory prednisone can reduce Ca concentrations. As discussed previously, methotrexate depletes folate and calcium in the treatment of cancer. Cisplatin has also been described as a chemotherapeutic medication that depletes magnesium. Vitamin B_6 is decreased by the antihypertensive medication hydralazine. Diuretics are famous for depleting ions. The most utilized agent, hydrochlorothiazide (HCTZ), is known to cause hypokalemia. Loop diuretics, represented by furosemide, deplete potassium as well as calcium and magnesium. The triamterene diuretic causes a folate deficiency. H_2 receptor antagonists such as cimetidine, which is used as an over-the-counter medication to reduce stomach acid production, produce B_{12} deficiencies. Proton pump inhibitors or metformin and pancreatic insufficiencies can also lead to vitamin B_{12} deficiencies by decreasing digestion and diseases of the ileum mucosal cells, leading to less absorption (Rufenacht et al., 2008). Laxatives also rob the system of vitamins. Mineral oil depletes carotene, retinol, and vitamins D and K. Others may just deplete potassium (phenolphthalein) or lipids and Ca (senna pod extracts). Estrogenic oral contraceptives for women deplete ascorbic acid (Rivers, 1975), vitamin B_6, and folate. The antipsychotic medication chlorpromazine is also known to deplete riboflavin (Roe, 1989).

Toxicant-Caused Nutritional Deficiencies

A number of toxicants also cause nutritional deficiencies. Some of the references on the subject of food and nutritional toxicology produced in the 21st century are the book by Omaye (2004) or individual articles as represented by Kordas et al. (2007). Raw soybeans contain a trypsin inhibitor that may be deadly if consumed in high quantities, because pancreatic function and protein digestion and absorption of essential amino acids are compromised. Alcohol decreases the active transport of both thiamine and folacin (Hathcock, 1982). Phytic acid, the main storage form of phosphorus in seeds, chelates metallic cations making Ca, Fe, K, Mg, Mn, and Zn insoluble and therefore unavailable for absorption (Bohn et al., 2008). Heavy metal toxicity appears to be related to a variety of nutrient deficiencies. Rats supplemented with 1.2% calcium, 0.6% phosphorous, 90 mg/kg iron, 50 mg/kg zinc, 0.08% magnesium, 70 mg/kg manganese, 0.2 mg/kg selenium, 5 mg/kg copper, 0.8 mg/kg molybdenum, 0.6 mg/kg iodine, and 3.0 mg/kg cobalt had lower liver enzymes in plasma (e.g., alkaline phosphatase) reflecting less liver toxicity and significantly lower blood lead levels than undernourished subjects (Herman et al., 2008). This phenomenon appears to be especially problematic in undernourished women and children in environmentally polluted areas of the world (Kordas et al., 2007). Blood lead levels appear to show an inverse relationship with calcium intake or protein intake in undernourished children (Elias et al., 2007). Certain cancers (e.g., breast) take part of their prognosis from nutritionally controlled proteins such as the zinc transporters (Levenson and Somers, 2008). Toxicant-induced deficiencies may lead to decreased nutrient absorption and/or activity. Additionally, the induced deficiency state is likely to increase the toxicity of the xenobiotic. This complex interaction is exemplified by the following example. Osteoporosis is a disease related to low Ca, while osteomalacia results from vitamin D deficiency. Phosphorus deficiency or high concentrations of aluminum or cadmium will also result in osteomalacia. Copper deficiency also increases bone metabolism and can lead to increased fractures. Excess fat-soluble vitamin A will reduce the absorption by competition with the other fat-soluble vitamins. Therefore, excess vitamin A may produce a deficiency in vitamin D and loss of bone mineral density. Excess vitamin D will lead to calcification of organs leading to mental disturbances (simplicity) and congenital heart disease (Hirota and Hirota, 2006). In this case, the switch from nutrient to toxicant depends on how the compound disrupts the balance of nutrients via absorption or action that leads to alterations in physiology or cellular homeostasis that becomes pathological rather than beneficial.

Overnutrition/Pharmacologic or Toxic Concentrations of Nutrients

Toxicity may also be observed in overnutrition. When does the toxicology biphasic curve indicate that intake of nutrients moves up from undernutrition to overnutrition? Clearly, too little of a nutrient or nutrients leads to deficiency states. This led to the development of RDAs, which now are called daily reference intakes (RDIs). However, these indicate how much is minimally needed to prevent clear deficiency states and do not consider stress, toxin exposure, genetic sensitivity, and so forth. A toxicologist might say that the point at which the morbidity curve increases due to excess nutrients is when a pharmacological or toxicological dose level is achieved. However, some nutritionists believe that most of the early signs of toxicity are reversible for most nutrients. Accordingly, excess nutrients exceeding the RDA or RDI in a stressed society exposed to toxicants and trying to prevent normal aging should be accepted as supernutritional or chemopreventive. This controversy is exemplified by the vitamin, mineral, and herbal supplements available at retail stores. Many products far exceed the RDA and RDI and claim health benefits. This is especially dangerous for products that are micronutrients, such as the metals, or for accumulating hydrophobic compounds. This will be clarified for certain categories of nutrients and their toxicities resulting from overnutrition. While it is clear that excess calories will result in obesity, there is a difference in the risk of cardiovascular disease, cancer, and other conditions related to inflammation if omega-3 fatty acids are consumed versus omega-6 fatty acids. These polyunsaturated fatty acids may also protect against environmental toxicants (Watkins et al., 2007). Obesity is problematic for development

of diabetes mellitus, fatty organ development, and other conditions. However, if resveratrol is given to a mouse fed a calorie-unrestricted diet, it becomes obese but does not appear to develop the diseases of aging such as fatty liver. In the steatosis model, this appears to be due to the inhibitory effect of resveratrol on tumor necrosis factor alpha (TNFα) and the promotion of antioxidant activities (increased superoxide dismutase, glutathione peroxidase, and catalase and decreased nitric oxide synthase in liver cells of the resveratrol group; Bujanda et al., 2008). This validates that it is just as important to know how overnutrition is achieved as the fact that it is accomplished via excess consumption of a nutrient or nutrients.

Fat-Soluble Vitamins

Excess fat-soluble vitamins will achieve toxicity. However, it is less obvious that toxicants or medications that lead to acute renal failure can also by lack of elimination lead to hypervitaminosis A (Lipkin and Lenssen, 2008). In a similar manner, the elderly human who takes in excess vitamin A supplementation has lower kidney function and experiences lower immune cell function as a result of vitamin A toxicity (Wardwell et al., 2008). Vitamin A toxicity must assume the entire retinoid signaling system that is involved in control of cell differentiation, proliferation, and apoptosis. Retinoid signal transduction occurs through the retinoic acid receptors (RARs) and the retinoid X receptors (RXRs) that work as RXR/RAR heterodimers or RXR/RXR homodimers. These receptors are ligand-dependent transcriptional regulators that inhibit transcription in the absence of the ligands and increase transcription in the presence of ligand binding. These effects are mediated through the aid of recruited coregulators that affect the acetylation of histones. The recruitment of corepressors NCoR and SMRT forms a complex with histone deacetylase (HDAC), resulting in increased HDAC activity. Ligand binding to the vitamin A receptors results in increased histone acetylase activity via recruitment of coactivators. RARs bind both all-*trans* retinoic acid (ATRA) and its 9-*cis* isomer, while RXRs only are stimulated by 9-*cis* retinoic acid. The vitamin A receptors' functions may be impeded by polycyclic aromatic hydrocarbons binding to the AH receptor (Benísek et al., 2008). Cells that are likely affected by excess vitamin A are embryonic/fetal cells, epithelial cells, immune cells, cells of the eye, and reproductive cells. Hypervitaminosis A has been known to cause embryotoxicity and developmental defects.

As indicated earlier, certain environmental pollutants can affect retinol concentrations and/or interfere with functions that are associated with vitamin A toxicity. Retinol plasma concentrations are elevated in frogs exposed to a breakdown product of DDT (p,p'-DDE), rats or mice exposed to TCDD, ducklings exposed to PCB 77, rats exposed to PCB 156 and 169, and juvenile sturgeon exposed to estradiol. Retinol concentrations drop and metabolism increases in trout exposed to PCBs (Novák et al., 2008). Certain species' livers such as that of the polar bear have extreme levels of vitamin A that when consumed cause hypervitaminosis A (Russell, 1967). Because vitamin A stores in the liver, hepatotoxicity including severe fibrosis, signs of portal hypertension, and marked hyperplasia of Ito cells results from vitamin A excess (Castaño et al., 2006). Vitamin A toxicity not only influences brain development, but apparently also affects behavior in adult humans. Other species, such as the zebrafish, show neuronal cell apoptosis in the presence of excess retinoic acid (Parng et al., 2007). In dogs, marmoset monkeys, and foxes, the kidney is also a storage site and possible target of excess vitamin A (Penniston and Tanumihardjo, 2006). Certain medications have been developed based on the retinoids. One such medication is isotretinoin that is used to treat acne based on the epithelial cell action of excess vitamin A. This medication can cause severe birth defects and also may cause psychiatric symptoms or suicidal thoughts (O'Donnell, 2004). Isotretinoin also shows another aspect of vitamin A toxicity—musculoskeletal alterations such as skeletal lesions, rheumatologic changes, and enthesopathy (pathologic, occasionally painful modifications at the insertion sites or entheses of tendons, ligaments, and articular capsules into bone; Stitik et al., 1999).

Vitamin D toxicity has been described by various authors (Chesney, 1989; Leu et al., 2008).

The articles cited here represent a nutritional journal and an endocrine journal. This is due to the view that vitamin D is both a vitamin and a prohormone that is converted by the liver and then the kidney enzyme to 1,25-dihydroxycholecalciferol (1,25[OH]$_2$ vitamin D3, Calcitriol), the active metabolite. The cellular or systemic toxicity associated with vitamin D excess relates to hypercalcemia. Azotemia (abnormal buildup of nitrogenous wastes such as creatinine and urea) and mild hypokalemia (kidney polyuria induction) appear to be a result of cellular disruptions. Toxicity to vascular cells and also the induction of apoptosis, G_0/G_1 arrest, differentiation induction, and modulating growth factor–mediated signaling make excess vitamin D both harmful to regular proliferating cells, but therapeutic in its antiproliferative actions on breast, lung, colorectal, and prostate cancer cells (Trump et al., 2006). The whole organism may experience vitamin D toxicity as feeding problems, irritability, lassitude, poor weight gain, and neurological problems including increased deep tendon reflexes. Bone resorption also results from the untoward effects of high calcium concentrations. This can lead to bone necrosis (Chesney, 1989). Another hypothesis for vitamin D toxicity is that it interferes with vitamin K similar to the medication warfarin. Vitamin K, other than its role in coagulation, aids nervous system function and prevents bone loss and calcification of the peripheral soft tissues. This hypothesis is further supported by the protective action of vitamin A against vitamin D toxicity, as vitamin A helps prevent toxicity of vitamin D by decreasing the expression of vitamin K–dependent proteins sparing vitamin K (Masterjohn, 2007).

The study of vitamin E toxicity must begin with an understanding of what defines vitamin E. Where the overwhelming studies only concentrate on α-tocopherol, natural vitamin E encompasses eight distinct molecules: α-, β-, γ-, and δ-tocopherols and α-, β-, γ-, and δ-tocotrienols. This is important for nutrition and for toxicity. Nanomolar concentrations of α-tocotrienol, but not α-tocopherol, are protective against neurodegeneration. The relative potency and toxicity of each form of vitamin E must be ascertained to assess what are nutritional, pharmacologic, and toxic doses of this antioxidant (Sen et al.,

2007). The predominant form of vitamin E in the diet without vitamin supplementation is γ-tocopherol at 2.5 times that of α-tocopherol. The γ-tocopherol form is an anti-inflammatory due to its inhibition of cyclooxygenase 2 (COX2) and prevention of prostaglandin E_2 (PGE_2) formation, which α-tocopherol does not do. The chemical structures of γ-tocopherol and other tocols are displayed in **Figure 12-2**. Note that the γ-tocopherol has an unsubstituted (-H) position on its benzene ring. This allows it, but not α-tocopherol, to react with reactive nitrogen species (RNS), including peroxynitrite (forms 5-nitro-γ-tocopherol). Macrophages form peroxynitrite due to their generation of ROS and reaction with stable nitric oxide radicals during the inflammatory process. This is increased by cigarette smoking, which yields twice the 5-nitro-γ-tocopherol. The anti-inflammatory action of γ-tocopherol also appears to explain its connection to cardiovascular disease. Unfortunately, supplements of vitamin E are usually of the α-tocopherol form. Humans who consume more than 200 IU daily of vitamin E supplements (i.e., 400 IU and above of α-tocopherol)

are at a greater risk of myocardial infarctions and other inflammatory-mediated problems due to decreased concentrations of γ-tocopherol. For example, a short duration of a high dose of vitamin E supplements (400 IU three times a day for 2 months) increases plasma α-tocopherol by 200–400% and decreases γ-tocopherol to 30–50% in unsupplemented humans. Although excess supplementation with vitamin E may yield benefits in antioxidant protection from toxicants that cause apoptosis or necrosis (Tannetta et al., 2008) and in macular degeneration or diabetic retinopathy (Bartlett and Eperjesi, 2008), this practice can lead to more inflammatory damage and also induce premature membrane rupture during pregnancy (Spinnato et al., 2008).

Vitamin K consists of two forms, namely phylloquinone (vitamin K_1, or simply K_1) and the menaquinones (vitamin K_2, or simply K_2). K_1 is converted into vitamin K_2 (MK4, menaquinone-4) and accumulates in tissues other than the liver. Menadione (2-methyl-1,4-naphthoquinone) is a catabolic product of vitamin K that is a probable intermediate in the synthesis of MK4, which is found in the arterial

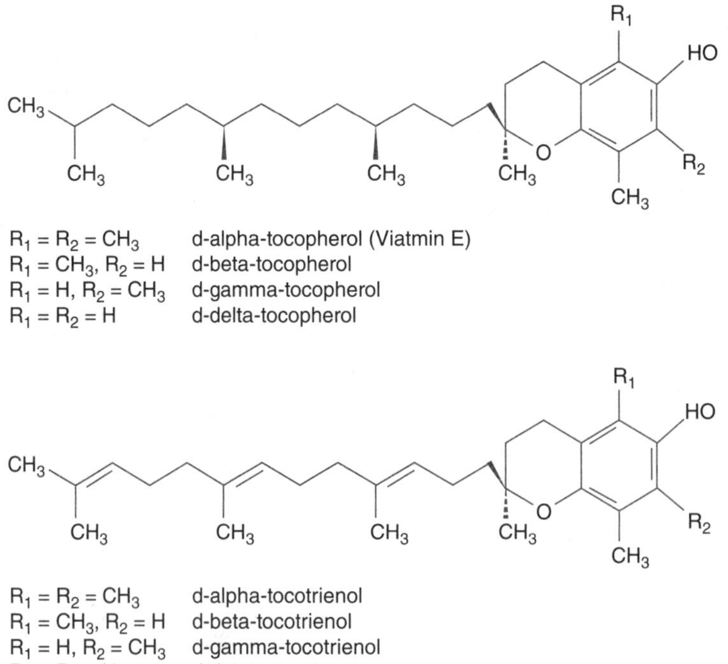

R₁ = R₂ = CH₃   d-alpha-tocopherol (Viatmin E)
R₁ = CH₃, R₂ = H   d-beta-tocopherol
R₁ = H, R₂ = CH₃   d-gamma-tocopherol
R₁ = R₂ = H   d-delta-tocopherol

R₁ = R₂ = CH₃   d-alpha-tocotrienol
R₁ = CH₃, R₂ = H   d-beta-tocotrienol
R₁ = H, R₂ = CH₃   d-gamma-tocotrienol
R₁ = R₂ = H   d-delta-tocotrienol

FIGURE 12-2 The Chemical Structures of the Tocols

vessel wall. It is difficult to find problems with high vitamin K intake as a nonprescription supplement. People with chronic liver disease will show cutaneous cell reactions around the site of injection of supplemental vitamin K (Bullen et al., 1978). Vitamin K's interference with the anticoagulant properties of warfarin or warfarin-induced arterial calcification is one negative and one positive side of the same interaction (Schurgers et al., 2007). Toxicity of vitamin K analogs has been reported since the late 1950s. Menadione generates oxygen radicals that cause DNA damage without cancer (Cojocel et al., 2006). Menadione toxicity is enhanced by pretreatment of mouse L929 cells with 50 Hz magnetic fields. Apoptosis, as indicated by cells participating in sub G_1 events of the cell cycle, was affected by a 100-μT magnetic field for 24 hours (decreased proportion of sub G_1 cells and increased cells in G_2/M phase) followed by 150 μM menadione for 1 hour. With a 300-μT magnetic field, the proportion of cells in the G_1 phase decreased (Markkanen et al., 2008). This is important, because toxicologists are not only concerned with chemical interactions, but also physical irradiative injury as well. Menadione at concentrations that are not overtly toxic on their own may also make other compounds like cyanide more toxic. For example, 20 μM menadione for 1 hour reduces rhodanese activity by 33%, 3-mercaptopyruvate sulfurtransferase by 20%, as well as the level of sulfane sulfur by about 23% and glutathione by 12% due to oxidative stress in U373 cells (Wróbel and Jurkowska, 2007).

Water-Soluble Vitamins

Vitamin C (ascorbic acid) is a beneficial antioxidant water-soluble vitamin. As such, concerns about bioaccumulation are not the same as for fat-soluble vitamins. Excess vitamin C is well tolerated up to doses (> 1 g) that would be toxic for many other substances. However, Nobel laureate Linus Pauling among others has encouraged mega-dosing of this vitamin (Pauling, 1970). High concentrations of sodium ascorbate prevent the biosynthesis of nitrosamines in the gastrointestinal tract from nitrates and nitrites in the diet and cancers that might result from sodium nitrite, ethylurea, and other similar compounds (Rustia, 1975). Although there were concerns of gastrointestinal disturbances by taking pharmacological doses of vitamin C, only mild gastrointestinal disturbances and diarrhea from the osmotic influence of unabsorbed ascorbic acid have been demonstrated clinically (Hathcock et al., 2005). However, the expected increase in iron absorption by ascorbic acid for humans with hemochromatosis warrants concern for hypersensitive populations (Herbert, 1999). Although vitamin C supplementation decreases cadmium-induced anemia in rats without affecting iron or cadmium concentrations in the liver (Fox and Fry, 1970), ascorbate may reduce Cu^{2+} to Cu^+, which is an oxidation state of copper that is less well absorbed (Lönnerdal, 1996). This is not the reason ascorbic acid decreases fulminant hepatitis in copper-accumulating Long Evans Cinnamon rats. Instead, the antioxidant role of vitamin C appears to play the key protective role in this animal model of Wilson's disease (Hawkins et al., 1995). The flipside of ascorbic acid's reducing power is its toxicity through diminishing high-altitude resistance in humans (Schrauzer et al., 1975). Extremely high (i.e., 80 g) intake of vitamin C also promotes the sensitivity to oxidation and hemolysis in the case of humans with a glucose-6-phosphate dehydrogenase deficiency (Rees et al., 1993). One of the most critical problems related to excess ascorbate is the acute renal failure associated with intrarenal oxalate crystal deposition (McHugh et al., 2008). Despite these and other hypothetical toxic concerns (e.g., systemic conditioning, uricosuria, vitamin B_{12} destruction, and mutagenicity), healthy cells and humans appear to tolerate high concentrations of vitamin C very well (Diplock, 1995; Rivers, 1989).

Thiamin (vitamin B_1) toxicity is only due to a hypersensitivity reaction as far as any scientific reports can determine. Thiamin may prevent ethylene glycol toxicity via prevention of the metabolic products (acidosis with anion gap) such as toxic oxalates (Andreelli et al., 1993). It is used in a "coma cocktail" with dextrose, oxygen, and the opiate antagonist naloxone due to the perceived low toxicity of this combination (Bartlett, 2004).

Riboflavin (vitamin B_2) toxicity is not considered a problem in human cells. Riboflavin through the activation of NADPH-flavin reductase aids in the reduction of methemoglobin caused by nitrite oxidation in human erythrocytes deficient in NADH-cytochrome b_5 reductase in the presence of glucose or 2-deoxy-D-glucose, but not lactate (Matsuki et al., 1978). However, the generation of hydrogen peroxide in the presence of light irradiation in cultured rat lens cells is enhanced by the presence of riboflavin (Jernigan, 1985).

Pantothenic (vitamin B_5) acid toxicity is minimal based on a lack of evidence of untoward effects. This vitamin accomplishes its protective actions on ototoxicity induced by the cancer cross-linking medication cisplatin (Ciges et al., 1996) or the antibiotic kanamycin (Moïseenok, 1984) via its role in mitochondrial energy production through the formation of coenzyme A.

Pyridoxine (vitamin B_6) toxicity is most problematic via a severe sensory neuropathy characterized by necrosis of dorsal root ganglion sensory neurons and degeneration of peripheral and central sensory projections. The neurons with large diameters appear to be the most sensitive (Perry et al., 2004). Pyridoxine causes histopathological changes in the rat testes (i.e., degeneration of germinal epithelial cells) and decreased sperm motility at doses exceeding 250 mg/kg for greater than 4 weeks of treatment (Tsutsumi et al., 1995). Vitamin B_6 has also been reported to cause subepidermal vesicular dermatosis (Bässler, 1989). Pyridoxine interferes with the action of levodopa in the treatment of Parkinson's disease through the formation of a Schiff-base with the medication followed by a non-enzymatic decarboxylation reaction. Similar reactions inactivate both the excess vitamin B_6 and medications such as the copper chelator penicillamine used in the treatment of Wilson's disease and the anti-arrhythmic agent quinidine. Pyridoxine is also a protective agent against isoniazid-induced convulsions, monosodium glutamate reactions of humans deficient in glutamic oxaloacetic transaminase (Ebadi et al., 1982), Gyromitra mushroom or false morel (monomethylhydrazine) poisoning, hydrazine exposure, and ethylene glycol poisoning (converts glyoxylic acid into glycine; Lheureux et al., 2005).

Cyanocobalamin (vitamin B_{12}) toxicity appears mainly via enhancing the cytotoxicity of other compounds used as antioxidants, such as vitamin C or thiols. Ascorbic acid in combination with cyanocobalamin generates hydrogen peroxide. Catalase can decrease the toxicity of this combination due to its metabolism of H_2O_2. Dithiothreitol in combination with vitamin B_{12} increases the formation of hydrogen peroxide. This leads to oxidative stress, lysosome destabilization, and DNA lesions and starts apoptotic mechanisms involving the activation of caspase-3 and release of cytochrome c. The oxidative burst was not prevented by iron chelation (deferoxamine and phenanthroline), but these chelators did reduce the genotoxicity and cytotoxicity (Solovieva et al., 2008). Although vitamin B_{12} and folic acid have been associated with increased prostate cancer risk (Hultdin et al., 2005), cyanocobalamin conversely shows protective effects against hepatic fibrosis induced by dimethylnitrosamine as indicated by the reduced expression of alpha-smooth muscle actin and heat-shock protein 47 (Isoda et al., 2008). The key role this nutrient plays in methylation reactions along with folic acid and synthesis of nucleic acids has been reported since the early 1950s, so its roles in both cellular function and cancer treatment continues to be of key interest (Gupta et al., 2008).

Biotin toxicity has not been observed despite supplementation in humans. It is of interest that there is an inverse relationship between plasma total lipid, cholesterol or phospholipid, and biotin status in inbred BHE rats. The obesity in BHE rats appears to be related to a reducing environment (i.e., accumulation of NADH) that is reversed by biotin injections and promotion of oxidative pathways (decreased pyruvate and lactate; Marshall et al., 1976). Pregnant rats injected with 10 mg biotin/100 g body weight at post-implantation stage (days 14 and 15 post-fertilization) inhibits fetal and placental growth with an accompanying decrease in uterine and placental glycogen, RNA, protein, and glucose-6-phosphate dehydrogenase activity. Hepatic G-6-PDH also decreases. This is reversed by estrogen supplementation but not by progesterone. This suggests that excess biotin causes an estrogen deficiency in the rat (Paul and

Duttagupta, 1976). The human implications of this result are unclear.

Folic acid (pteroylglutamic acid) neurotoxicity appears similar to that of thiamine (B$_1$) if injected directly into the cerebrospinal fluid of animals, inducing seizures and excitation. However, human neurotoxicity is rarely reported (Snodgrass, 1992). It is of importance to cancer chemotherapy that a metabolite of folic acid, folinic acid, increases the cytotoxic action of the cancer chemotherapy medication 5-fluorouracil (5-FU; Hartenstein et al., 1988), which inhibits thymidine monophosphate synthesis. This appears to be a result of 5,10-methylene tetrahydrofolate locking thymidylate synthase in an inhibited state in the presence of 5-FU (Showalter et al., 2008). Similarly, the methyltetrahydrofolate metabolite of folic acid is elevated in vitamin B$_{12}$ deficiency, which as indicated earlier results in neurotoxicity. There has been some suggestion that methyltetrahydrofolate is the toxic folate that causes neuronal destruction in a manner similar to the neurotoxic and stimulatory red marine alga *Digenea simplex* product kainic acid or Huntington's disease (Brennan et al., 1981). Folic acid also causes renal enlargement and acute renal failure. The enlargement of the kidney is associated with a direct inhibition of 5′-phosphodiesterase 16 hours following administration to rats and rebound stimulation of activity at 72 hours (Gaddis et al., 1982).

Choline, inositol, and p-aminobenzoic acid are not true essential vitamins, but may be considered more controversially as conditional B vitamins in that they are essential to animals other than humans, but may have some requirements under special conditions (Hathcock, 1982). Choline, a component of phosphatidylcholine or lecithin, toxicity appears to have some detrimental effect on male rat reproduction as indicated by decreased pachytene spermatocytes following 24 days of 25-mg doses (Vachhrajani et al., 1993). Intraperitoneal 50-mg doses of choline chloride (5 days per week for a total of 40 doses) produces lung lesions, including peripheral nodules of small cells, neoplastic bronchiolar epithelium, carcinomatous lesions, and changes in the pleural surface by 680 days in treated guinea pigs. Addition of asbestos fibers intraperitoneally results in synergistic enhancement of lesions of lung cancer (Sahu, 1989). Because phospholipids are important parts of cell signaling pathways in cancer cell–endothelial cell interaction, scientists have to consider both the direct toxicity of choline and the presence of phosphatidylcholine (PC) or the activity of cholinephosphotransferase (terminal enzyme in PC synthesis) and c-*fos* protein expression pathways as measures of breast cancer as induced by dimethylbenz(*a*)anthracene (Sinha Roy et al., 2008). Inositol seems to be well tolerated in humans, although inositol phosphates appear to inhibit uptake of zinc and iron by human intestinal cells (Han et al., 1994). The key interaction of the signaling molecule inositol 1,4,5-triphosphate (IP3) in calcium release should be considered with regard to calcium toxicity from apoptosis to necrosis (Rasmussen et al., 1990). Para-aminobenzoic acid (PABA), which has been used in older formulations of sunscreens, has literature from the 1940s and 1950s indicating both possible endocrine toxicity (Sullivan and Archdeacon, 1947) and allergic dermatitis (Greenwood, 1951). However, PABA is usually well tolerated in excess amounts and is protective against the toxicity of *cis*-diamminedichloroplatinum(II) in rats via its reaction with an aquated form of this toxic cross-linking reagent and its ability to reduce renal excretion of the platinum (Esposito et al., 1995).

Minerals

Ca excess not only calcifies organs and leads to apoptotic and necrotic mechanisms as discussed earlier, but also calcium loading in the heart and depressed repolarizing currents induce afterpolarizations and ventricular arrhythmias (Lazzara, 1988). Also, reperfusion injury following hypoxia in heart cells is mediated in part by excess calcium (Wang et al., 2007).

Iron overload has led to deaths especially in children who consume large quantities of iron-supplemented vitamins. Treatments involve both iron chelation by deferoxamine and exchange transfusion (Carlsson et al., 2008). The hepatotoxicity of iron involves the formation of hemosiderin rather than ferritin iron, which is a relatively nontoxic form (Bonkovsky,

1991). Administration of dicyclopentadienyl iron or ferrocene to mice shows the hepatonecrosis as measured by plasma alanine aminotransferase activity and the fibrosis as increased hepatic hydroxyproline content. Liver siderosis is indicated by the increased lipid peroxidation product malondialdehyde (Valerio and Petersen, 2000). Iron toxicity in the liver also appears to be a function of the iron particle size that determines the surface iron to core iron ratios (Bovell et al., 2009).

Phosphorus excess is related to calcium homeostasis. Treatment of calcium and phosphorus imbalances that occur with age or other factors leading to end-stage renal disease has had its own complications regarding bone mineralization. If calcium and phosphate are low, aluminum may start to be deposited into the bone (Brunier, 1994). The assumptions that growth will not be affected by an excess amount of a potentially limiting nutrient like phosphorus are not justified and miss harmful nutrient interactions (Boersma and Elser, 2006). Excess phosphate had a small effect on eggshell production in the laying hen likely due to the decreased intestinal availability of calcium (Boorman and Gunaratne, 2001). The main concern for excess phosphorus in healthy animals is the excretion of phosphorus and environmental eutrophication rather than direct toxicity to the animal or human. There appears to be some benefit from calcium and phosphorus (as well as iron, zinc, and copper) against lead poisoning (Levander, 1979).

It is well known that excess sodium causes dehydration and can lead to high blood pressure in humans and other animals. However, the acidosis that results from excess sodium chloride intake appears to increase bone resorption (Frings-Meuthen et al., 2008). Excess sodium chloride in spontaneously hypertensive rats increases superoxide generation and the activity of NADPH oxidase in the brain cortex and hippocampus. This indicates that blood pressure increases and oxidative stress both appear to increase the development of stroke (Kim-Mitsuyama et al., 2005). Excess sodium in the presence of D-aldosterone infusion (0.75 µg/hr sc) or deoxycorticosterone acetate (DOCA) administration (100 mg/kg/wk sc) in

the uninephrectomized rat results in myocardial fibrosis (Brilla and Weber, 1992). There is also a positive correlation between excess sodium intake and gastric cancer (Battarbee and Meneely, 1978).

Potassium excess is more dangerous, but is still hard to obtain with normal kidney function. It is associated with hyperkalemia. The heart develops abnormal electrocardiograms (ECGs). Muscle weakness and ascending paralysis occur. Nausea, vomiting, paralytic ileus, and local mucosal necrosis can lead to perforation of the gastrointestinal tract (Saxena, 1989). Some compounds increase the chances of hyperkalemia, such as phenothiazine overdose (Garnier et al., 2008), angiotensin-converting enzyme (ACE) inhibitors (Howes, 1995), acute beta-blocker poisoning (Delacour et al., 1986), taking seeds containing the steroid cardenolide (cardiac glycosides such as digoxin; Eddleston and Haggalla, 2008), glyphosate-surfactant herbicide intoxication (Lee, Shih, et al., 2008), *Bufo bufo gargarizans* bufadienolides and bufotoxins steroid toad poisons (Barrueto et al., 2006; Cheng et al., 2006; Steyn and van Heerden, 1998), and the antifreeze additive ethylene glycol (Hylander and Kjellstrand, 1996). The mechanisms for hyperkalemia include increased intake of potassium salts, inhibiting the $3Na^+$, $2K^+$-ATPase by cardiac glycosides, disrupted intermediate metabolism by cyanide, activation of K^+ channels by fluoride, and the presence of acidosis and muscle wasting especially in induced kidney failure (Bradberry and Vale, 1995). Alternatively, hyperkalemia can complicate the toxicity of other agents such as 3,4-methylenedioxymethamphetamine (ecstasy; Raviña et al., 2004).

Sulfur is usually provided by the amino acids methionine, cysteine, and taurine. Methionine deficiency leads to decreased protein synthesis and DNA hypomethylation (in concert with decreased folate), which is indicated as a risk factor in cancer formation. Polymorphisms of the transmethylation and transsulfuration pathways or hepatic dysfunction can lead to excess methionine concentrations as can excess intake in apparently normal infants. This can result in brain edema. Cysteine deficiency reduces GSH concentrations, which is critical in maintaining the redox states of cells and detoxication reactions. Ultrahigh doses of N-acCys have led to epileptic seizures and death (overdose with 2450 mg/kg N-acCys in 11.5 h instead of 208 mg/kg). Taurine deficiency can result in neuronal and particularly retinal dysfunctions. There have been no reports of toxic effects of taurine up to 1000 mg/L in energy drinks (van de Poll et al., 2006).

Hypermagnesemia is characterized by lethargy, confusion, arrhythmias, and muscle weakness known as quadriparesis (Moe, 2008). It is not an easy state to obtain without kidney damage and excess consumption of magnesium. However, patients with congestive heart failure have increased mortalities due to hypermagnesemia caused by excessive antacid and laxative use (Corbi et al., 2008). Excess magnesium also causes hypotension that reverses only after intravenous calcium and peritoneal dialysis (Mordes et al., 1975).

Manganese excess is associated with brain abscesses (Kumar et al., 2008), Parkinsonian-like symptoms accompanied by behavioral changes, and rarely seizures (Hsieh et al, 2007). Hepatic encephalopathy is usually associated with high ammonia levels resulting from liver cirrhosis induced by chronic excessive use of ethanol, psychoactive medications, and benzodiazepines. However, manganese chelation may be of benefit, indicating some role for hypermanganesemia in this link between hepatic damage and brain cell dysfunction (Dbouk and McGuire, 2006). It is of interest that most of the manganese in circulation is associated with the erythrocyte and can't be correlated with plasma concentrations, as most medicines and toxins are monitored (Smith et al., 2007).

Copper toxicity is frequently balanced by zinc, and imbalances in either decreases the status of the other. Liver damage and photosensitization secondary to hepatotoxicity was noted in cattle fed excess copper (Dawson and Laven, 2007). The hepatotoxicity of copper in the Long Evans Cinnamon rat, which accumulate copper similar to Wilson's disease in humans, is accompanied by increased polyploidy, delayed mitotic progression, and decreased nuclear protein phosphatase-1 (PP-1) activity (Yamada et al., 1998). Excess copper also leads to neurotoxicity

dependent on formation of a copper-dopamine complex that results in dopamine oxidation to aminochrome, dopamine-dependent copper uptake, and a one-electron reduction of adrenochrome (Paris et al., 2001).

Zinc is necessary for cell-mediated immunity. However, excess zinc is mostly toxic due to its ability to decrease copper status (i.e., reduced superoxide dismutase, ceruloplasmin, and cytochrome c oxidase; altered immunity; higher plasma free cholesterol; and high-density lipoprotein [HDL] cholesterol as well as HDL apolipoproteins; Lefevre et al., 1985). On its own, it is difficult to consume an amount of zinc that is lethal. There is an exception for pregnant animals, because zinc toxicity may be manifested by developmental defects during the embryonic period or embryolethality (Maret and Sandstead, 2006).

Selenosis can cause hepatic damage, skin and hair (loss) alterations, brittle fingernails, and foul breath (dimethylselenide exhaled versus trimethylselenonium ion in the urine). This is opposite to its role as an antioxidant in selenium-dependent glutathione peroxidase that prevents a cardiomyopathy (Keshan disease) in combination with coxsackievirus (Alexander, 2007). Neurological lesions have been described in swine from excess selenium (Raisbeck, 2000). Aquatic birds show vacuolar degeneration in liver cells progressing to centrolobular and panlobular necrosis, nephrosis, apoptosis of pancreatic exocrine cells, hypermaturity and avascularity of contour feathers of the head with atrophy of feather follicles, lymphocytic necrosis and atrophy of lymphoid organs, and severe atrophy and degeneration of fat (Green and Albers, 1997). Excess selenium's chemoprevention of cancer appears to result from increased apoptosis induced by selenodiglutathione in oral cancer cells compared with normal oral mucosal cells. This metabolite of selenium is associated with the induction of the FAS ligand and activation of stress kinase signaling pathways such as the key Jun NH2-terminal kinase (JNK). Heme oxygenase is also induced. A pharmacologic chemopreventive agent, 1,4-phenylenebis(methylene)selenocyanate, similarly induces FAS ligand, heme oxygenase, and stress kinase pathways, but is not JNK-dependent and is not tumor selective. These two different selenium compounds indicate that how selenium affects the redox state of the cell is crucial in mediating its effects (Fleming et al., 2001).

Chromium toxicity has been observed from excess chromium picolinate used to induce weight loss. Anemia, thrombocytopenia, hemolysis, hepatotoxicity, and kidney failure can result from excess chromium intake (Cerulli et al., 1998). Chromium causes apoptosis through generation of ROS and via p53 (Rana, 2008). Cr(III) has been associated with deletion mutations and DNA strand breaks from the hydroxyl radical produced by the Fenton reaction. It also produces skeletal disorders and neurotoxicity. The $[Cr(salen)(H_2O)_2]^+$ complex is an efficient inhibitor of transcription factors–DNA complex formation and transcription (Raja and Nair, 2008). There is also evidence for direct DNA binding of Cr(III) (Beyersmann and Hartwig, 2008).

Molybdenum excess is best measured similar to manganese in whole blood. However, this trace mineral requires an additional level of sensitivity afforded by detection via neutron activation and inductively coupled plasmamass spectrometry (Chan et al., 1998). Molybdenum exists as molybdopterin for the maintenance of activities of the enzymes sulfite oxidase, xanthine oxidase, and aldehyde oxidase. Excesses of molybdenum are most likely in ruminants and result in extensive kidney damage, reproductive failure, growth depression, decreased hemoglobin (Hb) and hematocrit (Hct), and interference with copper metabolism. In humans, excess molybdenum appears to be associated with hyperuricemia and gout, but this is based on a study without controls or proper follow-up (Novotny and Turnlund, 2007).

Vanadium has been of interest not only as a trace mineral, but also for its antidiabetic, insulin-promoting action and for its chemotherapeutic effect against cancer. The antitumor effects are either due to the apoptosis and/or activation of tumor suppressor genes through inhibition of the protein tyrosine phosphatases and/or activation of the tyrosine phosphorylases. Vanadium compounds also inhibit metastases via preventing the induction

of intracellular adhesive molecules (Faneca et al., 2008). It is the inhibition of the protein phosphatases that appears to be linked to vanadium's cytotoxicity (Beyersmann and Hartwig, 2008).

Boron deficiency in plants affects root elongation, indoleacetic acid (IAA) oxidase activity, sugar translocation, carbohydrate metabolism, nucleic acid synthesis, pollen tube growth, membrane potential, plasmalemma-bound enzymes and ion fluxes across membranes, cytoskeletal proteins, accumulation of phenolics and polyamines, and nitrogen metabolism. Boron toxicity results in altered metabolism, reduced root cell division, lower leaf chlorophyll contents and photosynthetic rates, and decreased lignin and suberin levels (Camacho-Cristóbal et al., 2008). In animals, boron damages both reproduction and development. It appears to reduce prostate cancer via inhibiting NAD^+ and $NADP^+$ and mechanically induced release of stored Ca^{2+} (Barranco et al., 2008). Boron is a member of the metalloids that also include silicon, germanium, arsenic, antimony, and tellurium. The metalloids range from essential as is the case for boron in higher plants, beneficial as represented by silicon and boron for yeast growth or mammalian cells throughout the lifecycle (*Xenopus* abnormal development, embryolethality in zebrafish, and impaired preimplantation development in two-cell mice embryo in low boron medium; Nielsen, 2000), to highly toxic as arsenic and antimony. However, even the most toxic metalloid (i.e., arsenic) has had some beneficial effects in treating infections such as syphilis and certain cancers. As shown in **Figure 12-3**, the membrane channels represented by the major intrinsic proteins including water-channeling aquaporins and glycerol-channeling aquaglyceroporins mediate both the cellular uptake of metalloids and their extrusion and detoxication (Bienert et al., 2008). Boron toxicity, even for subacute administration, causes degeneration of proximal tubular cells of the rat kidney (Sabuncuoglu et al., 2006). Considering that boron appears to reduce ROS and decreases fulminant hepatic failure, boron's toxicity must be balanced against its beneficial effects (Pawa and Ali, 2006). Boron's effects are still controversial and are not universally

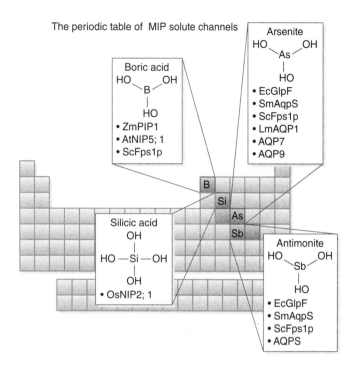

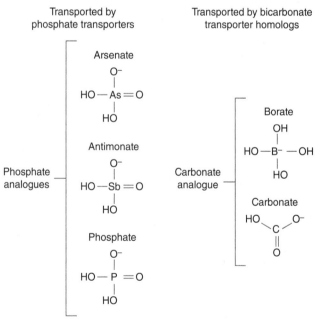

FIGURE 12-3 Transport Systems of Metalloids

Note: Metalloids form a group of chemical elements that exhibit characteristics between metals and non-metals — they occur naturally as poly-hydroxylated species. The tri-hydroxylated species arsenite [As(OH)$_3$] and antimonite [Sb(OH)$_3$] can be oxidized to form the respective oxyanions arsenate (H$_2$AsO$_4^-$) and antimonate (H$_2$SbO$_4^-$), whereas boric acid [B(OH)$_3$], as a weak Lewis acid, forms borate [B(OH)$_4^-$] at increasing pH. **(a)** The periodic table from the major intrinsic proteins (MIPs) point of view. The metalloid element group is highlighted in grey. Poly-hydroxylated uncharged species of some metalloids are channelled via MIPs and the chemical structures and the first pKa values are displayed for the four that are the primary focus of this article: boric acid (blue), silicic acid (green), arsenite (brown) and antimonite (red). The MIPs that facilitate the membrane diffusion of these compounds are listed below each structure. Abbreviations: *At, A. thaliana; Ec, E. coli; Lm, L. major; Os, O. sativa; Sc, S. cerevisiae; Sm, S. meliloti; Zm, Z. mays*. AQP7 and AQP9 are mammalian isoforms. AQP, aquaporin; Fps, fdp1 suppressor; GlpF, glycerol uptake factor; NIP, nodulin26-like intrinsic protein; PIP, plasma membrane intrinsic protein. **(b)** Oxyanions of metalloids transported by active transporters. The proximity between carbon and boron, as well as phosphorus and arsenic and antimony in the periodic system reflects the formation of chemically similar ions.

accepted as evidence for its inclusion as an essential mineral for animal cell function.

The discussion of iodine completes this section on mineral excess. Iodine excess by itself in humans is neither toxic to the thyroid nor to other organs. Japanese populations consume 5–14 times the upper safety limit of 1 mg set in the United States. In fact, molecular iodine (I_2) is effective in preventing hypothyroidism and fibrocystic breast disease, and iodine alone or in combination with progesterone has been demonstrated to shrink breast tumors in animals. Iodine toxicity may be of importance in contributing to Hashimoto's thyroiditis and Graves' disease, increasing nodule formation in euthyroid individuals taking more than 20 mg iodine or iodide, stimulating more cases of autoimmune thyroiditis, and may cause ocular damage (Patrick, 2008). Iodide in drinking water also becomes iodo-acids such as iodoacetic acid that is genotoxic in mammalian cells (Richardson et al., 2008). Iodinated radiocontrast media also yield kidney damage (Jost et al., 2008) and appear to be mutagenic (Deimling et al., 2009).

Protein Toxicity, Limiting Amino Acid Theory, Uremia

People are taking excess protein to build larger muscles. Their intake flies in the face of the ability of the gastrointestinal cells to absorb amino acids and the liver's ability to handle the excess nitrogen through synthesis of urea and exporting this nitrogenous waste to a functionally healthy kidney. Excessive protein can lead to hyperaminoacidemia, hyperammonemia, hyperinsulinemia nausea, diarrhea, and even death from a diet too high in lean protein known as the "rabbit starvation syndrome" (Bilsborough and Mann, 2006). Excess amino acids increase the catabolism of enzymes, signal the brain to alter food consumption and eating patterns, and may produce neurotransmitter differences by flooding the brain cells with precursors of those neurotransmitters. Plasma concentrations of amino acids can rise to toxic levels. Antagonisms arise for structurally related amino acids. Feeding limiting amino acids to a sufficiently fed animal makes other amino acids limiting, causing malnutrition that limits growth

(Munro, 1978). Certain animals may be able to overcome this problem with adaptation of their catabolic rate for the excess amino acids (Smith and Austic, 1978). Many cases of uremia involve kidney dysfunction. Other factors for chronic uremia include improper metabolism of proteins and amino acids that produce toxic metabolites and resulting negative nitrogen balance, rhabdomyolysis, decreased protein synthesis, and abnormally high intracellular free amino acid concentrations. There is usually an increase in plasma concentrations of conjugated amino acids, high levels of nonessential amino acids, and a decrease in essential amino acids. Metabolic perturbations and inter-organ exchange of amino acids may explain some of these effects. Encephalopathy may result from low tryptophan concentrations. Sulfur-containing amino acids are found in excess, including homocysteine (Fürst, 1989), which appears to be involved in atherogenesis of renal failure or other cardiovascular diseases (Perna et al., 2008).

Excess Carbohydrates

Excess carbohydrate intake may exacerbate metabolic syndrome, hyperinsulinemia, and increase insulin resistance. There is some concern about the glycemic index of various foods, how slowly glucose is released from carbohydrates, HDL-cholesterol, and the development of type 2 diabetes mellitus (Wolever, 2000). In combination with diabetes mellitus, hyperglycemia can lead to a number of detrimental outcomes for cardiovascular health, eye function, and the brain polyol pathway activity; neuronal structural changes; and impaired long-term spatial memory (Malone et al., 2008). There appears to be a link between hyperglycemia, ROS generation (via glycolysis, specific defects in the polyol pathway, uncoupling of nitric oxide synthase, xanthine oxidase, NAD(P)H oxidase, and advanced glycation), and mitochondrial/kidney dysfunction (Forbes et al., 2008).

Hyperlipidemia and Hypercholesterolemia

Apart from ethanol-induced fatty liver and hepatic cirrhosis, hyperlipidemia and hypercholesterolemia appear to induce liver steatosis, inflammatory changes, fibrosis, cirrhosis, and hepatocarcinoma. Liver failure may result from the last two factors, but the others do alter liver function in ways that are of importance to toxicologists who have to be concerned with the effects of medications and toxicants on hepatic cells (Pan et al., 2006). The effects of high lipid and cholesterol on the cardiovascular system should be obvious to all humans. The interactions of the toxicant N-nitrosodiethylamine and hypercholesterolemia are apparent in liver damage, liver lipid peroxidation, and fragility of erythrocytes (Mittal et al., 2006). Hypercholesterolemia also appears to induce atherosclerotic plaques similar to mechanisms involved in carcinogenesis via angiogenesis through increased vascular endothelial growth factor (VEGF) signaling (Kavantzas et al., 2006). It also appears that microcirculation changes as a result of excess cholesterol ingestion provoke decreases in nitric oxide, possibly through inactivation of NO via superoxide formation (Stokes et al., 2002).

Nucleic Acids

Nucleotide supplementation appears to decrease diarrhea and other symptoms of irritable bowel disease in humans, increase villi height and crypt depth of gastrointestinal cells of piglets, and may enhance immune cell function. However, constipation is increased with these viscous compounds (Dancey et al., 2006), and increased purine nucleotide synthesis or enhanced degradation may lead to excess uric acid production and gout. The cells affected are those associated with uric acid crystal formation (soft tissues, joints, and renal) and by increased free-radical formation and reduced synthesis of signal transducers as a result of purine degradation (García Puig and Mateos, 1994).

Naturally Occurring Toxicants in Food

Other than foodborne bacteria that most people usually associate with food poisoning, there are some natural products/contaminants in food that prove to be more toxic than infectious. That is the category under investigation here,

and it includes the usual toxicants important to the nutritional or food toxicologist.

Mycotoxins

Storage of food increases the possibility of mold formation. A listing of the important mold products that produce substantial toxicity in animal and human populations was determined in 1979 (International Programme on Chemical Safety, 1979). Cereal grains have been one large source of ochratoxigenic fungi produced by seven molds of the species *Penicillium* and six molds of the species *Aspergillus*. Ochratoxin A (R)-N-[(5-chloro-3,4-dihydro-8-hydroxy-3-methyl-1-oxo-1H-2-benzopyran-7yl)carbonyl]-L-phenyl-alanine) produces nephrotoxic, hepatotoxic, immunotoxic, teratogenic, and carcinogenic reactions in a number of species (Juan et al., 2008). Its mode of action is not abundantly clear, as there is no clear-cut evidence of DNA adduct formation or extensive ROS production. It may produce its genotoxic action via disruption of mitosis, yielding blocked or asymmetric cell division (Mally and Dekant, 2008). The furane and coumarin mycotoxins include the ochratoxins and aflatoxins. The aflatoxins have been described earlier as CYP-activated toxicants that form DNA adducts, cause cancer, and at high concentrations lead to liver damage and possibly failure due to fat infiltration, focal necrosis, and biliary hyperplasia. These effects may be prevented by high concentrations of a food preservative, butylated hydroxytoluene (BHT), and an antioxidant that inhibits ethoxy-resorufin O-deethylase (EROD) and methoxy-resorufin O-demethylase (CYP1A1 and CYP1A2 activities, respectively), but increases medication metabolism as indicated by the oxidation of nifedipine (Guarisco et al., 2008). Fruit of the varieties of apples, grapes, oranges, pears, and peaches are prone to having the cyclic lactone mycotoxin patulin (4-hydroxy-4H-furo {2, 3-C} pyron-2 {6H}-1; clavacin), which is produced by some species of *Penicillium*, *Aspergillus*, and *Byssochlamys*. Its topical genotoxicity is confirmed by a significant increase in the olive tail moment of the comet assay in mouse skin cells, significant G_1 and S-phase arrest, and induction of apoptosis as measured by annexin V and PI staining assay through a flow cytometer (Saxena et al., 2009). Zearalenone is another macrocyclic lactone associated with *Fusarium* contamination of corn products that has a high affinity for estrogen receptors, causing estrogenic effects in pigs and infertility and reduced milk production in cattle (Luongo et al., 2006). Alternariol (3,7,9-trihydroxy-1-methyl-6H-benzo[c] chromen-6-one) is a genotoxic mycotoxin formed by *Alternaria alternate* that causes DNA strand breaks through apparent inhibition of topoi-somerases I and II (Fehr et al., 2008).

Trichothecenes are another chemical class of mycotoxins produced by *Fusarium* infection of barley, corn, and wheat. Deoxynivalenol, or vomitoxin, is one of the type B trichothecene mycotoxins. The structure of trichothecenes is illustrated in **Figure 12-4**. Trichothecenes for the most part have a double bond at position C-9,10, a 12,13-epoxide ring, and some acetoxy and hydroxyl moieties. There are four types of trichothecenes (A-D) based on structural features. Oxygen at position C-8 defines the type A trichothecenes, such as T-2 (most potent mycotoxin; Dohnal et al., 2008) and HT-2 toxins. A carbonyl at C-8 indicates a Type B trichothecenes, such as the prevalent deoxynivalenol. A second epoxide group at C-7,8 or C-9,10 denotes a type C trichothecenes. A macrocyclic ring between C-4 and C-15 with two ester linkages is characteristic of type D trichothecenes. Trichothecenes in general and deoxynivalenol in particular affect immune cell function. At low concentrations, deoxynivalenol causes upregulation of transcription and post-transcription of chemokines, cytokines, and inflammatory mediator genes. High concentrations of trichothecenes induce apoptosis of leukocytes resulting in immune suppression. These agents also bind to ribosomes producing a "ribotoxic stress response." Quick activation of

mitogen-activated protein kinases via upstream activation of double-stranded RNA (dsRNA)–activated protein kinase (a serine/threonine protein kinase that can be normally activated by dsRNA or the cytokine interferon) and hematopoietic cell kinase (a nonreceptor–associated Src oncogene family kinase) yield this toxic response (Pestka, 2008).

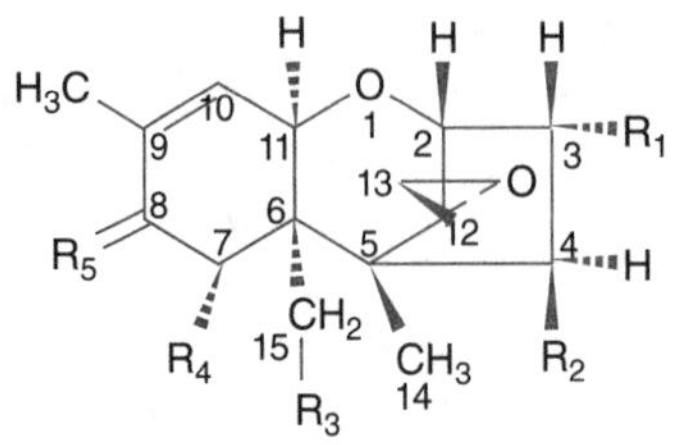

Fumonisins (eicosanoic carbocyclic esters) are another set of mycotoxins that are produced by *Fusarium* species. They affect both plant and animal species, producing fatal leukoencephalomalacia in horses and pulmonary edema and hepatic damage in pigs, and they are associated with human cancers and neural tube defects. Fumonisins interfere with sphingolipid metabolism through inhibition of ceramide synthesis. An extraction method has been developed to analyze the various fumonisins (B_1, B_2, and B_3), free sphingoid bases, and sphingoid base 1-phosphates to assess the impact of this class of mycotoxins (Zitomer et al., 2008). Moniliformin is another mycotoxin produced by *Fusarium* that is found as the sodium or potassium salt of 1-hydroxycyclobut-1-ene-3,4-dione. Its toxicity has been linked to inhibition of the enzymes pyruvate dehydrogenase, glutathione peroxidase, and glutathione reductase in heart cells. This changes free radical metabolism in the heart and may in combination with increased cardiac permeability lead to pathologies such as Keshan disease in humans.

Claviceps cyperi and *Claviceps purpurea* appear to be the major source for ergot alkaloids such as ergotamine, ergostine, and ergocristine that cause sleepy grass toxicosis in cattle by a similar mechanism to how lysergic acid diethylamide causes hallucinations in humans (decreased serotonin activity). Convulsive and gangrenous forms of ergotism are also found in humans and animals. The tremogens are indole trepenoids from ergot fungal species such as *Acremonium lolii* that cause neurotoxicity that induces shaking, hence the name of this class of mycotoxins (Hussein and Brasel, 2001).

Cyanide

There are many poisonous food items, such as the toxic natural licorice root and

FIGURE 12-4 The Structure of Trichothecenes

its glycyrrhizin that inhibits short-chain dehydrogenase reductases, mimicking mineralocorticoid-induced hypertensive action (Ghosh et al., 1994); truly poisonous plants such as those that harbor the belladonna alkaloids; poisonous and hallucinatory mushrooms; and poisonous animals such as the pufferfish. These are examined in more detail elsewhere, but it is worth looking at the intrinsic incidence of cyanide in foods. Cyanide inhibits oxidative phosphorylation and is responsible for the term *cyanosis*, which is associated with a bluish coloration due to hypoxic injury to animal tissues. Although some of the other toxicants found naturally in food denote a few species, 2500 plant species contain cyanogenic glucosides. These cyanide compounds taste bitter and can evolve hydrogen cyanide gas on tissue disruption. This defines them as phytoanticipins as a defense against herbivores. These compounds also serve as a nutrient storage form of nitrogen and sugar in plants that can be mobilized on demand at times of stress. Insect herbivores that preferentially feed on plants metabolize cyanogenic glucosides or store them in their own defense mechanisms against predation. Certain diplopods, chilopods, and insects can also synthesize these compounds on their own. In the organism *Zygaena filipendulae* (six-spot moth of the Lepidoptera order), cyanogenic glucosides are used in defense and in nitrogen metabolism, and the evolution of hydrogen cyanide is the gas used as part of the male attractant for mating (Zagrobelny et al., 2008). Modern North Americans and Western Europeans are not very cognizant of foods that contain these compounds, except for the peach pit and amygdalin. However, in Brazil and other parts of the world (Thailand, Nigeria, Democratic Republic of the Congo, and Indonesia, but especially in Africa) where the potato is not the key starch source, cassava (*Manihot esculenta*) of the family Euphorbiaceae has roots that are approximately 30% starch that can be cooked or made into flour, but raw cassava that has not been cooked or soaked contains toxic amounts of cyanogenic glucosides. The sweet or low-cyanogenic glucoside-containing varieties have as low as 20 mg cyanide/kg fresh roots. The bitter variety or those cassava roots harvested in drought

may contain 1 g cyanide/kg fresh roots. Fungal fermentation increases the protein and fat content while decreasing the cyanide content. This is especially true of the low-cyanide content cassava (Oboh and Oladunmoye, 2007).

Genetics and Nutrition/Nutritional Genomics

Sensitivity to toxicants is not just caused by genetics or nutrition; many times it is the result of a combination of both. The new field of nutritional genomics takes these factors into account. How this field intersects with toxicology is demonstrated by a set of workshops on nutrition-toxicology issues and genetics-toxicology topics. Nutrients influence the expression of genes. For example, polyunsaturated fatty acids (PUFA) upregulate oxidative gene expression via interaction of PUFA with the peroxisome proliferator activated receptor alpha (PPARα). PPARα is induced by PUFA, which coordinates with the lipid ligand–binding domain within the PPAR protein. PPARα then binds to a hexameric direct repeat sequence located in the 5′-flanking region of the genes that encode for lipid oxidative enzymes such as carnitine palmitoyltransferase-1 and acyl-CoA oxidase. PUFA also suppresses hepatic lipogenic gene expression through inhibition of endoplasmic reticulum proteolytic release of sterol regulatory element binding protein-1 and the DNA⁻ binding activity of the potent enhancing factor, Sp1. Amino acid nutrition/availability influences mRNA translation via up- or downregulation of the initiation of that process (binding of mRNA to the 40S ribosomal subunit followed by the 60S ribosomal subunit binding into a translationally competent 80 S ribosome). Zinc regulates the metal response element (MRE) transcription factor (MTF-1), which binds to the MREs of promoter for metallothionein. Zinc deficiency, on the other hand, causes induction of cholecystokinin and uroguanylin in small intestinal cells.

Cytochrome P450 (CYP) is of particular interest in the study of nutrients' interactions with genes and toxicants. Grilling meat produces heterocyclic amines that induce CYP1A2 and N-hydroxylation reactions followed by acetylation. Aflatoxin B_1 is activated and detoxified by CYP enzymes (3A4 and 1A2). One glass of grapefruit juice has enough furanocoumarins to inhibit CYP3A4 in a way that induces a 10-fold increase in AUC, which is important because dose–response in logarithmic. This could turn a medication into an overdose or alternatively result in 10-fold less toxicity for toxicants activated by this CYP isozyme. The popular herbal medicine St. John's wort has the opposite influence as an inducer of the same isozyme. In determining DNA damage as a result of oxidation by hydrogen peroxide, various antioxidants from kiwifruit, fried onions, and soya milk reduce the impacts as indicated by the comet assay. However, people who supplement with large doses of various antioxidants including β-carotene have shown no protection or just the opposite— increased cancer risk.

Caloric restriction appears to retard the aging process. One possible way this is accomplished is through reduced oxidative stress. Obesity leads to increased cardiovascular disease, diabetes mellitus, and the development of cancer that is augmented by other toxicants such as cigarette smoke. Ten percent of those who have diabetes mellitus have mutations in the mitochondrial genome. A sucrose-rich diet augments those with the mutations by decreasing adenosine triphosphate (ATP) synthesis efficiency, while vitamin A has the opposite effect. Folate intake has been linked to decreased risk of colorectal cancers. For that same cancer, diet and CYP play a role. Those people who consume well done meat and have rapid CYP1A2 and *N*-acetyltransferase 2 activity have more colorectal cancer. Genes and diet also affect breast cancer risk. MnSOD polymorphisms that would result in increased oxidative stress increased breast cancer risk especially in those premenopausal women who did not consume sources rich in the antioxidant vitamin C.

DNA microarray chips and transgenic and knockout mouse models are methods that are indicative of the role genetics and nutrition together play in causing sensitivities to toxicants but also possible protective mechanisms that may protect impacted cell populations, tissues,

and whole organisms (Archer et al., 2001). Using resources from diverse fields such as immunology, cell biology, and nutrition, toxicoproteomics has been measuring the global protein expression in tissue fluids such as plasma and tissues such as the liver to map the injury by model toxicants. By doing this research, it is hoped that better biomarkers of toxic injury will be discovered, toxicity signatures may be clarified under various conditions, and mechanisms of action more clearly described and understood (Merrick, 2008).

Questions

1. Why is nutritional toxicology the most important section of true toxicology in the current human population of the United States?

2. Why is ascorbic acid supplementation a good idea unless you are obese and eating a high-fat bacon or other high-fat meat product preserved with nitrates and nitrites?

3. Why does zinc deficiency result in problems with wound healing and ROS and increase heavy metal toxicity?

4. Why are metal-containing antacids problematic for Ca, Cu, folate, or phosphate, yet proton pump inhibitors and H_2 receptor antagonists result in less vitamin B_{12}? Why are the antacids also capable of yielding osteoporosis and osteomalacia (what is the difference)?

5. Vitamin A is a fat-soluble vitamin associated with normal vision. Why does its excess also produce birth defects, psychiatric effects, skin alterations, and liver toxicity, among other problems?

6. What mineral is associated with vitamin D toxicity?

7. What water-soluble vitamin shows toxicity in excess without any other compound assisting in its toxicity?

8. What does ferritin versus hemosiderin indicate in the liver?

9. Does diet or toxicants in food alter genes or gene expression?

References

Alexander J. 2007. Selenium. *Novartis Found Symp.* 282:143–149; discussion 149–153, 212–218.

Alsop D, Brown S, Van Der Kraak G. 2007. The effects of copper and benzo[a]pyrene on retinoids and reproduction in zebrafish. *Aquat Toxicol.* 82:281–295.

Andreelli F, Blin P, Codet MP, Fohrer P, Lambrey G, Massy Z. 1993. [Diagnostic and therapeutic management of ethylene glycol poisoning. Importance of crystalluria. Apropos of a case]. *Nephrologie.* 14:221–225.

Archer MC, Clarkson TW, Strain JJ. 2001. Genetic aspects of nutrition and toxicology: report of a workshop. *J Am Coll Nutr.* 20(2 Suppl):119–128.

Archer MC, Tannenbaum SR, Fan TY, Weisman M. 1975. Reaction of nitrite with ascorbate and its relation to nitrosamine formation. *J Natl Cancer Inst.* 54:1203–1205.

Barranco WT, Kim DH, Stella Jr SL, Eckhert CD. 2008. Boric acid inhibits stored Ca(2+) release in DU-145 prostate cancer cells. *Cell Biol Toxicol.* 25:309–320.

Bartlett D. 2004. The coma cocktail: indications, contraindications, adverse effects, proper dose, and proper route. *J Emerg Nurs.* 30:572–574.

Bartlett HE, Eperjesi F. 2008. Nutritional supplementation for type 2 diabetes: a systematic review. *Ophthalmic Physiol Opt.* 28:503–523.

Barrueto F Jr, Kirrane BM, Cotter BW, Hoffman RS, Nelson LS. 2006. Cardioactive steroid poisoning: a comparison of plant- and animal-derived compounds. *J Med Toxicol.* 2:152–155.

Bässler KH. 1989. Use and abuse of high dosages of vitamin B6. *Int J Vitam Nutr Res Suppl.* 30:120–126.

Battarbee HD, Meneely GR. 1978. The toxicity of salt. *CRC Crit Rev Toxicol.* 5:355–376.

Beattie O, Geiger J. 2005. *Frozen in time: the fate of the Franklin expedition.* Vancouver, British Columbia: Greystone Books.

Benísek M, Bláha L, Hilscherová K. 2008. Interference of PAHs and their N-heterocyclic analogs with signaling of retinoids in vitro. *Toxicol In Vitro.* 22:1909–1917.

Bienert GP, Schüssler MD, Jahn TP. 2008. Metalloids: essential, beneficial or toxic? Major intrinsic proteins sort it out. *Trends Biochem Sci.* 33:20–26.

Bilsborough S, Mann N. 2006. A review of issues of dietary protein intake in humans. *Int J Sport Nutr Exerc Metab.* 16:129–152.

Boersma M, Elser JJ. 2006. Too much of a good thing: on stoichiometrically balanced diets and maximal growth. *Ecology.* 87:1325–1330.

Bohn L, Meyer AS, Rasmussen SK. 2008. Phytate: impact on environment and human nutrition.

A challenge for molecular breeding. *J Zhejiang Univ Sci B.* 9:165–191.

Bonkovsky HL. 1991. Iron and the liver. *Am J Med Sci.* 301:32–43.

Boorman KN, Gunaratne SP. 2001. Dietary phosphorus supply, egg-shell deposition and plasma inorganic phosphorus in laying hens. *Br Poult Sci.* 42:81–91.

Bovell E, Buckley CE, Chua-Anusorn W, Cookson D, Kirby N, Saunders M, St Pierre TG. 2009. Dietary iron-loaded rat liver haemosiderin and ferritin: *in situ* measurement of iron core nanoparticle size and cluster structure using anomalous small-angle x-ray scattering. *Phys Med Biol.* 54:1209–1221.

Bradberry SM, Vale JA. 1995. Disturbances of potassium homeostasis in poisoning. *J Toxicol Clin Toxicol.* 33:295–310.

Bradman A, Eskenazi B, Sutton P, Athanasoulis M, Goldman LR. 2001. Iron deficiency associated with higher blood lead in children living in contaminated environments. *Environ Health Perspect.* 109:1079–1084.

Brennan MJ, van der Westhuyzen J, Kramer S, Metz J. 1981. Neurotoxicity of folates: implications for vitamin B12 deficiency and Huntington's chorea. *Med Hypotheses.* 7:919–929.

Brilla CG, Weber KT. 1992. Mineralocorticoid excess, dietary sodium, and myocardial fibrosis. *J Lab Clin Med.* 120:893–901.

Brunier GM. 1994. Calcium/phosphate imbalances, aluminum toxicity, and renal osteodystrophy. *ANNA J.* 21:171–177.

Bujanda L, Hijona E, Larzabal M, Beraza M, Aldazabal P, García-Urkia N, Sarasqueta C, Cosme A, Irastorza B, González A, Arenas JI Jr. 2008. Resveratrol inhibits nonalcoholic fatty liver disease in rats. *BMC Gastroenterol.* 8:40.

Bullen AW, Miller JP, Cunliffe WJ, Losowsky MS. 1978. Skin reactions caused by vitamin K in patients with liver disease. *Br J Dermatol.* 98:561–565.

Buu-Hoï NP, Hien DP. 1968. Potentiation of the anticoagulant effects of anti-vitamins K by 6-mercaptopurine. *Naturwissenschaften.* 55:134.

Beyersmann D, Hartwig A. 2008. Carcinogenic metal compounds: recent insight into molecular and cellular mechanisms. *Arch Toxicol.* 82:493–512.

Camacho-Cristóbal JJ, Rexach J, González-Fontes A. 2008. Boron in plants: deficiency and toxicity. *J Integr Plant Biol.* 50:1247–1255.

Canady RA, Coker RD, Egan SK, Krska R, Kuiper-Goodman T, Olsen M, Pestka J, Resnik S, Schlatter J. 2001. Deoxynivalenol. JECFA47. http://www.inchem.org/documents/jecfa/jecmono/v47je05.htm

Cannell JJ, Vieth R, Willett W, Zasloff M, Hathcock JN, White JH, Tanumihardjo SA, Larson-Meyer

DE, Bischoff-Ferrari HA, Lamberg-Allardt CJ, Lappe JM, Norman AW, Zittermann A, Whiting SJ, Grant WB, Hollis BW, Giovannucci E. 2008. Cod liver oil, vitamin A toxicity, frequent respiratory infections, and the vitamin D deficiency epidemic. *Ann Otol Rhinol Laryngol.* 117:864–870.

Carlsson M, Cortes D, Jepsen S, Kanstrup T. 2008. Severe iron intoxication treated with exchange transfusion. *Arch Dis Child.* 93:321–322.

Castaño G, Etchart C, Sookoian S. 2006. Vitamin A toxicity in a physical culturist patient: a case report and review of the literature. *Ann Hepatol.* 5:293–295.

Cavanagh JB. 1991. What have we learnt from Graham Frederick Young? Reflections on the mechanism of thallium neurotoxicity. *Neuropathol Appl Neurobiol.* 17:3–9.

Cerulli J, Grabe DW, Gauthier I, Malone M, McGoldrick MD. 1998. Chromium picolinate toxicity. *Ann Pharmacother.* 32:428–431.

Chan S, Gerson B, Subramaniam S. 1998. The role of copper, molybdenum, selenium, and zinc in nutrition and health. *Clin Lab Med.* 18:673–685.

Cheng CJ, Lin CS, Chang LW, Lin SH. 2006. Perplexing hyperkalaemia. *Nephrol Dial Transplant.* 21:3320–3323.

Cheng J, Yang Y, Ma J, Wang W, Liu X, Sakamoto M, Qu Y, Shi W. 2009. Assessing noxious effects of dietary exposure to methylmercury, PCBs and Se coexisting in environmentally contaminated rice in male mice. *Environ Int.* 35(3):619–625.

Chesney RW. 1989. Vitamin D: can an upper limit be defined? *J Nutr.* 119(12 Suppl):1825–1828.

Ciges M, Fernández-Cervilla F, Crespo PV, Campos A. 1996. Pantothenic acid and coenzyme A in experimental cisplatin-induced ototoxia. *Acta Otolaryngol.* 116:263–268.

Cojocel C, Novotny L, Vachalkova A. 2006. Mutagenic and carcinogenic potential of menadione. *Neoplasma.* 53:316–323.

Combet E, Paterson S, Iijima K, Winter J, Mullen W, Crozier A, Preston T, McColl KE. 2007. Fat transforms ascorbic acid from inhibiting to promoting acid-catalysed N-nitrosation. *Gut.* 56:1678–1684.

Combs GF Jr, Peterson FJ. 1983. Protection against acute paraquat toxicity by dietary selenium in the chick. *J Nutr.* 113:538–545.

Corbi G, Acanfora D, Iannuzzi GL, Longobardi G, Cacciatore F, Furgi G, Filippelli A, Rengo G, Leosco D, Ferrara N. 2008. Hypermagnesemia predicts mortality in elderly with congestive heart disease: relationship with laxative and antacid use. *Rejuvenation Res.* 11:129–138.

Dawson EB, Evans DR, Harris WA, Teter MC, McGanity WJ. 1999. The effect of ascorbic acid supplementation on the blood lead levels of smokers. *J Am Col Nutr.* 18:166–170.

Dawson C, Laven RA. 2007. Failure of zinc supplementation to prevent severe facial eczema in cattle fed excess copper. *N Z Vet J.* 55:353–355.

Dbouk N, McGuire BM. 2006. Hepatic encephalopathy: a review of its pathophysiology and treatment. *Curr Treat Options Gastroenterol.* 9:464–474.

Deimling LI, Machado FL, Welker AG, Peres LM, Santos-Mello R. 2009. Micronucleus induction in mouse polychromatic erythrocytes by an X-ray contrast agent containing iodine. *Mutat Res.* 672:65–68.

Delacour JL, Blanc PL, Wagschal G, Daoudal P. 1986. [Hyperkalemia in acute beta-blocker poisoning]. *Presse Med.* 15:1377.

Dancey CP, Attree EA, Brown KF. 2006. Nucleotide supplementation: a randomised double-blind placebo controlled trial of IntestAidIB in people with Irritable Bowel Syndrome [ISRCTN67764449]. *Nutr J.* 5:16.

Depeint F, Bruce WR, Shangari N, Mehta R, O'Brien PJ. 2006. Mitochondrial function and toxicity: role of B vitamins on the one-carbon transfer pathways. *Chem Biol Interact.* 163:113–132.

Dey SK, Nayak P, Roy S. 2001. Chromium-induced membrane damage: protective role of ascorbic acid. *J Environ Sci (China).* 13:272–275.

Diplock AT. 1995. Safety of antioxidant vitamins and beta-carotene. *Am J Clin Nutr.* 62(Suppl): 1510S–1516S.

Dohnal V, Jezkova A, Jun D, Kuca K. 2008. Metabolic pathways of T-2 toxin. *Curr Drug Metab.* 9:77–82.

Ebadi M, Gessert CF, Al-Sayegh A. 1982. Drug-pyridoxal phosphate interactions. *Q Rev Drug Metab Drug Interact.* 4:289–331.

Eddleston M, Haggalla S. 2008. Fatal injury in Eastern Sri Lanka, with special reference to cardenolide self-poisoning with Cerbera manghas fruits. *Clin Toxicol (Phila).* 46:745–748.

Elias SM, Hashim Z, Marjan ZM, Abdullah AS, Hashim JH. 2007. Relationship between blood lead concentration and nutritional status among Malay primary school children in Kuala Lumpur, Malaysia. *Asia Pac J Public Health.* 19:29–37.

Esposito M, Vannozzi M, Viale M, Pellecchia C, Civalleri D, Gogioso L. 1995. Effect of para-aminobenzoic acid on the pharmacokinetics and urinary excretion of cis-iamminedichloroplatinum(II) in rats. *Anticancer Res.* 15:2541–2547.

Faneca H, Figueiredo VA, Tomaz I, Gonçalves G, Avecilla F, Pedroso de Lima MC, Geraldes CF, Pessoa JC, Castro MM. 2008. Vanadium compounds as therapeutic agents: some chemical and biochemical studies. *J Inorg Biochem.* 103:601–608.

Fehr M, Pahlke G, Fritz J, Christensen MO, Boege F, Altemöller M, Podlech J, Marko D. 2008. Alternariol acts as a topoisomerase poison, preferentially affecting the IIalpha isoform. *Mol Nutr Food Res.* 53(4):441–451.

Fleming J, Ghose A, Harrison PR. 2001. Molecular mechanisms of cancer prevention by selenium compounds. *Nutr Cancer*. 40:42–49.

Flora SJS. 2009. Structural, chemical and biological aspects of antioxidants for strategies against metal and metalloid exposure. *Oxid Med Cell Longev*. 2:191–206.

Flora SJS, Tandon SK. 1986. Preventive and therapeutic effects of thiamine, ascorbic acid, and their combination on lead intoxication. *Acta Pharmacol Toxicol*. 58:374–378.

Forbes JM, Coughlan MT, Cooper ME. 2008. Oxidative stress as a major culprit in kidney disease in diabetes. *Diabetes*. 57:1446–1454.

Fox MR, Fry BE Jr. 1970. Cadmium toxicity decreased by dietary ascorbic acid supplements. *Science*. 169:989–991.

Frings-Meuthen P, Baecker N, Heer M. 2008. Low-grade metabolic acidosis may be the cause of sodium chloride-induced exaggerated bone resorption. *J Bone Miner Res*. 23:517–524.

Fürst P. 1989. Amino acid metabolism in uremia. *J Am Coll Nutr*. 8:310–323.

Gaddis RR, Louis-Ferdinand RT, Beuthin FC. 1982. Differential effects of folic acid on water content, protein and microsomal 5'-phosphodiesterase activity of the rat kidney. *Food Chem Toxicol*. 20:159–164.

García Puig J, Mateos FA. 1994. Clinical and biochemical aspects of uric acid overproduction. *Pharm World Sci*. 16:40–54.

Garnier F, Mathe A, Bruyeres R. 2008. Images in cardiology: electrical aspects of Brugada: hyperkalaemia and intoxication with phenothiazines. *Heart*. 94:1578.

Ghosh D, Erman M, Wawrzak Z, Duax WL, Pangborn W. 1994. Mechanism of inhibition of 3 alpha, 20 beta-hydroxysteroid dehydrogenase by a licorice-derived steroidal inhibitor. *Structure*. 2:973–980.

Green DE, Albers PH. 1997. Diagnostic criteria for selenium toxicosis in aquatic birds: histologic lesions. *J Wildl Dis*. 33:385–404.

Greenwood GJ. 1951. Toxic cutaneous manifestations of para-aminobenzoic acid derivatives. *Ann Allergy*. 9:72–73.

Guarisco JA, Hall JO, Coulombe RA Jr. 2008. Mechanisms of butylated hydroxytoluene chemoprevention of aflatoxicosis—inhibition of aflatoxin B1 metabolism. *Toxicol Appl Pharmacol*. 227:339–346.

Gupta Y, Kohli DV, Jain SK. 2008. Vitamin B12-mediated transport: a potential tool for tumor targeting of antineoplastic drugs and imaging agents. *Crit Rev Ther Drug Carrier Syst*. 25:347–379.

Guzeva VI, Chukhlovina ML, Chukhlovin BA. 2008. [Environmental factors and parkinsonian syndrome]. *Gig Sanit*. Mar-Apr(2):60–62.

Han O, Failla ML, Hill AD, Morris ER, Smith JC Jr. 1994. Inositol phosphates inhibit uptake and transport of iron and zinc by a human intestinal cell line. *J Nutr*. 124:580–587.

Hartenstein R, Wendt TG, Kastenbauer ER. 1988. 5-Fluorouracil/folinic acid/cisplatin-combination and simultaneous accelerated split-course radiotherapy in advanced head and neck cancer. *Adv Exp Med Biol*. 244:275–284.

Hathcock JN. 1982. *Nutritional toxicology*. Volume I. New York: Academic Press, p.6.

Hathcock JN, Azzi A, Blumberg J, Bray T, Dickinson A, Frei B, Jialal I, Johnston CS, Kelly FJ, Kraemer K, Packer L, Parthasarathy S, Sies H, Traber MG. 2005. Vitamins E and C are safe across a broad range of intakes. *Am J Clin Nutr*. 81:736–745.

Hawkins RL, Mori M, Inoue M, Torii K. 1995. Proline, ascorbic acid, or thioredoxin affect jaundice and mortality in Long Evans cinnamon rats. *Pharmacol Biochem Behav*. 52:509–515.

Herman DS, Geraldine M, Venkatesh T. 2008. Influence of minerals on lead-induced alterations in liver function in rats exposed to long-term lead exposure. *J Hazard Mater*. 166(2–3):1410–1414.

Herbert V. 1999. Hemochromatosis and vitamin C. *Ann Intern Med*. 131:475–476.

Heyer G, Simon M, Schell H. 1998. [Dose-dependent pellagroid skin reaction caused by carbamazepine]. *Hautarzt*. 49:123.

Hirota K, Hirota T. 2006. [Nutrition-related bone disease]. *Nippon Rinsho*. 64:1707–1711.

Howes LG. 1995. Which drugs affect potassium? *Drug Saf*. 12:240–244.

Hsieh CT, Liang JS, Peng SS, Lee WT. 2007. Seizure associated with total parenteral nutrition-related hypermanganesemia. *Pediatr Neurol*. 36:181–183.

Huff JD, Keung YK, Thakuri M, Beaty MW, Hurd DD, Owen J, Molnár I. 2007. Copper deficiency causes reversible myelodysplasia. *Am J Hematol*. 82:625–630.

Hultdin J, Van Guelpen B, Bergh A, Hallmans G, Stattin P. 2005. Plasma folate, vitamin B12, and homocysteine and prostate cancer risk: a prospective study. *Int J Cancer*. 113:819–824.

Hussein HS, Brasel JM. 2001. Toxicity, metabolism, and impact of mycotoxins on humans and animals. *Toxicology*. 167:101–134.

Hylander B, Kjellstrand CM. 1996. Prognostic factors and treatment of severe ethylene glycol intoxication. *Intensive Care Med*. 22:546–552.

Iezhitsa IN, Spasov AA. 2008. [Potassium magnesium homeostasis: physiology, pathophysiology, clinical consequences of deficiency and pharmacological correction]. *Usp Fiziol Nauk*. 39:23–41.

International Programme on Chemical Safety. 1979. No. 11: *Mycotoxins*. Environmental Health Criteria. Geneva: World Health Organization.

Isoda K, Kagaya N, Akamatsu S, Hayashi S, Tamesada M, Watanabe A, Kobayashi M, Tagawa Y, Kondoh M, Kawase M, Yagi K. 2008.

Hepatoprotective effect of vitamin B12 on dimethylnitrosamine-induced liver injury. *Biol Pharm Bull.* 31:309–311.

Jedrychowski W, Masters E, Choi H, Sochacka E, Flak E, Mroz E, Pac A, Jacek R, Kaim I, Skolicki Z, Spengler JD, Perera F. 2007. Pre-pregnancy dietary vitamin A intake may alleviate the adverse birth outcomes associated with prenatal pollutant exposure: epidemiologic cohort study in Poland. *Int J Occup Environ Health.* 13:175–180.

Jernigan HM Jr. 1985. Role of hydrogen peroxide in riboflavin-sensitized photodynamic damage to cultured rat lenses. *Exp Eye Res.* 41:121–129.

Jost G, Pietsch H, Sommer J, Sandner P, Lengsfeld P, Seidensticker P, Lehr S, Hütter J, Sieber MA. 2008. Retention of iodine and expression of biomarkers for renal damage in the kidney after application of iodinated contrast media in rats. *Invest Radiol.* 44(2):114–123.

Juan C, Pena A, Lino C, Moltó JC, Mañes J. 2008. Levels of ochratoxin A in wheat and maize bread from the central zone of Portugal. *Int J Food Microbiol.* 127:284–289.

Katsonis FN, Mackey MA, eds. 2002. *Nutritional Toxicology.* 2nd ed. Boca Raton, FL: CRC Press.

Kavantzas N, Chatziioannou A, Yanni AE, Tsakayannis D, Balafoutas D, Agrogiannis G, Perrea D. 2006. Effect of green tea on angiogenesis and severity of atherosclerosis in cholesterol-fed rabbit. *Vascul Pharmacol.* 44:461–463.

Kim YJ, Kim YS, Kim MS, Ryu JC. 2007. The inhibitory mechanism of methylmercury on differentiation of human neuroblastoma cells. *Toxicology.* 234:1–9.

Kim-Mitsuyama S, Yamamoto E, Tanaka T, Zhan Y, Izumi Y, Izumiya Y, Ioroi T, Wanibuchi H, Iwao H. 2005. Critical role of angiotensin II in excess salt-induced brain oxidative stress of stroke-prone spontaneously hypertensive rats. *Stroke.* 36:1083–1088.

Klevay LM. 2008. Alzheimer's disease as copper deficiency. *Med Hypotheses.* 70:802–807.

Klöcker N, Rudolph P, Verse T. 2004. Evaluation of protective and therapeutic effects of dexpanthenol on nasal decongestants and preservatives: results of cytotoxic studies *in vitro. Am J Rhinol.* 18:315–320.

Kordas K, Lönnerdal B, Stoltzfus RJ. 2007. Interactions between nutrition and environmental exposures: effects on health outcomes in women and children. *J Nutr.* 137:2794–2797.

Kumar N, Boeve BF, Cowl CT, Ellison JW, Kamath PS, Swanson KL. 2008. Hypermanganesemia, hereditary hemorrhagic telangiectasia, brain abscess: the hepatic connection. *Neurology.* 71:1118–1119.

Kuroiwa Y, Okamura T, Ishii Y, Umemura T, Tasaki M, Kanki K, Mitsumori K, Hirose M, Nishikawa A. 2008. Enhancement of esophageal carcinogenesis in acid reflux model rats treated with ascorbic acid and sodium nitrite in combination with or without initiation. *Cancer Sci.* 99:7–13.

Lazzara R. 1988. Electrophysiological mechanisms for ventricular arrhythmias. *Clin Cardiol.* 11(3 Suppl 2): II1–4.

Lee CH, Shih CP, Hsu KH, Hung DZ, Lin CC. 2008. The early prognostic factors of glyphosate-surfactant intoxication. *Am J Emerg Med.* 26:275–281.

Lee HJ, Paul S, Atalla N, Thomas PE, Lin X, Yang I, Buckley B, Lu G, Zheng X, Lou YR, Conney AH, Maehr H, Adorini L, Uskokovic M, Suh N. 2008. Gemini vitamin D analogues inhibit estrogen receptor-positive and estrogen receptor-negative mammary tumorigenesis without hypercalcemic toxicity. *Cancer Prev Res (Phila).* 1:476–484.

Lefevre M, Keen CL, Lönnerdal B, Hurley LS, Schneeman BO. 1985. Different effects of zinc and copper deficiency on composition of plasma high density lipoproteins in rats. *J Nutr.* 115:359–368.

Lepak JM, Kraft CE, Honeyfield DC, Brown SB. 2008. Evaluating the effect of stressors on thiaminase activity in alewife. *J Aquat Anim Health.* 20:63–71.

Leu JP, Weiner A, Barzel US. 2008. Vitamin D toxicity: caveat emptor. *Endocr Pract.* 14:1188–1190.

Levander OA. 1979. Lead toxicity and nutritional deficiencies. *Environ Health Perspect.* 29:115–125.

Levenson CW, Somers RC. 2008. Nutritionally regulated biomarkers for breast cancer. *Nutr Rev.* 66:163–166.

Lheureux P, Penaloza A, Gris M. 2005. Pyridoxine in clinical toxicology: a review. *Eur J Emerg Med.* 12:78–85.

Lipkin AC, Lenssen P. 2008. Hypervitaminosis a in pediatric hematopoietic stem cell patients requiring renal replacement therapy. *Nutr Clin Pract.* 23:621–629.

Lönnerdal B. 1996. Bioavailability of copper. *Am J Clin Nutr.* 63:821S–829S.

Luongo D, Severino L, Bergamo P, De Luna R, Lucisano A, Rossi M. 2006. Interactive effects of fumonisin B1 and alpha-zearalenol on proliferation and cytokine expression in Jurkat T cells. *Toxicol In Vitro.* 20:1403–1410.

Ma Y, Yu WD, Hershberger PA, Flynn G, Kong RX, Trump DL, Johnson CS. 2008. 1alpha, 25-dihydroxyvitamin D3 potentiates cisplatin antitumor activity by p73 induction in a squamous cell carcinoma model. *Mol Cancer Ther.* 7:3047–3055.

Mahaffey KR, Haseman JD, Goyer RA. 1973. Dose-response to lead ingested in rats fed low dietary calcium. *J Lab Clin Med.* 82:92–101.

Mally A, Dekant W. 2008. Mycotoxins and the kidney: modes of action for renal tumor formation by ochratoxin A in rodents. *Mol Nutr Food Res.* 53(4):467–478.

Malone JI, Hanna S, Saporta S, Mervis RF, Park CR, Chong L, Diamond DM. 2008. Hyperglycemia not hypoglycemia alters neuronal dendrites and impairs spatial memory. *Pediatr Diabetes*. 9:531–539.

Manzardo S, Coppi G. 1991. [Protective action of some compounds against the toxicity of acetaldehyde, acrolein and formaldehyde in the rat]. *Boll Chim Farm*. 130(10):399–401.

Maret W, Sandstead HH. 2006. Zinc requirements and the risks and benefits of zinc supplementation. *J Trace Elem Med Biol*. 20:3–18.

Markkanen A, Juutilainen J, Naarala J. 2008. Pre-exposure to 50 Hz magnetic fields modifies menadione-induced DNA damage response in murine L929 cells. *Int J Radiat Biol*. 84:742–751.

Marshall MW, Haubrich M, Washington VA, Chang MW, Young CW, Wheeler MA. 1976. Biotin status and lipid metabolism in adult obese hypercholesterolemic inbred rats. *Nutr Metab*. 20:41–61.

Masterjohn C. 2007. Vitamin D toxicity redefined: vitamin K and the molecular mechanism. *Med Hypotheses*. 68:1026–1034.

Matsuki T, Yubisui T, Tomoda A, Yoneyama Y, Takeshita M, Hirano M, Kobayashi K, Tani Y. 1978. Acceleration of methaemoglobin reduction by riboflavin in human erythrocytes. *Br J Haematol*. 39:523–528.

Medina D, Lane HW, Shepherd F. 1983. Effect of dietary selenium levels on 7,12-dimethylbenzanthracene-induced mouse mammary tumorigenesis. *Carcinogenesis*. 4:1159–1163.

McHugh GJ, Graber ML, Freebairn RC. 2008. Fatal vitamin C-associated acute renal failure. *Anaesth Intensive Care*. 36:585–588.

Merrick BA. 2008. The plasma proteome, adductome and idiosyncratic toxicity in toxicoproteomics research. *Brief Funct Genomic Proteomic*. 7:35–49.

Mittal G, Brar AP, Soni G. 2006. Impact of hypercholesterolemia on toxicity of N-nitrosodiethylamine: biochemical and histopathological effects. *Pharmacol Rep*. 58:413–419.

Mocchegiani E, Malavolta M, Marcellini F, Pawelec G. 2006. Zinc, oxidative stress, genetic background and immunosenescence: implications for healthy ageing. *Immun Ageing*. 3:6.

Moe SM. 2008. Disorders involving calcium, phosphorus, and magnesium. *Prim Care*. 35:215–237.

Moïseenok AG, Dorofeev BF, Sheĭbak VM, Khomich TI. 1984. [Antitoxic properties of pantothenic acid derivatives, precursors of coenzyme A biosynthesis, with regard to kanamycin]. *Antibiotiki*. 29:851–855.

Mordes JP, Swartz R, Arky RA. 1975. Extreme hypermagnesemia as a cause of refractory hypotension. *Ann Intern Med*. 83:657–658.

Munro HM. 1978. Nutritional consequences of excess amino acid intake. *Adv Exp Med Biol*. 105:119–129.

Neuvonen PJ. 1976. Interactions with the absorption of tetracyclines. *Drugs*. 11:45–54.

Nielsen FH. 2000. The emergence of boron as nutritionally important throughout the life cycle. *Nutrition*. 16:512–514.

Novák J, Benísek M, Hilscherová K. 2008. Disruption of retinoid transport, metabolism and signaling by environmental pollutants. *Environ Int*. 34:898–913.

Novotny JA, Turnlund JR. 2007. Molybdenum intake influences molybdenum kinetics in men. *J Nutr*. 137:37–42.

Nowak G, Carter CA, Schnellmann RG. 2000. Ascorbic acid promotes recovery of cellular functions following toxicant-induced injury. *Toxicol Appl Pharmacol*. 167:37–45.

Oboh G, Oladunmoye MK. 2007. Biochemical changes in micro-fungi fermented cassava flour produced from low- and medium-cyanide variety of cassava tubers. *Nutr Health*. 18:355–367.

O'Donnell J. 2004. Polar hysteria: an expression of hypervitaminosis A. *Am J Ther*. 11:507–516.

Omaye ST. 2004. *Food and nutritional toxicology*. Boca Raton, FL: CRC Press.

Osinubi AA, Daramola AO, Noronha CC, Okanlawon AO, Ashiru OA. 2007. The effect of quinine and ascorbic acid on rat testes. *West Afr J Med*. 26:217–221.

Pan SY, Yang R, Dong H, Yu ZL, Ko KM. 2006. Bifendate treatment attenuates hepatic steatosis in cholesterol/bile salt- and high-fat diet-induced hypercholesterolemia in mice. *Eur J Pharmacol*. 552:170–175.

Paris I, Dagnino-Subiabre A, Marcelain K, Bennett LB, Caviedes P, Caviedes R, Azar CO, Segura-Aguilar J. 2001. Copper neurotoxicity is dependent on dopamine-mediated copper uptake and one-electron reduction of aminochrome in a rat substantia nigra neuronal cell line. *J Neurochem*. 77:519–529.

Parng C, Roy NM, Ton C, Lin Y, McGrath P. 2007. Neurotoxicity assessment using zebrafish. *J Pharmacol Toxicol Methods*. 55:103–112.

Patrick L. 2008. Iodine: deficiency and therapeutic considerations. *Altern Med Rev*. 13:116–127.

Paul PK, Duttagupta PN. 1976. The effect of an acute dose of biotin at a post-implantation stage and its relation with female sex steroids in the rat. *J Nutr Sci Vitaminol (Tokyo)*. 22:181–186.

Pauling L. 1970. Evolution and the need for ascorbic acid. *Proc Natl Acad Sci USA*. 67:1643–1648.

Pawa S, Ali S. 2006. Boron ameliorates fulminant hepatic failure by counteracting the changes associated with the oxidative stress. *Chem Biol Interact*. 160:89–98.

Penniston KL, Tanumihardjo SA. 2006. The acute and chronic toxic effects of vitamin A. *Am J Clin Nutr*. 83:191–201.

Perna AF, Luciano MG, Pulzella P, Satta E, Capasso R, Lombardi C, Ingrosso D, De Santo NG. 2008. Is homocysteine toxic in uremia? *J Ren Nutr.* 18:12–17.

Perry TA, Weerasuriya A, Mouton PR, Holloway HW, Greig NH. 2004. Pyridoxine-induced toxicity in rats: a stereological quantification of the sensory neuropathy. *Exp Neurol.* 190:133–144.

Pestka JJ. 2008. Mechanisms of deoxynivalenol-induced gene expression and apoptosis. *Food Addit Contam.* 24:1–13.

Peterson FJ, Combs GF Jr, Holtzman JL, Mason RP. 1982. Effect of selenium and vitamin E deficiency on nitrofurantoin toxicity in the chick. *J Nutr.* 112:1741–1746.

Plecko B, Paul K, Paschke E, Stoeckler-Ipsiroglu S, Struys E, Jakobs C, Hartmann H, Luecke T, di Capua M, Korenke C, Hikel C, Reutershahn E, Freilinger M, Baumeister F, Bosch F, Erwa W. 2007. Biochemical and molecular characterization of 18 patients with pyridoxine-dependent epilepsy and mutations of the antiquitin (ALDH7A1) gene. *Hum Mutat.* 28:19–26.

Raisbeck MF. 2000. Selenosis. *Vet Clin North Am Food Anim Pract.* 16:465–480.

Raja NS, Nair BU. 2008. Chromium(III) complexes inhibit transcription factors binding to DNA and associated gene expression. *Toxicology.* 251:61–65.

Rana SV. 2008. Metals and apoptosis: recent developments. *J Trace Elem Med Biol.* 22:262–284.

Rasmussen H, Barrett P, Smallwood J, Bollag W, Isales C. 1990. Calcium ion as intracellular messenger and cellular toxin. *Environ Health Perspect.* 84:17–25.

Raviña P, Quiroga JM, Raviña T. 2004. Hyperkalemia in fatal MDMA ('ecstasy') toxicity. *Int J Cardiol.* 93:307–308.

Rees DC, Kelsey H, Richards JD. 1993. Acute haemolysis induced by high dose ascorbic acid in glucose-6-phosphate dehydrogenase deficiency. *BMJ.* 306:841–842.

Richardson SD, Fasano F, Ellington JJ, Crumley FG, Buettner KM, Evans JJ, Blount BC, Silva LK, Waite TJ, Luther GW, Mckague AB, Miltner RJ, Wagner ED, Plewa MJ. 2008. Occurrence and mammalian cell toxicity of iodinated disinfection byproducts in drinking water. *Environ Sci Technol.* 42:8330–8338.

Rivers JM. 1975. Oral contraceptives and ascorbic acid. *Am J Clin Nutr.* 28:550–554.

Rivers JM. 1989. Safety of high-level vitamin C ingestion. *Int J Vitam Nutr Res Suppl.* 30:95–102.

Roe DA. 1988. Drug and nutrient interactions in the elderly diabetic. *Drug Nutr Interact.* 5:195–203.

Roe DA. 1989. *Diet and drug interactions.* New York: Von Nostrand Reinhold.

Roussel AM, Andriollo-Sanchez M, Ferry M, Bryden NA, Anderson RA. 2007. Food chromium content, dietary chromium intake and related biological variables in French free-living elderly. *Br J Nutr.* 98:326–331.

Rufenacht P, Mach-Pascual S, Iten A. 2008. [Vitamin B12 deficiency: a challenging diagnosis and treatment]. *Rev Med Suisse.* 4:2212–2214, 2216–2217.

Russell FE. 1967. Vitamin A content of polar bear liver. *Toxicon.* 5:61–62.

Rustia M. 1975. Inhibitory effect of sodium ascorbate on ethylurea and sodium nitrite carcinogenesis and negative findings in progeny after intestinal inoculation of precursors into pregnant hamsters. *J Natl Cancer Inst.* 55:1389–1394.

Ryan EP, Holz JD, Mulcahey M, Sheu TJ, Gasiewicz TA, Puzas JE. 2007. Environmental toxicants may modulate osteoblast differentiation by a mechanism involving the aryl hydrocarbon receptor. *J Bone Miner Res.* 22:1571–1580.

Sabuncuoglu BT, Kocaturk PA, Yaman O, Kavas GO, Tekelioglu M. 2006. Effects of subacute boric acid administration on rat kidney tissue. *Clin Toxicol (Phila).* 44:249–253.

Sahu AP. 1989. Effect of choline and mineral fibres (chrysotile asbestos) on guinea-pigs. *IARC Sci Publ.* 90:185–189.

Sardesai VM. 1993. Molybdenum: an essential trace element. *Nutr Clin Pract.* 8:277–281.

Saxena K. 1989. Clinical features and management of poisoning due to potassium chloride. *Med Toxicol Adverse Drug Exp.* 4:429–443.

Saxena N, Ansari KM, Kumar R, Dhawan A, Dwivedi PD, Das M. 2009. Patulin causes DNA damage leading to cell cycle arrest and apoptosis through modulation of Bax, p(53) and p(21/WAF1) proteins in skin of mice. *Toxicol Appl Pharmacol.* 234:192–201.

Schrag D, Chung KY, Flombaum C, Saltz L. 2005. Cetuximab therapy and symptomatic hypomagnesemia. *J Natl Cancer Inst.* 97:1221–1224.

Schrauzer GN, Ishmael D, Kiefer GW. 1975. Some aspects of current vitamin C usage: diminished high-altitude resistance following overdosage. *Ann N Y Acad Sci.* 258:377–381.

Schurgers LJ, Spronk HM, Soute BA, Schiffers PM, DeMey JG, Vermeer C. 2007. Regression of warfarin-induced medial elastocalcinosis by high intake of vitamin K in rats. *Blood.* 109:2823–2831.

Sen CK, Khanna S, Rink C, Roy S. 2007. Tocotrienols: the emerging face of natural vitamin E. *Vitam Horm.* 76:203–261.

Sengottuvelan M, Deeptha K, Nalini N. 2009. Resveratrol attenuates 1,2-dimethylhydrazine (DMH) induced glycoconjugate abnormalities during various stages of colon carcinogenesis. *Phytother Res.* 23(8):1154–1158.

Séréni C, Degos CF. 1990. [Lesions of the brain stem and cerebellum of alcoholic and nutritional deficiency origin]. *Rev Prat.* 40:1193–1196.

Showalter SL, Showalter TN, Witkiewicz A, Havens R, Kennedy EP, Hucl T, Kern SE, Yeo CJ, Brody JR. 2008. Evaluating the drug-target relationship between thymidylate synthase expression and tumor response to 5-fluorouracil. Is it time to move forward? *Cancer Biol Ther.* 7:986–994.

Simamura E, Shimada H, Ishigaki Y, Hatta T, Higashi N, Hirai K. 2008. Bioreductive activation of quinone antitumor drugs by mitochondrial voltage-dependent anion channel 1. *Anat Sci Int.* 83:261–266.

Singh VK, Srinivasan V, Toles R, Karikari P, Seed T, Papas KA, Hyatt JA, Kumar KS. 2005. Radiation protection by the antioxidant alpha-tocopherol succinate. Proceedings of the Human Factors and Medicine Research Task Group NATO RTG 099 Radiation Bioeffects and Countermeasures. Armed Forces Radiobiology Research Institute, Bethesda, MD, June 21–23, pp. 16.1–16.10 published in AFRRI CD 05-02.

Sinha Roy S, Mukhopadhyay S, Mukherjee S, Das SK. 2008. Breast cancer is associated with an increase in the activity and expression of cholinephosphotransferase in rats. *Life Sci.* 83:661–665.

Smith D, Gwiazda R, Bowler R, Roels H, Park R, Taicher C, Lucchini R. 2007. Biomarkers of Mn exposure in humans. *Am J Ind Med.* 50:801–811.

Smith TK, Austic RE. 1978. The branched-chain amino acid antagonism in chicks. *J Nutr.* 108:1180–1191.

Snodgrass SR. 1992. Vitamin neurotoxicity. *Mol Neurobiol.* 6:41–73.

Soldin OP, Aschner M. 2007. Effects of manganese on thyroid hormone homeostasis: potential links. *Neurotoxicology.* 28:951–956.

Solovieva ME, Solovyev VV, Kudryavtsev AA, Trizna YA, Akatov VS. 2008. Vitamin B12b enhances the cytotoxicity of dithiothreitol. *Free Radic Biol Med.* 44:1846–1856.

Spinnato JA 2nd, Freire S, Pinto e Silva JL, Rudge MV, Martins-Costa S, Koch MA, Goco N, Santos Cde B, Cecatti JG, Costa R, Ramos JG, Moss N, Sibai BM. 2008. Antioxidant supplementation and premature rupture of the membranes: a planned secondary analysis. *Am J Obstet Gynecol.* 199:433.e1–8.

Stearns DM. 2000. Is chromium a trace essential metal? *Biofactors.* 11(3):149–162.

Steyn PS, van Heerden FR. 1998. Bufadienolides of plant and animal origin. *Nat Prod Rep.* 15:397–413.

Stitik TP, Nadler SF, Foye PM, Juvan L. 1999. Greater trochanter enthesopathy: an example of "short course retinoid enthesopathy": a case report. *Am J Phys Med Rehabil.* 78:571–576.

Stokes KY, Cooper D, Tailor A, Granger DN. 2002. Hypercholesterolemia promotes inflammation and microvascular dysfunction: role of nitric oxide and superoxide. *Free Radic Biol Med.* 33:1026–1036.

Sullivan CD, Archdeacon JW. 1947. The effects of a large dose of para-amino-benzoic acid on the body and endocrine gland weights of rats; toxic manifestations. *Endocrinology.* 41:325–327.

Tannetta DS, Sargent IL, Linton EA, Redman CW. 2008. Vitamins C and E inhibit apoptosis of cultured human term placenta trophoblast. *Placenta.* 29:680–690.

Trump DL, Muindi J, Fakih M, Yu WD, Johnson CS. 2006. Vitamin D compounds: clinical development as cancer therapy and prevention agents. *Anticancer Res.* 26:2551–2556.

Tsutsumi S, Tanaka T, Gotoh K, Akaike M. 1995. Effects of pyridoxine on male fertility. *J Toxicol Sci.* 20:351–365.

Uthus EO, Ross S. 2008. Dietary selenium (Se) and copper (Cu) interact to affect homocysteine metabolism in rats. *Biol Trace Elem Res.* 129(1–3):213–220.

Vachhrajani KD, Sahu AP, Dutta KK. 1993. Excess choline availability: a transient effect on spermatogenesis in the rat. *Reprod Toxicol.* 7:477–481.

Valentovic MA, Ball JG, Sun H, Rankin GO. 2002. Characterization of 2-amino-4,5-dichlorophenol (2A45CP) in vitro toxicity in renal cortical slices from male Fischer 344 rats. *Toxicology.* 172:113–123.

Valerio LG Jr, Petersen DR. 2000. Characterization of hepatic iron overload following dietary administration of dicyclopentadienyl iron (Ferrocene) to mice: cellular, biochemical, and molecular aspects. *Exp Mol Pathol.* 68:1–12.

van de Poll MC, Dejong CH, Soeters PB. 2006. Adequate range for sulfur-containing amino acids and biomarkers for their excess: lessons from enteral and parenteral nutrition. *J Nutr.* 136 (6 Suppl):1694S–1700S.

Vanhanen H. 1994. Cholesterol malabsorption caused by sitostanol ester feeding and neomycin in pravastatin-treated hypercholesterolaemic patients. *Eur J Clin Pharmacol.* 47:169–176.

Wang C, Brown S, Bhattacharyya MH. 1994. Effect of cadmium on bone calcium and 45Ca in mouse dams on a calcium-deficient diet: evidence of Itai-Itai-like syndrome. *Toxicol Appl Pharmacol.* 127:320–330.

Wang S, Radhakrishnan J, Ayoub IM, Kolarova JD, Taglieri DM, Gazmuri RJ. 2007. Limiting sarcolemmal Na+ entry during resuscitation from ventricular fibrillation prevents excess mitochondrial Ca2+ accumulation and attenuates myocardial injury. *J Appl Physiol.* 103:55–65.

Wardwell L, Chapman-Novakofski K, Herrel S, Woods J. 2008. Nutrient intake and immune function of elderly subjects. *J Am Diet Assoc.* 108:2005–2012.

Watkins BA, Hannon K, Ferruzzi M, Li Y. 2007. Dietary PUFA and flavonoids as deterrents for environmental pollutants. *J Nutr Biochem.* 18:196–205.

Wayment JR, Harris JM. 2009. Biotin-avidin binding kinetics measured by single-molecule imaging. *Anal Chem.* 81:336–342.

White WS, Kim CI, Kalkwarf HJ, Bustos P, Roe DA. 1988. Ultraviolet light-induced reductions in plasma carotenoid levels. *Am J Clin Nutr.* 47:879–883.

Wolever TM. 2000. Dietary carbohydrates and insulin action in humans. *Br J Nutr.* 83(Suppl 1): S97–S102.

Wróbel M, Jurkowska H. 2007. Menadione effect on l-cysteine desulfuration in U373 cells. *Acta Biochim Pol.* 54:407–11.

Xu DX, Wei W, Sun MF, Wu CY, Wang JP, Wei LZ, Zhou CF. 2004. Kupffer cells and reactive oxygen species partially mediate lipopolysaccharidein-duced downregulation of nuclear receptor pregnane x receptor and its target gene CYP3a in mouse liver. *Free Radic Biol Med.* 37:10–22.

Yamada T, Sogawa K, Kim JK, Izumi K, Suzuki Y, Mura-matsu Y, Sumida T, Hamakawa H, Matsumoto K. 1998. Increased polyploidy, delayed mitosis and reduced protein phosphatase-1 activity associated with excess copper in the Long Evans Cinnamon rat. *Res Commun Mol Pathol Pharmacol.* 99:283–304.

Zagrobelny M, Bak S, Møller BL. 2008. Cyanogenesis in plants and arthropods. *Phytochemistry.* 69:1457–1468.

Zitomer NC, Glenn AE, Bacon CW, Riley RT. 2008. A single extraction method for the analysis by liquid chromatography/tandem mass spectrometry of fumonisins and biomarkers of disrupted sphingolipid metabolism in tissues of maize seedlings. *Anal Bioanal Chem.* 391:2257–2263.

Toxic Reactions
of Tissues/Organs

Routes of Administration and Which Organs Are Most Likely Impacted Based on Route and Toxicokinetic Models

This is a chapter outline intended to guide and familiarize you with the content to follow.

I. Routes of administration

    A. Accidental exposure—see Figure 13-1

        1. Integument (dermal)

           a. Structure—see Figure 13-2

               (1) Entry points—small lipids through skin; other compounds through cracks, hair shafts, sweat glands/hydration

           b. Models of absorption

               (1) European Union (EU)—see Figure 13-3

               (2) Polycyclic aromatic hydrocarbon absorption—topostructural, topochemical, geometric descriptors, and molecular weight determine skin absorption

               (3) Organic solvent equation $Ks = k_e \times M[1\text{-exp}\,(-k_e \times t)]$; toluene absorption $= 34 \pm 9\ \mu g/cm^2$ through mouse skin, while more polar 1-propanol/isobutanol (15.5) and ethylene glycol (23.7) compounds have lower values as expected

               (4) For deposited films must consider evaporation and absorption ($\chi = hk_{evap}\rho/DC_{sat}$)—for topical applications such as the insect repellant DEET in ethanol would cause a fraction deposition ($f = h_{dep}/h$) = 0.1 for this moderately sized compound

               (5) Absorption also depends on the % relative humidity and temperature, which change circulation and perfusate flow (determined in pigs which don't perspire, adding another factor); perspiring humans ↑ herbicide parathion absorption only 17% when temp ↑ from 21–28°C and a huge 227% when temp ↑ from 21–40.5°C

        2. Ocular absorption (OU)

           a. Two- to threefold higher absorption in human eye as in pig; human sclera = ½ thickness of swine, but similar to rabbit. However, precorneal residence times for certain formulations (gum) exceed that of saline preparations, which is not similar to the rabbit

           b. P-glycoprotein plays a key role in the ocular/blood transfer of medications and toxicants as do ABCC2 and a drug efflux pump/cancer-resistance protein

           c. As the eye pumps out or transfers toxicants to the blood/brain, toxicity can result in animals with large eyes and smaller brains (e.g., cats, dogs, rabbits, infant humans) when compared to adult humans—respiratory depression of infant given adrenergic α2 agonist brimonidine and kidney failure of infant given adrenergic α1 agonist phenylephrine

CONCEPTUALIZING TOXICOLOGY 13-1

3. See inhalation under peak toxicity routes

4. Ingestion for contaminated food items and infants (GI tract + digestive juices + flora affecting slow lag phase with liver first pass makes this route unique)

B. Ingestion (PO)

1. More absorption with longer intestinal tracts—more acid hydrolysis in ruminants also due to digestion time; rats cannot vomit to remove any oral toxicants

2. Lag time between ingestion and plasma concentrations except for compounds that absorb through the oral mucosa (e.g., nitroglycerin)

3. Compare with intravenous route for bioavailability = $AUC_{0-\infty}$ oral × $100/AUC_{0-\infty}$ IV; for repeated administrations average plateau concentration = $C_{av,\infty} = f \times D_{oral} / V_d k_{el} \times \tau$; if severe liver or kidney damage occurs, C_{av} will not plateau but keep climbing with each new dose until animal/person dies; C_{max} determines if threshold toxicity is reached and AUC more concerned with effects over a duration of a toxic concentration—see Figure 13-4

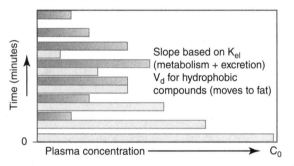

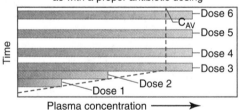

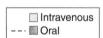

4. pH is important, because charged compounds are less likely to be absorbed orally

5. Toxicokinetics takes a compound from absorption through excretion; uses radiolabeled compound, the most likely route of administration and IV as a comparison; various tissues taken based on targets of toxicant action; humans should only be dosed with medications based on the dosage based on mg/kg; however, establishing dose from rats or mice should be based initially on mg/surface area between species (takes metabolic rate into account)

a. Enterohepatic recirculation of metabolites must be considered otherwise will mistakenly account for > 100% of the compound—see Figure 13-5

b. Resveratrol inhibits P-glycoprotein efflux of toxicants and inhibits CYP3A4 leading to increases in AUC and C_{max} of compounds such as nicardipine from oral but not IV administration (overdose)

c. Organic compound transporters (OAT, OCT) and peptide transporter-1 are also expressed in intestinal tract

CONCEPTUALIZING TOXICOLOGY 13-1 (*continued*)

     d. As, Cr, Mn, and Pb have specific carrier-mediated absorption; As, Cr, Hg, and Mn absorption affected by valence state; Al, As, Cr, Hg, Mn, and Pb toxicokinetics altered by biotransformation; organic forms of metals absorbed much easier; metals compete for absorption; Mn and Pb absorption affected by particle size

     e. Humans will have a higher peak for compounds equally well absorbed by the rat due to the higher rate of absorption and those poorly absorbed by the rat with have a higher AUC due to more complete absorption by the human; human stomach has lower pH (charge + acid degradation)

     f. Transporters—human intestine protects itself form toxicants by ABC transporters and CYPs, which vary from jejunum to ilium ($\approx 2/3$ of jejunal mRNA expression) to colon ($< 1/3$ of jejunal expression)

C. Peak toxicity routes

  1. Intravenous (IV)—route against which all routes are compared as the compound is immediately establishing blood/plasma concentration; first parenteral route considered

     a. As in the first figure above, $C_o =$ highest concentration at time zero and for hydrophobic compounds, then compound rapidly disperses into fat/fatty organs to determined apparent volume of distribution or V_d, then metabolism and kidney excretion usually determine the rest of the curve, slope of elimination curve $= -K_{el}/2.303$, where K_{el} is the elimination constant (inverse of half-life)

  2. Inhalation—route that gets to heart and brain rapidly for anesthesia, people inhaling drugs of abuse for maximum effect, and danger of inhalation of volatile compounds, small particles, etc.

     a. Solid toxicants experienced based on shape and composition; ultra-small particles such as carbon nanotubes must be considered in terms of cell signaling rather than absorption % as they rapidly pass into lung cells, the circulation, and vascular cells—see Figure 13-6

     b. Toxicants may cause lung damage → cardiovascular damage → CNS damage more readily by this route

     c. Mouse may be poor model of human or rat toxicity of trichloroethylene (TCE) toxicity as prevalence of non-ciliated Clara cells with high CYP concentrations (600-fold higher activity to TCE) → accumulation of chloral metabolite → aneuploidy

     d. Rat may be poor model for human based on lack of alveolarized or respiratory bronchioles

     e. Beagle dogs have five generations of respiratory bronchioles similar to human and offer better respiratory model

     f. Many compounds can use the IV pharmacokinetic equations

     g. Paraquat an unusual prooxidant toxicant as is transported into the lung via the polyamine uptake system even if it is not inhaled

  3. Sublingual (SL)—absorption of compounds such as nitroglycerin into the bloodstream through the oral mucosa

     a. Hydrophobic medications are rapidly absorbed, but have short duration of action through sublingual blood vessels (>buccal or cheek>palatal or roof of mouth) and bypasses liver first-pass metabolism giving reasonable bioavailability (nitroglycerin as model medication). Not a key route used for toxicology analysis but used for rapid medication delivery

D. Parenteral routes

  1. Intravenous—see previous

  2. Parenteral routes causing slower release for hydrophobic compounds

     a. Intramuscular (IM)—high protein content; binds drug procaine very well and releases slowly

     b. Subcutaneous (SC)—high fat content; lowest lethality for procaine

  3. Intraperitoneal—also absorbed through the peritoneum but on other side of the intestines and still is shunted through the liver first pass metabolism without the digestion or exclusion from absorption of the GI tract; this route may yield longer lasting influence of compounds such as cisplatin with lower peak for acute toxicity (good treatment for ovarian and similarly located cancers)

CONCEPTUALIZING TOXICOLOGY 13-1 (*continued*)

4. Intrathecal (cerebrospinal fluid or CSF entry by injection into the spinal column) or intracerebroventricular (brain CSF)

    a. Tertiary compounds such as atropine serve both as antidote to acetylcholinesterase inhibition and toxicant at higher concentration (antagonism of ACh), while quaternary compound lachesine did not penetrate the BBB (blood–brain barrier) into the CNS; if injected ICV lachesine is more toxic than the tertiary compounds

    b. Following fluoro-gold from CSF → choroid plexus of 3rd and lateral ventricles (2 minutes and traces in peripheral circulation) → forebrain ventricular organs, parenchymal tissues, hypophysis (15–20 minutes and peak in peripheral circulation at latter time)

    c. Radical scavengers and iron-chelating agent Desferal given ICV protect against Fenton reaction and neurodegeneration—not via protection against neurotoxic dopamine metabolite

CONCEPTUALIZING TOXICOLOGY 13-1 (*continued*)

The fields of physiology and pharmacology come into play when entering the arena of the intact complex organism. Because the requirements of each field involve the consideration of interactions of chemicals with organ systems, the interplay of effects on one organ system and the cascade of effects that are manifested throughout the organism require clinicians and scientists to know by which route the chemical or physical insult came and the adaptations made to adjust to the ensuing damage. Additionally, mammals must be considered as the reference animal, because government agencies require pharmaceutical products to be tested for their toxicity and toxicants for environmental dispersion have to attempt to model effects on animals of interest to humans including the *Homo sapiens* or model organisms that may provide information applicable to human risk assessment. The approach of this chapter is to indicate the most likely routes of administration or exposure first—accidental exposure to the skin or eyes (surface area and availability), oral, inhalation, and finally parenteral (injected internal) routes. Note the example given in **Figure 13-1** from the U.S. Environmental Protection Agency (EPA) for pesticides. This figure confirms the most likely routes of accidental exposure to most chemicals. Because the plasma concentrations are the standard for many exposures (except for those chemicals that do not show representative or indicative plasma concentrations, such as arsenic), intravenous injection is the standard to compare all routes against. Parenteral routes are more easily administered for determination of dose and response, including intravenous (IV), intraperitoneal (IP), subcutaneous (SC), intramuscular (IM), intracerebroventricular (ICV), and intrathecal. Except for injected medications, venoms, and other puncture wounds, these parenteral routes are unlikely routes of accidental exposure to environmental chemicals. However, for certain compounds such as ethylene glycol ether, dimethylmercury, and compounds dissolved in dimethyl sulfoxide, the dermal route in humans and similar animals is nearly equivalent to giving the compounds orally or by certain injection routes. This makes the route and the chemical properties of the toxicant important in modeling exposure and risk.

Transcutaneous Absorption

Structure of the Integument

Basic biology defines the integument as the outer protective cover of the body that provides a large surface area for contact with chemicals or physical agents. In other animals, the body covering may involve scales or other features (e.g., the exoskeleton of an insect). In a mammal, the integument involves skin, including the layers of the outer epidermis and the inner dermis, and associated structures such as the hair, nails, and the sebaceous and sweat

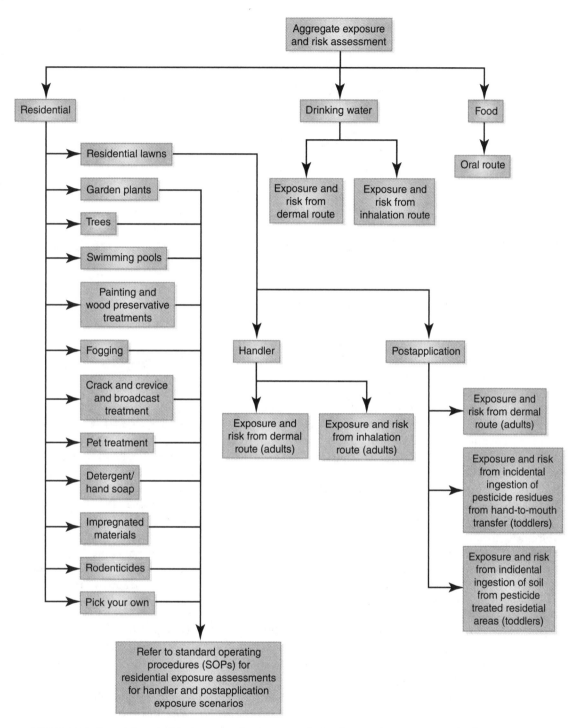

FIGURE 13-1 Example from the U.S. Environmental Protection Agency of Pathways and Routes to Be Considered in an Aggregate Exposure and Risk Assessment

Reproduced from U.S. Environmental Protection Agency. 2001. General Principles for Performing Aggregate Exposure and Risk Assessments. November 28, 2001. Office of Pesticide Programs, Office of Prevention, Pesticides, and Toxic Substances. U.S. EPA, Washington, D.C. http://www.epa.gov/pesticides/trac/science/aggregate.pdf

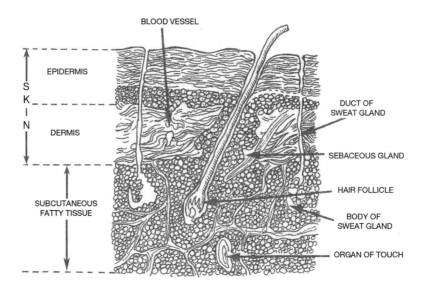

FIGURE 13-2 The Structure of the Skin and Fatty Subcutaneous Layer

glands, as shown in **Figure 13-2**. Some of these structures are important in monitoring long-term exposure to chemicals such as heavy metals (e.g., nails and hair). Others increase absorption of chemicals by providing gaps in the skin or entry points (hair shafts) and hydration of the skin (e.g., sweat glands). The most superficial layer of the five-layer epidermis is the stratum corneum, or horny layer. This multiple layer of dead cells that are shed in a continuous manner substitutes keratin for cytoplasm. These cells are held together by desmosomes to exclude water (and prevent dehydration) and provide a rugged exterior. This makes the absorption of water-soluble substances much more difficult, especially in adult dry skin. Skin cracks and wounds decrease the barrier. The next deeper clear layer, or stratum lucidum, of keratinocytes is absent in thin layers of skin, but has a cushion of eleidin that will eventually become keratin. This layer is thick in the palms of the hands and the soles of the foot, where absorption of compounds such as hydrocortisone cream is the lowest. The eleidin prevents water permeation due to protein-bound lipids. The stratum granulosum is the next layer deep in the epidermis. Cells are layered in two to four sheets deep and composed of granules consisting of keratohyalin. Lysosomal enzymes are prominent in the cytoplasm of these degenerating cells. Nuclei are absent or degraded. In thin layers of skin, this layer may also be absent. The next deep spiny layer, or stratum spinosum, is composed of eight to 10 layers of irregularly shaped cells with intercellular desmosomes. The high concentration of RNA in these cells allows for keratin synthesis. The deepest base layer, or stratum basale, is just a single row of columnar cells. These cells undergo mitosis and are responsible for skin cancers known as basal cell carcinoma. The thickness of the skin varies within the body of a mammal (more thickness on dorsum or back except for the cat and lateral surfaces of appendages) and between mammals.

Models of Skin Absorption

It is beyond the scope of this chapter to give a complete accounting for all the models of skin permeability of various classes of chemicals; this has been done more thoroughly elsewhere (Riviere, 2005). The European Commission Health and Consumer Protection Directorate-General (2004) gives guidance on how dermal absorption should be modeled as shown in **Figure 13-3**, which has used various scientific publications including those of the EPA (1996, 1999). Note that human and rodent

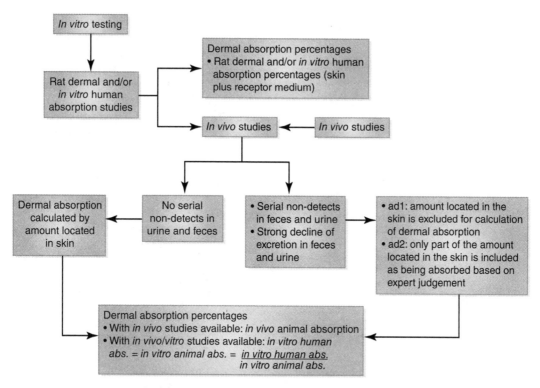

FIGURE 13-3 Dermal Percentage Absorption Determination from *in Vitro* Skin Preparations and Live Rat and Human Studies

(rat) models are preferred for determination of skin absorption. This section examines certain models for specific examples that indicate the importance of chemical properties on the ability of compounds to cross this barrier. It also examines a key component of hydration or perspiration on dermal absorption. Recall that the log P term indicates the hydrophobicity of a compound due to its preferential fractionation into the solvent octanol versus water. For quantitative structure–activity relationships, a number of structural and chemical features can be used. The dermal absorption of polycyclic aromatic hydrocarbons (PAHs) is well described by topostructural (planar, two-dimensional representation of the ring structures), topochemical (adding where the important functional groups on the planar rings interact), and geometric (overall shape and volume of the molecule including van der Waals volume) descriptors, and by the physicochemical property molecular weight. However, quantum chemical parameters such as charges, electronegativities, super delocalization, hardness, softness, and E_{LUMO} and E_{HOMO} (molecular orbital energies) do not predict dermal penetration of PAHs (Gute et al., 1999).

It is also important to model the dermal absorption of organic solvents, because they represent a smaller lipophilic liquid that may more easily find its way through the skin barrier. The skin absorption rate of an organic solvent at any time t, Ks, is a function of the amount remaining in the body, M, and the elimination rate, k_e. This leads to the equation Ks = k_e × M[1 − exp(−k_e × t)]. For example, the elimination rate for toluene (1/h) is 0.11. The permeation coefficient, Kp, for toluene in a mixture of organic solvents is determined by dividing Ks by the concentration of toluene in the solvent mixture. The μg of toluene absorbed per cm^2 of mouse skin in 30 min was determined to be 34.4 ± 9.1 (mean ± standard deviation). This number was lower for more polar alcohol or small glycol mixtures with toluene ranging from 15.5 for 1-propanol or isobutanol to 23.7 for ethylene glycol. Acetone and ether had similar effects on toluene absorption with a permeation of 24.8 and 25.4, respectively. The larger organic propylene glycol increased dermal permeation of toluene to 53.5. The Ks values ranged from 0.94 to 2.34 for the compounds mentioned so far. Organic solvents known to pass easily transcutaneously such as N,N-dimethylformamide, the low-molecular-weight methanol, and dimethyl sulfoxide increased the Ks to 8.54, 9.84, and 11.90, respectively. Thus, it is important in regard to the organic solvent and the solvent mixture (Tsuruta, 1996). This is also true for solutes dissolved or suspended in the solvents.

For a deposited film, it is necessary to consider both evaporation and absorption. The ratio of evaporation rate to absorption rate, χ, is represented by the equation: $\chi = hk_{evap}\rho/DC_{sat}$, where h is the thickness of the stratum corneum, ρ is the density of the liquid permeant, D is the diffusivity of the film in the stratum corneum, and C_{sat} is the film's solubility in the stratum corneum. For topical applications of a toxicant such as the mosquito repellant N,N-diethyl-3-methylbenzamide (DEET), there is postulated to be a deposition layer that is a relatively permeable layer of the stratum corneum into which a solute deposited by a solvent is rapidly dissolved. The equation for this phenomenon is $f = h_{dep}/h$ (f = fractional deposition depth, h_{dep} = permeable layer of stratum corneum that is the deposition layer associated with the desquamation process and loss of barrier lipids, and h = thickness of entire stratum corneum), where f varies from > 0 to < 1. A moderately sized compound like DEET or benzyl alcohol deposited by the solvent ethanol would have a value for f of approximately 0.1. It should be noted that the formulation of the compound is important as well. Microencapsulation drops the permeation into the skin by 25–35% (Kasting et al., 2008). For example, the effect of air temperature, % relative humidity, perfusate temperature, and perfusate flow was determined on the percutaneous absorption of the lipophilic organophosphate parathion through porcine skin *in vitro*. Because pigs do not perspire, this is a good test for interactions of physical factors on absorption. For the 4-mg dose, the factors that interacted to increase absorption were % relative humidity or air temperature and perfusate flow. Increased permeation was found for % relative humidity and perfusate flow for the 40-mg dose. At the highest dose of 400 mg, increased absorption could be found with interactions of % relative humidity or air temperature and perfusate flow, as well as air temperature and % relative humidity (Chang et al., 1994). In an animal that perspires, it would follow that the effect of temperature would be increased dramatically by increased sweating. Human volunteers were exposed to 2% parathion dust; the absorption followed by urinary excretion of the metabolite paranitrophenol peaked 5–6 hours following exposure. Raising the air temperature from 21°C to 28°C caused only a 17% increase in parathion absorption (paranitrophenol excretion). Increasing the temperature from 21°C to 40.5°C increased parathion absorption by an astonishing 227% (Funckes et al., 1963). This is an important finding, because the temperature and humidity are factors that affect absorption in animals that do not perspire. Although perspiration was not measured in this study, the combination of temperature, humidity, and perspiration act to increase absorption in a dramatic manner. Because parathion is also an acetylcholinesterase inhibitor, it would be expected to increase acetylcholine concentrations where it is absorbed at the highest concentrations. Acetylcholine activates sweat glands and so would increase the perspiration generated by heat. This would further enhance a possible toxic effect of dehydration from temperature as well as further enhance parathion absorption (Gordon, 2003). The subject of temperature or thermoregulation on the toxicity of chemicals has many aspects that show temperature as augmenting the toxicity or altered thermoregulation as a response, which is beyond the scope of the present discussion (Gordon et al., 2008).

Ocular Absorption

The eye has not been a highly studied model for absorption for toxicants, despite the frequency of accidents involving eye exposure to toxic substances in solid, liquid, or gas form and via the use of cosmetics and ocular pharmaceuticals.

There is a high degree of hydration of the eye, and the sclera is approximately 70% water. The thickness of the sclera is important in trans-scleral drug delivery. A model pharmaceutical agent for small-molecular-weight absorption is acetaminophen, 120 kDa dextran represents high-molecular-weight compounds, and insulin is the model protein. Because the human sclera is half the thickness of that of a pig, these model compounds exhibit two- to threefold increased absorption in the human (Nicoli et al., 2009). However, the rabbit cornea appears to have similar absorption of the immunosuppressant agent tacrolimus to the human eye (Van Eyk et al., 2007), but there are definite species differences in the retention of certain formulations of medications or toxicants. The human retains a gellan gum formulation (Gelrite) of technetium-99m labeled diethylenetriaminepentaacetic acid better than the same compound administered with 0.5% w/v hydroxyethyl cellulose solution or isotonic saline. This is not true for the precorneal residence of the rabbit eye (Greaves et al., 1990). The transporter P-glycoprotein is important in the blood versus ocular disposition of medications and toxicants (Senthilkumari et al., 2009). ABCC2 also aids in toxin and medication efflux in humans and rabbits leading to lower concentrations in the eye than expected unless efflux in considered along with low permeability to certain compounds across the corneal epithelium (Karla et al., 2007). There has also been demonstrated to be a breast cancer–resistance protein or drug efflux pump in human corneal epithelial cells (Karla et al., 2009). Because the size of eye is similar for dogs, cats, rabbits, infants, and adult humans, the area of the eye exposed to environmental chemicals is similarly large. The brain size behind that eye is not the same and can lead to differential toxicity. For example, an infant with congenital glaucoma who was given the adrenergic alpha-2 agonist brimonidine eye drops developed respiratory depression due to central nervous system (CNS) toxicity (Heimann et al., 2007). The same holds true for body weight differences, as an infant with low body weight and a history of renal failure given eye drops containing the adrenergic alpha-1 agonist phenylephrine experienced renal failure due to constriction of the renal blood vessels

(Shinomiya et al., 2003). These considerations have been important in which medication to choose, for instance, in inducing mydriasis (pupil dilation) in avian species to perform eye examinations without other apparent toxic effects (Ramer et al., 1996).

Oral Absorption

This is a key route of administration that is clearly used in toxicant and medication testing. Species differences are important; for example, the transit time for a compound in the gastrointestinal tract would be high in an elephant and low in a mouse. Ruminants digest for longer times and either do acid degradation or achieve more release of a toxic component (e.g., cyanide from amygdalin). Certain animals are famous for emesis (e.g., cats) and others for not being able to vomit (e.g., rats due to the presence of a limiting ridge; DeSesso and Jacobson, 2001). These are important differences to consider when modeling toxicant absorption from the per os (PO), or oral, route. The oral route will have a distinct lag time between administration and plasma concentrations unless the compound absorbs through the oral mucosa as is the case for nitroglycerin, for example. Bioavailability is important here. Bioavailability is the amount absorbed compared with the IV route:

$$\text{bioavailability} = \text{AUC}_{0-\infty}\text{oral} \times 100/\text{AUC}_{0-\infty}\text{IV},$$

where AUC is the area under the plasma concentration curve from time of administration to the time of complete elimination or in calculus the integral function. Because the IV route by definition has 100% of the compound in the plasma at time zero, then distributes the compound to the body volume, and then (metabolizes and) eliminates the compound, this is always the reference route. It is also the most toxic route along with inhalation, because the most rapid peak is achieved. After all, anesthesia is given via IV or inhalation to put someone out rapidly. IV antibiotics are only given in the case of the most dangerous infectious conditions. Most other medications are given orally and can stand to wait some time to have an effect. The oral route is also the usual route for repeated administration. The average plateau concentration in the plasma,

$$C_{av,\infty} = f \times D_{oral}/V_d k_{el} \times \tau,$$

where f = fraction absorbed, D = dose amount; V_d = the volume of distribution and involves other compartments, including the body fat or water depending on the hydrophobicity or hydrophilicity of the compound; k_{el} = the elimination constant, which is based on the slope of the elimination curve and is inversely related to the half-life or the time $(0.693/t_{1/2})$; and τ is the constant time interval between doses. Note the example shown in **Figure 13-4**. The single oral dose of a compound results in a lag, a peak, then a drop-off. In repeated administrations,

by the third or fourth dose, a relative steady state is achieved after a peak following each dose. This is important because the maximum concentration of C_{max} will determine a threshold for toxicity, while the AUC gives a measure of the chronic exposure of a mean concentration that is achieved with repeated doses. In antibiotic treatment, for example, the toxic effect of the first dose is not noted as much as the third or fourth dose that has a lethal impact on the microorganism in the host, because the first dose only achieves a killing effect at peak, while doses past the third one are in the toxic range for the bacteria from the minimum concentration or C_{min} to C_{max}. This is why in toxicology studies or in therapeutic treatments, missing an early dose is more important than a later one

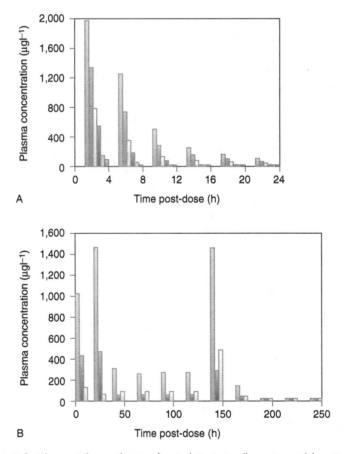

A

B

FIGURE 13-4 Human Male Volunteers' Pharmacokinetics of an Oral Matrix Metalloproteinase Inhibitor, Marimastat

Note: Mean marimastat plasma concentration-time profiles following single oral administration of 25, 50, 100, 200, 400 or 800 mg of marimastat to male volunteers. For clarity, error bars have not been included. Standard errors for C_{max} are representative; 16.4, 47.8, 44.7, 118.6, 149.3, and 164.7 for the 25 mg, 50 mg, 100 mg, 200 mg, 400 mg and 800 mg doses respectively. B. Mean marimastat plasma concentration-time profiles following repeat oral administration of 50, 100 and 200 mg of marimastat to male volunteers. For clarity, error bars have not been included. Standard errors for C_{max} and C_{minare} representative; 97.5, 67.9 and 339.2 for C_{maxat} last dose, 16.1, 11.7 and 42.4 for C_{minat} last dose, for 50 mg, 100 mg and 200 mg doses respectively.

due to the achieving of the steady state concentrations and the adjustment of the recipient's receptors to the action of the toxicant or medication after many repeated doses. These adaptations explain the tolerance achieved in alcohol consumption and the low impact of missing a dose or taking an extra dose of a medication after repeated use for months or years, unless a chronic toxic outcome is imminent.

The effect of pH cannot be overestimated. Henderson-Hasselbalch equation indicates that acids in acidic environments are uncharged and bases in basic environments are uncharged. It is the uncharged compound that is more likely to be absorbed orally unless the charged compound is properly chelated to a transporting molecule. Accordingly, weak acids are of less concern in the duodenum, for example, where bicarbonate is added in high quantities. Weak bases on the other hand are less likely to be charged moving from the acidic stomach to the more basic environment of the small intestine. The blood pH is even more basic and promotes transport of weak bases into tissues if they are not bound up to albumin in the plasma or transport in the red blood cell.

The paragraphs that follow examine how a toxicokinetic analysis should be done and then investigate how human and animal subjects absorb, distribute, metabolize, and eliminate an orally administered dose in a given study. The National Toxicology Program recommends that a toxicokinetic study be able to determine: (1) the rate and degree of absorption; (2) the body distribution of the chemical and its metabolites; (3) the site of metabolism, identification of the metabolites, and the rate of metabolism; (4) elimination routes and rates; and (5) dose effects on absorption, distribution, metabolism, and elimination. Other guidelines are to use the same species for toxicokinetic studies as were used originally to determine that there were toxic effects. Both sexes should be tested, and only one sex used unless sex differences arise. Radiolabelled chemicals are preferred to account for the original chemical and its metabolites through the organism and its excretion. Separation of compound from metabolite fractions should be done by high-pressure liquid chromatography or gas chromatography in a manner

that can account for any metabolite that represents more than 10% of the absorbed dose. The most common route of human exposure should be used along with the IV route. If the chemical is included in the food or drinking water, gavage should be used to insure that an accurate dose determination can be made. Doses should be given based on a log of the response after an LD_{50} curve is established at 0.1 LD_{50}, 0.01 LD_{50}, and 0.001 LD_{50}. More doses are recommended to establish a linear kinetic range or characterize a toxicant with nonlinear kinetics such as enterohepatic recirculation. Blood, fat, muscle, liver, kidney, and other target organs such as the brain should be sampled for the presence of the toxicant especially if central nervous system toxicity is anticipated or the heart sampled if cardiac toxicity is expected. Sampling times should be based on the limit of detection of the compound and represent 8-12 points. For example, 5, 10, 20, 40, and 60 minutes may be followed by 2, 4, 6, 8, and 24 hours for samples that reach their limit of detection in 24 hours. Excreta should be collected and analyzed over similar time intervals. Tissue–blood partition coefficients should be determined for a variety of tissues as indicated earlier and for possible storage sites. Rates of biotransformation may be more easily determine *in vitro*, but only at concentrations expected *in vivo* and related to findings in the intact animal, because complicated interactions may play a role in the living organism that do not occur with isolated enzymes, cell fractions, or cell or tissue preparations. When a toxicokinetic model is established, it should then be validated by choosing a different route of exposure, dose levels, or dose frequency to test predictions made by the model. Single dose models are considered adequate except for induction or suicide inhibition of metabolic pathways. In these cases, 5 days to 2 weeks may be necessary to determine the effects of multiple doses. Age testing may be important and may use naïve rodents of 3, 6, 12, and 18 months, where 2 years is their lifespan (Buchanan et al., 1997).

The application of these techniques can be observed by looking at a toxicokinetic paper and analyzing its design and data. The study examined here is true toxicokinetic analysis, because it analyzes the absorption through excretion of a flame retardant, tetrabromobisphenol A (TBBPA), in human volunteers and rats (Schauer et al., 2006). This is similar to another chemical currently in the literature, bisphenol A, that has generated concerns about toxicity to human infants drinking from hard polycarbonate plastic baby bottles. This European Union study was selected, because it is unusual for studies in the United States to use human volunteers for strictly toxic exposures—a practice generally reserved for testing pharmaceuticals. A single oral dose of TBBPA of 0.1 mg/kg was used in the five human volunteers, while rats were given 300 mg/kg. This makes sense, as the difference in metabolism from a rat to a human is based on body surface area (BSA) ratios. The dosages should be calculated in mg/kg for differences in body weight within a species for similarly aged animals and mg/cm² for determining dose equivalents between species. Because the "average" human has a BSA of approximately 18,500 cm² for a 70-kg subject and the rat has a BSA of 365 cm² for a 0.2-kg subject, the following calculations result:

rat dosage = 300 mg/kg; rat dose = 0.2 kg
    × 300 mg/kg = 60 mg
rat dosage per surface area = 60 mg/365 cm²
    = 0.16 mg/cm²
0.16 mg/cm² = first approximation at
    a human dosage per surface area
human dose = 0.16 mg/cm² × 18,500 cm²
    = 3,041 mg
human dosage = 3,041 mg/70 kg = 43 mg/kg

Because a human volunteer should not be given a chemical even at 0.1 LD_{50}, a safety factor of a log unit should be used for rat-to-human differences and then another log unit used for differences between humans for a factor of 100 (10 × 10). That would make the human dose 0.43 mg/kg. This is less than a logarithm from the dosage actually employed in this study. A short-cut to the actual human dose is to take the 300 mg/kg rat dosage and take off the kg for an approximate human dose of 300 mg. Divide that by the 70 kg to obtain 4.29 mg/kg for a human dose. Then, use a safety factor of 10 between species to get back to the 0.43 mg/kg figured previously. The study did not indicate how the low dose was selected for human subjects, but

indicated that the Declaration of Helsinki was followed along with the Regional Ethical Committee of the University of Würzburg, Germany. Health of the human subjects was assessed using a verbal medical history, and three healthy males and two healthy females were chosen for analysis. This supports the sex differences called for in toxicokinetics analysis but does not indicate the dose–response of the human or the animal. Twenty-three urine sampling times were indicated at 0, 3, 6, 9, 12, 15, 23, 27, 32, 36, 39, 47, 53, 58, 63, 71, 77, 82, 87, 95, 101, 124, and 178 hours. These exceeded the number suggested for analysis, but the times of sampling were not the standard, 24, 48, 72, 96, and 120 hours. The times were close, but the pre-selection of these unusual times was not discussed. Blood samples were taken at more uniform times of 0, 1, 2, 4, 6, 8, 12, 24, 32, 36, 48, 60, 72, 84, 96, 124, and 178 hours. Clearly, use of tissue samples would have been unethical, but fecal samples could have been instructive for oral doses.

For the rat portion of the analysis, six male rats were used, which assumes no sex difference in toxicokinetics. Urine and fecal samples were collected in individual metabolic cages for 4 days prior to dosing by gavage, which assured the full dose was received. Urine was collected for 6- and 12-hour intervals for 100 hours following dosing, while feces were collected every 12 hours. Blood samples were collected at predetermined time points representing 3- (early points) to 12 (later points)-hour intervals. Tissue samples were not taken, because each rat represented a repeated measure design after serving as its own control prior to dosing. Liquid chromatography–mass spectrometry (LC-MS) determined the TBBPA and it metabolites. TBBPA-sulfate and TBBPA-glucuronide conjugates were used as standards for rat fecal analysis by extraction and high-pressure liquid chromatography with ultraviolet detector (HPLC-UV) quantitation. These techniques followed recommendations for the use of sensitive methods that anticipate metabolites in various fractions. Fecal samples would more likely have the unmetabolized compound or biliary excreted conjugates. Results from the rats indicated that the key but low concentrations of metabolites at early time points were indeed the

TBBPA-diglucuronide, a TBBPA-glucuronide-sulfate, tribromobisphenol A, and tribromobisphenol A glucuronide. The low dose given to the humans could not confirm the presence of these metabolites due to the limit of detection (LOD) of the analytical method. That indicates that animal experiments yield more information unless the dose is higher in the human due to accidental exposure or the use of more expensive analysis with lower detection limits. However, species differences have to be considered. The peak of TBBPA in the rat plasma was at 3 hours post-administration at 103 µM. Greater than 80% of the unmetabolized compound was excreted in the feces of the rat 24 hours following dosing. The elimination followed first-order kinetics with an elimination half-life of 13 hours. The major metabolite of the TBBPA-sulfate peaked in the plasma at 3 hours with 700 µM, while the TBBPA-glucuronide was at 25 µM. The low bioavailability of TBBPA to the plasma appears to be due to its effective conjugation and elimination in the bile and enterohepatic recirculation that allows the liver to further conjugate and eliminate the medication. This is unusual as enterohepatic recirculation may account for more than 100% of a toxin or medication as the dose is encountered more than once (Schauer et al., 2006).

To illustrate this finding with another example, the toxicokinetics of a compound A that is involved in enterohepatic recirculation is illustrated in **Figure 13-5**. The model represented in the figure accounts for the compound absorption from the gastrointestinal (GI) tract, its movement to a central compartment, recirculation through the bile and reabsorption, and elimination. This figure also shows that IV administration goes directly to a rapid peak in the central compartment, but could also be subject to nonlinear kinetics as indicated by a recirculation model (Shou et al., 2005).

One of the key classes of chemicals for which oral absorption varies greatly depending on their chemical form is the metals. Arsenic, chromium, lead, and manganese have specific carrier-mediated processes. Arsenic, chromium, manganese, and mercury absorption is affected by valence state. Organic forms of arsenic, lead, and most famously mercury are known to be

much better absorbed than the inorganic metal. Absorption of lead and manganese is affected by particle size where these metals bind. Aluminum, arsenic, chromium, lead, manganese, and mercury have their toxicokinetics altered by biotransformation. These same factors also alter the effect or toxicodynamics (Yokel et al., 2006). Not only should absorption of compounds be measured as a result of simple exposure, but interactions with other chemicals may enhance or retard their absorption or retention. For example, metals compete for absorption and tend to antagonize each other. However, a compound such as resveratrol inhibits transporter P-glycoprotein efflux of toxicants and medications and also inhibits the medication-metabolizing isozyme CYP3A4. This combination of effects leads to increases in the plasma AUC and the C_{max} of medications such as the calcium-channel antagonist nicardipine from oral, but not IV, administration. This could lead to cardiovascular toxicity from an overdose if these factors are not taken into account (Choi et al., 2009). Absorption also

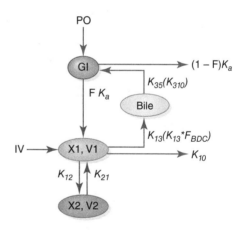

FIGURE 13-5 Illustration of Enterohepatic Recirculation (ERR) Model

Note: Population pharmacokinetic/toxicokinetic model containing EHR that comprises of four compartments: GI tract, central, peripheral and gallbladder. X1, V1, X2 and V2 are amounts (X) and volume of distribution (V) of Compound A in central (systemic circulation and liver) and peripheral (tissues) compartments, respectively. Rate constants for the individual compartments are Ka (absorption), K12, K21, K10 (elimination in central compartment), K13 (=K10 · FBILE), K31 (rate constant at no gallbladder emptying) and K310 (rate constant at gallbladder emptying at TGE, postdose time for gallbladder emptying). FBILE is a fraction of K10 for the compound excreted to bile from the central compartment. FBDC is a change in K13 in the presence of the bile-duct cannulation (BDC). F is the bioavailability of the compound.

depends on the part of the intestinal tract and the xenobiotic transporters present.

The effect of food and the anatomy and physiology of the gastrointestinal tract relate heavily to the absorption of toxic chemicals. Digestion and major absorption of nutrients, water, and electrolytes occur in the small intestine, although water and electrolytes are also absorbed in the large intestine. This is important when considering the rat as a model of human exposure to toxicants by the oral route. Although rats and humans masticate their food and produce saliva, there is no oropharynx in the rat as the epiglottis separates the nasal and oral cavity. The human stomach is totally secretory, while the rat stomach is divided into a forestomach lined with stratified epithelium as a site for bacterial digestion and a glandular stomach releasing acid and proenzymes. The acidity of the rat stomach is less (pH 3–5) than that of the human (pH 1–2). This difference in pH can affect the charge of certain molecules and absorption and may degrade acid-labile chemicals. This acidity is neutralized to a large degree by bicarbonate release from Brunner's glands upon entering the small intestine. The mucosal conduit (mouth, pharynx, esophagus, lower rectum, and anal canal) has stratified squamous epithelium with little vascularization that limits absorption to those substances that can readily cross barriers such as nitroglycerin; isosorbide dinitrate; and other medications, solvents, and toxicants that may be considered sublingual in their route of exposure. The absorbing regions of the GI tract have single columnar epithelium with structures that vastly increase the surface area (plicae, crypts, and villi) with richly vascularized lamina propria. The difference between the total length of the GI tract of the rat and human is only 5.5-fold, despite the enormous difference in their relative weights (0.25 kg vs. 70 kg). Both have a small intestine percentage of the total tract in the low 80s, but the rat has 90% jejunum compare to 38% for the human small intestine. The rats use the 26% of the large intestine that represents the cecum for microbial digestion, where the human cecum is 5% and considered vestigial. Although the human small intestine is only five times that of a rat, its surface area is 200 times greater. This is due to the presence of plicae

circulars (or Kerckring's folds) that increase the surface area threefold in the human, which are not found in the rat. The villi increase human proximal (duodenum and upper jejunum) small intestine surface area by fivefold in the rat and 10-fold in the human. Microvilli increase both rat and human proximal small intestine by another 20-fold. These are important features for modelers who wish to predict human absorption of toxicants from rat data. Clearly, the upper small intestine deserves the focus for absorption. Based on these data, the problems of increased human absorption have two different effects on the toxicokinetics. The rate of absorption will be higher to a more rapid peak in the human for toxicants equally well absorbed by both species. Additionally, toxicants poorly or less completely absorbed by the rat will find more absorption in the human (higher dose or AUC; DeSesso and Jacobson, 2001). The human intestine protects itself from toxicants by efflux via ATP-binding cassette (ABC) transporters and cytochrome P450 metabolism. This varies in the human intestine, especially for multi-drug resistance–associated protein 2 (MRP2 or ABCC2) mRNA expression, which decreases significantly from human jejunum samples to ileum ($^2/_3$ of jejunal expression) to colon ($< ^1/_3$ of jejunal expression). CYP3A4 similarly varies in these sections. P-glycoprotein also appears to follow a similar trend, but shows high variability between subjects. MRP1 (ABCC1) does not show any trend based on section (Berggren et al., 2007). For the specific case of the phytoestrogen resveratrol, there is significant metabolism of this health-promoting compound in the intestinal tract. The polar sulfate and glucuronide conjugates need specific carriers out of the intestinal epithelial cells. The glucuronide conjugate is transported out of enterocytes through MRP3 in the basolateral membrane and breast cancer resistance protein (BCRP, ABCG2) located in the apical membrane (van de Wetering et al., 2009). Certain transporters are found in the small intestine that mediate uptake of toxicants. Organic anion transporting polypeptides (rodents: Oatps, human: OATPs) are part of the *Slco/SLCO* gene superfamily. They transport amphipathic chemicals (e.g., medications, bile salts, steroids, and peptides). OATp1a5 has been studied and a QSAR analysis has been performed based on the substrate binding site of the protein (Yarim et al., 2005). Note also that in addition to the organic anion-transporting polypeptide family, the organic anion and organic cation transporters (OATs/OCTs; SLC22 family) and the peptide transporter-1 (PEPT1; SLC15 family) are expressed in the intestinal tract. They are also expressed in the liver, which would be the first stop for intestinally absorbed toxicants via the portal circulation. The kidney expression would also be of interest as the liver prepares toxicants in first-pass metabolism for renal excretion (Zaïr et al., 2008).

Inhalation

The next most likely route of exposure to toxicants is inhalation. Unless the subject spends little time inhaling a powder, liquid, gas, aerosol, or vapor, a dose or LD_{50} is not usually established. Rather an LC_{50} is more appropriate. Inhalation and IV administration lead to the fastest peaks and therefore represent the routes by which drugs of abuse are taken for the greatest impact. Toxicants in the solid form are based on shape (geometric radius and standard deviation) and composition; small spheres, for example, may exit the lung as fast as they enter, whereas asbestos fibers may essentially stay imbedded in the respiratory tract for a lifetime. Other substances cross across the alveoli for absorption into the bloodstream and head directly for the heart and then the brain. This makes this route extremely dangerous for lung damage, cardiovascular injury, and central nervous system toxicity. The toxicity also depends on the anatomy and physiology of the respiratory tract, because species have different tracheal diameters and length as well as the divisions into the bronchi. This has made the search for a species that represents the human dependent on the anatomy, physiology, and the biochemistry of the respiratory tract. Stenosis of the rat bronchiole has been used to investigate nitrogen dioxide–induced asthma (Juhos et al., 1980). The rat proves to be a better model for trichloroethylene (TCE) toxicity, because exposure to this compound has not caused lung cancer or acute lung toxicity

in the rat or the human. The mouse, however, has many non-ciliated Clara cells with high concentrations of cytochrome P450 (approximately 600-fold higher than the human activity toward TCE). This leads to accumulation of the chloral metabolite in the mouse and aneuploidy and a poor assumption of similar toxicity in other rodents and the human (Green, 2000). In a comparison of the rhesus monkey to the Sprague-Dawley rat, videomicrometry demonstrated that rats lack alveolarized or respiratory bronchioles in their most distal airway. Additionally, the rat proximal airways consist of simple cuboidal or columnar epithelium, differentiating it from the pseudostratified epithelium found in the monkey. Goblet cells, submucosal glands, and cartilage are lacking in the rat proximal airway as well. Despite these differences, hyperresponsiveness of the proximal airways of rats and monkeys to methacholine was similar. However, respiratory bronchioles of monkeys were not as responsive to methacholine as the proximal bronchi. Rats on the other hand had increased responsiveness of their distal bronchioles (Kott et al., 2002). Rats also show metabolism of the herbicide Acetochlor to a quinone-imine in their nasal epithelial cells leading to formation of protein adducts, cell death, compensatory hyperplasia, and subsequent adenoma development. This is not the metabolic cascade followed by the human (Green et al., 2000). These findings may indicate that the expensive use of monkeys is necessary to model certain toxicants in the air.

The beagle dog has been investigated as a better respiratory model than the rat. The respiratory bronchioles consist of five generations in the beagle dog and branch similarly to the human, making it a good toxicological model (Takenaka et al., 1998). The beagle dog has served as a model for many inhaled toxicants, from marijuana smoke (Sullivan and Willard, 1978) to the inhalation of insoluble radioactive Cerium-144 fused to aluminosilicate particles (Hahn et al., 2001).

Much has been learned about inhalation of agents and their plasma concentrations from anesthesia. The anesthesia model used is crucial for a volatile compound. The use of IV pharmacokinetic equations employing half-life and effect site concentrations may be utilized (Hendrickx and De Wolf, 2008). Another clinical model follows a Severinghaus relationship. That relationship indicates that nitrous oxide uptake proceeds as the inverse square root of the time profile. However, that relationship is an over-estimate of the amount of volatile substance that is necessary for anesthesia and can lead to overdose (Connor and Philip, 2009). This route does not depend on the activity of the trans-porter P-glycoprotein for inhaled medications such as digoxin, even though this transporter is present at low levels in rat lung cells (Madlova et al., 2009). However, the toxicology may reside in the lung itself. For example, the development of nanotechnology indicates that biomark-ers may have to be developed to look for the toxicity of carbon nanotubes. **Figure 13-6** indi-cates the cellular signals in the lungs as a result

of exposure to carbon nanotubes. Note that many cells and factors appear to be involved in the damage from these microscopic particles. The intimate involvement of blood vessels and immune cells in the lung is important in con-sidering absorption and lung damage. Also, gas exchange, oxidative injury, and inflammation are key mediators of lung toxicity.

One chemical that does not have to be inhaled to be taken up by the lung is Paraquat. Paraquat is absorbed from the plasma through a polyamine uptake system, which appears to be dependent to some degree on the presence of sodium ions (Dinis-Oliveira et al., 2006). However, its release indicates that Paraquat uptake and extrusion in the kidney and by inference other organs appear to involve human organic cation transporter hOCT2 (not hOCT1 or hOCT3), whose overexpression enhances

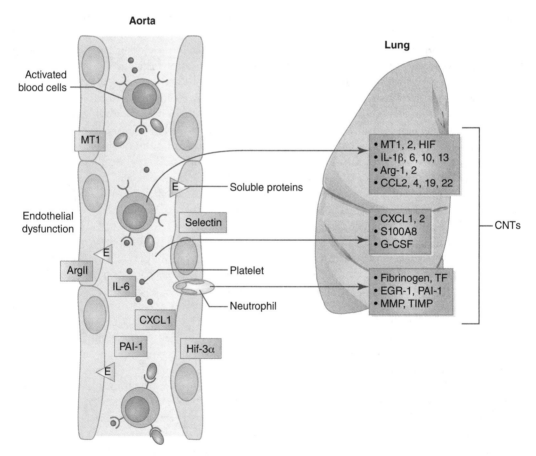

FIGURE 13-6 The Production of Lung and Endothelial Dysfunction by Carbon Nanotubes. Possible Mediators and Biomarkers of Toxic Damage

accumulation and toxicity of Paraquat. Similarly, expression of human multidrug and toxic compound extrusion (hMATE)1 also increases accumulation and cytotoxicity of Paraquat (Chen et al., 2007).

Parenteral Routes

Injected routes are likely in medicine and the exposure to venoms. They also represent all the toxicant in the organism. This section begins with the conduit and reference route, blood or plasma, and continues from there into slower release routes and the route that tests the effectiveness of the blood–brain barrier.

Intravenous

Intravenous is the reference route for other routes, for by definition at time zero of injection the concentration (C_0) is the highest in the blood or plasma. The toxicant might then move into blood cells or tissues and can be excreted by a variety of routes based on its hydrophilicity (kidney) or volatility (lung). Hydrophobic toxicants can find their way to fatty tissues and may be metabolized and excreted. Thus, it is important to consider volume of distribution, or V_d. Note in **Figure 13-7**, for example, that a compound appears to have its highest concentration at the time of injection as illustrated by

IV bolus administration of nerve agents Soman and Sarin to guinea pigs. The initial drop represents the apparent volume of distribution as hydrophobic compounds find their way into the fatty tissues in a one-compartment (classical plasma) model. There is then a slower log-linear phase of drop-off reflecting metabolism and excretion. Because concentration is equal to amount per volume, $C_0 = D_{IV}/V_d$, where D_{IV} represents the amount of injected compound. In a first-order equation, the slope of the line depends on the elimination rate constant k_{el}. The slope for a line is $y = mx + b$, where m represents the slope and b the y-intercept. Because the compound is decreasing over time, the slope is negative. The slope of a semilogarithmic curve is $-k_{el}/2.303$. Why is that? Because the falloff depends on a steady rate of elimination and is exponential, it should fall off as $e^{-k(el)t}$ with t being time. This equation has been modified to indicate the rate of falloff as k(el). Because $e^{-k(el)t}$ is also expressed as ln $k_{el}t$, the curve expressed in semilogarithmic fashion would have to be divided by 2.303, because $2.303 \log_{10} = $ ln. Ultimately, the data have a natural logarithmic falloff, with the slope $= -k_{el}/2.303$. The concentration C at a given time t would be represented by $C = C_0 e^{-k(el)t}$. This k_{el} function is the inverse of the half-life, $t_{1/2}$, which is the time it takes for the concentration to fall to ½ C_0. The mathematical expression is $k_{el} = 0.693/t_{1/2}$. Notice

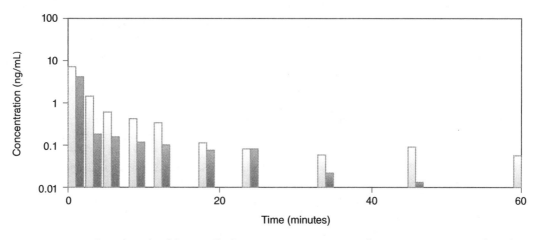

FIGURE 13-7 Semilogarithmic Plot of the Mean Blood Concentration (+SEM, n = 6) of Two Nerve Agents into Anesthetized, Atropinized, Restrained, and Mechanically Ventilated Guinea Pigs

Note: Dark bars represent intravenous one-time injection of 0.8 LD$_{50}$ s(-)sarin. Light bars represent 0.8 LD$_{50}$ soman.

that half-life does not depend on concentration theoretically, because it is only a function of the elimination rate. This is an absurd notion for toxicologists, for as doses approach lethality, it would be expected that compounds may affect kidney and liver function and drastically alter the rate of elimination. However, in a reasonable pharmacological or therapeutic range of a substance, this makes sense.

Calculus can also be to better understand toxicokinetics. The C_0 function would represent a possible toxic peak that would relate to threshold toxicity. However, if a threshold were not reached, the time the compound spent at each concentration would be more important. That is effectively the integral function from time 0 to the time of elimination and is known as the AUC. For the equation $V_d = D_{ivIV}/C_0$, that would yield another factor for C_0 since it would be very difficult to truly assess the concentration at the time of injection. Instead, consider two concentrations in the linear range over two times and curve fit. This extrapolates back to C_0. $C_0 = AUC_{0\to\infty} \times k_{el}$, where $AUC_{0\to last} = \Sigma\frac{1}{2}(c_1 \times c_2) + (t_2 - t_1)$ for concentrations (c) determined at sampling time 1 (t_1) and time 2 (last time taken). Next, it is possible to extrapolate from samples taken to ∞. $AUC_{0\to\infty} = AUC_{0\to t(last)} + C_{last}/k_{el}$. This reveals more compartments and enables advanced modeling of each compartment (e.g., liver or brain) from peak for an IV or inhalation dose to their first-order natural logarithm decline. It is also important to determine how much of the compound has actually left the body versus persists in the organism. This is a function of total body clearance $Cl_b = k_{el} \times Vd$. Substituting $D_{IV}/AUC_{0\to\infty} \times k_{el}$ for Vd, it is clear that $Cl_b = D_{IV}/AUC_{0\to\infty}$, so it appears that clearance is about how much was put into the body versus how much is left. If the compound effectively persists through a lifetime, then AUC rises and clearance is effectively zero. Otherwise, Cl_b is not based mathematically on rate of clearance or half-life. If more than 100% of the compound is found to be cleared, one must assume that the body experiences the same compound and its metabolites more than once as occurs in enterohepatic recirculation.

For chronic toxicity, it is necessary to know both the half-life and clearance for determining

bioaccumulation even though $t_{1/2}$ and Cl_b functions have no mathematical relationship. More complex modeling may lead to a two-compartment model or linking one-compartment models of multiple organs giving a new k_{el}. This type of modeling is important for compounds that are not represented by a straight line semi-logarithmically, but instead still show exponential behavior. A two-compartment model looks at both compartments as follows:

$$k_{21} = (\alpha B + \beta A)/(A + B); k_{el} = \alpha\beta/k_{21};$$
$$k_{12} = \alpha + \beta - k_{21} - k_{el}$$

In the one-compartment model, the terminal half-life or β is the same as the k_{el}, which it is not the two-compartment model. The intravenous route points to the plasma or blood concentration as the best model of toxicokinetics. This is also the method for therapeutic drug monitoring. For certain compounds such as the anti-arrhythmic $3Na^+,2K^+$-ATPase inhibitor, digitalis, plasma concentrations are required as part of the dosing regimen. For some medications such as the myeloablative medication for hemopoietic stem cell transplantation, busulfan, there is a threefold variation in exposure to the same IV dose in humans (Russell and Kangarloo, 2008).

Intraperitoneal

Intraperitoneal absorption is an unlikely route of absorption, although it provides a good avenue for evaluating toxicants. For example, the oral and IP route share the liver as the first organ to receive a high concentration. This is important as the acetylcholinesterase inhibitor Soman (methyl pinacolyl phosphorofluoridate), whose IV toxicokinetics were shown in Figure 13-7 compared with Sarin, has a higher murine LD_{50} via the IP route (0.425 mg/kg) than the subcutaneous route (0.165 mg/kg). This relates to Soman's detoxication in the liver. This route would also be good to compare with oral, as the acid and digestive enzymes would not be present to alter toxicity. This would be especially important for acid-labile toxic proteins or peptides. Intraperitoneal administration of the cancer chemotherapy agent cisplatin is considered a possible new option for treatment of ovarian cancer patients at the time of surgery. New toxicokinetics indicate a three-compartment model is necessary to account for changes in IP fluid and plasma platinum concentrations. From this a dose recommendation can be made based on prevention of renal toxicity and potency in treating the cancer cells (Royer et al., 2009). Another anticancer agent, paclitaxel, shows some benefits of IP administration versus IV administration for a toxic agent. The IV route in rabbits exhibited a rapid, high serum peak one-half hour after administration. The IP route showed higher concentrations when the IV route was waning, at 6 and 24 hours after injection. Additionally, omentum, mesenteric lymph nodes, ovary, and stomach had higher AUCs for IP paclitaxel (Soma et al., 2008). This indicates that a longer-lasting influence with a lower peak for acute host toxicity appears to be experienced for abdominal organs by IP administration. This supports the idea that this route may be a preferred method for treating ovarian and similarly located cancers. Because the liver is likely to have high residues of compounds given by the IP route, induction of liver metabolism should play a role in the increased toxic effects of bioactivated compounds. Divided doses of polychlorinated biphenyls given IP to immature female Sprague-Dawley rats had enhanced uterotropic potency compared with a single dose equal to the other doses combined possibly due to the induced pentoxyresorufin O-dealkylase (PROD) activity and increased toxic metabolites produced in the liver (Soontornchat et al., 1994).

Subcutaneous and Intramuscular

Now the discussion moves into the parenteral routes of slow release for fat-soluble chemicals that lead to the lowest toxicity or lethality. One area is associated with a fatty layer (SC) and one with high protein content for binding (IM). One medication that models this type of slow release due to protein binding is procaine, a drug banned for use in horse racing due to its local anesthetic action peripherally and stimulatory in the central nervous system. The pharmacokinetics in horses was clearly examined years ago, but still is used today in combination with penicillin to cause

slow absorption from the intramuscularly administered antibiotic. An IV dosage of 2.5 mg/kg procaine HCl into a horse results in an instant plasma peak of more than 1,000 ng/mL. This peak is followed by an initial drop representing a $t_{1/2\alpha}$ of 5 minutes. Procaine has a slower phase of elimination with a $t_{1/2\beta}$ of 50.2 minutes. This fits a two-compartment open model. Because it binds strongly to plasma protein (albumin), procaine has both an apparent $V_{d\beta}$ of 3,500 L in the horse and a true $V_{d\beta}$ of 6,500 L. A slightly larger SC injection (3.3 mg/kg) results in a lower peak of 400 ng/mL. The two-compartment open model was modified to account for the first-order absorption from the SC site ($K = 0.048$ min^{-1}), and a $t_{1/2}$ was calculated as 75 minutes. IM injection of a much higher dosage of procaine HCl (10 mg/kg) results in a rapid plasma peak of 600 ng/mL, which is much lower than the other parenteral routes considering the size of the dosage. The half-life was calculated as 2.5 hours. Giving procaine with penicillin IM (33,000 IU/kg) results in a lower peak of 270 ng/L procaine and a much enhanced half-life of 9 hours (Tobin and Blake, 1976). More than a decade earlier, the lethality of procaine was determined in mice. Note that the LD$_{50}$ values increase with delayed less bioavailable compound (p.o.) or sustained lower peak release with 45 mg/kg for IV, 230 mg/kg for IP, 500 mg/kg for oral, 630 mg/kg for IM, and the lowest lethality for the SC route at 800 mg/kg (Barnes and Eltherington, 1964). To discover the effect of procaine on penicillin administration intramuscularly in the horse, penicillin G procaine (22,000 units of penicillin G/kg) or penicillin G potassium (22,000 U/kg) or procaine hydrochloride (1.5 mg/kg) or a mixture of penicillin G with procaine HCl was injected. The IM-injected penicillin G procaine had almost twice the half-life in the horse (24.7 hours) of penicillin G alone (12.9 hours). The effect of penicillin compounding of the procaine was more dramatic on procaine's half-life, as penicillin G procaine had a half-life of 15.6 hours for the procaine portion. The half-life of a mixture of penicillin G and procaine HCl exhibited a 1-hour half-life for the procaine. This dramatic interaction is of therapeutic importance and toxicological significance (Uboh et al.,

2000). A sustained lower peak is more toxic to the microorganism invader and less toxic to the host than a large, fast peak would be.

Intrathecal or Intracerebroventricular

Injection into the spinal canal or into the cerebral ventricles delivers a medication or toxicant to the cerebrospinal fluid (CSF) and the central nervous system. This may determine whether a compound may be neurotoxic if it could cross the blood–brain barrier. Quaternary ammonium compounds are model agents that do not penetrate the barrier between the central nervous system and the rest of the body. This has toxicological significance. This phenomenon was studied in the early 1960s and found to be important in the development of what were then called cholinolytics (now referred to as cholinergic receptor antagonists, or more specifically muscarinic receptor antagonists). Three structures were studied for passage from the carotid artery into the brain of cats and their effect. Four (4) mg/kg dosages of two tertiary compounds (atropine—the sulfate of the tropine ester of tropic acid—and amizil—the hydrochloride of 2-ethylaminoethyl ester of benzilic acid) and one quaternary chemical (lachesine—N-ethyl-N,N-dimethyl-2-(benziloyloxy)ethylammonium chloride) were evaluated through injection into the carotid artery. Amizil had 9.00 ± 0.35 µg penetrate into the brain, while 4.60 ± 0.26 µg of the atropine penetrated. None of the quaternary compound lachesine penetrated the central nervous system. In contrast, the cholinergic antagonistic activity of the quaternary compound exceeds that of the other compounds if injected directly into the brain (Golikov and Pechenkin, 1963).

In the past, it would be inconceivable that the direct injection route into the central nervous system would be used except to produce a spinal anesthetic block. However, current therapies for hematological malignancies in the central nervous system are treated with intrathecal injections of the antimetabolite folic acid analog methotrexate, antimetabolite pyrimidine analog cytosine arabinoside (cytarabine), and anti-inflammatory corticosteroids. Use of methotrexate or cytarabine by this route of administration increases the half-life in the CSF and may lead to unwanted toxicities such as spinal cord lesions, seizures, and encephalopathy. The most likely toxicities are spinal cord lesions, leaving human patients with tetraplegia, paraplegia, and cauda equina syndrome that result in lack of control over muscles, bowel movements, and urination. Cytarabine is the most causal agent alone at high doses, in slow-release formulations, or in combination with methotrexate (Kwong et al., 2009). ICV administration of toxicants should take into account the distribution of fluoro-gold as an indicator of disposition with time. Two minutes following injection, most of the compound is found in the choroid plexus in the lateral and third ventricles. Fifteen to 30 minutes post-administration, fluoro-gold penetrated into the forebrain ventricular organs, parenchymal tissues, and the hypophysis. The peripheral circulation detected the compound at 2 minutes, a peak at 20 minutes, and a decline thereafter. This indicates the time course expected for compounds injected in this fashion into the rat brain (Li et al., 2006).

The use of ICV compounds to treat toxicity can yield unexpected results. For example, the injection of radical scavengers appears to protect against Parkinson's disease generated from neurodegeneration of dopaminergic neurons via the Fenton reaction. The iron-chelating agent Desferal (deferoxamine) injected ICV did not affect striatal tyrosine hydroxylase activity or dopamine metabolism. However, 6-hydrodopamine's induced decline in striatal and frontal cortex dopamine concentrations, dihydroxyphenylacetic acid, and homovanillic acid, as well as the left and right striatum tyrosine hydroxylase activity and dopamine turnover was prevented by Desferal pretreatment. The lowest protective dose was 1.3 µg Desferal, which was 200-fold lower than that of the 6-hydrodopamine. This indicated the iron chelation was the likely mechanism rather than interference with the neurotoxicity of the dopamine metabolite. This line of research led to a series of blood-brain barrier-penetrating iron chelators for possible uses in neurodegenerative diseases such as Parkinson's disease, Alzheimer's disease, Friedreich's ataxia, and Huntington's disease (Youdim et al., 2004). Thus, this route shows promise both in determination of toxicity and in prevention of toxic reactions leading to neurotoxicity.

Questions

1. What compounds pass the skin easily? Why?
2. Why is it unwise to give your pet cats or dogs or your infant eye drops meant for adults?
3. Why is oral toxicity a problem for the liver and GI tract but less problematic than an injected or inhaled toxicant?
4. Why is the variability of ABC transporters and CYPs important in the GI tract?
5. Why is the beagle dog but not rodents a better model of human respiratory toxicity?
6. Why might the nerve agent sarin be less toxic via the IP route compared with other parenteral routes?
7. Why is the anesthetic agent procaine most toxic by the IV route, less toxic by the IM route, and least toxic by the SC route?
8. How do we know that quaternary ammonium compounds do not pass the blood-brain barrier in intact adult humans?

References

Barnes CD, Eltherington LG. 1964. *Drug dosage in laboratory animals*. Berkeley, CA: University of California Press.

Berggren S, Gall C, Wollnitz N, Ekelund M, Karlbom U, Hoogstraate J, Schrenk D, Lennernäs H. 2007. Gene and protein expression of P-glycoprotein, MRP1, MRP2, and CYP3A4 in the small and large human intestine. *Mol Pharm*. 4:25-2257.

Buchanan JR, Burka LT, Melnick RL. 1997. Purpose and guidelines for toxicokinetic studies within the National Toxicology Program. *Environ Health Perspect*. 105:468-471.

Chang SK, Brownie C, Riviere JE. 1994. Percutaneous absorption of topical parathion through porcine skin: in vitro studies on the effect of environmental perturbations. *J Vet Pharmacol Ther*. 17:434-439.

Chen Y, Zhang S, Sorani M, Giacomini KM. 2007. Transport of paraquat by human organic cation transporters and multidrug and toxic compound extrusion family. *J Pharmacol Exp Ther*. 322:695-700.

Choi JS, Choi BC, Kang KW. 2009. Effect of resveratrol on the pharmacokinetics of oral and intravenous nicardipine in rats: possible role of P-glycoprotein inhibition by resveratrol. *Pharmazie*. 64:49-52.

Connor CW, Philip JH. 2009. Closed-form solutions for the optimum equivalence of first-order compartmental models and their implications for classical models of closed-circuit anesthesia. *Physiol Meas*. 30:N11-21.

DeSesso JM, Jacobson CF. 2001. Anatomical and physiological parameters affecting gastrointestinal absorption in humans and rats. *Food Chem Toxicol*. 39:v209-228.

Dinis-Oliveira RJ, De Jesús Valle MJ, Bastos ML, Carvalho F, Sánchez Navarro A. 2006. Kinetics of paraquat in the isolated rat lung: Influence of sodium depletion. *Xenobiotica*. 36:724-737.

Erdely A, Hulderman T, Salmen R, Liston A, Zeidler-Erdely PC, Schwegler-Berry D, Castranova V, Koyama S, Kim YA, Endo M, Simeonova PP. 2009. Cross-talk between lung and systemic circulation during carbon nanotube respiratory exposure. Potential biomarkers. *Nano Lett*. 9:36-43.

European Commission Health and Consumer Protection Directorate-General, Directorate E—Food Safety: plant health, animal health and welfare, international questions, E1—Plant health. 2004. Guidance document on dermal absorption. http://ec.europa.eu/food/plant/protection/evaluation/guidance/wrkdoc20_rev_en.pdf

Funckes AJ, Hayes GR Jr, Hartwell WV. 1963. Urinary excretion of paranitrophenol by volunteers following dermal exposure to parathion at different ambient temperatures. *J Agric Food Chem*. 11:455-457.

Golikov SN, Pechenkin VA. 1963. [Study of the penetration of some cholinolytic substances through the hemato-encephalic barrier by the cerebral ventricle perfusion method.] *Biull Eksp Biol Med*. 56:82-85.

Gordon CJ. 2003. Role of environmental stress in the physiological response to chemical toxicants. *Environ Res*. 92:1-7.

Gordon CJ, Spencer PJ, Hotchkiss J, Miller DB, Hinder-liter PM, Pauluhn J. 2008. Thermoregulation and its influence on toxicity assessment. *Toxicology*. 244:87-97.

Greaves JL, Wilson CG, Rozier A, Grove J, Plazonnet B. 1990. Scintigraphic assessment of an ophthalmic gelling vehicle in man and rabbit. *Curr Eye Res*. 9:415-420.

Green T. 2000. Pulmonary toxicity and carcinogenicity of trichloroethylene: species differences and modes of action. *Environ Health Perspect*. 108(Suppl 2):261-264.

Green T, Lee R, Moore RB, Ashby J, Willis GA, Lund VJ, Clapp MJ. 2000. Acetochlor-induced rat nasal tumors: further studies on the mode of action and relevance to humans. *Regul Toxicol Pharmacol.* 32:127–133.

Gute BD, Grunwald GD, Basak SC. 1999. Prediction of the dermal penetration of polycyclic aromatic hydrocarbons (PAHs): a hierarchical QSAR approach. *SAR QSAR Environ Res.* 10:1–15.

Hahn FF, Muggenburg BA, Snipes MB, Boecker BB. 2001. The toxicity of insoluble cerium-144 inhaled by beagle dogs: non-neoplastic effects. *Radiat Res.* 155:95–112.

Heimann K, Peschgens T, Merz U, Hoernchen H, Wenzl T. 2007. [Depression of respiration via toxic effects on the central nervous system following use of topical brimonidine in an infant with congenital glaucoma]. *Ophthalmologe.* 104:505–507.

Hendrickx JF, De Wolf A. 2008. Special aspects of pharmacokinetics of inhalation anesthesia. *Handb Exp Pharmacol.* (182):159–186.

Juhos LT, Green DP, Furiosi NJ, Freeman G. 1980. A quantitative study of stenosis in the respiratory bronchiole of the rat in NO -induced emphysema. *Am Rev Respir Dis.* 121:541–549.

Karla PK, Earla R, Boddu SH, Johnston TP, Pal D, Mitra A. 2009. Molecular expression and functional evidence of a drug efflux pump (BCRP) in human corneal epithelial cells. *Curr Eye Res.* 34:1–9.

Karla PK, Pal D, Quinn T, Mitra AK. 2007. Molecular evidence and functional expression of a novel drug efflux pump (ABCC2) in human corneal epithelium and rabbit cornea and its role in ocular drug efflux. *Int J Pharm.* 336:12–21.

Kasting GB, Bhatt VD, Speaker TJ. 2008. Microencapsulation decreases the skin absorption of N,N-diethyl-m-toluamide (DEET). *Toxicol In Vitro.* 22:548–552.

Kott KS, Pinkerton KE, Bric JM, Plopper CG, Avadhanam KP, Joad JP. 2002. Methacholine responsiveness of proximal and distal airways of monkeys and rats using videomicrometry. *J Appl Physiol.* 92:989–996.

Kwong YL, Yeung DY, Chan JC. 2009. Intrathecal chemotherapy for hematologic malignancies: drugs and toxicities. *Ann Hematol.* 88:193–201.

Li C, Marshall CT, Lu C, Ding J, Wang H, Roisen FJ, Xiao M. 2006. The dynamic distribution of fluoro-gold and its interrelation with neural nitric oxide synthase following intracerebroventricular injection into rat brain. *Biotech Histochem.* 81:41–50.

Madlova M, Bosquillon C, Asker D, Dolezal P, Forbes B. 2009. In-vitro respiratory drug absorption models possess nominal functional P-glycoprotein activity. *J Pharm Pharmacol.* 61:293–301.

Millar AW, Brown PD, Moore J, Galloway WA, Cornish AG, Lenehan TJ, Lynch KP. 1998. Results of single and repeat dose studies of the oral matrix metalloproteinase inhibitor marimastat in healthy male volunteers. *Br J Clin Pharmacol.* 45:21–26.

Nicoli S, Ferrari G, Quarta M, Macaluso C, Govoni P, Dallatana D, Santi P. 2009. Porcine sclera as a model of human sclera for in vitro transport experiments: histology, SEM, and comparative permeability. *Mol Vis.* 15:259–266.

Ramer JC, Paul-Murphy J, Brunson D, Murphy CJ. 1996. Effects of mydriatic agents in cockatoos, African gray parrots, and blue-fronted Amazon parrots. *J Am Vet Med Assoc.* 208:227–230.

Riviere JE. 2005. *Dermal absorption models in toxicology and pharmacology.* Boca Raton, FL: Taylor and Francis.

Royer B, Jullien V, Guardiola E, Heyd B, Chauffert B, Kantelip JP, Pivot X. 2009. Population pharmacokinetics and dosing recommendations for cisplatin during intraperitoneal peroperative administration: development of a limited sampling strategy for toxicity risk assessment. *Clin Pharmacokinet.* 48:169–180.

Russell JA, Kangarloo SB. 2008. Therapeutic drug monitoring of busulfan in transplantation. *Curr Pharm Des.* 14:1936–1949.

Schauer UM, Völkel W, Dekant W. 2006. Toxicokinetics of tetrabromobisphenol a in humans and rats after oral administration. *Toxicol Sci.* 91:49–58.

Senthilkumari S, Velpandian T, Biswas NR, Bhatnagar A, Mittal G, Ghose S. 2009. Evidencing the modulation of P-glycoprotein at blood-ocular barriers using gamma scintigraphy. *Curr Eye Res.* 34:73–77.

Shinomiya K, Kajima M, Tajika H, Shiota H, Nakagawa R, Saijyou T. 2003. Renal failure caused by eyedrops containing phenylephrine in a case of retinopathy of prematurity. *J Med Invest.* 50:203–206.

Shou M, Lu W, Kari PH, Xiang C, Liang Y, Lu P, Cui D, Emary WB, Michel KB, Adelsberger JK, Brunner JE, Rodrigues AD. 2005. Population pharmacokinetic modeling for enterohepatic recirculation in Rhesus monkey. *Eur J Pharm Sci.* 26:151–161.

Soma D, Kitayama J, Ishigami H, Kaisaki S, Nagawa H. 2008. Different tissue distribution of paclitaxel with intravenous and intraperitoneal administration. *J Surg Res.* 155(1):142–146.

Soontornchat S, Li MH, Cooke PS, Hansen LG. 1994. Toxicokinetic and toxicodynamic influences on endocrine disruption by polychlorinated biphenyls. *Environ Health Perspect.* 102:568–571.

Spruit HET, Langenberg JP, Trap HC, van der Wiel HJ, Helmich RB, van Helden HP, Benschop HP. 2000. Intravenous and inhalation toxicokinetics of sarin stereoisomers in atropinized guinea pigs. *Toxicol Appl Pharmacol.* 169:249–254.

Sullivan MF, Willard DH. 1978. The beagle dog as an animal model for marihuana smoking studies. *Toxicol Appl Pharmacol.* 45:445–462.

Takenaka S, Heini A, Ritter B, Heyder J. 1998. The respiratory bronchiole of beagle dogs: structural characteristics. *Toxicol Lett*. 96–97:301–308.

Tobin T, Blake JW. 1976. A review of the pharmacology, pharmacokinetics and behavioral effects of procaine in thoroughbred horses. *Br J Sports Med*. 10:109–116.

Tsuruta H. 1996. Skin absorption of solvent mixtures—effect of vehicles on skin absorption of toluene. *Ind Health*. 34:369–378.

Uboh CE, Soma LR, Luo Y, McNamara E, Fennell MA, May L, Teleis DC, Rudy JA, Watson AO. 2000. Pharmacokinetics of penicillin G procaine versus penicillin G potassium and procaine hydrochloride in horses. *Am J Vet Res*. 61:811–815.

U.S. Environmental Protection Agency. 1996. Health Effect Test Guidelines. Dermal Penetration (EPA 712-C-96-350). Washington, DC: U.S. Environmental Protection Agency.

U.S. Environmental Protection Agency. 1999. Proposed rule for *in vitro* dermal absorption rate testing of certain chemicals of interest to occupational safety and health administration. *Fed Regist*. 64(110):1999.

U.S. Environmental Protection Agency, Office of Pesticide Programs. 2001. *General principles for performing aggregate exposure and risk assessments.* Washington, DC: U.S. Environmental Protection Agency. http://www.epa.gov/pesticides/trac/science/aggregate.pdf

van de Wetering K, Burkon A, Feddema W, Bot A, de Jonge H, Somoza V, Borst P. 2009. Intestinal breast cancer resistance protein (BCRP)/Bcrp1 and multidrug resistance protein 3 (MRP3)/Mrp3 are involved in the pharmacokinetics of resveratrol. *Mol Pharmacol*. 75:876–885.

Van Eyk AD, Van Der Bijl P, Meyer D. 2007. In vitro diffusion of the immunosuppressant tacrolimus through human and rabbit corneas. *J Ocul Pharmacol Ther*. 23:146–151.

Yarim M, Moro S, Huber R, Meier PJ, Kaseda C, Kashima T, Hagenbuch B, Folkers G. 2005. Application of QSAR analysis to organic anion transporting polypeptide 1a5 (Oatp1a5) substrates. *Bioorg Med Chem*. 13:463–471.

Yokel RA, Lasley SM, Dorman DC. 2006. The speciation of metals in mammals influences their toxicokinetics and toxicodynamics and therefore human health risk assessment. *J Toxicol Environ Health B Crit Rev*. 9:63–85.

Youdim MB, Stephenson G, Ben Shachar D. 2004. Ironing iron out in Parkinson's disease and other neurodegenerative diseases with iron chelators: a lesson from 6-hydroxydopamine and iron chelators, Desferal and VK-28. *Ann N Y Acad Sci*. 1012:306–325.

Zaïr ZM, Eloranta JJ, Stieger B, Kullak-Ublick GA. 2008. Pharmacogenetics of OATP (SLC21/SLCO), OAT and OCT (SLC22) and PEPT (SLC15) transporters in the intestine, liver and kidney. *Pharmacogenomics*. 9:597–624.

CHAPTER 14

Forensic Toxicity Testing

This is a chapter outline intended to guide and familiarize you with the content to follow.

I. Forensic toxicity testing

A. Analytic chemistry melded with organ damage consistent with the compound and concentration found (consonance of data)

1. Most intentional poisoning deaths = suicide; most unintentional poisoning deaths from overdose of opioids and cocaine; toxicity from ethanol, drugs of abuse, overuse of medications lead car crash causes; unintentional nonfatal poisonings causes by opioids > benzodiazepines

2. Most exposures were oral

3. Sampling of tissues

   a. Living being is preferred as death results in tissue destruction, possible loss of toxicant, and redistribution of toxicant (from organ to plasma resulting in false poisoning indication if plasma is the key item utilized)

   For humans: take 15 mL of blood for ethanol/toxicants

   Take 30 mL urine for metabolites

   Hair samples (pulled not cut) for drugs of abuse (e.g., methamphetamine in child's hair from house manufacturing this drug) → extraction with HCl → enzymatic treatment (Pronase or β-glucuronidase) → hot CH_3OH extraction → hot NaOH disintegration and extraction

   Metals → urine, blood, and hair samples + possibly fingernails (As especially)

   Teeth for chronic exposure to Pb in children

   (1) Therapeutic drug monitoring

   (a) Required for highly lipophilic medications or pharmacokinetics, vary widely by patient

   (b) Also may be a function of a larger loading dose, long half-life, and narrow therapeutic range for action vs. toxicity (digitalis as loading dose needed to establish 0.5–1.5 or 2.0 ng/mL therapeutic range, 2 ng/mL toxicity, 1 h to achieve active plasma levels when taken orally, and a $t_{\frac{1}{2}} = 160$ h + interacts with many medications including Ca^{2+}-channel blockers, class III antiarrhythmic amiodarone, β-blockers, and NSAIDs)—see Table 14-2

   (c) C_{trough} (also known as C_{min}) works for HIV medication atazanavir or cancer chemotherapy medication methotrexate—see figure

CONCEPTUALIZING TOXICOLOGY 14-1

(d) For compounds such as the immunosuppressant mycophenolate mofetil used for kidney transplantation, the trough value doesn't correlate with dose or therapeutic effect so concentration at 2 h (C2) following dosing sampled

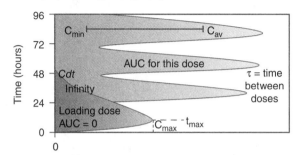

Plasma concentration, C

b. For dead people or animals, antemortem or postmortem collection of as many fluids as possible to reach results (peripheral blood, aqueous humors, urine, stomach contents, etc.), analyzing for original compound + metabolites:

50 g of brain, liver, kidney; 25 mL of heart blood; 10 mL of peripheral blood; and all available vitreous humors, bile, urine, and gastric contents

For specific toxicants, lung, intestine, or other specimens may be taken from other organs or larvae feeding on corpses as was done for malathion

4. Analysis of tissues (classic analytic chemistry)

a. Acid digestion → steam → volatiles (acetaldehyde, acetone, CO, CN, CH_3OH, CH_3CH_2OH, isopropanol, phenol, or anions such as Br^-, F^-, oxalate)

Acid fraction → leaches metals → atomic absorption (AA) or inductively coupled plasma emission spectroscopy (ICP)

b. Base digestion → aqueous phase-acidified + organic solvent → cleanup of proteins → barbiturate analysis

Base digestion → organic phase-acidified → aqueous (made basic and contains basic medications such as amphetamine) + organic phases (contains neutral medications such as simvastatin)

5. Analysis of tissues (modern extraction linked to GC-MS, LC-MS, or LC-[tandem] MS[/MS])

a. Tissue represents the aqueous phase continuously extracted in the presence of inert diatomaceous earth by liquid–liquid chromatography extraction wells robotically; organic eluate is evaporated and reconstituted for electrospray (tandem) LC-MS/MS analysis.

6. Rapid screening tests—see Table 14-1

a. Drugs of abuse are detectable in urine up to a few hours to days following use, while peptide hormones are undetectable in urine; injected steroids may be detectable for a month or more following use

b. Certain standards of indications for human urine involve correct urine temperature, pH, creatinine, specific gravity, and human IgG

c. Adulterants involve changing pH, oxidizing agents, fixatives (to ruin immunoassays), while diuretics are used to remove metabolites more rapidly prior to testing

d. Hair samples have ability to confirm use of drugs of abuse up to 90 days following use

e. Usual postmortem examination for toxicants—Figure 14-1; first considerations are CO poisoning (COHb), CN (from fire inhalation or plant ingestion), drugs of abuse or prescription medications, hypoglycemia (insulin overdose or other causes), uncontrolled diabetes mellitus, ethanol

CONCEPTUALIZING TOXICOLOGY 14-1 *(continued)*

Blood → COHb, CN, HbA$_{1c}$, drug analyses, ethanol

Urine → drug (metabolites), ethanol, glucose

Vitreous humor → ethanol, glucose

Bile → RIA for drugs where urine can't be collected

Gastric contents → drugs

Liver, skeletal muscle, spleen, lung, kidney, brain, heart → drugs, ethanol

CSF (if enough available) → drugs, ethanol

Problem is organ most protected on plane impact is kidney (80% available), while urine is not (80% unavailable)—see Figure 14-2

B. Signs/symptoms of exposure

　1. Toxidromes—symptoms consistent with exposure to a given agent

　　a. Ethanol use—ataxia, slurred speech, nystagmus on light exposure, etc.

　　b. Hg—triad of tremors, erethism, and gingivitis

　　c. Pediatric toxidromes and agents

　　　(1) Respiratory—difficult breathing for botulinum toxin, d-tubocurarine, organophosphates, carbamates, strychnine, CO, CN, metabolic acidosis, liver failure, heart failure, methemoglobinemia (metHb), salicylates

　　　(2) Hypoxia—CO, NO_3/NO_2-induced metHb formation (of G-6-PDH deficiency), CN

　　　(3) Wheezing—β-adrenergic antagonists, Cl (irritant) gas, hydrocarbons, isocyanates, organophosphates, carbamates, smoke inhalation, sulfites in food

　　　(4) Osmolarity gap—acetone, ethanol, ethyl ether, ethylene glycol, isopropanol, mannitol, methanol, renal failure, ketoacidosis

　　　(5) Anion gap—acetaminophen, β-adrenergic medications, CO, CN, Fe, isoniazid, salicylates, theophylline, toxic alcohols, valproic acid

　　　(6) Neuromuscular—antipsychotics, metoclopramide, amphetamines, anticholinergics, antihistamines, cocaine, γ-hydroxybutyrate, SSRIs and tricyclic antidepressants, malignant hyperthermia, phencyclidine (PCP)

　　　(7) CNS depression—opiates, ethanol/organic solvents, sedative-hypnotics, tricyclic antidepressants

　　　(8) Coma—alcohols/organic solvents, anticholinergics, As, β-adrenergic antagonists, cholinergic agents, CO, Pb, Li, opioids, PCP, phenothiazine antipsychotics, salicylates, sedative-hypnotics, tricyclic antidepressants

　　　(9) Miosis (pupil constriction)—opioids, cholinergic agents, clonidine (α2 adrenergic agonist), nicotine, phenothiazines, PCP

　　　(10) Mydriasis (pupil dilation)—anticholinergics, glutethimide, meperidine, sympathomimetics, withdrawal from alcohol or opioids

　　　(11) Seizures—amphetamines, cocaine, caffeine, theophylline, tricyclic antidepressants, venlafaxine, phenothiazines and butyrophenones, camphor, organophosphates, carbamates, ethylene glycol, isoniazid, meperidine, methanol, salicylates, withdrawal from depressants

　　　(12) Serotonin syndrome—monoamine oxidase inhibitors (MAOIs) + SSRIs

　　　(13) Sleepiness—antihistamines, any sedative hypnotic, alcohols, γ-hydroxybutyrate, tricyclic antidepressants, opioids, CO, CN, hypoglycemic agents

　　　(14) Withdrawal from depressants opposite to withdrawal from stimulants (effects of withdrawal opposite to action of agent)

　　　(15) Hyperthermia—serotonin syndrome, anticholinergics, MAOIs, metals, PCP, phenothiazines, salicylates, sympathomimetics, withdrawal from CNS depressants, malignant hyperthermia (halothane or succinyl choline)

CONCEPTUALIZING TOXICOLOGY 14-1 (*continued*)

(16) Hypothermia—β-blockers, CO, cholinergic agonists, ethanol, hypoglycemia-inducing agents, sedative-hypnotics

(17) Cardiovascular

(a) Hypertension—glycyrrhizin, mineralocorticoids, α-1 agonist, Cd

(b) Hypotension—CO, CN, hemorrhagic agents, Fe, opioids, nitrites, phenothiazine, sedative-hypnotics, tricyclic antidepressants, theophylline

(c) Bradycardia—β-blockers, Ca^{2+}-channel blockers, cardiac glycosides, clonidine, CN (high concentration), Li, nicotine, opioids, carbamates, organophosphates, parasympathomimetics

(d) Tachycardia—amphetamines, antihistamines, caffeine, clonidine, cocaine, theophylline, CO (lower concentrations), CN (lower concentrations), H_2S, anticholinergics, ethanol, PCP, sympathomimetics, withdrawal from CNS depressants, theophylline, thyroid hormone

(e) Torsade de pointes (dangerous ventricular arrhythmia)—amiodarone, As, chloroquine, quinine, quinidine, organophosphates, tricyclic antidepressants

(18) Hepatic—acetaldehyde, acetaminophen, aflatoxin, *Amanita phalloides*, CCl_4, other chlorinated hydrocarbons, halothane, phenol, phosphorus, valproic acid

(19) Renal—Hg, Au, Cd, statins via muscle wasting and creatinine formation

(20) Skin—Sulfonamides, aromatic antiepileptics, lamotrigine, penicillins, doxycycline, nevirapine, strong acids and bases, anilines, CO, cyanide, strychnine, metals

2. Toxicoproteomics

a. Develop biomarkers for organ = specific toxicity

b. Organ (e.g., liver) and plasma must be analyzed to detect proteins and peptides released or leaked from the organ

c. Use five levels of analysis:

(1) Match DNA microarrays with altered protein profiles

(2) Compare affected pathways from gene transcripts and proteins responsible for activation or repression events

(3) Posttranslational altered proteins analysis as reflective of gene expression of kinases, proteases, phosphorylases, conjugation enzymes

(4) Protein trafficking and signaling pathway determination in nuclei, mitochondria, endoplasmic reticulum, plasma membrane and cytosol

(5) Kinetic protein analysis of serum proteome over pretoxic, toxic, and recovery periods

CONCEPTUALIZING TOXICOLOGY 14-1 (*continued*)

This section includes forensic charts for each chapter describing an organ system. The most likely toxicants that primarily damage each organ are included in each chart. As tempting as it is to give a "laundry list" of toxicants that damage an organ, there usually is an organ through which the lethal effects are manifested. For example, an extremely high concentration of heavy metals given orally may strip off the cells of the intestinal tract and lead to hemorrhaging and death.

A lower oral dose may damage the liver, which stores metals. A lower dosage yet would likely damage the kidney, as this is the excretory organ. A lower dose might also cause central nervous system (CNS) damage. This forensic approach indicates that toxicant damage to organs may not be a lethal or even extremely toxic event with irreversible damage. All toxicants that affect these systems are characterized based on the ability to do significant damage or have the toxicant altered in a way that damages another organ (e.g., liver detoxication leading to kidney damage). This might appear to be a chapter on analytical chemistry, and in some ways it is an extension of this area. In another sense, there must be consonance of data. That means that the amount or concentration of toxicant at the target organ, the damage found, and the symptoms prior to death should all confirm the toxicity. For example, if a person had a high amount of cyanide in the intestinal tract but showed no cyanosis, this would not likely be the cause of death. A blunt trauma to the head may be more indicative of the brain damage that was found. A person found under water with no water in the lungs did not likely drown but died prior to that point. Similarly, it is necessary to have data that consistently point to the cause of death.

Most Likely Suspects

The toxicants that are usually tested in clinical or forensic toxicology laboratories are those most likely to kill or significantly affect function in humans. These toxicants have government programs to limit exposure such as drugs of abuse, overdose of medications, ethanol, carbon monoxide, lead poisoning, and a series of other toxicants. Most of the agents can be found in common use in the households of many Americans. The Centers for Disease Control (CDC), in 2008 reported that > 41,000 people died from poisoning. For the first time since 1980, poisoning was the leading cause of injury death and tripled over a 30 year period. Medication and illegal drug deaths in that period increased from a bare majority (60%) to almost the sole cause of poisoning deaths (90%; Warner, 2011). These mainly drug-related poisoning deaths in the U.S. are still mainly unintentional, while the remainder result from suicides or undetermined intent (CDC, 2015). Motor vehicle crashes were the first in unintentional deaths, and those related to intoxication from alcohol, drugs of abuse, overuse of medications, and so forth appear to lead that list. It is of interest that unintentional poisonings of people between the ages of 35 and 54 exceeded deaths from car accidents. The overwhelming majority of the 18% of intentional deaths from poisoning

in 2005 (5,833 people) were suicides rather than homicides (89 homicides). Ninety-five percent of all unintentional and undetermined deaths were related to opioid pain medication overdose followed by the drugs of abuse cocaine and heroin. Unintentional nonfatal poisonings came mainly from opioids followed by benzodiazepines (GABAergic sleeping pills). A more defined accounting for the year 2007 was a publication put forward from the American Association of Poison Control Centers (Bronstein et al., 2008). In 2007, 2,482,041 human exposures were reported (8.1/1,000 population). Nearly 65% of those calls were for children. Greater than 78% were oral exposures. Most cases resulted in no effect or minimal toxicity. Lethality was mostly experienced in adults over 19 years of age (0.2% of the 860,692 cases for that age group).

In 2007, 131,744 nonhuman exposures were reported, primarily for dogs (118,371) followed by cats (11,818). The top 25 exposures reported to U.S. poison control centers were analgesics (12.5%); cosmetics and personal care products (9.1%); household cleaning supplies (8.7%); sedative-hypnotics and antipsychotic medications (6.2%), foreign bodies, toys, and miscellaneous items (5.1%); topical preparations (4.5%); cold and cough medicines (4.5%); antidepressants (4.0%); pesticides (3.9%); cardiovascular medications (3.5%); alcohols (3.3%); antihistamines (3.2%); food products and food poisonings (3.1%); bites and envenomations (3.1%); antimicrobials (2.7%); vitamins (2.7%); plants (2.4%); hormones and hormone antagonists (2.2%); gastrointestinal preparations (2.2%); hydrocarbons (2.0%); chemicals (2.0%); stimulants and street drugs (1.9%); anticonvulsants (1.7%); arts, crafts, and office supplies (1.6%); and fumes, gases, and vapors (1.6%). People over 19 years of age were most likely exposed to cosmetics and personal care products (20.0%); cleaning supplies (14.3%); analgesics (13.4%); foreign bodies, toys, and miscellaneous items (11.1%); topical preparations (10.1%); cold and cough medicines (7.6%); vitamins (5.7%); pesticides (5.2%); plants (4.9%); antihistamines (4.6%); gastrointestinal preparations (4.3%); antimicrobials (4.0%); arts, crafts, and office supplies (3.4%); hormones and hormone antagonists (3.0%); cardiovascular medications

(2.8%); electrolytes and minerals (2.8%); alcohols (2.7%); food products and food poisonings (2.3%); deodorizers (2.0%); dietary supplements, herbals, and homeopathic preparations (2.0%); asthma therapies (1.9%); hydrocarbons (1.8%); other or unknown nondrug substances (1.8%); sedative-hypnotics and antipsychotic medications (1.7%); and antidepressants (1.6%). Exposures for children under 6 years of age involve cosmetics and personal care products (10.7%); cleaning supplies (7.6%); analgesics (7.2%); foreign bodies, toys, and miscellaneous items (6.0%); topical preparations (5.4%); cold and cough medicines (5.4%); vitamins (3.1%); pesticides (2.8%); plants (2.6%); antihistamines (2.5%); gastrointestinal preparations (2.3%); arts, crafts, and office supplies (2.2%); hormones and hormone antagonists (1.8%); cardiovascular medications (1.5%); electrolytes and minerals (1.5%); alcohols (1.5%); food products and food poisoning (1.3%); deodorizers (1.2%); dietary supplements, herbals, and homeopathic preparations (1.1%); asthma therapies (1.0%), hydrocarbons (1.0%); other or unknown nondrug substances (1.0%); sedative-hypnotics and antipsychotic medications (0.9%); and antidepressants (0.9%).

Which ones are the most lethal? For 2007, the most fatalities were reported for sedative-hypnotics and antipsychotic medications (377 people); opioids (331); antidepressants (220); acetaminophen in combination (208); cardiovascular medications (203); stimulants and other street drugs (188); alcohols (170); acetaminophen only (140); anticonvulsants (99); fumes, gases, and vapors (80); cyclic antidepressants (80); muscle relaxants (70); antihistamines (69); aspirin alone (63)l chemicals (45); unknown drug (44); other nonsteroidal anti-inflammatory drugs (NSAIDs; 44 people died); oral hypoglycemic (36); automotive, aircraft, and boat products (28); miscellaneous drugs (21); antihistamine/decongestants without phenylpropanolamine (21); hormones and hormone antagonists (20); anticoagulants (20); and diuretics (16). (Bronstein et al., 2012)

A real forensic toxicologist is not a television crime scene analyst looking at rare chemicals used by a clever murderer. They usually are employed to do head space analysis of blood collected by a police officer for a person arrested for driving under the influence of ethanol on a weekend or holiday. However, increasing numbers of children are having hair samples pulled from their scalps using gloves to detect methamphetamine as evidence against their parents (for having a drug lab in home). Note that it is going to be important to match signs and symptoms of exposure to sampling techniques and handling/storage of samples, and finally methods of analysis. Forensic analysis means a legal analysis that will be scientifically sound, meet specifications for chain of evidence and chain of custody (knowing each person responsible for the sampling or sample throughout the analysis), be free from contamination by samplers and analysis group, have confirming tests, and be consistent with medical knowledge as to cause of poisoning or death. The sections that follow examine each area to show the extent of scientific detective work that should ultimately yield a report on the agent or mixture of agents consonant with the observed toxicity.

Signs/Symptoms of Exposure

Some toxicities are easily diagnosed, because they come with a variety of unmistakable symptoms. Others are more difficult to assess, because the symptoms are common for a variety of agents. An example of a toxicology assessment is when a police officer stops a car for erratic driving, and then shines a light into the driver's eyes. If the eyes vibrate (nystagmus) in the light, the office will assume ethanol intoxication and test for ataxia via a walking test and having the drive touching his finger to his nose. If the eyes appear too constricted, the officer will assume that opiates may be involved. Toxidromes are a set of symptoms associated with a given agent or agents that may be used to evaluate a poisoned animal or person. Some of the most common toxidromes are for stimulants, sedative-hypnotic medications, opiates, anticholinergics, and cholinergic agents (Tomassoni et al., 2015). Certain toxidromes have been noted historically and in novels. For example, the mad hatter in Lewis Carroll's *Alice's Adventures in Wonderland* has the syndrome associated with mercury poisoning due to spraying of felt hats with mercury nitrate to preserve the fiber. The set of symptoms fit the fictional mad hatter with excitability (erethism), gum disease (gingivitis), and tremor. Excessive salivation was also part of the syndrome. A set of pediatric toxidromes is provided in the subsections that follow (Koren, 2007).

Respiratory

- Difficulty breathing: Neuromuscular blockade is achieved by botulinum toxin; neuromuscular blockers such as d-tubocurarine, organophosphates, and carbamates (AChE inhibition at high doses with tremor, muscle weakness, agitation, seizures, and coma, but at lower doses induce vomiting, diarrhea, abdominal cramping, bradycardia, miosis, drooling, respiratory hypersecretion, and diaphoresis); strychnine; and tetanus. CNS depression occurs with opiates, ethanol (or other alcohols), sedative-hypnotics, and tricyclic antidepressants. Other factors that may lead to labored breathing are carbon monoxide, cyanide, metabolic acidosis, liver failure, heart failure, methemoglobinemia, and salicylates.
- Hypoxia: carbon monoxide poisoning, nitrate poisoning or other methemoglobinemia, hemolysis caused by glucose-6-phophate dehydrogenase (G-6PDH) deficiency (favism), cyanide poisoning.
- Wheezing: beta-antagonists, irritant gases such as chlorine, hydrocarbons, isocyanates, organophosphates, carbamates, smoke inhalation, foodborne sulfites.

Changes in Osmolarity and Ion Balance

- Osmolarity gap: Because osmolarity should be 290 mOsm/kg (= $2 \times$ [Na$^+$ (mEq/L)] + glucose [mg/dL]/18 + blood urea nitrogen [mg/dL]/2.8), alterations in osmolarity may be caused by acetone, ethanol, ethyl ether, ethylene glycol, isopropyl alcohol, mannitol, methanol, renal failure, and ketoacidosis (type I diabetic and alcoholic).
- Anion gap: Calculated as Na$^+$ − ([Cl$^-$] + [HCO$_3^-$]), where normal ranges from 8–12

mEq/L, this may be caused by acetaminophen overdose (as would liver failure and jaundice), beta-adrenergic medications, carbon monoxide, cyanide, iron, isoniazid, salicylates, theophylline, toxic alcohols, and the antiseizure medication valproic acid.

Neuromuscular

- Acute movement disorder: Dystonia (twisting and repetitive movements) may be caused antipsychotics and metoclopramide. Dyskinesia (difficulty with/distortion of voluntary movements as in tic, chorea, spasm, or myoclonus) may be produced by amphetamines, anticholinergics, antihistamines, cocaine, gamma-hydroxybutyrate, selective serotonin reuptake inhibitors (SSRIs), and tricyclic antidepressants. Rigidity may be caused by malignant hyperthermia (dangerous increase in temperature that is a reaction to general anesthetic agents and succinylcholine), neuroleptic malignant syndrome, and phencyclidine.
- Coma: Alcohols, anticholinergics, arsenic, beta-receptor antagonists, cholinergic agents, carbon monoxide, lead, lithium, opioids, phencyclidine, phenothiazine antipsychotics, salicylates, sedative-hypnotics, and tricyclic antidepressants.
- Opioid overdose: CNS depression (sedation and lethargy to coma), respiratory depression, hypoxia, and miosis (no pupil constriction or miosis with other sedative-hypnotic agents). Miosis may also be caused by cholinergic agents, clonidine (adrenergic alpha-2 receptor agonist that decreases sympathetic outflow from the CNS), nicotine, phenothiazines, and phencyclidine (PCP). The opposite of miosis is dilation or mydriasis caused by anticholinergics (belladonna alkaloids), glutethimide, meperidine, sympathomimetics (mimic action of norepinephrine and epinephrine), and withdrawal from CNS depressants such as alcohol or opiates.
- Seizures: Amphetamines, cocaine, caffeine, theophylline, tricyclic antidepressants, venlafaxine, phenothiazines and butyrophenones,

camphor, organophosphates, carbamates, ethylene glycol, isoniazid, meperidine, methanol, salicylates and any withdrawal from psychoactive drug (likely depressants—see withdrawal symptoms).

- Serotonin syndrome (hot and confused): Monoamine oxidase inhibitors (MAOIs) in combination with SSRIs lead to akathisia-like restlessness, muscle twitches, myoclonus, hyperreflexia, diaphoresis (excess perspiration), penile erection, shivering, tremor, and with increased severity seizures and coma. Other agents that can increase temperature are anticholinergics (accompanied by dry flushed skin, dry mouth, mydriasis, delirium, hallucinations, tachycardia, ileus or decreased peristalsis, urinary retention, and in most severe poisonings coma and respiratory arrest), MAOIs, metals, phencyclidine, phenothiazines (accompanied by muscle rigidity, metabolic acidosis, and confusion for neuroleptic overdose), salicylates, sympathomimetics, and withdrawal from CNS depressants such as ethanol and opioids. Decreased temperature or hypothermia can be caused by beta-blockers, carbon monoxide, cholinergic agonists, ethanol, hypoglycemia-inducing agents, and sedative-hypnotics.

- Sleepiness: Antihistamines, any sedative-hypnotic, alcohols, gamma-hydroxybutyrate, tricyclic antidepressants, opioids, carbon monoxide, cyanide, and hypoglycemic agents.

- Withdrawal symptoms: Withdrawal from depressants or toxicity from high levels of stimulants leads to diaphoresis, diarrhea, fever, insomnia, hypertonia, hyperreflexia, lacrimation, respiratory distress, seizures, and tachycardia. Withdrawal from stimulants has the opposite effects such as bradycardia, depression, increased appetite (nicotine withdrawal), and sleepiness.

Cardiovascular

- Blood pressure:
  - Hypertension: Glycyrrhizin, mineralocorticoids, agents that may cause tachycardia, alpha-1 agonists such as phenylephrine, and cadmium or other heavy or metals (or other toxicants) that induce renal damage or lead to adrenal tumors.
  - Hypotension: Carbon monoxide, cyanide, hemorrhagic agents, iron, opioids, nitrites, phenothiazines, sedative-hypnotics, tricyclic antidepressants, and theophylline.

- Cardiac:
  - Bradycardia (too slow): Beta-receptor antagonists (especially beta-1 blockers), calcium-channel blockers, cardiac glycosides (e.g., digitalis), clonidine, cyanide, lithium, nicotine, opioids, carbamates and organophosphates (AChE inhibitors), and parasympathomimetics (mimics action of acetylcholine).
  - (Atrial) tachycardia (too fast): Amphetamines, antihistamines, caffeine, clonidine, cocaine, theophylline, carbon monoxide, cyanide, hydrogen sulfide, anticholinergics (antihistamines, phenothiazines, tricyclics and atropine), ethanol, phencyclidine, sympathomimetics, withdrawal from any depressive psychoactive drug, theophylline, and thyroid hormone.
  - Ventricular arrhythmias: Speeding from amphetamines, cocaine, caffeine, chloral hydrate, aromatic hydrocarbons, anticholinergics and theophylline. Q-T prolongation that can lead to torsade de pointes (polymorphic ventricular tachycardia that may become deadly ventricular fibrillation) may be caused by the antiarrhythmic medication amiodarone, arsenic, chloroquine, quinine, quinidine, organophosphates, and tricyclic antidepressants.

Hepatic

- Acetaldehyde (metabolite of ethanol), acetaminophen, aflatoxin, *Amanita phalloides* (death cap mushroom) or similar species, carbon tetrachloride, other chlorinated hydrocarbons that at lower doses may also lead to kidney failure, halothane, phenol, phosphorus, and valproic acid.

Renal

- Direct: Glomerulonephritis can be caused by mercury and gold compounds as indicated by proteinuria (Bigazzi, 1994). Heavy metal exposure as assessed by cadmium and other metals found in the urine appear to cause early kidney damage as indicated by an increase in urinary N-acetyl-β-D-glucosaminidase (Thomas et al., 2009).
- Indirect: Statins have caused rhabdomyolysis (muscle wasting) and ensuing renal failure (Omar et al., 2001).

Skin

- Stevens-Johnson syndrome and toxic epidermal necrolysis: Sulfonamides, aromatic antiepileptics, lamotrigine, penicillins, doxycycline, and nevirapine. Other skin problems can be found with strong acids and bases (chemical burns), anilines (darkening), carbon monoxide (cherry red coloration), cyanide (blue under finger nails, but if skin exposed may find a redness and a bitter almond-like smell), strychnine (dark face and neck), metals (certain metals give a metallic luster to the skin), vanadium (green tongue).

Toxicoproteomics

A new field worth examining is toxicoproteomics. Using model liver and kidney toxicants, biomarkers for organ-specific toxicity are being determined (Merrick and Witzmann, 2009). Samples can be subjected to two-dimensional gel electrophoresis and mass spectrometry, liquid chromatography of protein digests that are analyzed by tandem mass spectrometers, retentate chromatography-mass spectrometry (laser-based mass spectrum), and antibody arrays available for toxicoproteomic studies. Analysis of the liver must involve both liver cells and the plasma, because injured organs release peptides and proteins into the plasma. In the case of the liver, some of the plasma proteins are normally synthesized by the liver. Liver toxicants such as acetaminophen, bromobenzene, dichlorobenzenes, lipopolysaccharide, and monocrotaline serve as model agents for causing hepatic necrosis and inflammation. Male rats are treated with a vehicle as a control, a low dose to observe effects not expected to be associated with injury, and a high dose to cause injury. Rats are sampled at 6, 24, and 48 hours following administration of the toxic agent. These times are associated with changes in histopathology and serum chemistries (alanine aminotransferase [ALT] and aspartate aminotransferase [AST]) and account for the time necessary to overwhelm the reduced glutathione content from reactive metabolites. Five levels of analysis are possible by this approach. First is matching gene alterations detected by DNA microarrays with altered protein profiles. Second is to compare affected pathways through altered gene transcripts and proteins responsible for activation or repression events. Third is analysis of posttranslationally altered proteins as they are related to modified genes encoding for kinases, proteases, phosphorylases, conjugation enzymes, or others that facilitate those post-translational processes. Fourth is a proteomic determination of alterations of protein trafficking and signaling pathways or subcellular site(s) of injury in nuclei, mitochondria, endoplasmic reticulum, plasma membrane, and cytosol. Fifth is the kinetic protein analysis of the changes in the serum proteome over the pretoxic, toxic, and recovery periods (Merrick, 2006).

Sampling Techniques

Once a presumed diagnosis has been made, the sampling should be made easier unless the toxicity proceeds to lethality unnoticed and with no clear indication of cause. In that case, an autopsy is performed. A living being is always preferred, as death results in tissue destruction, possible loss of toxicant, and redistribution of toxicant. For instance, if the time of death is known, the amount of cyanide may be extrapolated back to the time of death based on the length of time the sample remained in the cadaver, length of storage time of the sample, preservation of the sample by addition of sodium fluoride, and storage conditions of the sample (McAllister et al., 2008). For example, antemortem and postmortem collection of vitreous humor, femoral vein and artery, left and right heart ventricles indicated that pigs given a high intravenous (IV) dose of morphine had significantly different free and total morphine values before and after death and by site of injection over time. Free morphine concentrations were higher in postmortem samples, but total morphine was similar to slightly lower in postmortem samples. Antemortem and postmortem values are not consistent based on IV dose. The femoral vein had the lowest values in either case, which is consistent with the site of metabolism (Crandall et al., 2006). In another example, two antipsychotic drugs, haloperidol and thioridazine, administered intraperitoneally redistribute from the rat lung to the blood following death as indicated by liquid chromatography—tandem mass spectrometry. This is important, because fatal arrhythmias may result from a high dose of these antipsychotics (Castaing et al., 2006). A variety of pre- and postmortem examinations revealed a variable redistribution of psychiatric medications into the blood (Rodda and Drummer, 2006). Although earlier reports (1970s) of redistribution following death are available in the literature, at least one publication indicates many of the difficulties of obtaining reliable samples in a critically ill poisoned patient (Boyle et al., 2009). The problems of the nature of the poison or poisons—gas, volatile liquid, corrosive chemical, metals, anions and nonmetals, nonvolatile organic substances (organic strong acids, organic weak acids, organic bases, organic neutral chemicals, organic amphoteric compounds), or mixtures of compounds that may react with each other or complex or disperse into living or dead tissue—is one factor. A second problem is associated with sample collection, transport, and storage, where little may be known of the toxic agent. The site where the victim is found may be remote or not ideally suited for sample collection or storage (e.g., battlefield conditions, car accident, fire, explosion). The analytical methodology employed may not be optimal based on the facilities available in that part of the country or world. The circumstances of the exposure may involve how the poison was encountered and for how long (multiple routes of exposure possible and many time sequences). Mechanical trauma or inhalation of stomach contents may complicate analysis (e.g., gunshot wounds, car accident). Tolerance or synergy due to prior or concurrent exposure may yield results that are initially not consistent with death (too low) or inconsistent with life (too high, especially in postmortem concentrations). For this reason, it is best to take as many fluids and tissues as possible postmortem, including peripheral blood, aqueous humors, urine, stomach contents, and so forth. Original compounds and metabolites will also give some indication of the total picture. As an example of the problems associated with sample collection and reliability, ethanol intoxication is a common poisoning in the population. Blood ethanol can be lost or produced especially in the presence of significant trauma, which happens often in alcohol-related deaths (Flanagan and Connally, 2005). What happens if only skeletal remains are found or the blood has been lost? One more recent publication indicates the possibility of bone as an indication of the presence of a medication or toxicant. The concentrations of the medications tested were generally higher in the bone than in the blood and some were not found in the bone. Thus, interpretation should be done cautiously. The encouraging factor is that there is at least one more possibility for the analyst when considering forensic determination of possible causes of death (McGrath and Jenkins, 2009). Sometimes the autopsy findings provide a toxicity not indicated previously by animal data. Two suicides by acetaminophen yielded rapid deaths without the usual hepatic centrilobular necrosis. Cardiac toxicity may cause death at high concentrations of acetaminophen in humans (Singer et al., 2007).

Live for Human Performance

The Society of Forensic Toxicologists (SOFT) and American Academy of Forensic Sciences (AAFS) (2006) produced a document titled "Forensic Toxicology Laboratory Guidelines," which describes in detail certified laboratory work in forensic toxicology including definitions, personnel, standard operating procedures, samples and receiving, security and chain of custody, analytical procedures, quality assurance and quality control, review of data, reporting of results, interpretation of toxicology results, and safety. This section focuses on the sampling portion. SOFT and AAFS recommend taking 15 mL of blood for ethanol and other toxicants that are needed to assess performance. The "reasonable complete" drug screen should only require 5 mL or less of blood. That requires sensitive and specific methodology development by forensic toxicology laboratories. Urine should have a minimum collection volume of 30 mL for analysis for detection of metabolites or the last tissue to indicate the presence of an illegal agent. Hair samples may be taken for exposure to drugs of abuse, but laboratory ability to analyze should meet the Society of Hair Testing proficiency for detection without false positives or negatives following extraction in hydrochloric acid, enzymatic treatment (Pronase followed by liquid–liquid extraction, or β-glucuronidase treatment and buffer extraction), hot methanol extraction (with or without sonication), and hot NaOH disintegration and extraction (Jurado and Sachs, 2003). Urine, blood, and hair have been used for heavy metals and especially arsenic analysis. The fingernails prove to indicate the chronic occupational exposure of workers to arsenic (Agahian et al., 1990). Lead concentrations in teeth have been studied since the 1970s and still serve to monitor environmental exposures in children in foreign countries (Arruda-Neto et al., 2009).

Postmortem

SOFT and AAFS (2006) recommend taking 50 grams of brain, liver, and kidney; 25 mL of heart blood; 10 mL of peripheral blood; and all available of the vitreous humor, bile, urine, and gastric contents as a start for all postmortem toxicology analyses. For specific toxicants lung, intestine, or other specimens may be taken. If a corpse has been deteriorating, even the organisms that are assisting in its decomposition can be sampled as was done for arthropod larvae *Chrysomya megacephala* (Fabricius) and *Chrysomya rufifacies* (Macquart) in a suspected case of malathion poisoning (Gunatilake and Goff, 1989).

Analysis Methodology

Classical Analytical Chemistry Approach

The classical approach involves making an acid or base digest of the tissue. The acidified portion may be subject to steam to release the volatile medications and poisons such as acetaldehyde, acetone, carbon monoxide, cyanide, ethanol, isopropanol, methanol, phenol, and so forth or anions such as bromide, borate, fluoride, and oxalate. The acid fraction leaches metals out of the tissues and can be analyzed by atomic absorption or inductively coupled plasma emission spectroscopy. The basic extract is separated into an aqueous and an organic phase. The aqueous phase is acidified and organic solvent is added. This yields the acidic medications such as the barbiturates (from barbituric acid). This step can be preceded by a precipitation of protein or similar cleanup procedure. The organic phase of the organic extract is extracted with acid and again separated into an aqueous and organic phase. The organic phase contains the neutral medications such as simvastatin. The aqueous phase is made basic and contains the basic medications such as amphetamine (the amine portion of the catecholamine structure produces its basic nature). In the past, volatiles were analyzed by gas–liquid chromatography. The medications or street drugs were determined by thin-layer chromatography techniques. Organic extracts of the tissues would also be used to analyze for hydrophobic compounds such as polycyclic aromatic hydrocarbons, polychlorinated biphenyls, and dioxins. If a chemical powder or unknown liquid is found near a corpse or stomach or intestinal contents yield a liquid, pill, or compound, they may be subjected to tests such as boiling point, melting point, and other physical determinations. These preparations may have a chemical added to it to form crystals. Chemical spot tests will be discussed later under rapid screening tests. Chromatography is the next topic, as it is the method of choice if specificity is required. The World Health Organization (2015) recommends that analytical toxicology laboratories contain the following equipment and have procedures to perform simple "spot" tests: Conway apparatus, Gutzeit apparatus, direct-reading spectrophotometer, ultraviolet (UV)/visible recording spectrophotometer, thin-layer chromatography—qualitative, thin-layer chromatography—quantitative, gas chromatography—packed columns, gas chromatography—capillary columns, gas chromatography—flame ionization detection, gas chromatography—nitrogen-phosphorus detection, gas chromatography—electron-capture detection, gas chromatography-mass spectrometry (GC-MS), high-performance liquid chromatography (HPLC)–UV detection, high-performance liquid chromatography-fluorescence detection, high-performance liquid chromatography-mass spectrometry (LC-MS), high-performance liquid chromatography-electrochemical detection, high-performance liquid chromatography–diode array UV detection, capillary electrophoresis, atomic emission spectrometry, atomic absorption spectrometry (flame), electrothermal atomic absorption spectrometry, inductively coupled plasma source spectrometry, radioimmunoassay—counting, enzyme immunoassay (e.g., enzyme-multiplied immunoassay technique), fluorescence immunoassay, enzyme-linked immunosorbent assay, fluorimetry, and infrared spectrometry. Pure standards are also required of the laboratory. Many of these techniques alone or in combination would not be trusted to identify an unknown. For example, SOFT/AAFS (2006) guidelines indicate that an identification by immunoassay followed by "confirmation" by flame ionization detectors and nitrogen-phosphorus detectors only give a range of suspects based on retention time of the columns and will not hold up in a court of law. Mass spectrometry (MS) gives structural features that may lead to identification of the unknown toxicant. The beam intensity for MS may be varied to change the amount of fragmentation of the compound, and low intensities may yield more of the molecular ion, which is the organic molecule with a positive charge due to removal of one electron.

Modern Extraction Linked to GC-MS, LC-MS, or LC-(Tandem) MS(/MS)

The gold standard for toxicology analyses currently is an extraction procedure followed by GC-MS analysis. Not all toxicants are volatile for gas chromatographic analysis, and newer methods employ liquid chromatography coupled with one or two mass spectrometers (Maurer, 2007). Because the sample matrix may be complicated with a variety of contaminants in the extract, mass spectra can now have a standardized computer program to subtract out interfering substances and provide evidence of the structure for unknown toxicants not available in standard MS libraries (Stimpfl et al., 2003). In June 1986, a poisoning epidemic in Sierra Leone was solved employing positive chemical ionization mass spectrometry and nuclear magnetic resonance spectroscopy. An unknown poison in bread samples proved to be the organophosphorus pesticide parathion (Hill et al., 1990). Note that two different methods of analysis were used as is recommended for determination and confirmation of an unknown toxicant. The development of LC-MS(/MS) has led to determination of unknown toxicants, and with the proper algorithms (e.g., SALSA [Stochastic Approach for Link-Structure Analysis]) it can yield epoxide adducts of proteins. Hemoglobin adducts are likely, such as those formed on incubation with styrene oxide, ethylene oxide, and butadiene oxide (Badghisi and Liebler, 2002). The biological sample in this case represents the aqueous phase and the organic solvent the second phase that involve high-throughput liquid–liquid extraction (LLE) methodology by robotic liquid handling of a 96-well LLE plate with inert diatomaceous earth particles for continuous and efficient extraction of analytes between the aqueous biological sample and the organic extraction solvent (Peng et al., 2001).

Rapid Screening Tests

The older color tests are used heavily by the law enforcement agencies for trafficking in illegal drugs. The U.S. Department of Justice, National Institute of Justice has a Standards and Testing

Program that has developed a list of Color Test Reagents/Kits for Preliminary Identification of Drugs of Abuse (NIJ Standard-0604.01), displayed in **Table 14-1**. There are also commercially available test kits for urine that measure 12 standard abused medications or street drugs and their metabolites using simple immunoassays to lateral flow-based immunoassays. For example, one commercially available kit uses sensitivities recommended by the National Institute on Drug Abuse to screen urine for the following compounds and their metabolites in urine: 25 ng/mL for phencyclidine, 50 ng/mL for marijuana (THC); 100 ng/mL for oxycodone, 300 ng/mL for cocaine, methadone, barbiturates, benzodiazepine, or propoxyphene; 500 mg/mL for MDMA (ecstasy), 1,000 mg/mL for amphetamine or methamphetamine; and 2,000 mg/mL for opiates.

Detection time is important in living beings. Peptide hormones are undetectable in urine. Cocaine detection may range from 1–4 days following administration. Propoxyphene can be detected from 6 hours to 2 days after use. Short-acting barbiturates may be detectable for 2 days. Amphetamines may be detected from 2–5 days after use. Clenbuterol can be found in urine 4–6 days following use. Nicotine may be observed in urine 4–10 days after a person ceases smoking. A 5–7 day detection time is common to euphorics such as ecstasy, the opiates, the dissociative anesthetic agent ketamine, and meth-amphetamines. Cannabinoids such as THC are detectable in urine for 5 days after one-time use to as high as 48–63 days in those using marijuana daily. Benzodiazepines may be detected in urine from 7–10 days following cessation of use. Oral anabolic steroids may be detected for 14–28 days, while injected steroids are detectable 1–3 months following use. People have employed diuretics to decrease the detectable concentration of the medication, but a specific gravity test and a test for diuretics indicate that a person is trying to avoid detection of a banned substance or indicate that use was below the legal limit for operating a motor vehicle or practicing medicine. Specific gravity is also altered by salts or detergents. Other compounds that may be attempted to be added to urine to avoid detection of banned substances or abused drugs

TABLE 14-1 Color Changes for Medications and Drug of Abuse Tests		
Reagent (#)	**Color Change**	**Drugs (form or solvent)**
Cobalt Thiocyanate (A.1)	Brilliant greenish blue	Benzphetamine HCl, brompheniramine maleate, chlordiazepoxide HCl, chlorpromazine HCl, doxepin HCl, hydrocodone tartrate, methadone HCl, methylphenidate HCl
	Strong greenish blue	Cocaine HCl, diacetylmorphine HCl, ephedrine HCl, meperidine HCl, phencyclidine HCl, procaine HCl, propoxyphene HCl, pseudoephedrine HCl
	Strong blue	Quinine HCl (all in CHCl$_3$)
Dille-Koppanyi Reagent. Modified (A.2)	Light purple	Amobarbital, pentobarbital, phenobarbital, secobarbital (all in CHCl$_3$)
Duquenois-Levine Reagent. Modified (A.3)	Strong reddish purple to very light purple	Mace (crystals)
	Pale reddish purple to light gray purplish red	Nutmeg (extract)
	Light yellow green	Tea (extract)
	Gray purplish blue to light purplish blue to deep purple	Tetrahydrocannabinol, THC (in ethanol)

(continues)

TABLE 14-1   Color Changes for Medications and Drug of Abuse Tests (*continued*)

Reagent (#)	Color Change	Drugs (form or solvent)
Mandelin Reagent (A.4)	Moderate olive	Acetaminophen ($CHCl_3$)
	Grayish olive green	Aspirin (powder)
	Brilliant yellow green	Benzphetamine HCl ($CHCl_3$)
	Strong orange	Brompheniramine maleate ($CHCl_3$), salt (crystals)
	Dark olive	Chlorpromazine HCl, codeine (both in $CHCl_3$), Excedrin (powder)
	Deep orange yellow	Cocaine HCl ($CHCl_3$)
	Strong yellow	Contac (powder)
	Moderate bluish green	d-Amphetamine HCl ($CHCl_3$)
	Dark yellowish green	d-Methamphetamine HCl ($CHCl_3$)
	Moderate reddish brown	Diacetylmorphine HCl ($CHCl_3$)
	Dark olive brown	Dimethoxy-meth HCl ($CHCl_3$)
	Dark reddish brown	Doxepin HCl, propoxyphene HCl (both in $CHCl_3$)
	Grayish olive	Dristan (powder)
	Moderate olive green	Mace (crystals)
	Bluish black	d,l-3,4-Methylenedioxyamphetamine HCl, MDA ($CHCl_3$)
	Dark yellowish brown	Mescaline HCl ($CHCl_3$)
	Dark grayish blue	Methadone HCl ($CHCl_3$)
	Very orange yellow	Methaqualone ($CHCl_3$)
	Brilliant orange yellow	Methylphenidate HCl ($CHCl_3$)
	Dark grayish reddish brown	Morphine monohydrate ($CHCl_3$)
	Dark brown	Opium ($CHCl_3$)
	Dark greenish yellow	Oxycodone HCl ($CHCl_3$)
	Deep orange	Procaine HCl ($CHCl_3$)
	Deep greenish yellow	Quinine HCl ($CHCl_3$)
Marquis Reagent (A.5)	Deep red	Aspirin (powder)
	Deep reddish brown	Benzphetamine HCl ($CHCl_3$)
	Deep purplish red	Chlorpromazine HCl, diacetylmorphine HCl (both in $CHCl_3$)
	Very dark purple	Codeine ($CHCl_3$)
	Strong reddish orange	d-Amphetamine HCl ($CHCl_3$)
	Deep reddish orange	d-Methamphetamine HCl ($CHCl_3$)
	Dark reddish brown	d-Amphetamine HCl, d-Methamphetamine HCl (both in $CHCl_3$)
	Moderate orange	Dimethoxy-meth HCl ($CHCl_3$)
	Blackish red	Doxepin HCl ($CHCl_3$)
	Dark grayish red	Dristan (powder)
	Dark red	Excedrin (powder)
	Olive black	Lysergic acid diethylamide. LSD ($CHCl_3$)
	Moderate yellow	Mace (crystals)
	Dark reddish brown	Dristan (powder)

TABLE 14-1   Color Changes for Medications and Drug of Abuse Tests (*continued*)

Reagent (#)	Color Change	Drugs (form or solvent)
Marquis Reagent (A.5) (*continued*)	Black	MDA ($CHCl_3$)
	Deep brown	Meperidine HCl ($CHCl_3$)
	Strong orange	Mescaline HCl ($CHCl_3$)
	Light yellowish pink	Methadone HCl ($CHCl_3$)
	Moderate orange yellow	Methylphenidate HCl ($CHCl_3$)
	Very deep reddish purple	Morphine monohydrate ($CHCl_3$)
	Dark grayish reddish Brown	Opium (powder)
	Pale violet	Oxycodone HCl ($CHCl_3$)
	Blackish purple	Propoxyphene HCl ($CHCl_3$)
	Dark brown	Sugar (crystals)
Nitric Acid (A.6)	Brilliant orange yellow	Acetaminophen ($CHCl_3$), Excedrin (powder), Morphine monohydrate ($CHCl_3$)
	Light greenish yellow	Codeine, MDA (both in $CHCl_3$)
	Pale yellow	Diacetylmorphine HCl ($CHCl_3$)
	Very yellow	Dimethoxy-meth HCl ($CHCl_3$)
	Brilliant yellow	Doxepin HCl ($CHCl_3$)
	Deep orange	Dristan (powder)
	Strong brown	Lysergic acid diethylamide (LSD) ($CHCl_3$)
	Moderate greenish yellow	Mace (crystals)
	Dark red	Mescaline HCl ($CHCl_3$)
	Dark orange yellow	Opium (powder)
	Brilliant yellow	Oxycodone HCl ($CHCl_3$)
Para-Dimethylamino-Benzaldehyde (A.7)	Deep purple	LSD ($CHCl_3$)
Ferric Chloride (A.8)	Dark greenish yellow	Acetaminophen (methanol)
	Deep orange	Baking soda (powder)
	Very orange	Chlorpromazine HCl (methanol)
	Moderate purplish blue	Dristan, Excedrin (both powder)
	Dark green	Morphine monohydrate (methanol)
Froede Reagent (A.9)	Grayish purple	Aspirin (powder)
	Very deep red	Chlorpromazine HCl ($CHCl_3$)
	Very dark green	Codeine ($CHCl_3$)
	Moderate olive brown	Contac (powder)
	Deep purplish red	Diacetylmorphine HCl, morphine monohydrate (both in $CHCl_3$)
	Very yellow green	Dimethoxy-meth HCl ($CHCl_3$)
	Deep reddish brown	Doxepin HCl ($CHCl_3$)
	Light bluish green	Dristan (powder)

(*continues*)

TABLE 14-1	Color Changes for Medications and Drug of Abuse Tests (*continued*)	
Reagent (#)	**Color Change**	**Drugs (form or solvent)**
Froede Reagent (A.9) (*continued*)	Brilliant blue	Excedrin (powder)
	Moderate yellow green	LSD (CHCl$_3$)
	Light olive yellow	Mace (crystals)
	Greenish black	MDA HCl (CHCl$_3$)
	Brownish black	Opium (powder)
	Strong yellow	Oxycodone HCl (CHCl$_3$)
	Dark grayish red	Propoxyphene HCl (CHCl$_3$)
	Brilliant yellow	Sugar crystals
Mecke Reagent (A.10)	Blackish red	Chlorpromazine HCl (CHCl$_3$)
	Very dark bluish green	Codeine, MDA HCl, morphine monohydrate (all in CHCl$_3$)
	Moderate olive brown	Contac (powder)
	Deep bluish green	Diacetylmorphine HCl (CHCl$_3$)
	Dark brown	Dimethoxy-meth HCl (CHCl$_3$)
	Very dark red	Doxepin HCl (CHCl$_3$)
	Light olive brown	Dristan (powder)
	Dark grayish yellow	Excedrin (powder)
	Dark bluish green	Hydrocodone tartrate Excedrin (CHCl$_3$)
	Greenish black	LSD (CHCl$_3$)
	Dark grayish olive	Mace (crystals)
	Moderate olive	Mescaline HCl, Oxycodone HCl (both in CHCl$_3$)
	Brownish black	Nutmeg (leaves)
	Olive black	Opium (powder)
	Deep reddish brown	Propoxyphene HCl (CHCl$_3$)
	Brilliant greenish yellow	Sugar (crystals)
Zwikker Reagent (A.11)	Light blue	Baking soda (powder)
	Light green	Excedrin (powder)
	Light purple	Pentobarbital, phenobarbital, secobarbital (all in CHCl$_3$)
	Moderate yellow green	Tea (leaves)
	Moderate yellowish green	Tobacco (leaves)
Simon's Reagent (A.12)	Dark blue	d-Amphetamine HCl, MDMA HCl (both in CHCl$_3$)
	Deep blue	Dimethoxy-meth HCl (CHCl$_3$)
	Pale violet	Methylphenidate HCl (CHCl$_3$)

Modified from National Institute of Justice Law Enforcement and Corrections Standards and Testing Program. 2000. Color test reagents/kits for preliminary identification of drugs of abuse (NIJ Standard 0604.01). Washington, DC: U.S. Department of Justice, Office of Justice Programs, National Institute of Justice. http://www.ncjrs.gov/pdffiles1/nij/183258.pdf

are acids and baking soda (change pH and can be detected by pH as well) and bleach to oxidize compounds or test components (odor and color test can detect these). If urine tampering is suspected, human physiological values of urine temperature (32.2–37.8°C), pH (4.5–8.0), and creatinine (> 20mg/dL) should be found. If urinary creatinine is < 20 mg/dL, it is diluted urine. Below 5 mg/dL creatinine, the sample is unlikely to be human urine. Specific gravity should be ≥ 1.003 g/mL and human IgG should be ≥ 0.5 mg/L. Some adulterants commonly used are glutaraldehyde (fixative that interferes with immunoassays and can be detected by gas chromatography), nitrite (oxidizing agent that can be detected colorimetrically), and pyridinium chlorochromate (oxidizing agent that can be detected by color, atomic absorption, or gas chromatography; Jaffee et al., 2008). Some "blocking agents" are more mythology than effective. For example, probenecid is a medication that decreases penicillin excretion. It does not work to retard anabolic steroid excretion and is also a banned substance in athletic competition even if it could do so. It is more difficult to alter professionally drawn blood samples, which are mostly useful for detection of toxicants and essential for therapeutic drug monitoring. Hair samples have increased longevity for substances and may detect use of drugs such as amphetamines, marijuana, cocaine, opiates, and phencyclidine for as long as 90 days following exposure. The combination of presence of a substance, its concentration at a given time following use, and its redistribution following death (determining minimum body burden may be more important in this case) is important, because the presence may indicate abuse, and excess leading to death may determine that a homicide was committed. This is especially true for injected substances that can only be legally obtained and administered by a medical practitioner. The investigation of the death of a very famous pop star headed in that direction as the number of medications and their concentrations were determined following autopsy (physician convicted of involuntary manslaughter due to administration of a fatal dose of the anesthetic agent propofol).

Confirmatory Tests

Confirmatory test usually require greater sensitivity and usually employ GC-MS or LC-MS as the gold standard for identification. For example, confirmatory tests require the sensitivity for marijuana at 15 ng/mL, cocaine at 150 ng/mL, and amphetamines at 500 ng/mL. However, phencyclidine and opiates remain at the screening values of 25 ng/mL and 2,000 ng/L, respectively.

Flow Chart of a Typical Postmortem Examination

An example where postmortems are common are crashes involving air transportation. The Federal Aviation Administration (FAA) has difficulty obtaining uniform samples from crashes, because explosions and other effects of impact may make recovery of certain biological fluids impossible. Note the flow chart in **Figure 14-1**. It is clear that esoteric toxicants are not considered in the first analysis. Clearly, carbon monoxide poisoning is a primary concern when a fire occurs in an enclosed plane or in vehicles powered by a combustion engine as indicated by the test for carboxyhemoglobin (COHb). That is also a concern in northern climates. The state of Minnesota now requires dwellings to contain carbon monoxide detectors by bedrooms in houses with furnaces that use combustion for heating purposes or contain a gas stove. Cyanide is another toxicant that occurs during a fire, and it may occur naturally in certain plants and has been employed in poisonings that could account for a plane crash. Alcohol or other volatile substances may render the pilot less capable of handling an aircraft safely due to the CNS effects of volatile solvents. Additionally, other possibly abused street drugs or prescription medications are of general concern during investigation of the reason for a plane or other crash involving the U.S. Department of Transportation. Glucose is important, because hypoglycemia may account for unconsciousness. Additionally, uncontrolled diabetes mellitus is a concern for pilots as indicated

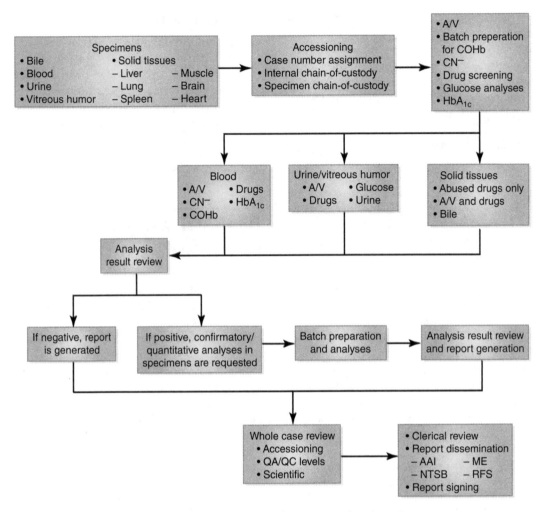

FIGURE 14-1 A Flowchart for a Typical Toxicological Processing of Postmortem Biological Samples

Reprinted from Characteristics and Toxicological Processing of Postmortem Pilot Specimens From Fatal Civil Aviation Accidents, August 2002. Office of Aerospace Medicine Washington, DC, http://www.hf.faa.gov/docs/508/docs/cami/0214.pdf

both by the glucose measurement and the use of the hemoglobin (Hb) A1c test which determines whether Hb is irreversibly glycated at the N-terminal valine of the β-chain (Nakanishi et al., 2003). The Civil Aerospace Medical Institute laboratory optimally requests 40 mL of blood in a green-top tube for COHb, blood CN^-, HbA_{1c}, and drug analyses. The same amount of blood in a grey-top tube is used for ethanol and drug analyses. Urine (100 mL optimally) is collected for drug, ethanol, and glucose analyses. Vitreous humor (2 mL optimally) is sampled for ethanol and glucose testing. Bile (10 mL) is analyzed by radioimmunoassay

(RIA) when urine cannot be collected. Gastric contents (100 mL) are used as necessary for drug analyses. Ethanol and drug analyses are also performed on 500 g of liver; 300 g of skeletal muscle; 150 g of spleen; 100 g of lung, kidney, and brain; and 50 g of heart. Spinal fluid will be sampled for the amount available and tested for ethanol and perhaps drugs if enough is present. The problem is that all these tissues may not be available or only available at suboptimal (adequate or less) volumes. This is demonstrated in **Figure 14-2**. The kidneys are found at the most protected portion (most dorsal) of the abdominal area and therefore had

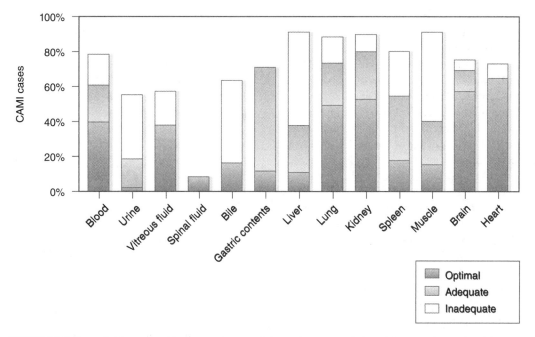

FIGURE 14-2 Optimal, Adequate, and Inadequate Amounts of Various Postmortem Biological Specimens Received at CAMI from the 1,891 Cases (Fatalities) of the United States Fatal Aviation Accidents that Occurred During 1996–2000

Reprinted from Characteristics and Toxicological Processing of Postmortem Pilot Specimens From Fatal Civil Aviation Accidents, August 2002. Office of Aerospace Medicine Washington, DC, http://www.hf.faa.gov/docs/508/docs/cami/0214.pdf

80% of the cases having optimal to adequate amounts of this tissue for examination for the years 1996–2000 (Chaturvedi et al., 2002). Uncontaminated spinal fluid is hardest to obtain, with less than 10% of the cases having optimal volumes for analyses. Urine is very useful in detecting metabolites of chemicals that may have already been excreted, but unfortunately appears to be inadequately available in more than 80% of the crashes. Blood is also heavily relied upon in toxicology for current levels of toxicants, the control of diabetes mellitus, and the clear indication of succumbing to fire (COHb and CN⁻). Unfortunately, optimal and adequate samples were only available in slightly more than 60% of the cases. It is interesting to note that gastric contents were more likely to be in optimal adequate volumes than blood. This is why it is important to consider all possible recoverable uncontaminated samples and what might be gained from their analyses.

Therapeutic Drug (Medication) Monitoring in Living Human Patients

On occasion, certain drugs carry a high danger of toxicity (small therapeutic index or LD_{50}/ED_{50}) and generally are so lipophilic that they require extensive monitoring. Other reasons for following plasma concentrations are that the pharmacokinetics vary widely by patient, plasma concentration is a better measure than dose for therapeutic and adverse effects, there is a plasma concentration that must be achieved to ensure proper onset of therapy (and must be kept close to that value), or the therapeutic effects are difficult to monitor. The last two points are similar to the determination of the international normalized ratio (INR), which is used to determine anticoagulant therapy with a medication such as warfarin (Anand and Yusuf, 2003). The target INR is 2–3. If the coagulation is too rapid, then dangerous clots may form. If coagulation is too low, hemorrhage may occur. This is specifically not therapeutic drug monitoring as the effect rather than the concentration of the medication is monitored. When effect is not well measured, then plasma concentration may be the next best option. Proper dosing is not possible without measuring resultant plasma concentrations. The journal *Therapeutic Drug Monitoring* is devoted to this area.

A number of factors must be considered regarding monitoring of medications. These include compliance (whether the patient is taking the medication as prescribed) and age, because neonates, children, and the elderly absorb, metabolize, and excrete differently than adults. The gender of the patient and pregnancy play important roles in pharmacokinetics/toxicokinetics. Hepatic disease may hamper metabolism. Renal disease can influence half-life and clearance. Cardiovascular disease can decrease or affect circulation and blood pressure, which is important regarding assumptions of speed of action, organ distribution, or filtration resulting in excretion. Respiratory disease affects circulation, blood pH, and is especially important in anesthetic gases and excretion of volatile components of the medication. Other medications clearly may interact in a toxic fashion with the medication or alter metabolism or elimination rate. Additionally, tolerance and dependence must be considered. There are a variety of environmental factors that influence drug metabolism. Genetic polymorphisms of drug metabolism also influence plasma concentrations. To do medication monitoring properly, the doctor takes a history that includes the patient's age, weight, sex, their genetic history of disease, the nature of their current disease, medications taken, doses, medication schedule, and for the specific medication(s) for which plasma concentrations must be determined the time of last dose, time of specimen, and the clinical status relevant to the drug used (e.g., blood pressure, ECG, EEG, plasma liver enzymes). Consider **Table 14-2**, where therapeutic ranges are reported for a variety of medications. The lowest value is the trough concentration (C_{trough})

below which no therapeutic value is indicated for the medication alone. This trough concentration works well for antibiotics and antivirals, as the C_{trough} for the HIV medication atazanavir, for example, is associated with efficacy (de Requena et al., 2005). Other medications may indeed change this value significantly, as is the case for certain combinations of protease inhibitors used to treat HIV infection (Guiard-Schmid et al., 2003). For anti-epileptic medications, the plasma concentration of lamotrigine varies fourfold when comparing joint anti-seizure therapy with the metabolic enzyme inhibitor valproic acid as opposed to inducers phenytoin or carbamazepine (Morris et al., 1998). The high peak concentration should represent a toxic threshold of sorts that would endanger the patient and have less therapeutic value. Note that for the cancer chemotherapy agent methotrexate, only the trough may be relevant. This indicates that all concentrations that are therapeutic are toxic as well, but hopefully more so to cancer cells. Toxicity to normal tissues is to be monitored carefully, so this may obviate the need for a peak value. Some compounds have controversial values or published articles indicating the lack of need for therapeutic drug monitoring for certain medications. Rapid metabolism of the medication may lead to a difficult match between therapeutic effect and plasma concentration of the unaltered drug. This is true for the immunosuppressant purine anti-metabolite azathioprine (Lin et al., 1980). Also, binding to the plasma protein albumin in the blood makes the compound unavailable for activity. Certain compounds such as the anti-seizure medication valproic acid and the anti-inflammatory salicylate have non-linear protein binding in their therapeutic range (Birkett, 1994). Other compounds have uncertain therapeutic value, such as may be the case for a person who has had HIV long enough to experience mutations in the virus that renders the protease inhibitor less effective. Some compounds may be well described by their area under the curve value, which requires many points and appears to be impractical. One such compound is the immunosuppressant mycophenolate mofetil, which is used in kidney transplant patients. The selection of a sampling time is difficult

TABLE 14-2   Therapeutic Drug Monitoring Based on Class of Drugs, Concentration Range, Monitoring Method, and Interaction with Other Medications

Class of Medication	Generic Name	Therapeutic Plasma Concentration Range
Aminoglycoside antibiotics	Amikacin	15–25 μg/mL
	Gentamicin	5–10 μg/mL
	Tobramycin	5–10 μg/mL
Other toxic antibiotics	Chloramphenicol	10–20 μg/mL
	Vancomycin	5–10 μg/mL or 10–20 μg/mL trough (30 min prior to next dose = controversial)
Anti-arrhythmics	Amiodarone	0.5–2.0 μg/mL
	Digoxin	0.5–2.0 ng/mL
	Digitoxin	10–30 ng/mL
	Flecainide	0.2–1.0 μg/mL
	Lidocaine	1.5–5.0 μg/mL
	Mexiletine	0.5–2.0 μg/mL
	Procainamide	4.0–8.0 μg/mL
	N-Acetyl procainamide (metabolite)	10–20 μg/mL
	Quinidine	2.0–5.0 μg/mL
Anti-arthritis or anti-inflammatory	Salicylates	100–250 μg/mL
Antiepileptics	Carbamazepine	5–12 μg/mL
	Ethosuximide	40–100 μg/mL
	Gabapentin	2–10 μg/mL
	Lamotrigine	3–14 μg/mL
	Phenobarbital	10–30 μg/mL
	Phenytoin	10–20 μg/mL
	Valproic acid	50–100 μg/mL
Bronchodilators	Caffeine	10–20 μg/mL
	Theophylline	10–20 μg/mL
Cancer chemotherapy	Methotrexate	> 0.01 μmol/L
HIV treatments — protease inhibitors	Atazanavir	150–850 ng/mL
	Indinavir	0.15 μg/mL trough, 10 μg/mL peak
	Lopinavir	3–8 μg/mL
	Nelfinavir	0.7–1.0 μg/mL (trough)
	Ritonavir	1.1–6.3 μg/mL (trough)
	Saquinavir	100 ng/mL (trough minimum for wt virus)
Immunosuppressants	Azathioprine	20–90 ng/mL at peak (mercaptopurine metabolite)
	Cyclosporine	C2 (conc 2 hours after dosing) > 800 ng/dL
	Mofetil mycophenolate	1–3.5 μg/mL (C2 trough)
	Sirolimus	4–20 ng/mL (C2 trough less on initiation, more for maintenance)
	Tacrolimus	5–20 ng/mL
Psychiatric medications	Lithium	0.8–1.2 mEq/L
	Amitriptyline	120–150 ng/mL
	Desipramine	150–300 ng/mL
	Doxepin	50–200 ng/mL

for this medication as the trough value has little correlation with the dose or therapeutic effect. The plasma concentration 2 (C2) hours following dosing may be the best measure for this medication (Jirasiritham et al., 2004). Note this C2 approach is also used for the immunosuppressant agent cyclosporine (Marcén et al., 2005). The methods for assessment of the plasma concentration include HPLC, GC/MS (or tandem MS), and automated immunoassays. Both accuracy and cost effectiveness must be considered for large-scale clinical use (Touw et al., 2005). Many of the automated immunoassay units focus on digoxin (ng/mL) and theophylline (mg/mL). Digitalis has difficult onset to effects (1 hour post administration) and a very narrow therapeutic range (0.5–1.5 or 2.0 ng/mL, a long half-life (160 hours) and interacts with many medications, so it must be monitored often and carefully. Any overdose may affect the heart and nervous system severely ($3Na^+$, $2K^+$-ATPase inhibition), so a digitalis antibody is used to avoid plasma concentrations in excess of 2.0 ng/mL. Automated methods in therapeutic drug monitoring reflect clearly established guidelines for use in a widespread and diverse population. Other medications have controversial aspects of when to measure or whether to measure at all. That is an easier decision to make if the therapeutic activity is more easily determined than previously thought when monitoring was considered. Additionally, the toxicity may be easily observed and does not endanger the patient more than the adverse effects of other medications that are not monitored by plasma concentrations. This is the reason that some doctors in rural areas use the effect of digitalis on heart rate alone as an inexpensive alternative to testing.

Questions

1. How would you use to toxidromes to discern the difference between someone driving under the influence of alcohol (ethanol) versus Vicodin (hydrocodone = opioid + acetaminophen)? How would CO poisoning look different from CN poisoning?

2. What samples should be taken for: (a) a child living in a house manufacturing methamphetamine but not taking any of the drug, (b) monitoring the level of digitalis in a patient, (c) a living person to show that they had used illegal drugs in the recent past, (d) a corpse buried in the ground that might have been poisoned with an organophosphate nerve agent, and (e) chronic exposure of a child to pica (Pb in paint chips)?

3. Why not test for original toxicant, medications, or peptide hormones in urine?

4. In plane crash cases, why not use the urine as this fluid is most likely to contain metabolites of drugs, ethanol, and other prescription medications used before the crash as well as whether the person had diabetes mellitus under control?

5. In therapeutic drug monitoring, when is C_{trough} appropriate to use for dosing versus C2 versus establishing a range with maximum and minimum plasma concentrations?

References

Agahian B, Lee JS, Nelson JH, Johns RE. 1990. Arsenic levels in fingernails as a biological indicator of exposure to arsenic. *Am Ind Hyg Assoc J.* 51:646–651.

Anand S, Yusuf S. 2003. Oral anticoagulants in patients with coronary artery disease. *J Am Coll Cardiol.* 41:62S–69S.

Arruda-Neto JD, de Oliveira MC, Sarkis JE, Bordini P, Manso-Guevara MV, Garcia F, Prado GR, Krug FJ, Mesa J, Bittencourt-Oliveira MC, Garcia C, Rodrigues TE, Shtejer K, Genofre GC. 2009. Study of environmental burden of lead in children using teeth as bioindicator. *Environ Int.* 35:614–618.

Badghisi H, Liebler DC. 2002. Sequence mapping of epoxide adducts in human hemoglobin with LC-tandem MS and the SALSA algorithm. *Chem Res Toxicol.* 15:799–805

Bigazzi PE. 1994. Autoimmunity and heavy metals. *Lupus.* 3:449–453.

Birkett DJ. 1994. Pharmacokinetics made easy 9: non-linear pharmacokinetics. *Aust Prescr.* 17:36–38.

Boyle JS, Bechtel LK, Holstege CP. 2009. Management of the critically poisoned patient. *Scand J Trauma Resusc Emerg Med.* 17:29.

Bronstein AC, Spyker DA, Cantilena LR Jr, Green JL, Rumack BH, Heard SE. 2008. 2007 annual report of the American Association of Poison Control Centers' National Poison Data System (NPDS): 25th annual report. *Clin Toxicol (Phila)*. 46:927–1057.

Bronstein AC, Spyker DA, Cantilena LR Jr, Rumack BH, Dart RC. 2012. 2011 Annual report of the American Association of Poison Control Centers' National Poison Data System (NPDS): 29th Annual Report. *Clin Toxicol (Phila)*. 50:911–1164.

Castaing N, Titier K, Canal-Raffin M, Moore N, Molimard M. 2006. Postmortem redistribution of two antipsychotic drugs, haloperidol and thioridazine, in the rat. *J Anal Toxicol*. 30:419–425.

Centers for Disease Control and Prevention. Web-based Injury Statistics Query and Reporting System (WISQARS) [Online]. 2015. National Center for Injury Prevention and Control, Centers for Disease Control and Prevention (producer). http://www.cdc.gov/injury/wisqars/fatal.html .

Chaturvedi AK, Smith DR, Soper JW, Canfield DV, Whinnery JE. 2002. Characteristics and toxicological processing of postmortem pilot specimens from fatal civil aviation accidents. Washington, DC: U.S. Department of Transportation, Federal Aviation Administration, Office of Aerospace Medicine, DOT/FAA/AM-02/14. http://www.hf.faa.gov/docs/508/docs/cami/0214.pdf.

Crandall CS, Kerrigan S, Aguero RL, Lavalley J, McKinney PE. 2006. The influence of collection site and methods on postmortem morphine concentrations in a porcine model. *J Anal Toxicol*. 30:651–658.

de Requena DG, Bonora S, Canta F, Marrone R, D'Avolio A, Sciandra M, Milia M, Di Garbo A, Sinicco A, Di Perri G. 2005. Atazanavir Ctrough is associated with efficacy and safety: definition of therapeutic range. NATAP, 12th CROI, Poster 645, Alexandria, VA.

Flanagan RJ, Connally G. 2005. Interpretation of analytical toxicology results in life and at postmortem. *Toxicol Rev*. 24:51–62.

Guiard-Schmid JB, Poirier JM, Meynard JL, Bonnard P, Gbadoe AH, Amiel C, Calligaris F, Abraham B, Pialoux G, Girard PM, Jaillon P, Rozenbaum W. 2003. High variability of plasma drug concentrations in dual protease inhibitor regimens. *Antimicrob Agents Chemother*. 47:986–990.

Gunatilake K, Goff ML. 1989. Detection of organophosphate poisoning in a putrefying body by analyzing arthropod larvae. *J Forensic Sci*. 34:714–716.

Hill RH Jr, Alley CC, Ashley DL, Cline RE, Head SL, Needham LL, Etzel RA. 1990. Laboratory investigation of a poisoning epidemic in Sierra Leone. *J Anal Toxicol*. 14:213–216.

Jaffee WB, Trucco E, Teter C, Levy S, Weiss RD. 2008. Focus on alcohol & drug abuse: ensuring validity in urine drug testing. *Psychiatr Serv*. 59:140–142.

Jirasiritham S, Sumethkul V, Mavichak V, Na-Bangchang K. 2004. The pharmacokinetics of mycophenolate mofetil in Thai kidney transplant recipients. *Transplant Proc*. 36:2076–2078.

Jurado C, Sachs H. 2003. Proficiency test for the analysis of hair for drugs of abuse, organized by the Society of Hair Testing. *Forensic Sci Int*. 133:175–178.

Koren G. 2007. A primer of paediatric toxic syndromes or 'toxidromes.' *Paediatr Child Health*. 12:457–459.

Lin SN, Jessup K, Floyd M, Wang TP, van Buren CT, Caprioli RM, Kahan BD. 1980. Quantitation of plasma azathioprine and 6-mercaptopurine levels in renal transplant patients. *Transplantation*. 29:290–294.

Marcén R, Villafruela JJ, Pascual J, Teruel JL, Ocaña J, Tenorio MT, Burgos FJ, Ortuño J. 2005. Clinical outcomes and C2 cyclosporin monitoring in maintenance renal transplant recipients: 1 year follow-up study. *Nephrol Dial Transplant*. 20:803–810.

Maurer HH. 2007. Analytical toxicology. *Anal Bioanal Chem*. 388:1311.

McAllister JL, Roby RJ, Levine B, Purser D. 2008. Stability of cyanide in cadavers and in postmortem stored tissue specimens: a review. *J Anal Toxicol*. 32:612–620.

McGrath KK, Jenkins AJ. 2009. Detection of drugs of forensic importance in postmortem bone. *Am J Forensic Med Pathol*. 30:40–44.

Merrick BA. 2006. Toxicoproteomics in liver injury and inflammation. *Ann N Y Acad Sci*. 1076:707–717.

Merrick BA, Witzmann FA. 2009. The role of toxicoproteomics in assessing organ specific toxicity. *EXS*. 99:367–400.

Morris RG, Black AB, Harris AL, Batty AB, Sallustio BC. 1998. Lamotrigine and therapeutic drug monitoring: retrospective survey following the introduction of a routine service. *Br J Clin Pharmacol*. 46:547–551.

Nakanishi T, Iguchi K, Shimizu A. 2003. Method for hemoglobin A(1c) measurement based on peptide analysis by electrospray ionization mass spectrometry with deuterium-labeled synthetic peptides as internal standards. *Clin Chem*. 49:829–831.

National Institute of Justice Law Enforcement and Corrections Standards and Testing Program. 2000. Color test reagents/kits for preliminary identification of drugs of abuse. NIJ Standard 0604.01. U.S. Department of Justice, Office of Justice Programs, National Institute of Justice. http://www.ncjrs.gov/pdffiles1/nij/183258.pdf

Omar MA, Wilson JP, Cox TS. 2001. Rhabdomyolysis and HMG-CoA reductase inhibitors. *Ann Pharmacother*. 35:1096–1107.

Peng SX, Branch TM, King SL. 2001. Fully automated 96-well liquid-liquid extraction for analysis of biological samples by liquid chromatography with tandem mass spectrometry. *Anal Chem.* 73:708–714.

Rodda KE, Drummer OH. 2006. The redistribution of selected psychiatric drugs in post-mortem cases. *Forensic Sci Int.* 164:235–239.

Singer PP, Jones GR, Bannach BG, Denmark L. 2007. Acute fatal acetaminophen overdose without liver necrosis. *J Forensic Sci.* 52:992–994.

Society of Forensic Toxicologists, American Academy of Forensic Sciences. 2006. Forensic toxicology laboratory guidelines. http://www.soft-tox.org/files/Guidelines_2006_Final.pdf.

Stimpfl T, Demuth W, Varmuza K, Vycudilik W. 2003. Systematic toxicological analysis: computer-assisted identification of poisons in biological materials. *J Chromatogr B Analyt Technol Biomed Life Sci.* 789:3–7.

Thomas LDK, Hodgson S, Nieuwenhuijsen M, Jarup L. 2009. Early kidney damage in a population exposed to cadmium and other heavy metals. *Environ Health Perspect.* 117:181–184.

Tomassoni AJ, French RN, Walter FG. 2015. Toxic industrial chemicals and chemical weapons: exposure, identification, and management by syndrome. *Emerg Med Clin North Am.* 33:13-36.

Touw DJ, Neef C, Thomson AH, Vinks AA. 2005. Cost-effectiveness of therapeutic drug monitoring: a systematic review. Cost-Effectiveness of Therapeutic Drug Monitoring Committee of the International Association for Therapeutic Drug Monitoring and Clinical Toxicology. *Ther Drug Monit.* 27:10-17.

Warner M, Chen LH, Makuc DM, Anderson RN, Miniño AM. 2011. Drug poisoning deaths in the United States, 1980-2008. National Center for Health Statistics Data Brief, December: 1-8. http://www.cdc.gov/nchs/data/databriefs/db81.pdf

World Health Organization. 2015. Guidelines for poison control. http://www.who.int/ipcs/publications/training_poisons/guidelines_poison_control/en/index4.html.

CHAPTER 15

The Skin and Eye: Most Likely Exposure Routes and Toxicities Due to Contact Exposure and Dose Toxicities

This is a chapter outline intended to guide and familiarize you with the content to follow.

I. Most likely routes of accidental exposure

A. Skin

1. Examples from life—sunburn, contact dermatitis

2. Provides barrier to charged substances (epidermis + degree or keratinization forms barriers as dermis is more permeable) and fluid barrier, metabolic barrier (contains enough CYPs to biotransform dermally applied 3-MC → carcinogenic metabolites → skin neoplasms), temperature regulation through blood flow alterations + hair + perspiration (horses, humans, but not pig), influences expression of immune system, mechanical support for internal organs (collagen type + amount → integrity + flexibility), neurosensory receptors + self-regulatory neuro-endocrine system, synthesizes vitamin D_3 (UV irradiation) + parathyroid hormone related protein

3. Types of damage—see Table 15-1

a. Burns from corrosive chemicals, desiccants, oxidants, reducing agents, protoplasmic poisons, and vesicants based on reactive nature of chemical, concentration, exposure time, regional skin properties, % skin burned, subsequent treatment

(1) pK_a → acid damage limited by necrotic eschar formed; HF = protoplasmic poison as well due to chelation of divalent ions such as Ca^{2+} and direct action of F^- on cardiac cells

pK_a → alkaline damage → liquefaction necrosis → saponification of lipids + denatured proteins—see Figure 15-1

(2) White phosphorus +oxygen → burn → renal failure from changing calcium/phosphorus ratio

(3) Strong solvents (hydrophobic and anesthetic phenol) → high penetration and removal of essential fats and oils (loss of hydration) → kidney damage

b. Contact dermatitis—see Figure 15-2

(1) Irritants (acids, bases, solvents, microtrauma by fiberglass or abrasive chemicals or detergents), allergic reaction (low-molecular-weight haptens → delayed-type hypersensitivity by T cells as recruited by skin-homing receptor binding to endothelial- and platelet-selectin such as occurs with poison ivy), or UV light → proinflammatory cytokine released from keratinocytes (e.g., IL1 and TNFα → inflammation; IL8 and IL10 → chemotaxis; IL6, IL7, IL12 (growth promotion), IL10, IL12, IL18 (lymphocyte stimulation)

c. Acneiform reactions

(1) Corticosteroids → Toll-like receptor 2 mediated response

(2) Isoniazid (used to treat tuberculosis) inhibits MAO and induces acne

CONCEPTUALIZING TOXICOLOGY 15-1

(3) Calcineurin blockers such as cyclosporine suppress immunity and lead to acne

(4) Li used to treat bipolar disorder leads to acne via neutrophil induction

(5) Blocking epidermal growth factor → acne

(6) Ionizing radiation has been used to treat acne, but can also induce skin damage and acne

(7) Aromatic antiseizure compounds (phenytoin) and nonaromatic antiseizure drug valproic acid (also causes oligomenorrhea and hyperandrogenism) → acne

(8) Chloracne formed by 2,3,7,8-TCDD-induced AhR dimerization with aryl hydrocarbon nuclear translocation protein—see Figure 15-3; EGF can repress CYP1A1 induction and chloracne; other aromatic hydrocarbons also induce hyperkeratinization via AhR binding

d. Toxic alopecia (hair loss)

(1) Dihydrotestosterone appears to induce hair loss as does overexpression of androgen receptors

(2) Poisoning of hair follicles (cytotoxic cancer chemotherapy agents) may be modified by induction of heat stress protein by geldanamycin analogues

(3) Heparanase overexpression by transit-amplifying cells helps with anticancer drug and heparin (heparanase inhibitor)-induced alopecia as this enzyme helps release heparin sulfate-bound growth factors

(4) Decreased biotinidase activity also associated with alopecia—biotin supplementation may prevent this dermal toxicity

(5) Nutritional deficiencies (e.g., Se, Zn) or Se, Tl, As, boric acid, vitamin A excess → alopecia; cholesterol-lowering drugs cause diffuse alopecia via interference with keratinization similar to excess Tl or vitamin A

e. Toxic epidermal necrosis (TEN)—see Figure 15-4

(1) Progression of Stevens-Johnson Syndrome (SJS) to a serious and occasionally fatal (25–40% mortality) condition depending on treatment involving vesicular eruptions of at least two mucosal surfaces (bullous disease characterized by epidermal cell death)

(2) Found in elderly with HIV infection or other infections (Epstein-Barr, herpes simplex, *Mycoplasma pneumoniae*, measles, mycobacterium, smallpox vaccination, group A streptococci, *Yersinia*, enterovirus), medication-induced (antibiotics, anticonvulsants, NSAIDs)

(3) SJS/TEN commonality = epidermal cell apoptosis induced by cytotoxic T-cells, Fas-Fas ligand interaction, TNFα, and NO synthase

f. Vesiculobullous and pemphigus (see Figure 15-5)

(1) IgA bullous autoimmune reactions to the skin which can be linked to antibiotic use (amoxicillin-clavulanic acid combination used for sinus infections)

g. Maculopapular eruptions—see Figure 15-6

(1) Rash with many small bumps caused by reaction to viruses or medications

(2) TH1 CD4 T-lymphocytes with cytotoxic properties or TH0 mediates the response as stimulated by skin homing chemokines CCL20, CCL27, CXCL9, CXCL10, and their receptors

(3) Enhanced by oxidative stress

h. Fixed drug reactions (drug-induced dermatosis)

(1) Associated with CD8(+) intraepidermal T cells with effector memory phenotype that occurs on reuse of a medication (antibiotics sulfonamides and tetracyclines) on the same skin area

i. Other immune reactions

(1) Lupus erythematosus-like syndrome (sulfonamides, anticonvulsants)

j. Phototoxicities and photoallergies

(1) UV-B usually associated with sunburns on Earth, but UV-A may cause most phototoxicities and photoallergies

CONCEPTUALIZING TOXICOLOGY 15-1 (*continued*)

(2) Photosensitivities = dyschromia (discoloration), pseudoporphyria (bullous), photo onycholysis (nail plate separation), lichenoid (bands parallel to epidermis) and telangiectatic (permanent dilation of preexisting blood vessels); augmented by ROS and RNS generated in skin cells or xenobiotics forming toxic quinones → O_{2^-}; UV-A and UV-B enhanced by photosensitizers generate lipid peroxides, singlet oxygen, superoxide, and NO → peroxynitrite

k. Skin cancers

(1) UV (primary cause) and genetic susceptibility, X-rays + some viruses + strong mutagenic chemicals (e.g., metabolites of 3-MC) → basal cell carcinomas (90%) followed by squamous cell carcinoma followed by most fatal of all—malignant melanoma; Kaposi's sarcoma caused by herpes virus ($\frac{1}{3}$ of HIV patients)

(2) UV-B → cyclobutane pyrimidine dimers → mutations in tumor suppressor genes and suppression of immune system (photolyase-containing liposomes removes dimers and reverses immune suppression) → clustering of growth factor receptors on plasma membrane of keratinocytes → MAP kinase activation → transcription factor → gene expression; high doses of UV-B → apoptosis; osmolyte loading of keratinocytes appears to inhibit damaging signal transduction induced by UV-B as both use similar pathway of hyperosmotic stress response (osmolyte transport system in human keratinocytes)

(3) UV-A → oxidative function starts with ceramide formation (also prevented by osmolyte loading) → mitochondria release cytochrome c without starting apoptosis in cytosol → transcriptional AP-2 oxidation → ICAM-1 expression and other UV-A inducible genes

(4) AhR involved in skin cancer formation from PAHs (chimney sweep scrotal cancers) but also critical in normal skin homeostasis (AhR-deficient mice → interfollicular and follicular epidermal hyperplasia with hyperkeratosis and acanthosis with dermal fibrosis); AhR pathway activated by UV

(5) HA-*ras* oncogene initiates skin cancer (A-T transversions in codon 61 by DMBA → papillomas and carcinomas); *p53* tumor suppressor gene involved in skin cancer progression; lipoxygenase (LOX) enzymes of arachidonic acid cascade (inflammatory mediators through COX and LOX enzymes) involved in formation of etheno adducts of DNA

l. Systemic toxicities

(1) Systemically reactivated allergic contact dermatitis—happens within hours of ingestion, it is not T-cell–mediated type IV delayed-type hypersensitivity; can be autoimmunity (Type III reaction) or IgE-mediated type I immediate hypersensitivity if accompanied by urticaria (wheal and flare) and anaphylaxis (drop in blood pressure and constricted bronchioles caused by histamine release)

(2) Cyanosis (dangerous to lethal) due to CN, generation of metHb due to nitrite, H_2S, or pseudocyanosis with Ag, Pb, amiodarone, chloroquine, phenothiazines, or blue food coloring ingestion

(3) Diaphoresis (excessive perspiration) associated with myocardial infarction, drugs of abuse withdrawal, pain and stress, or acetylcholinesterase inhibition (also accompanied by salivation, miosis, headaches, nausea, night-waking, diarrhea, labored breathing, incoordination, mental confusion)

(4) Skin flushing from allergic reaction, scombrotoxic fish poisoning (histamine), or niacin excess

(5) Jaundice—yellowing of skin due to hemolysis (e.g., As, oxidative medications, crotalid snake venoms) or liver damage (e.g., acetaminophen, ethanol, antiretrovirals)

(6) Hyperpigmentation due to Ag, As, Au, Bi, Fe, Pb, Tl, NSAIDs, antimalarials, amiodarone, cytotoxic anticancer medications, tetracyclines, psychotropic drugs

(7) Skin reactions from keloids, fat atrophy, gangrene, contractions, arthralgias, neuritis, hyperpigmentation, corneal ulcerations, vasospasm, post-envenomation herpes simplex or granuloma annulare with recurrent skin eruptions, distant-site eruptions, persistent lesions, or urticaria + jellyfish nematocyst toxin

CONCEPTUALIZING TOXICOLOGY 15-1 (*continued*)

(8) Pruritus (itching)—and vasculitis—iron-deficiency anemia, myeloproliferative disorders, monoclonal gammopathy and multiple myeloma, lymphoma, uremia secondary to renal toxicity, cholestasis secondary to liver damage, disorders of the thyroid, dry skin (xerosis), eczema or scabies

4. Percutaneous absorption

   a. S = significant absorption (> 100 chemicals according to Finland)

   b. LD_{50} < 1.0 g/kg = acute dermal toxicant according to ACGIH

   c. Most compound much less than 100% absorption

   d. Absorption follows Fick's law of diffusion: $K_p = J/\Delta C$

   e. Metals absorbed based on molecular volume (function of ionic radius + counter ion that diffuses with a given metal rather than polarity reflects metals' absorption)—for example, Cr(III)2(SO$_4$)$_3$ not absorbed (strong affinity for epithelial and dermal tissues) while the nitrate is only slightly better absorbed (counterion influence); Cr(VI) does not similarly bind to organic substrates; for Ni salts penetration for counterions follow the order acetate > nitrate > sulfate > chloride; organic metal acts like organic nonelectrolyte

   f. Skin metabolism should not only be considered for compounds such as PAHs, but also for metals (e.g., conversion of Cr(VI) → Cr(II) by sulfhydryl groups

   g. Dimethyl sulfoxide and petrolatum increase skin absorption

5. Skin toxicity tests—see Table 15-2

   a. Historic and controversial (with animal rights groups) Draize test—expose 10% of intact skin by shaving or clipping fur off of rabbit (preferred although more sensitive than human), rat, or mouse

   b. Acute dermal toxin = one applied to that area increases mortality with dose (e.g., dimethyl mercury)

   c. Erythema (redness), edema (raised surface), eschar (depth of tissue injury), and skin dryness determined 1, 24, 48, and 72 h after treatment

   d. Guinea pig maximization test (skin sensitization)—shaved and exposed dermally or intradermally for 14 days → 10–14 day recovery period → lower challenge dose given → evaluate edema and erythema 24, 48, and 72 h following challenge dose (e.g., 2,4-dinitrochlorobenzene, *p*-nitrodimethylaniline, or *p*-phenylenediamine); murine lymph node lymphocyte threefold proliferation also used as a cutoff value to assess sensitizers; photoallergy employs similar sensitization schedule and challenge dose excepting lower doses and use of light (UV-A); phototoxicities more likely caused by compounds with benzene rings (acute = enhanced sunburn → vesicles → healing with hyperpigmentation)

   e. Irritation could also be assessed by IL-1α cytokine response; allergic contact dermatitis also determined by IL-8 or B7 (adhesion molecule) or T-lymphocyte activation in dendritic cells

B Eye—see Figure 15-7

1. Examples from life—sunburn (cornea, lens, retinal damage), irritation by shampoo or particles, vascularization caused by excess contact lens use, lacrimation by cutting onion

2. Collagen (parallel formations necessary for opacity)

3. Types of damage—see Table 15-3

   a. Corneal damage—provides 48 diopters of refraction if undamaged and normal thickness

      (1) Layers: epithelium → Bowman layer → stroma (90%) → Descemet membrane → endothelium

      (2) SJS similar to skin caused by SNP in Toll-like receptor 3 gene, especially SNP 299698T/G and genotype patterns 293248A/A and 299698T/T; inflammation due to CXC chemokines (attract neutrophils)

      (3) Damage to collagen→ scar (absorbs UV maximum sensitivity = 270 nm, but UV-C absorbed by Earth's atmosphere so UV-B → photokeratitis with stromal swelling); oxygen + UV-B → ROS (from heme oxygenase-1 + NADPH cytochrome P450 reductase) and RNS— defended by cellular and extracellular SODs

CONCEPTUALIZING TOXICOLOGY 15-1 (*continued*)

(4) Damage through CO-induced mitochondrial dysfunction

(5) Metabolism of 1,2-dichloroethane → milky white opacity—see Figure 15-8

(6) Acids and bases burn (limbal stem cell deficiency)

(7) Cationic detergents = most irritating

(8) Injury progression from necrotic lesions → debridement → influx of neutrophils → secrete metalloproteinases which aid debridement but damage ocular structures → ischemic cells secrete VEGF, TGF, and FGF → angiogenesis which promotes conjunctiva but ↓ corneal transparency

b. Lens damage

(1) Cataracts—see Figure 15-9, as caused by diabetes mellitus (conversion of glucose conversion by aldose reductase → sorbitol and ↑ osmotic pressure and ↓ expression of caveolin-1 → apoptosis); naphthalene → dihydrodiol (also aldose reductase); UV-B and ROS (activation of NF- κB)

(2) Mitochondrial damage (CCCP, SDS) → decreased mitochondria length → swelling → changing from short to round mitochondria → cytotoxicity, and decreased mitochondria with aging lenses leads to lens damage

(3) Apoptosis of lens epithelial cells → less posterior capsule opacification; simvastatin or EGF ↓ apoptosis → ↑ opacity

c. Retinal damage

(1) Aging → retinal tears or attachment, oxidative damage and inflammation, rod and cone degeneration, pigmentation alterations, neurological deficits; UV-B (photochemical, mechanical thermal) and O_2 promote aging

(2) Quinolones and acridines accumulate in retinal pigment epithelium (affect lysosomal degradation) → "bulls-eye" pigmentation and depigmented ring

(3) Cardiac glycosides which inhibit $3Na^+,2K^+$-ATPase affect color vision by changing ion fluxes

(4) Mitochondrial DNA damage or other mitochondrial function inhibitors affect retina due to high ATP demand of retina; also prone to blindness from formic acid formed by alcohol dehydrogenase from methanol

(5) Choroidal circulation makes retina more prone to damage from cytotoxic agents (alkylating agents, antimetabolites, mitotic inhibitors); organic solvents can disrupt color vision (n-hexane and dying-back axonopathy) as do perchloroethylene, CS_2, and Hg

(6) Inhibition of AChE by diazinon in fish embryos → necrotic cells within inner nuclear layer and isolated pyknotic cells in ganglion layer of the retina

(7) NSAID indomethacin reduces ocular blood flow via COX-1 inhibition, but also may form a quinone imine via metabolism. Similarly, tamoxifen and thioridazine oxidation via CYPs and myeloperoxidase → oxidative stress

(8) Phosphodiesterase (PDE) inhibition by erectile dysfunction medication → ischemic disorders of optic disc (where optic nerve enters retina); PDE-6 especially important as it converts light signals → electrical signals

(9) Pb^{2+} targets L-type Ca^{2+} channels and neurotransmitter release, intracellular Ca^{2+} concentrations, Ca^{2+} regulatory proteins, mitochondrial function—causes blindness by neural toxicity/microvascular alterations and loss of neuromuscular control of eye; similarly, diabetes mellitus destroys blood/retinal barrier—see diabetic retinopathy in Figure 15-10; microvascular also altered by canthaxanthin → retinopathy

d. Optic nerve damage

(1) Cigarette smoke contains carcinogens such as catechol and hydroquinone which auto-oxidize → semiquinone and HO·; other toxicants in smoke are alkaloids, aromatic hydrocarbons and amines, phenols, terpenes, carboxylic acids, indole, benzofurans, inorganic particulates, and tar → optic chiasma degeneration in chick embryos, demyelination, and swollen mitochondria

CONCEPTUALIZING TOXICOLOGY 15-1 (*continued*)

(2) Gliosis (astrocyte proliferation) accompanies CNS structural damage as kainic acid produces in brain and retina

(3) Mitochondrial damage is also critical to optic nerve function such as done by rotenone

(4) Dichloromethane → direct toxicity + conversion to carbon monoxide

(5) Antioxidant lycopene or protein and B vitamin deficiencies (especially riboflavin) → ↑ optic neuropathy susceptibility

(6) Acrylamide and CS_2 → axonopathies

e. Central visual system lesions

(1) Pb alters conduction velocities of visual, auditory, and somatosensory impulses through CNS neurons

(2) Methylmercury causes constriction of the visual field, paresthesias, impairments of hearing and speech, mental disturbances, diaphoresis, hypersalivation

4. Eye toxicity tests—see Table 15-4

a. Draize test—very controversial among animal rights groups

(1) Adapted Friedenwald's quantitative scale of ocular damage including animal blinks or wipes (discomfort level), mucosal and epithelial effects, redness of conjunctiva, corneal edema/opacity, iritis, discharge, lacrimation, blepharitis (eyelid inflammation) by biomicroscopy, and fluorescein staining + recorded systemic effects. Can also look for cataracts and retinal damage by classic ophthalmic examination and a color vision panel (subtle retinal damage)

CONCEPTUALIZING TOXICOLOGY 15-1 (*continued*)

Many humans experience sunburn at some point in their lives. People use tanning salons without thinking of the future danger of melanomas from ultraviolet (UV) irradiation damage. Chemicals of all sorts are spilled on the skin. People have contact dermatitis and other skin reactions. Similarly, excess radiation can burn the cornea or damage lens or retinal cells. The eyes become red and irritated when accidentally exposed to shampoo, a large particle that does not clear on blinking, or eye drops that contain allergens. People went blind during the years of Prohibition in the United States by drinking methanol, which initially appeared to have the same effects as ethanol. Cataracts develop with age in animals and humans, but are hastened by diabetes mellitus (aldose reductase conversion to sorbitol; Dvornik, 1992) and chemical agents. Glaucoma induces blindness and is hastened by certain chemicals. Even something apparently minor, such as the oxygen permeation of contact lenses or how solvents may travel under contact lenses and damage or cause vascularization of the cornea, becomes important in examining toxicity. On occasion, the high permeability of a large, exposed surface such as the skin can lead to toxicity, as is the case in people who over-apply a muscle pain relief agent containing methyl salicylate, for example. In the laboratory, a small amount of dimethyl mercury may be absorbed easily across the skin and cause death. Health practitioners stress the use of skin and eye protection against sun radiation and chemical exposure for those using adhesives, paints, solvents, and hazardous chemicals. Those with latex allergies must also protect themselves from exposure to latex gloves or balloons. It is important to select the correct protection that prevents skin or eye contact, while allowing the person to thermoregulate and the eye cells to obtain the oxygen and other substances they need for proper function. The Occupational Safety and Health Administration (OSHA, 2015) indicates that the choice of glove, for instance, is determined by whether one is trying to prevent abrasions; avoid lacerations by sharps; prevent chemicals and fluids from coming in contact with the skin (type dependent on the chemical permeation rate); deal with extremes of hot and cold; provide general duty protection; prevent the contamination of products with one's skin bacteria, DNA (forensic work), and so forth; and avoid the damage of ionizing radiation.

Forensic Analysis of Skin Damage

Dermatologists specialize in skin damage and look for the most dangerous signs, such as melanomas or other skin cancers. **Table 15-1** provides a list of agents that can cause skin damage. The pH of a compound may cause damage to the skin, with bases with pH > 11.5 inflicting the most damage. With an acid, the amount of a neutralizing compound that it takes to bring the pH back to neutral is a better indicator of the damage done than the absolute pH. The damage done is a function of the concentration of the substance (i.e., pH), the substances' nature (reducing agent, oxidizer, corrosive, protoplasmic poison, vesicants, and desiccants), percentage burn, time of exposure, regional skin properties (age, race, location, preexisting skin disturbances such as dermatitis), and management of the burn following damage (Ahmadi et al., 2008). This is important, because the skin (especially the epidermis in mammals) is normally a good barrier that prevents diffusion

TABLE 15-1   Forensic Chart of Dermal Toxicity

Skin Toxicity	Toxic Agents
Acne-Causing	
Antibiotics	Isoniazid (Oliwiecki and Burton, 1988)
Aromatic anticonvulsants	Phenytoin and androgen excess (Derman, 1995)
Calcineurin blockers	Cyclosporine (Gaber et al., 2008)
Chloracne	2,3,7,8-TCDD and other halogenated aromatics—AH-mediated and reversed by EGF (Hankinson, 2009)
Epidermal Growth Factor (EGF) blockers	Cetuximab antibody to EGF (Labianca et al., 2007)
Psychotropic medications	Lithium and neutrophils (Chan et al., 2000), biopsychosocial model of skin disorders (Gupta and Gupta, 2003)
Radiation	Ionizing (Carrotte-Lefebvre et al., 2003)
Sebaceous gland effects	Sex steroids (George et al., 2008)
Toll-like receptor 2 induction	Corticosteroids (Shibata et al., 2009)
Allergic Contact Dermatitis—true allergic response experienced by those who react and must be sensitized resulting in redness, itching, small blisters → widespread large overlapping fluid-filled blisters treated by corticosteroids	Antiseptics/topical medications—bacitracin, benzalkonium chloride, benzocaine, lanolin, neomycin, propylene glycol
	Glues—acrylic monomers, bisphenol A, glutaraldehyde (fixative)
	Metals—chromium, nickel
	Pesticides—benomyl, captafol, captan, cresol, 2,4,-dichloro-4'-nitrophenyl ether (TOK), dichlorvos, formaldehyde, malathion (OP), maneb, naled, natural pyrethroids (some), parathion (OP), pentachloronitrobenzene (PCNB fungicide), thiram, triazine, zineb
	Rubber compounds—diphenylguanidine, hydroquinone, p-phenylenediamine
	Flowers—chrysanthemum, English ivy, narcissus bulb, primrose, tulip bulb
	Plants—celery, garlic, liverwort, onions, *Toxicodendron* species (poison ivy, oak, sumac), rhus
	Trees—cashew, cedar, lichens, pine
Blistering (bullous) disorders including vesiculobullous and autoimmune pemphigus	Linear IgA bullous (autoimmune) disease is produced by diuretics, NSAIDs, vancomycin (Ho et al., 2007)

(continues)

TABLE 15-1 Forensic Chart of Dermal Toxicity (*continued*)	
Skin Toxicity	**Toxic Agents**
Burns	Reducing agents—tissues bind these free electrons causing their intermolecular bonds to become unstable (hydrazine, hydroxylamine)
	Oxidants—disrupt covalent bonds and architecture (chromic acid). The byproducts of the oxidation reaction are often toxic themselves and continue to react (e.g., lipid peroxidation products).
	Corrosives—denature proteins (alkalis such as NaOH and CaOH)
	Protoplasmic poisons—bind to organic ions and inhibiting the action required for tissue function (hydrofluoric acid)
	Vesicants—produce anoxic necrosis at contact site (mustard gas)
	Desiccants—produce exothermic reactions simultaneously heating and dehydrating tissue (sulfuric acid; from Ahmadi et al., 2008)
Contact Phototoxic Photosensitization—common occupational exposure in humans and coming in contact with plant or fungus product that is absorbed into the skin resulting in redness, pain, blistering, and hyperpigmentation after recovery similar to sunburn	Plants—buttercup, carrots, celery, dill, figs, Klamath weed, lime, mustard (with *Gliocladium* or pink rot)
Phototoxic Photosensitization Dermatitis—common in domestic animals after ingestion of a compound making them sensitive to UV light	Antifungals—fenticlor, Jadit
	Antimicrobials/antiseptics—bithionol, chlorhexidine
	Copper toxicosis in sheep
	Cosmetics/dyes—acridine, fluorescin, methyl blue/violet, trypaflavin
	Cyanobacteria (blue-green algae) poisoning
	Deodorant soaps—halogenated carbanilides/phenols
	Fluorescent brightening agent for fibers—Blankophor
	Food additive—cyclamates (artificial sweetener)
	Hepatic injury—jaundice coloration
	Herbal supplements—*Ginkgo biloba*, *Hypericum* sp. (St. John's wort)
	Medications—antihistamines, coal tar and derivatives, NSAIDs, oral contraceptives and estrogens, phenothiazines, sulfonamides, sulfonylureas, tetracyclines, thiazide diuretics, tricyclic antidepressants
	Melanogenics—furocoumarins
	Perfumes and toiletries—cedar, citron, lavender oils, *Rutaceae*, *Umbelliferae*
	Plants—*Lechuguilla*, *Lantana*, *Kochia*, St. John's wort, *Tetradymia* sp. (horsebrush), *Tribulus terrestris* (goathead)
	Psoralens—methoxsalen, trioxsalen
	Tattoos—cadmium sulfide
	(Colorado Department of Public Health and Environment Consumer Protection Division, 2001)
Fixed Drug Eruption	Sulphonamides, tetracyclines, mefenamic acid, terbinafine induce a relapse drug-induced dermatosis via effector memory T cells (Mizukawa and Shiohara, 2009)

TABLE 15-1   Forensic Chart of Dermal Toxicity (*continued*)

Skin Toxicity	Toxic Agents
Hair Loss	
Androgens	Hyperandrogenism from intake or syndromes (Essah et al., 2006)
Anticancer drugs	Anthracyclines (e.g., Adriamycin), taxanes (e.g., Taxol), alkylating compounds (e.g., cyclophosphamide), and the topoisomerase inhibitor etoposide prevented by induction of a hair stress protein by heat or subcutaneous/intradermal injection of geldanamycin or 17-(allylamino)-17-demethoxygeldanamycin (Jimenez et al., 2008)
Anticoagulants	Heparin (Heully et al., 1964)
Anti-epileptics	Valproic acid
Metals	Various metal deficiencies and toxicity of selenium (Srivastava et al., 1995) and thallium (Zhao et al., 2008)
Nutrients	Excess vitamin A or other retinoids
Other medications	Amphetamines, bromocryptine, levodopa, cimetidine, topical beta-blockers, oral contraceptives, some hypocholesterolemic and anti-infectious agents, NSAIDs (Llau et al., 1995)
Irritant Contact Dermatitis	Acids, animal entrails and secretions, artificial fertilizers, bases, cement, clay, cleansers, coal and stone dusts, cutting oils, disinfectants, fibers, flour, glues, meat, petroleum-based organic solvents, oxidants, paints, pesticides, plants (asparagus, cucumber, orange peel), plaster, reducing agents, soldering fluxes, water (Canadian Centre for Occupational Safety and Health, 2015)
Maculopapular Eruptions (due to cytokine responses [TH0 or TH1 pattern])	Barbiturates, penicillins, phenytoin, sulfonamides (Fernández et al., 2009)
Skin Cancers	
Basal cell carcinoma (90%)	UV irradiation and the generation of reactive oxygen species and reactive nitrogen species from xenobiotics (Bickers and Athar, 2006)
Squamous cell carcinoma (second most common)	
Malignant melanoma (most serious)	
Paget's disease (seen in nipple, groin, or anus)	
Kaposi's sarcoma (herpes virus-linked)	
Systemic Toxicity	
Contact dermatitis from ingestion	Asteraceae, balsam of Peru, botanicals, foods (e.g., garlic and onions), drugs, formaldehyde, metals (cobalt, copper, gold, mercury, nickel), *Parthenium hysterophorus* ("parthenium weed"), propylene glycol (Nijhawan et al., 2009)
Cyanosis	Cyanide, oxidation of hemoglobin by nitrates/nitrites (Carpenter, 1993)
Diaphoresis (ACh stimulated eccrine sweat glands)	Organophosphates
Flushing	Scombrotoxic fish (histamine), allergic responses to toxicants/medications
Jaundice	Liver damaging chemicals such as chronic alcohol abuse (cirrhosis), hemolytic agents such as metals (arsenic), nitrofurantoin, quinine, hemolytic snake venoms (hyperbilirubinemia with scleral lesions)
Metallic pigmentation	Arsenic hyperpigmentation, bismuth lines, gold (chrysiasis), iron staining, lead hue, silver (argyria)

(continues)

TABLE 15-1   Forensic Chart of Dermal Toxicity (*continued*)

Skin Toxicity	Toxic Agents
Urticaria (weal and flare)	Allergic IgE-mediated anaphylaxis to toxins and medications, non-immune-mediated mast cell degranulation by benzoic acid and jellyfish nematocyst venom (can also cause keloids, fat atrophy, gangrene, contractions, arthralgias, neuritis, hyperpigmentation, corneal ulcerations, vasospasm and post-envenomation herpes simplex or granuloma annulare; Burnett, 1991)
Toxic Epidermal Necrolysis (severe variant of Stevens-Johnson syndrome characterized by epidermal scalding; Shay et al., 2009) Erythema multiforme (minor and major)—another variant of Stevens-Johnson syndrome	Medications—allopurinol, barbiturates, bortezomib, and carbamazepine (*HLA* allele *B*1502* in Han Chinese; Ferrell and McLeod, 2008), corticosteroids (including dexamethasone), hydantoins, imatinib, isoniazid, NSAIDs, penicillins, procainamide, quinolones, rituximab, sulfonamides in first 2 months of treatment (Castaneda et al., 2009)
Vasculitis (also serum sickness and Arthus) immune complex disease (Breathnach, 1995)	Allopurinol, cefaclor, colony-stimulating factors, hydralazine, isotretinoin, methotrexate, minocycline, D-penicillamine, phenytoin, propylthiouracil (ten Holder et al., 2002)

Data from Extension Toxicology Network. 1993. Cutaneous toxicity: toxic effects on skin. http://pmep.cce.cornell.edu/profiles/extoxnet/TIB/cutaneous-tox.html.

of many substances readily through this layer. Once the epidermis is breached, the dermis provides a much more permeable layer for entrance of toxicants, infectious agents, escape of needed physiological fluids (water loss prevention), and so forth. The skin also provides a metabolic barrier. In addition, it provides a surface for temperature regulation through regulation of blood flow, degree of hair or fur covering, and perspiration for animals such as the human or the horse (not the pig). Skin exposure to chemicals also influences the expression of the immune system and vice versa. The skin provides mechanical support for internal organs. It is the organ having numerous and varied neurosensory receptors. It also consists of a self-regulatory neuro-endocrine system involving paracrine or autocrine mechanisms. Systemic effects of the skin endocrine system are observed by the formation of vitamin D_3 and parathyroid hormone–related protein (PTHrP). UV radiation is both an environmental stressor of note and affects cutaneous endocrine system function (Slominski and Wortsman, 2003). Secretions of the skin originate from apocrine, eccrine, and sebaceous glands. Other

than vitamin D metabolism, other metabolic components involve keratinization of the outermost layer. Collagen (type and amount) determines the structural integrity and flexibility of skin layers. In the eye, the collagen structure also determines whether a layer is opaque or passes light easily. Melanin colors the upper layer based on ethnic heritage and sun exposure. Lipids are metabolized in skin, as are carbohydrates. The cells of the skin respire if they are not of the top layer. They also contain enough cytochrome P450 and other xenobiotic metabolic enzymes to transform chemicals such as 3-methylcholanthrene (3-MC) into active carcinogenic metabolites, which then transform skin cells into neoplasms. Even in burn wounds, consideration has to be made of the chemical agent that caused the burn and the possible ensuing systemic toxicity of the absorbed chemical. Special note should be made of cement (wet), hydrofluoric acid, phenol, and white phosphorus. The sections that follow examine more closely each category of skin toxicity. Some reactions are so severe that they require discontinuing an important medication for treatment of a life-threatening illness, such as cancer.

Many of the skin reactions that do not cause direct damage involve an immune response to the chemical agent or the chemical agent bound to a component of skin. Genetic differences in response explain susceptibility to sulfonamides used to treat infections and anticonvulsants, including lupus erythematosus–like syndrome. Immune reactions appear to play a role in exanthematous reactions. Cell-mediated reactions involving the skin's immune system include erythema multiforme, fixed drug eruptions, lichenoid reactions, lupus erythematosus–like syndrome, Stevens-Johnson syndrome, and toxic epidermal necrosis. Anaphylactoid reactions, anaphylaxis, and angioedema appear to be mediated by Type I or Type III immunoglobulin (Ig)–mediated hypersensitivity, but may also arise form non-allergic pharmacological mechanisms. Arthus, serum sickness, and vasculitis are immune complex reactions. Drug-induced pemphigus, a condition in which people develop an autoimmune reaction to their skin, also involves dysregulation of the immune system. Antibody-independent acantholysis can also occur directly for thiol-containing medications (Breathnach, 1995).

Burns

Most people have experienced burns at some point in their lives and are often familiar with their appearance, the danger of infection, and the resultant scarring. Many burns are the result of excess temperature (or low temperatures as in frostbite). As indicated, in Table 15-1 burns also can originate from exposure to corrosive chemicals, desiccant, oxidants, reducing agents, protoplasmic poisons, and vesicants. A person exposed to an alkaline chemical for too long a time without treatment is shown in **Figure 15-1**. The important portion is the reactive nature of the agent with the skin as just enumerated, its concentration, time of exposure, regional skin properties (vary with age and

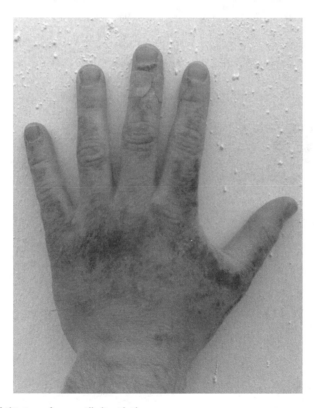

FIGURE 15-1 Effects of Skin Burns from an Alkaline Fluid

Courtesy of Blazius

degree or keratinization and hydration, race, location such as the thick stratum corneum of the plantar surface of the foot versus the thin face epidermis, and whether the person already had an existing dermatitis of some sort), percentage of skin burned, and subsequent treatment. The concentration of the acid or base is measure by pH, but is better assessed by the pK_a, which indicates the strength of an acid or the conjugate acid formed from a strong base. The alkaline damage shown in the figure is due to alkaline damage that causes liquefaction necrosis progressing to saponification of lipids and denatured proteins, such as occurs in people exposed to liquid cement. Acids generally form a less problematic coagulation necrosis and a necrotic eschar that is a physical barrier limiting the advancement of the burn. Hydrofluoric acid (HF) acts as a protoplasmic poison as well as an acid, as it chelates calcium (and other divalent cations) leading to necrosis. The inhibition of the $3Na^+,2K^+$-ATPase results in efflux of K^+ causing extreme pain with concentrations > 20% HF. Hypocalcemia and hypomagnesia lead to cardiac arrhythmias with Fl^- ions causing direct irritation and poisoning to cardiac cells that may be hard to manage and fatal. Another chemical of interest is white phosphorus, as it ignites in atmospheres containing oxygen.

It continues to burn the skin as long as it is allowed access to air. Moisture attenuates this effect. Systemic toxicity can result from reversal of the calcium/phosphorus ratio in the plasma, resulting in renal failure and mortality. It may be difficult to see that strong solvents such as phenol can produce burns as well. Due to the hydrophobicity of phenol and its anesthetic effect, it can penetrate deeply into tissue before untoward effects are experienced. Intravascular hemolysis caused by excretion of unconjugated phenol progresses from damage to kidney glomeruli and tubules (Ahmadi et al., 2008).

Contact Dermatitis

Another form of skin toxicity is also familiar to many people. Contact dermatitis is a localized skin inflammatory response. Acids, bases, and lipophilic solvents that led to burns can also cause irritation at the site of exposure. It has the usual inflammatory reactions of heat, pain, redness, and swelling. Both irritant and allergic contact dermatitis occur when repeated contact with low-molecular-weight xenobiotics/haptens produce an immunological reaction. The visible effects of an irritant contact dermatitis are shown in **Figure 15-2**. The innate immune system produces a reaction that results in

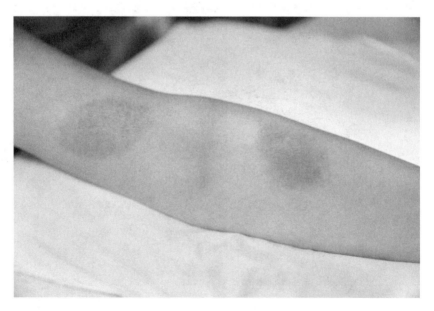

FIGURE 15-2 Irritant Contact Dermatitis
© Jodi Jacobson/Getty Images

proinflammatory cytokines being released from keratinocytes in response to repeated insults from the chemical agent. Something as apparently innocuous as repeatedly washing the hands with soap and water can produce this phenomenon. Hydrophobic solvents remove essential fats and oils from skin, promote transepidermal loss of hydration, and make the skin more susceptible to reaction to chemicals and conditions that previously showed no observable untoward effects. Microtrauma can be induced by fiberglass fibers and irritation by abrasive chemicals and detergents. Even UV light can cause keratinocytes to produce cytokines such as IL1 and TNFα (inflammation), IL8 and IL10 (chemotaxis), IL6, IL7, IL15 granulocyte-macrophage colony-stimulating factor, transforming growth factor (TGF) α (growth promotion), and IL10, IL12, and IL18 (lymphocyte-mediated specific adaptive immunity). Intercellular adhesion molecule 1 starts the infiltration of white blood cells into the epidermis for cutaneous inflammation (Hogan, 2014). Allergic contact dermatitis differentiates from irritant contact dermatitis by the delayed-type hypersensitivity produced by hapten-specific T lymphocytes (Nosbaum et al., 2009). People are also familiar with allergic contact dermatitis caused by common toxic plants (poison ivy, oak, and sumac) that produce these reactions, which spread upon vigorous scratching due to the intense itching. The use of calamine lotion with an antihistamine is a classic over-the-counter treatment for this type of malady.

Acneiform Chemicals

Teenagers are acutely aware that hormonal changes may cause the development of acne. Drug-induced acne is not bona fide acne, but rather forms of folliculitis. The causes of acneiform reactions are multifold (Scheinfeld, 2009). Corticosteroids induce toll-like receptor 2 and acneiform reactions (Shibata et al., 2009). This may be closest to the teenager example, except for the sebaceous gland effects of excess sex hormones usually taken as oral contraceptives or anabolic steroids for rapid development of muscle tissue (George et al., 2008). However, if one considers the biopsychology of the stressed

teenager, it is not surprising that stress reactions and psychotropic medications also induce acneiform eruptions (Gupta and Gupta, 2003). An antibiotic that inhibits the catecholamine and indoleamine catabolic enzyme monoamine oxidase (MAO) is isoniazid. This unusual antibiotic used in tuberculosis therapy also leads to acne (Oliwiecki and Burton, 1988). Immune system modulation also leads to acneiform reactions including calcineurin blockers such as the immunosuppressant cyclosporine (Gaber et al., 2008). Lithium induces neutrophils (Chan et al., 2000). Blocking another signaling pathway, specifically epidermal growth factor (EGF) blockers, also leads to acneiform reactions (Labianca et al., 2007). Ionizing radiation has been used to treat extreme forms of acne, but the damage induced in other cases leads to acneiform development (Carrotte-Lefebvre et al., 2003). Aromatic anti-seizure compounds, especially phenytoin, also result in drug-induced acne. Valproic acid also appears to cause oligomenorrhea, hyperandrogenism, and acneiform reactions (Scheinfeld, 2009). Chloracne, exhibited in **Figure 15-3**, appears to originate through the aryl hydrocarbon receptor (AhR) dimerization with the aryl hydrocarbon nuclear translocator protein as do other 2,3,7,8-p-tetrachlorodibenzodioxin (TCDD)-mediated toxicities. EGF represses induction of CYP1A1 by TCDD by preventing the recruitment of transcriptional coactivation protein p300 to the CYP1A1 gene in cultured human keratinocytes. EGF also inhibits chloracne development mechanisms in those same cells (Hankinson, 2009). Aromatic hydrocarbons that bind to AhR, such as TCDD and β-naphthoflavone, induce hyperkeratinization of keratinocytes lining the sebaceous follicles in differentiating human skin cultures, similar to that found during chloracne. Halogenated hydrocarbons such as TCDD show transglutaminase cross-linking that mediates the hyperkeratinization characteristic of chloracne. Retinoids (vitamin A analogs) affect epidermal differentiation and AhR-dependent alteration of enzymes that metabolize retinoids (Du et al., 2006). Earlier reports suggest that altered vitamin A metabolism in the skin may be a cause of chloracne via halogens of all types including fluoride in toothpaste to the halogenated aromatics usually associated with this

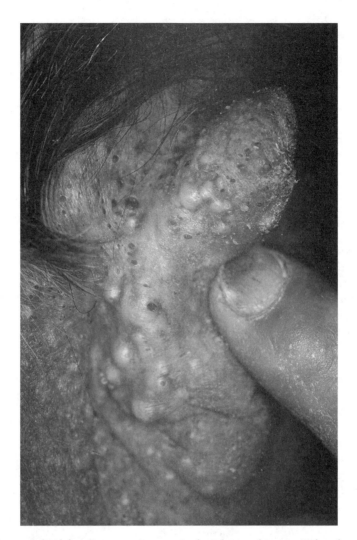

FIGURE 15-3 Chloracne Outbreak from Exposure to Dioxins or Similar Halogenated Aromatic Hydrocarbons
© DermNetNZ

disease (Coenraads et al., 1994). The concern is the exposure to an agent that has strong carcinogenic properties rather than the chloracne that develops.

(Toxic) Alopecia-Inducing Chemicals

Also familiar to the general population is the hair loss that develops during abuse of anabolic steroids or from toxic cancer chemotherapeutic agents. Hair development is dependent on the presence of testosterone and its active metabolites. Androgenic alopecia appears to be related to local androgen production at hair follicles. Dihydrotestosterone production increases through hyperactivity of 5α-reductase and 17β-hydroxysteroid dehydrogenase. Overexpression of the androgen receptors appears to accompany testosterone-related hair loss (Essah et al., 2006). Poisoning of the hair follicle by a variety of cytotoxic anti-cancer medications was usually prevented toxicokinetically by a scalp tourniquet of cooling, limiting blood flow, and the concentration of the agent into the area. This did not always work, especially for taxane. More recently the induction of heat stress protein (HSP) by pretreatment with heat or injection of geldanamycin or 17-(allylamino)- 17-demethoxygeldanamycin prior to chemotherapy protected against alopecia without limiting the effectiveness of the chemotherapy agent to cancer cells (Jimenez et al., 2008). Another study shows the effectiveness of heparanase expressed by transit-amplifying (TA) cells in releasing heparin sulfate–bound growth factors. This process helps repopulate the lower follicle of the hair shaft by TA cells and helps promote follicle vascularization. This appears to explain how mice that overexpress heparanase are resistant to the alopecia induced by anti-cancer drugs and the heparanase inhibitor heparin (Zcharia et al., 2005). This may also explain the alopecia induced by other anticoagulants reported in the 1960s (Heully et al., 1964). It appears that biotinidase enzyme activity of rats treated with valproic acid decreased in liver and serum and was associated with alopecia development. Biotin supplementation may prevent this dermal toxicity (Arslan et al., 2009). Other nutritional deficiencies, such as selenium or zinc deficiency, have been associated with alopecia. Selenium is also an element that in excess can result in alopecia areata, which progresses to alopecia universalis (Srivastava et al., 1995). The skin and fingernails are also affected by selenosis, as is the liver (Alexander, 2007). Thallium poisoning causes a nail dystrophy and alopecia in addition to neurotoxicity (Zhao et al., 2008). Arsenic poisoning is also associated with an exfoliative dermatitis, alopecia, nail lesions, polyneuritis, and serious cardiovascular, blood, and digestive disturbances. Boric acid can also result in alopecia in addition to erythema and digestive disorders, but hyperthermia and convulsions are of greater concern. Although retinoic acid is important in hair follicle formation and in patterning through homeobox gene proteins Hox C8 and Hox C6 (Bergfeld, 1998), excess vitamin A produces skin abnormalities and nail dystrophy in addition to liver damage (Cheruvattath et al., 2006). Medications other than the ones mentioned previously usually produce a diffuse non-scarring alopecia, which quickly reverses on discontinuation of the offending drug. Antimitotic agents are the most likely causes of generalized hair loss via interference with replication of hair matrix cells (anagen phase of hair growth interrupted).

Lithium causes hair thinning (Llau et al., 1995). Cholesterol-lowering medications produce a diffuse alopecia via interference with keratinization similar to thallium and vitamin A poisoning (Yardley, 1969).

Toxic Epidermal Necrosis

This section moves out of the realm of toxic reactions familiar to lay people on to dangerous skin conditions that may rapidly lead to mortality. Toxic epidermal necrosis (TEN), as shown in **Figure 15-4**, is a condition that makes humans very ill and can lead rapidly to death. TEN is a continuum of blistering or bullous conditions and an extreme variant of Stevens-Johnson syndrome (SJS). SJS was reported in the early 1920s with boys who had eruptive fever, stomatitis, and ophthalmalgia. Toxic epidermal necrolysis results from extensive epidermal scalding. Because stroking the skin in either condition may lead to subepithelial separation (positive Nikolsky sign), SJS and toxic epidermal necrolysis are variants of a serious bullous disease with epidermal cell death. Both diseases are defined by vesicular eruption of at least two mucosal surfaces. The milder SJS involves < 10% of the total body surface area and 3% lethality. Overlapping SJS/TEN involves 10–30% of the body surface area, while TEN must include > 30% of the skin surface and 25–40% mortality. TEN occurs mostly in the elderly or people with HIV infection. Causes of TEN are medications (antibiotics, anticonvulsants, and nonsteroidal anti-inflammatory drugs [NSAIDs]) and infections (Epstein-Barr virus, herpes simplex, *Mycoplasma pneumoniae*, measles, mycobacterium, smallpox vaccination, group A streptococci, *Yersinia*, and enterovirus). Epidermal cell apoptosis is one noted commonality with SJS/TEN and may involve cytotoxic T cells, Fas-Fas ligand interaction, TNFα, and nitric oxide synthase. The skin and eye are both important targets of the immune reactions that lead to these bullous disorders (Shay et al., 2009).

Other Bullous Eruptions

Other blistering reactions may involve linear IgA bullous autoimmune diseases of the

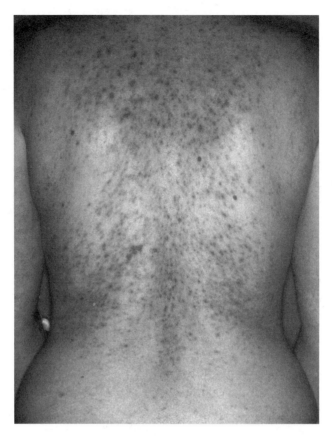

FIGURE 15-4 Toxic Epidermal Necrolysis Occurring from a Severe Form of Stevens-Johnson Syndrome

© ISM/Phototake

skin including vesiculobullous disease and pemphigus. The serious nature of an autoimmune reaction to the skin is clear based on the area of involvement. Blisters are large in autoimmune pemphigus, shown in **Figure 15-5**. Pemphigus is usually a disease of the elderly, whereas the linear IgA disease has been described for children sensitive to certain antibiotics (Ho et al., 2007).

Maculopapular Eruptions

Various medications and viruses cause a unique type of rash characterized by macules (spots) and papules (bumps) as illustrated in **Figure 15-6**. The appearance is usually red with many small bumps. The cytokine patterns for this type of eruption are TH1, involving CD4 T-lymphocytes with cytotoxic properties, or TH0. Skin-homing receptor binding to endothelial- and platelet-selectin recruits T cells into inflamed skin in allergic contact dermatitis (Gainers et al., 2007). In maculopapular rash development, different chemokines and their receptors, including CCL20, CCL27, CXCL9, or CXCL10, mediate skin homing. Oxidative stress also can enhance these reactions (Fernández et al., 2009).

Fixed Drug Eruptions

Although many skin reactions involve the immune system, fixed drug eruption lesions appear to be associated with the presence of CD8(+) intraepidermal T cells with the effector memory phenotype. This is a form of drug-induced dermatosis that results from a relapse of a skin reaction to the same or structurally similar medication in the same region (Mizukawa and Shiohara, 2009).

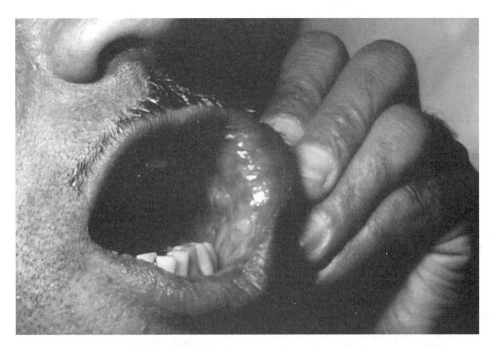

FIGURE 15-5 This 1964 image depicted a Tehrani man who was being treated for what was diagnosed as **pemphigus vulgaris**. He presented with a painful, long-standing intraoral lesions of 3 years duration. In this particular view, the lesions can be seen on the interior surface of his left cheek.

CDC/ Dr. J. Lieberman; Dr. Freideen Farzin, Univ. of Tehran.

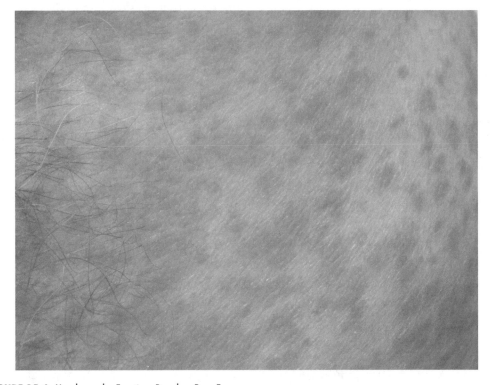

FIGURE 15-6 Maculopapular Eruptions Based on Drug Exposure

© DermNetNZ

The "usual suspects" for immune reactions such as the antibiotics represented by the sulphonamides and the tetracyclines head the list of reactive agents.

Phototoxicities and Photoallergies

Medications applied to the skin or taken orally can interact with sunlight to produce an allergic reaction or skin toxicity. Where sunburns have usually been associated with UV light within the 280–320 nm range (UV-B = 280–315 nm), there has been increased concern that most phototoxicities and photoallergies occur due to the UV-A range of sunlight (315–400 nm). UV-C (germicidal UV of 100–280 nm) might do significant damage to astronauts, but it is usually well absorbed by the Earth's atmosphere. Photosensitivities due to medications encompass dyschromia (discoloration of the skin), pseudoporphyria (bullous photosensitivity that mimics porphyria cutanea tarda in adults), photo onycholysis (nail disorder characterized by separation of the nail plate from underlying and lateral support structures), and lichenoid (banded configuration parallel to the epidermis) and telangiectatic (permanent dilation of preexisting blood vessels causing red lesions to appear) reactions (Stein and Scheinfeld, 2007). Skin cells also generate reactive oxygen (Haber-Weiss and Fenton reactions) and nitrogen species (nitric oxide synthase) due to metabolic activity.

Xenobiotics may form toxic quinones via CYPs, which yield superoxide anion. UV-A and UV-B radiation also form lipid peroxidation products, singlet oxygen, and superoxide, and with NO they generate peroxynitrite. The presence of photosensitizers increases the absorption of UC radiation and the generation of reactive oxygen species (ROS) and reactive nitrogen species (RNS) (Bickers and Athar, 2006).

Skin Cancers

The generation of oxidative stress in phototoxicities just mentioned links to some types of cutaneous malignancy. UV irradiation is the primary cause of skin cancer followed by genetic susceptibility, X-irradiation treatment, and some viral causes. However, some strongly mutagenic chemicals are also topical carcinogens (e.g., 3-methylcholanthrene following metabolic activation). Fair skin, time spent exposed to UV without sunscreen, history of prior skin damage by sun, a family history of skin cancer, many moles, advanced age, congenital melanocytic nevus (large dark-colored birthmarks), actinic keratosis (precancerous skin lesion), and HIV infection (Kaposi's sarcoma) increase the risk of skin cancer development. Basal cell carcinomas comprise 90% of all human skin cancers. As indicated by the name, the skins at the base of the epidermis are transformed by long-term exposure to UV irradiation. Clinically, this is quite treatable. Squamous cell carcinoma is the second most likely skin cancer. This one starts in the epidermis, but may penetrate to deeper layers of the skin or metastasize to other organs. Malignant melanoma is the skin cancer most associated with fatalities. Kaposi's sarcoma is a skin cancer caused by a herpes virus and is associated with one-third of AIDS patients. It also has a slower growing form in elderly men with Italian or Jewish genetics. Paget's disease is a rare skin cancer that may arise from breast cancer or start in the groin or near the anus. This cancer may originate with sweat glands.

UV irradiation is implicated in premature skin aging (wrinkling, dryness, thinning, seborrheic keratoses), phototoxicity, photoallergy, and autoimmune diseases (lupus erythematosus, polymorphous light eruption, solar urticaria) in addition to skin cancer. UV-B causes the formation of cyclobutane pyrimidine dimers, which is linked to generation of mutations in the tumor suppressor genes and suppression of the skin's immune system. Topically administered photolyase-containing liposomes remove some of the UV-generated dimers and prevent skin immune suppression. DNA repair is clearly involved, because providing a DNA repair enzyme in a liposomal lotion prevents precancerous and cancerous lesions in patients with *Xeroderma pigmentosum* (DNA repair deficiency syndrome). UV-B appears to affect cell signaling; this is indicated by the fact that UV-B radiation's effects can only be prevented by inhibition of the DNA damage and the clustering of growth factor receptors on the plasma membrane of keratinocytes. The clustering of growth factor receptors ultimately leads to activation of mitogen-activated protein (MAP) kinase, transcription factor, and gene expression. At high doses of UV-B radiation, apoptosis is induced. A similar signaling pathway is caused by hyperosmotic stress, which is assisted by an osmolyte transport system in human keratinocytes. Interestingly, osmolyte loading of keratinocytes appears to inhibit many of the damaging signal transduction changes induced by UV-B. UV-A's oxidative function in skin cells starts with the generation of the second messenger ceramide from cell membrane sphingomyelin involving singlet oxygen. This causes the mitochondria to release cytochrome c into the cytoplasm without starting apoptosis. A transcriptional factor AP-2 is then oxidized by cytochrome c, which causes the expression of ICAM-1 and other UV-A-inducible genes. It is worth noting that cholesterol in the membrane appears to provide protection against this process and identifies signal-transducing microdomains or rafts as an important target for UV-A. Osmolytes also prevent this process by preventing ceramide formation. As far as chemical carcinogens, testicular skin cancers in chimney sweeps were the first known occupational skin cancer (squamous cell tumor) hazard identified. Activation of procarcinogens by CYPs has been identified in skin cells, especially keratinocytes. Cytoplasmic constitutive expression of CYP1A1, 1B1, 2B6, 2E1 and 3A5 and induction of CYP3A4 by dexamethasone has been described. CYP1A1 is particularly implicated in the activation of PAHs such as benzo(a)pyrene. AhR is definitely involved in skin tumor formation from these compounds, as mice that lack the receptor are resistant to skin tumorigenesis. UV irradiation does in fact also activate the AhR pathway. However, AhR-deficient mice display interfollicular and follicular epidermal hyperplasia with hyperkeratosis and acanthosis with dermal fibrosis. This indicates that AhR plays a critical role in regulation of skin homeostasis. The *p53* tumor suppressor gene does not appear to play a role in skin cancer initiation, but rather seems to be involved in skin cancer progression. This is indicated by *p53* null mice that were not prone to skin cancer without application of a chemical mutagen. Instead, it appears that activation of Ha-*ras* oncogene is the critical initiating event in skin cancer. A-T transversions in codon 61 by dimethylbenzanthracene (DMBA) activate Ha-*ras* and correlate with papillomas and carcinomas. Additionally, transgenic mice having a v-Ha-*ras* oncogene fused to the regulatory region of the human keratin K1 gene can develop skin tumors just on application of a chemical promoter. The CYP enzymes are also involved also in detoxication and may also mediate some allergic functions of skin. These cells are also capable of expression of multidrug resistance through proteins such as P-glycoprotein. This may make them resistant to treatment by chemotherapeutic agents. The promotion of skin tumors appears to be mediated through the arachidonic acid cascade. Lipoxygenase enzymes such as 8S-LOX and 12S-LOX are expressed in human and murine skin cells. These enzymes are overexpressed in papillomas and squamous cell cancers. Formation of HETE products by these enzymes correlates with etheno adducts of DNA. Overexpression of cyclooxygenase enzyme COX-2 is found in various cancers including squamous cell skin cancer. COX-2 inhibitors appear to suppress the prostaglandin-production and tumor-promotion effects of the clot-dissolving stimulator tissue plasminogen activator (TPA). This combination of factors indicates the complex interaction of phototoxicity, CYP induction pathways, and inflammatory mediates (leukotrienes and prostaglandins) in the multistage development of skin tumors (Merk et al., 2004).

Systemic Toxicities

Contact dermatitis has already been described earlier in this chapter. However, on ingestion of an allergen, especially the metals nickel, cobalt, chromate, or Balsam of Peru; garlic; food coloring; or preservatives, a skin eruption is discovered that represents a systemic rather than a simple skin reaction (Nijhawan et al., 2009). This reaction is more properly termed systemically reactivated allergic contact dermatitis. A topical exposure has already sensitized the skin, and ingestion reactivates this reaction. Usually the skin reaction (flares at site of previous dermatitis or patch test such as atopic eczema, diaper dermatitis, or medication-induced) is accompanied by headache, fever, and physical discomfort (malaise). Because the reaction occurs within hours of ingestion, the usual T cell–mediated type IV delayed-type hypersensitivity cannot be the prime mover. A type III immunological reaction may mediate reactivity to these haptens (similar to one type of autoimmunity). IgE-mediated type I immediate hypersensitivity is expected in urticaria and anaphylaxis (Bajaj and Saraswat, 2006).

The cellular hypoxia generated by cyanide poisoning is termed *cyanosis*. However, the generation of methemoglobin by oxidation of hemoglobin gives a similar color and hypoxic injury. Sulfhemoglobin formation from hydrogen sulfide poisoning (sulfur binds to hemoglobin) also generates the low oxyhemoglobin associated with cyanosis. Pseudocyanosis can be generated by silver, lead, medications (anti-arrhythmic amiodarone, antimalarial chloroquine, antipsychotic phenothiazines), or even excess blue food coloring ingestion. Accordingly, pulse oximetry or arterial blood pO_2 should be monitored to avoid incorrect attribution of the blue coloration to true cyanosis (Carpenter, 1993).

Excessive perspiration or diaphoresis is usually associated with a myocardial infarction, withdrawal from drugs of abuse, and extreme pain or stress. When accompanied by miosis due to pupil constriction, excess salivation, headaches, nausea, night-waking, diarrhea, labored breathing, incoordination, and mental confusion, these symptoms indicate systemic poisoning by an acetylcholinesterase inhibitor represented by organophosphates such as the formerly restricted (now discontinued) use insecticide methyl parathion (Edwards and Tchounwou, 2005).

Flushing of the skin can result from an allergic reaction (Fasano, 2006), pharmaceutical to toxic concentrations of niacin (Guyton, 2007), and scombrotoxic fish poisoning (Attaran and Probst, 2002). This involves changes in blood vessels associated with histamine or niacin. The differences in causes are important as immune reactions are different from histamine poisoning alone (scombroid fish) or the liver damage and flushing associated with toxic doses of niacin.

Liver damage is a good point to finish the discussion of flushing, because it is the likely cause of jaundice. Widely studied are the cases of medication overdoses or toxic reactions such as acetaminophen overdose or chronic statin use. Alcohol abuse leads to cirrhosis of the liver. Other causes of jaundice are hemolytic. Intrahepatic cholestatic jaundice can arise from antiretroviral medications (Varriale et al., 2004). Hemolysis can result from arsenic poisoning, oxidative medications such as nitrofurantoin or quinine, and crotalid snake venoms. One review examined the Heinz body hemolysis produced by methylene blue in humans (Sills and Zinkham, 1994). In either the case of liver damage or hemolysis, toxic concentrations of bilirubin—degraded hemoglobin—causes systemic poisoning of nerve cells (Fernandes and Brites, 2009).

Hyperpigmentation of skin can be caused by gold (preferentially taken up by the dermis in UV-irradiated skin and stimulates melanin production; Leonard et al., 1986), arsenic (Hall, 2002), bismuth, lead, iron, silver, thallium (Aasly 2007), and medications (NSAIDs, antimalarials, amiodarone, cytotoxic anticancer drugs, tetracyclines, and psychotropic drugs; Dereure, 2001). Identification of metallic substances can be made by microscopic techniques (light, electron, and X-ray energy spectroscopy; Bergfeld and McMahon, 1987).

Urticaria, as indicated earlier, comes from IgE-mediated processes and can originate from rapid immune reactions to medications and toxicants that result in anaphylaxis. An interesting case is the reaction to jellyfish nematocyst toxin. Anaphylaxis is a rare reaction. However, the immune and toxic responses may involve keloids, fat atrophy, gangrene, contractions, arthralgias, neuritis, hyperpigmentation, corneal ulcerations, vasospasm, post-envenomation herpes simplex or granuloma annulare with recurrent skin eruptions, distant-site eruptions, persistent lesions, or urticaria. Immune reactions can be B cell or T cell mediated on previous exposure to the jellyfish toxin. Systemic poisoning not involving the immune reaction can result from cardiac block, ventricular arrhythmia, coronary artery vasoconstriction, and Purkinje fiber network disturbances at high doses based on affected Na^+ and $Ca2^+$ ionic transfer. Moderate doses depress the respiratory center of the central nervous system (CNS). Lower doses can cause renal failure via acute tubular necrosis (Burnett, 1991).

Pruritus

Systemic toxicity mainly surfaces as generalized pruritus (itching) and cutaneous vasculitis. Pruritus may originate from iron-deficiency anemia, myeloproliferative disorders, monoclonal gammopathy and multiple myeloma, lymphoma, uremia secondary to renal toxicity, cholestasis secondary to liver damage, and disorders of the thyroid. Dry skin (xerosis) may also be a cause of pruritus. Eczema or scabies must be eliminated as a cause before causes of possible systemic toxicity are investigated (Lee, 2009).

Percutaneous Absorption

Percutaneous absorption is one of three routes evaluated for human occupational exposure to toxicants. The other two are inhalation and ingestion, which are covered elsewhere. With less inhalation exposure occurring, skin is becoming more important in assessing the total picture of occupational exposure. The Scientific Committee on Occupational Exposure Limit Values assigns an S to compounds that have significant dermal absorption (Sartorelli, 2002; Foà, 2009). In Finland, more than 100 chemicals carry an S or approximately one-fifth of the listed compounds. The Swedish National Board of Occupational Safety and Health (Johanson, 1999:13) has given an S to 70 of 300 listed agents based on the ease of percutaneous absorption. The American Conference of Governmental Industrial Hygienists (ACGIH, 2015) uses threshold limit values (TLVs) for inhaled compounds, and similarly sets a standard of $LD_{50} < 1.0$ g/kg as an acute dermal toxicant. The percutaneous absorption can be compared with TLV–time-weighted average (TWA) as is done in the Netherlands. If the amount of a chemical absorbed from the arms and legs exceeds 10% of that amount absorbed in 8 hours by inhalation at the occupational exposure limit, then the toxicant is assigned as S. This is an historic value

since it was the assumed percent absorption for compounds that had no dermal absorption data in the 1970s. This was changed by the U.S. Environmental Protection Agency's Office of Pesticides Program's Scientific Advisory Panel in 1983 to a worst case assumption of 100% absorption for chemicals with no dermal application data and acute dermal toxicity test methodologies were published (Environmental Protection Agency, 1998). Because dermal application to human volunteers has questionable ethics, an animal whose skin has similar properties to human percutaneous absorption may be used or new alternative approaches should be test (due to animal rights concerns). Data for porcine skin, for example, show that this 100% absorption worst case assumption is quite conservative. Of six radiolabelled compounds dissolved in ethanol and administered topically to pigs compared with intravenous injection, the highest percutaneous absorption was 25.7% for the small aromatic acid benzoic acid followed by the female steroid progesterone (16.2%), the methylxanthine caffeine (11.8%), the male steroid testosterone (8.8%), and lastly the organophosphates parathion (6.7%) and malathion (5.2%; Carver and Riviere, 1989). This is as expected, because more hydrophobic compounds have higher absorption than charged chemicals.

Metals are an interesting case, because they can change permeability based on charge/valence, hydrophobic groups, molecular volume/counterion, protein reactivity, solubility at various pHs, time of exposure, dose, vehicle of administration, age of skin, region of skin, homeostatic regulation of ions, skin layers and shunt, and oxidation-reduction reactions in skin. The permeability coefficient K_p based on Fick's law of diffusion is related to the flux through the stratum corneum or outer layer of the skin. As a reminder, the equation for steady-state conditions is $K_p = J/\Delta C$, where ΔC is the concentration gradient across the skin. However, not all substances observe Fick's law perfectly. Sodium chromate appears to have similar K_ps for concentrations < 0.005 M and above 0.753 M. However, a fourfold increase in K_p (cm/h) occurs at 0.261 M (apparent peak) across guinea pig skin. Potassium chromate appears to decrease percutaneous absorption across human abdominal skin with increasing concentration (> 20-fold decrease from 10^{-5} to 2.1 M). Mercury (II) chloride appeared to have a maximum absorption at 16 mg Hg/mL across guinea pig skin. Vehicles that can increase absorption of metals include dimethyl sulfoxide and petrolatum (increases skin hydration and promotes hydrophilic chemical absorption), although petrolatum leaves metals suspended in fine particles that may not uniformly be in skin contact. Molecular volume (ionic radius of elemental species and counterion that diffuses with it) correlates with the absorption of metals, rather than polarity. The metals counter-influence penetration rates. For example, Cr(III) sulfate does not appear to be absorbed, and the nitrate is only slightly better in penetrating skin. For nickel salts, the counterion concentration gradient between superficial and deep layers of the stratum corneum appears to influence penetration in the following order acetate → nitrate → sulfate → chloride. As metals are covalently bonded to organic molecules, they act like organic nonelectrolytes rather than their former ionic character. Dimethyl mercury exhibited permeation through latex gloves and the human skin as demonstrated with fatal results in an academic researcher (Endicott, 1998). Only 40 µL of methyl mercury on the skin would result in severe systemic human toxicity. Lead compounds have been studied heavily ranging from the lead acetate formed from old wine (vinegar or acetic acid stored in lead wine canisters in Roman times) to former gasoline additives such as the anti-knock tetraethyl lead. When 10 mg of lead is placed on 2 cm² skin and the amount of lead diffusion is measured 24 hours later, the lead(II) oxide is least absorbed (< 1.0 µg Pb), followed by lead(II) acetate (5 µg Pb), lead(II) naphthenate (30 µg Pb), lead(II) nuolate (130 µg Pb), and tetrabutyl lead (632 µg Pb; Bress and Bidanset, 1991). The valence of the metals also changes the diffusion, electrophilicity, and protein reactivity. Trivalent chromium is prevented from being absorbed as indicated by the 20-fold higher dose it takes to sensitize skin to Cr(III) sulfate compared with potassium Cr(VI). Part of the lack of permeation of Cr(III) is that it shows a strong affinity for epithelial and dermal tissues and forms stable complexes, which limit the rate of diffusion. Negatively charged chromate and dichromate ions such as oxo-complexes of Cr(VI) do not similarly bind to organic substrates. The protein-reactivity mentioned earlier that can occur with different valence states of metals usually occurs with Ag(I), Al(III), As(III), Hg(II), and Ni(II). These complexes can be irreversible or reversible. For instance, Zn binding to metallothionein is released on metabolic demand. Hg vapor has a high skin permeability coefficient at approximately 1 cm/h. It appears that about half the mercury can be removed from skin by stripping the outer layer with adhesive cellophane tape. This interaction makes Hg vapor inhalation the most toxic exposure route. Metal diffusion rates through skin may be predicted by electrophilicity values of individual cations, use of tape stripping to determine the metal content of each layer of skin removed, or an *in vitro* analysis of human full thickness of skin exposed to metals. Additionally, the pH will affect the solubility and penetration of metals. Cr(III) salts have poor aqueous solubility, which decreases with increasing skin pH. On the other hand, Cr(VI) exists as a dichromate at pHs between 2 and 6 and chromate at pH > 6. The permeability for chromate-dichromate increased with alkaline pH (8–12.7) rather than acidic pH (1.4–5.6) due to the smaller CrO_4^{2-} ion predominating at high pH and the larger $Cr_2O_7^{2-}$ ion at low pH. Another important factor is the time the metal remains in contact with the skin. The highest percutaneous absorption of Hg is in the first 5 hours, with the final 36–48 hour time period usually being 25–35% of the initial rate and occasionally only 1% of the initial absorption rate.

Age of skin plays a role in percutaneous absorption. Infant skin appears to be more permeable to lipophilic compounds than adult human skin. Aging skin (~60 years of age) has significantly lower diffusivity to metals than young skin (in mid-teens). This may due to diminished blood supply or diminished surface lipid content. There also appears to be a regional skin penetration of metals and other xenobiotics with scrotum > forehead > post-auricular > abdomen > forearm > leg > back. This is mainly a function of the intercellular lipid composition as in aging, but also the thickness of the stratum corneum and shunt density play some role. The shunts can be sweat ducts that allow metals to avoid the least permeable stratum corneum. This indicates that hair follicles (and hair itself) and sweat ducts affect penetration of metals. This is a "two-way street" as toxic metals can enter and micronutrients such as Na, Fe(II), Zn(II), and Cu(II) can be lost from the body into sweat. Homeostatic control of essential metals in the skin such as Na, K, Ca, or Zn also plays a role in regulating the body burden of xenobiotics. Metallothionein (Zn-binding) and ceruloplasmin (Cu-binding) bind toxic metals. Calmodulin regulates Ca^{2+}-dependent processes. Metabolic processes play a role. CYPs clearly affect organic compounds. Metals are also subject to oxidation and reduction in the skin. For example, Cr(VI) is reduced to Cr(II) by tissue proteins containing sulfhydryl moieties. Nickel bio-oxidation from the II to III or IV states may occur due to ROS (H_2O_2 or ClO^-) during inflammatory reactions. This is an important reaction as the immunogenic form of nickel is Ni(III), not Ni(II) (Hostynek, 2003).

Although a quantitative structure-activity relationships (QSAR) approach based on physicochemical properties would be best, the experimental protocols for experimental dermal absorption do not match the QSAR approach. The compounds of interest should be nonionic, < 750 Da molecular weight, and moderately hydrophobic. The exposure period should encompass only pseudo-steady-state conditions. The purpose is to propose dermal occupational exposure limits (DOELs). The variability of skin and exposure conditions limits the ability to obtain these values (generalized dermal exposure measurements; extent of skin contamination; regional skin permeability differences; need for percutaneous penetration data; conditions of exposure related to the behavior of workers and their use, misuse, or lack or use of proper safety equipment and procedures; presence of preexisting skin diseases). Biological monitoring may give some useful information despite the lack of good physiological-based pharmacokinetic modeling for skin absorption. There are a number of accepted biological exposure indices that can be used to assess risk of dermal exposure (Sartorelli, 2002).

Dermal Toxicity Tests

Except for the LD_{50}, it appears that dermal and eye toxicity tests draw the most criticism from animal rights organizations. The animal may have the fur clipped or shaved and the toxicity is evident. Cosmetics manufacturers advertise their lack of animal testing to alleviate customers' concerns about animal welfare. Alternative models are moving rapidly to replace many of the classical dermal toxicity tests. However, the systemic and immune system involvement in tests makes animal models still important.

Pesticides and biocides are exposed to humans primarily via the dermal route, and the European Union's RISKOFDERM project indicates that risk of chemical exposure via this route is important in current occupations, where inhalation has been severely curtailed (Buist et al., 2009). Dermal toxicity testing starts with the acute dermal toxicity test, as shown in **Table 15-2**. The method reflects a mortality testing protocol, but does not carefully insist on the standard 5-point LD_{50} determination. Rather, it gives a sense of the dose that when evenly exposed to 10% of intact skin with clipped or shaved fur, but not abraded (changes permeability), causes increasing deaths with increased doses. As this is an acute dose, cumulative irritants or similar substances may not produce a skin or systemic response. However, the first concern is for a chemical such as dimethyl mercury that may be easily absorbed and lead to CNS toxicity and death. Skin reactions are a benefit of the study but not the initial concern.

The next test is the skin irritation (Draize) test, which has been the target of much of the controversy. The animals are again clipped or carefully shaved and exposed to the chemical for determination of redness (erythema), edema (raised surface), depth of tissue injury (eschar), and dryness of skin. An intact site is also located for exposure (no preparation). Either 0.5 mL liquid or 0.5 g solid or solid dissolved in physiological saline or 1.0% carboxymethylcellulose is applied and sealed in with impervious plastic

TABLE 15-2   Dermal Toxicity Tests

Testing For	Individual Assays
Acute Dermal Toxicity (U.S. Environmental Protection Agency OPPTS 870.1200)	Preferred: albino rabbit 12 weeks old (ease of handling, skin permeability, and extensive database).
	Others: 5- to 6-week-old rat, guinea pig. Five/dose level naïve to exposure and healthy intact skin—both sexes. Three doses with 24 h exposure to establish dose-response and ability to determine median lethal dose.
	Vehicle—aqueous or oil, then gum arabic, ethanol and water, carboxymethylcellulose, glycerol, propylene glycol, PEG vegetable oil, and mineral oil. Vehicle should be considered in effects. Fur clipped from dorsal area of trunk (10% body surface) or shaved 24 h prior to dosing. Uniformly applied toxicant and porous gauze dressing and nonirritating tape. Prevent animal from oral ingestion of applied material. Remove with solvent after 24 h and observe 14 days with behavioral, skin, and weight assessed with final gross necropsy.
Skin irritation—Draize test (animal and human; Basketter et al., 1994), alternative (Eskes et al., 2007)	Erythema (redness) and eschar (injury in depth) formation and edema (raised skin)
Skin sensitization (Yuan et al., 2009)	Guinea pig maximization test—intradermal administration ± Freund's adjuvant and occluded topical application 1 week later. Subjective analysis of sensitized/nonsensitized.
	Murine local lymph node assay—application to a site with defined lymph nodes draining the site. EC3 (threefold simulation index of lymphocyte proliferation) equals a sensitizer.
	Buehler—Three (days 1, 7, and 14) 6-h duration exposures followed by a nonirritating challenge dose (Maurer, 2007)
	Draize—10 daily injection and challenge dose 25 days after last exposure (Maurer et al., 1975)
	Other similar tests—optimization test (10 injections using Freund's complete adjuvant in weeks 2 and 3 and challenge dose on day 35), Freund's complete adjuvant test (days 1, 5, and 9 intradermal shoulder injections followed by challenge doses to flank), split adjuvant test (5–10 sec of dry ice exposure following shaving, test agent applied and covered, reapplied on day 3, day 4 adjuvant is applied to edges of test site, on day 7 test agent reapplied and left for 2 days then uncovered with challenge dose given topically to a different shaved site occluded for 24 h on day 22).
Photoallergy and Phototoxicity	Rabbit or guinea pig administered orally or intravenously small dose for 10–14 days, rest period of 14–21 days, animals then given challenge dose + defined wavelength of light (UV or visible; Dubakiene and Kupriene, 2006) Phototoxicity is more a function of damage to the skin resulting from absorption of damaging light energy forming reactive intermediates.
Alternative (*in vitro assays*; Goldberg and Maibach, 1998)	Irritation assessed in cell cultures or reconstituted tissue equivalents (RTE) and skin explants by 3[4,5-dimehtylthiazol-2yl]-2,5-diphenyltetrazolium bromide, arachidonic acid, prostaglandins, IL1-α, and histochemistry and bioengineering measures such as transepithelial water loss for RTE and skin explants. Corrosion assessed in the same models by arachidonic acid, prostaglandins for corrosion along with histochemistry for RTE and skin explants. Allergic contact dermatitis determined by IL-8 and B7 for the same models and histochemistry for RTE and skin explants. T-lymphocyte activation can be measured as a response to allergic contact dermatitis in blood monocytes (dendritic cells/models)

to retard evaporation of volatile liquids. The animal is restrained for 4 hours to allow the chemical time to irritate the skin but not allow grooming by the animal. The areas are then cleaned with warm, soapy water. The albino rabbit skin is assessed 1, 24, 48, and 72 hours after treatment as the best animal predictor of human skin irritation (monkeys are too expensive and difficult to handle). Unfortunately, the rabbit can give false-positives as its skin can be more sensitive than that of the human. Because so much controversy surrounds this test's use in animals, a human patch test has been devised where corrosive chemicals are screened out for human exposures (Basketter et al., 1994). Alternatives of the EpiDerm, EPISKIN, and SIFT methods have been evaluated as possible replacements of the Draize test (Eskes et al., 2007).

The classic skin sensitization test is the guinea pig maximization test. A guinea pig is shaved and exposed to the chemical in an appropriate vehicle injected dermally or intradermally daily for 14 days. The chemical may also be given 4–5 days/week for 2 weeks. Following a 10–14 day rest period, a lower concentration is given as a challenge dose. The edema and erythema are evaluated 24, 48, and 72 hours following the challenging dose and compared to the sensitizing dose. Freund's adjuvant is used to maximize the immune response for those substances that may require more of a boost that cannot be done in this short time period. Good examples of allergens are 2,4-dinitrochlorobenzene, p-nitrodimethylaniline, or p-phenylenediamine. Other guinea pig models exist as modifications of the methods in the Draize test (Maurer et al., 1975; Mauer, 2007). There is also a mouse model, in which murine lymph node responses are monitored for those nodes that drain the site of application. This gives more quantitative values, as a threefold induction of lymphocyte proliferation is the cutoff used to assess a sensitizing agent. Again, these tests are costly and raise difficult ethical issues. An alternative approach is a quantitative structure-activity relationship based on the two animal models and using a support vector machine that can analyze high dimensionality of data points. Certain molecular descriptors of the compounds are more important than others in determining

sensitizing potential. The program uses a particle swarm optimization algorithm to optimize molecular parameters that correlate well with sensitization (Yuan et al., 2009).

Alternative methods involve using cell cultures, reconstituted tissue equivalents, skin explants, or dendritic cells and models to assess irritation, corrosion, or allergic contact dermatitis. Here the reactions are monitored biochemically for cell cultures. Changes in arachidonic acid or prostaglandin responses could signal either an irritant or corrosive event. However, IL-1α is a better measure of irritation. Allergic contact dermatitis is signaled by the appearance of IL-8, an 8-kDa heparin-binding basic polypeptide that is a T lymphocyte chemotactic agent, or B7, an adhesion molecule expressed in antigen-presenting cells that is required for optimal T cell activation. The same signals can also be measured in reconstituted tissue equivalents or skin explants with the addition of confirmatory histochemistry. Allergic contact dermatitis may be assessed by T cell activation in dendritic cells and models. *In vitro* phototoxicity and photoirritation models are being evaluated by the European Union (Goldberg and Maibach, 1998). Regarding photoallergy, the sensitization schedule and the challenge dose procedure look similar to other allergic sensitization, except for the need for lower doses and the use of light. The earliest agent that showed evidence of immune-mediated photosensitivity is 3,3′,4′,5-tetrachlorosalicylanilide (allergic contact sensitivity). Usually a delay in response is observed. UV-A light appears to mediate most photoallergy or phototoxicity responses as it penetrates deeper into the skin. Phototoxicities are more likely produced by compounds with benzene rings that absorb light energy with wavelengths < 320 nm. For acute phototoxic reactions, rapidly developing enhanced sunburn is determined. Vesicles are noted with more severe reactions. Lesions heal with hyperpigmentation. Occasionally, phototoxicity is elicited with pigmentary changes, such as blue-gray for amiodarone or brown for compounds containing psoralen. Lichen planus–like eruptions and pseudoporphyria may appear in the light-exposed area. Tetracyclines and other medications may cause a photo-onycholysis visible on nails that would not necessarily appear on the claws of test animals. However, histological examination of the skin of animals should look for dermal edema, dyskeratosis, and necrosis of keratinocytes. Also, epidermal spongiosis with dermal edema and a mixed infiltrate of immune cells (lymphocytes, macrophages, and neutrophils) may be present (Dubakiene and Kupriene, 2006).

Forensic Analysis of Eye Damage

The dermal toxicities indicated earlier can also visit the eye to dramatic effect. The Draize eye test is also considered inhumane by animal rights organizations. The difference is that skin scars may not have large impacts on functions if large areas are not involved. The way collagen is laid down in the eye for transparency is important in vision. Scarring may lead to blindness or at least impaired sight. Additionally, the corneal cells obtain oxygen from the air, and limiting that exchange can lead to vascularization of that outermost layer. Also of concern are the humors of the eye and the proper maintenance of eye pressure. Excessive pressure can lead to blindness via glaucoma. Thus, the iris muscle and pupil constriction versus dilation must be considered in eye toxicity. The clarity of

the lens (versus cataracts) and its ability to focus light is an important target for toxicant action. The retina of the eye is the next area to focus on for toxicity. Vision may also be affected by damage to the optic nerve. The eye is similar to skin with regard to corneal damage, but has other areas that respond to perturbations of cells, neural/neurotransmitter inputs, and processing of afferent signals.

Review the eye structure as portrayed in **Figure 15-7**. Note the structures already mentioned. The ones depicted early on up until the lens mainly are involved in the proper refraction of light. The receptors for vision are located on the retina through which signals are passed to the optic nerve into the central nervous system for decoding and formation of the image. Not only do toxicants induce reversible or irreversible damage to these eye structures, but medications can induce eye problems as well. Consider all structures of the eye, including the eyelids and lacrimal glands. Inflammatory or immune hypersensitivity reactions or dermatitis can lead to eyelid swelling or partial closure. Lacrimators, such as tear gas, can induce redness and irritation. Medications such as drug preservatives many times cause conjunctival hyperemia (red eye), which may or may

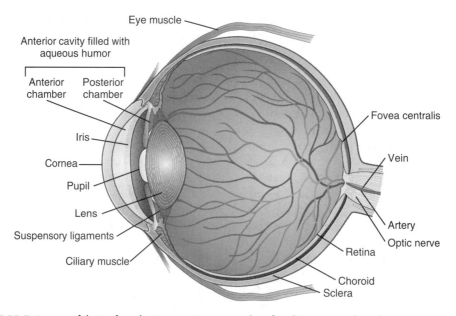

FIGURE 15-7 Structure of the Eye from the Outermost Structures to the Left and Innermost to the Right

not involve the cornea depending on severity. Botulism toxin is used to paralyze muscles to treat "aging lines" and can cause drooping of the eyelid if used to treat uncontrolled twitching of the eyelid (blepharospasm). Older men who have benign prostatic hyperplasia are frequently given the α-adrenergic blocker tamsulosin. This causes serious postoperative adverse effects in cataract surgery (intraoperative floppy iris syndrome). The sulfa antibiotics may cause angle-closure glaucoma via swelling of the ciliary body. Also, muscarinic antagonists such as atropine, scopolamine, or β_2 adrenergic agonist dilate the pupil and may yield angle-closure glaucoma. Open-angle glaucoma is induced by increased intraocular pressure by the steroidal anti-inflammatory cortisol or hydrocortisone administered on the skin or injected into the eye (intravitreally). Cancer chemotherapeutic compounds that augment microtubule formation such as paclitaxel also induce this type of glaucoma. The steroidal anti-inflammatory agents also induce clouding of the lens (subcapsular cataract), which does not reverse on removal of the drug. The antipsychotic phenothiazines cause clouding of the lens by alterations in the anterior cortex, while the alkylating anticancer medication busulfan alters the posterior cortex. Retinopathies develop from agents that make their way to the eye through the delicate vasculature of the posterior eye such as antimalarial aminoquinolines (bull's eye maculopathy). Phenothiazines (bind melanin granules causing severe phototoxic retinopathy) and weak estrogenic anticancer tamoxifen (crystalline deposits on inner retina) damage the eyes and skin through deposits. Treatment of cancer, lupus nephritis, and other ailments with retinoids can decrease night vision and alter dark adaptation. The antiarrhythmic medication amiodarone is associated with bilateral optic neuropathy. The oxazolidinone antibiotic linezolid may cause a swollen or pale optic disc where the optic nerve inserts into the retina (anoptic neuropathy), and other changes in vision such as sharpness (acuity) and color. The medications that are used to treat erectile disfunction (cGMP-specific phosphodiesterase type 5 inhibitors) usually carry a warning about decreased vision resulting from decreased color vision and blurriness

and increased light sensitivity. Ethambutol, a medication used in the treatment of mycobacterium including tuberculosis may cause bilateral, retrobulbar optic neuropathy (loss in visual acuity or color and changes in visual field). Note that medications may cause more than one part of the eye to be damaged as is also true for toxicants (Li et al., 2008).

The history of antipersonnel devices in warfare and unregulated, untested cosmetic products and medications and their association with significant eye damage led to the development of the Draize eye test, which is now much maligned. World War I used mustard gas with the *bis*-(2-chloroethyl) sulfide being the most irritating. It causes denaturation of enzymes and cross-links DNA strands. Epithelial sloughing of the conjunctiva occurs rapidly (minutes to hours) with epidermal blistering exacerbated by ischemic ulceration. The cornea may become cloudy (opacification), with corneal limbal stem-cell dysfunction and ultimately ulcerative keratitis. Another event in history that shook the cosmetics industry occurred when women used a cosmetic product in 1944 that contained a coal-tar derivative, paraphenylenediamine. This chemical is capable of causing allergic blepharitis (inflammation of the eyelash follicle and edge of eyelid), toxic keratoconjunctivitis, and a secondary bacterial keratitis. The women reacted in both eyes with a keratitis that developed into corneal scars. This led to the newspapers of the day exhorting Congress for consumer product testing and protection (Wilhelmus, 2001). The subsections that follow examine the forensic chart for eye damage and go structure by structure through the effects noted in **Table 15-3**.

Corneal Damage

Inflammation of the type seen in SJS and similar problems discussed for the skin are also part of damage to the outermost area of the eye. Single-nucleotide polymorphisms (SNPs) in the Toll-like receptor 3 gene, especially SNP 299698T/G and genotype patterns 293248A/A and 299698T/T, were strongly associated with SJS and toxic epidermal necrolysis in Japanese patients (Ueta et al., 2007). The inflammation

TABLE 15-3   Forensic Chart of Ocular Toxicity

Ocular Toxicity	Toxic Agents
Cornea	
Burns	Acids, ammonia, bases, bleach, compounds of chlorine, detergents, pesticides, solvents (Merle et al., 2008)
Inflammation — Toll-like receptors	Allergens (Pearlman et al., 2008)/compounds causing Stevens-Johnson Syndrome (Ueta et al., 2007)
Irritation/opacity	Solvents, acids, alkali, detergents (Ubels et al., 2000), dichloroethane in dogs (Kuwabara et al., 1968)
Oxidative damage	Metals, Paraquat (Shoham et al., 2008)
Photokeratitis	UV-B (Cejka et al., 2007)
Lens	
Cataracts	UV-B, reactive oxygen species (Yao et al., 2009), mitochondrial poisons (Bantseev et al., 2008), corticosteroids, phenothiazines (Li et al., 2008)
Posterior capsule opacification following cataract surgery	Statin, epidermal growth factor (Zhang et al., 2009)
Retina	
Cone disruption	Inhibition of 3Na+,2K+-ATPase (cardiac glycosides), inhibition or carbonic anhydrase (methazolamide; Widengård et al., 1995); phosphodiesterase inhibition and sildenafil citrate (Carter, 2007)
Lysosomal function impairment	Chloroquine, hydroxychloroquine, and quinacrine accumulation (Browning, 2004)
Mechanical	Lasers (Glickman, 2002)
Mitochondrial respiration disruption	Anticancer agents, mitochondrial poisons (Ebringer, 1990)
Neurotoxicity	Heavy metals and mitochondrial toxicity — lead toxicity or calcium overload and rod damage (He et al., 2000), methanol and mitochondria (Eells et al., 2000), organic solvents (Viaene et al., 2009), styrene, perchloroethylene, carbon disulfide, mercury (Gobba and Cavalleri, 2003)
Oxidative Toxicity	Light (Glickman, 2002), iron (He et al., 2007)
Thermal	Light (Glickman, 2002)
Vascular alterations	Canthaxanthin (Kim et al., 2009)
Eye Pressure	
Glaucoma	Atropine, cortisol (Li et al., 2008)
Optic Nerve	Cigarette smoke condensate toxicants in developing eye (Ejaz et al., 2009), mitochondrial disruptors (Rojas et al., 2008), organic solvents (Kobayashi et al., 2008), amiodarone, ethambutol, digitalis, isoniazid, perhexiline maleate, chloroquine, monoamine oxidase inhibitors, cyclosporine A, anticancer medications, interferon, vigabatrin, disulfiram, tetracycline, lithium, nalidixic acid, corticosteroids, nutritional deficiencies, methanol, tobacco-alcohol (Orssaud et al., 2007), acrylamide (Godin et al., 2000), carbon disulfide (Peters et al., 1986)
Visual Centers of CNS	Lead (Langauer-Lewowicka and Kazibutowska, 1991), methylmercury (Murata et al., 2007)

that results from these receptors occurs due to the production of CXC chemokines that have paired cysteines separated by an amino acid. These CXC chemokines cause neutrophil but not monocyte chemotaxis. This is an essential element in pathogen defense, but neutrophils cause extensive tissue damage including keratitis and noninfectious corneal inflammation associated with contact lens wear (Pearlman et al., 2008).

Damage to the collagen of the cornea and the development of scar tissue limits sight. Avian corneas have type V and type I striated heterotypic fibrils that regulate fibril diameter, as essential feature to corneal transparency. Similar associations have been found for the human. Type V collagen is found in disrupted corneal preparations as the interaction with the other collagen type makes it difficult to detect in the intact cornea. Type III collagen is not found in the cornea, but found in the subepithelial layers of the limbus and the stroma (White et al., 1997). This collagen structure allows light of wavelength ranges from high UV (310 nm) through the infrared (2,500 nm). It also bends light waves (refraction) significantly. Diopters measure the strength of refraction equaling the reciprocal of the focal length in meters. The human cornea provides 48 diopters of refraction if undamaged and normal thickness. This feature has become more important as humans correct vision problems with laser *in situ* keratomileusis (LASIK surgery). Corneas with a central thickness of < 500 µm were considered at risk for this type of surgery and may be more prone to damage of deeper eye structures from exposure to UV light or other toxicants. In surgical terms, a residual stroma of < 250 µm following LASIK surgery is to be avoided, or those with a central corneal thickness < 400 µm should avoid this type of procedure. However, a study has shown that people did well post-LASIK surgery with a thickness of 438–499 µm representing 41.1 to 46.3 diopters in thickness (de Benito-Llopis et al., 2009). The five major zones of the cornea are the epithelium, Bowman layer, stroma (90% of thickness), Descemet membrane, and endothelium. The cells exposed to air are squamous and apoptotic. The cornea absorbs most

UV radiation below 280 nm with a maximum sensitivity of 270 nm (Zuchlich, 1998). While most UV-C is effectively absorbed by the Earth's atmosphere, UV-B is most problematic for the cornea, able to cause photokeratitis with swelling of the corneal stroma, thinning of the corneal epithelium, and a decrease in antioxidants. The increase in corneal hydration, changing to a more grayish color (decreased transparency), and increased protein content with UV exposure makes the cornea more susceptible to further UV-B damage (Cejka et al., 2007). The decrease in antioxidants is important to corneal diseases. The exposure to UV light and high oxygen tensions requires the cornea to defend against ROS and RNS. CuZn-SOD or SOD1, MnSOD, and extracellular SOD or EC-SOD or SOD3 are found in the corneal epithelial, stromal, and endothelial cells. The cornea also has heme oxygenase-1 (HO-1) and NADPH cytochrome P450 reductase in sufficient quantities to develop oxygen radicals. Because the mammalian *ho-1* promoter is inducible by heme, β-amyloid, TH1 cytokines, dopamine, hydrogen peroxide, lipopolysaccharides, UV light, transition metals, and prostaglandins, these factors either provide protection by inducing HO-1 (breakdown of prooxidant heme or carbon monoxide production that stimulates antioxidant gene expression) or increase oxidative stress via carbon monoxide-induced mitochondrial dysfunction. Aging corneal cells have less antioxidant activity and are less capable of wound healing. UV-B induces metabolic changes in the cornea and can cause erythema, blistering, photoconjunctivitis, and chemosis and causes hydroxyl radical formation via homolytic fission of H_2O_2. UV-A and UV-B are capable of severe burning of the corneal epithelium as exemplified by unshielded arc welding. Metallic particles in the cornea form rust rings within 24 hours of exposure if not removed. Oxidative damage, induction of proteolytic enzymes by iron, and liquefaction necrosis can result. Methyl viologen (Paraquat) splashed into the eye is reduced by NADPH cytochrome P450 reductase and undergoes oxidation to produce superoxide radical, deplete NADPH, and alter calcium homeostasis. Serious inflammatory damage results (Shoham et al., 2008).

Corneal opacity, as indicted by exposure of dogs to 1,2-dichloroethane, appears to occur as a result of necrosis of the corneal endothelium, partially denuded Descemet's membrane, formation of excess basement membrane, and swelling of the corneal stroma (Kuwabara et al.,1968). Corneal opacity is displayed in **Figure 15-8**. Other irritants appear to cause opacities if they damage the corneal epithelial cells without loss of epithelium from the ocular surface. Hydration may increase the effect slightly, but does not appear to be the critical factor (Ubels et al., 2000). Some of the agents that cause irritation for shorter periods cause more severe damage for longer periods. Ocular burns may be classified by the limbal stem cell deficiency resulting from the injury. The destruction of limbic cells results in recurrent epithelial ulcerations, chronic stromal ulcers, deep stromal revascularization, and conjunctival overlap, and may cause corneal perforation. The most frequently observed burns occur from acids and bases in 1.6% and 0.6% of eye injuries, respectively. The severity of the burn is indicated by the nature of the chemical, the exposure duration, concentration, quantity, and pH of the agent. Bases include ammonia (becomes ammonium hydroxide), sodium hypochlorite (due to presence of caustic soda), soda (NaOH), potash (KOH), and lime (Ca(OH)$_2$). The last compound adheres to the conjunctiva, providing a pool of toxicant to damage to cornea. Alkaline substances penetrate rapidly due to their cationic charge and cause collagen denaturation. The saponified anionic fatty acids of cell membranes produced by alkaline degradation also are immediately lethal to epithelial cells. Sulfuric acid is responsible for the most severe acid damage (acid and oxidizer), but strong acids (pH $\leq$ 2.5) all can produce deep necrosis by denaturing and coagulating proteins. The coagulation limits further penetration of the acid. Hydrophobic solvents may damage the corneal epithelium and cause stromal swelling. Cationic detergents also serve as the most irritating of the surfactants. All share certain elements as the injury progresses. Following the initial injury (minutes to hours), a phase of debridement of necrotic lesions occurs along with healing. Debridement is accompanied by the influx

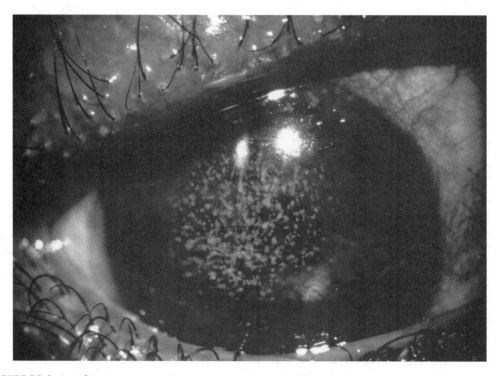

FIGURE 15-8 Corneal Opacity

© Bob Masini/Phototake

of inflammatory cells that are attracted by the degradation products produced in the cornea and conjunctiva. Neutrophils constitute the majority of inflammatory white blood cells and secrete metalloproteinases (collagenases, gelatinases, and stromelysin) that aid the debridement process while destroying ocular structures. The persistence of healthy cells around the damaged tissue participates in the healing process. The ischemic cells produced by the injury secrete growth factors such as vascular endothelial growth factor (VEGF), TGF, and fibroblast growth factor (FGF) that promote angiogenesis in the burned tissue. This vascularization may be beneficial to the conjunctiva while being injurious to the transparency of the cornea. Fibroblast proliferation by FGF and stem cell division promote the healing of the conjunctiva and cornea. Fibroblasts form the symblepharon that clouds the cornea. Tissue may also fill the iridocorneal angle and produce ocular hypertension. Stem cells originating from the corneal limbal cells or conjunctival fornix layers provide healthy replacements for reconstructing the corneal epithelium or conjunctiva. As seen in most functional laboratories, water flushing is the universal initial emergency treatment for eye contact by chemicals. However, hypertonic solutions are preferable as they create a flow from the inside to the outside of the eye (Merle et al., 2008).

Lens Damage

The ability to focus light onto the retina is an important function of the lens, and the ability to change diopters to achieve near focus (accommodation) is an important feature. This ability declines with age (presbyopia) as people over 50 years old can attest. Again, transparency is important. This can also decline with age as cataracts develop (**Figure 15-9**). Diabetes mellitus can also change the pressure in the lens, which causes cataracts. UV-B again penetrates and does damage to the lens cells. It damages the proteins of the eye (α, β, and γ-crystallins). Mutations in the crystallin genes along with environmental factors, such as continual UV light and ROS, cause changes in the protein structure. The γ-crystallins are the

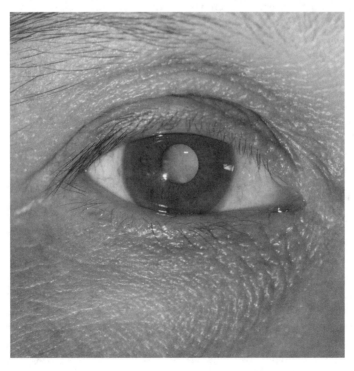

FIGURE 15-9 Human Cataract

most stable of these eye proteins and appear to concentrate mostly in the central region of the lens. Changes in this protein, especially a G18V point mutation in the less stable γS-crystallin, have been associated with progressive cortical cataracts in a Chinese family (Ma et al., 2009). UV-B also generates ROS in lens cells via NADPH oxidase as indicated by the prevention by diphenyleneiodonium (NADPH oxidase inhibitor) and antioxidant epigallocatechin gallate. The ROS appear to be essential in activation of NF-κB, which modulates the activities of metalloproteinases MMP-2 and MMP-9. These mechanisms are involved in the cell migration induced by UV-B in human lens epithelial cells (Yao et al., 2009).

For the effects of mitochondrial poisons, the unusual mitochondria of the lens cells must be described. All cell organelles may scatter light and must be degraded, especially toward the center of the lens. The use of a fluorescent dye specific for metabolically active mitochondria, rhodamine-123, has made mitochondrial analysis in the lens cells possible. Mammalian lens epithelial cells have dense filamentous mitochondria up to 5 μm long in a calyx surrounding individual epithelial nuclei. Fiber cells appose epithelial cells on the apical side of epithelial cells. In this side, longer mitochondria (≤ 15 μm) exist. The calyx of mitochondria is undone at the lens equator due to the differentiation of epithelial cells in fiber cells. The mitochondria of the superficial cortex are not as dense or do not have much connection to the nuclei but are much longer (≤ 100 μm). The mitochondria disappear more rapidly in aging lenses. For example, rat lenses show no mitochondria at a depth of 170 μm at 1 week of age and 30 μm at 22 months. There is likely a hypoxic state in the lens core due to the decrease in density of mitochondria in this region. Toxic chemicals also decrease mitochondrial number, allowing more oxygen to penetrate to the core. This may lead to lens opacities. The continual development of the lens from embryogenesis until death and the high concentration of protein make the lens sensitive to damage. This is clear from the effects of UV-B on the lens. However, it is of interest to note that the mitochondrial depolarizing agent *m*-chlorophenyl hydrazone (CCCP) to bovine lenses *in vitro*

caused a concentration and time-dependent loss of sharp focus. The number and length of mitochondria decreased with CCCP treatment. The surfactant sodium dodecyl sulfate (SDS) also caused a loss of sharp focus and a three-phased change in mitochondria. The first phase included a loss in mitochondrial length. This was followed by a phase of swelling and change from short to round mitochondria. The third cytotoxic phase resulted in the absence of metabolically active mitochondria as indicated by lack of rhodamine-123 fluorescence (Bantseev et al., 2008). Signaling pathways can also lead to cell damage or apoptosis. High levels of glucose are associated with less expression of caveolin-1 and increased apoptosis of lens epithelial cells. Because apoptosis of these cells reduces posterior capsular opacification, the increase in caveolin-1 expression and decreased apoptosis by 3-hydroxy-3-methylglutaryl coenzyme A (HMG-CoA) reductase inhibitor simvastatin or EGF is of concern for posterior capsular opacification (Zhang et al., 2009). Some historic chemicals that produce cataracts are those such as naphthalene, which has a literature back to the early 1930s. The enzyme aldose reductase responsible for converting glucose to sorbitol in diabetes mellitus–induced cataracts is also the enzyme that converts naphthalene to the dihydrodiol that leads to cataracts (Dvornik, 1992). There is a marked and faster progression of naphthalene-induced cataracts in brown Norway rats with pigmented eyes compared with albino Sprague-Dawley rats (Murano et al., 1993).

Retinal Damage

The retina is a very sensitive organ for damage. Aging alone produces changes that can cause blindness such as microvascular alterations, shrinkage that can cause retinal tears or detachment, oxidative damage and inflammation, rod and cone degeneration, changes in pigmentation, and neurological deficits (Xu et al., 2009). Again, the exposure to light (especially UV-B) and oxygen are some of the key agents that promote aging. Chemicals that augment this process clearly enhance the damage to the retina. These effects are hard to parcel out as many agents can have multiple causes of retinal damage. For example, light damages via photochemical, mechanical, and thermal effects depending on the wavelength and duration of exposure. The photochemical damage occurs due to absorption of the photons and generation of oxidative reactions. However, if the deposition of energy is faster than thermal diffusion, temperatures may reach the critical 10°C above basal and yield thermal damage. Laser pulses may also deposit energy faster than mechanical relaxation can occur. This causes a thermoelastic pressure wave and tissue disruption by shear forces or cavitation-nonlinear effects (Glickman, 2002). Nutrients can also turn into toxicants. Iron is required for the phototransduction cascade. Constant shedding and synthesis characterize the outer segments of photoreceptor cells. Disc membranes of the newly synthesized cells require lipid synthesis through iron containing fatty acid desaturase. Iron serves as a cofactor for guanylate cyclase, which synthesizes the second messenger of the phototransduction cascade (cGMP). Retinal pigment epithelium contains an iron-containing isomerohydrolase in the endoplasmic reticulum that converts all-*trans*-retinyl ester to 11-*cis*-retinol in the visual cycle. Excess iron catalyzes the Fenton reaction generating hydroxyl radical, causing lipid peroxidation, DNA strand breaks, and degradation of macromolecules. High oxygen tensions and high concentrations of polyunsaturated fatty acids in photoreceptors make them highly susceptible to this type of attack. Excess iron appears to cause ocular siderosis (interocular foreign bodies or intraocular hemorrhage). Retinal degeneration and age-related macular degeneration also occur in iron overload. Because these conditions are related to the generation of ROS, antioxidants and iron chelators may prevent or treat these disorders (He et al., 2007).

Certain chemicals accumulate in the retinal pigment epithelium, including quinolones and acridines such as chloroquine, hydroxychloroquine, and quinacrine (antimalarials). These chemicals are thought to interfere with lysosomal degradation of various substances. These conditions start with a paracentral scotomata (isolated area of diminished vision within a visual field) and a classic "bulls-eye" by a pigmented area surrounded by a depigmented ring and another ring of pigmentation. If no fundus changes are evident, this condition is reversible. Otherwise, it progresses to parafoveal retinal pigment epithelial atrophic lesions followed by peripheral retinal pigment epithelial mottling. In advanced conditions, arteriolar narrowing and disk pallor develop (Browning, 2004).

Cones and color vision appear to be affected by alterations of ion fluxes across the membranes of photoreceptors. That appears to be why inhibitors of the $3Na^+,2K^+$-ATPase, such as the cardiac glycosides digitalis from the foxglove plant and digitoxin, impair color vision. Similarly, inhibition of carbonic anhydrase by methazolamide caused disturbances in the color vision of 8 of 14 human volunteers exposed to this compound based on the Lanthony New Color Test. Acidosis of other effects was not significantly correlated with effects on color vision (Widengård et al., 1995).

The genome of the organelles and especially the mitochondria (tenfold more labile) is more susceptible to DNA damage than nuclear DNA. Due to the high demand for ATP synthesis in the retina (as well as in brain, heart, and skeletal muscle), chemotherapeutic agents used in the treatment of cancers are more disruptive to mitochondrial genes and function (Ebringer, 1990). The choroidal circulation also makes the retina more prone to damage. Cytotoxic agents including alkylating agents, antimetabolites, and mitotic inhibitors lead the list of agents that damage the retina. Topical administration of these agents is the best way of treating a tumor of the iris, because the highest concentrations are attained this way. However, choroidal and retinal tumors are best treated with intravenous injection. This indicates that toxicities are also likely to develop from systemic administration of chemotherapeutic agents such as 1,3-bis(2- chlorethyl)-1-nitrosourea (Ueno et al., 1982). The mitochondria are also prone to disruption by the formation of formic acid by alcohol dehydrogenase. Formic acid results in acidemia, metabolic acidosis, and blindness in primates and a rat model using an inhibitor of formate oxidation. Toxicity is noted by reductions in electroretinogram and flash-evoked cortical potential with increasing blood formate. Mitochondria show visible disruption and vacuolation in the retinal pigmented epithelium, photoreceptor inner segments, and the optic nerve (Eells et al., 2000). Organic solvents (aliphatic and aromatic lipophilic compounds that are more or less volatile) also show a remarkable diversity of neurotoxicity. Some of these compounds interact with neuronal membranes to produce anesthetic/narcotic effects (e.g., the older discontinued anesthetics of ethyl ether or chloroform or newer Propofol, which is 2,6-diisopropylphenol). These agents can cause a reversible prenarcotic syndrome of headache, dizziness, and light-headedness also frequently associated with irritation of the mucous membranes. At much higher concentrations, this can lead to unconsciousness, seizures, and death. If > 5 years of high-exposure conditions or > 10 years of lower exposure conditions are experienced, this is where the eye and other neurological functions are impaired such as anosmia (loss of smell), loss of hearing, color vision alterations (blue-yellow deficits), peripheral neuropathy, and depression. This can progress to irreversible toxic encephalopathy (severe cognitive impairment, memory problems, attention deficits, psychomotor function alterations). This can lead to less mental flexibility, mood changes, personality changes, diffuse pain, and sleep disorders (Viaene et al., 2009). There also appears to be at least an increased sensitivity of female workers to color disturbances due to exposure to low concentrations of toluene (Zavalić et al., 1996). Other neurotoxic agents such as styrene, perchloroethylene, carbon disulfide, and mercury also affect color vision similarly with blue-yellow deficits or less often red-green loss as well. Köllner's rule suggests that the retinal location of the toxicity causes the effects on vision. Some chemicals or metabolites affect cone function directly or interfere with dopamine neurotransmission. Dying-back or distal axonopathy may occur for agents such as n-hexane (Gobba and Cavalleri, 2003). Organophosphates such as diazinon inhibit acetylcholinesterase (AChE). Exposure of medaka (teleost fish model for toxicity) embryos to diazinon inhibited how embryo or retinal AChE and small foci of necrotic cells appeared between days 5 and 7 later with the inner nuclear layer and isolated pyknotic

cells in the ganglion layer of the retina. The organophosphate diisopropyl phosphorofluoridate similarly produced large foci of necrotic cells at the same sites (Hamm et al., 1998).

Systemic administration of the NSAID indomethacin reduces ocular blood flow, likely through inhibition of COX-1 (Ogawa et al., 2009). However, one article suggests that this drug's metabolite is a quinone imine that could cause oxidative stress that would damage the retinal pigmented epithelium. This same article indicates that oxidation in the retina via CYPs and myeloperoxidase may also be responsible for the tamoxifen and thioridazine (Toler, 2004). High doses of tamoxifen may indeed be oxidative. Human patients show that chronic use of tamoxifen may be related to retinal nerve fiber atrophy or macular edema (Baget-Bernaldiz et al., 2008).

Another enzyme of interest is phosphodiesterase (PDE) in retinal function. An inhibitor of PDE type 5 aids in erectile dysfunction and causes rare ischemic disorders of the optic disc (Fraunfelder and Fraunfelder, 2008). PDE metabolizes cGMP and cAMP. PDE-4 is expressed in immune cells and may be related to asthma, rheumatoid arthritis, and atopic dermatitis. PDE-5 is a cGMP-specific enzyme not only located in the vasculature of the penis, but also in the lung, platelets, and vascular and visceral smooth muscle. PDE-6 is of importance in this section due to its unique localization in the retinal rod and cone outer segments. It plays a key role in the conversion of light stimulation to electrical signals. Sildenafil is a very strong inhibitor of PDE-5, but has 10% inhibition activity toward PDE-6. Other PDE isozymes bind much more weakly to sildenafil (100–10,000 times less active). Visual alterations caused by this medication are changes in color perception, blue tinge to the environment, and brightness perception deficits that may be attributed to PDE inhibition (Carter, 2007).

Neural toxicity in humans as a result of exposure to inorganic lead (Pb) was one of the earliest conclusions drawn regarding this heavy metal during the era of Roman rule. As a divalention, Pb^{2+} also targets L-type calcium channels, which recognize the dihydropyridine family of calcium channel antagonists. Cultured skeletal muscle cells but not neural retinal cells from embryonic chicks caused a significant dose-dependent reduction in dihydropyridine receptors at concentrations > 1 μM and incubation times > 12 hours (Luo and Berman, 2004). Similarly, inorganic lead also targets acetylcholinesterase in skeletal muscle cultures but not retinal cells cultures in the chick embryo (Luo and Berman, 1997). If these mechanisms are not in play for lead in the CNS, what actually causes the neurotoxicity? The effects on calcium channels are still considered important, but the effects of lead are on neurotransmitter release, intracellular calcium concentrations, and calcium-regulatory proteins, which are also pertinent to the neurotoxic action. Lead substitutes for calcium in protein kinase C (PKC) and increases membrane-associated PKC pools in astroglial and microvascular endothelial cells. There is a causal relationship between PKC activation and inhibition of astroglial-induced microvessel formation *in vitro* (Laterra et al., 1992). Thus, it appears that blindness due to lead comes from two sources, neural toxicity/microvascular alterations and loss of neuromuscular control of the eye. This appears to be the case in lead-exposed workers. Calcium overload or lead toxicity appears to have the same action in rods, which are sensitive to chemically induced or inherited retinal degenerations. They both induce rod-selective apoptosis with mitochondrial depolarization, swelling, and cytochrome c release. Caspase-9 and caspase-3 are sequentially activated. An inhibitor of the mitochondrial permeability transition pore cyclosporin A prevents the effects of calcium or lead, which are additive. The calcineurin inhibitor FK506 has no effect on this toxicity. Two different caspase inhibitors, carbobenzoxy-Leu-Glu-His-Asp-CH_2F and carbobenzoxy-Asp-Glu-Val-Asp-CH_2F (but not carbobenzoxy-Ile-Glu-Thr-Asp-CH_2F), could prevent the post-mitochondrial events. Oxidation does not appear to play a role as glutathione and pyridine nucleotides remain unchanged (He et al., 2000).

The delicate retinal vasculature must also be considered. The effects of diabetes mellitus on destroying the blood/retinal barrier are well known (Kim et al., 2009). Toxic chemicals such as canthaxanthin also affect the vasculature causing a retinopathy (see **Figure 15-10** for

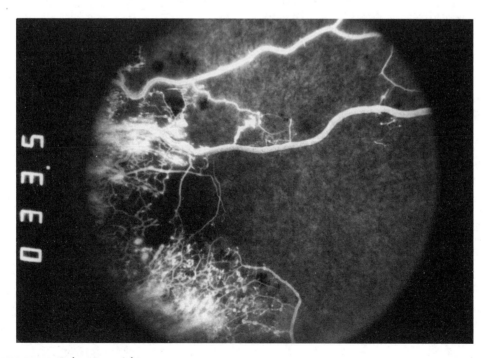

FIGURE 15-10 Diabetic Retinopathy
© William Feig/Phototake

diabetic retinopathy). This pigment, which is used in medications and as a food and cosmetic colorant, interacts with lipid membranes and aggregates in the macula. Crystal formation in the macular lutea damages the blood vessels in the area of deposition (Sujak, 2009).

Optic Nerve Damage

Cranial nerve II originates in the optic disc of the retina, where there are no rods or cones. That is why it is referred to as the blind spot. If retinal reattachments or tear repairs are performed using a laser, other blind spots will appear. The developmental damage done to the optic nerve and other eye structures by cigarette smoke condensate was tested in the chick embryo. Smoke contains carcinogens such as catechol and hydroquinone, which auto-oxidize to produce semiquinone and hydroxyl radicals. Other toxic particulate matter in smoke are alkaloids, naphthalene, other aromatic hydrocarbons, phenols, terpenes, carboxylic acids, indoles, benzofurans, aromatic amines, inorganic particulate matter such as silicates, and tar. Treatment of chick embryos with cigarette smoke condensate causes optic chiasma degeneration, extensive myelin thickness inconsistency, demyelination of nerve fibers, and swollen mitochondria (Ejaz et al., 2009). Damage to CNS structures is frequently accompanied by proliferation of astrocytes known as gliosis. The neurotoxicant kainic acid ($C_{10}H_{15}NO_4$), an analogue of glutamate derived from the red alga *Digenea simplex*, induces gliosis in the brain (hippocampal CA1, CA3, dentate gyrus) and the retina. This was performed in transgenic mice expressing a green fluorescent protein when the glial fibrillary acid protein promoter was activated (Ho et al., 2009). For some compounds, it is difficult to tease apart retinal damage from toxicity experienced by the optic nerve. For example, a compound (ethambutol) used for the treatment of a *Mycobacterium avium-intracellulare* infection resulted in bitemporal visual field effects. This suggests optic chiasm damage. Multifocal electroretinography indicated marked low-amplitude responses as taxation and in the regions corresponding to the visual field effects. These data give an alternative

explanation that ethambutol damages the retina (Liu et al., 2008). Mitochondrial disruptors mentioned as altering vision via damage to other eye structures damage the optic nerve as well. Rotenone is a well known specific complex I inhibitor used in lakes to control invasive fish populations. It is of interest that treatment with a certain wavelength range of light ($\lambda = 630$–1000 nm or near-infrared) that activates the cultured neuronal cells without damage alleviates mitochondrial optic neuropathies caused by rotenone. Near-infrared light also prevents the decline in ATP concentrations, increased ROS and nitric oxide, and increased apoptosis of rotenone-treated cells. If the near-infrared light is used *in vivo* via light-emitting diodes, it also exerts neuroprotective effects against rotenone (Rojas et al., 2008). Some compounds exert a dual effect that makes them more neurotoxic than toxic to the retina. Dichloromethane exerts direct toxic effects and, via metabolism to carbon monoxide, contributes two ways to the optic neuropathy observed in a patient exposed to a significant challenge of inhalation of dichloromethane while cleaning a tank containing dichloromethane (Kobayashi et al., 2008).

Another difficulty is separating optic nerve damage that results from nutritional deficiencies versus toxic compounds. Both appear to involve alterations of cellular energy production, correction of oxidative stress, and quenching of free radicals. At times, there is a mixture of nutritional deficiency with toxicity as observed in Cubans between 1991 and 1993. Cubans who used tobacco and alcohol (tobacco-alcohol amblyopia or "lazy eyes"—the lack of ability to see details) were more prone to optic neuropathy caused by nutritional deficiencies. Deficiency in the antioxidant carotenoid lycopene was most associated with susceptibility to optic neuropathy. Low consumption of protein and B vitamins (especially riboflavin, which is a cofactor for glutathione synthesis) appeared to increase the risk of neuropathy. The amblyopia presents as a retrobulbar optic neuropathy, classic cecocentral scotoma ("champagne-cork" appearance), and dyschromatopsia in the "red-green" axis. Nicotine is a clearly harmful agent here. The role of cyanide in smoke has not been proven to be detrimental in animal models. Riboflavin may provide antioxidant protection, but it is disrupted by ethanol intake. The progression from blurriness to blindness may be slow over months. This progression does not involve pain and is usually bilateral. A unilateral deficit is usually observed for recent nutritional deficiencies combined with intoxication. A difference in pupil size or anisocoria may be absent. The pupillary light reflex (direct and consensual) may be paired to an afferent pupillary defect (Marcus Gunn phenomenon), which confirms optic nerve damage. Methanol toxicity by formation of formic acid from drinking wood alcohol is considered both nutritional and toxic. Brief spots of light or phosphenes precede or accompany visual acuity loss in methanol toxicity that may cause optic nerve atrophy. The aspect of the optic fundus (interior of the eye including the retina, optic disc, macula, fovea, and posterior pole) is not relevant to nutritional optic neuropathies. Peripapillary hemorrhages or papilledema may indicate nutritional deficiencies coupled to toxic exposures. A pure optic neuropathy may be experienced by vegans who do not take nutritional supplements or those engaged in rapid weight-loss regimens. Medications can also couple to nutritional deficiencies to produce neuropathy. The anti-tuberculosis medication isoniazid couples to pyridoxine deficiency (vitamin B_6). Ethambutol mentioned earlier appears to chelate zinc, which is required for cytochrome oxidase activity. Some medications cause either direct toxicity to the optic nerve or increase intracranial hypertension (amiodarone, chloroquine, cisplatin, corticosteroids, cyclosporine A, digitalis, disulfiram, ethambutol, 5-fluorouracil, interferon, isoniazid, lithium, MAO inhibitors [MAOIs], methotrexate, nalidixic acid, perhexiline maleate, tetracycline, vigabatrin). The antiseizure compound vigabatrin is responsible for ~30% of toxic–nutritional optic neuropathies. It presents in elderly tobacco users as a decrease in isopters (areas of equal visual acuity in the field of vision) with a scotoma in the central 30° of the nasal hemifield. The alcohol abuse prevention medication disulfiram produces retrobulbar optic neuropathy that mimics alcoholic optic neuropathy (Orssaud et al., 2007).

There are two other toxicants worth mentioning for their neurotoxicity. These are acrylamine monomer and carbon disulfide. One cannot image doing molecular biology without the aid of polyacrylamide gel electrophoresis. The distal axonopathies have been observed in response to acrylamide monomer. It is of interest that cattle were accidentally exposed to monomeric acrylamide and N-methylolacrylamide. They showed progressive retinal degeneration and optic nerve heads (Godin et al., 2000). Grain storage workers exposed to carbon tetrachloride/carbon disulfide (80/20 fumigants) showed classic CS_2 toxicity (of rayon workers) with dysfunction of optic nerve, auditory nerve, peripheral axons, extrapyramidal system, and altered behavior (psychotic mania) and cognition changes (Peters et al., 1986). CS_2- and 2,5-hexanedione-induced axonopathies are characterized by formation of neurofilaments with enlarged preterminal regions of central and peripheral axons via increased neurofilament transport (models of giant axonal neuropathies; Pappolla et al., 1987).

Central Visual System Lesions

Two classic heavy metals come to mind when blindness and behavioral alterations are mentioned with changes in the visual system. Pb poisoning can affect higher functions of cognition and attention (Hirata et al., 2004). Lead alters the conduction velocity of visual, auditory, and somatosensory impulses. Copper and zinc protect workers from high Pb concentrations by lowering Pb blood concentrations and reducing lead's impact on neural structures and red blood cell heme (Langauer-Lewowicka and Kazibutowska, 1991). Methylmercury poisoned many people in Minamata Bay, Japan and continues to be a problem for people who consume too much seafood as their major source of protein, including the much publicized poisoning of an actor from the United States. Neuropathological lesions are found in the visual, auditory, and post- and pre-central cortex areas. Neurological signs of methylmercury poisoning are constriction of visual field, paresthesias (tingling, tickling, pricking, burning sensations without visual cause), impairments of hearing and speech, mental disturbances, excessive sweating, and hypersalivation (Murata et al., 2007). The triad of mercury poisoning effects derived from those who worked in the felt hat industry ("mad hatter") and inhaled large quantities of mercury nitrate are gingivitis, tremor, and erethism or abnormal excitability.

Eye Toxicity Tests

Eye toxicity has an interesting history that has affected which tests are used to assess damage. Human toxicity was noted first in women using cosmetics with coal tar or soldiers returning from World War I with mustard gas injuries (mentioned earlier in the discussion of eye toxicity). Ida C. Mann was an ophthalmologist in London during World War II who studied the effects of mustard gas on the eye due to government concerns of the possible use of these agents again. She developed a qualitative test using a rabbit model. Jonas S. Friedenwald undertook a study for the U.S. military in the same period for the development of a quantitative scale (more than + or −) of ocular damage. Conjunctival redness was given a 0–2 scale and corneal edema from 0–4. John H. Draize adapted Friedenwald's scale in his system of ocular toxicity during the same era for the military for antipersonnel chemical agents. He then joined the Food and Drug Administration's Division of Pharmacology and tested the adverse effects of cosmetics. He headed the Dermal and Ocular Branch in 1940 and studied beauty aids, as they were known back then. He studied acute, intermediate, and chronic exposures to rabbit skin, penis, and eyes to these untested products. This method was expanded to testing insecticides, sunscreens, antiseptics, and British anti-Lewisite (2,3-dimercaptopropanol used as an antidote to Lewisite or 2-chlorovinyldichloroarsine and further developed as a chelator of arsenic, mercury, lead, and gold). The Draize technique became the Draize test in the early 1960s. In the early 1970s, the Consumer Product Safety Commission used a uniform grading for product testing using the Draize test. The tests used for the eye are indicated in **Table 15-4**. The animal model was the rabbit, because its large eyes enabled ease of use for the Draize test. Statistics indicate three animals minimum for testing, while

biologic variation may indicate the need for more animals (six maximum). Animal welfare issues indicated that the fewest animals that could give reliable results should be employed. Liquids are most easily tested, but ointments, pastes, solids, gases, vapors, and aerosols all require testing. The product should be tested in the concentrations used, but individual ingredients can be tested alone or in vehicle as well. Although the initial researchers back in the 1940s used 0.1 mL, later research showed that 0.01 ml (10 μL) was more appropriate based on most day-to-day human exposures. Dose-responses were done to establish a minimum strength of toxicity threshold. The solution is placed in the lower conjunctival sac or dropped directly onto the cornea. Effects are determined with magnification with loupes or slit-lamp biomicroscopy. Fluorescein staining and photodocumentation better record the damage. The number of times the animal blinks or wipes its treated eye may also indicate discomfort level. Mucosal and epithelial effects mark the endpoints that are expected to be evaluated (density and area of corneal opacification [score 0–80]; severity of iritis [score 0–10]; and conjunctival redness, edema, and discharge [score 0–20] for a total score of 0–110), even though systemic effects are to be recorded. Other measures can be scored such as lacrimation and blepharitis. The threshold for irritation for the Draize test was a corneal opacity score ≥ 1, iritis score ≥ 1, or conjunctival redness score ≥ 2 or swelling ≥ 2.5. Corrosive ocular destruction was scored as dangerous. Corneal involvement for > 1 week was characterized as hazardous. Mild or brief ocular surface involvement marked a product as suspect. The criticisms of this test indicate that the exposure is not necessarily consistent with human accidental exposure. The number of variables that must be scored does not lend itself to reproducibility and is most problematic for moderately irritating compounds. The rabbit eye has relatively low tear production, blink frequency, ocular surface sensitivity, a nictitating membrane, genus-specific constituents of tear film, a relatively larger corneal surface area, a thinner cornea without a Bowman's layer, and different ocular pigmentation from human eyes.

TABLE 15-4   Ocular Toxicity Tests

Testing For	Individual Assays
Topical eye exposure resulting in eye irritation or damage	Draize test — New Zealand white (albino) rabbits, 3–6/dose, one eye = test and the other = control, 0.1 mL/eye (former due to topical application or intraocular injection) changed to 0.04 mL in lower conjunctival cul de sac; external visual examination with scope or slit-lamp biomicroscopy at 1, 23, 48, and 72 hours; corneal and iris scoring; can do histopathological evaluation of enucleated eyes
Other morphological tests	Corneal epithelial dye staining, corneal dye permeability, corneal thickness, corneal opacification (light transmission), lens optics, stromal haze, corneal electrical conductivity, corneal endothelial specular microscopy following topical instillation or anterior-chamber perfusion, confocal microscopy, laser flare-cell meter, intraocular pressure, Scheimpflug photography of crystalline lens, electroretinography, impression and exfoliative cytology, histopathology
Physiology	Cornea epithelial regeneration rate after debridement or superficial keratectomy, corneal stromal wound tensile strength or bursting threshold, corneal and conjunctival water content, blinking rate, tear flow, tear constituents, conjunctival vascular blood flow, conjunctival and iris capillary permeability of intravenous dye, conduction of long ciliary nerve, corneal protein profile, ileal contractility, release of cytokines (inflammation)
Cell culture alternatives (e.g., Kruszewski et al., 1997)	
Morphology	Cell density, cell size and shape, cell–cell contacts, nuclear size/shape/appearance, cytoplasmic appearance
Viability	Crystal violet uptake or trypan blue exclusion, cell mitosis and replication
Adhesion	Cell attachment, cell–cell adhesion
Proliferation	Colony formation and efficiency, DNA/RNA alterations
Membrane integrity	Fluorescein and neutral red leakage, ethidium bromide uptake, release of cellular enzymes or tagged molecules
Metabolism	Intracellular protein content, neutral red uptake, glucose or calcium utilization, protein synthesis rate, ATP/NADPH concentrations, ion concentrations, enzyme activities, C-reactive protein (inflammation), pH changes, mitochondrial function, mRNA synthesis
Uptake of labeled precursors	Thymidine/DNA synthesis, uridine/RNA synthesis, amino acid incorporation
Regeneration	Wound healing
Gene expression	Stress-response proteins (HO-1)
Modeling	Structure–activity relationships
Clinical measures in human volunteers/patients Ocular surface	OSDI (vision-related function, ocular symptoms, environmental triggers), National Eye Institute Visual Functioning Questionnaire (NEI VFQ-25), the McMonnies Dry Eye Questionnaire, the Short Form-12 (SF-12) Health Status Questionnaire, and an ophthalmic examination including Schirmer tests, tear breakup time, and fluorescein and lissamine green staining (Schiffman et al., 2000)
Color vision	Desaturated Panel D-15 test for color vision loss (Lanthony, 1978)
Retinal damage	Electroretinogram, electro-oculogram, and visual evoked potential (Leibu et al., 2006)
Optic nerve damage	Optic nerve head stereophotography, confocal scanning laser ophthalmoscopy, scanning laser polarimetry, and optical coherence tomography to distinguish normal eyes from those with early to moderate glaucomatous visual field defects (Greaney et al., 2002)

Modified from Wilhelmus KR. 2001. The Draize eye test. *Surv Ophthalmol.* 45:493–515.

As shown in Table 15-4, there are many morphological tests that can be performed with dye confirming damage. Electrical examinations also indicate morphological alterations that may not be picked up easily by visual methods. In animals, histopathologies can be assessed. Tissue and cell function can be assessed for physiology of the cells or the whole organism reaction (e.g., blinking, tearing). Cell cultures can be assessed for morphological changes and viability. Apoptotic cells can also be assessed by flow cytometry. Adhesion, proliferative responses to injury, membrane integrity, and metabolism can also be determined. Uptake of precursors may give the DNA, RNA, and protein synthesis profile of a cell experiencing serious toxicity. Expression of stress-response or inflammatory factors can be performed as well. Wound healing may be assessed. However, care must be taken to see how wound healing and scarring may lead to deficits in visual acuity. Toxicologists may also model the effects via QSARs for well-known functions and structurally related toxicants (Wilhelmus, 2001). Human volunteers or patients have various imaging devices that can assess where the damage is occurring (Greaney et al., 2002) and a variety of electrical measures to confirm the functional damage (Leibu et al., 2006). There are also forms and simple stains that help a clinician assess the problem a patient may be having from an accidental or occupational exposure to toxic chemicals, such as the Ocular Surface Disease Index (OSDI) questionnaire (vision-related function, ocular symptoms, environmental triggers); National Eye Institute Visual Functioning Questionnaire (NEI VFQ-25); the McMonnies Dry Eye Questionnaire; the Short Form-12 (SF-12) Health Status Questionnaire; and an ophthalmic examination including Schirmer tests, tear breakup time, and fluorescein; and lissamine green staining (Schiffman et al., 2000). The classic ophthalmic examination gives some conclusive evidence of dramatic injury. Additionally, a color vision panel may indicate more subtle retinal damage (Lanthony 1978). Although vision tests were first designed to look for surface irritation or damage, they have evolved to include systemic toxicity that affects visual perception. Human cell lines may offer an alternative approach to testing ocular irritants (Kruszewski et al., 1997).

Questions

1. Why is a burn from alkaline substances such as concrete more dangerous than one caused by acid?
2. How can one differentiate between irritant contact dermatitis and allergic contact dermatitis?
3. Why do steroids generate acne?
4. Why do some anticoagulants or anticancer drugs cause hair loss?
5. Link the following reactions to their mechanisms:

Diseases	Letter(s) of Mechanism(s)	Possible Mechanistic Choices
(1) toxic epidermal necrosis	_____	(a) IgA autoimmune response
(2) pemphigus	_____	(b) chemokines
(3) maculopapular eruptions	_____	(c) + CD4 T-lymphocytes
(4) fixed drug reactions	_____	d) CD8(+) intraepidermal T cells
	_____	(e) epidermal cell apoptosis.

6. How does UV-B light yield skin cancers?
7. Why does skin coloration indicate some toxicities?
8. Why is Cr(III) not absorbed well, yet Cr(VI) is?
9. How is acute skin toxicity different from a skin sensitization test?
10. Corneal damage involves UV light and oxygen. What is the protection offered in corneal cells?
11. What are the major causes of cataracts?
12. Why do cardiac glycosides affect color vision?
13. Ethanol and methanol cause optic nerve damage via toxic metabolites. How is damage by carbon disulfide and other similar agents characterized?
14. Which metals are famous for affecting central sensory processing, including alterations/lesions in the central visual system?
15. Why does the Draize test mainly test acute damage to external structures of the eye?

References

Aasly JO. 2007. Thallium intoxication with metallic skin discoloration. *Neurology.* 68:1869.

Ahmadi H, Durrant CAT, Sarraf KM, Jawad M. 2008. Chemical burns: a review. *Curr Anaesth Crit Care.* 19:282–286.

Alexander J. 2007. Selenium. *Novartis Found Symp.* 282:143–149.

American Conference of Governmental Industrial Hygienists. 2015. TLV®/BEI® development process. https://www.acgih.org/tlv-bei-guidelines/policies-procedures-presentations/tlv-bei-development-process.

Arslan M, Vurucu S, Balamtekin N, Unay B, Akin R, Kurt I, Ozcan O. 2009. The effects of biotin supplementation on serum and liver tissue biotinidase enzyme activity and alopecia in rats which were administrated to valproic acid. *Brain Dev.* 31:405–410.

Attaran RR, Probst F. 2002. Histamine fish poisoning: a common but frequently misdiagnosed condition. *Emerg Med J.* 19:474–475.

Baget-Bernaldiz M, Soler Lluis N, Romero-Aroca P, Traveset-Maeso A. 2008. [Optical coherence tomography study in tamoxifen maculopathy]. *Arch Soc Esp Oftalmol.* 83:615–618.

Bajaj AK, Saraswat A. 2006. Systemic contact dermatitis. *Indian J Dermatol Venereol Leprol.* 72:99–102.

Bantseev V, McCanna DJ, Driot JY, Sivak JG. 2008. The effects of toxicological agents on the optics and mitochondria of the lens and the mitochondria of the corneal epithelium. *Semin Cell Dev Biol.* 19:150–159.

Basketter DA, Whittle E, Griffiths HA, York M. 1994. The identification and classification of skin irritation hazard by a human patch test. *Food Chem Toxicol.* 32:769–775.

Bergfeld WF. 1998. Retinoids and hair growth. *J Am Acad Dermatol.* 39:S86–S89.

Bergfeld WF, McMahon JT. 1987. Identification of foreign metallic substances inducing hyperpigmentation of skin: light microscopy, electron microscopy and x-ray energy spectroscopic examination. *Adv Dermatol.* 2:171–183.

Bickers DR, Athar M. 2006. Oxidative stress in the pathogenesis of skin disease. *J Invest Dermatol.* 126:2565–2575.

Breathnach SM. 1995. Mechanisms of drug eruptions: Part I. *Australas J Dermatol.* 36:121–127.

Bress WC, Bidanset JH. 1991. Percutaneous in vivo and *in vitro* absorption of lead. *Vet Hum Toxicol.* 33:212-214.

Browning DJ. 2004. Bull's-eye maculopathy associated with quinacrine therapy for malaria. *Am J Ophthalmol.* 137:577–579.

Buist HE, Schaafsma G, van de Sandt JJ. 2009. Relative absorption and dermal loading of chemical substances: consequences for risk assessment. *Regul Toxicol Pharmacol.* 54:221-228.

Burnett JW. 1991. Clinical manifestations of jellyfish envenomation. *Hydrobiologia.* 216–217:629–635.

Canadian Centre for Occupational Safety and Health. 2015. Dermatitis, irritant contact. http://www.oshcanada.com/oshanswers/diseases/dermatitis.html.

Carpenter KD. 1993. A comprehensive review of cyanosis. *Crit Care Nurse.* 13:66–72.

Carrotte-Lefebvre I, Delaporte E, Mirabel X, Piette F. 2003. [Radiation-induced skin reactions (except malignant tumors)]. *Bull Cancer.* 90:319–325.

Carter JE. 2007. Anterior ischemic optic neuropathy and stroke with use of PDE-5 inhibitors for erectile dysfunction: cause or coincidence? *J Neurol Sci.* 262:89–97.

Carver MP, Riviere JE. 1989. Percutaneous absorption and excretion of xenobiotics after topical and intravenous administration to pigs. *Fundam Appl Toxicol.* 13:714–722.

Castaneda CP, Brandenburg NA, Bwire R, Burton GH, Zeldis JB. 2009. Erythema multiforme/Stevens-Johnson syndrome/toxic epidermal necrolysis in lenalidomide-treated patients. *J Clin Oncol.* 27:156–157.

Cejka C, Plátenik J, Guryca V, Sirc J, Michálek J, Brůnová B, Cejková J. 2007. Light absorption properties of the rabbit cornea repeatedly irradiated with UVB rays. *Photochem Photobiol.* 83:652–657.

Chan HH, Wing Y, Su R, Van Krevel C, Lee S. 2000. A control study of the cutaneous side effects of chronic lithium therapy. *J Affect Disord.* 57:107–113.

Cheruvattath R, Orrego M, Gautam M, Byrne T, Alam S, Voltchenok M, Edwin M, Wilkens J, Williams JW, Vargas HE. 2006. Vitamin A toxicity: when one a day doesn't keep the doctor away. *Liver Transpl.* 12:1888–1891.

Coenraads PJ, Brouwer A, Olie K, Tang N. 1994. Chloracne. Some recent issues. *Dermatol Clin.* 12:569–576.

Colorado Department of Public Health and Environment Consumer Protection Division. 2001. 6 CCR 1010-22. State Board of Health rules and regulations for body art establishments. (Adopted July 18, 2001, effective August 30, 2001). https://www.colorado.gov/pacific/sites/default/files/Rules%20and%20Regulations%20for%20Body%20Art%20Establishments.pdf.

de Benito-Llopis L, Alió JL, Ortiz D, Teus MA, Artola A. 2009. Ten-year follow-up of excimer laser surface ablation for myopia in thin corneas. *Am J Ophthalmol.* 147:768–73, 773.e1–2.

Dereure O. 2001. Drug-induced skin pigmentation. Epidemiology, diagnosis and treatment. *Am J Clin Dermatol.* 2:253–262.

Derman RJ. 1995. Effects of sex steroids on women's health: implications for practitioners. *Am J Med.* 98:137S–143S.

Du L, Neis MM, Ladd PA, Keeney DS. 2006. Differentiation-specific factors modulate epidermal CYP1-4 gene expression in human skin in response to retinoic acid and classic aryl hydrocarbon receptor ligands. *J Pharmacol Exp Ther.* 319:1162–1171.

Dubakiene R, Kupriene M. 2006. Scientific problems of photosensitivity. *Medicina (Kaunas).* 42:619–624.

Dvornik D. 1992. Aldose reductase inhibitors as pathobiochemical probes. *J Diabetes Complications.* 6:25–34.

Ebringer L. 1990. Interaction of drugs with extra-nuclear genetic elements and its consequences. *Teratog Carcinog Mutagen.* 10:477–501.

Edwards FL, Tchounwou PB. 2005. Environmental toxicology and health effects associated with methyl parathion exposure—a scientific review. *Int J Environ Res Public Health.* 2:430–441.

Eells JT, Henry MM, Lewandowski MF, Seme MT, Murray TG. 2000. Development and characterization of a rodent model of methanol-induced retinal and optic nerve toxicity. *Neurotoxicology.* 21:321–330.

Ejaz S, Adil M, Oh MH, Anjum SM, Ashraf M, Lim CW. 2009. Detrimental effects of cigarette smoke constituents on physiological development of extraocular and intraocular structures. *Food Chem Toxicol.* 47:1972–1979.

Endicott K. 1998. *Dartmouth Alumni Magazine.* April 1998. Available at: http://www.udel.edu/OHS/dartmouth/drtmtharticle.html (16 January 2008).

Eskes C, Cole T, Hoffmann S, Worth A, Cockshott A, Gerner I, Zuang V. 2007. The ECVAM international validation study on *in vitro* tests for acute skin irritation: selection of test chemicals. *Altern Lab Anim.* 35:603–619.

Essah PA, Wickham EP 3rd, Nunley JR, Nestler JE. 2006. Dermatology of androgen-related disorders. *Clin Dermatol.* 24:289–298.

Fasano MB. 2006. Dermatologic food allergy. *Pediatr Ann.* 35:727–731.

Fernandes A, Brites D. 2009. Contribution of inflammatory processes to nerve cell toxicity by bilirubin and efficacy of potential therapeutic agents. *Curr Pharm Des.* 15:2915–2926.

Fernández TD, Canto G, Blanca M. 2009. Molecular mechanisms of maculopapular exanthema. *Curr Opin Infect Dis.* 22:272–278.

Ferrell PB Jr., McLeod HL. 2008. Carbamazepine, HLA-B*1502 and risk of Stevens-Johnson syndrome and toxic epidermal necrolysis: US FDA recommendations. *Pharmacogenomics.* 9:1543–1546.

Foà V. 2009. The SCOEL work and decision-making process. http://www.baua.de/de/Themen-von-A-Z/Gefahrstoffe/Tagungen/Grenzwert-Tagung/pdf/Vortrag-06.pdf?__blob=publicationFile&v=3.

Fraunfelder FW, Fraunfelder FT. 2008. Central serous chorioretinopathy associated with sildenafil. *Retina.* 28:606–609.

Gaber AO, Kahan BD, Van Buren C, Schulman SL, Scarola J, Neylan JF; Sirolimus High-Risk Study Group. 2008. Comparison of sirolimus plus tacrolimus versus sirolimus plus cyclosporine in high-risk renal allograft recipients: results from an open-label, randomized trial. *Transplantation.* 86:1187–1195.

Gainers ME, Descheny L, Barthel SR, Liu L, Wurbel MA, Dimitroff CJ. 2007. Skin-homing receptors on effector leukocytes are differentially sensitive to glyco-metabolic antagonism in allergic contact dermatitis. *J Immunol.* 179:8509–8518.

George R, Clarke S, Thiboutot D. 2008. Hormonal therapy for acne. *Semin Cutan Med Surg.* 27:188–196.

Glickman RD. 2002. Phototoxicity to the retina: mechanisms of damage. *Int J Toxicol.* 21:473–490.

Gobba F, Cavalleri A. 2003. Color vision impairment in workers exposed to neurotoxic chemicals. *Neurotoxicology.* 24:693–702.

Godin AC, Dubielzig RR, Giuliano E, Ekesten B. 2000. Retinal and optic nerve degeneration in cattle after accidental acrylamide intoxication. *Vet Ophthalmol.* 3:235–239.

Goldberg AM, Maibach HI. 1998. Dermal toxicity: alternative methods for risk assessment. *Environ Health Perspect.* 106(Suppl 2):493–496.

Greaney MJ, Hoffman DC, Garway-Heath DF, Nakla M, Coleman AL, Caprioli J. 2002. Comparison of optic nerve imaging methods to distinguish normal eyes from those with glaucoma. *Invest Ophthalmol Vis Sci.* 43:140–145.

Gupta MA, Gupta AK. 2003. Psychiatric and psychological co-morbidity in patients with dermatologic disorders: epidemiology and management. *Am J Clin Dermatol.* 4:833–842.

Guyton JR. 2007. Niacin in cardiovascular prevention: mechanisms, efficacy, and safety. *Curr Opin Lipidol.* 18:415–420.

Hall AH. 2002. Chronic arsenic poisoning. *Toxicol Lett.* 128:69–72.

Hamm JT, Wilson BW, Hinton DE. 1998. Organophosphate-induced acetylcholinesterase inhibition and embryonic retinal cell necrosis in vivo in the teleost (*Oryzias latipes*). *Neurotoxicology.* 19:853–869.

Hankinson O. 2009. Repression of aryl hydrocarbon receptor transcriptional activity by epidermal growth factor. *Mol Interv.* 9:116–118.

He L, Poblenz AT, Medrano CJ, Fox DA. 2000. Lead and calcium produce rod photoreceptor cell apoptosis by opening the mitochondrial permeability transition pore. *J Biol Chem.* 275:12175–12184.

He X, Hahn P, Iacovelli J, Wong R, King C, Bhisitkul R, Massaro-Giordano M, Dunaief JL. 2007. Iron homeostasis and toxicity in retinal degeneration. *Prog Retin Eye Res.* 26:649–673.

Heully F, Reng DE, Taillandier M, Meyer D, Simon G. 1964. [Anticoagulant medication and alopecia.] *Ann Med Leg Criminol Police Sci Toxicol.* 44:474–480.

Hirata M, Kosaka H, Yoshida T. 2004. A study on the effect of lead on event-related potentials among lead-exposed workers. *Ind Health.* 42:431–434.

Hogan DJ. 2014. Irritant contact dermatitis. http://emedicine.medscape.com/article/1049353-overview

Ho G, Kumar S, Min XS, Kng YL, Loh MY, Gao S, Zhuo L. 2009. Molecular imaging of retinal gliosis in transgenic mice induced by kainic acid neurotoxicity. *Invest Ophthalmol Vis Sci.* 50:2459–2464.

Ho JC, Ng PL, Tan SH, Giam YC. 2007. Childhood linear IgA bullous disease triggered by amoxicillin-clavulanic acid. *Pediatr Dermatol.* 24:E40–E43.

Hostynek JJ. 2003. Factors determining percutaneous metal absorption. *Food Chem Toxicol.* 41:327–345.

Jimenez JJ, Roberts SM, Mejia J, Mauro LM, Munson JW, Elgart GW, Connelly EA, Chen Q, Zou J, Goldenberg C, Voellmy R. 2008. Prevention of chemotherapy-induced alopecia in rodent models. *Cell Stress Chaperones.* 13:31–38.

Johanson G. 1999:13 Criteria document for Swedish Occupational Standards: Ethylene glycol monomethyl ether and ethylene glycol monomethyl ether acetate. https://gupea.ub.gu.se/bitstream/2077/4217/1/ah1999_13.pdf

Kim JH, Kim JH, Yu YS, Min BH, Kim KW. 2009. Clusterin inhibits blood-retinal barrier breakdown in diabetic retinopathy. *Invest Ophthalmol Vis Sci.* 51(3):1659–1665.

Kobayashi A, Ando A, Tagami N, Kitagawa M, Kawai E, Akioka M, Arai E, Nakatani T, Nakano S, Matsui Y, Matsumura M. 2008. Severe optic neuropathy caused by dichloromethane inhalation. *J Ocul Pharmacol Ther.* 24:607–612.

Kruszewski FH, Walker TL, DiPasquale LC. 1997. Evaluation of a human corneal epithelial cell line as an *in vitro* model for assessing ocular irritation. *Fundam Appl Toxicol.* 36:130–140.

Kuwabara T, Quevedo AR, Cogan D. 1968. An experimental study of dichloroethane poisoning. *Arch Ophtalmol.* 79:321–330.

Labianca R, La Verde N, Garassino MC. 2007. Development and clinical indications of cetuximab. *Int J Biol Markers.* 22(1 Suppl 4):S40–S46.

Langauer-Lewowicka H, Kazibutowska Z. 1991. [Value of the studies of multimodal evoked potentials for evaluation of neurotoxic effects of combined exposure to lead, copper and zinc]. *Neurol Neurochir Pol.* 25:715–719.

Lanthony P. 1978. The desaturated panel D-15. *Doc Ophthalmol.* 46:185–189.

Laterra J, Bressler JP, Indurti RR, Belloni-Olivi L, Goldstein GW. 1992. Inhibition of astroglia-induced endothelial differentiation by inorganic lead: a role for protein kinase C. *Proc Natl Acad Sci USA.* 89:10748–10752.

Lee A. 2009. Skin manifestations of systemic disease. *Aust Fam Physician.* 38:498–505.

Leibu R, Jermans A, Hatim G, Miller B, Sprecher E, Perlman I. 2006. Hypotrichosis with juvenile macular dystrophy: clinical and electrophysiological assessment of visual function. *Ophthalmology.* 113:841–847.e3.

Leonard PA, Moatamed F, Ward JR, Piepkorn MW, Adams EJ, Knibbe WP. 1986. Chrysiasis: the role of sun exposure in dermal hyperpigmentation secondary to gold therapy. *J Rheumatol.* 13:58–64.

Li J, Tripathi RC, Tripathi BJ. 2008. Drug-induced ocular disorders. *Drug Saf.* 31:127–141.

Liu Y, Dinkin MJ, Loewenstein JI, Rizzo JF 3rd, Cestari DM. 2008. Multifocal electroretinographic abnormalities in ethambutol-induced visual loss. *J Neuroophthalmol.* 28:278–282.

Llau ME, Viraben R, Montastruc JL. 1995. [Drug-induced alopecia: review of the literature]. *Therapie.* 50:145–150.

Luo ZD, Berman HA. 1997. The influence of Pb2+ on expression of acetylcholinesterase and the acetylcholine receptor. *Toxicol Appl Pharmacol.* 145:237–245.

Luo ZD, Berman HA. 2004. Pb2+-mediated down-regulation of dihydropyridine receptors in skeletal muscle. *Toxicol Lett.* 152:167–173.

Ma Z, Piszczek G, Wingfield PT, Sergeev YV, Hejtmancik JF. 2009. The G18V CRYGS mutation associated with human cataracts increases γS-crystallin sensitivity to thermal and chemical stress. *Biochemistry.* 48:7334–7341.

Maurer T. 2007. Guinea pigs in hypersensitivity testing. *Methods.* 41:48–53.

Maurer T, Thomann P, Weirich EG, Hess R. 1975. The optimization test in the guinea-pig. A method for the predictive evaluation of the contact allergenicity of chemicals. *Agents Actions.* 5:174–179.

Merk HF, Abel J, Baron JM, Krutmann J. 2004. Molecular pathways in dermatotoxicology. *Toxicol Appl Pharmacol.* 195:267–277.

Merle H, Gérard M, Schrage N. 2008. [Ocular burns]. *J Fr Ophtalmol.* 31:723–734.

Mizukawa Y, Shiohara T. 2009. Fixed drug eruption: a prototypic disorder mediated by effector memory T cells. *Curr Allergy Asthma Rep.* 9:71–77.

Murano H, Kojima M, Sasaki K. 1993. Differences in naphthalene cataract formation between albino and pigmented rat eyes. *Ophthalmic Res.* 25:16–22.

Murata K, Grandjean P, Dakeishi M. 2007. Neurophysiological evidence of methylmercury neurotoxicity. *Am J Ind Med.* 50:765–771.

Nijhawan RI, Molenda M, Zirwas MJ, Jacob SE. 2009. Systemic contact dermatitis. *Dermatol Clin.* 27:355–364.

Nosbaum A, Vocanson M, Rozieres A, Hennino A, Nicolas JF. 2009. Allergic and irritant contact dermatitis. *Eur J Dermatol.* 19:325–332.

Occupational Safety and Health Administration. 2015. Personal protective equipment. https://www.osha.gov/SLTC/personalprotectiveequipment/index.html.

Ogawa N, Mori A, Hasebe M, Hoshino M, Saito M, Sakamoto K, Nakahara T, Ishii K. 2009. Nitric oxide dilates rat retinal blood vessels by cyclooxygenase-dependent mechanisms. *Am J Physiol Regul Integr Comp Physiol.* 297:R968–R977.

Oliwiecki S, Burton JL. 1988. Severe acne due to isoniazid. *Clin Exp Dermatol.* 13:283–284.

Orssaud C, Roche O, Dufier JL. 2007. Nutritional optic neuropathies. *J Neurol Sci.* 262:158–164.

Pappolla M, Penton R, Weiss HS, Miller CH Jr, Sahenk Z, Autilio-Gambetti L, Gambetti P. 1987. Carbon disulfide axonopathy. Another experimental model characterized by acceleration of neurofilament transport and distinct changes of axonal size. *Brain Res.* 424:272–280.

Pearlman E, Johnson A, Adhikary G, Sun Y, Chinnery HR, Fox T, Kester M, McMenamin PG. 2008. Toll-like receptors at the ocular surface. *Ocul Surf.* 6:108–116.

Peters HA, Levine RL, Matthews CG, Sauter S, Chapman L. 1986. Synergistic neurotoxicity of carbon tetrachloride/carbon disulfide (80/20 fumigants) and other pesticides in grain storage workers. *Acta Pharmacol Toxicol (Copenh).* 59 (Suppl 7):535–546.

Rojas JC, Lee J, John JM, Gonzalez-Lima F. 2008. Neuroprotective effects of near-infrared light in an in vivo model of mitochondrial optic neuropathy. *J Neurosci.* 28:13511–13521.

Sartorelli P. 2002. Dermal exposure assessment in occupational medicine. *Occup Med (Lond).* 52:151–156.

Scheinfeld N. 2009. Drug-induced acne and acneiform eruptions: a review. *Skin and Aging.* 17. http://www.skinandaging.com/content/drug-induced-acne-and-acneiform-eruptions-a-review.

Schiffman RM, Christianson MD, Jacobsen G, Hirsch JD, Reis BL. 2000. Reliability and validity of the Ocular Surface Disease Index. *Arch Ophthalmol.* 118:615–621.

Shay E, Kheirkhah A, Liang L, Sheha H, Gregory DG, Tseng SC. 2009. Amniotic membrane transplantation as a new therapy for the acute ocular manifestations of Stevens-Johnson syndrome and toxic epidermal necrolysis. *Surv Ophthalmol.* 54(6):686–696.

Shibata M, Katsuyama M, Onodera T, Ehama R, Hosoi J, Tagami H. 2009. Glucocorticoids enhance Toll-like receptor 2 expression in human keratinocytes stimulated with *Propionibacterium acnes* or proinflammatory cytokines. *J Invest Dermatol.* 129:375–382.

Shoham A, Hadziahmetovic M, Dunaief JL, Mydlarski MB, Schipper HM. 2008. Oxidative stress in diseases of the human cornea. *Free Radic Biol Med.* 45:1047–1055.

Sills MR, Zinkham WH. 1994. Methylene blue-induced Heinz body hemolytic anemia. *Arch Pediatr Adolesc Med.* 148:306–310.

Slominski A, Wortsman J. 2003. Self-regulated endocrine systems in the skin. *Minerva Endocrinol.* 28:135–143.

Srivastava AK, Gupta BN, Bihari V, Gaur JS. 1995. Generalized hair loss and selenium exposure. *Vet Hum Toxicol.* 37:468–469.

Stein KR, Scheinfeld NS. 2007. Drug-induced photoallergic and phototoxic reactions. *Expert Opin Drug Saf.* 6:431–443.

Sujak A. 2009. Interactions between canthaxanthin and lipid membranes—possible mechanisms of canthaxanthin toxicity. *Cell Mol Biol Lett.* 14:395–410.

ten Holder SM, Joy MS, Falk RJ. 2002. Cutaneous and systemic manifestations of drug-induced vasculitis. *Ann Pharmacother.* 36:130–147.

Toler SM. 2004. Oxidative stress plays an important role in the pathogenesis of drug-induced retinopathy. *Exp Biol Med (Maywood).* 229:607–615.

Ueno N, Refojo MF, Liu LH. 1982. Pharmacokinetics of the antineoplastic agent 1,3-bis(2-chloroethyl)-1-nitrosourea (BCNU) in the aqueous and vitreous of rabbit. *Invest Ophthalmol Vis Sci.* 23:199–208.

Ubels JL, Pruis RM, Sybesma JT, Casterton PL. 2000. Corneal opacity, hydration and endothelial morphology in the bovine cornea opacity and permeability assay using reduced treatment times. *Toxicol In Vitro.* 14:379–386.

Ueta M, Sotozono C, Inatomi T, Kojima K, Tashiro K, Hamuro J, Kinoshita S. 2007. Toll-like receptor 3 gene polymorphisms in Japanese patients with Stevens-Johnson syndrome. *Br J Ophthalmol.* 91:962–965.

U.S. Environmental Protection Agency. 1998. Health effects test guidelines OPPTS 870.1200 acute dermal toxicity. Washington, DC. http://nepis.epa.gov/Exe/ZyPDF.cgi/P100G6SW.PDF?Dockey=P100G6SW.PDF.

Varriale M, Salvio A, Giannattasio F, d'Errico T, Montone L, Borgia F, Gentile I, Reynaud L, Borgia G, Rossiello R, Visconti M. 2004. Intrahepatic cholestatic jaundice related to administration of ranitidine. A case report with histologic and ultramicroscopic study. *Minerva Gastroenterol Dietol.* 50:339–343.

Viaene M, Vermeir G, Godderis L. 2009. Sleep disturbances and occupational exposure to solvents. *Sleep Med Rev.* 13:235–243.

White J, Werkmeister JA, Ramshaw JA, Birk DE. 1997. Organization of fibrillar collagen in the human and bovine cornea: collagen types V and III. *Connect Tissue Res.* 36:165–174.

Widengård I, Mandahl A, Törnquist P, Wistrand PJ. 1995. Colour vision and side-effects during treatment with methazolamide. *Eye (Lond).* 9:130–135.

Wilhelmus KR. 2001. The Draize eye test. *Surv Ophthalmol.* 45:493–515.

Xu H, Chen M, Forrester JV. 2009. Para-inflammation in the aging retina. *Prog Retin Eye Res.* 28:348–368.

Yardley HJ. 1969. Sterols and keratinization. *Br J Dermatol.* 81(Suppl 2):29–38.

Yao J, Liu Y, Wang X, Shen Y, Yuan S, Wan Y, Jiang Q. 2009. UVB radiation induces human lens epithelial cell migration via NADPH oxidase-mediated generation of reactive oxygen species and up-regulation of matrix metalloproteinases. *Int J Mol Med.* 24:153–159.

Yuan H, Huang J, Cao C. 2009. Prediction of skin sensitization with a particle swarm optimized support vector machine. *Int J Mol Sci.* 10:3237–3254.

Zavalić M, Turk R, Bogadi-Sare A, Skender L. 1996. Colour vision impairment in workers exposed to low concentrations of toluene. *Arh Hig Rada Toksikol.* 47:167–175.

Zcharia E, Philp D, Edovitsky E, Aingorn H, Metzger S, Kleinman HK, Vlodavsky I, Elkin M. 2005. Heparanase regulates murine hair growth. *Am J Pathol.* 166:999–1008.

Zhang Z, Yao K, Jin C. 2009. Apoptosis of lens epithelial cells induced by high concentration of glucose is associated with a decrease in caveolin-1 levels. *Mol Vis.* 15:2008–2017.

Zhao G, Ding M, Zhang B, Lv W, Yin H, Zhang L, Ying Z, Zhang Q. 2008. Clinical manifestations and management of acute thallium poisoning. *Eur Neurol.* 60:292–297.

Zuchlich JA. 1998. The cornea—ultraviolet action spectrum for photokeratitis. In: *Measurement of optical radiation hazards,* ed. D. Sliney, 143–160. Oberschleißheim: International Commission for Non-ionizing Radiation Protection.

CHAPTER 16

Gastrointestinal System Toxicity and Oral Exposure (GI Tract, Pancreas, Liver)

This is a chapter outline intended to guide and familiarize you with the content to follow.

I. Gastrointestinal (GI) system

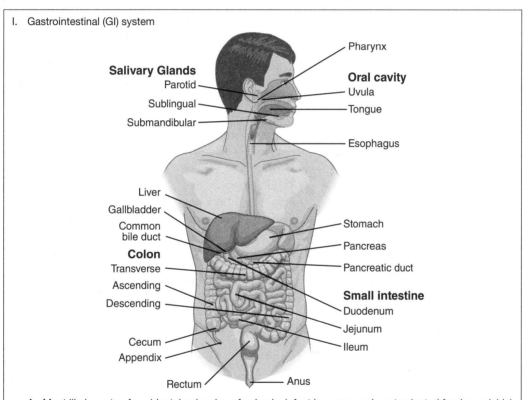

A. Most likely route of accidental poisoning of animals, infant humans, and contaminated food or suicidal ingestions

B. Damage to GI structures (proximal → distal)—see Table 16-1

   1. Mouth

      a. Teeth—stain with food products (coffee, tea), tetracycline, chlorhexidine (in prescription mouthwash), fluoride; TCDD arrests molar development (AhR stimulation → apoptosis) and formation of enamel; cleft palate caused by cell cycle progression and proliferation disruption (TCDD, mycotoxin, glucocorticoids, secalonic acid, retinoic acid)

CONCEPTUALIZING TOXICOLOGY 16-1

2. Bone—osteonecrosis of jaw by bisphosphonates via ↑ infection, ischemia, low bone turnover, direct bone toxicity, soft tissue toxicity

3. Tongue—discoloration by V_2O_5, edema by 30% H_2O_2; paralysis of tongue = D-tubocurarine (reversible) and *Clostridium botulinum* toxin (months to reversal due to destroyed mechanisms of ACh release or fatal)

   a. Mucositis—anticancer medications

   b. Strong H_2O_2 solutions (> 30%) → irritation and burns and tissue emphysema (blood or tissue protein contact) → hypoxanthine-guanine phosphoribosyltransferase mutations in human T lymphocytes (genotoxicity)

   c. Radiation → dry mouth, sore throat, altered taste, dental decay, voice quality alterations, chewing and swallowing difficulties (salivary glands affected) → cancer; ethanol (via ADH) → acetaldehyde → cancer; tobacco (via CYP) → active metabolites → cancer

   d. Anticholinergic medications also lead to dry mouth

   e. Bitter yields reflex rejection due to bitter taste receptors (quinine) or high concentration of salt/acid (affect K^+ channels)

   f. Mercury leads to gingivitis (one of triad of symptoms of Hg poisoning) → damage to salivary gland DNA

4. Esophagus

   a. See 1 g for effects of radiation on swallowing

   b. Bullae and vesicles in mouth caused by anticancer medication methotrexate leads to difficulties in swallowing

   c. Anticholinergic atropine → inhibits cough reflex in dogs

   d. Strong acids and alkali (pH > 11.5) → strictures which inhibit swallowing

   e. NSAIDs exacerbates gastric reflux or KCl + quinidine → strictures → cytokine-mediated esophagitis → leads to esophageal cancer

   f. Antibiotic tetracycline → transient, self-limiting esophagitis

   g. Bisphosphonates → severe injury when taken by person without water who then lies down

   h. Oxidative stress → lipid peroxidation (malondialdehyde) and ↓ SOD → esophageal mucosa injury

   i. Bile acids → ROS and RNS induction → DNA damage with short-term apoptosis and long term apoptosis resistance → cancers of esophagus, stomach, small intestine, liver, biliary tract, pancreas, and colon/rectum

   j. Hyperglycemia due to diabetes mellitus induced by natural chemical streptozotocin → RNS → nitrosative stress (peroxynitrite) + glycoconjugates of epithelial barrier → esophageal injury

   k. Mycophenolic acid (immunosuppressant) → apoptosis and GI disturbances

   l. Ethanol via ADH → acetaldehyde (and worse with CYP activation of tobacco products) → G:C > T:A transversions → TP53 mutations (exons 4–10) → oral and esophageal cancers

5. Stomach

   a. NSAIDs (via COX inhibition and ↓ formation of PGE2 and PGI_2 resulting in less mucus and increased acid and pepsin secretion) or *Helicobacter pylori* infection (H_2S generation usually anti-inflammatory and cytoprotective but actually proinflammatory in the presence of *H. pylori* + NO generation through macrophage L-arginine/nitric oxide pathway → nitrosating compounds) → ulcers (type I–IV) + duodenal ulcers

   b. Formation of nitrosamines from nitrates → nitrites and cancer (prevented by antioxidants); isothiocyanates in cruciferous vegetables protect gastric mucosal cells from genotoxicity related to *H. pylori* infection

   c. Chronic ethanol damage to stomach prevented by lupeol and NAC (restore non-protein sulfhydryl depletion), however this gastroprotection reversed by COX inhibition (indomethacin) or NO-synthase inhibition (L-NAME), Ca^{2+} also plays a role in ethanol toxicity as indicated by action of Ca^{2+}-channel blockers

CONCEPTUALIZING TOXICOLOGY 16-1 (*continued*)

d. Three models of stomach ulceration: HCl/ethanol $\pm$ omeprazole (proton pump inhibitor to prevent acid secretion); indomethacin (strong NSAID) + bethanechol (muscarinic agonist); mice undergoing cold stress

e. Cancer from thiophenes in coal-tar fumes; road workers exposed to bitumen fumes → overexpression of TNF-related apoptosis-inducing ligand, DR5 death receptor, and caspase-3 and TUNEL

6. Duodenal toxicity

a. Acute ethanol administration ↑ lipid absorption, while chronic ethanol use ↓ lipid absorption and interferes with Na^+ and H_2O absorption due to ↓ ATP and effects on ATPase and secretion of antidiuretic hormone; EtOH also ↑ Mg^{2+} and ↓ Ca^{2+} absorption and causes necrosis of villus epithelium + lymphocyte and plasma cell infiltration

b. Cancer chemotherapy agents → DNA strand breaks, clonogenic death of basal epithelial cells, ↑ ROS → lipid peroxidation → NF-κB, Wnt, p53 signaling pathways → ceramide pathway → cell death and activated macrophage metalloproteinases; TNF can amplify NF-κB signaling → MAPK signaling → signal overload and ulceration → bacterial invasion → cytokine inflammation or sepsis; anticancer drug methotrexate also damages via nitrosative stress

c. NSAIDs still damage the duodenum via COX-1 inhibition

d. Immunosuppressive medication mycophenolate mofetil → ulcerative esophagitis, reactive gastropathy, duodenal and ileal graft-versus-host disease

e. Heavy metals compete for absorption in this part of the small bowel → transport across luminal membrane → transport across basolateral membrane (this portion determines residence time in mucosal epithelial cytoplasm → mucosal sloughing); Ca^{2+} mainly absorbed here; Hg^{2+} absorbed in proximal jejunum; Zn^{2+} mainly absorbed in jejunum and ilium; selenomethionine absorbed in entire intestinal tract

(1) Pb → tissue desiccation and mucosal damage (damage from neurotoxicity)

(2) Hg → sloughing of intestinal mucosa + edema in capillary walls (also affects hematopoiesis) → shock and peripheral vascular collapse (high Hg levels; death usually neurotoxicity)

(3) Cr(VI) → oral cancer in rats, small intestine cancer in mice

(4) Carcinogenic sodium arsenite → stimulates pregnane X receptor and forms heterodimer with retinoid X receptor α → induces CYP3A4

(5) Iron transport mediated by intramembrane divalent metal transporter 1 and then by ferroportin (concentrates in liver)

f. Accidental ingestion of plastic hardener methyl ethyl ketone peroxide → oxidative damage → ulceration of proximal GI tract (death from liver necrosis)

g. Bacterial and fungal toxins—*Clostridium perfringens* β-toxin → hemorrhagic luminal fluid in small intestine (mainly jejunum and ilium); *Staphylococcus aureus* toxins A–E + enterotoxins G and I → toxic shock; *Fusarium* mycotoxins → ↓ villus height in turkey duodenum

h. Immune reactivity—LPS → ↓ duodenal and ileal proline transport in Meishan pigs (not Yorkshire), ↑ glycyl sarcosine transport in both pig breeds

7. Jejunum

a. In this region, nutrient mineral deficiencies (i.e., Fe) increase carcinogenic Ni absorption due to less Ni export from jejunal mucosa

b. D-glucose addition to mucosal side of voltage clamped intestinal sections yielded highest current increases in jejunum—interference with glucose transport by deoxynivalenol or vomitoxin most important here and duodenum; Cd inhibits D-galactose transport in the presence of Ca; also transports toxic glycosides such as prunasin from amygdalin

c. Ouabain or vanadium inhibition of $3Na^+,2K^+$-ATPase leads to ↓ amino acid and H_2O transport

d. Jejunum produces more ROS and RNS than many other organs (duodenum, kidney, ileum, blood, cerebellum, brain, heart, liver), so GSH important

CONCEPTUALIZING TOXICOLOGY 16-1 (*continued*)

8. Ileum

    a. Bacterial toxins—this region and jejunum succumbs to *C. perfringens* type A toxin in chickens due to contaminated wheat- and barley-based diets; *S. aureus* α toxin and *C. perfringens* NetB → jejunal and ileal necrosis; *C. difficile* toxins A (antibiotic-induced diarrhea and pseudomembranous colitis—prevented by A2A adenosine receptor agonist) and B → pathogenesis in this area; bacterial flora also can activate a cancer chemotherapy prodrug irinotecan → toxic SN-38 via β-glucuronidase activity → diffuse small and large intestinal damage (higher flora in large bowel in normal humans); cholera toxin → secretory diarrhea (controlled by 2-thioxo-4-thiozolidinone cystic fibrosis transmembrane conductance regulator)

    b. Endotoxin or LPS decrease jejunal radical formation and activate phospholipase A_2 → increased permeability of ileal wall to bacterial invasion and sepsis; high concentrations of the herbicide glyphosate also increases permeability and disrupt actin cytoskeleton; Cd^{2+} also disrupts the paracellular barrier increasing its own absorption and toxicity

    c. Okadaic acid → tumor-promoting specific cell-permeating inhibitor of protein phosphatases → diarrhetic shellfish poisoning and genotoxicity in ileum, liver and kidney

    d. Immune system—IP injection of zymosan → neutrophil migration → increased myeloperoxidase activity in ileum and lung → IL-1 and TNF-α (controlled by TNF-α- soluble inhibitor etanercept) → ileal and pancreatic injury; depleted U ingestion → ↑ COX-2 expression, IL-1β and IL-10 → inflammation via neutrophil response (short-term hypersensitivity), but ↓ macrophage function (CCL-2 mRNA) = chronic poisoning of immune response

    e. Chronic cocaine → ischemia/infarction and hemorrhage in distal ileum

    f. Bacterial bile acids include lithocholic acid, which is prevented by vitamin D-induced metabolism by CYP3A1 and CYPA2; however, liver-derived chenodeoxycholic bile acids prevent the induction of CYP3A in rat liver and increase the toxicity of lithocholic acid

    g. Isoliquiritigenin, a licorice flavonoid → muscarinic receptor agonist-related spasmogenic action on rat stomach fundus, but an opposite Ca^{2+} channel antagonism-related spasmolytic effect on rabbit jejunum, guinea pig ileum, and atropine-treated rat stomach fundus (change in motility)

    h. Mycotoxin aflatoxin B_1 → release of ACh → ileal spasms

9. Colon

    a. Excess Fe → free radicals and lipid peroxidation → cecum and proximal colon cancer (prevented by difluoromethylornithine which inhibits ornithine decarboxylase = less polyamine synthesis for inflammation and NSAIDs as anti-inflammatory agents via COX inhibition)

    b. Dimethylhydrazine metabolized → azoxymethane → DNA methylation and cell signaling changes (upregulation of Wnt-β catenin, phospholipase A_2, MAPK) associated with colon cancer

    c. Crohn's colitis from bacterial infections, ischemia, autoimmunity → chronic inflammation and cancer

    d. Mesenteric vessel effects of alosetron, amphetamines, cocaine, ergotamine, estrogen, pseudoephedrine, sodium polystyrene, and vasopressin → colonic ischemia

    e. Colon pseudo-obstruction caused by atropine, narcotics, nifedipine, phenothiazines, tricyclic antidepressants, vincristine (↓ motility)

    f. Antibiotics → pseudomembranous colitis; ampicillin → hemorrhagic colitis

    g. Cancer chemotherapy agents → neutropenic colitis

    h. Au, α-methyldopa, and NSAIDs → cytotoxic colitis (allergic reaction, antimetabolite action or mucosal cytotoxicity)

    i. Lymphocytic colitis produced by altered immune response due to cyclo 3 fort, flutamide, lansoprazole, NSAIDs, or ticlopidine

C. Pancreatic damage—see Table 16-2

    1. Soybean trypsin inhibitor (heat labile) → pancreatic damage

    2. Ethanol → acetaldehyde → acinar atrophy and fibrosis; ↑ permeability of intestinal wall → endotoxemia and necroinflammation → stellate cell activation → progressive deterioration of pancreas

CONCEPTUALIZING TOXICOLOGY 16-1 (*continued*)

3. Choline deficiency + ethionine → ↑ IL-6 → serotonin 5-HT_{2A} receptor activation (blocked by risperidone) → necrotic pancreatitis

4. Mercaptopurine immunosuppressants → inflammatory bowel disease (IBD)

5. Estrogens → ↑ VLDL and ↓ triglyceride lipase in liver → hypertriglyceridemia → pancreatitis

6. Diuretics furosemide and hydrochlorothiazide + ACE inhibitor lisinopril → necrotizing pancreatitis

7. Medications classed by cases: class I (> 20), class II (> 10), class III (any pancreatitis); oral toxic medications may cause pancreatitis in sensitive individuals

8. Oleic acid → mitochondrial membrane dysfunction (prevented by topiramate, an antiseizure compound ↑ expression of nutrient sensor PPARα and mitochondrial fatty acid carrier CPT-1-which leads to β-oxidation of the lipid) → exocrine pancreas ↑ secretion of H_2O and HCO_3^- and endocrine ↓ insulin response to glucose

9. Alloxan reduction → dialuric acid → redox cycling → $O_2^{-\cdot}$ + ↑ cytosolic Ca^{2+} → β-cell damage → ↓ insulin

10. Streptozotocin → GLUT2 glucose transporter → gains entrance to pancreatic β-cells → alkylates DNA → activation of poly ADP-ribosylation → depletes cellular NAD^+ and ATP → ATP dephosphorylation → substrate for xanthine oxidase → $O_2^{-\cdot}$ (and Fenton to H_2O_2 + HO·); also ↑ NO-inhibiting aconitase activity → DNA damage

11. Pancreatic cancers from DNA damage in exocrine pancreas from compounds such a DMBA and other PAHs activated by cells of pancreatic duct: preneoplastic acidophilic atypical acinar cell foci and nodules → growth mediated by cholecystokinin-A receptors

12. 4-nitroquinoline-1-oxide → 4-hydroxyaminoquinoline-1-oxide metabolite → DNA adducts →↑ apoptosis and induction of p53 proliferative gene(s)

13. Rat pancreas → acinar adenomas and adenocarcinomas while human develops ductal adenocarcinomas as is seen in hamster exposed to *N,N*-dipropylnitrosamine → β-oxidation → *N*-nitrosamines

D. Liver damage—see Table 16-3

1. A study of biochemical anatomy (zones 1–3; see Figure 16-1)

a. Zone 1 = periportal = high direct and oxidative toxicity (high O_2) but high GSH

(1) Metals highest here and bile outflow in this area

(2) Fe oxidation products → lipid peroxidation

(3) Cu → generates GSSG + $O_2^{-\cdot}$ → mitochondrial ↓ Mn SOD and thiol/disulphide ratio → ↓ ATP → collapse of mitochondrial membrane potential → induction of mitochondrial permeability transition → hepatocellular apoptosis

(4) Doxorubicin reduced by CYP reductase → generates ROS → interferes with macromolecule synthesis → covalently binds to and X-links DNA, inhibits topoisomerase II, arrests cells in G^2 phase → induces apoptosis → attracts inflammatory cells → periportal fibrosis (fibrosis is precursor to cirrhosis and then liver cancer if survive the severely compromised liver function)

(5) Cisplatin → CYP activation → cross-links DNA → G^2 phase arrest → apoptosis → periportal fibrosis

(6) Methapyrilene → S-oxidation of thiophene group → depletes periportal GSH but ↑ GSH centrilobular region →↑ HO-1 and glutamate cysteine ligase catalytic subunit → apoptosis → necrosis → hepatic cancer if animal survives liver damage

(7) Allyl alcohol → model oxidation activation in periportal region

(8) Ethanol metabolized extensive periportal and inhibits gluconeogenesis decreases O_2 uptake

(9) Aflatoxin → CYP activation → diffuse and severe hydropic (intracellular edema) degeneration, bile duct hyperplasia, periportal fibrosis

(10) Dexamethasone → fat accumulation in periportal region and causes liver enlargement by increased excretion of p-glycoprotein expressed in this region → microvesicular steatosis (fatty)

CONCEPTUALIZING TOXICOLOGY 16-1 (*continued*)

(11) α-naphthyl isothiocyanate attracts neutrophils via β2-integrin CD18 → periportal inflammation, wide-spread hepatic necrosis, acute cholestatic hepatitis

b. Zone 3 = reductive metabolic radical formation (low O_2), more CYP, less GSH

(1) Fe damage from iron-supplemented vitamins → hemosiderin → centrilobular fibrosis

(2) Acetaminophen → CYP activation → N-acetyl-p-benzoquinone imine + GSH → GSH depletion, covalent adduct formation, initiates mitochondrial damage → ↓ ATP → massive centrilobular necrosis + extensive inflammatory cell infiltration; NAC protective (bolstering GSH) early but later delays recovery by impairing glucose metabolism (periportal hepatocyte vacuolation)

(3) Ethanol in this region →↑ endotoxin, plasma aminotransferase (leakage), CYP2E1, lipid peroxidation, NF-κB, TNF-α, iNOS, COX-2, procollagen-I + hypoxia generated by EtOH → acetaldehyde → Na^+ influx and decreased hepatocyte pH

(4) CCl_4 model of centrilobular necrosis, increased halogens draw electrons away from electropositive carbon → CYP2E1 → reductive dehalogenation → electron withdrawal stabilizes radical formation (carbon-centered) → necrosis + steatosis (via protein synthesis inhibition at the ribosome which is protected by cycloheximide), however if protein synthesis is inhibited then steatosis increases and necrosis decreases

(5) Tienilic acid → CYP2C9 → electrophilic reactive intermediates bind covalently to macromolecules → ↓ GSH and ↑ lipid peroxidation → upregulation of GSH synthase and glutamate-cysteine ligase (attempts to ↑ GSH synthesis), HO-1 and NAD(P)H dehydrogenase quinone 1 (oxidative stress), GSH-transferase and UDP glycosyltransferase 1A6 (phase II drug metabolism); inhibition of glutamine-cysteine ligase by buthionine-(S,R)-sulfoximine → extensive centrilobular necrosis from tienilic acid

c. Kupffer cells

(1) Produce cytokines mediating hepatic acute phase response and cholestasis to LPS in circulation → bile acid transport sensitivity resides with regulation of Ntcp by retinoid X receptor-retinoid acid receptor nuclear heterodimer and liver-enriched transcription factor hepatocyte nuclear factor 1α inhibited by cytokine release

2. Sex-linked damage

a. Female human and animals have higher rates of certain liver toxicities related to:

(1) Continuous release of growth hormone from the pituitary (vs. male stochastic release) → activate STATs (signal transducers and activators of transcription) genes

(2) Males involve DNA methylation in gene expression and ↑ CYP7B1 (oxysterol 7α-hydroxylase) expression in males represses androgen biosynthesis (↓ bioavailability of DHEA precursor to testosterone)

(3) Women who take estrogen-containing birth control → activate estrogen receptor → regulates *CYP7b1* expression → inflammation and hepatotoxicity including intrahepatic cholestasis (most frequent liver toxicity of pregnancy)

(4) PCBs, PBBs, hexachlorobenzene → induce CYP1A1 (ethoxyresorufin O-deethylase) which is already high in centrilobular region of female fats → development of uroporphyria

b. Males sensitive to liver production of vitellogenin (egg yolk protein) by environmental estrogens → hypertrophy of the fish liver; formamide → hemangiosarcoma of the liver in male mice

3. Apoptosis/necrosis

a. CYP metabolites from pharmaceuticals (especially acetaminophen and statins) → apoptosis → severe damage = necrosis—worse with ethanol

b. Diversity of damage leads to death of cells including cholestasis, viral hepatitis, ischemia or reperfusion injury, liver preservation for transplantation, and direct toxicity of medications or industrial chemicals

c. Mitochondrial permeability changes and dysfunction lead to apoptosis (requires sufficient ATP synthesis to initiate a death program through Fas → caspase cascade) or necrosis

CONCEPTUALIZING TOXICOLOGY 16-1 (*continued*)

    d. Invasion of neutrophils → centrilobular necrosis (macrophages and natural killer cells also promote injury via TNF-α, IL-1β, and NO), while monocyte infiltration (especially M2s) → phagocytosis of apoptotic cells, resolves inflammation and promotes tissue repair (via Il-10, IL-6, and IL-18)

4. Steatosis (fatty liver)

    a. Obesity, insulin resistance, ethanol → triglyceride accumulation

    b. CCl_4 especially with protein synthesis inhibitor puromycin → steatosis (↓ triglyceride secretion via VLDL and other triglyceride transfer proteins)

5. Fibrosis/cirrhosis

    a. Ethanol → macrocyte involvement (M1) and stellate liver cells, which are activate by CD8+ T cells

    b. WBCs responsible for fibrosis vary based on the development of hepatic damage

6. Neoplasms

    a. Develop from severe DNA modification or multiple insults (mutations in tumor suppressor genes [p53 mutations present in 30–60% of liver cancer patients], proto-oncogenes, and DNA mismatch genes); aflatoxin B_1 forms an epoxide via CYP → mutates p53 at codon 249 (promoter of cancer), but aflatoxin is also an initiator (does not require cirrhotic damage) and works synergistically with hepatitis B virus (incorporates in host DNA and activates promoters of several oncogenes, inhibits apoptosis, viral protein ↑ expression of epidermal growth factor receptor and potentiates TGF-α, fibrosis stimulated by upregulating expression of TGF-β, inflammation)

    b. Inflammation → fibrosis or cirrhosis or cancer (hepatitis C model)

    c. Vinyl chloride monomer → CYP oxidation to chloroethylene oxide → exocyclic etheno adducts form with DNA (and generate lipid peroxidation and oxidative stress) → promutagenic and affect proto-oncogenes and tumor suppressor genes

    d. Stimulating the AhR (dioxins and PCBs), constitutive androstane receptor (phenobarbital), or peroxisome proliferators (plasticizers = phthalates) → cancer without gene mutation (mitogens)

    e. Obesity → cancer may be due to fatty liver, gallstone development, or related to food ingredients, excessive calories, loss of protective factors due to ↓ exercise, or signaling factors from adipose tissue

7. Cytoskeleton toxicity

    a. Ethanol affects α-tubulin (hyperacetylation) and microtubule stability

    b. Macrolactones of marine toxins target actin cytoskeleton → severe hepatotoxicity

    c. Microcystins from cyanobacteria (agricultural lakes) → inhibit phosphatases 1 and 2A—disrupts cytoskeleton → hepatic hemorrhage

    d. As disrupts cytoskeleton (soundness, shape, and movement)

    e. Anticancer medication paclitaxel (diterpenoid) → binds to β-tubulin and prevents disassembly of microtubules → mitotic arrest; opposite mechanism of vinca alkaloids that prevent polymerization of microtubules by binding to β-tubulin and not allowing α-tubulin interaction → mitotic arrest (same endpoint)

8. Sinusoidal injury

    a. Binge ethanol intake + acetaminophen → cytoskeletal injury → sinusoidal epithelial cells swell and lose ability to endocytose FITC-FSA → fenestrae form → RBC penetration into Space of Disse → sinusoidal collapse and ↓ blood flow (similar to veno-occlusive disease caused by pyrrolizidine alkaloids of the toxic *Crotalaria* plant species)

9. Immune and inflammatory damage

    a. Metabolic liver injury from medications formation of active metabolites damaging organelles → initiate immune response

CONCEPTUALIZING TOXICOLOGY 16-1 (*continued*)

b. Immune liver injury from anti-medication antibodies or autoimmune antibodies are generated by anesthetic halothane or diuretic tienilic acid (rapid onset on subsequent challenge) or slow-developing autoimmunity in brown Norway rats exposed to anti-arthritis drug penicillamine or cats exposed to the medication for hyperthyroidism propylthiouracil

c. Medications such as antibiotics minocycline and nitrofurantoin, and discontinued antihypertensive medication α-methyldopa develop a condition resembling idiopathic (unknown cause) autoimmune hepatitis—may also involve autoimmune reactions resembling lupus, autoimmune-hemolytic anemia, or vasculitis as well

d. Liver prone to infiltration by immune cells (lymphocytes and neutrophils) due to two vascular supplies, lack of certain adhesion molecule (P-selectin) to prevent infiltration and presence of chemoattractant molecules/receptors (VAP1 and osteoponin among others)

e. Neutrophils generate hypochlorous acid $\rightarrow$ ROS $\rightarrow$ cell mortality

10. Cholestasis and bile duct toxicity

a. Retention of toxic bile salts due to damage to drug transporting proteins on hepatocyte canalicular membrane

b. Inhibition of ATP-dependent bile salt transport proteins $\uparrow$ damage by medications/toxicants—e.g., anti-diabetic, anti-inflammatory troglitazone + ACE inhibitor (hypertension medication) lisinopril

c. Direct damage to cholangiocytes (epithelial cells of bile duct) sustain direct damage by medications such as the antibiotic flucloxacillin

d. Usually liver cells sense toxic products of metabolism and $\uparrow$ elimination (xenobiotic receptors CAR and PXR = members of NR1I nuclear receptor family) induced by phenobarbital (as are some CYPs)

E. GI tests—see Table 16-4

1. DNA analysis of cheek swabs; micronucleus assay of buccal cells

2. ^{13}C-sucrose breath test for small intestinal sucrase activity; ^{13}CO$_2$ breath evolution test for mucositis (cancer chemotherapy and jejunal sucrase activity)

3. NSAIDs and cancer chemotherapy $\rightarrow$ GI permeability probes, oxidative phosphorylation (direct measures + mitochondrial DNA analysis), ROS formation (direct measures + COX-2 mRNA expression)

4. Cell and tissue preparations analyzed for organelle damage + biochemical measures (e.g., keratin in epithelial cells, enzyme markers for brush border, lysosomes)

5. Intact animals assessed by nutrient and toxicant absorption—compared with ulcer model of MPTP in rat, EtOH-induced colitis, 1,2-dimethylhydrazine-induced colon cancer, enterohepatic recirculation in monkey (has gall bladder)

6. Zebrafish GI motility alternative to mammalian testing

F. Pancreatic tests—see Table 16-5

1. Leakage of digestive (exocrine) enzymes amylase and lipase into plasma

2. Endocrine cell damage monitored by insulin and glucagon (β-cells and α-cells, respectively), direct examination of Islets of Langerhans cells (β-cell mass), anti-insulin antibody immunohistochemical staining, or effects of lack of insulin ($\uparrow$ blood or urine glucose or glucose tolerance test if minor damage)

3. Inflammatory reactions assessed via IL-6, TNF-α + histological grading of vacuolization, inflammation, lobular disarray, and edema

4. Pancreatic cancer from agents such as TCDD need examination of apoptotic bodies, immunohistochemistry of CYP1A1, CCK, AhR, CCKAR, amylase, proliferation of cell nuclear antigen, and development/incidence of lesions

G. Liver tests—see Table 16-6

1. Leakage of enzymes into plasma (ALT = hepatocyte necrosis and AST less indicative as may be $\uparrow$ with muscle and heart damage, body mass changes, blood diseases, and pancreatic

CONCEPTUALIZING TOXICOLOGY 16-1 (*continued*)

injury)—transaminases should be 3 × normal activity and coupled to ↑ serum bilirubin (jaundice indicative of lack of liver processing of this hemoglobin degradation product)

2. Plasma GST-α indicative of centrilobular damage as occurs with acetaminophen

3. γ-Glutamyl transpeptidase indicates hepatobiliary damage

4. Paraoxygenase-1 (metabolizes organophosphates) reduction in serum is consistent with liver injury as it is transported there by HDL (cholesterol mobilizing lipoprotein)

5. Leakage of purine nucleotide phosphorylase into hepatic sinusoids = marker for necrosis prior to ALT leakage

6. Liver mitochondrial malate dehydrogenase in plasma = necrosis and cirrhosis

7. Leakage of sorbitol dehydrogenase = necrotic liver

8. Leakage of alkaline phosphatase = cholestatic hepatobiliary injury

9. Function aspects of liver damage = ↑ ammonia (urea cycle not functional), jaundice (bilirubin not conjugated to glucuronic acid and sent on in the bile to be converted to other products by gut flora), lack of plasma proteins albumin, and clotting factors prothrombin and fibrinogen

10. Liver organ weight may be useful in assessing damage but more specific information derived from fatty tissue, glycogen, and bile acid content as does examination for periportal, midzonal, and centrilobular necrosis or random damage

11. Centrilobular hypertrophy may accompany CYP induction

12. Steatosis (fatty liver) can be microvesicular or macrovesicular

13. Liver cancer or precancerous lesions may be divided into hepatocellular alterations, hepatic hyperplasias/adenoma, or primary hepatocyte carcinoma

CONCEPTUALIZING TOXICOLOGY 16-1 (*continued*)

Oral exposure from ingesting contaminated food or water is the next most likely route of exposure after skin and eye exposure. Consider babies' instinctive behavior of putting objects in their mouths for examination. There are a number of structures that deserve closer examination here. The toxicity to absorption structures is the major focus in this chapter. It is appropriate that this chapter be reviewed after the skin chapter, because the skin and the gastrointestinal (GI) tract both have high cell turnover that can be exacerbated by conditions that cause skin (e.g., psoriasis) or GI cell sloughing (e.g. *Helicobacter pylori* infection [Abdalla et al., 1998], stress, or Crohn's disease [Boudry et al., 2007]). Two of the areas that suffer the highest toxicity on exposure to external ionizing radiation are the skin and the GI tract. The radiological treatment of prostate cancer, for example, is indeed limited by concerns of GI damage (Sefrová et al., 2009). This chapter could then warrant the same considerations as the coverage of the skin regarding mechanisms of damage and toxicity

as the GI tract is considered "external" to the body. However, the important structures in each area of the tract that involve taste and part of speech, mastication, saliva secretion, swallowing, peristalsis, acid and enzyme production and secretion, specialized absorption, and finally the portal vein processing by the first pass through the liver are essential to consider for activation of toxicants, detoxication, nutrient processing, and conversion of waste products for excretion by the kidneys. The liver is the last structure covered in this chapter, because it represents the final processing of intestinal contents prior to becoming part of the bloodstream.

Forensic Analysis of GI Damage

Table 16-1 is a forensic table for GI toxicity and liver damage resulting from portal vein transport. Note that it is separated into regions for examination of specific problems resulting from toxicity to a given area.

TABLE 16-1 Forensic Chart of GI Toxicity

GI Toxicity	Toxic Agents
Mouth	
Bone	Bisphosphonates (Reid, 2009), tetracycline, TCDD (Alaluusua and Lukinmaa, 2006), mycotoxins, secalonic acid D, cortisol, retinoic acid (Dhulipala et al., 2006)
Burns	Concentrated acids, alkali, peroxides (Naik et al., 2006)
Cancer	Radiation, tobacco, ethanol (McCullough and Farah, 2008)
Edema/irritation	Oxalates (Zhong and Wu, 2006)
Gingivitis	Inorganic mercury (Schmid et al., 2007)
Mucositis	Anticancer (Keefe and Gibson, 2007)
Muscle paralysis	Botulinum toxin (Braun, 2006)
Paresthesias (numbness)	Topical Na^+-channel blockade (local anesthetics), systemic Na^+ channel poisoning (Watkins et al., 2008)
Salivary glands	Radiation (Bhide et al., 2009), anticholinergic medications (psychotropic; Smith et al., 2008)
Esophagus	
Mucosal injury	Caustic agents, aspirin/NSAIDs (Sugimoto et al., 2010), cytokines (Souza et al., 2009), oxidative stress (Liu et al., 2009), tetracycline, KCl^+ quinidine SO_4, bisphosphonates taken without water at high doses (Zografos et al., 2009), diabetes mellitus and generation of RNS/glyco-oxidation (Zayachkivska et al., 2008)
Cancer	Acid, bile refluxes (Bernstein et al., 2009), ethanol, tobacco compounds (Szymańska, 2010)
Swallowing	Atropine (Tsubouchi et al., 2008), caustic agents and strictures (Doo et al., 2009), chemoradiotherapy (Lazarus, 2009)
Stomach	
Cancer	Nitrates forming nitroso compounds with *H. pylori* (Izzotti et al., 2009), bitumen fume condensates (Binet et al., 2002)
Hemorrhage	NSAIDs (Lim et al., 2009), *Panicum maximum* cultivars Mombasa, Tanzania, and Maasai (Cerqueira et al., 2009)
Mucosal damage	Salt (Izzotti et al., 2009), ethanol (Lira, 2009)
Ulcers	NSAIDs (Lim, 2009), *H. pylori* with mutagens (Izzotti et al., 2009)
Duodenum	
Bleeding ulcers	Aspirin (Yeomans et al., 2009)
Cancer	Cr(VI) (Stout et al., 2009)
CYP expression	As and metabolites (Medina-Díaz et al., 2009)
Graft versus host disease	Mycophenolate mofetil (Parfitt et al., 2008)
Hemorrhage	*Clostridium perfringens* beta-toxin (Vidal et al., 2008)
Malabsorption of nutrients	Ethanol (Krawitt, 1977), avidin (White et al., 1992)
Mucositis	Anticancer, radiation (Sonis, 2009b)

TABLE 16-1   Forensic Chart of GI Toxicity (*continued*)

GI Toxicity	Toxic Agents
Duodenum (*continued*)	
Nitrosative stress	Methotrexate (Kolli et al., 2008)
Sloughing	Acute mercury poisoning (Iino et al., 2009)
Ulcers	Methyl ethyl ketone peroxide (van Enckevort et al., 2008)
Villus height reduction	*Fusarium* mycotoxins (Girish and Smith, 2008)
Jejunum	
Glutathione depletion	Buthionine sulfoximine (Mårtensson et al., 1990)
Increased toxicant absorption	Fe deficiency increasing Ni absorption (Müller-Fassbender et al., 2003)
Inhibited transport of simple sugars	Deoxynivalenol (Awad et al., 2007), Cd (Mesonero et al., 1996)
Nerve-mediated Na and fluid loss	Ethanol (Hallbäck et al., 1990)
ROS and RNS	Intrinsically high and decreased by endotoxin challenge (Kozlov et al., 2003)
Sodium-potassium	Ouabain, vanadium (vanadate; Hajjar et al., 1989)
ATPase inhibition	
Transport of toxic glycosides	Prunasin (amygdalin metabolite; Strugala et al., 1995)
Ileum	
Acetylcholine release	Aflatoxin B_1 (Luzi et al., 2002)
Antagonism at Ca^{2+} channels	Isoliquiritigenin (Chen, Zhu, et al., 2009)
Bacterial prodrug activation	Irinotecan (Brandi et al., 2006)
CYP3A expression	Chenodeoxycholic acid enhance toxicity of lithocholic acid (Khan et al., 2010)
Enteritis	*Clostridium perfringens* type A toxins (Cooper and Songer, 2009), *Clostridium difficile* toxin A (Cavalcante et al., 2006)
Genotoxicity	Okadaic acid (Le Hégarat et al., 2006)
Inflammatory alterations	Depleted uranium (Dublineau et al., 2007)
Ischemia, infarction, and hemorrhage	Cocaine (Lingamfelter and Knight, 2010)
Multiple-organ dysfunction syndrome	Zymosan induction of TNF-α (Malleo et al., 2008)
Permeability changes/sepsis	Luminal phospholipase A2 activation by LPS (Zayat et al., 2008), glyphosate (Vasiluk et al., 2005), Cd^{2+} (Duizer et al., 1999)
Colon	
Cancer/clastogenesis	*N*-nitroso compounds (Pearson et al., 2009)
Cancer/lipid peroxidation	Fe (Lund et al., 2001)
Cancer/polyamine synthesis and inflammation	Single nucleotide polymorphism in ornithine decarboxylase promoter (Rial et al., 2009)
Chloride secretion	Trimethyltin chloride (Yu et al., 2009)
Colitis models	Dextran sodium sulfate (Whittem et al., 2010) 2,4,6-trinitrobenzene sulfonic acid (Fichtner-Feigl et al., 2008)
Cytotoxicity	Cobalt-doped tungsten carbide nanoparticle suspensions (Bastian et al., 2009)
DNA methylation/cell signaling	Dimethylhydrazine/azoxymethane (Davidson et al., 2009; Likhachev et al., 1978;

Mouth Toxicity

Dentists can provide information about what might be toxic to structures in the mouth. The dental profession is concerned with the combined effects of high sugar on mouth bacteria and the degradation of teeth by low-pH beverages (carbonic acid) such as soda pop. Certain compounds also discolor teeth. Coffee, tea, and red wine can discolor teeth, as does the use of tobacco products. The antibiotic tetracycline binds strongly to calcium and can produce a blue-gray stain. Fluoride used by dentists to guard against tooth decay also can stain from chalky white to brown. Minocycline similarly stains teeth a green/grey or blue/gray. This discoloration appears to be permanent. Another antibiotic of the quinolones, ciprofloxacin, has caused a greenish discoloration of teeth if given to infants prior to teething. Chlorhexidine used in prescription antiseptic mouthwashes cause yellow-brown stains. Iron can also stain the teeth and cause colon cancer or liver damage depending on the dose (Addy and Moran, 1985). The tongue may be discolored from systemic poisoning; for example, green tongue is observed in workers heavily exposed to vanadium pentoxide (Kawai et al., 1989). More disturbing than coloration changes alone, certain compounds cause cancer and disturb tooth and enamel development. 2,3,7,8-Tetrachlorodibenzo-p-dioxin (TCDD) through the aryl hydrocarbon receptor (AhR) and epidermal growth factor receptor increases apoptosis of cells. In the developing rat (or Finnish children), mineralization of teeth is decreased by TCDD exposure resulting in arrests in molar development. Polychlorinated dibenzodioxins/polychlorinated dibenzofurans (PCDDs/PCDFs) appear to affect the formation of the protective enamel layer of teeth (Alaluusua and Lukinmaa, 2006). Some chemicals also disturb proper developmental bone fusion in the mouth. Cleft palate results from chemicals that disrupt cell-cycle progression and proliferation such as TCDD, mycotoxin, secalonic acid D, glucocorticoids, and retinoic acid (Dhulipala et al., 2006).

It is appropriate to look at the mouth for the first signs of toxicity or DNA damage, because it represents the route for ingestion and inhalation. Because 90% of all cancers originate from epithelial cells, it is worth examining the oral epithelium. It has four layers: the lamina propria composed of connective tissue, stratum basale or the basal cell layer, the stratum spinosum or prickle cell layer, and the keratinized layer at the surface. Rete pegs project from the lamina propria into the epidermal layer. The basal cell layer has a high mitosis rate, producing new cells that migrate to the surface to replace those shed from continual use. It has CYPs and is capable of activating/metabolizing toxic compounds. This can transform the stem cells in the basal layer, which can be examined for chromosome breakage and loss (Holland et al., 2008). Mucosal injury or mucositis occurs dramatically as mouth ulcers or diarrhea in lower parts of the GI tract with targeted anticancer therapies (Keefe and Gibson, 2007). Because teeth- whitening products contain either hydrogen peroxide or carbamide peroxide, toxicity is of concern for repeated use of high concentrations in the mouth. Animal studies have shown that 30% H_2O_2 causes severe irritation or burns. If the peroxide comes in contact with blood or tissue proteins, the effervescence releases oxygen and causes tissue emphysema. Thirty percent H_2O_2 results in edema of the tongue and subsequent intraepithelial and subepithelial vesiculation. Hydrogen peroxide rinses can result in mouth irritation, dryness, loss of taste, elongation of filiform papillae, and diffuse mucosal whitening. Cellular studies indicate that 0.34–1.35 µM H_2O_2 induces a dose-dependent increase in hypoxanthine-guanine phosphoribosyltransferase mutations in human T lymphocytes and other measures of increased genotoxicity (cytokinesis block micronucleus assay and sister chromatid exchanges [Naik et al., 2006]).

Some plants have a high concentration of nonsoluble calcium oxalate crystals including *Anthurium* species, *Arisaema* species, *Caladium bicolor, Zantedeschia* species, *Aglaonema* species, *Dieffenbachia* species, *Monstera deliciosa, Syngonium podophyllum, Philodendron* species, *Epipremnum aureum*, and *Symplocarpus foetidus*. The stalk of the *Dieffenbachia* plant is the most potent it this regard. Oxalate needlelike crystals produce pain and edema when an animal tries to ingest the toxic plant (lips, tongue, oral mucosa) or if they contact their face (conjunctiva or skin). The oxalates cause direct trauma from physical action of the crystals resulting in edema and secondarily from bradykinins and enzymes released from the plant cells (Zhong and Wu, 2006).

Radiation for head and neck cancer in humans may induce dry mouth or xerostomia, sore throat, altered taste, dental decay, changes in voice quality, and impaired chewing and swallowing leading to decreased nutritional intake and weight loss. This is due to damage to the parotid (purely serous and produces most of saliva in stimulated state) and submandibular glands (predominantly serous with 10% mucus-secreting acini and produces most of saliva in unstimulated state) responsible for most of salivary flow. The salivary glands contain secretory units consisting of acinar cells (secrete serous/protein and mucous/mucin portions of saliva), myoepithelial cells, intercalated duct, striated duct, and excretory duct. Parasympathetic stimulation via acetylcholine release to postsynaptic M3 muscarinic receptors activates inositol-1,4, 5-trisphosphate, which mobilizes intracellular calcium stores, triggering a watery saliva flow low in amylase for digestion of polysaccharides from acinar cells. Sympathetic activation via β_2 adrenergic receptors activates protein kinase A throughout the cAMP pathway and causes exocytosis of secretory granules (scant, viscous saliva) high in amylase. Salivary flow reductions (50–70% after 10–16 Gy radiation) or loss (after 40–42 Gy radiation) is a phased process, which has been studied in the rat. Days 0–10 or phase I cause a 40% reduction in water without altering amylase secretion or producing cell loss. In 10–120 days, plasma membrane destruction leads to acinar cell death and lack of amylase secretion. Progenitor cell and stem cell death occur during phase III (120–240 days). Radiation changes the saliva to thick, tenacious, and acidic. Additional chemotherapy (not cetuximab, which is an epidermal growth factor receptor inhibitor) results in increased acute toxicity, especially for mucositis (Bhide et al., 2009). Another reason for dry mouth can be the effect of anticholinergic compounds like atropine (used for dental surgery for that reason) or

the adverse effects of psychotropic medications (Smith et al., 2008).

Radiation is also a predisposing factor to oral cancer as any dental patient is made aware during their cancer screening for chronic cumulative effects of dental X-rays. Also, it makes sense that because CYPs are present in the cells of the mouth, tobacco chewing or smoking also lead to activated metabolites that result in oral carcinogenesis. Many people do not know that their antiseptic mouthwashes or the consumption of ethanol and tobacco increases the risk of oral cancers. Those who smoke and drink alcohol increase the penetration of the oral mucosa by the carcinogens in smoke in the presence of ethanol. Ethanol can eliminate the lipid component of the barrier present in the oral cavity and increase the permeability of the human ventral tongue mucosa. Chronic ethanol exposure results in epithelial atrophy and decreased basal cell size in rat esophageal mucosa and hyper-regeneration, making the tissues more sensitive to chemical carcinogens. Short-term exposure of rabbit oral mucosa to ethanol caused dysplastic changes with keratoses (premalignant lesions), increased density of basal cell layer, and increased mitotic figures. Alcohol dehydrogenase present both in the epithelial cells and in people with aerobic oral flora including *Streptococcus salivarius*, *S. intermedius*, and *S. mitis* produce high amounts of the primary metabolite of ethanol, acetaldehyde. Acetaldehyde is mutagenic and appears to be covalently bound to protein and DNA in patients with oral cancer and dysplasia, with lipid peroxidation products as well (McCullough and Farah, 2008).

Bone toxicity may result from some toxicants and medications. Bisphosphonates (zoledronate and/or pamidronate) used in cancer management cause osteonecrosis of the jaw. They probably do so via increased infection, ischemia (decreased proliferation of endothelial cells), low bone turnover, direct toxicity to the bone (inhibition of farnesyl pyrophosphate synthase in the mevalonate and ultimately cholesterol result in apoptosis in osteoclasts), and toxicity to soft tissue. Non-osteoclasts may suffer toxicity through inhibition of the mevalonate pathway in the absence of a bone surface.

The presence of a bone surface adjacent to the soft tissue may cause toxicity due to binding and accumulation of the bisphosphonate at the bone surface (Reid, 2009).

Muscle paralysis may result from a variety of toxicants including D-tubocurarine. However, ingestion of the toxin from *Clostridium botulinum* is first indicated by paralysis of the tongue and the muscles of mastication, although death comes from respiratory paralysis (Braun, 2006).

Taste is a discriminator used by a variety of species for initial indication of toxicity. A bitter taste results in reflex rejection. What is bitter taste though? A physiology book might indicate that bitter taste results from blocking potassium channels and downstream activation of a G protein known as transducin. It appears that bitter ligands activate "B-best" neurons in the nucleus of the solitary tract and parabrachial nucleus (PBN). However, the PBN B-best units are activated by intense salt and acid. This indicates a strong bitter rejection that can result from a compound such as quinine due to its bitter nature or a high concentration of salt/acid (Travers and Geran, 2009).

Some systemic toxicities are also diagnosed by signs from damage to mouth cells. A likely example is the "mad hatter's" disease experienced by occupational exposure of workers in the felt hat industry to mercury nitrate. The triad for determining exposure is gingivitis or gum disease, tremor, and erethism or an abnormal form of excitability. Although this represents mainly a neurotoxic action of inorganic mercury, silver-colored amalgam fillings for cavities contain mercury in an inorganic state that can evolve by volatilization or physical grinding and corrosion. Chronic exposure to mercury vapor and/or inorganic mercury leads to oral cavity lesions, tremor, decreased coordination, decreased sensation, and psychiatric symptoms including anxiety, excessive timidity, and pathological fear of ridicule (note triad of symptoms is part of this overall picture). Although methyl mercury has been viewed as more toxic, inorganic mercury can damage salivary gland DNA (Schmid et al., 2007).

Some toxicants cannot be deciphered by taste. Sodium-channel blockade by local anesthetics (as used in dental work) can cause loss of feeling on the lips, mouth, and other oral structures. Brevetoxins (10 lipid-soluble cyclic polyethers) from the dinoflagellate *Karenia brevis* cause neurotoxic shellfish poisoning by binding to receptor site 5 on the voltage-gates sodium channel and induce a channel-mediated sodium influx. Nausea and vomiting occur with paresthesias (burning or tingling sensations) or numbness of mouth, lips, and tongue (and distal paresthesias, ataxia, slurred speech, and dizziness [Watkins et al., 2008]). Mercury poisoning can also result in a metallic taste.

Esophageal Toxicity

Swallowing is a key function mediated by a variety of structures from the top of the esophagus to the sphincter at the entrance to the stomach. Chemoradiotherapy for head and neck cancers not only influences the mouth, but also impairs swallowing and voice (Lazarus, 2009). Even a relatively benign antimetabolite such as methotrexate if taken at toxic concentrations causes development of bullae and vesicles in the mouth and makes swallowing difficult (Bookstaver et al., 2008). Atropine used in oral surgery to dry the area of the mouth also induces a swallowing disorder that inhibits the cough reflex in dogs. This may lead to aspiration pneumonia (Tsubouchi et al., 2008). Caustic agents apparently are readily available in Asia and many children have taken in strong alkali and acids. Swallowing is made difficult by the esophageal strictures that form following injury, but can be repaired surgically with balloon dilatation. However, the caustic injury or the surgical repair attempt can result in esophageal rupture (Doo et al., 2009). Aspirin augments the effects of gastric reflux for those with a lower intragastric pH (Sugimoto et al., 2010). Drug-induced esophageal injury occurs mainly where the esophagus narrows (middle third behind left atrium). Tetracycline-induced injury is transient and self-limiting and represents one class of agents that produces esophagitis. Persistent esophagitis with stricture occurs in patients taking nonsteroidal anti-inflammatory drugs (NSAIDs) enhanced by gastroesophageal reflux or those supplementing KCl while taking quinidine sulfate. Severe injury has been observed with osteoporosis patients on biphosphonates who have taken high doses without water and then lie down (Zografos et al., 2009). On the other end of the pH range, for example, 2.25% ethyl ammonium chloride was intentionally ingested by a 60-year-old woman. She developed a persistent cough, copious oral secretions, worsening hoarseness, and had poor esophageal motility in the mid to lower third of the esophagus in addition to systemic mild hypotension, nonanion gap metabolic acidosis, and oliguria (Hammond et al., 2009). For NaOH, the toxic pH for esophageal injury is > 11.5 and is time- and pH-dependent (Atug et al., 2009).

Gastroesophageal reflux has been related to development of esophageal cancer. A current alternative to the caustic damage theory for development of esophagitis is a cytokine-mediated mechanism as studied in rats (Souza et al., 2009). Oxidative stress as indicated by an increase in malondialdehyde and decrease in superoxide dismutase content also appears to play a role in esophageal mucosa injury (Liu et al., 2009). What is not generally well known is that bile acids may be involved in cancers of the esophagus, stomach, small intestine, liver, biliary tract, pancreas, and colon/rectum. The untoward effects of bile acids are reactive oxygen species (ROS) and (RNS) induction, DNA damage, increased mutation, short-term induction of apoptosis, and selection for long-term apoptosis resistance (Bernstein et al., 2009). Diabetes mellitus is a condition that also causes damage to the esophagus. In an experimental animal model of uncontrolled hyperglycemia induced by streptozotocin, there is an excess production of RNS initiating nitrosative stress. This stress depends upon the balance of pro- and antioxidative activity, paracrine regulation (NO/NOS and PG/COS signaling pathways), and pre-epithelial and epithelial cellular homeostasis. Identification alterations of glycoconjugates of the epithelial barrier and generation of peroxynitrite are important in the pathophysiology of diabetes mellitus–induced esophageal injury (Zayachkivska et al., 2008). Certain medications other than aspirin have untoward effects on the GI tract. The immunosuppressive medication mycophenolic acid causes increased apoptotic counts in the esophagus in 57% of patients taking the medication between 1 month and 10 years posttransplant. Similar findings were found in the duodenum (82%), but less in gastric biopsies (28%). The symptoms associated with these apoptosis increases were diarrhea (55%), nausea (45%), abdominal pain (35%), vomiting (25%), GI bleed (15%), dysphagia (difficulty swallowing for 10%), dyspepsia, anemia, and hematemesis (5% for each; Nguyen et al., 2009).

Esophageal cancers resulting from TP53 mutations (exons 4–10) are common in South America and appear to involve the same risk factors as oral cancer—ethanol and tobacco product use. Mutations inactivate this gene, which normally makes the tumor protein 53. This protein binds directly to DNA and determines whether damaged regions will be repaired or to signal the process of apoptosis. The mutation rate of this gene increased from 38% in nonsmokers to 66% in current smokers, with G:C > T:A transversions in 15% of smokers alone. Alcohol drinkers were observed to have more G:C > A:T transitions. G:C > A:T transitions at CpG sire occurred in nonexposed individuals (Szymańska et al., 2010).

It is of interest that some toxic substances may also be of therapeutic use in the esophagus. Spasms of the lower esophageal sphincter between the esophagus and the stomach or achalasia make swallowing difficult and painful. Intrasphincteric botulinum toxin (80 U) appears to provide better results than balloon dilation for pregnant Thai women for swallowing and adequate nutrition (Wataganara et al., 2009).

Stomach Toxicity

Ulcers are known to originate from chronic use of NSAIDs and from *H. pylori* infections. NSAIDs have been used therapeutically to relieve pain (analgesia), decrease inflammation, and prevent strokes and heart attacks via its anticoagulant properties. Other factors influencing gastric toxicity are age- and sex-related or determined by use of tobacco products and ethanol as noted earlier for other sections of the GI tract. One of the most serious NSAID interactions is the age-related decrease in gastric mucosal prostaglandin synthesis (PGE_2 and PGI_2 produced by the cytoprotective constitutively expressed cyclooxygenase enzyme COX-1) with age, when these medications are used more intensively for arthritis relief (anti-inflammatory role more of a function of inhibition of the inducible COX-2 enzyme) and prevention of myocardial infarctions. Because most NSAIDs have pKas from 3–5, their acidity directly induces cellular dehydration and mortality. Normally, acid does not penetrate well into cells with pH values close to neutral or slightly higher. However, the stomach pH makes NSAIDs with a pKa of 4–5 easily ionized and enhances their entry into gastric mucosal cells. In the cells, the slightly alkaline pH makes them exist primarily in the nonionized state. NSAIDs intracellularly become ionized and less hydrophobic, making them accumulate in what has been referred to as the "chemical greenhouse effect." Their accumulation leads to focal mucosal pallor followed by hemorrhagic foci and ulceration simultaneously with decreased mucosal blood flow. The chemical association with acidic derivatives of NSAIDs and surface phospholipids appears to explain a decline observed in mucosal lipophilicity. Acutely, these medications inhibit cell proliferation but have the opposite effect chronically to cells of fundic and duodenal mucosa. NSAIDs also initiate or exacerbate stomach inflammation despite their systemic anti-inflammatory activity through upregulation of adhesion molecules (increased cytokine TNF-α, leukotriene LTB_4, and intracellular adhesion molecule-1 [ICAM-1]) with leukocyte adherence to the vascular endothelium in the microcirculation of the stomach. NSAIDs also uncouple mitochondrial oxidative phosphorylation leading to decreased adenosine triphosphate (ATP) and increased cell death. The endoplasmic reticulum (ER) also experiences stress by induction of glucose-regulated protein-78 (adapts to accumulation of unfolded proteins with some stress) and C/EBP homologous transcription factor (induces apoptosis with overwhelming stress). If the stress is increased to the ER, apoptosis can be initiated via activating transcription factor 6 (ATF6), ATF4, and X-binding protein. Increased intracellular calcium is also caused by celecoxib ("safer"

on GI system COX-2 inhibitor), which activates the ER stress response.

Another reaction of interest in the stomach (and in the brain, cardiovascular system, liver, and kidney) is the generation of hydrogen sulfide. H_2S can be damaging (pro-inflammatory, vasodilatory) or protective (anti-inflammatory, atherosclerotic) depending on the concentration generated—as are other signaling molecules such as NO or CO. The gastric mucosa expresses two enzymes that mediate H_2S generation, cystathionine β-synthase, and cystathionine γ-lyase. H_2S protects endogenously to mucosal injury, but contributes to the inflammation produced by *H. pylori*. H_2S induces anti-inflammatory and cytoprotective genes in the presence of NSAIDs including heme oxidase-1 (HO-1), vascular endothelial growth factor, insulin-like growth factor receptor, and several genes associated with the transforming growth factor (TGF)-β receptor signaling pathway. It is of interest that the induction of HO-1 may produce more CO, which is cytoprotective and anti-inflammatory at endogenous concentrations via inhibition of NF-κB and inducible nitric oxide synthase. NSAIDs also increase the amplitude and frequency of gastric contractions/motility. This increases microvascular permeability and promotes cellular damage (Lim et al., 2009). NSAIDs also induce matrix metalloproteinases (MMPs), especially MMP-9 and MMP3, in a dose-dependent manner along with infiltration of inflammatory cells and disruption of the gastric mucosa. Melatonin downregulates both MMPs and heals acute gastric ulcers. Melatonin also provides antioxidant activities that protect against NSAID-induced gastric damage (inhibits protein oxidation, lipid peroxidation, hydroxyl radical formation, and SOD-2 expression [Ganguly and Swarnakar, 2009]).

The gram-negative rod *H. pylori* is another major contributor to stomach ulcers. However, alone it is not the threat that a cursory examination might indicate. In almost all infected people, a chronic gastritis develops starting with introduction by 10 years of age (90% of children). The progression of the disease to ulcers or other clinical outcomes depends on the genotype of the infection, host health status, and exposure to environmental factors. This last portion is the focus of toxicology interest. Adequate nutritional status (high consumption of fruit, vegetables, and vitamins) appears to prevent the pathology associated with infection. Chronic *H. pylori* infection may be accompanied by normal, decreased, or increased acid secretion (via direct inhibition by the bacterial vacuolating cytotoxin, lipopolysaccharide, or acid- inhibiting factor or indirect inhibition of parietal cell function via cytokines, hormonal, paracrine, and neural control mechanisms), all of which may progress to gastric ulcer. Type I ulcers occur in the gastric body and appear to occur in people with low night acid secretion. Type II ulcers occur in the antrum and appear irrespective of acid secretion. Type III ulcers are found within 3.0 cm of the pylorus, associate with duodenal ulcers, and occur with high acid secretion. Type IV ulcers are observed in the gastric cardia and low acid secretion. Antral-predominant gastritis correlates with duodenal ulcer development. Corpus-predominant gastritis increases the risk of development of gastric ulcers, gastric atrophy, intestinal metaplasia, and gastric adenocarcinoma. Oddly, a systemic infection with *H. pylori* increases vascular inflammation as well and is correlated with increases in coronary artery disease, atherosclerosis, and stroke. This organism has also been connected to idiopathic Parkinson's disease or Alzheimer's disease. Glaucoma, especially open-angle glaucoma and pseudo-exfoliation glaucoma, may also involve *H. pylori* infection. The reason for mentioning these diseases is due to the generation of ROS and other inflammatory mediators. Toxic substances share some of these mechanisms as a key to their impact. For example, *H. pylori* infection stimulates macrophages through L-arginine/nitric oxide pathways. In the stomach, the generation of NO will yield the nitrosating compounds N_2O_3 and N_2O_4. These compounds in turn can produce nitrosamines and yield DNA damage. Nitrosating organisms in the GI tract can also catalyze the reaction between nitrite and organic nitrogen compounds in the stomach contents to form genotoxic *N*-nitroso compounds. The nitrite is formed in the stomach during hypochlorhydria occurring from *H. pylori*–induced atrophic gastritis. Stomach bacteria convert dietary nitrate to nitrite. Nitrate

absorbed in the upper GI tract can also be concentrated by the salivary glands, and buccal bacteria convert the secreted nitrate to nitrite. This explains why diets high in fruits and vegetables high in antioxidant carotenoids, vitamin C, and vitamin E avoid nitrosamine formation and prevent the toxic action of nitrosamides. Similarly, polyphenols or catechins from the popular green tea brews also inhibit intragastric nitrosation. These protective mechanisms yield less cancer of the GI tract in individuals with *H. pylori* infection. Regarding noncancer diseases of the stomach, the high-salt diet of Americans consuming processed food destroys the mucosal barrier and favors *H. pylori* colonization. Salt has been found to cause gastritis and increase the genotoxic action of *N*-methyl-*N*-nitro-*N*-nitrosoguanidine. The combination of high salt and low antioxidants (fresh fruits) aids the progression of atrophic gastritis. The combination of bacterial colonization, increased nitrite concentrations, and depletion of vitamin C yield more formation of *N*-nitroso compounds. Vitamin E also protects the tract from *H. pylori* (in male Mongolian gerbils) by reducing the accumulation of activated neutrophils as indicated by reduced myeloperoxidase activity and mouse keratinocyte-derived chemokine in gastric mucosal cells compared with a tocopherol-deficient group. Although antioxidants do not protect against chronic gastritis from *H. pylori*, cruciferous vegetables contain phytochemicals that are converted to anticancer isothiocyanates such as sulforaphane by the GI flora, which in turn protect gastric mucosal cells from genotoxicity related to *H. pylori* infection. A source of antioxidants and cytotoxic chemicals that may aid in reducing infection is a combination of wild blueberry and other berry derivatives. It is also important to note that the atrophic gastritis caused by *H. pylori* also decreases vitamin B_{12} and folic acid absorption reducing methylation reactions, including the homocysteine to methionine reactions. This increases plasma homocysteine in infected patients (Izzotti et al., 2009).

Ethanol damages the stomach; this is found to be most problematic in chronic alcoholism. It is worth looking at the protective effects of a natural pentacyclic triterpene, lupeol, and

N-acetylcysteine (NAC) on ethanol-induced gastric damage to elucidate ethanol toxicity. Lupeol and NAC restore nonprotein sulfhydryl depletion/oxidation caused by ethanol. Lupeol's gastroprotection was decreased by indomethacin, a potent COX inhibitor, and L-NAME, an NO-synthase inhibitor, indicating key roles for these mechanisms on ethanol toxicity or increased ethanol toxicity with COX-inhibiting NSAIDs. Interfering with Ca^{2+} channels (verapamil) profoundly affected lupeol protection, indicating similar action in ethanol's disruptive effects. However, presynaptic adrenergic (α_2) antagonism by yohimbine or K(ATP)-channel blocker glibenclamide had weak activity in undoing lupeol's protection, indicating little sympathetic activity or K^+ channel activity in ethanol's gastric toxicity (Lira et al., 2009).

It is of importance that three different models of stomach ulceration exist for testing the effects of agents that might prevent those ulcers. One includes giving 0.2 mL of 0.3 M HCl/60% ethanol solution to mice. A proton pump inhibitor (omeprazole) is given to indicate a protection control group for comparison purposes. Another mouse model is 100 mg/kg indomethacin (strong NSAID) given *per os* (PO) and 5 mg/kg bethanechol intraperitoneally (IP; muscarinic agonist). Stress induced by restraining mice for 4 hours in a cold environment (4°C) is a third model. The human equivalent toxicities were discussed earlier. Because toxicology is also the study of antidotes, it is of interest that an alkaloid extract of the bark of the Bolivian plant *Galipea longiflora* (Rutaceae family) was more potent in preventing stomach ulcers in the three murine models due to decreased acid secretion and increased gastric mucus content than was 2-phenylquinolone, which was also isolated from this plant (Zanatta et al., 2009).

Cancer of the stomach can result from exposure to the agents mentioned earlier or from the classic toxicants such as polycyclic aromatic hydrocarbons (PAHs). Road workers or roofers who work with asphalt are exposed to it via the skin and to bitumen fumes via the lung, stomach, and circulation to the bone marrow. This increases the risk of cancers to all these regions. Bitumen fumes contain PAHs. Nitrogen-, sulfur-, and/or oxygen-containing PAHs or their alkyl-substituted analogues may also lead to the mutagenicity and carcinogenicity of bitumen fumes. Polar adducts of DNA are observed in rats treated with coal-tar fume condensates. Thiophenes also appear to play an important role in the carcinogenicity of the fumes with some less mutagenic than the corresponding isomeric PAH and others potent carcinogens. It is of interest that sulfur analogues of PAHs in bitumen fumes have a higher concentration than the PAH of similar molecular weight, where the opposite is true for coal-tar fumes. This explains why more polar adducts of DNA are found in animals exposed to bitumen fumes (Binet et al., 2002). Road pavers show increased activation of the intrinsic pathway apoptosis–regulating proteins BAX and BCL-2 due to exposure to bitumen fumes from the hot asphalt. Their skin cells activate the extrinsic pathway for apoptosis with overexpression of tumor necrosis factor–related apoptosis-inducing ligand (TRAIL) and its death receptor, DR5, and caspase-3 as well as enhanced terminal deoxynucleotidyl transferase-mediated dUTP nick-end labeling (TUNEL) in chronically bitumen-exposed skin (Rapisarda et al., 2009).

Some "stomach" poisons are actually metabolic inhibitors and are used to control ants and similar pest populations (distinct from insect growth regulators and neurotoxins). These agents include hydramethylnon, sulfuramid, and sodium tetraborate decahydrate. Boric acid has also been used to poison rodents. In feeding studies in mice, boric acid causes hyperkeratosis and acanthosis (precancerous thickening) with hyperplasia and/or dysplasia of the stomach at high doses (25,000–100,000; National Toxicology Program, 1987). Plaster of Paris mixed 1:1 with sugar, cornmeal, cornstarch, oatmeal, and cocoa powder has been used as a homemade rodenticide by hardening in the stomach of the rodent and not passing through, causing starvation. An interesting compound that is really an anticoagulant was first used to disrupt the stomach and GI tract of rodents. Sweet clover (*Melilotus* sp.) was a good food source for milk cattle in Wisconsin at the beginning of the 20th century. However, spoiled sweet clover caused internal hemorrhaging and the death of dairy cattle. This is due to the release of plant enzymes that, when the clover is cut, act on the glycoside component melilotoside, liberating a sugar moiety and coumarin. *Penicillium* and *Aspergillus* contamination results in metabolism to dicoumarol. This agent inhibits vitamin K epoxide reductase, which prevents clotting. Karl Link of the University of Wisconsin synthesized warfarin as a more potent derivative (the WARF name comes from his source of funding from the Wisconsin Alumni Research Foundation) and a rodenticide. After many years of use, rats and mice apparently were selected for spontaneous mutations in the gene synthesizing the vitamin K epoxide reductase (VKORC1) that conferred resistance to this "stomach" toxicant (hemorrhaging ulcer formation [Rost et al., 2009]).

Not everything that affects the GI tract has a known mechanism of action. For example, *Panicum maximum* cultivars Mombaça, Tanzânia, and Massai cause severe colic and death in horses and mules through severe hemorrhages and some mucosal erosions and ulcerations but the cause of this toxicity is unknown (Cerqueira et al., 2009).

Duodenal Toxicity

The specialized cells for absorption are found in the duodenum with villi and other sensitive structures. This is similar to the brush border also associated with the proximal tubule of the kidney where similar mechanisms occur for reabsorption of important nutrients that are filtered through the glomerulus. Problems with the duodenum or other sections of the small intestine (jejunum and ileum) may also involve pancreatic damage, because the pancreatic duct provides digestive enzymes into the proximal duodenum. Liver involvement may also prevent the formation or release of the bile salts into the proximal duodenum. Other internal organ toxicities may also impair absorption as certain transport molecules may not be formed. Additionally, changes in the microflora and nutritional deficiencies can augment or decrease absorption or nutrients or toxic substances. Also, inflammatory reactions may alter intestinal absorption. Even water absorption is crucial here, because toxicity may result in dehydrating diarrhea. One of the substances

recognized early for many of these influences is ethanol. Acute ethanol administration increases the absorption of lipids, while chronic ethanol abuse yields decreased lipid absorption. Ethanol also diminishes ATP content and the activities of various catabolic enzymes (hexokinase, fructose-1- phosphate aldolase, fructose-1, 6-diphosphate aldolase, and fructose-1, 6-diphosphase). However, in the jejunum the activities of adenylate cyclase (producing signaling molecule cAMP) and pyruvate kinase are increased. Also, the small intestine as a whole has less amino acid, carbohydrate, vitamin B_{12}, and vitamin B_1 absorption. There has always been a controversy as to whether the caloric intake of alcoholics due to the alcohol itself and poor nutrition were both contributors to their poor nutritional status or whether alcohol toxicity affected absorption of nutrients. All appear to contribute to the problems of chronic alcohol administration. Ethanol also interferes with sodium and water absorption—possibly related to its effects on ATP or ATPase content—and causes less pituitary secretion of antidiuretic hormone, allowing further dehydration. Ethanol increases magnesium absorption but decreases calcium absorption. The calcium picture is complex as calcium absorption is related to vitamin D absorption. The hydrophobic vitamin D absorption is decreased in steatorrhea (or fatty stool production) or poor fat absorption. Steatorrhea may be related to pancreatic damage, liver damage/bile salt formation, cholestasis, intestinal bacterial overgrowth, small intestinal lesions caused by nutritional deficiencies (folic acid), or toxic insults. Ethanol might be that toxic insult, because giving high doses of ethanol by intragastric but not intraperitoneal administration reduces calcium absorption while causing necrosis of the villus epithelium and infiltration of lymphocytes and plasma cells in the remaining crypts (Krawitt, 1977).

Cytotoxic cancer chemotherapy agents cause cells with a high turnover rate to be affected. Mucositis is the key reaction that results in diarrhea from either anticancer medications or ionizing radiation (Sonis, 2009a). The five-stage process leading to mucositis involves initiation by DNA strand breaks, clonogenic death of basal epithelial cells, and the generation of ROS. The primary damage response is the next phase involving signal transduction pathways, especially NF-κB, Wnt, p53, and associated canonical pathways, triggered by the DNA strand breaks and lipid peroxidation. Cytotoxic agents and radiation can activate NF-κB directly or indirectly via ROS. Two hundred genes are expressed as a result of this signal transduction molecule including cytokines, cytokine modulators, COX-2, inducible NO-synthase, SOD, and cell adhesion molecules. Normal cells will become apoptotic due to NF-κB formation. Radiation and chemotherapy also stimulate the ceramide pathway. This produces cell death via activation of matrix metalloproteinases from macrophages that respond to the fibrinolysis due to connective tissue damage from radiation or cytotoxic agents. Signal amplification can occur in a third phase as TNF has a positive feedback response on NF-κB, initiating MAPK signaling. This is followed by a signaling overload response that progresses to the next phase of ulceration. Bacteria may then invade, stimulating more pro-inflammatory cytokines or producing sepsis. If the worst does not occur, there is spontaneous ulcer healing from signaling produced by the submucosa's extracellular matrix and involving the activation of the intrinsic tyrosine kinase (Sonis, 2009b). One cancer chemotherapeutic antimetabolite to folic acid is methotrexate. Its toxicity appears to be manifested through nitrosative stress. In the rat, nitrate was elevated fivefold 12 hours following methotrexate administration. Also, nitrotyrosine was elevated in all parts of the small intestine, with the most found in the duodenum (Kolli et al., 2008).

NSAIDs still induce gastroduodenal damage, but even low-dose acetylsalicylic acid for prevention of cardiovascular disease appears to be toxic via its inhibition of COX-1, aspirin-specific alterations of the gastroduodenal mucosa, and reduction in platelet aggregation (Yeomans et al., 2009). As mentioned earlier, other medications can also cause GI disturbances. The immunosuppressive medication mycophenolate mofetil causes ulcerative esophagitis, reactive gastropathy, duodenal and ileal graft-versus-host disease with crypt architectural disarray, lamina propria inflammation, dilated damaged crypts, and crypt epithelial apoptosis (Parfitt et al., 2008).

Heavy metals also cause GI disturbances to differing degrees. Metals compete for absorption and damage, so localization of the sites of metal absorption and the presence of other metals have profound influences on toxicity. Metal absorption across the intestinal wall involves two steps. The first step involves transport over the luminal membrane into the epithelial cytoplasm. The second step is important as the timing of the transport over the basolateral membrane into the serosal fluid determines the metal's residence time in the mucosal epithelial cytoplasm. Slow movement out of this area makes the rate of mucosal sloughing a key factor in damage versus absorption. All metals are not absorbed in the same area of the intestine equally. For example, divalent cadmium is absorbed mainly in the duodenum, Zn^{2+} in the jejunum and ileum, Hg^{2+} in the proximal jejunum, and selenomethionine in the entire intestinal tract (Andersen et al., 1994). Acute heavy metal poisoning of the GI tract varies based on the metal. Lead causes tissue desiccation and mucosal damage to the GI tract, but death results from neurological damage. At lesser concentrations, lead affects hematopoiesis or the formation of blood cells. Mercury binds more strongly to proteins, and acute oral toxicity results in sloughing of the intestinal mucosa to a degree that pieces can be found in the stools. Significant water is lost in this way. Hg also induces edema via damage to the capillary walls. Shock and peripheral vascular collapse can occur; however, for those doses of Hg that do not cause shock or renal failure, neurological damage usually defines mercury poisoning (Iino et al., 2009). Certain metals also cause cancer. Cr(VI) in drinking water appears to be carcinogenic to the cells of the oral cavity in rats, but appears to shift to sensitivity to oncogenesis in the small intestine of mice (Stout et al., 2009). Another carcinogenic metal is arsenic and its metabolites monomethylarsonous acid and dimethylarsinous acid. Usually, metals are not considered to be CYP inducers that may mediate carcinogenic mechanisms. Also, the intestine is rarely considered to be a large source of metabolism, because the portal circulation to the liver usually has profound effects on metabolism. Sodium arsenite and its metabolites induce CYP3A4 via increasing the pregnane X receptor (forms a heterodimer with retinoid X receptor alpha) in the small intestine and Ub-protein conjugates tempering the induction mechanism (Medina-Díaz et al., 2009). Iron toxicity may be noted in the liver, but its transport/absorption in the duodenum is mediated by the intramembrane divalent metal transporter 1. Iron export from a variety of cells is mediated by ferroportin, which is regulated by a circulating hormone hepcidin. This combination, along with plasma membrane transferrin and iron regulatory proteins 1 and 2 receptor, influences iron regulation from nutrient to toxic concentrations (Valerio, 2007).

Oxidative damage can also ulcerate the proximal GI tract as occurs due to ingestion of the plastic hardener methyl ethyl ketone peroxide; this has occurred accidentally in humans. Death usually results from liver necrosis, which can be prevented by the free radical scavenger N-acetylcysteine. Severe metabolic acidosis also occurs in response to the formation of formic acid similar to methanol intoxication and can cause optic nerve lesions (van Enckervort et al., 2008).

Bacterial toxins also can cause fatal reactions via intestinal damage. *Clostridium perfringens* type B and C isolates produce beta-toxin that causes significant hemorrhagic luminal fluid in the small intestine. Jejunum and ileal damage are more severe than damage to the duodenum (Vidal et al., 2008). *Staphylococcus aureus* produces toxins A–E and toxic shock syndrome toxin-1, causing food poisoning and toxic shock syndrome; it also produces enterotoxins G and I (scarlet fever and toxic shock). These enterotoxins produce villous atrophy with abnormal brush border. More detailed analysis implicates these toxins in microvilli destruction, mitochondrial damage (dilation), and lysosomes with cellular debris (Naik et al., 2008). Fungus-contaminated feed may be toxic to various organs or at least reduce feed efficiency in animals via intestinal alterations. For example,

feed contaminated with *Fusarium* mycotoxins decreased the villus height in the duodenum of turkeys (Girish and Smith, 2008).

Immune responses to intestinal contents can also affect nutrient transport as a more subtle toxic reaction but is species and segment related. Lipopolysaccharide (LPS; gram-negative bacteria membrane component) infusion into pig intestines causes decreased ileal glucose transport in Yorkshire breeds but increased in the Meishan breed. Duodenal and ileal proline transport is decreased by LPS in Meishans but unaffected in Yorkshires. Glycylsarcosine transport is increased by LPS in both pig breeds. Resistance of the paracellular pathway between cells (barrier function) is increased in Yorkshires but not Meishans by LPS (Albin et al., 2007). Damage caused by flavonoids, diterpenes, and terpenes in *Ginkgo biloba* extract to the calciform cells in the duodenum may be responsible for less uptake of these cells of a diagnostic radiobiocomplex sodium pertechnetate ($^{99m}TcO_4Na$). This reduced uptake may also be due to oxidative stress generating inflammatory cell infiltration (Moreno et al., 2007). Certain food substances also prevent absorption of important nutrients. For example, in the original *Rocky* movie with Sylvester Stallone, there is a training scene where he eats a number of raw eggs prior to his morning run. There is a substance known as avidin in raw egg whites that has a high affinity for biotin binding, making this nutrient unavailable (White et al., 1992).

Jejunal Toxicity

Many of the toxicants that affect the tract proximal to the jejunum will also affect this more distal structure. Its length and the completion of the digestion process in this area make transport of nutrients and toxicants more important in this region. For example, it is important to note that certain mineral deficiencies increase the absorption of other toxic minerals, as is the case for Fe deficiency and Ni absorption due to less Ni export from the jejunal/intestinal mucosa (Müller-Fassbender et al., 2003). Also, studies using the chicken intestine indicate that addition of addition of D-glucose to the mucosal side of voltage-clamped intestinal sections exhibited the highest current increases in the jejunum. This makes Na^+-glucose symport most important in this region. Any toxin that interferes with this transporter mainly affects duodenal and jejunum sections of the small intestine, as does deoxynivalenol or vomitoxin (type B trichothecene is especially prevalent in *Fusarium* fungal species; Awad et al., 2007). Cd is found to inhibit D-galactose transport in the presence of Ca in the rabbit jejunum (Mesonero et al., 1996). Unfortunately, this sodium-linked cotransport of sugars can also be utilized to transport toxic glycosides, such as prunasin (D-mandelonitrile-beta-D-glucoside), which is the primary metabolite of amygdalin (Strugala et al., 1995). Poisoning the $3Na^+,2K^+$-ATPase by ouabain or vanadium (vanadate) also has the effect of altering amino acid and water absorption (Hajjar et al., 1989). It is of interest that the jejunum on its own produces more ROS and RNS prior to insult than many other organs (jejunum > duodenum > kidney > ileum > blood > cerebellum > brain > heart > liver) as detected by electron paramagnetic resonance imaging of a nontoxic spin probe, 1-hydroxy-3-carboxy pyrrolidine. Endotoxin challenge as a model of toxic shock increases radical formation in the rat liver, heart, lung, and blood, but actually decreases ROS and RNS in the jejunum. This indicates that radical formation shifts result in the expected toxicity, decreased blood pressure due to NO formation or $ONOO^-$ production, and extensive oxidative damage (Kozlov et al., 2003). Oxidative injury may be important also due to the requirement for glutathione for prevention of severe degeneration of epithelial cells of the jejunum and colon as occurs with buthionine sulfoximine (Mårtensson et al., 1990). This protective function of reduced glutathione will become extremely important in maintaining liver function against toxic metabolites. Another aspect of small intestinal function is nerve-mediated toxicity via Na and fluid secretion. The rat jejunum, for example, responds to 8% ethanol perfusion by a net secretion of fluid and sodium. This is prevented by ganglionic blockade by hexamethonium, but does not interfere with ethanol absorption (Hallbäck et al., 1990).

Ileal Toxicity

The ileum is the last chance of the small intestine to absorb many nutrients. The jejunum and ileum succumb to the toxicity of *Clostridium perfringens* type A. The energy-rich, protein-rich, wheat- and barley-based diets of chickens causes growth of this pathogenic organism as opposed to diets rich in corn. Toxins such as alpha toxin and NetB may play a role in the development of jejunal and ileal necrotic enteritis. This disease is characterized by lesions that are focal-to-confluent, often with tightly adhered pseudomembrane (Cooper and Songer, 2009). *Clostridium difficile* produces toxins A and B that are responsible for its pathogenesis. Toxin A causes the antibiotic-induced diarrhea and pseudomembranous colitis. A selective A2A adenosine receptor agonist, ATL 313, appears to prevent some of the most damaging influences of toxin A on the ileum by reducing secretion and edema, myeloperoxidase activity (neutrophil infiltration), TNF- α production, adenosine deaminase activity, and cell death (Cavalcante et al., 2006). Where endotoxin and LPS decrease jejunal radical formation, they also activate phospholipase A_2 and increase the permeability of the ileal/intestinal wall to bacterial invasion and sepsis by cleaving the phosphatidylcholine protective layer of the surface of the GI tract. Specific inhibitors of phospholipase A_2 protect against this permeability change (Zayat et al., 2008). Permeability increases are also caused by other toxicants, such as the widely used herbicide glyphosate (at > 10 mg/mL), as determined by reductions in transmembrane electrical resistance and increased permeability to [³H]-mannitol. Glyphosate also disrupts the actin cytoskeleton of ileal cells at the same high concentrations (Vasiluk et al., 2005). Cd^{2+} disrupts the paracellular barrier, increasing its toxicity to and absorption between ileal cells (Duizer et al., 1999). Bacteria can also activate a pro-drug as is the case of the antiproliferative cancer medication irinotecan. Carboxylesterases of the gastrointestinal cells, liver, serum, and cancer cells activate this drug to the toxic SN-38. The liver conjugates this metabolite to a nontoxic glucuronide. Bacteria flora β-glucuronidase is capable of releasing large amounts of active SN-38.

Germ-free mice had a lethal dose of ≥ 150 mg, while holoxenic mice succumbed to a dose range of 60–80 mg irinotecan. Normal mice with a good bacterial flora also had diffuse small and large intestinal damage, while germ-free mice had significantly less damage, mostly centered in the ileum. Diarrhea was found in 19 of 20 normal mice given 60 mg of the anticancer medication, while holoxenic mice had no diarrhea at that dose and sporadic diarrhea between 80 and 100 mg (Brandi et al., 2006). Diarrhea is also produced by ingestion of other toxins, such as that produced by the black sponge *Halichondria okadai*. Okadaic acid, responsible for diarrhetic shellfish poisoning, is a tumor promoter that is a specific cell-permeating inhibitor of protein phosphatases. It also induces micronuclei formation indicating genotoxicity. Also, apoptosis was observed by the TUNEL assay in mouse ileum, liver, and kidney (Le Hégarat et al., 2006). Secretory diarrhea is responsible for death from cholera toxin exposure. Inhibition of the cystic fibrosis transmembrane conductance regulator by 2-thioxo-4-thiozolidinone inhibits intestinal fluid loss and may be a useful toxicant for use in an animal model of cystic fibrosis (Ma et al., 2002). Zymosan, a yeast cell wall preparation consisting of protein–carbohydrate complexes, is used as a mouse model of multiple organ dysfunction syndrome of nonseptic origin. Zymosan IP injection causes peritoneal exudation and migration of neutrophils, pancreatic and ileal injury, an increase in myeloperoxidase activity of the ileum and the lung, and the formation of IL-1β and TNF-α. The mediation of injury by TNF-α formation is indicated by reversal of these effects by a specific TNF-α–soluble inhibitor, etanercept (Malleo et al., 2008).

Chronic cocaine use can cause significant intestinal damage. For example, in one case report, ischemia/infarction and hemorrhage were noted in the distal ileum on autopsy (Lingamfelter and Knight, 2010). Metabolism in the ileum may not parallel that in the liver by CYP3A isoenzymes. For example, vitamin D receptor is known to induce the formation of CYP3A1 and CYPA2 by 1,25-dihydroxy-vitamin D_3. However, this activated form of vitamin D induces vitamin D receptor expression in the ileum of the rat or the human, but only in the rat liver. This indicates differences in CYP regulation for human ileum enzymes. What role does this play in toxicity? The bile acids from human liver are represented by chenodeoxycholic acid, while the more toxic forms from bacterial metabolism are represented by lithocholic acid. It appears that vitamin D promotes the metabolism of the toxic lithocholic acid. However, chenodeoxycholic acid appears to "short-circuit" this mechanism in the rat ileum by preventing the induction of the CYP3A isoenzymes by higher vitamin D receptor expression and may increase the toxicity of lithocholic acid (Khan et al., 2010). Motility is also important in this portion of the small intestine. Isoliquiritigenin, a flavonoid extract of licorice (*Glycyrrhiza glabra*), inhibits charcoal meal travel at low doses and increases the travel speed at high doses. It is of interest that the section of the GI tract is also important in the effects of this flavonoid. Isoliquiritigenin produces an atropine-sensitive concentration-dependent spasmogenic action in rat stomach fundus, but a spasmolytic/opposite action on the rabbit jejunum, guinea pig ileum, and atropine-treated rat stomach fundus. The spasmogenic effect appears likely via muscarinic receptor agonism, while antagonizing calcium channels produce the spasmolytic effect (Chen, Zhu, et al., 2009). Aflatoxin B_1 produces ileal spasms via release of acetylcholine as indicated by atropine antagonism, although death occurs via liver damage (Luzi et al., 2002). Changes in the immune response in the small intestine also occur in the ileum. Depleted uranium ingestion in drinking water in rats causes increased responses of the inflammatory pathway (increased COX-2 expression for formation of prostaglandins, increased IL-1β and IL-10 cytokines, induced neutrophils) while decreasing other parameters associated with macrophage function (the previously mentioned changes in interleukins accompanied by decreased expression of CCL-2 mRNA) or the NO pathway (reduced expression of endothelial NO synthase mRNA, inductive NO synthase activity, and NO_2^-/NO_3^- concentrations). This indicates possibilities for chronic poisoning of the immune response or alternatively producing short-term hypersensitivity (Dublineau et al., 2007).

Colon Toxicity

Colon cancer is a scourge of well-fed carnivorous humans. It has been suspected that red meat consumers have an iron-rich diet that increases the risk of colon cancer. A feeding study of iron-fortified diets to rats at levels appropriate for human consumption indicated an increase in free radical–generating capacity and lipid per-oxidation with the cecum/proximal colon as the site of highest risk (Lund et al., 2001). Difluoro-methylornithine and NSAIDs prevent colorec-tal cancer development in mice. Polyamine synthesis is stimulatory of inflammation and colorectal cancer. The first enzyme in the syn-thesis of polyamines is ornithine decarboxylase, which is inhibited by difluoromethylornithine. NSAIDs by definition are anti-inflammatory agents. The role of polyamine synthesis is con-firmed by recurring adenomas in colon polyps accompanied by a single nucleotide polymor-phism of the ornithine decarboxylase promoter (Rial et al., 2009). Dimethylhydrazine is a selec-tive colon cancer–causing agent. Its metabo-lism to azoxymethane (Likachev et al., 1978) has made the metabolite a modern model for DNA methylation and cell-signaling changes indicative of cancer development. The discover-ies that various plant flavonoids released into the colon during digestion, such as quercetin, reduce various cancer formations, including colon cancer, yielded mechanistic questions (Deschner et al., 1991). Gene expression analyses via high-density microarrays indicate that Wnt-beta catenin, phospholipase A_2-eicosanoid, and mitogen-activated protein kinase appear to be upregulated during development of colon can-cer from azoxymethane (Davidson et al., 2009). Mutations in *APC*, *Ras*, *DCC*, and *p53* genes are also associated with precancerous tumors or polyps that may develop into malignant tumors. As mentioned previously, consumption of red meat can increase colorectal cancer risk by 12–20%, as opposed to a diet rich in fish, which may lower the risk by 40%. The heme iron may play a role as indicated previously, but also cho-lesterol, fatty acids, and products formed from preservation and cooking, including *N*-nitroso chemicals and heterocyclic amines, are possible contributors to these cancers. Increased protein

in the diet increases the amount of *N*-nitroso compounds, which is true of meat eaters. DNA-alkylation is catalyzed by the intestinal micro-flora, inducing colitis-linked colorectal cancer. These changes may be monitored by fecal water biomarker analysis. Bile acids are produced from cholesterol metabolism. The secondary bile acids produced by bacteria stimulate the proliferation of colonic cells and induce apop-tosis. These bile acids also cause single-stranded DNA breaks and base oxidation and alter the barrier function. This may lead to mutations that are resistant to apoptosis, forming tumors that metastasize to other areas. Fortunately, consumption of foods rich in phenolic com-pounds (tea, red wine, chocolate) are antioxi-dant, anti-inflammatory, and anticarcinogenic by preventing promotion of tumorigenesis and inducing apoptosis. Calcium also is thought to protect against heme iron and colorectal cancer. Probiotics and prebiotics affect the microflora to decrease the risk of cancer and promote host health (Pearson et al., 2009).

Conditions that may lead to cancer forma-tion but are problematic on their own involve colon inflammation. Bacterial infections, isch-emia, and autoimmunity can yield ulcerative colitis or Crohn's colitis. Supplementation of drinking water with low-molecular-weight dextran sodium sulfate yields epithelial dam-age and enhanced colonic inflammation in mice, which can be visualized in a journal devoted to exhibiting videos (Whittem et al., 2010). A truly opposite approach is to use a weekly enema or intrarectal administration of 2,4,6- trichlorobenzene sulfonic acid. This coli-tis type yields an initial T helper type 1 response in BALB/c mice, including cytokines IL-12p70 and interferon-γ. After 3 weeks, this reaction decreases and is replaced by an increase in IL-23/IL-25 at 4 to 5 weeks. This is followed by higher IL-17 and interleukins normally associated with a T helper type 2 response, especially an IL-13 peak between 8 and 9 weeks. IL-13 induces the IL-13Rα$_2$ receptor key to synthesis of TGF-β$_1$ and fibrosis (Fichtner-Feigl et al., 2008).

Trimethyltin chloride increases chloride secre-tion regulated by the basolateral Ca^{2+}-sensitive K^+ channels (Yu et al., 2009). Nanotechnology is a new source of potential toxicants, especially those coupled to metals. Cobalt-doped tungsten carbide nanoparticle suspensions induced highest toxicity to astrocytes and colon epithelial cells due to the ionic cobalt content of the particles (Bastian et al., 2009).

Clinically, a number of medications and chemicals cause common colonic toxicity. Alosetron, amphetamines, cocaine, ergotamine, estrogen, pseudoephedrine, sodium polystyrene, and vasopressin have been linked cases of colonic ischemia due to effects on mesenteric vessels (shunting of blood away from mesentery, thrombogenesis, and vasospasm). Colonic pseudo-obstruction has been found in patients taking atropine, various narcotic agents, nifedipine, phenothiazines, tricyclic antidepressants, and vincristine by either antagonizing neurotransmitters that increase intestinal motility, stimulating neurotransmitters that decrease motility, binding to receptors that cause dysmotility, relaxing smooth muscle, and increasing toxicity to enteric neurons. Antibiotics can lead to pseudomembranous colitis. If people use cathartics over a long period of time, lower colonic motility may occur along with abdominal distention. There is an association between ampicillin and hemorrhagic colitis. Anticancer medications may cause neutropenic colitis. The iron-chelating agent deferoxamine has been linked to patients with *Yersinia* enterocolitis.

These diseases result from either from altering the bowel flora and allowing pathogenic microorganisms to develop or become more virulent, or reduced immune system function or altering the mucosal barrier to bacterial invasion. Cytotoxic colitis occurs with α-methyldopa, gold compounds, and NSAIDs due to an allergic reaction, antimetabolite action, or mucosal cytotoxicity. A toxic colitis is found in people who administer corrosive chemicals intrarectally. Lymphocytic colitis is associated with an activated or attenuated immune response due to the use of cyclo 3 fort, flutamide, lansoprazole, NSAIDs, or ticlopidine (Cappell, 2004).

Forensic Analysis of Pancreatic Damage

This sections returns to dietary causes of toxicity. For example, lectins from beans (such as *Phaseolus vulgaris*) may cause toxicity via damage to cells of the GI tract. In the Upper Midwest, corn and soybeans are the key crops. Soybeans are toxic if not processed with significant heating, which people in this area know well from the smells of soybean plants. Soybeans produce trypsin inhibitors that can cause lethality by significant damage to the pancreas (Liener, 1983). Damage to the pancreas by agents listed in **Table 16-2** may affect exocrine (most of the

---

TABLE 16-2   Forensic Chart of Pancreatic Toxicity

Pancreatic Toxicity	Toxic Agents
Increased HCO_3 and water secretion/decreased protein	Oleic acid (Laugier and Sarles, 1977)
Mitochondrial membrane dysfunction	Oleate (Frigerio et al., 2006)
Pancreatic cancer	Alcohol (Apte et al., 2009), azaserine (Povoski et al., 1993), 7,12-dimethylbenzo[*a*]anthracene (Harris et al., 1977), 4-hydroxyaminoquinoline-1-oxide (Imazawa et al., 2003), *N*-nitrosamines (Scarpelli et al., 1984)
Pancreatitis	Alcohol (Apte et al., 2009), ethionine (Yamaguchi et al., 2009), medications (Trivedi and Pitchumoni, 2005)
Reactive oxygen species	Alloxan, streptozotocin (Szkudelski, 2001)
Trypsin inhibition	Soybean trypsin inhibitors (Liener, 1983)

digestive enzyme functions of the GI tract) and endocrine (insulin and glucagon and diabetes mellitus) functions of this key small organ. Usually, the exocrine function is more sensitive to these agents, especially via the oral route of administration. Alcohol has been mentioned earlier for other GI disturbance, and it plays a role in acute and chronic pancreatitis with acinar atrophy and fibrosis. The increase in the permeability of the intestinal wall leads to endotoxinemia, necroinflammation, and progressive deterioration of the pancreas via activation of stellate cells. This environment is then facilitatory for production of cancer stroma (Apte et al., 2009). A good article to help start thinking about toxicity to the pancreas beyond these more likely toxicities was published in the 1980s (Scarpelli, 1989). Severe necrotic pancreatitis develops from diets that are deficient in choline and supplemented with ethionine. Initial observations of changes in S-adenosylmethionine and methionine adenosyltransferases did not give a clear linkage between toxicity/lethality and observed decreases in these parameters (Lu et al., 2003). However, it appears that IL-6 is a good indicator of the inflammatory reaction that precedes the toxicity from an ethionine-rich diet, and the serotonin 5-HT$_{2A}$ receptor may mediate the damage as indicated by the protection offered by an 5-HT$_{2A}$ antagonist risperidone (Yamaguchi et al., 2009).

Medications can also cause pancreatitis. Inflammatory bowel disease has higher occurrences of acute pancreatitis with azathioprine/mercaptopurine immunosuppressants (Bermejo et al., 2008). Estrogens can increase hypertriglyceridemia by increasing very low-density lipoprotein (VLDL) and reducing triglyceride lipase in the liver. Severe hyperglyceridemia leads to pancreatitis (Lee and Goldberg, 2008). Diuretics such as furosemide and hydrochlorothiazide (with the angiotensin-converting enzyme [ACE] inhibitor lisinopril) can cause an acute or fatal necrotizing pancreatitis (Bedrossian and Vahid, 2007). The list of medications based on risk of pancreatitis has been separated into classes. Class I is reserved for those medications with > 20 reported cases and includes didanosine (antiretroviral), asparaginase (anticancer), azathioprine, valproic acid (antiseizure), pentavalent antimonials (antiparasitic for leishmaniasis), pentamidine (antiprotozoal), mercaptopurine, mesalamine (anti-inflammatory), estrogens, opioid analgesics, tetracycline (antibacterial), cytarabine (anticancer), steroids, trimethoprim-sulfamethoxazole (antibacterial), sulfasalazine (anti-inflammatory), furosemide (loop diuretic), and sulindac (analgesic). Class II medications indicate > 10 cases of pancreatitis and include rifampin (antibacterial), lamivudine (antiretroviral), octreotide (somatostatin analog), carbamazepine (antiseizure), acetaminophen (analgesic), phenformin (banned in U.S. antidiabetic medication due to fatal lactic acidosis), interferon alfa-2b (immunomodulator/anticancer), enalapril (ACE inhibitor), hydrochlorothiazide (diuretic), cisplatin (anticancer), erythromycin (macrolide antibacterial), and cyclopenthiazide (another thiazide diuretic). Class III represents the rest of medications with any reported incidence of pancreatitis. Considered together, it appears that many medications taken orally and causing toxicity may yield pancreatitis in patients prone to this disease (Trivedi and Pitchumoni, 2005). The fatty acid oleate was shown in the 1970s to induce the exocrine pancreas to secrete more water and bicarbonate on an acute infusion. Protein output first increased then was inhibited below basal values. An anti-cholecystokinin-pancreozymin factor was proposed (Laugier and Sarles, 1977). A 3-day treatment with oleic acid causes mitochondrial membrane dysfunction and low insulin response to a stimulatory concentration of glucose. These lipotoxic effects appear to be counteracted by topiramate, an antiseizure medication that increases expression of the nutrient sensor PPARα and the mitochondrial fatty acid carrier CPT-1, which is associated with an increased β-oxidation rate of the lipid (Frigerio et al., 2006). ROS can be generated to damage the pancreas as a whole and the B cells more specifically that produce the insulin. Alloxan is reduced to dialuric acid, forming a redox cycle that generates superoxide radicals. Hydrogen peroxide is then generated by SOD, and hydroxyl radicals form via the Fenton reaction. These ROS and a large increase in cytosolic Ca^{2+} concentrations rapidly damage the B cells. Streptozotocin gains entrance to the pancreas via the GLUT2 glucose transporter. It alkylates DNA and induces activation of poly ADP-ribosylation. The poly ADP-ribosylation depletes cellular NAD^+ and ATP. Subsequent ATP dephosphorylation provides a substrate for xanthine oxidase, which generates superoxide and, via dismutation and Fenton reaction, hydrogen peroxide and hydroxyl radical. Streptozotocin also increases nitric oxide, which inhibits aconitase activity and produces more DNA damage. B cells then undergo necrosis (Szkudelski, 2001). DNA damage results in the exocrine pancreas carcinomas that are so difficult to treat. There are questions as to factors that mediate the progression from damage to cancer. Acidophilic atypical acinar cell foci and nodules represent preneoplastic lesions that are generated by azaserine (α-diazoketone). Their growth appears to be mediated by cholecystokinin-A receptors (Povoski et al., 1993). 7,12-Dimethylbenz[a]anthracene (DMBA) and other similar PAHs can be metabolized by cells of the pancreatic duct to active DNA-reactive compounds found as adducts. The reason this compound has been employed is that the amount of adducts formed is higher with DMBA than benzo[a]pyrene (Harris et al., 1977). It is clear that some agents such as 4-hydroxyaminoquinoline-1-oxide (a metabolite of 4-nitroquinoline-1-oxide) produce cancer via adduct formation, increased apoptosis, and the induction of proliferative genes, particularly p53 (Imazawa et al., 2003). The model system used for these studies is important. For example, the rat pancreas responds to carcinogens with acinar adenomas and adenocarcinomas, but not with ductal adenocarcinomas as occurs in humans. N,N-dipropylnitrosamine undergoes β-oxidation to N-nitrosamines that cause pancreatic ductal adenocarcinomas in the Syrian golden hamster (Scarpelli et al., 1984).

Forensic Analysis of Liver Damage

The liver is the filter and processing organ for nutrients and toxicants that are absorbed by the intestinal tract through the portal vein. It is under low oxygen tension because it filters venous blood. It can metabolize the toxic components for excretion by the kidney or pass them out through the bile duct. The liver should be viewed as the biochemical anatomy organ due to the distribution of important metabolic enzymes and cofactors in the liver acini. **Figure 16-1** shows the biochemical anatomy of the liver moving from portal vein or hepatic artery to central vein (terminal hepatic vein). The zones and the formation of a hypoxic zone by the central vein (zone 3) are important for toxic reductive mechanisms and the increased presence of CYPs for bioactivation. The high glutathione concentration in the liver (10 mM) lessens into zone 3, which could manifest the toxicity of metabolites. However, metals would be expected to be highest coming in from the intestine into zone 1 and exert their largest influence there. Bile outflow also occurs in zone 1. Kupffer cells, stellate cells, and sinusoidal endothelium should also be considered in addition to hepatocytes in zones or bile duct cells. Liver damage is the reason many people succumb to an overdose of many over-the-counter medications, prescription medications, and/or drugs of abuse. The relationship between alcoholism and cirrhosis of the liver is a well understood phenomenon. Moldy feed has caused fatalities in animals (aflatoxin) as well as ingestion of blue-green algae–contaminated water (microcystins). This section focuses first on the areas or sites of the liver susceptible to toxicants and then the toxicity associated with a variety of toxicants due to specific types of injury as listed in **Table 16-3**.

Anatomical Localization of Liver Injury

Periportal Toxicity (Zone 1)

Periportal (zone 1) damage occurs more often than people care to consider based on the availability of iron-supplemented children's vitamins. Children who are not mature enough to understand the difference between medicines, vitamins, and candy should only have access to vitamins not supplemented with minerals. Consuming an entire bottle of Fe-supplemented vitamins would be fatal. The liver can store iron in ferritin and in an insoluble toxic hemosiderin form causing centrilobular (zone 3)

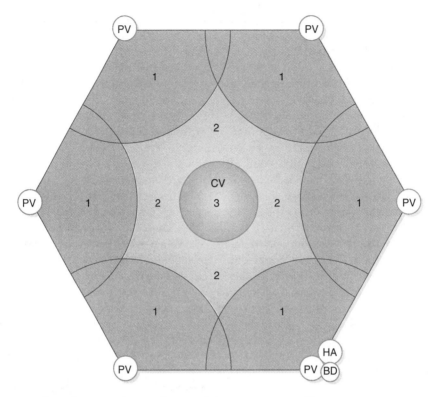

FIGURE 16-1 Biochemical Anatomy Schematic of a Liver Lobule in a Hexagon (Variable in Size)

Note: A liver acinus would stretch from one central vein (CV) or terminal hepatic vein to another CV. The flow direction is from portal vein (PV) or hepatic artery (HA) to central vein, so the oxygenation of the tissue decreases into the hexagon (zone 1 → zone 3). The bile duct (BD) is there to remove primary bile acids and conjugated compounds into the duodenum possibly for enterohepatic recirculation. Zone 3 has the highest CYP activities for activation and least glutathione for conjugation/detoxication.

fibrosis as indicated by hepatic hydroxyproline content (collagen deposition). Hepatocellular necrosis is also involved as indicated by plasma alanine aminotransferase activity (leaked out of liver cells). Lipid peroxidation also results from ROS generated by excess iron (Valerio and Petersen, 2000). The oxygen-rich environment of the periportal region also is responsible for copper-induced hepatocellular apoptosis. Cu catalyzes the generation of oxidized glutathione (GSSG) from the reduced form (GSH) and superoxide. Degradation of the Cu-Zn SOD causes decreased dismutation of $O_2^{-\cdot}$. The mitochondria in zone 1 show decreased Mn SOD function, reduced thiol/disulphide ratio, and increased superoxide resulting in loss of ATP, collapse of the mitochondrial membrane potential, and induction of the mitochondrial permeability transition (Roy et al., 2009). Anticancer agents damage here as well for a

variety of reasons. Doxorubicin is activated by P-450 reductase, generates ROS consistent with the oxygenation of zone 1 but also interferes with synthesis of macromolecules, binds covalently to and cross-links DNA, inhibits topoisomerase II, arrests cells in G_2 phase, and induces apoptosis. It also attracts the accumulation of inflammatory cells. Cisplatin is activated by metabolism and forms DNA adducts, also causing G_2 phase arrest and apoptosis. These two anticancer agents induce periportal fibrosis, focal inflammation, and degeneration of hepatic cords in addition to apoptosis. 5- Fluorouracil causes less damage than the other agents but still can lead to apoptosis, invasion by inflammatory cells, and damaged cytoplasmic organelles with collagenous fibrils in necrotic cells. This agent is first metabolized to 5-fluoro-deoxyuridine-monophosphate prior to inhibition of thymidylate synthase

TABLE 16-3   Forensic Chart of Hepatic Toxicity

Hepatic Toxicity	Toxic Agents
Anatomical	
Periportal (zone 1)	Fe (Valerio and Petersen, 2000), Cu (Roy et al., 2009), anticancer (El-Sayyad et al., 2009), allyl alcohol (Campion et al., 2009), signs of N-acetylcysteine-induced delayed acetaminophen recovery (Yang et al., 2009), ethanol metabolism and effects on gluconeogenesis and oxygen uptake—lactate decreasing ketogenesis (Lopez et al., 2009), aflatoxin (Kiran et al., 1998), dexamethasone (Micuda et al., 2007), α-naphthyl isothiocyanate (Kodali et al., 2006)
Centrilobular (zone 3)	Acetaminophen overdose (Yang et al., 2009), atenolol-induced inflammation + prednisone (Dumortier et al., 2009), tienilic acid enhanced by buthionine-(S,R)-sulfoximine (Nishiya et al., 2008), alcohol cirrhosis (Tipoe et al., 2008)
Kupffer cells	Lipopolysaccharide-induced cholestasis, clodronate (Sturm et al., 2005)
Disease	
Sex-linked	Estrogen-induced intrahepatic cholestasis (Leuenberger et al., 2009), estrogen-induced steatosis (Elias et al., 2007), formamide-induced hemangiosarcoma (National Toxicology Program, 2008), PCBs, PBBS, and hexachlorobenzene induction of uroporphyria development via CYP1A1 induction (Smith et al., 1990)
Apoptosis/necrosis	Acetaminophen (Holt et al., 2008), CCl_4 (Weber et al., 2003)
Steatosis	Obesity, ethanol, CCl_4 puromycin (Pan et al., 2007)
Fibrosis/cirrhosis	Ethanol, CCl_4, bile duct ligation/destruction, α-naphthyl isothiocyanate, dietary 3,5-diethoxycarbonyl-1,4-dihydrocollidine, thioacetamide, dimethylnitrosamine, infection (Henderson and Iredale, 2007)
Neoplasms	Aflatoxin, ethanol (Cha and Dematteo, 2005), dioxins, PCBs, phenobarbital (Oliver and Roberts, 2002), vinyl chloride (Bolt, 2005), CCl_4 (Weber et al., 2003), di(2-ethylhexyl)phthalate (Butterworth et al., 1987), sex hormones (Kalra et al., 2008), tamoxifen (Brown, 2009)
Cytoskeleton toxicity	Ethanol (Shepard and Tuma, 2009), pectenotoxins (Espiña and Rubiolo, 2008), As (Bernstam and Nriagu, 2000), vinca alkaloids, paclitaxel (Hruban et al., 1989), microcystins (Dawson, 1998)
Sinusoidal injury	Acetaminophen augmented by ethanol binge (McCuskey, 2006)
Immune/inflammatory	Isoniazid, ketoconazole, troglitazone, pyrazinamide, halothane, tienilic acid, penicillamine, propylthiouracil, procainamide, minocycline, α-methyldopa, hydralazine, propylthiouracil, phenytoin, statins, zafirlukast, CCl_4, acetaminophen, ethanol, Con A, α-naphthyl isothiocyanate (Adams et al., 2010)
Cholestasis/bile duct injury	Indomethacin, statins, digoxin, enalapril, midazolam, tamoxifen, diclofenac, methotrexate, troglitazone, lisinopril, itraconazole, verapamil, bosentan, glyburide, flucloxacillin (Grattagliano et al., 2009)

(El-Sayyad et al., 2009). Methapyrilene (N,N-dimethyl-N′-pyridyl-N′[2-thienylmethyl]-1,2-ethanediamine) has become a model hepatotoxin for observing the effect of S-oxidation of the thiophene group. It depletes the rich concentration of GSH in the periportal region while increasing reduced glutathione in the centrilobular region. Heme-oxygenase 1 and glutamate cysteine ligase catalytic subunit are increased as a cellular defense mechanism. Cytotoxicity progresses via apoptosis and is followed by necrosis and hepatic cancer development if the animal survives the initial liver damage (Mercer et al., 2009). Allyl alcohol is a model periportal toxicant dependent on oxidative mechanism for activation. Along with the toxicity to periportal cells, a marked upregulation of multidrug resistance–associated protein 4 is noted in protected centrilobular hepatocytes (Campion et al., 2009). Ethanol is extensively metabolized in the periportal region and inhibits gluconeogenesis and decreases oxygen uptake more in the periportal region. Lactate decreases ketogenesis more in this region as well (Lopez et al., 2009). The moldy feed aflatoxin produces diffuse and severe hydropic degeneration, bile duct hyperplasia, and periportal fibrosis in broiler chicks. This was reduced to slight or moderate hydropic degeneration by inclusion of polyvinylpolypyrrolidone in the diet (Kiran et al., 1998).

Because fibrosis is a precursor to cirrhosis, it is worth investigating how model hepatotoxicants affect the regional manifestation of fibrotic damage. Thioacetamide, dimethylnitrosamine, and carbon tetrachloride were reinvestigated for the damage they cause when administered orally or by IP injection. Thioacetamide caused little fibrosis. Instead, it resulted in inflammatory infiltration in the periportal region and bile duct proliferation. The Histological Activity Index indicated fibrosis 6 weeks after administration. Dimethylnitrosamine produced piecemeal necrosis with little necrosis and 100% lethality 5 weeks after administration. Carbon tetrachloride resulted in a periportal fibrosis at 8–10 weeks and a septal fibrosis at 12–14 weeks. This study indicated a concern about the reproducibility of the toxic results of these chemicals between laboratories and individual researchers (Jang et al., 2008). Fat accumulation in the periportal region is induced by dexamethasone treatment. p-Glycoprotein is expressed primarily in the periportal region. The corticosteroid dexamethasone may cause enlargement of the liver at least in part by increased excretion of p-glycoprotein substrates in the bile and microvesicular steatosis (Micuda et al., 2007). Another periportal susceptibility is the attraction of neutrophils via beta2-integrin CD18. Alpha-naphthyl isothiocyanate causes periportal inflammation, widespread hepatic necrosis, and acute cholestatic hepatitis in wild-type or in partially CD18-deficient mice, but not in CD18-null type mice (Kodali et al., 2006). From these examples, it is apparent that oxygen-mediated toxicity, the unequal distribution of metabolic enzymes and transporting moieties, the proximity to the circulation and inflammatory cells, the highest concentrations of toxicants entering from the portal circulation, and the presence of the bile ducts in the periportal region all lead to damage in this region.

Centrilobular Toxicity (Zone 3)

Many women succumb to liver damage caused by using acetaminophen for pain relief, supposing it to be a safe analgesic. At high concentrations, the N-acetyl-p-benzoquinone imine metabolite conjugation with GSH depletes glutathione concentrations, forms covalent adducts, and initiates mitochondrial damage (increased membrane permeability transition and collapse of mitochondrial membrane potential). The reduction in ATP results in massive centrilobular necrosis (high CYP and low GSH) and extensive inflammatory cell infiltration. N-acetylcysteine (NAC; precursor to GSH) is the antidote early in this process to support the glutathione-based protection. However, if given later, NAC actually delays recovery by impairing glucose metabolism and endangering the endogenous GSH recovery. The liver is an odd organ in that it is known to regenerate tissue even following partial liver surgical removal. The cells that are least affected by acetaminophen and may serve as sources for recovery are found in the periportal region. That is also the source of extended toxicity if NAC is given too late as indicated by periportal hepatocyte vacuolation (Yang et al., 2009).

The other big looming disease of the liver that has brought down many people is chronic alcohol-induced cirrhosis. In a voluntary feeding model, rats show increased damage if ethanol is accompanied by fish oil as the source of dietary fatty acids. Ethanol does generate steatosis or fatty liver. It also causes necrosis, inflammation, and centrilobular collagen deposition indicating fibrosis. The extent of liver damage and modulation of metabolism by toxic metabolites are observed as increased endotoxin, alanine aminotransferase in plasma, CYP2E1, and lipid peroxidation. NF-κB and proinflammatory TNF-α, iNOS, and COX-2 increase on ethanol toxicity as does procollagen-I, especially in the centrilobular regions (Tipoe et al., 2008). Part of the reason for the centrilobular damage induced by ethanol is the hypoxia generated by the metabolism to acetaldehyde and beyond in an area that is already oxygen poor. An increase in intracellular Na^+ is observed in hepatocytes exposed to ethanol and hypoxia. Na$^+$ influx does not occur when the metabolic inhibitors are used, during the incubation of cells in a bicarbonate-free buffer, or in the presence of 5-(N,N-dimethyl)-amiloride, a Na$^+$/H$^+$ exchange antagonist (Carini et al., 2000). Ethanol metabolism decreased the hepatocyte pH. Inhibition of ethanol metabolism by 4-methylpyrazole and acetaldehyde oxidation by cyanamide prevented this toxic effect. The immune system can also be involved in centrilobular damage as well. A patient on the beta-blocker atenolol exhibited an acute hepatitis with portal and centrilobular inflammatory lesions. The immunosuppressant steroid prednisone was given and resolved the periportal lesions but worsened the centrilobular damage (Dumortier et al., 2009). Carbon tetrachloride is another model of centrilobular necrosis. The CYP2E1 enzyme initiates the process in the hepatocytes near the central vein. Mice deficient in this enzyme are resistant to the liver damage associated with CCl$_4$. Downregulation of the gene responsible for expression of this enzyme is a protective mechanism against CCl$_4$ hepatotoxicity. However, it is interesting that age may increase the toxicity of this compound, possibly by influencing circadian rhythms. Not only are there sex-differences in toxicity, but also periods of the day/night cycle when animals and humans are more susceptible to toxicity. Period 2 is an important part of the core clock oscillator and plays a protective role in CCl$_4$-induced liver damage through inhibiting uncoupling protein-2 gene expression in mice via a PPARα signaling pathway. The presence of Period 2 gene expression keeps ATP levels higher and decreases production of toxic metabolites (Period 2–null mice have decreased ATP concentrations and increased toxic metabolites; Chen, Li, et al., 2009). This last study is not only important to consider for the site specificity of the liver damage but to encourage young researchers to consider that the rodent model uses an animal during the light period that normally sleeps during the daylight hours and may not be the best toxicity model for a human during waking hours.

A diuretic medication tienilic acid was withdrawn from the marker based on fulminant hepatic failure. Tienilic acid is metabolized by CYP2C9 to electrophilic reactive intermediates that bind covalently to macromolecules including the CYP enzyme. It decreases hepatic GSH content and causes lipid peroxidation. When hepatic gene expression was analyzed by microarrays, glutathione synthase and glutamate-cysteine ligase were upregulated indicating increased glutathione synthesis. Oxidative stress was indicated by increased expression of heme oxygenase-1 and NAD(P)H dehydrogenase quinone 1. Phase II drug metabolism was also elevated as indicated by glutathione S-transferase and UDP glycosyltransferase 1A6 expression. When an inhibitor of glutamate-cysteine ligase, buthionine-(S,R)-sulfoximine, was given with tienilic acid, extensive centrilobular necrosis was observed (Nishiya et al., 2008).

Kupffer cells produce cytokines that mediate the hepatic acute phase response and cholestasis to a circulating lipopolysaccharide known as endotoxin during sepsis. The sensitivity to transport of bile acids resides in the regulation of basolateral Na$^+$-taurocholic acid cotransporting polypeptide (Ntcp) by retinoid X receptor-retinoid acid receptor nuclear heterodimer and the liver-enriched transcription factor hepatocyte nuclear factor 1α. Cytokine release by the Kupffer cells inhibits the regulatory factors binding and transactivation of the Ntcp gene. The studies used to identify Kupffer cells as the cause of certain toxicities such as hepatic acute phase response use the phagocytic nature of the Kupffer cells to accumulate the toxin dichloromethylene-bisphosphonate, known as clodronate in liposomes, which depletes the liver of these cells (Sturm et al., 2005).

Toxicity Associated with Liver Damage

Sex-Linked Damage

It is important to address why female humans and animals display higher rates of certain liver toxicities. This is an important feature in women's health. For example, women activate STATs genes in the liver by continuously secreting growth hormone from the pituitary, as opposed to the stochastic (more random pulses) distribution of male growth hormone production. Sexually dimorphic liver gene expression occurs for processes such as androgen metabolism, energy production, and inflammation. Males involve DNA methylation and methylation-sensitive transcription factors in hepatic gene expression (*Slp* and *Cyp2d9* promoters). CYP7B1 (oxysterol 7α-hydroxylase) has increased expression in males and represses androgen biosynthesis by decreasing the availability of DHEA, the key precursor to testosterone. Clearance of the estrogen receptor antagonist hydroxycholesterol by CYP7B1 metabolism activates the estrogen receptor. Women who use estrogen-containing medications for birth control of menopausal symptoms activate the estrogen receptor, which also regulates *Cyp7b1* expression. This can lead to estrogen-induced inflammation and hepatotoxicity, including intrahepatic cholestasis. However, if PPARα (peroxisome proliferator-activated receptor) is stimulated, this activates heteromeric transcription factors GABPs (especially GABPα) bound to the *Cyp7b1* promoter. This represses expression of the enzyme and decreases intrahepatic cholestasis, which is the most frequently observed liver toxicity of pregnancy (Leuenberger et al., 2009). Changes in liver enzyme induction and resultant toxicity are also sex-dependent. Development of uroporphyria in response to polychlorinated biphenyls (PCBs), polybrominated biphenyls, or hexachlorobenzene treatment appears to be a significant factor for female rats. Ethoxyresorufin O-deethylase associated with CYP1A1 is higher in female rats, and the induction of CYP1A1 and CYP1A2 is highly induced in the centrilobular region. The association between CYP1A1 and uroporphyria development is consistent with the metabolic activity and induction of this enzyme in female rats (Smith et al., 1990).

Conversely, males can be very sensitive to the effects of environmental estrogens as the liver is called to make vitellogenin (egg yolk protein) with essentially no place to transport it. For example, male fish exposed to high concentrations of 17α-ethynylestradiol show gross hypertrophy of the liver (accumulation of fat and disruption of acinar organization) and kidney and high mortalities (Elias et al., 2007). Male

mice (B6C3F1), but not female mice or either sex of rats (F344/N), exhibit hemangiosarcoma of the liver in response to formamide (National Toxicology Program, 2008).

Apoptosis/Necrosis

Apoptosis is probably the likely form of cell mortality becoming necrosis only in severe damage. CYP metabolites are the usual chemical toxic species that may yield problems, especially from pharmaceuticals (Gómez-Lechón et al., 2008). However, the death of liver cells can come from diverse mechanisms such as cholestasis, viral hepatitis, ischemia or reperfusion injury, liver preservation for transplantation, and direct toxicity of medications or industrial chemicals. Both apoptosis and necrosis occur due to mitochondrial permeabilization and dysfunction. Apoptosis still requires sufficient ATP synthesis or stores to initiate a death program through Fas ligand with Fas, leading to stimulation of the caspase activation cascade. Necrosis requires acute ATP depletion as a result of metabolic damage consistent with the perturbations that occur with ischemia or reperfusion injury or medication-induced toxicity (Malhi et al., 2006). The model medication for apoptosis or necrosis is still the over-the-counter analgesic acetaminophen. Acetaminophen or paracetamol (European generic name for the same drug) is the leading cause of acute liver failure in the United States and the widely used model for hepatic toxicity in the mouse. As discussed previously, the quinone imine metabolite is responsible for the depletion of glutathione and adduct formation. A centrilobular necrosis results with extreme invasion of neutrophils. It appears that the toxic species and the infiltration of the polymorphonuclear leukocytes participate in the progression of acetaminophen hepatotoxicity. The benefit of removal of apoptotic neutrophils from inflammatory sites stems from the leaking of their proinflammatory and toxic intracellular contents that harm surrounding less damaged or healthy tissue. However, circulating monocyte infiltration appears to lead to phagocytosis of apoptotic cells and helps resolve inflammation while promoting tissue repair. This dichotomy of white blood cell function in toxicity and repair is important in understanding mechanisms that lead to either apoptosis/necrosis or recovery. Hepatic macrophages, natural killer cells, and neutrophils can all contribute to cellular injury via TNF-α, IL-1β, and NO. The macrophages conversely provide protection to liver cells via Il-10, IL-6, and IL-18. The way this may be possible is that macrophages can be divided into two populations. Classically activated M1s generate proinflammatory cytokines. Alternatively activated M2s down-regulate inflammation, participate in tissue remodeling, remove tissue debris and apoptotic cells, and induce new blood vessel formation (Holt et al., 2008).

A former medication and industrial solvent is carbon tetrachloride. The haloalkanes are toxic based on how well they form a stable carbon-centered radical. The more halide groups there are, the more electron-withdrawing capacity from the carbon center that becomes more electropositive. This makes a radical formation more likely. CCl_4 is dependent on oxygen in an interesting manner for lipid peroxidation. Too high pressures (> 100 mm Hg) prevents lipid peroxidation, as does the anoxic state. However, hypoxic states between 5 and 35 mm Hg favor lipid peroxidation and the reductive dehalogenation of carbon tetrachloride by CYP2E1, CYP2B1, CYP2B2, and possibly CYP3A to form a trichloromethyl radical, CCl_3 ·. This reactive intermediate binds to macromolecules (lipid, nucleic acids, protein) and disrupts lipid metabolism/fatty degeneration leading to steatosis (fatty liver). DNA adducts lead to hepatic cancer. Reactions with oxygen lead to trichloromethylperoxy radical CCl_3OO·, which initiates lipid peroxidation of polyunsaturated fatty acids (especially phospholipids). This alters the permeability of mitochondrial, endoplasmic reticulum, and plasma membranes. Calcium sequestration is lost and leads to apoptosis and necrosis. Additionally, the fatty acids degrade to toxic reactive aldehydes (particularly 4-hydroxynonenal) that inhibit enzymes. Hypomethylation of cellular components due to CCl_4 toxicity inhibits protein synthesis (RNA hypomethylation) or lipoprotein secretion (phospholipid hypomethylation). Together these processes lead to cell death.

Activation of TNF-α leads to apoptosis, while TGF-α proceeds to fibrosis. The formation of IL-6 and IL-10 helps the cells not too damaged toward recovery. CYP inducers increase toxicity, while inhibitors decrease CCl_4 toxicity (Weber et al., 2003). Ketones and ketogenic compounds (alcohols) potentiate CCl_4 hepatotoxicity (Pilon et al., 1988). Because carbon tetrachloride can damage membranes in the cell, the damage to the ER is assumed from the location of the CYPs; however, the ribosomes are part of the rough ER. While CCl_4 inhibits protein synthesis, it does not do so by damaging the membranes of the ER. Actually, it appears that the damage to protein synthesis occurs via disruption of the ribosomes, because cycloheximide protects against the protein synthesis inhibition by CCl_4. An antioxidant N,N'-diphenyl-p-phenylenediamine protects against membrane and ribosomal injury (Farber et al., 1971).

Steatosis

Fatty liver, or steatosis, can be generated by a simple process, such as overfeeding geese to make a fatty liver, which is used in the French cuisine pâté de foie gras. Obesity, insulin resistance, and ethanol can lead to triglyceride accumulation that is the basis of steatosis. CCl_4 can also lead to steatosis, especially in the presence of puromycin. CCl_4 3 hours after administration in rats decreases the secretion of triglycerides as part of VLDL. The failure of the Golgi has been implicated in this accumulation of fat. Why would a protein synthesis inhibitor such as puromycin increase steatosis yet decrease necrosis? There are a number of transporting proteins that are important for export of triglycerides. Triglycerides are secreted due to lipoproteins, which depend on the function of apolipoprotein B (apoB) and microsomal triglyceride transfer protein (MTP). ApoB is a structural protein, while MTP is a required chaperone for assembling the triglyceride-lipoprotein complexes. That is why protein synthesis inhibition by either carbon tetrachloride or specific agents that bind to ribosomes cause steatosis (Pan et al., 2007). A further elucidation shows that there are hyperlipidemic stages for rats given CCl_4 and experiencing acute liver damage or given puromycin amino nucleoside and developing nephrotic syndrome. In both pathological states, the hyperlipidemic state is associated with an increase in high-density lipoprotein (HDL) and steady-state levels of apo A-1 mRNA. Early stages of these diseases show increases in total cholesterol and triacylglycerols but no induction of HDL and apo A-1 mRNA. Further examination of these secondary hyperlipidemia models shows that small viscosity changes below the physiological range induce apo A-1 gene expression at the mRNA level, but inhibit apo A-1 gene expression when viscosity returns to physiological values (Nuño et al., 1997). Mice also lacking phosphatidylinositol transfer proteins also lead to spinal cerebellar degeneration, intestinal and hepatic steatosis, and hypoglycemia (Alb et al., 2003).

Fibrosis/Cirrhosis

Many of the mechanisms already mentioned can lead to fibrosis and cirrhosis of the liver. The chief cause is clearly ethanol. However, the chronic nature of the disease may give some hint that mechanisms other than direct toxicity play key roles in the development of fibrosis and its progression to cirrhosis. The infiltration of immune cells appears to be vitally important in the development of liver fibrosis. However, not all immune cells play a vital role in models of liver fibrosis development. First, consider innate immunity. Bile duct ligation causes the infiltration of neutrophils. This would appear on first glance to implicate neutrophils in fibrosis. However, if neutrophils are depleted or faulty transgenic ones lacking IL-8 expression are present, fibrosis is little affected. Similarly, the α-naphthyl isothiocyanate model of liver fibrosis is little affected by neutrophils with a poor chemokine receptor (CXCR2[-/-]) for recruitment to the site of toxic injury. Mast cells also do not play a role in fibrosis as indicated by CCl_4 or by a pig serum challenge in mast-cell-deficient mutant Ws/Ws rats or W/Wv mice. As indicated for carbon tetrachloride, there are at least two populations of macrophages—one that is engaged in injury that leads to fibrosis (M1s) and one that leads to repair (M2s). For example, a 3-day dimethylnitrosamine treatment of rats resulted in activated hepatic stellate cells and marked fibrosis thereafter. However, when a mutated form of monocyte chemoattractant protein 1 was given, the infiltration by macrophages was reduced considerably and activated stellate cells were not found (no fibrosis). In support of these findings of macrocyte involvement in fibrosis, thioacetamide-induced fibrosis is reduced in rats by treatment with gadolinium chloride ($GdCl_3$). $GdCl_3$ inhibits ED1-immunolabelled cells (exudates macrophages) and ED2-immunolabelled cells (Kupffer cells). If the stellate cells are important in fibrosis, then natural killer cell (lymphocyte subclass) activation should eliminate activated stellate cells and decrease fibrosis. This is exactly what occurred in mice fed a 3,5-diethoxycarbonyl-1, 4-dihydrocollidine (DDC) diet or injected with carbon tetrachloride to generate liver fibrosis. Addition of a Toll-like receptor 3 ligand, poly-inosinic-polycytidylic acid, activated natural cells and interferon gamma as part of stimulation of innate immunity.

Next, consider adaptive immunity and B and T lymphocytes. The T cells comprise the cell-mediated immunity and the B cells provide antibody-producing or humoral immunity. CCl_4- or thioacetamide-treated mice, which were genetically modified to express rat IL-10, had decreased fibrosis. IL-10 reduces the CD8+ T cell activation of stellate cells. In a parasite (schistosomiasis) model of hepatic fibrosis mediated by T-helper type 2 cytokine release, an inhibitor of IL-13 (sIL-13Ralpha2-Fc) reduced procollagen I and procollagen III mRNA expression by fibroblasts and the development of fibrosis. Another researcher found that in CCl_4-treated mice B cells appeared to play more of a role in the laying down of collagen in the development of fibrosis and did so independent of any T cells. A schistosomiasis model conversely caused more liver fibrosis in B cell–deficient mice. Thus, it appears that inflammation and white blood cells play a role in hepatic fibrosis and necrosis, but the immune cells and cytokines responsible for these effects may vary based on the nature of the development of hepatic damage (Henderson and Iredale, 2007).

Neoplasms

As previously examined, genotoxic agents, both activation-independent and metabolically activated, play a role in the development of cancer, as do similar epigenetic mechanisms of cancer formation. However, what is unique to liver cancer? Is it simply its location as the filter of food-borne toxicants? Is it the liver's metabolic activity? Perhaps it is a function of its stem cell population and regeneration capacity. On closer examination, numerous mechanisms lead to the formation of various primary liver tumors. Hepatocellular carcinoma clearly can come from either a severe event of DNA modification/damage or multiple insults. CCl_4 reveals the carbon-centered radical that initiates hepatic cancer (Weber et al., 2003). Mutations in tumor suppressor genes, proto-oncogenes, and DNA mismatch repair genes all produce cancers. The most widely studied tumor suppressor gene is p53. Mutations in this gene are present in 30–60% of patients with liver cancer. Point mutations in one allele or deletion in another one in the p53 gene help the promotion of cancers, but not initiation. Here is where a contaminant of spoiled (moldy) food has a role in hepatocarcinogenesis. Aflatoxin B_1 from *Aspergillus flavus* contamination of stored food items (peanuts, corn, rice) forms an epoxide, which forms a p53 mutation in codon 249 (G → T; arginine → serine). The aflatoxin B_1 mutation is also considered a tumor initiator because it is found in normal patients without any signs of cirrhotic damage. Hepatitis B virus acts synergistically with aflatoxin B_1 in hepatic cancer. On its own, this virus is associated with chronic liver cancer development. Hepatitis B integrates into the host DNA 80% of the time and may cause direct effects. It may activate promoters of several oncogenes (c-jun and c-fos) and inhibit apoptosis (inhibits p53 protein) through a protein of 154 amino acids that it produces. This viral protein increases expression of the epidermal growth factor receptor and potentiates TGF-α. Liver fibrosis is also stimulated by upregulating TGF-β signaling. The inflammatory reactions to the virus also appear to be proportional to the development of cancer. Inflammatory reactions are now thought to play a role in cancer as well as fibrosis and cirrhosis, as hepatitis C generates more liver inflammation and more frequent cirrhosis than hepatitis B. Cirrhosis increases dramatically the frequency of liver cancer in chronically hepatitis-infected patients. Cirrhosis indicates that alcohol is a key factor in chronic liver cancers. Another sign that a tumor suppressor gene has aided in cancer development is loss of heterozygosity.

Proto-oncogenes may be overexpressed in a variety of cancers. However, in liver cancers, Ras, c-fos, and c-erbB-2 mutations are not frequent in hepatic tumors. c-Myc is overexpressed in < 50% of liver cancers, but signals intrahepatic metastases and shorter survival. One classic agent that is a known human carcinogen that directs its activity toward hepatic endothelial/sinusoidal cells and parenchymal cells is vinyl chloride. It is oxidized to a chloroethylene oxide and then exocyclic etheno adducts form with DNA. These adducts are pro-mutagenic and affect proto-oncogenes and tumor suppressor genes and the gene and gene product levels. Lipid peroxidation and oxidative stress also play a role here (Bolt, 2005).

Although signaling pathways are not in common to all hepatic cancer development, mutations in the Wnt/beta-catenin pathway are seen as an early marker for 25% of liver cancer cases. Other important signaling pathway alterations are those involved in interferon response and TGF-β/IGF2R/Smad pathway (Cha and Dematteo, 2005).

Some liver cancers develop from stimulating the proliferation of liver cells and inhibition of apoptosis. These events can be modified by the aryl hydrocarbon receptor (dioxins and PCBs), constitutive androstane receptor (phenobarbital) without resorting to gene mutation (Oliver and Roberts, 2002). Peroxisome proliferators such as the ubiquitous plasticizing agent di(2-ethylhexyl)phthalate cause liver cancers in female rats and male and female mice at high doses. These agents also are known as hypolipidemic carcinogens. Although these chemicals may produce ROS as a result of peroxisome proliferation, it is their ability to act as mitogenic stimulators that correlates with their carcinogenic potency (Butterworth et al., 1987).

Obesity alone appears to be a risk factor for development of various organ cancers including liver tumors. The role of food intake may be linked to carcinogenic food ingredients, excessive calories, loss of protective factors by reduced exercise, signaling factors from the adipose tissue itself, and other injurious conditions such as the development of a fatty liver or gallstones (Percik and Stumvoll, 2009). The role of sex hormone receptors in hepatocellular carcinoma is not well known despite the understanding of a male predominance in chronic liver diseases such as hepatitis B, hepatitis C, alcoholic liver disease, and alcoholic steatohepatitis progressing to cirrhosis and further on to liver cancer. The increase in hepatic neoplasms and oral contraceptives indicates a role for the estrogen receptor, and so does the presence of androgen receptors in hepatic cancer, which indicates a stimulatory role for testosterone, especially in the intrahepatic recurrence of tumors (Kalra et al., 2008). A note of interest is that tamoxifen, a weak estrogenic medicinal compound used to treat breast cancer, causes liver tumors in rats. This appears to involve metabolism rather than hormonal action, as tamoxifen is α-hydroxylated and then conjugated to a sulfate in the rat liver. This is a reactive species of this compound that binds to DNA at the N(2)-position of guanine, yielding pro-mutagenic lesions. It is unclear whether this is species-specific or occurs in female patients (Brown, 2009).

Cytoskeleton Toxicity

Again, ethanol plays a role in liver injury. Ethanol induces hyperacetylation of proteins including histone H3 (one of five main histone proteins), p53 (tumor suppressor), PGC-1α (energy metabolism regulator), SREPB-1c (lipid homeostasis), AceCS2 (soluble mitochondrial matrix protein), and α-tubulin (constitutive protein of microtubules). This includes cytoskeletal proteins such as α-tubulin and affects microtubule stability (Shepard and Tuma, 2009). Marine toxins of the macrolactone chemical group target the actin cytoskeleton in liver causing severe hepatotoxicity (pectenotoxins of dinoflagellate genus *Dinophysis*; Espiña and Rubiolo, 2008). Another water-borne toxin that is becoming a large problem in lakes contaminated with phosphorus runoff from fertilization of farm fields and lawns is the freshwater cyanobacterium *Microcystis aeruginosa*, which is released into the water and causes toxicity upon ingestion. Microcystins are heptapeptides with a unique structure that are potent inhibitors of phosphatases 1 and 2A. Inhibition of these enzymes disrupts the cytoskeleton and results in gross hepatic hemorrhage (Dawson, 1998). Arsenic disrupts the cytoskeletal structures responsible for structural soundness of cells, their shape, and movement. Changes in liver and skin have been studied but have not provided a molecular mechanism as of yet (Bernstam and Nriagu, 2000).

Cytoskeleton toxicity is not just the mode of agents known to damage the liver with little therapeutic value. It is also the mechanism used in the treatment of metastatic cancers as cell division is impaired. The anticancer drug paclitaxel was isolated from the bark of the Western yew tree in 1971. It is a diterpenoid compound that binds to the β-tubulin subunit of microtubules and prevents their disassembly, resulting in mitotic arrest of cancer cells and normal cells of the esophagus, stomach, small intestine, colon, liver, and bone marrow. Another set of antimitotic medications for treating neoplasms are the vinca alkaloids from the Madagascar periwinkle plant. They also bind to β-tubulin, but prevent polymerization with α-tubulin (Hruban et al., 1989).

Sinusoidal Injury

A topic related to cytoskeletal injury is the early damage to sinusoidal endothelial cells due to acetaminophen toxicity. This is especially apparent following binge ethanol intake. Sinusoidal epithelial cells swell and lose their ability to endocytose FITC-FSA (scavenger receptor ligand). Gaps in the cells form by damage to fenestrae prior to any signs of observed histological changes to parenchymal cells. Red blood cells penetrate into the space of Disse and may be followed by sinusoidal collapse and decreased blood flow. The gaps observed are larger with acetaminophen plus ethanol—similar to hepatic veno-occlusive disease caused by pyrrolizidine alkaloids of the toxic *Crotalaria* plant species. NO donor administration or inhibition of iNOS decreases toxicity, while inhibitors of eNOS increase toxicity to these cells. That suggests a protective role for constitutive NO originating from sinusoidal epithelial cells. Inhibitors of

MMP-2 and MMP-9 also minimize toxicity to these cells. Taken together it appears that the cytoskeleton is the target of the toxicity, because this structure aids in the formation and maintenance of the fenestrae (McCuskey, 2006).

Immune and Inflammatory Damage

Immune mechanisms that can lead to fibrosis and ultimately to cirrhosis have already been examined. Acute and idiosyncratic drug-induced liver injuries are important contributors to sickness and death of patients. The idiosyncratic responses are more prone to develop into fulminant liver failure (25% of intensive care unit cases). It is easy in toxicology to focus on the formation of active metabolites and their direct toxicity to macromolecules or organelles. Idiosyncratic drug-induced liver injury of this type is classified as metabolic. Medications such as isoniazid (anti-tuberculosis), ketoconazole (anti-fungal), troglitazone (banned antihyperglycemic agent), and pyrazinamide (anti-tuberculosis) fit into the metabolic group. However, it appears that the direct toxicity may initiate the immune response. Idiosyncratic reactions that generate a fever, rash, a 1- to 4-week onset of symptoms, and a rapid onset on another challenge dose are classified as immune. Drugs that yield anti-medication or autoimmune antibodies include halothane (anesthetic) or tienilic acid (diuretic). However, some medications that yield auto-immunity in brown Norway rats, such as the anti-arthritis medication penicillamine or propylthiouracil (treats Graves' disease–induced autoimmunity in cats), do not have a rapid onset on a subsequent challenge. Similarly, heparin-induced, antibody-mediated thrombocytopenia does not reemerge once the antibodies are no longer present. Those that develop clear autoimmune antibodies such as procainamide-induced lupus-like syndrome usually resolve rapidly if the reaction is not severe and no re-challenge occurs. Some medications, such as the antibiotics minocycline and nitrofurantoin and discontinued anti-hypertensive α-methyldopa, develop a condition resembling idiopathic autoimmune hepatitis. Development of idiopathic drug-induced liver injury may take as long as a year or more and involve autoimmune reactions such as lupus-like syndrome,

autoimmune-hemolytic anemia, or vasculitis. Isoniazid, minocycline, α-methyldopa, hydralazine, propylthiouracil, phenytoin, statins, and zafirlukast are representative of this group.

There are 10^{10} resident lymphocytes in the human liver that can initiate an innate immune response. The total lymphocyte population is represented by the T cells, the B cells, the natural killer (NK) cells, and the natural killer T (NKT) cells. Inflammation and intrahepatic localization of lymphocytes increase lymphocyte recruitment. The degree of damage to hepatocytes and cholangiocytes is associated with the scale of lymphocyte infiltration and inflammatory response. The liver's two sources of blood supply (portal vein and hepatic arteries) make it more prone to immune-mediated damage. The immune cells migrate across the sinusoidal epithelial cells just discussed. These sinusoidal cells lack the P-selectin adhesion molecule and have very low levels of E-selectin expression. The portal vascular endothelium expresses selectins when inflamed. ICAM-1 is a constitutively expressed adhesion receptor in the sinusoidal epithelium that mediates leukocyte adhesion to hepatic sinusoids. VAP-1 is another sinusoidal adhesion receptor that mediates lymphocyte recruitment. VAP-1 has an enzymatic activity that, on provision of a substrate, leads to NF-κB-dependent upregulation of VCAM-1 and ICAM-1. This enhances lymphocyte adhesion from the blood flow. CD44 is an adhesion molecule that causes the sequestration of neutrophils in sinusoids during sepsis due to deposition of hyaluronan (HA)-associated protein on sinusoidal cells. During inflammatory bowel disease, MAdCAM-1 is expressed as an adhesion molecule that is normally confined to the mucosal endothelium of the GI tract. This adhesion molecule can also be induced in the liver resulting in T cell infiltration that leads to immune cell–mediated toxicity. Chemokine secretion by liver cells leads to lymphocyte recruitment. CCR5 ligands CCL3–5 are expressed in high amounts in portal vascular endothelium. This leads to graft-versus-host disease, immune-mediated liver disease, and graft rejection. The parenchymal infiltration occurs in the periportal area in active hepatitis and in the hepatic lobules in lobular hepatitis. Viral infection and autoimmune liver injury are associated with expression of CXCR3 ligands CXCL9–11 on sinusoidal epithelium. Chemokines can also be expressed by cholangiocytes, hepatocytes, and stellate cells during inflammation and transported from the basolateral to luminal endothelial surface by transcytosis from hepatocytes and stellate cells or captured by the proteoglycan-rich endothelium glycocalyx from the flow from cholangiocytes. Stellate and Kupffer cells are activated by ROS and innate immune signaling pathways triggered by toxicants. Once the lymphocytes infiltrate, they can establish tertiary lymphoid structures for continued recruitment in the liver, including neovessels in the portal tracts that exhibit features of endothelial venules in secondary lymphoid tissue. In autoimmunity, the cytokine IL-17 appears to be produced by a subset of the helper T cell, known as the Th17 cell due to the secretion of this cytokine. The role of the macrophages in fibrosis due to various agents including acetaminophen has already been covered. Osteopontin (OPN) is an acidic member of the small integrin-binding ligand N-linked glycoprotein family and appears to be responsible for macrophage chemotaxis in a number of diseases. OPN is expressed in Kupffer cells exposed to CCl_4. This macrophage chemoattractant factor appears to be involved in the concanavalin A (Con A)–induced hepatitis model in the mouse. OPN appears in the Con A model to involve lymphocytes and neutrophils. OPN appears to be involved in alcoholic liver disease causing increased neutrophilic inflammation and necrosis. The neutrophils mentioned here and previously cause additional damage via generation of hypochlorous acid, leading to increased ROS and ultimately cell mortality. The drugs most associated with these mechanisms are α-naphthyl isothiocyanate and halothane (Adams et al., 2010).

Cholestasis and Bile Duct Toxicity

Cholestasis, or retention of toxic bile salts in the liver cells, is enhanced by damage to proteins on the hepatocyte canalicular membrane that transports drugs. Examples of drug substrates for these transport proteins are indomethacin, statins, digoxin, enalapril, midazolam, tamoxifen, diclofenac, methotrexate, and troglitazone. Inhibition of ATP-dependent bile salt transport proteins makes coadministration of other medications more likely to cause cholestasis. Pairs of medications that become problematic are troglitazone plus lisinopril, itraconazole plus verapamil, and bosentan plus glyburide. Cholangiocytes, epithelial cells of the bile duct, may sustain direct injury by medications such as flucloxacillin, an isoxazolyl-penicillin (Grattagliano et al., 2009). Usually, the liver cells are able to sense toxic products caused by metabolism and enhance their elimination. Xenobiotic receptors CAR and PXR are key members of the NR1I nuclear receptor family. A ligand for these receptors is phenobarbital, which has been used to treat cholestatic liver disease. A Chinese herbal medicine, Yin Zhi Huang, treats or prevents neonatal jaundice and is a CAR ligand. This action increases the speed of bilirubin clearance (Kakizaki et al., 2009).

GI Toxicity Tests

GI toxicity tests as indicated by research publications are listed in **Table 16-4**. DNA analysis of humans has been performed on cells on the inside of the cheek. Buccal cells are also used in a minimally invasive test for those who use chewing tobacco or are exposed systemically to mutagens. The micronucleus assay in exfoliated buccal cells has been used since the 1980s to determine cytogenetic damage caused by environmental and occupational exposures to toxicants. The human micronucleus project (www.humn.org) is an international project to validate the methodology (staining), scoring (inter- and intra-individual differences), and interpretation of this test. Its variability currently limits its usefulness (Holland et al., 2008).

The buccal test is truly noninvasive, as is the ^{13}C-sucrose breath test for small intestinal sucrase activity. Mucositis can be assessed by the evolution of $^{13}CO_2$ in the breath as a measure of enzymatic activity. This has been found to correlate well with damage of chemotherapy and repair and jejunal sucrase activity (Butler, 2008). Exposing rats is a classic way of assessing

TABLE 16-4   GI Toxicity Tests

Testing For	Individual Assays
Mouth/systemic DNA damage	Buccal cell micronucleus assay (Holland et al., 2008)—exfoliated buccal mucosal cells are collected by a tongue depressor, spatula, or cytobrush (preferred) moistened with water. Cells are shaken in a saline solution to release cells and then centrifuged to wash the cells in a buffer solution. Pipette or cytocentrifugation transfer to slides is followed by fixation in methanol-glacial acetic acid. Staining (Feulgen-Fast Green preferred for specificity of DNA specificity) is followed by light microscopy and scoring.
Complete GI toxicity based on rat mechanistic model	Cell models—ultrastructural and biochemical models
	Intact animals—nutrient and toxicant absorption, microscopic examination (check liver and pancreas as well)
	Permeation, mitochondrial DNA, and COX-2 analyses (Yáñez et al., 2003)
	Toxicant models—MPTP-induced ulcers (Deng and Zheng, 1994), trinitrobenzene sulfonic acid-induced colitis (Fitzpatrick et al., 2010), 1,2-dimethylhydrazine-induced colon cancer (Moreira et al., 2009), enterohepatic recirculation in animal that has a gall bladder (Shou et al., 2005)
Noninvasive small intestinal damage/mucositis	^{13}C-sucrose breath test (Butler, 2008)—intestinal sucrase activity is determined by ingesting ^{13}C-sucrose and determining breath $^{13}CO_2$ levels.
Intestinal motility—alternative	Zebrafish (*Danio rerio*; Eimon and Rubinstein, 2009)

toxicity. Because NSAIDs and chemotherapy agents are a key group of toxicants of the GI tract and affect GI permeability, oxidative phosphorylation, generation of ROS and mitochondrial DNA, GI permeability probes, mitochondrial DNA analysis, and COX-2 mRNA expression may give many of the parameters that need to be evaluated. In the human patient, symptoms of diarrhea frequency, stomach and abdominal pain, and visualization of gross abnormalities of the upper and lower GI through a flexible scope give some information, such as the development of precancerous polyps or ulcers. However, mechanistic analyses indicate that other techniques mentioned earlier may be beneficial to understanding the cause of the inflammation that can result in mucositis (Yáñez et al., 2003). Clearly there are different levels of analysis. Cell or tissue preparations can be used to look for damage to organelles and biochemical markers of damage (e.g., keratin in epithelial cells, enzyme markers for brush border, lysosomes, peroxisomes, mitochondria, and ER). Intact animals can be used to assess absorption of nutrients and the toxicant itself. The liver and pancreas can also be indicated as organs for assessing puzzling effects not directly related to cellular damage in the tract. Microscopic examination is also important in these models. Results should be compared with known toxicants such as ulcers produced by 1-methyl-4-phenyl-1,2,3,6-tetrahydopyridine (MPTP destruction of mucus bicarbonate via dopaminergic neuron damage; Deng and Zheng, 1994) in the rat; bile acid-, ethanol-, or trinitrobenzene sulfonic acid (immunologically; Fitzpatrick et al., 2010)-induced colitis; 1,2-dimethylhydrazine-induced colon cancer (Moreira et al., 2009); and enterohepatic recirculation in a species that has a gall bladder (such as monkeys [Shou et al., 2005] but not deer, rats, and horses).

An alternative approach to GI toxicity *in vivo* is through the use of zebrafish (*Danio rerio*) to evaluate toxic effects on GI motility, because the clear view of development and ease of use of adults makes drug toxicity evaluation relatively easy (Eimon and Rubinstein, 2009).

Pancreas Toxicity Tests

Organ damage is usually assessed by leakage of enzymes normally sequestered in the organ into the plasma as indicated in **Table 16-5**. For the pancreas, exocrine enzymes should not be found in appreciable amounts/activities in the plasma. Amylase and lipase are clinically relevant markers of pancreatic damage (Arafa et al., 2009). Inflammatory reactions that may lead to (cerulein-induced) pancreatitis may be examined by cytokines IL-6 and TNF-α, and histological grading of vacuolization, inflammation, lobular disarray, and edema (Jo et al., 2008). When inducing pancreatic cancer using agents such as 2,3,7,8-TCDD, it is also useful to examine apoptotic bodies, immunohistochemistry of CYP1A1, CCK, AhR, CCKAR, amylase, and proliferating cell nuclear antigen, and looking for the development/incidence of lesions (Yoshizawa et al., 2005). Toxicants that damage the acinar cells affect the exocrine pancreas. Chemicals that damage the endocrine pancreas may be monitored by plasma hormones insulin (beta-cells) or glucagon (alpha-cells) and blood/urine glucose levels as diabetes mellitus is manifested. A glucose tolerance test may also be done to see similar dysfunctions. Additionally, direct damage to the Islets of Langerhans indicates endocrine dysfunction and can be measured by β-cell mass (point counting method) anti-insulin antibody immunohistochemical staining (Kim et al., 2009).

Liver Toxicity Tests

Enzymes leaking out of cells again has served the clinical community well in assessing liver damage in human patients as shown in **Table 16-6**. Liver enzymes alanine aminotransferase (ALT) and aspartate aminotransferase (AST) have served has indicators of liver damage. Increasing serum ALT levels indicate hepatocyte necrosis. AST may be elevated in muscle damage, heart injury, body mass alterations, blood diseases, or pancreatic injury and so may not be the best indicator of liver dysfunction alone. Hy's law should be considered as a good indicator of severe hepatotoxicity. Transaminases should be three times normal activity coupled to increases in serum bilirubin concentrations at two times normal levels. However, this threshold is too high for treatment, because irreversible changes may have already occurred. Leakage of other enzymes may also be good biomarkers for liver damage. α-Glutathione-S-transferase (GST-α) is a conjugation enzyme protective against activated metabolites such as those derived from acetaminophen. It is found primarily in the centrilobular region of the liver, so it indicates necrosis close to the hypoxic central vein region. γ-Glutamyl transpeptidase indicates hepatobiliary damage, particularly cholestasis, as it is localized in the bile ducts. It is also expressed in the kidney and the pancreas. Paraoxygenase-1 (PON-1) is an HDL-associated esterase that metabolizes organophosphates. It is mostly a

TABLE 16-5	Pancreas Toxicity Tests
Testing For	**Individual Assays**
Plasma (exocrine)	Amylase and lipase (clinical; Arafa, 2009)
	Glucose tolerance test, serum insulin levels (Kim, 2009).
Organ damage	Pancreatic myeloperoxidase, glutathione-S-transferase, nitric oxde, malondialdehye (Arafa, 2009)
	Pancreatic IL-6,TNF-α, histological examination/grading of vacuolization, inflammation, lobular disarray, edema (Jo, 2008)
	Apoptotic bodies in pancreatic sections, immunohistochemistry of CYP1A1, CCK, AhR, CCKAR, amylase, proliferating cell nuclear antigen, incidence of lesions (Yoshizawa, 2005)
	Anti-insulin antibody immunohistochemical staining of β-cells, point counting β-cell mass determination, insulin mRNA expression, TUNEL staining for apoptosis, caspase-3 activity (Kim, 2009)

TABLE 16-6 Liver Toxicity Tests	
Testing For	**Individual Assays**
Plasma	Alanine aminotransferase (3x normal) + bilirubin (2x normal; hepatocyte necrosis according to Hy's law), aspartate aminotransferase, α-glutahione-S-transferase (centrilobular necrosis), γ-glutamyl transpeptidase (hepatobiliary/cholestasis), paraoxygenase-1 (decreased = liver damage), purine nucleotide phosphorylase (hepatic necrosis released to sinusoids), malate dehydrogenase (necrosis/cirrhosis; Marrer, 2010), sorbitol dehydrogenase, glutamate dehydrogenase, alkaline phosphatase (cholestatic), albumin, glucose, coagulation factors, ammonia, urea nitrogen (Ramaiah, 2007)
Organ damage	Histological determination of periportal, midzonal, and centrilobular, or random damage, microvesicular and macrovesicular steatosis, glycogen accumulation, CYP induction accompanied by centrilobular hypertrophy, hepatocellular alterations, hepatic hyperplasia/adenoma, carcinoma (Ramaiah, 2007)

liver enzyme, although the brain, kidney, and lung express this enzyme. It is not leaked but is released in conjunction with HDL. Its reduction in serum is consistent with liver injury in conjunction with other markers, but can also signal atherosclerosis and vasculitis. Purine nucleotide phosphorylase is located in the cytoplasm of endothelial cells, Kupffer cells, and hepatocytes. Its leakage into hepatic sinusoids is a marker for necrosis, which occurred prior to ALT leakage in endotoxin-challenged rat livers. Malate dehydrogenase of the tricarboxylic acid cycle is found at highest activity in the mitochondria of the liver and less in the heart, skeletal muscle, and brain. It is an indication of necrosis and cirrhosis. Enzyme data should be interpreted carefully and in combination with other data that are consonant with the liver toxicity to avoid embarrassment associated with finding that a genetic population expresses certain polymorphisms that may be mistaken for injury or lower normal activities that mask damage (e.g., PON-1 and GST-α; Marrer and Dieterle, 2010). Other leakage enzymes are sorbitol dehydrogenase and glutamate dehydrogenase for necrotic livers and alkaline phosphatase for cholestatic hepatobiliary injury. Other factors that can indicate liver injury include a reduced ability to produce albumin for the plasma oncotic pressure, coagulation factors such as prothrombin and fibrinogen, and waste conversion functions as monitored by plasma ammonia and urea nitrogen concentrations (Ramaiah, 2007). According to the Society of Toxicology, organ weights

may be helpful in assessing certain types of organ damage (Sellers et al., 2007). More specific parameters, such as the accumulation of fatty tissue, glycogen, or bile acids in the liver, may yield more specific information. A set of reference histology slides on various types of liver damage are available from the Internet Pathology Laboratory for Medical Education, Mercer University School of Medicine (Klatt, 2015). Examination should be able to determine periportal, midzonal, and centrilobular necrosis or random damage. Steatosis can be microvesicular or macrovesicular. CYP induction may be accompanied by centrilobular hypertrophy. Cancer or precancerous lesions may be indicated by hepatocellular alterations, hepatic hyperplasias/adenoma, or primary hepatocyte carcinoma (Ramaiah, 2007).

Questions

1. Bisphosphonates taken orally with little or no water do what kinds of damage to the mouth and esophagus? Why?
2. How do NSAIDs and *H. pylori* lead to stomach damage?
3. Why does chronic ethanol ingestion lead to the opposite of acute ingestion in the duodenum?
4. Why is GSH so important in the jejunum (importance in liver is understood based on metabolic role)?

5. Why is phospholipase A_2 activity important to pathogenesis of the ileum?

6. Why is chronic red meat consumption a problem for the colon?

7. How is alloxan destruction of pancreatic cells mediated?

8. Indicate which kinds of mechanisms mediate damage in zones 1 versus 3 in the liver.

9. Which toxicant appears to be sex-linked; leads to steatosis, cirrhosis, and cytoskeletal changes; and is associated with liver cancer?

10. Why is taking acetaminophen for a headache following binge drinking similar to poisoning oneself with pyrrolizidine alkaloids from eating toxic plants of the *Crotalaria* species?

11. What factors makes liver cells prone to immune infiltration-induced damage?

12. What would be a test for an intact human with mucositis?

13. What are tests for intact animals or humans of exocrine and endocrine pancreatic damage?

14. Why is liver damage indicated by someone's eyes and skin turning yellow?

References

Abdalla AM, Krivosheyev V, Hanzely Z, Holt PR, Perez-Perez GI, Blaser MJ, Moss SF. 1998. Increased epithelial cell turnover in antrum and corpus of *H pylori*-infected stomach, irrespective of CagA status. *Gastroenterology*. 114:A50–A51.

Adams DH, Ju C, Ramaiah SK, Uetrecht J, Jaeschke H. 2010. Mechanisms of immune-mediated liver injury. *Toxicol Sci*. 115:307–321.

Addy M, Moran J. 1985. Extrinsic tooth discoloration by metals and chlorhexidine. II. Clinical staining produced by chlorhexidine, iron and tea. *Br Dent J*. 159:331–334.

Alaluusua S, Lukinmaa PL. 2006. Developmental dental toxicity of dioxin and related compounds—a review. *Int Dent J*. 56:323–331.

Alb JG Jr., Cortese JD, Phillips SE, Albin RL, Nagy TR, Hamilton BA, Bankaitis VA. 2003. Mice lacking phosphatidylinositol transfer protein-alpha exhibit spinocerebellar degeneration, intestinal and hepatic steatosis, and hypoglycemia. *J Biol Chem*. 278:33501–33518.

Albin DM, Wubben JE, Rowlett JM, Tappenden KA, Nowak RA. 2007. Changes in small intestinal nutrient transport and barrier function after lipopolysaccharide exposure in two pig breeds. *J Anim Sci*. 85:2517–2523.

Andersen O, Nielsen JB, Sorensen JA, Scherrebeck L. 1994. Experimental localization of intestinal uptake sites for metals (Cd, Hg, Zn, Se) in vivo in mice. *Environ Health Perspect*. 102(Suppl 3): 199–206.

Apte M, Pirola R, Wilson J. 2009. New insights into alcoholic pancreatitis and pancreatic cancer. *J Gastroenterol Hepatol*. 24(Suppl 3):S51–S56.

Arafa HM, Hemeida RA, Hassan MI, Abdel-Wahab MH, Badary OA, Hamada FM. 2009. Acetyl-L-carnitine ameliorates caerulein-induced acute pancreatitis in rats. *Basic Clin Pharmacol Toxicol*. 105:30–36.

Atug O, Dobrucali A, Orlando RC. 2009. Critical pH level of lye (NaOH) for esophageal injury. *Dig Dis Sci*. 54:980–987.

Awad WA, Razzazi-Fazeli E, Böhm J, Zentek J. 2007. Influence of deoxynivalenol on the D-glucose transport across the isolated epithelium of different intestinal segments of laying hens. *J Anim Physiol Anim Nutr (Berl)*. 91:175–180.

Bastian S, Busch W, Kühnel D, Springer A, Meissner T, Holke R, Scholz S, Iwe M, Pompe W, Gelinsky M, Potthoff A, Richter V, Ikonomidou C, Schirmer K. 2009. Toxicity of tungsten carbide and cobalt-doped tungsten carbide nanoparticles in mammalian cells in vitro. *Environ Health Perspect*. 117:530–536.

Bedrossian S, Vahid B. 2007. A case of fatal necrotizing pancreatitis: complication of hydrochlorothiazide and lisinopril therapy. *Dig Dis Sci*. 52:558–560.

Bermejo F, Lopez-Sanroman A, Taxonera C, Gisbert JP, Pérez-Calle JL, Vera I, Menchén L, Martín-Arranz MD, Opio V, Carneros JA, Van-Domselaar M, Mendoza JL, Luna M, López P, Calvo M, Algaba A. 2008. Acute pancreatitis in inflammatory bowel disease, with special reference to azathioprine-induced pancreatitis. *Aliment Pharmacol Ther*. 28:623–628.

Bernstam L, Nriagu J. 2000. Molecular aspects of arsenic stress. *J Toxicol Environ Health B Crit Rev*. 3:293–322.

Bernstein H, Bernstein C, Payne CM, Dvorak K. 2009. Bile acids as endogenous etiologic agents in gastrointestinal cancer. *World J Gastroenterol*. 15:3329–3340.

Bhide SA, Miah AB, Harrington KJ, Newbold KL, Nutting CM. 2009. Radiation-induced xerostomia: pathophysiology, prevention and treatment. *Clin Oncol (R Coll Radiol)*. 21:737–744.

Binet S, Pfohl-Leszkowicz A, Brandt H, Lafontaine M, Castegnaro M. 2002. Bitumen fumes: review of work on the potential risk to workers and the present knowledge on its origin. *Sci Total Environ.* 300:37–49.

Bolt HM. 2005. Vinyl chloride-a classical industrial toxicant of new interest. *Crit Rev Toxicol.* 35:307–323.

Bookstaver PB, Norris L, Rudisill C, DeWitt T, Aziz S, Fant J. 2008. Multiple toxic effects of low-dose methotrexate in a patient treated for psoriasis. *Am J Health Syst Pharm.* 65:2117–2121.

Boudry G, Jury J, Yang PC, Perdue MH. 2007. Chronic psychological stress alters epithelial cell turn-over in rat ileum. *Am J Physiol Gastrointest Liver Physiol.* 292:G1228–G1232.

Brandi G, Dabard J, Raibaud P, Di Battista M, Bridonneau C, Pisi AM, Morselli Labate AM, Pantaleo MA, De Vivo A, Biasco G. 2006. Intestinal microflora and digestive toxicity of irinotecan in mice. *Clin Cancer Res.* 12:1299–1307.

Braun U. 2006. [Botulism in cattle]. *Schweiz Arch Tierheilkd.* 148:331–339.

Brown K. 2009. Is tamoxifen a genotoxic carcinogen in women? *Mutagenesis.* 24:391–404.

Butler RN. 2008. Measuring tools for gastrointestinal toxicity. *Curr Opin Support Palliat Care.* 2:35–39.

Butterworth BE, Loury DJ, Smith-Oliver T, Cattley RC. 1987. The potential role of chemically induced hyperplasia in the carcinogenic activity of the hypolipidemic carcinogens. *Toxicol Ind Health.* 3:129–149.

Cavalcante IC, Castro MV, Barreto AR, Sullivan GW, Vale M, Almeida PR, Linden J, Rieger JM, Cunha FQ, Guerrant RL, Ribeiro RA, Brito GA. 2006. Effect of novel A2A adenosine receptor agonist ATL 313 on Clostridium difficile toxin A-induced murine ileal enteritis. *Infect Immun.* 74:2606–2612.

Campion SN, Tatis-Rios C, Augustine LM, Goedken MJ, van Rooijen N, Cherrington NJ, Manautou JE. 2009. Effect of allyl alcohol on hepatic transporter expression: zonal patterns of expression and role of Kupffer cell function. *Toxicol Appl Pharmacol.* 236:49–58.

Cappell MS. 2004. Colonic toxicity of administered drugs and chemicals. *Am J Gastroenterol.* 99:1175–1190.

Carini R, De Cesaris MG, Spendore R, Albano E. 2000. Ethanol potentiates hypoxic liver injury: role of hepatocyte Na(+) overload. *Biochim Biophys Acta.* 1502:508–514.

Cerqueira VD, Riet-Correa G, Barbosa JD, Duarte MD, Oliveira CM, de Oliveira CA, Tokarnia C, Lee ST, Riet-Correa F. 2009. Colic caused by *Panicum maximum* toxicosis in equidae in northern Brazil. *J Vet Diagn Invest.* 21:882–888.

Cha C, Dematteo RP. 2005. Molecular mechanisms in hepatocellular carcinoma development. *Best Pract Res Clin Gastroenterol.* 19:25–37.

Chen G, Zhu L, Liu Y, Zhou Q, Chen H, Yang J. 2009. Isoliquiritigenin, a flavonoid from licorice, plays a dual role in regulating gastrointestinal motility in vitro and in vivo. *Phytother Res.* 23:498–506.

Chen P, Li C, Pang W, Zhao Y, Dong W, Wang S, Zhang J. 2009. The protective role of Per2 against carbon tetrachloride-induced hepatotoxicity. *Am J Pathol.* 174:63–70.

Cooper KK, Songer JG. 2009. Necrotic enteritis in chickens: a paradigm of enteric infection by *Clostridium perfringens* type A. *Anaerobe.* 15:55–60.

Davidson LA, Wang N, Ivanov I, Goldsby J, Lupton JR, Chapkin RS. 2009. Identification of actively translated mRNA transcripts in a rat model of early-stage colon carcinogenesis. *Cancer Prev Res (Phila).* 2:984–994.

Dawson RM. 1998. The toxicology of microcystins. *Toxicon.* 36:953–962.

Deschner EE, Ruperto J, Wong G, Newmark HL. 1991. Quercetin and rutin as inhibitors of azomethanol-induced colonic neoplasia. *Carcinogenesis.* 12:1193–1196.

Deng XY, Zheng ZT. 1994. [An animal model of peptic ulcer induced by destruction of dopaminergic neurons]. *Zhonghua Nei Ke Za Zhi.* 33:313–316.

Dublineau I, Grandcolas L, Grison S, Baudelin C, Paquet F, Voisin P, Aigueperse J, Gourmelon P. 2007. Modifications of inflammatory pathways in rat intestine following chronic ingestion of depleted uranium. *Toxicol Sci.* 98:458–468.

Dhulipala VC, Welshons WV, Reddy CS. 2006. Cell cycle proteins in normal and chemically induced abnormal secondary palate development: a review. *Hum Exp Toxicol.* 25:675–682.

Doo EY, Shin JH, Kim JH, Song HY. 2009. Oesophageal strictures caused by the ingestion of corrosive agents: effectiveness of balloon dilatation in children. *Clin Radiol.* 64:265–271.

Duizer E, Gilde AJ, Versantvoort CH, Groten JP. 1999. Effects of cadmium chloride on the paracellular barrier function of intestinal epithelial cell lines. *Toxicol Appl Pharmacol.* 155:117–126.

Dumortier J, Guillaud O, Gouraud A, Pittau G, Vial T, Boillot O, Scoazec JY. 2009. Atenolol hepatotoxicity: report of a complicated case. *Ann Pharmacother.* 43:1719–1723.

Eimon PM, Rubinstein AL. 2009. The use of in vivo zebrafish assays in drug toxicity screening. *Expert Opin Drug Metab Toxicol.* 5:393–401.

Elias EE, Kalombo E, Mercurio SD. 2007. Tamoxifen protects against 17alpha-ethynylestradiol-induced liver damage and the development of urogenital papillae in the rainbow darter (*Etheostoma caeruleum*). *Environ Toxicol Chem.* 26:1879–1889.

El-Sayyad HI, Ismail MF, Shalaby FM, Abou-El-Magd RF, Gaur RL, Fernando A, Raj MH, Ouhtit A. 2009. Histopathological effects of cisplatin, doxorubicin and 5-flurouracil (5-FU) on the liver of male albino rats. *Int J Biol Sci.* 5:466–473.

Espiña B, Rubiolo JA. 2008. Marine toxins and the cytoskeleton: pectenotoxins, unusual macrolides that disrupt actin. *FEBS J.* 275:6082–6088.

Farber E, Liang H, Shinozuka H. 1971. Dissociation of effects on protein synthesis and ribosomes from membrane changes induced by carbon tetrachloride. *Am J Pathol.* 64:601–617.

Fichtner-Feigl S, Strober W, Geissler EK, Schlitt HJ. 2008. Cytokines mediating the induction of chronic colitis and colitis-associated fibrosis. *Mucosal Immunol.* 1(Suppl 1):S24–S27.

Fitzpatrick LR, Meirelles K, Small JS, Puleo FJ, Koltun WA, Cooney RN. 2010. A new model of chronic hapten-induced colitis in young rats. *J Pediatr Gastroenterol Nutr.* 50:240–250.

Frigerio F, Chaffard G, Berwaer M, Maechler P. 2006. The antiepileptic drug topiramate preserves metabolism-secretion coupling in insulin secreting cells chronically exposed to the fatty acid oleate. *Biochem Pharmacol.* 72:965–973.

Ganguly K, Swarnakar S. 2009. Induction of matrix metalloproteinase-9 and -3 in nonsteroidal anti-inflammatory drug-induced acute gastric ulcers in mice: regulation by melatonin. *J Pineal Res.* 47:43–55.

Girish CK, Smith TK. 2008. Effects of feeding blends of grains naturally contaminated with *Fusarium* mycotoxins on small intestinal morphology of turkeys. *Poult Sci.* 87:1075–1082.

Gómez-Lechón MJ, O'Connor JE, Lahoz A, Castell JV, Donato MT. 2008. Identification of apoptotic drugs: multiparametric evaluation in cultured hepatocytes. *Curr Med Chem.* 15:2071–2085.

Grattagliano I, Bonfrate L, Diogo CV, Wang HH, Wang DQ, Portincasa P. 2009. Biochemical mechanisms in drug-induced liver injury: certainties and doubts. *World J Gastroenterol.* 15:4865–4876.

Hajjar JJ, Dobish MP, Tomicic TK. 1989. Effect of chronic vanadate ingestion on amino acid and water absorption in rat intestine. *Arch Toxicol.* 63:29–33.

Hallbäck DA, Eriksson M, Sjöqvist A. 1990. Nerve-mediated effect of ethanol on sodium and fluid transport in the jejunum of the rat. *Scand J Gastroenterol.* 25:859–864.

Hammond K, Graybill T, Speiss SE, Lu J, Leikin JB. 2009. A complicated hospitalization following dilute ammonium chloride ingestion. *J Med Toxicol.* 5:218–222.

Harris CC, Autrup H, Stoner G, Yang SK, Leutz JC, Gelboin HV, Selkirk JK, Connor RJ, Barrett LA, Jones RT, McDowell E, Trump BF. 1977. Metabolism of benzo[a]pyrene and 7,12-dimethylbenz[a]anthracene in cultured human bronchus and pancreatic duct. *Cancer Res.* 37:3349–3355.

Henderson NC, Iredale JP. 2007. Liver fibrosis: cellular mechanisms of progression and resolution. *Clin Sci (Lond).* 112:265–280.

Holland N, Bolognesi C, Kirsch-Volders M, Bonassi S, Zeiger E, Knasmueller S, Fenech M. 2008. The micronucleus assay in human buccal cells as a tool for biomonitoring DNA damage: the HUMN project perspective on current status and knowledge gaps. *Mutat Res.* 659:93–108.

Holt MP, Cheng L, Ju C. 2008. Identification and characterization of infiltrating macrophages in acetaminophen-induced liver injury. *J Leukoc Biol.* 84:1410–1421.

Hruban RH, Yardley JH, Donehower RC, Boitnott JK. 1989. Taxol toxicity. Epithelial necrosis in the gastrointestinal tract associated with polymerized microtubule accumulation and mitotic arrest. *Cancer.* 63:1944–1950.

Iino M, O'Donnell CJ, Burke MP. 2009. Post-mortem CT findings following intentional ingestion of mercuric chloride. *Leg Med (Tokyo).* 11:136–138.

Imazawa T, Nishikawa A, Toyoda K, Furukawa F, Mitsui M, Hirose M. 2003. Sequential alteration of apoptosis, p53 expression, and cell proliferation in the rat pancreas treated with 4-hydroxyaminoquinoline 1-oxide. *Toxicol Pathol.* 31:625–631.

Izzotti A, Durando P, Ansaldi F, Gianiorio F, Pulliero A. 2009. Interaction between *Helicobacter pylori*, diet, and genetic polymorphisms as related to non-cancer diseases. *Mutat Res.* 667:142–157.

Jang JH, Kang KJ, Kim YH, Kang YN, Lee IS. 2008. Reevaluation of experimental model of hepatic fibrosis induced by hepatotoxic drugs: an easy, applicable, and reproducible model. *Transplant Proc.* 40:2700–2703.

Jo YJ, Choi HS, Jun DW, Lee OY, Kang JS, Park IG, Jung KH, Hahm JS. 2008. The effects of a new human leukocyte elastase inhibitor (recombinant guamerin) on cerulein-induced pancreatitis in rats. *Int Immunopharmacol.* 8:959–966.

Kakizaki S, Takizawa D, Tojima H, Yamazaki Y, Mori M. 2009. Xenobiotic-sensing nuclear receptors CAR and PXR as drug targets in cholestatic liver disease. *Curr Drug Targets.* 10:1184–1193.

Kalra M, Mayes J, Assefa S, Kaul AK, Kaul R. 2008. Role of sex steroid receptors in pathobiology of hepatocellular carcinoma. *World J Gastroenterol.* 14:5945–5961.

Kawai T, Seiji K, Wantanabe T, Nakatsuka H, Ikeda M. 1989. Urinary vanadium as a biological indicator of exposure to vanadium. *Int Arch Occup Environ Health.* 61:283–287.

Keefe DM, Gibson RJ. 2007. Mucosal injury from targeted anti-cancer therapy. *Support Care Cancer*. 15:483–490.

Khan AA, Dragt BS, Porte RJ, Groothuis GM. 2010. Regulation of VDR expression in rat and human intestine and liver—consequences for CYP3A expression. *Toxicol In Vitro*. 24:822–829.

Kim JW, Yang JH, Park HS, Sun C, Lee SH, Cho JH, Yang CW, Yoon KH. 2009. Rosiglitazone protects the pancreatic beta-cell death induced by cyclosporine A. *Biochem Biophys Res Commun*. 390:763–768.

Kiran MM, Demet O, Ortatath M, Oğuz H. 1998. The preventive effect of polyvinylpolypyrrolidone on aflatoxicosis in broilers. *Avian Pathol*. 27:250–255.

Klatt EC. 2015. The internet pathology laboratory for medical education. Mercer University School of Medicine, Savannah, Georgia. Hosted by the University of Utah Eccles Health Sciences Library. http://library.med.utah.edu/WebPath/webpath .html#MENU.

Kodali P, Wu P, Lahiji PA, Brown EJ, Maher JJ. 2006. ANIT toxicity toward mouse hepatocytes in vivo is mediated primarily by neutrophils via CD18. *Am J Physiol Gastrointest Liver Physiol*. 291:G355–G363.

Kolli VK, Abraham P, Rabi S. 2008. Methotrexate-induced nitrosative stress may play a critical role in small intestinal damage in the rat. *Arch Toxicol*. 82:763–770.

Kozlov AV, Szalay L, Umar F, Fink B, Kropik K, Nohl H, Redl H, Bahrami S. 2003. Epr analysis reveals three tissues responding to endotoxin by increased formation of reactive oxygen and nitrogen species. *Free Radic Biol Med*. 34:1555–1562.

Krawitt EL. 1977. Ethanol and development of disease and injury to the alimentary tract. *Environ Health Perspect*. 20:71–73.

Laugier R, Sarles H. 1977. Action of oleic acid on the exocrine pancreatic secretion of the conscious rat: evidence for an anti-cholecystokinin- pancreozymin factor. *J Physiol*. 271:81–92.

Lazarus CL. 2009. Effects of chemoradiotherapy on voice and swallowing. *Curr Opin Otolaryngol Head Neck Surg*. 17:172–178.

Lee J, Goldberg IJ. 2008. Hypertriglyceridemia-induced pancreatitis created by oral estrogen and in vitro fertilization ovulation induction. *J Clin Lipidol*. 2:63–66.

Le Hégarat L, Jacquin AG, Bazin E, Fessard V. 2006. Genotoxicity of the marine toxin okadaic acid, in human Caco-2 cells and in mice gut cells. *Environ Toxicol*. 21:55–64.

Leuenberger N, Pradervand S, Wahli W. 2009. Sumoylated PPARalpha mediates sex-specific gene repression and protects the liver from estrogen-induced toxicity in mice. *J Clin Invest*. 119:3138–3148.

Liener IE. 1983. Naturally occurring toxicants in foods and their significance in the human diet. *Arch Toxicol Suppl*. 6:153–166.

Likhachev AIa, Petrov AS, P'rvanova LG, Pozharisski KM. 1978. [Mechanism of methylation of DNA bases by symmetrical dimethylhydrazine]. *Biull Eksp Biol Med*. 86:679–681.

Lim YJ, Lee JS, Ku YS, Hahm KB. 2009. Rescue strategies against non-steroidal anti-inflammatory drug-induced gastroduodenal damage. *J Gastroenterol Hepatol*. 24:1169–1178.

Lingamfelter DC, Knight LD. 2010. Sudden death from massive gastrointestinal hemorrhage associated with crack cocaine use: case report and review of the literature. *Am J Forensic Med Pathol*. 31:98–99.

Lira SR, Rao VS, Carvalho AC, Guedes MM, de Morais TC, de Souza AL, Trevisan MT, Lima AF, Chaves MH, Santos FA. 2009. Gastroprotective effect of lupeol on ethanol-induced gastric damage and the underlying mechanism. *Inflammopharmacology*. 17:221–228.

Liu F, Jiang MZ, Shu XL, Zhang XP. 2009. [Role of oxidative stress in the pathogenesis of esophageal mucosal injury in children with reflux esophagitis]. *Zhongguo Dang Dai Er Ke Za Zhi*. 11:425–428.

Lopez CH, Suzuki-Kemmelmeier F, Constantin J, Bracht A. 2009. Zonation of the action of ethanol on gluconeogenesis and ketogenesis studied in the bivascularly perfused rat liver. *Chem Biol Interact*. 177:89–95.

Lu SC, Gukovsky I, Lugea A, Reyes CN, Huang ZZ, Chen L, Mato JM, Bottiglieri T, Pandol SJ. 2003. Role of S-adenosylmethionine in two experimental models of pancreatitis. *FASEB J*. 17:56–58.

Lund EK, Fairweather-Tait SJ, Wharf SG, Johnson IT. 2001. Chronic exposure to high levels of dietary iron fortification increases lipid peroxidation in the mucosa of the rat large intestine. *J Nutr*. 131:2928–2931.

Luzi A, Cometa MF, Palmery M. 2002. Acute effects of aflatoxins on guinea pig isolated ileum. *Toxicol In Vitro*. 16:525–529.

Ma T, Thiagarajah JR, Yang H, Sonawane ND, Folli C, Galietta LJ, Verkman AS. 2002. Thiazolidinone CFTR inhibitor identified by high-throughput screening blocks cholera toxin-induced intestinal fluid secretion. *J Clin Invest*. 110:1651–1658.

Malhi H, Gores GJ, Lemasters JJ. 2006. Apoptosis and necrosis in the liver: a tale of two deaths? *Hepatology*. 43:S31–S44.

Malleo G, Mazzon E, Genovese T, Di Paola R, Muià C, Caminiti R, Esposito E, Di Bella P, Cuzzocrea S. 2008. Etanercept reduces acute tissue injury and mortality associated to zymosan-induced multiple organ dysfunction syndrome. *Shock.* 29:560–571.

Marrer E, Dieterle F. 2010. Impact of biomarker development on drug safety assessment. *Toxicol Appl Pharmacol.* 243:167–179.

Mårtensson J, Jain A, Meister A. 1990. Glutathione is required for intestinal function. *Proc Natl Acad Sci USA.* 87:1715–1719.

McCullough MJ, Farah CS. 2008. The role of alcohol in oral carcinogenesis with particular reference to alcohol-containing mouthwashes. *Aust Dent J.* 53:302–305.

McCuskey RS. 2006. Sinusoidal endothelial cells as an early target for hepatic toxicants. *Clin Hemorheol Microcirc.* 34:5–10.

Medina-Díaz IM, Estrada-Muñiz E, Reyes-Hernández OD, Ramírez P, Vega L, Elizondo G. 2009. Arsenite and its metabolites, MMA(III) and DMA(III), modify CYP3A4, PXR and RXR alpha expression in the small intestine of CYP3A4 transgenic mice. *Toxicol Appl Pharmacol.* 239:162–168.

Mercer AE, Regan SL, Hirst CM, Graham EE, Antoine DJ, Benson CA, Williams DP, Foster J, Kenna JG, Park BK. 2009. Functional and toxicological consequences of metabolic bioactivation of methapyrilene via thiophene S-oxidation: induction of cell defence, apoptosis and hepatic necrosis. *Toxicol Appl Pharmacol.* 239:297–305.

Mesonero JE, Yoldi MC, Yoldi MJ. 1996. Calcium-cadmium interaction on sugar absorption across the rabbit jejunum. *Biol Trace Elem Res.* 51:149–159.

Micuda S, Fuksa L, Mundlova L, Osterreicher J, Mokry J, Cermanova J, Brcakova E, Staud F, Pokorna P, Martinkova J. 2007. Morphological and functional changes in p-glycoprotein during dexamethasone-induced hepatomegaly. *Clin Exp Pharmacol Physiol.* 34:296–303.

Moreira AP, Sabarense CM, Dias CM, Lunz W, Natali AJ, Glória MB, Peluzio MC. 2009. Fish oil ingestion reduces the number of aberrant crypt foci and adenoma in 1,2-dimethylhydrazine-induced colon cancer in rats. *Braz J Med Biol Res.* 42:1167–1172.

Moreno SR, Carvalho JJ, Nascimento AL, Pereira M, Rocha EK, Olej B, Caldas LQ, Bernardo-Filho M. 2007. Experimental model to assess possible medicinal herb interaction with a radiobiocomplex: qualitative and quantitative analysis of kidney, liver and duodenum isolated from treated rats. *Food Chem Toxicol.* 45:19–23.

Müller-Fassbender M, Elsenhans B, McKie AT, Schümann K. 2003. Different behaviour of 63Ni and 59Fe during absorption in iron-deficient and iron-adequate jejunal rat segments ex vivo. *Toxicology.* 185:141–153.

Naik S, Smith F, Ho J, Croft NM, Domizio P, Price E, Sanderson IR, Meadows NJ. 2008. Staphylococcal enterotoxins G and I, a cause of severe but reversible neonatal enteropathy. *Clin Gastroenterol Hepatol.* 6:251–254.

Naik S, Tredwin CJ, Scully C. 2006. Hydrogen peroxide tooth-whitening (bleaching): review of safety in relation to possible carcinogenesis. *Oral Oncol.* 42:668–674.

National Toxicology Program. 1987. NTP toxicology and carcinogenesis studies of boric acid (CAS No. 10043-35-3) in B6C3F1 mice (Feed Studies). *Natl Toxicol Program Tech Rep Ser.* 324:1–126.

National Toxicology Program. 2008. NTP Toxicology and carcinogenesis studies of formamide (CAS No. 75-12-7) in F344/N Rats and B6C3F1 Mice (Gavage Studies). *Natl Toxicol Program Tech Rep Ser.* (541):1–192.

Nguyen T, Park JY, Scudiere JR, Montgomery E. 2009. Mycophenolic acid (cellcept and myofortic) induced injury of the upper GI tract. *Am J Surg Pathol.* 33:1355–1363.

Nishiya T, Mori K, Hattori C, Kai K, Kataoka H, Masubuchi N, Jindo T, Manabe S. 2008. The crucial protective role of glutathione against tienilic acid hepatotoxicity in rats. *Toxicol Appl Pharmacol.* 232:280–291.

Nuño P, Hernández A, Mendoza-Figueroa T, Panduro A. 1997. Viscosity regulates apolipoprotein A-1 gene expression in experimental models of secondary hyperlipidemia and in cultured hepatocytes. *Biochim Biophys Acta.* 1344:262–269.

Oliver JD, Roberts RA. 2002. Receptor-mediated hepatocarcinogenesis: role of hepatocyte proliferation and apoptosis. *Pharmacol Toxicol.* 91:1–7.

Pan X, Hussain FN, Iqbal J, Feuerman MH, Hussain MM. 2007. Inhibiting proteasomal degradation of microsomal triglyceride transfer protein prevents CCl4-induced steatosis. *J Biol Chem.* 282:17078–17089.

Parfitt JR, Jayakumar S, Driman DK. 2008. Mycophenolate mofetil-related gastrointestinal mucosal injury: variable injury patterns, including graft-versus-host disease-like changes. *Am J Surg Pathol.* 32:1367–1372.

Pearson JR, Gill CI, Rowland IR. 2009. Diet, fecal water, and colon cancer—development of a biomarker. *Nutr Rev.* 67:509–526.

Percik R, Stumvoll M. 2009. Obesity and cancer. *Exp Clin Endocrinol Diabetes.* 117:563–566.

Pilon D, Brodeur J, Plaa GL. 1988. Potentiation of CCl4-induced liver injury by ketonic and ketogenic compounds: role of the CCl$_4$ dose. *Toxicol Appl Pharmacol.* 94(2):183–190.

Povoski SP, Zhou W, Longnecker DS, Roebuck BD, Bell RH Jr. 1993. Stimulation of growth of azaserine-induced putative preneoplastic lesions in rat pancreas is mediated specifically by way of cholecystokinin-A receptors. *Cancer Res.* 53:3925–3929.

Ramaiah SK. 2007. A toxicologist guide to the diagnostic interpretation of hepatic biochemical parameters. *Food Chem Toxicol.* 45:1551–1557.

Rapisarda V, Carnazza ML, Caltabiano C, Loreto C, Musumeci G, Valentino M, Martinez G. 2009. Bitumen products induce skin cell apoptosis in chronically exposed road pavers. *J Cutan Pathol.* 36:781–787.

Reid IR. 2009. Osteonecrosis of the jaw: who gets it, and why? *Bone.* 44:4–10.

Rial NS, Meyskens FL, Gerner EW. 2009. Polyamines as mediators of APC-dependent intestinal carcinogenesis and cancer chemoprevention. *Essays Biochem.* 46:111–124.

Rost S, Pelz HJ, Menzel S, MacNicoll AD, León V, Song KJ, Jäkel T, Oldenburg J, Müller CR. 2009. Novel mutations in the VKORC1 gene of wild rats and mice—a response to 50 years of selection pressure by warfarin? *BMC Genet.* 10:4.

Roy DN, Mandal S, Sen G, Biswas T. 2009. Superoxide anion mediated mitochondrial dysfunction leads to hepatocyte apoptosis preferentially in the periportal region during copper toxicity in rats. *Chem Biol Interact.* 182:136–147.

Scarpelli DG. 1989. Toxicology of the pancreas. *Toxicol Appl Pharmacol.* 101:543–554.

Scarpelli DG, Rao MS, Reddy JK. 1984. Studies of pancreatic carcinogenesis in different animal models. *Environ Health Perspect.* 56:219–227.

Schmid K, Sassen A, Staudenmaier R, Kroemer S, Reichl FX, Harréus U, Hagen R, Kleinsasser N. 2007. Mercuric dichloride induces DNA damage in human salivary gland tissue cells and lymphocytes. *Arch Toxicol.* 81:759–767.

Sefrová J, Paluska P, Odrázka K, Jirkovský V. 2009. [Chronic gastrointestinal toxicity after external-beam radiation therapy for prostate cancer]. *Klin Onkol.* 22:233–241.

Sellers RS, Morton D, Michael B, Roome N, Johnson JK, Yano BL, Perry R, Schafer K. 2007. Society of Toxicologic Pathology position paper: organ weight recommendations for toxicology studies. *Toxicol Pathol.* 35:751–755.

Shepard BD, Tuma PL. 2009. Alcohol-induced protein hyperacetylation: mechanisms and consequences. *World J Gastroenterol.* 15:1219–1230.

Shou M, Lu W, Kari PH, Xiang C, Liang Y, Lu P, Cui D, Emary WB, Michel KB, Adelsberger JK, Brunner JE, Rodrigues AD. 2005. Population pharmacokinetic modeling for enterohepatic recirculation in Rhesus monkey. *Eur J Pharm Sci.* 26:151–161.

Smith FA, Wittmann CW, Stern TA. 2008. Medical complications of psychiatric treatment. *Crit Care Clin.* 24:635–656, vii.

Smith AG, Francis JE, Green JA, Greig JB, Wolf CR, Manson MM. 1990. Sex-linked hepatic uro-porphyria and the induction of cytochromes P450IA in rats caused by hexachlorobenzene and polyhalogenated biphenyls. *Biochem Pharmacol.* 40:2059–2068.

Sonis ST. 2009a. Regimen-related gastrointestinal toxicities in cancer patients. *Curr Opin Support Palliat Care.* 4(1):26–30

Sonis ST. 2009b. Mucositis: The impact, biology and therapeutic opportunities of oral mucositis. *Oral Oncol.* 45:1015–1020.

Souza RF, Huo X, Mittal V, Schuler CM, Carmack SW, Zhang HY, Zhang X, Yu C, Hormi-Carver K, Genta RM, Spechler SJ. 2009. Gastroesophageal reflux might cause esophagitis through a cytokine-mediated mechanism rather than caustic acid injury. *Gastroenterology.* 137:1776–1784.

Stout MD, Herbert RA, Kissling GE, Collins BJ, Travlos GS, Witt KL, Melnick RL, Abdo KM, Malarkey DE, Hooth MJ. 2009. Hexavalent chromium is carcinogenic to F344/N rats and B6C3F1 mice after chronic oral exposure. *Environ Health Perspect.* 117:716–722.

Strugala GJ, Stahl R, Elsenhans B, Rauws AG, Forth W. 1995. Small-intestinal transfer mechanism of prunasin, the primary metabolite of the cyanogenic glycoside amygdalin. *Hum Exp Toxicol.* 14:895–901.

Sturm E, Havinga R, Baller JF, Wolters H, van Rooijen N, Kamps JA, Verkade HJ, Karpen SJ, Kuipers F. 2005. Kupffer cell depletion with liposomal clodronate prevents suppression of Ntcp expression in endotoxin-treated rats. *J Hepatol.* 42:102–109.

Sugimoto M, Nishino M, Kodaira C, Yamade M, Ikuma M, Tanaka T, Sugimura H, Hishida A, Furuta T. 2010. Esophageal mucosal injury with low-dose aspirin and its prevention by rabeprazole. *J Clin Pharmacol.* 50:320–330.

Szkudelski T. 2001. The mechanism of alloxan and streptozotocin action in B cells of the rat pancreas. *Physiol Res.* 50:537–546.

Szymańska K, Levi JE, Menezes A, Wünsch-Filho V, Eluf-Neto J, Koifman S, Matos E, Daudt AW, Curado MP, Villar S, Pawlita M, Waterboer T, Boffetta P, Hainaut P, Brennan P. 2010. TP53 and EGFR mutations in combination with lifestyle risk factors in tumours of the upper aerodigestive tract from South America. *Carcinogenesis.* 31:1054–1059.

Tipoe GL, Liong EC, Casey CA, Donohue TM Jr, Eagon PK, So H, Leung TM, Fogt F, Nanji AA. 2008. A voluntary oral ethanol-feeding rat model associated with necroinflammatory liver injury. *Alcohol Clin Exp Res.* 32:669–682.

Travers SP, Geran LC. 2009. Bitter-responsive brain-stem neurons: characteristics and functions. *Physiol Behav.* 97:592–603.

Trivedi CD, Pitchumoni CS. 2005. Drug-induced pancreatitis: an update. *J Clin Gastroenterol.* 39:709–716.

Tsubouchi T, Tsujimoto S, Sugimoto S, Katsura Y, Mino T, Seki T. 2008. Swallowing disorder and inhibition of cough reflex induced by atropine sulfate in conscious dogs. *J Pharmacol Sci.* 106:452–459.

Valerio LG Jr, Petersen DR. 2000. Characterization of hepatic iron overload following dietary administration of dicyclopentadienyl iron (Ferrocene) to mice: cellular, biochemical, and molecular aspects. *Exp Mol Pathol.* 68:1–12.

Valerio LG. 2007. Mammalian iron metabolism. *Toxicol Mech Methods.* 17:497–517.

van Enckevort CC, Touw DJ, Vleming LJ. 2008. N-acetylcysteine and hemodialysis treatment of a severe case of methyl ethyl ketone peroxide intoxication. *Clin Toxicol (Phila).* 46:74–78.

Vasiluk L, Pinto LJ, Moore MM. 2005. Oral bioavailability of glyphosate: studies using two intestinal cell lines. *Environ Toxicol Chem.* 24:153–160.

Vidal JE, McClane BA, Saputo J, Parker J, Uzal FA. 2008. Effects of *Clostridium perfringens* beta-toxin on the rabbit small intestine and colon. *Infect Immun.* 76:4396–4404.

Wataganara T, Leelakusolvong S, Sunsaneevithayakul P, Vantanasiri C. 2009. Treatment of severe achalasia during pregnancy with esophagoscopic injection of botulinum toxin A: a case report. *J Perinatol.* 29:637–639.

Watkins SM, Reich A, Fleming LE, Hammond R. 2008. Neurotoxic shellfish poisoning. *Mar Drugs.* 6:431–455.

Weber LW, Boll M, Stampfl A. 2003. Hepatotoxicity and mechanism of action of haloalkanes: carbon tetrachloride as a toxicological model. *Crit Rev Toxicol.* 33:105–136.

White HB 3rd, Orth WH 3rd, Schreiber RW Jr, Whitehead CC. 1992. Availability of avidin-bound biotin to the chicken embryo. *Arch Biochem Biophys.* 298:80–83.

Whittem CG, Williams AD, Williams CS. 2010. Murine colitis modeling using dextran sulfate sodium (DSS). *J Vis Exp.* (35):ii. doi: 10.3791/1652.

Yamaguchi I, Hamada K, Yoshida M, Isayama H, Kanazashi S, Takeuchi K. 2009. Risperidone attenuates local and systemic inflammatory responses to ameliorate diet-induced severe necrotic pancreatitis in mice: it may provide a new therapy for acute pancreatitis. *J Pharmacol Exp Ther.* 328:256–262.

Yáñez JA, Teng XW, Roupe KA, Fariss MW, Davies NM. 2003. Chemotherapy induced gastrointestinal toxicity in rats: involvement of mitochondrial DNA, gastrointestinal permeability and cyclooxygenase-2. *J Pharm Pharm Sci.* 6:308–314.

Yang R, Miki K, He X, Killeen ME, Fink MP. 2009. Prolonged treatment with N-acetylcystine delays liver recovery from acetaminophen hepatotoxicity. *Crit Care.* 13:R55.

Yeomans ND, Hawkey CJ, Brailsford W, Naesdal J. 2009. Gastroduodenal toxicity of low-dose acetylsalicylic acid: a comparison with nonsteroidal anti-inflammatory drugs. *Curr Med Res Opin.* 25:2785–2793.

Yoshizawa K, Marsh T, Foley JF, Cai B, Peddada S, Walker NJ, Nyska A. 2005. Mechanisms of exocrine pancreatic toxicity induced by oral treatment with 2,3,7,8-tetrachlorodibenzo-p-dioxin in female Harlan Sprague-Dawley Rats. *Toxicol Sci.* 85:594–606.

Yu H, Chen S, Yang Z, Pan A, Zhang G, Shan J, Tang X, Zhou W. 2009. Trimethyltin chloride induced chloride secretion across rat distal colon. *Cell Biol Int.* 34:99–108.

Zanatta F, Gandolfi RB, Lemos M, Ticona JC, Gimenez A, Clasen BK, Cechinel Filho V, de Andrade SF. 2009. Gastroprotective activity of alkaloid extract and 2-phenylquinoline obtained from the bark of *Galipea longiflora* Krause (Rutaceae). *Chem Biol Interact.* 180:312–317.

Zayachkivska O, Gzregotsky M, Ferentc M, Yaschenko A, Urbanovych A. 2008. Effects of nitrosative stress and reactive oxygen-scavenging systems in esophageal physiopathy under streptozotocin-induced experimental hyperglycemia. *J Physiol Pharmacol.* 59(Suppl 2):77–87.

Zayat M, Lichtenberger LM, Dial EJ. 2008. Pathophysiology of LPS-induced gastrointestinal injury in the rat: role of secretory phospholipase A2. *Shock.* 30:206–211.

Zhong LY, Wu H. 2006. [Current researching situation of mucosal irritant components in Araceae family plants]. *Zhongguo Zhong Yao Za Zhi.* 31:1561–1563.

Zografos GN, Georgiadou D, Thomas D, Kaltsas G, Digalakis M. 2009. Drug-induced esophagitis. *Dis Esophagus.* 22:633–637.

CHAPTER 17

The Lung and Gill Exposures Representing Toxic Concentrations— Model for Environmental Toxicology

This is a chapter outline intended to guide and familiarize you with the content to follow.

I. Respiratory organs—models of environmental toxicology

    A. Lung

        1. Air concentrations and time of exposure more important than dose

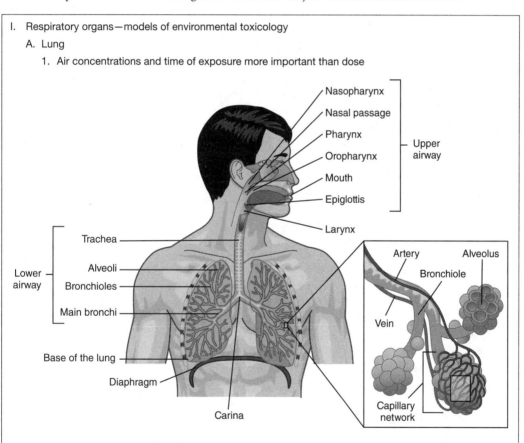

        2. Damage can occur anywhere dust, particles, fibers, aerosols, vapors, and gases contact structures and only transfer into circulation at level of respiratory bronchioles and alveoli where normal gas exchange occurs

        3. Best model of human respiratory tract in animals is the beagle dog (monkeys too expensive), which has five generations of respiratory bronchioles similar to human; rodents lack bronchioles

CONCEPTUALIZING TOXICOLOGY 17-1

4. N-nitrosamines from cigarette snuff → liver genotoxicity and similar damage to nasal cavity of rats, while in humans snuff use leads to no observed cancer of the mouth or lung, but increased pancreatic cancer

5. Nasal epithelial toxicity—see Table 17-1

   a. Human is a nose breather (can use either nose or mouth), but can the same be said of a dog (can use either but pants)? Humans are microsmatic (weak sense of smell), while dogs are macrosmatic (highly developed sense of smell). Rodents are obligate nose breathers

   b. Highest velocity of air movement and highly accelerated by sneeze (toxic particle protection)

   c. Nose humidifies, warms, and filters (somewhat) air and has simple turbinates in human (complex branching turbinates in dog, mouse, rabbit, and rat)

   d. Squamous epithelium lines the lumen of the nasal chambers (rats have more olfactory epithelium than humans—see Figure 17-2); hair cells in lamina propria contain fibroblasts, lymphocytes, mast cells, etc.; mucus is an antioxidant secreted by goblet cells that protect against ozone, O_3 (mucus-soluble chemicals and particles)

   e. Particles trapped in mucous → oral dose

   f. Formaldehyde (HCHO) damages transitional and respiratory epithelium (cross-links DNA) of vestibule and is a function of airflow; cigarette smoke and chronic HCHO → squamous cell hyperplasia and epithelial cell proliferation; nasal cancer from HCHO due to epithelial degeneration, regenerative cell replication, and inflammation

   g. Caustic chemicals (dimethylamine, glutaraldehyde, ammonia, HCl) damage squamous epithelium and lesions by fumigant methyl bromide

   h. Cl_2 gas and O_3 → inflammation → epithelial and mucous cell hyperplasia (can be protective at low acute exposures of O_3 as provides antioxidant factors)

   i. Lectin-binding chitinase gene product may be key factor for allergen-induced inflammation and cellular injury

   j. Cl_2, HCHO, and O_3 → respiratory epithelial damage and cilia loss

   k. Olfactory epithelial damage separated into:

      (1) Necrosis from direct irritation by Cl_2, SO_2

      (2) Sensory cell injury by β, β′-iminopropionitrile (and metabolites)

      (3) Toxicity to sustentacular cell degeneration and necrosis of sensory cells by metabolites of refined dimethyl esters of adipic, glutaric, and succinic acids due to nasal carboxylesterase activity → support cell death

      (4) CYP-mediated necrosis and atrophy of olfactory epithelial cells by metabolites of acetaminophen, ferrocene, 3-methylfuran, nitrosodiethylamine

      (5) Mitochondrial poisoning by H_2S—loss of nasal respiratory epithelium as well and at lethal concentrations poison sensory cells as well

6. Larynx

   a. High-velocity airflows in this region as well

   b. Asbestos fiber irritation starts the cancer series here (larger fibers at this level and smaller at deeper levels)

   c. Ethanol via ADH → acetaldehyde and free radicals by CYP2E1 → DNA adducts, destroying folate → secondary hyperproliferation

   d. Smoking cannabis → tongue and laryngeal cancers (tetrahydrocannabinol) rather than cigarettes and lung cancer (PAHs)—however, unfiltered cigarettes → aromatic DNA adducts, N7-alkylated guanosines and oxidative DNA damage (PAHs, aromatic amines, N-nitrosamines and ROS) → laryngeal cancer

   e. Metalworking fluids (diethanolamine) → laryngeal, tracheal, pancreatic, and rectal cancers

   f. TDIC—low concentrations → nasal damage; high concentrations → laryngeal, tracheal, and lung damage

CONCEPTUALIZING TOXICOLOGY 17-1 (*continued*)

g. Necrosis by cisplatin chemotherapy combined with radiation for nasopharyngeal cancer

h. Caustic agents damage vocal cords

i. Laryngeal spasms caused by tear gas (2-chlorobenzylidene malononitrile)

7. Tracheal/bronchiolar tree

a. Epithelial-mesenchymal trophic unit = model of tracheobronchial airway tree consisting of an epithelial layer (including submucosal cells) with underlying interstitium of fibroblasts, smooth muscle, cartilage, and vascular + intertwining nerves + immunological cells (inflammatory and migratory such as macrophages)

(1) Infants (lack of repair) and women (cancer and autoimmunity) more susceptible to damage; in female mice opposite is true (protected from fibrosis by bleomycin)

b. Tracheal ciliated mucosal cells affected by *Bordetella* species (whooping cough), production of adenylate cyclase toxin (depletes ATP and ↑ IL-6), dermonecrotic toxin, tracheal cytotoxin

c. Cilia paralysis by nicotine and ciliostasis also by alkylated phenols in cigarette smoke

d. Asbestos—size of fiber determines where it damages—10 μm in tracheobronchial region, 3 μm lower and upper lobe regions, < 3 μm into lung tissue and lining, and < 0.25 μm for asbestosis and mesothelioma (cancer of lining of the lung). Ultrathin, short fibers (more potent if straight or amphiboles) are only ones that cross the pulmonary–pleural barrier and cause mesothelioma and pleural plaques → intercepted by cells → macrophage attracted → immune-mediated oxidant injury → induced *fos/jun* proto-oncogenes

e. O_3 or allergens → induce myofibroblasts, smooth muscle hypertrophy, interstitial fibrosis, basement membrane zone thickening

f. Bronchiole constriction and inflammation key to COPD and asthma—5-HT, ACh, histamine → constriction; Cl_2 → bronchospasms

g. Nanotechnology (carbon nanotubes) → interstitial pulmonary fibrosis, allergic asthma and asbestos-like inflammation; Cd-containing nanotubes → lung cancer, pleural fibrosis/mesothelioma along with kidney and liver injury

8. Respiratory bronchioles/alveoli (respiratory zone)

a. Gas exchange occurs in this region

b. Movement of diaphragm (and intercostal muscles and abdominal muscles for rapid forced exhalation) and lung compliance with change in pressures and presence of pulmonary surfactant responsible for changes in lung volume (as modified by temperature and pressure of the air—Boyle's Law and humidity = BTPS correction factor) necessary to achieve exchange of gases in respiratory zone—see respiratory volumes

c. Respiration in clinic usually assessed by respirometry/spirogram (see Figure 17-2) and mainly the $FEV_{1.0}$ (forced expiratory volume at 1 second) and classified into obstructive disorders (blocks airway such as asthma, allergy and ↓ $FEV_{1.0}$ and $FEV_{1.0}$/FVC ratio; where FVC = forced vital capacity), restrictive (fibrosis normal or ↑ $FEV_{1.0}$/FVC ratio) or both (emphysema ↓ $FEV_{1.0}$ and $FEV_{1.0}$/FVC ratio); asbestos ↓ $FEV_{1.0}$ and $FEV_{1.0}$/FVC + pulmonary plaques on X-ray analysis

d. O_3 alone or in combination with peroxyacyl nitrate (lung irritant in smog) produced changes in lung volumes, but not peroxyacyl nitrate alone; ozone's damage exacerbated by nitrogen dioxide exposure

e. $PM_{2.5}$ airborne particulate matter is most damaging to this area of the lung and mainly due to combustion products containing metals; small particles like this can even be generated in homes during cooking a meal; diesel associated particles or electron transfer compounds, ROS, and other radical species → irritation and inflammation → asthma, COPD, and cancer; Co, Cr, Ni, Pt (especially chlorinated platinum compounds) → induce airway narrowing and are asthma sensitizers; $Cr(IV)O_2$ causes lung lesions → hyperplastic Type II pneumocytes and collagenized fibrosis; Cr → bronchiolar epithelium appearance in alveoli by terminal

CONCEPTUALIZING TOXICOLOGY 17-1 (*continued*)

bronchioles, foamy macrophage response, cholesterol granulomas, alveolar proteinosis, and minute fibrotic pleurisy in rats; Cd, Cr(VI), Ni → lung cancer (Cd also alters lung barrier function by direct effects on adherens junction proteins)

f. Mineral dust → pneumoconiosis (miner's lung) and interstitial fibrosis

g. Nicotine → α-hydroxylation pathways via CYPs → reactive intermediates → DNA adducts → lung cancer; smoke products cause excess of G → T transversions (PAH adduct sites on *p53* gene); smoking or Al dust or Cd → emphysema (Al also produces pulmonary granulomatosis)

h. The herbicide Paraquat (oxidation/reduction indicator methyl viologen) is reduced by NADPH cytochrome P450 reductase and then easily transfers the electron to oxygen to produce O_2^-. Paraquat does not need to be inhaled to be damaging to the lung as alveolar cells I, II and Clara cells use the polyamine transport system to accumulate and prolong the $t_{1/2}$ and oxidative damage of this compound

i. Phosgene gas ($COCl_2$) produces lipid peroxidation and stimulates leukotriene formation leading to increased capillary permeability and edema

j. Agricultural gas anhydrous NH_3 → NH_4OH in contact with tissue → hemoptysis (cough up blood), pharyngitis, bronchiectasis, and pulmonary edema

k. Developing lung more sensitive—case of *Stachybotrys chartarum* mycotoxin and hemolytic activity → pulmonary hemorrhage in infants of Cleveland, OH area due to furnace design that took air from basement

B. Gill

1. Concentration in water and time of exposure more important than dose

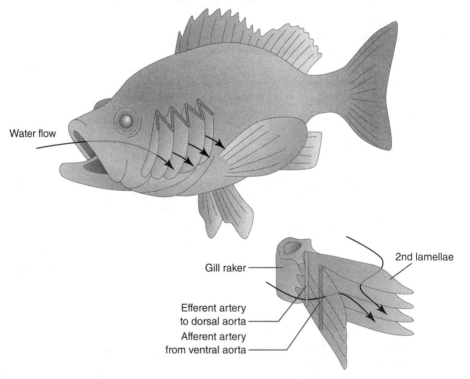

Water flow

Gill raker

2nd lamellae

Efferent artery to dorsal aorta

Afferent artery from ventral aorta

2. Accumulation of the toxicant from the gill is based on the concentration of the compound in the water, hydrophobicity of the compound (K_{OW}), and factors related to fish physiology such as organic composition of the fish, metabolic rate of the fish (or zooplankton), growth rate of the fish, and total gill area and activity of the gill. See FGETS model in the chapter

CONCEPTUALIZING TOXICOLOGY 17-1 (*continued*)

3. Toxic effects on gill—see Table 17-2

    a. Small particles affect the gill as they do the lung; Ag nanoparticles of 10 nm are most concentrated in the rainbow trout (active gill sensitive surface water species) and induce CYP1A2 (induction of oxidative metabolism); TiO_2 nanoparticles → ↓ oxidant defense and ↑ lipid peroxidation

    b. Cd, Cu, Zn → Oxidative membrane damage and perturbations of acid–base balance of Eastern oyster

    c. Enzyme inhibition

        (1) $NaAsO_2$ → inhibited acid phosphatase, alkaline phosphatase, glutamate oxaloacetate transaminase, glutamate pyruvate transaminase, AChE in gill of mollusc *Lamellidens marginalis*, and reduced level of GSH-S-transferase and catalase

        (2) Pesticide chlorpyrifos-ethyl → AChE inhibition (+ butyrylcholinesterase at higher concentrations) in gills and hepatopancreas of Mediterranean crab

        (3) Analgesic acetaminophen → inhibits AChE in gill and ↑ liver lipid peroxidation

        (4) Anticonvulsant carbamazepine → inhibited antioxidant enzymes, $3Na^+$, $2K^+$-ATPase, + ↓ GSH in rainbow trout

    d. CYP induction

        (1) PAHs or PCBs → gill tissue CYP1A induction

    e. Other enzyme induction

        (1) Beta-blocker propranolol → gill GSH-S-transferase

        (2) 17β-estradiol in water → induces catalase in juvenile sea bass gills, while intraperitoneal injection ↓ a variety of antioxidant enzyme activities

    f. Histopathological damage

        (1) $NaAsO^2$ affected gas exchange, filter feeding, and immune protection

        (2) Hg and crystalline granular inclusions in mitochondria of prawn gills

        (3) Diesel fuel and unleaded gasoline → epithelial hyperplasia of gill and esophagus + liver damage in larvae

        (4) NaClO (bleach) → hypertrophy, lamellar fusion, increase in goblet cell size and number

        (5) AChE-inhibiting pesticide carbaryl → rupture of basal laminae, abnormal infiltrations of hematocytes in hemocoelic space of gill lamellae and interstitial spaces of hepatopancreas, fused gill lamellae, and necrosis-like histopathology of gill lamellae and tubules of hepatopancreas of juvenile prawns

        (6) $NaNO_3$, KNO_3, and KCl → lamellar swelling, epithelial thickening, pillar cell disruption, necrosis, and distortion to juvenile blue swimmer crab

        (7) Pesticide 2,4-D → developing gill abnormalities (agenesis) in South American toad

    g. Gill functional damage

        (1) Mn → dopaminergic inhibition of lateral cilia movement in gill of bivalve mollusc *Crassostrea virginica*

        (2) 2,2′,4,4′-tetrabromodiphenyl ether → loss of cell viability, disruption of redox status, mitochondrial membrane lipid peroxidation, and apoptosis

        (3) Zebrafish more sensitive to ammonia and urea exposure due to expression of transport proteins (Rh for NH_3 and UT for urea)—exposure of zebrafish to high external NH_3 or phloretin (phenolic ketone inhibition of monosaccharide and anion transport) → NH_3 and urea tissue concentrations in adult and juvenile zebrafish, respectively (age-dependent); NH_3 → ↑ Rh mRNA expression in embryo and larvae gills and UT mRNA in both adults and developing zebrafish; phloretin → ↑ UT mRNA only in developing gill tissue; nonlethal NH_3 → ↑ oxidative stress in gills and brain of mudskipper

CONCEPTUALIZING TOXICOLOGY 17-1 (*continued*)

C. Lung toxicity tests—see Table 17-3

    1. Aerodynamic diameter and mass change particle behavior so models for human must reflect similar deposition in various portion of the respiratory tract (dose metrics)

Region	Particle/Fiber (3:1 Length/Width) Size	Type of Deposition
Nasopharyngeal	30 µm down to 5 µm	Inertial impaction region or simple interception for long fibers
Bronchiolar region	5 µm down to 1 µm	Gravitational sedimentation
Alveolar region	1 µm to nanoparticles	Brownian diffusion

    2. For diffusible particles with a mass median < 0.3 µm, diameter is used to model rather than aerodynamic diameter. Metal nanoparticles greatly increase surface area for oxidative reactions. Electrostatic forces, thermal phoresis (movement along a thermal gradient applies mainly to aerosols), vapor pressure, interaction with applied magnetic field, and Raleigh-Taylor gas effects (instability that occurs with fluid interactions such as oil/water interfaces) also affect toxicant movements in lung tissue

    3. Fluids also follow nonlinear Navier-Stokes equations such as described by:

$$\rho\left(\frac{\partial v}{\partial t} + \mathbf{v} \cdot \nabla\mathbf{v}\right) = -\nabla p + \nabla \cdot \mathbf{T} + \mathbf{f},$$

Where $\mathbf{v}$ = flow velocity, ρ = fluid density, p = pressure, $\mathbf{T}$ = deviatoric component of total stress tensor (which has order 2), $\mathbf{f}$ = body forces per unit volume acting on the fluid, and ∇ = the del operator (partial derivatives of a vector in a gradient) and for the lung assuming laminar flow the equation can become:

$$\frac{\partial}{\partial xj}(uiuj) = -1\,\rho\,\frac{\partial p}{\partial xi} + \nu\,\frac{\partial 2ui}{\partial xj\partial xj}$$

where Here u = air phase velocity, p = the pressure, ρ = the air density, and ν is the kinematic viscosity. This model was used to model particles deposition in lung (Walters and Luke, 2011)

    4. Start with general timed exposures of concentrations of the toxicant to rodents, then more complicated mammalian species (dog) to confirm results (nonhuman primates very expensive), then to specialized models of cats and other species as necessary

    5. If compound too precious, then intratracheal or intrabronchial instillation necessary to avoid dense hair coat of a rodent. Also, one lobe of the lung may be treated leaving the other lung as a control. These studies may overestimate the effect in humans. Despite its problems, the instillation approach has yielded important data, such as the 12-month lag time for detection of instilled asbestos fiber fragments in pleural epithelium and development of pulmonary carcinomas and malignant pleural mesothelioma and earlier incidence of tumors in animals also treated with benzo(a)pyrene

    6. Alternative approaches using human respiratory tract epithelial cell cultures at body temperature and close to 100% humidity have to resolve cell-type responses, dose, procedures for exposure, and applicability of results to human respiratory tract damage prior to acceptance as a valid approach to pulmonary toxicity testing. A single system such as this does not reasonably test all parameters of intact animal inhalation toxicity

D. Gill toxicity tests—see Table 17-4

    1. Fish biotransform toxicants at much slower rates than mammals (10^6 rat hepatocytes have clearance value for herbicide atrazine at 3.81 ± 1.96 mL/h, while 10^6 trout hepatocytes only clear at 0.002 mg/h which is ~1000 fold slower)

    2. Gill also represents a significant extrahepatic metabolic site and cultured gill cells have been used to assess metabolism as well as cell damage

    3. Whole fish assays indicate damage to and metabolism by gill tissue. Isolated gill or gill cells indicate similar parameters as well as uptake studies in pavement and mitochondria-rich cells. Fish embryos represent the European Union's alternative approach and also yield developmental and bioaccumulation data

CONCEPTUALIZING TOXICOLOGY 17-1 (*continued*)

The lung is the next area, following skin, eyes, and gastrointestinal tract, in which damage associated with environmental exposure to toxicants can occur. Concentrations are more important than dose over long periods of time, because equilibrium will likely occur between the concentration in the air (or water in the case of fish) and the concentration in the body unless toxicity leads to organ damage and decreased exchange with the environment or decreased metabolism and excretion. For short periods of time, the breathing style is important, which is rarely expressed in toxicology or physiology texts. How a person (respiratory depth versus anatomical dead space) or fish respires (% active gill) is as important. When gas chambers still existed in the United States, execution personnel would instruct persons being executed to wait to hear the cyanide gas evolve and take a deep breath rather than more slowly panting and extending their suffering. For high concentrations of toxic substances, this is an essential part of the dose taken in the first breath and lethality. Otherwise, for lower concentrations, the concentration of the gas, vapor, aerosol, or particle; particle sizes; and respiratory volumes must be considered along with damage to the respiratory organ (lung or gill), exchange across the respiratory organ, cardiac output for speed of delivery through the circulation, and the disposition and target organs. This is important for the "canary in the mine" technique. The higher heart rate of the canary versus the human heart increases the rapid circulation of the toxic substances exchanged from the air into the blood and makes the canary the first to succumb to mine gas as a warning to the human. This is similar to environmental toxicology, because particles may have different sizes and shapes that are inhaled or taken through the gill and retained or intercepted by the wall of the respiratory pathway cells. Some are excluded or exhaled in subsequent breaths and have little effect on respiration of the organism. Thus, there is a form of dispersion, deposition, sink, and so forth that explains the toxicokinetics that is a microcosm of an external air/water environmental toxicology assessment.

Forensic Analysis of Lung Damage

Prior to examining the impact of toxicants on the lung, a brief review of comparative anatomy and physiology of the respiratory tracts and how they are measured is important. While less expensive rodents are preferred toxicology models, the respiratory tract size and architecture make the beagle (dog) a better model for human inhalation exposure when human data are lacking. Certainly, monkeys are closer to humans but are very expensive for use in this regard. Regarding beagles as a respiratory model, they have respiratory bronchioles that branch up to five generations in patterns similar to the human. Rodents on the other hand lack bronchioles and similar small laboratory animals may only have a single short generation (Takenaka et al., 1998). After all, when people used inhaled snuff (tobacco powder), it is not the same part of the rat or mouse respiratory tract that will respond due to trapping relatively large particles. Additionally, there is much too intimate a connection between the rat mouth and nasal passages. Oral administration of N-nitrosamines from cigarette snuff, especially 4-(N-methyl-N-nitrosamino)-1-(3-pyridyl)-1-butanone (NNK), not only caused liver genotoxicity, but had similar effects on the nasal cavity in rats (Pool-Zobel et al., 1992). In a Swedish human population who use wet snuff, or snus, there were no observed cancers of the mouth or lung. Rather, pancreatic cancer was increased (Luo et al., 2007). Thus, it is necessary to be careful in interpreting rodent data for extrapolation to human inhalation toxicity risks, because aquaporin (moisture; King and Agre, 2001) and other species and sex-specific differences exist between human and rodent responses, even for genotoxic agents such as 1,3-butadiene and its reactive epoxy metabolites (Walker et al., 2009).

Lung Anatomy and Physiology

Nasal Epithelium

It makes good sense to start with the first organ to encounter the toxicant, the nose. This is true at rest unless an organism is mainly a mouth-breather. The differences in impacts between lab animals and humans must be made clear so as not to generalize toxic impacts. It is the area with the highest velocity of air movement as opposed to deep within the lung. This can be greatly increased by a sneeze, which is a toxic particle protection mechanism. The nose provides humidifying, warming, and filtering of inhaled air. It has been described as a scrubber that catches a certain amount of chemicals to prevent deeper damage. The nose is composed of two elongated tubes from the nostril to the nasopharynx separated by a nasal septum. Air passes through the nares into a slight dilation known as the vestibule. The nasal chambers pass through flexible cartilage prior to bone and toward the soft palate. Squamous epithelium lines the lumen, some containing hairs in humans under which lie the lamina propria containing the fibroblasts, lymphocytes, mast cells, and so forth (mesenchymal). Mucus originating from goblet cells in the epithelium and subepithelial glands continuously covers these cells, which are supplied with vasculature and nervous innervations. There is an increase in mucosal substances going from the tip of the nose into the nasal turbinates. Because mucus has an antioxidant action, ozone from air pollution affects regions of the human, rat, and monkey with little mucosubstances as indicated in **Table 17-1**. The high surface area (4 × tracheal area) to catch particulate matter from and provide moisture and heat to air is provided by bony protrusions (turbinates). Humans have three relatively simple turbinates, as opposed to complex branching structures in the dog, mouse, rabbit, and rat. Humans are microsmatic, or have a weak sense of smell, and may breathe either with the nose or through the mouth. Dogs are macrosmatic, or have a highly developed sense of smell, and can also use either pathway. Rats, mice, hamsters, and guinea pigs are obligate nose breathers due to the close anatomical juxtaposition of the epiglottis and the soft palate. Particles captured in the mucus are moved out by breathing action, sneezing, and the movement of the cilia. The cilia move slowly over the olfactory mucosa (turnover in days) to fast over the transitional and

respiratory epithelium (turnover in minutes for a rat). The cilia cause the mucus laden with air contaminants to become an oral dose as the material is beaten into the nasopharynx and oropharynx. Cells lining the nose are the ones that will first experience the concentrations that will cause toxicity to the respiratory tract. Species differences are important for toxicity analysis. As shown in **Figure 17-1**, the

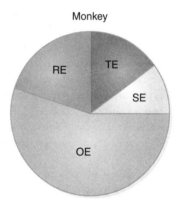

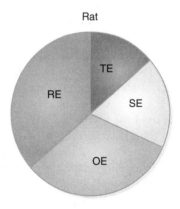

FIGURE 17-1 Distribution of the Surface Epithelia Lining the Nasal Lateral Wall of the Monkey and Rat

Note: Four distinct epithelial cell populations line both mammalian species — SE = squamous epithelium; TE = transitional epithelium; RE = respiratory epithelium; OE = olfactory epithelium. However, considerably more olfactory epithelium (OE) lines the intranasal surface of the rat compared to the monkey.

Data from Harkema JR, Carey SA, Wagner JG. 2006. The nose revisited: a brief review of the comparative structure, function, and toxicologic pathology of the nasal epithelium. *Toxicol Pathol.* 34:252–269.

TABLE 17-1   Forensic Chart of Respiratory System Toxicity

Respiratory Toxicity	Toxic Agents
Nasal Epithelium (Harkema et al., 2006)	
Cancer	Formaldehyde, nickel dust, ionizing radiation, wood dust, leather dust, cigarette smoke
Oxidant injury	Ozone
Septal necrosis with perforation	Cocaine
Olfactory epithelial damage	Methyl bromide, chlorine, sulfur dioxide, beta-beta´-iminodipropionitrile, acetaminophen, ferrocene, 3-methylfuran, nitrosodiethylamine, hydrogen sulfide (Roberts et al., 2008)
Olfactory sensory neurons	Vinca alkaloids, mycotoxin, trichothecene, satratoxin
Squamous epithelial ulceration/erosion	Dimethylamine, glutaraldehyde, ammonia, HCl
Squamous cell metaplasia	Cigarette smoke, formaldehyde
Transitional/respiratory epithelial damage	Formaldehyde, ozone, chlorine, hydrogen sulfide (Roberts et al., 2008)
Larynx	
Cancer	Asbestos (Brusis et al., 2007), ethanol (Pöschl and Seitz, 2004), metalworking fluids (Mirer, 2003), cannabis (Carriot and Sasco, 2000), cigarette smoke (Szyfter et al., 1999)
Noncancerous cell damage	Toluene diisocyanate (Collins, 2002)
Laryngeal necrosis	Cisplatin + radiation (Baron-Hay et al., 1999)
Spasms	2-chlorobenzylidene malononitrile (Davey and Moppett, 2004)
Trachea/Bronchioles	
Cancer	Asbestos (Anttila et al., 1993)
Cilia beat rate	Nicotine (Hahn et al., 1992), alkylated phenols (Pettersson et al., 1985)
Constriction	Chlorine (Winder, 2001)
Infection/inflammation	*Bordetella* species toxins (Vojtova et al., 2006)
Respiratory Bronchioles and Alveoli	
Asthma	Diesel exhausts (Just et al., 2006), Cr, Ni, Pt, Co (Rüegger, 1995)
Cancer	Cigarette smoke (Pfeifer et al., 2002), Cr (VI), Ni, Cd (Beveridge et al., 2010)
Edema	Paraquat (Wyatt, 1981), phosgene (Sciuto and Hurt, 2004), ammonia (Amshel et al., 2000)
Emphysema	Cigarette smoke (Vallyathan and Hahn, 1985), aluminum dust (Chen et al., 1978), cadmium (Forti et al., 2010)
Fibrosis	Asbestos (Warheit, 1989), mineral dust (Schenker et al., 2009), Paraquat (Wyatt et al., 1981), aluminum dust (Chen et al., 1978), coal dust (McCunney et al., 2009), silicon dust (Cohen et al., 2008), chromium (Lee et al., 1989), nanotechnology (Bonner, 2010)
Metal fume fever	Zinc (Rüegger, 1995)
Necrosis	Napthalene (Lin et al., 2009)
Surfactant	ROS, agents that activate protease or leak plasma proteins (Cepkova and Matthay, 2009)
Mesothelium	
Cancer	Asbestos (Chiappino, 2005)
Developing Lung	
Airway narrowing	Passive cigarette smoke (Elliot et al., 1998)
Nicotine metabolism	*In utero* exposure to nicotine and gene mutations (Poetsch et al., 2010)
Pulmonary hemorrhage	*Stachybotrys chartarum* (Yike et al., 2007)

rat has more olfactory epithelium compared with the monkey or human. This is also true unfortunately for other lab animal models such as the mouse, rabbit, and dog. This sensory part of the epithelium must be able to sense odor molecules, so it contacts the air and toxicants suspended in the air stream. These cells can regenerate (neurogenesis) following injury.

Toxicants may be separated by region of the nose affected. The preservative formaldehyde injures the transitional and respiratory epithelium especially of the vestibule (anterior regions) and is more a function of airflow. Caustic chemicals in the airflow, such as dimethylamine, glutaraldehyde, ammonia, and HCl, damage the squamous epithelium. The fumigant methyl bromide causes lesions in the olfactory epithelium. Chronic exposure to the disinfectant chlorine and the pollutant ozone show certain tissue-specific activity and airflow dynamics causing inflammation followed by epithelial hyperplasia (increased DNA synthesis and accumulation of a proteinaceous material containing Ym 1/2 chitinase) in the supra- or sub-nuclear cytoplasm of nonciliated cuboidal/columnar epithelial cells and mucous cell metaplasia (overexpression of mucin-specific gene *MUC5AC*) in rats and monkeys. Respiratory epithelial damage and cilia loss also result from chlorine, formaldehyde, and ozone exposures. Formaldehyde-induced DNA cross-links are found in rat respiratory and transitional epithelium but not in the olfactory mucosa or the bone marrow. Acute exposures to ozone have the effect of antioxidant protection originating from the mucus cell metaplasia indicating that further damage undermines the initial protective mechanisms of the nasal cells. The appearance of the lectin-binding chitinase gene product may be a key factor in allergen-induced inflammation and cellular injury. Cigarette smoke and chronic formaldehyde inhalation cause squamous cell metaplasia and epithelial cell proliferation. It appears that the nasal cancer from formaldehyde results from epithelial degeneration, regenerative cell replication, and inflammation. Olfactory epithelial damage may result from necrosis resulting from direct irritation (chlorine, sulfur dioxide), sensory-cell

injury alone (beta-beta′-iminodipropionitrile), toxicity to sustentacular cell and degeneration and necrosis of sensory cells followed by support cell mortality, and CYP-mediated necrosis and atrophy of olfactory epithelial cells by metabolites of acetaminophen, ferrocene, 3-methylfuran, and nitrosodiethylamine. In addition to the chemicals that can cause direct damage and those metabolites just mentioned such as acetaminophen, CYP-linked metabolism of chlorthiamid and beta-beta′-iminodipropionitrile also are responsible for other nasal damage of these inhaled chemicals. Nasal carboxylesterase activity is linked to olfactory epithelial sustentacular cell toxicity of dibasic ester (refined dimethyl esters of adipic, glutaric, and succinic acids used in paints, adhesives, crop protection, etc.; Harkema et al., 2006).

The National Toxicology Program has discerned different cancers that result from chemical exposure (Brown, 1990). Squamous cell carcinomas of the anterior nasal cavity arise from inhalation of 1,2-dibromo-3-chloropropane (rat and mouse), 1,2-dibromoethane (rat), dimethylcarbamyl chloride (rat), α-epichlorhydrin (rat), or HCl/paraformaldehyde (rat) or drinking dimethylvinyl chloride in water (rat). Transitional and respiratory epithelial papillary adenomas and/or carcinomas include inhalation of 1,2-dibromo-3-chloropropane (rat and mouse), 1,2-dibromoethane (rat and mouse), 1,2-epoxybutane (rat), and propylene oxide (rat), or oral/gavage of dimethylvinyl chloride and 2,6-xylidine, or skin painting with 2,3-dibromo-1-propanol or intraperitoneal (IP) injection of nitrosaminoketone. Olfactory epithelial or Bowman's glands tumors were produced by inhalation or injection of bis(chloromethyl)-ether (rat), oral/dietary administration of *p*-cresidine, dimethylvinyl chloride, or 2,6-xylidine, or IP injection of nitrosaminoketone, procarbazine, or tris(aziridinyl)-phosphine sulfide. Nasal rhabdomyomas and rhabdosarcomas were induced in rats by 1, 4-dioxane in drinking water, dietary 2,6-xylidine, oral gavage of dimethylvinyl chloride, or safrole/corn oil, or IP injection of nitrosaminoketone. Nasal vascular tumors accompanied mouse inhalation or 1,2-dibromo-3-chloropropane or propylene oxide.

It is also of interest that neurotoxicity may be mediated for airborne particles through the olfactory nerves. Olfactory sensory neurons can be directly targeted for apoptosis by tubulin-targeting cancer chemotherapy medications such as the vinca alkaloids or toxins such as mycotoxin, trichothecene, or satratoxin (black mold *Stachybotrys chartarum*) followed by olfactory epithelial loss (Harkema et al., 2006). A neurotoxin that damages the nasal respiratory and olfactory epithelial cells is hydrogen sulfide. It has been noted that people who have experienced a lethal dose of this gas lose their ability to smell the rotten egg odor. Hydrogen sulfide is a mitochondrial toxicant and the inhibition of cytochrome oxidase, similar to cyanide poisoning, appears to be the key feature in its toxic effects. It seems odd then that a study found that H_2S-poisoned Sprague-Dawley rats showed no significant changes in gene expression of cytochrome oxidase or bioenergetics, but did find alterations in cell cycle regulation, protein kinase regulation, cytoskeletal organization, and biogenesis (Roberts et al., 2008).

Larynx

The larynx and trachea still have high-velocity airflows that may cause impact of dense particles or interception of fibers. Laryngeal cancer starts the problem with asbestos fiber that also leads to lung cancer, mesothelioma, and asbestosis for deeper structures (Brusis et al., 2007). Alcohol is still problematic as it is in the breath of intoxicated individuals as indicated by the forensic evidence provided by breathalyzer tests. It is still the metabolism to acetaldehyde by alcohol dehydrogenase and generation of free radicals via CYP2E1 induction that are most problematic, generating DNA adducts, destroying folate, and producing secondary hyperproliferation. Acetaldehyde may also arise from the action of oral (and fecal) bacteria, especially due to smoking coupled with poor oral health (Pöschl and Seitz, 2004). Smoking tobacco is more likely to lead to lung cancers, but smoking cannabis leads to tongue and laryngeal cancers. It appears that the Δ9-tetrahydrocannabinol appears to produce cancer in a different manner from that of the result of burn products such as polycyclic aromatic hydrocarbons (PAHs;

Carriot and Sasco, 2000). However, in cigarettes with less filtering and higher percentage of genotoxic agents coupled with the number of cigarettes smoked (dose), laryngeal cancers in Poland appear to be linked to aromatic DNA adducts, N7-alkylated guanosines, and oxidative DNA damage from direct interactions and metabolism of PAHs, aromatic amines, N-nitrosamines, and reactive oxygen species (ROS) in the smoke stream (Szyfter et al., 1999). Metalworking fluids, particularly diethanolamine, appear to induce cancers of the larynx, pancreas, rectum, bladder, skin, and scrotum (Mirer, 2003). Toluene diisocyanate (TDIC) at lower concentrations (> 0.1 ppm) causes nasal damage (rhinitis and epithelial hyperplasia), but affects the larynx, trachea, and lung at higher concentrations. This leads to body weight changes and decreased survival (Collins, 2002). Laryngeal necrosis produced by chemotherapy (cisplatin) combined with radiation for treatment of nasopharyngeal cancer is a life-threatening complication (Baron-Hay et al., 1999). Caustic and other inhaled agents can damage the vocal cords. Even a relatively benign exposure to helium changes the pitch of the voice by its influence on the vocal cords. Laryngeal spasms can be problematic as indicated by marked laryngospasm following removal of a tracheal tube in a surgical patient exposed a few hours earlier to an incapacitating tear gas (2-chlorobenzylidene malononitrile or CS gas; Davey and Moppett, 2004).

Tracheal/Bronchiolar Airway Tree

Tracheal ciliated mucosal cells are affected by *Bordetella* species that produce whooping cough and other persistent respiratory infections. All species of this bacterium produce adhesions and toxins including adenylate cyclase toxin (CyaA), dermonecrotic toxin (DNT), and a tracheal cytotoxin (TCT). The CyaA toxin not only depletes cells of ATP by conversion to cAMP, but aids in the adhesion of the bacterium to the ciliated mucosa and induces formation of IL-6 (Vojtova et al., 2006). Cilia of the trachea and other mucosal cells have reduced beat frequency due to the direct action of nicotine. This would increase the exposure times of respiratory tissues to toxic particulate matter (Hahn et al., 1992).

The alkylated phenols in cigarette smoke also cause ciliostasis (Pettersson et al., 1985). The size of fiber or particle and its number and residence time become a major contributor to where it damages in the lung. The presence of more than 3 million large anthophyllite asbestos fibers (> 3 μm in length) cause lower and upper lobe cancers, and anthophyllite fibers of 10 μm in length are expected to deposit higher up into the tracheobronchial region, with only rare cancers of the lining of the lung or mesothelioma, which is the defining cancer related to asbestos exposure (Anttila et al., 1993). Short asbestos fibers (< 3 μm long) move into the lung tissue and into the lining surrounding the lung. Thin fibers < 0.25 μm appear to be strongly associated with lung cancer, mesothelioma, and asbestosis as they may need to be transported via the lymph to other tissues. Although long fibers > 10 μm appear to cause lung cancer, there have been discussions that fibers of ~ 5 μm may cause mesothelioma and ~ 2 μm produce asbestosis. However, there are some inconsistent data for fiber length and asbestosis (Stayner et al, 2008). The ultrathin short fibers appear to be the only ones that can cross the pulmonary-pleural barrier, so this confirms their ability to induce mesothelioma and pleural plaques (Chiappino, 2005). It appears that fiber shape is important as well. Serpentine or chrysotile asbestos are curled and are less potent than amphiboles or long, straight fibers in causing mesothelioma. The toxicity from asbestos is still considered an immune-mediated oxidant toxicity, because larger fibers resist ingestion by macrophages, which become lodged in the area where the fiber was intercepted. Tracheal and mesothelial cells have induced *fos/jun* proto-oncogenes by reactions to asbestos fibers due to aberrant signal transduction from redox-dependent/oxidant injury (Heintz et al., 2010).

The epithelial-mesenchymal trophic unit is a model for the tracheobronchial airway tree. Cellular differences and branch points are considered differently sensitive or responsive to toxic insult. The complexity of the airway cellular architecture is indicated by an epithelial layer of epithelial and submucosal cells covering an interstitial compartment comprised of fibroblasts, smooth muscle, cartilage, and vasculature in the basement membrane zone. Nerve processes intertwine between the smooth muscle, subepithelial matrix, and the epithelium. Immunological cells (inflammatory and migratory cells) comprise an important part of the toxic response as seen in asbestos exposure and may vary in response throughout the airway (even though this is difficult to prove). Cellular injury induces effects in multiple compartments, as may occur in ozone exposure or exposure to allergens, such as induction of myofibroblasts, smooth muscle hypertrophy, interstitial fibrosis, and thickening of the basement membrane zone. Proximal and distal airways are differentially affected by oxidant gases and aryl hydrocarbons activated by xenobiotic metabolism. This point is important, as metabolic enzyme activities, antioxidant enzyme activities, intracellular glutathione (GSH) concentrations, response to GSH depletion, and returning to normal GSH concentrations varies in the tracheobronchial airway. Infants are more prone to injury than adults, reflecting both their target cell population/induction of activating and detoxifying enzymes and the failure of repair mechanisms. In regard to lack of repair, there are proliferative and squamation phases in which infants have surviving cuboidal cells that do not differentiate and remaining squamated cells that do not form a normal cuboidal epithelium pattern. There are also sex differences, as women disproportionately form lung cancer and experience autoimmune diseases. In mice, an opposite effect is noted as female C57BL/6J mice are less likely to develop fibrosis from the anticancer agent bleomycin. This last effect may be related to CYPs (isoenzymes and induction), GSH (or GST activity), and possibly other metabolic differences in the male versus female lung tissues (Plopper et al., 2001). Bronchiole constriction and inflammation play key roles in chronic obstructive pulmonary disease (COPD) and asthma. Various physiological substances can cause bronchoconstriction, including serotonin, acetylcholine, and histamine. They are not equivalent as a nitric oxide donor molecule 1,2,3,4-oxatriazolium, 3-(3-chloro-2-methylphenyl)-5-[[(methylphenyl)sulphonyl]amino], hydroxide inner salt (GEA 3175) reverses (dilates) the action of 5-HT more than the other agents (Laursen et al., 2006). Chlorine is one among a number of irritating gases that causes bronchospasms (Winder, 2001). The use of nanotechnology also presents both new potential avenues for treatment of disease but also pulmonary toxicity. Pleural and interstitial lung disease has been reported, such as carbon nanotubes and interstitial pulmonary fibrosis, allergic asthma, and asbestos-like inflammation. However, if the nanotubes contain heavy metals such as cadmium, other endpoints such as lung cancer, pleural fibrosis/mesothelioma, and systemic toxicity (kidney and liver) may be possible as well (Bonner, 2010).

Respiratory Bronchioles/Alveoli

This is a "working" area of the lung as gas exchange occurs in this respiratory zone. It is now worth mentioning the lung physiology of gas exchange, respirometry, and prevalent lung diseases. Respiratory volumes are non-invasive ways of measuring lung function. Another noninvasive method for determining gas (oxygen) exchange to hemoglobin is to use a pulse oximeter. These methods are followed by X-rays, blood arterial oxygen determination, and finally biopsies, which are more invasive techniques. Normal inspiration at rest occurs mainly through the movements of the diaphragm as assisted by external intercostal muscles that cause increased volume and therefore decreased pressure of the thoracic cavity as indicated by Boyle's Law ($pV = nRT$, where p = pressure, V = volume, n = number of moles of a gas, R = universal gas constant, and T = temperature). Normal expiration at rest occurs via the movements of the diaphragm up into the thoracic cavity as assisted by the internal intercostal muscles, which decrease the volume and increase pressure of the thoracic cavity. The abdominal muscles can assist during forced expiration. The normal volumes associated with inspiration and expiration and the clinical measurement of the tidal volume and forced expiratory volume are shown in **Figure 17-2**. Normal respiration at rest is measured by the tidal volume. All volumes are dependent on the height, sex, and age of the subject. The tidal volume is also dependent on the weight as this volume also represents metabolism. For this reason, the thyroid function greatly influences the tidal volume as well, and thyroid disruptors may be seen with decreases in the tidal volume due to hypothyroidism. A minute of

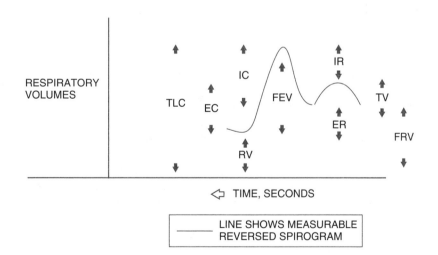

FIGURE 17-2 Normal Lung Volumes

Note: TV = tidal volume at rest, IR = inspiratory reserve volume, ER = expiratory reserve volume, IC = inspiratory capacity (= IR + TV as capacities all include TV), EC = expiratory capacity (= ER + TV); FEV = forced expiratory volume and represents a forced vital capacity or FVC; FEV_1 = FEV at one second, FEV_{25-75} = 25−75% of FVC, RV = residual volume and cannot be measured without lung collapse from pneumothorax and is part of FRV (functional residual volume = ER + RV), and total lung capacity (IR + TV + ER + RV) or TLC = total lung capacity (FEV + RV).

tidal volumes or other respiratory volumes under activity is the ventilator minute volume (VE). The ability to inhale (inspiratory reserve volume [IRV] or inspiratory capacity [IC]) and exhale (expiratory reserve volume [EVR], expiratory capacity [EC], vital capacity [VC], or forced expiratory volume [FEV]) requires an open airway and can greatly be affected by obstructive inflammatory disorders such as chronic bronchitis or asthma. Tumors, secretions, mucosal thickening, contraction of the smooth muscle, edema, and decreased elastic recoil due to parenchymal destruction (emphysema) can all be obstructive disorders. The ability of the lung to allow gas exchange, maintain proper surface tension, prevent small alveoli from collapsing, and thereby thwart respiratory distress syndrome on inhalation is facilitated by the secretion of pulmonary surfactant by type II alveolar cells. This allows the lung to be compliant or follow the pressure gradient by a proportional change in volume. The clinical evaluation usually occurs via a forced expiratory volume. Inspiration and expiration require elasticity of the lung that can be altered by fibrotic conditions that are part of restrictive disorders (decreased compliance). Restrictive disorders occur when effective lung volume or total lung capacity is decreased below 80% of normal. This can result from surgical removal of part of the lung, abnormal structures in the lung, weakness of inspiratory muscles of respiration, and lung parenchymal damage. Emphysema, for example, fits both a restrictive and obstructive disorder of the lung that occurs after chronic smoking or other chronic insults. The FEV at 1 second ($FEV_{1.0}$) is a very reproducible parameter that is ~80% of forced vital capacity (FVC) for normal young humans (~20 years of age) that is reduced to ~70% of FVC at age 70. FEV_1 is used frequently to evaluate obstructive disorders. The $FEV_{25-75\%}$ is a better measure of small airway flow limitations than the $FEV_{1.0}$, but is much less reproducible in the clinical setting. The $FEV_{1.0}$ is decreased for obstructive, severe restrictive disorders, or mixed disorders but can be normal or elevated for less severe restrictive disorders. The $FEV_{1.0}$/FVC ratio or Tiffeneau-Pinelli index is normal or increased for purely restrictive disorders, but decreased for obstructive or mixed

disorders (O'Brien 2009). The following study of respiratory volumes and specific respiratory toxicants is a helpful example. Young adult men were exposed to filtered air (control), 0.3 ppm peroxyacyl nitrate (photochemically produced smog irritant), 0.45 ppm ozone, and a mixture of O_3 and peroxyacyl nitrate. The human subject alternated 15-minute rest and 20-minute bicycle ergometer exercise periods at a workload that elicited at a VE = 27 L/min BTPS (adjusted to standard temperature, pressure, and humidity). FRC and FVC were determined before and after exposure with an additional FVC measurement 5 minutes after each exercise period. Heart rate was monitored through exposure, because cardiac output is an important factor in oxygen/carbon dioxide circulation and exchange. VE, oxygen uptake, respiratory rate, and tidal volume were measured the last 2 minutes of each exercise period. Filtered air or peroxyacyl nitrate (PAN) exposure elicited no observed alterations in any measured parameter. Ozone alone or mixed with PAN decreased V_T and concomitantly increased respiratory rate and significantly reduced FVC, $FEV_{1.0}$, $FEV_{2.0}$, $FEV_{3.0}$, $FEF_{25-75\%}$, IC, ERV, and TLC (Drechsler-Parks et al., 1984).

For forensic analysis of asbestos, asbestosis can be assessed by occupational exposure records combined with an X-ray indication of diaphragmatic pleural plaques and FEV/FVC analyses. Reductions in $FEV_{1.0}$, forced end-expiratory flow 75–80% ($FEF_{75-80\%}$), and $FEV_{1.0}$/FVC accompanied by increases in thoracic gas volume (TGV) and RV/TGV ratios in nonsmoking shipyard and construction workers exposed to asbestos (Kilburn and Warshaw, 1990). The dust formation caused by the World Trade Center collapse following the September 11, 2001 terrorist attacks has had long-term effects on rescue and recovery workers and volunteers. Reduced FVC was found along with lower respiratory disease. There was an additional association with reflux disorders (gastroesophageal, nonerosive, nonacid, or laryngopharyngeal reflux diseases) and lower airway disease suggesting air trapping (de la Hoz et al., 2008).

These studies (de la Hoz et al., 2008; Kilburn and Warshaw, 1990) show the importance of particulates in the air on lower respiratory functions. Respiratory bronchioles (and large airway carinas) collect particulate matter at 25–100 times that observed in the mainstem bronchus, resulting in toxicity at this critical portion of respiratory gas exchange. Airborne particulate matter of $PM_{2.5}$ (< 2.5 µm diameter) is the most damaging to health and usually is mainly metals from combustion products (Churg and Brauer, 2000). Even cooking (Chinese-style in the cited Hong Kong study) can increase ultrafine particles (14.6–100 nm), accumulation mode (100–661.2 nm), and $PM_{2.5}$ in homes during and following (90 minutes in the kitchen and 60 minutes in the living room) cooking emission episodes (Wan et al., 2011).

As mentioned earlier, asbestosis occurs with the smallest of the fibers that damage and lead to fibrosis in the same terminal airways and alveolar regions as gaseous toxicants such as O_3 and NO_2 (Warheit, 1989). Mineral dust in agricultural workers leads to higher rates of pneumoconiosis and interstitial fibrosis. Farm workers also had higher incidences of COPD, including emphysema, chronic bronchitis, and small airways disease (Schenker et al., 2009). Type II and Clara cells of the alveoli have the ability to biotransform nicotine-derived smoke products 4-(methylnitrosamino)-1-(3-pyridyl)-1-butanone (NNK) and N'-nitrosonornicotine (NNN) via α-hydroxylation pathways to reactive intermediates that form DNA adducts and subsequently lung cancer. Human CYP2A13 and 2B6, rat CYP2A3, and mouse CYP2A5 are most important in converting NNK to the O^6-methyl-dGuo adduct-forming metabolite (Hecht, 2008). Additionally, there are more agents capable of causing lung cancer in cigarette smoke that may involve *p53* mutations. Smoking-associated lung cancers have an excess of G → T transversions (30% of smokers' lung cancers compared with 12% in lung cancers of nonsmokers). Preferential PAH adduct sites on the *p53* account for these G → T transversion hot spots. G → A transitions appear almost exclusively in cancer not related to tobacco use. Thus, it appears that nicotine and aromatic hydrocarbons have the most impact following metabolism in this region of the lung. However, there are other pulmonary carcinogens in smoke such as azaarenes,

1,3-butadiene, ethyl carbamate, ethylene oxide, hydrazine, and heavy metals (arsenic, cadmium, chromium, nickel, ^{210}Po [radioactive]; Pfeifer et al, 2002). Acute ozone exposure induces injury to the ciliated cells of the airway and to type I epithelial cells in the alveolar region. Nitrogen dioxide causes additive or synergistic damage with ozone (Mustafa, 1990). Particles associated with diesel exhausts in urban settings appear to provide the irritation for increased cases of asthma. This may be due to chronic oxidative injury and elicited inflammatory reactions (Just et al., 2006). Another source links electron transfer compounds (aromatic nitro compounds, conjugated iminium ions, quinones, metal complexes), ROS, and other radical species to lipid peroxidation, oxidation or adduct formation of DNA, and mechanisms for the formation of asthma, COPD, and cancer (Kovacic and Somanathan, 2009). One electron transfer compound is the herbicide Paraquat (1,1'-dimethyl-4,4'-bipyridilium), also known as the oxidant-reduction indicator methyl viologen. When instilled into the bronchus of male rats, Paraquat had an enormous half-life of 76 hours with 10^{-10} g or as low as 11 hours at 10^{-5} g. The lower half-life was due to the formation of pulmonary edema. It can also produce fibrosis 7 days after dosing if the animal survives the initial damage (Wyatt et al., 1981). Paraquat does not have to be inhaled to target the lung, because alveolar cells I and II and Clara cells selectively take up Paraquat into the lung via the polyamine transport system. The toxicity other than the selective uptake and long half-life is due to redox cycling and production of superoxide and subsequently other ROS (Dinis-Oliveira et al., 2008). World War I poisonous antipersonnel phosgene gas ($COCl_2$) also produces lipid peroxidation and leukotrienes that lead to increased capillary permeability and edema (Sciuto and Hurt, 2004). Coal miners have oxidant toxicity associated with the iron content of coal dust and resulting fibrosis (McCunney et al., 2009). Returning to asthma, chromium, nickel, platinum, and cobalt are known to induce airway narrowing, and chlorinated platinum salts are potent asthma sensitizers (Rüegger, 1995). In one study, $Cr(IV)O_2$ caused lung lesions in rats with thickened hyperplastic

Type II pneumocytes and collagenized fibrosis. Cr also caused bronchiolar epithelium to appear in the alveoli next to terminal bronchioles, foamy macrophage response, cholesterol granulomas, alveolar proteinosis, and minute fibrotic pleurisy primarily in female rats. A small percentage of only the female rats developed keratin cysts, and a smaller group also had keratinized squamous cell carcinoma. This might not be relevant to human cancer (Lee et al., 1989). However, chromium (VI), cadmium, and nickel increase the incidence of lung cancers in nonsmokers (Beveridge et al., 2010). Miners and scientists manufacturing or reconstituting high-pressure liquid chromatography columns should be aware that pneumoconiosis may lead to a massive fibrosis due to chronic inhalation of silicon dust or small beads (Cohen et al., 2008). A more relevant poison to agricultural areas is that of inhaled anhydrous ammonia. The ammonia becomes ammonia hydroxide on contact with tissue producing a liquefaction necrosis on the skin and due to its affinity for mucous membranes causes exposed individuals to cough up blood from the respiratory tract (hemoptysis), pharyngitis, bronchiectasis, and pulmonary edema (Amshel et al., 2000). Chronic cigarette smoking may lead to emphysema, but so does exposure to aluminum dust. In the case of aluminum, pulmonary granulomatosis may develop in humans similar to exposed rabbits (Chen et al., 1978). Although there does not initially appear to be an obvious link between cigarette smoke and aluminum dust, aluminum and silicon lung concentrations are increased in heavy smokers (Vallyathan and Hahn, 1985). Cadmium (part of long-lasting batteries) inhalation also causes emphysema, pneumonitis, and lung cancer (as indicated earlier in the section on heavy metals as part of the components of cigarette smoke). $CdCl_2$ appears to affect lung barrier function by direct effects on adherens junction proteins at noncytotoxic concentrations (Forti et al., 2010). Zinc is an interesting metal due to its low overall toxicity, but produces an influenza-like metal fume fever (Rüegger, 1995). Other dusts (e.g., kaolin from pottery making, textiles, talc) also cause acute and chronic lung damage, as do other gases, vapors, and aerosols. Some do

so directly via toxicity or corrosion. Others are more often related to inflammation and irritation. Some require metabolism (e.g., naphthalene and its conversion to epoxide resulting in bronchiole epithelial cell necrosis with some bronchiole and alveolar adenomas; Lin et al., 2009). A number of other lung disorders can occur, but the presence of pulmonary surfactant is vital in lung inflation at low transpulmonary pressures. Artificial surfactants or natural surfactant (80% phospholipids, 8% neutral lipids, and 12% proteins) have been used successfully in treating premature infants with respiratory distress syndrome, which is a form of edema and inflammation that if survived can progress to a fibrosis. This substance, vasodilator nitric oxide, anti-inflammatory/immune suppressant glucocorticoids, and anti-inflammatory lysofylline (reduces TNF-α, IL-1, and IL-6 responses and releases oxidized free fatty acids from cell membranes) are used as therapeutic agents to mediate the negative effects of acute lung injury or acute respiratory distress syndrome (Cepkova and Matthay, 2006).

Developing Lung

Surfactant broaches the end of the fetal period and beginning of the neonate and the progression toward the adult lung. Developing lungs respond more sensitively to the toxicants already mentioned, including cigarette smoke. Infants exposed to passive cigarette smoke had increased asthma severity, lower respiratory infections, sudden infant death syndrome (SIDS), and a narrowing of the airway due to a thickening of the walls (Elliot et al., 1998). In utero exposure to nicotine and mutagenic cigarette smoke metabolites appears to affect flavin-containing monooxygenase 3 polymorphisms in infants born to heavy-smoking mothers, favoring the homozygote 472AA genotype in SIDS cases. This gene–environment interaction indicates the airborne toxicants should be avoided during pregnancy and also during the development of the neonate (Poetsch et al., 2010). The developing lung is also forming new blood vessels. Toxicants from *Stachybotrys chartarum*, an indoor air mold, were distributed to infants in the Cleveland, Ohio area due to a design of furnace that used the air in the basement as part of its air supply. Pulmonary hemorrhage appeared in the infants starting in 1993 due to spore toxicity (trichothecene mycotoxins) and hemolytic activity (hemolysins and proteinases). The proteinases appear to contribute to lung inflammation and injury in rat pups (Yike et al., 2007).

Forensic Analysis of Gill Damage

The gill is the respiratory and a major excretory organ of aquatic organisms. These structures are normally associated with vertebrates such as fish, where they are appendages of the visceral arches. Invertebrates have gills in some situations. As with the lung of air-breathing animals, concentrations of toxicants and time yield damage and then become a dose internally or damage the respiratory structure. The lung is only an excretory organ for volatile substances such as ethanol, dimethyl sulfoxide, and dimethylselenide (a metabolite of selenium). Water-soluble substances pass through the gill if small enough. The lung is an active organ involving respiratory muscles and changing volumes. The gill may be passive such as in the shark or active as in trout. This makes a considerable difference in the bioaccumulation of organic toxicants. The U.S. Environmental Protection Agency (EPA) developed Food and Gill Exchange of Toxic Substances (FGETS), which examines the kinetic exchange of nonpolar, nonmetabolized organic chemicals across fish gills and from contaminant food. In this program, the fish species, its growth rate, and the activity of the gill are extremely important factors in bioaccumulation of organic compounds. Fish growth is modeled by: $dW/dt = F \times E \times R \times SDA$, where F = g/day fish's feeding flux, E = g/day egestive fluxes, R = g/day respiratory fluxes, and SDA = fish's specific dynamic action. Note that the respiratory portion is just one consideration through the gill. The total body burden of B_f = µg chemical/fish is modeled as $dB_f/dt = S_g J_g + J_1 = S_g k_w (C_w - C_a) + J_1$, where S_g = total gill area in cm², J_g = the net diffusive flux across the gill in µg/cm²/day, J_1 = net mass exchange across the fish's intestine from food in µg/day, k_w = chemicals' mass conductance through the

interlamellar water of the gills in cm/day, C_w = chemical's environmental water concentration, and C_a = chemical's concentration in the fish's blood. So, as in the lung, the surface area for gas exchange/chemical exchange is important, and the rates of transfer of the chemical are based on concentration gradients based on Fick's first law of diffusion. The fish is visualized as a three-phase solvent composed of water, lipid, and structural organic matter with the chemical in rapid equilibrium between all three phases. The whole body concentration or $C_f = B_f/W = (P_1 + P_1 K_1 + P_S K_S) C_a$, where P_a = aqueous fraction of fish, P_1 = lipid fraction of fish, K_1 = lipid/water partition coefficient similar to K_{OW}, P_s = structural organic fraction of fish, K_S = lipid/structural organic matter partition similar to $K_{OC} = 0.4 K_{OW}$. The bioconcentration factor or $BCF = C_f/C_w = P_a + P_1 K_1 = P_S K_S$. Substituting into the body burden equation, the modelers derived $dB_f/dt = S_g k_w (C_w - C_f/BCF) + J_1 = S_g k_w (C_w - B_f[W\ BCF]) = J_1$. Inputs to the model are fish species and genus to insure proper modeling of gill morphological parameters (estimate net exchange rate of $S\ k_w$), chemical molecular weight, molar volume, melting point, log P (log K_{OW}), fish's initial live weight, fish's initial whole body concentration of the chemical, aqueous concentration of the chemical, and chemical concentration in the fish's prey. The program calculates for a species the S = total gill area in cm² = $s_1 W^s 2$ and ρ = # lamellae (mm gill filament) $- 1 = r_1 W^r 2$, where W = fish's live weight. Another factor that is an important input is the active gill parameter between 0.33 and 1.0. This corrects the difference between the anatomical surface area and the physiological area of the fish (Barber et al., 1988). The surface area of the intestine may favor the absorption of metals such as zinc (Sappal et al., 2009). Organic compounds usually associate with sediment and depending on the size of the particle may be taking in orally or via the branchial route. For fish, invertebrates, and even for zooplankton, the metabolic rate drives the ventilation rate or G_v in L/day. Then factoring in G_v with Fick's law of diffusion and the respiratory surface area, the uptake clearance constant or $k_1 = E_w \times G_v/W_B$, where E_w = gill chemical uptake efficiency

TABLE 17-2 Forensic Chart of Gill Toxicity	
Gill Toxicity	**Toxic Agents**
Acid–base balance	Heavy metals (Macey et al., 2010)
Agenesis (developmental abnormalities)	2,4-D (Aronzon et al., 2010)
CYP induction	10-nm silver nanoparticles (Scown et al., 2010), PCBs (Calò et al., 2009)
Enzyme inhibition	Arsenic (Chakraborty et al., 2010), chlorpyrifos-ethyl (Ghedira et al., 2009), acetaminophen, propanolol (Solé et al., 2010)
Epithelial hyperplasia	Diesel fuel, gasoline (Rodrigues et al., 2010)
Histopathological damage	Arsenic (Chakraborty et al., 2010), carbaryl (Bhavan and Geraldine, 2009), sodium hypochlorite (López-Galindo et al., 2010), nitrates, KCl (Romano and Zeng 2007)
Mitochondrial damage	Hg (Yamuna et al., 2009), PBDEs (Shao et al., 2010)
Oxidative stress	Ammonia (Ching et al., 2009), estrogen (Ahmad et al., 2009), TiO^2 (Hao et al., 2009), carbamazepine (Li et al., 2009)
Transporter induction	Ammonia, phloretin (Braun et al., 2009)

(a function of log P) and W_B = wet weight of the animal (Arnot and Gobas, 2004).

Now consider damage to the gill and its effects as described in **Table 17-2**. Similar to the lung, small particles are expected to have some toxic influence on the gill. Silver nanoparticles of 10-nm diameter (as compared with 35 nm and 600–1,600 nm particles) were most highly concentrated in rainbow trout (*Oncorhynchus mykiss*) gill. They did not cause lipid peroxidation at the concentrations tested. However, the 10-nm silver nanoparticles induced CYP1A2, indicating a possible induction of oxidative metabolism (Scown et al., 2010). Oxidative membrane damage by heavy metals Cu, Zn, and Cd correlates with perturbations in the acid-base balance in the Eastern oyster, *Crassostrea virginica* (Macey et al., 2010). Similarly, TiO_2, a nanoparticle associated with sunscreens, soaps, and a host of other products, causes significant decreases in oxidative protection (SOD, catalase, peroxidase) and increased lipid peroxidation in juvenile carp (*Cyprinus carpio*; Hao et al., 2009). A more toxic metal, sodium arsenite, inhibited acid phosphatase, alkaline phosphatase, glutamate oxaloacetate transaminase, glutamate pyruvate transaminase, and acetylcholinesterase based on time and concentration in the gill of the mollusc *Lamellidens marginalis*. Untoward

effects on immunity were likely indicated by NO depletion and reduced phenoloxidase activity. The conjugation enzyme glutathione-S-transferase was reduced, as was the antioxidant enzyme catalase. Histopathological damage was severe, compromising gas exchange, filter feeding, and immune protection (Chakraborty et al., 2010).

Mercury is a ubiquitous aquatic toxic metal. Due to its volatility, it is found in the atmosphere and then descends in rainwater. Mercury's high density makes it drop to bottom of lakes, rivers, and oceans into an anaerobic environment where microbial methylation yields hydrophobic methylmercury. However, even inorganic granules of Hg appear to damage the benthic aquatic organisms such as the prawn *Macrobrachium malcolmsonii*. Mitochondrial damage is noted in Hg-exposed prawn gills as well as crystalline granular inclusions (Yamuna et al., 2009). Manganese is neurotoxic to people and affects dopaminergic inhibition of lateral cilia movement in the gill of the bivalve mollusc, *Crassostrea virginica*, with no effect of the excitation to the cilia by serotonin, producing cilia paralysis (Martin et al., 2008).

Another likely contamination of aquatic species, such as the marine pejerrey *Odontesthes argentinensis* and especially sensitive developing larvae, arises from oil spills. Diesel fuel and unleaded gasoline caused epithelial hyperplasia of the gill and esophagus as well as liver damage in the larvae (hepatic sinusoid dilation, hepatocytomegaly, bi-nucleated and nuclear degeneration of hepatocytes; Rodrigues et al., 2010). A ubiquitous flame-retardant class of compounds, polybrominated diphenyl ethers, is found in fish, other wildlife, and also in humans. Rainbow trout gill cells (RTgill-W1 cells) exposed to µM concentrations of 2,2′,4,4′-tetrabromodiphenyl ether caused a loss of cell viability and a disruption of redox status as indicated by less NAD(P)H autofluorescence during flow cytometry. Additionally, mitochondrial membrane lipid peroxidation was detected by reduced nonyl acridine orange fluorescence. Apoptosis was found through altered cellular forward-angle light scatter (change in cell size) and side light scatter properties (alterations in internal cellular complexity) and sub-G1 DNA content (Shao et al., 2010). The antifouling compound sodium hypochlorite (chlorine bleach) released from power plants affects juvenile *Solea senegalensis*, causing gill pathologies (hypertrophy, lamellar fusion, increase in goblet cell number and size) at nonlethal concentrations (López-Galindo et al., 2010). Induction of CYP1A is also still caused by aromatic hydrocarbons such as PAHs from car exhausts or PCBs from transformers (Calò et al., 2009). Agricultural runoff also affects aquatic species. Pesticides such as the acetylcholinesterase (AChE)-inhibiting insecticide carbaryl exhibit rupture of the basal laminae, abnormal infiltration of hematocytes in hemocoelic space of the gill lamellae and in interstitial spaces of the hepatopancreas, fused gill lamellae, and necrosis-like histopathology of the gill lamellae and the tubules of the hepatopancreas in juvenile prawns (Bhavan and Geraldine, 2009). Chlorpyrifos-ethyl similarly inhibits AChE and at higher concentrations butyrylcholinesterase as well in the gills and hepatopancreas of the Mediterranean crab, *Carcinus maenas* (Ghedira et al., 2009). Ammonia and urea fertilizer run off from farm fields and are very water soluble. The teleost zebrafish (*Dania rerio*) have the most concentrated transport of ammonia (Rh proteins) and urea (UT proteins) transporters in their gills. The UT proteins have diffuse expression with $3Na^+,2K^+$-ATPase-type mitochondrion-rich cells. The pillar cells surrounding the blood spaces of the lamellae express Rhag, while the outer layer of the lamellae and the filament express Rhbg. High external ammonia or phloretin (phenolic ketone inhibitor of monosaccharide and anion transport) increased ammonia and urea tissue concentrations in adult and juvenile zebrafish, respectively (age-dependent). Ammonia increased Rh mRNA expression in embryo and larvae gills but not adults. Phloretin induced UT mRNA expression similarly, only in the developing gill tissue. Both the adult and developing zebrafish respond to high ammonia by inducing UT mRNA expression, while phloretin induced Rh mRNA expression. This indicates that the transport of ammonia and urea excretion (nitrogenous waste products) is tightly linked—at least in this fish species (Braun et al., 2009). Nonlethal ammonia concentrations also induce a transient oxidative stress in the gills and brain of the mudskipper (*Boleophthalmus boddarti*) as quantified by lipid peroxidation products and decreased GSH, glutathione peroxidase activity, glutathione reductase activity, and catalase activity (Ching et al., 2009). Nitrates and potassium are other nutrients (found in fertilizers) that can affect the gill. $NaNO_3$, KNO_3, and KCl induced lamellar swelling, epithelial thickening, pillar cell disruption, necrosis, and distortion to juvenile blue swimmer crab (*Portunus pelagicus* Linnaeus) gills (Romano and Zeng, 2007). An emerging class (due to heightened awareness) of aquatic pollutants arises from the use of medications and personal care products. The analgesic acetaminophen inhibits AChE in the gill and increases liver lipid peroxidation, while the beta-blocker propanolol increases gill glutathione-S-transferase activity (Solé et al., 2010). Hormones in the water, especially estrogenic compounds, are of grave concern for liver and kidney toxicity and proper reproductive function. The gill responds to 17β-estradiol in water with an increase in catalase in the juvenile sea bass (*Dicentrarchus labrax* L.), while IP injection decreases antioxidant enzymatic activities (catalase, glutathione peroxidase, glutathione reductase, glutathione-S-transferase; Ahmad et al., 2009). The anticonvulsant carbamazepine leads to oxidative stress in the gill of the rainbow trout (inhibited SOD, catalase, glutathione reductase, glutathione peroxidase, and $3Na^+$, $2K^+$-ATPase, reduced GSH concentration; Li et al., 2009).

Development of the gill must also be considered similar to the developing lung. For example, a widely employed herbicide, 2,4-dichlorophenoxyacetic acid (2,4-D), causes agenesis (abnormal development) of gills along with other developmental toxicity in the South American toad (*Rhinella arenarum*; Aronzon et al., 2010).

Lung Toxicity Tests

The tests of inhaled gases, aerosols, vapors, and fibers/particles usually involve a rodent model. However, humans do not have a furry coat to trap air contaminants. Humans live much longer than rodents and have symmetrical branching of the bronchioles and respiratory bronchioles. This requires testing in larger mammals with a similar body mass. Dose metrics are important factors in the deposition of material in various portions of the respiratory tract. Particles behave differently based on their aerodynamic diameter and mass. This is especially true for rapidly dissolving substances. For easily diffusible particles with a mass median aerodynamic diameter < 0.3 µm, the physical diameter is used for modeling rather than the aerodynamic diameter. Otherwise, physical properties such as particle area and particle count play a larger role. Metal nanoparticles greatly increase the surface area for oxidative reactions. For example, a metal coin may have a surface area in cm^2, while a similar mass of nanoparticles would have a surface area in acres. The toxicity is clearly different for these examples. Deposition of particles occurs by a variety of physical interactions such as gravitational sedimentation, inertial impaction, Brownian diffusion, simple interception for long fibers and large particles, electrostatic forces, thermal phoresis/Ludwig-Soret effect (usually applies to aerosols), vapor pressure, interaction with an applied magnetic field, and Raleigh-Taylor gas effects (instability of an interface between two fluids when one fluid is accelerating into the other, such as oil–water interface). Fluid dynamics of the tract must also

TABLE 17-3 Lung Toxicity Tests	
Testing For	**Individual Assays**
Lethality, reproductive toxicity, developmental toxicity, motor effects, metabolism, toxicokinetics, cancer	Rodent models — varied concentrations with timed exposures (conc × time = dose)
Confirmatory tests	Dogs, nonhuman primates tested using varied concentrations and timed exposures.
Specialized animal models	Cattle, cats, ferrets, goats, guinea pigs, hamsters, horses, pigs, rabbits, sheep as specialized model systems (Phalen et al., 2008)
Intratracheal and intrabronchial instillation	Particles are dissolved or suspended in small volume of water and administered under anesthesia with a catheter into a restrained animal (rodent). Accounting for toxicity of the invasive procedure and the vehicle are important factors. One lung may be exposed leaving the other as a control, or both lungs may be exposed having sham- and vehicle-exposed control animals instead (Driscoll et al., 2000).
Alternative/cellular	Cultured human airway epithelial cells are exposed to atmospheres of toxicants via air/liquid interactions at body temperature (37°C) and 90–100% relative humidity with the cells supplied nutrients on porous membranes leaving apical/superficial surfaces for toxicant damage/absorption (Aufderheide et al., 2003).

be properly modeled such as by using the Navier-Stokes equations (nonlinear partial differential equations yielding a velocity field = velocity of a fluid at a given point in space and time). Clearance of the particles must then be calculated as well. As shown in **Table 17-3**, the exposure of rodents, more complicated mammalian species, or specialized animal models is done as a concentration and time of exposure scenario for the most basic data necessary for toxicological evaluation (Phalen et al., 2008). However, some compounds are too precious to waste or too toxic to test in this manner. Additionally, the dense hair coat on a rodent may serve to lower the toxicity to a small concentration of a particle due to adsorption or physical trapping or cause toxicity to the tester when the animal is examined. Thus, intratracheal or intrabronchial instillation may be a favored approach. The dose is clear, as are the portions of lung affected. The dose–response can also help the researcher define a more appropriate concentration range and time of exposure for more standard inhalation studies. Instillation also limits the toxicity to the tester. One lobe of the lung may also be exposed, leaving the other lung as a control as well. Long fibers or highly water-soluble compounds that may be caught earlier in the respiratory tract of an obligate nose-breathing rodent, but not in a human breathing through the mouth, may also reach the lung of the model animal in this manner. Instillation is performed using a catheter with the material suspended or dissolved in water if possible and given under anesthesia. Unfortunately, bypassing the upper respiratory tract may leave potential target tissues unexposed. Also, the invasive nature of the procedure and danger of inflammation due to the vehicle is ever present. Additionally, the high dose does not necessarily represent well the human chronic exposure situation (Driscoll et al., 2000), and critical evaluations indicate that intratracheal repetitive administration of 19 granular dusts ("19-dust-studies") is not a good human exposure model of cancer risk. The dose given is an overload for the lung, as it represents a lifetime of human exposure. The rodent response to this high dose is unique to the species employed (rat). Low-dose studies are not utilized over longer time periods. The cancer developed in

the high-dose rat studies results from a different/inflammatory mechanism rather than a particle-specific toxicity. The high percentage of rats that develop cancer (~50%) is not representative of the cancer incidence of miners breathing lower doses of similar particles over a lifetime of working in dust-laden and diesel fume–filled environments (Valberg et al., 2009). Despite the pitfalls of the instillation approach, useful data regarding residence time in the lung and transit time to the mesothelium come from intrabronchial instillation of asbestos fibers. Small chrysotile B asbestos and benzo[a]pyrene were administered by polyvinyl catheter into the right lower lobe of the lung of anesthetized 6-week-old Wistar rats. Pulmonary carcinomas and malignant pleural mesotheliomas developed 12–31 months after application. This is interesting, because 12 months was the earliest time point that small asbestos fragments were detected in the pleural epithelium. Benzo[a]pyrene does not increase the tumor incidence, but does make them appear earlier (4.5 months for adenocarcinomas of the lung and 7.7 months for pleural mesotheliomas; Fasske, 1988).

Alternative approaches using human respiratory tract epithelial cell cultures at body temperature (37°C) and 90–100% relative humidity and nutrients supplied through porous membranes have been described (Aufderheide et al., 2003). The European Union requires alternative testing under the Registration, Evaluation, Authorisation and Restriction of Chemicals (REACH). However, there is no standard accepted procedure for *in vitro* testing of airborne toxicants. Cell type, dose, and fundamental study procedures have yet to be established and represent true obstacles to alternative testing. Also, a single system does not currently appear to test all parameters of an intact animal inhalation toxicity test (Costa, 2008).

Gill Toxicity Tests

The fish offers more stumbling blocks for assessing toxicity to the gill and bioaccumulation of toxic substances. This is especially problematic for Canadian and European scientific communities that are required to assess bioaccumulation

TABLE 17-4	Gill Toxicity Tests
Testing For	**Individual Assays**
Whole fish assays	Histological damage and metabolism studies
Isolated gill or gill cells	Histological damage, metabolism, and uptake studies in pavement and mitochondria-rich cells
Fish embryos ("*in vitro*" European alternative)	Histological damage, developmental and organ toxicity, and metabolism/bioaccumulation studies (Weisbrod et al., 2009)

in fish. Fish biotransform toxicants via mono-oxygenation reactions (CYPs) at much slower rates than mammals. This is especially true for the herbicide atrazine, which has a clearance value of 3.81 ± 1.96 mL/h in 10^6 rat hepatocytes but only at high cellular concentrations reports a lethargic 0.002 mL/h in 10^6 trout hepatocytes. The chemical uptake by the gill versus the intestine provides additional complications based on the chemical's hydrophobicity and where the fish resides (benthic vs. pelagic). There is not a standard fish cell line similar to the human CaCo-2 line to determine toxicant uptake. The gill itself may represent a significant extrahepatic metabolic site, such as the presystemic branchial metabolism of the ubiquitous plasticizer di-2-ethylhexyl phthalate, limiting its bioaccumulation in fish (Barron et al., 1989). The isolated gill or perfused intestinal preparation has found some usefulness in assessing fish uptake and branchial metabolism that may cause toxicity or limit uptake. Fish embryos are considered *in vitro* systems in Europe and have been useful alternatives to acute adult fish toxicity testing. Culture gill cells (pavement cells and mitochondria-rich cells) have been used to assess toxicant metabolism and cell damage (Weisbrod et al., 2009). Gill assessments occur via whole fish assays, isolated gill or gill cells, and fish embryos, as displayed in **Table 17-4**.

Microcosm for Environmental Toxicology

The lung is a dispersion model for various aerodynamic particles, aerosols, vapors, and gases. The wind speed is the velocity of the air in various parts of the respiratory tract. Target cells and deposition on, adsorption on, or absorption into those cells represents in small the various organisms in an air pollution model. The most sensitive of those cells may model the biomarker organism for monitoring the earliest effects. The air–liquid interactions in the lung are akin to the air–rain (humidity in the lung) or air–water interactions.

The gill is a good model for bioaccumulation of toxicants up a food web from water pollution. Active and passive mechanisms must be considered along with behavior of the organism in the water column. Taken together, this is a good time to think about the interaction among cellular models, animal models, and ecological models. After all, what is gained or lost by using a reductionist approach favored by research scientists to investigate the ultimate molecular mechanism(s) for a toxic action? When do models fail in the other direction to address true population or ecological impacts? What other information is needed to develop a better model of realistic exposure scenarios and impacts? Just the differences in how various mammalian respiratory tracts differ and the resultant toxicity of a given chemical or fiber give cause to reexamine assumptions that field testing or animal testing is too expensive or inhumane. Predictive accuracy is important, because unexpected result occasionally occur. Such is the case for endometriosis in a primate study looking for reproductive toxicity of 2,3,7,8-TCDD (Rier et al., 1993). Because dioxins are part of air pollutants from diesel fuel, were former models capable of predicting this toxicity? Most likely, the models were not, because it was not known to look at endometriosis as a toxic endpoint. It is necessary to be careful when describing the parameters and assumptions of the models used. It is important to know what a model can detect and those things it will miss or cannot predict based on the test systems used.

Questions

1. Why are the lung and the gill different in determining toxicity from exposure when compared to the GI tract dose–response paradigm?
2. Why is a beagle dog a better respiratory model than a rodent?
3. What common toxicant causes cancer of the nose tract entry, and how does it accomplish this action?
4. What is the difference in toxicity between chronically smoking filtered cigarettes versus smoking unfiltered cannabis or cigarettes?
5. What size, shape, and thickness does asbestos have to be to cause mesothelioma, and what are the mechanisms involved?
6. The Chinese population of 2013 is being exposed to very high levels of air pollutants that may ultimately affect lung cancer incidence. Is ozone or peroxyacyl nitrate more responsible for changes in current breathing volumes of exposed individuals?
7. Why is Paraquat always a lung toxicant by any route of administration?
8. What effect might an oil spill, such as the one that occurred in the Gulf of Mexico in 2010, have on gill function?
9. Why might the zebrafish be a sensitive marker for exposure to agricultural fertilizer?
10. Explain why lung tissue is insufficient to test all of respiratory toxicity. Give examples.
11. Why is bioaccumulation a major concern in fish studies of gill toxicity?

References

Ahmad I, Maria VL, Pacheco M, Santos MA. 2009. Juvenile sea bass (*Dicentrarchus labrax* L.) enzymatic and non-enzymatic antioxidant responses following 17beta-estradiol exposure. *Ecotoxicology*. 18:974–982.

Amshel CE, Fealk MH, Phillips BJ, Caruso DM. 2000. Anhydrous ammonia burns case report and review of the literature. *Burns*. 26:493–497.

Anttila S, Karjalainen A, Taikina-aho O, Kyyrönen P, Vainio H. 1993. Lung cancer in the lower lobe is associated with pulmonary asbestos fiber count and fiber size. *Environ Health Perspect*. 101:166–170.

Arnot JA, Gobas FA. 2004. A food web bioaccumulation model for organic chemicals in aquatic ecosystems. *Environ Toxicol Chem*. 23:2343–2355.

Aronzon CM, Sandoval MT, Herkovits J, Pérez-Coll CS. 2010. Stage-dependent toxicity of 2,4-dichlorophenoxyacetic on the embryonic development of a South American toad, *Rhinella arenarum*. *Environ Toxicol*. 26:373–381.

Aufderheide M, Knebel JW, Ritter D. 2003. Novel approaches for studying pulmonary toxicity in vitro. *Toxicol Lett*. 140–141:205–211.

Barber MC, Suarez LA, Lassiter RR. 1988. Project summary. FGETS (food and gill exchange of toxic substances): a simulation model for bioaccumulation of nonpolar organic pollutants by fish. Washington, DC: U.S. Environmental Protection Agency. EPA'/600/S3-87/038.

Baron-Hay S, Clifford A, Jackson M, Clarke S. 1999. Life threatening laryngeal toxicity following treatment with combined chemoradiotherapy for nasopharyngeal cancer: a case report with review of the literature. *Ann Oncol*. 10:1109–1112.

Barron MG, Schultz IR, Hayton WL. 1989. Presystemic branchial metabolism limits di-2-ethylhexyl phthalate accumulation in fish. *Toxicol Appl Pharmacol*. 98:49–57.

Beveridge R, Pintos J, Parent ME, Asselin J, Siemiatycki J. 2010. Lung cancer risk associated with occupational exposure to nickel, chromium VI, and cadmium in two population-based case-control studies in Montreal. *Am J Ind Med*. 53:476–485.

Bhavan PS, Geraldine P. 2009. Manifestation of carbaryl toxicity on soluble protein and histopathology in the hepatopancreas and gills of the prawn, *Macrobrachium malcolmsonii*. *J Environ Biol*. 30:533–538.

Bonner JC. 2010. Nanoparticles as a potential cause of pleural and interstitial lung disease. *Proc Am Thorac Soc*. 7:138–141.

Braun MH, Steele SL, Perry SF. 2009. The responses of zebrafish (*Danio rerio*) to high external ammonia and urea transporter inhibition: nitrogen excretion and expression of rhesus glycoproteins and urea transporter proteins. *J Exp Biol*. 212:3846–3856.

Brown HR. 1990. Neoplastic and potentially preneoplastic changes in the upper respiratory tract of rats and mice. *Environ Health Perspect*. 85:291–304.

Brusis T, Michel O, Schmidt W, Metternich FU. 2007. [Chance or causality: problems recognizing laryngeal carcinoma as a result of occupational exposition to noxious substances of blue collar worker employed in the rubber industry]. *Laryngorhinootologie*. 86:714–722.

Calò M, Bitto A, Lo Cascio P, Polito F, Lauriano ER, Minutoli L, Altavilla D, Squadrito F. 2009. Cytochrome P450 (CYP1A) induction in sea bream (*Sparus aurata*) gills and liver following exposure to polychlorobiphenyls (PCBs). *Vet Res Commun.* 33(Suppl 1):181-184.

Carriot F, Sasco AJ. 2000. [Cannabis and cancer]. *Rev Epidemiol Sante Publique.* 48:473-483.

Cepkova M, Matthay MA. 2006. Pharmacotherapy of acute lung injury and the acute respiratory distress syndrome. *J Intensive Care Med.* 21:119-143.

Chakraborty S, Ray M, Ray S. 2010. Toxicity of sodium arsenite in the gill of an economically important mollusc of India. *Fish Shellfish Immunol.* 29:136-148.

Chen WJ, Monnat RJ Jr, Chen M, Mottet NK. 1978. Aluminum induced pulmonary granulomatosis. *Hum Pathol.* 9:705-711.

Chiappino G. 2005. [Mesothelioma: the aetiological role of ultrathin fibres and repercussions on prevention and medical legal evaluation]. *Med Lav.* 96:3-23.

Ching B, Chew SF, Wong WP, Ip YK. 2009. Environmental ammonia exposure induces oxidative stress in gills and brain of *Boleophthalmus boddarti* (mudskipper). *Aquat Toxicol.* 95:203-212.

Churg A, Brauer M. 2000. Ambient atmospheric particles in the airways of human lungs. *Ultrastruct Pathol.* 24:353-361.

Cohen RA, Patel A, Green FH. 2008. Lung disease caused by exposure to coal mine and silica dust. *Semin Respir Crit Care Med.* 29:651-661.

Collins MA. 2002. Toxicology of toluene diisocyanate. *Appl Occup Environ Hyg.* 17:846-855.

Costa DL. 2008. Alternative test methods in inhalation toxicology: challenges and opportunities. *Exp Toxicol Pathol.* 60:105-109.

Davey A, Moppett IK. 2004. Postoperative complications after CS spray exposure. *Anaesthesia.* 59:1219-1220.

Dinis-Oliveira RJ, Duarte JA, Sánchez-Navarro A, Remião F, Bastos ML, Carvalho F. 2008. Paraquat poisonings: mechanisms of lung toxicity, clinical features, and treatment. *Crit Rev Toxicol.* 38:13-71.

de la Hoz RE, Christie J, Teamer JA, Bienenfeld LA, Afilaka AA, Crane M, Levin SM, Herbert R. 2008. Reflux symptoms and disorders and pulmonary disease in former World Trade Center rescue and recovery workers and volunteers. *J Occup Environ Med.* 50:1351-1354. [Erratum in: 2009. *J Occup Environ Med.* 51:509.]

Drechsler-Parks DM, Bedi JF, Horvath SM. 1984. Interaction of peroxyacetyl nitrate and ozone on pulmonary functions. *Am Rev Respir Dis.* 130:1033-1037.

Driscoll KE, Costa DL, Hatch G, Henderson R, Oberdorster G, Salem H, Schlesinger RB. 2000. Intratracheal instillation as an exposure technique for the evaluation of respiratory tract toxicity: uses and limitations. *Toxicol Sci.* 55:24-35.

Elliot J, Vullermin P, Robinson P. 1998. Maternal cigarette smoking is associated with increased inner airway wall thickness in children who die from sudden infant death syndrome. *Am J Respir Crit Care Med.* 158:802-806.

Fasske E. 1988. Experimental lung tumors following specific intrabronchial application of chrysotile asbestos. Longitudinal light and electron microscopic investigations in rats. *Respiration.* 53:111-127.

Forti E, Bulgheroni A, Cetin Y, Hartung T, Jennings P, Pfaller W, Prieto P. 2010. Characterisation of cadmium chloride induced molecular and functional alterations in airway epithelial cells. *Cell Physiol Biochem.* 25:159-168.

Ghedira J, Jebali J, Bouraoui Z, Banni M, Chouba L, Boussetta H. 2009. Acute effects of chlorpyriphos-ethyl and secondary treated effluents on acetylcholinesterase and butyrylcholinesterase activities in *Carcinus maenas.* *J Environ Sci (China).* 21:1467-1472.

Hahn HL, Kleinschrot D, Hansen D. 1992. Nicotine increases ciliary beat frequency by a direct effect on respiratory cilia. *Clin Investig.* 70:244-251.

Hao L, Wang Z, Xing B. 2009. Effect of sub-acute exposure to TiO_2 nanoparticles on oxidative stress and histopathological changes in Juvenile Carp (*Cyprinus carpio*). *J Environ Sci (China).* 21:1459-1466.

Harkema JR, Carey SA, Wagner JG. 2006. The nose revisited: a brief review of the comparative structure, function, and toxicologic pathology of the nasal epithelium. *Toxicol Pathol.* 34:252-269.

Hecht SS. 2008. Progress and challenges in selected areas of tobacco carcinogenesis. *Chem Res Toxicol.* 21:160-171.

Heintz NH, Janssen-Heininger YM, Mossman BT. 2010. Asbestos, lung cancers, and mesotheliomas: from molecular approaches to targeting tumor survival pathways. *Am J Respir Cell Mol Biol.* 42:133-139.

Just J, Nisakinovic L, Laoudi Y, Grimfeld A. 2006. [Air pollution and asthma in children]. *Arch Pediatr.* 13:1055-1060.

Kilburn KH, Warshaw RH. 1990. Abnormal pulmonary function associated with diaphragmatic pleural plaques due to exposure to asbestos. *Br J Ind Med.* 47:611-614.

King LS, Agre P. 2001. Man is not a rodent: aquaporins in the airways. *Am J Respir Cell Mol Biol.* 24:221-223.

Kovacic P, Somanathan R. 2009. Pulmonary toxicity and environmental contamination: radicals, electron transfer, and protection by antioxidants. *Rev Environ Contam Toxicol*. 201:41-69.

Laursen BE, Stankevicius E, Pilegaard H, Mulvany M, Simonsen U. 2006. Potential protective properties of a stable, slow-releasing nitric oxide donor, GEA 3175, in the lung. *Cardiovasc Drug Rev*. 24:247-260.

Lee KP, Ulrich CE, Geil RG, Trochimowicz HJ. 1989. Inhalation toxicity of chromium dioxide dust to rats after two years exposure. *Sci Total Environ*. 86:83-108.

Li ZH, Zlabek V, Velisek J, Grabic R, Machova J, Randak T. 2009. Responses of antioxidant status and Na$^+$-K$^+$-ATPase activity in gill of rainbow trout, *Oncorhynchus mykiss*, chronically treated with carbamazepine. *Chemosphere*. 77:1476-1481.

Lin CY, Wheelock AM, Morin D, Baldwin RM, Lee MG, Taff A, Plopper C, Buckpitt A, Rohde A. 2009. Toxicity and metabolism of methylnaphthalenes: comparison with naphthalene and 1-nitronaphthalene. *Toxicology*. 260:16-27.

López-Galindo C, Vargas-Chacoff L, Nebot E, Casanueva JF, Rubio D, Solé M, Mancera JM. 2010. Biomarker responses in *Solea senegalensis* exposed to sodium hypochlorite used as antifouling. *Chemosphere*. 78:885-893.

Luo J, Ye W, Zendehdel K, Adami J, Adami HO, Boffetta P, Nyrén O. 2007. Oral use of Swedish moist snuff (snus) and risk for cancer of the mouth, lung, and pancreas in male construction workers: a retrospective cohort study. *Lancet*. 369:2015-2020.

Macey BM, Jenny MJ, Williams HR, Thibodeaux LK, Beal M, Almeida JS, Cunningham C, Mancia A, Warr GW, Burge EJ, Holland AF, Gross PS, Hikima S, Burnett KG, Burnett L, Chapman RW. 2010. Modelling interactions of acid-base balance and respiratory status in the toxicity of metal mixtures in the American oyster *Crassostrea virginica*. *Comp Biochem Physiol A Mol Integr Physiol*. 155:341-349.

Martin K, Huggins T, King C, Carroll MA, Catapane EJ. 2008. The neurotoxic effects of manganese on the dopaminergic innervation of the gill of the bivalve mollusc, *Crassostrea virginica*. *Comp Biochem Physiol C Toxicol Pharmacol*. 148:152-159.

McCunney RJ, Morfeld P, Payne S. 2009. What component of coal causes coal workers' pneumoconiosis? *J Occup Environ Med*. 51:462-471.

Mirer F. 2003. Updated epidemiology of workers exposed to metalworking fluids provides sufficient evidence for carcinogenicity. *Appl Occup Environ Hyg*. 18:902-912.

Mustafa MG. 1990. Biochemical basis of ozone toxicity. *Free Radic Biol Med*. 9:245-265.

O'Brien JM. 2009. Airflow, lung volumes, and flow-volume loop. http://www.mymerck.com/mmpe/sec05/ch046/ch046b.html

Pettersson B, Curvall M, Enzell C. 1985. The inhibitory effect of tobacco smoke compound on ciliary activity. *Eur J Respir Dis Suppl*. 139:89-92.

Pfeifer GP, Denissenko MF, Olivier M, Tretyakova N, Hecht SS, Hainaut P. 2002. Tobacco smoke carcinogens, DNA damage and p53 mutations in smoking-associated cancers. *Oncogene*. 21:7435-7351.

Phalen RF, Oldham MJ, Wolff RK. 2008. The relevance of animal models for aerosol studies. *J Aerosol Med Pulm Drug Deliv*. 21:113-124.

Plopper CG, Buckpitt A, Evans M, Van Winkle L, Fanucchi M, Smiley-Jewell S, Lakritz J, West J, Lawson G, Paige R, Miller L, Hyde D. 2001. Factors modulating the epithelial response to toxicants in tracheobronchial airways. *Toxicology*. 160:173-180.

Poetsch M, Czerwinski M, Wingenfeld L, Vennemann M, Bajanowski T. 2010. A common FMO3 polymorphism may amplify the effect of nicotine exposure in sudden infant death syndrome (SIDS). *Int J Legal Med*. 124:301-306.

Pool-Zobel BL, Klein RG, Liegibel UM, Kuchenmeister F, Weber S, Schmezer P. 1992. Systemic genotoxic effects of tobacco-related nitrosamines following oral and inhalational administration to Sprague-Dawley rats. *Clin Investig*. 70:299-306.

Pöschl G, Seitz HK. 2004. Alcohol and cancer. *Alcohol Alcohol*. 39: 155-165.

Rier SE, Martin DC, Bowman RE, Dmowski WP, Becker JL. 1993 Endometriosis in rhesus monkeys (*Macaca mulatta*) following chronic exposure to 2,3,7,8-tetrachlorodibenzo-p-dioxin. *Fundam Appl Toxicol*. 21(4):433-441.

Roberts ES, Thomas RS, Dorman DC. 2008. Gene expression changes following acute hydrogen sulfide (H$_2$S)-induced nasal respiratory epithelial injury. *Toxicol Pathol*. 36:560-567.

Rodrigues RV, Miranda-Filho KC, Gusmão EP, Moreira CB, Romano LA, Sampaio LA. 2010. Deleterious effects of water-soluble fraction of petroleum, diesel and gasoline on marine pejerrey *Odontesthes argentinensis* larvae. *Sci Total Environ*. 408:2054-2059.

Romano N, Zeng C. 2007. Acute toxicity of sodium nitrate, potassium nitrate, and potassium chloride and their effects on the hemolymph composition and gill structure of early juvenile blue swimmer crabs (*Portunus pelagicus* Linnaeus, 1758) (Decapoda, Brachyura, Portunidae). *Environ Toxicol Chem*. 26:1955-1962.

Rüegger M. 1995. [Lung disorders due to metals]. *Schweiz Med Wochenschr*. 125:467-474.

Schenker MB, Pinkerton KE, Mitchell D, Vallyathan V, Elvine-Kreis B, Green FH. 2009. Pneumoconiosis from agricultural dust exposure among young California farmworkers. *Environ Health Perspect.* 117:988–994.

Sappal R, Burka J, Dawson S, Kamunde C. 2009. Bioaccumulation and subcellular partitioning of zinc in rainbow trout (*Oncorhynchus mykiss*): crosstalk between waterborne and dietary uptake. *Aquat Toxicol.* 91:281–290.

Sciuto AM, Hurt HH. 2004. Therapeutic treatments of phosgene-induced lung injury. *Inhal Toxicol.* 16:565–580.

Scown TM, Santos EM, Johnston BD, Gaiser B, Baalousha M, Mitov S, Lead JR, Stone V, Fernandes TF, Jepson M, van Aerle R, Tyler CR. 2010. Effects of aqueous exposure to silver nanoparticles of different sizes in rainbow trout. *Toxicol Sci.* 115:521–534.

Shao J, Dabrowski MJ, White CC, Kavanagh TJ, Gallagher EP. 2010. Flow cytometric analysis of BDE 47 mediated injury to rainbow trout gill epithelial cells. *Aquat Toxicol.* 97:42–50.

Solé M, Shaw JP, Frickers PE, Readman JW, Hutchinson TH. 2010. Effects on feeding rate and biomarker responses of marine mussels experimentally exposed to propranolol and acetaminophen. *Anal Bioanal Chem.* 396:649–656.

Stayner L, Kuempel E, Gilbert S, Hein M, Dement J. 2008. An epidemiological study of the role of chrysotile asbestos fibre dimensions in determining respiratory disease risk in exposed workers. An epidemiological study of the role of chrysotile asbestos fibre dimensions in determining respiratory disease risk in exposed workers. *Occup Environ Med.* 65:613–619.

Szyfter K, Banaszewski J, Jałoszyński P, Pabiszczak M, Szyfter W, Szmeja Z. 1999. Carcinogen: DNA adducts in tobacco smoke-associated cancer of the upper respiratory tract. *Acta Biochim Pol.* 46:275–287.

Takenaka S, Heini A, Ritter B, Heyder J. 1998. The respiratory bronchiole of beagle dogs: structural characteristics. *Toxicol Lett.* 96–97:301–308.

Valberg PA, Bruch J, McCunney RJ. 2009. Are rat results from intratracheal instillation of 19 granular dusts a reliable basis for predicting cancer risk? *Regul Toxicol Pharmacol.* 54:72–83.

Vallyathan V, Hahn LH. 1985. Cigarette smoking and inorganic dust in human lungs. *Arch Environ Health.* 40:69–73.

Vojtova J, Kamanova J, Sebo P. 2006. Bordetella adenylate cyclase toxin: a swift saboteur of host defense. *Curr Opin Microbiol.* 9:69–75.

Walker VE, Walker DM, Meng Q, McDonald JD, Scott BR, Seilkop SK, Claffey DJ, Upton PB, Powley MW, Swenberg JA, Henderson RF; Health Review Committee. 2009. Genotoxicity of 1,3-butadiene and its epoxy intermediates. *Res Rep Health Eff Inst.* (144):3–79.

Walters DK, Luke WH. 2011. Computational fluid dynamics simulations of particle deposition in large-scale, multigenerational lung models. *J Biomech Eng.* 133:011003.

Wan M-P, Wu C-L, Sze To G-N, Chan T-C, Chao T-C. 2011. Ultrafine particles, and $PM_{2.5}$ generated from cooking in homes. *Atmos Environ.* 45:6141–6148.

Warheit DB. 1989. Interspecies comparisons of lung responses to inhaled particles and gases. *Crit Rev Toxicol.* 20:1–29.

Weisbrod AV, Sahi J, Segner H, James MO, Nichols J, Schultz I, Erhardt S, Cowan-Ellsberry C, Bonnell M, Hoeger B. 2009. The state of in vitro science for use in bioaccumulation assessments for fish. *Environ Toxicol Chem.* 28:86–96.

Winder C. 2001. The toxicology of chlorine. *Environ Res.* 85:105–214.

Wyatt I, Doss AW, Zavala DC, Smith LL. 1981. Intrabronchial instillation of paraquat in rats: lung morphology and retention study. *Br J Ind Med.* 38:42–48.

Yamuna A, Bhavan PS, Geraldine P. 2009. Ultrastructural observations in gills and hepatopancreas of prawn *Macrobrachium malcolmsonii* exposed to mercury. *J Environ Biol.* 30:693–699.

Yike I, Rand T, Dearborn DG. 2007. The role of fungal proteinases in pathophysiology of *Stachybotrys chartarum*. *Mycopathologia.* 164:171–281.

CHAPTER 18

The Cardiovascular System as Conduit for a Dose Becoming a Dosage: Exposure and Toxicities

This is a chapter outline intended to guide and familiarize you with the content to follow.

I. The cardiovascular system

  A. Blood circulation

    1. Blood as a diagnostic tool—see Table 18-1

      a. Anemias—reduced and/or dysfunctional hemoglobin (Hb)

        (1) Iron deficiency or metals that interfere with Fe uptake into heme (Al, Cd, $Ga[NO_3]_3$, Zn, or $Na_2Cr_2O_7 \cdot 2H_2O$ in rodents and gossypol = microcytic hypochromic)

        (2) Pb poisoning and Cu deficiency = sideroblastic anemia (nucleated RBCs + Fe granules in perinuclear mitochondria)

        (3) Vitamin B_{12} or folic acid deficiency or chronic ethanol's effects on erythropoiesis = megaloblastic anemia

        (4) Nitro-derivatives or aromatic or aliphatic compounds, carcinogenic dyes, alloxan, saponins, surfactants, metformin (autoimmune antibodies) in many species, and organosulfoxides from onions for dogs = hemolytic (toxic) anemia and Heinz body formation (Hb damage from oxidation or mutation → small, round inclusions in RBC)

        (5) NO_2/NO_3 from fertilizer runoff, hydroxylamine metabolite of dapsone = metHb; chronic metHb occurs from metHb reductase deficiency (RBC soluble = Type I; RBC soluble + membrane-bound = Type II)

        (6) Coumadin, aspirin, hemorrhagic disease toxins or venoms (anticoagulants), streptokinase (clot dissolution) → hemorrhage

        (7) Benzene benzoquinone formation, radiation → bone marrow damage → aplastic anemia/pancytopenia (other less familiar mostly chemotherapy agents are busulfan, chloramphenicol, paclitaxel, methotrexate, azathioprine, albendazole)

      b. Hemoglobin mutations + DNA adducts—test for exposure to compounds such as acrylamide, aflatoxin B1, agaritine, aristolochic acid, pyrrolizidines, safrole → metHb formation more likely when certain amino acids are altered and stability of globin protein in oxyHb form at risk

      c. H_2S + other toxic sulfur-containing gases, medications, paints = sulfhemoglobin, which lasts the lifetime of the RBC (~21 days in human)

      d. Carboxyhemoglobin—CO binds 245 × stronger than O_2 to Hb → red but hypoxic organs especially the CNS (MRI results = diffuse bifrontal white matter T2 hyperintensities as well as partial necrosis of the right globus pallidus), heart and pulmonary effects. Glutamate, neutrophil activation, peroxynitrite formation, and reduced oxygen species may mediate CO's effects. Low CO levels are seen by cyt c binding rather than COHb

CONCEPTUALIZING TOXICOLOGY 18-1

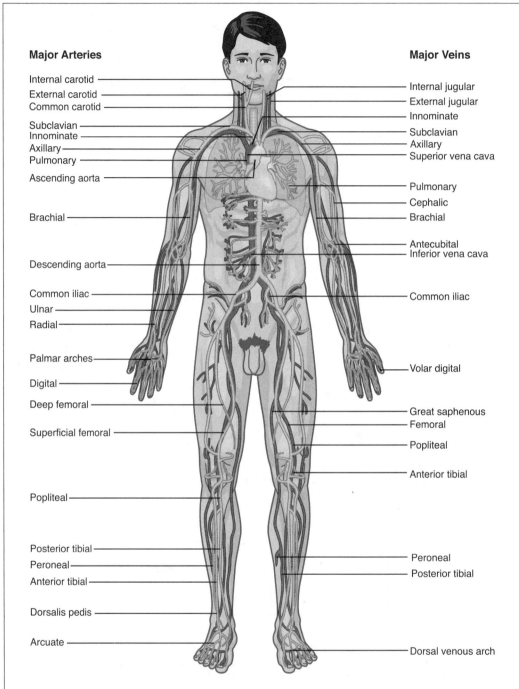

Major Arteries

- Internal carotid
- External carotid
- Common carotid
- Subclavian
- Innominate
- Axillary
- Pulmonary
- Ascending aorta
- Brachial
- Descending aorta
- Common iliac
- Ulnar
- Radial
- Palmar arches
- Digital
- Deep femoral
- Superficial femoral
- Popliteal
- Posterior tibial
- Peroneal
- Anterior tibial
- Dorsalis pedis
- Arcuate

Major Veins

- Internal jugular
- External jugular
- Innominate
- Subclavian
- Axillary
- Superior vena cava
- Pulmonary
- Cephalic
- Brachial
- Antecubital
- Inferior vena cava
- Common iliac
- Volar digital
- Great saphenous
- Femoral
- Popliteal
- Anterior tibial
- Peroneal
- Posterior tibial
- Dorsal venous arch

e. Cyanosis—CN does not bind to hemoglobin unless it is oxidized to metHb but blocks cellular respiration at cytochrome oxidase

f. Excess NaCl (↑ osmolarity), ethanol (decreases antidiuretic hormone secretion), or other agents or conditions leading to H_2O loss → dehydration → polycythemia (not enough plasma with crenated/shrunken RBCs) versus high altitude, chronic hypoxia (such as low CO exposures),

CONCEPTUALIZING TOXICOLOGY 18-1 (*continued*)

high erythropoietin possibly related to hazardous material exposure → polycythemia vera (increased RBC formation)

g. Halogenated hydrocarbons (hexachlorobenzene, TCDD), metals, biocides, hydrophobic medications, steroids → activation of nuclear receptor pair constitutively active receptor (CAR) and pregnane xenobiotic receptor (PXR) → production of 5-aminolevulinate synthase → overloads ("interferes with") heme synthesis pathway → porphyria (overproduction of heme precursors)

h. Thrombocytopenia (too few platelets causing hemorrhaging) caused by natural antithrombin medication heparin or agents that affect bone marrow (pancytopenia) such as benzene, large heavy metals such as Au (poisoning various cell types) and psychoactive medications (or estrogen excess in dogs); combines with a hemolytic anemia with microvascular thrombosis and tissue ischemia and infarction for medications such as clopidogrel, cyclosporine, micafungin, mitomycin C, quinine, and ticlopidine (immune-mediated via ADAMTS13 metalloproteinase or endothelial damage)

i. Blood sampling—especially important for As, as it is taken up by RBCs; clonogenic assays predict future possible problems in blood cell formation/hematopoiesis

B. Vascular—blood vessel damage that leads to plaque formation, aneurism, rupture—see Table 18-2

1. Smoking, hypertension, obesity/high cholesterol, and triglycerides are major causes of human disease

a. Nicotine → coronary spasm and ischemia

b. PAHs → reactive metabolites → adducts to vascular wall → atherosclerotic plaque development; allylamine and benzo(a)pyrene → damage endothelial cells and/or medial smooth muscle → migration of inflammatory cells → mediators invade vascular wall → smooth muscle cells grow → cellular lipid accumulation

2. Inflammatory agents

a. Caveolae (lipid rafts of 50–100 nm rich in cholesterol and sphingolipids and involved in signal transduction related to endocytosis, cancer formation, and uptake of pathogenic microorganisms) responsible for uptake of organic pollutants and mediate inflammation via caveolin-1 gene protein product (responsible for formation and maintenance of caveolae)

b. Homocysteine → binds to NMDA receptor → oxidative stress → Ca^{2+} influx → inhibits function of important electron acceptor in O_2 metabolism (thiolactonyl derivative of homocysteine) in mitochondria and endoplasmic reticulum → atherogenic and carcinogenic actions; autoantibodies to peptide-bound homocysteine and oxidized LDL and microbial products of homocysteinylated LDL aggregates in atherosclerotic plaques → acute inflammation

c. Toxic advanced glycation end-products formed during diabetes mellitus or Alzheimer's disease → RAGE immunoglobulin superfamily receptor binding → ROS → vascular dysfunction

d. Vascular endothelial—metals

(1) Cd → encodes for ZIP8 $Mn^{2=}/HCO_3^-$ symporter → transports Cd into vasculature → hemorrhage of testicular vessels

(2) As → liver sinusoidal endothelial capillarization → fibrosis

(3) Pb → ROS formation, inactivates endogenous NO, downregulates soluble guanylate cyclase ↓ NO signaling → damage + alters vasoactive function that ↑ blood pressure

(4) Hg → host of damage to SH groups → mitochondrial toxicity, ↓ GSH, ↑ lipid peroxidation and oxidative stress, inflammation, thrombosis, endothelial dysfunction, vascular smooth muscle dysfunction, dyslipidemia, and immune dysfunction

(5) Oxidative stress → opens transient receptor potential 2 cation channel → ↑ Ca^{2+} → apoptosis and endothelial hyperpermeability

(6) Nitroglycerin not only is vasodilatory but also → NO_x species by aldehyde dehydrogenase → uncouples oxidative phosphorylation → ↑ ROS → rebound ischemia, endothelial and autonomic dysfunction, and oxidation of key thiol group in aldehyde dehydrogenase

CONCEPTUALIZING TOXICOLOGY 18-1 (*continued*)

(7) Toxic cancer chemotherapy agents are usually injected intravenously and cause significant damage to the vasculature at or close to the site of injection; vascular endothelial growth factor (VEGF) antibodies (bevacizumab) leads either to hemorrhage or hypertension, and renal and cardiac toxicity depending on the person's response to decreased angiogenesis (blood vessel formation); formaldehyde and methylglyoxal are also endothelial cytotoxins

(8) Radiation → inflammation → delayed fibroproliferation → microvascular injury; endothelial damage related to loss of vascular thromboresistance → clots

e. Blood flow alterations

(1) Histamine or α-adrenergic receptor antagonists or toxic levels of tricyclic antidepressants → vasodilatory → anaphylactic shock; may be enhanced by erectile dysfunction medications

(2) Catecholamines → ↑ capillary pressure → proinflammatory cytokines → capillary leak; similar leaks occur due to plant toxins abrin and ricin (both inhibit protein synthesis)

(3) IL-2 and immunotoxin therapies → endothelial cell damage, ↑ cytokines and other proinflammatory agents, altered cell–cell and cell–matrix adhesion, cytoskeletal alterations → vascular leak syndrome

(4) Minoxidil → localized blood flow changes (augmentation of coronary blood flow sixfold in dogs) → vascular lesions

(5) PM2.5 and smoke products → endothelin type A receptor expression → vasoconstriction; more problematic still for TiO_2 nanoparticles → ↑ vascular tone and damaged endothelium-dependent, flow-induced dilation related to ROS formation

(6) Cancer chemotherapy medications and herbal toxic pyrrolizidine alkaloids → vascular lesions to fatal hepatic veno-occlusive disease via a variety of mechanism

f. Detection of vascular damage

(1) Willebrand Factor (or propeptide, endothelin and NO) → deeper find caveolin-1 (linked to ↑ cAMP) and smooth muscle α-actin

C. Cardiac

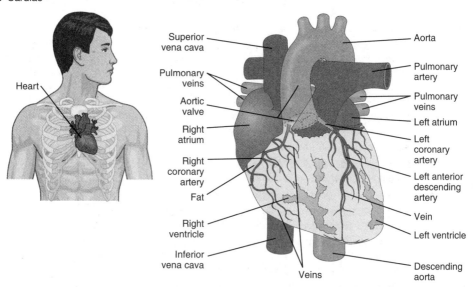

1. Pump for circulating toxicants to target organs, especially water-soluble ones as hydrophobic compounds may travel in the larger lymphatic system; dose in the GI tract or intravenous injection becomes a dosage here as rapid distribution to the body turns an amount into a concentration

2. Heart extremely sensitive to hypoxic damage unlike skeletal muscle. Also differentiates from skeletal muscle by lack of recruitment (all atria myocytes contract together as do all ventricular

myocytes due to gap junctions—see Figure 18-1). Also external Ca^{2+} rather than SR Ca^{2+} starts the signaling for the autorhythmic cell pacemaker and the contractility of the heart (SR activated later in the process via the ryanodine receptors). Overstretching/heart enlargement (hypertrophy) causes congestive heart failure (CHF). Also, heart that is in tachycardia or atrial fibrillation may be contracting too fast to allow complete filling giving a CHF-like action unless ventricular rate is controlled by medication or cardioversion/pacemaker. Cardiac output (CO) = heart rate (HR) × stroke volume (SV) = measure of heart performance

3. Cardiac damage (see Table 18-3 Myocardial Damage) may involve the heart muscle (myocardial damage) or heart conduction and rhythm dysfunction

   a. Muscular damage

      (1) Hypoxia versus oxidant damage (e.g., low Se, mycotoxins, anthracyclines, zidovudine and reperfusion injury) → hypoxic ischemia (infarcts) or apoptosis (necrosis from nitrite, oxidative phosphorylation inhibitors) versus oxidant stress and cardiomyopathy (generation of oxygen radicals). Ionophore antibiotics used in cattle also cause mitochondrial dysfunction due to abnormal movements of Na^+, K^+, and Ca^{2+} into muscle cells

      (2) Androgen–androgen receptor system (upregulation of mitochondrial transcription factor A and phosphorylation of serine-threonine kinase) plays an important role in cardiac growth, remodeling after angiotensin II's adverse effects (↑ blood pressure), and protects against doxorubicin toxicity, while the chemotherapy medication paclitaxel (microtubules targeted) increases toxic metabolites of anthracyclines

      (3) Chronic ethanol use generates lipid peroxidation, but dilated cardiomyopathy apparently linked to apoptotic mechanisms

      (4) Passive smoking → neurohormonal activation, ↑ ROS, activation of MAPK → cardiac remodeling

      (5) Cardiac hypertrophy generated by chronic toxicity of hypoxic or pro-oxidative compounds (acetaldehyde, azide, cocaine, doxorubicin, monocrotaline). Angiotensin II, catecholamines, and endothelin 1 → G protein activation and/or ↑Ca^{2+} signaling, and/or stimulation of 3 MAP kinases (ERKs, p38, c-Jun terminal kinase) → hypertrophy

      (6) Catecholamine excess generated via chronic stress (↑ adrenergic activity) affects microcirculation (hypoxia), causes Ca^{2+} overload, and creates toxic catecholamine oxidation products. Isoproterenol (β_1 and β_2 adrenergic agonist medication) → ↓ dystrophin → loss of sarcolemmal integrity → ischemia. Similarly, methamphetamine → reversible cardiomyopathy → irreversible myocyte hypertrophy and fibrosis (increased use). Other more "benign" overused stimulants such as caffeine and ephedrine at high doses → hemorrhagic myocardial necrosis in rats

      (7) TCDD → activate AhR → cardiovascular lesions/cardiomyopathy possibly via induction of CYP1A1, 1A2, 1B1 → ROS, DNA adducts, ↑ pro-inflammatory products of arachidonic acid cascade. Other halogenated chemicals, such as bis(2-chloroethyoxy)methane, → 2-chloracetaldehyde appears to the cardiotoxic metabolite (more like ethanol toxicity than AhR receptor activator) → mitochondrial damage → myocardial inflammation, myofiber vacuolation, and/or myofiber necrosis

      (8) Heavy metals (Au, Co, Cr, Hg, Sb) can cause chronic toxicity and may be highly elevated by infection → idiopathic dilated cardiomyopathy. Coxsackie B2 virus also ↑ concentration and toxicity (inflammatory lesions) of Cd, Ni, and methylmercury. Ni and methylmercury → alter natural killer cell function and ↓ macrophage mobilization directly. ↑ Ca^{2+} and ↓ Zn^{2+} in the heart may explain severity of inflammatory lesions

4. Heart rhythm/conduction—see Figure 18-2

   a. Starts at SA node in autorhythmic/pacemaker cells with Na^+ bringing cells to threshold

      (1) Blocks Na^+ channel with tetrodotoxin, saxitoxin, tricyclic antidepressants

      (2) Persistent activation (keep Na^+ channel open) by aconitine and mesaconitine (site 2) → increased force of cardiac contractions but hypotensive and bradycardic (slow heart beat) due to stimulation of ventromedial nucleus of hypothalamus

CONCEPTUALIZING TOXICOLOGY 18-1 (*continued*)

(3) Digitalis toxicity (Na^+, K^+-ATPase inhibition) → ↑ Na^+ and hypokalemia symptoms → classic "scooped out" ST segment, sinus bradycardia, and prolonged PR interval, but can also cause junctional tachycardia, atrial tachycardia, and bidirectional ventricular tachycardia depending on which node is blocked (SA or AV)

(4) Halogenate hydrocarbons obtund SA node and cause AV node autorhythmicity

(5) Ethanol causes sinus node automaticity in naïve rats

(6) Scorpion venom→ catecholaminergic storm (neurotoxicity) → atrial flutter and subsequent adrenergic myocarditis, toxic myocarditis, or myocardial ischemia

(7) Caffeine (↑ cAMP) and atropine (block muscarinic receptors) and methamphetamine → atrial tachycardia (and other damage depending on potency, dose, and chronic use)

b. External Ca^{2+} allows heart to beat and depolarizes pacemaker cells (then allows SR to release internal Ca^{2+} for contractility). Hypocalcemia→ QT prolongation or intermittent QTc prolongation→ life-threatening torsades de pointes (ventricular tachycardia which can deteriorate to fibrillation). Hypercalcemia→ tachycardia (short QT interval and widening T wave) and heart spasms (can mimic acute MI ECG)

c. K^+ efflux repolarizes pacemaker and contractile cells. Decreasing K^+ (hypokalemia) leads to more arrhythmias (caused by diuretics, certain antibiotic/antifungal compounds, and emetics) → prolonged repolarization of ventricular Purkinje fibers → prominent U wave (also flattened T wave, ST depression, and wide PR interval). Hyperkalemia caused by spironolactone (K^+-sparing diuretic) → widened QRS merging with T wave → stop heart if sufficiently high

d. Arrhythmia agents—see Table 18-3 Heart Conduction and Rhythm Dysfunction

(1) Agents that speed atria → atrial flutter → atrial fibrillation (doesn't contract) → blood clots → MI or pulmonary embolism. These supraventricular tachycardias are more likely in people or animals with an anesthetized SA node or atrial ectopic centers in right atrium

(2) Agents that speed ventricle (*much* more dangerous) → ventricular tachycardias → circus rhythm → ventricular fibrillation → rapidly developing hypoxia, asystole, death

(a) Organophosphates → ↑ cholinergic activity → QT prolongation → late-onset ventricular tachycardia

(b) Pt and anthracycline chemotherapy medications → QTc alterations

(3) Channelopathies—see Figure 18-3

(a) I_{Kr} blockers associated with long QT syndrome including Zn^{2+} and Ba^{2+}

(b) Antiarrhythmic amiodarone associated with inhibition of hERG (K^+ channel), but cytotoxicity related to altering mitochondrial membrane potential

(c) Testosterone ↓ $I_{ca,L}$ and ↑ I_{Kr} resulting in a greater repolarization reserve (shorter QT, therefore less susceptibility to torsades de pointes)—opposite to estrogen

(d) Toxicants can affect ryanodine receptor-Ca^{2+} release channel complex 2m FK-506 binding protein, cardiac SR Ca^{2+} ATPase, and phospholamban, which result in arrhythmias. Heightened filament Ca^{2+} sensitivity is both the basis for cardiomyopathies and ventricular arrhythmias

(e) Taxines of the yew plant block Na^+ and Ca^{2+} channels → ventricular tachycardia → stop heart in diastole

e. ECG analysis

(1) PR interval determines block (> 0.2 sec) in conduction pathway from atria through ventricles (AV node, AV bundle, bundle branches, Purkinje fibers)

(2) ST interval elevation = ischemia

f. Cardiac enzymes

(1) Creatine phosphokinase, troponin signal damage to myocardium

CONCEPTUALIZING TOXICOLOGY 18-1 (*continued*)

The cardiovascular system is the conduit for food-borne toxicants, especially those that are water soluble. The lymphatic system can also circulate fat-soluble chemicals, but is not easily sampled. The heart and vascular cells are sensitive to hypoxia and so chronic toxicity such as occurs in cigarette smokers may be manifested by continued hypoxic insult, resulting in atherosclerosis (buildup of plaque in an artery) and myocardial infarction (MI; ischemic heart disease resulting from hypoxic injury). The blood is an essential internal tissue for sampling to determine the presence of toxicants and toxicokinetics. This is where a dose becomes a concentration and distributes to the body. The distribution to target tissues makes the dose a dosage. Some toxicants (and some therapeutic concentrations of medications) bind strongly to red blood cells (RBCs), which makes their toxicity easily assessed. Blood "poisoning" is mainly a misnomer meaning bacterial infection to the point of sepsis. Very few agents are hemolytic and even those that are really damage neurological structures first by lack of oxygen or blood pressure. Those agents that deny oxygen binding to hemoglobin are still not truly blood poisons, because the toxicity is experienced by lack of oxygen in the heart and nervous tissue first. Some agents also damage hematopoiesis in the bone marrow and affect immune function first, followed by formation of platelets for clotting and RBCs for cellular respiration. This function is beyond the scope of this chapter, but the blood as a diagnostic tool is addressed in this chapter. Accordingly, agents that cause aplastic anemia or pancytopenia (bone marrow damage) are addressed here. It is also important to note that the albumin portion of plasma is known to bind a variety of mediations and toxicants, making them less available for action or toxicity. Depending on how the toxicant travels in blood (RBC-bound, albumin-bound, or in free circulation in the plasma), different fractions are important for determination of toxicity such as whole blood, plasma, or serum (liquid portion of clotted blood).

Forensic Analysis of Blood as a Diagnostic Tool

Table 18-1 indicates some uses of blood as a diagnostic tool. One of the most common problems in humans is the development of anemia. It is normally thought of as a nutritional problem, which is usually correct. There are various forms of anemia that can be generated by toxicants. Even medications at therapeutic doses can cause nutritional deficiencies.

Anemias

Anemias involve low RBC counts and low hemoglobin levels. Hemoglobin is determined in clinical laboratories by the methemoglobin cyanide method, which uses a reagent solution to convert the hemoglobin to the hemiglobincyanide (HiCN) and is determined by the equation: $A_{540} = \varepsilon c_{HiCN} l$, where $\varepsilon = 11$ L mmol^{-1} cm^{-1} and l = light path length in cm. Other hemoglobin forms can interfere with this reading, because they either do not convert to the HiCN form or become another form with a different extinction coefficient. Such is the case with sulfhemoglobin, which forms SulfHiCN with an $\varepsilon = 8.0$ at 540 nm (Zwart, 1993). This method is perfectly suitable for detecting microcytic (small RBC), hypochromic (low color) anemia associated with Fe or Cu deficiencies.

Microcytic Hypochromic Anemia and Sideroblastic Anemia

Iron deficiency is indicated by an increase in free RBC protoporphyrin concentrations (Brown, 1991). Lead is well known for producing this form of anemia and stippling of RBCs (Papanikolaou et al., 2005). The production of sideroblasts (abnormal, atypical nucleated RBCs with Fe granules in perinuclear mitochondria) characterizes lead poisoning and copper deficiency as differentiated from a straightforward Fe deficiency. Both lead poisoning and copper deficiency result in ferritin accumulation

TABLE 18-1	Forensic Chart of Blood Analysis for Systemic Toxicity			
Toxicity	**Microscopic Examination**	**Spectrophotometric Readings**	**Pathophysiology**	**Toxicants**
Anemias				
Fe/Cu deficiency	Microcytic, hypochromic	↓ Fe, or Cu by AA ↓ A_{540} HiCN	↑ Free protoporphyrin	Pb, Al, Cd, Zn, $Ga(NO_3)_3 \cdot 9H_2O$, gossypol, $Na_2Cr_2O_7 \cdot 2H_2O$, 1,3-dichloropropane
B_{12}/folic acid deficiency	Megaloblastic	Also decreased Hb	Increased LDH (intermedullary megaloblast precursor destruction)	As, benzene, chlordane, nitric oxide
Hemolysis	Pink plasma + Heinz bodies (species specific) Immature cells/Low blood cells	↑Hb and Hb degradation products in plasma and RBC		As, Cd, Hg, methyl chloride, napthalene, Pb, gossypol, phenols, saponins, surfactants, autoimmunity medications, organosulfoxides (dogs)
Methemoglobin	May have some cell lysis	+CN at 540 nm or 0-crossing point 1st-derivative	Hypoxia—bluish skin color (cyanotic)	NO_2/NO_3, aromatic amino and nitro compounds, catechol, phenol
Sulfhemoglobin	Possible hemolysis and Heinz body formation	↑620 nm (+CN to eliminate metHb interference)	Cyanotic, odor rotten eggs on breath, chocolate brown blood color	Sulfur-containing medications, H_2S and other sulfur-containing gases, and paints
Hemoglobin mutations	Some hypoxic shape irregularities, lysis, and Heinz bodies			Mutagens such as acrylamide, aflatoxin B1, agaratine, aristolochic acid, pyrrolizidines, safarole in food
Hemorrhage	Low blood cells, high immature cells			Anticoagulants, thrombolytics, ricin, bacterial toxins, mycotoxins, venoms
Pancytopenia/ aplastic anemia	Low blood cells		Bone marrow damage	As, Cd, Cu, anticancer medications, benzene, busulfan, ionizing radiation, methotrexate, pesticides
Carboxyhemoglobin	Cherry red	CO-oximetry and COHb at 540 nm with 555 nm as isosbestic point, other measures are important as very low CO may not show as COHb and postmortem Hb can become metHB	Headache, fatigue, weakness, muscle cramps, nausea, vomiting, upset stomach, diarrhea, confusion, memory loss, incoordination, chest pain, rapid heartbeat, difficult or shallow breathing, altered sensitivity to sound, light, smell, taste or touch	CO, $Ni(CO)_4$, stress/induction of heme oxygenase-1
Cyanosis	Blue tissue	Oxidation of Hb with sodium nitrite yields CNmetHb	Rapid (seconds) neurological damage	CN compounds such as sodium cyanide, amygdalin, smoke

TABLE 18-1	Forensic Chart of Blood Analysis for Systemic Toxicity (*continued*)			
Toxicity	**Microscopic Examination**	**Spectrophotometric Readings**	**Pathophysiology**	**Toxicants**
Dehydration/ polycythemia	Crenated RBCs and high RBC counts or hematocrit		High RBC count/concentrated urine, sunken eyes, low BP, fast HR, low skin elasticity, low blood flow to extremeties	NaCl (too much salt in diet), ethanol
Polycythemia vera	Too many RBCs		JAK2 617V > F	Mutagenic compounds
Porphyria	Anemia with enlarged spleen (erythropoi-ectic) or hepatic (liver function deficits or cancer)		Porphyrin products prior to heme (coproporphyrin) in urine and stool with neurological symptoms	Halogenated hydrocarbons, metals
Thrombocytopenia	Too few platelets		Immune-mediated of endothelium damage leading to ischemia and infarction	Medications, estrogen, snake venoms, metals (e.g., Au, Hg)
Plasma concentration			Tissue enzymes or microRNAs (leaking/damaged organs)	Toxicants that are water soluble or bind to plasma proteins
Blood concentration			RBC uptake limits usefulness of plasma	Toxicants that are accumulated in RBCs (e.g., As)
AA = atomic absorption, HiCN = hemoglobin determination by methemoglobin cyanide method (Zwart, 1993)				

in erythrocyte precursors due to the disruption of heme synthesis. Copper deficiency does not allow the formation of ceruloplasmin, which oxidizes iron from Fe^{2+} to Fe^{3+}, the state necessary for incorporation of iron into transferrin. Lead inhibits several enzymes involved in heme synthesis (Klauder and Petering, 1977). A key biomarker for lead exposure in heme synthesis is the inhibition of δ-aminolevulinic acid dehydratase (Sakai, 2000). Sodium dichromate dihydrate given via drinking water also causes a microcytic, hypochromic anemia in rodents, with more sensitivity in rats than mice (Bucher, 2007). Other metals such as aluminum (Abreo et al., 1991), zinc (Yanagisawa et al., 2009), anticancer gallium nitrate (Seligman et al., 1992), and environmental sludge contaminant cadmium interfere with iron and/or copper uptake or metabolism into heme and cause this form of anemia as well (Osuna et al., 1981). Gossypol is a cottonseed toxicant occasionally used as a male contraceptive in certain portions of the world. It prevents dissociation of oxygen from oxyhemoglobin, is hemolytic, and leads to microcytic hypochromic anemia. In rats, gossypol increases heme oxygenase activity in the liver and kidney, while having the opposite effect in the spleen (Aneja et al., 2003). Dogs become anemic when exposed to 1,3-dichloropropene (Stott et al., 2001).

Occupational exposures cause a number of other blood disorders including production of too much heme as occur in porphyrias, or they cause various types of anemias such as the microcytic hypochromic anemia, megaloblastic anemia, aplastic anemia/pancytopenia, hemolytic anemia, and reductions of immunity/immune cells (or conversely induction of autoimmunity and leukemia; Lisiewicz, 1993). The following subsections cover the anemias first and then address the metabolic disorders associated with porphyria. Immunological effects are covered elsewhere.

Megaloblastic Anemia

Megaloblastic anemia is normally caused by low vitamin B_{12} (or an autoimmune reaction known as pernicious anemia) or low folic acid or a combined deficiency of both nutrients. Megaloblastic anemia has been closely associated with chronic alcohol intake. Those who have folate deficiencies usually reflect undernutrition, yet alcoholics with good nutritional intake have megaloblastic anemia due to the toxic action of alcohol on erythropoiesis (Airoldi et al., 1987). Vitamin B_{12} also provides a detoxication route for low-level cyanide poisoning as indicated by the relationship between low vitamin B_{12} levels, cyanide in cigarette smoke, and blindness. Heavy smoking may put a strain on hematological versus the detoxification roles of vitamin B_{12} and can result in hematological changes in addition to blindness (Editorial, 1970). Arsenic has been shown to interfere with DNA synthesis in humans producing megaloblasts, but is more likely to affect young, proliferating marrow nucleated erythroid precursor cells in mice (Morse et al., 1980). Benzene biotransformation to an epoxide is more often associated with bone marrow damage and aplastic anemia than megaloblastic anemia, although it can produce both depending on the dose and degree of disturbance of DNA synthesis. NO can also produce megaloblastic anemia (as well as other anemias such as the microcytic form). However, its inhibition of methionine synthase can produce a functional vitamin B_{12} deficiency leading more likely to the megaloblastic anemia (Pradhan,

2009). The insecticide chlordane has been associated with blood dyscrasias including megaloblastic anemia (Furie and Trubowitz, 1976).

Hemolytic Anemias

The following used to be called the toxic anemias, which were usually defined by hemolysis. They were also linked to the species-specific formation of Heinz bodies. Agents of this class were nitro-derivatives of aromatic or aliphatic compounds, carcinogenic dyes, and alloxan (Fertman and Fertman, 1955). Later, these toxic anemias were thought to be oxidative and include formation of brown or green pigments including choleglobin, hemochromes, vergoglobin, sulfhemoglobin or methemoglobin formation and the water-insoluble, stainable granules that were called Heinz bodies (Jandl et al., 1960). Various inheritable or mutated unstable hemoglobins also form Heinz bodies from intracellular precipitation of degradation products (Winterbourn and Carrell, 1974). Heinz bodies appear to form more often in species other than the human and more often in neonatal humans than adults. It appears that Heinz bodies form based on the amount of hemoglobin bound by the erythrocyte membrane (Tillmann et al., 1973). Oxidative damage to hemoglobin even occurs during the storage of blood due to the generation of reactive oxygen species (ROS; Kanias and Acker, 2010). Saponins from plants cause hemolysis via hydrolysis of glycosidic bond and disruption of the erythrocyte membrane (Segal et al., 1974). Surfactants (soaps/detergents) cause osmotic lysis of the RBC plasma membrane due to increasing permeability (Shalel et al., 2002). Many compounds such as heavy metals, medications, and phenols (especially catechol) are metabolized to species that generate oxygen radicals. The oxidation of hemoglobin can yield methemoglobin (Fe^{3+} rather than Fe^{2+}) formation. Methemoglobin does not carry oxygen and must be reduced by methemoglobin reductase (cytochrome b_5 reductase) and NADH, which is lacking in the human fetus or infant. Further, oxidation of hemoglobin can lead to lysis of the RBC (Bukowska and Kowalska, 2004). Dogs respond to *Allium* species due to the presence of organosulfoxides, especially alk(en) ylcysteine sulfoxides, with oxidative hemolysis. This means that cooked onions or similar aromatic leeks, chives, garlic, shallots, and scallions that humans like to flavor their cooking can be fatal in their pets (cats and especially dogs; Tang et al., 2008). Autoimmune antibodies can also cause fatal hemolysis such as occurs with the diabetes medication metformin (Packer et al., 2008). Hemolysis also increases bilirubin concentrations. Therefore, it is of interest that high bilirubin concentrations that may occur from liver dysfunction or hemolytic damage to intact erythrocytes via loss of membrane lipids (inner phospholipids such as phosphatidylethanolamine and phosphatidylserine, which redistributed to the surface of the RBC; Brito et al., 2002).

Methemoglobin

Methemoglobin (metHb) may be associated with hemolysis, but the formation of this hemoglobin species alone is problematic to human and animal populations due to the induced hypoxia. Babies exposed to nitrate in drinking water or fetuses of mothers exposed to nitrates or nitrites form metHb and are susceptible to hypoxia. Because the formation of metHb is an oxidative process, it follows that other oxidative stress indicators are present. This includes lipid peroxidation, reduced compounds that maintain the redox state (such as glutathione [GSH]), and even immune system impairment (Rodríguez-Estival et al., 2010). At times, it is not the substance itself but rather the metabolite that causes the toxic effects. The hydroxylamine metabolite of the medication dapsone (4,4'-diaminoidiphenylsulfone) causes the metHb formation, hemolysis, and anemia associated with treatment of leprosy and other diseases of the skin (Orion et al., 2005). Hb species are difficult to characterize without use of special reagents to change them into another species. MetHb is found at 406 nm, which does not well separate it from oxyHb (414 nm) or Hb (430). MetHb also has a band at 630 nm, but can be mistaken for methylene blue, a treatment for metHb. The old method of Evelyn and Malloy (1938) converts the metHb to cyanometHB, which is read at 540 nm (hemoglobin does not bind CN). A newer, more sensitive method

has been developed using the first-derivative spectrum recorded at 405 and then 425 nm. At the exact point where the first-derivative spectrum or oxyHb is zero, the first-derivative value of oxyHb and metHb is proportional to the metHb in a mixture of the two species (Taulier et al., 1987).

Sulfhemoglobin

Sulfhemoglobin forms on exposure to hydrogen sulfide gas, other toxic sulfur-containing gases, or medications (e.g., acetanilide, sulfonamide, phenacetin), or it can occur via consumption of paint containing toxic sulfur-containing compounds (Wu and Kenny, 1997). Sulfhemoglobin (sulfHb) lasts the lifetime of the RBC and does not get converted back to hemoglobin (Chatfield and La Mar, 1992). Bacteria located in the colon can also produce hydrogen sulfide on their own utilizing inorganic sulfite and sulfite additives via fermentation of cysteine and methionine and sulfomucin metabolism of sulfate-reducing bacteria (Goubern et al., 2007). Some separation between metHb formation and sulfHb formation is not always possible, because it may depend on the subject for certain chemicals more than the chemical agent itself. This is why some animals and humans have a mixture of metHb and sulfHB in the blood during hemoxidative events leading to hemolysis and Heinz body formation (Chu et al., 1999).

Hemoglobin Mutations

Hemoglobin mutations (as well as DNA adducts and hemoglobin adducts) have been used to evaluate exposure to agents such as those found in food or herbal medicines (acrylamide, aflatoxin B1, agaritine, aristolochic acid, pyrrolizidines, safrole) and other DNA-altering substances (Jeffrey and Williams, 2005). Some of the hemoglobins formed by a single-nucleotide polymorphism (e.g., HbS) change shape and lyse under hypoxic conditions (George Priya Doss and Rao, 2009). It is of importance to toxicologists also to know that certain amino acid changes in the four chains of hemoglobin (two α and two β in the adult) make oxidation of the heme iron more likely, because the globin protein is then less likely to stabilize the oxyHb form of each chain (four O_2 molecules/Hb).

Therefore, metHb is more likely to form in these variants. Hb contains 141 or 146 amino acid residues per globin chain and a heme prosthetic group. Porphyrin, protoporphyrin IX, and an Fe^{2+} in the center are the components of the heme. When oxygen binds to form oxyHb, the pyrrole nitrogens of the porphyrin ring and a "proximal" histidine (His 87 at F8) from the α-globin chain coordinate with molecular oxygen. The His87 at F8 of the α-globin chain is also found in the hydrophobic heme pocket, which allows the oxygen molecule to bind reversibly to the heme iron. In this oxyHb structure, the Fe^{2+} is nearly coplanar with the pyrrole nitrogens in the porphyrin ring and is smaller due to the presence of molecular oxygen. This displaces the His and causes a shift in the F helix. This alters the conformation of the three-dimensional structure of Hb, allowing other oxygen molecules to bind more effectively (oxyHb dissociation curve). This will be of importance for hypoxic states such as generated by more effective binding of carbon monoxide, as they "rob" the more effective bind portion of the sigmoid curve (increased slope indicating better binding with saturation). This elaborate structure prevents extensive metHb formation in the presence of oxygen, but some does form due to some $O_2^{-\bullet}$ formation on the release of oxygen. As mentioned earlier, adults have sufficient metHb reductase and NADH to keep the iron in the ferrous rather than the ferric (nonoxygen binding) state. However, if the globin chains (α, β, or fetal γ) are modified by mutation to Hb Ms (HbM) by replacement of the histidines with tyrosine or asparagine, then spontaneous oxidation of Hb to metHb is possible and will form an anemic state due to lack of oxygen binding. Other groups are also important as the substitution of β-chain of the glutamic acid for valine at position 67 (E11) or methionine for leucine at position 28 (B10).

Another problem that can result in congenital methemoglobinemia is a deficiency in the metHb reductase. In type I (deficiency in the RBC-soluble form of the enzyme) there is cyanosis, while in Type II (deficiency in the soluble and membrane-bound forms of the enzyme) there is cyanosis and impaired brain/neurological development (severely developmentally delayed individuals). More than 30 mutations of the *cytb5r* gene have been reported in exons 2–9, with most being missense mutations. Mutations that result in a truncated protein ($< \frac{1}{3}$ of mutations) are associated with the severe Type II disease (Percy et al., 2005).

Hemorrhage can result from interference with clotting factors such as thrombin (heparin), vitamin K (coumadin/warfarin and inhibition of vitamin K 2,3-epoxide reductase; Ishizuka et al., 2008), ADP (clopidogrel bisulfate), and thromboxane A_2 (COX-1 inhibitors such as aspirin), or dissolution of a clot by tissue plasminogen activator or streptokinase (Guidry et al., 1991). There are toxins in certain diseases that are hemorrhagic (e.g., the hemorrhagic toxin or TcsH of the gram-positive bacterium *Clostridium sordellii*; Aronoff and Ballard, 2009) or factors in venoms of terrestrial snakes (e.g., that found in the venom of *Bothrops alternates* of Argentina; Lanari et al., 2010). Certain molds produce hemorrhagic compounds (Steyn, 1995). One of the most toxic lectins in the world, ricin, is found in the castor bean plant. Castor oil cakes used for soil conditioning cause hemorrhagic diarrhea in dogs and do not require mastication to release the toxic components as the bean itself requires (Hong et al., 2011). Hemorrhagic necrosis of the basic nucleus, cerebellum, and pallium is also noted in children who consume multiple tablets of diphenoxylate-atropine (Xiao et al., 2011). If enough skin is lost to toxic epidermal necrolysis, then hemorrhagic shock can develop as has been reported in patients taking the antimalarial compounds dihydroartemisinin with chloroquine or with amodiaquine (Ugburo et al., 2009). Other oxidative compounds such as the herbicide diquat also can cause cerebral hemorrhagic lesions (Vanholder et al., 1981). People develop hematuria from the anticancer alkylating agent cyclophosphamide due to hemorrhagic cystitis (bladder cell damage/inflammation; Ayhanci et al., 2010). The effects of toxicants that damage the vascular endothelium and promote hemorrhage are discussed in the vascular toxicants section later in this chapter. It is important to note that in toxicological assessment of preclinical safety studies the degree of hemorrhage is classified by the number of sites affected (single versus multiple sites; McGrath, 1993).

Bone Marrow Damage/Pancytopenia

Pancytopenia or aplastic anemia (immune-mediated destruction) occurs when the bone marrow pluripotent stem cells become damaged and do not make blood cells. Immune deficiency may be one of the first and fatal signs of this toxicity. Direct toxicity to the cells is the most studied cause of this disorder, but autoimmune pancytopenia is a known clinical problem. Benzene metabolism into the epoxide and from there to the hydroquinone and benzoquinone is thought to damage bone marrow stromal cells. The stromal cells cannot produce the cytokines necessary to maintain normal hematopoietic cell survival and proliferation. Mice have less glutathione and quinone reductase than rats and so are more sensitive to benzene toxicity in the bone marrow. Giving mice 1,2-dithiole-3-thione to induce GSH and quinone reductase protects against hydroquinone toxicity, while an inhibitor of quinone reductase (dicoumarol) increases hydroquinone toxicity. This is due to the finding that giving mice recombinant murine IL1A prior to benzene exposure prevents the bone marrow depression. Bone marrow damage usually occurs at high acute doses rather than low chronic doses, which are more likely to form leukemias. Similarly, ionizing radiation at higher doses produces severe and fatal bone marrow damage as occurred in people exposed to > 5 Grays (500 REM—measures of absorbed radiation dose) following the explosion of the Chernobyl nuclear reactor in 1986 (Organisation for Economic Co-operation and Development Nuclear Energy Agency, 2003).

Medications can also cause bone marrow damage. Busulfan is an alkylating anticancer medication that damages hematopoietic stem cells and decreases their proliferation. The antibiotic chloramphenicol deteriorates the stromal environment of the marrow and suppresses the growth of granuloid-committed progenitor cells and fibroblast colonies (Chen, 2005). Other anticancer agents, such as the medication that does not allow the disassembly of microtubules (paclitaxel), may result in pancytopenia from a single dose following increased mitotic granulocytic and erythroid cells (and hypoplasia) in CBA/CaLac mice (Churin et al., 2008). One anticancer medication that also serves as a treatment for rheumatoid arthritis is methotrexate. This antimetabolite impairs tetrahydrofolate status, which causes liver toxicity and a possibly fatal pancytopenia. The pancytopenia can be successfully treated with granulocyte colony-stimulating factor (Yoon and Ng, 2001). Azathioprine is an immune suppressant agent that also has adverse effects including infections, allergy, anemia, thrombocytopenia, and pancytopenia (La Mantia et al., 2007). These findings alert toxicologists and clinicians that agents that influence blood-forming cells may in certain people at high chronic doses produce pancytopenia. Additionally, certain patients with compromised liver function may experience increased bone marrow toxicity of medications. Albendazole is a broad-spectrum anthelmintic (antiparasitic) benzimidazole that has caused a death in a patient with cirrhosis due to prolonged pancytopenia (Opatrny et al., 2005).

Carboxyhemoglobin

Carboxyhemoglobin formation is a classic feature that results from high levels of carbon monoxide in the atmosphere. CO binds 245 times more strongly to hemoglobin (Hb) than does oxygen, so 1% CO in the atmosphere will bind 50% of the Hb, providing a lethal dose. Although the toxicity is due to interference with the oxidative phosphorylation chain, it is detected easily in the blood with an increase in COHb spectral peak at 540 nm (also recording 555 nm as the isosbestic point) and with CO-oximetry. However, on postmortem it must be considered that metHb might have formed from oxidation of Hb (Olson et al., 2010). If a human patient survives CO poisoning, a brain MRI should reveal new diffuse bifrontal white matter T2 hyperintensities and partial necrosis of the right globus pallidus. At COHb levels $< 25\%$, headache is the most common symptom. It is easier to diagnose at dangerously high concentrations, where changes in mental status occur ($25\% < COHb < 50\%$) followed by myocardial ischemia, ventricular arrhythmias, pulmonary edema, lactic acidosis, hypotension, coma, seizures, and ultimately death (50-60% COHb). CO poisoning to various organs can be mediated by glutamate release (starts an ischemic cascade in the brain), activation of neutrophils (oxygen radicals and brain lipid peroxidation/reversible demyelination), production of peroxynitrite (oxidative vascular damage and neuronal death), and reduced oxygen species (which are formed during hyperbaric reoxygenation and oxidize essential proteins and nucleic acids; Quinn et al., 2009). A complicating factor of low-level chronic CO poisoning is the phenomenon of stress-induced COHb formation. It appears that induction of heme oxygenase-1 may be an important protective mechanism in disease, but excessive induction during severe illness or stress appears to yield higher COHb due to the formation of carbon monoxide during the oxidative degradation of Hb. This explains the finding where low minimum or high maximum levels of arterial COHb in human patients were associated with increased intensive care mortality. Increased inflammatory markers correlated with higher arterial COHb levels (Melley et al., 2007). Very low chronic CO poisoning may also not show well in the blood, because CO may be found binding to cytochromes (especially cytochrome c oxidase; Alonso et al., 2003) or myoglobin. Additionally, it appears that some of the cardiac effects may be manifested by disruption of the NO pathways. Specifically, CO increases nitrosative stress by increased peroxynitrite formation (preventive effect of N-acetylcysteine and FeTPPS) without NO formation (no preventive effect of NO synthase inhibitor L-NAME). This would increase cardiac fiber calcium sensitivity. Additionally, the lack of NO will cause some vasoreactivity loss. CO then acts as a partial guanylate cyclase agonist, causing disequilibrium between cGMPc/cAMP pathways (increase in cAMP levels and enhanced contractility). This combination of effects would lead to the cardiac ischemic response noted in the living animal or human patient (Wattel et al., 2006).

Cyanosis

Cyanide poisoning has on occasion been linked to carbon monoxide due to the hypoxia generated. However, CN does not bind to Hb unless it is in the oxidized (metHb) state. CN usually presents with dilated pupils, while CO poisoning usually does not. CN takes seconds to work,

while CO usually takes hours unless the pure form is accidentally inhaled. CN induces three steps in alteration of the cardiovascular system: tachycardia and hypertension ("catecholamine rush"), followed by tachycardia and hypotension, and ultimately hypotension to cardiac arrest. The respiratory effects of CO are indicated by an increase in the rate of breathing, while CN causes an early phase tachypnea and hyperpnea reflecting the acidosis followed by a decrease in respiratory rate and central apnea. While the treatment of CO poisoning is either normobaric or hyperbaric oxygen, CN must be bound off cytochrome oxidase. This requires normobaric oxygen only to sustain the oxygenation of Hb, while the other treatments deal with CN toxicity directly. Four antidotes to CN are usually used including metHg inducers (e.g., amyl nitrite, sodium nitrite, 4-dimethylaminophenol), sodium thiosulfate, dicobalt EDTA, and hydroxocobalamin. The metHb must reach 20–40% to be effective in the binding of CN. Sodium thiosulfate is a substrate of rhodanese that converts CN into a less toxic thiocyanate (eliminated in urine). The last two antidotes are cobalt compounds. Dicobalt EDTA can chelate two CN ions, but is toxic to the cardiovascular system. Similarly, hydroxocobalamin binds CN, forming cyanocobalamin (eliminated in urine). This compound is a favored antidote, because it is well tolerated (Baud, 2007).

Polycythemia and Polycythemia Vera

Dehydration is another condition that leads to blood test alterations (polycythemia) due to less plasma with a high osmotic pressure. Two easily considered agents that Western society has encountered that lead to dehydration in excess are salt (NaCl) and ethanol. Many bars and fast food restaurants offer free snacks (popcorn, pretzels, peanuts) or inexpensive items (French fries) that are often loaded in salt. This causes dehydration via osmotic stress and makes patrons thirsty, which typically drives them to buy the establishments' frequently high-priced drinks. Ethanol is another dehydrating agent that has been shown following exercise to delay the return of plasma viscosity and plasma fibrinogen to normal levels (El-Sayed, 2001).

Its chronic use decreases vasopressin (antidiuretic hormone [ADH]) mRNA synthesis by hypothalamic cells of the brain (Gulya et al., 1991). Because alcohols are converted to aldehydes as part of the metabolic process, it is of interest that aldehyde dehydrogenase 7A1 (ALDH7A1) protects mammals against salinity, dehydration, and osmotic stress, similar to what occurs plants. ALDH7A1 generates osmolytes and metabolizes aldehydes as its protection against hyperosmotic stress (Brocker et al., 2010). Other than hyperosmotic stress or effects on ADH or ALDH, many bacterial toxins cause dehydration, with changes in membrane permeability. Occasionally, the bacterial flora can produce a toxin through metabolic action such as ammonia that leads to increased permeability of the cells of the gastrointestinal tract (Sharkey et al., 2006). Overdose of medications, such as the antibiotic rifampin, causes dehydration in addition to other toxic effects (Rechciński et al., 2006). Clearly, damaging medications such as anticancer medications lead to fluid loss in the gastrointestinal tract via damaged cells or emesis/vomiting; radiation treatment or burns can also lead to blood or fluid loss (Wolff et al., 2001). In wildlife toxicology, exposure of birds to oil via their feathers can result in dehydration accompanied by emaciation and hypothermia in addition to the toxicity of the polycyclic aromatic hydrocarbons (PAHs) in oil (Troisi et al., 2006).

Polycythemia vera is a myeloproliferative (malignancy) disease that includes erythrocytosis, leukocytosis, and thrombocytosis. Normally, an overproduction of RBCs may occur with chronic exposure to high altitude, chronic hypoxia (similar to low CO levels that occur in tunnel workers), or on overproduction of the kidney hormone erythropoietin. Patients with polycythemia vera appear more likely to develop vascular thrombosis, polycythemia vera–related myelofibrosis, and acute leukemia. These disorders are clonal in origin and appear to be linked to a hypersensitivity to cytokines. The role of toxic environmental chemicals in causing this condition has not been well studied. However, the use of a molecular probe (JAK2 617V > F) has indicated that a cluster of people close to hazardous material (waste-coal power plants and U.S. Environmental Protection Agency

Superfund sites) in three counties in eastern Pennsylvania may indeed have polycythemia vera due to toxic waste exposure (Seaman et al., 2009). Since leukemias are also myeloproliferative diseases known to develop from radiation or benzene, it is likely that mutagenic agents also lead to polycythemia vera.

Porphyria

Interference in the heme synthesis pathway in genetically sensitive individuals yields porphyria, which leads to overproduction of specific heme precursors and accumulation in tissues. Porphyria cutanea tarda is a form or porphyria associated with a skin condition that may not only be inherited, but can be acquired from chronic exposure to halogenated hydrocarbons and metals and associated with the activity of uroporphyrinogen decarboxylase. Classic cases of acquired porphyria, which manifest with neurological symptoms (peripheral neuropathy), are the thousands of inhabitants of Turkey exposed to the fungicide hexachlorobenzene. They also had moderate to high coproporphyrin in their urine and stool, but were abnormally low in uroporphyinogen-1-synthase associated with an acute porphyria rather than porphyria cutanea tarda. 2,3,7,8-Tetrachlorodibenzo-p-dioxin (TCDD) is the most potent porphyrogenic agent; it has been linked to disease outbreaks in Vietnam veterans exposed to Agent Orange and a worker at a chemical plant in Seveso, Italy exposed to TCDD. Hormones, medications, infections, traumas, and dietary factors may also activate the disease. This is emphasized in the veterans of many wars including the Gulf War, where exposure to stress, sun, fires, inoculations, and other chemicals may initiate the disease. Deficiencies in aminolevulinate acid (ALA) dehydratase, uroporphyrinogen decarboxylase, coproporphyrinogen oxidase, and protoporphyrinogen oxidase may cause porphyria (Downey, 1999). A more recent paper (Thunell, 2006) suggests in the abstract (page S43) that acute porphyric attack is due to the "toxic proximal overload of the enzyme-deficient heme-biosynthetic pathway." The focus is on transcription control of the gene that is responsible for production of 5-aminolevulinate synthase (ALAS1). Activation of the nuclear receptor pair constitutively active receptor (CAR) and pregnane xenobiotic receptor (PXR) by alcohols, biocides, hydrophobic medications, solvents, and steroid hormones is the key to controlling transcription of this gene and leads to porphyria and development of apoCYPs. Also, the stress hormone cortisol binds to the glucocorticoid receptor and augments the expression of CAR and PXR, indicating a role for stress in the development of the disease process as indicated earlier for war veterans. The promoter regions of ALAS1 and apoCYPs are also activated by ligand-dependent growth hormone pulse-controlled hepatocyte nuclear factor 4 (HNF4), insulin-responsive forkhead box class O-(FOXO) protein pathway (infection/stress), and the proliferator-activated receptor γ co-activator 1 α (PGC-1 α) circuit (fasting and glucagon). Sex-dependent control of growth hormone and other activities indicates the sex differences in porphyria development. Also, crosstalk in the genomic circuits controlling ALAS1-transcription may account for high individual variations in the severity of the disease induced by chemical or other insults. Porphyrias affect the RBC count (anemia) if they originate in the bone marrow (erythropoietic), but mainly affect the liver if the porphyrin compounds accumulate there (decreased liver function and hepatic cancer development).

Thrombocytopenia

Thrombocytopenia or too few platelets may result in mortality if not caught early and treated adequately. Anticoagulants such as heparin may cause thrombocytopenia (Cines et al., 2004). Those agents mentioned earlier that cause bone marrow damage will likely also lead to low platelet counts. For example, benzene is capable of bone marrow damage that affects all blood cells. Large heavy metals such as gold (orally administered triethylphosphine gold for rheumatoid arthritis) also affect numerous cell types resulting in depression of white blood cells (responsible for the therapeutic and a toxic effect of the compound), thrombocytopenia, dermatitis, stomatitis, and proteinuria and aplastic anemia for the injection route (Tozman and Gottlieb, 1987). This is of interest, because the immune system can be involved in tissues that bind large metals to their surfaces as happens for gold and mercury (hapten binding causes autoimmune reactions when attached to larger carriers/proteins; Fuortes et al., 1995). Thrombocytic thrombocytopenic purpura involves a hemolytic anemia and thrombocytopenia with microvascular thrombosis leading to tissue ischemia and infarction. Medications leading to this disease are clopidogrel, cyclosporine, micafungin, mitomycin C, quinine, and ticlopidine, which may act via immune-mediated toxicity via ADAMTS13 metalloproteinase or damage to the endothelium (Nazzal et al., 2011). Linezolid is a medication developed for the treatment of tuberculosis whose adverse effects include thrombocytopenia and anemia with peripheral neuropathy (Schecter et al., 2010). Psychoactive medications such as lithium, clozapine, carbamazepine, valproic acid, and selective serotonin reuptake inhibitor (SSRI) antidepressants appear to affect blood counts and function, including thrombocytopenia, interference with clotting/platelet function, aplastic anemia, hemolytic anemia, leukopenia, agranulocytosis, leukocytosis, eosinophilia, and thrombocytosis (Mazaira, 2008). An anticancer medication, gemcitabine, has also been found to cause reduced platelet counts in patients with severe hepatic dysfunction (Teusink, 2010). Combination radiation treatment and chemotherapy for cancer treatment may also lead to thrombocytopenia (Tans et al., 2011). Estrogen from medications or excess production by functional Sertoli cell or ovarian granulose cell tumors causes bone marrow toxicity in dogs involving thrombocytopenia, anemia, and leukocytosis or leukopenia (Sontas et al., 2009). As mentioned earlier, snake venoms can be hemorrhagic as well as neurotoxic. Thrombocytopenia is generated by the C-lectin type protein venom of the snake *Bothrops asper*. Additionally, two enzymes in the venom lead to defibrination (Gutiérrez et al., 2009). Bacteria can produce toxins that famously affect the blood system. Shiga toxin (serotype O 157:H7) produced by enterohemorrhagic *E. coli* from contaminated food products causes hemolytic uremic syndrome with the triad of thrombocytopenia, hemolytic anemia, and acute renal failure (Scheiring et al., 2008).

Plasma and Blood Analysis

Certain toxicants that either bind to plasma protein or are water soluble are found appropriately in plasma. Organochlorine pesticides and polychlorinated biphenyls can be analyzed in plasma of affected organisms despite the distribution to fat. This is especially true for recent exposures or continued exposures of animals high up in the food web such as vultures or humans (Dhananjayan et al., 2011). Although plasma enzymes are also used to assess organ damage, relatively stable microRNAs may prove much more organ specific, sensitive, and quantitative toxicity biomarkers as real-time polymerase chain reaction allows for amplification of the signal prior to extensive irreversible damage (Laterza et al., 2009). Plasma composition may be affected by damage to the liver, because albumin, prothrombin, and fibrinogen have hepatic origins. Oxidative damage can also be assessed in plasma by various lipid peroxidation products (Møller et al., 2010). Blood is more important for elements such as arsenic that, once metabolized in the liver (arsenic methylation), is taken up by erythrocytes or excreted into the urine (Shiobara et al., 2001). Blood sampling also affords the toxicologist the analyses listed here for alterations of blood cells.

Clonogenic Analysis

One of the most telling predictors of blood cells problems is the clonogenic assay. Separate analyses can be performed beyond or prior to animal testing for effects on hematopoiesis—granulopoiesis (formation of granulocytes), megakaryopoiesis (formation of precursor of platelets), and erythropoiesis (formation of RBCs; Parent-Massin, 2001).

Forensic Analysis of Vascular Toxicants

Many people are aware that chronic smoking leads to damage to the vasculature. Also, hypertension appears to damage the endothelial lining, making the vasculature more subject to plaque formation in people with high cholesterol and triglycerides, as occurs with obesity. This would make NaCl a major overdose toxicant in humans eating processed food. The sensitivity of the vascular endothelium to direct action of toxicants, hypoxic insult, uptake of toxicants, and inflammation is extremely important in atherosclerosis development. Because vascular disease is the number one human killer in Western industrialized nations, this is a major concern in medicine.

Inflammation

The toxicants that damage the vasculature are listed in **Table 18-2**. Environmental pollutants only are a major consideration in wildlife or in human populations after smoking behavior, alcohol intake, high fat consumption, salt ingestion, and medication use are considered as primary factors in vascular disease. Nicotine causes toxicity to vascular endothelial cells, starts the adhesion pathway, and causes inflammation of the vasculature that leads to high blood pressure and atherosclerosis. Nicotine also causes coronary spasm and ischemia that yields coronary artery disease and MI (Balakumar and Kaur, 2009). PAHs in smoke are biotransformed in vascular cells to reactive metabolites that form adducts to vessel wall, leading to the development of atherosclerotic plaques (Ramos and Moorthy, 2005). Lipid rafts and particularly caveolae (carriers of exocytic and endocytic pathways of the plasma membrane that perform mechanosensing and lipid regulation; Parton and Simons, 2007) are plentiful in vascular endothelium. They appear to be involved in the uptake of organic pollutants and mediation of the inflammatory response, which looks to involve the caveolin-1 gene (Majkova et al., 2010). The stimulation growth and development of aortic smooth muscle cells by agents such as allylamine and benzo[*a*]pyrene are important in the development of atherosclerotic lesions (damage to endothelial cells and/or medial smooth muscle cells → migration of inflammatory cells → mediators find their way into vascular wall → smooth muscle cells grow → cellular lipid accumulation). Oxidative metabolism of these compounds by CYPs, effects on phospholipid turnover,

TABLE 18-2　Forensic Chart of Vascular Toxicity	
Toxicity	**Toxicants**
Angiostatic: Chemotaxis inhibition and tube formation in endothelium	Cd
Apoptosis	Ionizing radiation, NO, peroxynitrite, anticancer agents
Blood flow changes	
Capillary leak	Catecholamines, abrin, ricin (inflammation or cell death), immunotherapy
Localized ↑ coronary blood flow	Endothelin receptor antagonists
Vascular tone decreases → reflex tachycardia →↑coronary blood flow	High-dose medications
Veno-occlusive disease	Anticancer, hormones, pyrrolizidine alkaloids
Capillarization of hepatic sinusoidal endothelium	As
Hemorrhage	Cd
Hypertension	Cd, Pb
Inflammation/caveolin-1 gene expression	Organic pollutants, nicotine
ROS	Various toxicants including particulate matter, Hg, organic nitrates, diabetes mellitus, Alzheimer's disease

activity of protein kinase C, ras-related signal transduction, and matrix interactions all appear to have a role in the toxic responses of the vasculature (Ramos et al., 1994). The toxicity of homocysteine may explain how many of these factors interrelate. Homocysteine binds to the N-methyl-D-aspartate (NMDA) receptor, leading to oxidative stress (failed ATP synthesis and ROS formation), calcium influx (depletes cell phosphate stores due to calcium apatite deposition and increases apoptosis), and inhibits thioretinaco ozonide (homocysteine thiolactonyl derivative acts as electron acceptor in oxygen metabolism) function in mitochondria and the endoplasmic reticulum (key to carcinogenic and atherogenic effects). Acute inflammation results from autoantibodies to proteins containing peptide-bound homocysteine and oxidized low-density lipoprotein (LDL) and microbial products derived from homocysteinylated LDL aggregates trapped in the vaso vasorum of atherosclerotic plaques. The trapped lipoprotein aggregates and obstructed lumen enhanced by high tissue pressure and endothelial dysfunction from lumen narrowing and

hyperplasic endothelial cells creates vulnerable plaques as a precursor to heart disease and stroke (McCully, 2009). Diabetes mellitus and Alzheimer's diseases lead to the formation of advanced glycation end products (AGEs) such as glyceraldehyde-derived AGEs. The toxic AGEs (mostly the glyceraldehyde-derived forms) bind to a receptor (RAGE of immunoglobulin superfamily) and generate ROS, which may explain in part diabetic or Alzheimer's vascular dysfunction (Takeuchi and Yamagishi, 2009).

Direct and Secondary Toxicity to Endothelial Cells

Metals can induce a variety of vascular toxicities. Cd-sensitive strains of mice express the Sic39a8 gene, which encodes for the ZIP8 $Mn^{2+}//HCO_3^-$ symporter. This transports Cd into the vasculature (and into the kidney for damage there) and induces hemorrhage in the testicular vessels. Cd also damages the heart muscle. Cd is also angiostatic in that it interferes with vascular endothelium cadherin (Ca^{2+}-dependent adhesion molecule). Liver sinusoidal endothelium capillarization by As leads to the development of fibrosis. Lead, as with cadmium, leads to damage that sustains increases in blood pressure. Perinatal exposure to a susceptible animal appears more important for the effects of Pb on blood pressure (Prozialeck et al., 2008). Lead also leads to ROS formation, inactivates endogenous NO, and downregulates soluble guanylate cyclase by ROS, decreasing NO signaling. This alters the vasoactive function of endothelium and is now considered the main target organ for the effect of Pb (Nemsadze et al., 2009). Oxidative stress by itself stimulates ADP-ribose formation, which opens transient receptor potential (melastatin) 2 cation channel. Calcium then enters, generating apoptosis and endothelial hyperpermeability (Hecquet and Malik, 2009). Organic nitrates, such as nitroglycerin, are unexpected vascular toxicants that are used therapeutically for their rapid vasodilatory activity. Nitroglycerin is converted by aldehyde dehydrogenase to a NO_x species and simultaneously uncouples oxidative phosphorylation yielding a burst of ROS. These events lead to rebound ischemia, endothelial and autonomic dysfunction, and oxidation of a key thiol group in aldehyde dehydrogenase (decreased nitrate metabolism; Gori and Parker, 2008). Cancer chemotherapy agents are often injected and cause significant damage at the high concentrations resulting at or close to the injection site. Cisplatin causes vascular disease in addition to toxicity in the kidneys, nerves, and lungs (Pliarchopoulou and Pectasides, 2010). Even angiogenesis inhibition for cancer treatment using vascular endothelial growth factor (VEGF) antibodies (bevacizumab) or tyrosine kinase inhibitors targeting VEGF receptors has led to hypertension and renal and cardiac toxicity (Kappers et al., 2009) or to hemorrhage based on lack of repair of vessels. Radiation also generates microvascular injury starting with inflammation and a delayed fibroproliferative phase. The endothelial damage appears to be linked to a deficiency of thrombomodulin, which yields a loss of vascular thromboresistance, excessive activation of thrombin receptors on cells by thrombin, and too little activity of plasma protein C (anticoagulant, anti-inflammatory, cytoprotective; Wang et al., 2007). Hg causes a variety of damage from binding to sulfhydryl groups. It causes mitochondrial toxicity, depletion of glutathione, heightened lipid peroxidation, and oxidative stress. Inflammation, thrombosis, endothelial dysfunction, vascular smooth muscle dysfunction, dyslipidemia, and immune dysfunction are other toxicities of this heavy metal (Houston, 2007). Anticancer medications, ionizing radiation, hormones, oxidized lipids, hyperoxia, NO, peroxynitrite, and viruses can be signals for apoptosis that leads to endothelial dysfunction (Mallat and Tedgui, 2000). Certain chemicals such as the fixative formaldehyde and methylglyoxal are endothelial cell cytotoxins. When people are exposed to methylamine or aminoacetone, their metabolism by semicarbazide-sensitive amine oxidase (SSAO) localized in the vascular smooth muscle layer to formaldehyde and methylglyoxal, respectively, will increase the toxicity of these compounds. Patients with diabetes mellitus have elevated activity of SSAO and are more likely to experience toxicity via production of these metabolic products (Yu, 1998).

Blood Flow Changes

Drug-induced changes in vascular tone (vasodilation) that result in decreased blood pressure, reflex tachycardia, and increases in coronary blood flow are the key indicators that vascular toxicity is occurring. Agents such as histamine cause anaphylactic shock via vasodilatory effects, as do alpha-adrenergic receptor blockade by alpha-blockers and toxic levels of tricyclic antidepressants (Thanacoody and Thomas, 2005). Blood pressure is of concern especially with the introduction of erectile dysfunction medications and their interaction with other vasodilative agents. However, localized changes in blood flow appear similarly damaging as occurs in dog coronary blood flow augmentation by minoxidil, for example (endothelin receptor antagonist; Brott et al., 2005). When air pollutants were exposed to mice (including PM 2.5 and smoke products), this induced a vasoconstriction related to endothelin type A receptor expression (Matsumoto et al., 2010). Nanoparticles have a larger surface area per unit of weight and may represent a greater problem. Inhaled TiO_2 nanoparticles increased spontaneous tone in coronary arterioles and also damaged endothelium-dependent, flow-induced dilation. Vascular tone changes, resistance to ACh-induced vasodilation, and blood flow around the heart appear are related to ROS formation (inhibited by tetramethylpiperidine-N-oxyl and catalase) and are consistent with findings of increased cardiac problems associated with exposure to particle pollution (LeBlanc et al., 2009). Catecholamines may lead to pulmonary edema via increased capillary pressure and activation of proinflammatory cytokines, causing capillary leak (Rassler, 2007). Similar leakage can occur via other toxicants, such as abrin (toxic protein of the jequirity bean *Abrus precatorius*) and its ability to inhibit protein synthesis in endothelial cells (Dickers et al., 2003) or ricin (Lord et al., 2003). Vascular lesions are prominent in endothelial damage and apoptosis caused by Shiga toxins (Cherla et al., 2003). IL-2 and immunotoxin therapies are limited by the production of vascular leak syndrome (increased vascular permeability and extravasation of fluids and proteins yielding interstitial edema and organ failure via a complex series of events involving activation or damage to endothelial cells and white blood cells [WBCs], cytokines and other inflammatory substances, changes in cell–cell and cell–matrix adhesion, and cytoskeletal function; Baluna and Vitetta, 1997). Some toxicants, such as those used in chemotherapy for cancer or hormone therapy (Doll and Yarbro, 1994) or traditional herbal mixtures containing pyrrolizidine alkaloids (Kumana, 1985), cause a variety of vascular toxicities from relatively minor asymptomatic venous lesions to fatal hepatic veno-occlusive disease. Mechanisms may involve direct medication-induced endothelial cell toxicity, influencing the clotting cascade, platelet activation and aggregation, changing the balance of thromboxane-prostacyclin (arachidonic acid cascade), and unregulated cytokine stimulation.

Detection of Vascular Damage

One glycoprotein that prevents blood loss from vascular damage via activation of platelets is von Willebrand Factor. Its increase in plasma indicates that the endothelial cells are likely to be experiencing some form of toxicity and precedes more gross alterations found by histology. Other factors that can also indicate similar damage are von Willebrand Factor propeptide, endothelin, and NO. Deeper in the vasculature is smooth muscle, whose injury can be monitored by caveolin-1 (cav-1) and smooth muscle α actin. As mentioned earlier, cav-1 has been linked to vascular insult and vasodilation. Intracellular increases in cAMP occur in endothelial and smooth muscle cells in response to this injury. The caveolae localized in the endothelial and smooth muscle cells contain both adenylyl cyclase and nitric oxide synthase (NOS) and are co-localized with and regulated by cav-1. The increase in NO from NOS activation would clearly cause vasodilation (Brott et al., 2005).

Forensic Analysis of Cardiac Toxicants

The heart is a complex organ that is a muscle and contains a nervous system. All must work together to give the contraction strength necessary to circulate the blood into the lungs and provide the systemic circulation at the proper rate to maintain blood pressure and tissue oxygenation as well as transfer nutrients, waste products, hormones, and so forth to their target organs for a variety of active states.

Heart Muscle

While it is useful to look at a figure of the heart such as might be found in an anatomy book, it is more helpful in the context of this section to look at the heart muscle at the ultrastructural level. Similar to skeletal muscle, striations can be seen with clear overlapping thin filaments of actin and thick filaments of myosin as illustrated in **Figure 18-1**. Because of this structure, this muscle is susceptible to many of the toxicants that affect skeletal muscle. However, the electron micrograph of the cardiac myocyte shows that it is extremely enriched with mitochondria and is severely damaged under hypoxic conditions, unlike skeletal muscle. The cardiac mitochondria are easily isolated and have served as the basis for much of the mitochondrial

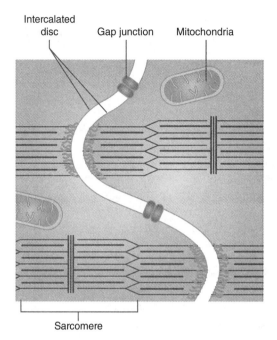

Intercalated disc   Gap junction   Mitochondria

Sarcomere

FIGURE 18-1 Representative Electron Micrograph of Sarcomere Ultrastructure in Adult Mouse Ventricular Cardiac Myocyte

energetic research over the decades. The gap junctions make all cardiac myocytes contract at once in the atria and then in the ventricles. Skeletal muscle allows motor units to contract separately and recruit. Calcium causes all muscle cells of the body to contract, but the skeletal muscle saturates myosin cross-bridges with influx from the sarcoplasmic reticulum in an all-or-none action. External calcium concentrations play a larger role in the contractility of the heart muscle, because the action potential that initiates a contraction causes voltage-sensitive L-type Ca^{2+} channels to open. Calcium moves from the extracellular fluid, raising cytosolic Ca^{2+} concentrations adjacent to the sarcoplasmic reticulum (SR). This Ca^{2+} binds to ryanodine receptors on the external surface of the SR. These receptors open intrinsic channels and allow the SR's calcium to contract the sarcomere based on the amount of Ca^{2+} released. This means that more external calcium entry stimulates more Ca^{2+}-induced contractility. This is essential in linking the toxicity of chronic use of calcium-channel blockers (especially of the

nifedipine class) to the induction of congestive heart failure (weak contraction). As with skeletal muscle, stretch also determines the strength of contraction, known as the Frank-Starling mechanism of the heart. This means that as the heart fills with blood, the stretch of the end-diastolic volume (end of ventricular filling) also determines the force of contraction and leads to an increased stroke volume on systole or contraction of the ventricles. Overstretch of the heart on the right side induced by pulmonary hypertension (caused by agents such as the banned diet medications fen-phen or fenfluramine combined with phentermine) or more likely systemic hypertension-induced left side hypertrophy (caused by a chronic excess of a variety of dietary substances, mineralocorticoids, and toxicants) is the leading cause of congestive heart failure. Lack of contraction force or a very slow heartbeat lowers blood pressure to dangerous levels due to the lack of cardiac output (stroke volume × heart rate).

Note the cardiac toxicities associated with myocardial damage listed in **Table 18-3**. Chemical agents may lead to a number of problems with severe damage (ischemia and necrosis) with acute exposures at high doses. Cardiomyopathies are weakening of the heart muscle (myocardial fiber degeneration or necrosis, inflammation, fibrosis), while congestive heart failure and hypertrophies may result from cardiomyopathies or chronic systemic hypertension or pulmonary hypertension, among other factors. Apoptosis may also accompany and augment direction oxidant damage and other damage.

Oxygen is a key factor affecting the health of myocytes. Too little oxygen leads to hypoxic/ischemic damage, and oxidative stress leads to cardiomyopathy or apoptosis/necrosis, depending on the severity and chronicity of the damage. For example, selenium deficiency in humans (Keshan disease in China) leads to less oxidative protection via decreased selenium-dependent glutathione peroxidase and coxsackievirus and results in dilated cardiomyopathy (Alexander, 2007). Other agents that increase oxidative stress, such as mycotoxins (e.g., citreoviridin), may also cause a cardiomyopathy in combination with dietary deficiencies inselenium, proteins, and antioxidant vitamins

TABLE 18-3   Forensic Chart of Cardiac Toxicity

Toxicity	Toxicants
Myocardial Damage	
Ischemia	Hypoxic agents or coagulants (infarct) at high dose–acute
Cardiomyopathy	Chronic exposure to oxidative agents (anthracyclines, ethanol, AZT), stimulants, aryl hydrocarbon receptor activation, heavy metals + inflammation
Apoptosis/necrosis	Nitrite, inhibitors of oxidative phosphorylation, fluoroacetate, ethanol, caffeine + ephedrine, bis(2-chloroethyoxy)methane, monensin
Congestive heart failure/hypertrophy	Calcium-channel blockage (nifedipine), fen-phen, acetaldehyde, azide, cocaine, doxorubicin, monocrotaline
Cardiac remodeling	Toxicities listed above if repaired lead to remodeling—an important toxicity of passive smoke
Heart Conduction and Rhythm Dysfunction	
Assorted dysrhythmias/arrhythmias	Thiazide and loop diuretics, carbenicillin, gentamicin, amphotericin B, glycyrrhetinic acid, dehydrating agents, fluorouracil
Asystole/cardiac standstill	Organophosphates, K^+-sparing diuretics, ACE inhibitors, renal toxicants/aging
Atrial flutter	Catecholaminergic storm following scorpion venom
Atrial tachycardia	Atropine, caffeine, Tl, methamphetamine, taxanes
Bradycardia	Aconitine, β_1 antagonism, hypoxia , taxanes
Brugada syndrome (ST elevation + T-wave inversion)	Aluminum phosphide
Depressed pacemaker function	Na^+-channel blockers, anesthetic halogenated hydrocarbons, ethanol
Ventricular tachycardia	Taxines, organophosphates
Ventricular fibrillation	K^+-sparing diuretics, ACE inhibitors, renal toxicants, quinine, aging
Torsades de pointes (I_{Kr} blockade)	Quinidine, sotalol, dofetilide, tefernadine or cisapride + CYPsA4 inhibitors, astermizole metabolite, thioridazine especially + CYPsD6 inhibitors, organophosphates, Ba, hormones/anti-hormones, Pt, anthracyclines

(Sun, 2010). This dichotomy is functionally relevant in the heart, where MI and reperfusion injury occur often in clinical practice due to the lack of oxygen and then the generation of oxygen radicals during reintroduction of oxygen to highly reduced tissues. This high oxygen demand makes the heart sensitive not only to ischemia infarcts, but also to apoptosis/ myocardial necrosis from nitrite (oxidizes hemoglobin to methemoglobin), mitochondrial respiratory chain inhibitors such as sodium azide (complex IV inhibition and apoptosis of rat cardiac myocytes prevented by calcium channel inhibitors; Inomata and Tanaka, 2003), rotenone (complex I), antimycin A (complex III), cyanide, carbon monoxide (complex IV), uncoupling dinitrophenols, and agents such as fluoroacetate that interfere with generating ATP upstream in carbohydrate metabolism (glycolysis and the Krebs cycle). The flipside of this coin is the danger of generation of oxygen radicals. It has been known for years that the anticancer anthracyclines such as doxorubicin have limited use due to their cardiac toxicity. Doxorubicin used to generate acute cardiac damage, but protocols have since been adjusted to avoid this result. Anthracyclines appear to cause myofibrillar loss through selectively inhibiting the expression of α-actin, troponin, myosin lightchain 2, and the M isoform of creatine kinase. The generation of ROS and lipid peroxidation through the generation of the semiquinone is not the complete picture, as pathways unrelated to oxygen radical generation have been examined to explain cardiac damage. β-Adrenergic receptors are found in downregulated anthracycline-linked ventricular abnormalities. Increases in macrophage-generated TNFα and IL-2 from monocytes may lead to dilated cardiomyopathy (Shan et al., 1996). Calcium influx may increase apoptosis and necrosis. Autophagy and senescence appear as other possible influences in chronic doxorubicin toxicity (Zhang et al., 2009). The use of an ionophore antibiotic in the dairy and beef industry has led to myocardial necrosis due to impaired mitochondrial function induced by abnormal movement of sodium, potassium, and calcium into muscle cells (Divers et al., 2009). It is of interest that the androgen–androgen receptor system plays an important role in cardiac growth, remodeling after angiotensin II's adverse effects, and protection against doxorubicin cardiotoxicity. This protective effect of testosterone was illustrated by upregulation of the mitochondrial transcription factor A and phosphorylation of the serine-threonine kinase in normal mice as contrasted with much decreased transcription and prominent vacuole formation in mitochondria of androgen receptor knockout mice treated with doxorubicin. This leads to increased apoptosis of cardiomyocytes (Ikeda et al., 2010). Anthracyclines are not at all tolerated in children. Other cancer chemotherapy agents also increase the cardiotoxicity of doxorubicin with mechanisms distinct from anthracyclines. The anti-HER2 antibody Trastuzumab prevents the heart from using particular survival factors to resist toxic stressors. Paclitaxel interferes with microtubule disassembly and causes more toxic anthracycline metabolites to form (Gianni et al., 2007). The antiretroviral medication AZT (zidovudine) also generates cardiomyopathy via mitochondrial oxidative stress and is attenuated in mice genetically engineered to overexpress mitochondrial superoxide dismutase or mitochondria-targeted catalase (Kohler et al., 2009).

Ethanol is another agent whose chronic use has led to heart disease. A controversy existed for years whether the ethanol itself or the dietary deficiencies generated by alcoholism damaged the muscle. Biopsies of human patients indicated that skeletal muscle injury or myopathy and cardiomyopathy were indeed directly linked to ethanol's direct action rather than to dietary deficiencies (Fernández-Solà et al., 1994). Although ethanol is known to generate lipid peroxidation during metabolism, apoptotic mechanisms again figure centrally in its chronic generation of dilated cardiomyopathy (Fernández-Solà et al., 2006). Both hypoxic agents and pro-oxidative compounds including acetaldehyde, azide, cocaine, doxorubicin, and monocrotaline can generate cardiac hypertrophy as a result of chronic toxicity. Agents known as model hypertrophy-inducing agents are angiotensin II, catecholamines, and endothelin 1. G-protein activation, increases in Ca^{2+} signaling, stimulated phosphoinositide-3-kinase activity, specific constituents of the protein kinase C family, and the three mitogen-activated protein kinases (MAPKs—ERKs, p38, and c-Jun N-terminal kinases) appear to be responsible for hypertrophic responses (Chen et al., 2001). The effects of cigarette smoking have focused mainly on the vascular damage. However, passive smoke inhalation leads to cardiac remodeling likely via increased neurohormonal insult, ROS, and increased activity of MAPK (Minicucci et al., 2009).

Notice that when examining some of the toxicants, increasing adrenergic activity damages the myocardium. This damage has been linked to multiple factors for some time, including hypoxia (especially microcirculation effects), calcium overload, and toxic catecholamine oxidation products (Rona, 1985). Isoproterenol (a β_1 and β_2 adrenergic agonist) represents catecholamines that cause a loss of sarcolemmal integrity through decreased dystrophin (part of the dystrophin–glycoprotein complex that along with integrins is part of the contractile and extracellular structure of the cell joining actin and laminin) leading to ischemia (Campos et al., 2008). In the same light, stimulants such as methamphetamine can cause relatively reversible cardiomyopathy or more irreversible myocyte hypertrophy and fibrosis (Lopez et al., 2009). Even natural stimulatory substances some consider safer, such as caffeine and ephedrine, cause hemorrhagic myocardial necrosis in rats exposed at high doses (Nyska et al., 2005).

Do agents normally associated with liver damage and aryl hydrocarbon receptor activation negatively affect the heart? Some small chlorinate hydrocarbons used as anesthetic agents are discussed later in regard to rhythm disturbances. TCDD and a pentachlorobiphenyl with dioxin-like action cause cardiovascular lesions/cardiomyopathy and chronic active arteritis (Jokinen et al., 2003). Although the exact mechanisms of aryl hydrocarbon receptor activation and cardiotoxicity are not completely clear, it is possible that induction of CYP1A1, 1A2, and 1B1 leads to increased ROS, DNA adducts, and increased pro-inflammatory substances synthesized form arachidonic acid (responsible for prostanoids and leukotrienes; Korashy and El-Kadi, 2006). A smaller chlorinated chemical, bis(2-chloroethyoxy)methane (CEM), that is absorbed through the skin causes myocardial inflammation, myofiber vacuolation, and/or myofiber necrosis. Mitochondrial damage appears central to CEM's toxic action (Nyska et al., 2009). This compound is more similar to ethanol than to the aryl hydrocarbon receptor activators in terms of toxicity, as 2-chloracetaldehyde appears to the cardiotoxic metabolite (2-chloroethyl fragments → 2-chloracetaldehyde + GSH → thiodiglycolic acid; Black et al., 2007).

Certain heavy metals also damage the myocardium. Some are seen to affect rhythm as they act like calcium; these are discussed later. Cobalt was used to keep the head on beer after it was poured, which used to be valued. A "beer drinker's cardiomyopathy" as indicated by the appearance of pericardial effusion, increased hemoglobin, and congestive heart failure appeared in Quebec City, Canada for those who drank heavily of this beverage with the cobalt additive (Barceloux, 1999). Excess iron also causes a cardiomyopathy, whose distribution to the heart appears to be linked to non-transferrin-bound iron, the plasma hepcidin concentration (lower leads to more transfer), the presence of growth differentiation factor 15, and low levels of heme oxygenase (Porter, 2009). Heavy metal toxicity may be elevated by certain infections. Idiopathic dilated cardiomyopathy appears in hearts with significantly increased levels of Hg (22,000-fold higher than normal),

Sb (12,000 × normal), Au (11 × normal), Cr (13 × normal), and Co (4 × normal; Frustaci et al., 1999). Coxsackie B3 virus increased the concentration and toxicity of Cd, Ni, and methylmercury in hearts and inflammatory lesions. Ni and methylmercury appear to alter natural killer cell function and reduce macrophage mobilization directly. Calcium increased and zinc decreased in the heart in response to methylmercury, which may partially explain the severity of the observed lesions (Ilbäck et al., 1995).

Heart Rhythm/Conduction

The heart is not only a muscle; it has its own conduction system and autorhythmic cells that allow it to beat on its own. Note that **Figure 18-2** includes the normal electrocardiogram (ECG) and some agents that have been instrumental in altering heart rhythms. The heart rhythm should originate by sodium entering the pacemaker/autorhythmic cells of the sinoatrial node and bringing the cells to threshold (Na^+ channel can be blocked by tetrodotoxin and saxitoxin or by the tricyclic antidepressants). Altering the sodium channel can have a variety of arrhythmic consequences as demonstrated by aconitine and related alkaloids. Aconitine and mesaconitine have high affinity for the open state of the voltage-sensitive sodium channels at site 2 leading to a persistent activation. The channels then become refractory to excitation. This leads to increased force of heart contractions (positive inotropic effect), but is also hypotensive and bradycardic due to stimulation of the ventromedial nucleus of the hypothalamus (decreased quantal release of acetylcholine). However, depending on patient and dose, these toxic alkaloids can lead to bradycardia, sinus tachycardia, ventricular ectopics (extra or skipped beats due to altered conduction system), ventricular tachycardia, and ultimately asystole (no cardiac activity; Chan, 2009). This contributes to the difficulty of characterizing an arrhythmic agent as is done in Table 18-3. An agent may cause most of the arrhythmias listed depending on subject, dose, and other conditions such as ionic balance and other chemicals in the body. The table gives likely outcomes for some agents. However, those that speed the

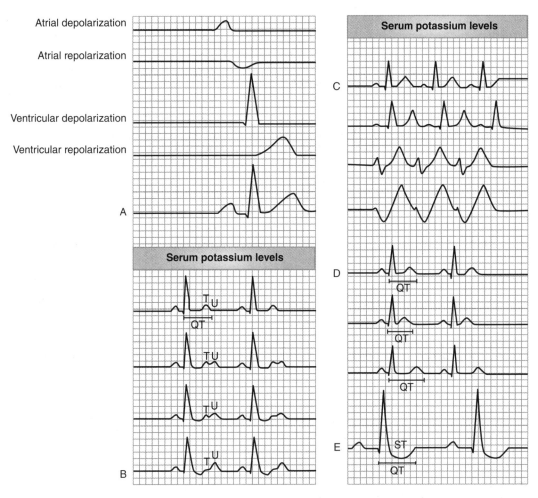

FIGURE 18-2 A. Normal Electrical Activity of the Heart. B. Effect of Low K$^+$ (hypokalemia). C. Effect of Excess K$^+$ (hyperkalemia). D. Effects of low and high Ca^{++}. E. Effect of digitalis.

atria are likely to cause atrial flutter followed by atrial fibrillation where the atria appear to spasm and not contact at all, leading to possible other arrhythmias and blood clots. These supraventricular tachycardias are more likely in people or animals with an anesthetized SA node or atrial ectopic centers in the right side of the heart. Ventricular tachycardias are likely in people or animals with ectopic centers in the ventricles, which override the AV nodal control. Ventricular tachycardia can deteriorate to the apparent spasm of ventricular fibrillation where the ventricles do not contract and blood flow ceases. This leads to rapid hypoxia, asystole, and death if not immediately remedied.

Calcium plays a role in the depolarization of pacemaker cells. External calcium enters these cells to depolarize them fully. Potassium efflux then repolarizes the cells. The ECG is the most sensitive way of determining the agents that damage the myocardium (e.g., ischemia elevates the ST interval off baseline), the causes of conduction problems (e.g., heart block and the PR interval), and the diagnosis of other dysrhythmias. Other signs of cardiac toxicity may be assessed by cardiac enzymes in the plasma (creatine phosphokinase), the appearance of the protein troponin, blood pressure monitoring, oximeter readings, and cardiac output determination. Altering external ion concentrations—especially calcium concentrations and potassium concentrations—and poisoning the $3Na^+,2K^+$-ATPase with digitalis from the foxglove plant, for example, lead to arrhythmias as indicated in Figure 18-2 Arrhythmias similar to the hyperkalemia induced by digitalis are noted with cardiotoxic cardenolides such as neriifolin transmitted to humans of New Caledonia via the double-lethal coconut crab (*Birgus latro* L.), which consumes *Cerbera manghas* fruit (Maillaud et al., 2010). Spironolactone and similar potassium-sparing diuretics, angiotensin-converting enzyme (ACE) inhibitors, and renal toxicants/aging can cause hyperkalemia with a widened QRS merging with the T wave to produce a curve resembling a sine wave. At 7.5 mEq K^+/L may generate cardiac standstill or ventricular fibrillation at 10–12 mEq/L. Thiazide and loop diuretics, antibiotics/antifungal compounds (carbenicillin, gentamicin, amphotericin B), licorice (glycyrrhetinic acid) along with emetics (vomiting), agents that cause dehydration (ethanol and caffeine) usually deplete potassium and can lead to hypokalemia with accompanying widening of the QRS complex, ST segment depression, T wave flattening, and enhanced U wave that may fuse with the T wave. Various "missed" beats and various types of arrhythmias result with low potassium levels. The contractile potentials in the myocardial cells use sodium to depolarize calcium to maintain a plateau as K^+ efflux starts. Then, as calcium channels close, potassium efflux continues to repolarize the contractile cells of the heart (Martin and Furnas, 1997). Ventricular fibrillation leading to death has been reported for people with quinine infusion for malaria (Busari and Busari, 2008).

Before further investigation into subsets of receptors, it is important to examine the channels that are related to cardiac channelopathies; both congenital and induced are indicated in **Figure 18-3**. Altering the flow of sodium and potassium affects all potentials, and here calcium also plays a crucial role in the heart. The heart seems uniquely sensitive to ion imbalances from diet or from medications and other toxic substances. Many medications can alter the ECG, occasionally with fatal consequences. Some conditions are congenital and do not require drug action such as long QT syndrome and Brugada syndrome. Long QT syndrome leads to sudden death and is caused by a malfunctioning or blocked delayed rectifier current of the heart, I_{Kr}. Expression of the Human Ether-a-go-go (named after flies shaking following ether anesthesia) Related Gene (*hERG*, an inwardly rectifying potassium channel coding gene) generates this current as modulated by *MiRP1*. Congenital long QT results from mutations of either gene producing or modulating the current and is produced by medications as torsades de pointes (formerly known as associated with non-sustained polymorphic ventricular tachycardia) that are I_{Kr} blockers. The activity of the frequently used antiarrhythmic medication amiodarone (following an MI) is toward inhibition of the hERG channel. Amiodarone's cytotoxicity results from changes noted in the mitochondria (altered mitochondrial membrane potential; Waldhauser et al., 2008). Various divalent metal cations also affect the E-4031-sensitive repolarization current (I_{Kr}) in rabbit ventricular myocytes. Cd^{2+}, Co^{2+}, Mn^{2+}, and Ni^{2+} shift the I_{Kr} activation curve to the right along the voltage axis, augment the maximum amplitude of I_{Kr}, and increase the speed of the current kinetics of I_{Kr}. Ca^{2+}, Mg^{2+}, and Sr^{2+} do not appreciably influence I_{Kr}, and Zn^{2+} or Ba^{2+} blocks I_{Kr} (Paquette et al., 1998). The influence of many conditions that cause arrhythmias may, therefore, originate from disturbances in K^+ homeostasis, which draws together what has already been mentioned for hypokalemia (due to increased $3Na+,2K+$-ATPase activity caused by β_2 agonists, theophylline, insulin shock; Ba^{2+} or chloroquine block of K^+ channels, GI losses of K^+, or alkalosis) and hyperkalemia (due to digitalis's inhibition of $3Na+,2K+$-ATPase, increased absorption of K^+ salts, inhibited metabolism [CN^-], activated K^+ channels [Fl^-], or acidosis with rhabdomyolysis, especially if this generates severe kidney damage; Bradberry and Vale, 1995). Tl^+ has been shown to cause arrhythmias based on its action at the SA node, causing either more or less spontaneous beat frequency dependent on the dose (Achenback et al., 1982)—more likely tachycardia based on poisonings reported in the literature (Meggs et al., 1994).

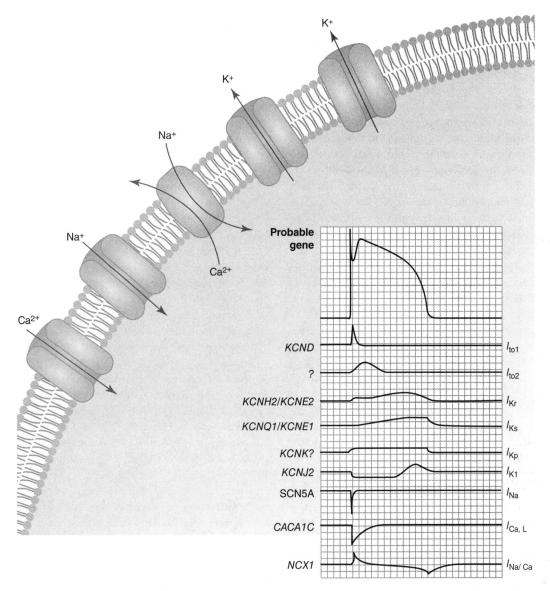

FIGURE 18-3 The Key Ion Channels (and an Electrogenic Transporter) in Cardiac Cells. K⁺ Channels Mediate K⁺ Efflux from the Cell; Na⁺ Channels and Ca²⁺ Channels Mediate Na⁺ and Ca²⁺ Influx, Respectively

Hypokalemia, mentioned earlier, increases the QT interval and indeed can augment the ability of certain medications to cause torsades de pointes by fast inactivation of I_{Kr}. The antiarrhythmic drug quinidine was characterized as one of the first medications that potently (low dose and first dose) caused this problem. At higher concentrations, quinidine blocks sodium and calcium currents. Other less potent antiarrhythmic medications (e.g., sotalol, dofetilide) cause torsades de pointes in a dose-dependent manner. Terfenadine is a drug that causes I_{Kr} blockade; its active metabolite is fexofenadine, a relative nontoxic antihistamine. Giving terfenadine with CYP3A4 inhibitors (macrolide antibiotics clarithromycin or erythromycin or azole antifungal agents itraconazole or ketoconazole) clearly augments this medication's cardiac toxicity. Similarly, the gastric prokinetic medication cisapride should not be given with CYP3A4 inhibitors due to QT interval changes induced by I_{Kr} blockade of the parent drug. In the case of an antihistamine withdrawn from the U.S. market, astemizole, one of its active metabolites blocks I_{Kr}. The antipsychotic agent thioridazine also blocks this current, especially with CYP2D6 inhibitors such as quinidine (unlikely combination) or more likely the SSRIs and tricyclic antidepressants. Other conditions increase the risk of torsades de pointes by reducing the net repolarizing current, such as being female, rapid intravenous injection of a medication, recent electrical conversion from atrial fibrillation, hypomagnesemia, and congestive heart failure or cardiac hypertrophy (Roden, 2001). As odd as some of these factors sound, they have relationships to the potassium current. For instance, testosterone and less so progesterone suppress $I_{ca,L}$ and increase I_{Kr} resulting in a greater repolarization reserve. Estrogen has an opposing influence, possibly explaining altered sensitivity to drug-induced torsades de pointes during the menstrual period (Jonsson et al., 2010). This indicates that hormones can represent arrhythmia-inducing toxicants or at least synergizing agents. This includes oral antidiabetic medications, drugs that treat hyperlipidemias/obesity, somatostatin analogues, thyroid effectors, and adrenal steroids (Gonzalez et al., 2010). Organophosphates that raise central and peripheral cholinergic activity result in QT interval prolongation followed by late-onset ventricular tachycardia. Following recovery from the acute effects of organophosphate poisoning, asystole can occur (Chacko and Elangovan, 2010). Cancer patients are highly prone to fatal arrhythmic episodes based on the electrolyte imbalances, starvation, and medications utilized. Especially problematic are the platinum compounds and anthracyclines, which cause QTc alterations. Other ECG disturbances with fluorouracil have been observed as bradyarrhythmias and tachyarrhythmias with taxanes (Bagnes et al., 2010).

Cardiac arrhythmias can occur with ion channelopathies or malignant arrhythmias from ventricular hypertrophy. Key channels of abnormalities or toxicant-induced changes are the ryanodine receptor-calcium release channel complex (RyR)2, FK-506 binding protein (FKBP 12.6), cardiac sarcoplasmic reticulum calcium ATPase (SERCA2a), and phospholamban (PLB). These proteins give a sense of what factors lead to arrhythmias as well as targets for antiarrhythmic medications (Dai, 2005). Heightened myofilament Ca^{2+} sensitivity is the basis of many cardiomyopathies and cardiac/ventricular arrhythmias (Huke and Knollmann, 2010).

Halogenated hydrocarbons obtund the SA node and cause AV node autorhythmicity (Bazaugour et al., 1974). Ethanol was considered a primitive anesthetic agent and causes sinus node automaticity in naïve rats (positive chronotropic effect = increased heart rate; Carpentier and Gallardo-Carpentier, 1987). Both of these agents make the presence of amphetamine or other sympathomimetic amines yield more tachyarrhythmias. Taxines are toxic alkaloids of the yew plant that block sodium and calcium channels and produce ventricular tachycardia (Panzeri et al., 2010), and at high doses they can cause the heart to stop in diastole. Atrial flutter (supraventricular arrhythmia) results from a catecholaminergic storm following scorpion envenomization. Heart damage may ensue due to adrenergic myocarditis, toxic myocarditis, or myocardial ischemia (Deman et al., 2009). Simple stimulants such as caffeine can lead to atrial tachycardia, as can blockade of muscarinic receptors with atropine (Bogan et al., 2009). Clearly, some potent stimulants such as methamphetamine are capable of generating tachycardia and other atrial and ventricular arrhythmias and myocardial ischemia (Islam et al., 2009). Cocaine and other drugs of abuse affect the heart rate and rhythm severely, as can withdrawal from drug dependence. A rodenticide, aluminum phosphide, causes a toxic myocarditis that can lead to sudden death via Brugada syndrome. Brugada syndrome is an inherited autosomal-dominant trait with a characteristic ECG pattern of ST-segment elevations in leads V_1 through V_3, as well as right bundle branch block and T wave inversion (Nayyar and Nair, 2009).

It is clear from this section and the prevalence of heart disease as the number one killer of humans in Western societies that cardiotoxicity is a genuine problem, especially in obese populations with attendant problems of hypertension and diabetes mellitus. Add smoking and heavy alcohol consumption to the list and cardiovascular damage is assumed in a large portion of the population. Coupled to this are legal and illegal drug use, which increase cardiac and vascular damage. Air pollution and stress are also aggravating factors in cardiovascular diseases. As people live longer, diseases of aging require aggressive treatments that carry high cardiovascular risk (damage to the vasculature, especially for injection of chemotherapy and cardiac damage/arrhythmia). Western society has become the largest ongoing experiment for cardiovascular toxicity; therefore, it appears unnecessary for this section to provide toxicity tests, despite the myocyte and node cultures used to assess the action of certain medications and other toxic substances indicated in the references cited in this section. ECG and clinical chemistry provide adequate information on living animals and humans, while autopsy allows for investigation of fatal reactions.

Questions

1. What differentiates anemia caused by Pb poisoning from straight Fe deficiency?
2. How is methemoglobin formed from nitrate poisoning, and how might this be different from other anemias?
3. Why are amino acid alterations in the chains of hemoglobin and subsequent metHb formation an indication of mutation rather than an oxidant toxicant?
4. How does pancytopenia (aplastic anemia) occur?
5. How is high-concentration, acute CO poisoning different from low-concentration, chronic CO poisoning?
6. What is the mechanism of CN poisoning? Does it involve hemoglobin?
7. What is the signaling mechanism for porphyria (overproduction of heme precursors)?
8. Arsenic can cause thrombocytopenia. How would that be diagnosed by a functional assay and also a blood test to confirm the presence of As?

9. What vascular structure rich in protein is responsible for uptake of organic pollutants and mediation of inflammation?
10. Why can damage to the vascular endothelium either increase or lower blood pressure as occurs with Pb or oxidative stress?
11. Why are particles so likely to induce vasoconstriction, especially nanoparticles?
12. What are shallower versus deeper factors signaling vascular toxicity?
13. How can hypoxia in the heart when reversed cause oxidant injury?
14. How can chronic stress and use of stimulants to stay awake damage the heart?
15. How can digitalis poisoning be distinguished from spironolactone poisoning?

References

Abreo K, Jangula J, Jain SK, Sella M, Glass J. 1991. Aluminum uptake and toxicity in cultured mouse hepatocytes. *J Am Soc Nephrol.* 1:1299–1304.

Achenbach C, Wiemer J, Ziskoven R, Winter U. 1982. Tl+-ions: effects on the automaticity of sinoatrial tissue and dV/dtmax and iK2 of cardiac Purkinje fibres. *Z Naturforsch C.* 37:1006–1014.

Airoldi M, Fantasia R, Aloigi-Luzzi D, Stefanetti C, Deserò D, Chiodini E, Gobbi A. 1987. [Macrocytosis, megaloblastosis and folate status in chronic alcoholics]. *Minerva Med.* 78:739–743.

Alexander J. 2007. Selenium. *Novartis Found Symp.* 282:143–149; discussion 149–153, 212–218.

Alonso JR, Cardellach F, López S, Casademont J, Miró O. 2003. Carbon monoxide specifically inhibits cytochrome c oxidase of human mitochondrial respiratory chain. *Pharmacol Toxicol.* 93:142–146.

Aneja R, Dass SK, Chandra R. 2003. Modulatory influence of tin-protoporphyrin on gossypol-induced alterations of heme oxygenase activity in male Wistar rats. *Eur J Drug Metab Pharmacokinet.* 28:237–243.

Aronoff DM, Ballard JD. 2009. *Clostridium sordellii* toxic shock syndrome. *Lancet Infect Dis.* 9:725–726.

Ayhanci A, Yaman S, Sahinturk V, Uyar R, Bayramoglu G, Senturk H, Altuner Y, Appak S, Gunes S. 2010. Protective effect of seleno-L-methionine on cyclophosphamide-induced urinary bladder toxicity in rats. *Biol Trace Elem Res.* 134:98–108.

Bagnes C, Panchuk PN, Recondo G. 2010. Antineoplastic chemotherapy induced QTc prolongation. *Curr Drug Saf.* 5:93–96.

Balakumar P, Kaur J. 2009. Is nicotine a key player or spectator in the induction and progression of cardiovascular disorders? *Pharmacol Res.* 60:361–368.

Baluna R, Vitetta ES. 1997. Vascular leak syndrome: a side effect of immunotherapy. *Immunopharmacology.* 37:117–132.

Barceloux DG. 1999. Cobalt. *J Toxicol Clin Toxicol.* 37:201–206.

Baud FJ. 2007. Cyanide: critical issues in diagnosis and treatment. *Hum Exp Toxicol.* 26:191–201.

Bazaugour R, Ollagnier M, Evreux JC, Perrot E, Michel AJ, Faucon G. 1974. [Effects of some anesthetic halogenated hydrocarbons on various levels of cardiac automatism]. *Anesth Analg (Paris).* 31:411–417.

Black SR, Decosta KS, Patel PR, Mathews JM. 2007. [14C]bis(2-chloroethoxy)methane: comparative absorption, distribution, metabolism and excretion in rats and mice. *Xenobiotica.* 37:427–440.

Bogan R, Zimmermann T, Zilker T, Eyer F, Thiermann H. 2009. Plasma level of atropine after accidental ingestion of *Atropa belladonna. Clin Toxicol (Phila).* 47:602–604.

Bradberry SM, Vale JA. 1995. Disturbances of potassium homeostasis in poisoning. *J Toxicol Clin Toxicol.* 33:295–310.

Brito MA, Silva RF, Brites D. 2002, Bilirubin induces loss of membrane lipids and exposure of phosphatidylserine in human erythrocytes. *Cell Biol Toxicol.* 18:181–192.

Brocker C, Lassen N, Estey T, Pappa A, Cantore M, Orlova VV, Chavakis T, Kavanagh KL, Oppermann U, Vasiliou V. 2010. Aldehyde dehydrogenase 7A1 (ALDH7A1) is a novel enzyme involved in cellular defense against hyperosmotic stress. *J Biol Chem.* 285:18452–18463.

Brott D, Gould S, Jones H, Schofield J, Prior H, Valentin JP, Bjurstrom S, Kenne K, Schuppe-Koistinen I, Katein A, Foster-Brown L, Betton G, Richardson R, Evans G, Louden C. 2005. Biomarkers of drug-induced vascular injury. *Toxicol Appl Pharmacol.* 207(2 Suppl):441–445.

Brown RG. 1991. Determining the cause of anemia. General approach, with emphasis on microcytic hypochromic anemias. *Postgrad Med.* 89:161–164, 167–170.

Bucher J. 2007. NTP toxicity studies of sodium dichromate dihydrate (CAS No. 7789-12-0) administered in drinking water to male and female F344/N rats and B6C3F1 mice and male BALB/c and am3-C57BL/6 mice. *Toxic Rep Ser.* (72):1–G4.

Bukowska B, Kowalska S. 2004. Phenol and catechol induce prehemolytic and hemolytic changes in human erythrocytes. *Toxicol Lett.* 152:73–84.

Busari O, Busari O. 2008. Ventricular fibrillation in a 5-year-old child on therapeutic dose of quinine dihydrochloride infusion for acute malaria. *J Natl Med Assoc.* 100:1063–1065.

Campos EC, Romano MM, Prado CM, Rossi MA. 2008. Isoproterenol induces primary loss of dystrophin in rat hearts: correlation with myocardial injury. *Int J Exp Pathol.* 89:367–381.

Carpentier RG, Gallardo-Carpentier A. 1987. Acute and chronic effects of ethanol on sinoatrial electrophysiology in the rat heart. *J Cardiovasc Pharmacol.* 10:616–621.

Chacko J, Elangovan A. 2010. Late onset, prolonged asystole following organophosphate poisoning: a case report. *J Med Toxicol.* 6:311–314.

Chan TY. 2009. Aconite poisoning. *Clin Toxicol (Phila).* 47:279–285.

Chatfield MJ, La Mar GN. 1992. 1H nuclear magnetic resonance study of the prosthetic group in sulfhemoglobin. *Arch Biochem Biophys.* 295:289–296.

Chen J. 2005. Animal models for acquired bone marrow failure syndromes. *Clin Med Res.* 3:102–108.

Chen QM, Tu VC, Purdon S, Wood J, Dilley T. 2001. Molecular mechanisms of cardiac hypertrophy induced by toxicants. *Cardiovasc Toxicol.* 1:267–283.

Cherla RP, Lee SY, Tesh VL. 2003. Shiga toxins and apoptosis. *FEMS Microbiol Lett.* 228:159–166.

Chu L, Ebersole JL, Holt SC. 1999. Hemoxidation and binding of the 46-kDa cystalysin of Treponema denticola leads to a cysteine-dependent hemolysis of human erythrocytes. *Oral Microbiol Immunol.* 14:293–303.

Churin AA, Gol'dberg VE, Karpova GV, Voronova OL, Feodorova EP, Kolotova OV, Skurikhin EG, Pershina OV. 2008. Reaction of bone marrow hematopoiesis to the toxic effect of paclitaxel. *Bull Exp Biol Med.* 145:213–217.

Cines DB, Bussel JB, McMillan RB, Zehnder JL. 2004. Congenital and acquired thrombocytopenia. *Hematology Am Soc Hematol Educ Program.* 2004:390–406. [Erratum in: *Hematology Am Soc Hematol Educ Program.* 2005:543. Dosage error in article text.]

Dai DZ. 2005. Two patterns of ion channelopathy in the myocardium: perspectives for development of anti-arrhythmic agents. *Curr Opin Investig Drugs.* 6:289–297.

Deman AL, Lerecouvreux M, Miandrisoa MR, Klein I, Romain H, Dubourdieu D, David S, Deroche J, Berbari H, Heno P. 2009. [Cardiac damage due to scorpion envenomation: case involving atrial flutter]. *Med Trop (Mars).* 69:309–310.

Dhananjayan V, Muralidharan S, Jayanthi P. 2011. Distribution of persistent organochlorine chemical residues in blood plasma of three species of vultures from India. *Environ Monit Assess.* 173:803–811.

Dickers KJ, Bradberry SM, Rice P, Griffiths GD, Vale JA. 2003. Abrin poisoning. *Toxicol Rev.* 22:137–142.

Divers TJ, Kraus MS, Jesty SA, Miller AD, Mohammed HO, Gelzer AR, Mitchell LM, Soderholm LV,

Ducharme NG. 2009. Clinical findings and serum cardiac troponin I concentrations in horses after intragastric administration of sodium monensin. *J Vet Diagn Invest.* 21:338–343.

Doll DC, Yarbro JW. 1994. Vascular toxicity associated with chemotherapy and hormonotherapy. *Curr Opin Oncol.* 6:345–350.

Downey DC. 1999. Porphyria and chemicals. *Med Hypotheses.* 53:166–171.

Editorial. 1970. Tobacco amblyopia. *Can Med Assoc J.* 102:420.

El-Sayed MS. 2001. Adverse effects of alcohol ingestion post exercise on blood rheological variables during recovery. *Clin Hemorheol Microcirc.* 24:227–232.

Evelyn KA, Malloy HT. 1938. Microdetermination of oxyhemoglobin, methemoglobin and sulfhemoglobin in a single sample of blood. *J. Biol. Chem.* 126:655–662.

Fernández-Solà J, Estruch R, Grau JM, Pare JC, Rubin E, Urbano-Marquez A. 1994. The relation of alcoholic myopathy to cardiomyopathy. *Ann Intern Med.* 120:529–536.

Fernández-Solà J, Fatjó F, Sacanella E, Estruch R, Bosch X, Urbano-Márquez A, Nicolás JM. 2006. Evidence of apoptosis in alcoholic cardiomyopathy. *Hum Pathol.* 37:1100–1110.

Fertman MH, Fertman MB. 1955. Toxic anemias and Heinz bodies. *Medicine (Baltimore).* 34:131–192.

Frustaci A, Magnavita N, Chimenti C, Caldarulo M, Sabbioni E, Pietra R, Cellini C, Possati GF, Maseri A. 1999. Marked elevation of myocardial trace elements in idiopathic dilated cardiomyopathy compared with secondary cardiac dysfunction. *J Am Coll Cardiol.* 33:1578–1583.

Fuortes LJ, Weismann DN, Graeff ML, Bale JF Jr, Tannous R, Peters C. 1995. Immune thrombocytopenia and elemental mercury poisoning. *J Toxicol Clin Toxicol.* 33:449–455.

Furie B, Trubowitz S. 1976. Insecticides and blood dyscrasias. Chlordane exposure and self-limited refractory megaloblastic anemia. *JAMA.* 235:1720–1722.

George Priya Doss C, Rao S. 2009. Impact of single nucleotide polymorphisms in HBB gene causing haemoglobinopathies: in silico analysis. *N Biotechnol.* 25:214–219.

Gianni L, Salvatorelli E, Minotti G. 2007. Anthracycline cardiotoxicity in breast cancer patients: synergism with trastuzumab and taxanes. *Cardiovasc Toxicol.* 7:67–71.

Gonzalez CD, de Sereday M, Sinay I, Santoro S. 2010. Endocrine therapies and QTc prolongation. *Curr Drug Saf.* 5:79–84.

Gori T, Parker JD. 2008. Nitrate-induced toxicity and preconditioning: a rationale for reconsidering the use of these drugs. *J Am Coll Cardiol.* 52:251–254.

Goubern M, Andriamihaja M, Nübel T, Blachier F, Bouillaud F. 2007. Sulfide, the first inorganic substrate for human cells. *FASEB J.* 21:1699–1706.

Guidry JR, Raschke RA, Morkunas AR. 1991. Toxic effects of drugs used in the ICU. Anticoagulants and thrombolytics. Risks and benefits. *Crit Care Clin.* 7:533–554.

Gulya K, Dave JR, Hoffman PL. 1991. Chronic ethanol ingestion decreases vasopressin mRNA in hypothalamic and extrahypothalamic nuclei of mouse brain. *Brain Res.* 557:129–135.

Gutiérrez JM, Escalante T, Rucavado A. 2009. Experimental pathophysiology of systemic alterations induced by *Bothrops asper* snake venom. *Toxicon.* 54:976–987.

Hecquet CM, Malik AB. 2009. Role of H_2O_2-activated TRPM2 calcium channel in oxidant-induced endothelial injury. *Thromb Haemost.* 101:619–625.

Hong IH, Kwon TE, Lee SK, Park JK, Ki MR, Park SI, Jeong KS. 2011. Fetal death of dogs after the ingestion of a soil conditioner. *Exp Toxicol Pathol.* 63(1–2):113–117.

Houston MC. 2007. The role of mercury and cadmium heavy metals in vascular disease, hypertension, coronary heart disease, and myocardial infarction. *Altern Ther Health Med.* 13:S128–S133.

Huke S, Knollmann BC. 2010. Increased myofilament Ca2+-sensitivity and arrhythmia susceptibility. *J Mol Cell Cardiol.* 48:824–833.

Ikeda Y, Aihara KI, Akaike M, Sato T, Ishikawa K, Ise T, Yagi S, Iwase T, Ueda Y, Yoshida S, Azuma H, Walsh K, Tamaki T, Kato S, Matsumoto T. 2010. Androgen receptor counteracts doxorubicin-induced cardiotoxicity in male mice. *Mol Endocrinol.* 24:1338–1348.

Ilbäck NG, Lindh U, Fohlman J, Friman G. 1995. New aspects of murine coxsackie B3 myocarditis—focus on heavy metals. *Eur Heart J.* 16(Suppl O):20–24.

Inomata K, Tanaka H. 2003. Protective effect of benidipine against sodium azide-induced cell death in cultured neonatal rat cardiac myocytes. *J Pharmacol Sci.* 93:163–170.

Ishizuka M, Tanikawa T, Tanaka KD, Heewon M, Okajima F, Sakamoto KQ, Fujita S. 2008. Pesticide resistance in wild mammals—mechanisms of anticoagulant resistance in wild rodents. *J Toxicol Sci.* 33:283–291.

Islam MN, Khan J, Jaafar H. 2009. Leave methamphetamine to be alive—Part II. *Leg Med (Tokyo).* 11(Suppl 1):S143–S146.

Jandl JH, Engle LK, Allen DW. 1960. Oxidative hemolysis and precipitation of hemoglobin. I. Heinz body anemias as an acceleration of red cell aging. *J Clin Invest.* 39:1818–1836.

Jeffrey AM, Williams GM. 2005. Risk assessment of DNA-reactive carcinogens in food. *Toxicol Appl Pharmacol.* 207(2 Suppl):628–635.

Jokinen MP, Walker NJ, Brix AE, Sells DM, Haseman JK, Nyska A. 2003. Increase in cardiovascular pathology in female Sprague-Dawley rats following chronic treatment with 2,3,7,8-tetrachlorodibenzo-p-dioxin and 3,3',4,4',5-pentachlorobiphenyl. *Cardiovasc Toxicol*. 3:299–310.

Jonsson MK, Vos MA, Duker G, Demolombe S, van Veen TA. 2010. Gender disparity in cardiac electrophysiology: implications for cardiac safety pharmacology. *Pharmacol Ther*. 127:9–18.

Kanias T, Acker JP. 2010. Biopreservation of red blood cells—the struggle with hemoglobin oxidation. *FEBS J*. 277:343–356.

Kappers MH, van Esch JH, Sleijfer S, Danser AH, van den Meiracker AH. 2009. Cardiovascular and renal toxicity during angiogenesis inhibition: clinical and mechanistic aspects. *J Hypertens*. 27:2297–2309.

Klauder DS, Petering HG. 1977. Anemia of lead intoxication: a role for copper. *J Nutr*. 107:1779–1785.

Kohler JJ, Cucoranu I, Fields E, Green E, He S, Hoying A, Russ R, Abuin A, Johnson D, Hosseini SH, Raper CM, Lewis W. 2009. Transgenic mitochondrial superoxide dismutase and mitochondrially targeted catalase prevent antiretroviral-induced oxidative stress and cardiomyopathy. *Lab Invest*. 89:782–790.

Korashy HM, El-Kadi AO. 2006. The role of aryl hydrocarbon receptor in the pathogenesis of cardiovascular diseases. *Drug Metab Rev*. 38:411–450.

Kumana CR, Ng M, Lin HJ, Ko W, Wu PC, Todd D. 1985. Herbal tea induced hepatic veno-occlusive disease: quantification of toxic alkaloid exposure in adults. *Gut*. 26:101–104.

La Mantia L, Mascoli N, Milanese C. 2007. Azathioprine. Safety profile in multiple sclerosis patients. *Neurol Sci*. 28:299–303.

Lanari LC, Rosset S, González ME, Liria N, de Roodt AR. 2010. A study on the venom of *Bothrops alternatus* Duméril, Bibron and Duméril, from different regions of Argentina. *Toxicon*. 55:1415–1424.

Laterza OF, Lim L, Garrett-Engele PW, Vlasakova K, Muniappa N, Tanaka WK, Johnson JM, Sina JF, Fare TL, Sistare FD, Glaab WE. 2009. Plasma MicroRNAs as sensitive and specific biomarkers of tissue injury. *Clin Chem*. 55:1977–1983.

LeBlanc AJ, Cumpston JL, Chen BT, Frazer D, Castranova V, Nurkiewicz TR. 2009. Nanoparticle inhalation impairs endothelium-dependent vasodilation in subepicardial arterioles. *J Toxicol Environ Health A*. 72:1576–1584.

Lisiewicz J. 1993. Immunotoxic and hematotoxic effects of occupational exposures. *Folia Med Cracov*. 34:29–47.

Lopez JE, Yeo K, Caputo G, Buonocore M, Schaefer S. 2009. Recovery of methamphetamine associated cardiomyopathy predicted by late gadolinium

enhanced cardiovascular magnetic resonance. *J Cardiovasc Magn Reson*. 11:46.

Lord MJ, Jolliffe NA, Marsden CJ, Pateman CS, Smith DC, Spooner RA, Watson PD, Roberts LM. 2003. Ricin. Mechanisms of cytotoxicity. *Toxicol Rev*. 22:53–64.

Maillaud C, Lefebvre S, Sebat C, Barguil Y, Cabalion P, Cheze M, Hnawia E, Nour M, Durand F. 2010. Double lethal coconut crab (*Birgus latro* L.) poisoning. *Toxicon*. 55:81–86.

Majkova Z, Toborek M, Hennig B. 2010. The role of caveolae in endothelial cell dysfunction with a focus on nutrition and environmental toxicants. *J Cell Mol Med*. 14:2359–2370.

Mallat Z, Tedgui A. 2000. Apoptosis in the vasculature: mechanisms and functional importance. *Br J Pharmacol*. 130:947–962.

Marbán E. 2002. Cardiac channelopathies. *Nature*. 415:213–218.

Martin CM, Furnas MD. 1997. Identifying drug-induced changes in electrocardiogram results of elderly individuals. *Consult Pharm*. 12:37-48.

Matsumoto G, Nakagawa NK, Vieira RP, Mauad T, da Silva LF, de André CD, Carvalho-Oliveira R, Saldiva PH, Garcia ML. 2010. The time course of vasoconstriction and endothelin receptor A expression in pulmonary arterioles of mice continuously exposed to ambient urban levels of air pollution. *Environ Res*. 110:237–243.

Mazaira S. 2008. [Haematological adverse effects caused by psychiatric drugs]. *Vertex*. 19:378–386.

McCully KS. 2009. Chemical pathology of homocysteine. IV. Excitotoxicity, oxidative stress, endothelial dysfunction, and inflammation. *Ann Clin Lab Sci*. 39:219–232.

McGrath JP. 1993. Assessment of hemolytic and hemorrhagic anemias in preclinical safety assessment studies. *Toxicol Pathol*. 21:158–163.

Meggs WJ, Hoffman RS, Shih RD, Weisman RS, Goldfrank LR. 1994. Thallium poisoning from maliciously contaminated food. *J Toxicol Clin Toxicol*. 32:723–730.

Melley DD, Finney SJ, Elia A, Lagan AL, Quinlan GJ, Evans TW. 2007. Arterial carboxyhemoglobin level and outcome in critically ill patients. *Crit Care Med*. 35:1882–1887.

Minicucci MF, Azevedo PS, Paiva SA, Zornoff LA. 2009. Cardiovascular remodeling induced by passive smoking. *Inflamm Allergy Drug Targets*. 8:334–339.

Møller P, Jacobsen NR, Folkmann JK, Danielsen PH, Mikkelsen L, Hemmingsen JG, Vesterdal LK, Forchhammer L, Wallin H, Loft S. 2010. Role of oxidative damage in toxicity of particulates. *Free Radic Res*. 44:1–46.

Morse BS, Conlan M, Giuliani DG, Nussbaum M. 1980. Mechanism of arsenic-induced inhibition of erythropoiesis in mice. *Am J Hematol*. 8:273–280.

Nayyar S, Nair M. 2009. Brugada pattern in toxic myocarditis due to severe aluminum phosphide poisoning. *Pacing Clin Electrophysiol.* 32:e16–e17.

Nazzal M, Safi F, Arma F, Nazzal M, Muzaffar M, Assaly R. 2011. Micafungin-induced thrombotic thrombocytopenic purpura: a case report and review of the literature. *Am J Ther.* 18:e258–e260.

Nemsadze K, Sanikidze T, Ratiani L, Gabunia L, Sharashenidze T. 2009. Mechanisms of lead-induced poisoning. *Georgian Med News.* (172–173):92–96.

Nyska A, Cunningham M, Snell M, Malarkey D, Sutton D, Dunnick J. 2009. The pivotal role of electron microscopic evaluation in investigation of the cardiotoxicity of bis(2-chloroethoxy)methane in rats and mice. *Toxicol Pathol.* 37:873–877.

Nyska A, Murphy E, Foley JF, Collins BJ, Petranka J, Howden R, Hanlon P, Dunnick JK. 2005. Acute hemorrhagic myocardial necrosis and sudden death of rats exposed to a combination of ephedrine and caffeine. *Toxicol Sci.* 83:388–396.

Organisation for Economic Co-operation and Development, Nuclear Energy Agency. 2003. Chapter V: Health impact. In: *Chernobyl: Assessment of radiological and health impact. 2002 Update of Chernobyl: Ten Years On.* https://www.nea.fr/rp/reports/2003/nea3508-chernobyl.pdf.

Olson KN, Hillyer MA, Kloss JS, Geiselhart RJ, Apple FS. 2010. Accident or arson: is CO-oximetry reliable for carboxyhemoglobin measurement postmortem? *Clin Chem.* 56:515–519.

Opatrny L, Prichard R, Snell L, Maclean JD. 2005. Death related to albendazole-induced pancytopenia: case report and review. *Am J Trop Med Hyg.* 72:291–294.

Orion E, Matz H, Wolf R. 2005. The life-threatening complications of dermatologic therapies. *Clin Dermatol.* 23:182–192.

Osuna O, Edds GT, Popp JA. 1981. Comparative toxicity of feeding dried urban sludge and an equivalent amount of cadmium to swine. *Am J Vet Res.* 42:1542–1546.

Packer CD, Hornick TR, Augustine SA. 2008. Fatal hemolytic anemia associated with metformin: a case report. *J Med Case Reports.* 2:300.

Panzeri C, Bacis G, Ferri F, Rinaldi G, Persico A, Uberti F, Restani P. 2010. Extracorporeal life support in a severe *Taxus baccata* poisoning. *Clin Toxicol (Phila).* 48:463–465.

Papanikolaou NC, Hatzidaki EG, Belivanis S, Tzanakakis GN, Tsatsakis AM. 2005. Lead toxicity update. A brief review. *Med Sci Monit.* 11:RA329–RA336.

Paquette T, Clay JR, Ogbaghebriel A, Shrier A. 1998. Effects of divalent cations on the E-4031-sensitive repolarization current, I(Kr), in rabbit ventricular myocytes. *Biophys J.* 74:1278–1285.

Parent-Massin D. 2001. Relevance of clonogenic assays in hematotoxicology. *Cell Biol Toxicol.* 17:87–94.

Parton RG, Simons K. 2007. The multiple faces of caveolae. *Nat Rev Mol Cell Biol.* 8:185–194.

Percy MJ, McFerran NV, Lappin TR. 2005. Disorders of oxidised haemoglobin. *Blood Rev.* 19:61–68.

Pliarchopoulou K, Pectasides D. 2010. Late complications of chemotherapy in testicular cancer. *Cancer Treat Rev.* 36:262–267.

Porter JB. 2009. Pathophysiology of transfusional iron overload: contrasting patterns in thalassemia major and sickle cell disease. *Hemoglobin.* 33(Suppl 1):S37–S45.

Pradhan P. 2009. Malarial anaemia and nitric oxide induced megaloblastic anaemia: a review on the causes of malarial anaemia. *J Vector Borne Dis.* 46:100–108.

Prozialeck WC, Edwards JR, Nebert DW, Woods JM, Barchowsky A, Atchison WD. 2008. The vascular system as a target of metal toxicity. *Toxicol Sci.* 102:207–218.

Quinn DK, McGahee SM, Politte LC, Duncan GN, Cusin C, Hopwood CJ, Stern TA. 2009. Complications of carbon monoxide poisoning: a case discussion and review of the literature. *Prim Care Companion J Clin Psychiatry.* 11:74–79.

Ramos KS, Bowes RC 3rd, Ou X, Weber TJ. 1994. Responses of vascular smooth muscle cells to toxic insult: cellular and molecular perspectives for environmental toxicants. *J Toxicol Environ Health.* 43:419–440.

Ramos KS, Moorthy B. 2005. Bioactivation of polycyclic aromatic hydrocarbon carcinogens within the vascular wall: implications for human atherogenesis. *Drug Metab Rev.* 37:595–610.

Rassler B. 2007. The role of catecholamines in formation and resolution of pulmonary oedema. *Cardiovasc Hematol Disord Drug Targets.* 7:27–35.

Rechciński T, Plewka M, Kurpesa M, Kidawa M, Peruga Z, Łopaciński B, Kołaciński Z, Krzemińska-Pakuła M. 2006. [Clinical presentation of ST-elevation acute coronary syndrome in the course of intoxication with megadose of rifampicin. A case report]. *Kardiol Pol.* 64:994–998.

Roden DM. 2001. Pharmacogenetics and drug-induced arrhythmias. *Cardiovasc Res.* 50:224–231.

Rodríguez-Estival J, Martínez-Haro M, Martín-Hernando MA, Mateo R. 2010. Sub-chronic effects of nitrate in drinking water on red-legged partridge (*Alectoris rufa*): oxidative stress and T-cell mediated immune function. *Environ Res.* 110:469–475.

Rona G. 1985. Catecholamine cardiotoxicity. *J Mol Cell Cardiol.* 17:291–306.

Sakai T. 2000. Biomarkers of lead exposure. *Ind Health.* 38:127–142.

Schecter GF, Scott C, True L, Raftery A, Flood J, Mase S. 2010. Linezolid in the treatment of multidrug-resistant tuberculosis. *Clin Infect Dis.* 50:49–55.

Scheiring J, Andreoli SP, Zimmerhackl LB. 2008. Treatment and outcome of Shiga-toxin-associated hemolytic uremic syndrome (HUS). *Pediatr Nephrol.* 23:1749–1760.

Seaman V, Jumaan A, Yanni E, Lewis B, Neyer J, Roda P, Xu M, Hoffman R. 2009. Use of molecular testing to identify a cluster of patients with polycythemia vera in eastern Pennsylvania. *Cancer Epidemiol Biomarkers Prev.* 18:534–540.

Segal R, Shatkovsky P, Milo-Goldzweig I. 1974. On the mechanism of saponin hemolysis—I. Hydrolysis of the glycosidic bond. *Biochem Pharmacol.* 23:973–981.

Seligman PA, Moran PL, Schleicher RB, Crawford ED. 1992. Treatment with gallium nitrate: evidence for interference with iron metabolism in vivo. *Am J Hematol.* 41:232–240.

Shalel S, Streichman S, Marmur A. 2002. The mechanism of hemolysis by surfactants: effect of solution composition. *J Colloid Interface Sci.* 252:66–76.

Shan K, Lincoff AM, Young JB. 1996. Anthracycline-induced cardiotoxicity. *Ann Intern Med.* 125:47–58.

Sharkey LC, DeWitt S, Stockman C. 2006. Neurologic signs and hyperammonemia in a horse with colic. *Vet Clin Pathol.* 35:254–258.

Shiobara Y, Ogra Y, Suzuki KT. 2001. Animal species difference in the uptake of dimethylarsinous acid (DMA(III)) by red blood cells. *Chem Res Toxicol.* 14:1446–1452.

Sontas HB, Dokuzeylu B, Turna O, Ekici H. 2009. Estrogen-induced myelotoxicity in dogs: a review. *Can Vet J.* 50:1054–1058.

Steyn PS. 1995. Mycotoxins, general view, chemistry and structure. *Toxicol Lett.* 82–83:843–851.

Stott WT, Gollapudi BB, Rao KS. 2001. Mammalian toxicity of 1,3-dichloropropene. *Rev Environ Contam Toxicol.* 168:1–42.

Sun S. 2010. Chronic exposure to cereal mycotoxin likely citreoviridin may be a trigger for Keshan disease mainly through oxidative stress mechanism. *Med Hypotheses.* 74:841–842.

Takeuchi M, Yamagishi S. 2009. Involvement of toxic AGEs (TAGE) in the pathogenesis of diabetic vascular complications and Alzheimer's disease. *J Alzheimers Dis.* 16:845–858.

Tang X, Xia Z, Yu J. 2008. An experimental study of hemolysis induced by onion (*Allium cepa*) poisoning in dogs. *J Vet Pharmacol Ther.* 31:143–149.

Tans L, Ansink AC, van Rooij PH, Kleijnen C, Mens JW. 2011. The role of chemo-radiotherapy in the management of locally advanced carcinoma of the Vulva: single institutional experience and review of literature. *Am J Clin Oncol.* 34:22–26.

Taulier A, Levillain P, Lemonnier A. 1987. Determining methemoglobin in blood by zero-crossing-point first-derivative spectrophotometry. *Clin Chem.* 33:1767–1770.

Teusink AC, Hall PD. 2010. Toxicities of gemcitabine in patients with severe hepatic dysfunction. *Ann Pharmacother.* 44:750–754.

Thanacoody HK, Thomas SH. 2005. Tricyclic antidepressant poisoning: cardiovascular toxicity. *Toxicol Rev.* 24:205–214.

Thunell S. 2006. (Far) Outside the box: genomic approach to acute porphyria. *Physiol Res.* 55(Suppl 2):S43–S66.

Tillmann W, Menke J, Schröter W. 1973. The formation of Heinz bodies in ghosts of human erythrocytes of adults and newborn infants. *Klin Wochenschr.* 51:201–203.

Tozman EC, Gottlieb NL. 1987. Adverse reactions with oral and parenteral gold preparations. *Med Toxicol.* 2:177–189.

Troisi GM, Bexton S, Robinson I. 2006. Polyaromatic hydrocarbon and PAH metabolite burdens in oiled common guillemots (*Uria aalge*) stranded on the east coast of England (2001–2002). *Environ Sci Technol.* 40:7938–7943.

Ugburo AO, Ilombu CA, Temiye EO, Fadeyibi IO, Akinolai OI. 2009. Severe idiosyncratic drug reaction (Lyells syndrome) after ingesting dihydroartemisinin. *Niger J Clin Pract.* 12:224–227.

Vanholder R, Colardyn F, De Reuck J, Praet M, Lameire N, Ringoir S. 1981. Diquat intoxication: report of two cases and review of the literature. *Am J Med.* 70:1267–1271.

Waldhauser KM, Brecht K, Hebeisen S, Ha HR, Konrad D, Bur D, Krähenbühl S. 2008. Interaction with the hERG channel and cytotoxicity of amiodarone and amiodarone analogues. *Br J Pharmacol.* 155:585–595.

Wang J, Boerma M, Fu Q, Hauer-Jensen M. 2007. Significance of endothelial dysfunction in the pathogenesis of early and delayed radiation enteropathy. *World J Gastroenterol.* 13:3047–3055.

Wattel F, Favory R, Lancel S, Neviere R, Mathieu D. 2006. [Carbon monoxide and the heart: unequivocal effects?] *Bull Acad Natl Med.* 190:1961–1974; discussion 1974–1975.

Westfall MV, Pasyk KA, Yule DI, Samuelson LC, Metzger JM. 1997. Ultrastructure and cell-cell coupling of cardiac myocytes differentiating in embryonic stem cell cultures. *Cell Motil Cytoskeleton.* 36:43–54.

Winterbourn CC, Carrell RW. 1974. Studies of hemoglobin denaturation and Heinz body formation in the unstable hemoglobins. *J Clin Invest.* 54:678–689.

Wolff RA, Evans DB, Gravel DM, Lenzi R, Pisters PW, Lee JE, Janjan NA, Charnsangavej C, Abbruzzese JL. 2001. Phase I trial of gemcitabine combined with radiation for the treatment of locally advanced pancreatic adenocarcinoma. *Clin Cancer Res*. 7:2246–2253.

Wu C, Kenny MA. 1997. A case of sulfhemoglobinemia and emergency measurement of sulfhemoglobin with an OSM3 CO-oximeter. *Clin Chem*. 43:162–166.

Xiao L, Lin X, Cao J, Wang X, Wu L. 2011. MRI findings in 6 cases of children by inadvertent ingestion of diphenoxylate-atropine. *Eur J Radiol*. 79:432–436.

Yanagisawa H, Miyakoshi Y, Kobayashi K, Sakae K, Kawasaki I, Suzuki Y, Tamura J. 2009. Long-term intake of a high zinc diet causes iron deficiency anemia accompanied by reticulocytosis

and extra-medullary erythropoiesis. *Toxicol Lett*. 191:15–19.

Yoon KH, Ng SC. 2001. Early onset methotrexate-induced pancytopenia and response to G-CSF: a report of two cases. *J Clin Rheumatol*. 7:17–20.

Yu PH. 1998. Deamination of methylamine and angiopathy; toxicity of formaldehyde, oxidative stress and relevance to protein glycoxidation in diabetes. *J Neural Transm Suppl*. 52:201–216.

Zhang YW, Shi J, Li YJ, Wei L. 2009. Cardiomyocyte death in doxorubicin-induced cardiotoxicity. *Arch Immunol Ther Exp (Warsz)*. 57:435–445.

Zwart A. 1993. Spectrophotometry of hemoglobin: various perspectives. *Clin Chem*. 39:1570–1572.

CHAPTER 19

Bone Marrow and Immune Organ Toxicity via Lymphatic and Blood Transport

This is a chapter outline intended to guide and familiarize you with the content to follow.

I. Immunotoxicology

    A. Blood → spleen and bone marrow (origin of immune cells)

        1. Myeloid progenitor cells → dendritic cells (majority of dendritic cells), neutrophils, macrophages, eosinophils, basophils (also origin of erythrocytes and thrombocytes)

        2. Lymphoid progenitor cells → T lymphocytes, B lymphocytes, lymphoid dendritic cells (minority of dendritic cells)

    B. Lymph → nodes, thymus (child)

    C. FDA tests for immunotoxicity—see Figure 19-1

        1. Topical application first test—innate immune defense

        2. Lung/inhalation—allergic reactions

        3. Circulation—immunosuppression

        4. Tiered approach—Tier 1 = immunotoxicity (cell-mediated immunity, humoral immunity, and immunopathology), Tier 2 = defining immune components (delayed-type hypersensitivity models, IgG responses to sheep RBCs, number of splenic B and T cells, macrophage measure of nonspecific immunity, host resistance to bacterial/viral challenge measured by death), Tier 3 = mode of action; also need a developmental immunotoxicity assay

    D. Small chemicals—form haptens to be recognized by binding to proteins/cells

    E. Innate immune defense

        1. Immediate maximal response but results in no immunological memory

        2. Neutrophils, monocytes/macrophages, eosinophils, natural killer cells, basophils

        3. Humoral/secreted responses

            a. Complement system damages membranes of pathogenic organisms and finishes antibody (Ab) response of B cell adaptive immunity

            b. Cytokines recruit immune cells to augment or complete work of mobile macrophages, granulocytes, and natural killer cells—see Table 19-1

                (1) IL-1 indicates a monocyte product that initiates the adaptive immune response

                (2) IL-2 indicates a lymphocyte product that generates cytotoxic T cells and stimulates B cell proliferation

                (3) Cytokines work at pM concentrations—more potent than hormones

                (4) Proinflammatory cytokines are in the IL-1 family; hepatic acute phase proteins are in the IL-6 family

---

CONCEPTUALIZING TOXICOLOGY 19-1

(5) Anti-inflammatory cytokines are in the IL-10 family

(6) Chemokines (CC and CX) stimulate cell migration from blood to tissues

(7) A complex series of cytokines and other proteins signal asthma. Chemokines, IL6, IL4, IL8, and Acyl CoA increase Th2 phenotype and help develop asthma, while IFNγ, Fox-P2, IL2, and iNOS genes are silenced in this process

F. Adaptive immune system—see Figure 19-2

  1. Antigen-dependent and antigen-specific, has lag phase for maximal response, establishes memory or contact with specific antigen

  2. Lymphocytes—establish self versus foreign via class I major histocompatibility complex (MHC)—class I on all nucleated cells in the human, while class II on presenting cells (macrophages, dendritic cells, activated B cells)

    a. Starts when T lymphocytes migrate to thymus → CD4$^+$ T helper cells (bind to class II MHC molecules) and CD8$^+$ pre-cytotoxic cells (bind to class I MHC molecules)

    b. Naïve T0 helper cells recruited by IL-1 secretion of antigen-presenting cell (APC) → T0 becomes Th1 by IL-12 and IL-18 secretions of dendritic cells → Th1 cells secrete IL-2, IFNγ, and lymphotoxin (stimulate CD8$^+$ pre-cytotoxic cells → cytotoxic cells that clear intracellular pathogens via two distinct pathways and produce immunologic memory); Th1 cells express Stat4, Stat1, and T-box transcription factor (maintains T and B cells)—see Figure 19-4 for T cell differentiation

    c. Lymphoid cells secreting IL-4 cause development of Th2 (cause B lymphocytes → antibody-producing plasma cells), upregulation of MHCII and B cell production of IgE (allergy pathway) and clear extracellular organisms; Th2 cells express Gata3; Th1 pathways suppress Th2 pathways and vice versa

    d. TGFβ stimulates development of Treg cells, which maintain immune tolerance and suppress autoimmune reactions

    e. IL-6 prevents T cell differentiation by TGFβ and stimulates Th17 (pathogenic T cell) → -IL-17 → stimulates autoimmune reactions; T17 cells retinoid-related orphan receptor

    f. Regulatory T cells (express Foxp2)

      (1) IL-2 induction → nTreg cells = contact-dependent, antigen-nonspecific and inhibit activation of other T cells

      (2) GFβ stimulates T cell receptor → iTreg cells

      (3) Dendritic cells → IL-10 and TGFβ → T0 → Tr1 → IL-10 → immunosuppression

      (4) Th3 → TGFβ and do not express CD25+ on surface as do other Treg cells

      (5) Memory regulatory T cells found in ovarian tumors, which produce high levels of inflammatory cytokines—subdivided into conventional CCR7$^+$ central memory and the CCR7$^-$ effector memory T cells

    g. Tfh reinforces diagnosis of angioimmunoblastic T cell lymphoma (depending on expression of master regulator transcription factor Bcl6) and provides specialized help to B cells

    h. Th9 (secretes IL-9, IL-10), Th17 (secretes IL-17), and Th22 (secretes IL-22) promote local tissue inflammation while nTreg cells and iTreg cells decrease allergen response

    i. CD28 interaction with B7 ligands → potent positive signal for cytokine synthesis and secretion, clonal expansion, increased survival of T cells, and recruiting B cells

    j. CTLA-4 interaction with B7 ligands → negative signal (ends T cell responses); CLA-4 deficient mice → die from autoimmunity

    k. B cells

      (1) Memory cells

      (2) Plasma cells make humoral antibodies/immunoglobulins (Abs/Igs)

        (a) IgA—entry points of the body (mucosa of respiratory, GI, and urogenital tracts)

        (b) IgD—antigen receptor on B cells

CONCEPTUALIZING TOXICOLOGY 19-1 (*continued*)

(c) IgE—on mast cells and basophils → histamine release → allergic reaction

(d) IgG—majority of Ab-based immunity to pathogens

(e) IgM—precedes IgG response to attack circulating pathogens

G. Effects of toxicants

1. Innate immunity—elimination of barriers to infection—see Table 19-2

a. Chemical/thermal burns, DMSO, changing pH of skin, radiation (including tear ducts and salivary glands)

b. Paralysis of respiratory tract cilia by cigarette smoke

c. Change pH of stomach with proton pump inhibitors and antacids

d. Anti-inflammatory medications such as steroids that can prevent inflammatory barrier and suppress immunity internally depend on dose and route of administration; physiological barriers may also be affected such as interferon for inducing antiviral protection of uninfected cells, complement lysis of microorganisms and facilitation of phagocytosis, Toll-like receptors for recognition of foreign molecules such as the lipopolysaccharide (LPS) on gram-negative bacteria and stimulate cell to release immunostimulatory cytokines; surfactant collectins disturb microbial cell wall

(1) Arsenic ↑ viral load by 50-fold and bacterial load by 17-fold (innate immunity effects such as ↓ respiratory burst of phagocytic cells and interferon); also ↓ IL-1β and TNFα

(2) Similar ↓ in phenoloxidase, ROS generation, phagocytosis found in green mussels in response to Cu or Hg toxicity

e. Asthma initially caused by dysregulation of epithelial-mesenchymal trophic unit (expression of profibrogenic growth factors such as EGF and CXCL8/IL-8 which attracts neutrophils) rather than just a Th2 cell inflammatory response—see Figure 19-3

f. Naphthalene model agent for modeling barrier disruption (epithelial cell damage)

2. Innate immunity—macrophages

a. M1—proinflammatory and cytotoxic macrophages stimulating by type I cytokines (IFNγ, TNFα) or LPS, double-stranded RNS or lipoteichoic acid (pathogenic organisms) → release IL-12 → Th1 adaptive immune responses → ROS, RNS, and proinflammatory cytokines IL-1, IL-6, and TNFα

(1) M1 macrophages found in hepatotoxicity associated with acetaminophen, CCl_4, phenobarbital or endotoxin. Corticosteroids or macrophage inhibitor $GdCl_3$ ↓ toxicity of these and other hepatic toxicants (e.g., allyl alcohol, $CdCl_2$). M1 activation by Toll-like receptor agonists ↑ hepatotoxicity of these agents

(2) M2—wound healing macrophages that suppress immune and inflammatory responses stimulated by IL-4 and IL-13 (M2a) or IL-1β or LPS combined with immune complexes (M2b) or IL-10, TGFβ or glucocorticoids (M2c) → Th2 immune response, but T cell proliferation is suppressed by IL-10 → phagocytosis of neutrophils by M2 macrophages, ↓ pro-inflammatory cytokines and lead to vascular growth. Targeting M2 macrophages with clodronate liposomes ↑ acetaminophen toxicity

3. Innate immunity—neutrophils (polymorphonuclear cells, or PMNs)

a. Recruited by inhaled O_3 or endotoxin → clearance of bacteria but also ↑ ROS and pro-inflammatory cytokines. $NiSO_4$ inhalation→ transpulmonary PMN infiltration and inflammation. Chronic smoking → leukocytosis + ↑ neutrophil sequestration in the lung (inhibition of leukotriene A_4 hydroxylase that cleaves neutrophil chemoattractant proline-glycine-proline) → ROS → COPD

b. Chronic ethanol → osteopontin → recruitment of neutrophils → steatohepatitis

c. Pb → immunosuppressant that ↓ phagocytic activity of PMNs

4. Innate Immunity—Eosinophils

a. Organophosphate malathion → ↑ eosinophils and lymphocytes in cricket frogs → tissue damage (similar to humans consuming denatured rapeseed oil)

CONCEPTUALIZING TOXICOLOGY 19-1 (*continued*)

    b. Tryptophan product → eosinophilia myalgia

    c. Dichlorodiphenylethylene → ↓ eosinophilic granula in children

    d. AMDRO contains a terpenoid → leucopenia in cattle including ↓ eosinophils and lymphocytes

5. Innate immunity—basophils/mast cells

    a. Anaphylactoid reactions (not adaptive immunity IgE-mediated allergy) caused by iodinated benzene ring derivatives → ↑ osmolarity → histamine release from mast cells → dangerous angioedema, bronchiole constriction and ↓ blood pressure

6. Innate immunity—natural killer (NK) cells

    a. Sulfur mustard gases → initial leukocytosis → years to malignancies → ↓ NK cells

    b. Surgical stress → ↓ NK cell cytotoxicity

    c. Purine metabolites and toxins from pertussis or cholera → ↓ proliferation of NK cells

    d. ↑ NK cells and IL-2 to treat metastatic renal cell carcinoma → headache, shaking, chills, fever, and leukocytosis (NK toxicity) and IL-2-induced fever, fluid retention, and eosinophilia

    e. Bacterial DNA → NK cells produce IFN γ → ↑ toxicity of LPS

7. Adaptive immunity—T lymphocytes—see Figure 19-5 and Table 19-3 for Type IV response

    a. Galectin-9 stimulates apoptosis in eosinophils, cancer cells, and T cells (especially CD4$^+$ T cells through Ca^{2+} influx-calpain-caspase 1 pathway) and stimulates T0 cells → Treg and suppressed Th17 = reduces impact of autoimmune arthritis in mouse model

    b. *Ehrlichia* → CD8$^+$T-cells → fatal toxic shock via liver damage, ↑ bacterial burden, ↓ CD4$^+$ T cell numbers (apoptosis), ↓ *Ehrlichia*-specific CD4$^+$ Th1 cells, and overproduction of TNFα and IL-10

    c. Gender-linked allergic response to cigarette smoke → Th2 cytokines are significantly ↑ in females compared with allergic males

    d. Type IV reactions = T cells (antigen-specific) aided by macrophages (antigen-nonspecific) → CD4 T cells → lymphokines, monokines → lymphocyte and macrophage infiltration → formation of a granuloma or cytotoxic T lymphocytes in response to exposure to poison ivy, pesticides, Au, Hg, Ni, Co, Cr, formaldehyde, parabens, topical antihistamines and estrogens, EDTA, TDIC, trimellitic anhydrides, antibiotics, quinidine, subcutaneous heparin

8. Adaptive immunity—B lymphocytes—see Figure 19-5 and Table 19-3 for Type I–III responses

    a. Cells of allergy and inflammation—activated by a surface Ig, CD40 protein surface protein and Toll-like receptors; memory B cells only require the Ig receptor response to cognate antigens = basis of vaccines or autoimmune immunoglobulins

    b. Myeloid cells mediate cytokine formation and secretion → inflammation tissue (e.g., diabetes mellitus type II or periodontal disease and disease severity = number of CD5-expressing infiltrating B cells) and other harmful effects on healthy tissue such as autoimmune diabetes mellitus type I and lupus

    c. B cells can activate T cells independent of Ig or cytokine response via surface expression of CD83

    d. The toxicity of obesity (overdose of fat/calories) → first infiltration of B cells into adipose tissue then T cells and macrophages (appears backward to most immune responses). B cells ↑ inflammation and insulin resistance via CD4$^+$ (protective)/CD8$^+$ (↑ insulin resistance) and T effector/Treg cell (protective) balance

    e. Regulatory B cells (Bregs) exist and are stimulated by surface Ig alone in conjunction with CD40 → secretion of IL-10 (from B10 or Breg cells) → anti-inflammatory activity

    f. Type I reactions are classic IgE-mediated allergic reactions to phthalates, B. *subtilis* (detergents), pesticides, azo dyes, BHA, BHT, TDIC, trimellitic anhydrides, Pt, Ni, Be, penicillin, cephalosporins, vaccines, allergen extracts, latex → histamine release → anaphylactic shock (↓ blood pressure and bronchoconstriction)

CONCEPTUALIZING TOXICOLOGY 19-1 (*continued*)

g. Type II reactions involve IgG (mainly with some IgM) and are cytotoxic in reaction to modification of tissue by Au, Hg, erythromycin estolate, nitrofurantoin, sulfonamides, antitubercular agents

h. Type III reactions result from formation of an antigen-antibody complex that activates complement (serum sickness and other immune complexes) due to exposure to Au, Hg (Hg-induced autoimmunity dependent on MHC class II susceptibility genes—see complex mechanism in Figure 19-6), hydralazine, heparin, quinidine, ticarcillin, valproate, pyramidon, procainamide, minocycline, thiazides, ACE inhibitors, Ca^{2+}-channel blockers, statins (medication-induced autoimmunity mechanism in Figure 19-7)

9. Immune suppression

a. TCDD and heavy metals → low dose autoimmunity (↑ autoreactive Vβ+CD4+17a and Vβ+CD3+ T cells in mice exposed at mid-gestation to TCDD) → higher dose immune suppression → wasting syndrome (TCDD-induced thymic atrophy, lipolysis, and altered intermediary metabolism—must have AhR present to affect NF-κB pathway and Foxp3 → induce Tregs); TCDD ↑ T cell stimulatory capacity of dendritic cells via a variety of factors including MHC class II while ↓ spleen and bone marrow–derived dendritic cell populations via Fas-mediated apoptosis; heavy metals have direct toxic action on portions of the immune system (high-dose anergy) and disturb antigen tolerance (downregulation of TGFβ mRNA expression and less oral tolerance to dietary ovalbumin as indicated by ↑ IFNγ)

CONCEPTUALIZING TOXICOLOGY 19-1 (*continued*)

The transport of toxicants in the blood can damage the immune organ of the spleen and be transported into the bone marrow where immune cells originate. Agents that cause aplastic anemia or pancytopenia, such as benzene and radiation, are usually first noticed by the developing immune deficiency. Transport of hydrophobic substances through the lymphatic system can cause damage to the lymph nodes or a child's thymus. The lymphatic system holds many immune cells and is also where human immunodeficiency virus (HIV) develops prior to it spilling into the blood. This is a large circulatory system that is often ignored even though it has more fluid than the blood and returns fluid to the blood that has leaked out of cells into the interstitium. Not only must immune deficiency be considered but also immune stimulation that might lead to a cytokine storm or an autoimmune or allergic reaction. This chapter begins by addressing tests. This is different from other chapters as the complexity of the immune response is indicated by tests which try to address the toxicity of an enhanced or deficient immune response or immune enhancement of direct toxicity. How does the U.S. Food and Drug Administration (FDA) test new investigative drugs for immunotoxicity? **Figure 19-1** shows that topical administration is the first avenue for testing the chemical agent.

Innate immune defenses are first responders in the barriers to pathogen entry. Allergic reactions (hypersensitivity) are then considered, beginning with all reactions at the surface of the body followed by allergic reactions in the lungs. When the chemical goes into blood and lymph circulation, immunosuppression becomes a concern. Then treatment of immune-suppressed individuals who have HIV infection and immune suppression during pregnancy are discussed. Accumulation of a drug or its metabolites may lead to autoimmunity as the compound may modify certain proteins or cause immunosuppression with high concentrations. Finally, toxicity tests are examined in more detail. It is important to note that model systems discussed elsewhere such as the Draize test come from immunotoxicology.

Recognition of Foreign Antigens

What are the mechanisms that an organism uses to recognize that a foreign substance has attached itself to the skin structures, is working its way through the skin, or is absorbed through the gastrointestinal (GI) tract or lung? In the

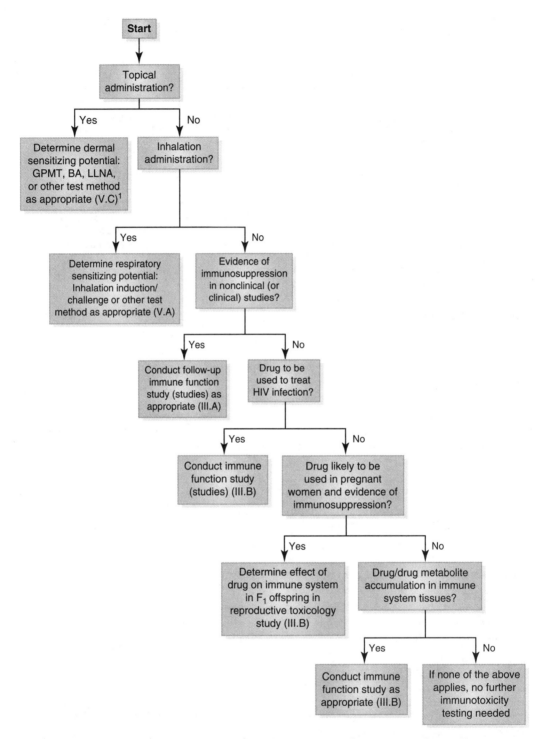

FIGURE 19-1 U.S. Food and Drug Administration's Flow Chart for Determination of Immunotoxicity of New Medications

Note: [1]GMPT = guinea pig maximization test; BA = Buehler assay; LLNA = murine local lymph node assay.

Reproduced from Center for Drug Evaluation and Research. 2002. *Guidance for industry. Immunotoxicology evaluation of investigational new drugs.* U.S. Department of Health and Human Services. Food and Drug Adminstration. Rockvillle, MD, USA. http://www.fda.gov/downloads/Drugs/GuidanceComplianceRegulatoryInformation/Guidances/ ucm079239.pdf.

circulation, foreign chemicals are fast moving and yet are still recognized. Binding of small-molecular-weight molecules to proteins may be necessary for recognition (forming haptens). The signaling pathways that recruit immune cells to analyze whether a chemical is sufficiently foreign to be processed are essential in having an appropriate response. It is also important to realize how immune cell function is activated to make cells more "sticky" so that their movement is altered and they might adhere to foreign molecules. Some fairly recent articles in the field of immunotoxicology indicate new tests for enhanced or suppressed immune function (Corsini and Roggen, 2009; Luster and Gerberick, 2010). There are a number of detailed books on immunotoxicology involving clinical aspects. However, for those interested in effects of environmental chemicals on immune function, an excellent overview of immunotoxicology and biological markers has been done by the National Academy of Sciences and is available for free download online (Committee on Biologic Markers, 1992).

Innate Immune Defenses

Consider the first and second lines of defense of the body from toxic substances and pathogens. The first line of defense is the innate immune defense followed by the adaptive immune system. The innate immune system is antigen independent, gives an immediate maximal response, and results in no immunologic memory. Conversely, the adaptive immune system is antigen dependent and antigen specific, has a lag phase before it reaches its maximal response, and is characterized as having memory of contact with each specific antigen. The immune responses are mediated by cells and their secretions (humoral). All immune cells originate from stem cells of the bone marrow. Myeloid cells include dendritic cells (majority of dendritic cells), neutrophils, macrophages, eosinophils, and basophils (and mast cells). Myeloid progenitor cells also give rise to the erythrocytes and thrombocytes. The lymphoid cells are the T lymphocytes, the B lymphocytes, natural killer cells, and lymphoid dendritic cells (minority of dendritic cells). There appear to be some differences among sources

of what constitutes cells for innate or adaptive immunity. If the reaction has no memory and does not differ by increasing cell numbers/responsiveness or have a T cell receptor, it may be considered innate. Therefore, a basophil that participates in the allergic response, but does not make the IgE that causes its reactivity, may be considered innate. In the same vein, a natural killer cell would be part of innate immunity while a natural killer T cell is a T lymphocyte and would be considered adaptive immunity. Adaptive immunity starts when T cells migrate to the thymus and differentiate into $CD4^+$ T helper cells and $CD8^+$ pre-cytotoxic cells. T helper cells become two populations, the Th1 cells that stimulate the $CD8^+$ pre-cytotoxic cells to become cytotoxic cells and the Th2 cells that cause the B lymphocytes to develop into the antibody-producing plasma cells (discovery of this process reviewed in Coffman et al., 1988). Innate and adaptive immunity are shown in **Figure 19-2**. Note that the innate immune response is indicated to the left in the figure in the (a) section. Note also that there are humoral/secreted agents mediating the immune response for innate immunity including the complement system (serum proteins activated to damage the membranes of pathogenic organisms by components of the microbial cells walls in innate immunity and by antibody binding in adaptive immunity) and cytokines (recruit immune cells) augmenting or completing the work of the highly mobile macrophages, granulocytes (including plentiful phagocytic neutrophils, antiparasitic and asthma-producing eosinophils, and the histamine-secreting basophils), and natural killer cells.

Cytokine Signaling and Linkage of Innate to Acquired Immune System

The role of cytokines must be examined prior to proceeding with further discussion of the innate immune system as these signaling agents recruit and link the innate and acquired immune systems. Cytokines are signaling molecules secreted from one cell to affect another (cytokines labeled interleukins were initially developed to indicate the multiple biological roles of cytokines) that can be

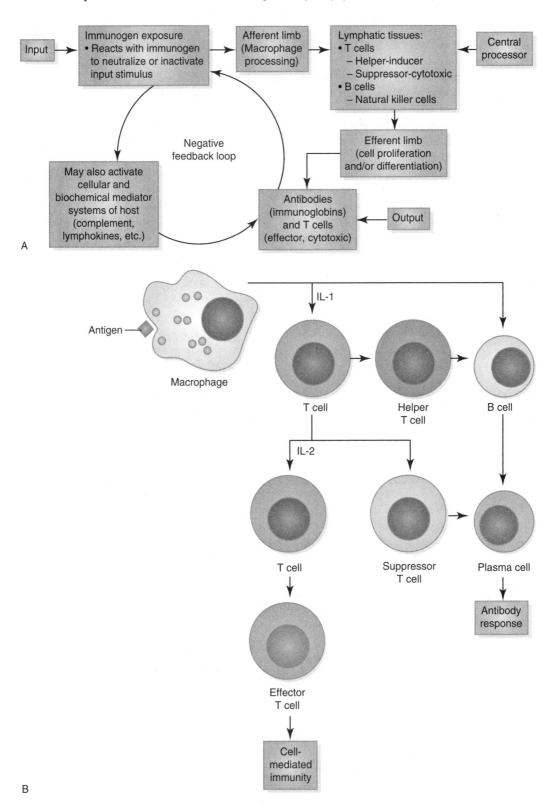

FIGURE 19-2 A. Processing of Foreign Matter by the Immune System. B. The Specific Immune Responses

divided into: (1) primarily lymphocyte growth factors, (2) pro-inflammatory agents, (3) anti-inflammatory molecules, and (4) polarization of the immune response to antigens. Evolution indicates that cytokines started as signaling agents inside cells prior to receptors or signaling cascades. Host defense and repair are properties of cytokines in starfish and *Drosophila* and temperature rise in poikilothermic lizards as a means of survival. The toxicology problem of cytokines is that they play a key role in innate defense such as interferon-γ (IFNγ) and protection from the organism that produces tuberculosis. However, this same cytokine can also stimulate several autoimmune diseases. So enough cytokines are necessary to stimulate immune reactions, but a storm of cytokines can be lethal. For example, sufficient interleukin 2 (IL-2) is needed to generate cytotoxic T cells to fight infections within cells, but not so much that graft-versus-host disease develops. How much is enough or too much? Cytokines are much more potent than hormones that work at nM concentrations. The cytokine released by monocytes/macrophages to recruit T helper cells to start the acquired immune response, IL-1, only needs to be 10 pM to induce gene expression and synthesis of COX-2. Similarly, IL-12 induces IFNγ at 20 pM. IL-1 was given that number as defining a monocyte product, while IL-2 indicated a lymphocyte product. However, IL-1 caused fever, induced acute phase protein synthesis, activated B lymphocytes, and was a cofactor in T lymphocyte proliferation when antigens or mitogens were present. IL-2 provided a further stimulation to T lymphocyte proliferation and activated B lymphocytes (IL-15 has similar functions). Thirty-three ILs were identified in 2007. The IL-1 family has 11 members and is proinflammatory (e.g., IL-1α, IL-1β, IL-18, IL-33). The IL-6 family includes hepatic acute phase proteins such as IL-6, leukemia inhibitory factor, IL-11, oncostatin, ciliary neurotropic factor, and cardiotropin-1. In contrast, the IL-10 family, which includes IL-22, is anti-inflammatory and decreases immune responses. Colony-stimulating factors (CSF) include IL3, granulocyte CSF, granulocyte-macrophage CSF, and macrophage CSF. They are distinct gene products with specific receptors despite their overlapping functions. Chemokines (structurally classes into CC, CXC, C and CX3C chemokines) are a very large group with 48 individual human genes (28 Scya genes for CCLs, 16 Scyb genes and one VCC1 gene for CXCLs, two Scyc1 genes for XCLs, and one Scyd1 gene for CX3CL1) that regulate cell migration from the blood into the tissue. (Dinarello, 2007). View **Table 19-1** as a guide to cytokine function.

Next, it is essential to examine asthma and cytokine responses (as well as other protein responses). It would appear logical that there would be a straightforward distinct group of pro-inflammatory interleukins involved in the process. However, immunity is a complicated process. Chemokine ligands (CCL8, CCL5, CCL11, and CCL24 attract Th2 lymphocytes), SERPINs (SERPINB2, SERPINB4, and SERPINA1 are serine protease inhibitors and protect the lower respiratory tract from proteolytic enzymes), and carboxypeptidase A3 (CPA3; asthma-associated protease present in lung epithelium as a mast cell marker which is upregulated in asthma) are genes serving as biomarkers of asthma. Retnla or Fizz (bronchial epithelial cell protein) and NOS2A (encodes for inducible NO synthase) are other possible indicators of asthma. If external toxicants are included along with stimulants of asthma, such as allergens, cigarette smoke, traffic exhaust, and folate-rich diet, then the methylation and silencing of genes such as IFNγ, Fox-P2, IL2, and iNOS and hypomethylation/activation of genes such as IL6, IL4, IL8, and Acyl CoA increase the Th2 phenotype and help develop asthma (Sircar et al., 2014). Secondhand smoke is sufficient to stimulate asthma as indicated by the T2 response of a mouse model (Seymour et al., 1997).

Acquired-immunity humoral agents are antibodies (Abs)/immunoglobulins (Igs) that are secreted by B lymphocyte plasma cells. These Abs include: (1) IgA found in mucosal areas of body entry routes such as the respiratory tract, GI tract, and urogenital tract; (2) IgD functioning as an antigen receptor of B cells; (3) allergic-stimulating IgE (promotes release of histamine from mast cells and basophils); (4) IgG providing majority of Ab-based immunity to pathogens; and (5) secreted IgM to eliminate circulating

TABLE 19-1   Functional Classes of Cytokines

Functional Class	Primary Property	Other Effects	Examples[a]
Lymphocyte growth factors	Clonal expansion	Th1/Th2/Th17 polarization	IL-2, IL-4, IL-7, IL-17, IL-15
Th1 cytokines	↑ Th1 response	Clonal expansion of CTL*	IFNγ, IL-2, IL-12, IL-18
Th2 cytokines	↑ Th2 responses	↑ antibody production	IL-4, IL-5, IL-18, IL-25, IL-33
Th17 cytokines	↑ Th17 responses, IFNγ	Autoimmune responses	IL-17, IL-23, IFNγ
Pro-inflammatory cytokines	↑ inflammatory mediators	↑ innate immune responses	IL-1α, IL-1β, TNFα, IL-12, IL-18, IL-23
			MIF, IL-32, IL-33, CD40L
Anti-inflammatory cytokines	↓ inflammatory genes	↓ cytokine-mediated lethality	IL-10, IL-13, TGFβ, IL-22, IL-1Ra, IFNα/β
Adipokines	Pro-inflammatory	↓ autoimmune disease pro-atherogenic	IL-1α, TNFα, IL-6, leptin, adiponectin, resistin
gp130 signaling cytokines	Growth factors	B-cell activation, acute phase	IL-6, CNTF, IL-11, LIF, CT-1
Nerve growth factors	↑ nerve/Schwann cells	B-cell activation	BNDF, NGF
Osteoclast activating cytokines	Bone resorption	Immune stimulation	RANK L
Colony-stimulating factors	Hematopoiesis	Pro- and anti-inflammatory	IL-3, IL-7, G-CSF, GM-CSF, M-CSF
Angiogenic cytokines	Neovascularization	Pro-metastatic	VEGF, IL-1, IL-6, IL-8
Mesenchymal growth factors	Fibrosis	Pro-metastatic	FGF, HGF, TGFβ, BMP
Type II interferon	Macrophage activation	Increase class II MHC	IFNγ
Type I interferons	Antiviral; ↑ class I MHC	Anti-inflammatory, anti-angiogenic	IFNα, IFNβ
Chemokines[†], others	↑ cellular emigration	↑ cell activation	IL-8, MCP-1, MIP-1α,

[a]does not include soluble cytokine receptors such as sTNFRp55, sTNFRp75, sIL-1R type II, IL-18 binding protein, osteoprotegerin.
*CTL = cytotoxic T-cell; BMP = bone morphogenic protein.
[†]The chemokine family includes CC, CXC, C and CX3C chemokines with more than 48 members.

Reproduced from Dinarello CA. 2007. Historical insights into cytokines. *Eur J Immunol.* 37(Suppl 1):S34–S45; Edwards TM, Myers JP. 2007. Environmental exposures and gene regulation in disease etiology. *Environ Health Perspect.* 115:1264–1270.

pathogens prior to sufficient IgG present. Cellular components of the adaptive immune system are the cell-mediated immune response fighting infections within cells mediated by the T cells. The humoral immune response fights infections/toxicants outside of cells mediated by the B cells. Because the antigen-presenting cells that activate both humoral and cell-mediated immunity through the Th cell include the B cells and granulocytes of the dendritic cells and the macrophages, the line between innate and acquired immunity starts to blur. This is as it should be because there is an important interplay between the two systems in achieving immune defense. The most potent presenting cell appears to be the dendritic cell, as this cell is required to activate resting T cells (Austyn, 1987). Any antigen-presenting cell may stimulate a sensitized T cell and can be done likely by tissue macrophages from normal routes of entry. This is displayed in Figure 19-2b as indicated by the secretion of IL-1 by the macrophage to recruit and initiate the T cell response that initiates the two types of adaptive immunity.

The commonality of these presenting cells is the presence of the major histocompatibility complex II for binding of a processed antigen on its surface for the Th cell to interact with/recognize.

Barriers

Barriers are the first line of defense so that chemicals or other foreign agents do not require recognition. Chemicals and physical alterations can eliminate these barriers. Many microorganisms will not readily penetrate intact skin, but the skin barrier can be made permeable by chemical and thermal burns, abrasions, dimethyl sulfoxide (DMSO), and other agents. A pH of 3–5 retards the growth of many bacteria, but changes in pH by use of skin products may alter that protection. Salivary glands and tear ducts secrete antimicrobial chemicals (antibodies, lysozyme for cleaving bacterial cell wall, lactoferrin), but can be damaged by radiation. Hairs and mucus intercept particles that may be inhaled and then swallowed. Cigarette smoke (nicotine) can paralyze the cilia. Phagocytosis by tissue macrophages takes place in these areas. These macrophages are the presenting cells mentioned earlier that can attract the adaptive immune defenses. Other phagocytic cells are monocytes for pathogens that enter the blood and neutrophils (the most plentiful of the white blood cells). Physiological barriers include body temperature (normal and fever), low pH of the stomach for swallowed microorganisms (altered by bases and proton-pump inhibitors), and chemical mediators (interferon for inducing antiviral protection of uninfected cells, complement lysis of microorganisms and facilitation of phagocytosis, Toll-like receptors for recognition of foreign molecules such as the lipopolysaccharide [LPS] on gram-negative bacteria and stimulation of cells to release immunostimulatory cytokines, surfactant collectins that disturb microbial cell wall). Inflammatory processes also represent a barrier to pathogens, which can be suppressed by medications (antihistamines, nonsteroidal anti-inflammatory drugs [NSAIDs], and steroidal anti-inflammatory agents) and toxicants.

The penetration of the barrier by biologically active allergens, air pollutants, irritants, environmental tobacco smoke, and respiratory viruses appears to be a key factor in the development of asthma via dysregulation of the epithelial-mesenchymal trophic unit. Susceptibility genes in the epithelium (*ESE 1* and *3*, *DPP10*, *NPSR1*, *PCDH1*, *CHI3L1*, *GSTP1*, *GSDML*, *OPN3*, and *HLA-G*) and mesenchyme (*ADAM33*, *KCNMB1*, *MYLK*, and *C/EBPα*) indicate that asthma may not be a Th2 cell inflammatory response so much as a problem of epithelium-mesenchymal homeostasis. The defect in the repair of epithelium in asthma appears to be related to the overexpression of profibrogenic growth factors such as epidermal growth factor (EGF) and leads to a chronic wounding. Naphthalene-induced epithelial damage appears to be a good mouse model of this phenomenon as indicated in **Table 19-2**. Severe asthma shows a link between epithelial expression of EGF receptors and immunoreactive CXCL8 (IL-8), which attracts neutrophils. Neutrophils form oxidants that amplify the damage as shown in **Figure 19-3**. The early development of asthma appears to be related to inflammatory events started by antigen-presenting airway dendritic cells recruited to disrupted epithelial cells (Holgate et al., 2009). Overall innate immunity may be compromised by heavy metals such as arsenic. Exposure of zebrafish to 2–10 ppb of arsenic ("safe" by drinking water standards) increases viral load by 50-fold and bacterial load by 17-fold. Respiratory burst activity is reduced (oxidant activity of phagocytic cells) along with interferon (13-fold) and Mx RNA (1.5-fold reduction in expression of interferon-induced members of the dynamin superfamily of guanosine triphosphates which display antiviral activity). IL-1β is reduced 2.5-fold and TNFα is decreased 4-fold, and their peak expression is delayed by arsenic treatment followed by bacterial challenge (Nayak et al., 2007). Similar reductions in phenoloxidase, reactive oxygen species (ROS) generation, and phagocytosis were discovered in the marine green mussel, *Perna viridis*, exposed to sublethal concentrations of Cu (20 µg/L) or Hg (10 µg/L; Thiagarajan et al., 2006).

Macrophages

This subsections moves to the discussion of individual components of innate immunity.

TABLE 19-2 Forensic Chart of Innate Immunity Alterations			
Tissue/Cell	**Function**	**Effect**	**Toxicants**
Epithelial-mesenchymal trophic unit	Barrier, antibacterial peptide, and cytokine formation	Disruption—leading to chronic wounding	Naphthalene
Neutrophils	Phagocytes	Oxidant production	Increases toxicity of endotoxin, ozone, and inhaled heavy metals Activity is decreased by lead in circulation (heavy metals)
Macrophages	Mobile phagocytes	M1 class: ROS, RNS, and pro-inflammatory cytokines—decreased by GdCl$_3$ M2: wound healing—decreased by clodronate liposomes	Augments hepatotoxic compounds (e.g., acetaminophen) Decreases hepatotoxicity
Eosinophils	Antiparasitic phagocytes	Tissue damage and pain	Eosinophilia-myalgia induced by L-tryptophan, malathion Reduced eosinophils in response to dichloro-diphenylethylene, combination of isopropyl (2E,4E,7S)-11-methoxy-3,7,11-trimethyl-2,4-dodecadienoate, and tetrahydro-5,5-dimethyl-2(1H)-pyrimidinone [3-[4(trifluoromethyl) phenyl]-1-[2-[4-(trifluoromethyl) phenyl]ethenyl]-2-propenylidene] hydrazone
Basophils	Allergy via IgE-mediated histamine release	Hives, itching, angioedema, bronchoconstriction, hypotension	Penicillin, cephalosporin
Mast cells	Anaphylactoid response		Iodinated radiocontrast agents, various antibiotics, dextran, muscle relaxants, heparin, NSAIDs
Natural killer cells	Antiviral and tumor cell killer	Headache, shaking, chills, fever, leukocytosis	Reduced—cancers associated with mustard gas exposure, purine metabolites, cholera toxin, pertussis toxin Increased by IL-2, bacterial DNA and increases the toxicity of LPS

LPS = lipopolysaccharide; NSAIDs = nonsteroidal anti-inflammatory drugs; RNS = reactive nitrogen species; ROS = reactive oxygen species.

The most mobile of the presenting cells are the tissue macrophages. They well represent a presenting phagocytic cell with reactive properties. One article likens the macrophage to that of the war of soldiers in the film *Star Wars* (Laskin, 2009). The M1 macrophages are cytotoxic and proinflammatory representing the Dark (toxic) Side of the (immune) Force, while the M2 macrophages may be likened to the rebel heroes who suppress immune and inflammatory responses, and lead to wound healing and new blood vessel formation. The toxic M1 macrophages are stimulated by type I cytokines (IFNγ, TNFα) or LPS, lipoproteins, double-stranded

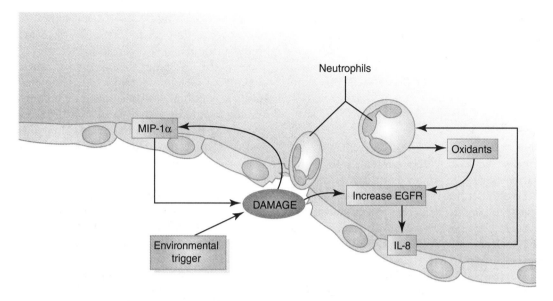

FIGURE 19-3 Amplification of Epithelial Injury via Stimulation of Epidermal Growth Factor Receptor (EGFR), Stimulation of Interleukin-8 Release (IL-8), Recruitment of Neutrophils, and Stimulation of Macrophage Inflammatory Protein-1 α (MIP-1α [CCL3])

RNA, or lipoteichoic acid associated with pathogenic organisms or internal signals of stress such as heat shock proteins or the alarmin high-mobility group box protein 1 (HMGB1). They go on to release IL-12, stimulating Th1 adaptive immune responses, and release ROS, reactive nitrogen species (RNS), and proinflammatory cytokines IL-1, IL-6, and TNFα. M2 macrophages are either activated by IL-4 and IL-13 (M2a macrophages) or IL-1β or LPS combined with immune complexes (M2b macrophages), IL-10, or transforming growth factor-β (TGFβ) or glucocorticoids (M2c macrophages). M2 macrophages aid the Th2 immune response. T lymphocyte proliferation is suppressed by the release of IL-10. M2 macrophages phagocytize apoptotic neutrophils, reduce pro-inflammatory cytokines, and lead to vascular growth and tissue/wound repair similar to tumor-associated macrophages. M1 macrophages would then be expected to increase the toxicity of toxicants when increased macrophages are found in hepatotoxicity associated with treatment by acetaminophen, CCl_4, phenobarbital, or endotoxin. Immunosuppression with corticosteroids prevents the toxicity, as do macrophage inhibitors gadolinium chloride ($GdCl_3$) and dextran

sulfate or by the macrophage depletion agent liposome-encapsulated dichloromethylene diphosphonate. M1 macrophage inhibition or depletion also guards the liver from allyl alcohol, cadmium chloride, concanavalin A, diethyldithiocarbamate, fumonisin, and thioacetamide toxicity. Alternatively, Toll-like receptor agonists that activate M1 macrophages such as LIP or polyinosinic-polycytidylic acid enhances the toxicity of acetaminophen, carbon tetrachloride, halothane, trovafloxacin, galactosamine, and *Corynebacterium parvum*. Because $GdCl_3$ depletes larger M1 macrophages around the periportal area of the liver and clodronate liposomes targets M2 macrophages of the larger Kupffer cells and smaller macrophages in midzonal and centrilobular regions, it would be expected to have opposite results in acetaminophen toxicity. This is exactly what happens as $GdCl_3$ decreases and clodronate liposomes increase acetaminophen-associated liver damage (Laskin, 2009). Certain compounds such as cytotoxic cancer chemotherapeutic agents damage bone marrow, resulting in decreased leukocytes of various sorts. Carbamazepine is a compound that has also been associated with severe hematopoietic adverse effects due to inhibition of bone marrow–derived granulocyte macrophage, erythroid, and megakaryocyte progenitor cells. Lithium has opposite/antidotal effects to carbamazepine, resulting in leukocytosis/increased white blood cells (WBCs; Gallicchio and Hulette, 1989).

Neutrophils

The phagocytic neutrophils (polymorphonuclear cells, or PMNs) and their oxidative enzymes/functions have been described elsewhere. Inhaled toxicants such as endotoxin and ozone initiate recruitment of neutrophils to the airspace. The positive side of this action would be in clearance of bacteria, while the negative end is similar to M1 macrophage infiltration—generation of ROS and pro-inflammatory cytokines. It is not always clear that the neutrophils are causal to the damage observed, as some high exposures may actually result in neutrophil depletion (Hollingsworth et al., 2007). Alcoholic steatohepatitis appears to occur due to osteopontin recruitment of neutrophils followed by parenchymal injury (Apte et al., 2005). Conversely, lead is an immunosuppressant agent that decreases the phagocytic activity of neutrophils in toad, *Bufo arenarum* (Rosenberg et al., 2003). However, heavy metal inhalation (e.g., nickel sulfate) increases inflammation and transpulmonary PMN infiltration (Hirano, 1996). In tobacco smokers, the pathogenesis of chronic obstructive pulmonary disease may be related to leukocytosis, increased neutrophil sequestration in the lung, and generation of ROS by those neutrophils (Sharma et al., 1997). Smoke products also lead to chronic obstructive pulmonary disease (COPD) through the recruitment of neutrophils. It appears that smoke products selectively inhibit leukotriene A_4 hydroxylase activity, an enzyme that cleaves the neutrophil chemoattractant proline-glycine-proline. The accumulation of this tripeptide leads to neutrophil invasion and lung cell inflammation (Snelgrove et al., 2010).

Eosinophils

Eosinophils and lymphocytes were found to be elevated in cricket frogs (*Fejervarya limnocharis*) exposed to the organophosphate insecticide malathion, resulting in tissue damage (Kundu and Roychoudhury, 2009). Similar effects are found in humans who consumed denatured rapeseed oil in Spain during 1981 (Gabriel et al., 1986). A famous outbreak of eosinophilia-myalgia syndrome developed in humans consuming tryptophan supplements or medications containing tryptophan employed as sleep aids and antidepressants. High eosinophil counts were accompanied by weight loss, pruritus (itchiness), fever, dyspnea (shortness of breath), and sensory abnormalities. Skin lesions, muscle pain, and other symptoms persisted for more than 17 months after discontinuing tryptophan use (Szeimies and Meurer, 1993). Decreased eosinophilic granula content was found in children exposed to dichloro-diphenylethylene (Karmaus et al., 2005). The fire ant bait mound treatment AMDRO contains (S)-methoprene (isopropyl (2E,4E,7S)-11-methoxy-3,7,11-trimethyl-2,4-dodecadienoate; a terpenoid) and hydramethylnon (tetrahydro-5,5-dimethyl-2(1H)-pyrimidinone [3-[4(trifluoromethyl) phenyl]-1-[2-[4-(trifluoromethyl)phenyl] ethenyl]-2-propenylidene]hydrazone; an amidinohydrazone). AMDRO fed to weanling castrated Holstein calves for 7 weeks experienced leucopenia by 2 weeks into the regimen, including significant reductions of eosinophils and lymphocytes (Evans et al., 1984).

Basophils/Mast Cells

Changes in basophils are usually associated with allergy, which is an adaptive immune response to be covered shortly. Turpentine elicits an inflammatory response in chickens with leukocytosis and heterophilia (increased granular leukocytes in animals that correspond to neutrophils in humans). Basophil and eosinophil populations show erratic counts. Toxic heterophil responses are noted with intense left shifts characterized by cell swelling, degranulation, cytoplasmic vacuolation, and cytoplasmic basophilia (Latimer et al., 1988). The classic allergic reaction to penicillin or sulfa medications involves an IgE-mediated release of histamine from basophils that is part of adaptive immunity. Alongside true allergic reactions or apart from allergic reactions, anaphylactoid reactions are caused by release of histamine from mast cells leading to the classic itching, skin flush, hives (urticaria), angioedema (swelling of tongue and airway leading to laryngeal blockage or GI tract causing intestinal pain and bowel obstruction), bronchiole constriction or spasm, and dangerous reduction in blood pressure that may lead to shock. Iodinated benzene ring derivatives with higher osmolality or higher ionicity have a rate of anaphylactoid reactions ranging from 4–12% (nonionic forms have a 1–3% rate; Nayak et al., 2009). The osmotic effects on mast cells or stimulation of complement receptors on mast cells can yield reactions to a variety of agents including those eliciting true allergic reactions or antibiotics such as sulfa drugs, vancomycin, ciprofloxacin, polymyxin B, volume-expansion agent dextran, muscle relaxants used during surgery, anticoagulants heparin and NSAIDs, acetaminophen, and so forth. Clinicians are most concerned about fatalities resulting from IgE-mediated angioedema and anaphylaxis versus non IgE-mediated angioedema and anaphylactoid reactions (Greenberger, 2006).

Natural Killer Cells

Natural killer cells can also be affected by toxic chemicals. Sulfur mustard gases used in the Iran–Iraq conflict lead to damage to the eye and respiratory tract, with increased asthma, COPD, and fibrosis. Following an initial leukocytosis, increased malignancies 16–20 years following exposure were associated with significantly decreased natural killer cells (Balali-Mood and Hefazi, 2006). Surgical stress also depresses natural killer cell cytotoxicity by direct toxic action (Pollock et al., 1991). Infection that produces toxins such as pertussis and cholera suppresses natural killer cell proliferation, as do purine metabolites (Miller, 1999). Artificially raising lymphokine-activated killer cells and IL-2 for treatment of metastatic renal cell carcinoma resulted in killer cell toxicity (headache, shaking, chills, fever, and leukocytosis) and IL-2-induced fever, fluid retention, and eosinophilia (Nakano et al., 1991). Bacterial DNA presents a stimulus for natural killer cells to produce IFNγ and increases the toxicity of LPS (Cowdery et al., 1996).

Adaptive Immunity

The important cells in adaptive immunity are the lymphocytes, represented by the B lymphocytes, the T (thymus) lymphocytes, and the null cells (the majority of null cells are the large, granular natural killer cells). In basic physiology, cell-mediated immunity is described as fighting infections inside cells mediated by the T cells. Humoral immunity represents fighting infections on the outside of cells mediated by antigen recognition of the B cells, forming antibody-producing plasma cells. These T and B cells have receptors to foreign antigens. However, the presence of T cells is necessary for T-dependent antigens that stimulate the release of IL-2 and production of the memory B cells and plasma. Some antigens are large and have repeated subunits such as the polysaccharide coat of bacteria. They bind directly to B lymphocytes and stimulate plasma cell antibody protection without stimulating the memory B cells. These T-independent antigens only generate a primary immune response (less antibody development than would occur as a secondary response), because the immune system does not develop memory of this type of antigen. Vaccines are based on B cell development of antibodies via the T cells' stimulation of immunological memory. So these T cells, developed during childhood from formation in the bone marrow and transferred to the thymus, are vitally important in development of immunity. This is clear from HIV infection, in which one of the T cells, the T helper cell, has a surface protein (CD4+) that the virus uses to gain entry and destroy the adaptive immune system.

T Lymphocytes

Before examining the B lymphocyte more closely, the development of subsets of T cells is crucial in understanding how toxicants may affect most or part of adaptive immunity by affecting populations of these key cells. Because the T lymphocytes appear to be programmed in the thymus, it is essential to know how self versus foreign is determined. Humans use human leukocyte antigens to mark self, class I, and class II major histocompatibility complex

(MHC) molecules. All nucleated cells in the human express class I MHC proteins on their surfaces, while class II MHC are found in the presenting cells (macrophages, dendritic cells, activated B cells) and the interior of the thymus. T cell development in the thymus only allows for proliferation of those cells that have the correct affinity for the body's own MHC I and II proteins. Those that bind to class II MHC molecules become the T helper cells mentioned earlier, and those that bind to class I MHC molecules become cytotoxic T cells. From here the complexity grows along with some major confusion as to the designation of all the T cell subsets. The confusion arises as to molecular markers on the cell surface, function, and T cell receptors. For example $CD4^+$ is expressed on the T helper cells and $CD8^+$ is expressed on the cytotoxic T cell. The $CD4^+$ is considered the helper T cell, but it can be cytotoxic in certain assays. The genetics of the receptor are clearly only $\gamma\delta$ or $\alpha\beta$ (Cobbold, n.d.). As shown in **Figure 19-4**, the T cells can be further differentiated into Th1, Th2, Th17, Tfh, and iTreg.

This figure represent some of the major T cell subsets, but not all of them. The differentiation of T cells is dependent on the cytokines that these cells express. The initial naïve T0 helper cell is recruited to the antigen-presenting cell by the secretion of IL-1 by the antigen-presenting cells (APC). Dendritic cell secretion of IL-12 and IL-18 turns the T0 into a Th1 cell that secretes IL-2, IFNγ, and lymphotoxin and produces immunological memory as indicated earlier and helps clear intracellular pathogens. Lymphoid populations of cells that secrete IL-4 cause development of Th2 cells, upregulation of MHC II, and B lymphocyte production of IgE. This is an allergy pathway and clears extracellular organisms. Stimulation of Th1 decreases Th2, and similarly Th2 stimulation yields inhibition of Th 1 pathways. $CD4^+CD25^+Foxp3^+$ T regulatory (Treg) cells, once known as suppressor T cells, help maintain immune tolerance and suppress autoimmune reactions. TGFβ appears to be a crucial factor in Treg development. Conversely, IL-6 prevents the differentiation of T cells stimulated by TGFβ and stimulates the formation of a pathogenic T cell known as Th17 in combination with TGFβ. The cell Th17 that produces

IL-17 appears to be distinct from the other T cells already described and plays a critical role in stimulating autoimmune reactions (Bettelli et al., 2006). This is important, for it shows toxicologists that induction of one subset of T cells or suppression of another may lead to similar pathogenic endpoints such as autoimmune reactions. For example, the pro-inflammatory cytokines TNFα, IL-1β, and IL-6 would be expected to cause damage to bone and cartilage such as occurs in rheumatoid arthritis. A β–galactoside binding animal lectin, galectin-9, stimulates apoptosis in eosinophils, cancer cells, and T cells, especially $CD4^+$ T cells through the $Ca2^+$ influx-calpain-caspase 1 pathway. It also stimulates naïve T cells to differentiate in Treg cells. Th17 cells are also suppressed by this lectin. This substance was then able to reduce the impact of experimentally induced autoimmune arthritis in a mouse model system (Seki et al., 2008). Natural regulatory T cells (nTreg) or innate regulatory T cells are a distinct subset of T cells dependent on the transcription factor forkhead box p3 or Foxp3. Without Foxp3, there are no Treg cells and uncontrolled inflammation. These nTreg cells are contact dependent and antigen nonspecific, and they inhibit activation of other T cells. The nTreg cells also do not make IL-2 but are dependent on IL-2 for their induction. Inducible Treg cells (iTreg) arise from stimulation of the T cell receptor by TGFβ (Murai et al., 2010). Other regulatory T cells are Tr1 cells that produce the immunosuppressive IL-10 and originate from naïve T cells in response to IL-10 and TGFβ produced by dendritic cells. Th3 cells are also regulatory T cells that synthesize TGFβ and do not express $CD25^+$ on their surface, as do the other Treg cells mentioned previously. Memory regulatory T cells have also been described in ovarian tumors, which express high levels of inflammatory chemokine receptors. These memory Tregs may be subdivided into expression of lymphoid chemokine receptor CCR7, with those containing the conventional $CCR7^+$ central memory and the $CCR7^-$ effector memory T cells. The effector memory T cells are more prominent in ovarian tumors, but both share a role in immune tolerance in lymphoid and peripheral locations of the body including tumor sites (Tosello et al.,

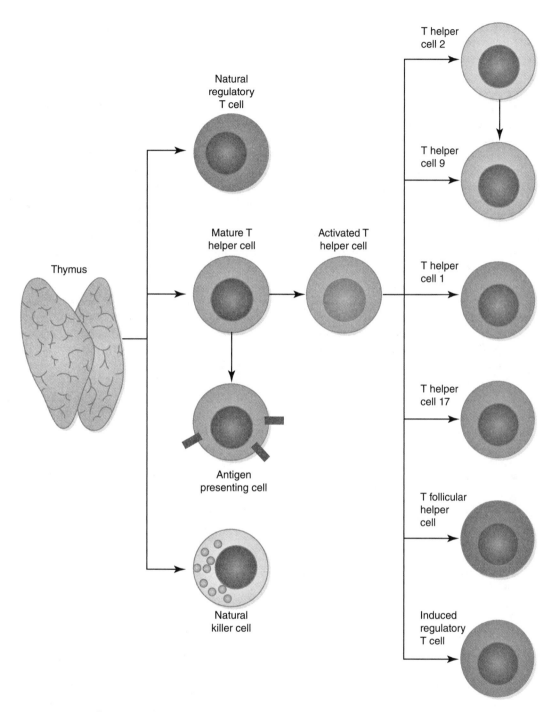

FIGURE 19-4 Differentiation of the T (Thymus-Programmed) Helper Cell Populations

2008). It becomes apparent that groups of cells are becoming subdivided by function and expression of cell surface markers. The complexity can be confusing and "the forest can get lost in the trees." However, the precise mechanism of toxicant injury via immune stimulation or suppression is important in antidotal therapy or preventive action. Also, treatments for diseases of aging such as cancer and rheumatoid arthritis are direct applications of this research (e.g., the presence of Treg cells and poor clinical outcomes of an immunotherapeutic regimen in metastatic renal cell carcinoma; Flörcken et al., 2012). Returning to T helper cells subsets in Figure 19-4, the follicular T helper cells (Tfh) are used to reinforce the diagnosis of angioimmunoblastic T cell lymphoma (and provide specialized help to B cells; Crotty, 2011). They differ from the other T helper cells if expression of factors/receptors is considered. Th1 involves the expression Stat4, Stat1, and T-box transcription factor/T-bet, the last of which is important in maintenance of T and B lymphocytes, dendritic cells, and natural killer cells as well as several autoimmune diseases (Peng, 2006). Th2 cells express Gata3, Th17 cells secrete IL-17 and express retinoid-related orphan receptor (RORγt), and regulatory T cells (Treg) express Foxp2. Other cells determined by the IL secretion are Th9 (IL-9 and IL-10) and Th22 (IL-22). The Th9, Th17, and Th22 cells' proinflammatory cytokines regulate local tissue inflammation, while the nTreg cells and iTreg type I IL-10-expressing cells maintain homeostasis by decreased allergen response (Akdis, 2010). Where IFNγ-secreting Th1 cells were considered the mediators of autoimmunity, more recent studies reveal that cells such as Th17 can produce diseases such as experimental autoimmune encephalomyelitis. Th9 also has encephalitogenic activity, but not Th2 cells. Thus, CD4$^+$ or CD8$^+$ lineages are not the only characterizations, because the specific IL expression determines much of their function (Jäger et al., 2009). This is important even for cytotoxic CD8$^+$ T cells, as two pathways exist for their function. One is by perforin-dependent TNF/TNFR pathways or by Fas/Ras ligand (FasL) interactions that destroy pathogen-infected cells. The other is via secretion of IFNγ and TNFα, which limit

pathogen replication and at high levels produce toxicity apart from foreign toxicants. This is important as the presence of CD8$^+$ T cells appear to mediate fatal toxic shock reactions to *Ehrlichia* by causing liver damage, increasing bacterial burden, reducing CD4$^+$ T cell numbers via apoptotic mechanisms, decreasing *Ehrlichia*-specific CD4$^+$ Th1 cells, and overproducing TNFα and IL-10 (Ismail et al., 2007).

It is not only important to understand the T cell subsets, but the activation of T cells. Costimulatory pathways, positive or negative, are necessary for activation or inhibition of T cells, respectively. Following T cell receptor binding to the antigen bound to the MHC molecule (signal one) on the surface of APC, a second signal occurs via interaction of T cell surface receptors with specific ligands on the APC. The most elucidated pathway for T cell activation is via the CD28/CTLA4-B7 pathway. CD28 is present on T cells and has two ligands, B7-1 (CD80) and B7-2 (CD86), found on the outside of activated APCs. The activated T cells produce more CTLA-4, which is similar to CD28 in structure and binds both B7 ligands. Where CD28 interaction with the B7 ligands is a potent positive signal results in cytokine synthesis and secretion, clonal expansion, increased survival of T cells, and recruiting B cells, CTLA-4's increased affinity for the B7 ligands ends T cell responses (negative signal). This is important, because CTLA-4-deficient mice die from autoimmunity to a variety of organs resulting from overdevelopment of lymphocytes. Blockade of the CD28-B7 pathway reduces autoimmunity. CD154 is also expressed in T cells and CD40 on APC, including B cells. Interaction of these two proteins provides activation for T and B cells. CD40 is vital for Ig (antibody) switching. Absence of CD154 results in hyper IgM X-linked syndrome. If this protein is blocked, then transplant rejection is ameliorated and autoimmune diseases related to B cell activation, such as systemic lupus erythematosus, are prevented. Additionally, blockade of CD154 prevents the autoimmune development of diabetes mellitus in rodents. Other costimulatory pathways are ICOS-B7RP-1 and PD-1-PD-L pathways (related to CD28-B7 family) and CD514-CD40 (members of TNF-TNF-R superfamily; Yamada et al., 2002). In asthmatic subjects, responses to stimulation of T cells are important in the disease process. IFNγ[+] T cells increase in response to antigen-independent or CD3[+]CD28-mediated stimulation in peripheral blood lymphocytes from atopic asthmatic patients. There is a sex-specific response as well. Women with atopic asthma produce more IL-13-secreting T cells when peripheral blood lymphocytes are subjected to antigen-independent stimulation than do male asthma patients or male and female atopic non-asthmatic subjects (Loza et al., 2010). This sex difference is due to increased Th2 cytokine elevation in females compared with allergic males (Seymour et al., 2002).

B lymphocytes

B cells are engaged in allergy and inflammation. Naïve B cells use a surface immunoglobulin or the CD40 protein surface protein with other ligands to activate. The Toll-like receptor (TLR) provides a third signal for activation. TLRs recognize certain patterns and activate the innate immune response. TLR1, TLR2, TLR4, and TLR5 are expressed on the cell surface and are activated by non-nucleic acid components of microbes. TLR1 together with TLR1 and TLR6 are stimulated by lipopeptides. TLR4 is activated by LPS, while TLR5 recognizes flagellin. Endocytic TLRs are 3, 7, 8 and 9, which are used to identify double-stranded RNA, single-stranded RNA, and CpG-containing DNA. All TLRs mentioned, except TLR3, signal adaptor molecule myeloid differentiation primary response gene 88 and IL-1 receptor-associated kinase. Further downstream, signaling occurs via interferon regulatory factor and/or nuclear factor-κB-dependent induction of type I interferon, IL-6, TNFα, and IL-12 (Crampton et al., 2010). Memory B cells require only one of these three signals (surface Ig, CD40, TLR) to activate. The immunoglobulin receptor responds to cognate antigens. Plasma B cells secrete antibodies that bind cognate antigens outside of cell contact and are the basis of vaccine development. Inflammatory disorders may involve the development autoimmune antibodies that damage host tissue. Ligation of Fc receptors on myeloid cells can drive a toxic/pathogenic

inflammatory response. Otherwise, Ig/antigen complexes stimulate complement proteins that bind to complement receptors on myeloid cells. In either case, myeloid cells mediate cytokine formation and secretion, inflammation, and untoward effects on healthy tissue.

Antibodies play a role in autoimmune reactions such as lupus and diabetes mellitus type I mentioned earlier in the discussion of T cell functions. B cells are also involved in inflammation not related to autoimmunity, such as diabetes mellitus type II and periodontal disease. In these non-autoimmune reactions, especially periodontal disease, neutrophils and monocytes infiltrate, followed by B lineage cells. These lineage cells contain the antibody-secreting plasma cells. The disease severity (lesions) is related to the number of infiltration B cells. The expression of CD5 on the surface of B cells is found in lesion sites and indicates an activated phenotype. The antibodies produced have dual functions, for those subjects that have high expression are protected from infection but may have increased autoimmunity as well.

Similar to T cells, the cytokines produced also indicate function, both pro- and anti-inflammatory. TNFα and IL-1 are secreted by human B cells even without induction. However, those humans who show inflammatory conditions such as periodontal disease overproduce these pro-inflammatory cytokines in response to TLR stimulation. B cells can also activate T cells independent of an Ig or cytokine response via the surface expression of CD83. B cells do not necessarily require T cells to damage tissue as may be suggested by the cytotoxic T cell designation. RANKL is a factor secreted by B cells that promotes osteoclasts to cause bone resorption. In diet-induced obesity, it is the B cell that first infiltrates into adipose tissue, followed by the T cells and then macrophages in a process that looks to be backward when compared to other immune function. Although some have through this infiltration a protective mechanism to prevent inflammation, it appears from more recent reports (summarized in Winer et al., 2014) that the B cell is capable of increasing inflammation and insulin resistance via the CD4[+]/CD8[+] and T effector/Treg cell balance. CD4[+] T cells/regs are protective, while CD8$^+$ T cells escalate insulin resistance. The B cells involved in inflammation have subsets based on cytokine expression such as the T cells. Simulation of B cells through surface Ig alone in conjunction with CD40 leads to the production of IL-10 secreting B cells termed B10 cells or regulatory B cells (Bregs). These are anti-inflammatory protective cells of various phenotypes (DiLillo et al., 2010) for the most part, unless upregulation of surface TLR2 is elicited. These cells were first discovered as transitional B cells that protect against inflammation and are similar to CD27-IL-10-producing naïve B cells that repopulate multiple sclerosis patients or humans with lupus or rheumatoid arthritis following B cell depletion. The experimental autoimmune arthritis and encephalomyelitis models mentioned with the T cells are ameliorated by B cell IL-10 secretion as indicated by prevention of Th1 differentiation. This secretion of IL-10 must be mediated by both TLRs and MyD88 adapter protein to prevent T cell differentiation and inflammation. However, TLR2 is the more important of the TLRs to stimulate IL-10 production in those patients with periodontal disease, because TLR2 induction upregulated IL-10 (not in healthy patients). TLR4 costimulation produced less IL-10. Patients with diabetes mellitus type II do not increase IL-10 in response to TLR2, TLR4, or TLR9 simulation. Inflammation may be due then to changes in IL-10 production elicited by genetic factors, diet, toxic insults, or other disease processes.

IL-6 is another B cell cytokine. However, the research literature (summarized in Erta et al., 2012) indicates a more complex picture for the multiple functions of this secretion. It can be pro-inflammatory and produce glucose intolerance depending on the polymorphisms of human IL-6. However, non-diabetic (type II) patients secrete more IL-6 than diabetic patients (Jagannathan et al., 2010; Larsen et al., 2007). Additionally, patients with periodontal disease may be protected against tissue destruction by IL-6's ability to induce IL-1 receptor antagonist (Irwin and Myrillas, 1998; Tilg et al., 1994) or conversely others have thought that Il-6 plays a key role in periodontal disease (Słotwińska, 2012). Th2 cells also secrete IL-6.

The combination of these studies indicates that one should be careful when assigning IL-6 to the pro- or anti-inflammatory cytokines or to only one lymphocyte population. This dichotomy is very apparent in muscle tissue (Muñoz-Cánoves et al., 2013) However, IL-8 secretion from B cells may be important in chronic inflammation as occurs in Crohn's disease. This also appears to be exacerbated by TLR2 stimulation. Mouse cells have B effector 1 and B effector 2 subsets with similar cytokine production to Th1 and Th2, respectively. IL-12 stimulates human B cells to produce IFNγ. This cytokine is also a secretion of murine B effector 1 and Th1 cells (Nikolajczyk, 2010). Other B cell subtypes respond by pathways linked to TLRs. Marginal zone B cells ("innate-like" B cells) respond more to TLR3 and TLR4 ligands than transitional or follicular B cells. Memory B cells mentioned earlier have higher surface expression of CD180, a protein that cooperates with TLR4 in recognition of LPS. TLRs appear to upregulated on memory versus naïve B cells. As complex as this appears, it is important as agonism at a TLR such as TLR7 by resiquimod induces IgM and IgG secretion without T cell activation *in vitro*. However, naïve B cells need some IL-2 with IL-10 to generate a biologically significant response. B cells limit their development via a population division destiny. Humans with loss-of-function mutations in positive regulators of TLR signaling (IRAK4, UNC-93B, or MyD88) have autoreactive B cells/autoimmunity at 5–10 times those of healthy patients (Crampton et al., 2010). In summary, it appears that there are not only classifications of T-dependent production of antibodies and T-independent, CD40L-independent, but BCR/CD19-dependent pathways for segregation of B cell clones. The B1 B cell subset is enriched in the CD21^{high} marginal zone compartment or recirculates with the B cell follicles. The abilities of B cells of the marginal zone of the spleen and the B1B cells to generate effector cells in the early stages of the immune response and B cell follicles (formed in conjunction with follicular dendritic cells) to become memory and plasma B cells for the late stage of recognition and antibody development are important in the development of the full immune response (Martin and Kearney, 2000).

Hypersensitivity Reactions (Allergy and Autoimmunity)

The Gell and Coombs's (1963) classification of hypersensitivity reactions has been used for more than 50 years to determine four types of immune reactions found in **Figure 19-5** and **Table 19-3**. This classification serves a useful purpose if used with a modern view of the workings of the immune system knowing that various medications and toxicants can generate several of these reactions simultaneously (Descotes and Choquet-Kastylevsky, 2001).

Type I

As shown in Table 19-3 and Figure 19-5, Type I allergies are linked to IgE-mediated release of histamine from basophils and mast cells and are also linked to leukotrienes and tryptase. This immediate hypersensitivity may lead to urticaria, pruritus, and bronchospasm/dyspnea associated with anaphylaxis and cardiogenic shock due to an abrupt drop in blood pressure. A common example of this response is people who respond to pollen with runny noses and congestion, more prevalent with increased CO_2 in the atmosphere and increased plant growth. Dust mites, animal dander, molds, and food products (e.g., peanuts) provide allergies that research indicates may be overcome by tolerance induced by introducing subthreshold amounts of the allergen. Medicines (especially antibiotics), chemicals found in cleaning products, metals, amines, and anhydrides also may elicit a Type I response. This reaction may chronically develop into asthma or elicit an asthmatic episode. Atopic dermatitis can also be a symptom of Type I hypersensitivity. A fairly important allergy is that to natural rubber latex isolated from the sap of the *Hevea brasiliensis* tree. Eleven of the 256 proteins are potential allergens. This latex allergy is seen in dental practice with contact to the skin or thin epithelial layer of the mucous membranes. Nonallergic contact dermatitis and delayed Type IV hypersensitivity are possible in addition to the critical Type I hypersensitivity. The Type I response may yield in addition to the conditions mentioned previously erythema, edema, rhinoconjunctivitis, palpitations, dizziness, vasodilation, GI cramps,

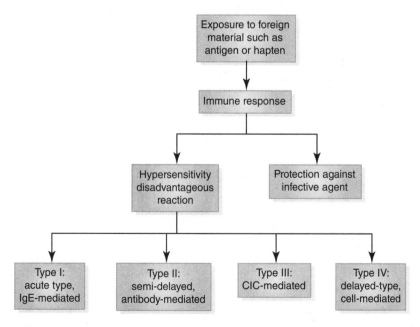

FIGURE 19-5 Hypersensitivity Reactions Based on the Gell and Coombs Classification. This Has Been Called into Question by Medicines that Can Elicit a Combination of all the Types Indicated Above and the Modern Understanding of the Immune System Including Non-Immune-Mediated Anaphylactoid Reactions

TABLE 19-3   Immunologic Hypersensitivity Reactions — Types I–IV

Gell and Coombs Classification*	Onset	Antibody (Ab)	Principal Cell	Site of Reaction	Biochemical Reaction/Effect	Routes	Toxicants
Type I — Ab-dependent Anaphylaxis (atopic reaginic)	Sec → min	Th1↑ → IgE (tonsils, bronchial lymph nodes, GI lymphatic Peyer's patches)	Basophil/mast cell (Fc receptor) → IL3-6, GM-CSF cytokines released (looks like Th2 reaction)	Dependent with antigen entry route: wheal + flare, hay fever, rhinitis, conjunctivitis, asthma, anaphylaxis	Histamine (↓ BP + bronchoconstriction), serotonin, platelet-activating factor, leukotrienes, prostaglandins (inflammation), thromboxanes	Dermal, respiratory, GI	Phthalates, *B. subtilis* (detergents), pesticides, azo dyes, BHA, BHT, TDIC, trimellitic anhydrides, Pt, Ni, Be, penicillin, cephalosporins, vaccines, allergen extracts, latex
Type II — Complement-independent lysis or complement-mediated immune adherence	Min → h	Th1 → IgM/IgG Tissue associated antigen	Thymus R-E cells Cytotoxic cell* attaches to Fc portion of Ig Complement fixes to receptors on target cell membrane	Vascular sinuses, reticuloendothelial system	Cytotoxic granules from cytotoxic cells lyses Ig-recognized cell Complement activation C3 to C3b, or C5b-9 MAC binds to target cell surface	All routes that become circulating antigen that attaches to cells	Au, Hg, erythromycin estolate, nitrofurantoin, sulfonamides, antitubercular agents
Type III — Immune complex	30 min → 2 h	Th1 → IgM/IgG Soluble antigen in serum	Neutrophil, macrophage, platelet attracted to deposition site	Lung, joints, kidney (immune complex deposition)	Complement chemotactic factors Neutrophil lysosomal hydrolytic enzymes	All routes — haptenized circulating antigen	Au, Hg, hydralazine, heparin, quinidine, ticarcillin, valproate, pyramidon, procainamide, minocycline, thiazides, ACE inhibitors, Ca²⁺-channel blockers, statins
Type IV — T cell reactions Contact tuberculin	18 → 72 h	Th2 → None	Responder T cell and monocyte/macrophage	Varies with antigen localization	Soluble lymphokines from antigen-stimulated T cell	Epidermal Intradermal	Pesticides, Au, Hg, Ni, Co, Cr, formaldehyde, parabens, topical antihistamines and estrogens, EDTA, TDIC, trimellitic anhydrides, antibiotics, quinidine, subcutaneous heparin

*Gell, 1963; Th1 are T helper cells (expressing CD4 protein) that initiate direct cell killing via proinflammatory cytokines IFN-γ and IL-2 that activate B cells, macrophages, cell-mediated immunity, and natural killer cells; Th2 are T helper cells that generate IL 4, 5, and 13 associated with IgE promotion and eosinophilic responses (atopy) and IL-10, which inhibits inflammatory responses of Th1; †Macrophage, neutrophil, eosinophil.

Modified from Committee on Biologic Markers, Board on Environmental Studies and Toxicology, National Research Council. 1992. *Biological markers in immunotoxicology.* Washington, DC: National Academies Press.

vomiting, and death. People who have a history of IgE-linked allergies (atopy), and especially fruit allergies (cross-reactive antibodies), and occupational or surgical exposure to latex are more likely to develop the allergic reaction. Females also have an increased risk (Kean and McNally, 2009). There also appears to be cross-sensitization between people with allergies to goldenrod (*Soliadgo virgaurea*) and latex (Bains et al., 2010).

Chemicals that induce type I allergic reactions are also a broad category. A solvent that results in significant occupational exposure from ure-thane foam–producing facilities and induces asthma and allergic rhinitis is 2,4-toluene diisocyanate (TDIC). IgE is elevated on chronic inhalation. IgE release from B cells is stimulated by IL-4 formation. TDIC causes Jurkat cells (immortalized T cell line) and human WBCs to release IL-4, which can be inhibited in Jurkat cells by an intracellular calcium chelator, N,N,N′,N′-tetraacetic acid. Both TNFα and IL-4 mRNA transcripts are increased by TDIC in Jurkat cells (Chiung et al., 2010). Beryllium exposure from the aerospace industry, nuclear applications, making precision instruments, and high-speed electronic circuit manufacture generates an irritant response at high concentrations and a Type I allergy at lower chronic exposures resulting in a progressive lung disease. A lymphocyte proliferation test indicates a sensitization to beryllium (Middleton and Kowalski, 2010). Metals as a group are irritants of the respiratory tract and also lead to allergic sensitization. Compounds containing Pt appear to be especially allergenic and have an adjuvant effect causing more severe allergic reactions (Burastero et al., 2009). Over the years, food additives such as azo dyes, benzoates, monosodium glutamate, sorbates, butylated hydroxyanisole (BHA), and butylated hydroxytoluene (BHT) have been suggested as linked to anaphylaxis.

More common chemicals that humans contact may be more well-known for other toxicities they produce. All agents listed in Table 19-3 are putative Type I allergy sensitizers due to supporting literature. However, a more recent analysis of the medical literature establishes only a clear causal link between sulfites used to preserve wines and asthma and anaphylaxis

(Reus et al., 2000). Other agents may enhance ongoing problems resulting from other allergic reactions (Goodman et al., 1990). Formaldehyde is more well-known as a carcinogen yet is a also a contact allergen that anatomists have been aware of for years. However, cosmetics appear to be the leading cause of dermatitis from exposure to formaldehyde in the general population (Lundov et al., 2010). The reason formaldehyde is not listed as a Type I allergen is that IgE responses in rodents and humans have not been reported associated with simple formaldehyde exposure. However, similar to the action of Pt, formaldehyde causes an inflammatory reaction and appears to act as an adjuvant to allergens (Wolkoff and Nielsen, 2010). Detergent enzymes isolated from *Bacillus subtilis* also exhibit Type I hypersensitivity intradermally with concentrations > 1 pg/mL or skin prick tests (1 mg/mL) in sensitized humans (Belin and Norman, 1977). The ubiquitous plasticizing agents such as the phthalates are listed as Type I agents, although the literature is equivocal on this issue. Epidemiological evidence has not provided adequate dose–response data, but appears to find a correlation between exposure to plasticizers and allergies or asthma (Kimber and Dearman, 2010).

Listing pesticides with a broad brush as Type I allergens may be somewhat misleading regarding their unique properties and actions. For example, Paraquat is an herbicide that generates oxygen radicals and either is an immune suppressant and lethal at high doses or has little effect at low doses (Riahi et al., 2010). Most sprayed pesticides have the potential to enter the respiratory tract and may then elicit allergic rhinitis and bronchial asthma-like diseases. When applied dermally or into the respiratory tract of mice, herbicide 2,4-dichlorophenoxy-acetic acid (2,4-D) was found to be a respiratory allergen inducing immediate hypersensitivity by all parameters (IgE production, influx of immune cells, and chemokine levels) while BRP (organophosphosphate) and furathiocarb (carbamate) insecticides elicited responses characteristic of contact allergens (increased MHC class II–positive B cells and Th1 cytokines in auricular lymph node cells; Fukuyama et al., 2009). Trimellitic anhydride is a reference respiratory allergen (Dearman et al., 2003), but can also provoke a T cell–dependent Type IV contact hypersensitivity as well (Schneider et al., 2009).

Type II

Crossing from Type I to Type II and III hypersensitivities, the discussion moves from more common allergic reactions to rare autoimmune disorders as modified tissue becomes recognized by the immune system. The presence of autoimmune antibodies is the key diagnostic indication of an autoimmune condition such as occurs with the well-known rheumatoid arthritis. Type II hypersensitivity is also known as cytotoxic hypersensitivity. It is not due to IgE, but mainly IgG, and involves K cells (antibody-dependent cell-mediated toxicity) instead of basophils and mast cells. Complement may bind to the cell-bound antibody and lead to tissue damage. Modification of host cells leads to autoimmune recognitions as occurs when IgG antibodies recognize intracellular substances between epidermal cells (pemphigus) or bind to the surface of RBCs (autoimmune hemolytic anemia) or glomerular basement membrane (glomerulonephritis as part of Goodpasture's syndrome). Myasthenia gravis and Graves' disease fall under Type II hypersensitivity. Large metals such as gold produce Type II or III hypersensitivity. Mercury vapor exposure to humans has caused pemphigoid and autoimmune anti-fibrillarin antibodies in some scleroderma patients. Similar anti-fibrillarin autoantibodies are found in the mouse model of mercury autoimmune disease (Schiraldi and Monestier, 2009). Mercury appears more associated with Type III immune complex hypersensitivity and that type of glomerulonephritis, but has in the past been identified as an agent that may also produce Type II reactions. Other metals discussed earlier such as Co, Cr, Ni, Pt, or Rh are more associated with Type I reactions and allergic asthma (Kusaka, 1993). Penicillin is also primarily known for its Type I reactions, while sulfa medications, nitrofurantoin, erythromycin, and antituberculosis medications are known for their Type II response (Charlier and Plomteux, 1997). Chlorpromazine, phenytoin, and sulfonamides are also known for producing Type II hypersensitivity.

Type III

Type III hypersensitivity has classically been defined as an Arthus reaction, which is characterized as an immediate nonatopic hypersensitivity resulting from the formation of an antigen–antibody complex that activates complement. This is a rare but severe condition for an injected compound that is accompanied by local inflammation, edema, hemorrhage, and necrosis. Serum sickness is a well-known Type III hypersensitivity, arising from antitoxin antibodies forming immune complexes that deposit in tissues. Mercury, gold, and cadmium are heavy metals associated with autoimmune reactions including the immune complexes associated with Type III hypersensitivity. Hg-associated skin creams have caused membranous nephropathy and minimal change disease. As mentioned earlier, occupational exposures to Hg have resulted in T cell proliferation and anti-laminin and anti-nucleolar autoantibodies. Wegener's granulomatosis, scleroderma, and lupus have been increased in Hg-exposed individuals. Gold therapy for rheumatoid arthritis has resulted in autoimmune glomerulonephritis. The genetic susceptibility to mercury-induced autoimmunity appears to be dependent upon the MHC class II susceptibility genes. The RT-1 locus appears to exert some control in rats, which exhibit autoimmunity with Hg exposure only if they have the RT-1^n > RT-$1a,b,c,f,k$ (decreasing susceptibility) but not the RT-1^l haplotype. The mouse is susceptible to Hg-induced autoimmunity if the I-A region of the MHC class II locus is modified with sensitivity based on the following order: H-2^s > H-2^q or H-2^f while H-2^a, H-2^b, and H-2^d are resistant haplotypes.

The complex mechanisms for mercury-induced autoimmunity are shown in **Figure 19-6**.

Note that the usual mercury-induced necrosis of somatic cells results in the proteasome processing a nucleoprotein and production of peptides that may be recognized. The Hg also affects T cell receptors with downstream enzyme activity effects and binds to intracellular proteins. IL-4 secretion is caused by the binding of Hg to glutathione. Autoreactive T cells are

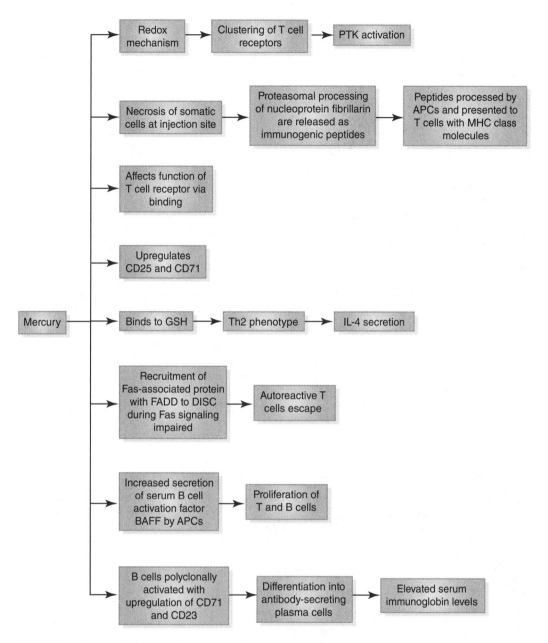

FIGURE 19-6 Putative Mechanisms of Mercury-Induced Autoimmunity.

allowed to escape T cell signaling that would normally cause them to die because Hg interferes with this process (Type IV hypersensitivity). The effects of Hg on the antigen-presenting cell allow the proliferation of T and B cells. Hg subsequently stimulates the upregulation of proteins in the B cells and production of antibodies such as IgG (Type II and III hypersensitivity) and IgE (Type I hypersensitivity; Schiraldi and Monestier, 2009).

A number of medications are listed under Type III hypersensitivity/autoimmunity. Since 1962, drug-induced lupus accompanied by arthritis, arthralgias, and possible fever has been observed with aromatase inhibitors (anastrozole, exemestane, letrozole), hydralazine, isoniazid, methyldopa, minocycline, procainamide, quinidine, statins, and sulfasalazine. Autoimmune hepatitis (minocycline), autoimmune thyroiditis (minocycline), vasculitis (hydralazine, sulfasalazine, sicca syndrome (aromatase inhibitors), Sjogren's syndrome (aromatase inhibitors), inflammatory arthropathies (aromatase inhibitors), dermatomyositis (statins), polymyositis (statins), lichen planus pemphigoides (statins), and autoimmune hemolytic anemia (methyldopa) have been reported in humans. In the rat GVH disease was associated with use of an immunosuppressant medication (cyclosporine), which also induced a scleroderma-like disease. The two high-risk medications are the antiarrhythmic medication procainamide and the antihypertensive agent hydralazine, with the antiarrhythmic drug quinidine at moderate risk of producing autoimmunity.

The mechanisms involved in the medication-induced development of autoimmunity are also complex, involving inhibition of central tolerance, inhibition of peripheral tolerance, defects in apoptosis, macrophage activation, and the haptenized therapeutic agent stimulating antibody production by the B cell as shown in **Figure 19-7**. The metabolites of procainamide represent medications that work to decrease central tolerance mechanisms with the development of antinuclear antibodies and autoantibodies to histone proteins (H2A/H2B dimer target). Procainamide results in ROS formation via unstable reactive metabolites such as procainamide-hydroxylamine. These products may damage the cells of the thymus and cause the formation of IgM anti-denatured DNA antibodies followed weeks later by serum anti-chromatin (H2A/H2B target) IgG. This procainamide metabolite disrupts anergy (immune unresponsiveness) in mature T cells and prevents thymocytes from developing tolerance to low-affinity self-antigens. It also has DNA-demethylating activity. DNA methylation regulates gene expression via formation of

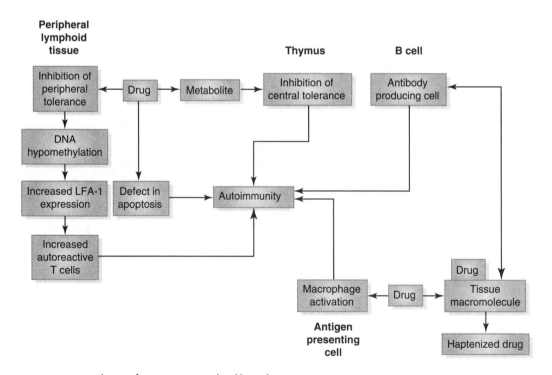

FIGURE 19-7 Mechanisms for Autoimmunity Induced by Medications

5-methylcytosines on the fifth carbon of the cytosine residues in CpG dinucleotides. Human CpG dinucleotides are usually methylated, which decreases DNA transcription. Abnormal T cell DNA methylation appears to be involved in systemic lupus erythematosis pathogenesis as indicated by the effect of 5-azacytidine, a model DNA methylation inhibitor. Procainamide decreases methylation of DNA via competitive inhibition of DNA methyltransferase. Hydralazine inhibits the ERK signaling pathway via interfering in protein kinase Cδ phosphorylation, and thus decreases the expression of the DNA methyltransferase. Both procainamide and hydralazine upregulate poly(ADP-ribosyl)polymerase. This polymerase is bound to chromatin and has the potential of affecting DNA methylation and apoptosis. The undermethylation leads to overexpression of LFA-1 (CD11a/CD18) causing T cell autoreactivity. This LFA overexpression in cloned Th2 cells in mice induced lupus-like reactions including anti-dsDNA antibodies and pulmonary and glomerular disease.

The tetracycline class of antibiotics includes minocycline, which has another method to induce autoimmunity. Reactive metabolites of minocycline may cause the development of antibodies against cross-reacting microsomal cytochromes, resulting in an immune response that includes chromatin degradation without directly stimulating the formation of anti-histone antibodies. Patients may be identified for minocycline-induced lupus by anti-neutrophil cytoplasmic antibodies (anti-myeloperoxidase and/or anti-elastase antibodies). Genetically, patients who test as HLA-DR4 and HLA-DR2 positive and have an HLA-DQB1 allele with a tyrosine at position 30 of the first domain are susceptible to this form of drug-induced lupus. The arthritis drug D-penicillamine indicates that autoimmunity can form in humans and rats via activation of macrophages. The medication forms an irreversible covalent bond with an aldehyde moiety on the macrophage that can form a reversible Schiff base with the amine on T cells, which may be the basis of T cell interaction with macrophages. A signaling pathway is stimulated by this interaction with the aldehyde group on the macrophage. Hydralazine or the anti-tuberculosis medication isoniazid can

also react with this aldehyde group forming a hydrazone. The macrophage increases expression of allele 3 of the solute carrier family 11 member a1 (SLC11A1) yielding autoimmunity. IL-15 and IL-1β synthesis occurs downstream and causes NK cell proliferation and the secretion of macrophage activators IFNγ and GM-CSF. Proinflammatory cytokines TNFα, IL-6, and IL-23 are released by the activated macrophages stimulating an autoimmune response in susceptible individuals. This overproduction of TNFα is not only a proinflammatory cytokine that promotes the development of autoimmune disorders such as ankylosing spondylitis, Crohn's disease, psoriasis, refractory asthma, and rheumatoid arthritis, but is also a master regulator of immune function. TNFα inhibitors, such as infliximab (monoclonal antibody to TNFα used to treat autoimmune diseases), are associated with autoantibody production to ds-DNA (not the histone proteins), but very little lupus of a self-limiting type. TNF inhibitors may induce this specific type of autoimmunity via decreased apoptosis and the proliferation of autoreactive T and B cells. Also, nucleosomes including nuclear material may accumulate due to the decreased clearance of cellular waste and result in autoantibody development.

Minocycline's inhibition of caspase-dependent or caspase-independent apoptosis is another way of developing autoimmunity. A more complicated mechanism is that lack of production of TNFα increases Th2 cytokines (IL-4, -5, -6, -10, -13) that increase Ig production. IFNα (type I interferon) is also increased, augmenting Th1 inflammation while inhibiting inflammation resulting from Th1 and Th17. TNFα inhibition also increases infections, and unmethylated bacterial CpG bacterial motifs activate B cells. Cytokine alterations and changes in signaling pathways can also play a role in autoimmunity. In a murine Sjogren's model (NFS/sld mice), low-dose 2,3,7,8-tetrachlorodibenzo-p-dioxin (TCDD) caused autoimmune lesions in the salivary glands along with other organs accompanied by stimulated production of IL-2 and IFNγ by splenic T cells. This is associated with upregulation of the AhR in the thymus of mice. Humans given IL-2 and lymphokine-activated killer cells for treatment of cancer developed goiter, hypothyroidism, and autoimmune thyroiditis. IL-2 treatment for cancer has also been associated with inflammatory arthritis. Melanoma treatment with IFNα-2b or anti-cytotoxic T lymphocyte antigen yielded auto-antibodies as well. This indicates that blocking T cell regulation leads to a better result against cancer and the development of autoimmunity.

Another possible mechanism for autoimmunity is provided by the actions of quinidine and pro-cainamide. Inhibition of macrophage clearance of apoptotic cell particles may lead to autoan-tibodies and to nucleosome degradation prod-ucts. Statins that reduce cholesterol synthesis via inhibition of 3-hydroxy-3-methylglutaryl coenzyme A (HMG-CoA) reductase may decrease autoimmunity via this activity and disruption of signaling pathways originating in T cell membranes. However, the statins have been associated with increased autoimmunity which may results from proapoptotic mecha-nisms leading to release of nuclear antigens while shifting T helper cells from a Th1 to a Th2 bias. This would result in more antigens and more autoantibody development. Chlorproma-zine also increases apoptosis, so it is important to sort out how an agent that decreases apopto-sis can produce autoimmunity yet the opposite mechanism is also problematic for development of the disease. Cyclosporine is an immune sup-pressant via calcineurin inhibition in the T cell. It would be expected to decrease autoimmunity, but also inhibits apoptosis of thymocytes that would have been eliminated by negative selec-tion. In combination with peripheral ultraviolet (UV) irradiation (but not without it as insuf-ficient autoreactive T cells are developed), cyclo-sporine induces autoimmunity.

Anticancer agents cause autoimmunity as well. The alkylating agent cyclophosphamide damages the function of Treg cells and generates autoimmunity. Methyldopa causes hemolytic anemia. Autoantibodies to RBCs and thrombo-cytes or Evan's syndrome exhibit decreased T4 and increased T8 cells and have CD4$^-$/CD8$^-$ T cells. In a small group of Evan's syndrome patients, this is associated with treatment by oxaliplatin, fludarabine, and ramipril. In an addition to medications, Hg (as mentioned

previously), iodine, vinyl chloride, canavanine, organic solvent, L-tryptophan, anilides, vaccines (influenza vaccine used during swine flu epidemic), microbials, particulate silica, ozone, and UV are factors that have also been associ-ated with autoimmune reactions (Chang and Gershwin, 2010). Heparin-induced thrombocy-topenia is another medication causing a serious condition based on immune complex forma-tion. The heparin–antiheparin/platelet factor 4 IgG immune complexes activate FcγRIIa (CD32) receptors on platelets, causing endothelial lesions accompanied by thrombocytopenia and blood clots (thrombosis; Castelli et al., 2007).

Type IV

Type IV represents cell-mediated immunity or delayed-type hypersensitivity mediated by the T cells (antigen specific) aided by macrophages (antigen nonspecific). There are two different T cell hypersensitivities recognized currently. One involves CD4 T cells, lymphokines, and monokines leading to lymphocyte and macro-phage infiltration of a tissue and the formation of a granuloma. The other involves cytotoxic T lymphocytes and damage ensuing from the actions of these active T cells. These reac-tions span not only contact dermatitis, but also graft or organ rejection, granulomatous disease, Hashimoto's thyroiditis, and insulin-dependent (Type I) diabetes mellitus. Notice the long list of agents in Table 19-3 that cause Type IV hypersensitivity. Those compounds listed under Type I to Type III hypersensitiv-ity as contact allergens or inducing contact dermatitis are Type IV allergens. The most common agents that induce contact dermatitis are poison ivy, fragrances, and the heavy metal nickel (Usatine and Riojas, 2010). Because skin disease ranks second in occupational illnesses, it is not surprising that dermal exposures to a variety of fungicides, insecticides, herbicides, and fumigants are associated with externally observable immune reactions (O'Malley, 1997). Chemicals such as the plasticizer bisphenol A, 4-nonylphenol (derived from nonionic sur-factants), and 4-*tert*-octylphenol (ingredient in detergents and wetting agents) increase the

T lymphocyte allergic reactions as indicated by an increase in IL-4 m-RNA expression in murine T-cells. The mechanism for IL-4 expression involves the nuclear factor of activated T cells or NFAT that binds to the IL-4 promoter. NFAT signaling in T cells involves the Ca^{2+}-dependent calcineurin signaling pathway that is inhibited by the immune suppressant medication cyclosporine (Edwards and Myers, 2007). It is expected that people with autoimmune disorders such as multiple sclerosis, psoriasis, systemic lupus erythematosus, and atopic eczema also show T cell reactivity to heavy metals such as inorganic mercury (from mercury amalgam fillings) and nickel. T cell hypersensitivity is especially prominent in women and can be studied with the lymphocyte transformation test, LTT-MELISA (Hybenova et al., 2010). Gold fillings have similarly led to contact allergies (Möller, 2010). Cell phone parts are newer ways that people can develop contact dermatitis from close long-term contact with metals (Rajpara and Feldman, 2010). Orthopedic implants (metal-on-metal bearing in hip arthoplasty) have resulted in Type IV cobalt hypersensitivity (Perumal et al., 2010). Formaldehyde has caused contact dermatitis in anatomists and morticians over the years, but is also a source of this disease based on permanent-press fabrics containing formaldehyde-based resins since the 1920s (Reich and Warshaw, 2010). Clearly, cosmetics can also cause problems, inducing allergic contact dermatitis due to positive patch-tests with nail lacquer and lipstick allergens, alkyl glucosides, copolymers, glycols, idebenone, octocrylene, protein derivatives, and shellac (Pascoe et al., 2010). p-Phenylenediamine of hair dyes, colophony (pine resin), lanolin alcohol, parabens (derivatives of p-hydroxybenzoic acid in cosmetics), and preservatives such as Kathon CG (isothiazolinone derivative) are other skin sensitizers for Type IV allergic reactions as indicated by testing of a Japanese population (Minamoto, 2010). In addition to these agents, organic mercury products such as thimerosal, quaternary ammonium bases (preservative), diguanides (phenoxyethanol preservative combinations), antioxidants (propyl gallate, BHA, BHT), and emulsifiers

such as wood alcohols to propylene glycol have shown to have some incidence of allergic skin sensitizing ability especially in patients with chronic eczema and women (Dastychová et al., 2008). It would appear odd that agents used to treat allergic reactions can indeed yield allergic responses. Type IV hypersensitivity to topical antihistamines, NSAIDs, and corticosteroids have been observed. Other dermal preparations of antibiotics and anesthetic agents used currently in over-the-counter antiseptic preparations also have yielded contact dermatitis (Davis, 2009). Although quinidine is usually associated with immune complexes associated with Type III allergies due to its method of administration, Type IV reactions are possible. Estrogen-containing creams and subcutaneously administered heparin make these applications more likely to stimulate Type IV hypersensitivity (Charlier and Plomteux, 1997). Some chemical agents are models of contact hypersensitivity. A strong contact sensitizer is 1-chloro-2,4-dinitrobenzene. A model skin contact sensitizer is 2-phenyl-4-ethoxymethylene-5-oxazolon, while toluene 2,4-diisocyanate sensitizes via the skin or respiratory route. Chemical sensitizers work by forming haptens via conjugating with macromolecular skin proteins. These sensitizing compounds upregulate the expression of allergic inflammation-related genes Oasl2 and Zbp1, while allergic sensitizers and a classic irritant (croton oil) increase the expression of 48 genes related to cytokine and cytokine receptors interactions in mouse ear skin. Only Cxcl9 and Cxcl10 expression appear related to skin sensitizer–induced skin inflammation (Ku et al., 2009). Trimellitic anhydride is another respiratory sensitizer, but can also cause reaction via dermal sensitization in mice as indicated by increases in antigen-specific IgE levels (immediate hypersensitivity) in serum and bronchioalveolar lavage fluid; proliferation of eosinophils and MCP-1, eotaxin, and MIP-1β chemokines (inflammatory mediators) in bronchioalveolar lavage fluid; and proliferation of IL-4, IL-10, and IL-13 (Th2 cytokines) indicating a T cell reaction in lymph nodes (Fukuyama et al., 2008).

Autoimmunity Versus Immune Suppression

Frequently, agents such as TCDD and heavy metals generate autoimmunity at lower chronic doses while causing outright immune suppression at high sublethal doses. For example, TCDD at high doses leads to a wasting syndrome that includes thymic atrophy, lipolysis, and altered intermediary metabolism. At lower doses, reproductive and developmental toxicity, cancer, and immune suppression are its toxic hallmarks. The immune system suppression involves a host of functions such as thymic involution, decreased pathogen resistance, inhibited fetal lymphocyte development and maturation, and suppressed adaptive immune responses (i.e., decreased antibody production, cytotoxic T lymphocyte activity, and delayed hypersensitivity responses). The lack of the aryl hydrocarbon receptor prevents the immune suppressant action of TCDD. TCDD increases the T cell stimulatory capacity of dendritic cells (increased MHC class II, ICAM-1, CD24, costimulatory molecule CD40, IL-12, enhanced T cell proliferation in a mixed lymphocyte reaction in splenic dendritic cells; increased MCCII, CD86, CD40, and CD54 [ICAM-1] in bone marrow–derived dendritic cells) while conversely depleting the spleen and bone marrow–derived dendritic cell populations via stimulation of Fas-mediated apoptosis. AhR binding appears to affect the NF-κB pathway as AhR absence leads to increased inflammatory responses. The noncanonical NF-κB pathway is linked to the induction of indoleamine 2,3-dioxygenase, an enzyme catalyzing the initial and rate-limiting step of tryptophan catabolism. T cell suppression is caused by the generation of tolerogenic dendritic cells that induce Tregs. TCDD stimulation of AhR induces IDO1 and IDO-like protein in the lung and spleen of C57BL/6 mice (this strain has a high-affinity AhR). Foxp3 transcripts in the spleen were also increased 2.5-fold by TCDD induction. Because Tregs' functions and phenotypes are controlled by Foxp3, these effects of TCDD give evidence for a role of aryl hydrocarbons in stimulating Treg functions. The interactions of TCDD with CD4+ and CD8+ cells are more complex, with changes occurring in T cell activation during extensive chromatin remodeling including AhR-DRE (dioxin-responsive enhancer)-mediated effects on a variety of genes (lineage-specific transcription factors, cytokines, cytokine receptors, signaling kinase families). TCDD suppresses allograft responses, allergic responses, and autoimmune responses of autoimmune encephalomyelitis and type I diabetes mellitus. Th1, Th2, and Th17 T cell responses (CD4+) are likely suppressed based on the inhibition of these disease states (Marshall and Kerkvliet, 2010).

There is an increased autoimmune reaction of mice exposed prenatally to TCDD. Midgestational exposure to TCDD to C57BL/6 mice resulted in elevated autoreactive Vβ+CD4+17a and Vβ+CD3+ T cells at 24 weeks of age after birth, with females being more reactive than males. Cytokine expression differences were noted by sex, as IFNγ increased in the females compared with higher IL-10 levels in male mice. Additionally, B-lineage cells present in bone marrow and the spleen showed phenotypic alterations and autoantibodies were found in the circulation. Male mice have biologically relevant levels of anti-IgG and anti-C3 deposition in their kidneys, indicating the likely inception of autoimmune nephritis. The SNR(1) mice that have a low-affinity AhR but spontaneously develop autoimmune responses in their kidney also exhibit increased peripheral Vβ+ cells and IFNγ in females exposed prenatally to TCDD. Both sexes have increased autoantibodies. Males also have the increased anti-IgG and anti-C3 deposition in their kidneys in this strain of mice. The autoimmune reaction may occur in these mice as opposed to immune suppression by altering T cell selection. The thymic epithelial cell targeting suggests that TCDD may change the epithelial-dependent deletion of autoreactive thymocytes. Both the change in MHCII molecules in thymic epithelial cells and the enhanced thymic negative selection of T cells and increased autoreactive T cells by TCDD treatment indicate how AhR stimulation at levels that are not immune suppressive can influence a selection process toward autoimmunity (Holladay et al., 2010).

Heavy metals are another good source for examining mechanisms of immune suppression, immune tolerance, and autoimmunity. Various metals, such as the ubiquitous lead or mercury compounds, work in an antigen-nonspecific fashion. They exert direct toxic action on portions of the immune system leading to immune suppression due to systemic malfunctions or dysregulation that cause autoimmune reactions. This moves the discussion into immune tolerance and especially oral tolerance, because this is an important function that may decrease the function of the immune system as the system reacts less to an agent over time. Clearly, lower doses are more effective here in producing this tolerance as higher consumption may stimulate immune function, and higher yet may cause outright cytotoxic actions of the metals. Oral tolerance is not a programmed function but is acquired as antigen-reactive clones are deleted or inactivated. Active suppression, clonal anergy, and clonal deletion are mechanisms that lead to antigen-driven tolerance. High doses usually result in anergy as differentiated from low-dose, cell-mediated active suppression. Regulatory cells mediate active suppression through secretion of immunosuppressive cytokines TGFβ and IL-4 following stimulation by the low dose of tolerogen. Tolerance is disturbed by heavy metal exposure. For example, 10 days of oral lead chloride exposure cause downregulation of TGFβ mRNA expression and less oral tolerance to the dietary antigen ovalbumin as indicated by increased IFNγ and other cytokine bias toward Th1 (Mishra, 2009). As indicated earlier, Au, Cd, and Hg induce autoimmune glomerulonephritis. Mechanisms of mercury-induced autoimmunity have also been mentioned in the preceding sections, but mercury's clear dependency on MHC class II susceptibility genes needs to be reemphasized to generate its responses. Mercury's ability to dysregulate immune tolerance occurs via prevention of the recruitment of adaptor protein, Fas-associated protein with a death domain (FADD), into the death-inducing signaling process in CD95 (another term for Fas-mediated apoptosis). With this apoptotic mechanism, lymphocyte deletion of autoreactive T cells does not occur. Diseases associated with this type of disruption are systemic lupus erythematosis and rheumatoid arthritis (Schiraldi and Monestier, 2009).

Toxicity Tests

The discussion returns to a more detailed examination of the FDA's guidance (Center for Drug Evaluation and Research, 2002) on testing new medications for immunotoxicity. Following a 28-day daily exposure of the agent to rodents, various parameters are measured. Hematology requires total and absolute differential leukocyte counts as a gross measure of immunotoxicity in the blood. Clinical chemistry parameters measured are globin levels and A/G ratios as indications of serum immunoglobulin changes, although this is not a good signal of immunosuppression. Liver damage and nephrotoxicity are other factors that must be considered to explain serum globin alterations. Gross pathology of lymphoid organs/tissues is indicated. Organ weight of the thymus and spleen are recorded with an option of lymph node weight measurements. Thymuses of young animals are preferable for analysis, because the thymus atrophies with age. Histology of the thymus, spleen, draining lymph node and one additional lymph node, bone marrow, Peyer's patch, bronchus-associated lymphoid tissues, and nasal-associated lymphoid tissues are performed. Peyer's patches of the rodent may be too difficult to isolate. If dogs or monkeys are used, the blood must be drained at necropsy to decrease spleen weight variability. Histopathology of the spleen and thymus are considered indicators of immunotoxicity. Route of administration of the toxicant/medication must be considered in evaluating tissues, because inhaled substances should use more nasal- and bronchus-associated lymphoid tissue, while compounds injected intravenously should consider the spleen as the target draining lymph organ. When using other routes, toxicologists should consider the closest lymph node that obtains the highest concentration as the key indicator of damage. When studying high doses approaching lethal concentrations, toxicologists should consider the stress response and corticosteroids (as indicated by adrenal cortical hyperplasia) as influencing immune functions such as increases in circulating neutrophils, decreased lymphocytes in circulation, lower thymus weight and cortical cellularity of the thymus, and altered spleen and lymph node cellularity. T cell–dependent antibody response should involve the stimulus of a recognized T cell–dependent antigen such as sheep red blood cells or keyhole limpet hemocyanin, which generate strong antibody production. Adjuvants should not be used to bolster the response. Mice or rat strain and numbers are important as variability within a strain for outbred species or differences between strains in T cell–dependent antibody response are well known. Serial collection of blood and enzyme-linked immunosorbent assay (ELISA) quantitation of antibody provide kinetics of responses that can be variable especially when using monkeys. The sum of the antibody response or area under the curve (AUC) can be reported in this case. Flow cytometry using antibodies or immunohistochemistry can be used to identify and/or quantitate the leukocyte subsets (immunophenotyping). Immunohistochemistry has some advantages over flow cytometry in retrospective analysis of tissues if immunotoxicity is noted along with alterations in cell types in specific compartments of lymphoid tissue. However, fixation is important as formaldehyde may interfere with certain lymphocyte marker localization. If a change in viral infection rates is observed or immunophenotyping demonstrates a change in natural killer cell number, then functional assays of natural killer cells are warranted. The *ex vivo* assays of natural killer cell activity utilize tissues or blood of treated animals co-incubated with target cells labeled with ^{51}Cr. Not only should viral (influenza or cytomegalovirus) resistance studies be performed with toxicant-treated host animals, but bacterial (*Listeria monocytogenes* or *Streptococcus pneumoniae*), fungal (*Candida albicans*), and parasitic (*Plasmodium yoelii* or *Trichinella spiralis*) challenges should be administered. Cancer is another resistance that can be determined utilizing B16F10 melanoma or PYB6 sarcoma tumor cell lines implanted into mice. Macrophage and neutrophil functions may be assessed using the methods of *in vitro* or *ex vivo* analysis of phagocytosis, oxidative burst, chemotaxis, and cytolytic activities. An *in vivo* method is also available using the reticuloendothelial cell of exposed animals to assess whether a radiolabeled or fluorescently labeled target was phagocytized. Cell-mediated immunity is a much more useful function to assay as antibody and complement-mediated Arthus reactions must be ruled out. Protein immunization and challenge have been used in rodent models of delayed-type hypersensitivity. Contact sensitizers in mice are not sufficiently validated models for the FDA. Cytotoxic T cell responses in mice using a virus, tumor cell line, or allograft as antigen challenge have been used in mice as assays of cell-mediated immunity. Monkeys have problems with consistency/reproducibility.

Tier Approach: Advantages and Drawbacks

A tiered approach to immunotoxicology can be used as suggested by the National Toxicology Program (Dean, 2004; Germolec, 2009). Tier 1 only provides basic information such as cell-mediated immunity (lymphocyte mitogen responsiveness), humoral immunity (plaque-forming cells), and immunopathology (hematology, organ weights including immune, kidney and liver organs, body weight, cellularity of the spleen, and histology of the spleen, thymus, and lymph node; Schuurman et al., 1994) that cannot be used to indicate specificity of the immune problem or unique host response. Tier 2 is more in depth, involving mechanisms of immunotoxicity. Cell-mediated immunity is assayed by delayed hypersensitivity models. Humoral-mediated immunity is determined by IgG responses to sheep RBCs. Immunopathology at this tier level involves quantitation of splenic B and T cells. Macrophage function is used as a measure of nonspecific (innate) immunity. Death is the measure of host resistance to bacterial or viral challenge, while tumor incidence and parasitemia are how tumor cell and parasite challenge are determined, respectively. Three tiers may involve screening for immunotoxic agents (Tier 1), defining immune components affected by toxic compounds (Tier 2), and mode of action of those toxic chemicals (Tier 3). The tier system has been analyzed by the National Academy of Sciences (National Research Council, or NRC; Subcommittee on Immunotoxicology, Committee on Biologic Markers, Board of Environmental Studies and Toxicology, National Research Council, 1992) and the World Health Organization (WHO Collaborating Center for Immunotoxicology and Hypersensitivity, 2008). Tier 1 under the NRC involves serum antibodies (IgG, IgM, IgA, IgE), natural antibody levels to ubiquitous antigens, secondary antibody responses to proteins and polysaccharides, immunophenotyping, secondary delayed-type hypersensitivity, and autoantibody titers (DNA, mitochondria). The WHO desired a Tier 1 including a hematological profile, antibody-mediated immunity, immunophenotyping, delayed hypersensitivity response, C-reactive protein, autoantibody titers (DNA, mitochondria), IgE to common allergens, natural killer cells activity or numbers, phagocytosis, and clinical chemistry. Historically, the guinea pig has served as the skin sensitization model dating back to Draize in the 1930s. Intradermal and/or epicutaneous administration of chemicals to 10–20 guinea pigs ± adjuvant over a 2- to 3-week period was used to induce sensitization followed by a 1- to 2-week rest period. This was followed by a challenge dose) and a 24- to 48-hour evaluation period for erythema (control = 5–10 sham-treated animals challenged). The Local Lymph Node Assay (LLNA) is considered a valid alternative for skin sensitization in which lymph node cell proliferation of four animals per group and three test concentrations (with a vehicle control) is determined in response to skin exposures to chemical agents. A ≥ 3-fold increase in draining lymph node cell proliferation (Stimulation Index) is considered the threshold for indication of a skin-sensitizing agent. Many of these older models either lack specificity or have an immune bias. For example, the brown Norway rat and BALB/c and C3H/HeJ murine models used to assess food allergies measure the Th2 allergic phenotype and elevated IgE production. This problem also applies to respiratory allergens, with the additional difficulty of designing an inhalation study. The clinical symptoms of rodent models for food allergies do not imitate human responses. Dogs and pigs are better models but provide greater expense and animal welfare issues. Newer models using cytokine and gene expression assays may be more specific, but need additional validation. Autoimmune/immune stimulatory models exist, but are not complete for all diseases that may exist in the human. For example, the popliteal lymph node assay measures nonspecific stimulation and proliferation in lymph nodes draining chemically exposed tissues, but fails in determination of the potential to produce a specific disease. It is also important to measure the effects of immunosuppressant or other immunomodulatory medications, because affecting one part of the immune cascade may lead to adverse responses in other portions of the immune response (Luster and Gerberick, 2010).

In Vitro Alternative Approaches

In vitro methods for immunotoxicology have been promoted by the European Centre for the Validation of Alternative Methods (EVCAM). EVCAM stresses the use of quantitative structure–activity relationship (QSAR) models and cell and tissue culture methods for assessment of toxicity. The QSAR model stresses the use of the deductive estimation of risk from existing knowledge (DEREK) rule base as a screen for skin sensitization. Human dendritic cell cultures can be used to induce IL-1β as a screen for skin sensitizers. This should include methods for introducing lipophilic chemicals into the culture medium and a skin-metabolizing system. EVCAM stresses that pivotal events in the immune system rather than the entire cascade should be identified and used in testing. Induction of immunotoxic effects rather than factors influencing the expression of these effects is the initial focus of the research in this area. Human tissues (lymphocytes, lymphoid tissue, blood, skin) and cytokines should be studied rather than animal responses. This immunotoxicology testing should be integrated with knowledge gained clinically from occupational, clinical, voluntary, accidental, and environmental exposures to estimate true human risks (Balls and Sabbioni, 2001).

Developmental Immunotoxicity Testing

Developmental immunotoxicology methods have also been considered. The effects of TCDD and diethylstilbestrol indicate that perinatal exposure is qualitatively and quantitatively different from adult animal exposure. Windows of vulnerability have been described for animals based on immune system development. For mice and rats, gestational days 7–9 involve hematopoietic stem cell formation. Gestational days 9–19 define tissue migration and progenitor cell expansion. Bone marrow and thymus colonization occur from gestational day 13 until parturition. Following birth until day 30, perinatal immune maturation occurs. Immune memory is established 30–60 days following birth. Humans have similar periods of immune sensitivity, but there are differences based on portions of gestation or postnatal development. Even rodents have differences in responses. For example, Pb affects macrophage and T cell function in rodents if exposed for the full gestational period. In contrast, rats exposed to Pb for the first half of embryonic development only appear to exhibit persistent macrophage alterations. Later, exposures to Pb influence both macrophage and T-dependent functional deficiencies. Chickens exhibit decreased inflammatory mediators with early embryonic exposures to lead, while exposures later in development inhibit T cell function. These differences are useful in identifying mechanisms of action but not hazard identification based on windows of vulnerability. The rat was selected as the developmental immunotoxicity model for hazard identification based on the reproductive toxicity data for this species. However, murine models may be better suited for mechanism identification as methods, reagents, and transgenic mouse models are much better defined for this purpose. There are differences in species responses here as well. Mice show antibody responses as the better measure of prenatal TCDD exposure, while rats exhibit thymus weight alterations as a more sensitive indicator. Differences with the human are also important, as human neonates exhibit weak immune responses that are predominated by Th2 rather than Th1 immunity. These developmental stage differences are important, because different immune cell responses may not be expressed at the time of exposure or testing. As an example, the immunosuppressant agent hydrocortisone, if administered late in rodent gestation, exhibits no inhibited antibody response 14 days following birth, but will be inhibited by postnatal day 28. A design that allows for toxicity evaluation of the immune, neurological, and reproductive systems simultaneously would expose pregnant dams from gestational day 12 until 7 days after delivery of the pups to ensure that the breast milk transfer was also of interest. On postnatal day 8, the pups are dosed directly daily until they reach 42 days of age (end of puberty). One male and one female would be used at this point to assess immune function, while other pups would serve as reproductive, lactational, and necropsy subjects. Plasma concentrations of the compound would be determined in the pups to indicate that placental or milk transfer did occur. The immune endpoint that would best serve to illustrate a number of functions simultaneously and have reproducibility as the T-dependent antigen response involving Th2 cells, B lymphocytes, and antigen-presenting cells as well as TNF, IL-1, IL-4, IFNγ, and adhesion molecules. Sheep RBCs would serve as the antigen, because those responses are clear in the rat. Thymus, spleen, and lymph node weights should be taken even though vaccination in humans can influence spleen and lymph weights. The weight of the thymus appears more reliable information than the cellularity of this organ and is a reproducible indicator of developmental immune system toxicity. Blood counts are additional useful data, especially because the neonate has significant blood development. The complete blood count or the differential count may be affected by toxicant exposure. Because the T-dependent antigen response does not assess Th1 function, a cytotoxic T cell assay or delayed (Type IV) hypersensitivity assay appears warranted. It is not clear what purposes would be served as of yet by macrophage function tests, complement analysis, or surface marker analysis as clinical consequences or changes are not clear and add to the expense of more detailed analysis. This is good mechanistic data, but may exceed the regulatory need to establish a hazard (Luster et al., 2003).

Questions

1. Which part of the immune defense system is considered indicative of asthma (innate or acquired and which component)? How does barrier breakdown play a role in asthma?
2. How can heavy metals such as arsenic lead to increased infection by altering the innate immune defense system?
3. What would be the effect of acetaminophen's hepatotoxicity when giving M1 macrophage inhibitor GdCl$_3$ or targeting M2 macrophages with clodronate liposomes?
4. How do smoke products cause COPD via innate immunity?
5. How can iodinated benzene derivatives mimic true IgE-mediated allergic reactions?
6. How can the cells be grouped based on their functions?
7. Why might females develop more allergies to cigarette smoke than males?
8. Why does insulin resistance related to obesity appear to be a backward immune response?
9. The Gell and Coombs's classification has one allergy, two autoimmune and one T cell reaction. What are they?

References

Akdis M. 2010. The cellular orchestra in skin allergy; are differences to lung and nose relevant? *Curr Opin Allergy Clin Immunol.* 10:443–451.

Apte UM, Banerjee A, McRee R, Wellberg E, Ramaiah SK. 2005. Role of osteopontin in hepatic neutrophil infiltration during alcoholic steatohepatitis. *Toxicol Appl Pharmacol.* 207:25–38.

Austyn JM. 1987. Lymphoid dendritic cells. *Immunology.* 62:161–170.

Bains SN, Hamilton RG, Abouhassan S, Lang D, Han Y, Hsieh FH. 2010. Identification of clinically relevant cross-sensitization between *Soliadgo virgaurea* (goldenrod) and *Hevea brasiliensis* (natural rubber latex). *J Investig Allergol Clin Immunol.* 20:331–339.

Balali-Mood M, Hefazi M. 2006. Comparison of early and late toxic effects of sulfur mustard in Iranian veterans. *Basic Clin Pharmacol Toxicol.* 99:273–282.

Balls M, Sabbioni E. 2001. Promotion of research on *in vitro* immunotoxicology. *Sci Total Environ.* 270:21–25.

Belin LG, Norman PS. 1977. Diagnostic tests in the skin and serum of works sensitized to *Bacillus subtilis* enzymes. *Clin Allergy.* 7:55–68.

Bettelli E, Carrier Y, Gao W, Korn T, Strom TB, Oukka M, Weiner HL, Kuchroo VK. 2006. Reciprocal developmental pathways for the generation of pathogenic effector TH17 and regulatory T cells. *Nature.* 441:235–238.

Burastero SE, Paolucci C, Fabbri M. 2009. Ambient pollutants as adjuvant for allergic sensitization: the emerging role of platinum group elements. *J Biol Regul Homeost Agents.* 23:207–215.

Castelli R, Cassinerio E, Cappellini MD, Porro F, Graziadei G, Fabris F. 2007. Heparin induced thrombocytopenia: pathogenetic, clinical, diagnostic and therapeutic aspects. *Cardiovasc Hematol Disord Drug Targets.* 7:153–162.

Center for Drug Evaluation and Research. 2002. Guidance for industry. *Immunotoxicology evaluation of investigational new drugs.* U.S. Department of Health and Human Services. Rockvillle, MD: Food and Drug Administration. http://www.fda.gov/downloads/Drugs/GuidanceComplianceRegulatoryInformation/Guidances/ucm079239.pdf.

Chang C, Gershwin ME. 2010. Drugs and autoimmunity—a contemporary review and mechanistic approach. *J Autoimmun.* 34:J266–J275.

Charlier CJ, Plomteux GJ. 1997. [Immunotoxicity of drugs]. *J Pharm Belg.* 52:196–200.

Chiung YM, Kao YY, Chang WF, Yao CW, Liu PS. 2010. Toluene diisocyanate (TDI) induces calcium elevation and interleukine-4 (IL-4) release—early responses upon TDI stimulation. *J Toxicol Sci.* 35:197–207.

Cobbold S. n.d. *T cell subsets.* http://users.path.ox.ac.uk/~scobbold/Teaching/TSUBSETS.pdf.

Coffman RL, Seymour BW, Lebman DA, Hiraki DD, Christiansen JA, Shrader B, Cherwinski HM, Savelkoul HF, Finkelman FD, Bond MW, Mossman, TR. 1988. The role of helper T cell products in mouse B cell differentiation and isotype regulation. *Immunol Rev.* 102:5–28.

Committee on Biologic Markers, Board on Environmental Studies and Toxicology, National Research Council. 1992. *Biological markers in immunotoxicology.* Washington, DC: National Academies Press. http://books.nap.edu/catalog.php?record_id=1591.

Corsini E, Roggen EL. 2009. Immunotoxicology: opportunities for non-animal test development. *Altern Lab Anim.* 37:387–397.

Cowdery JS, Chace JH, Yi AK, Krieg AM. 1996. Bacterial DNA induces NK cells to produce

IFN-gamma in vivo and increases the toxicity of lipopolysaccharides. *J Immunol.* 156:4570–4575.

Crampton SP, Voynova E, Bolland S. 2010. Innate pathways to B-cell activation and tolerance. *Ann N Y Acad Sci.* 1183:58–68.

Crotty S. 2011. Follicular helper CD4 T cells (TFH). *Annu Rev Immunol.* 29:621–663.

Dastychová E, Necas M, Vasku V. 2008. Contact hypersensitivity to selected excipients of dermatological topical preparations and cosmetics in patients with chronic eczema. *Acta Dermatovenerol Alp Panonica Adriat.* 17:61–68.

Davis MD. 2009. Unusual patterns in contact dermatitis: medicaments. *Dermatol Clin.* 27:289–297.

Dean JH. 2004. A brief history of immunotoxicology and a review of the pharmaceutical guidelines. *Int J Toxicol.* 23:83–90.

Dearman RJ, Skinner RA, Humphreys NE, Kimber I. 2003. Methods for the identification of chemical respiratory allergens in rodents: comparisons of cytokine profiling with induced changes in serum IgE. *J Appl Toxicol.* 23:199–207.

Descotes J, Choquet-Kastylevsky G. 2001. Gell and Coombs's classification: is it still valid? *Toxicology.* 158:43–49.

DiLillo DJ, Matsushita T, Tedder TF. 2010. B10 cells and regulatory B cells balance immune responses during inflammation, autoimmunity, and cancer. *Ann NY Acad Sci.* 1183:38–57.

Dinarello CA. 2007. Historical insights into cytokines. *Eur J Immunol.* 37(Suppl 1):S34–S45.

Edwards TM, Myers JP. 2007. Environmental exposures and gene regulation in disease etiology. *Environ Health Perspect.* 115:1264–1270.

Erta M, Quintana A, Hidalgo J. 2012. Interleukin-6, a major cytokine in the central nervous system *Int J Biol Sci.* 8:1254–1266

Evans DL, Jacobsen KL, Miller DM. 1984. Hematologic and immunologic responses of Holstein calves to a fire ant toxicant. *Am J Vet Res.* 45:1023–1027.

Flörcken A, Takvorian A, Van Lessen A, Singh A, Hopfenmüller W, Dörken B, Pezzutto A, Westermann J. 2012. Sorafenib, but not sunitinib, induces regulatory T cells in the peripheral blood of patients with metastatic renal cell carcinoma. *Anticancer Drugs.* 23:298–302.

Fukuyama T, Tajima Y, Ueda H, Hayashi K, Shutoh Y, Harada T, Kosaka T. 2009. Allergic reaction induced by dermal and/or respiratory exposure to low-dose phenoxyacetic acid, organophosphorus, and carbamate pesticides. *Toxicology.* 261:152–161. Erratum in: *Toxicology.* 262:272.

Fukuyama T, Ueda H, Hayashi K, Tajima Y, Shuto Y, Saito TR, Harada T, Kosaka T. 2008. Use of long term dermal sensitization followed by intratracheal challenge method to identify low-dose chemical-induced respiratory allergic responses in mice. *Toxicol Lett.* 181:163–170.

Gabriel LC, Escribano LM, Villa E, Leiva C, Valdes MD. 1986. Ultrastructural study of blood cells in toxic oil syndrome. *Acta Haematol.* 75:165–170.

Gallicchio VS, Hulette BC. 1989. In vitro effect of lithium on carbamazepine-induced inhibition of murine and human bone marrow-derived granulocyte-macrophage, erythroid, and mega-karyocyte progenitor stem cells. *Proc Soc Exp Biol Med.* 190:109–116.

Gell PGH, Coombs RRA. 1963. The classification of allergic reactions underlying disease. In: Coombs RRA, Gell GH, Eds., *Clinical aspects of immunology.* Oxford, UK: Blackwell Science.

Germolec D. 2009. *Levels of evidence criteria for NTP immunotoxicology studies.* Society of Toxicology Meeting, Baltimore, MD, March 17. http://ntp.niehs .nih.gov/ntp/test_info/germolecitoxcriteriasotfinal _508.pdf.

Greenberger PA. 2006. Anaphylactic and anaphylactoid causes of angioedema. *Immunol Allergy Clin North Am.* 26:753–767.

Hirano S. 1996. [Evaluation of pulmonary toxicity of heavy metal compounds]. *Nippon Eiseigaku Zasshi.* 50:1013–1025.

Goodman DL, McDonnell JT, Nelson HS, Vaughan TR, Weber RW. 1990. Chronic urticaria exacerbated by the antioxidant food preservatives, butylated hydroxyanisole (BHA) and butylated hydroxytoluene (BHT). *J Allergy Clin Immunol.* 86:570–575.

Holgate ST, Roberts G, Arshad HS, Howarth PH, Davies DE. 2009. The role of the airway epithelium and its interaction with environmental factors in asthma pathogenesis. *Proc Am Thorac Soc.* 6:655–659.

Holladay SD, Mustafa A, Gogal RM Jr. 2010. Prenatal TCDD in mice increases adult autoimmunity. *Reprod Toxicol.* 31:312–318

Hollingsworth JW, Kleeberger SR, Foster WM. 2007. Ozone and pulmonary innate immunity. *Proc Am Thorac Soc.* 4:240–246.

Hybenova M, Hrda P, Procházková J, Stejskal V, Sterzl I. 2010. The role of environmental factors in autoimmune thyroiditis. *Neuro Endocrinol Lett.* 31:283–289.

Irwin CR, Myrillas TT. 1998. The role of IL-6 in the pathogenesis of periodontal disease. *Oral Dis.* 4:43–47.

Ismail N, Crossley EC, Stevenson HL, Walker DH. 2007. Relative importance of T-cell subsets in monocytotropic ehrlichiosis: a novel effector mechanism involved in Ehrlichia-induced immunopathology in murine ehrlichiosis. *Infect Immun.* 75:4608–4620.

Jagannathan M, McDonnell M, Liang Y, Hasturk H, Hetzel J, Rubin D, Kantarci A, Van Dyke TE, Ganley-Leal LM, Nikolajczyk BS. 2010. Toll-like receptors regulate B cell cytokine production in patients with diabetes. *Diabetologia.* 53:1461–1471.

Jäger A, Dardalhon V, Sobel RA, Bettelli E, Kuchroo VK. 2009. Th1, Th17, and Th9 effector cells induce experimental autoimmune encephalomyelitis with different pathological phenotypes. *J Immunol.* 183:7169–7177.

Karmaus W, Brooks KR, Nebe T, Witten J, Obi-Osius N, Kruse H. 2005. Immune function biomarkers in children exposed to lead and organochlorine compounds: a cross-sectional study. *Environ Health.* 4:5.

Kean T, McNally M. 2009. Latex hypersensitivity: a closer look at considerations for dentistry. *J Can Dent Assoc.* 75:279–282.

Kimber I, Dearman RJ. 2010. An assessment of the ability of phthalates to influence immune and allergic responses. *Toxicology.* 271:73–82.

Ku HO, Jeong SH, Kang HG, Pyo HM, Cho JH, Son SW, Yun SM, Ryu DY. 2009. Gene expression profiles and pathways in skin inflammation induced by three different sensitizers and an irritant. *Toxicol Lett.* 190:231–237.

Kundu CR, Roychoudhury S. 2009. Malathion-induced sublethal toxicity on the hematology of cricket frog (*Fejervarya limnocharis*). *J Environ Sci Health B.* 44:673–680.

Kusaka Y. 1993. [Occupational diseases caused by exposure to sensitizing metals]. *Sangyo Igaku.* 35:75–87.

Larsen CM, Faulenbach M, Vaag A, Vølund A, Ehses JA, et al. 2007. Interleukin-1-receptor antagonist in type 2 diabetes mellitus. *N Engl J Med.* 356:1517–1526.

Laskin DL. 2009. Macrophages and inflammatory mediators in chemical toxicity: a battle of forces. *Chem Res Toxicol.* 22:1376–1385.

Latimer KS, Tang KN, Goodwin MA, Steffens WL, Brown J. 1988. Leukocyte changes associated with acute inflammation in chickens. *Avian Dis.* 32:760–772.

Loza MJ, Foster S, Bleecker ER, Peters SP, Penn RB. 2010. Asthma and gender impact accumulation of T cell subtypes. *Respir Res.* 11:103.

Lundov MD, Johansen JD, Carlsen BC, Engkilde K, Menné T, Thyssen JP. 2010. Formaldehyde exposure and patterns of concomitant contact allergy to formaldehyde and formaldehyde-releasers. *Contact Dermatitis.* 63:31–36.

Luster MI, Dean JH, Germolec DR. 2003. Consensus workshop on methods to evaluate developmental immunotoxicity. *Environ Health Perspect.* 111:579–583.

Luster MI, Gerberick GF. 2010. Immunotoxicology testing: past and future. *Methods Mol Biol.* 598:3–13.

Marshall NB, Kerkvliet NI. 2010. Dioxin and immune regulation: emerging role of aryl hydrocarbon receptor in the generation of regulatory T cells. *Ann NY Acad Sci.* 1183:25–37.

Martin F, Kearney JF. 2000. B-cell subsets and the mature preimmune repertoire. Marginal zone and B1 B cells as part of a "natural immune memory". *Immunol Rev.* 175:70–79.

Middleton D, Kowalski P. 2010. Advances in identifying beryllium sensitization and disease. *Int J Environ Res Public Health.* 7:115–124.

Miller JS, Cervenka T, Lund J, Okazaki IJ, Moss J. 1999. Purine metabolites suppress proliferation of human NK cells through a lineage-specific purine receptor. *J Immunol.* 162:7376–7382.

Minamoto K. 2010. [Skin sensitizers in cosmetics and skin care products]. *Nippon Eiseigaku Zasshi.* 65:20–29.

Mishra KP. 2009. Lead exposure and its impact on immune system: a review. *Toxicol In Vitro.* 23:969–972.

Möller H. 2010. Contact allergy to gold as a model for clinical-experimental research. *Contact Dermatitis.* 62:193–200.

Muñoz-Cánoves P, Scheele C, Pedersen BK, Serrano AL. 2013. Interleukin-6 myokine signaling in skeletal muscle: a double-edged sword? *FEBS J.* 280:4131–4148.

Murai M, Krause P, Cheroutre H, Kronenberg M. 2010. Regulatory T-cell stability and plasticity in mucosal and systemic immune systems. *Mucosal Immunol.* 3:443–449.

Nakano E, Iwasaki A, Seguchi T, Sugao H, Tada Y, Matsuda M, Sonoda T. 1991. [Usefulness and limitation of immunotherapy of metastatic renal cell carcinoma with autologous lymphokine-activated killer cells and interleukin 2]. *Nippon Hinyokika Gakkai Zasshi.* 82:395–404.

Nayak AS, Lage CR, Kim CH. 2007. Effects of low concentrations of arsenic on the innate immune system of the zebrafish (*Danio rerio*). *Toxicol Sci.* 98:118–124.

Nayak KR, White AA, Cavendish JJ, Barker CM, Kandzari DE. 2009. Anaphylactoid reactions to radiocontrast agents: prevention and treatment in the cardiac catheterization laboratory. *J Invasive Cardiol.* 21:548–551.

Nikolajczyk BS. 2010. B cells as under-appreciated mediators of non-auto-immune inflammatory disease. *Cytokine.* 50:234–242.

O'Malley MA. 1997. Skin reactions to pesticides. *Occup Med.* 12:327–345.

Pascoe D, Moreau L, Sasseville D. 2010. Emergent and unusual allergens in cosmetics. *Dermatitis.* 21:127–137.

Peng SL. 2006. The T-box transcription factor T-bet in immunity and autoimmunity. *Cell Mol Immunol.* 3:87–95.

Perumal V, Alkire M, Swank ML. 2010. Unusual presentation of cobalt hypersensitivity in a patient with a metal-on-metal bearing in total hip arthroplasty. *Am J Orthop (Belle Mead NJ).* 39:E39–E41.

Pollock RE, Lotzová E, Stanford SD. 1991. Mechanism of surgical stress impairment of human perioperative natural killer cell cytotoxicity. *Arch Surg.* 126:338–342.

Rajpara A, Feldman SR. 2010. Cell phone allergic contact dermatitis: case report and review. *Dermatol Online J.* 16:9.

Reich HC, Warshaw EM. 2010. Allergic contact dermatitis from formaldehyde textile resins. *Dermatitis.* 21:65–76.

Reus KE, Houben GF, Stam M, Dubois AE. 2000. [Food additives as a cause of medical symptoms: relationship shown between sulfites and asthma and anaphylaxis; results of a literature review]. *Ned Tijdschr Geneeskd.* 144:1836–1839.

Riahi B, Rafatpanah H, Mahmoudi M, Memar B, Brook A, Tabasi N, Karimi G. 2010. Immunotoxicity of paraquat after subacute exposure to mice. *Food Chem Toxicol.* 48:1627–1631.

Rosenberg CE, Fink NE, Arrieta MA, Salibián A. 2003. Effect of lead acetate on the in vitro engulfment and killing capability of toad (*Bufo arenarum*) neutrophils. *Comp Biochem Physiol C Toxicol Pharmacol.* 136:225–233.

Schuurman HJ, Kuper CF, Vos JG. 1994. Histopathology of the immune system as a tool to assess immunotoxicity. *Toxicology.* 86:187–212.

Seki M, Oomizu S, Sakata KM, Sakata A, Arikawa T, Watanabe K, Ito K, Takeshita K, Niki T, Saita N, Nishi N, Yamauchi A, Katoh S, Matsukawa A, Kuchroo V, Hirashima M. 2008. Galectin-9 suppresses the generation of Th17, promotes the induction of regulatory T cells, and regulates experimental autoimmune arthritis. *Clin Immunol.* 127:78–88.

Schiraldi M, Monestier M. 2009. How can a chemical element elicit complex immunopathology? Lessons from mercury-induced autoimmunity. *Trends Immunol.* 30:502–509.

Schneider C, Döcke WD, Zollner TM, Röse L. 2009. Chronic mouse model of TMA-induced contact hypersensitivity. *J Invest Dermatol.* 129:899–907.

Schwaab T, Schwarzer A, Wolf B, Gui J, Fisher JL, Crosby NA, Seigne JD, Ernstoff MS. 2008. Characterization of nTreg in patients with metastatic renal cell carcinoma (RCC) undergoing DC-vaccination and cytokine therapy. *J Clin Oncol.* 26:abstr 16038.

Seymour BW, Friebertshauser KE, Peake JL, Pinkerton KE, Coffman RL, Gershwin LJ. 2002. Gender differences in the allergic response of mice neonatally exposed to environmental tobacco smoke. *Dev Immunol.* 9:47–54.

Seymour BW, Pinkerton KE, Friebertshauser KE, Coffman RL, Gershwin LJ. 1997. Second-hand smoke is an adjuvant for T helper-2 responses in a murine model of allergy. *J Immunol.* 159:6169–6175.

Sharma RN, Deva C, Behera D, Khanduja KL. 1997. Reactive oxygen species formation in peripheral blood neutrophils in different types of smokers. *Indian J Med Res.* 106:475–480.

Sircar G, Saha B, Bhattacharya SG, Saha S. 2014. Allergic asthma biomarkers using systems approaches. *Front Genet.* 4:308.

Słotwińska SM. 2012. Cytokines and periodontitis. Part I: interleukin-1 and interleukin-1 receptor antagonism. *Centr Eur J Immunol.* 37:173–177.

Snelgrove RJ, Jackson PL, Hardison MT, Noerager BD, Kinloch A, Gaggar A, Shastry S, Rowe SM, Shim YM, Hussell T, Blalock JE. 2010. A critical role for LTA4H in limiting chronic pulmonary neutrophilic inflammation. *Science.* 330:90–94.

Subcommittee on Immunotoxicology, Committee on Biologic Markers, Board of Environmental Studies and Toxicology, National Research Council. 1992. *Biologic Markers in Immunotoxicology.* Washington, DC: National Academies Press.

Szeimies RM, Meurer M. 1993. [The tryptophan-associated eosinophilia-myalgia syndrome. A clinical follow-up of 8 patients]. *Dtsch Med Wochenschr.* 118:213–220.

Thiagarajan R, Gopalakrishnan S, Thilagam H. 2006. Immunomodulation the marine green mussel *Perna viridis* exposed to sub-lethal concentrations of Cu and Hg. *Arch Environ Contam Toxicol.* 51:392–399.

Tilg H, Trehu E, Atkins MB, Dinarello CA, Mier JW. 1994. Interleukin-6 (IL-6) as an antiinflammatory cytokine: induction of circulating IL-1 receptor antagonist and soluble tumor necrosis factor receptor p55. *Blood.* 83:113–118.

Tosello V, Odunsi K, Souleimanian NE, Lele S, Shrikant P, Old LJ, Valmori D, Ayyoub M. 2008. Differential expression of CCR7 defines two distinct subsets of human memory CD4+CD25+ Tregs. *Clin Immunol.* 126:291–302.

Usatine RP, Riojas M. 2010. Diagnosis and management of contact dermatitis. *Am Fam Physician.* 82:249–255.

WHO Collaborating Center for Immunotoxicology and Hypersensitivity. 2008. International Programme on Chemical Safety. Project on the Harmonization of Approaches to the Assessment of Risk from Exposure to Chemicals. WHO/IPCS Scoping Meeting for the Development of Guidance for Immunotoxicology Risk Assessment for Chemicals, RIVM, Bilthoven, The Netherlands, 28-29 February.

Winer DA, Winer S, Chng MHY, Shen L, Engleman EG. 2014. B Lymphocytes in obesity related adipose tissue inflammation and insulin resistance. *Cell Mol Life Sci.* 71: 1033–1043.

Wolkoff P, Nielsen GD. 2010. Non-cancer effects of formaldehyde and relevance for setting an indoor air guideline. *Environ Int.* 36:788–799.

Yamada A, Salama AD, Sayegh MH. 2002. The role of novel T cell costimulatory pathways in autoimmunity and transplantation. *J Am Soc Nephrol.* 13:559–575.

CHAPTER 20

The Nervous System and Exposure to Lipophilic Toxicants or Transported Neurotoxic Agents

This is a chapter outline intended to guide and familiarize you with the content to follow.

I. Neurotoxicology

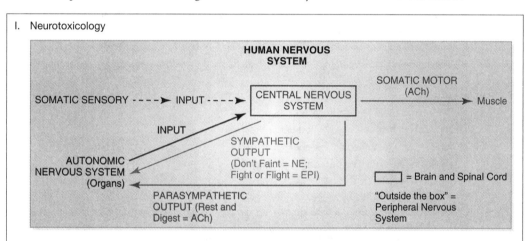

HUMAN NERVOUS SYSTEM

SOMATIC SENSORY ----> INPUT ----> CENTRAL NERVOUS SYSTEM

SOMATIC MOTOR (ACh) ------> Muscle

INPUT

AUTONOMIC NERVOUS SYSTEM (Organs)

SYMPATHETIC OUTPUT (Don't Faint = NE; Fight or Flight = EPI)

PARASYMPATHETIC OUTPUT (Rest and Digest = ACh)

☐ = Brain and Spinal Cord

"Outside the box" = Peripheral Nervous System

A. Divisions

   1. Central (CNS) = Integrating Center

   2. Peripheral = Sensory Inputs and Motor and Autonomic Outputs + Neurohormones

B. CNS Toxicity—see Table 20-1

   1. Blood-brain barrier (BBB)—specialized endothelial cells providing a barrier (usually excludes molecules > 400 Da) and electrical resistance of 2000 Ωcm^2

      a. Broaching the barrier by magnetic nanoparticles, hypovascularity, fibrosis, or necrosis—see Figure 20-2

      b. Ultrasonic radiation can temporarily allow passage of molecules up to 150 kDa

      c. ROS can damage endothelial lining and tight junctional structures creating damaged protein, polyunsaturated lipids, and nucleic acids despite protection offered by GSH, GSH peroxidase, SOD, and catalase—specific uptake of paraquat to generate ROS decreased by L-valine (neutral amino acid transport) or low Na^+ (usually used for secondary active transport)

      d. Pb^{2+} is an historic neurotoxic heavy metal causing learning problems to lethality. Pb^{2+} causes protein leakage from capillary endothelium of the BBB → cerebral hemorrhage. Pb^{2+} uses L-type Ca^{2+} channels via store-operated Ca^{2+} channels and Ca^{2+} permeable acid-sensing channels to enter cells. Certain cells transport more lead (RBE4 model), while other retain more (BMEC model). Retaining lead interferes with Ca^{2+}-dependent signaling pathways affecting vascular resistance, hypertension, and cellular inflammation

e. Malathion damages by malaoxon metabolite inhibiting AChE, especially in RBE4 model

f. Damage to astrocytes can also cause leakage through the BBB (e.g., 3-chloropropanediol → focal lesions via astrocyte death, but not neuronal death)

g. Choroid plexus (generates CSF)—metal damage separated

(1) Direct damage = Hg and Cd

(2) Pathway affected = Pb (affects regulatory pathway of transthyretin production and secretion—also affects thyroid hormone transport into brain) and Mn (Fe/transferrin-dependent and independent pathways → involving store operated Ca^{2+} channels to accumulate Mn = Parkinson-like syndrome)

(3) Sequestered as CNS defense mechanism = Fe, Ag, Au

(4) As, Cd, and Pb act synergistically on developing rat brain starting with BBB disruption →↑ apoptosis in astrocytes, cerebral cortex, and cerebellum (proximal ERK signaling → downstream JNK signaling →↑ intracellular Ca^{2+} and ROS)

h. Kainic acid (mainly hippocampus damage) breaches BBB

i. Experimental allergic encephalomyelitis (multiple sclerosis model) involves disruption of BBB + bipiperidyl mustard or triamine → necrotizing vasculitis and parenchymal necrosis

j. Aurothioglucose → damages brain blood vessels → necrosis and thrombosis

k. Development of the BBB important as it limits damage by hexachlorophene and unconjugated bilirubin (more problematic in children)

2. Metabolic barrier = oxidative enzymes of endothelial cells' cytosol (MAO, xanthine oxidase, NADPH-cytochrome P450 reductase)

3. Mechanisms of neurotoxicity beyond blood-brain barrier

a. Altered calcium homeostasis—see Figure 20-3

(1) 10,000-fold gradient outside/inside cells

(2) Ca^{2+} removed by Ca^{2+}-ATPase and Na^+/Ca^{2+} exchanger + sequester in endoplasmic reticulum and mitochondria + calmodulin binding

(3) Ca^{2+} causes structural damage and signals cell death, but also plays major roles in release of neurotransmitters, neuronal excitability, integrations of electrical signals, synaptic plasticity, cellular metabolism, and gene expression

(4) ↑ $[Ca]_i$ → capsaicin-activated receptors → conductance permeability to Ca^{2+} (and other heavy metal cations such as Co^{2+}) → peripheral nerve damage

(5) Activating NMDA receptors (by kainic acid at type II receptors as type I only increase Na^+ permeability), EAA receptors (ionotropic—directly activate ion channels and metabotropic—enzymatic process) → Ca^{2+} influx. This NMDA receptor induction may be related to methylmercury (MeHg) neurotoxicity in a mink model

(6) Ammonia neurotoxicity related to formation of glutamine and NMDA/nitric oxide/cGMP pathway and mitochondrial dysfunction (conversion back to ammonia → Krebs cycle and malate-aspartate shuttle enzyme interference)—see Figure 20-3

b. Altered protein structure and function

(1) Protein kinase C—activation by phorbol ester or MeHg → ↑ PKC activity → neurodegeneration due to over-phosphorylation. Similarly, inhibition of serine/threonine protein phosphatases 1 and 2A by okadaic acid → neurodegeneration

(2) Calpain I (Ca^{2+}-activated neural cysteine protease) is a downstream site that ↑ Ca^{2+} may activate and is present in neurons susceptible to excitotoxins (including organophosphorus compounds that inhibit AChE → ↑ ACh → Ca^{2+} through L-type channels → calpain activation) or ischemia induced neural degeneration. This enzyme's substrates are neurofilament polypeptides, microtubule-associated proteins, tubulin, and spectrin (structural proteins). Linked to spinal and head trauma, peripheral nerve injury, demyelination disease, muscular atrophy, lens cataract formation, and cerebral ischemia

CONCEPTUALIZING TOXICOLOGY 20-1 (*continued*)

(3) Phospholipase A$_2$ activation (by compounds such as MeHg apart from its lipid peroxidation activity, ischemia, chemical anoxia, or cytolytic toxins) → deacylate the sn-2 fatty acyl position of membrane phosphatides → activation of second messenger systems → uncontrolled influx of Ca^{2+} → cell death

(4) Lysosomal acid hydrolases

    i. Direct toxicity elicited by ischemia, radiation poisoning, acrylamide, triorthocresyl phosphate, Al, and neurodegenerative disorders such as ALS and Creutzfeldt-Jakob disease with minimum morphological changes in neuronal lysosomal system

    ii. A late stage ↑ secondary lysosomes accompanies axotomy, chromatolysis, guanethidine, n-hexane, malnutrition, radiation, and Wobbler mutation

    iii. Early lysosomal alteration occurs with secondary lysosome alteration and accumulation of lipofuscin (old antimalarial chloroquine), ceroid, and storage bodies

(5) Nerve growth factor (NGF) deprivation—toxicants or aging factors such as β-amyloid, τ and mutated presenilin proteins, free radicals and oxidative stress (as from heavy metal poisoning), and pro-inflammatory cytokines that activate TNFα ↑ apoptosis similarly to withdrawal of NGF

(6) Persistent organic pollutants and AhR signaling—polyhalogenated compounds such as PCBs → numbness, limb weakness, ↓ conduction velocities of peripheral nerves, developmental deficiencies, and speech disturbances (affects dopaminergic and cholinergic neurotransmission as well as affects thyroid hormone and other signaling pathways and GABAergic via Notch signaling pathway during development and *SOX11* regulation of neuronal differentiation)

c. Alterations of gene expression

(1) Following trimethyltin toxicity research—from silver stains for neurodegeneration (hippocampus and limbic cortex) the research team moved onto cDNA or antibody probes (cellular) moving to protein and gene expression (molecular)—uncovered a protein product stannin. Found less stannin antibody reactivity in rat hippocampus, entorhinal cortex, and amygdala structures treated with trimethyltin (more binding)

(2) Neurodegenerative diseases and environmental agents

    i. Alzheimer's disease—amyloidβ peptides → microglia activation and inflammatory cytokine release, excessive release of excitotoxic glutamine from glial cells, inhibition of axonal and dendritic transport, peptides bind to reactive metals and may damage mitochondria

        (a) Hg → ↑ β-amyloid secretion (in brain cultures) and τ (tau is part of the microtubule-associated proteins) hyperphosphorylation; Mn also leads to τ hyperphosphorylation; MeHg → ↑ ROS

        (b) Pb ↑ β-amyloid in a mouse hippocampal cell line and ↓ chaperone activity in astrocyte cultures

        (c) Microgliosis (inflammatory reaction) due to exposure to Hg, Pb, trimethyltin, parathion

    ii. Parkinson's disease—mutations in α–synuclein gene (PARK1 and PARK4) → cytoplasmic inclusions (Lewy bodies) in dopaminergic neurons + oxidative stress + impaired proteasome activity

        (a) MPTP model agent for causing dopaminergic neurotoxicity and affects mitochondria complex I (both neurodegenerative diseases appear to affect mitochondrial function)

        (b) Dithiocarbamate fungicide → preferential injury to dopaminergic neurons and ↑ α-synuclein while inhibiting ubiquitin E1 ligase in primary ventral mesencephalic cultures

        (c) Al, Cu, Fe, and certain pesticides initiate fibrillation of α-synuclein mimicking Parkinson's disease

CONCEPTUALIZING TOXICOLOGY 20-1 (*continued*)

(3) Hypoxia via thromboembolic stroke or cardiac arrest and ubiquitins

    i.   Focal ischemia from stroke, while cardiac arrest causes global ischemia

    ii. CA-1 sector of hippocampus most sensitive to delayed neuronal death from global ischemia. Cells function for 2 days then neuronal death occurs over next 4 days unless protein synthesis is inhibited. $\uparrow$ Ubiquitin is key in this process because it is engaged in degradation of short-lived, denatured, or damaged proteins involving an ATP-dependent protease complex

(4) Cellular immediate-early genes—see Figure 20-4

    i.   Excitatory neurotoxins (kainic or domoic acids) that work via $\uparrow$ Ca^{2+} via glutamate subclasses or convulsants (pentylenetetrazol or lindane) that work via suppression of $GABA_A$ receptor $\rightarrow$ hyperactivity via L-type Ca^{2+} channels (or cerebral ischemia or surgical lesions) all activate transcription of cellular immediate-early genes in the brain which can precede cell death. These genes follow the transcription-independent phosphorylation of ion channels, enzymes, receptors, and cytoskeletal proteins by protein kinases. These cellular immediate-early genes cause longer-lasting effects via Fos and Jun (turn brief excitatory signals into enduring changes in cellular phenotype via altered expression of target genes)

    ii. There are ionotropic and metabotropic glutamate receptors (mGluR)—mGluR selective agonist trans-1-aminocyclopentane-1,3-dicarboxylate or quisqualate prevents the neurotoxic action of glutamate and kainate (ionotropic receptor agonists) to rat cerebellar granule cells. IP_3 via phospholipase C appears to be the pathway that prevents neurodegenerative diseases via activation of ionotropic glutamate receptors

    iii. MDMA (ecstasy) $\rightarrow$ apoptotic damage to 5-HT fibers and $\uparrow$ expression of brain-derived neurotrophic factor, neurotrophin-3, and nerve growth factor (repair)

(5) Heat shock/stress protein expression

    i.   Neuronal hsp72 expressed in a variety of brain injury models including global ischemia and kainic acid. Hyperthermic states $\rightarrow$ glial and vascular expression of this protein (less neuronal involvement)

    ii. Phencyclidine, ketamine, and MK801 $\rightarrow$ $\uparrow$ hsp70 mRNA and HSP72 protein in cingulate neurons of rats. Antipsychotic medications reduce brain injury and heart shock proteins (may indicate that drug-induced brain injury may lead to psychotic states)

(6) Developmental gene expression affected by neurotoxic chemicals

    i.   Different chemicals alter expression of different markers—for example mercury chloride, valproic acid, and trimethyltin chloride downregulated mRNA for NF-68, NF-200, NMDA glutamate receptor, and GABA receptor, while Pb $\downarrow$ expression of GFAP (see II. B.) mRNA

  d. Oxidative stress

    (1) Fe^{2+}, Mn^{2+}, and Cu^{2+} $\rightarrow$ oxygen radicals ($O_2^{-\cdot}$ $\rightarrow$ lipid peroxidation) via Haber-Weiss reaction catalyzed by MAO (dopaminergic neurotoxicity) $\rightarrow$ disrupts oxidative phosphorylation $\rightarrow$ loss of ion homeostasis $\rightarrow$ neuronal cell death

    (2) Paraquat $\rightarrow$ ROS generation $\rightarrow$ accelerated autophagy by ASK1 overexpression $\rightarrow$ endoplasmic reticulum stress $\rightarrow$ neuronal apoptosis

    (3) Neuroinflammatory side to oxidative stress involves NO + $O_2^{-\cdot}$ release from macrophages and microglia $\rightarrow$ peroxynitrite and other RNS $\rightarrow$ nitrosative stress $\rightarrow$ pro-inflammatory gene transcription in glia $\rightarrow$ unfolded and misfolded proteins $\rightarrow$ neurodegeneration and mitochondrial disruption (respiratory chain or mitochondrial DNA unprotected by histone proteins)

  e. Anoxia

    (1) KCN $\rightarrow$ histotoxic hypoxia in corpus striatum and hippocampus of rats $\downarrow$ NE, DA, and 5-HT neurotransmitters

CONCEPTUALIZING TOXICOLOGY 20-1 (*continued*)

f. Environmental causes of neurodegenerative diseases

   (1) ALS/PDC (amyotrophic lateral sclerosis/Parkinson-dementia complex) caused by a toxic amino acid (β-methylamino-L-alanine) made by cyanobacteria that contaminate many lakes with agricultural runoff

   (2) Parkinson's disease caused by dopaminergic neuron destruction by the widely used herbicide glyphosate

g. Solvent-induced CNS depression versus CS_2 toxicity

   (1) K_{OW}-based CNS depression and anesthesia

   (2) Fetal solvent syndrome

   (3) Toluene ↓ ACh in striatum and hippocampus (learning and memory), ↑ extracellular glutamine (neurogenesis and mature function of CNS) and taurine in hippocampus and dopamine in rat prefrontal cortex. Toluene also inhibits excitatory NMDA (except with chronic treatment of hippocampal neurons) and nicotinic receptors and enhances inhibitory $GABA_A$ and glycine receptors. Neuroimmune function affected neurotrophins used to support survival, differentiation, and maintenance of neuronal populations. Neurotrophins are upregulated in mouse hippocampus and allergic stimulation ↓ sensitivity to toluene. Toluene (and other solvents) may ↑ allergic reactions and alter neurogenesis and neuronal migration. Toluene also affects catecholamines → autonomic dysfunction. See Figure 20-5

II. Nerve toxicity tests—see Table 20-2

A. *In situ* sea lamprey model

   1. Giant Muller and Mauthner neurons in the brain and spinal cord

B. Gliosis and glial fibrillar acidic protein (GFAP)

   1. Proliferation of astrocytes following nervous system damage (reactive gliosis) with accumulation of glial fibrillary acidic protein in surviving astrocytes and respond to various neurotoxic chemicals such as 3-acetylpyridine, amino-adipate, bilirubin, cadmium, colchicines, 5,7-dihydroxytryptamine, domoic acid, 6-hydroxydopamine, IDPN, kainate, MDA, MDMA, methamphetamine, MeHg, MPTP, tributyltin, triethyltin, and trimethyltin. Area of brain affected important based on chemical and can differentiate between excitatory neurotoxin analogs (NDMA-receptor antagonist dizocilpine blocked ↑ GFAP of D-MDMA in corpus striatum but other amphetamine analog D-flenfluramine did not affect striatal GFAP and was not affected by pretreatment with dizocilpine)

C. Neurite outgrowth and neurofilament protein levels

   1. A mouse NB41A3 neuroblastoma cell line in culture exhibits less neurite outgrowth and levels of neurofilament proteins in the presence of excitotoxins β-N-methylamino alanine (BMAA) and kainate

D. Inflammatory brain injury and quinolinic acid

   1. Kynurenine pathway → quinolinic acid (HIV-linked dementia) damages in order of sensitivity hippocampus > striatum > cerebral cortex > thalamus

E. Dopaminergic neurotoxicity gene expression

   1. MPTP + MAOB → MPP^+ → dopamine reuptake pump transfers this toxic species into dopaminergic neurons; this substance mainly acts by damaging mitochondrial via oxidative processes

F. Demyelination versus neuronal membrane damage

   1. Hexachlorophene, Pb, Te damage myelin and can be detected centrally by release of myelin basic protein inducing mitogenicity of astrocytes to remyelinate. Damage to the neuronal membrane may be detected by release of fibroblast growth factor

G. Spinal cord damage

   1. Must differentiate glial (C6 glioma cells) versus neuronal (Neuro-2a cells) cell damage—this shows differential effect of plasticizer *N*-butylbenzenesulfonamide → progressive spastic myelopathy

CONCEPTUALIZING TOXICOLOGY 20-1 *(continued)*

(neuroaxonal degeneration) in New Zealand white rabbits (Neuro-2a cells more sensitive—10-fold lower concentrations affected uptake of ^{3}[H]-thymidine)

H. Sulfated glycoprotein-2 (SGP-2)

1. SPG-2 co-localizes to β-amyloid plaques within the parenchyma of brains of patients with Alzheimer's disease, especially in the hippocampus. Also found in human glioma, retinitis pigmentosa, spongiform encephalitis (sheep and goats), transformed neuroretinal cells (quail). Kainic acid → rapid hippocampal pyramidal neuron degeneration and two- to threefold ↑ SPG-2 RNA and protein concentrations. SPG-2 may play roles in apoptosis and clearance of debris following neurodegeneration

I. Laminated-binding protein (LBP)

1. Laminin found in basement membrane of undisturbed brain cells. Ischemia or similar injury → laminin-like molecules associated with reactive glial cells. However, LBP-positive staining astrocytes = early predictors for brain structures where permanent neuron loss would occur. Laminin only stained the somata of reactive astrocytes but not in glial processes = astrogliosis

J. Silver staining during neural degeneration

1. Damaged neurons stain with higher affinity for Ag than intact neurons

K. Noninvasive magnetization transfer techniques in magnetic resonance imaging (MRI)

1. Alterations in white matter can be visualized in normal MRIs of intact humans, and axonal degeneration is at least determinable in cats by changes in magnetization transferred on the lesioned side of the brain

L. Urine nerve growth factor receptor-truncated

1. Humans may have urine tested for nerve growth factor-truncated (degradation product of nerve growth factor) as a measure of neuropathy in diabetic patients

M. Human neurobehavioral tests

1. Blood (e.g., Mn) or hair samples (e.g., MeHg) must be used to assess presence of toxic chemical combined with Stanford-Binet Intelligence Test (especially copying as a visuospatial measure) and appearance of tremor plus effects on attention, fine motor performance, verbal learning, and memory performance. These tests are less mechanistic and more risk assessment for the human population. For children, the pediatric environmental neurobehavioral test may be substituted for the usual adult neurotoxicity screens. Years of exposure may ↑ the toxicity even if the intensity is ↓

CONCEPTUALIZING TOXICOLOGY 20-1 (*continued*)

This chapter covers the sensory, decision-making, and control portion of animals. The complex relationships between portions of the central nervous system and the peripheral nervous system, plasticity of various functional regions, effects of hormones and medications on behavior, ravages of age, disease, toxicant exposure, and so forth make this a difficult area to study. Embryonic and fetal development periods are more sensitive to effects of neurotoxic agents, and learning during childhood also is a complex process and sensitive time to determine the effect of chemicals. Intelligence and degree of learning may make an organism more resilient by establishing more neural integration that suffers less from small deficits induced by chemicals and the early stages of progressive neurological degenerative disease such as Alzheimer's disease. Some chemicals may also cause neural degeneration resembling Alzheimer's or Parkinson's disease. In a recent study, it was revealed that neurodegenerative toxic metabolites such as β-amyloid were removed from the brain during sleep (60% increase in interstitial space resulting in a convective exchange of cerebrospinal fluid with interstitial fluid; Xie et al., 2013)! It is important to also examine the development and function of the blood–brain barrier and the disposition of toxicants based on their charge and lipophilicity. For example, methylmercury may reach a brain easier than a mercuric or mercurous salt if given orally or injected into the bloodstream, while intrathecal injection may yield similar damage. This is all pertinent to the ultimate toxicity observed. Toxicants that affect energy functions, such as cyanide or hydrogen sulfide, are especially damaging to the nervous system, because the brain uses much of its energy in maintaining memory functions. The action potential and its dependence on the membrane potential maintained by the sodium-potassium ATPase also exhibits the dependence of neural integrity on the generation of adenosine triphosphate (ATP) from glucose and oxygen. Swelling that other organs might tolerate to a degree can be lethal to an entire organ like the brain or to individual neurons. Pain and loss of neurons must be considered, because dysfunction may be as problematic as loss of function.

Central Nervous System Toxicity

The central nervous system (CNS) as may be recalled from anatomy is the decision-making function of an animal comprised of the brain and spinal cord. In complex beings such as humans, dysfunctions of that system are considered mental illness. However, toxic insults that may cause behavioral abnormalities are rarely considered even in modern medicine. History cites the central neurotoxic influences of chemicals, especially heavy metals. Roman rulers exhibited signs of lead poisoning from chronic exposure to lead in drinking water, utensils, and wine. Ludwig van Beethoven showed similar bouts of mania and depression that may have been related to lead poisoning as indicated by analysis of hair and bone samples taken from the corpse of this famous composer. Vincent Van Gogh famously cut off his own ear and in his paintings indicated halo-like circles surrounding objects, indicating retinal swelling from severe lead poisoning. There is some indication that intelligence quotient (IQ) deficits or criminal activity may be related to lead exposure as a child. The "mad hatter syndrome" characterized the bizarre behavior of

laborers in the felt hat industry using mercury nitrate to preserve the garments dating back to the 1600s. Even modern cases of mercury poisoning have made the news, such as the case of an actor who ate an exclusive fish protein diet or a young student who exhibited strange behavior. Pesticides, industrial solvents, and mold are common agents inducing depression, memory disturbances, sleep problems, difficulties with concentration, and other behavioral dysfunctions. Ongoing developmental exposure in developed countries such as the United States and Canada is indicated by cord blood analyses (Genuis, 2008). It is important to characterize all exposures to human and animal populations to prevent, treat, and monitor toxic effects leading to everything from learning deficits to neurodegeneration.

Blood–Brain Barrier

The blood–brain barrier is a very selective diffusion barrier whose integrity is vitally important for normal function as indicated by problems from disruption by ischemic stroke, traumatic brain injury, multiple sclerosis, and Alzheimer's disease. It is composed of specialized endothelial cells that line the cerebral microvessels. These specialized cells interact with astrocytes, pericytes, and neuronal processes, forming not only a barrier to many charged molecules but also providing an electric resistance of 2,000 Ωcm^2 *in vivo* and 700 Ωcm^2 *in vitro* (Balbuena et al., 2010). A schematic of how the barrier is usually constructed and its broaching using magnetic nanoparticles and microbubbles with a low-energy burst tone, focused ultrasound shows how diagnostic and therapeutic agents may be delivered to a normal brain or one marked by hypovascularity, fibrosis, or necrosis **Figure 20-1**.

The brain usually excludes molecules > 400 Da from entering, thereby excluding toxic agents. However, this also excludes beneficial therapeutic agents and diagnostic imaging chemicals. It is interesting how focused ultrasonic radiation can temporarily allow passage of substances up to 150 kDa to pass. Those of 2,000 kDa weight or 55 nm in diameter still would be hampered in passage unless significant damage is done to this barrier (Liu et al., 2010).

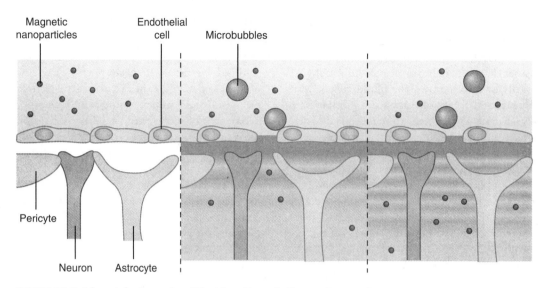

FIGURE 20-1 Schematic for Penetration of Blood-Brain Barrier by Magnetic Nanoparticles

Note: Intact CNS capillaries depicted in the left frame block magnetic nanoparticle delivery into the brain parenchyma. The middle frame displays the presence of microbubbles and low-energy burst tone, focused ultrasound temporarily disrupts the BBB, enhancing passive influx of therapeutic magnetic nanoparticles at the target location. The right frame shows combining magnetic nanoparticles with low-energy burst tone, focused ultrasound actively moves the therapeutic magnetic nanoparticles into the brain.

Damage of course can come from reactive oxygen species (ROS) as these are specialized blood vessels with an endothelial lining including tight junctional structures that make up the physical barrier. The metabolic barrier consists of enzymes of the cytosol of endothelial cells, including monoamine oxidase (MAO), xanthine oxidase, and NADPH-cytochrome P450 reductase (twofold higher in brain microvessels than in brain homogenate). This set of enzymes produces oxygen radicals on their own or reduces a redox cycling compound that yields superoxide when exposed to oxygen. The oxygen free radicals created damage protein, polyunsaturated lipids (rich in brain microvessels), and nucleic acid, yielding cell damage and mortality despite protection by glutathione (GSH), GSH peroxidase, superoxide dismutase (SOD), and catalase (Lagrange et al., 1999). Another way toxicants that generate free radicals such as Paraquat may cross the barrier is via a specific uptake/transport system. It appears that L-valine (neutral amino acid transport) or low Na^+ decreased Paraquat penetration through the blood–brain barrier (Shimizu et al., 2001).

The effects of a heavy metal (Pb acetate) and an organophosphate acetylcholinesterase inhibitor (malathion) on bovine brain microvascular endothelial cells (BMEC), rat brain microvascular endothelial cells (RBE4), and a neuroblastoma cell line (SH-SY5Y) provide some insight into the effects of how certain classes of chemicals may gain entry into the brain and then have selective damaging action. Pb is a known neurotoxic substance in humans that causes a variety of learning problems and can be lethal. It causes protein leakage from capillary endothelium cells of the blood–brain barrier (BBB), which leads to cerebral hemorrhage. Pb^{2+} is capable of using the L-type Ca^{2+} channels via store-operated calcium channels and Ca^{2+}-permeable, acid-sensing channels to enter cells. The BMEC model showed no effects of Pb, indicating that either these cells possess protective mechanisms or lack the enzymes that are subject to Pb inhibition. The RBE4 model was negatively impacted by Pb at concentrations $\geq 10^{-7}$ M. Astrocytes are very sensitive to lead poisoning. Transendothelial electrical resistance (TEER) was affected by lead or malathion in a concentration-dependent fashion. The RBE4 model had higher basal TEER measurements. Although malathion damage appears to be dependent on degree of metabolism to the active oxon and inhibition of cholinesterase by the cells, the transport was similar. However, lead transport varied based on cell type. The RBE4 model transported more Pb (five times the abluminal side concentration of the BMEC cells and twice the luminal concentration), while the BMEC model was tolerant of higher concentrations and retained more Pb. This retention of lead by the BMEC model can lead to interference with calcium-dependent signaling pathways that influence vascular resistance, hypertension, and cellular inflammation. The RBE4 model also exhibited higher acetylcholinesterase (AChE) inhibition than the BMEC model, indicating that rat cells may have a higher rate of conversion of the malathion to the inhibitory malaoxon form. This may be due to increased monooxygenase activity or decreased carboxylesterase activity in RBE4 cells (Balbuena et al., 2010). Damage to astrocytes alone can lead to leakage through the BBB. 3-Chloropropanediol induces focal lesions via astrocyte death. This is not accompanied by neuronal death (Prior et al., 2004).

The choroid plexus is also of interest in the BBB protection of the brain, because this is the source of the cerebrospinal fluid (CSF) from a network of capillaries. Metal damage here is separated into three groups as the choroid plexus may provide some protection from these agents. Hg and Cd are among the directly damaging metals. Pb on the other hand affects the plexus regulatory pathway of transthyretin production and secretion. Because transthyretin is the major carrier for thyroxine in the CSF, this will impair the transport of thyroid hormone across the BBB and affect brain metabolism and may lead to depression. Manganese uses an iron pathway (transferrin-dependent) and transferrin-independent pathways that may involve store-operated Ca channels to accumulate Mn in the brain causing a Parkinson-like syndrome. A third class of metal such as Fe, Ag, or Au is sequestered in the choroid plexus as a CNS defense mechanism (Zheng, 2001). Mixtures of As, Cd, and Pb are synergistically toxic to the developing (rat) brain. Disruption of the BBB started the toxicity. Astrocytes experienced toxic effects, as did the cerebral cortex and cerebellum. Increased apoptosis marked changes in

these structures. As described in the following sections of this chapter, other changes marked toxicity to astrocytes. Proximal activation of ERK signaling and downstream activation of JNK pathway occurred. Intracellular calcium (Ca_i^{2+}) concentrations and ROS generated by these metals also resulted in hastened apoptosis (Rai et al., 2010). Kainic acid, which mainly damages the hippocampus via inotropic glutamate receptors, is also known to breach the BBB (Benkovic et al., 2006).

A model of multiple sclerosis, experimental allergic encephalomyelitis involves disruption of the BBB. This interacts with other toxicants such as bipiperidyl mustard or triamine with increased development of necrotizing vasculitis and parenchymal necrosis. Gold thioglucose, which causes damage to the control of eating behavior via damage to the ventromedial nucleus of the hypothalamus, also achieves some of its neurotoxicity through brain blood vessel damage (necrosis and thrombosis result). This interaction does not occur with another neurotoxin, dipiperidinoethane. The reason the median eminence of the hypothalamus and area postrema of the dorsal medulla show damage from these other compounds may be that they lack a BBB and have greater penetration of these damaging agents. The experimental allergic encephalomyelitis lesions with the reduced BBB may be analogous to the areas lacking the barrier in the necrotic damage of these toxic agents (Levine and Sowinski, 1982). The development of the BBB is important, because chemicals toxic to developing organisms, such as hexachlorophene (Brandt et al., 1983) and unconjugated bilirubin (Ghersi-Egea et al., 2009), would not be as damaging later at lower concentrations with more exclusion from the CNS.

Brain Injury Mechanisms

There are a number of ways of viewing brain injury by toxicants. One approach is to define the type of injury as involving an axonopathy (axon degenerates with myelin sheath), myelinopathy (separation of myelin from nerve or demyelination), damage to specific cells types such as the astrocytes, neuropathy (damage and loss of neurons), or neurotransmission dysfunction. The most classical approach is the last of these categories, defining agents that decrease synthesis of neurotransmitters (e.g., styryl pyridines for acetylcholine, or ACh), affect exocytosis of neurotransmitter (botulinum toxin endopeptidase affects SNARE proteins' ability to release ACh from peripheral nerve endings [Gul et al., 2010] or increase release by black widow spider venom), act as a neurotransmitter agonist/antagonist/analog, inhibit synaptic degradation enzymes (e.g., organophosphates AChE or MAO inhibitors), or block reuptake of neurotransmitters (as with dopamine reuptake block by cocaine) causing abusive stimulation of a receptor (e.g., serotonin syndrome or glutamate receptor-linked neurodegeneration). Any of these brain injury mechanisms may be monitored by magnetic resonance imaging (MRI) analysis coupled to enzyme work (creatine kinase). For example, hexachlorophene exposure or similar agent should yield damage to myelin-rich tissues. This is picked up by enlargement of the olfactory tract, optic nerve, and pyramidal tract with diffuse swelling of the brain. On the other hand, axonopathies caused by acrylamide monomer used in creating a gel for electrophoresis shows ataxia and bilateral hindlimb weakness associated with enlarged lateral ventricles on both sides of the brain and a similar enlargement of the third ventricle, aqueduct, and cisterns. No swelling of the brain is noted in this type of neurotoxicity. Primary motor areas of the cortex decrease in size with some indications of primary and secondary sensory area reductions (Igisu and Kinoshita, 2007). These methods are wonderful for diagnosis of the type of injury and consideration of links between involved areas and deficits of neurological function (e.g, short-term memory and damage to the hippocampus), but the mechanism of damage and therefore possible prevention measures or antidote are unclear without specific exposure information. These measures may also miss a definitive diagnosis of a neurodegenerative disorder such as Alzheimer's disease, which requires a postmortem brain analysis for confirmation. Additionally, neurodegenerative disorders are almost never attributed to environmental causes by health practitioners. Another possibility for defining neurotoxicities is related to specific mechanisms of action such as altered calcium homeostasis, modified protein structure and function, changes in gene expression, and biological indicators of neuronal damage (neural degeneration, neuronal injury, metabolic damage, non-neuronal indicators). Brain regions and functions may be examined regarding toxicant injury. All classifications of neurotoxicity have their benefits. Because the second approach is more the research approach of a meeting (Mattson et al., 1993), this is the modern biological approach that will be favored in this chapter's examination of neurotoxicity and is reflected in **Table 20-1**.

Newer articles will also be used to provide further enlightenment on approaches that elucidate signaling pathways and so forth that mediate neurotoxicity.

Altered Calcium Homeostasis

Although many mechanisms may initiate neuronal death, such as amyloid mismetabolism in Alzheimer's disease, abusive stimulation of the N-methyl-D-aspartate (NMDA) receptor by glutamate, or changes in the signaling pathways including growth factors, alterations in calcium homeostasis are where these mechanisms share a common endpoint. Normally, a complex series of controls keep Ca^{2+} concentrations high outside of the neuron compared with inside the nerve cells (10,000-fold concentration gradient). Voltage-dependent and ligand-gated calcium channels provide access to the cell while the plasma membrane Ca^{2+}-ATPase and the Na^+/Ca^{2+} exchanger remove calcium via active transport mechanisms. The endoplasmic reticulum and mitochondria have mechanisms to sequester excess calcium from the cytoplasm. Proteins such as calmodulin help keep the Ca^{2+} in a bound state where less toxic activity may occur. Protein kinase C, Ca^{2+}/calmodulin-dependent protein kinase II, and calpains (protease) respond to alterations in Ca^{2+} concentrations. Ca^{2+} alters neuronal architecture by yielding structural damage and begins the process of cell death. The mechanisms of calcium-mediated neuronal injury are shown in **Figure 20-2**.

Ca^{2+} has a key role in neuronal cells, because it mediates the release of neurotransmitters and

TABLE 20-1	Forensic Chart of Nervous System Toxicity
Nervous System Toxicity	**Toxic Agents**
Blood–brain barrier	
Oxygen radicals	Quinones, bipyridinium ions, nitroheterocyclic compounds (Lagrange et al., 1999)
Specific transport and cytotoxic action	Paraquat (Shimizu et al., 2001), heavy metals (Pb), organophosphates (malathion, chlorpyrifos; Balbuena et al., 2010)
Astrocyte damage	3-Chloropropanediol (Prior et al., 2004)
Disruption of choroid plexus	Metals via three mechanisms of action (Zheng, 2001)
Experimental allergic encephalomyelitis	Bipiperidyl mustard, triamine, gold thioglucose (Levine and Sowinski, 1982)
Ca^{2+} disruption	
NMDA receptor	Glutamate, methyl mercury, ammonia
Non-NMDA receptor	AMPA, kainic acid, domoic acid (Gibbons et al., 1993)
Protein disruption	
Protein kinase C increased activity	Phorbol ester, methyl mercury (Sarafian and Verity, 1993)
Calpain I activation	NMDA, kainic acid (Robert-Lewis and Siman, 1993), organophosphates (el-Fawal and Ehrich, 1993)
Lysosomal acid hydrolase inhibition	Leupeptin, chloroquine, ROS, chronic irradiation (Nixon and Cataldo, 1993)
Phospholipase A_2 activation	Methylmercury, anoxic and cytolytic toxicants (Verity, 1993)
Lysosomal rupture	Silica or sodium urate crystals, photosensitive dyes $+ O_2 +$ light, weakly basic amines (Nixon and Cataldo, 1993)
Nerve growth factor deprivation and/or TNF-α activation	Heavy metals' oxidative toxicity (Deckwerth and Johnson, 1993; Pappas et al., 2003)
AHR signaling	Ca homeostasis, IP and ryanodine receptors, membrane phospholipases, protein kinases (Kodavanti, 2006), dioxin $+$ estrogen and apoptosis (Kajta et al., 2009), developmental disruption of inhibitory GABAergic pathways (Gohlke et al., 2009)
Alterations in gene expression	
Immediate-early gene stimulation	Glutamate, kainic acid, domoic acids, lindane (Vendrell et al., 1993), MDMA (Dzietko et al., 2010)
Heat shock/stress protein genes	ROS, anoxia, aglycemia (Nowak, 1993), phencyclidine, ketamine, MK801 as prevented by antipsychotics (Sharp et al., 1993)
Stannin expression	Trimethyltin (Toggas et al., 1993)
Ubiquitin expression	Ischemia (hypoxia; Caday et al., 1993)
Developmental gene expression *in vitro*	Methylmercury chloride, lead chloride, valproic acid, trimethyltin chloride (Hogberg, et al., 2010)
Oxidative stress	Paraquat, ammonia/glutamine, heavy metals
Mitochondrial disruption	Ammonia/glutamine (Albrecht et al., 2010); see ALS agents, CN (Hariharakrishnan et al., 2010)
Slow-developing neurodegeneration (ALS, Alzheimer's, Parkinson's)	Aluminum (Strong et al., 1993), Cycad, cyanobacteria (Bradley and Mash, 2009), glyphosate (Barbosa et al., 2001), bromphenylacetylurea, and dying-back axonopathy (see solvent section; Shi et al., 2010)
Solvent-induced anesthesia or CNS depression vs. CS_2	Toluene, ethanol (Matsuoka, 2007; Win-Shwe and Fujimaki, 2010)

AHR = aryl hydrocarbon; ALS = amyotrophic lateral sclerosis; AMPA = α-amino-3-hydroxy-5-methyl-4-isoxazolepropionic acid; CN = cyanide; CNS = central nervous system; ROS = reactive oxygen species; MDMA = 3,4-methylenedioxy-methamphetamine; NMDA = N-methyl-D-aspartate

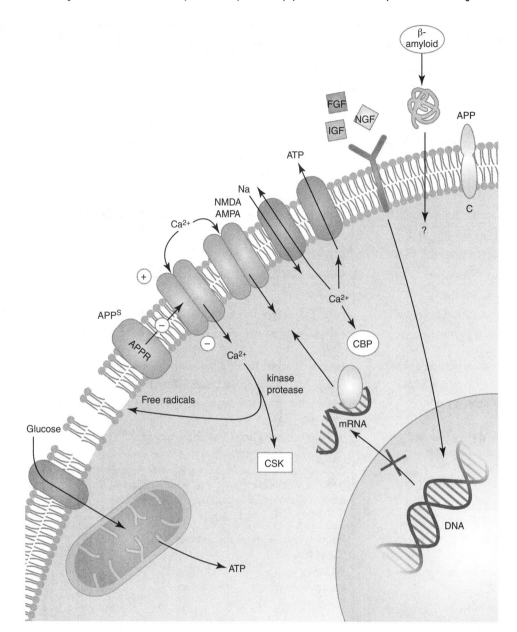

FIGURE 20-2 Ca²⁺ Signaling in Neuronal Cells Affected by Excitatory Amino Acids (EAA), Growth Factors, and Amyloid Precursor Protein (APP) Products

Note: NMDA and AMPA are receptors for EAA such as glutamate or the toxic kainic acid or domoic acid from seaweed, respectively. These receptors and voltage-gated Ca²⁺ channels are key sites of Ca²⁺ influx into regions of the brain that are vulnerable in ischemic stroke and Alzheimer's disease such as the short-term memory center, the hippocampus. Ca²⁺ is rapidly removed normally by the Na⁺/Ca²⁺ exchanger or slowly by the Ca²⁺-ATPase, storage in the endoplasmic reticulum or mitochondria, or Ca²⁺-binding proteins (CBP). Glucose is the sole energy source for neurons in the production of ATP. in the presence of oxygen. High, sustained, internal Ca²⁺ concentrations [Ca]$_i$ result in overstimulation of kinases and proteases and the generation of free radicals. All of these factors lead to cytoskeletal disruption and membrane damage. The growth factors bFGF, NGF, and IGFs stabilize [Ca]$_i$ and prevent disruption of [Ca]$_i$ homeostasis. As an example, bFGF suppresses the expression of a 71 kDa NMDA receptor protein which resuls in reduced vulnerability to excitotoxicity. Normal proteolytic cleavage of APP results in liberation of secreted forms of APP (APP^S) which bind to cell surface receptors and cause a reduction of [Ca]$_i$. The APP^S can protect neurons against insult such as hypoglycemia. Aberrant APP processing results in both a disruption of the normal neuroprotective action of APP^S and the deposition and aggregation of b-amyloid which destabilizes [Ca] and makes neurons vulnerable to 1excitotoxic/ischemic insults. CSK referes to non-receptor tyrosine kinase Csk, an intergral negative regulator of the Src family tyrosine kinases (SFKs) that specifically phosphorylates the negative regulatory site of SFKs inhibiting their potential to form cancer cells.

Data from Altered calcium signaling and neuronal injury: stroke and Alzheimer's disease as examples. Mattson MP, Rydel RE, Lieberburg I, Smith-Swintosky VL. Ann N Y Acad Sci. 1993 May 28;679:1-21.

controls neuronal excitability, integrations of electrical signals, synaptic plasticity, cellular metabolism, and gene expression. Elevated free intracellular calcium concentration or $[Ca^{2+}]_i$ also results in peripheral nerve damage as mediated by the capsaicin (8-methyl-N-vanillyl-6-monemaide; spicy portion of hot peppers used in certain muscle rub ointments)-activated receptors. These receptors cause conductance permeability to cations including Ca^{2+} and Co^{2+}. Some heavy metal neuronal toxicity may be mediated by this mechanism. Capsaicin affected the subpopulation of dorsal root ganglion neurons of the Aδ and C-fiber type. The receptors mentioned earlier of the NMDA class are not the only way that calcium influx may occur. The excitatory amino acid (EAA) receptors are grouped into ionotropic receptors (directly activate ion channels) and metabotropic (enzymatic process or modulation of other EAA receptors or voltage-sensitive ion channels). These have examples of G-protein-mediated activation of phospholipase C producing IP3 and opening of K^+ conductances and enhanced effectiveness of non-NMDA receptors, respectively. The ionotropic receptors may be the NMDA type described earlier that are highly permeable to calcium. The non-NMDA receptors are activated by kainite and α-amino-3-hydroxy-5-methyl-4-isoxazolepropionate (AMPA) as shown in Figure 20-2. These channels may act indirectly via Na^+-dependent depolarization of the cell membrane. This leads to opening of the voltage-gated Ca^{2+} channels. This is the type I kainate receptor class, which is Na^+-permeable but Ca^{++}-impermeable as contrasted with the type II kainate receptor class that has Ca^{2+}-permeability as its hallmark. Cells not having Ca^{2+}-permeable receptors still may be responsive to glutamate or capsaicin. Additionally, the presence of Ca^{2+}-permeable receptors does not necessarily make a neuronal cell prone to excitotoxins. Cultured astroglia or CA3 pyramidal cells die in response to kainate but not NMDA agonists and do not express Co^{2+}-permeable non-NMDA receptors (but do express type II non-NMDA receptors; Gibbons et al., 1993).

The role of Ca^{2+} in low-dose methylmercury (MeHg) neurotoxicity may be linked to the induction of NMDA receptors in a mink model. Similarly, a human SH-SY 5Y neuroblastoma cell line should increase NMDA receptors preceding an increase in caspase-3 activity 4 hours following exposure to 0.25–1.0 μM MeHg. NMDA receptor antagonists dizocilpine (((+)-5-methyl-10,11-dihydro-5H-dibenzo[a,d] cyclohepten-5,10-iminemaleate [(+)-MK801]) and memantine (1-amino-3,5-dimethyl-adamantane; 10 μM) completely blocked and a Ca^{2+} chelator 1,2-bis(o-aminophenoxy)ethane-N,N,N′,N′-tetraacetic acid (BAPTA; 1.0 μM) partially reduced neuronal cell damage (Ndountse and Chan, 2008). Ammonia neurotoxicity is also linked to hepatic encephalopathy via formation of glutamine and the NMDA/nitric oxide/cGMP pathway. Excess ammonia not turned into urea by a dysfunctional liver will accumulate in the brain. However, glutamine synthetase located in the astrocytes converts the ammonia plus glutamic acid to glutamine, the NDMA receptor activator. Inhibition of this enzyme by methionine sulfoximine prevents ammonia-induced brain edema and increased cranial pressure despite elevated ammonia concentrations.

Glutamine itself produces the oxidative stress and cell swelling associated with ammonia toxicity. Glutamine is excessively accumulated in mitochondria and impairs mitochondrial function, which is deadly to high metabolic rates of brain cells. Astrocytes given glutamine induce mitochondrial permeability transition (mPT) and mitochondrial swelling, which is inhibited by mPT inhibitor cyclosporine A or by histidine, an inhibitor of mitochondrial glutamine uptake (prevents brain edema associated with thioacetamide-induced hepatic failure). Histidine completely prevents the overexpression of astrocytic aquaporin-4, nuclear factor κB (NF-κB), and mitogen-activated protein kinases (MAPKs) that mediate neuronal swelling. The "Trojan Horse" hypothesis for brain mitochondrial dysfunction from glutamine is that the glutamine crosses into the mitochondria and is deaminated back into ammonia. This is confirmed by preventing this toxicity by a glutaminase inhibitor, 6-diazo-5-oxo-L-norleucine. The ammonia then interferes with the Krebs cycle and malate-aspartate shuttle enzymes. This is not the only toxicity of ammonia as NMDA receptor blockers and scavengers of ROS and reactive nitrogen species (RNS) prevent swelling of cerebral cortical slices. This strongly implicates glutamine as the toxin in brain cells. However, things are not as clear as they appear here. In fact, extracellular glutamine causes a decrease in NO and cGMP production in normal and ammonia-exposed brains, likely due to limited transport of NO precursor arginine. It is uncertain whether this disruption of the NO/cGMP signal transduction is protective or toxic to the cell. It is possible to hypothesize that in acute hepatic encephalopathy this disruption may be protective as less ROS and RNS may be generated. However, in the chronic form of the disease this may be damaging as cGMP concentrations are observed to decline. The events of ammonia toxicity as mediated through glutamine (Gln) are displayed in **Figure 20-3** (Albrecht et al., 2010).

A further complication is the neuroprotective effect to excess glutamate or 1-methyl-4-phenylpyridinium (MPP$^+$) by preincubation of cerebellar granule cells to subtoxic concentrations of glutamate or NMDA. This is not due to a tolerance mechanism and is blocked by NMDA receptor antagonists or protein or RNA synthesis inhibitors. Thus, it is possible that subtoxic increases in calcium in the cell can provide a mechanism via protein synthesis that protects neuronal cells from a larger surge of calcium via the three glutamate receptors: NMDA, quisqualate, or kainite (Marini and Paul, 1993).

Another target that can influence Ca^{2+} homeostasis is the inositol(1,4,5)P$_3$ kinase. Cerebral ischemia exacted a time-dependent reduction in this enzyme's activity in two phases—early and 6 hours following insult. Once the 3-kinase clears the IP$_3$ second messenger signal, there is an increase in signal at about 8 hours following ischemia prior to the development of tissue infarct. This enzyme could serve as an indication of this kind of damage (Sun, Lin, et al., 1993).

Altered Protein Structure and Function

Protein Kinase C

One of the biggest problems with contamination of seafood is the presence of methylmercury. A severe instance of an inorganic form of mercury waste being dumped into a food source occurred in Minamata Bay in Japan. The mercury as a result of its high density reaches the bottom of a lake, ocean, or riverbed where anaerobic conditions predominate. Methylation by bacteria produces a lipophilic mercury form that is more easily absorbed across the intestinal tract. People need to avoid eating too much ahi, bigeye tuna, tilefish, swordfish, shark, king mackerel, marlin, orange roughy, and fish caught in any waters that are subject to a mercury advisory. This is especially true for pregnant women and children, because developing systems are more subject to mercury poisoning. The neurological damage is the key toxicity of methylmercury. The appearance of Minamata disease occurred in animals and people eating from catch from the Shiranui Sea. The first indication was cats appearing to be behaviorally abnormal and falling into the sea. People in town soon thereafter had parasthesia (numbness in the limbs and lips). Blindness and deafness appeared in exposed humans. Some developed tremors, had difficulty with walking, and others shouted uncontrollably. These are the symptoms prior to coma and death that follow methylmercury poisoning. If large contamination by foodborne MeHg is not the culprit, it is likely that the oral "silver" dental amalgams that are ~50% mercury are a large source of mercury vapor that readily reaches the brain as well (unless the teeth are capped). The basis of this poisoning resides on where mercury binds in the brain. It appears that the granule layer of the cerebellum is highly sensitive to MeHg poisoning, resulting in ataxia (loss of coordination).

As indicated earlier, NMDA receptors and Ca^{2+} entry may be a portion of the toxicity observed. However, proteins regulating cell-signaling pathways internally in the cell are also affected by MeHg. For example, protein phosphorylation is essential in activation of various signaling pathways of various cells and especially neurons (neurotransmitter synthesis by phosphorylated neurotransmitter enzymes, neurotransmitter release by phosphorylated synaptic vesicle proteins, membrane/action potential maintained by phosphorylated ion channel proteins, neuritogenesis by phosphorylated cytoskeletal proteins). An example of a

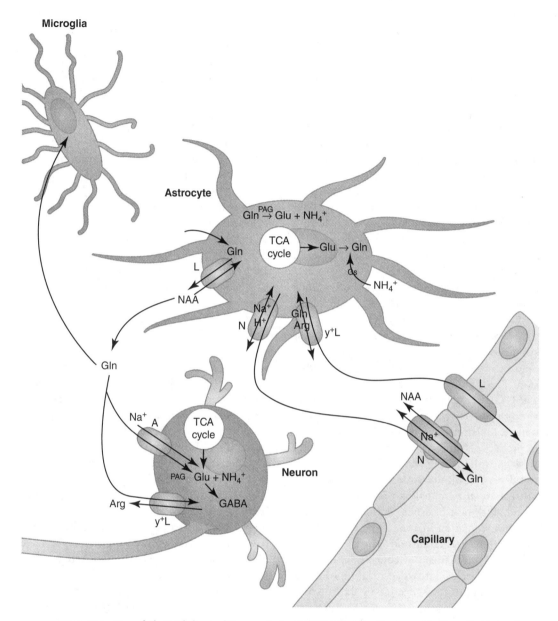

FIGURE 20-3 Major Steps of Gln Metabolism and Transport in the CNS Which May Contribute to, or Modulate, Gln-Mediated Ammonia Toxicity

Note: Ammonia (NH_4^+ ammonium ion in water) is incorporated ("detoxified") into glutamine (Gln) in astrocytes (and perhaps microglia) by the amidation of glutamate (Glu) to glutamine (Gln), a process catalyzed by glutamine synthase (GS). Gln accumulated in astrocytes (i) crosses the mitochondrial membrane and is hydrolyzed by phosphate-activated glutaminase (PAG) to glutamate (Glu) and NH_4^+, and (ii) exits astrocytes preferably by the system N (the SNAT3 transporter) which is controlled by extracellular Glu, and partly by system L in exchange for large neutral amino acids (NAA). The Gln that leaves astrocytes enters neurons mainly via system A to be converted to the amino acid neurotransmitters Glu and GABA, and possibly by system y^+L (the y^+LAT2 transporter) in exchange of Arg, which serves the purpose of modulating the availability of Arg for NO synthesis and thus may influence the rate of the NO/cGMP pathway. A portion of Gln derived from astrocytes leaves the CNS via the L and N systems that are localized in capillary endothelial cells that forms the blood–brain barrier, some of the Gln may enter the microglial cells and modulate their function.

genetic abnormality in protein phosphorylation is the Dunce mutant of the fruit fly, *Drosophila melanogaster*. As can be guessed from the designation of this mutation, the mutation of one of three genes encoding for cAMP phosphodiesterase enzymes leads to major memory problems. Protein kinase C (PKC) is important in neurotoxic action as indicated by the damage to cultured hippocampal neurons or retinal neurons by 10–100 nM phorbol ester (phorbol-12-myristate 12-acetate), which is a specific activator of PKC. A double mutant of rdg that causes a form of PKC (eye PKC) to lack expression, which results in functional neurons following light exposure, identifies this enzyme as mediating a form of neurodegeneration. There is an association between glutamate-mediated excitotoxicity and PKC in cultured cerebellar granule neurons. The exposure of these neuronal cells to 50 μM glutamate caused elevated Ca_i^{2+}, activation of phosphatidyl inositol turnover, and sustained activation of PKC resulting in 85–95% neuron mortality 24 hours into the incubation. The inclusion of PKC inhibitor ganglioside GT1b in the incubation medium appears to almost completely ameliorate the effects of glutamate. MeHg causes a dose-dependent increase in protein phosphorylation and increased inositol phospholipid turnover. During the neuron degeneration, PKC remains active and the proteolytic enzyme calpain is inhibited. This would allow over-phosphorylation and prevent the downregulation that the proteolytic enzyme would produce (Sarafian and Verity, 1993).

Another mechanism of concern with MeHg exposure is the oxidative degeneration of dopaminergic neurons as occurs in Parkinson's disease. The nematode *Caenorhabditis elegans* indicates that MeHg exposure induces antioxidant protection via glutathione-S-transferase induction (*gst-4* and *gst-38*) that is linked to antioxidant transcription factors SKN-1/Nrf2. Additionally, reduction in the SKN-1 gene augments MeHg toxicity and dopaminergic neuron vulnerability (VanDuyn et al., 2010).

Abnormal phosphorylation may also play a role in the cerebellar neurotoxicity of the polyether toxin of marine dinoflagellates, okadaic acid. It appears that okadaic acid is a specific inhibitor of serine/threonine protein phosphatases 1 and 2A. A specific target of phosphorylation, such as the microtubule-associated protein, tau, must be inferred, because other protein phosphorylation by cAMP-dependent protein kinase does not appear to lead to neurodegeneration (Fernández et al., 1993).

Calpain I (μ-Calpain)

The Ca^{2+}-activated neutral cysteine protease or calpain I is a downstream site that increasing calcium levels may activate, thus leading to neural degeneration. It is an enzyme that is localized in neurons selectively susceptible to excitotoxin- or ischemia-induced degeneration. Neurofilament polypeptides, microtubule-associated proteins, tubulin, and spectrin serve as structural proteins of the neurons that are favored substrates of this protease. It is not hard to imagine that many diseases and neuropathologies have been linked to activation of calpain I due to the cellular degeneration that results. Spinal and head trauma, peripheral nerve injury, demyelination disease, muscular atrophy, lens cataract formation, and cerebral ischemia are all linked to increased calpain I activity. Spectrin proteolysis in the hippocampus is a good indication that this enzyme has been activated as infusion of excitatory amino acid analogs (kainic acid, NMDA) leads to spectrin degradation within 3 hours of inception of treatment as indicated by Western blot analysis. It is of interest that both receptor pathways lead to similar downstream endpoints. They have different starting points as carboxypiperazin-4-yl-propylphosphonate, a selective and potent NMDA receptor antagonist, blocked the spectrin degradation by NMDA but not by kainate (Roberts-Lewis and Siman, 1993). Organophosphorus-induced delayed neuropathy modeled in White Leghorn chickens appears to be mediated via increases in intracellular concentrations of calcium mediated through the L-type calcium channel. Dihydropyridine and phenylalkylamine calcium-channel blockers prevent these actions. Calpain activation appears to play a role in this neurotoxicity as calcium influx through the dihydropyridine channel is connected with calpain activation (el-Fawal and Ehrich, 1993).

Phospholipase A$_2$ (PLA$_2$) Activation

Prolonged unusual activation of PLA$_2$ enzymes deacylate the sn-2 fatty acyl position of membrane phosphatides, activate second messenger systems, cause uncontrolled influx of Ca^{2+}, and ultimately result in cell death. Again, MeHg has a role here. It appears that the activation PLA$_2$ is independent of the lipid peroxidation that results from heavy metal exposure. The antioxidant α-tocopherol (vitamin E) prevents the lipid peroxidation associated with MeHg exposure without affecting PLA$_2$ activation. Increases in [Ca$_i^{2+}$] can activate PLA$_2$, as may a G-protein-coupled mechanism related to the H-*ras* oncogene. This mechanism was determined by the stimulation of PLA$_2$ by microinjection of the H-*ras* oncogene into fibroblasts without affecting phosphoinositide metabolism. It appears that ischemia, chemical anoxic, and cytolytic toxins all can play a role in PLA$_2$ activation leading to cell death (Verity, 1993).

Lysosomal Acid Hydrolases

Primary and secondary lysosomes are involved in the neural degeneration process. The question of the primary role of the release of acid hydrolases into the cell on toxicant exposure indicates whether the lysosomes initiate the degeneration process or are just used to clean up cellular debris following other damage yielding apoptosis or necrosis (normal process of end-stage cell death). Among the latter that involve a primary toxic action followed by minimal morphological changes in the neuronal lysosomal system are natural neuronal cell death during development, peripheral deprivation during development, Purkinje cell degeneration (Pcd mutation), Werdnig Hoffman disease, ischemia, experimental hypertensive injury, acute radiation poisoning, acrylamide neurotoxicity, triorthocresyl phosphate neurotoxicity, aluminum neurotoxicity, amyotrophic lateral sclerosis, and Creutzfeldt-Jakob disease. A late-stage increase in secondary lysosomes accompanying apoptosis and necrosis is observed with axotomy, chromatolysis, guanethidine, n-hexane, malnutrition, radiation, and Wobbler mutation. However, the more important toxicities that are mediated via early lysosomal alterations including storage disease of lysosomes due to inhibition of hydrolases are secondary lysosome alteration (Alzheimer's disease, chloroquine, natural cell death—*Anuran*, nutritional deprivation—*Anuran*), accumulation of lipofuscin (a type of lipopigment) granules (Alzheimer's disease, chloroquine, chronic irradiation, leupeptin, medial frontal epilepsy, motor neuron degeneration involving late-onset mouse mutation, Parkinson's disease, vitamin E deficiency), accumulation of ceroid (another type of lipopigment caused by Hermansky-Pudlak syndrome, myoclonus epilepsy, neuronal ceroid lipofuscinosis), and accumulation of storage bodies (acid lipase deficiency as in Wolman disease, glycogenoses type II as in Pompe disease, glycoproteinoses as in mannosidoses, mucolipidoses, mucopolysaccharidoses as in Hurler disease, and sphingolipidoses as in Tay-Sachs disease). One example from this last list is leupeptin—an inhibitor of lysosomal protease cathepsins and other cysteine proteases. It increases the formation of ceroid lipofuscin and dense bodies. Purkinje cells are most vulnerable, exhibiting cell degeneration, while lipofuscin accumulation in neocortical pyramidal cells is similar to normal aging in that cells do not die. Chloroquine, a favored antimalarial medication, diffuses into lysosomes and is protonated and trapped. The pH becomes more alkaline and exceeds the optimum for acid proteases. Multilamellar bodies appear with lipofuscin buildup. Purkinje cells are again susceptible and degenerate, with axonal dystrophy possible in other neuronal cells. ROS formation during Parkinson's disease occurs during the synthesis of neuromelanin in the substantia nigra and oxidation of dopamine by MAOB. These dopaminergic neurons in vitamin E deficiency have exacerbated free radical formation and increased lipid peroxidation. Lipopigment accumulates making them less subject to catabolism by lysosomal hydrolases. Chronic irradiation of the electric organ of the fish *Torpedo californica* also increases lipofuscin in neuronal lysosomes.

Lysosomal rupture is a consequence that results in rapid cell death by releasing the degrading hydrolase enzymes. Silica or sodium urate crystals are phagocytosed by macrophages or other phagocytic white blood cells and eventually rupture the lysosomal membrane.

Similar action is noted if photosensitive dyes are allowed to accumulate in the lysosomes, which in the presence of molecular oxygen and distinct wavelengths of light generate a peroxidation reaction. Weakly basic amines also concentrate several hundred-fold in lysosomes, leading to leakage of lysosomal hydrolases. In contrast, the antipsychotic medication chlorpromazine stimulates the formation of autophagic vacuoles in cultured rat dorsal root ganglion neurons by concentrating in lysosomes, but does not cause degeneration (Nixon and Cataldo, 1993).

Nerve Growth Factor Deprivation

The mechanism that is important in nerve growth or degeneration is the presence or absence of nerve growth factor (NGF), respectively. During normal neuroblast development and connection to a neighboring target, the target neuron secretes small amounts of neurotrophic factors that determine survival of a population of neurons. Those neurons not receiving this input die. During normal neuronal development, this process of neural degeneration occurs in half of the developing neurons. The degeneration process may be marked by DNA fragmentation (Deckwerth and Johnson, 1993). It appears that toxicants or aging factors that activate TNFα promote apoptosis and cell death similarly to withdrawal of NGF. Thus, β-amyloid, τ and mutated presenilin proteins, free radicals and oxidative stress (as from heavy metal poisoning), and pro-inflammatory cytokines lead to degeneration of neurons. Neurotrophic factors in this regard are linked to rescue of damaged neurons (Pappas et al., 2003).

Persistent Organic Pollutants and Ah Receptor Signaling

A number of organic pollutants with ability to bioaccumulate due to resistance to metabolism (polyhalogenate) are neurotoxic. From accidental exposures, polychlorinated biphenyls (PCBs) are known to cause in addition to a skin reaction (chloracne) the more severe problems of numbness, weakness in the limbs, decreased conduction velocities of peripheral nerves, developmental deficiencies (hypoactivity and lower IQ), and speech disturbances. Prenatal exposure in animals leads to symptoms similar to attention-deficit/hyperactivity

disorder. Impaired cognitive development, motor problems, and sensory (auditory) deficiencies have also been noted. Changes in dopaminergic neurotransmission may account for some of the effects (especially activity and motor functions), possibly through inhibition of vesicular dopamine (monoamine) transport. Also results a study (Juarez de Ku et al., 1994) demonstrated effects on cholinergic neurotransmission in the hippocampal and forebrain system that may indicate learning problems and cognitive impairment. Ca homeostasis and activity of PKC also appear to be affected by PCBs, indicating changes in cell signaling. Some neurological effects may also be mediated via dramatic decreases in thyroid hormone produced by PCBs. PCBs also generate oxidative stress as indicated by less damage when nitric acid synthase and phospholipase A2 are inhibited. Additionally, a variety of other signaling pathways are affected (Kodavanti, 2006). The Ah receptor (AhR) is a key consideration for any aryl hydrocarbon, including PCBs, PAHs, dioxins, and dibenzofurans. AhR stimulation via beta-naphthoflavone induces damage in neocortical and hippocampal cells of mouse primary neural cell cultures via apoptotic pathways as indicated by caspase-3 activity and lactate dehydrogenase release (Kajta et al., 2009). Estrogen signaling appears to be involved in this AhR-mediated neurotoxicity as indicated by enhanced apoptosis by the high-affinity estrogen receptor (ER) antagonist ICI 182,780 or selective estrogen receptor modulator tamoxifen. Raloxifine (selective estrogen receptor modulator) and methylpiperidino pyrazole (ERα antagonist) did not affect caspase-3 activity but did reduce the late release of lactate dehydrogenase induced by β-naphthoflavone (Kajta et al., 2009). Developmentally, the AhR stimulation by TCDD especially damages inhibitory GABAergic pathway development in the ventral telencephalon in mice via activation of the Notch signaling pathway. This Notch pathway maintains the neural progenitor population through activation of Hes1 and Hes5, which decrease DNA binding of proneural bHLH transcription factors ngn2 and Mash1. The gene *SOX11*, which is a key regulator of neuronal differentiation, may be directly regulated by AhR (Gohlke et al., 2009).

Alterations in Gene Expression

Benefit of a Molecular Approach to Neurotoxicology — Stannin and Organotin

If the neurotoxicity of organotin compounds is made based on morphological data alone, it is only clear that trimethyltin causes accumulation of dense bodies and autophagic vacuoles in the cytoplasm, vacuoles in the Golgi apparatus, and cell necrosis of neuronal cells. This is not produced by elemental tin or metabolites of trimethyltin. Triethyltin produces a different array of toxicity to the myelin with interstitial brain edema as a clinical result. Unfortunately, this does not indicate the mechanism by comparing two closely related structures, which produce either neuropathy or myelinopathy. If a toxicologist is meant to provide antidotes or at least understand how the toxicities are manifested, then the molecular approach is a more appropriate characterization.

It may be fruitful to follow how one research team mapped trimethyltin toxicity (Toggas et al., 1993). Initially, regional mapping was done via silver stains for neurodegeneration. This focused the research on the hippocampus and limbic cortex of the rat brain. cDNA or antibody probes (cellular level) provide the next layer of analysis proceeding to protein and gene expression analyses (subcellular level). The research team hypothesized first that sensitive neurons must express a gene product or products that make them more sensitive to trimethyltin. Subtractive hybridization allows removal of mRNAs common to all cells and focuses on enriching cDNAs preferentially expressed by sensitive cells. By this method, a unique cDNA was isolated and identified as pr9T-19-37. Its protein product was given the name of stannin. A full-length clone was made for sequencing. The amino acid sequence of the protein was determined. Antibodies were also made to the N-terminal of stannin and used to identify neurons with high stannin expression. A stannin fusion protein was constructed in a bacterium (*Escherichia coli*). This served three purposes. The first was an affinity ligand for antibody production. The second was production of large quantities of stannin. The third was the most intriguing: determination of whether stannin

expression in a cell that has no such previous expression becomes sensitive to trimethyltin exposure (lower IC_{50}). One experiment possible from these approaches is to show that stannin immunoreactivity would decrease in cells following trimethyltin exposure, as the protein would be bound and not available. This was indeed found in coronal brain sections of treated rats in hippocampus, entorhinal cortex, and amygdala structures. The *E. coli* that had stannin expression showed a decreased curve in response to 100 μM trimethyltin exposure as monitored by optical density. Eukaryotic cells were also transfected with stannin cDNA to see if they also became more sensitive to trimethyltin exposure. This would move from a demonstration that cells more appropriate for mammalian modeling were similar to bacterial sensitivity when stannin was expressed. Because developing rat brain cells appear to be more sensitive, the expression of stannin mRNA should reflect that sensitivity. In fact, on postnatal day 1, expression is seen throughout the hippocampal region, which reorganizes to an adult pattern by postnatal day 20. As is demonstrated here, the designation of trimethyltin toxicity as stannin related gives much more information for molecular analysis and antidote development than does a neuronopathy designation (Toggas et al., 1993).

Neurodegenerative Diseases — Genes and Environmental Agents

Neurodegenerative diseases associated with aging include Alzheimer's disease and Parkinson's disease. Alzheimer's disease is known to involve some amyloid precursor protein gene missense mutations leading to cleavage products such as amyloidβ (Aβ) peptides Aβ40 and Aβ40 found in amyloid plaques. The toxicity of Aβ involves activation of microglia, which initiates an inflammatory response via cytotoxic cytokine release. There is also excessive release of excitatory amino acids such as glutamate from glial cells that damage neurons via excitotoxicity. Aβ also appears to inhibit axonal and dendritic transport. These mutant peptides also generate free radicals by binding to redox-reactive metals and may injure mitochondria. These protein aggregates do not form in normal healthy neurons due to molecular chaperones (heat shock proteins that keep proteins from misfolding and aggregating), ubiquitin-proteasome system (ubiquitin attaches to misfolded or truncated proteins and is recognized for proteasomal digestion), and autophagy/lysosomal degradation. Parkinson's disease is associated with mutations in the α-synuclein gene (PARK1 and PARK4) leading to cytoplasmic inclusions known as Lewy bodies in dopaminergic neurons. Oxidative stress and impaired proteasome activity are other factors leading to Parkinson's disease involving mutations in the ubiquitin carboxy-terminal hydroxylase L1 gene (PARK5), in the parkin gene (PRK2), and in the DJ-1 gene (PARK7). MPTP is discussed later as an agent causing dopaminergic neurotoxicity and used to model Parkinson's disease. This agent ultimately affects mitochondrial complex I. Mitochondrial disruption also occurs through inhibition of oxidative phosphorylation through the use of rotenone, which also appears to affect dopaminergic neurotransmission. Notice that mitochondrial damage appears to be a common problem in neurodegenerative disorders, with alterations in ATP generation, protein phosphorylation, and regulation of calcium. Some toxins mimic some of these features. Al, Cu, Fe, and certain pesticides initiate fibrillation of α-synuclein. Hg elicits an increase in β-amyloid secretion and τ (tau is part of the microtubule-associated proteins) hyperphosphorylation. Manganese also leads to τ hyperphosphorylation via the activation of ERK MAPK (Cai et al., 2011) and neurological degenerative disorders. Amyloid precursor protein levels increase with Hg in brain cell cultures or Pb in a mouse hippocampal cell line. Pb causes a decrease in chaperone activity (glucose-related protein 78 kDa) in astrocyte cultures. A dithiocarbamate fungicide preferentially injures dopaminergic neurons and increases α-synuclein and inhibits ubiquitin E1 ligase in primary ventral mesencephalic cultures. Methylmercury increases the formation of ROS and in combination with copper and ascorbate or glutathione depletion enhances its neurotoxicity and ROS formation. Additionally, brain inflammatory pathways are excited via microgliosis and astrogliosis (increased glial cell reactivity) via mercury, lead, trimethyltin, and parathion. It is clear that many chemicals stimulate various cascades that lead to brain cell damage via cell signaling involving inflammatory pathways, energy pathways, oxidative damage, cytoskeletal changes, and excitotoxicity that can involve the interactions of various cell types. *In vitro* methods that model these toxicities should make sure that all cell–cell interactions are properly examined such as neuron-glial cell or between neurons or glial cells (Zurich and Monnet-Tschudi, 2009).

Hypoxia via Thromboembolic Stroke or Cardiac Arrest and Ubiquitins

Hypoxia, lack of nutrients (especially aglycemia), and lack of blood pressure produce significant, although not identical, damage to the central nervous system. When a thromboembolic stroke (blood clot in coronary or vertebral artery) causes damage, it usually is localized and characterized as focal ischemia. On the other hand, cardiac arrest leads to delayed neuronal death known as global ischemia. It is important to differentiate how this global ischemia occurs. A global forebrain occlusion results from a gerbil with a 5–10 minute induced occlusion in both coronary arteries. The CA-1 sector of the hippocampus appears most sensitive to this delayed neuronal death. It is of interest that the neurons appear quite functional for up to 2 days following the procedure, showing electrical excitability and synthesize proteins. Within the next 4 days, the neurons die unless protein synthesis is inhibited. This suggests a process similar to apoptosis rather than a necrotic degeneration. Because the protein ubiquitin is upregulated during apoptosis that occurs during development, this was a likely candidate for molecular analysis during global ischemia. Ubiquitin appears to be involved in processes such as protein degradation, cell cycle control, ribosome biogenesis, induced mutagenesis, DNA repair, and cellular responses to stress or damage. Ubiquitin is found in all eukaryotic cells and has two basic classes. Class I ubiquitin genes encompass the monoubiquitin fusion genes (single sequence fused to a tail peptide sequence) that are highly expressed as mRNA during early stages of development. Class II ubiquitin genes cover the polyubiquitin genes that express primarily during mature and later stages of development. In a yeast cell, the polyubiquitin gene is only critical to the survival of cells during stress or trauma, not for normal functioning. Some heat shock factors to be discussed more fully later in this section of the chapter appear to be coded for by the 5′-flanking region of some polyubiquitin genes. Ubiquitins usually operate via conjugating with other proteins. Protein ubiquitination is key factor in speedy degradation of short-lived, denatured, or damaged proteins involving an ATP-dependent protease complex. This puts ubiquitin in the role of regulating (1) the cell cycle such as cyclin degradation, (2) activity of regulatory proteins, and (3) elimination of nonfunctional or dysfunctional proteins. Elevated total ubiquitin mRNA is present following induction of transient global ischemia in the gerbil, for example. This is mainly a result of upregulation of 3.6-kb and possibly 2.2-kb transcripts of *polyubiquitin* mRNAs for 4 hours following ischemia induction, which only lasts for ~24 hours. The expression of these transcripts decreases thereafter. In the hippocampus, the polyubiquitin gene expression reached is maximal prior to the inception of delayed neuronal death. Even though it is not clear whether ubiquitin is aiding survival or inducing apoptotic mechanisms, ubiquitin immunoreactivity initially declines, then preferentially rises in gerbil hippocampal regions such as CA-3 that do ultimately survive the insult of transient global ischemia. An *in situ* hybridization study was proposed to answer that question (Caday et al., 1993). However, a later analysis by another research group that did an *in situ* hybridization using a rat model showed similar results of one polyubiquitin (UbC) mRNA expression showing maximal expression 4 hours after occlusion of the distal middle cerebral artery that remained high at 24 hours. This preceded the expression of heat shock protein 70. This other group saw UbC as the most stress inducible of the three ubiquitin genes and considered it a marker of ischemic stress rather than an indicator of survival or predetermined death in focal ischemia (Noga et al., 1997).

Cellular Immediate-Early Genes

Many of the excitatory neurotoxins, such as kainic or domoic acids, work via increases of calcium caused by the glutamate receptor subclasses mentioned earlier. Convulsants such as pentylenetetrazol or lindane (γ-hexachlorocyclohexane) work via suppression of the γ-aminobutyric acid receptor (GABA$_A$), resulting in hyperactivity/depolarization of the neurons. In this case, L-type voltage-dependent Ca^{2+} channels open, which still elevates calcium concentrations in the cells. These events and processes such as cerebral ischemia or surgical lesions lead to activation of transcription of cellular immediate-early genes in the brain, which can precede cell death. Rapid, short-lived changes occur in neurons that are transcription independent such as phosphorylation of ion channels, enzymes, receptors, or cytoskeletal proteins by protein kinases. The longer-lasting effects come from transcription-dependent responses, such as those mediated by cellular immediate-early genes encoding for nuclear proteins. These proteins are known for putative transcription factors such as Fos and Jun. Fos is a product of the proto-oncogene *c-fos*, which forms a dimer with Jun. Jun is a product of the proto-oncogene *c-jun*. This complex binds to the DNA sequence TGACTCA known to be the binding site of the transcription factor activator protein-1. Because these proteins contain a leucine zipper, they are classed as a basic-zipper superfamily, which consists of activating transcription factor and cAMP response element to bind protein families. These proteins act as third messengers linking relatively brief excitatory signals external to the cell into enduring changes in cellular phenotype via altering the expression of target genes (Vendrell et al., 1993). These events are summarized in **Figure 20-4**. This figure gives a good schematic of the role of cellular immediate-early genes in cell death. However, there needs to be a little clarification in light of a publication (Pizzi et al., 1993) that defines the distinction between glutamate ionotropic receptors and metabotropic glutamate receptors (mGluR). It appears that the mGluR selective agonist trans-1-aminocyclopentane-1,3-dicarboxylate or quisqualate prevents the

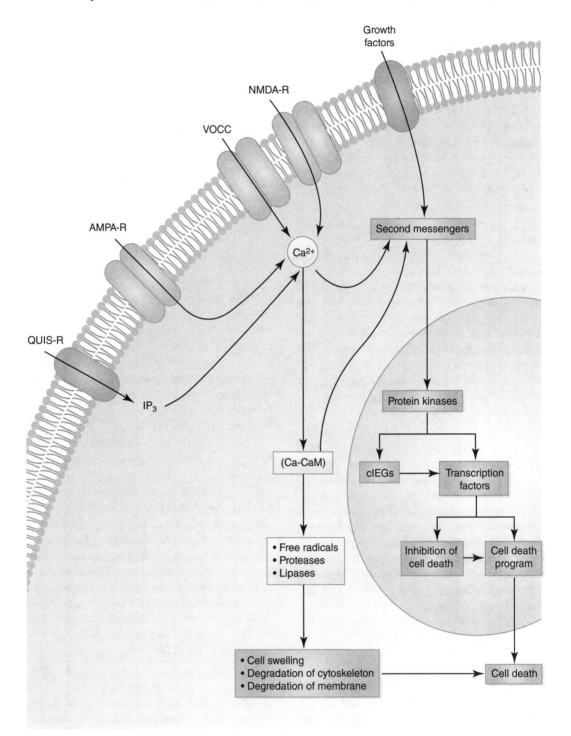

FIGURE 20-4 Model for Cellular Immediate-Early Genes (cIE) Response in Cell Death

Note: VOCC: voltage operated calcium channels; NMDA-R: NMDA receptors; AMPA-R: AMPA receptor; QUIS-R quisqualate receptor; IP$_3$: inositol 1,4,5-triphosphate; CaM: calmodulin

neurotoxic action of glutamate and kainate (ionotropic receptor agonists) to rat cerebellar granule cells. mGluR-evoked responses are potentiated by aniracetam, which blocks cell death caused by glutamate, kainate, or α-amino-3-hydroxy-5-methyl-4-isoxazoleproprionic acid. If this is truly the case, the IP_3 generation via phospholipase C may be a pathway that leads to decreased toxicity and a possible treatment of neurodegenerative diseases via activation of ionotropic glutamate receptors. Excitatory neurotransmitters can cause damage as well. For example, ecstasy (3,4-methylenedioxymeth-amphetamine, or MDMA) is known to cause apoptotic damage to serotonergic fibers in the adult rat brain and damage the cortex, septum, thalamus, hypothalamus, and the cornu ammonis 1 region of the developing rat. It is of interest that MDMA increased the expression of brain-derived neurotrophic factor (BNDF), neurotrophin-3, and nerve growth factor. These serve as markers that damage is occurring and also indicate repair. This last point is supported by the increased sensitivity to CNS damage by MDMA in P7 CD1/BDNF knockout mice as opposed to those wild-type mice that could express these protective neurotrophins (Dzietko et al., 2010).

Heat Shock/Stress Protein Expression

It appears that neuronal hsp72 is expressed in a variety of brain injury models, including global ischemia. In contrast, hyperthermic stress elicits a glial and vascular expression of this protein with less neuronal participation in the response. ROS or damaged proteins can start the stress response. In cultures, anoxia and aglycemia deplete ATP stores and activate heat shock factors. Hsp72 increases in hypothalamic cells and other brain regions in response to kainic acid. Selective loss of CA3 neurons appears to be linked to expression of nsp72 in CA1 (Nowak, 1993). Heat shock protein induction (hsp70 mRNA and HSP72 protein) and vacuole formation following phencyclidine, ketamine, and MK801 in cingulate neurons or rats indicated that the molecular expression was indicative of the tissue injury. It is of interest that antipsychotic medications such as haloperidol reduced this brain injury and induction of the heat shock proteins. From this finding, it can be inferred that certain psychotic states induced by drug abuse or endogenous compounds might be mediated through neuronal injury via the sigma or other receptors. This leads to a possible neurotoxicological link between chemical exposure and schizophrenia. It also indicates the possible antidotal use of antipsychotic medications in preventing certain types of neural degeneration (Sharp et al., 1993).

Developmental Gene Expression Affected by Neurotoxic Chemicals

As with the adult organism, it is important to develop sensitive *in vitro* approaches to developmental neurotoxicity. It is also vital to know if the same mechanisms that signal damage in the adult are relevant to the developing organism. Rat cerebellar granule cells in primary culture responded to mercury chloride, valproic acid, and trimethyltin chloride with downregulation of mRNA levels for NF-68, NF-200, NMDA glutamate receptor, and GABA receptor as neuronal markers; however, interestingly, astrocyte markers of GFAP and S100β appeared unaffected. Lead chloride is known to cause significant neurological deficits in animals and humans during development, including memory and learning functions. This heavy metal indeed did decrease the expression of GFAP mRNA, while the other neuronal markers were less altered. This *in vitro* mRNA expression system shows that differences in gene expression for developmental neurotoxins can be helpful in classifying the activity of these agents, including neuronal versus glial cell damage (Hogberg et al., 2010).

Oxidative Stress

In the preceding sections, it is clear that metals induce oxygen radicals, as do a number of other toxicants, including agents from Paraquat to ammonia/glutamine. One such metal is the trace nutrient manganese. High levels of Mn exposure yield disorientation, memory impairment, acute anxiety, and hallucination. Chronic Mn poisoning yields permanent damage to the nigrostriatal system with depletion of dopamine similar to Parkinson's disease. Oxygen radicals can be produced by Fe^{2+}, Mn^{2+}, and Cu^{2+} in a Haber-Weiss reaction catalyzed by MAO as discussed in the section on dopaminergic neurotoxicity. Superoxide is the first radical produced and leads to lipid peroxidation. In combination with disrupting oxidative phosphorylation/energy metabolism, this produces a loss of ion homeostasis and neuronal cell death (Sun, Yang, et al., 1993). The redox cycling compound Paraquat induces apoptosis signal-regulating kinase 1 (ASK1) as it induces autophagy (autophagic vacuoles, activation of beclin-1, accumulation of LC3 II, p62 degradation, mammalian target of rapamycin dephosphorylation). Although autophagy is somewhat of a protective response, the acceleration of autophagy by ASK1 overexpression and endoplasmic reticulum stress created by Paraquat ROS generation induces neuronal apoptosis (Niso-Santano et al., 2011). In neurodegenerative and neuroinflammatory disorders, it is important to indicate which diseases result from oxidative stress and those that represent the outcome of the disease state. Alzheimer's disease, amyotrophic lateral sclerosis (ALS), Huntington's disease, multiple sclerosis, and Parkinson's disease all have evidence for a primary role of oxidative stress in neuronal death. There is a neuroinflammatory side to oxidative stress involving NO release from macrophages and microglia in the CNS along with superoxide. The NO + $O_2^{\cdot-}$ combination leads to the formation of peroxynitrite and other RNS or nitrosative stress. This stimulates pro-inflammatory gene transcription in glia and elevates the stress tremendously. In combination with this series of events, there is an accumulation of unfolded or misfolded proteins in brain cells of neurodegenerative disorders. Additionally, redox-active ions such as Cu or Fe and redox-inactive metal ions such as Zn become imbalanced. Mitochondrial disruption is the final feature in common in these disorders as stated earlier. These are not separate phenomena as oxidative stress can cause proteins to assemble improperly or damage the mitochondria via the respiratory chain or mitochondrial DNA unprotected by histone proteins (Sayre et al., 2008). One of the biggest obstacles to looking at lower order oxidative damage in nondividing cells is the methodology for detection of DNA oxidation. The formation of the thymine glycol would allow detection that

is specific for double-stranded DNA damage. This chemical can then be converted to 2-methylglyceric methyl ester by base hydrolysis and sodium borohydride reduction followed by methanolysis. Following derivatization to the di-(tertiary butyl-dimethylsilyl) ether, gas chromatography–mass spectrometry identification and quantitation can be performed with sensitivity for small tissue sections or cell cultures (Markey et al., 1993).

Determination of oxidative injury to brain mitochondria is not a function of lipid peroxidation assays as many sources can yield these products. Mitochondria have MAO forms on their outer membrane that can generate oxygen radicals. Glutathione is high in mitochondria and acts as a reducing cofactor for removal of hydroperoxides by (reduced GSH) glutathione peroxidase and (oxidized) glutathione reductase. Oxidative damage that leads to mitochondrial dysfunction can be assessed via oxidized glutathione (glutathione disulfide or GSSG; Werner and Cohen, 1993). The developing brain has fewer radical scavengers and high availability of iron, so it is more likely to have free radical damage in mitochondria. Neurons are more sensitive to free radical attack than glial cells. In infants born extremely prematurely, oligodendrocyte progenitors and immature oligodendrocytes are selectively vulnerable populations of cells to this type of ROS and RNS damage. Apoptosis is more likely started by this damage in the developing brain. The mitochondrial permeability transition may be a good target to prevent this damage (Blomgren and Hagberg, 2006).

Mitochondrial Function Disruption, Energy Production, and Anoxia

Examination of neurotoxicity now moves in the opposite direction from oxygen radicals to low-oxygen tensions that are clearly damaging, such as occurs in stroke. The action of ammonia and glutamine on mitochondrial swelling, mTP, and inhibition of the Krebs cycle and malate-aspartate shuttle enzymes in the earlier section on altered Ca^{2+} homeostasis have already been described. However, further examination of the effects of anoxia on the developing and the adult brain should disclose other mechanistic information. Cyanide poisoning is a function of disrupted oxidative phosphorylation forming histotoxic hypoxia. For example, potassium cyanide was most potent in the corpus striatum and hippocampus of rats, decreasing the neurotransmitters norepinephrine (NE), dopamine (DA), and 5-hydroxytryptamine (5-HT or serotonin). This was resolved by alpha-ketoglutarate treatment or sodium thiosulfate antidotal therapy (Hariharakrishnan et al., 2010). The developing brain has increased sensitivity to respiratory chain disruption or hypoxia-ischemia.

Environmental Causes of Neurodegenerative Diseases

Some disorders such as Alzheimer's disease and ALS appeared to be diseases of aging with no environmental cause. ALS was the first to have clear linkage to an area of the southern Pacific region (Guam). Low calcium in the soil with high aluminum levels appeared to offer an explanation as animals also given sublethal chronic aluminum levels had cytoskeletal features associated with ALS (Strong et al., 1993). However, it was later thought that the seeds of the cycad *Cycas micronesica* had a neurotoxic non-protein amino acid, β-methylamino-L-alanine (BMAA), which appeared to cause ALS. More recently, it was discovered that symbiotic cyanobacteria within specialized roots of the cycad produced this toxic amino acid. This suggests worldwide that cyanobacteria have a product that can biomagnify up the food chain. People dying from ALS/PDC (Parkinson-dementia complex) in Guam had average brain concentrations of 5.0 mM BMAA. North American patients dying from Alzheimer's disease had an average BMAA concentration of 0.8 mM. It is possible that many slow-progressing neurodegenerative diseases considered heretofore to originate from age alone may have an environmental toxicant as one possible cause (Bradley and Mash, 2009). The neurodegeneration associated with Parkinson's disease may also be related to the use of the herbicide glyphosate, because this glycine derivative appeared to cause symmetrical Parkinsonian syndrome in a man 1 month after he accidentally sprayed himself with it (Barbosa et al., 2001).

Solvent-Induced CNS Depression Versus Carbon Disulfide Toxicity

Most volatile gases and solvents induce generalized depression and anesthesia of the central nervous system based on their K_{ow}. Many hypotheses concerning their actions, including alterations of Ca-induced release of neurotransmitters, have been postulated without a definitive answer. Alcohol's disinhibition of certain behaviors followed by ataxia and slurred speech progressing to coma and death are signs of many solvent-induced depressive actions. Toluene is an example of a solvent that produces a depression of the CNS similarly to ethanol or sedative-hypnotics (benzodiazepines and barbiturates). It rapidly crosses the blood–brain barrier and has been measured in the brains of test animals using a cannula. Its effects are an increase in sleep, headaches, eye irritation, memory impairment, dizziness, depression, and fatigue. Low chronic concentrations affect spatial learning and memory, while high concentrations lead to cerebellar dysfunction (ataxia or lack of coordinated movement), cerebral and hippocampal atrophy, and loss of brain volume. Exposure during pregnancy yields an embryopathy referred to as fetal solvent syndrome with growth retardation, microencephaly, deep-set eyes, low-set ears, a flat nasal bridge, micrognathia (small lower jaw that interferes with feeding the affected infant), and cognitive deficits. Toluene's effects on neurotransmitters are similar to other solvents, affecting stimulatory neurotransmitters such as decreased acetylcholine in the striatum and hippocampus (main excitatory neurotransmitter in CNS and involved in learning and memory). Extracellular glutamine (responsible for neurogenesis and mature function of CNS) and taurine increased in the mouse hippocampus in response to toluene, but not dopamine (excitatory) or glycine (inhibitory). However, in the rat prefrontal cortex but not the nucleus accumbens, toluene increased extracellular dopamine. In combination with cocaine, the location of the dopamine increases reverses with the nucleus accumbens, showing the elevated levels of this excitatory neurotransmitter. It is of interest that toluene in *Xenopus* oocytes potentiates the serotonergic currents. Receptor function is also altered by solvents. Toluene inhibits the excitatory NMDA and nicotinic (ACh) receptors and enhances inhibitory GABAA and glycine receptors in the increased glutamate, as well as more inhibitory neurotransmitters such as GABA (main inhibitory neurotransmitter of CNS) and serotonin. However, chronic treatment of rat hippocampal neurons with toluene exhibited an upregulation of NMDA receptors, which may increase NO and peroxynitrate concentrations. Neuroimmune functions also appear to be affected by solvents. Toluene appears to generate a T cell deficiency by altering the neuroimmune crosstalk. Neurotrophins, used to support survival,

differentiation, and maintenance of neuronal populations, appear also to be affected by toluene exposure. Neurons of the hippocampus are under control of neurotrophins such as nerve growth factor, brain-derived neurotrophic factors, and the tyrosine kinase family of neurotrophin receptors. Toluene upregulates these neurotrophins in mouse hippocampus based on strain of mouse, and allergic stimulation lowers the threshold for toluene sensitivity in C3H/HeN mice. Toluene and similar solvents therefore may increase allergic reactions as well as alter neurogenesis and neuronal migration. It appears that developmental exposure may have a variety of systems improperly interact

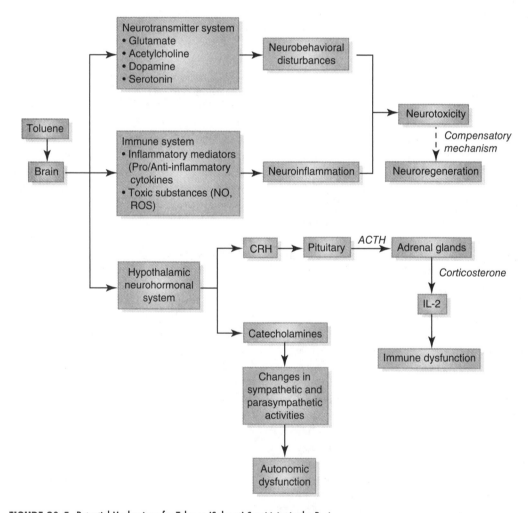

FIGURE 20-5 Potential Mechanisms for Toluene (Solvent) Sensitivity in the Brain

Note: NO = nitric oxide; ROS = reactive oxygen species; CRH = corticotropin releasing hormone; ACTH = adrenocorticotropic hormone

prompting problems in neurons, immune cells, and neurotrophins that persist into later life. Additionally, solvents provide a stress that appears to act via the hypothalamus → pituitary → adrenal axis leading to adrenocortical hypertrophy. Disturbances of the catecholamines within the hypothalamus may also influence autonomic nervous system function as indicated by heart and GI disturbances. The process of toluene interactions that influence the nervous system is delineated in **Figure 20-5** (Win-Shwe and Fujimaki, 2010).

It appears that certain solvents at low chronic levels also induce a behavioral disorder known by a variety of names such as organic solvent syndrome, painters' syndrome, psycho-organic syndrome, or chronic solvent encephalopathy. One famous agent in this regard is carbon disulfide. These agents differentiate from toluene and styrene in that the latter two agents are more defined by sensorineural hearing loss and acquired color vision disturbances. Carbon disulfide also famously causes psychotic behavior. Other agents such as chlorofluorocarbons, 2-bromopropane, and 1-bromopropane were considered to be peripheral nerve agents until more recent research uncovered CNS intoxication and damage from 1-bromopropane from occupational exposure (Matsuoka, 2007). This divergence between CNS and PNS toxicity is important for other agents as well. Chlorphenyl acetyl urea was a very good antiseizure medication affecting mainly the CNS, while a derivative bromphenylacetylurea has served as a model of peripheral nerve dying-back axonopathy, which may be a model for mitochondrial dysfunction that leads to ALS (Shi et al., 2010).

Nerve Toxicity Tests

Table 20-2 summarizes some nervous system toxicity tests.

In Situ Sea Lamprey Model

The squid giant axon and the sea lamprey (*Petromyzon marinus*) offer good alternative models for neuronal injury done to single neurons.

TABLE 20-2 Nervous System Toxicity Tests

Testing For	Individual Assays
Single neuron damage	Sea lamprey model (Hall, 1993)
Generic nervous system damage	Gliosis and glial fibrillary acidic protein (O'Callaghan, 1993)
	Sulfated glycoprotein-2 expression (May, 1993)
	Neurite outgrowth and neurofilament protein levels (Abdulla and Campbell, 1993)
	Silver staining techniques (Switzer, 1993)
Inflammatory injury	Quinolinic acid (Heyes, 1993)
Dopaminergic neurotoxicity	MAOB, dopamine reuptake pump, and tyrosine hydroxylase expression (Toggas et al., 1993) MPTP-goldfish model (Pollard et al., 1993) on other gene expression (Jones et al., 2013)
Myelin and neuronal cell membrane damage	Mitogenicity of astrocytes associated with myelin basic protein release to microglial cells or macrophages or fibroblast growth factor mitogenesis (De Vries et al., 1993)
Spinal cord damage (myelopathy)	DNA synthesis in Neuro-2a and glioma cells (Nerurkar et al., 1993)
Noninvasive early axonal degeneration	Magnetization transfer changes in MRI (Lexa et al., 1993)
Diabetic neuropathy	Nerve growth factor-truncate in urine (Hruska et al., 1993)
Neurobehavioral tests	A battery of adult tests and child analyses that tests various functions, learning, and lifelong exposures leading to neurodegeneration coupled to measures of prenatal, childhood, or adult exposures (Rohlman et al., 2008)

MAOB = monoamine oxidase B; MPTP = 1-methyl-4-phenyl-1,2,3,6-tetrahydropyridine; MRI = magnetic resonance imaging

The easily identifiable giant Muller and Mauthner neurons in the brain and spinal cord of the larval sea lamprey are fairly unique in the mature vertebrate central neurons as they exhibit rapid sprouting following axotomy and recognize some spinal cord targets. They have appropriate dendritic and axonal morphology and can be used to generate precise lesions. Pharmacological/toxicological intervention via injection into a single soma can be done, because the size (60–100 μm) and accessibility of this structure are advantageous for single-cell exposure. The lack of intrinsic vasculature makes the larval sea lamprey resistant to ischemic injury present in higher vertebrates that may complicate discernment of direct neuronal damage (Hall, 1993).

Gliosis and Glial Fibrillary Acidic Protein

Astrocytes in the brain tend to proliferate and hypertrophy following nervous system damage. This is called reactive gliosis or astrogliosis. Accumulation of glial fibrillary acidic protein (GFAP) is a generic measure of gliosis in surviving astrocytes following neuronal injury, because GFAP is a major intermediate in filament protein of astrocytes. Toxicants such as 3-acetylpyridine, amino-adipate, bilirubin, cadmium, colchicines, 5,7-dihydroxytryptamine, domoic acid, 6-hydroxydopamine, IDPN (β,β′-iminodipropionitrile), kainate, MDA, MDMA, methamphetamine, methylmercury, MPTP (dicussed later under dopaminergic gene expression), tributyltin, triethyltin, and trimethyltin induce reactive gliosis. Injuries such as aging (elderly), brain heating, genetic mutations, nerve cut, nocardia infection, and stab wounds also yield gliosis (O'Callaghan, 1993). GFAP analysis can also be used to follow the developmental damage sequence of brain areas following exposure to a toxicant such as trimethyltin (Barone, 1993). This method indicates injury as opposed to depletion of neurotransmitters, which may or may not indicate damage. It is also important to determine the damaged area, because different excitatory neurotoxicants may produce different patterns of damage. For example, D-methamphetamine or D-3,4-methylenedioxymethamphetamine (D-MDMA) causes increases in GFAP in the corpus striatum, but not in the hippocampus or cerebral cortex. Pretreatment with dizocilpine (MK-801), a noncompetitive NMDA-receptor antagonist, substantially blocked the increases in GFAP by D-methamphetamine and completely prevented the raised GFAP concentrations associated with D-MDMA. The amphetamine analog D-fenfluramine had no effect on striatal GFAP, nor was affected by dizocilpine pretreatment. This indicates that GFAP can model differential effects of excitatory neurotoxin analogs (Miller and O'Callaghan, 1993). There are different areas of the brain that are more sensitive to certain neurotoxins eliciting a gliosis response. GFAP for PCBs is most elevated in the optic lobe of the Atlantic tomcod fish (Evans et al., 1993). Other factors also increase upon ischemia or other brain injury. Some are more specific to the cell type. For example, insulin-like growth factor (IGF)-I mRNA and peptide are expressed in reactive astrocytes following experimental demyelination along with GFAP. However, IGF-II and IGFBP-2 mRNA and peptide are expressed in activated macrophages converging around the infarct and in the meninges, blood vessels, and choroid plexus of the brain following ischemic insult (Lee and Bondy, 1993).

Neurite Outgrowth and Neurofilament Protein Levels

Another use of neurofilament proteins employs a mouse NB41A3 neuroblastoma cell line in culture to monitor neurite outgrowth as a measure of healthy cells and the level of two neurofilament proteins, 68 kDa and 160 kDa in size. Two excitatory toxicants affect neurite outgrowth and decrease the concentrations of the two neurofilament proteins, β-N-methylamino alanine (BMAA) and kainate. The effects of kainate have been mentioned earlier in this chapter. BMAA is the postulated exogenous excitotoxin responsible for Guam disease or ALS (Abdulla and Campbell, 1993).

Inflammatory Brain Injury and Quinolinic Acid

Quinolinic acid is an excitotoxic kynurenine pathway metabolite found in inflammatory neurological diseases. Induction of enzymes of the kynurenine pathway such as indoleamin-2,3-dioxygenase may cause an increase in this intrinsic neurodegenerative toxicant. IFNγ and TNFα appear to stimulate synthesis of quinolinic acid. HIV infection was one very important disease associated with a 3.5-fold increase in quinolinic acid production in early stages. Basal ganglia lesions and motor deficits correlated with quinolinic acid concentrations. Inflammatory lesions following transient cerebral ischemia appear to be related to quinolinic acid formation with the following hierarchy of susceptibility: hippocampus > striatum > cerebral cortex > thalamus. The cerebellum showed little change in this excitatory neurotoxicant in gerbils following transient cerebral ischemia and an absence of pathology (Heyes, 1993).

Dopaminergic Neurotoxicity Gene Expression

MPTP (1-methyl-4-phenyl-1,2,5,6-tetrahydropyridine) causes dopaminergic neurodegeneration due to expression of the adrenergic neurotransmitter metabolizing enzyme MAOB (first gene product that converts MPTP into MPP^+) and the dopamine reuptake pump (second gene product), which transfers the toxic chemical species into the dopaminergic neurons. The damage is then seen via the expression of tyrosine hydroxylase (third gene product) in damaged neurons. These three gene products may be a measure of MPTP toxicity (Toggas et al., 1993). However, more recent studies indicate that the expression of three other genes (Mtap2, Lancl 1, and Kansl1l) is highly correlated by principal component analysis for MPTP exposure, and they could be markers for this chemical's neurotoxicity (Jones et al., 2013). The actual target of MPP^+ is the mitochondria and depletion of ATP. It is of interest that most species used to study neurotoxicity in primates do not respond similarly, because rats and many mice species are resistant to MPTP. However, the goldfish appears to alter movement to MPTP and show the beneficial effects of medications that may be used to treat Parkinson's disease using MPTP toxicity as the model without the use of primates (Pollard et al., 1993).

Because MPTP toxicity is essentially an oxidative process, it may be important to indicate in a living organism how much oxygen radical formation is occurring in the brain. MPTP analogs were assayed for their ability to form ˙OH free radicals via salicylate hydroxylation (hydroxyl radical trapping) in the striatum of rats (Chiueh et al., 1993).

Demyelination Versus Neuronal Membrane Damage

Demyelination of the neuron by agents such as hexachlorophene, lead, or tellurium may be monitored peripherally or centrally. Myelin basic protein is found either in peripheral or central nervous system myelin sheaths, but is higher centrally. The release of this protein to the peripheral macrophages or the central microglial cells is suspected to induce the mitogenicity (of astrocytes) necessary for remyelination and may be a good marker of myelin damage. However, damage to the neuronal membrane may be indicated by the release of fibroblast growth factor (De Vries et al., 1993).

Spinal Cord Damage (Myelopathy)

A method of analyzing for spinal cord injury determines more specifically glial versus neuronal cell damage through the use of cultures of neuronal cells (Neuro-2a) and glioma (C6) cells. This system was used to assay the differential effect of the plasticizer N-butylbenzenesulfonamide (NBBS). NBBS causes a progressive spastic myelopathy distinguished by neuroaxonal degeneration in New Zealand white rabbits. The 70% reduction in the uptake of $^3[H]$-thymidine occurred at a 10-fold lower concentration for Neuro-2a cells (20 μM) than C6 glioma cells (250 μM) in the presence of NBBS. These cells were also examined microscopically for detaching from substrate or lack of trypan blue exclusion and release of lactate dehydrogenase (signs of cell death). Glioma cells were also monitored for decreased staining for glial fibrillary acidic protein and S-100 protein, while Neuro-2a cells were assayed for decreased 160-kDa neurofilament subunit protein. This multipronged molecular approach allowed the nature of the differential sensitivity to be accurately measured apart from a designation of myelopathy (Nerurkar et al., 1993).

Sulfated Glycoprotein-2

Sulfated glycoprotein-2 (SGP-2) is a protein that co-localizes to β-amyloid plaques within the parenchyma of brains of patients with Alzheimer's disease, especially in the hippocampus. Clones of this gene have also been detected in human glioma and retinitis pigmentosa. Hamsters infected with scrapie (fatal transmissible neurodegenerative spongiform encephalopathy usually associated with sheep and goats) or quails with transformed neuroretinal cells also have clones of this gene. Experimental toxicity indicates that kainic acid causes rapid (days) hippocampal pyramidal neuron degeneration and a two- to threefold increase in SGP-2 RNA and protein concentrations. *In situ* hybridization localized the induction mainly to reactive astrocytes. The protein was found in degenerated CA3 and CA4 pyramidal neurons of the hippocampus and hilus of the dentate gyrus by immunocytochemical means. The expression of SGP-2 may play a role in apoptosis as gleaned from the peripheral action of a similar protein in the prostate. SGP-2 may increase clearance of debris following neurodegeneration by promoting cell–cell interactions (activating microglia). It may also serve neurotrophic (growth and repair of neurites) and neuroprotective roles (similar to complement lysis inhibitor) as well (May, 1993).

Laminin-Binding Protein

Laminin is usually found in the basement membrane of undisturbed brain cells. During injury such as ischemia, laminin-like molecules are associated with reactive glial cells. As indicated earlier, glial fibrillary acidic protein has served as a measure of transient ischemia with intense immunostaining of astrocytes in the CA1 region of the hippocampus where delayed neuronal cell loss occurred. Staining for laminin-binding protein (LBP) occurs in the first few days following transient ischemia in astrocytes of the CA3 region of the hippocampus. The LBP-positive

staining astrocytes were fairly early predictors for areas of the brain or substructures where permanent neuron loss would occur. This staining was found to persist up to at least 160 days post-injury as this was the latest data point taken in a rat study. Laminin on the other hand only stained the somata of reactive astrocytes and was not found in glial processes. Thus, it appears that LBP immunohistochemical staining is another good marker of astrogliosis after transient ischemia or other damage to the CNS (Jucker et al., 1993).

There are some expressions linked to adhesive factors such as laminin and the trophic agents following brain injury. One labeled G41 appeared primarily as brain localization, and specifically its highest expression was in the cerebellum, hippocampus, hypothalamus, and cerebral cortex with moderate to low expression in the striatum, midbrain, and pons (Quach et al., 1993). It is likely in the future that careful use of analysis of the proper array of factors released following toxic insult may indicate the area(s) affected and time course of injury. It may be easier then to determine agents that act similarly and their mechanisms of action.

Silver Staining During Neural Degeneration

Pretreatment of neurons prior to injury will yield a damaged tissue that has a higher affinity for binding silver than normal, intact neurons. Chemical reduction then leaves black deposits that indicate the sites of neural degeneration (Switzer, 1993).

Noninvasive Magnetization Transfer Techniques in MRI

For humans, a less invasive test for neurotoxicity may involve the use of MRI. Regular MRI scans can be better than computed tomography scans for alterations in white matter such as those that may be caused by multiple sclerosis. Early axonal (Wallerian) degeneration is not discernable by conventional MRI, but is visualized in cats by changes in magnetization transfer in the lesioned side (Lexa et al., 1993).

Urine Nerve Growth Factor Receptor-Truncated

Another noninvasive technique for measuring neuropathies is the use of nerve growth factor-truncated (NGFR-t) in urine samples of human patients. Nerve growth factor receptor is localized on the neuronal cell surface and binds nerve growth factor as discussed earlier. Nerve biopsies would be problematic, and so trophic factors indicating injury and possible repair cannot be determined directly in intact animals or human patients. However, the cleavage product of nerve growth factor receptor known as NGFR-t can be determined in the rat (found elevated after rat sciatic nerve section) or the human through the use of monoclonal antibodies. Means for NGFR-t normalized to creatinine concentrations in urine were < 110 ng NGFR-t/ mg creatinine for normal and diabetic human patients, but > 120 ng/mg for diabetic patients with neuropathy (Hruska et al., 1993).

Human Neurobehavioral Tests

Because neurobehavioral tests in children offer a very sensitive tool for assessing exposures to toxic chemicals, this must also be considered a valuable tool for neurotoxicity monitoring. It must be accompanied by some measure of the chemical (blood Mn or hair methylmercury) as well to insure that amounts of the toxicant are consonant with the observed toxicity. Mercury has a dose–response indication between hair concentration and Stanford-Binet copying (visuospatial), tremor, attention, fine motor performance, verbal learning, and memory performance. For manganese, blood concentrations appear to match well with aiming, finger tapping, symbol digit, digit span, additions, coordinated movements, learning, recall, executive function, memory, sustained concentration and sequencing, verbal ability, cognitive flexibility, visuospatial construction ability, and visual contrast sensitivity. The questions for these tests are less mechanistic than assessing risk to a population. For example, what drop in function such as IQ scale is sufficient to indicate a dysfunctional deficit that gets labeled as an environmental disease? How many people have to experience these effects to be of concern? These questions suggest that a threshold for effect must be reached in an exposed population. It also indicates that dose–response is important. Pesticide exposure may be determined by a questionnaire completed by the exposed adult or parent of an exposed child, community of residence (in exposed area), occupation (exposure through work), or maternal blood for metabolites. Although the blood measure would appear best, the delay between exposure during embryonic or fetal development and testing may be such that only former parenteral occupation may be currently relevant to a past heavy exposure. Which battery of tests is adequate and reasonable to screen a population? One such assessment may be the pediatric environmental neurobehavioral test, or perhaps it is easier to use and evaluate commonly used adult neurotoxicity screens in children. Lifetime exposure also becomes an issue for neurodegenerative diseases. Additionally, Haber's law indicates that exposure is a function of both intensity and duration. Thus, the exposure throughout a lifetime may be sufficient to cause toxicity even if the intensity is lessened over the years (Rohlman et al., 2008).

Questions

1. How does lead damage the BBB?
2. How is heavy metal damage to peripheral nerves related to the action of muscle rubs containing hot pepper extract?
3. How is ammonia experienced in astrocytes and neurons based on Figure 20-3?
4. Overstimulation of the brain by glutamine is plainly neurotoxic and generates neurodegeneration over time. Are there other signals that also can lead to similar neurotoxicity?
5. How does the discovery of stannin change the mechanistic viewpoint of trimethyltin neurotoxicity?
6. In global ischemia, what process needs to be inhibited to prevent neuronal death?
7. What mechanism appears to prevent glutamate and kainate neurodegeneration?

8. How does toluene affect neurotoxicity while causing immune and autonomic nervous system dysfunction (Figure 20-5)?

9. Why are GFAP increases in a specific brain area indicative of a certain type of neurotoxicity?

10. Because MPTP mainly damages mitochondria, why are dopaminergic neurons more sensitive to its toxic actions?

11. What options exist for testing humans for neurotoxic actions of chemicals?

References

Abdulla EM, Campbell IC. 1993. Use of neurite outgrowth as an in vitro method of assessing neurotoxicity. *Ann NY Acad Sci.* 679:276–279.

Albrecht J, Zielińska M, Norenberg MD. 2010. Glutamine as a mediator of ammonia neurotoxicity: a critical appraisal. *Biochem Pharmacol.* 80:1303–1308.

Balbuena P, Li W, Magnin-Bissel G, Meldrum JB, Ehrich M. 2010. Comparison of two blood-brain barrier in vitro systems: cytotoxicity and transfer assessments of malathion/oxon and lead acetate. *Toxicol Sci.* 114:260–271.

Barbosa ER, Leiros da Costa MD, Bacheschi LA, Scaff M, Leite CC. 2001. Parkinsonism after glycine-derivate exposure. *Mov Disord.* 16:565–568.

Barone S Jr. 1993. Developmental differences in neural damage following trimethyl-tin as demonstrated with GFAP immunohistochemistry. *Ann NY Acad Sci.* 679:306–316.

Benkovic SA, O'Callaghan JP, Miller DB. 2006. Regional neuropathology following kainic acid intoxication in adult and aged C57BL/6J mice. *Brain Res.* 1070:215–231.

Blomgren K, Hagberg H. 2006. Free radicals, mitochondria, and hypoxia-ischemia in the developing brain. *Free Radic Biol Med.* 40:388–397.

Bradley WG, Mash DC. 2009. Beyond Guam: the cyanobacteria/BMAA hypothesis of the cause of ALS and other neurodegenerative diseases. *Amyotroph Lateral Scler.* 10(Suppl 2):7–20.

Brandt I, Dencker L, Larsson KS, Siddall RA. 1983. Placental transfer of hexachlorophene (HCP) in the marmoset monkey (*Callithrix jacchus*). *Acta Pharmacol Toxicol (Copenh).* 52:310–313.

Caday CG, Sklar RM, Berlove DJ, Kemmou A, Brown RH Jr, Finklestein SP. 1993. Polyubiquitin gene expression following cerebral ischemia. *Ann NY Acad Sci.* 679:188–194.

Cai T, Che H, Yao T, Chen Y, Huang C, Zhang W, Du K, Zhang J, Cao Y, Chen J, Luo W. 2011. Manganese

induces tau hyperphosphorylation through the activation of ERK MAPK pathway in PC12 cells. *Toxicol Sci.* 119:169–177.

Chiueh CC, Murphy DL, Miyake H, Lang K, Tulsi PK, Huang SJ. 1993. Hydroxyl free radical (·OH) formation reflected by salicylate hydroxylation and neuromelanin. In vivo markers for oxidant injury of nigral neurons. *Ann NY Acad Sci.* 679:370–375.

Deckwerth TL, Johnson EM Jr. 1993. Neurotrophic factor deprivation-induced death. *Ann NY Acad Sci.* 679:121–131.

De Vries GH, Neuberger TJ, Baichwal RR, Bigbee JW, Zane L, Yoshino JE. 1993. Release of membrane-associated growth factors during neural injury. *Ann NY Acad Sci.* 679:217–225.

Dzietko M, Sifringer M, Klaus J, Endesfelder S, Brait D, Hansen HH, Bendix I, Felderhoff-Mueser U. 2010. Neurotoxic effects of MDMA (ecstasy) on the developing rodent brain. *Dev Neurosci.* 32:197–207.

el-Fawal HA, Ehrich MF. 1993. Calpain activity in organophosphorus-induced delayed neuropathy (OPIDN): effects of a phenylalkylamine calcium channel blocker. *Ann NY Acad Sci.* 679:325–329.

Evans HL, Little AR, Gong ZL, Duffy JS, Wirgin I, el-Fawal HA. 1993. Glial fibrillary acidic protein (GFAP) indicates in vivo exposure to environmental contaminants: PCBs in the Atlantic tomcod. *Ann NY Acad Sci.* 679:402–406.

Fernández MT, Zitko V, Gascón S, Torreblanca A, Novelli A. 1993. Neurotoxic effect of okadaic acid, a seafood-related toxin, on cultured cerebellar neurons. *Ann NY Acad Sci.* 679:260–269.

Genuis SJ. 2008. Toxic causes of mental illness are overlooked. *Neurotoxicology.* 29:1147–1149.

Ghersi-Egea JF, Gazzin S, Strazielle N. 2009. Blood-brain interfaces and bilirubin-induced neurological diseases. *Curr Pharm Des.* 15:2893–2907.

Gibbons SJ, Brorson JR, Bleakman D, Chard PS, Miller RJ. 1993. Calcium influx and neurodegeneration. *Ann NY Acad Sci.* 679:22–33.

Gohlke JM, Stockton PS, Sieber S, Foley J, Portier CJ. 2009. AhR-mediated gene expression in the developing mouse telencephalon. *Reprod Toxicol.* 28:321–328.

Gul N, Smith LA, Ahmed SA. 2010. Light chain separated from the rest of the type a botulinum neurotoxin molecule is the most catalytically active form. *PLoS One.* 5:e12872.

Hall GF. 1993. Cellular responses of identified lamprey central neurons to axonal and dendritic injury. An *in situ* model for studying cellular injury on the single cell level in the vertebrate CNS. *Ann NY Acad Sci.* 679:43–64.

Hariharakrishnan J, Satpute RM, Bhattacharya R. 2010. Cyanide-induced changes in the levels of neurotransmitters in discrete brain regions of rats and their response to oral treatment with alpha-ketoglutarate. *Indian J Exp Biol.* 48:731–736.

Heyes MP. 1993. Quinolinic acid and inflammation. *Ann NY Acad Sci.* 679:211–216.

Hogberg HT, Kinsner-Ovaskainen A, Coecke S, Hartung T, Bal-Price AK. 2010. mRNA expression is a relevant tool to identify developmental neurotoxicants using an *in vitro* approach. *Toxicol Sci.* 113:95–115.

Hruska RE, Chertack MM, Kravis D. 1993. Elevation of nerve growth factor receptor-truncated in the urine of patients with diabetic neuropathy. *Ann NY Acad Sci.* 679:349–351.

Igisu H, Kinoshita Y. 2007. Magnetic resonance for evaluation of toxic encephalopathies: implications from animal experiments. *Neurotoxicology.* 28:252–256.

Jones BC, Miller DB, O'Callaghan JP, Lu L, Unger EL, Alam G, Williams RW. 2013. Systems analysis of genetic variation in MPTP neurotoxicity in mice. *Neurotoxicology.* 37:26–34.

Juarez de Ku LM., Sharma-Stokkermans M, Meserve LA. 1994. Thyroxine normalizes polychlorinated biphenyl (PCBP dose-related depression of choline acetyltransferase (ChAT) activity in hippocampus and basal forebrain of 15-day old rats. *Toxicology.* 94:19–30.

Jucker M, Bialobok P, Kleinman HK, Walker LC, Hagg T, Ingram DK. 1993. Laminin-like and laminin-binding protein-like immunoreactive astrocytes in rat hippocampus after transient ischemia. Antibody to laminin-binding protein is a sensitive marker of neural injury and degeneration. *Ann NY Acad Sci.* 679:245–252.

Kajta M, Wójtowicz AK, Maćkowiak M, Lasoń W. 2009. Aryl hydrocarbon receptor-mediated apoptosis of neuronal cells: a possible interaction with estrogen receptor signaling. *Neuroscience.* 158:811–822.

Kodavanti PR. 2006. Neurotoxicity of persistent organic pollutants: possible mode(s) of action and further considerations. *Dose Response.* 3:273–305.

Lagrange P, Romero IA, Minn A, Revest PA. 1999. Transendothelial permeability changes induced by free radicals in an *in vitro* model of the blood-brain barrier. *Free Radic Biol Med.* 27:667–672.

Lee WH, Bondy C. 1993. Insulin-like growth factors and cerebral ischemia. *Ann NY Acad Sci.* 679:418–422.

Levine S, Sowinski R. 1982. Localization of toxic encephalopathies near lesions of experimental allergic encephalomyelitis. *Am J Pathol.* 107:135–141.

Lexa FJ, Grossman RI, Rosenquist AC. 1993. Detection of early axonal degeneration in the mammalian central nervous system by magnetization transfer techniques in magnetic resonance imaging. *Ann NY Acad Sci.* 679:336–340.

Liu HL, Hua MY, Yang HW, Huang CY, Chu PC, Wu JS, Tseng IC, Wang JJ, Yen TC, Chen PY, Wei KC. 2010. Magnetic resonance monitoring of focused ultrasound/magnetic nanoparticle targeting delivery of therapeutic agents to the brain. *Proc Natl Acad Sci USA.* 107:15205–15210.

Marini AM, Paul SM. 1993. Induction of a neuroprotective state in cerebellar granule cells following activation of N-methyl-D-aspartate receptors. *Ann NY Acad Sci.* 679:253–259.

Markey SP, Markey CJ, Wang TC. 1993. Oxidative damage in double-stranded genomic DNA as measured by GC/MS assay of a thymine glycol derivative. *Ann NY Acad Sci.* 679:352–357.

Matsuoka M. 2007. [Neurotoxicity of organic solvents--recent findings]. *Brain Nerve.* 59:591–596.

Mattson MP, Rydel RE, Lieberburg I, Smith-Swintosky VL. 1993. Altered calcium signaling and neuronal injury: stroke and Alzheimer's disease as examples. *Ann NY Acad Sci.* 679:1–21.

May PC. 1993. Sulfated glycoprotein-2: an emerging molecular marker for neurodegeneration. *Ann NY Acad Sci.* 679:235–244.

Miller DB, O'Callaghan JP. 1993. The interactions of MK-801 with the amphetamine analogues D-methamphetamine (D-METH), 3,4-methylenedioxymethamphetamine (D-MDMA) or D-fenfluramine (D-FEN): neural damage and neural protection. *Ann NY Acad Sci.* 679:321–324.

Ndountse LT, Chan HM. 2008. Methylmercury increases N-methyl-D-aspartate receptors on human SH-SY 5Y neuroblastoma cells leading to neurotoxicity. *Toxicology.* 249:251–255.

Nerurkar VR, Wakayama I, Rowe T, Yanagihara R, Garruto RM. 1993. Preliminary observations on the in vitro toxicity of N-butylbenzenesulfonamide: a newly discovered neurotoxin. *Ann NY Acad Sci.* 679:280–287.

Niso-Santano M, Bravo-San Pedro JM, Gómez-Sánchez R, Climent V, Soler G, Fuentes JM, González-Polo RA. 2011. ASK1 overexpression accelerates paraquat-induced autophagy via endoplasmic reticulum stress. *Toxicol Sci.* 119:156–168.

Nixon RA, Cataldo AM. 1993. The lysosomal system in neuronal cell death: a review. *Ann NY Acad Sci.* 679:87–109.

Noga M, Hayashi T, Tanaka J. 1997. Gene expressions of ubiquitin and hsp70 following focal ischaemia in rat brain. *Neuroreport.* 8:1239–1241.

Nowak TS Jr. 1993. Synthesis of heat shock/stress proteins during cellular injury. *Ann NY Acad Sci.* 679:142–156.

O'Callaghan JP. 1993. Quantitative features of reactive gliosis following toxicant-induced damage of the CNS. *Ann NY Acad Sci.* 679:195–210.

Pappas TC, Decorti F, Macdonald NJ, Neet KE, Taglialatela G. 2003. Tumour necrosis factor-alpha- vs. growth factor deprivation-promoted cell death: different receptor requirements for mediating nerve growth factor-promoted rescue. *Aging Cell*. 2:83–92.

Pizzi M, Fallacara C, Arrighi V, Memo M, Spano PF. 1993. Attenuation of excitatory amino acid toxicity by metabotropic glutamate receptor agonists and aniracetam in primary cultures of cerebellar granule cells. *J Neurochem*. 61:683–689.

Pollard HB, Adeyemo M, Dhariwal K, Levine M, Caohuy H, Markey S, Markey CJ, Youdim MB. 1993. The goldfish as a drug discovery vehicle for Parkinson's disease and other neurodegenerative disorders. *Ann NY Acad Sci*. 679:317–320.

Prior MJ, Brown AM, Mavroudis G, Lister T, Ray DE. 2004. MRI characterisation of a novel rat model of focal astrocyte loss. *MAGMA*. 17:125–132.

Quach TT, Schrier BK, Duchemin AM. 1993. Gene expression in brain injury: identification of a new cDNA structurally related to adhesive and trophic agents. *Ann NY Acad Sci*. 679:423–430.

Rai A, Maurya SK, Khare P, Srivastava A, Bandyopadhyay S. 2010. Characterization of developmental neurotoxicity of As, Cd, and Pb mixture: synergistic action of metal mixture in glial and neuronal functions. *Toxicol Sci*. 118:586–601.

Roberts-Lewis JM, Siman R. 1993. Spectrin proteolysis in the hippocampus: a biochemical marker for neuronal injury and neuroprotection. *Ann NY Acad Sci*. 679:78–86.

Rohlman DS, Lucchini R, Anger WK, Bellinger DC, van Thriel C. 2008. Neurobehavioral testing in human risk assessment. *Neurotoxicology*. 29:556–567.

Sarafian TA, Verity MA. 1993. Changes in protein phosphorylation in cultured neurons after exposure to methyl mercury. *Ann NY Acad Sci*. 679:65–77.

Sayre LM, Perry G, Smith MA. 2008. Oxidative stress and neurotoxicity. *Chem Res Toxicol*. 21:172–188.

Sharp FR, Butman M, Wang S, Koistinaho J, Graham SH, Sagar SM, Berger P, Longo FM. 1993. *Ann NY Acad Sci*. 679:288–290.

Shi P, Gal J, Kwinter DM, Liu X, Zhu H. 2010. Mitochondrial dysfunction in amyotrophic lateral sclerosis. *Biochim Biophys Acta*. 1802:45–51.

Shimizu K, Ohtaki K, Matsubara K, Aoyama K, Uezono T, Saito O, Suno M, Ogawa K, Hayase N,

Kimura K, Shiono H. 2001. Carrier-mediated processes in blood–brain barrier penetration and neural uptake of paraquat. *Brain Res*. 906:135–142.

Strong MJ, Wakayama I, Garruto RM. 1993. The neuronal cytoskeleton in disorders of late onset and slow progression. *Ann NY Acad Sci*. 679:388–393.

Sun AY, Yang WL, Kim HD. 1993. Free radical and lipid peroxidation in manganese-induced neuronal cell injury. *Ann NY Acad Sci*. 679:358–363.

Sun GY, Lin TA, Wixom P, Zoeller RT, Lin TN, He YY, Hsu CY. 1993. Effects of focal cerebral ischemia on expression and activity of inositol 1,4,5-trisphosphate 3-kinase in rat cortex. *Ann NY Acad Sci*. 679:382–387.

Switzer RC 3rd. 1993. Silver staining methods: their role in detecting neurotoxicity. *Ann NY Acad Sci*. 679:341–348.

Toggas SM, Krady JK, Thompson TA, Billingsley ML. 1993. Molecular mechanisms of selective neurotoxicants: studies on organotin compounds. *Ann NY Acad Sci*. 679:157–177.

VanDuyn N, Settivari R, Wong G, Nass R. 2010. SKN-1/Nrf2 inhibits dopamine neuron degeneration in a *Caenorhabditis elegans* model of methylmercury toxicity. *Toxicol Sci*. 118:613–624.

Vendrell M, Curran T, Morgan JI. 1993. Glutamate, immediate-early genes, and cell death in the nervous system. *Ann NY Acad Sci*. 679:132–141.

Verity MA. 1993. Mechanisms of phospholipase A_2 activation and neuronal injury. *Ann NY Acad Sci*. 679:110–120.

Werner P, Cohen G. 1993. Glutathione disulfide (GSSG) as a marker of oxidative injury to brain mitochondria. *Ann NY Acad Sci*. 679:364–369.

Win-Shwe TT, Fujimaki H. 2010. Neurotoxicity of toluene. *Toxicol Lett*. 198:93–99.

Xie L, Kang H, Xu Q, Chen MJ, Liao Y, Thiyagarajan M, O'Donnell J, Christensen DJ, Nicholson C, Iliff JJ, Takano T, Deane R, Nedergaard M. 2013. Sleep drives metabolite clearance from the adult brain. *Science*. 342:373–377.

Zheng W. 2001. Toxicology of choroid plexus: special reference to metal-induced neurotoxicities. *Microsc Res Tech*. 52:89–103.

Zurich MG, Monnet-Tschudi F. 2009. Contribution of *in vitro* neurotoxicology studies to the elucidation of neurodegenerative processes. *Brain Res Bull*. 80:211–216.

CHAPTER 21

Toxicity to Neuroendocrine Organs and Endocrine Disruption

This is a chapter outline intended to guide and familiarize you with the content to follow.

I. Neuroendocrine organ toxicity and endocrine disruption—see Table 21-1

   A. Example—the female Sprague-Dawley rat model of breast cancer indicated atrazine increased cancer incidence. However, the disruption of the hypothalamic control of pituitary and ovarian function in the rat would have an opposite reaction in menopausal women. This indicated that atrazine was not necessarily a human carcinogen but was a case of endocrine disruption (a developing toxicology field at the time)

   B. Hypothalamus—posterior pituitary—see Figure 21-1

      1. Involved in control of water (ADH), milk letdown response (oxytocin), reproduction (GnRH), stress regulation (CRH), growth (GHRH), metabolism (TRH), and lactation (leading to pituitary release of prolactin)

      2. Cycad poisoning → hypersomnolent behavior in rats due to ↓ orexin-A neurons

      3. Dieldrin antagonizes $GABA_A$ inhibitory neurotransmission and so targets bony fish hypothalamic cells as they have a high density of GABA-producing cells. Dieldrin also causes neurodegeneration via affecting a variety of proteins involved in neuron architecture (e.g., tau) as well as energy functions (oxidative phosphorylation)

      4. Cocaine affects medial preoptic area of anterior hypothalamus → ↓ oxytocin and ↑ aggression in female rats

      5. Reproduction

         a. TCDD → AhR → affects lateral preoptic area and septal region of hypothalamus → less GnRH release (ability to transport hormone out of hypothalamic cells into blood)

         b. PCBs (especially Aroclor 1221) → AhR → ↑ GnRH at low doses blocked by nuclear estrogen receptor antagonist (PCBs also affect DA, NE, and 5-HT receptors) and ↑ mating behavior in treated dams

         c. Chlorpyrifos → ↑ neurite outgrowth and cell confluence similarly to estradiol, while methoxychlor does not

         d. Glutamate or KCl → ↑ GnRH release from hypothalamic neurons: o,p'-DDT ↑ glutamate-evoked GnRH release more than bisphenol A, while methoxychlor and the breakdown product of DDT, p,p-DDE had no such effects; TCDD exposure during development ↓ KCl-evoked GnRH release (but more GnRH peptide in cells)

         e. Bisphenol A and phytoestrogen genistein → ↑ immunoreactivity of the sexually dimorphic rat hypothalamus to Ca^{2+}-binding protein calbindin (hyper-masculinizing); genistein ↑ anterior periventricular nucleus in male rats (involved in ovulation in females and GnRH in both sexes); genistein also suppresses the GNRH pulse generator → less LH pulses

CONCEPTUALIZING TOXICOLOGY 21-1

    f. Chlordecone → ↑ lordosis quotients in females (feminization), while also masculinizing males and females (↑ mounting behavior); coumestrol ↓ male or female sexual behaviors; 4-methylbenzylidene camphor ↓ proceptive (courting), lordosis quotients, and receptivity behaviors in the female animals

    g. Atrazine affects hypothalamus and reproductive hormones

    h. Bisphenol A (contained in hard plastic bottles) affects NO-cGMP pathway in medial preoptic nucleus and ventromedial subdivision of the bed nucleus of stria terminalis → affecting reproductive and sexual behavior; differentiated from organophosphate insecticide methoxychlor in pregnant sheep as both chemicals ↓ GnRH and ESR2 mRNA, but only bisphenol A ↑ expression of ESR1 mRNA in medial preoptic area

    i. Anabolic steroids such as 17α-methyltestosterone ↑ $GABA_A$ tone onto downstream GnRH neurons → smaller testes size

    j. Pulp mill effluents influence DA transmission and spawning behavior of fish

    k. Sewage sludge applied to grazing lands affected GnRH and galaninergic (sleep-active neurons) of pregnant animals and offspring

6. Energy, thyroid control, feeding

    a. PBDEs → ↓ thyroxine; bisphenol A → transient ↑ thyroxine

    b. DES → reproductive tumors in offspring and obesity (↑ feeding behavior and obesogens that affect peroxisome proliferator-activated receptors and nuclear hormone receptors involved in lipolysis)

    c. Bacterial toxin LPS → ↓ eating behavior (may be related to ↓ Fos expression in melanin-concentrating hormone neurons), selective partitioning of energy for fat (may be related to ↑ expression of Fos in orexin neurons) and fever; LPS also ↓ appetite by ↑ atypical protein kinase Czeta/λ activity expressed in arcuate and paraventricular nuclei; destruction of the arcuate nucleus of the hypothalamus by MSG treatment → ↑ fat accumulation and ↓ energy production

    d. Amphetamine and endotoxin anorectic effects related to catecholamine neurotransmission in the perifornical hypothalamus

    e. Al affects via ↑ acetyl CoA and AChE inhibition (binds to –SH groups)—causes adipsia (lack of thirst), aphagia (loss of swallowing), hypokinesia (↓ bodily movement), fatigues, seizures, etc.

    f. Pb ↓ GHRH release (but prolactin elevated)

    g. Pb ↓ thyroid hormone

    h. SSRI fluoxetine bioaccumulates in goldfish → ↑ expression of CRH and ↓ expression of neuropeptide Y → anorexigenic effects

    i. MDMA → hyperthermia in animals only with intact hypothalamus and thyroid; ↓ hyperthermia if antagonize DA, 5-HT, and $α_1$-adrenergic receptors or ↑ hyperthermia in presence of caffeine, PDE-4 inhibition, or adenosine receptors $A_{1/2}$ or A_{2A} antagonists but not A_1 receptor antagonism

C. Anterior pituitary

1. Place where hormones outside the brain are produced and stimulated to release by releasing hormones of the hypothalamus

2. ACTH (regulates adrenal stress functions) is encoded by proopiomelanocortin (PMOC) gene as detected by green fluorescent protein gene (EGFP)—affected expression by the synthetic steroid dexamethasone or oppositely by inhibitor of steroid synthesis, aminoglutethimide

3. Triazine herbicide simazine and a PCB congener (3,3′,4,4′,5-pentachlorobiphenyl) interfere with PMOC-EGFP and interrenal development in the zebrafish; another triazine herbicide atrazine inhibits growth hormone secretion due to binding to GHRH receptor

4. Cd enters via L-type voltage and receptor-mediated Ca^{2+} channels → accumulates in cell → chronotoxic effect on secretory timing of pituitary (ACTH and TSH) by altering amino acid peaks (disappearance of nocturnal peak of amino acid content and appearance of glutamate peak during resting phase of photoperiod)

5. Al damages hypothalamus and affects anterior pituitary → ↓ prolactin levels

CONCEPTUALIZING TOXICOLOGY 21-1 (*continued*)

6. $Cr^{VI} \rightarrow$ hypertrophy of corticotrophs in pituitary of teleost disrupting pituitary $\rightarrow$ interrenal axis in freshwater fish (analogous to pituitary $\rightarrow$ adrenal axis of mammals)

7. 3-Methyl-4-nitrophenol from diesel exhaust $\downarrow$ FSH and LH in rats and LH in quail

8. Organophosphates (dimethoate) $\rightarrow \downarrow$ LH (and testosterone) in developing mouse

9. MEHP (phthalate) disrupts murine gonadotrope LβT2 cells by inhibiting 11β-hydroxysteroid dehydrogenase type 2 mRNA expression and enzyme activity

10. Stress hormone corticosterone inhibits proliferation of gonadotrope cells, which is reversed by mifepristone (anti-progestin abortion drug)

11. Lack of negative feedback from thyroid (exposed to radioactive iodine) $\rightarrow$ adenohypophysis hypertrophy $\rightarrow \uparrow$ TSH (clinical sign of hypothyroidism)

12. Environmental estrogens $\rightarrow$ pituitary tumors and $\uparrow$ prolactin secretion (this hormone and pituitary adenomas $\downarrow$ by dopamine agonists such as bromocriptine)

13. Pituitary tumors are classified by size and hormonal activity. Prolactinoma is the most common tumor subtype. 30% are nonfunctional adenomas $\rightarrow$ headaches, visual alterations, hypopituitarism; GH-secreting adenomas = 10–20%; corticotroph adenomas (10–15%) leading to $\uparrow$ ACTH $\rightarrow$ adrenal hypertrophy $\rightarrow$ Cushing's disease; thyrotroph adenomas rare $\rightarrow$ hyperthyroidism. Most pituitary tumors are monoclonal and half are aneuploid (unstable genetics) but not modeled on oncogenes or tumor suppressor genes. Other events leading to tumors are cell-cycle gene mutation, p53 mutation (carcinoma), altered bcl-2 family expression, $\downarrow$ expression of pituitary apoptosis gene, and growth signaling factors and cytokine stimulation of oncogenesis

D. Stress axis (HPA)

1. Malathion $\uparrow$ sensitivity of negative feedback from corticosterone/cortisol $\rightarrow \uparrow$ iNOS mRNA $\downarrow$ corticotropin RH mRNA $\rightarrow$ insulin resistance

2. Ethanol affects HPA axis ($\uparrow$ ACTH and corticosterone proestrus) and gonadal axis ($\uparrow$ basal and stress estradiol proestrus, but $\downarrow$ GnRH mRNA in diestrus)—only $\uparrow$ agouti-related protein in binge-drinking mice (addiction pathway)

3. Adrenals

   a. Cortex

      (1) Pb $\rightarrow$ parenchymal damage, altered corticosterone + $\downarrow$ cytosolic and nuclear glucocorticoid receptor binding

      (2) Adrenal most susceptible to chemically induced lesions—outer layer (zona glomerulosa produces aldosterone to regulate blood pressure) least likely to be affected, but lesions found in zona fasciculata (produces immune suppression and $\uparrow$ plasma glucose via corticosterone/cortisol) and zona reticularis (androgens); all three layers have plentiful mitochondria and are susceptible to mitochondrial poisons. The adrenal's high degree of vascular architecture and high degree of unsaturated fatty acids in membranes of mammals make this organ subject to lesions and lipid peroxidation. CYPs are in high concentration in this organ as well (susceptible to CCl_4 poisoning similar to liver)

      (3) Adrenal toxicity caused by short-chain aliphatic chemicals, amphiphilic/surfactant chemicals, steroids, and toxic chemicals that interfere with hydroxylation/steroidogenesis. Its high degree of vascular architecture and high degree of unsaturated fatty acids in membranes of mammals make this organ subject to lesions and lipid peroxidation. CYPs are in high concentration in this organ as well. Also concentrates hydrophobic chemicals methacrylonitrile, DDT metabolites, and PCBs

   b. Medulla

      (1) Sympathetic stimulation of epinephrine (adrenalin), norepinephrine (noradrenalin), chromogranin, and neuropeptide release from chromaffin cells

      (2) Excess GH or prolactin from the pituitary, excess stimulation of cholinergic nerves, and diet-induced hypercalcemia $\rightarrow$ chromaffin cell growth

      (3) Retinoids $\rightarrow$ hypercalcemia and medullary tumors

      (4) Reserpine (depletes catecholamines and 5-HT from brain and adrenal medulla) $\rightarrow$ hyperplasia and pheochromocytoma (growths in medullar)

CONCEPTUALIZING TOXICOLOGY 21-1 (*continued*)

E. Pineal gland

1. Circadian rhythms maintained by melatonin (as regulated by calmodulin-regulated adenylyl cyclase1) → regulates gonadal function (hypothalamic GnRH pulse generator) and controls cancer function; disrupted by electrical fields from high-tension power lines

F. Thyroid

1. Follicular cells

a. Produce the long-acting thyroxine (T_4) and the potent but short-acting T_3—see Figure 21-2. Many disruptors of thyroid including effects on serum levels of thyroid hormones, thyroperoxidase inhibition, perchlorate discharge test, iodine uptake inhibition, changes in the activity of iodothyronine deiodinases, modifying the action of thyroid hormones, and effects on binding proteins

b. Amphibian metamorphosis (tadpole → frog) important model of disrupting effects of pesticides. Goitrogens (chemicals that cause hypertrophy of the thyroid due to lower production of thyroid hormone → lack of negative feedback on pituitary → ↑ TSH secretion stimulating growth of thyroid → possible cancer

2. C-Cells

a. Produce calcitonin

b. Source of medullary thyroid cancer—can be produced in aging rats exposed to hypercalcemia over a long period of time

G. Parathyroid

1. Produces parathyroid hormone to regulate calcium levels in blood and activates kidney enzyme to produce 1,25-hydroxy vitamin D_3 (also plays roles in Mg reabsorption in kidney and cAMP levels)

2. Hyperphosphatemia → secondary hyperparathyroidism; hyperparathyroidism → uremic toxicity and kidney failure; bisphosphonate treatment for bone metastases → hyperparathyroidism → hypocalcemia → jaw bone degeneration

3. L-asparaginase (enzyme medication given to leukemia patients) given to rabbits → parathyroid oxyphilic necrosis and hypocalcemia tetany

4. Amifostine (cancer chemotherapy protective agent) → dramatic ↓ parathyroid hormone while furosemide (loop diuretic used to treat congestive heart failure) → nephrocalcinosis (↑ parathyroid hormone)

5. Some heavy metals may also ↓ parathyroid hormone (damage Ca^{2+}-sensing system), while Cd (in aged female rats) and fluorosis yield the opposite effect

6. Certain pesticides (diazinon, heptachlor) damage chief cells → degranulation → vacuolation → ↓ serum Ca^{2+}

H. Gonads

1. Male—testes

a. Bisphenol A and estradiol → ↓ plasma and testicular hormonal levels and plasma LH and ↓ number of Leydig cells due to ↓ expression of ERα mRNA

b. Phthalates (plasticizers) → androgen receptor antagonism

c. Ovatestes (cells looking like ovarian cells) and vitellogenin (egg yolk protein) sometimes found when exposed to environmental estrogens; too much vitellogenin synthesis in male liver may lead to liver damage as well

d. Flutamide (antiandrogen) → spermatocyte degeneration and necrosis; fungicide vinclozolin also antiandrogen

e. MDMA affects brain and also causes DNA damage in sperm and interstitial edema of testes

f. CCl_4 is liver toxicant but also causes oxidative stress in gonad → degeneration of germ and Leydig cells and sperm deformities

g. Organophosphates disrupt pituitary-gonadal axis not affected by antioxidants, except for lindane's ability to shrink and distort seminiferous tubules, ↓ Leydig cell density and atrophy of tissue

CONCEPTUALIZING TOXICOLOGY 21-1 (*continued*)

h. Tributyltin affects various gonadal (testosterone and estradiol) and pituitary hormones (LH) based on timing of assay and post treatment time

i. Plant steroidal glycoalkaloids → ↑ relative weights of seminal vesicles and testes

2. Female—ovaries

a. Accumulate Pb in granulosa cells → delayed growth and puberty

b. 4-Vinylcyclohexene in mice → biotransformation to diepoxide → targets primordial and primary follicles—ovotoxicity related to apoptosis/atresia mediated through Bcl-2 and MAP kinase family signaling

c. Methyltestosterone causes precocious ovarian development in catfish and ↑ LH in pituitary, ↓ GnRH transcripts in preoptic area of hypothalamus, and ↑ dopamine (transmitter which inhibits gonadotropin synthesis) = neurohormonal disruption

d. Tamoxifen (weak estrogen used to treat breast cancer) and methyldihydrotestosterone → oocyte atresia

e. Continuous androgen exposure affects the hypothalamus-pituitary-gonad axis (affects GnRH and GnRH receptor expression, androgen receptors, but not a stress response) as does the herbicide atrazine

f. TCDD targets developing ovary → delayed puberty and acyclicity (19 genes upregulated while 31 ovarian genes downregulated)

g. Bromocryptine = dopaminergic agonist → ↓ prolactin secretion from anterior pituitary (affects corpus luteum maintenance along with LH) → ↓ progesterone → ↑ ovarian weight and histopathology

h. Methylmercury affects fecal estradiol in post-fledgling white ibises

I. Thymus

1. Normally considered an immune organ with the key feature being its programming of T lymphocytes, however, the creation of ovarian follicular cysts by estrogen is prevented by thymectomy. This occurs via estrogen ↑ permeability of blood vessels of thymus → prevention of final stages of Treg cell development. Treg cells prevent ovarian follicular cysts

2. Organochlorines lead to autoimmunity, which affects thyroid and ↓ thymus volume

3. Tributyltin → ↓ thymus volume and interferes with interrenal tissues involved in steroidogenesis, peroxisome proliferator-activating receptors, and CYP3a/PXR

4. Antipsychotic medications (olanzapine and risperidone) affect thymus and spleen

5. Endocrine disruption of adrenal medulla and anterior pituitary → ↑ corticosterone and prolactin → thymus suppression. Similar damage to the thymus occurs with a nine-pesticide mixture exposure to larval *Xenopus laevis*

J. Pancreas

1. Is an exocrine and endocrine organ, with the major concern the production of insulin, which can be eliminated by autoimmunity (diabetes mellitus type 1) or reduced in effectiveness by obesity/aging (insulin resistance and diabetes mellitus type 2)

2. β-cells which produce insulin are susceptible to oxygen radicals (very low antioxidant activity as indicate by susceptibility to alloxan and streptozotocin). The autoimmune production of diabetes mellitus type 1 is mediated through cytokines IL-1, IL-1β, TNFα, IFNγ, superoxide radicals, H_2O_2, and NO (this last agent assists IL-1β-induced insulin secretion. NFκB is a critical factor mediating damage to β-cells. Pineal gland may assist in protection of β-cells as melatonin confers protection against ROS

3. Heavy metal damage here may be prevented by Zn induction of metallothionein induction. Arsenic alters signal transduction factors NFκB, p38 MAPK, TNFα, PI3K (↓ glucose-induced insulin secretion), PKB/Akt, and insulin-stimulated glucose uptake in fat or skeletal muscle cells. Cd induces hyperglycemia that appears to be associated with lipid peroxidation, decreased insulin release, activation of gluconeogenic enzymes, and insulin receptor dysfunction. It also causes a dose-dependent ↓ in glucose transporter 4 (GLUT4) protein and mRNA (key factor activated by

CONCEPTUALIZING TOXICOLOGY 21-1 (*continued*)

insulin and affected by As or Cd). Hg causes oxidative stress and disrupts Ca^{2+} homeostasis and ↓ insulin secretion. Ni also generates oxygen radicals ↓ insulin and glucagon (α-cells)

4. Type 2 diabetes is associated with persistent organic pollutants via mitochondrial damage (susceptible DNA)

5. Alcohol damages via a non-oxidative metabolism pathway → fatty acid ethyl esters → pancreatic edema, trypsin activation, vacuolization of the pancreas, and fragility of lysosome in acinar cells (along with production of NFκB and AP-1), and the production of acetaldehyde via alcohol dehydrogenase → interferes with PPAR-γ. There appears to be a link between obesity and alcohol as ethanol, long-chain fatty acids (↓ protein processing), and fatty ester activities increase cytosolic Ca^{2+} as a result of mitochondrial disruption (ATP depletion) → apoptosis and induction of CHOP-10

6. Glucotoxicity → oxidative stress, endoplasmic reticulum stress, and protein glycation

K. Secondary endocrine organs

1. Heart

a. Produces ANP related to membrane guanylyl cyclase (GC) receptors. GC-B receptors mediate autocrine/paracrine cGMP → cardiac hypertrophy and fibrosis—affected by steroids, catecholamines, arginine vasopressin, angiotensin II, endothelin

2. Kidney

a. Erythropoietin (maintains RBCs) drops on creatinine overload → anemia

3. Stomach and small intestine

a. Gastrin from stomach and secretin, cholecystokinin, and glucose-dependent insulinotropic peptide by small intestine—affected by disruption of suprachiasmatic nucleus of the hypothalamus or low melatonin level and is especially problematic for those with sleep disruption and inflammatory bowel disease

4. Liver

a. Insulin-like growth factors (IGF)—overexpression of IGF binding protein-1 in mice → altered brain development (hydrocephalus and motor disorders, reduced width of cerebral cortex including disorganized neural layers, underdeveloped corpus callosum, and short and thick dentate gyrus in the smaller hypothalamus plus ante- and perinatal mortality and post-natal reductions in growth

5. Skin, liver (revisited), kidney

a. Related to 1,25-dihydroxyvitamin D_3 formation and effects of parathyroid disruptors + cancer cell formation

II. Endocrine organ disruption tests

A. Hypothalamus-pituitary-gonadal axis and thyroid

1. Pubertal male and female assays (Tier 1) test entire reproductive axis and thyroid function as it may affect that axis

B. Anterior pituitary tumor models

1. Rodent prolactinomas may be hormonally stimulated (estrogen), implanted as a prolactin-secreting tumor cell line, or sporadic adenomas (3 models). DES can help produce lactotroph hyperplasias. Aged Sprague-Dawley rats may spontaneously develop pituitary tumors. Pituitary adenomas may be marked by production of polysialylated neural cell adhesion molecule. GH3 cells implanted into Wistar/Furth rats are also models of prolactinomas. GH hypersecretion occurs via a mutation of G_s protein. Intermediate lobe tumors produce ACTH and express proopiomelanocortin mRNA

C. Adrenal

1. Proposed tests involve ACTH challenge. ACTH and corticosteroids need to be monitored as ACTH may not change. Gossypol ↓ cortisol secretion and causes an increase in ACTH and adrenal weight due to lack of negative feedback. Organochlorides in the polar bear may be related to alterations in plasma cortisol levels. Fecal glucocorticoid metabolites may indicate adrenal disruption and adrenal medulla toxicity may be modeled by adrenal tumors

CONCEPTUALIZING TOXICOLOGY 21-1 (*continued*)

D. Thyroid (revisited)

1. Amphibian metamorphosis bioassay with tadpoles is a recent and reliable test for thyroid disruption. May be coupled to measuring TSH, T_3 and T_4 for more information on where on the pituitary-thyroid axis the disruption occurred. Enzyme activities of deiodinases and thyroid peroxidases may give more information *in vitro*, but cultured thyroid may be a better assay of effects on the entire thyroid

E. Parathyroid

1. Parathyroid gland isolated from miniature pigs = model

F. Testes

1. Hershberger assay (Tier 1 employing castrated male rat) tests for androgens and antiandrogens

G. Ovaries/uterus

1. Immature or ovariectomized rats given estrogenic compounds → uterotrophic effects (enlargement)

CONCEPTUALIZING TOXICOLOGY 20-1 (*continued*)

Prior to 1995, a major concern of the U.S. Environmental Protection Agency was the development of cancer from chronic exposure to toxic agents. That is still a concern, but in the time that has elapsed since 1995, the field of endocrine disruption has erupted into its own concern for survival of species due to reproductive effects of environmental estrogens and androgens. However, the estrogen and androgen receptors are not the only concerns: Other agents affect various neuroendocrine organs or produce endocrine-like action or antagonize the action or hormones. It is easy to see how the hypothalamic-pituitary-adrenal (HPA) axis may be affected by toxic substances, because this is the classic stress pathway. One good example of this switch in focus is the rat breast cancer model. Rats have a different response to aging than human females. Scientists have used this fact to argue that the postulated breast cancer–causing action of atrazine reflected this unusual increase in estrogen in female rats via changes in hormone secretion. Thus, it appears that by trying to prove that atrazine was not a probable human carcinogen based on the rat breast cancer model, it put that herbicide squarely in the endocrine disruption area. Continuing with atrazine as an example, this finding came around 1995 and has been further elucidated since then. It appears that the endocrine control of the central nervous system (CNS) through the hypothalamus is indeed disrupted and leads to estrogen-induced surges of luteinizing hormone (LH) and prolactin in ovariectomized Sprague-Dawley and Long-Evans hooded rats treated with atrazine (Cooper et al., 2000). Other researchers have shown an opposite dose-dependent suppression of LH in female Sprague-Dawley or Wistar rats that may in part be due to protein adducts in the pituitary and the hypothalamus of the major metabolite of atrazine, diaminochlorotriazine (Dooley et al., 2010). In either instance, these actions of atrazine are cases for effects of chemical agents on the hypothalamus-pituitary-ovary pathway. This chapter examines each endocrine organ's effects as important findings have emerged for thyroid disruptors including animal models of those effects as well as agents that target other endocrine systems. Physiology indicates that the endocrine designation means that a given organ system produces a hormone that is secreted into the blood and then targets other organs. By that definition, prostaglandins that come from multiple organs cannot be considered endocrine despite their endocrine-like action. However, changes in prostaglandin function that would influence one or more endocrine organ can and should be considered in this endocrine disruption approach. Agents that disrupt the brain also have some influence on endocrine organs. Some agents that affect brain and endocrine function alike are metals such as As, Cd, Hg, Mn, Pb, and Zn (Iavicoli et al., 2009). Unless it is clear that this effect is directed against the hypothalamus or similar neuroendocrine organ, this chapter will not reiterate the effects of neurotoxic agents. As each endocrine organ is examined in order, refer to **Table 21-1** for specific examples of endocrine disruption. Note that the classes of endocrine-disrupting agents are pesticides, which were first represented historically by the effects of dichlorodiphenyltrichloroethane (DDT) on the condor; industrial chemicals, especially those like polychlorinated biphenyls (PCBs) and dioxins (organohalogens) that bind strongly to the Ah receptor; cytotoxic metals at sublethal concentrations; the ubiquitous plasticizers; alkylphenols; medicines such as steroid hormones found in birth control or the now banned diethylstilbestrol; and phytoestrogens as found in soybeans. Another type of agent flame-retardant polybrominated diphenyl ethers (PDBEs) have direct neurotoxicity and yet, due to their close structural similarity to thyroid hormone, bind to the thyroid hormone receptor and suppress thyroid receptor–mediated transcription (Ibhazehiebo et al., 2011). These agents are part of a growing list of chemicals that either are potent in their influences on endocrine organs or are ubiquitous or persistent and therefore exert a chronic influence on endocrine function.

TABLE 21-1 Forensic Chart of Endocrine System Toxicity	
Endocrine System Toxicity	**Toxic Agents**
Hypothalamus — posterior pituitary	Al^{3+} (Yellamma et al., 2010), atrazine (Cooper et al., 2000), bisphenol A and NO system (Gotti et al., 2010), PCBs (Jolous-Jamshidi et al., 2010), cycad (McDowell et al., 2010), fluoxetine (Menningen et al., 2010), methoxychlor (Mahoney and Padmanabhan, 2010), quinolinic acid (Obukuro et al., 2010), MDMA (Sprague et al., 2003; Vanattou-Saïfoudine et al., 2010), dieldrin (Martyniuk et al., 2010), pulp and paper mill effluents (Popesku et al., 2010), cocaine (Johns et al., 2010), anabolic steroids (Penatti et al., 2010), TCDD (Clements et al., 2009), chlorpyrifos, PCBs, DDT, dioxin, genistein, PDBEs, DES (Gore, 2010), sewage sludge (Bellingham et al., 2010), malathion (Rezg et al., 2010), ethanol (Cubero et al., 2010), LPS (Hollis et al., 2010), amphetamine, endotoxin (Adamson et al., 2010), AChE inhibitors (Umegaki et al., 2009), PFOS (Shi et al., 2009), monosodium glutamate (Leitner and Bartness, 2009), Pb (Doumouchtsis et al., 2009), ethanol (Lan et al., 2009)
Anterior pituitary	Aminoglutethimide, dexamethasone, simazine, 3,3′,4,4′,5-pentachlorobiphenyl (Sun et al., 2010), Cd (Caride et al., 2010b; Hachfi and Sakly, 2010), atrazine (Fakhouri et al., 2010), Al^{3+} (Calejo et al., 2010), 3-methyl-4-nitrophenol (Li et al., 2009), organophosphates (Verma and Mohanty, 2009), DEHP/MEHP (Hong et al., 2009), PFOS (Shi et al., 2009), Cr^{VI} (Mishra and Mohanty, 2009)
Pineal gland	Electromagnetic fields (Henshaw et al., 2008)
Adrenal cortex	Pb (Doumouchtsis et al., 2009), Hg (Tan et al., 2009), Cd, organochlorides, ketoconazole, etomidate, gossypol, DMBA, spironolactone, Pb, digitalis (Hinson and Raven, 2006), α-[1,4-dioxido-3-methylquinoxalin-2-yl]-N-methylnitrone, organophosphates, triparanol, aniline, chlorphentermine, captopril, excess corticosteroids (Rosol et al., 2001)
Adrenal medulla	Excess GH, excess prolactin, excess dietary calcium, reserpine, excess sugars and sugar alcohols, retinoids (Rosol et al., 2001)
Thyroid Follicular cells	Perfluorononanoate (Liu et al., 2011), methimazole, 6-propylthiouracil, perchlorate (Hornung et al., 2010), thiocyanate, aminotriazole, sulfonamides, Li, amiodarone, FD&C Red No. 3, iopanoic acid, liver microsomal metabolism inducers (Capen, 1992), PCB (Gore, 2010), PFOS (Shi et al., 2009), N-bis(2-hydroxypropyl)-nitrosamine (Hoshi et al., 2009), organochlorines (Langer, 2010), $KBrO_3$ (Stasiak et al., 2009), PDBEs (Ibhazehiebo et al., 2011), Hg (Tan et al., 2009), bisphenol A (Zoeller, 2010)
C-Cells	Hypercalcemia, aging, Cd + ethanol (Piłat-Marcinkiewicz et al., 2004)

TABLE 21-1   Forensic Chart of Endocrine System Toxicity (*continued*)

Endocrine System Toxicity	Toxic Agents
Parathyroid	U (McDiarmid et al., 2011), L-asparaginase (rabbits; Chisari et al., 1972), amifostine (Fouladi et al., 2001), aminoglycosides (Kang et al., 2000), furosemide (Pattaragarn et al., 2004), diazinon (Rangoonwala et al., 2005), heptachlor (Rangoonwala et al., 2004), carbendazim (Barlas et al., 2002), heroin (Barai et al., 2009), excess phosphate (Almaden et al., 2009), cyclosporine A (Wada et al., 2006), bisphosphonate (Ardine et al., 2006), iron lactate (Matsushima et al., 2005), Cd (Brzóska and Moniuszko-Jakoniuk, 2005), Sr (Oste et al., 2005), Al (Cannata-Andía and Fernandez-Martin 2002), dipropylene glycol (Hooth et al., 2004), F (Huang et al., 2002), endotoxemia (Nakamura et al., 1998), ozone (Atwal, 1979)
Testes	Bisphenol A, estradiol (Nakamura et al., 2010), MDMA (Barenys et al., 2010), flutamide (Jensen et al., 2004), organophosphates (Verma and Mohanty, 2009), DEHP (Hong et al., 2009), Pb (Doumouchtsis et al., 2009), CCl_4 (Khan and Ahmed, 2009), Hg (Tan et al., 2009), lindane, glyphosate (Hinson and Raven, 2006), ionizing and radiofrequency radiation (Esmekaya et al., 2011), tributyltin (Si et al., 2011), steroidal glycoalkaloids (Soares-Mota et al., 2010)
Ovaries	Atrazine (Tillitt et al., 2010), TCDD (Jablonska et al., 2010; Valdez et al., 2009), androgens (Feng et al., 2009; Swapna and Senthilkumaran, 2009), tamoxifen (Cevasco et al., 2008), Pb (Doumouchtsis et al., 2009), bromocriptine (Kumazawa et al., 2009), Hg (Tan et al., 2009), 4-vinylcyclohexene (Hoyer and Sipes, 2007)
Thymus	Estrogen (Chapman et al., 2009), organochlorines (Langer, 2010), tributyltin (Pavlikova et al., 2010), antipsychotics (Mishra and Mohanty, 2010), pesticides (Hayes et al., 2006)
Pancreas	Ethanol (Clemens and Mahan, 2010), di-desulfo-yessotoxin (Tubaro et al., 2010), excess lipid (Kusminski et al., 2009)
β cells	Oxygen radicals (including from hyperglycemia; Brunner et al., 2009; alloxan and streptozotocin; Peschke, 2008), heavy metals (Chen et al., 2009), persistent organic pollutants (Lim et al., 2010), long-chain saturated fatty acids (Morgan, 2009)
Secondary endocrine organs	
Heart	Glucocorticoids, catecholamines (Kuhn, 2004)
Kidney	From high creatinine to heavy metals (all renal toxicants that cause renal failure)
Stomach and small intestine	Compounds that cause disruption are pineal toxicants, hypothalamic toxicants, pro-oxidants taken orally and other inflammatory mediators of the gut
Liver	Neurological effects of overexpression of insulin-like growth factor binding protein-1 (Doublier et al., 2000)
Skin, liver, kidney	Cancer formation and decreased vitamin $1\alpha,25(OH)_2D_3$ formation (Kemmis and Welsh, 2008)

Primary Endocrine Organs

Hypothalamus

Posterior Pituitary (Brain)

The hypothalamus is the major source of control for endocrine and autonomic function as summarized in **Figure 21-1**. Normally, six groups of cells are recognized as affecting neuroendocrine function from the hypothalamus involving reproduction (gonadotropin-releasing hormone [GnRH]), sugar, inflammatory control, blood pressure and aggressive behavior during stress (corticotropin-releasing hormone [CRH]), growth (growth hormone–releasing hormone [GHRH]; somatostatin inhibits the secretion of growth hormone), metabolism (thyrotropin-releasing hormone [TRH]), and lactation (dopamine inhibits lactation, while TRH [Jacobs et al.,

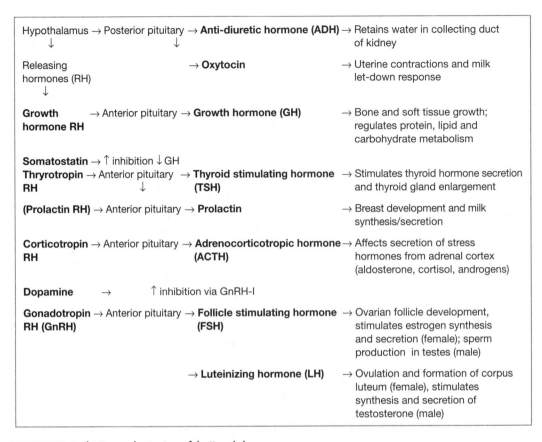

FIGURE 21-1 The Neuroendocrine Axes of the Hypothalamus

Note: Hormones indicated by bold letters. Parentheses means uncertain as hormone. Arrows indicate stimulation unless marked as inhibition.

1971] and possibly other prolactin-releasing hormones/peptides increase lactation; Hinuma et al., 1998). Additionally, connections of the neurons of the hypothalamus and the mainly ductal cells of the posterior pituitary are responsible for fluid regulation either directly or via uterine contractions preventing blood loss (vasopressin/antidiuretic hormone [ADH] and oxytocin).

Hormones are released on different schedules. Most are secreted during the animals' active period (day for humans), but those involved in growth and sexual/reproductive function are highest during the sleep cycle. Clearly, this is reversed for rodents who are active during the night. This is important, for if rodents are dosed as toxicology models during the daylight for ease of the researcher, then toxicants and

medications are being given during the time of rest and sleep. This is an unlikely scenario for exposure related to humans except for sleeping pill interactions or carbon monoxide poisoning in a house heated by some method of incomplete combustion such as flame.

The literature is rife with endocrine disruption articles. However, endocrine disruption is just the effect of fungicides, herbicides, insecticides, industrial chemicals, plastics, plasticizers, and pharmaceuticals and phytoestrogens in the environmental waste streams on hormone regulation of homeostatic functions. This means that any effect on hormones or hormone receptors (e.g., effects of PCBs on estrogen receptors or Ah receptor found actively expressed in the brain or thyroid receptor, phthalates' antagonism of androgen receptor) represents disruption that should be addressed. A profound effector of the Ah receptor is 2,3,7,8-tetrachlorodibenzo-p-dioxin (TCDD). Developmental exposure to TCDD disrupts growth, reproduction, spatial learning, and memory. Rats exposed *in utero* to TCDD had their hypothalamic explants analyzed using an *in vitro* superfusion system to evaluate effects on the GnRH release. Exposed rats showed larger mediobasal hypothalamus/preoptic area GnRH content. However, the cellular structures of the lateral preoptic area and septal region showed distinct pathology related to exposure. It appeared that there was less GnRH release, indicating that the damage involved the ability to transport the hormone out of the hypothalamic cells and into the blood (which is the definition of endocrine function; Clements et al., 2009).

Another example of Ah receptor activation involves the hypothalamic-pituitary-gonadal axis and the effects of different PCBs. In an immortalized hypothalamic cell line, GT1-7, the specific PCB mixtures represented by Aroclor 1221 and Aroclor 1254 both elevated GnRH gene expression starting at low doses. A nuclear estrogen receptor antagonist, ICI 182,780, blocked some of the effects of the PCBs. It is important to note that normal mammalian hypothalamic neurons express only one form of the estrogen receptor, ERβ, but these immortalized cells have more than one estrogen receptor so this may not be the best model system. However, this immortalized hypothalamic cell line only increased GnRH peptide release and caused morphological changes in GT1-7 cells, including more cellular confluence and neurite extension in the presence of Aroclor 1221 but not with Aroclor 1254 (Gore, 2010). Aroclor 1254 caused only small neurite retraction and neurotoxicity. It is important to note that some endocrine disruptors show differential effects based on dose. One such example is the action of the estrogenic organochlorine pesticides methoxychlor and chlorpyrifos, which increase GnRH gene expression at low doses and inhibit expression at high doses in GT1-7 cells. However, these two chemicals do not cause exactly the same toxicity: Chlorpyrifos increased neurite outgrowth and cell confluence similarly to estradiol, while methoxychlor did not. Not only can expression be changed, but release mechanisms may also be affected. For example, glutamate or KCl can be used to evoke GnRH release from hypothalamic neurons. The old persistent insecticide *o,p'*-DDT stimulated glutamate-evoked GnRH release more than bisphenol A, while methoxychlor and the breakdown product of DDT, *p,p*-DDE had no such effects. Dioxin exposure during development caused the rat hypothalamus to release less GnRH in response to KCl. Because the hypothalamic cells exposed to dioxin showed increased GnRH peptide, this suggested that the hormone was synthesized but not released in these affected animals. Endocrine disruptors also may impact neurotransmission (another mechanism of the effects of PCBs on hypothalamic cells by affecting dopamine, norepinephrine, and serotonin receptors).

Development is a key sensitive period, especially for estrogens and androgens on the brain that develops in a sexually dimorphic manner. This developmental sensitivity may be a result of direct action on steroid receptors, altered P450 aromatase activity (converts testosterone to estradiol), circulating alpha-fetoprotein (protects brain from mother's estradiol *in utero*), and apoptosis (hypothalamic nuclei programmed death plays a role in sexual differentiation). Even in cell preparations (GT1-7) or adult hypothalamic cells, the effects of substances such as PCBs may be partially due to apoptosis at lower concentrations and necrosis at higher concentrations (affecting, for example, the viability of cells that produce releasing hormones such as GnRH).

The size of a region of the hypothalamus and its expression of certain genes can signal disruptive changes during development. For example, bisphenol A, a famous endocrine-disrupting chemical component of hard plastic water bottles, and phytoestrogen genistein increased the immunoreactivity of the sexually dimorphic nucleus of the male rat hypothalamus to the calcium-binding protein calbindin (hypermasculinizing). Additionally, the anterior periventricular nucleus involved in ovulation in females and possibly linked to release of GnRH in both sexes was increased by genistein in male rats. The pulse generator in the hypothalamus may also be affected by treatment.

Genistein appears to suppress hypothalamic electrical activity, and therefore the 30- to 90-minute intervals of the GnRH pulse generator. This results in fewer LH pulses than would have occurred from the anterior pituitary due to GnRH pulses from the hypothalamus.

Behavior is also modified by treatment as PCBs increased mating behavior in the female offspring of treated dams. Similarly, male and female rat offspring from pregnant females treated with the estrogenic pesticide chlordecone had increased lordosis quotients indicating feminization. Surprisingly, both males and females also indicated that they were simultaneously masculinized as both exhibited higher mounting behavior. Certain chemicals also decrease sexual functioning, such as the phytoestrogen coumestrol given following birth, which decreases male or female sexual behaviors. Similarly, a compound found in ultraviolet filters, 4-methylbenzylidene camphor, diminished the apparent attractiveness of exposed females to normal males possibly due to decreasing proceptive (courting), lordosis quotients, and receptivity behaviors in the female animals.

This endocrine disruption issue becomes more complicated as it is understood that brain development is highly dependent on certain hormones, such as thyroid hormone. Also, some agents disrupt more than one hormone axis. Polybrominated diphenyl ethers (PBDEs) given to pregnant dams reduce thyroxine concentrations in the mothers and their pups, while bisphenol A causes transient increases in thyroxine in pups treated during development. Because bisphenol A is considered primarily an estrogenic compound, other axes must be considered when studying the full neuroendocrine disruptive action of an agent. Delayed effects must also be considered, such as is the case with the estrogenic compound diethylstilbestrol (DES), which became infamous when reproductive tumors were found in the female offspring of women who took this now banned medication. However, the obesity that developed as a result of developmental exposure to DES (as well as ovarian dysfunction and pituitary tumors in female mice; Ohta et al., 2014) indicates that not only does the hypothalamus control metabolism and energy through the thyroid axis but also has circuits that alter feeding behavior, adipocytes, and adipokines such as leptin. Some researchers have postulated that obesogens may be related to changes in the peroxisome proliferator-activated receptors and nuclear hormone receptors involved in lipolysis.

Disruptions of neuroendocrine functions are not just limited to the exposed animal. For example, some neuroendocrine problems appear to transfer down generations following exposure, such as was observed when vinclozolin exposure yielded less attractive female animals in the F3 generation. The mechanisms for these effects are not always clear, but may involve epigenetic factors. One example of multigenerational effects involves the HPA (stress) axis and the DNA methylation of the glucocorticoid promoter. These stress-sensitive, disrupted animals may have the disruption reversed by providing a methyl donor. Similar results were found for DNA methylation of the estrogen receptor alpha (ERα) promoter. Rat pups that are groomed to excess by their mothers have lower indices of sexual behavior, less sensitivity of GnRH neurons to feedback from steroid hormones, and lower expression of ERα in the anteroventral periventricular nucleus of the hypothalamus (Gore, 2010).

A toxin from bacteria, lipopolysaccharide (LPS), produces changes in the eating behavior (hypophagia), selective partitioning of fat for energy, and fever. IL-10 reduces the hypophagia or under-eating in rats exposed during the dark phase of the light-dark cycle. LPS causes an increase in Fos (marker of transcriptional activity) expression in orexin neurons and a decrease in Fos expression in cells of the caudal arcuate nucleus, which is ameliorated by IL-10 intracerebroventricular injection. However, IL-10 or LPS both decrease Fos expression in melanin-concentrating hormone neurons. The parts of the hypothalamus that regulates energy expenditure and food intake are the orexin and melanin-concentrating neurons. Changes in transcriptional activity indicate inhibition of function, which can result in less releasing hormone being produced (such as CRH) and changes in behavior (Hollis et al., 2010). In contrast, c-Fos exhibits increased expression following treatment of rats with donezepil, an acetylcholinesterase (AChE) inhibitor used in the treatment of Alzheimer's disease. This is accompanied by an increase in adrenocorticotropic hormone (ACTH) secretion from the anterior pituitary. These effects may at least partially explain the transient (2-week) loss of appetite that is experienced on inception of drug treatment (Umegaki et al., 2009). Another research team has found that greatly increased atypical protein kinase Czeta/lambda activity expressed in the arcuate and paraventricular nuclei (sites of LPS, leptin, and insulin action) of the hypothalamus appears to be related to the decreased appetite due to LPS. Inhibition of this enzyme blocks the anorexic effect of LPS, inflammation, and fever (Thaler et al., 2009). Anorectic effects of toxicants such as amphetamine and endotoxin appear to be related to catecholamine neurotransmission in the perifornical hypothalamus. Increases in dopamine and epinephrine were found in this area of the hypothalamus in response to endotoxin treatment of lean Zucker rats (Adamson et al., 2010).

It is also important to consider sympathetic outflow from the hypothalamus as a control of metabolism and stress. Neonatal administration of the taste-enhancing food additive monosodium glutamate (MSG) destroys the arcuate nucleus of the hypothalamus and is associated with increased fat accumulation and decreased production of energy. In the Siberian hamster model, MSG causes reduced Nissl and neuropeptide staining in the arcuate nucleus and similar effects on neuropeptide fiber staining in the paraventricular nucleus of the hypothalamus. This indicates significant deletions in the central sympathetic outflow circuits. However, the inability of these animals to sustain their thermogenesis through the brown adipose tissue is not related to the sympathetic outflow. An endocrine disruption effect could still be responsible, because the cause does not lie in the adipose tissue itself (Leitner and Bartness, 2009). A stressor of HPA axis is the organophosphate, malathion. In this disruption, malathion predisposes the rat to type 2 diabetes mellitus. Malathion accomplishes this action by an increased sensitivity of negative feedback from corticosterone, a hormone of the adrenal cortex that increases glucose in the bloodstream.

Hypothalamic inducible NO synthase mRNA is increased by malathion, and corticotropin RH mRNA is decreased. These changes along with hypertriglyceridemia lead to a condition that increases the likelihood of insulin resistance. So a perturbation in one axis of the hypothalamus disrupts how cells respond to insulin secretion by the pancreas as stimulated by glucose (carbohydrates) in the diet (Rezg et al., 2010).

Ethanol would normally be considered just an overall neurotoxic and especially a developmental toxicant, but it is also an endocrine disruptor. The hypothalamic-pituitary-gonadal axis and the HPA axis are both affected in female pups of ethanol-treated female rats. The reproductive axis exhibited higher basal and stress estradiol in proestrus as related to other phases of the cycle and decreased GnRH mRNA levels compared to control females in diestrus. Ethanol exposure also caused higher LH variability across the estrous cycle and a surge in LH after a stress. The stress axis indicated that ACTH and corticosterone were elevated in proestrus. Arginine vasopressin mRNA is also elevated in rat hypothalamus. This last finding is important when considering the role of vasopressin in water homeostasis, memory, and especially sexual/reproductive behavior (Lan et al., 2009).

When other agents are examined that affect the hypothalamus, it is clear that the herbicide atrazine affects the hypothalamus. It should not be surprising that metals also have an influence here due to their neurotoxicity. In some cases, neurotransmission is increased for certain stimulatory neurotransmitters rather than increased by metal toxicity. For example, aluminum toxicity increases acetylcholine (due to increased acetyl CoA and AChE inhibition due to Al binding to enzyme SH groups) according to the following hierarchy in the rat brain: hippocampus > pons-medulla > cerebral cortex > hypothalamus > cerebellum. The hippocampus as the link between the limbic (emotional) brain and the cerebral cortex (higher level decision making) is a major focus. Here, the interest is in changes in behavior that may reflect changes in hypothalamic functions. Al causes adipsia (absence of thirst), aphagia (loss of ability to swallow), hypokinesia (decreased bodily movement), fatigue, seizures, and so forth (Yellamma et al., 2010).

Pb is a metal that is mainly considered a neurotoxic or blood toxic agent. However, lead appears to affect a variety of endocrine organs directly based on dose and length of exposure. Lead decreases growth hormone (GH) release due to either reduced synthesis of GHRH or inhibition of GHRH release indicating a hypothalamic effect. Another possibility is reduced somatotrope response (GH producing cells of pituitary). In any case, the hypothalamic-pituitary axis is affected as blunted thyroid-stimulating hormone (TSH), GH, a follicle-stimulating hormone (FSH)/LH to TRH, GHRH, and GnRH stimulation, respectively, have been reported. Interestingly, prolactin appears to be elevated in Pb poisoning. At the gonad level, the testes appear to first develop subclinical damage preceding hypothalamic and pituitary disruption that causes no increased FSH and LH release due to low plasma testosterone concentrations. The ovaries accumulate Pb in the granulosa cells, delaying growth and pubertal development and decline in fertility. The adrenals are affected by lead as indicated by parenchymal damage, altered corticosterone concentrations at rest or during stress, and reduced cytosolic and nuclear glucocorticoid receptor binding. Thyroid hormone actions are also decreased by lead (Doumouchtsis et al., 2009).

At the very least, the first toxic symptoms that may be attributed to hypothalamic function are thirst, hydration, water preservation, appetite/feeding, salt appetite, bladder function, ovarian and testicular function, body temperature regulation, metabolism, energy levels, sleep cycles, wakefulness, blood pressure regulation, heart rate, hormonal/neurotransmitter regulation, mood and behavioral functions, and pituitary gland regulation, because they are wholly or in part under the control of the hypothalamus. Affecting specific receptors results in more specific action on the hypothalamic-pituitary axis, because neurokinin 1, 2, and 3 receptor antagonism by an experimental agent (SCH 206272) results in testicular toxicity in beagle dogs due to decreases in pulsatility and magnitude of LH and testosterone. This was associated with changes in the hypothalamus with increase in the number of gonadotropin-releasing hormone–containing neurons (Enright et al., 2010). Cycad poisoning (possibly due to a toxic amino acid from some species of cyanobacteria) not only causes loss of dopaminergic function in the limbic system of the brain (Parkinsonism), but also appears to decrease orexin-A neurons in the hypothalamus altering wakefulness (hypersomnolent behavior) in Sprague-Dawley rats (McDowell et al., 2010) The selective serotonin reuptake inhibitor antidepressant fluoxetine is a very commonly prescribed medication that has environmental relevance because it is commonly found in wastewater and bioaccumulates in fish. For example, fluoxetine exposure to goldfish (*Carassius auratus*) caused increased expression of CRH and decreased expression of neuropeptide Y, which may explain the anorexigenic (lowered feeding behavior) effects of this medication. Additionally, genes involved in glucose metabolism of liver fructose-1,6,-bisphosphatase had decreased expression, and muscle hexokinase had increased expression with impacts on overall energy functions (Mennigen et al., 2010). These examples of hypothalamic neurotoxicity exhibit the complexity of the neuroendocrine system as direct toxicity or indirect feedback influences the function of many components of a given axis.

One of the cellular systems that appear to co-localize with the gonadal hormone systems is NO-cGMP signaling (nitrergic neurons). It appears that NO synthase expression either in the adult or during development is highly sensitive to estrous cycles in the female rat. Bisphenol A affects the NO-cGMP pathway in the medial preoptic nucleus, and the ventromedial subdivision of the bed nucleus of the stria terminalis affects reproductive and sexual behavior (Gotti et al., 2010). This is of interest because most endocrine-disrupting chemicals described in the extant literature are not expected to act directly through the hypothalamus but directly or indirectly through the estrogen receptor to be discussed later in this chapter under ovarian function (Shanle and Xu, 2011). However, even in this discussion, it appears that the developmental effects on the hypothalamus of bisphenol A can be differentiated from the organophosphate insecticide methoxychlor even though they are thought to have estrogenic and antiandrogenic endocrine-disrupting action. Pregnant sheep exposed to either of these endocrine-disrupting chemicals, for example, had offspring with decreased GnRH mRNA as determined by *in situ* hybridization. Estrogen receptor 1 (ESR1) mRNA expression in the medial preoptic area was increased by prenatal treatment with bisphenol A but not methoxychlor. Both chemicals reduced ESR2 mRNA expression in the same area of the hypothalamus. These differences in estrogen receptor expression may indicate the reason behind the impact of bisphenol A on LH surge amplitude and the alteration of LH surge timing by methoxychlor, which appears to confirm some aspects of the bisphenol A effects alluded to earlier (Mahoney and Padmanabhan, 2010).

Exposure to chemicals such as PCBs not only affects neural systems, but also affects hormonal levels and animal behavior. This results in deficits in context or experience-dependent modulation of social approach and investigation in rats that could be similar to disorders such as autism in acutely socially isolated animals. The behavior disorders were correlated with changes in the areal measurements of the periventricular nucleus of the hypothalamus (Jolous-Jamshidi et al., 2010). One should take caution in interpretation of studies done with isolated brain cultures or slices. For example, quinolinic acid may be responsible for neurodegeneration in the CNS. One study used rat hypothalamic slice cultures and observed that N-methyl-D-aspartate (NMDA) receptor activation caused selective loss of orexin neurons. This might suggest a link between quinolinic acid and narcolepsy, a sleep disturbance in which people fall asleep suddenly without warning. However, injection of quinolinic acid into the lateral hypothalamus of male C57BL/6 mice caused selective loss of melanin-concentrating hormone neurons (involved in paradoxical or REM sleep; Peyron et al., 2009) instead of orexin neurons. This loss of melanin-concentrating hormone neurons was blocked by an NMDA receptor antagonist. It is of interest that orexin neurons were reduced by injection during the dark (active for rodents) phase of the diurnal cycle, but melanin-concentrating

hormone neurons were still more sensitive to reduction by quinolinic acid. However, while the *in vivo* mouse model did not support the *in vitro* rat culture model and did not indicate that narcolepsy and quinolinic acid are linked, it was able to demonstrate that cell populations activating different hormone responses in the hypothalamus are differentially sensitive to chemical disruption (Obukuro et al., 2010).

Some chemicals that cause significant damage of the CNS, such as ecstasy (MDMA) discussed in the former chapter really focus their toxicity on the hypothalamus. In hypophysectomized and thyroparathyroidectomized Sprague-Dawley rats, MDMA did not cause the hyperthermia observed in intact animals (just the opposite with hypothermia). In fact, the serotonergic neurotoxicity did not develop in animals with these neuroendocrine organs removed (Sprague et al., 2003). The receptors for this action have been further elucidated involving the exacerbation of the hyperthermic influence of MDMA by caffeine. It appears that dopamine, serotonin (5-HT$_2$), α_1-adrenergic receptor antagonists (Shering 23390, ketaserin, and prazosin, respectively) prevent MDMA-induced hyperthermia and its increase by caffeine. However, phosphodiesterase (PDE)-4 inhibitor rolipram and adenosine A$_{1/2}$ receptor antagonist 9-chloro-2-(2-furanyl)-[1,2,4]triazolo[1,5-C]quinazolin-5-amine 15943 or the A$_{2A}$ receptor antagonist SCH 58261, but not the A$_1$ receptor antagonist DPCPX, increased hyperthermia caused by MDMA. This research suggested that serotonin and catecholamines regulate hyperthermia from MDMA exposure, while adenosine A$_{2A}$ receptor antagonism and PDE inhibition are the mechanisms underlying caffeine's exacerbating influence (Vanattou-Saïfoudine et al., 2010).

In the CNS toxicity chapter, the action of the banned persistent pesticide dieldrin could have been mentioned due to its ability to antagonize inhibitory GABA$_A$ receptor-mediated neurotransmission. The increased ubiquitin-proteasome activity, oxidative stress, inflammation, and DNA damage would fit well into the categories used in that chapter. However, it is mentioned here since it targets the teleostean (fish with bony skeletons) hypothalamus due to a high density of GABA-producing cells. In the process in also affects pituitary function. It appears that dieldrin affects both neural functions and hormonal activities. In the hypothalamus, dieldrin affects proteins associated with neurodegeneration such as apolipoprotein E, microtubule-associated tau (τ) protein, enolase 1, stathmin 1a, myelin basic protein, and parvalbumin. It also affects proteins involved in oxidative phosphorylation (energy), differentiation, proliferation, and cell survival (Martyniuk et al., 2010). Anabolic steroid use also affects neuroendocrine function. In this case, the GABAergic neurons remain the focus. 17α-Methyltestosterone treatment of adolescent male mice reduced the action potential frequency in GnRH neurons, lowered the serum gonadotropin concentrations, and resulted in smaller testes size. It appears that this effect is a consequence of increasing the activity of steroid-sensitive presynaptic neurons of the medial preoptic area of the hypothalamus. This effect increases GABA$_A$ receptor–mediated inhibitory tone onto downstream GnRH neurons (Penatti et al., 2010).

In contrast, pulp and paper mill effluents affect dopaminergic neurotransmission and spawning behavior of fish (fathead minnow is the premier model for freshwater environmental toxicity). The hypothalamus of treated fathead minnow indicated that these effluents affected gene expression for cholecystokinin, RevErbbeta2, and urotensin I (Popesku et al., 2010). A hormone that comes from the medial preoptic area of the anterior hypothalamus is the hormone that causes uterine contractions and the milk letdown response—oxytocin. Chronic and intermittent cocaine administration to female rats caused increased aggression and lower oxytocin levels in this area of the hypothalamus. It is of interest that only the intermittently cocaine-treated females drank more water than other rats (Johns et al., 2010).

Mixtures of chemicals also affect mammals in a realistic environmental assessment. Sewage sludge applied to pasture land caused a disruption of the neuroendocrine axis, especially the GnRH and galaninergic (sleep-active neurons in the ventrolateral preoptic area of

the mammalian brain) systems, of pregnant grazing animals and their offspring. The hypothalamus of animals exposed *in utero* to chemicals of the sewage sludge exhibited decreased GnRH mRNA expression and decreased mRNA expression for the GnRH receptor and galanin receptor. The pituitary showed similar effects of the expression of the receptor mRNAs. The mothers only paralleled the findings in the offspring for the galanin receptor mRNA expression in the hypothalamus and pituitary (Bellingham et al., 2010). Differential disruption of the hypothalamus may also explain certain addictive behaviors. For example, acute ethanol administration caused a dose-dependent elevation of agouti-related protein in the arcuate nucleus of the hypothalamus of C57BL/6J mice that binge drink ethanol but not 129/SvJ mice. This indicates a positive feedback loop for ethanol consumption related to disruption of the hypothalamus in genetically sensitive strains of mice (Cubero et al., 2010).

Sometimes it is difficult to distinguish a stress response from a true biochemical disruption of an endocrine organ. For instance, the persistent industrial chemical perfluorooctane sulfonate (PFOS) in zebrafish embryos upregulated the expression of corticotrophin-releasing factor/hormone. This finding could either be a stress reaction or sign of disruption of signaling in the hypothalamus. Conversely, TSH gene expression in the anterior pituitary was downregulated. This appears to be a disruption, because CRF should increase TSH synthesis and release. Additionally, the sodium/iodide symporter and iodothyronine deiodinase1 genes of the thyroid were upregulated, which is contrary to the finding of reduced TSH expression unless the TSH was responding to the negative feedback of increased thyroid hormone secretion. However, transthyretin gene expression was downregulated, while the thyroid hormone receptors TRα had increased expression and TRβ had decreased expression. These data, taken together with an unchanged thyroxine whole body content and triiodothyronine increases, indicate that more disruption occurs here than normally adjusting physiology to PFOS exposure (Shi et al., 2009). The complexity of these hormonal interactions and feedbacks makes interpretation difficult and at times faulty.

Anterior Pituitary

The anterior pituitary is the site of hormone production stimulated by releasing hormones of the hypothalamus. One of the more critical hormones for managing stress is ACTH. ACTH is encoded in the proopiomelanocortin (POMC) gene, which can be discerned in a transgenic line of zebrafish linked to a green fluorescent protein gene (EGFP). The disruption by chemicals in the expression of this gene has been followed in the zebrafish. Dexamethasone, a potent synthetic steroid used in the treatment of adrenal insufficiency and Addison's disease, and aminoglutethimide, which has the opposite action by blocking steroid synthesis, both affected the expression of POMC:EGFP and interrenal development as determined by the expression of the ftz-fl gene (ff1b). The triazine herbicide simazine (related to atrazine) and a PCB congener (3,3',4,4',5-pentachlorobiphenyl) interfered with POMC expression in the anterior pituitary of zebrafish and interrenal development in zebrafish (Sun et al., 2010). Atrazine's effects can be revisited in the pituitary. Isolated pituitary cells from postnatal day 7 male rats exposed to atrazine show inhibited GH secretion due to atrazine binding to the GHRH receptor (Fakhouri et al., 2010).

Metals also alter the function of the anterior pituitary. Cadmium is a metal that enters cells through L-type voltage and receptor-mediated Ca^{2+} channels. It accumulates in the cell by binding to cytoplasmic and nuclear components. Cd is a chronotoxin in that it affects the secretory timing of pituitary. In male Sprague-Dawley rats given cadmium in their drinking water, ACTH and TSH medium levels were affected around the clock and altered the timing of ACTH and GH peak levels (Caride et al., 2010b). Part of the timing of the hypothalamus is the appearance of amino acid peaks. Cd in the drinking water at a lower concentration (25 mg/L for 30 days) caused disappearance of the nocturnal peak of the anterior pituitary amino acid content and the appearance of a glutamate peak during the resting phase of the photoperiod, while in the posterior pituitary a peak of aspartate and glutamate occurred at 12:00 h and a disappearance of the glutamate peak at 16:00 h. Doubling the Cd in the drinking water caused the anterior pituitary amino acid content peak to disappear at 12:00 and 00:00 h, while for the two minimum values at these hours a peak appeared at 08:00 h. In the posterior pituitary, this higher Cd concentration caused two maximum values for aspartate and glutamate between 00:00 and 04:00 h and abolished the glutamine daily pattern (Caride et al., 2010a). Cd also appears to target the hypothalamic-pituitary axis, because it affects reproductive function in the male rat. FSH drops in response to Cd, which decreases spermatozoa number in the testes. LH does not vary despite an increase in testosterone. This indicates a disruption of negative feedback control in the hypothalamic-pituitary axis (Hachfi and Sakly, 2010). Aluminum is another metal that not only damages the hypothalamus, but has deleterious effects on pituitary cells resulting in decreased serum prolactin levels (Calejo et al., 2010). Cr^{VI} causes a hypertrophy of corticotrophs in the pituitary of the teleost (fish), *Channa punctatus*. This disrupts the pituitary-interrenal axis in freshwater fish (equivalent to the pituitary-adrenal axis of mammals). Hypertrophy and degranulation of intrarenal cells and increased plasma cortisol concentrations were noted in exposed fish (Mishra and Mohanty, 2009).

Other toxic organic chemicals also affect anterior pituitary functions. A component of diesel exhaust, 3-methyl-4-nitrophenol, has effects on the accessory structures of the testes and the anterior pituitary of treated castrated immature rats. Weights of seminal vesicles and Cowper's glands increased but plasma FSH and LH decreased, although levels of testosterone were unchanged by treatment with a low dose of this aromatic chemical (1 mg/kg). This indicates a disruption of the function of the anterior pituitary that is confirmed by similar reductions in LH levels in quail by 3-methyl-4-nitrophenol (Li et al., 2009). Organophosphate as represented by dimethoate exposure especially in the developing mouse causes weak immunointensity staining of LH cells, reduction in their size and number, and lower plasma LH and testosterone concentrations. Direct action on the testes was also noted in male neonates, indicating effects on Leydig cells and inhibition of steroidogenesis (Verma and Mohanty, 2009). Di-(2-ethylhexyl) phthalate (DEHP) and mono-(2-ethylhexyl) phthalate (MEHP) affect the testes, with MEHP being 10-fold more toxic. MEHP also disrupts murine pituitary gonadotrope LβT2 cells by inhibition of 11β-hydroxysteroid dehydrogenase type 2 mRNA and enzyme activity with very low concentrations (10^{-7} M). Corticosterone inhibits the proliferation of these gonadotrope cells, which is reversed by the glucocorticoid receptor antagonist RU486 (abortion medication). However, MEHP lowers the concentration of corticosterone by 10-fold that it takes to affect the glucocorticoid receptor, and RU486 is no longer able to completely block this action. This shows an interaction between a metabolite of a toxicant (MEHP), a product of the HPA axis (corticosterone), and the pituitary-gonadal (testes) axis (Hong et al., 2009). This is important, because it illustrates that a disruptive effect may lead to irreversible organ damage or at least be less likely to be influenced by medications due to profound biochemical alterations.

Certain parts of the pituitary may enlarge in response to a lack of negative feedback from the organ it controls such as the thyroid. If the thyroid is disrupted sufficiently by a compound such as radioactive iodine, the thyrotrophic cells in the part of the pituitary known as the adenohypophysis cause hypertrophy and produce more TSH (a clinical sign of hypothyroidism). Environmental estrogens can produce pituitary tumors in certain animal models and increase prolactin secretion from the rat pituitary. One treatment for this condition is dopamine agonist administration. Dopamine agonists such as bromocriptine, pergolide, cabergoline, and quinagolide have the ability to reduce excess prolactin, because dopamine is the neurotransmitter (and neurons) used to control (reduce) prolactin and the pituitary adenomas that develop without that control (Gillam et al., 2004). Pituitary tumors are the most frequently observed intracranial growths, most of which are nonmetastatic adenomas. They are classified by size (micro- through macroadenomas) and hormonal activity (overproduction of prolactin, GH, ACTH, FSH, LH, or TSH

or non-functioning if no clinical symptom is noted). As indicated earlier, the prolactinoma is most common pituitary tumor subtype and is found in women to induce oligomenorrhea or amenorrhea and galactorrhea. GH-secreting pituitary adenomas represent 10–20% of pituitary growths and cause acromegaly and overgrowth of many tissues via sustained high levels of insulin-like growth factor I. Corticotroph adenomas (10–15% of pituitary tumors) release ACTH and other proopiomelanocortin-derived peptides causing Cushing's disease and adrenal hyperplasia. Thyrotroph adenomas are infrequently observed (0.5–2%) and are mostly macroadenomas leading to signs of hyperthyroidism. Thirty percent of all adenomas are nonfunctioning and are also mostly macroadenomas. These mainly produce headaches, visual alterations, and hypopituitarism. Most pituitary adenomas are monoclonal, and approximately half are aneuploid, which represents unstable genetics. Few are modeled on the mutations of oncogenes and tumor suppressor genes. A small group of inheritable prolactinomas arise out of the multiple endocrine neoplasia type I syndrome. Carney's complex is an autosomal-dominant genetic disorder that develops from protein kinase A regulatory subunit 1 germ-line mutations and leads to pituitary tumors. Cell-cycle gene mutation appear to be linked to pituitary tumors such as loss of function of growth suppressor genes Rb, p16, p27, and GaDD46 γ. Mutations of p53 indicate a pituitary carcinoma rather than a benign adenoma. Pituitary tumor transforming gene is an oncogene that is overexpressed in most tumors and is involved in sister chromatid separation that occurs in cell division and induction of apoptosis (p53-dependent or p53-independent). Altered expression of the bcl-2 family (bcl-2 and bax) also may underlie pituitary tumor formation. Additionally, decreased expression of the pituitary tumor apoptosis gene may lead to oncogenic transformation in this endocrine organ.

As discussed earlier, various hormones may increase the size of various portions of the pituitary such as anterior pituitary hyperplasia by the hypothalamus producing too much GHRH and certain neurotransmitters such as dopamine working on the D_2 receptor may control prolactin and somatotropin-secreting tumors. However, growth signaling factors and cytokines are also potential oncogenic stimulators. Corticotropinomas appear to express epidermal growth factor and its receptor. Transforming growth factor alpha (TGFα) overexpression and loss of nerve growth factor mark the development and progression of prolactin-secreting tumors. Pituitary tumors also appear to be associated with the transforming growth factor beta (TGFβ) family, fibroblast growth factor family, and bone morphogenetic factors. Il-6, leukemia inhibitory factor, and constituents of the gp130 cytokine family are cytokines that appear to promote or develop pituitary tumors (Seilicovich et al., 2005).

Pineal Gland

Circadian rhythms are maintained by the secretion of melatonin from the pineal gland, and disruption of these rhythms may be monitored via melatonin levels. The pineal gland receives signals from the retinohypothalamic tract to the suprachiasmatic nuclei, which produce a signal to the pineal gland to regulate melatonin synthesis. Melatonin regulates gonadal function via altering the firing frequency of the hypothalamic GnRH pulse generator. This causes changes in the release of pituitary hormones LH and FSH and thereby stimulates testicular production of testosterone and estrogen production and release from the ovaries. Melatonin appears to have growth inhibition activity and cancer control function. Breast, prostate, and other tumors appear to have growth reductions in the presence of physiologic or pharmacologic levels of this hormone (Mirick and Davis, 2008). Melatonin has other properties as a free radical scavenger/antioxidant, cryoprotective agent, immunomodulator (pineal removal results in precocious involution and histological disorganization of the thymus), endocrine modulator, thermoregulator, and therapeutic agent (Ravindra et al., 2006). Something as simple as power line corona ions (electrical fields) appear to disrupt melatonin in rats and may increase the risk of leukemia in adults and children living near high-voltage power lines (Henshaw et al., 2008). Calmodulin-regulated adenylyl cyclases

play a large role in cross-talk and plasticity of the CNS. Among these enzymes, adenylyl cyclase 1 activity is the "gatekeeper" of melatonin synthesis in the pineal gland. Changes in calmodulin and/or adenylyl cyclase activity by toxicants would drastically change melatonin synthesis (Wang and Storm, 2003).

Adrenal Cortex

Although the adrenal cortex may be considered an organ to mediate stress, it is the endocrine gland most likely to suffer chemically induced lesions. The cortex has three layers and a medullary region. The outermost layer of the cortex, the zona glomerulosa, produces aldosterone that helps maintain blood pressure via sodium retention. This layer is the least likely to experience toxicity. The next two layers in order are the zona fasciculata and the zona reticularis, which produce cortisol/corticosterone (dependent on species of animal) and androgens, respectively. These layers produce the most lesions. A lack of cortisol or corticosterone is truly problematic, because it maintains blood sugar during stress, reduces inflammation, and feeds back on the hypothalamus and the pituitary to affect ACTH release. All three layers have plentiful mitochondria, so mitochondrial poisons clearly impact adrenal function. Compounds that cause adrenal toxicity are usually short-chain aliphatic chemicals, agents that produce lipidosis, amphiphilic/surfactant chemicals, steroids, and medications and toxic chemicals that interfere with hydroxylation and especially steroidogenesis. Vacuolar (impaired steroidogenesis from triaryl phosphates or other organophosphates or α-[1,4-dioxido-3-methylquinoxalin-2-yl]-N-methylnitrone; DMNM) and granular degeneration (mitochondrial damage from agents such as DMNM or amphenone), necrosis, and hemorrhage can result from high-dose (acute) toxic insult. Chronic damage yields atrophy, fibrosis, and nodular hyperplasia. The adrenal pathology is related to inhibition of enzymes in specific organelles such as the mitochondrial CYP11B1 11β-hydroxylase and smooth endoplasmic reticulum (SER) CYP17 (17α-hydroxylase) and CYP21 (steroid 21-hydroxylase). Endothelial (parenchymal) cell damage can also have organelle-specific toxicity as exemplified by DMNM (mitochondria), triparanol (SER), and aniline (lipid aggregation in cytoplasm) or chlorphentermine (phospholipid aggregation in cytoplasm). Even some medications have toxic effects related to their pharmacological activity. Captopril is an angiotensin-converting enzyme (ACE) inhibitor, which inhibits the formation of the vascular constricting agent angiotensin II from angiotensin I formed and released from the kidney. As angiotensin II induces CYP11B2 to form aldosterone, aldosterone levels drop. Atrophy of the zona glomerulosa can occur due to the decreased stimulation of angiotensin II. If too much cortisol is used to treat inflammatory disorders, the feedback mechanism decreases ACTH secretion, which will decrease CYP11A1. As cholesterol is not metabolized, accumulation of fat vacuoles will occur in cortical cells and lead to atrophy of the zona fasciculata and reticularis (Rosol et al., 2001).

It is important to differentiate stress-producing chemicals from those that have direct toxic action on the adrenal cortex. For example, Hg is a very toxic metal that accumulates in endocrine organs, such as the adrenal, the thyroid, and reproductive organs. It has effects on wildlife and humans. Whereas most of the actions would be expected to be inhibitory in action, mercury's toxicity is also a stressor. However, mercury's toxicity is greater than its stress-inducing effects and disrupts the HPA (stress) axis and the gonadal axis, precipitating pathophysiological changes in these endocrine organs (Tan et al., 2009). For example, fecal cortisol concentrations were significantly altered in post-fledgling white ibises (*Eudocimus albus*) exposed to environmentally relevant doses of methylmercury (Adams et al., 2009). Although the HPA axis may be affected anywhere along its pathway, it is normally regulated by arginine vasopressin and CRH in the hypothalamus and then ACTH release from the pituitary. Cortisol (human) or corticosterone (animal such as rat, which lacks CYP17) then is released from the adrenal cortex with two other hormones resulting in a negative feedback function on the hypothalamus and the pituitary.

The adrenal cortex itself is highly susceptible to toxic chemicals due to its high degree of vascular architecture, especially in mammals (less so in the interregnal organ of birds and fish). It also has a high degree of unsaturated fatty acids in its membranes, which makes it subject to lipid peroxidation. CYPs are found in high concentration and activity in this organ (it was where the first CYP activity was noted historically). These aforementioned two factors explain the adrenal's susceptibility to CCl_4, which is similar in the liver. The adrenal cortex has a mechanism for taking up lipoproteins that allows lipophilic toxicants to concentrate hydrophobic chemicals such as methacrylonitrile and metabolites of DDT and PCBs. The adrenal cortex has receptors, transcription factors, enzymes, and other targets for toxic action. There are free radicals generated during steroid hydroxylation reactions. Taken together, it is not surprising that adrenal lesions may result from heavy metals such as Cd, organochlorides, and complex aromatic hydrocarbons (e.g., ketoconazole, etomidate). One example of an adrenal effect resulted from the sedative etomidate, which was used in the early 1980s. In a trauma unit, all severely injured patients given this sedative died, compared to a 66% mortality rate for those given benzodiazepines (Leddingham and Watt, 1983). Adrenal insufficiency was caused in these patients due to inhibition of CYP11B1, which is responsible for cortisol synthesis (Harvey, 2014).

Other medications that inhibit steroidogenic enzymes are cardiac glycosides digoxin and digitoxin, antifungal ketoconazole, antibiotic nitrofurantoin, luteolytic azaserine, and aminoglutethimide (formerly developed as an anticonvulsant but used primarily to inhibit steroid formation). Some of these agents are so effective in this regard that they have been used in the treatment of adrenal tumor production of excess corticosteroids (Cushing's syndrome). One pesticide mitotane, which is a derivative of DDT (*o,p′*-DDD), is used as an antineoplastic agent in the treatment of adrenocortical carcinoma due to its inhibitory action on steroidogenic enzymes and damages the mitochondria (leading to severe, acute necrosis and hemorrhage). Certain CYPs (e.g., CYP1B1) activate the toxicity of adrenal toxicants such as 7,12-dimethylbenz[α]anthracene (DMBA). The potassium-sparing diuretic spironolactone (via aldosterone antagonism) causes adrenal lesions once activated by adrenal CYPs. It also inhibits the transcription of the gene responsible for coding for synthesis of the steroidogenic acute regulatory (StAR) protein, which provides the rate-limiting step in steroid hormone synthesis in the adrenals and the gonads via translocation of the cholesterol from the cytosol to the inner mitochondrial membrane (the pesticide lindane and glyphosate inhibit the formation of this protein in the testes). Induction of CYPs can also lead to adrenal toxicity such as CYP11B2 induction of aldosterone (increased blood pressure via sodium retention in the distal convoluted tubule of the kidney) biosynthesis by PCB 126. This same PCB congener at high concentration makes the AT1 (angiotensin II) receptor more responsive, leading to increased aldosterone synthesis. Similarly, Pb appears to increase synthesis of aldosterone. 2-Chloro-s-triazine herbicides induce CYP19 (aromatase) that may cause the adrenal cortex to secrete estrogen.

There are more than 60 compounds currently known that impact adrenal function. Once damaged, the lack of corticosteroids has deleterious effects on surviving stress. However, the picture of adrenal disruption does not stop with adrenal hormone synthesis and secretion. The corticosteroid-binding globulin has decreased binding capacity in the plasma in the presence of nonsteroidal anti-inflammatory drugs (NSAIDs). This makes cortisol more bioavailable. Liver metabolism of steroids also affects cortisol levels. Metyrapone inhibits adrenal 11β-hydroxylase, which decreases cortisol synthesis. It also increases extra-adrenal metabolism of cortisol to inactive cortisone. This would have profound effects by decreasing plasma cortisol concentrations. The kidney also regulates the effects of cortisol. The mineralocorticoid receptor of the kidney cannot distinguish between aldosterone, the true mineralocorticoid, and cortisol. That is why 11β-hydroxylase activity in the kidney is important to metabolize much higher (by 1,000-fold) cortisol levels rapidly. However, a toxic ingredient in natural licorice contains glycyrrhetinic acid, which inhibits this enzyme and causes hypertension from what appears to be an excess of aldosterone, but really is an excess of active cortisol. Another medication used to induce abortions, RU486 or mifepristone, works via progesterone antagonism but also antagonizes glucocorticoid and thereby alters circulating cortisol levels (Hinson and Raven, 2006).

Adrenal Medulla

The medullary cells are stimulated directly by the sympathetic nerve to produce epinephrine (the historic adrenalin), norepinephrine (noradrenalin), chromogranin, and neuropeptides from the chromaffin cells, where the discussion of endocrine disruption must center. There are also ganglion cells. The rat often develops diffuse or nodular hyperplasia and benign and malignant pheochromocytomas. These chromaffin cell growths can result from excess GH or prolactin from the pituitary, excess stimulation of cholinergic nerves, and diet-induced hypercalcemia. Other dietary factors such as the sugars and sugar alcohols xylitol, sorbitol, lactitol, and lactose produce medullary tumors if chronically present at 10–20% in the diet. They do this likely via increased absorption and urinary excretion of calcium. Because hypercalcemia increases catecholamine synthesis in response to stress, renal tumors may be reduced in xylitol-treated rats by limiting calcium intake. Retinoids (related to vitamin D) or conditions such as nephrocalcemia also produce hypercalcemia and medullary tumors. Reserpine, a medication that depletes stores of catecholamines and serotonin from the brain and adrenal medulla, is used to treat hypertension. Reserpine is another way of stimulating hyperplasia and pheochromocytoma in the rat (Rosol et al., 2001).

Thyroid

Follicular

The follicular cells of the thyroid produce the thyroid hormones triiodothyronine (T_s) and tetraiodothyronine (T_4), which regulate cellular metabolism. T_4 is the longer acting thyroxine, while T_3 has the shorter half-life but higher potency. There are chemicals that disrupt the thyroid to produce reduced hormone synthesis and therefore increase TSH production by the pituitary due to lack of negative feedback in the complicated hypothalamus-pituitary-thyroid axis, shown in **Figure 21-2**. Extra TSH stimulates an increase in thyroid size similar to less iodine in the diet causing a condition known as goiter. Chemicals that decrease thyroid function (hypothyroidism) via a variety of mechanisms are known as goitrogens. There are also chemicals that produce a hyperthyroid condition via increasing T_3 levels such as perfluorononanoate, which increases circulating T_3 concentrations, thyroid-associated gene expression, and liver protein transthyretin in zebrafish (Liu et al., 2011).

Chemicals that interfere with thyroxine synthesis and release are methimazole, 6-propylthiouracil, and perchlorate. In thyroid gland explant cultures from prometamorphic *Xenopus laevis* tadpoles, perchlorate was the most potent inhibitor of T_4 release (Hornung et al., 2010). Many goitrogenic chemicals cause thyroid tumors as the decrease in thyroid function leads to an increase in TSH and an enlarged thyroid. If these cells decrease in function due to damage to the cells, and especially if they activate oncogenes via mutations, then cancers are much more likely. Goitrogens such as thiocyanate and perchlorate inhibit the iodine-trapping mechanism of thyroid, which normally concentrates iodine 1,000-fold from plasma. Aminotriazole, methimazole, sulfonamides, and thiourea prevent organic binding of iodine and iodine coupling to iodothyronines to form T_4 and T_3. Lithium and excess iodine inhibit thyroid

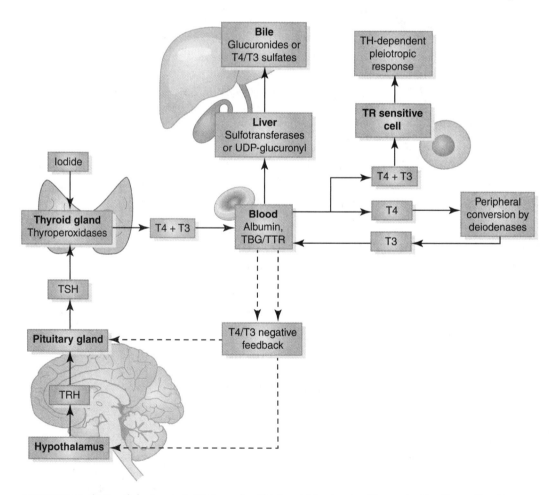

FIGURE 21-2 The Hypothalamic–anterior Pituitary–thyroid Axis and Other Associated Factors that Contribute to Thyroid Function and Disruption

hormone secretion by action on proteolysis of active hormone from the colloid. Because T_3 is more potent than T_4, chemicals that inhibit the conversion enzyme (5′-monodeiodinase) such as amiodarone, FD&C Red No. 3 (erythrosine), and iopanoic acid also produce thyroid tumors by lack of negative feedback on pituitary release of TSH and resulting follicular cell overstimulation.

Thyroid function may be secondarily compromised by increasing liver microsomal metabolism of thyroid hormones by a variety of chemicals including the medications phenobarbital, benzodiazepines, calcium-channel blockers, steroids, and retinoids. The usual array of CYP inducers such as chlorinated hydrocarbons and polyhalogenated biphenyls also affect thyroid hormone metabolism. Of course, iodine deficiency or natural goitrogens in food, surgical removal of part of the thyroid, or implanting TSH-secreting pituitary tumor cells can also disrupt the thyroid and increase thyroid tumors in rats (Capen, 1992). High-dose erythrosine also produces a change in thyroid hormone economy by a significant increase in reverse T_3 (an inactive hormone to clear excess T_4 from the system to conserve energy during stress or illness), decreased T_3, and increased serum TSH (Capen, 1998). Thyroid tumor formation is also dependent on the NKX2-1 homeodomain transcription factor as demonstrated by Nkx2-1-thyroid-conditional hypomorphic mice that have a greater than twofold higher constitutive cell proliferation rate and develop more thyroid adenomas compared with wild-type mice in response to the genotoxic carcinogen N-bis(2-hydroxypropyl)-nitrosamine (DHPN), followed by sulfadimethoxine (SDM) but not to the nongenotoxic carcinogen amitrole (3-amino-1,2,4-triazole; Hoshi et al., 2009). Oxidative stress generated by potassium bromate can also generate thyroid follicular cell tumors in rats (Stasiak et al., 2009). PCBs, depending on the mixture or dose, yield thyroid hormone receptor activation or suppression (Gore, 2010). Another ubiquitous chemical, bisphenol A, not only binds weakly to the estrogen receptor, it also antagonizes T_3 activation of the thyroid hormone receptor (Zoeller, 2010). Persistent organochlorines have been found in an eastern Slovakia population to increase thyroid volume as a sign of autoimmune reactions such as positive thyroperoxidase antibodies in the blood and/or hypoechogenicity image (Langer, 2010).

C-Cells

The C-Cells synthesize and release calcitonin to regulate calcium deposition into bone, which lowers plasma-free Ca^{2+} levels. The neural crest-derived parafollicular C-Cells of the thyroid are a source of medullary thyroid cancer (~4% of all thyroid cancers; Cakir and Grossman, 2009). This can happen to aging rats or those exposed to long-duration hypercalcemia. It is also important to note that male Wistar rat C-Cells exhibit increased activity in response to simultaneous exposure of Cd and ethanol (Piłat-Marcinkiewicz et al., 2004).

Parathyroid

The parathyroid gland produces parathyroid hormone to regulate calcium levels in the blood and activates the formation of vitamin D_3 by the 25-vitamin D_3 1α-hydroxylase of the kidney. Parathyroid hormone also aids in the reabsorption of Mg in the distal convoluted tubule and the formation of cAMP. Certain protein synthesis–inhibiting antibiotics such as the aminoglycosides interfere with Mg reabsorption and cAMP formation, and hypomagnesia can lead to a variety of disease states (Kang et al., 2000). It makes sense that changes in free calcium levels or phosphate or vitamin D or other factors that lead to bone formation affect parathyroid function as part of this endocrine gland's homeostatic mechanisms. Hyperphosphatemia is an important risk factor in the development of secondary hyperparathyroidism, which can be treated by medications that increase intracellular calcium of parathyroid cells (calcimimetics; Almaden et al., 2009). Not surprisingly, compounds with additional phosphate molecules given chronically to rats such as sodium hexametaphosphate (chelating agents in cosmetics) cause parathyroid hypertrophy and hyperplasia, inorganic phosphaturia, hepatic focal necrosis, muscle fiber alterations, increased kidney weight with calcium deposition and desquamation, and growth inhibition (Lanigan, 2001).

No matter how hyperparathyroidism occurs, chronically elevated parathyroid hormone can lead to uremic toxicity that is normally associated with kidney failure (Rodriguez and Lorenzo, 2009). It is of interest that hyperphosphaturia can be generated by excess parathyroid hormone secretion as occurs in acute-phase endotoxemia in rats (Nakamura et al., 1998). Agents that raise parathyroid hormone levels may also increase osteoporosis (along with osteocalcin), as does the immunosuppressive medication cyclosporine A (Wada et al., 2006).

Another condition related to secondary hyperparathyroidism is osteonecrosis of the jaw. Apparently, patients treated with bisphosphonate for bone metastases have hypocalcemia associated with hyperparathyroidism prior to development of the degeneration of the jawbone (Ardine et al., 2006). One of the earliest reported toxicities was found in one species of test animals, but not humans, to a medication to treat leukemia. Rabbits given L-asparaginase isolated from the bacteria *Escherichia coli* showed a delayed effect of parathyroid oxyphilic necrosis and hypocalcemia tetany (Chisari et al., 1972). An aminothiol prodrug medication, amifostine, used to provide cellular protection from the ravages of cancer chemotherapy and radiation has a rather dramatic and immediate effect on reducing parathyroid hormone. Fifteen minutes from the time of infusion, parathyroid hormone levels drop from an average of 38 ng/L to 2 ng/L (Fouladi et al., 2001). The loop diuretic, furosemide, has the opposite action by inducing nephrocalcinosis in humans and animals that appears to be prevented by either parathyroidectomy or calcimimetic agents such as NPS R-467 (Pattaragarn et al., 2004). Industrial fluorosis appears to yield increased levels of parathyroid hormone and calcitonin (Huang et al., 2002).

Some heavy metals may again yield toxicity as calcium sensing is a key component of this system. Exposure of Gulf War veterans to depleted uranium increased urinary uranium levels. Those with increased urinary uranium also had a significant reduction in serum intact parathyroid hormone and elevated urinary calcium and sodium excretion (McDiarmid et al., 2011). Strontium also appears to reduce serum parathyroid hormone levels and cause osteomalacia

in rats with chronic renal failures (Oste et al., 2005). Aluminum overload during kidney dialysis affects bone formation directly and also decreases normal release of parathyroid hormone. Al inhibits parathormone synthesis at the transcriptional level and changes the relationship between the hormone and calcium as well as calcium and phosphorus (Cannata-Andía and Fernández-Martín, 2002). Conversely, lifetime Cd exposure in aged female rats led to increases in parathyroid hormone (parathormone) and calcitonin, while also impacting the kidney (Brzóska and Moniuszko-Jakoniuk, 2005). Iron lactate administered intravenously to Sprague-Dawley rats first increased parathyroid hormone release, then over a 3- to 6-day period caused storage granule area reductions and moderate atrophy of the chief cells. This would initially yield an increase in osteoclasts and an osteopenia (reduced bone mineral density in bone, but not enough to be classified as osteoporosis; Matsushima et al., 2005).

Other chemicals shown to affect the parathyroid include the pesticide diazinon, which caused degranulation, vacuolation, and loss of secondary granules and lipid droplets in parathyroid chief cells with an attendant drop in free serum calcium levels (Rangoonwala et al., 2005). The insecticide heptachlor similarly damages chief cells with degranulation, vacuolation, loss of secretory granules and lipid droplets, reduction in chromatin, and degeneration of the endoplasmic reticulum as well as the cristae of the mitochondria (Rangoonwala et al., 2004). The systemic fungicide carbendazim at high daily doses yields histopathological alterations in the parathyroid, thyroid, and adrenal glands of rats, but not the pituitary (Barlas et al., 2002). High sublethal concentrations of an opiate, heroin, also caused cytoplasmic vacuolization, increased pycnotic nuclei, and development of patchy areas among the chief cells in the rat parathyroid gland (Barai et al., 2009). Secondary lesions of the parathyroid and the forestomach of the rat accompany the hepatic and renal (and testicular in the male) toxicity of the component of a number of commercial products, dipropylene glycol (Hooth et al., 2004). One interesting observation is the inhalation of ozone producing parathyroiditis with morphological alterations in chief cells. This toxicity appears to have an inflammatory element with specific lesions as well as endothelial proliferation of the capillary bed, formation of platelet thrombi, extravasation of erythrocytes, and disruption of basal lamina of the epithelial cells (Atwal, 1979).

Another regulatory substance of clinical interest is parathyroid hormone–related peptide (PTHrP). PTHrP is associated with poor prognosis in cancer cells. It appears that this peptide interferes with death receptor signaling from CD95, TNF-R, and TRAIL-R in Saos human osteosarcoma cells. PTHrP also downregulates expression of pro-apoptotic Bcl-2 family members (Bax, PUMA) and upregulates the expression of anti-apoptotic factors Bcl-2 and Bcl-xl. Resistance to cancer chemotherapy appears to result from the blocking action of PTHrP on p53 family-dependent apoptosis signaling pathways (Gagiannis et al., 2009).

Testes

The effect of bisphenol A and estradiol cause reproductive toxicity in prepubertal male rats. Both estrogenic substances decreased plasma and testicular hormonal levels and plasma LH, but did not decrease intrinsic estradiol and FSH levels. Leydig cells (number) of the testes appeared more affected than pituitary function by decreased expression of ERα mRNA. Leydig cells also showed decreased expression of steroidogenic enzymes and cholesterol carrier protein (Nakamura et al., 2010). Some researchers have found ovatestes (cells that look like ovarian cells). Many link the production of vitellogenin (egg yolk protein) in the liver as a sign of estrogenic activity in the male, which can lead to signs of histological damage at high concentrations (Elias et al., 2007). An antiandrogen model endocrine-disrupting chemical is flutamide, which decreases testicular function causing spermatocyte degeneration and necrosis. Interestingly, male fathead minnows also exhibited increases in vitellogenin and beta-estradiol (Jensen et al., 2004).

A substance that is more typically considered a CNS function disruptor is the amphetamine derivative MDMA. MDMA not only affects brain function, but also reproductive

function in males. Developmental exposure to MDMA in Sprague-Dawley rats causes DNA damage in sperm and interstitial edema in the testes. Sperm count and motility are also decreased in a dose-dependent manner by ecstasy. A delay in preputial (exocrine glands in genitals of some mammals) separation was found in treated animals (Barenys et al., 2010). Ubiquitous plasticizer phthalates cause androgen receptor antagonism. The fungicide vinclozolin is an antiandrogen as well (Gore, 2010). One would expect the toxicity of a radical-forming chemical on metabolism such as CCl_4 to reside in the liver, which of course it does. However, the oxidative stress affects hormone levels (decreases testosterone, LH, and FSH and increases estradiol and prolactin) in male rats, which would be expected to be feminizing. Partial degeneration of germ and Leydig cells accompanied by deformities in spermatogenesis was also noted. These effects were prevented by augmentation of the antioxidant defenses (Khan and Ahmed, 2009). Of the more interesting effects are the dose-related male–male pairing behavior and decreases in egg production in white ibises (Frederick and Jayasena, 2011).

It would be expected that ionizing radiation would cause injury to the reproductive organs as radiologists attempt to protect them from X-irradiation during diagnostic procedures. However, it appears that dosing rats with 900 MHz pulse-modulated radiofrequency fields induces oxidative injury and decreases antioxidant defense mechanisms in the testes, liver, lung, and heart tissues (Esmekaya et al., 2011). Although oxidative stress may be the cause of many different types of toxicities to tissues including the testes, it appears that the organophosphorus insecticide dichlorvos induced declines in sperm motility, testosterone levels, and ultimately necrosis, edema, and cellular damage to testicular tissues that was not protected by added antioxidant vitamins C or E (Dirican and Kalender, 2012). Organophosphates appear to disrupt the pituitary-gonadal axis from weak immunointensity staining of LH to testicular integrity (Verma and Mohanty, 2009). However, the organochlorine insecticide/medication lindane's ability to shrink and distort seminiferous tubules, decrease the density of Leydig cells and blood vessels, and atrophy the tissue was protected by antioxidants vitamin C, vitamin E, and α-lipoic acid (Nagda and Bhatt, 2011). Tributyltin's effects on male mice depend on the dose and the time post treatment. Initially, there is a decrease in intratesticular and serum testosterone concentrations that recovers by 84 days following exposure. These same mice also exhibited decreased serum 17β-estradiol concentrations by 49 days post treatment, which became a dose-dependent increase by day 84. Additionally, day 84 revealed a decreased serum LH level and intratesticular 17β-estradiol concentrations. This indicates that endocrine disruptors have a complex effect on hormone homeostasis that may not be easily dissected into single organ or toxicity timing assays (Si et al., 2011). This has also been observed in steroidal glycoalkaloids, such as can be found in the plant *Solanum lycocarpum* St. Hill that caused reductions in the weights of the thymus, adrenal gland, spleen, heart, and kidneys and increased relative weights for heart, epididymises, lungs, seminal vesicles, and testicles in treated male rats. Exposed female rats experienced no observed differences in organ weights and few differences in relative organ weights, although both sexes had reduced triglyceride concentrations. Females also had increased albumin and aminotransferase activity and reduction of total protein in serum samples compared with untreated controls. This indicates that sex differences also complicate the detection of endocrine disruption using animal models (Soares-Mota et al., 2010).

Ovaries

4-Vinylcyclohexene appears to affect the ovaries directly in rodents, especially in mice. This murine sensitivity appears to be related to biotransformation to the damaging diepoxide. This chemical species appears to target the primordial and primary follicles (small pre-antral follicles). This ovotoxicity is related to the increase in apoptosis (atresia) as mediated through Bcl-2 and mitogen-activated protein kinase family signaling and usually follows repeated exposure (Hoyer and Sipes, 2007). Some chemicals affect the ovaries directly but also influence the hypothalamus-pituitary-gonad axis.

Methyltestosterone caused precocious ovarian development in female catfish (*Clarias gariepinus*), but also increased LH immunoreactivity of the pituitary gland and decreased GnRH transcripts in the preoptic area of the hypothalamus. Additionally, the transmitter that inhibits gonadotropin synthesis, dopamine, was increased while serotonin and norepinephrine decreased in the preoptic area of the hypothalamus by methyltestosterone in female catfish (Swapna and Senthilkumaran, 2009). Tamoxifen is a weak estrogen that blocks much of the action of estrogen in females and disrupts in a fashion that causes oocyte atresia similarly to methyldihydrotestosterone (Cevasco et al., 2008). Continuous androgen exposure to adult female rats causes a condition known as polycystic ovary syndrome. It may be easy to see how this could be the direct effect of a male hormone on a key female reproductive structure. However, this exposure has effects on the rest of the hypothalamus-pituitary-gonad axis. Hypothalamic medial preoptic androgen receptor expression and the number of androgen receptor and GnRH-immunoreactive cells were increased by 5α-dihydrotestosterone. This was not a stress nor was it disruptive of the stress axis as CRH was unaffected. GnRH receptor expression was also downregulated in the pituitary and the hypothalamus. However, it is of interest that low-frequency acupuncture restored the estrous cyclicity that was disrupted by androgen treatment within 1 week and elevated hypothalamic GnRH and androgen receptor expression levels (these two factors co-localize in the hypothalamus), but did not alter GnRH receptor or CRH expression (Feng et al., 2009).

The herbicide atrazine also affects the entire hypothalamus-pituitary-gonad axis. Atrazine exposure to fathead minnows causes gonadal abnormalities in male and female fish. Atrazine appears to reduce egg production by changing the final maturation of oocytes (Tillitt et al., 2010). TCDD appears to target the developing ovary for damage and produces delayed puberty and acyclicity (Jablonska et al., 2010). It appears that 19 genes with known functions are upregulated, while 31 ovarian genes are downregulated $\geq$ 1.5-fold, including 17α-hydroxylase, the one responsible for estradiol synthesis. However, serum progesterone was unaffected in female Sprague-Dawley rats chronically exposed from development (Valdez et al., 2009). There are effects on the production of progesterone in female rats treated with a medication used in the treatment of Parkinson's disease, bromocriptine. This occurs because bromocriptine is a dopaminergic agonist. This in turn reduces prolactin secretion by the anterior pituitary. Prolactin, along with LH, is important in maintaining the corpus luteum early in rat pregnancy and progesterone falls. Toxicity can be noted in rats in as little as 2 weeks with this medication as indicated by increased ovarian weights and histopathological changes (Kumazawa et al., 2009). Methylmercury also affects fecal estradiol in post-fledgling white ibises (Adams et al., 2009).

Thymus

Normally, the thymus is viewed as an immune organ of major import but not as an endocrine organ. However, the thymus is engaged in certain endocrine-disruption activities. Estrogen causes ovarian follicular cysts in injected female mice and rats. This is not due to the hypothalamus-pituitary-gonadal axis but rather to the presence of the thymus. Thymectomy prevents the formation of cysts and ovulation occurs. Estrogen appears to increase the permeability of the blood vessels of the thymus leading to prevention of final stages of Treg cell development. In the absence of these regulatory immune cells, cyst formation proceeds (Chapman et al., 2009). Organochlorines have disrupted the immune system of humans, causing autoimmunity that affects other organs (see thyroid) and decreases the thymus volume (Langer, 2010). Tributyltin also causes thymus reduction in addition to interference with interrenal tissues involved in steroidogenesis, peroxisome proliferator-activating receptors, and CYP3a/PXR (Pavlikova et al., 2010). Thus, it appears that disruption of one organ may impact a second in addition to any direct effects. Another example is the thymus and spleen histopathology associated with antipsychotic medication treatment (olanzapine and risperidone). Not only may direct effects lead to thymus suppression, but elevated corticosterone and prolactin levels due to disruption of other endocrine organs (adrenal medulla and anterior pituitary,

respectively; Mishra and Mohanty, 2010). Similarly, increases in corticosterone during toxic stress could explain the damage to the thymus induced by a nine-pesticide mixture in larval exposure of *Xenopus laevis* (Hayes et al., 2006).

Pancreas

The pancreas is an exocrine and endocrine organ involved in digestive functions and maintenance of blood glucose levels, respectively. It is of interest that when exocrine enzymes such as amylase are found in the plasma instead of the exocrine pancreas or intestinal contents, this is a sign of pancreatic damage similar to finding low insulin as a sign of β-cell dysfunction. Diabetes mellitus results from a number of factors such as autoimmune destruction of pancreatic β-cells (type 1) or obesity and/or low insulin receptor responses (insulin resistance or type 2). In toxicity to the β-cells, oxygen radicals appear to play a significant role. The autoimmune response appears to be mediated through the cytokines IL-1, IL-1β, TNFα, IFNγ, superoxide radicals, H_2O_2, and NO. Nitric oxide assists in the IL-1β-induced inhibition of insulin secretion by β-cells. NFκB appears to be a critical factor mediating β-cell damage. The role of antioxidant in preventing pancreatic damage or less release of insulin during hypoglycemia points to the use of N-acetyl-L-cysteine, ascorbic acid, and d-α-tocopherol in the prevention of damage. This also hints that other toxicants that cause oxidative stress such as heavy metals may be prevented by induction of metallothionein by zinc, which does appear to prevent diabetes in rat models. Conversely, zinc deficiency is associated with increased type 1 and type 2 diabetic responses. It appears that the zinc transporter ZnT-8 is responsible for zinc accumulation and regulating insulin secretion in β-cells.

Heavy metals cause a variety of organ damage including the pancreas. For instance, arsenic induces cancer, nervous system dysfunctions, peripheral vascular disease, and endocrine disruption. Human epidemiology points to a dose-dependent increase in diabetes mellitus in villages of Taiwan exposed to arsenic in their drinking water. Arsenic changes signal transduction factors such as NFκB, p38 MAPK, TNFα, PI3K, PKB/Akt, and insulin-stimulated glucose uptake in fat or skeletal muscle cells. PI3K may be the important factor here, because this signaling appears to reduce glucose-induced insulin secretion from β-cells. At high doses, arsenic increases PI3K-mediated PKB/AKt phosphorylation in pancreatic β-cells. Cd induces hyperglycemia that appears to be associated with lipid peroxidation, decreased insulin release, activation of gluconeogenic enzymes, and insulin receptor dysfunction. It also causes a dose-dependent decrease in glucose transporter 4 (GLUT4) protein and mRNA, which is a key factor activated by insulin and affected by As or Cd. Hg is more well known for its nervous system and renal toxicity. However, Hg does damage β-cells. In isolated primary murine pancreatic islet cell cultures, mercury yielded a disruption of calcium homeostasis and reduced secretion of insulin. Oxidative stress is a key mechanism of Hg-induced damage, including apoptosis of death of β-cells. Ni also generates oxygen radicals (elevated iNOS and cGMP) that appear to damage islet cells, yielding hypoinsulinemia (β-cells) and hypoglucagonemia (α-cells; Chen et al., 2009).

Type 2 diabetes appears to increase with persistent organic pollutants. They may mediate their damage via the dysfunction of mitochondria, which has highly susceptible DNA. Mitochondrial DNA abnormalities yield β-cell damage, insulin resistance, and diabetes mellitus (Lim et al., 2010). Ethanol is usually associated with oxidative metabolism by alcohol dehydrogenase and CYP2E1 to acetaldehyde and reactive oxygen species (ROS) by the liver. In the pancreas, the non-oxidative pathway is favored, producing fatty acid ethyl esters (FAEEs). FAEEs infused into rats yields pancreatic edema, trypsin activation, and vacuolization of the pancreas, including increasing the fragility of lysosomes in acinar cells. Pro-inflammatory cytokines NFκB and AP-1 are activated as well. Stellate cell damage leads to the necroinflammatory response. These stellate cells do express alcohol dehydrogenase, so acetaldehyde formation may be important here. Acetaldehyde interferes with the peroxisome proliferator-activated receptor-γ (PPAR-γ) inhibition of stellar cells, causing stellate cells to activate. Profibrogenic actions of acetaldehyde were found to be related

to increased PPAR-γ phosphorylation at a mitogen-activated protein (MAP) kinase. It also appears that ethanol may interfere with vitamin A metabolism, which appears to be necessary to reduce activation of stellate cells (Clemens and Mahan, 2010). These nonoxidative pathways appear also to be important in lipotoxicity (cellular dysfunction) and lipoapoptosis, because excess lipid is processed in the pancreas in obesity, linking obesity to type 2 diabetes (Kusminski et al., 2009). Linking ethanol, fatty acid, and fatty acid ester toxicities may be the increase in cytosolic Ca^{2+} concentrations due to inhibition of mitochondrial function (ATP depletion) and resulting reduced Ca^{2+}-activated ATPase activity in the endoplasmic reticulum and plasma membrane (Petersen et al., 2009). Not all fatty acids are toxic (monosaturated and polyunsaturated from tolerated to cytoprotective); however, it appears the long-chain saturated fatty acids are most toxic to β-cells by a decrease in protein processing. This leads to an apoptotic response and induction of CHOP-10 (a bZIP protein involved in differentiation and apoptosis) synthesis (Morgan, 2009).

Returning to ROS, chronic hyperglycemia involves oxidative stress as one of the mechanisms of glucotoxicity worsening type 2 diabetes by altering the reduction-oxidation balance, formation of advanced glycation products, protein kinase C activation, and increased production of superoxides by the mitochondria. Other factors in glucotoxicity are stress of the endoplasmic reticulum (expression of endoplasmic reticulum-chaperone proteins Bip and Grp94, as well as apoptosis proteins CHOP and GADD34) and protein glycation (Maillard reaction as posttranslational modification). Pancreatic islet cells exhibit large reductions in insulin secretion in response to long-term high blood glucose concentrations that appear to be linked to downregulation of proteins and reduced insulin mRNA expression. The degradation of the insulin gene promoter and PDX-1 and MafA transcription factors appears to be a key factor in this regard (Brunner et al., 2009). Oxidative stress cannot be overemphasized for the β-cells, as they have very low antioxidant capacity. Alloxan and streptozotocin are chemicals usually used to selectively destroy pancreatic β-cells as they accumulate in these cells and generate oxygen radicals. The circadian rhythm hormone melatonin has been found to reduce insulin secretion via high-affinity, pertussis-toxin-sensitive, G_i protein-coupled MT_1 and MT_2 receptors that inhibit cAMP and cGMP pathways. However, pharmacological levels of melatonin confer protection against ROS. Furthermore, plasma melatonin and arylalkylamine-N-acetyltransferase activity are reduced in diabetic rats when compared with nondiabetic rats or humans. Thus, it appears that the pineal gland may also be linked to the control and/or toxicant protection of these susceptible pancreatic cells (Peschke, 2008). Other signaling factors such as H_2S and substance P in caerulein induce acute pancreatitis and may also be mediating factors in pro-inflammatory reactions that have a role in sepsis (Shanmugam and Bhatia, 2010). Yessotoxins (polycyclic ether compounds of phytoplanktonic dinoflagellates) yield cardiac toxicity. However, di-sulfo-yessotoxin causes fatty degeneration in the liver and the pancreas (Tubaro et al., 2010).

Secondary Endocrine Organs

Heart

The heart produces atrial natriuretic peptide (ANP), or hormone. This hormone is linked to membrane guanylyl cyclase (GC) receptors. ANP maintains blood pressure and volume as well as antihypertrophic effects on the heart through its receptor GC-A. GC-B receptors appear to mediate autocrine/paracrine cGMP actions involving cellular proliferation and differentiation in a variety of organs. Altering this receptor or factor will result in cardiac hypertrophy and fibrosis. The intestinal peptide uroguanylin activates GC-C and helps control kidney handling of a salt load. The effects of GC-C in the apical, brush-border membrane of intestinal epithelial cells are observed by increased activity of cGMP-dependent protein kinase II and subsequent increased cystic fibrosis transmembrane conductance regulator-dependent chloride and bicarbonate secretion. This drives sodium ions into the intestinal lumen and is stimulated by *E. coli* heat-stable enterotoxins producing

diarrhea. Compounds that can affect ANP production or secretion are anti-inflammatory steroids (glucocorticoids), catecholamines, arginine vasopressin, angiotensin II, and endothelin. (Kuhn, 2004)

Kidney

Toxicity to the kidney is pretty straightforward. It is known that any factor that may result in kidney failure, such as creatinine overload, produces a drop in the red blood cell count (anemia) due to lower secretion of erythropoietin by the kidney. Any toxicity that is substantial will likely have this result.

Stomach and Small Intestine

Gastrin is a hormone produced by the stomach, and secretin, cholecystokinin, and glucose-dependent insulinotropic peptide are produced in the small intestine. However, inflammatory diseases of the gastrointestinal (GI) tract can be manifested in a variety of ways. Endocrine disruption can come from disruption of the suprachiasmatic nucleus of the hypothalamus (see discussion of hypothalamic disruptors earlier in this chapter) or low melatonin levels (see discussion of pineal gland disruptors earlier in this chapter). Both help regulate the circadian clocks. Disruption of sleep alone will have dramatic GI effects, especially in sensitive individuals with inflammatory diseases of the bowel (such as inflammatory bowel syndrome or IBS). Melatonin not only sets the rhythms but also combats ROS or reactive nitrogen species (RNS) generation by compounds taken in orally. GI hormones motilin and ghrelin activate the migrating motor complex that starts in the stomach, while gastrin, ghrelin, cholecystokinin, and serotonin generate spikes on slow waves causing peristalsis in the small and large intestines (Konturek et al., 2011).

Liver

Insulin-like growth factors (IGFs) are made by the liver. In the important fish toxicology species, the fathead minnow, hepatic expression of IGF-1 (as well as growth hormone receptor and the receptor for IGF-1) was much more in males than females and possibly related to sexual dimorphism in this species (Filby and Tyler, 2007). This makes interpretation of changes and problems associated with these changes more difficult. However, it was noted that hepatic overexpression of IGF binding protein-1 in mice appears to have endocrine effects on brain development and also causes ante- and perinatal mortality and postnatal reductions in growth. Some of the brain effects were hydrocephalus and motor disorders, reduced width of cerebral cortex including disorganized neural layers, underdeveloped corpus callosum, and short and thick dentate gyrus in the smaller hypothalamus (Doublier et al., 2000). This is of interest, because toxicologists are mainly concerned with liver metabolism and neurological toxicity as a result of failures in those systems (e.g., urea formation from ammonia).

Skin, Liver, Kidney

The formation of the active form of vitamin D, 1,25-dihydroxyvitamin D_3, is a shared function of the skin (UV-irradiation), 25-hydroxylation in the liver, and controlled 1-hydroxylation in the kidney. Parathyroid hormone controls the kidney function, so the parathyroid disruptors mentioned in the earlier discussion of parathyroid function are important here. It is also of importance to note that $1\alpha,25(OH)_2D_3$ mediates growth inhibitory signaling. Cancer cell formation results in decreased formation of this important growth regulator. Cancer cells are also less sensitive to its growth inhibitory effects. This occurs early in the process of oncogenesis so may be important in the action of mutagenic or other cancer-causing agents (Kemmis and Welsh, 2008).

Endocrine Organ Disruption Tests

The U.S. Environmental Protection Agency (EPA) and the Organisation for Economic Co-operation and Development's (OECD; a European Union [EU] organization) task force on Endocrine Disruptor Testing and Assessment have suggested a tiered system for endocrine

disruption. Some of the assays discussed in this section reflect the *in vivo* tests for screening for endocrine disruptors as shown in **Table 21-2** (Clode, 2006).

Hypothalamus-Pituitary-Gonadal (HPG) Axis and Thyroid

The pubertal female and male assays (Tier 1 tests) are more appropriate for testing the entire reproductive axis and also thyroid function as it may affect that axis. Although the female test is the preferred method for detecting effects on the whole axis (testing thyroid hormone status, HPG function, estrogens, and antiestrogens), the pubertal male assay provides an alternative test (thyroid function, HPG maturation, steroidogenesis, steroid hormone function). The exposure time is a 30-day period, which is approximately the 28-day subacute OECD guideline for oral toxicity in rodents. In this TG 407 study design (Tier 1 test) body weight, food intake, and clinical observations are made with motor activity, grip strength, and auditory startle determined during the last week of treatment. Prior to necropsy, hematology and clinical chemistry are assessed. Organ weights are determined for liver, kidneys, adrenals, testes, epididymides, thymus, spleen, brain, and heart, and histopathology is noted for these organs and on spinal cord, stomach, small and large intestines, thyroid, trachea, lungs, gonads, accessory sex organs, urinary bladder, lymph nodes, and bone marrow. To make this more of an endocrine disruptor assay, the weights are recorded for each testis, seminal vesicles with coagulating gland, prostate, ovaries, thyroid, and uterus. Additionally, histopathology examination is required on pituitary, vagina (female), one epididymis and coagulating gland (male), and mammary glands (female). Thyroid hormones are quantitated; semen analyzed (male); and estrous cycles are monitored for 5 days prior to necropsy to insure that necropsy occurred during estrous. Tier 2 tests require a two-generation exposure. In this design, the male and female are exposed for 10 weeks, mated, and the next generation is allowed full gestation. The resulting litter is the F_{1a} generation that goes to weaning and selection of

TABLE 21-2   Endocrine Organ Toxicity Tests

Testing For	Individual Assays
Hypothalamus → pituitary → gonadal axis + thyroid	Tier 1 tests: Pubertal female assay (preferred) – following exposure measure body weight, age of vaginal opening, estrous cycle, serum TSH and T_4, weights of uterus, ovaries, thyroid, liver, kidneys, pituitary, adrenals and histopathology of uterus, ovaries, vagina, and thyroid
	Pubertal male assay - following exposure body weight, food intake, age or preputial separation, T_4, TSH, weights of seminal vesicles with coagulating gland, ventral prostate, testes, epididymides, thyroid, liver, kidneys, pituitary, and adrenals and histopathology of thyroid, testes, epdiymides, Cowper's gland, levator and bulbocavernosus muscles
	Tier 2 tests: Two generation exposure (EPA OPPTS 870.3800; OECD TG416) gives the substance to young male and female rats for 10 weeks prior to mating, during paring period and until necropsy. F_1 exposure through weaning and maturation, during paring period and until necropsy. F_{2a} rear offspring to weaning. Record body weights, food intakes, estrous cycles (female), age of preputial separation (male) and vaginal opening (female), sex ratio at time of puberty, and anogenital distance, and following necropsy of both generations weights of uterus, ovaries, testes, epididymides, prostate, seminal vesicle, brain, liver, kidneys, spleen, pituitary, thyroid, adrenals and target organs, semen analyses and histopathology of vagina, uterus with cervix, ovary, testis, epididymis, seminal vesicle, prostate, and coagulating glands (Clode, 2006)
Pituitary tumor models	Estrogen (or DES or estrone)-treated rats, implanted prolactin-secreting tumor cells, aged rats, GH hypersecreting Gs protein mutation, ACTH-secreting Cushing's syndrome-like mice, single retinoblastoma gene causing multiple neuroendocrine neoplasia modified to produce gonadotropinomas or pineal gland tumors (Seilicovich et al., 2005)
Adrenal cortex	ACTH challenge and use of H295R human adrenocortical carcinoma line (Harvey et al., 2007), adrenal weight coupled to ACTH and glucocorticoid concentrations, measuring corticosteroid metabolites in feces in animals in the wild (Hinson and Raven, 2006)
Adrenal medulla	Adrenal tumors (Rosol et al., 2001), bovine chromaffin cells as model of delayed neuropathy by organophosphorus compounds (Romero et al., 2006)
Thyroid disruption	Amphibian metamorphosis, cultured thyroid, thyroid enzymes, pituitary and thyroid hormone levels coupled to histology (van den Berg, 2010)
	Fish reproduction and development (Blanton and Specker, 2007)
Parathyroid	Isolated miniature pig parathyroid (Soshin et al., 2010)
Estrogenic effects	Tier 1 tests: Immature rats exposed to 17β-estradiol (or DES or ethinyl estradiol; positive control), vehicle (negative control) or three test groups and mark body weight, clinical observations (uterine growth), and vaginal openings (Clode, 2006)
Androgenic/ antiandrogenic effects	Tier 1 tests: Hershberger assay uses castrated male rats + vehicle (negative control) + testosterone (positive control) + chemical or mixture for androgenic effects + chemical and testosterone for antiandrogenic effects and monitored for body weight, food intake, clinical observations (accessory sex organs weights along with liver, kidney and adrenals); serum LH and testosterone levels), and pre-putial separation (Clode, 2006)

F_1 generation. Another 10-week exposure is followed by mating and another gestation and littering event leading to the F_{2a} generation. These rats would be allowed to go to weaning then the F_1 and F_{2a} generations are necropsied. The results reflect mostly tissue examination (Clode, 2006).

Anterior Pituitary Tumor Models

Sheep and monkeys are large animal models that may be stimulated to provide expensive but comparable pituitary results to those of the human and can be used in developing gene transfer technologies to treat pituitary tumors.

The rodent is still the preferred animal model. For prolactinomas, hormonal stimulation (estrogen-stimulated Fisher 344 rat or chronic estrogen treatment of male Sprague-Dawley rats), implantation of prolactin-secreting tumor cell lines, and sporadic adenomas are the three model systems. Diethylstilbestrol (DES) or estrone implants and injections of 17β-estradiol all appear to be good models of lactotroph hyperplasias. Aged female or male Sprague-Dawley and Wistar strains may spontaneously develop pituitary tumors as well (as indicated by problems associated with these old animals as a measure of cancer produced by atrazine or similar agent). MMQ cells are derived from rat pituitary 7315a and only secrete prolactin. These cells implanted in the Buffalo rat model for chronic hyperprolactinemia. The 235-1 cell line derived from this tumor inoculated into athymic mice and rats of the Buffalo following culture of the cell line caused enlarged mammary glands. Prolactin-secreting tumor 7315b has been used as a model of severe hyperprolactinemia on the pituitary gonadal axis in rats. Wistar/Furth rats with transplantable SMtTW prolactin tumors represent human prolactinomas that are sensitive to dopamine agonists and express a marker (polysialylated neural cell adhesion molecule) that may be diagnostic of malignant pituitary adenomas. Similarly, GH3 cells implanted into the flanks of Wistar/Furth rats are an *in vivo* model of prolactinomas. GH hypersecretion occurs in a mutation of the G_s protein (gsps) in which G_s α is in a constitutively active state in a transgenic animal model or GH3 cell transplants. The AVP-SV40T antigen model expresses the SB40 T antigen controlled by the arginine vasopressin (AVP) gene promoter. These animals develop anterior pituitary tumors constituted by undifferentiated somatotrophs. Intermediate lobe tumors exhibit immunoreactivity for ACTH and express proopiomelanocortin mRNA. Transgenic animals upregulating the expression of CRF show symptoms similar to adrenal tumors (Cushing's syndrome). Transgenic mice with the polyoma early region promoter coupled to a cDNA encoding polyoma T antigen develop ACTH-secreting pituitary tumors. Cytokines are also involved in the differentiation, proliferation, and secretory

functions of pituitary cells that secrete ACTH as they were involved in many pituitary tumors. It appears that leukemia inhibitory factor is especially significant for cells that synthesize ACTH. A lethal phenotype with a complex Cushing's syndrome–like pathology is noted in mice not expressing neuroendocrine-specific protein 7B2. This 7B2 protein is essential for synthesis of prohormone convertase 3, which is an endoprotease that processes neuroendocrine precursor proteins. Multiple neuroendocrine neoplasia develops in mice with a single retinoblastoma gene. Melanotroph cells prevented from developing neoplasia in this animal model (by transgenic expression of the human retinoblastoma gene to melanotrophs) develop anterior lobe tumors more rapidly. Tumors of the pituitary and pineal glands develop in another model involving the Cre-LoxP-mediated somatic inactivation of the retinoblastoma gene. Null cell adenomas and gonadotropinomas were developed in transgenic mice. Null cell adenomas exhibit no pituitary hormone production but express genes related to gonadotrophin synthesis. Anterior pituitary nodules secreting FSH develop in mice with a temperature-sensitive mutant of simian virus 40T antigen linked to human FSHβ regulatory elements (Seilicovich et al., 2005).

Adrenal

Toxicants target the adrenal more than other endocrine organs, yet it is a much-ignored, important piece of endocrine disruption. Proposed tests involve an *in vivo* rodent model using an ACTH challenge. Additionally, the H295R human adrenocortical carcinoma line can be used to indicate molecular targets and measure steroids, enzyme activities, and gene expression (Harvey et al., 2007). If the adrenal were affected, it would be expected that ACTH would be elevated. However, even when steroid hormone synthesis in the adrenal is compromised, it is not unusual for basal ACTH concentrations in the blood to be unchanged. Thus, ACTH and corticosteroids are both measured as a measure of adrenal function. Gossypol, for instance, causes seemingly opposite findings of an increase in adrenal weight and decreased cortisol secretion. This is due to a lack of cortisol feedback on the HPA axis resulting in increased ACTH release. Unlike many other endocrine organs, the corticosteroid hormones are not stored and then released upon stimulation. Rather, the adrenal synthesizes them on stimulation from a cholesterol precursor so the synthetic capacity is a better measure here of toxicity. Adrenal weight alone is not a good measure as stress alone can yield this result and may not reflect a toxic stress. Because the hormone shows circadian patterns of synthesis, it is difficult to assess basal function and easier to determine what occurs with an ACTH challenge. However, in the polar bear (*Ursus maritimus*) in the wild, persistent organochlorides and plasma cortisol concentrations could be related. Short-lived toxicants provide a larger challenge to the toxicologist who now has to think as an endocrinologist. In the wild, the use of fecal glucocorticoid metabolites provides evidence of adrenal disruption and is noninvasive, which is especially important in endangered or protected species (Hinson and Raven, 2006). Toxicity to the adrenal medulla may be modeled by tumor development in this organ. Additionally, bovine chromaffin cells are an interesting model for organophosphorus-induced delayed neuropathy, because they are rich in neuropathy target esterase (Romero et al., 2006).

Thyroid

The amphibian metamorphosis bioassay with tadpoles such as *Xenopus laevis* is the EPA standard for looking for thyroid-disrupting pesticides and other toxic chemicals. The delay in metamorphosis and increased size of the tadpole indicate more subtle damage, while higher concentrations lead to outright lethality. Regarding the complicated hypothalamus-pituitary-thyroid axis (discussed previously in the thyroid disruption section), determination of where thyroid function is compromised by a given chemical or mixture is extremely difficult, especially considering species differences in thyroid hormone homeostasis and sensitivity to disruption. Histology may be coupled to thyroid hormone levels, TSH levels, and T_3 or T_4 to further elucidate changes related to thyroid

function. *In vitro* tests may employ enzymes used in thyroid hormone synthesis such as deiodinases and thyroid peroxidases. These miss the whole organ function. Cultured thyroid would be a way of determining direct effects on the whole thyroid, but miss the whole axis from the hypothalamus that may be the cause of the disruption or enhance thyroid disruption in the living organism (van den Berg, 2010). Another model is fish development and reproduction as a measure of thyroid development (Blanton and Specker, 2007). However, many additional targets could be analyzed, because thyroid disruption could involve alterations in serum levels of thyroid hormones, thyroperoxidase inhibition, perchlorate discharge test, iodine uptake inhibition, changes in the activity of iodothyronine deiodinases, modifying the action of thyroid hormones, and effects on binding proteins (Zoeller et al., 2007). This indicates that compounds ranging from radioactive iodine to medications to pesticides have been implicated in thyroid disruption. One major concern with a damaged thyroid is the development of hyperplasia (goiter) that can be a result of lower thyroid hormone levels (lack of negative feedback to pituitary causing higher TSH stimulation of the thyroid gland) that may result in thyroid cancer. There have been a number of models of thyroid disruption including the amphibian. Thioureas are drugs used to treat hyperthyroidism (Manna et al., 2013) and thiourea itself is part of the *Xenopus laevis* tadpole model to arrest and synchronize tadpole development to improve detection of thyroid hormone disruption (Gutleb et al., 2007).

Parathyroid

An alternative test model for parathyroid toxicity studies employs parathyroid gland isolated from miniature pigs. These pigs appear to be finding increased use in toxicity studies as a mammal that is not a rodent (Soshin et al., 2010).

Testes

The Hershberger assay (Tier 1 test) can be used to test for androgens or antiandrogens. A castrated male rat given a chemical or mixture will only develop if the androgen is in the test substance. For antiandrogens, testosterone is given subcutaneously to castrated males that are then monitored for lack of sexual development (Clode, 2006).

Ovaries/Uterus

Immature or ovariectomized rats exposed to estrogenic substances will have rapid growth of the uterus or uterotrophic effects (Tier 1 test). This is the basis for the assay considered primary in detecting environmental estrogens. The rat uterus development from birth through day 16 is estrogen independent. During its quiescent period from days 17 to 26 is the time to expose the rat to possible estrogenic compounds or mixtures. Past day 26, the uterus will show the estrogenic effects as this period is when endogenous 17β-estradiol signals the onset of puberty (Clode, 2006).

Questions

1. How do the chlorinated organic compounds DDT, DDE, and TCDD show differential action on the hypothalamus mechanisms of GnRH release?
2. Why is eating the flavor enhancer MSG problematic during pregnancy?
3. How is MDMA hyperthermia mediated and enhanced by caffeine?
4. How can Cd affect a variety of hormones in the anterior pituitary?
5. How can the effects of environmental estrogens on the pituitary be reduced by neurotransmitter analogs?
6. Why can high-tension power lines affect sleep cycles, reproductive function, and cancer development?
7. Why is the adrenal gland so susceptible to chemically induced lesions?
8. Reserpine depletes catecholamines and 5-HT in the brain and adrenal medulla. What effect does this have on the adrenal?
9. Why are goitrogens important in amphibians and mammals?
10. Calcium is usually considered an important physiological nutrient. Why is chronic

overconsumption an issue for the thyroid, especially in aging rats?
11. Why might heavy metals decrease the function of the parathyroid, while phosphate compounds have the opposite effect?
12. What do the differing effects of tributyltin indicate about gonadal toxicity assays?
13. What does estrogenic endocrine disruption in the ovary have to do with thymus function?
14. How does mitochondrial damage versus ROS separate two forms of damage to the pancreas?
15. What direct effect does blocking the estrogen receptor with the weak estrogen tamoxifen or the exposure to the androgen methyldihydrotestosterone indicate about direct effects on the ovaries? How might the endocrine disruption be enlarged to other organs by continuous exposure to an androgen?

References

Adams EM, Frederick PC, Larkin IL, Guillette LJ Jr. 2009. Sublethal effects of methylmercury on fecal metabolites of testosterone, estradiol, and corticosterone in captive juvenile white ibises (*Eudocimus albus*). *Environ Toxicol Chem.* 28(5):982–989.

Adamson TW, Carll C, Svec F, Porter J. 2010. Role of the perifornical hypothalamic monoamine neurotransmitter systems in anorectic effects of endotoxin. *Neuroendocrinology.* 91:48–55.

Almaden Y, Rodriguez-Ortiz ME, Canalejo A, Cañadillas S, Canalejo R, Martin D, Aguilera-Tejero E, Rodríguez M. 2009. Calcimimetics normalize the phosphate-induced stimulation of PTH secretion *in vivo* and *in vitro. J Nephrol.* 22:281–288.

Ardine M, Generali D, Donadio M, Bonardi S, Scoletta M, Vandone AM, Mozzati M, Bertetto O, Bottini A, Dogliotti L, Berruti A. 2006. Could the long-term persistence of low serum calcium levels and high serum parathyroid hormone levels during bisphosphonate treatment predispose metastatic breast cancer patients to undergo osteonecrosis of the jaw? *Ann Oncol.* 17:1336–1337.

Atwal OS. 1979. Ultrastructural pathology of ozone-induced experimental parathyroiditis. IV. Biphasic activity in the chief cells of regenerating parathyroid glands. *Am J Pathol.* 95:611–632.

Barai SR, Suryawanshi SA, Pandey AK. 2009. Responses of parathyroid gland, C cells, and plasma calcium and inorganic phosphate levels in rat to sub-lethal heroin administration. *J Environ Biol*. 30(5 Suppl):917–922.

Barenys M, Gomez-Catalan J, Camps L, Teixido E, de Lapuente J, Gonzalez-Linares J, Serret J, Borras M, Rodamilans M, Llobet JM. 2010. MDMA (ecstasy) delays pubertal development and alters sperm quality after developmental exposure in the rat. *Toxicol Lett*. 197:135–142.

Barlas N, Selmanoglu G, Koçkaya A, Songür S. 2002. Effects of carbendazim on rat thyroid, parathyroid, pituitary and adrenal glands and their hormones. *Hum Exp Toxicol*. 21:217–221.

Bellingham M, Fowler PA, Amezaga MR, Whitelaw CM, Rhind SM, Cotinot C, Mandon-Pepin B, Sharpe RM, Evans NP. 2010. Foetal hypothalamic and pituitary expression of gonadotrophin-releasing hormone and galanin systems is disturbed by exposure to sewage sludge chemicals via maternal ingestion. *J Neuroendocrinol*. 22:527–533.

Blanton ML, Specker JL. 2007. The hypothalamic-pituitary-thyroid (HPT) axis in fish and its role in fish development and reproduction. *Crit Rev Toxicol*. 37:97–115.

Brunner Y, Schvartz D, Priego-Capote F, Couté Y, Sanchez JC. 2009. Glucotoxicity and pancreatic proteomics. *J Proteomics*. 71:576–591.

Brzóska MM, Moniuszko-Jakoniuk J. 2005. Effect of low-level lifetime exposure to cadmium on calciotropic hormones in aged female rats. *Arch Toxicol*. 79:636–646.

Cakir M, Grossman AB. 2009. Medullary thyroid cancer: molecular biology and novel molecular therapies. *Neuroendocrinology*. 90:323–348.

Calejo AI, Rodriguez E, Silva VS, Jorgacevski J, Stenovec M, Kreft M, Santos C, Zorec R, Gonçalves PP. 2010. Life and death in aluminium-exposed cultures of rat lactotrophs studied by flow cytometry. *Cell Biol Toxicol*. 26:341–353.

Cannata-Andía JB, Fernández-Martín JL. 2002. The clinical impact of aluminium overload in renal failure. *Nephrol Dial Transplant*. 17(Suppl 2):9–12.

Capen CC. 1992. Pathophysiology of chemical injury of the thyroid gland. *Toxicol Lett*. 64–65: 381–388.

Capen CC. 1998. Correlation of mechanistic data and histopathology in the evaluation of selected toxic endpoints of the endocrine system. *Toxicol Lett*. 102–103:405–409.

Caride A, Fernández-Pérez B, Cabaleiro T, Lafuente A. 2010a. Daily pattern of pituitary glutamine, glutamate, and aspartate content disrupted by cadmium exposure. *Amino Acids*. 38:1165–1172.

Caride A, Fernández-Pérez B, Cabaleiro T, Tarasco M, Esquifino AI, Lafuente A. 2010b. Cadmium chronotoxicity at pituitary level: effects on plasma ACTH, GH, and TSH daily pattern. *J Physiol Biochem*. 66:213–220.

Cevasco A, Urbatzka R, Bottero S, Massari A, Pedemonte F, Kloas W, Mandich A. 2008. Endocrine disrupting chemicals (EDC) with (anti) estrogenic and (anti)androgenic modes of action affecting reproductive biology of *Xenopus laevis*: II. Effects on gonad histomorphology. *Comp Biochem Physiol C Toxicol Pharmacol*. 147:241–251.

Chapman JC, Min SH, Freeh SM, Michael SD. 2009. The estrogen-injected female mouse: new insight into the etiology of PCOS. *Reprod Biol Endocrinol*. 7:47.

Chen YW, Yang CY, Huang CF, Hung DZ, Leung YM, Liu SH. 2009. Heavy metals, islet function and diabetes development. *Islets*. 1:169–176.

Chisari FV, Hochstein HD, Kirschstein RL, Seligmann EB. 1972. Parathyroid necrosis and hypocalcemic tetany induced in rabbits by L-asparaginase. *Am J Pathol*. 68:461–468.

Clemens DL, Mahan KJ. 2010. Alcoholic pancreatitis: lessons from the liver. *World J Gastroenterol*. 16:1314–1320.

Clements RJ, Lawrence RC, Blank JL. 2009. Effects of intrauterine 2,3,7,8-tetrachlorodibenzo-p-dioxin on the development and function of the gonadotrophin releasing hormone neuronal system in the male rat. *Reprod Toxicol*. 28:38–45.

Clode SA. 2006. Assessment of *in vivo* assays for endocrine disruption. *Best Pract Res Clin Endocrinol Metab*. 20:35–43.

Cooper RL, Stoker TE, Tyrey L, Goldman JM, McElroy WK. 2000. Atrazine disrupts the hypothalamic control of pituitary-ovarian function. *Toxicol Sci*. 53:297–307.

Cubero I, Navarro M, Carvajal F, Lerma-Cabrera JM, Thiele TE. 2010. Ethanol-induced increase of agouti-related protein (AgRP) immunoreactivity in the arcuate nucleus of the hypothalamus of C57BL/6J, but not 129/SvJ, inbred mice. *Alcohol Clin Exp Res*. 34:693–701.

Dirican EK, Kalender Y. 2012. Dichlorvos-induced testicular toxicity in male rats and the protective role of vitamins C and E. *Exp Toxicol Pathol*. 64:821–830.

Dooley GP, Ashley AK, Legare ME, Handa RJ, Hanneman WH. 2010. Proteomic analysis of diaminochlorotriazine (DACT) adducts in three brain regions of Wistar rats. *Toxicol Lett*. 199:17–21.

Doublier S, Duyckaerts C, Seurin D, Binoux M. 2000. Impaired brain development and hydrocephalus in a line of transgenic mice with liver-specific expression of human insulin-like growth factor binding protein-1. *Growth Horm IGF Res*. 10:267–274.

Doumouchtsis KK, Doumouchtsis SK, Doumouchtsis EK, Perrea DN. 2009. The effect of lead intoxication on endocrine functions. *J Endocrinol Invest.* 32:175–183.

Elias EE, Kalombo E, Mercurio SD. 2007. Tamoxifen protects against 17alpha-ethynylestradiol-induced liver damage and the development of urogenital papillae in the rainbow darter (*Etheostoma caeruleum*). *Environ Toxicol Chem.* 26:1879–1889.

Enright BP, Leach MW, Pelletier G, LaBrie F, McIntyre BS, Losco PE. 2010. Effects of an antagonist of neurokinin receptors 1, 2 and 3 on reproductive hormones in male beagle dogs. *Birth Defects Res B Dev Reprod Toxicol.* 89:517–525.

Esmekaya MA, Ozer C, Seyhan N. 2011. 900 MHz pulse-modulated radiofrequency radiation induces oxidative stress on heart, lung, testis and liver tissues. *Gen Physiol Biophys.* 30:84–89.

Fakhouri WD, Nuñez JL, Trail F. 2010. Atrazine binds to the growth hormone-releasing hormone receptor and affects growth hormone gene expression. *Environ Health Perspect.* 118:1400–1405.

Feng Y, Johansson J, Shao R, Mannerås L, Fernandez-Rodriguez J, Billig H, Stener-Victorin E. 2009. Hypothalamic neuroendocrine functions in rats with dihydrotestosterone-induced polycystic ovary syndrome: effects of low-frequency electroacupuncture. *PLoS One.* 4:e6638.

Filby AL, Tyler CR. 2007. Cloning and characterization of cDNAs for hormones and/or receptors of growth hormone, insulin-like growth factor-I, thyroid hormone, and corticosteroid and the gender-, tissue-, and developmental-specific expression of their mRNA transcripts in fathead minnow (*Pimephales promelas*). *Gen Comp Endocrinol.* 150:151–163.

Fouladi M, Stempak D, Gammon J, Klein J, Grant R, Greenberg ML, Koren G, Baruchel S. 2001. Phase I trial of a twice-daily regimen of amifostine with ifosfamide, carboplatin, and etoposide chemotherapy in children with refractory carcinoma. *Cancer.* 92:914–923.

Frederick P, Jayasena N. 2011. Altered pairing behaviour and reproductive success in white ibises exposed to environmentally relevant concentrations of methylmercury. *Proc Biol Sci.* 278:1851–1857.

Gagiannis S, Müller M, Uhlemann S, Koch A, Melino G, Krammer PH, Nawroth PP, Brune M, Schilling T. 2009. Parathyroid hormone-related protein confers chemoresistance by blocking apoptosis signaling via death receptors and mitochondria. *Int J Cancer.* 125:1551–1557.

Gillam MP, Fideleff H, Boquete HR, Molitch ME. 2004. Prolactin excess: treatment and toxicity. *Pediatr Endocrinol Rev.* 2(Suppl 1):108–114.

Gore AC. 2010. Neuroendocrine targets of endocrine disruptors. *Hormones (Athens).* 9:16–27.

Gotti S, Martini M, Viglietti-Panzica C, Miceli D, Panzica G. 2010. Effects of estrous cycle and xenoestrogens expositions on mice nitric oxide producing system. *Ital J Anat Embryol.* 115:103–108.

Gutleb AC, Schriks M, Mossink L, Berg JH, Murk AJ. 2007. A synchronized amphibian metamorphosis assay as an improved tool to detect thyroid hormone disturbance by endocrine disruptors and apolar sediment extracts. *Chemosphere.* 70:93–100.

Hachfi L, Sakly R. 2010. Effect of Cd transferred via food product on spermatogenesis in the rat. *Andrologia.* 42:62–64.

Harvey PW. 2014. Adrenocortical endocrine disruption. *J Steroid Biochem Mol Biol.* Oct 18. Epub ahead of print.

Harvey PW, Everett DJ, Springall CJ. 2007. Adrenal toxicology: a strategy for assessment of functional toxicity to the adrenal cortex and steroidogenesis. *J Appl Toxicol.* 27:103–115.

Hayes TB, Case P, Chui S, Chung D, Haeffele C, Haston K, Lee M, Mai VP, Marjuoa Y, Parker J, Tsui M. 2006. Pesticide mixtures, endocrine disruption, and amphibian declines: are we underestimating the impact? *Environ Health Perspect.* 114(Suppl 1):40–50.

Henshaw DL, Ward JP, Matthews JC. 2008. Can disturbances in the atmospheric electric field created by powerline corona ions disrupt melatonin production in the pineal gland? *J Pineal Res.* 45:341–350.

Hinson JP, Raven PW. 2006. Effects of endocrine-disrupting chemicals on adrenal function. *Best Pract Res Clin Endocrinol Metab.* 20:111–120.

Hinuma S, Habata Y, Fuj2R, Kawamata Y, Hosoya M, Fukusumi S, Kitada C, Masuo Y, Asano T, Matsumoto H, Sekiguchi M, Kurokawa T, Nishimura O, Onda H, Fujino M. 1998. A prolactin-releasing peptide in the brain. *Nature.* 393:272–276. Erratum in: 1998. *Nature.* 394:302.

Hollis JH, Lemus M, Evetts MJ, Oldfield BJ. 2010. Central interleukin-10 attenuates lipopolysaccharide-induced changes in food intake, energy expenditure and hypothalamic Fos expression. *Neuropharmacology.* 58:730–738.

Hong D, Li XW, Lian QQ, Lamba P, Bernard DJ, Hardy DO, Chen HX, Ge RS. 2009. Mono-(2-ethylhexyl) phthalate (MEHP) regulates glucocorticoid metabolism through 11beta-hydroxysteroid dehydrogenase 2 in murine gonadotrope cells. *Biochem Biophys Res Commun.* 389:305–309.

Hooth MJ, Herbert RA, Haseman JK, Orzech DP, Johnson JD, Bucher JR. 2004. Toxicology and carcinogenesis studies of dipropylene glycol in rats and mice. *Toxicology.* 204:123–140.

Hornung MW, Degitz SJ, Korte LM, Olson JM, Kosian PA, Linnum AL, Tietge JE. 2010. Inhibition of thyroid hormone release from cultured amphibian thyroid glands by methimazole, 6-propylthiouracil, and perchlorate. *Toxicol Sci.* 118:42–51.

Hoshi S, Hoshi N, Okamoto M, Paiz J, Kusakabe T, Ward JM, Kimura S. 2009. Role of NKX2-1 in N-bis(2-hydroxypropyl)-nitrosamine-induced thyroid adenoma in mice. *Carcinogenesis.* 30:1614–1619.

Hoyer PB, Sipes IG. 2007. Development of an animal model for ovotoxicity using 4-vinylcyclohexene: a case study. *Birth Defects Res B Dev Reprod Toxicol.* 80:113–125.

Huang Z, Li K, Hou G, Shen Z, Wang C, Jiang K, Luo X. 2002. [Study on the correlation of the biochemical indexes in fluoride workers]. *Zhonghua Lao Dong Wei Sheng Zhi Ye Bing Za Zhi.* 20:192–194.

Iavicoli I, Fontana L, Bergamaschi A. 2009. The effects of metals as endocrine disruptors. *J Toxicol Environ Health B Crit Rev.* 12:206–223.

Ibhazehiebo K, Iwasaki T, Kimura-Kuroda J, Miyazaki W, Shimokawa N, Koibuchi N. 2011. Disruption of thyroid hormone receptor-mediated transcription and thyroid hormone-induced Purkinje cell dendrite arborization by polybrominated diphenyl ethers. *Environ Health Perspect.* 119:168–175.

Jablonska O, Shi Z, Valdez KE, Ting AY, Petroff BK. 2010. Temporal and anatomical sensitivities to the aryl hydrocarbon receptor agonist 2,3,7,8-tetrachlorodibenzo-p-dioxin leading to premature acyclicity with age in rats. *Int J Androl.* 33:405–412.

Jacobs LS, Snyder PJ, Wilber JF, Utiger RD, Daughaday WH. 1971. Increased serum prolactin after administration of synthetic thyrotropin releasing hormone (TRH) in man. *J Clin Endocrinol Metab.* 33:996–998.

Jensen KM, Kahl MD, Makynen EA, Korte JJ, Leino RL, Butterworth BC, Ankley GT. 2004. Characterization of responses to the antiandrogen flutamide in a short-term reproduction assay with the fathead minnow. *Aquat Toxicol.* 70:99–110.

Johns JM, McMurray MS, Joyner PW, Jarrett TM, Williams SK, Cox ET, Black MA, Middleton CL, Walker CH. 2010. Effects of chronic and intermittent cocaine treatment on dominance, aggression, and oxytocin levels in post-lactational rats. *Psychopharmacology (Berl).* 211:175–185.

Jolous-Jamshidi B, Cromwell HC, McFarland AM, Meserve LA. 2010. Perinatal exposure to polychlorinated biphenyls alters social behaviors in rats. *Toxicol Lett.* 199:136–143.

Kang HS, Kerstan D, Dai L, Ritchie G, Quamme GA. 2000. Aminoglycosides inhibit hormone-stimulated Mg2+ uptake in mouse distal convoluted tubule cells. *Can J Physiol Pharmacol.* 78:595–602.

Kemmis CM, Welsh J. 2008. Mammary epithelial cell transformation is associated with deregulation of the vitamin D pathway. *J Cell Biochem.* 105:980–988.

Khan MR, Ahmed D. 2009. Protective effects of *Digera muricata* (L.) Mart. on testis against oxidative stress of carbon tetrachloride in rat. *Food Chem Toxicol.* 47:1393–1399.

Konturek PC, Brzozowski T, Konturek SJ. 2011. Gut clock: implication of circadian rhythms in the gastrointestinal tract. *J Physiol Pharmacol.* 62:139–150.

Kuhn M. 2004. Molecular physiology of natriuretic peptide signaling. *Basic Res Cardiol.* 99:76–82.

Kumazawa T, Nakajima A, Ishiguro T, Jiuxin Z, Tanaharu T, Nishitani H, Inoue Y, Harada S, Hayasaka I, Tagawa Y. 2009. Collaborative work on evaluation of ovarian toxicity. 15) Two- or four-week repeated-dose studies and fertility study of bromocriptine in female rats. *J Toxicol Sci.* 34(Suppl 1):SP157–165.

Kusminski CM, Shetty S, Orci L, Unger RH, Scherer PE. 2009. Diabetes and apoptosis: lipotoxicity. *Apoptosis.* 14:1484–1495.

Lan N, Yamashita F, Halpert AG, Sliwowska JH, Viau V, Weinberg J. 2009. Effects of prenatal ethanol exposure on hypothalamic-pituitary-adrenal function across the estrous cycle. *Alcohol Clin Exp Res.* 33:1075–1088.

Langer P. 2010. The impacts of organochlorines and other persistent pollutants on thyroid and metabolic health. *Front Neuroendocrinol.* 31:497–518.

Lanigan RS. 2001. Final report on the safety assessment of sodium metaphosphate, sodium trimetaphosphate, and sodium hexametaphosphate. *Int J Toxicol.* 20(Suppl 3):75–89.

Leddingham IM, Watt I. 1983. Influence of sedation on mortality in multiple trauma patients. *Lancet.* 1:1270.

Leitner C, Bartness TJ. 2009. Acute brown adipose tissue temperature response to cold in monosodium glutamate-treated Siberian hamsters. *Brain Res.* 1292:38–51.

Li X, Li C, Suzuki AK, Watanabe G, Taneda S, Taya K. 2009. Endocrine disruptive effect of 3-methyl-4-nitrophenol isolated from diesel exhaust particles in Hershberger assay using castrated immature rats. *Biosci Biotechnol Biochem.* 73:2018–2021.

Lim S, Cho YM, Park KS, Lee HK. 2010. Persistent organic pollutants, mitochondrial dysfunction, and metabolic syndrome. *Ann NY Acad Sci.* 1201:166–176.

Liu Y, Wang J, Fang X, Zhang H, Dai J. 2011. The thyroid-disrupting effects of long-term perfluorononanoate exposure on zebrafish (*Danio rerio*). *Ecotoxicology.* 20:47–55.

Mahoney MM, Padmanabhan V. 2010. Developmental programming: impact of fetal exposure to endocrine-disrupting chemicals on gonadotropin-releasing hormone and estrogen receptor mRNA in sheep hypothalamus. *Toxicol Appl Pharmacol.* 247:98–104.

Manna D, Roy G, Mugesh G. 2013. Antithyroid drugs and their analogues: synthesis, structure, and mechanism of action. *Acc Chem Res.* 46:2706–2715.

Martyniuk CJ, Kroll KJ, Doperalski NJ, Barber DS, Denslow ND. 2010. Genomic and proteomic responses to environmentally relevant exposures to dieldrin: indicators of neurodegeneration? *Toxicol Sci.* 117:190–199.

Matsushima S, Tsuchiya N, Fujisawa-Imura K, Fujisawa-Imura K, Hoshimoto M, Takasu N, Torii M, Ozaki K, Narana I, Kotani T. 2005. Ultrastructural and morphometrical evaluation of the parathyroid gland in iron-lactate-overloaded rats. *Toxicol Pathol.* 33:533–539.

McDiarmid MA, Engelhardt SM, Dorsey CD, Oliver M, Gucer P, Gaitens JM, Kane R, Cernich A, Kaup B, Hoover D, Gaspari AA, Shvartsbeyn M, Brown L, Squibb KS. 2011. Longitudinal health surveillance in a cohort of gulf war veterans 18 years after first exposure to depleted uranium. *J Toxicol Environ Health A.* 274:678–691.

McDowell KA, Hadjimarkou MM, Viechweg S, Rose AE, Clark SM, Yarowsky PJ, Mong JA. 2010. Sleep alterations in an environmental neurotoxin-induced model of parkinsonism. *Exp Neurol.* 226:84–89.

Mennigen JA, Sassine J, Trudeau VL, Moon TW. 2010. Waterborne fluoxetine disrupts feeding and energy metabolism in the goldfish *Carassius auratus*. *Aquat Toxicol.* 100:128–137.

Mirick DK, Davis S. 2008. Melatonin as a biomarker of circadian dysregulation. *Cancer Epidemiol Biomarkers Prev.* 17:3306–3313.

Mishra AK, Mohanty B. 2009. Effect of hexavalent chromium exposure on the pituitary-interrenal axis of a teleost, *Channa punctatus* (Bloch). *Chemosphere.* 76:982–988.

Mishra AC, Mohanty B. 2010. Effects of lactational exposure of olanzapine and risperidone on hematology and lymphoid organs histopathology: a comparative study in mice neonates. *Eur J Pharmacol.* 634:170–177.

Morgan NG. 2009. Fatty acids and beta-cell toxicity. *Curr Opin Clin Nutr Metab Care.* 12:117–122.

Nagda G, Bhatt DK. 2011. Alleviation of lindane induced toxicity in testis of Swiss mice (*Mus musculus*) by combined treatment with vitamin C, vitamin E and alpha-lipoic acid. *Indian J Exp Biol.* 49:191–199.

Nakamura T, Mimura Y, Uno K, Yamakawa M. 1998. Parathyroid hormone activity increases during endotoxemia in conscious rats. *Horm Metab Res.* 30:88–92.

Nakamura D, Yanagiba Y, Duan Z, Ito Y, Okamura A, Asaeda N, Tagawa Y, Li C, Taya K, Zhang SY, Naito H, Ramdhan DH, Kamijima M, Nakajima T. 2010. Bisphenol A may cause testosterone reduction by adversely affecting both testis and pituitary systems similar to estradiol. *Toxicol Lett.* 194:16–25.

Obukuro K, Takigawa M, Hisatsune A, Isohama Y, Katsuki H. 2010. Quinolinate induces selective loss of melanin-concentrating hormone neurons, rather than orexin neurons, in the hypothalamus of mice and young rats. *Neuroscience.* 170:298–307.

Ohta R, Ohmukai H, Toyoizumi T, Shindo T, Marumo H, Ono H. 2014. Ovarian dysfunction, obesity and pituitary tumors in female mice following neonatal exposure to low-dose diethyl-stilbestrol. *Reprod Toxicol.* 50:145–151.

Oste L, Bervoets AR, Behets GJ, Dams G, Marijnissen RL, Geryl H, Lamberts LV, Verberckmoes SC, Van Hoof VO, De Broe ME, D'Haese PC. 2005. Time-evolution and reversibility of strontium-induced osteomalacia in chronic renal failure rats. *Kidney Int.* 67:920–930.

Pattaragarn A, Fox J, Alon US. 2004. Effect of the calcimimetic NPS R-467 on furosemide-induced nephrocalcinosis in the young rat. *Kidney Int.* 65:1684–1689.

Pavlikova N, Kortner TM, Arukwe A. 2010. Modulation of acute steroidogenesis, peroxisome proliferator-activated receptors and CYP3A/PXR in salmon interrenal tissues by tributyltin and the second messenger activator, forskolin. *Chem Biol Interact.* 185:119–127.

Penatti CA, Davis MC, Porter DM, Henderson LP. 2010. Altered GABAA receptor-mediated synaptic transmission disrupts the firing of gonadotropin-releasing hormone neurons in male mice under conditions that mimic steroid abuse. *J Neurosci.* 30:6497–6506.

Peschke E. 2008. Melatonin, endocrine pancreas and diabetes. *J Pineal Res.* 44:26–40.

Petersen OH, Tepikin AV, Gerasimenko JV, Gerasimenko OV, Sutton R, Criddle DN. 2009. Fatty acids, alcohol and fatty acid ethyl esters: toxic Ca²⁺ signal generation and pancreatitis. *Cell Calcium.* 45:634–642.

Peyron C, Sapin E, Leger L, Luppi PH, Fort P. 2009. Role of the melanin-concentrating hormone neuropeptide in sleep regulation. *Peptides.* 30:2052–2059.

Piłat-Marcinkiewicz B, Brzóska MM, Kasacka I, Sawicki B. 2004. Histological evaluation of the thyroid structure after co-exposure to cadmium and ethanol. *Rocz Akad Med Bialymst.* 49(Suppl 1): 152–154.

Popesku JT, Tan EY, Martel PH, Kovacs TG, Rowan-Carroll A, Williams A, Yauk C, Trudeau VL. 2010.

Gene expression profiling of the fathead minnow (*Pimephales promelas*) neuroendocrine brain in response to pulp and paper mill effluents. *Aquat Toxicol*. 99:379–388.

Rangoonwala SP, Kazim M, Pandey AK. 2005. Effects of diazinon on serum calcium and inorganic phosphate levels as well as ultrastructures of parathyroid and calcitonin cells of *Rattus norvegicus*. *J Environ Biol*. 26:217–221.

Rangoonwala SP, Suryawanshi SA, Pandey AK. 2004. Responses of serum calcium and inorganic phosphate levels, parathyroid gland and c cells of *Rattus norvegicus* to heptachlor administration. *J Environ Biol*. 25:75–80.

Ravindra T, Lakshmi NK, Ahuja YR. 2006. Melatonin in pathogenesis and therapy of cancer. *Indian J Med Sci*. 60:523–535.

Rezg R, Mornagui B, Benahmed M, Chouchane SG, Belhajhmida N, Abdeladhim M, Kamoun A, El-fazaa S, Gharbi N. 2010. Malathion exposure modulates hypothalamic gene expression and induces dyslipidemia in Wistar rats. *Food Chem Toxicol*. 48:1473–1477.

Rodriguez M, Lorenzo V. 2009. Parathyroid hormone, a uremic toxin. *Semin Dial*. 22:363–368.

Romero D, Quesada E, Sogorb MA, García-Fernández AJ, Vilanova E, Carrera V. 2006. Comparison of chromaffin cells from several animal sources for their use as an *in vitro* model to study the mechanism of organophosphorous toxicity. *Toxicol Lett*. 165:221–229.

Rosol TJ, Yarrington JT, Latendresse J, Capen CC. 2001. Adrenal gland: structure, function, and mechanisms of toxicity. *Toxicol Pathol*. 29:41–48.

Seilicovich A, Pisera D, Sciascia SA, Candolfi M, Puntel M, Xiong W, Jaita G, Castro MG. 2005. Gene therapy for pituitary tumors. *Curr Gene Ther*. 5:559–572.

Shanle EK, Xu W. 2011. Endocrine disrupting chemicals targeting estrogen receptor signaling: identification and mechanisms of action. *Chem Res Toxicol*. 24:6–19.

Shanmugam MK, Bhatia M. 2010. The role of pro-inflammatory molecules and pharmacological agents in acute pancreatitis and sepsis. *Inflamm Allergy Drug Targets*. 9:20–31.

Shi X, Liu C, Wu G, Zhou B. 2009. Waterborne exposure to PFOS causes disruption of the hypothalamus-pituitary-thyroid axis in zebrafish larvae. *Chemosphere*. 77:1010–1018. Erratum in: *Chemosphere*. 81:821.

Si J, Wu X, Wan C, Zeng T, Zhang M, Xie K, Li J. 2011. Peripubertal exposure to low doses of tributyltin chloride affects the homeostasis of serum T, E2, LH, and body weight of male mice. *Environ Toxicol*. 26:307–314.

Soares-Mota MR, Schwarz A, Bernardi MM, Maiorka PC, Spinosa Hde S. 2010. Toxicological evaluation of 10% *Solanum lycocarpum* St. Hill fruit consumption in the diet of growing rats: hematological, biochemical and histopathological effects. *Exp Toxicol Pathol*. 62:549–553.

Soshin T, Takai H, Kato C, Fujii E, Matsuo S, Ito T, Suzuki M. 2010. A method for sampling and tissue preparation of the parathyroid glands in miniature pigs for toxicity studies. *J Toxicol Sci*. 35:235–238.

Sprague JE, Banks ML, Cook VJ, Mills EM. 2003. Hypothalamic-pituitary-thyroid axis and sympathetic nervous system involvement in hyperthermia induced by 3,4-methylenedioxymethamphetamine (Ecstasy). *J Pharmacol Exp Ther*. 305:159–166.

Stasiak M, Lewiński A, Karbownik-Lewińska M. 2009. [Relationship between toxic effects of potassium bromate and endocrine glands]. *Endokrynol Pol*. 60:40–50.

Sun L, Xu W, He J, Yin Z. 2010. *In vivo* alternative assessment of the chemicals that interfere with anterior pituitary POMC expression and interrenal steroidogenesis in POMC: EGFP transgenic zebrafish. *Toxicol Appl Pharmacol*. 248:217–225.

Swapna I, Senthilkumaran B. 2009. Influence of ethynylestradiol and methyltestosterone on the hypothalamo-hypophyseal-gonadal axis of adult air-breathing catfish, *Clarias gariepinus*. *Aquat Toxicol*. 95:222–229.

Tan SW, Meiller JC, Mahaffey KR. 2009. The endocrine effects of mercury in humans and wildlife. *Crit Rev Toxicol*. 39:228–269.

Thaler JP, Choi SJ, Sajan MP, Ogimoto K, Nguyen HT, Matsen M, Benoit SC, Wisse BE, Farese RV, Schwartz MW. 2009. Atypical protein kinase C activity in the hypothalamus is required for lipopolysaccharide-mediated sickness responses. *Endocrinology*. 150:5362–5372.

Tillitt DE, Papoulias DM, Whyte JJ, Richter CA. 2010. Atrazine reduces reproduction in fathead minnow (*Pimephales promelas*). *Aquat Toxicol*. 99:149–159.

Tubaro A, Dell'ovo V, Sosa S, Florio C. 2010. Yessotoxins: a toxicological overview. *Toxicon*. 56:163–172.

Umegaki H, Yamamoto A, Suzuki Y, Iguchi A. 2009. Responses of hypothalamo-pituitary-adrenal axis to a cholinesterase inhibitor. *Neuroreport*. 20:1366–1370.

Valdez KE, Shi Z, Ting AY, Petroff BK. 2009. Effect of chronic exposure to the aryl hydrocarbon receptor agonist 2,3,7,8-tetrachlorodibenzo-p-dioxin in female rats on ovarian gene expression. *Reprod Toxicol*. 28:32–37.

van den Berg M. 2010. The use of cultured amphibian thyroid glands to detect thyroid hormone disruptors. *Toxicol Sci*. 118:4–6.

Vanattou-Saïfoudine N, McNamara R, Harkin A. 2010. Mechanisms mediating the ability of caffeine to influence MDMA ('Ecstasy')-induced hyperthermia in rats. *Br J Pharmacol*. 160:860–877.

Verma R, Mohanty B. 2009. Early-life exposure to dimethoate-induced reproductive toxicity: evaluation of effects on pituitary-testicular axis of mice. *Toxicol Sci.* 112:450–458.

Wada C, Kataoka M, Seto H, Hayashi N, Kido J, Shinohara Y, Nagata T. 2006. High-turnover osteoporosis is induced by cyclosporin A in rats. *J Bone Miner Metab.* 24:199–205.

Wang H, Storm DR. 2003. Calmodulin-regulated adenylyl cyclases: cross-talk and plasticity in the central nervous system. *Mol Pharmacol.* 63:463–468.

Yellamma K, Saraswathamma S, Kumari BN. 2010. Cholinergic system under aluminium toxicity in rat brain. *Toxicol Int.* 17:106–112.

Zoeller TR. 2010. Environmental chemicals targeting thyroid. *Hormones (Athens).* 9:28–40.

Zoeller RT, Tyl RW, Tan SW. 2007. Current and potential rodent screens and tests for thyroid toxicants. *Crit Rev Toxicol.* 37:55–95.

CHAPTER 22

Toxicity to Reproductive Organs and Developmental Toxicity

This is a chapter outline intended to guide and familiarize you with the content to follow.

I. Reproductive organ and developmental toxicity—see Table 22-1

A. Mutagenic damage

1. Dominant lethal assay—one-fifth of LD_{50} given to male rats mated to untreated females → mutagenic index = number of early fetal deaths/total implants $\times$ 100

2. Toxicogenomics—more recent ability to detect/predict toxic outcomes

B. Epigenetic developmental disruption—see Figure 22-1

1. Many toxicants affect DNA expression without necessarily altering DNA sequences or causing other DNA damage/clastogenesis

2. Most sensitive period is embryonic period of high cell division and epigenetic alterations (DNA is most demethylated at this stage with exception of imprinting genes—remethylated after blastocyst stage based on DNA methyltransferases)

3. Epigenetic factors that can be monitored include non-coding RNA expression, DNA methylation patterns, and alterations of histone proteins

4. Genomic imprinting = one parental allele is inhibited from expressing its allele at one single locus in parental germ stem cells. Angelman's, Beckwith-Wiedemann, and Prader-Willis syndromes; some cancers; and other diseases are associated with dysregulation of imprinted genes. Imprinting genes in primordial germ cells → sperm and egg in male and female, respectively. When these cells enter genital ridge, both imprinted and non-imprinted genes are demethylated prior to sex-specific remethylation of imprinted genes during formation of haploid sperm and oocytes during meiosis. Males develop imprinted pattern at birth, while females wait until egg growth during the arrested time of meiotic prophase I. Following this time, the females eliminate this pattern in the primordial germ cells of next generation

5. Methylation at C-5 position of CpG dinucleotides = best characterized epigenetic alterations (interferes with binding of transcriptional proteins and serves as site for methyl-DNA binding proteins to attach and recruit chromatin remodeling proteins)

6. Arsenic → ↑ pathways associated with NF-κB signaling → inflammation-driven tumor progression and apoptosis → liver cancers of organisms exposed *in utero*; promoter methylation of tumor suppressor gene RASSF 1A = possible cause of human bladder tumors. Hypomethylation of leukocyte DNA ↑ risk of skin lesions

7. BPA (hard plastics) → hypomethylation of phosphodiesterase Type 4 variant → ↑ expression of adult prostate cells (cancer in male rats)

8. Phthalates (soft plastics such as butyl benzyl phthalate) → demethylation of estrogen receptor alpha promoter-associated CpG islands of MCF7 breast cancer cells

---

CONCEPTUALIZING TOXICOLOGY 22-1

9. PAHs → DNA adducts + steroid-like receptor action → ↓ fetal growth and effects on brain development and behavior (AhR alterations); hypomethylation of white blood cell DNA hypermethylation of 5′-CpG islands involved in expression of acyl-CoA synthetase long-chain family member 3 and asthma

10. Tobacco smoke exposure in womb → lower overall DNA methylation in children buccal cells → gene instability and increased mutations but increased methylation of tumor suppressor genes

C. Early male developmental toxicity

1. Sperm development and delivery

a. Genetic variation of CYP19 (aromatase gene encoding for enzyme that converts androgens → estrogen) or paraoxonase gene (encoding for enzyme that prevents LDL oxidation) ↓ sperm counts

b. PAH-exposed Chinese population exhibited affected DNA in tail without altering sperm quality or morphology

c. Combination chemotherapy for cancer (cisplatin, vinblastine, bleomycin) → azoospermia (no measurable sperm) in one-fourth of treated male patients

d. Nonylphenol (environmental estrogen) + ionizing radiation → ↑ abnormal spermatozoa and DNA damage → dead implantations + skeletal malformations in developing organisms when mated to normal females

e. BPA based on hormonal action + oxidative stress → ↓ spermatogenesis and semen quality; phthalate metabolites active in reducing semen quality

f. PCB congener CB-153 → ↓ sperm counts in men with short androgen receptor CAG repeat length

g. Antidepressant SSRI fluoxetine → ↓ spermatogenesis

h. Pb-exposed workers had ↑ plasma inhibin B produced by Sertoli cells in the testes → correlated with ↓ sperm concentration without altering FSH and estradiol; lead exposure to cynomolgus monkeys affected sperm chromatid structure rather than sperm count, viability, or morphology

i. Pesticide agricultural workers → morphological abnormalities of sperm and offspring

j. Sperm effects are not just reproductive concerns as men with poor sperm characteristics → ↑ risk testicular cancer

k. Environmental toxicants gain access to spermatogenesis structures via focal adhesion protein (disrupts junctions by altering signaling pathways via oxidative stress)—see Figure 22-2; other mechanisms affect sperm as indicated by Ca^{2+}-channel blockers, anti-hormone gossypol from cotton seeds (↓ serum testosterone, LH, FSH and testicular 17β-hydroxysteroid dehydrogenase, and 17-ketosteroid reductase in male rat), organophosphates (inhibit AChE and generate ROS), metallothionein induction by Cd (causing Zn deficiency or Zn depletion by a phthalate)

l. Environmental toxicants can disrupt the apical ectoplasmic specialization that prevents spermatids from being released prior to full development (lack acrosomal tip necessary for fertilization and/or tail for motility)

m. Complicating reproductive problems in male are sperm-delivery problems (achieving erection [related to age, hormonal alterations, diabetes mellitus, surgical damage to neurons, antihypertensive medications, radiation therapy, psychogenic agents], emission, and ejaculation)—intact nervous system (CS_2 poisoning) with reasonable blood pressure, and proper libido (altered by tamoxifen or drugs of abuse). Arsenic may play a role here by generating ROS → inactivating NO needed for vasodilation that causes erectile response. Erectile function also is affected by end-stage renal disease (asymmetric dimethylarginine accumulation). Cimetidine (H_2 antagonist used to treat GERD) → impotence

D. Early female developmental toxicity

1. Egg development, maturation, and release—famous effects of old insecticide DDT (and metabolite DDE) → egg shell thinning

CONCEPTUALIZING TOXICOLOGY 22-1 (continued)

2. Concentration dependence

a. 100% effluent from kraft mill (metals + chlorinated organic compounds) → less egg production in fathead minnows while 1% effluent created ovipositors in male fish (feminization), enhanced egg production in females (↑ vitellogenin = egg yolk protein)

b. Sodium hypochlorite bleach had similar toxicity to eggs of *Daphnia* and marine brine shrimp, but glutaraldehyde fixative only had defined LC_{90} to brine shrimp eggs and erratic concentration–response curve to *Daphnia* eggs. Aquatic eggs of this type are exposed directly to toxicants

c. Oviposition (laying eggs) also important in amphibians (decline worldwide) — African clawed frogs exposed to organochlorine pesticide methoxychlor → delay in gonadotropin-induced oviposition and ↓ number of fertilized eggs, with ↑ gonadosomatic index, estradiol/progesterone and estradiol/testosterone ratios. Vitellogenin ↓ at highest concentration of the pesticide

d. ROS appear to be responsible for the mitochondrial damage done to mouse oocytes by As_2O_3 (reversed by N-acetyl-cysteine). They are also toxic to ovarian follicle development and early embryonic toxicity in viviparous organisms. This is true for animals lacking certain genes (*Gpx4*, *SOD1* null, *Ggt1*, *Gclm* null) or exposed to GSH depletion agent buthionine sulfoximide or oxidative chemicals such as H_2O_2, Cr(VI), DMBA, or the cancer chemotherapy alkylating agent cyclophosphamide, and radiation

e. Vinylcyclohexene diepoxide does not work via ROS to cause ovarian damage but rather affects key apoptotic signaling pathways

f. Organophosphates malathion and diazinon → ↓ fetal mouse oocyte survival and regulation of genes involved in transcription (BP75), translation (ribosomal protein S5), and mitochondrial energy production (cytochrome oxidase subunits I and III)

E. Fertilization

1. Pb and other heavy metals affect sperm DNA and have other untoward effects on fertilization; Pb inhibits mannose-induced acrosome reaction and ↓ ability of sperm to penetrate/fertilize egg

2. *p,p′*-DDE → failed fertilization after *in vitro* fertilization, also ↑ aromatase activity and therefore premature estradiol production, which affects oocyte maturation

3. DES or other organic solvents → ↓ implantation rate of *in vitro* fertilization; smoking also ↓ outcomes of *in vitro* fertilization

4. Benzo[a]pyrene prevents conception

5. Dibenzodioxins and dibenzofurans → ↑ lethality at eight-cell stage of embryo, but ↑ blastocyst formation in a dose-dependent manner in survivals

6. ROS (from heavy metals and other compounds) → disrupts cell membrane integrity → alters receptor binding, steroidogenesis and hormone production; ROS also affect sperm DNA ↓ sperm count (fertilizing capacity)

F. Embryo toxicity/fetal toxicity

1. Not specific to stage of development

a. The A/D ratio and the Relative Teratogenic Index assumed that most chemicals caused maternal toxicity in viviparous animals that led to developmental effects. This is too simplistic as the fungicide dinocap in the mouse → cleft palate, otolith defects, and fetal weight deficits at doses < those that affected maternal health. There are chemical differences as well — dimethyltriazine yields malformations when given at day 14 but not day 10 of rat development, while diethyltriazine gives opposite results (affects at day 10 but not day 14). In birds a complicating factor is that heavy metals, petrochemicals, and pesticides affect the avian embryos more than the adults due to bioaccumulation in the yolk

b. Nonspecific effects would affect all stages of development, and organisms develop anatomically from superior (brain) to inferior (heart → limbs → external genitalia). Late development may involve fusion of bones (such as the palate). Sensitive embryonic periods in the human would be 3–5 weeks in womb (heart = 3.5–6.5 weeks, legs 4.5–8 weeks at

CONCEPTUALIZING TOXICOLOGY 22-1 (*continued*)

beginning of fetal period, ear 4th–14th week of gestation, eyes 4.5–10 weeks, teeth and palate 6th–12th week, external genitalia 7th–15th week). Chemicals that may affect all periods are DNA-damaging alkylating agents, intercalating agents, amino acid antagonists, and microtubule poisons

2. Specific to stage of development

   a. Thalidomide and limb deformities—amelia (loss of limbs) or phocomelia (reduction in long bones) associated with binding to cereblon protein (E3 ubiquitin ligase complex), preventing limb outgrowth and expression of fibroblast growth factor Tgf8 in zebrafish and chickens

   b. Glucocorticoids and cleft palate—dexamethasone passes the maternal blood–placental barrier and binds to the glucocorticoid cytoplasmic receptor → ↓ proliferation of mesenchymal cells of the palate due to ↑ lactate, alanine CH_3, acetate glutamine, glutamate, lipid $CH_2CH_2CH=CH$, choline $N(CH_3)^{3+}$, and creatine, while arginine, valine, lipid $-C=C-CH_2-C=C$, aspartic acid, and myo-inositol ↓. These amino acid alterations reflect changes in maternal methyl group metabolism, with S-adenosyl methionine being the key methyl donor. ↑ Creatine → ↑ ATP → alters the methylation of methionine to homocysteine (maternal factor accounting for cleft palate)

   c. DES and reproductive abnormalities—vaginal cancers in female offspring caused by direct binding to ERα and ERβ as well as indirect effects on the hypothalamic-pituitary-adrenal axis. Male effects appear to be related to ↓ expression of genes *GATA4* and *ID2* associated with sexual maturation

   d. Ethanol and fetal alcohol syndrome—neurological effects mediated through redistribution of L1 cell adhesion molecule in lipid rafts at concentrations similar to those that prevent L1-mediated neurite outgrowth. Kidney effects mediated through disruption of action of vitamin A as retinoic acid (↓ ureteric branch bud point tips and alters receptor tyrosine kinase signaling pathway in those bud tips). However, acetaldehyde (ethanol metabolite via alcohol dehydrogenase) can act as a nonspecific DNA-damaging agent apart from the specificity of alcohol's direct effects. Maternal genes play a significant role in the developmental effects of ethanol. Changes in the dopaminergic mesolimbic system in combination with genetic and epigenetic alterations in the developing organism may also play a role in alcohol addiction and reinforcement behavior. Some also point to the role of oxidative stress in the developmental neural toxicity of ethanol as indicated by the restoration of alterations on the expression of transcription factor nuclear factor (erythroid derived 2)-like 2 by the antioxidant resveratrol acting on redox-regulating proteins in rodents

   e. Cocaine—most damage to dopamine (DA)-rich and subcortical brain regions. Parvalbumin immunostaining (expressed in inhibitory neurons and is very susceptible to oxidative stress) in layers two and/or three of prefrontal cortex are observed. ↑ Apical dendrite length in pyramidal neurons in DAergic tracts of cortical areas. DA D1 receptor (coupled to Gsα that activates adenylyl cyclase) involved in cocaine developmental neurotoxicity. Cocaine also appears to be embryotoxic (↓ number embryos surviving past morula stage) and genotoxic (more micronuclei)

   f. Retinoids—especially (*E*)-4[2-(5,6,7,8-tetrahydro-5,5,8,8-tetramethyl-2-naphthalenyl)-1-propenyl]benzoic acid—bind to retinoic acid receptor preventing embryonic stem cell differentiation into cardiomyocytes. Toxicity prevented by retinoic acid receptor antagonist Ro 41-5253. Abnormalities involve microphthalmia, encephalopathy, spina bifida, limb abnormalities, and cleft palate. Last toxicity produced by ↓ expression of Bone Morphogenetic Protein Receptor-1B and Smad5 (Smad 5 is a key factor in the signal transduction mediating TGFβ inhibition of the proliferation of human hematopoietic progenitor cells) mRNA induced by osteogenic medium in the differentiation of mouse embryonic palate mesenchymal cells

   g. Valproic acid—antiepileptic compound induces incomplete closure of neural tube (spina bifida aperta) in humans. Cardiac, limb, and neurodevelopmental problems also found in humans exposed during development. Cardiomyocyte differentiation and gene expression tests uncovered that myosin heavy chain gene and cardiac tissue-specifying homeobox gene Nkx2.5 were affected by valproic acid and analogues with the exception of (±)-2-ethyl-4-methyl pentanoic acid. Microarrays in a mouse embryo model also found genes encoding for CYP26A1 (regulates retinoic acid by 4- and 18-hydroxylation), Fgf15 (fibroblast growth

CONCEPTUALIZING TOXICOLOGY 22-1 (*continued*)

factor 15 regulates the expression of Otx2 in developing mouse brain), Gja1 (gap junction protein), Hap1 (Huntingtin-associated protein 1 binds to mutant huntingtin protein based on glutamine content), H1f0 (a histone protein expressed during differentiation), Lin7b (helps establish and maintain the unequal distribution of channels and receptors in polarized cells' plasma membranes), Otx2 (homeobox protein OTX 2 involved in brain development whose overexpression found in childhood brain cancers), and Sall2 (zinc finger protein). Altered expression of these genes may be responsible for malformations and/or cancer in developing organisms

  h. Partial AChE inhibition and sensory neuron development—a lower nonlethal dose of chlorpyrifos-oxon exposure to zebrafish embryos caused a significant inhibition of AChE and aberrant peripheral axon extension and gene expression profiling in Rohon-Beard sensory neurons

G. Late male developmental toxicity

  1. Famous study of alligators in Lake Apopka, Florida due to a spill of dicofol contaminated with DDT and metabolites → ↓ penis size in male alligators and ↑ plasma testosterone in males and females (+ ↓ egg mass in females, hatchling mass and snout vent—female hatchlings had smaller spleens)

  2. Atrazine exposure to *Xenopus laevis* larvae → genetic male amphibians to be hermaphroditic and have less masculine features on the larynges

  3. Estrogenic organochlorine pollutants affect behavior of breeding gulls. Similar estrogenic compounds also result in behavioral abnormalities affecting precopulatory pairs of amphipods or fish. This change in behavior is also found in mammals (rats) exposed to BPA or TCDD. Increased male mating behavior also may result from PCB exposure in the kestrel (falcon). Fathead minnows exposed to estrogen or sewage treatment plant effluent were less likely to compete for a nest with competing males and had ↑ vitellogenin and ↓ 11-ketotestosterone as physiological signs of feminization

H. Late female developmental toxicity

  1. Species differences—many animals such as rats have estrous periods ("heat") that are not similar to the human. Additionally, some animals give birth to litters (cats, dogs, rats, etc.), while human females rarely have multiple births. The rabbit, alpaca, ferrets, mink, cat, and otters do not have an estrous cycle but will release an egg on sexual stimulation and/or mating call of the male. In birds the default sex produced is a male following fertilization, barring any other hormonal signals, while human females default to making a female in the absence of testosterone production by the fetus. These differences indicate difficulties in interpreting animal models for prediction of human female late developmental toxicity

  2. Estrogenic agents—gulls respond to *o,p′*-DDT, methoxychlor, and DES in a manner similar to estrogen. Hydroxylated PCB congeners have similar activity in birds based on induction of liver microsomal enzymes and trapping more water-soluble metabolites in avian eggs. Alkyl phenols cause fish to synthesize vitellogenin

  3. Decreased nest attentiveness and reduced incubation of the eggs can follow exposures of the dove to DDE/PCB mixtures resulting in poor reproductive outcomes

I. Reproductive/developmental tests—see Table 22-2

  1. Reproductive indices/tests—mating index, fertility index, gestation index, live birth index, sex ratio, 4-day survival index, lactation index, preweaning index. Other concerns are human sperm counts, male hypospadias (unusual urethral opening), cryptorchidism (undescended testicle), and testicular cancer. Rise in infertility is a key concern of the EPA. There are single and multigenerational tests to insure that toxicity is observed in subsequent generations. Reproductive organs are weighed and examined for histopathology following exposure. Exposing one sex versus the other is important, as are prenatal and postnatal exposures. Following through the preweaning period may lead to effects occurring due to transfer of toxicants in the milk. Sexual behavior endpoints (such as lordosis in female rats) are necessary to indicate neurotoxicity or endocrine action of toxicants. Couple-mediated endpoints are mating rate and time to mating/time to pregnancy, pregnancy rate, delivery rate, gestation length, total and

CONCEPTUALIZING TOXICOLOGY 22-1 (*continued*)

living litter size, number of live and dead offspring or fetal death rate, offspring gender or sex ratio, birth weight, postnatal weights, offspring survival, external malformations and variations, and offspring reproduction for multigenerational studies. Other endpoints for reproductive toxicity are ovulation rate, fertilization rate, pre-implantation loss, implantation number, internal malformations and variations, and postnatal structural and functional development. Male-specific endpoints are weights, visual examination, and histopathology of testes, epididymides, seminal vesicles, prostate, and pituitary. Sperm count, morphology, and motility are included. Mounting, intromissions, and ejaculations round out the behavioral tests for male reproductive toxicity. LH, FSH, testosterone, estrogen, and prolactin are the measured hormones that may be disrupted. Testis descent, preputial separation, sperm production, ano-genital distance, and structure of external genitalia complete the male-specific endpoints. Female-specific endpoints involve organ weights, visual examination, and histopathology of the ovaries, uterus, vagina, and pituitary. However, the visual examination and histopathology also extend to the oviducts and mammary glands. Vaginal smear cytology indicates estrous cycle normality. Lordosis, time to mating, vaginal plugs, and sperm are measures of sexual behavior. LH, FSH, estrogen, progesterone, and prolactin are measured hormone levels that may be disrupted in the female. Offspring growth, milk quantity, and milk quality quantify affected lactation. Normality of external genitalia, vaginal opening, vaginal smear cytology, and onset of menstruation mark development problems, while vaginal smear cytology and ovarian histology (menopause) indicate senescence and the completion of female-specific reproductive testing. Rounding out other possibilities for testing are *in vitro* studies (e.g., sperm, egg) and human epidemiology reports

2. Developmental toxicity endpoints—developmental toxicity encompasses the death of a developing organism, structural abnormality, altered growth, or functional deficiency. Maternal toxicity endpoints are mortality, mating index, fertility index, gestation length, body weight (day 0, during gestation, day of necropsy), body weight change (throughout gestation, during treatment and discrete periods during treatment, post-treatment to euthanizing, maternal weight corrected for weight of gravid uterus, and litter weight), organ weights (absolute, relative to body weight, relative to brain weight), food and water consumption if relevant, clinical measurements (types, incidence, degree, and duration of clinical signs of toxicity, enzyme markers, and clinical chemistries), and gross necropsy and histopathology. Behavioral endpoints (conditioned learning) indicate developmental neurotoxicity. Establish a reference concentration for developmental toxicity of an oral dose (RfD_{DT}) or inhalation (RfC_{DT}), no-observed-adverse-effect level (NOAEL) and/or lowest-observed-adverse-effect level (LOAEL). A benchmark dose (BD) is also established similar to other toxicity modeling by the EPA. This is done by assessing where a 10% ↑ in abnormalities of development is found. This is divided by the uncertainty factor to establish the RfD_{DT} or RfC_{DT}, depending on the route of administration

3. Sperm chromatid structure assay—denatured and acridine orange–stained DNA used in combination with flow cytometry indicate DNA fragmentation (red staining single-stranded and green staining double-stranded DNA). Biological significance reached at ≥ 30% DNA fragmentation

4. Fish assay—Fish early life-stage test requires 360 fish and 1–3 months of analysis. A full lifecycle of toxicity is evaluated/predicted but mechanisms not necessarily provided. See model for strong AhR agonist (TCDD), neurotoxic AChE inhibitor (chlorpyrifos), and narcotic surfactant (linear alkylbenzene sulfonate) in Figure 22-3

5. *In vitro* models—the European Union has validated three *in vitro* models—the rat micromass test, the post-implantation rat whole-embryo culture test, and the embryonic stem cell test (embryonic fibroblasts, BALB/c-3T3, and embryonic stem cells, ES-D3, examining cell proliferation and cytotoxicity). First two tests require animal tissue for analysis

6. ToxCast high-throughput screening data—chemical library of 309 unique structures based on *in vivo* data supporting chronic/cancer, multigenerational/reproductive, or prenatal effects. Each compound was overwhelmingly soluble in the solvent DMSO, commercially available with > 90% purity and a molecular weight of 250–1,000 (fits pesticides well). Developmental defects caused by these chemicals were included into the ToxCastDB database from ToxRefDB *in vivo* (mainly from studies of pregnant rats and rabbits and reproductive and cancer studies including specific abnormalities and developmental LEL and categorical LEL) or ToxCast *in vitro* assay results. The

CONCEPTUALIZING TOXICOLOGY 22-1 (*continued*)

ToxCast high-throughput model includes platforms such as real-time cell electronic sensing in human A549 cells, transcriptional activity with multiplexed reporter genes in human HepG2 liver cells, primarily evaluating inflammatory responses using ELISA in a mixture of human primary cells, cellular HCS evaluating markers such as stress pathways, mitochondrial involvement, cell cycle, cell loss, mitotic arrest, the cytoskeleton in human HepG2 liver cells, transcriptional upregulation of genes involved in metabolism using primary human hepatocytes, nuclear receptor activity (gene reporter assays) in human embryonic kidney HEK 293 cell lines, biochemical enzyme inhibition and receptor-binding assays in a cell-free format, and MESC cytotoxicity and cardiomyocyte differentiation. Six hundred sixty-two *in vitro* high-throughput assays were compared to a training set of chemicals. The statistical results indicated better than a 70% accuracy in predicting the potential to cause developmental toxicity *in vivo*, but also reinforced the need to have individual species-specific models for predicting developmental toxicity in rats and rabbits, determining specific effects on signal transduction mechanisms or other cellular targets that can be linked to a specific developmental toxicity endpoint, clustering toxicity endpoints based on similar biological or developmental processes/stages, establishing role of xenobiotic metabolism in these developmental toxicity endpoints (as it does impact toxicity), and having a clear *in vivo* dose–response in the assay characteristics

CONCEPTUALIZING TOXICOLOGY 22-1 (*continued*)

This chapter explores the application of data regarding the effects of toxicants on the ovaries and testes and endocrine disruption to gain an understanding reproductive function. Oviparous animals need to lay eggs with intact shells, but this can be disrupted by the infamous pesticide used in the mid-20th century, dichlorodiphenyltrichloroethane (DDT). Viviparous organisms need intact maternal physiological systems and placental transfer of nutrients and oxygen. These disruptions plus disruption of embryonic and fetal development are examined in this chapter. Also, agents that cause lack of fertilization, inability of an embryo to implant in the womb, and inability of the mother to deliver the organism must be considered. Indices of reproduction are also investigated, including mating index, fecundity, male fertility, female fertility, incidence of parturition, resorptions, live organisms at birth, and survival up to 21 days postpartum. Additionally, malformations (used to be called teratology for the "study of monsters") are discussed.

Formation of the sperm and delivery of the nuclear material within is the most important function of the male. Also, using activated enzymes on the sperm tip to have one sperm gain entrance to the egg for fertilization is important. See **Table 22-1** for reproductive system and developmental toxicity.

TABLE 22-1 Forensic Chart of Reproductive System/Developmental Toxicity	
Reproductive System Toxicity	**Toxic Agents**
Genetic	Mutagens that may act based on the genes expressed or available for attack at that time or delayed based on effects on germ cell genes that will be nonfunctional later
Epigenetic	Gene expression changes during development caused by a variety of agents that act as signals or change signaling via DNA methylation patterns, including mutagens such as products of combustion/smoke such as PAHs acting similar to steroids, heavy metals such as As, chemicals used in the manufacture of plastics (bisphenol A, phthalates; Perera and Herbstman, 2011)

(*continues*)

TABLE 22-1   Forensic Chart of Reproductive System/Developmental Toxicity (*continued*)

Reproductive System Toxicity	Toxic Agents
Male sperm	
DNA	PAHs (Han et al., 2011), nonylphenol, X-irradiation (Dobrzyńska, 2011), Pb (Foster et al., 1996)
Spermatogenesis and semen quality	Bisphenol A (Li et al., 2011), phthalates (Hauser et al., 2006), DDE and PCB congener CB-153 (Bonde et al., 2008), fluoxetine (Bataineh and Daradka, 2007), Pb (Mahmoud et al., 2005), pesticides (Hanke and Jurewicz, 2004), medications such as sulfasalazine (Linares et al., 2011), nifedipine (Waghmare et al., 2011), gossypol (El-Sharaky et al., 2010), electromagnetic radiation (Agarwal et al., 2008), oxidative stress from bisphenol A, TCDD, Cd and disruption of cell junctions and adhesions of Sertoli cells and seminiferous tubules (Wong and Cheng, 2011), Zn deficiency induced by metallothionein inducers and other agents interfering with testicular Zn absorption (Daston et al., 1994; Thomas et al., 1982), cytotoxic cancer chemotherapy (Hansen, 1992), organophosphates (Bustos-Obregón and Recardo, 2008)
Male impotence	
Libido	Tamoxifen and aromatase inhibitors (Visram et al., 2010)
Erectile dysfunction	Medications, ionizing radiation, As (Hsieh et al., 2008), drugs of abuse (kava; Rychetnik and Madronio, 2011), CS2 (Frumkin, 1998), asymmetric dimethylarginine (Kielstein and Zoccali, 2005), cimetidine (Sawyer et al., 1981)
Female	
Oviparous: eggshell fragility	DDT/DDE (Bernanke and Köhler, 2009)
Egg production/viability	Kraft mill effluent (Werner et al., 2010), sodium hypochlorite, glutaraldehyde (Raikow et al., 2007), methoxychlor (Pickford and Morris, 2003)
Viviparous: Oocyte	As (mitochondrial damage; Zhang et al., 2011), organophosphates (Bonilla et al., 2008), Buthionine sulfoximide, 4-vinylcyclohexene diepoxide, cyclophosphamide, ionizing radiation, Cr, PAHs, methoxychlor (Devine et al., 2012)

Developmental System Toxicity	Toxic Agents
Fertilization	Heavy metals, organochlorines, PAHs, DES, organic solvents (Kumar and Mishra, 2010)
Nonspecific embryo toxicity/GLEMEDS	Heavy metals, petrochemicals, pesticides, dioxins (organochlorines; Fry, 1995)
Specific embryonic/fetal development	Thalidomide (Ito et al., 2010), glucocorticoids (Zhou et al., 2011), DES (Alwis et al., 2011; Larocca et al., 2011; Nakamura et al., 2008), ethanol (Alfonso-Loeches and Guerri, 2011; Gilliam et al., 2011; Gray et al., 2011; Kumar et al., 2011; Langevin et al., 2011; Tang et al., 2011), cocaine (Del Valle et al., 2008; Thompson et al., 2010), retinoids (Chen et al., 2010; Louisse et al., 2011), valproic acid (de Jong et al., 2011; Kultima et al., 2010)
Late male development	DDT and testosterone enhancement/reduced alligator penis size (Milnes et al., 2005), atrazine and hermaphroditism of amphibians (Hayes et al., 2002)
Behavior	DDT, mirex, PCBs, lindane, ethinyl estradiol, bisphenol A, endosulfan, octylphenol, phenol, vinclozolin, methoxychlor, bisphenol A, TCDD (Clotfelter et al., 2004), sewage effluent, estradiol, methyltestosterone (Martinović, 2007)
Feminizing (germ cells in cortex), vitellogenin synthesis	o,p′-DDT, methoxychlor, DES, estrogen, alkyl phenols, isoflavonoid phytoestrogens (Fry, 1995)
Late female development	
Behavior	DDT/DDE, PCBs, dioxins (Clotfelter et al., 2004)
Right oviduct partial regression	o,p′-DDT, methoxychlor, DES, estrogen (Fry, 1995)

Mutagenic Damage

One of the earliest ways of detecting genetic mutations in the sperm was the dominant lethal assays. A high dose (one-fifth of the LD_{50}) was given to male mice or rats that were then mated to untreated females. Fourteen days following mating the females were examined for early and late fetal deaths, corpora lutea, and total implantation. The mutagenic index was equal to the number of early fetal deaths/total implants $\times$ 100 (Epstein, 1973). Now, it is possible to predict many other toxic outcomes through toxicogenomics using gene expression analyses (Daston and Naciff, 2010).

Epigenetic Developmental Disruption

A good model of an epigenetic analysis of critical periods in development is presented in **Figure 22-1**. In this case, gene expression is altered apart from any changes in DNA sequence. Here critical periods in development appear early during the embryonic period of high cell division and epigenetic alterations. Epigenetic factors that can be monitored include non-coding RNA expression, DNA methylation patterns, and alterations of histone proteins. One of the best understood mechanisms involving epigenetics during mammalian development is that of genomic imprinting, in which one parental allele is inhibited from expressing its allele at one single locus in parental germ stem cells. This allows only one chromosome of the XX associated with the human female karyotype to be inactivated at the very start of embryogenesis. Angelman's, Beckwith-Wiedemann, and Prader-Willis syndromes; some cancers; and other diseases are associated with dysregulation of imprinted genes. The best characterized epigenetic alterations include the addition of a methyl group to the C-5 position of cytosine in CpG dinucleotides (DNA methylation), although histone

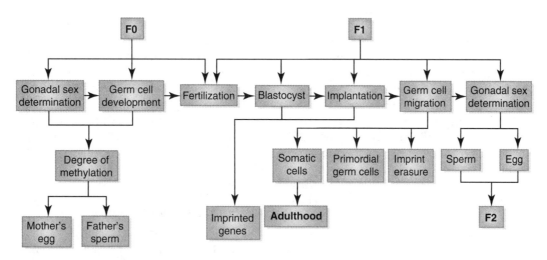

FIGURE 22-1 Developmental Toxicity Periods from an Epigenetics Approach

Note: F_0 is the parental generation for formation of the father's sperm (solid blue line) and mother's ovum (solid red line) and a time when methylation of DNA is reprogrammed. After fertilization/conception, the F_1 offspring's embryonic development starts. During this period, all genes excepting imprinted genes are demethylated. Male genes (dotted blue lines) precede female genes (dotted red line) in demethylation rate. Meanwhile, imprinted genes' (solid purple line) consistent methylation pattern confers parental-specfici monoallelic expression to the new generation's somatic tissues through their adult life. At the blastocyst stage, remethylation of non-imprinted genes occurs. Determination of gonadal sex of this embryo occurs with the epigenetic reprogramming of primordial germ cells as the parental imprinting is eradicated. The sperm (solid blue) and egg (solid pink) allow for normal gamete development. Abnormal development favors secondary sexual characteristics of female despite male genes as indicated by the pink line prior to sex differentiation. The gonadal cells of the fetus represent the F_2 generation's genetic starting points. However, the F_3 generation is necessary to study any true multigenerational inherited disorders from toxicant exposure.

protein posttranslational modifications and micro-RNA-induced suppression of gene expression during development are important as well. As proximal gene promoter regions overlap with CpG regions, DNA methylation becomes a form of gene regulation by interfering with binding of transcription proteins. It also serves to provide a site for methyl-DNA binding proteins to attach and recruit chromatin remodeling proteins. Demethylation of DNA following fertilization and prior to the blastocyst stage allows access of the embryo to many genes with the exception of imprinted genes, which maintain the parents' pattern for the life of the organism. This is necessary for normal development. However, the activity of DNA methyltransferases DNMT3a and DNMT3b remethylate the DNA after the blastocyst stage. Normal development also depends on DNMT1, which maintains the methylation patterns and returns hemimethylated CpG sites to full methylation status.

The imprinted genes in primordial germ cells will ultimately become sperm and egg in male and female mammals, respectively. When they enter the genital ridge, this time the imprinted along with the non-imprinted genes are demethylated prior to sex-specific remethylation of imprinted genes during formation of the haploid sperm and oocytes during meiosis. The males develop their imprinted pattern around birth, while females do so during egg growth during the arrested time of meiotic prophase I. The females then eliminate this pattern in the primordial germ cells of the next generation.

When scientists examine the periods when DNA is less protected, it appears that the early embryonic period is most susceptible, followed by the period following birth when somatic cell methylation patterns may be altered by exogenous chemicals in conjunction with childhood developmental patterns of the organism. The chemicals that do epigenetic damage show the following patterns of toxicity (Perera and Herbstman, 2011).

Arsenic

Arsenic is known for liver cancers of organisms exposed *in utero*. It appears that umbilical cord blood in children born to arsenic-exposed mothers shows a substantial increase in pathways associated with NF-κB signaling. This would promote inflammation-driven tumor progression as well as apoptosis. Promoter methylation of the tumor suppressor gene RASSF 1A suggests a possible cause for As-linked human bladder tumors. Hypomethylation of leukocyte DNA appears to increase risk of As exposure and skin lesions.

Bisphenol A

Bisphenol A (BPA) is used in the manufacture of hard plastics and has recently been viewed as a potential hazard to babies drinking from bottles that leach BPA into their drinks. Exposure to BPA during development has increased prostate intraepithelial (male) cancer in rats and shows methylation changes possibly consistent with this disease (hypomethylation of phosphodiesterase Type 4 variant resulting in increased expression in adult prostate cells).

Phthalates

These plasticizers are known for their endocrine disruption (antiandrogen and proestrogen). One effect that seems to fit this profile is the demethylation of estrogen receptor alpha (ERα) promoter-associated CpG islands in MCF7 breast cancer cells exposed to butyl benzyl phthalate. Exposure of rats to di(2-ethylhexyl) phthalate during sexual differentiation caused male reproductive tract malformations associated with abnormal expression of insulin-like growth factor, *c-kit ligand*, and leukemia inhibitory factor genes.

Polycyclic Aromatic Hydrocarbons

In addition to the direct formation of DNA adducts by metabolically activated polycyclic aromatic hydrocarbons (PAHs), these chemicals appear to be similar in molecular size and action to hormones synthesized from cholesterol on steroid receptors. PAHs have been associated with a wide variety of disorders including decreased fetal growth and effects on brain development and behavior (may be related to altered expression of glutamate receptor subunits, which is involved in long-term potentiation as a cellular expression of learning and memory). Also, recall the effects of PAHs as inducers of the AhR with regard to the metabolic activation in the adult liver. AhR alterations have developmental implications for the brain cells (benzo[*a*]pyrene altered neurotransmitters dopamine, norepinephrine, and serotonin and their metabolites in specific brain areas; reduced expression of NMDA receptor subunit *NMDAR2B*; reduced long-term potentiation across the hippocampal perforant path granular cell synapses; and upregulated the pro-inflammatory and reactive oxygen species [ROS]–generating enzyme COX-2 in rat astrocytes) and lymphocytes (increase pro-inflammatory cytokines such as interleukin-1 beta [IL-1β], tumor necrosis factor alpha [TNFα], interferon gamma [IFN-γ]. and chemokine CCL1). Umbilical cord blood of exposed newborns indicates hypomethylation of white blood cell DNA, which appeared to persist through at least 3 years of age. Asthma was also analyzed via methylation-sensitive restriction fingerprinting. It appears that the acyl-CoA synthetase long-chain family member 3 involved in fatty acid metabolism contains 5′-CpG islands that are sensitive to methylation alterations. Hypermethylation appears to be the problem in asthmatic children exposed to PAHs *in utero*.

Tobacco Smoke

DNA methylation patterns in genomic DNA from buccal cells in children exposed to tobacco smoke in the womb indicate much lower overall DNA methylation leading to gene instability and increased mutations, but some increased methylation in gene-specific regions such as tumor suppressor genes. This trend seems to be found in various cancers. Also, asthma seems to be indicated in the grandchildren of women who smoked during pregnancy. This type of multigenerational effect is similar to the effects of diethylstilbestrol on uterine cancer of the F_2 generation.

Early Male Developmental Toxicity

Male developmental toxicity may start with sperm formation for the next generation and proceed into the embryonic development and organogenesis that lead to fetal development. As the sex hormones play a role, then the development of sex organs and gametes completes the cycle for that generation.

Sperm Development and Delivery

Male infertility can come from numerous sources such as not making sperm, having dysfunctional sperm, inability to achieve erection, and so forth. For example, semen quality has indeed been seen to drop since the early 1980s in a nonindustrialized human population of Spain as indicated by decreased semen volume with increased sperm motility, yet decreased motile density per ejaculate (Corrales et al., 2011). This kind of effect between people can either be genetic or induced by changes in gene expression. For example, a genetic variant in the CYP19 (aromatase) gene that encodes for the enzyme that converts testosterone (androgens) into estrogen(s) creates men with lower sperm counts and lower sperm motility (Lazaros, Xita, Kaponis, et al., 2011). Variants in the paraoxonase gene encoding for an enzyme that prevents low-density lipoprotein (LDL) oxidation appears to be associated with oligospermic (low sperm counts) men (decreased PON1 55L/L, PON1 192Q/Q, and PON2 311S/S genotypes and increased PON1 55M, PON1 192R, and PON2 311C alleles). Correlates include PON1 55M and PON1 192R with lower sperm motility and PON2 311C with decreased concentration as indicators of semen quality alterations by genetic variants (Lazaros, Xita, Hatzi, et al., 2011).

The toxicologist's challenge is decipher the basis of the decrease in sperm counts reported in this and other Western human populations during the 20th century and whether it represents chemical exposure, stressful living, or a combination of factors (te Velde et al., 2010). Some chemicals do indeed affect sperm DNA and not semen quality or sperm morphology as indicated by analysis of human sperm DNA comet assay. In a PAH-exposed population in China, urinary 2-hydroxynaphthalene was associated with increased percentage of DNA in the tail (tail%) and 1-hydroxypyrene with increased tail% (Han et al., 2011). It would be expected that combined chemotherapy for germ cell cancer with DNA adduct-forming agent cisplatin, microtubule formation inhibitor vinblastine, and induction of DNA strand-breaks by bleomycin would lead to serious damage to sperm formation and induce azoospermia (no measurable sperm in semen samples) in more than one-fourth of the male patients and low sperm counts and subclinical Leydig cell dysfunction of the majority of males treated with this combination (in addition to the more serious damage done to the kidney, nervous system, and terminal arterioles; Hansen, 1992). Nonylphenol is an environmental estrogen that may not look on first glance like it should cause DNA damage. However, when nonylphenol (50 mg/kg) ± 0.05 Gray of ionizing radiation (X-rays) was given as a subchronic 8-week exposure to male mice, the percentage of abnormal spermatozoa increased and DNA damage was noted. The sperm also decreased the percentage of pregnant females, although the fertilizing ability did not decrease. Instead, it was noted that dead implantations per pregnant female and skeletal malformations were manifested in the developing organisms (Dobrzyńska, 2011). Therefore, it is not so easy to predict effects of chemicals based on their expected mutagenicity, such as ionizing radiation, or epigenetic effects that a steroid hormone-like substance may have.

BPA has been shown to reduce spermatogenesis and semen quality (sperm concentration, counts, vitality, and motility) in humans and animals. It appears that this chemical is known to have estrogenic and antiandrogenic (androgen receptor antagonist) effects, and a proposed mechanism of oxidative stress has been put forward to explain some of its untoward actions (Li et al., 2011). Urinary metabolites of dibutyl phthalate (monobutyl phthalate) and butyl benzyl phthalate (monobenzyl phthalate) were correlated with semen quality of human males. The monobutyl phthalate was associated with low sperm concentration and motility, while the highest concentrations of monobenzyl phthalate appeared to reduce sperm concentration (Hauser et al., 2006). Persistent organic pollutants (p,p'-DDE and polychlorinated biphenyl [PCB] congener CB-153) also had correlations of effects on human semen quality. For example, PCB congener CB-153 was associated with low sperm counts in men with short androgen receptor CAG repeat length. This PCB congener was also found in higher concentration in men exhibiting low sperm motility, and may indicate post-testicular effects of lower α-glucosidase activity. European men also had more frequent damage to their sperm chromatin integrity than Inuit in response to p,p'-DDE and CB-153. This did not noticeably affect fertility in European men, but the presence of these chemicals appeared to affect Inuit fertility more (Bonde et al., 2008).

A medication that affects spermatogenesis is the famous antidepressant selective serotonin reuptake inhibitor fluoxetine. When this drug is administered at 200 mg/kg to rats over a 60-day period, it highly reduced spermatogenesis in seminiferous tubules of the testes and lower sperm motility and density (lower primary and secondary spermatocytes and spermatids) in the cauda epididymides and testes. The testes, epididymides, ventral prostate, and seminal vesicle were also smaller in treated rats. Testosterone and follicle-stimulating hormone (FSH) were also lower. Fluoxetine also caused the male to impregnate fewer females, resulting in fewer implantations and viable fetuses (Bataineh and Daradka, 2007).

It is expected that metals affect male reproduction. Lead is a toxic metal usually associated with neurological or blood cell effects. However, lead workers at a smelter in Belgium had higher plasma levels of inhibin B produced by Sertoli cells in the testes. This correlated with decreased sperm concentration without significantly affecting FSH or estradiol levels (Mahmoud et al., 2005). However, environmentally relevant levels of lead exposure to cynomolgus monkeys caused no significant effects on circulating testosterone levels or sperm count, motility, viability, or morphology (semen quality). Instead, disturbing changes in sperm chromatid structure were noted (Foster et al., 1996). Agricultural workers had specific morphological abnormalities of sperm with decreased sperm count and percentage of viable sperm. Also, more malformations of their offspring occurred, including orofacial cleft, hemangioma birthmarks, and defects in the musculoskeletal and nervous systems consistent with pesticide exposure (Hanke and Jurewicz, 2004). Infertility and abnormal semen analysis indicate more severe cellular problems as human men with these poor characteristics also have a 20-fold increase in the risk of testicular cancer (Raman et al., 2005). Chemicals alone may not be the sole cause of changes in semen quality: Increased cell phone use (non-ionizing radiation) appears to decrease sperm count, motility, viability, and normal morphology. The electromagnetic waves may do so via specific effects, a thermal molecular effect, or both (Agarwal et al., 2008).

Mechanistically, how do scientists separate infertility caused by a variety of environmental chemicals? The migration of the developing sperm is complex and offers many points for chemical influence. The spermatogonia ($2n$) migrate through the gateway of the tight junctions that open for them to travel between Sertoli cells toward the lumen of the seminiferous tubule. Once past this juncture, they are considered primary spermatocytes ($2n \times 2$) and mature via meiotic division (meiosis I) into secondary spermatocytes ($n \times 2$). After a second meiotic division (meiosis II) further down through the channel between the Sertoli cells, the spermatids (n) mature into spermatozoa with a head, midpiece, and tail. They then are released into the seminiferous tubules. They remain immotile for approximately 20 days in the human and acquire motility as they mature through the seminiferous tubules to the epididymis. They move via peristalsis from the epididymis to the vas deferens where they await sexual arousal, emission, and ejaculation. This process is controlled by the hormones FSH, testosterone, and estrogen, which are produced by the pituitary gland, and the Leydig and Sertoli cells of the testes, respectively. This makes the process very susceptible to not only mutagens during the division process but also to endocrine disruptors.

The blood–testes barrier prevents circulating antibodies from recognizing the sperm and damage to this barrier would be problematic for normal sperm formation. The barrier consists of tight junction, desmosome, gap junction, and testis-specific adherens junction (basal ectoplasmic specialization composed of actin filament bundles between layers of plasma membrane and the cisternae of endoplasmic reticulum of two neighboring Sertoli cells). The presence of focal adhesion protein unfortunately makes this a gateway for environmental toxicants. The apical ectoplasmic specialization anchors the developing spermatids in the seminiferous epithelium until they are completely developed. Environmental toxicants can disrupt this anchoring, prematurely releasing morphologically incomplete sperm that lack an acrosomal tip necessary for fertilization and/or a tail for motility.

Discerning the nature of each chemical is difficult, because, for example, BPA or PAHs act as endocrine receptors (endocrine disruptors) and can activate non-genomic membrane estrogen receptor–initiated signal transduction pathways. However, compounds such as BPA, 2,3,7,8-tetrachlorodibenzo-p-dioxin (TCDD), or cadmium can also generate oxidative stress pathways in the testes by initially downregulating antioxidant enzymes such as catalase, Se-dependent glutathione peroxidase, and catalase. ROS generate damage to various macromolecules such as carbohydrates, DNA, lipids, and proteins. This oxidative stress also is implicated in damage to the cell junctions and adhesion between neighboring Sertoli cells and/or Sertoli-germ cells through altered phosphatidylinositol 3-kinase (PI3K)/c-Src/focal adhesion kinase, which mediates the ability of epithelial cells to lose their junctional structure and polarity so that they can migrate similar to mesenchymal cells. This alteration in PI3K occurs in oxidative stress due to the translocation of the regulatory subunit PI3K p85 from the cytosol to the cell–cell interface. PI3K then stimulates a nonreceptor tyrosine kinase c-Src located at the blood–testes barrier and apical endoplasmic specialization. This localization allows this pathway to interact with connexin43/plakofilin-2 and β1-integrin/lamininα3β3γ3 protein complexes at the cell junctions. Other untoward effects may be manifested through the mitogen-activated protein kinase (MAPK) signaling pathway and cytokine signaling with cross-talk through internalization of polarity proteins.

The whole complex scheme for disruption of cell junctions via oxidative stress and altered signaling pathways is illustrated in **Figure 22-2**. The phosphorylation of adherens junction proteins through the PI3K/c-Src/FAK pathway by any mechanism leads to the internalization of the adherens junction proteins and breaks them loose from their adaptors. The association of c-Src and Par6/Pals complex keeps them apart from JAM-C rendering the Jam-C-based adhesion protein complexes unstable. This is a molecular mechanism underlying the premature release of incomplete sperm mentioned earlier. These chemicals have other actions as well. Cd activates MAPK p38 and decreases cell

proliferation, while increasing DNA damage and apoptosis in primary pig Sertoli cells. BPA stimulates MAP kinases ERK, ZJNK, and p38 and increases the activity of aromatase and COX-2, increasing PGE2, while decreasing the testosterone level and activation of protein kinases A and B in rat Leydig cells. TCDD influences the same three MAP kinases in mouse testes while decreasing the activity of antioxidant enzymes or Smad2 activation, but increases c-Jun and ATF3. PAHs affect mouse testes by decreasing spermatid number, testosterone, and the antioxidant enzyme superoxide dismutase (SOD). The summary of these chemicals' action usually is separated into epigenetic effectors such as vinclozolin or endocrine disruptors such as BPA, cadmium, or TCDD. However, it appears that many of their actions through oxidative

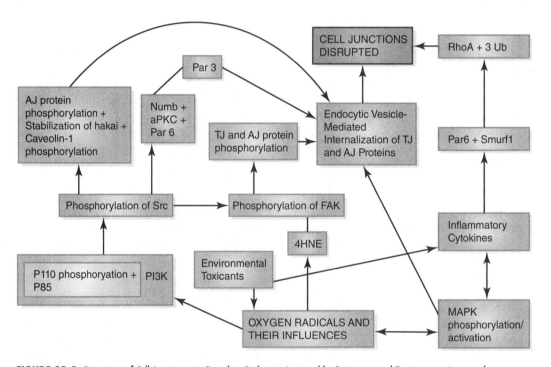

FIGURE 22-2 Disruption of Cell Junctions via Signaling Pathways Activated by Environmental Toxicants via Increased Oxidative Stress

Note: Disruption of cell junctions via signaling pathways activated by environmental toxicants via increased oxidative stress. Oxidative stress activates PI3K/c-Src/FAK pathway→caveolin-1 phosphorylation, tight junctions &/or adherens junctions proteins, stability of E3 ubiquitin ligase Hakai, & interaction of polarity proteins with endocytic adaptor Numb→ internalization of tight junctions (TJ) & adherens junctions (AJ) proteins at cell–cell interface. Another oxidative stress pathway: down-regulation &/or inactivation of integrins at apical ES, a testis-specific anchoring junction type→ feedback mechanism to dephosphorylate FAK. Aldehydes (e.g. 4-OH-2-nonenal) produced during oxidative stress inactivate FAK. Another pathway involves production of cytokines regulated by the activation of MAPK via oxidative stress. Cytokines→ ↑ROS from leukocytes to further increase oxidative stress. Cytokines & activation of MAPK together→ endocytic vesicle-mediated internalization of TJ & AJ proteins. Polarity proteins (e.g.)Par6 are also involved in mediating the action of cytokines to recruit E3 ubiquitin ligase Smurf1 for polyubiquitination and degradation of RhoA, which is important for disruption of cell junctions. This illustrates that crosstalk exists between the PI3K/c-Src/FAK and cytokines/MAPK pathways via polarity proteins as their common downstream signaling mediators.

stress and altered signal transduction disrupt the integrity of the Sertoli and seminiferous cells via targeting the polarity proteins (Wong and Cheng, 2011).

Sperm motility can be affected reversibly by oxidative stress such as induced by sulfasalazine (Linares et al., 2011), calcium-channel blockers such as nifedipine (Waghmare et al., 2011), and by natural toxic agents such as gossypol $(1,1',6,6',7,7'$-hexahydroxy-5,5′ diisopropyl-3,3′dimethyl-[2,2′] binaphthalenyl-[8,8′] dicarbaldehyde) isolated from cotton seeds. Gossypol has been considered as a natural antifertility agent but should not be considered benign because it causes decreased sperm count, sperm motility, serum levels of testosterone, and luteinizing hormone (LH) and FSH in male albino rats, while it increased the activities of testicular 17β-hydroxysteroid dehydrogenase and 17-ketosteroid reductase. It also damages testicular and hepatic tissue (El-Sharaky et al., 2010). Organophosphates that inhibit acetylcholinesterase (AChE) will affect sperm via a number of mechanisms. Necrospermia and teratozoospermia primarily of the tail are found in organophosphate toxicity with increased apoptotic cells and vacuolization of the seminiferous epithelium and with most profound influence on primary spermatocytes. Organophosphates also lead to chromatin damage that may be related to their generation of ROS (as in parathion biotransformed into paraoxon; Bustos-Obregón and Recardo, 2008).

Cadmium's effects, if given to the pregnant mother during development, may also be explained by Zn deficiency caused by metallothionein induction in the liver of the mother. Inducers of metallothionein such as α-hederin, urethane, or Cd may at least partially explain their toxicity to the developing organism and male testes function by causing Zn deficiency (not the cancer induced directly but deficiency states would augment dysplasias of the gonads; Daston et al., 1994). One plasticizer famous for this depletion of Zn from the rat testes is di(2-ethylhexyl) phthalate and its resultant damage to the sensitive (more so than the mouse) rat prostate gland (Thomas et al., 1982).

The delivery of sperm via emission and ejaculation depends on an intact nervous system, correct hormones and behavior on desire and ability to mate, and blood pressure/vasodilatory mechanisms for erection. The importance of the intact nervous system is made by chronic exposure of a human to carbon disulfide poisoning, which led to impotence, irritability, and problems with balance as part of olivopontocerebellar (multiple-system) atrophy (Frumkin, 1998). Impotence may be the label given to a variety of disorders of sexual reproductive function in the male. It may make sense that surgical or medication treatment for prostate cancer has led to male impotence. However, a weak estrogen (tamoxifen) given for male breast cancer led to decreased libido in ~13% and erectile dysfunction in ~8% of human males treated with this medication at an Ottawa, Canada cancer center over a 20-year period. Third-generation aromatase inhibitors anastrozole and letrozole had fewer reported effects on libido and overall toxicity despite disruption of the endocrine system (Visram et al., 2010). Erectile dysfunction is mostly associated with age, hormonal alterations/disruption (such as androgen deprivation therapy for treatment of nonmetastatic prostate cancer; Higano, 2003), diabetes mellitus, surgical damage to neurons, adverse effects of medication (such as antihypertensive drugs such as beta-blockers and thiazide diuretics), radiation therapy, and psychogenic agents/factors. The key enzyme for erection appears to be nitric oxide synthase (NOS) isoforms in the corpus cavernosum as NO mediates the dilation of the vascular smooth muscle. Drugs of abuse, such as kava, also play a role in loss of sexual drive or impotence in males (Rychetnik and Madronio, 2011).

It may not be obvious how the toxic heavy metal As may play a role in impotence. However, its role in cardiovascular disease may be related to NOS activity. It appears that As-exposed human males in Taiwan had higher rates of erectile dysfunction associated with lower testosterone levels. It may be that oxygen radicals generated by As inactivate NO and reduce its physiological action (Hsieh et al., 2008). Certain other cardiovascular toxicants, such as asymmetric dimethylarginine accumulation in end-stage renal disease, also lead to problems with erectile function and fertility in addition to their more serious effects on cardiovascular function (that may lead to death), cerebral blood and neural function, insulin resistance, thyroid dysfunction, and bone homeostasis (Kielstein and Zoccali, 2005). Cimetidine, a histamine (H_2) antagonist that decreases acid production, was found in the early 1980s to cause cardiovascular, central nervous system (CNS), dermatologic, endocrine, gastrointestinal (GI), hematological, or renal damage on overdose and these effects alone would have reproductive implications. However, its effects on impotence and oligospermia in older men made the concern for younger men with unimpaired hepatic or renal function a concern for long-term treatment of gastroesophageal reflux disease (Sawyer et al., 1981).

Early Female Developmental Toxicity

Female developmental toxicity is more complex than that of males, because the eggs develop in the fetus prior to birth in viviparous organisms; therefore, influences on the maternal system may be more profound for female development and multigenerational effects. Because mitochondrial inheritance is only through a matrilineal system, energy metabolism that leads to the egg cleavage rate and later proper aerobic metabolism of the neonate and onward may be attributable to alterations in female development.

Egg Development, Maturation, and Release

In oviparous animals, especially birds, chemicals such as DDT/DDE cause eggshell thinning and reduce the ability of the organism to reproduce via this mechanism alone (Bernanke and Köhler, 2009). The production of eggs can also be influenced in oviparous fish for instance. For example, fathead minnows exposed to 100% effluent from a bleached kraft mill containing various metals and chlorinated organic compounds that produce endocrine disruption produced fewer eggs. On the other hand, exposure to 1% effluent created ovipositors in male fish and enhanced the production of eggs and liver somatic index due to increased deposition of vitellogenin, a key protein of egg production and index of

estrogenic activity of chemicals or chemical mixtures. This indicates that effects can increase or decrease production of eggs or reproduction based on dose and chemical composition of the exposure fluid to the maternal system while having negative consequences associated with the endocrine disruption in either case (Werner et al., 2010). Chemical biocides appear to cause variable toxicity to invertebrate species' eggs. For example, while sodium hypochlorite (bleach) was similarly toxic to resting eggs to *Daphnia mendotae* and marine brine shrimp (*Artemia* sp.), glutaraldehyde had a defined LC_{90} to the brine shrimp eggs but caused an erratic concentration–response curve with *Daphnia* (Raikow et al., 2007). The environment the egg is released into is also important for both oviparous and viviparous organisms. An aquatic egg can contact pesticides or other environmental chemicals directly (Pašková et al., 2011). A normal egg, sperm, zygote, or blastocyst from a mammal placed in the uterus of an animal or human with diabetes mellitus increases the risk that this developing organism will experience this disease (Ahmed, 2011). This shows that the egg's environment is important to its ability to develop outside the organism in oviparous organisms and inside the uterine horn or uterus of mammals. It is also important to assess the effects of endocrine disruptors on the oviposition (laying eggs) of amphibians, which appear to be in decline worldwide. Exogenous gonadotropin-induced oviposition was determined in *Xenopus laevis* females exposed to 0.5–500 μg methoxychlor (pesticide)/L. There was a delay in the gonadotropin-induced oviposition and reduced numbers of fertilized eggs in African clawed frogs exposed to the highest concentration of this pesticide. The reduced egg output reflected the increased gonadosomatic index in treated frogs. Estradiol/progesterone and estradiol/testosterone ratios were elevated post-oviposition and progesterone synthesis in ovarian explants (*ex vivo*) of methoxychlor-treated frogs. The egg yolk protein vitellogenin was significantly reduced at the highest concentration of the pesticide. In total, it appears the endocrine disruption led to reproductive toxicity in these amphibians (Pickford and Morris, 2003).

Arsenic is a metal whose toxicity has been described earlier. An oxidized form of arsenic, As_2O_3, is a compound that does severe mitochondrial damage with a 3867 base pair deletion in the susceptible mitochondrial DNA. ROS is apparently responsible for this damage as N-acetyl-cysteine eliminated the ROS, decreased the mitochondrial DNA damage, and restored more adenosine triphosphate (ATP) content in mouse oocytes (Zhang et al., 2011). Organophosphates malathion (250 μM) and diazinon (900 nM) affected cultured 10-day fetal mouse oocyte survival after 24 hours of exposure and the regulation of genes encoding for proteins involved in transcription (BP75), translation (ribosomal protein S5), and mitochondrial energy production (cytochrome oxidase subunits I and III; Bonilla et al., 2008).

The entire ovarian follicle should be considered in viviparous organisms. ROS play a major role in the toxicity for follicle development and early embryonic toxicity. Transgenic mice lacking the antioxidant enzyme glutathione peroxidase gene (Gpx4) yielded embryo lethality, while those only lacking the nuclear or mitochondrial form of this enzyme did not affect female fertility. It is interesting that lacking mitochondrial Gpx4 caused males to have highly reduced spermatogenesis and male fertility. Mice lacking superoxide dismutase (SOD1 null) show either reduced pre-ovulatory follicles and corpora lutea or increased postimplantation embryonic lethality depending on the species. Mice without the γ-glutamyl transpeptidase 1 (Ggt1) are affected in their ability to have a normal lifespan and have complete female infertility with decreased "ovarian large antral follicles, corpora lutea, and ovulatory response to exogenous gonadotropins" (Devine et al., 2012, page 27). Cysteine replacement works to reverse the lack of Ggt1. The inability of mice to synthesize glutathione (GSH) due to the absence of glutamate cysteine ligase (Gclm null) causes embryos to die prior to gestational day 8.5. However, the oocyte concentrations of the females of this mouse strain have much lower fertility and fewer than one-fifth of the oocytes of normal mice. Further evidence for the role of GSH on protection of the antral follicles is provided by treatment of adult cycling

rats with two doses of 5 mmol/kg of buthionine sulfoximide. GSH dropped by > 50%, and there was an increase in atretic antral follicles. Hydrogen peroxide at concentrations ≥ 3 mM caused pyknotic cell development in an ovarian culture system, but did not show morphological changes in the primary and small primary follicles until concentrations exceeded 6 mM H_2O_2.

4-Vinylcyclohexene diepoxide—a metabolite of the volatile byproduct of chemical synthesis 4-vinylcyclohexene that causes reductions in primordial and smallest primary follicles possibly via apoptotic signaling pathways, MAPK/AP-1 signaling, and KIT/KIT ligand signaling. Generating ROS or other oxidative stress do not seem to be how vinylcyclohexene diepoxide causes ovarian damage. However, the cancer chemotherapy alkylating medication cyclophosphamide appears to not only cause double-stranded DNA breaks, but also generates ROS. There have been reports in humans of depletion of the ovarian follicle pool causing permanent infertility (Meirow and Nugent, 2001; Howell and Shalet, 1998). In mice cyclophosphamide damages primordial and primary follicles, which does not appear to be related to apoptosis. On the other hand, adult rats exposed to this alkylating agent show damage to secondary and antral follicles via an apoptotic mechanism. It is of interest that human granulosa cells also show this apoptosis-induced toxicity via ROS generation from cyclophosphamide exposure. Because ROS appear to be involved in ovarian damage, it is of no surprise that ionizing radiation destroys small and antral follicles in rats, mice, and the rhesus monkey. Radiation treatment of women will produce a temporary lack of menstrual periods by damaging growing follicles, but not complete loss of fertility by sparing some of the primordial follicle pool. Chromium (especially Cr[VI] in drinking water) generates oxidative stress and follicular atresia in adult mice.

Other compounds show that apoptosis pathways lead to follicle damage. In rat granulosa cells, Cr stimulates the expression of proapoptotic BCL2 family proteins and phosphorylation of TRP53 and MAPK3/1, while reducing expression of antiapoptotic BCL2 family proteins and AKT. These events lead to caspase 3 and PARP cleavage and time-dependent increase in apoptotic cell death. PAHs appear to damage primordial and primary follicles via an increase in apoptosis and generating ROS. The compound 9,10-dimethyl-1,2-benzanthracene (DMBA) in the presence of antiapoptotic concentrations of FSH is toxic to antral follicles at ≥ 1 µM in culture. DMBA stimulates expression of proapoptotic protein BAX and caspase 3 activation. DNA fragmentation is also noted by TUNEL staining 48 hours into DMBA exposure. Treatment of mice with an organochlorine pesticide methoxychlor at ≥ 32 mg/kg for 20 days induced atresia of antral follicles without similarly affecting primordial, primary, or secondary follicles. Apoptosis played a role as indicated by an increase in *Bax* mRNA prior to atresia. Signs of ROS-induced damage were indicated by increased hydrogen peroxide, oxidative protein (nitrotyrosine immunostaining), and DNA damage (8-hydroxy-2′-deoxyguanosine immunostaining; Devine et al., 2012).

Fertilization

Human seminal fluids contain Na, Mg, P, K, Ca, Fe, Cu, Zn, Se, Rb, and Sr. More than 75% of seminal fluids also contain V, Mn, Co, As, Mo, Cd, Sn, and Ba. Pb, Cd, Hg, nicotine and/or cotinine, and trichloroethylene and its metabolites (chloral and trichloroethanol in the semen of mechanics) were also found in specific individuals, especially with occupational exposure or cigarette exposure. Follicular fluids of females were found in a similar manner to contain cotinine, benzo[*a*]pyrene, PCBs (isomers with 3–7 atoms of chlorine), *p,p′*-DDE, mirex, hexachloroethane, 1,2,4-trichlorobenzene, Cd, BPA, and dioxins and benzofurans. This means that many toxic substances may interfere with the environment in which fertilization occurs. It should not be surprising therefore to find that lead and other heavy metals affect *in vitro* fertilization through sperm DNA damage and other toxicity. Pb levels are higher in non-pregnant patients compared with successful pregnancies, and lead negatively impacts sperm biomarkers such as mannose receptors and mannose-induced acrosome reactions. *p,p′*-DDE leads to failed fertilization after *in vitro* fertilization. Diethylstilbestrol (DES) exposure *in utero* decreases the implantation rate

of *in vitro* fertilization. Similar results of poor implantations were found in women partnered to men exposed occupationally to high concentrations of organic solvents. Pesticides appear to have the opposite effect, resulting in a higher implantation rate. Benzo[*a*]pyrene appears to prevent conception. Smoking also decreases the outcomes of *in vitro* fertilization. It appears the dioxins and benzofurans are lethal to a population of eight-cell stage embryos, but the survivors accelerated blastocyst formation in a dose-dependent manner. Thus, early embryonic development rather than fertilization per se appears to be affected. DDE stimulates the aromatase enzyme leading to premature production of estradiol, which is known to affect oocyte maturation. One can anticipate either a positive or negative consequence of this action complicating the prediction of fertility outcomes.

Some of the mechanisms behind poor fertilization take the discussion back to the generation of ROS related to heavy metal exposure. The gametes certainly are susceptible to this kind of damage. But if the whole organism is taken into consideration, ROS disrupt membrane integrity of cells. This can lead to changes in receptor binding, steroidogenesis, and hormone production. DNA damage of sperm and apoptosis of these cells lead to decreased ability to generate sufficient normal sperm to fertilize. Add to this the ability of Pb to interfere with the mannose-induced acrosome reaction and fertilization becomes impossible or at the least far less likely. In conclusion, effects on gametes, fertilization mechanisms, implantation, and early embryonic development all appear as decreases in fertility that are difficult to tease out in a human population (Kumar and Mishra, 2010).

Embryo Toxicity/Fetal Toxicity

Not Specific to Stage of Development

Back in the 1980s there was some belief that the adult-to-development (A/D) ratio could explain the effects of most chemicals that caused developmental damage. The assumption of this and the relative teratogenic index was that most chemicals caused maternal toxicity in viviparous organisms that resulted in embryonic or fetal effects. Unfortunately, this was too simple, because some chemicals confounded the A/D ratio. For example, the fungicide dinocap in the CD-1 mouse caused cleft palate, otolith defects, and fetal weight deficits at doses considerably lower than those that caused maternal toxicity. It would be expected from Sprague-Dawley rats and Syrian golden hamsters that the A/D ratio would be 1. However, the mouse has an A/D ratio of 8–16, meaning that the developmental toxicity develops at a dose 8- to 16-fold below that which causes adult toxicity (Rogers, 1987). Thus, the species selected and the specific chemical are important in determination of which chemicals indeed are more cytotoxic and therefore less stage-specific and those that are more dependent on specific mechanisms that are more susceptible to attack during certain periods of development than overall toxicity to the maternal adult animal. Because the animal develops effectively from superior to inferior, the brain development would be influenced first followed by heart and so on to the reproductive functions and the limbs. However, late functions may also involve fusion of some bones such as the palate (and the development of cleft palate in those exposed to a nonspecific cytotoxic agent at that point in the fetal period).

In the late 1970s, an article indicated that the first 2 weeks of human development involve the developing zygote and implantation of the bilaminar embryo and that this was not usually a period during which developmental toxicants have an impact (Harbison, 1978). Major morphological deformities would be expected in the embryonic period from 3–7 weeks post-fertilization. The most sensitive period for CNS development would be between 3 and just beyond 5 weeks in the womb. The sensitive heart formation period would be from 3.5 weeks to just beyond 6.5 weeks. The arms and legs would be most sensitive to toxic influences from 4.5 weeks to the beginning of the fetal period at 8 weeks. The ear has the longest sensitive period from a little beyond the 4th week to the 14th week of gestation. From 4.5 to about 10 weeks the eyes are most sensitive (goes a couple of weeks into the fetal period). The

teeth and palate are nearly the same, starting their sensitive periods at somewhere late in the 6th week and proceeding into the 12th week. The external genitalia are last starting their most sensitive period at the 7th week and proceeding to 15 weeks post-conception. Following the embryonic period, the fetal period from 8 weeks to full term (38 weeks) may have physiological alterations and more minor changes in organ size or structure. However, arresting the development of the brain is always noticeable, because lead poisoning in children shows that the ability to learn extends beyond birth. The development of the eyes and secondary sex characteristics also proceeds to full term, so changes may yield some deficits in these areas as well. Now, the term *cytotoxic* may indicate to some that all these agents that inhibit DNA or RNA or protein synthesis have the same action and the same effect at the same developmental period. However, in pregnant rats dimethyltriazine yields malformations when given on gestational day 14 but not day 10, while diethyltriazine is developmentally toxic on day 10 but not day 14. It appears that one cannot truly make a good correlation between the LD50, carcinogenicity, and developmental toxicity. Some agents are both mutagenic and cause developmental deformities, such as DNA-damaging alkylating agents (e.g., cyclophosphamide and nitrogen mustard), electrophiles (although some mainly damage the liver based on metabolism, e.g., aflatoxin), antimetabolites (e.g., methotrexate and azathioprine), intercalating agents (e.g., actinomycin D, chloroquine), amino acid antagonists (e.g., asparaginase, azaserine), and microtubule poisons (e.g., colchicine or vinca alkaloids or miscellaneous chemicals such as the preservative formaldehyde or the paint additive urethane). Less problematic would be caffeine (Harbison, 1978).

In birds, there is a classification of embryo malformations from toxic chemicals exposure in the wild. More toxic agents such as heavy metals, petrochemicals, and pesticides affect avian embryos more than adults due to bioaccumulation in the yolk. Dioxins (or organochlorines as a whole) and selenium appear to fit the bioaccumulation model. Toxicity seen for sublethal doses is found subcutaneously (edema) and in the heart (edema and malformations), malformed beaks, and axial skeleton abnormalities termed GLEMEDS (Great Lakes embryo mortality, edema, and deformity syndrome; Fry, 1995).

Specific to Stage of Development

Thalidomide and Limb Deformities

Back in the 1950s and early 1960s, a sedative medication used for treating morning sickness in pregnant women started showing startling signs of limb malformations in children born to these women, including loss of limbs (amelia) or reduction in long bones of the limbs (phocomelia). There were other reported effects on the heart, eye, GI tract, and kidney. For 50 years, it was unclear as to the mechanism involved, and there were reports of interference with nutrients, energy metabolism, nucleic acid synthesis, oxidative stress, and antiangiogenic activity. A more recent report (Ito et al., 2010) identified cereblon as a thalidomide-binding protein. Cereblon is part of an E3 ubiquitin ligase complex with damaged DNA binding protein 1 and another protein (Cul4A). This ubiquitin ligase activity, which is inhibited by thalidomide, is necessary for limb outgrowth and expression of fibroblast growth factor Tgf8 in zebrafish and chickens (Ito et al., 2010).

Glucocorticoids and Cleft Palate

The palate closes late in fetal development. A number of factors and toxicants can generate cleft palate including smoking, overdoses of vitamin A, and deficiency in folic acid and B vitamins. Glucocorticoid-induced palate was reported more than 40 years ago (Sato, 1963; Pinsky and Di George, 1965) and continues to be studied through dexamethasone receptor levels as they influence palatal and lung fibroblasts. This investigation has taken on some new techniques such as metabonomics or the combination of ^{1}H-NMR spectroscopy and multivariate statistics to examine dynamic multivariate metabolic responses to toxicity or genetic expression alterations. Key events that can be interrupted causing cleft palate are growth, elevation, contact, and fusion (no longer can find

the medial edge epithelial cells). Dexamethasone is a glucocorticoid that passes the maternal blood–placental barrier and binds to its (glucocorticoid) cytoplasmic receptor. This activation of the receptor reduces proliferation of mesenchymal cells in the palate. The cleft arises from the small size of the palate halting development of bilateral palates. In the 21-day gestation of the mouse, plate shelves grow and elevate to a horizontal position by day 14. By day 17, fusion should have been completed in the absence of a toxic or genetic influence. Some mice are more susceptible to cleft palate, which may be due to high maternal plasma homocysteine concentrations or reduced 11β-hydroxysteroid dehydrogenase type 2 (glucocorticoid pre-receptor metabolizing enzyme) in placental trophoblastic cells. The metabonomic analysis revealed alterations of maternal metabolites that correlate with cleft palate formation in a specific mouse strain (C57BL/6J). The shift in the ^{1}H-NMR spectrum indicated increases in the metabolites lactate, alanine CH_3, acetate, glutamine, glutamate, lipid $CH_2CH_2CH=CH$, choline $N(CH_3)^{3+}$, and creatine, while arginine, valine, lipid $-C=C-CH_2-C=C$, aspartic acid, and myo-inositol decreased in the dexamethasone group. The decreases in arginine and increases in alanine, N-acetyl glycoprotein, choline, and creatine may result from an alteration of maternal methyl group metabolism. The key methyl-donating amino acid is S-adenosyl methionine, which is formed from methionine. ATP may increase from increased creatine, which would then influence methylation from methionine to homocysteine. These alterations may account for cleft palate formation (Zhou et al., 2011).

DES and Reproductive Abnormalities

DES can disrupt the maternal system in a number of ways. It directly causes the female hamster to have changes in uterine and cervical dimensions, ovarian polyovular follicles, vaginal hypospadias, and endometrial hyperplasia/dysplasia. Indirectly, DES induces ovarian/oviductal salpingitis and cystic ovarian follicles. Changing endocrine status is a combination of direct and indirect influences of DES (circulating levels of 17β-estradiol, LH, and FSH). The lack of corpora lutea in hamsters due to DES was of unclear origin. In human females who were exposed to DES *in utero*, various reproductive abnormalities of a similar nature resulted, including neoplasia, infertility, and poor pregnancy outcomes. It is clear from this study that direct changes to reproductive organs are possible along with key indirect effects on the hypothalamic-pituitary-adrenal axis that could explain these developmental results (Alwis et al., 2011). DES appears to bind at low concentrations (10^{-10} M) to for ERα and ERβ. The female mouse exposed in the womb to DES shows disorganized uterine musculature, ovary-independent vaginal epithelial cell proliferation, and persistent EGF- and IL-1-related genes due to binding of DES to ERα as indicated by the effects of ERα agonist propyl pyrazole thiol. Polyovular follicles appear to be mediated by both ERα and ERβ as indicated by effects of the ERα agonist and ERβ agonist diarylpropionitrile at 10^{-9} M (Nakamura et al., 2008). The male reproduction system appears to be altered by DES, but not BPA, exposure by reduced expression of genes *GATA4* and *ID2* associated with sexual maturation (Sertoli cell differentiation; Larocca et al., 2011).

Ethanol and Fetal Alcohol Syndrome

Fetal alcohol syndrome occurs via a variety of mechanisms. However, many of its neurological effects appear to be mediated through redistribution of the L1 cell adhesion molecule in lipid rafts at concentrations similar to those that prevent L1-mediated neurite outgrowth (Tang et al., 2011). Ethanol's effects on kidney development may be through disrupting the action of vitamin A as retinoic acid is a key to renal development and prevents the ethanol-induced reduction in ureteric branch point tips. Gene expression shows that ethanol alters enzyme expression involved in metabolism of ethanol and kidney development, including cRET (receptor tyrosine kinase signaling pathway expression at ureteric bud tips; Gray et al., 2011). However, some support the role of the ethanol metabolite acetaldehyde as a nonspecific DNA-damaging agent that results in a variety of effects that are known as fetal alcohol syndrome. It appears that Aldh2 (aldehyde dehydrogenase 2 is the critical metabolism enzyme

of this toxicant) is essential for development of Fanconi anemia DNA repair pathway-deficient embryos (Fancd2(-/-); Langevin et al., 2011). This last finding is of interest, because it seems that the maternal genes in mice determine the skeletal (shortened digits) and perhaps kidney and vertebral (fusions) effects of ethanol. Transferring ethanol-susceptible or more resistant mice into the womb of a susceptible maternal system made that mouse more susceptible as if it shared the maternal genes. This indicates that the environment in the womb (how the mother responds to ethanol or metabolizes ethanol) appears to have the most effect on the outcome of the developing organism (Gilliam et al., 2011). This does not downplay the direct or indirect roles of ethanol and its metabolite acetaldehyde on excitotoxicity, free radical formation, and neuroinflammatory damage. In adult and adolescent brains, activation of the innate immune system appears to mediate neuroinflammatory reactions via TLR4 receptors. Membrane proteins are affected by ethanol and influence neurotransmitter receptors such as NMDA and GABA-A, ion channels such as L-type Ca^{2+} channels and GIRKs, and signaling pathways such as PKA and PKC signaling. For example, changes in the dopaminergic mesolimbic system in combination with genetic and epigenetic alterations may be responsible for alcohol addiction and reinforcement behaviors (Alfonso-Loeches and Guerri, 2011). Some also argue for a prooxidant effect of ethanol as indicated by the neuroprotection offered by resveratrol (3,5,4'-trihydroxy-trans-stilbene), an antioxidant phytoalexin found in red grapes and blueberries, against ethanol's neural developmental toxicity. Resveratrol restores the changes caused by ethanol on the expression of transcription factor nuclear factor-erythroid derived 2-like 2 (nfe2l2 or Nrf2) by acting on redox-regulating proteins in rodents (Kumar et al., 2011).

Cocaine

"Crack cocaine babies" are very irritable and have neurobehavioral deficits. A variety of animal models including a rabbit model of intravenous prenatal cocaine exposure indicate problems with brain development. Specifically, dopamine-rich and subcortical brain regions suffer the most toxicity. Cellular alterations include increased dendritic-expressed parvalbumin immunostaining (inhibitory neurons express this substance and are highly susceptible to oxidative stress) in layers two and/or three of the prefrontal cortex. Apical dendrite length is increased in pyramidal neurons in dopaminergic tracts of the cortical areas. The interneurons that express parvalbumin appear to be the ones affected by this medication/drug of abuse. It appears that dopamine D1 receptor is involved in this toxicity. More distinctly, it appears that Gsα (heterotrimeric G protein subunit that activates adenylyl cyclase) coupling to the D1 receptor is reduced due to the sequestration of the dopamine receptor (Thompson et al., 2010). A two-cell stage mouse embryo bioassay appeared to reveal that cocaine base paste was embryotoxic (reduced number of embryos progressing through the compacted morula stage) and genotoxic (produced more micronuclei as determined by Tarkowski's technique; Del Valle et al., 2008).

Retinoids

Retinoids prevent embryonic stem cell differentiation into cardiomyocytes based on their concentration in the medium. The most potent of the retinoids appears to be (E)-4[2-(5,6,7,8-tetrahydro-5,5,8,8-tetramethyl-2-naphthalenyl)-1-propenyl]benzoic acid compared with retinol, all-*trans*-retinoic acid, 13-*cis*-retinoic acid, 9-*cis*-retinoic acid, etretinate, and acitretin. Similar findings for potencies occurred in the limb bud micromass assay and the post-implantation whole-embryo culture system. These appear to be related to binding to the retinoic acid receptor, because Ro 41-5253, a retinoic acid receptor antagonist, prevented these *in vitro* developmental toxicities. Similar findings for producing any malformations in the rat, mouse, or rabbit were found for the comparative potencies of retinoids. It appears that the *in vitro* assays are good at interpreting *in vivo* findings of all malformations (e.g., microphthalmia, encephalopathy, spina bifida, limb abnormalities) or cleft palate only when the species differences in absorption, distribution, metabolism, and excretion are known (Louisse et al., 2011). Retinoids, such as all-*trans*-retinoic acid appear to work during the organogenesis process. For example, all-*trans*-retinoic acid inhibited the expression of Bone Morphogenetic Protein Receptor-1B and Smad5 (Smad 5 is a key factor in the signal transduction mediating TGFβ inhibition of the proliferation of human hematopoietic progenitor cells) mRNA induced by osteogenic medium in the differentiation of mouse embryonic palate mesenchymal cells. This is a model for palatogenesis or the induction of cleft palate by certain developmental toxicants (Chen et al., 2010). In all cases, it appears that retinoids interfere with signal pathways that mediate differentiation of cells.

Valproic Acid

The exposure during pregnancy of antiepileptic medication valproic acid yields incomplete closure of the neural tube (exencephaly and anencephaly in mice, spina bifida aperta in humans). In rats, cardiac malformations have been found as well. Humans exposed during development also show cardiovascular, limb, and neurodevelopmental problems. The last is most expected during to the pharmacological action of valproic acid. More recent models such as the embryonic stem cell test have screened for the potencies of various valproic acid analogues on cardiomyocyte differentiation and gene expression. Myosin heavy-chain gene and cardiac tissue-specifying homeobox gene Nkx2.5 were affected by valproic acid and analogues with the exception of (±)-2-ethyl-4-methyl pentanoic acid (de Jong et al., 2011). More molecular markers are able to be identified using microarrays in a mouse embryo model of valproic acid–induced developmental toxicity. Candidate target genes included CYP26A1 (encodes for a cytochrome P450 superfamily member that regulates retinoic acid levels by 4-hydroxylatiion and 18-hydroxylation; retinoic acid is involved in embryonic and adult gene expression), Fgf15 (fibroblast growth factor 15 regulates the expression of Otx2 in developing mouse brain), Gja1 (gap junction protein), Hap1 (Huntingtin-associated protein 1 binds to mutant huntingtin protein based on glutamine content), H1f0 (a histone protein expressed during differentiation), Lin7b (helps establish and maintain the unequal distribution of channels and receptors in polarized cells' plasma membranes), Otx2 (homeobox protein OTX 2 involved in brain development whose overexpression is found in childhood brain cancers), and Sall2 (zinc finger protein). The importance of the identification of these genes indicates developmental roles of key genes whose disruption (under- or overexpression) can lead to pathologies such as cancer or malformations (cleft palate that may be surgically ameliorated) or both (Kultima et al., 2010).

Partial AChE Inhibition and Sensory Neuron Development

Inhibition of AChE, if severe enough, should trigger many abnormalities from the overload of acetylcholine or the oxidative stress caused by organophosphates. For example, at a lower, nonlethal dose of chlorpyrifos-oxon, zebrafish embryos caused a significant inhibition of AChE and aberrant peripheral axon extension and gene expression profiling in Rohon-Beard sensory neurons. However, general development, muscle fiber development, and nicotinic ACh receptor cluster formation was sufficiently too close to controls to be considered nonspecifically teratogenic (Jacobson et al., 2010).

Late Male Developmental Toxicity

Sperm formation and testosterone synthesis in the human male depend on the release of gonadotropin-releasing hormone from the pituitary and follicle-stimulating hormone (spermatogenesis) and LH (testosterone synthesis) from the anterior pituitary in mammals. Endocrine disruptors have multiple actions that make them reproductive toxicants.

One finding reported first in 1996 (Guillette, 1996) that has been of interest even to the U.S. Congress is the reduction of penis size of alligators in Lake Apopka, Florida due to a spill of dicofol (contaminated with DDT and its metabolites) and sulfuric acid. As the lead researcher of this study (Guillette personal communication at Society of Toxicology meeting, 2004, Baltimore, MD) pointed out, it is not the penis size that is the primary toxicological concern; it is the endocrine disruption of the entire

organism. This study also involved reproductive and developmental measurements of hatching success, primary sex determination, egg mass, hatchling mass, and snout vent length in addition to male phallus size and female oviduct epithelial cell height. Hatching success did not appear to be affected. Mean egg mass was lower in the contaminated lake compared with one less contaminated (Lake Woodruff). Liver and thyroid masses appeared similar between lakes. Female hatchlings of Lake Apopka, however, had smaller spleens than male and female alligators of the control lake. Plasma testosterone was higher for males or females located in the contaminated lake, although changes in aromatase activity due to contamination were not found. The researchers stressed that the resultant effects on hormone level are apparently postembryonic and relate to the early juvenile development of the alligator (Milnes et al., 2005). In another study, the effects of atrazine on *Xenopus laevis* larvae indicated that residual concentrations of this herbicide caused genetic male amphibians to be hermaphroditic and have less masculine features on the larynges (Hayes et al., 2002).

One type of toxicity that may appear very late is behavioral toxicity. For example, abnormal behavior in breeding gulls indicated estrogenic effects of organochlorine pollutants such as *o,p'*-DDT, mirex, and some PCBs. Separation of precopulatory pairs may affect amphipods as indicated by chemicals such as the pesticide lindane, the birth control pill ethinyl estradiol, or the plasticizer BPA. Male courtship is negatively affected by endosulfan (cichlid), estradiol (goldfish, guppy, and medaka), octylphenol or phenol (medaka), and PCBs (dove). Male mating behavior is similarly affected by the hormones DES and ethinyl estradiol (quail), vinclozolin or methoxychlor (quail), and BPA and TCDD (rat). Increased male mating behavior may be another outcome of PCB exposure in a different species (kestrel; Clotfelter et al., 2004). Competing for nests and females appears to be important in reproductive behavior. While spawning behavior appears unaffected, fathead minnows exposed to competing males were less likely to compete for a nest or female when exposed to estradiol or sewage treatment plant effluent as indicated by increased physiological feminization (increased vitellogenin and decreased 11-ketotestosterone), yet they were more able to compete when exposed to methyltestosterone. It appears as if reproductive outcome may also depend on the parents exhibiting proper mating, nesting, incubation, and other reproductive-related behavior especially in oviparous animals (Martinović et al., 2007). Also important were proper nurturing following birth and lack of consumption of young that appear deformed such as occurs in rats and other species.

Late Female Developmental Toxicity

In contrast to the human male, human females' hormonal signals are follicle-stimulating hormone for estrogen synthesis and follicle maturation and LH for egg release. Most of the rodent models (as well as cats and other domestic animals) have estrous cycles with a period of heightened arousal ("heat") that scientists refer to as estrous, which is important in reproductive success. Human females have changes in basal body temperature when they release an egg and a menstrual cycle, but no period of estrous per se. Most of these animal models also give birth to litters from uterine horns, while humans rarely have multiple births without medication and have fallopian tubes in which life-threatening ectopic implantations can occur. The rabbit, alpaca, ferret, mink, cat, and otter in domestic breeding situations do not have an estrous cycle but will release an egg on sexual stimulation and/or mating call of the male. The default in the human is to produce a female with homogametic sex chromosomes unless testosterone is synthesized. In contrast, in birds the default sex is the male unless estrogen is synthesized as the heterogametic sex (ZW) is female and the homogametic sex is male (ZZ). These differences make animal models for human reproduction difficult to interpret unless parallel mechanisms and problems develop from interference with similar reproductive processes.

The development of the gonads and migration of germ cells offer some helpful similarities. For example, in birds and mammals the development of the gonad from the indifferent genital ridge is similarly positioned in the dorsal body cavity superior to the kidneys. In mammals, the Y chromosome causes condensation of cells into the early seminiferous tubules. Primordial germ cells of birds and mammals have their inception in the extraembryonic cells in the yolk sac and migrate into indifferent gonads at mid-gestation. In animals, these germ cells are found in the ovarian cortex of females and become primary spermatogonia in the human male due to the presence of testosterone. The primordial germ cells migrate into the seminiferous tubules in male birds. Estradiol synthesis helps create the ovarian structures such as the left oviduct and shell gland from the left Mullerian duct and the presence of primordial germ cells in the left ovary in female birds, while the right gonad regresses with the decreased production of a glycoprotein. Oviducts do not develop in males due to Mullerian regression factor in the absence of estrogen. Male birds are more influenced in dose-dependent manner by estrogen than their mammalian counterparts, as the number of primordial germ cells that are found in the cortex is dependent on this female hormone. The largest doses of estrogen make the cortical layer of primordial germ cells close to that of an ovary. These cortical germ cells differentiate in a meiotic prophase more typical of ovarian germ cells, while the gonadal medulla contains lower primordial germ cells in the seminiferous tubules in estrogen-exposed male bird embryos. Female embryos show alterations in oviducts due to estrogen exposure, but not the ovarian structure. Estrogen in male gulls and chickens in a dose-dependent fashion also increases the likelihood that the left oviduct may remain along with the vasa deferens. In females, estrogen may result in a large right oviduct. These same female chicks will also lay eggs with abnormal shells that may be thin or soft. In mammals, testosterone is the driver of sexual differentiation, so estrogen's effects are not the same as in birds. Maternal estrogen is not usually a problem, because α-fetoprotein does a good job of protecting the fetus via its strong estrogen-binding capacity. Androgens would be expected to have greater effects on mammals than estrogens. However, species differences in maternal estrogen levels and blood levels of α-fetoprotein make estrogen's effects more dependent on the chosen mammalian model. Exogenous estrogen would be expected to affect the uterus and brain based on the effects of DES more than other primary sexual organs.

Estrogenic Agents

Gulls respond to *o,p′*-DDT, methoxychlor, and DES in a manner similar to estrogen. Males will have primordial germ cells localized in the cortex, while in females the right oviduct may not completely regress. Hydroxylated PCB congeners may have similar activity in birds based on induction of liver microsomal enzymes and trapping these more water-soluble metabolites in the avian eggs. Alkyl phenols have caused fish to synthesize vitellogenin, indicating feminization. Isoflavonoid phytoestrogens have affected the reproduction of wild quail and have become increasingly used by human populations such as is found in soy products. (Fry, 1995).

Female behavior is also affected in various species such as how *o,p′*-DDT increases female reproductive behavior in the rat. Additionally, decreased nest attentiveness in the dove (DDE/PCB mixture), gull (PCBs), and falcons (DDT/DDE) and reduced incubation of egg by the dove (DDE/PCB mixture), tern (PCBs, dioxins), or gull (PCBs, dioxins) can lead to poor reproductive outcomes (Clotfelter et al., 2004).

Reproductive/Developmental Tests

The first indication of toxicity is reproductive in origin and involves the classic indexes listed in the sections that follow. See **Table 22-2** for a list of reproductive and developmental toxicity tests. Specific models for development are also discussed.

TABLE 22-2 Reproductive and Developmental Toxicity Tests	
Testing For	**Individual Assays**
Classical Indeces	Mating index, fertility index, gestation index, live birth index, sex ratio, 4-day survival index, lactation index, preweaning index (US EPA, 1996)
Nationally-Recognized Reproductive Tests	EPA multigenerational test, National Toxicology Program's Fertility/Reproductive Assessment by Continuous Breeding; Screening tests from NTP and OECD; Dominant lethal assay, subchronic toxicity tests, couple-specific, male-specific, and female-specific endpoints (US EPA, 1996)
Nationally-Recognized Reproductive Tests	EPA Developmental Toxicity tests using dose-response, maternal endpoints, litters with implants, litters with live births (including malformations and variations), and functional competence evaluation. Less expensive screens involve two dose levels (maternally toxic + lower dose) and examination of maternal toxicity and litter examination for prioritization purposes. OECD exposure and evaluation of exposure from 2 weeks prior to mating to 4 days postnatal. (US EPA, 1991)
Sperm DNA Fragmentation	Male infertility can be assessed by acidic denaturation of sperm DNA, acridine orange staining for ssDNA (fluoresces red) and dsDNA (fluoresces green), and flow cytometry determination of % fragmented DNA with >30% fragmentation leading to 2-fold increased spontaneous abortions in human population (Evenson, 2005)
Fish Development	AHR-responses/cardiotoxicity, axonal growth, and gill assays (Volz, 2011)
	Embryotoxicity and malformations coupled to a dioxin activity assay and genotoxicity assay as well as GC-MS analysis (Gustavsson, 2007)
In Vitro Tests	EC_{50}s assessed for rat limb micromass test, postimplantation rat whole-embryo culture and embryonic stem cell test (Louisse, 2011)
Predicting Developmental Toxicity	Toxcast high throughput screening data using data from pregnant rats and rabbits and *in vitro* assays (Sipes, 2011)

Reproductive Indices/Tests

The U.S. Environmental Protection Agency (EPA) has approved a set of guidelines for reproductive toxicity risk assessment. They may vary from other sources that have fecundity (ability to produce an offspring in a given period of time) listed or number of resorptions and live pups at 1, 4, 12, and 21 days postpartum in exposed rodents.

$$\text{Mating Index} = \frac{\text{Number of males or females mating}}{\text{Number of male or females cohabited}} \times 100$$

Vaginal plug or sperm in a vaginal smear is evidence of copulation. This index can also involve determination of estrous cycles:

$$\text{Fertility Index} = \frac{\text{Number of cohabited females becoming pregnant}}{\text{Number of non-pregnant couples cohabited}} \times 100$$

The EPA does not prefer this index, because real-world (as opposed to the toxicology testing lab) exposures may involve both sexes to agents. In this case, female and male fertility indexes may be preferred. The definition of fertility is simply the ability to conceive and not a successful outcome of that fertilization.

$$\text{Gestation (Pregnancy) Index} = \frac{\text{Number of females delivering live young}}{\text{Number of females with evidence of pregnancy}} \times 100$$

$$\text{Live Birth Index} = \frac{\text{Number of live offspring}}{\text{Number of offspring delivered}} \times 100$$

$$\text{Sex Ratio} = \frac{\text{Number of males offspring}}{\text{Number of female offspring}}$$

$$\text{4-Day Survival Index (Viability Index)} = \frac{\text{Number of live offspring at lactation day 4}}{\text{Number of live offspring delivered}} \times 100$$

This last index does not assume any normalization to a certain litter size until 4 days after delivery and the determination of this index.

$$\text{Lactation Index (Weaning Index)} = \frac{\text{Number of live offspring at day 21}}{\text{Number of live offspring born}} \times 100$$

In this index if the number of offspring per litter were standardized, then the number of offspring following that standardization should be used in place of the number of live offspring born.

$$\text{Preweaning Index} = \frac{\text{Number of live offspring born} - \text{number of offspring weaned}}{\text{Number of live offspring born}} \times 100$$

Again, if a normalization/standardization were performed, then number of offspring remaining after that normalization should be used in the denominator of this index as well (EPA, 1996).

The EPA has been concerned with the reported decline in human sperm counts and male hypospadias (opening of urethra on underside of penis rather than distal end), cryptorchidism (undescended testicle), and testicular cancer. In females endometriosis prevalence and possible link to halogenated aromatic hydrocarbons are of concern. Rise in infertility is also a multifaceted, developing problem. Adverse outcomes during pregnancy also fit into the reproductive toxicity area. Developmental toxicity to the next generations' reproductive organs is also of note, such as steroidogenic or anti-steroidogenic compounds that may influence the onset of puberty or reproductive function as an adult. Because these effects may occur as a result of long-term treatment of a male for showing appreciable concentrations of the compound of interest in the ejaculate, due to bioaccumulation in either sex, or due to a compensatory mechanism of chronic exposure, the dosing protocols are supposed to take into account the varied pharmacokinetics and pharmacodynamic data that inform dose levels and duration of treatment.

Mating periods are 21 days for rodents, because females have 4- or 5-day estrous cycles and should have cycled four to five times during this period. The EPA is interested in using one male per female or 20 males to produce 20 pregnancies per dose group. This requires quite a few animals for a complete generation or multigenerational test to get a dose–response, which may not be linear at all due to different adaptations to chronic dosing that may affect reproductive outcome. The single-generation test involves exposing F_1 and F_2 offspring continuously *in utero* from conception until parturition and through the preweaning period when milk transfer of toxicant may occur or change behavior of dams to the offspring. The EPA uses this design to follow effects into the peripubertal and young adult phases following birth. Generational comparisons may not be possible, because each generation will have different exposure histories. Parental age, sexual experience, and parity of the females come into play for future litters that also may affect the outcome of chemical exposures. Both generations may be examined for weights and histopathology of testes, epididymides, and accessory sex organs for males, and vagina, uterus, cervix, ovaries, and mammary glands for females. For sex-specific effects, it may be necessary to couple sperm or ovarian changes to crossover matings—that is, mating treated one sex with the other untreated sex and vice versa. A two-generation test is optional, because it will identify effects caused by prenatal and postnatal exposure, alterations of germ cells transmitted from the earlier generation's exposure to expression in the next generation, and those delayed effects requiring a latent period prior to expression (including epigenetic expression changes).

Alternatives to this reproductive toxicity design include the Reproductive Assessment by Continuous Breeding, which was developed as a one-generational test by the National Toxicology Program (NTP) but has been extended into a two-generational test to be in concert with the EPA's recommendations. This has as its unique feature cohabitation of male–female pairs in the initial parent's generation for 14 weeks, producing up to five litters of pups removed at birth. Treatments are initiated in both sexes 1 week prior to cohabitation and proceed for the following 2 weeks. Viability, litter and/or pup weight, sex, and external abnormalities are recorded from the pups prior to being euthanized. The last groups of pups can be followed through the preweaning period to assess effects following birth and during milk transfer of toxicants. This design may pick up cumulative effects and subfertility (producing fewer pups per litter or fewer litters). In the mouse, this test has been modified to also examine sperm measures such as sperm number, morphology, and motility and look for the presence of abnormal cells in vaginal smears. Another alternative combines continuous breeding of rats with exposure of more than one generation, germ cell tests, and reproductive hormone levels to determine effects of environmental androgens or estrogens. Treatment is continuous through breeding, pregnancy, and lactation. Crossover mating is also done for sex-specific effects. Combining continuous breeding with sex-specific multiple endpoints gives some advantages in detecting endocrine disruption as it has come to be understood currently.

Screening tests involve shorter exposures such as the Organisation for Economic Co-operation and Development (OECD) Reproductive/Developmental Toxicity Screening Test of the Screening Information Data Set protocol and NTP's Short-Term Reproductive and Developmental Toxicity Screen. These establish priorities rather than regulatory exposure limits because further testing is required. A mutagenesis assay that may be considered reproductive toxicity is the dominant lethal assay where high dosing over a 1- to 5-day period of males is followed by mating and euthanizing the females to look for early fetal deaths indicating some mutagenesis of the sperm DNA (analysis of pre- and post-implantation loss). A female oogenesis equivalent dominant lethal assay is also available. The main problem is that embryo deaths may not indicate a genetically transferrable toxicity; however, it would still be considered a reproductive toxicant. Subchronic tests involve a detailed reproductive analysis exposing rats for 90 days initiating at weeks 6 through 8. Starting at 8 weeks has the advantage of observing a more mature stage of sexual development for reproductive structure abnormalities (visual examination of reproductive organs and weights and histopathology of testes, epididymides, and accessory sex glands for the male and vagina, uterus, cervix, ovaries, and mammary glands for the female). Sexual behavioral endpoints that may indicate neurotoxicity or endocrine action of toxicants are lordosis (receptivity to male mating) in female rats and copulatory activity of males. Impairment that is caused by rear leg motor function deficits or general lethargy should not be considered as reproductive toxicity but rather systemic toxicity.

Endpoints for toxicity tests are divided into couple mediated (involving both mated sexes), female specific, and male specific. Couple-mediated endpoints are mating rate and time to mating/time to pregnancy, pregnancy rate, delivery rate, gestation length, total and living litter size, number of live and dead offspring or fetal death rate, offspring gender or sex ratio, birth weight, postnatal weights, offspring survival, external malformations and variations, and offspring reproduction for multigenerational studies. Other endpoints for reproductive toxicity are ovulation rate, fertilization rate, pre-implantation loss, implantation number, internal malformations and variations, and postnatal structural and functional development. Male-specific endpoints are weights, visual examination, and histopathology of testes, epididymides, seminal vesicles, prostate, and pituitary. Sperm count, morphology, and motility are included. Mounting, intromissions, and ejaculations round out the behavioral tests for male reproductive toxicity. LH, FSH, testosterone, estrogen, and prolactin are the measured hormones that may be disrupted. Testis descent, preputial separation, sperm production, anogenital distance, and structure of external genitalia complete the male-specific endpoints.

Female-specific endpoints involve organ weights, visual examination, and histopathology of the ovaries, uterus, vagina, and pituitary. However, the visual examination and histopathology also extend to the oviducts and mammary glands. Vaginal smear cytology indicates estrous cycle normality. Lordosis, time to mating, vaginal plugs, or sperm are measures of sexual behavior. LH, FSH, estrogen, progesterone, and prolactin are measured hormone levels that may be disrupted in the female. Offspring growth, milk quantity, and milk quality quantify affected lactation. Normality of external genitalia, vaginal opening, vaginal smear cytology, and onset of menstruation mark development problems, while vaginal smear cytology and ovarian histology (menopause) indicate senescence and the completion of female-specific reproductive testing. Rounding out other possibilities for testing are *in vitro* studies (e.g., sperm, egg) and human epidemiology reports.

Developmental Toxicity Endpoints

Another EPA (1991) document should be considered for developmental endpoints. Developmental toxicity encompasses the death of a developing organism, structural abnormality, altered growth, or functional deficiency. Maternal toxicity endpoints are mortality, mating index, fertility index, gestation length, body weight (day 0, during gestation, day of necropsy), body weight change (throughout gestation, during treatment and discrete periods during treatment, post-treatment to euthanizing, maternal weight corrected for weight of gravid uterus and litter weight), organ weights (absolute, relative to body weight, relative to brain weight), food and water consumption if relevant, clinical measurements (types, incidence, degree, and duration of clinical signs of toxicity, enzyme markers, and clinical chemistries), and gross necropsy and histopathology. Evaluations are also made for litters with implants and litters with live offspring. Litters with implants are examined for number of implantation sites/dam, number of corpora lutea (follicle that develops during pregnancy to maintain pregnancy through progesterone secretion)/dam, percent pre-implantation loss (number of corpora lutea – implantations × 100/number of corpora lutea), number and percentage of live offspring/litter, number and percentage of resorptions/litter, number and percentage of litters with resorptions, number and percentage of later fetal deaths/litter, number and percentage of nonlive (later fetal deaths + resorptions) implants/litter, number and percentage of litters with nonlive implants, number and percentage of affected (nonlive + malformed) implants/litter, number and percentage of litters with affected implants, number and percentage of litters with total resorptions, number and percentage of stillbirths/litter, and number and percentage of litters with live offspring. Litters with live offspring end the other evaluation and start the evaluation of number and percentage live offspring/litter; viability of offspring; sex ratio/litter; mean offspring body weight/litter; mean male and female body weight/litter; number and percentage of offspring with external, visceral, or skeletal malformations/litter; number and percentage of malformed offspring/litter; number and percentage of litters with malformed offspring; number and percentage of malformed males or females/litter; number and percentage of offspring with external, visceral, or skeletal variations/litter; number and percentage of offspring with variations/litter; number and percentage of litters having offspring with variations; types and incidence of individual malformations; types and incidence of individual variations; individual offspring and their malformations and variations (grouped by litter and dose); clinical signs (type incidence, duration, and degree); and gross necropsy and histopathology.

Beyond recording basic reproductive outcomes, functional deficits may indicate more subtle but still important damage done during development. For example, behavioral tests including types of learning (conditioning) may be tested for developmental neurotoxicity. Other systems (cardiovascular, digestive, endocrine, immune, respiratory, and reproductive) may also change their functional competence or experience delays in functional competence. Evaluating these functional deficits requires dose–response curves, replicating studies to increase confidence in results, a pharmacology or physiological challenge that may uncover a lack of competence of an organ system (especially relevant to those with reserve functional capacity such as a large liver or two kidneys), functional tests with some individual variability among individuals (because those with little variability may become lethal on challenge to that function), battery of functional tests and at several ages (increases confidence that the full range of function is tested and changes with maturation), defining critical periods for disruption of functional competence (prenatal and postnatal and how these periods are altered by time and degree of exposure), and maternal-pup interaction analysis for postnatal studies (maternal behavior; milk compositions; pup suckling behavior; possible exposure through feed, water, or other means).

Pregnant mice, rats, or rabbits are the usual models for developmental toxicity testing. The oral administration (unless other route is considered more valid) of the test compound is followed through organogenesis as a major feature of developmental abnormalities or delays. The maternal system is monitored throughout pregnancy (the exposure period). The dam and her uterine contents are examined just prior to term to evaluate developmental consequences of exposure. One or both of the mating pair may also be exposed prior to conception and may follow results over several generations as well. Less expensive screens involve exposing maternal system (mouse or rat) to a dose that shows maternal toxicity and one lower dose to prevent detection of false positives. The outcomes are general maternal toxicity, litter size, pup viability and weight, and gross malformations of offspring. This allows prioritization for further testing but does not stand on its own. The OECD (European Union) screen involves exposure 2 weeks prior to mating to 4 days postnatal and then evaluating adults of the mating pairs (general toxicity and reproductive organ damage) and pups (counts, weights, gross physical malformations, and clear behavioral abnormalities). This OECD test spans both the developmental and reproductive areas as a toxicity screen. At the time of the EPA's (1991) developmental toxicity testing document, the *in vitro* tests were not thoroughly examined but were considered insufficient by themselves for a thorough risk assessment establishing reference concentrations for developmental toxicity of an oral dose (RfD_{DT}) or inhalation (RfC_{DT}), no-observed-adverse-effect level (NOAEL), and/ or lowest-observed-adverse-effect level (LOAEL). However, these are listed later in their own section (*in vitro* models) for consideration as alternative testing. Establishing the benchmark dose (BD) is similar to other toxicity modeling by the EPA. The excess proportion of abnormal responses (Y axis) is plotted against the dose (log dose). The true dose–response is plotted to find where the LED_{10} exists (10% lower bound of ED or "true" 10% abnormality above normal as best can be obtained with statistical bounds of uncertainty defined) or a 10% increase in abnormalities of development (for example increasing abnormalities by 10% = effective dose at a specified response level [10%] or ED_{10}). Then an upper confidence is established for this risk (shifts curve to left and provides a safety factor). The 10% increase is found on this shifted curve and established as the LED_{10} or BD. This LED_{10} is then divided by the uncertainty factory (UF) to establish the RfD_{DT} or RfC_{DT}, depending on the route of administration.

Sperm Chromatin Structure Assay

Fresh semen samples frozen in liquid nitrogen or dry ice are shipped to a lab for the Sperm Chromatin Structure Assay. Samples are thawed and diluted to 1 to 2×10^6 sperm/mL and treated for 30 seconds with a pH 1.2 detergent buffer to denature DNA at the sites of DNA strand breaks. Acridine orange is then used to stain single-stranded DNA or double-stranded DNA, which fluoresce red and green, respectively. Flow cytometry is then used to determine the extent of DNA fragmentation and the ratio of red to green sperm. Reproductive toxicants usually cause DNA fragmentation in rodent assays of germ cells isolated by taking them from the epididymis or ejaculate. Some samples could result in successful *in vitro* fertilization, but yield a high degree of failure at the embryonic stage. Human males living in a town with heavy smog and a high rate of infertility and spontaneous abortions (miscarriages) exhibited sperm DNA fragmentation by this assay. Young men who sprayed pesticides without protective equipment also showed a higher risk of DNA fragmentation. It is biologically significant if $\geq$ 30% of the sperm have DNA fragmentation, because the egg is incapable of repairing this damage, causing approximately twofold increases in spontaneous abortions (Evenson and Wixon, 2005).

Fish Assay

The fish early life-stage (FELS) test is a bioassay for aquatic risk assessment. The test requires 360 fish and 1–3 months of analysis. A full lifecycle of toxicity is evaluated/predicted but mechanisms are not necessarily provided. Adverse outcome pathways may be a way to turn an ecotoxicity test into a developmental framework that serves mechanistic developmental ends and ecotoxicity endpoints at the same time. The chemicals tested in a proposed fish analysis of early life stages were the cardiotoxic strong aryl hydrocarbon receptor (AhR) agonist or TCDD, a neurotoxic AChE inhibitor or chlorpyrifos, and a narcotic surfactant or linear alkylbenzene sulfonate. Three tiers were used in this testing scheme as displayed in **Figure 22-3**. The effects of TCDD should be obvious in terms of mechanism affecting CYP1A, NAD(P)H:quinone oxidoreductase, aldehyde dehydrogenase 3, UDP glucuronosyltransferase, and glutathione transferase. However, the zebrafish shows the functional changes following embryonic exposure in heart malformations and cardiotoxicity prior to systemic effects. For the AChE-inhibiting chlorpyrifos, exposure during embryogenesis decreases baseline locomotor activity and choice accuracy that persist into adulthood even if the fish are transferred into clean water. Chlorpyrifos appears to inhibit axonal growth or primary and secondary motoneurons as well as Rohon-Beard and dorsal root ganglia sensory neurons affecting the neural circuitry through AChE inhibition. These effects also include the microtubules as indicated by the occurrence of altered

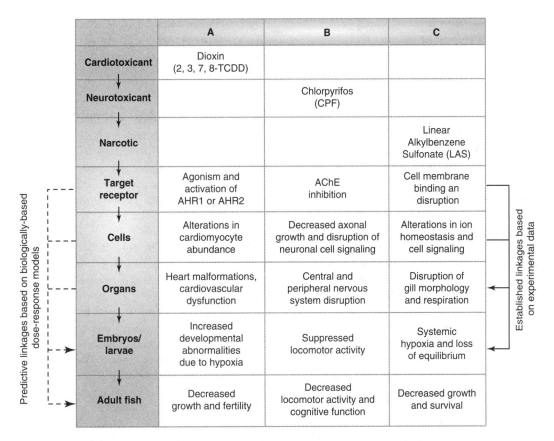

FIGURE 22-3 The development of: (A) cardiac myocytes challenged by TCDD; (B) axonal growth and neuronal cell signaling by chlorpyrifos; (C) disruption of the cell membrane and cell signaling by linear alkylbenzene sulfonate.

phosphorylation. The last model compound, linear alkylbenzene sulfonate (LAS), has the structure of many anionic laundry and dish detergents. This compound binds to cellular membranes compromising membrane integrity and fluidity. This effect in turn changes ion homeostasis and signal transduction, and can yield necrosis at high concentrations of LAS. This change is similar in action to narcotic and/ or anesthetic medications. Because the gill is the first structure this hydrophobic chemical encounters in the fish, it is also the site of toxicity. The epithelium or primary and secondary lamellae exhibit hypertrophy and edema, which can lead to decreased respiration, systemic hypoxia, loss of equilibrium, and mortality. Fish embryos and larvae are the most susceptible phases of development for a variety of fish species (including the well-studied model

of the fathead minnow as well as smallmouth bass, northern pike, and white sucker). These effects excepting the most severe are reversible. The tiers approach relies on these named effects with tier 1 involving AhR-specific reporter assays, axonal growth assays, and gill viability assays. Additionally, fish-specific hepatocyte lines are exposed to chemicals to determine their metabolism (half-life and metabolites). Tier 2 would then involve medium-to-high-throughput screening of fish embryos (3- to 5-day zebrafish embryo toxicity assay). This is important, because multiple target organs may be evaluated simultaneously, which involves the developing physiology of the organism in all its complexity. This may be problematic in some jurisdictions, as some countries protect certain fish stages and require alternative cell-based models. If both tiers prove positive, then a low-throughput FELS test would be necessary to evaluate persistent chronic toxicity of low concentrations of chemicals that do not bio-degrade well (persistent halogenated organic pollutants or metals) or are constantly released from sewage treatment plants into waters such as pharmaceutical agents and their metabolites (Volz et al., 2011).

To detect specific types of extremely toxic organic chemicals, other assays may be used in concert with the early life-stage development assay (of zebrafish or *Danio rerio*). For example, organic solvent extracts can be cleaned up and fractionated and dissolved in DMSO for application to CALUX® cells in culture on a 96-well plate that determines TCDD-like activity via exposure, lysation of the cells, adding luciferin, and quantitation in a luminometer. This can be compared to the chemical analysis via gas chromatography–mass spectrometry. Genotoxicity can also be assessed via ISO protocol for the umu-C genotoxicity assay (ISO/TC 147/SC 5/WG9 N8) utilizing *Salmonella typhimurium* TA1535/pSK1002. Positive genotoxicity may determine some of the reasons for the embryotoxicity or later malformations that occur from a mixture of compounds such as nitroaromatics in sludge. These kinds of protocols are favored in the European Union (Gustavsson et al., 2007).

In Vitro Models

Three *in vitro* assays have been validated to be used in the testing of developmental toxicity for industrial chemicals under the European Union's (European Centre for the Validation of Alternative Methods) Registration, Evaluation, Authorisation, and Restriction of Chemicals (REACH) regulation: the rat limb micromass test, the post-implantation rat whole-embryo culture test, and the embryonic stem cell test. The rat limb micromass test and the post-implantation rat whole-embryo culture require primary animal tissue for analysis. The embryonic stem cell assay involves cell growth inhibition of embryonic fibroblasts (BALB/c-3T3) and embryonic stem cells (ES-D3) for effects on cell proliferation and cytotoxicity. Additionally, the ES-D3 cells' ability to differentiate into cardiomyocytes in the presence of the potential

developmental toxicant is assessed. All have EC_{50}s determined and are then determined to have little influence, weak influence, or strong embryotoxicity (Louisse et al., 2011).

Toxcast High-Throughput Screening Data

The EPA's ToxCast phase I employs a chemical library of 309 unique structures. The selection was based on *in vivo* data supporting chronic/cancer, multigenerational/reproductive, or prenatal effects. Each compound was overwhelmingly soluble in the solvent DMSO, commercially available with > 90% purity and of a molecular weight of 250–1000. These criteria fit the active ingredients of pesticides. Developmental defects caused by these chemicals were entered into the ToxCastDB database from ToxRefDB *in vivo* (mainly from studies of pregnant rats and rabbits and reproductive and cancer studies including specific abnormalities and developmental lowest effect level or dLEL and categorical LEL) or ToxCast *in vitro* assay results. The ToxCast high-throughput model includes platforms such as real-time cell electronic sensing in human A549 cells, transcriptional activity with multiplexed reporter genes in human HepG2 liver cells, primarily evaluating inflammatory responses using enzyme-linked immunosorbent assay (ELISA) in a mixture of human primary cells, cellular high-content screening evaluating markers such as stress pathways, mitochondrial involvement, cell cycle, cell loss, mitotic arrest, the cytoskeleton in human HepG2 liver cells, transcriptional upregulation of genes involved in metabolism using primary human hepatocytes, nuclear receptor activity (gene reporter assays) in human embryonic kidney HEK 293 cell lines, biochemical enzyme inhibition and receptor-binding assays in a cell-free format, and murine embryonic stem cell (MESC) cytotoxicity and cardiomyocyte differentiation. Altogether, 662 *in vitro* high-throughput assays were compared to a training set of chemicals. Positive and negative developmental toxicity outcomes were made for 17 categorical endpoints. Pearson's correlation test (comparing AC50 assay potency values to *in vivo* categorical developmental toxicity) and Student's t-test were used for continuous and the chi-squared test for dichotomous (comparing *in vitro* positive/negative results with *in vivo* categorical developmental toxicity) statistical methods. The results of this analysis indicated the need to use individual species-specific models for predicting developmental toxicity in rats and rabbits, determine specific effects on signal transduction mechanisms or other cellular targets that can be linked to a specific developmental toxicity endpoint, cluster toxicity endpoints based on similar biological or developmental processes/stages, and establish the role of xenobiotic metabolism in these developmental toxicity endpoints (because it does impact toxicity). In vivo dose–response appears to be lacking in the assay characteristics, and this statistical approach at least has better than a 70% accuracy in predicting the potential to cause developmental toxicity *in vivo* (Sipes et al., 2011).

Questions

1. What purpose did the dominant lethal assay serve in toxicity testing? How has toxicogenomics refined and replaced it as a toxicity measure?

2. What signaling events appear to be associated with: a) liver cancer, b) bladder cancer, and c) skin lesions associated with epigenetic alterations from arsenic exposure?

3. How do environmental toxicants gain access to male spermatogenesis structures?

4. What are the mechanisms underlying the toxicity of chemicals to sperm?

5. Why are oocytes in ovarian follicles exquisitely sensitive to ROS?

6. What are three distinct ways Pb can interfere with fertilization?

7. Why is time of development important for nonspecific developmental toxicants such as alkylating agents or other compounds that damage DNA, prevent protein synthesis, or cause mitotic arrest?

8. How does thalidomide prevent limb growth?

9. Why do glucocorticoids induce cleft palate?

10. How does ethanol cause developmental neurological and kidney damage?

11. How might retinoids and valproic acid toxicity be linked?

12. Why was Guillette correct that reduced penis size is not the key finding of alligator studies in a pesticide-contaminated lake in Florida?

13. Why is it important to perform reproductive assays through the preweaning period?

14. What is the benchmark dose for developmental toxicity?

References

Agarwal A, Deepinder F, Sharma RK, Ranga G, Li J. 2008. Effect of cell phone usage on semen analysis in men attending infertility clinic: an observational study. *Fertil Steril.* 89:124–128.

Ahmed RG. 2011. Evolutionary interactions between diabetes and development. *Diabetes Res Clin Pract.* 92:153–167.

Alfonso-Loeches S, Guerri C. 2011. Molecular and behavioral aspects of the actions of alcohol on the adult and developing brain. *Crit Rev Clin Lab Sci.* 48:19–47.

Alwis ID, Maroni DM, Hendry IR, Roy SK, May JV, Leavitt WW, Hendry WJ. 2011. Neonatal diethylstilbestrol exposure disrupts female reproductive tract structure/function via both direct and indirect mechanisms in the hamster. *Reprod Toxicol.* 32:472–483.

Bataineh HN, Daradka T. 2007. Effects of long-term use of fluoxetine on fertility parameters in adult male rats. *Neuro Endocrinol Lett.* 28:321–325.

Bernanke J, Köhler HR. 2009. The impact of environmental chemicals on wildlife vertebrates. *Rev Environ Contam Toxicol.* 198:1–47.

Bonde JP, Toft G, Rylander L, Rignell-Hydbom A, Giwercman A, Spano M, Manicardi GC, Bizzaro D, Ludwicki JK, Zvyezday V, Bonefeld-Jørgensen EC, Pedersen HS, Jönsson BA, Thulstrup AM; INUENDO. 2008. Fertility and markers of male reproductive function in Inuit and European populations spanning large contrasts in blood levels of persistent organochlorines. *Environ Health Perspect.* 116:269–277. Review. Erratum in: 2008. *Environ Health Perspect.* 116:276.

Bonilla E, Hernández F, Cortés L, Mendoza M, Mejía J, Carrillo E, Casas E, Betancourt M. 2008. Effects of the insecticides malathion and diazinon on the early oogenesis in mice *in vitro*. *Environ Toxicol.* 23:240–245.

Bustos-Obregón E, Recardo, HB. 2008. Ecotoxicology and testicular damage (environmental chemical pollution). A review. *Int J Morphol.* 26:833–840.

Chen M, Huang HZ, Wang M, Wang AX. 2010. Retinoic acid inhibits osteogenic differentiation of mouse embryonic palate mesenchymal cells. *Birth Defects Res A Clin Mol Teratol.* 88:965–970.

Clotfelter ED, Bell AM, Leverin KR. 2004. The role of animal behavior in the study of endocrine-disrupting chemicals. *Anim Behav.* 68:665–676.

Corrales JJ, Cordero M, Galindo P, Burgo RM, Hernández J, Manuel Miralles J. 2011. [Trends in semen quality in a non-industrialized population from the Salamanca area, Spain, during the last 30 years]. *Med Clin (Barc).* 136:277–283.

Daston GP, Naciff JM. 2010. Predicting developmental toxicity through toxicogenomics. *Birth Defects Res C Embryo Today.* 90:110–117.

Daston GP, Overmann GJ, Baines D, Taubeneck MW, Lehman-McKeeman LD, Rogers JM, Keen CL. 1994. Altered Zn status by alpha-hederin in the pregnant rat and its relationship to adverse developmental outcome. *Reprod Toxicol.* 8:15–24.

de Jong E, Doedée AM, Reis-Fernandes MA, Nau H, Piersma AH. 2011. Potency ranking of valproic acid analogues as to inhibition of cardiac differentiation of embryonic stem cells in comparison to their *in vivo* embryotoxicity. *Reprod Toxicol.* 31:375–382.

Del Valle LJ, Pella R, Mercedes A, Velasquez LA, Orihuela PA. 2008. Embryotoxicity of serum from women smoking cocaine base paste (CBP). *Eur J Obstet Gynecol Reprod Biol.* 139:28–31.

Devine PJ, Perreault SD, Luderer U. 2012. Roles of reactive oxygen species and antioxidants in ovarian toxicity. *Biol Reprod.* 86:27.

Dobrzy´nska MM. 2011. Male-mediated F1 effects in mice exposed to nonylphenol or to a combination of X-rays and nonylphenol. *Drug Chem Toxicol.* 35:36–42.

El-Sharaky AS, Newairy AA, Elguindy NM, Elwafa AA. 2010. Spermatotoxicity, biochemical changes and histological alteration induced by gossypol in testicular and hepatic tissues of male rats. *Food Chem Toxicol.* 48:3354–3361.

Epstein SS. 1973. Use of the dominant-lethal test to detect genetic activity of environmental chemicals. *Environ Health Perspect.* 6:23–26.

Evenson DP, Wixon R. 2005. Environmental toxicants cause sperm DNA fragmentation as detected by the Sperm Chromatin Structure Assay (SCSA). *Toxicol Appl Pharmacol.* 207(2 Suppl):532–537.

Foster WG, McMahon A, Rice DC. 1996. Sperm chromatin structure is altered in cynomolgus monkeys with environmentally relevant blood lead levels. *Toxicol Ind Health.* 12:723–735.

Frumkin H. 1998. Multiple system atrophy following chronic carbon disulfide exposure. *Environ Health Perspect.* 106:611–613.

Fry, DM. 1995. Reproductive effects in birds exposed to pesticides and industrial chemicals. *Environ Health Perspect.* 103(Suppl 7):165–171.

Gilliam D, Valdez N, Branson S, Dixon A, Downing C. 2011. Maternal effects on ethanol teratogenesis in a cross between A/J and C57BL/6J mice. *Alcohol.* 45:441–449.

Gray SP, Cullen-McEwen LA, Bertram JF, Moritz KM. 2011. Mechanism of alcohol-induced impairments in renal development: could it be reduced retinoic acid? *Clin Exp Pharmacol Physiol.* 39:807–813.

Guillette LJ Jr, Pickford DB, Crain DA, Rooney AA, Percival HF. 1996. Reduction in penis size and plasma testosterone concentrations in juvenile alligators living in a contaminated environment. *Gen Comp Endocrinol.* 101:32–42.

Gustavsson L, Hollert H, Jonsson S, van Bavel B, Engwall M. 2007. Reed beds receiving industrial sludge containing nitroaromatic compounds. Effects of outgoing water and bed material extracts in the umu-c genotoxicity assay, DR-CALUX assay and on early life stage development in zebrafish (*Danio rerio*). *Environ Sci Pollut Res Int.* 14:202–211.

Han X, Zhou N, Cui Z, Ma M, Li L, Cai M, Li Y, Lin H, Li Y, Ao L, Liu J, Cao J. 2011. Association between urinary polycyclic aromatic hydrocarbon metabolites and sperm DNA damage: a population study in Chongqing, China. *Environ Health Perspect.* 119:652–657.

Hanke W, Jurewicz J. 2004. The risk of adverse reproductive and developmental disorders due to occupational pesticide exposure: an overview of current epidemiological evidence. *Int J Occup Med Environ Health.* 17:223–243.

Hansen SW. 1992. Late-effects after treatment for germ-cell cancer with cisplatin, vinblastine, and bleomycin. *Dan Med Bull.* 39:391–399.

Harbison RD. 1978. Chemical-biological reactions common to teratogenesis and mutagenesis. *Environ Health Perspect.* 24:87–200.

Hauser R, Meeker JD, Duty S, Silva MJ, Calafat AM. 2006. Altered semen quality in relation to urinary concentrations of phthalate monoester and oxidative metabolites. *Epidemiology.* 17:682–691.

Hayes TB, Collins A, Lee M, Mendoza M, Noriega N, Stuart AA, Vonk A. 2002. Hermaphroditic, demasculinized frogs after exposure to the herbicide atrazine at low ecologically relevant doses. *Proc Natl Acad Sci USA.* 99:5476–5480.

Higano CS. 2003. Side effects of androgen deprivation therapy: monitoring and minimizing toxicity. *Urology.* 61(2 Suppl 1):32–38.

Howell S, Shalet S. 1998. Gonadal damage from chemotherapy and radiotherapy. *Endocrinol Metab Clin North Am.* 27:927–943.

Hsieh FI, Hwang TS, Hsieh YC, Lo HC, Su CT, Hsu HS, Chiou HY, Chen CJ. 2008. Risk of erectile dysfunction induced by arsenic exposure through well water consumption in Taiwan. *Environ Health Perspect.* 116:532–536.

Ito T, Ando H, Suzuki T, Ogura T, Hotta K, Imamura Y, Yamaguchi Y, Handa H. 2010. Identification of a primary target of thalidomide teratogenicity. *Science.* 327:1345–1350.

Jacobson SM, Birkholz DA, McNamara ML, Bharate SB, George KM. 2010. Subacute developmental exposure of zebrafish to the organophosphate pesticide metabolite, chlorpyrifos-oxon, results in defects in Rohon-Beard sensory neuron development. *Aquat Toxicol.* 100:101–111.

Kielstein JT, Zoccali C. 2005. Asymmetric dimethylarginine: a cardiovascular risk factor and a uremic toxin coming of age? *Am J Kidney Dis.* 46:186–202.

Kultima K, Jergil M, Salter H, Gustafson AL, Dencker L, Stigson M. 2010. Early transcriptional responses in mouse embryos as a basis for selection of molecular markers predictive of valproic acid teratogenicity. *Reprod Toxicol.* 30:457–468.

Kumar S, Mishra VV. 2010. Review: toxicants in reproductive fluid and *in vitro* fertilization (IVF) outcome. *Toxicol Ind Health.* 26:505–511.

Kumar A, Singh CK, Lavoie HA, Dipette DJ, Singh US. 2011. Resveratrol restores Nrf2 level and prevents ethanol-induced toxic effects in the cerebellum of a rodent model of fetal alcohol spectrum disorders. *Mol Pharmacol.* 80:446–457.

Langevin F, Crossan GP, Rosado IV, Arends MJ, Patel KJ. 2011. Fancd2 counteracts the toxic effects of naturally produced aldehydes in mice. *Nature.* 475:53–58.

Larocca J, Boyajian A, Brown C, Smith SD, Hixon M. 2011. Effects of *in utero* exposure to bisphenol A or diethylstilbestrol on the adult male reproductive system. *Birth Defects Res B Dev Reprod Toxicol.* 92:526–533.

Lazaros LA, Xita NV, Hatzi EG, Kaponis AI, Stefos TJ, Plachouras NI, Makrydimas GV, Sofikitis NV, Zikopoulos KA, Georgiou IA. 2011. Association of paraoxonase gene polymorphisms with sperm parameters. *J Androl.* 32:394–401.

Lazaros L, Xita N, Kaponis A, Hatzi E, Plachouras N, Sofikitis N, Zikopoulos K, Georgiou I. 2011. The association of aromatase (CYP19) gene variants with sperm concentration and motility. *Asian J Androl.* 13:292–297.

Li DK, Zhou Z, Miao M, He Y, Wang J, Ferber J, Herrinton LJ, Gao E, Yuan W. 2011. Urine bisphenol-A (BPA) level in relation to semen quality. *Fertil Steril.* 95:625–630. e1–4.

Linares V, Alonso V, Domingo JL. 2011. Oxidative stress as a mechanism underlying sulfasalazine-induced toxicity. *Expert Opin Drug Saf.* 10(2):253–263.

Louisse J, Gönen S, Rietjens IM, Verwei M. 2011. Relative developmental toxicity potencies of retinoids in the embryonic stem cell test compared with their relative potencies in *in vivo* and two other *in vitro* assays for developmental toxicity. *Toxicol Lett.* 203:1–8.

Mahmoud A, Kiss P, Vanhoorne M, De Bacquer D, Comhaire F. 2005. Is inhibin B involved in the toxic effect of lead on male reproduction? *Int J Androl.* 28:150–155.

Martinović D, Hogarth WT, Jones RE, Sorensen PW. 2007. Environmental estrogens suppress hormones, behavior, and reproductive fitness in male fathead minnows. Environ Toxicol Chem. 26:271–278.

Meirow D, Nugent D. 2001.The effects of radiotherapy and chemotherapy on female reproduction. *Hum Reprod Update.* 7:535–43.

Milnes MR, Bermudez DS, Bryan TA, Gunderson MP, Guillette LJ Jr. 2005. Altered neonatal development and endocrine function in Alligator mississippiensis associated with a contaminated environment. *Biol Reprod.* 73:1004–1010.

Nakamura T, Katsu Y, Watanabe H, Iguchi T. 2008. Estrogen receptor subtypes selectively mediate female mouse reproductive abnormalities induced by neonatal exposure to estrogenic chemicals. *Toxicology.* 253:117–124.

Pašková V, Hilscherová K, Bláha L. 2011. Teratogenicity and embryotoxicity in aquatic organisms after pesticide exposure and the role of oxidative stress. *Rev Environ Contam Toxicol.* 211:25–61.

Perera F, Herbstman J. 2011. Prenatal environmental exposures, epigenetics, and disease. Reprod *Toxicol.* 31:363–373.

Pickford DB, Morris ID. 2003. Inhibition of gonadotropin-induced oviposition and ovarian steroidogenesis in the African clawed frog (*Xenopus laevis*) by the pesticide methoxychlor. *Aquat Toxicol.* 62:179–194.

Pinsky L, DiGeorge AM. 1965. Cleft palate in the mouse: a teratogenic index of glucocorticoid potency. *Science.* 147:402–403.

Raikow DE, Landrum PE, Reid DE. 2007. Aquatic invertebrate resting egg sensitivity to glutaraldehyde and sodium hypochlorite. *Environ Toxicol Chem.* 26:1770–1773.

Raman JD, Nobert CF, Goldstein M. 2005. Increased incidence of testicular cancer in men presenting with infertility and abnormal semen analysis. *J Urol.* 174:1819–1822; discussion 1822.

Rogers JM. 1987. Comparison of maternal and fetal toxic dose responses in mammals. *Teratog Carcinog Mutagen.* 7:297–306.

Rychetnik L, Madronio CM. 2011. The health and social effects of drinking water-based infusions of kava: a review of the evidence. *Drug Alcohol Rev.* 30:74–83.

Sato H. 1963. Effect of adrenocorticoids during pregnancy. *Lancet.* 2:1235–1236.

Sawyer D, Conner CS, Scalley R. 1981. Cimetidine: adverse reactions and acute toxicity. *Am J Hosp Pharm.* 38:188–197.

Sipes NS, Martin MT, Reif DM, Kleinstreuer NC, Judson RS, Singh AV, Chandler KJ, Dix DJ,

Kavlock RJ, Knudsen TB. 2011. Predictive models of prenatal developmental toxicity from ToxCast high-throughput screening data. *Toxicol Sci.* 124:109–127.

Tang N, Farah B, He M, Fox S, Malouf A, Littner Y, Bearer CF. 2011. Ethanol causes the redistribution of L1 cell adhesion molecule in lipid rafts. *J Neurochem.* 119:859–867.

te Velde E, Burdorf A, Nieschlag E, Eijkemans R, Kremer JA, Roeleveld N, Habbema D. 2010. Is human fecundity declining in Western countries? *Hum Reprod.* 25:1348–1353.

Thomas JA, Curto KA, Thomas MJ. 1982. MEHP/DEHP: gonadal toxicity and effects on rodent accessory sex organs. *Environ Health Perspect.* 45:85–88.

Thompson BL, Stanwood GD, Levitt P. 2010. Specificity of prenatal cocaine exposure effects on cortical interneurons is independent from dopamine D1 receptor co-localization. *J Chem Neuroanat.* 39:228–234.

U.S. Environmental Protection Agency. 1991. Guidelines for developmental toxicity risk assessment. *Federal Register.* 56:63798–63826.

U.S. Environmental Protection Agency. 1996. Guidelines for reproductive risk assessment. *Federal Register.* 61:56274–56322.

Visram H, Kanji F, Dent SF. 2010. Endocrine therapy for male breast cancer: rates of toxicity and adherence. *Curr Oncol.* 17:17–21.

Volz DC, Belanger S, Embry M, Padilla S, Sanderson H, Schirmer K, Scholz S, Villeneuve D. 2011. Adverse outcome pathways during early fish development: a conceptual framework for identification of chemical screening and prioritization strategies. *Toxicol Sci.* 123:349–358.

Waghmare A, Kanyalkar M, Joshi M, Srivastava S. 2011. In-vitro metabolic inhibition and antifertility effect facilitated by membrane alteration: search for novel antifertility agent using nifedipine analogues. *Eur J Med Chem.* 46:3581–3589.

Werner J, Ouellet JD, Cheng CS, Ju YJ, Law RD. 2010. Pulp and paper mill effluents induce distinct gene expression changes linked to androgenic and estrogenic responses in the fathead minnow (*Pimephales promelas*). *Environ Toxicol Chem.* 29:430–439.

Wong EW, Cheng CY. 2011. Impacts of environmental toxicants on male reproductive dysfunction. *Trends Pharmacol Sci.* 32:290–299.

Zhang W, Liu Y, An Z, Huang D, Qi Y, Zhang Y. 2011. Mediating effect of ROS on mtDNA damage and low ATP content induced by arsenic trioxide in mouse oocytes. *Toxicol In Vitro.* 25:979–984.

Zhou J, Xu B, Shi B, Huang J, He W, Lu S, Lu J, Xiao L, Li W. 2011. A metabonomic approach to analyze the dexamethasone-induced cleft palate in mice. *J Biomed Biotechnol.* pii: 509043.

CHAPTER 23

Excretion of Hydrophilic Toxicants and Metabolites and Kidney Toxicity

This is a chapter outline intended to guide and familiarize you with the content to follow.

I. Nephrotoxicity—see Figure 23-1 and Table 23-1 (nephron = basic physiological structure)

   A. Prerenal azotemia ($\uparrow$ blood urea nitrogen or BUN)

      1. Combining loop and thiazide diuretics or large dose of osmotic diuretics (or osmotic contract dye) stimulates NaCl uptake and renal vasoconstriction $\rightarrow$ tubular dysfunction and necrosis

      2. Agents that cause a sudden $\downarrow$ in blood pressure such as α_1-receptor blockers especially in combination with erectile dysfunction medications such as sildenafil citrate, nitroglycerin, Ca^{2+}-channel blockers, diazoxide, hydralazine, angiotensin-converting enzyme (ACE) inhibitors, and angiotensin receptor antagonists especially with compromised kidney autoregulation (lack vasodilatory response of glomerular afferent arteriole and vasoconstriction of efferent arteriole in response to $\downarrow$ renal perfusion) $\rightarrow$ prerenal azotemia

      3. Renal artery stenosis in elderly augments these toxicities

      4. NSAIDs $\downarrow$ vasodilatory prostaglandins (PGs), ACE inhibitors, or angiotensin receptor antagonists $\rightarrow$ $\downarrow$ ability of kidney to autoregulate $\rightarrow$ severe perfusion loss through vasoconstriction

   B. Vascular damage

      1. Damage to endothelial cell lining of blood vessels of kidney by immunosuppressant agents (e.g., cyclosporine) or antivirals (e.g., interferon, which also uses an immune reaction to produce thrombin) $\rightarrow$ release of thromboxane A_2 $\rightarrow$ initiates clot formation $\rightarrow$ thrombotic microangiopathy and renal vascular injury

      2. Especially damaging are cytotoxic cancer chemotherapy agents mitomycin C, cisplatin, bleomycin, and gemcitabine $\rightarrow$ thrombotic thrombocytopenic purpura-hemolytic uremic syndrome. This syndrome can also be produced by immune-mediated reactions to anticoagulant agents ticlopidine and clopidogrel, and antimalarial agent quinine

      3. Anticoagulants warfarin or heparin or clot-dissolving agent tissue plasminogen activator $\rightarrow$ reduce atherosclerotic plaques $\rightarrow$ cholesterol released from these plaques occludes small-diameter arcuate and interlobular arteries, terminal arterioles, and glomerular capillaries $\rightarrow$ ischemia, necrosis, and infarction of kidney

   C. Glomerular damage (filtration)

      1. Damage leads to proteinuria as the glomerulus normally keeps protein and blood cells out of the tubular filtrate

      2. Can be caused by inflammatory mediators such as lymphokines ($\uparrow$ by NSAIDs mefenamate and fenoprofen). White blood cells in filtrate = hypersensitivity reactions

      3. Lesions of filtration membrane by toxic rheumatoid arthritis medications, Au, and penicillamine, plus ACE inhibitors and foscarnet

CONCEPTUALIZING TOXICOLOGY 23-1

4. Heavy metals Ag, Au, Hg, and Li produce autoimmunity in various parts of the body but not always in human kidney (Au and Hg have been shown on chronic exposure to cause autoimmune glomerulonephritis). Cd produces autoimmunity in rodents. Progression of disease = thickening of glomerular basement membrane (BGM) → ↑ glomerular permeability (albumin = proteinuria and edema) → podocyte foot processes effaced and swelling of epithelial cells + some subendothelial deposits → capillary thickening → Igs cause granular deposits in BGM with thin argyrophilic projections → blood and albumin in urine (mixed nephrotoxic/nephritis form of nephrotic syndrome) with mesangial cell and matrix ↑ and capillary wall thickening). Lupus nephritis progresses from class I → class V membranous glomerulonephritis

D. Proximal convoluted tubule (PCT) injury

1. Immunosuppressive agents, radiocontrast agents, and antifungal amphotericin B → acute vasoconstriction → ischemic tubular injury

2. Chemotherapy agent methotrexate, antiretroviral nucleoside analogs, NSAID salicylates, and urate can concentrate in PCT due to human organic anion transporter (hOAT) in the basolateral membrane. Probenecid (medication to treat gout) blocks hOAT and ↓ penicillin excretion

3. Fanconi-type abnormality most associated with antiretroviral medications

4. Toxic tubular necrosis (loss of brush border) caused by bisphosphonates (incorporated into ATP analogs and inhibits 3Na$^+$, 2K$^+$-ATPase)

5. S_1 and S_2 segments of kidney usually damaged by overburdened lysosomes

   a. Aminoglycosides accumulated by binding proteins NSP73, calreticulin, CLIMP-53 → stimulation of caspases and Bcl-2 signal transduction

   b. Cd binds to metallothionein and is freed to do damage in lysosomes

6. S_3 segment damaged by metabolic activation, accumulation of compounds by specific transporters, and hypoxia/reperfusion injury

   a. Cisplatin biotransformed to aquated species → oxidative stress and heat shock protein–mediated damage (hydration and chloride stabilization of cisplatin structure largely prevents damage in this segment)

   b. Hexachlorobutadiene is conjugated by GSH in the liver and damages this segment of the kidney as it is transformed to a reactive thioketene

   c. Hg damage via organic anion transporter OAT1/Slc22a6

   d. Chlorinated anilines cause proximal renal necrosis of S_3 region. Oxidative stress is indicated as the ultimate toxic mechanism, but the involvement of prostaglandin H synthase activity indicates the role of non-microsomal enzymes in the toxicity of these compounds in the kidney

E. Interstitium

1. T lymphocytes predominate here = cellular immune responses → granulomas

2. Tubulitis associated with proinflammatory and profibrotic cytokine formation are induced by antibiotics, diuretics, H$_2$ antagonists, allopurinol (anti-gout), interferon, proton-pump inhibitors, and NSAIDs

F. Loop of Henle

1. Chronic renal damage from NSAID accumulation (countercurrent concentrator and subsequent effects on PGs) and acetaminophen (accumulation and GSH depletion). See Figure 23-2

G. Distal convoluted tubule (DCT)

1. Compounds that damage tubules of the nephron elsewhere damage here, such as calcineurin inhibitors that lead to PCT damage when damage here at DCT leads to Mg wasting, tubular collapse, vacuolization, and nephrocalcinosis. Amphotericin B also directly damages here → K$^+$ wasting, nonoliguric renal failure, and distal tubular acidosis. Foscarnet (acyclic nucleoside phosphonoformic acid → distal tubular acidosis and nephrogenic diabetes insipidus (lack of ADH action instead of lack of ADH). Cisplatin also damages here

CONCEPTUALIZING TOXICOLOGY 23-1 (*continued*)

H. Collecting duct

1. Similar to the distal convoluted tubule, toxic compounds such as aminoglycosides cause ion wasting (Mg) and resistance to the effects of ADH

2. Fluoride toxicity here is mediated through mitochondrial toxicity

I. Acid–base and electrolyte balance

1. Potassium balance

   a. Hypokalemia caused by diuretics, carboplatin, cisplatin, or gentamycin

   b. Hyperkalemia—spironolactone (K^+-sparing diuretic), ACE inhibitors, angiotensin receptor antagonists, cyclosporine, COX-2 inhibitors, the anticoagulant heparin, and NSAIDs; exacerbated by blocking Na^+ channel activity via pentamidine, trimethoprim, or NSAIDs or decreased adrenergic activity via use of beta-blockers—hyperkalemia also leads to acidosis via K^+/H^+ exchange in cells

2. Sodium balance

   a. Hyponatremia caused by thiazide diuretics with cyclophosphamide and vincristine cancer chemotherapy agent have similar action via antidiuretic effect in distal tubules. NSAIDs $\rightarrow \downarrow$ PGs $\rightarrow$ potentiating antidiuretic hormone (ADH) action $\rightarrow$ hyponatremia

   b. Hypernatremia—Li^+ and demeclocycline $\rightarrow$ nephrogenic diabetes insipidus $\rightarrow$ hypernatremia

3. Acid–base balance

   a. Acidosis—carbonic anhydrase inhibition by acetazolamide, dorzolamide, mafenide acetate, 6-mercaptopurine, and sulfanilamide $\rightarrow$ proximal tubular acidosis

J. Species-specific toxicity

1. Sustiva (efavirenz) $\rightarrow$ renal epithelial cell necrosis in rat (toxic glutathione-conjugated metabolites) but not in human or cynomolgus monkey

II. Kidney toxicity tests—see Table 23-2

A. The standard clinical indications of creatinine clearance or BUN may be delayed or not sensitive enough to pick up early, possibly reversible damage to the kidney

B. Histopathology has the most bearing on determining renal toxicity, but biopsies are not favored unless cancer may be present

C. Nephrotoxic acute kidney injury biomarkers—urinary albumin, αGST, α_1-microglobulin, β_2-microglobulin, clusterin, cystatin-C, heart-type L-fatty acid–binding protein (signals hypoxia), hepatocyte growth factor (prevents fibrosis), IL-18 (signals tubule-interstitial damage and kidney disease progression to more fatal outcomes in ICUs), KIM-1 (kidney injury protein-1 or transmembrane protein with Ig and mucin domains), liver-type fatty acid protein (involved in fatty acid transport to plasma membrane for β-oxidation, protects against oxidative stress and marks injury), N-acetyl-β-glucosaminidase (elevated in Cr), nertrin-1 (prevents inflammatory –associated lipocalin (expressed at low amounts normally but $\uparrow$ dramatically in injured kidney cells), osteopontin (upregulated in ischemia/perfusion injury and macrophage chemoattractant), retinol-binding protein, and Na^+/H^+ exchanger isoform 3 (most prevalent apical Na^+ transporter differentiating prerenal azotemia, acute tubular necrosis, and intrinsic acute renal failure other than acute tubular necrosis)

D. Ischemic injury—urinary albumin, α-GST, α_1-microglobulin, β_2-microglobulin, clusterin, cysteine-rich protein, cystatin-C, exosomal fetuin-A, heart-type fatty acid–binding protein, hepatocyte growth factor, IL-18, KIM-1, liver-type fatty acid protein, N-acetyl-β-glucosaminidase, netrin, neutrophil gelatinase-associated lipocalin, osteopontin, retinol-binding protein, and Na^+/H^+ exchanger isoform 3

E. Septic injury—urinary albumin, α-GST, α_1-microglobulin, β_2-microglobulin, cystatin-C, exosomal fetuin-A, hepatocyte growth factor, IL-18, KIM-1, liver-type fatty acid protein, N-acetyl-β-glucosaminidase, netrin-1, neutophil gelatinase-associated lipocalin, retinol-binding protein, and Na^+/H^+ exchanger isoform 3

F. Renal transplantation—urinary αGST, α_1-microglobulin, β_2-microglobulin, heart-type fatty acid–binding protein, hepatocyte growth factor, IL-18, KIM-1, liver-type fatty acid protein, N-acetyl-β-glucosaminidase, retinol-binding protein, and Na^+/H^+ exchanger isoform 3

CONCEPTUALIZING TOXICOLOGY 23-1 (*continued*)

G. Proximal tubule

    1. Pars convolute region (S_1 and S_2)—p-aminohippuric acid uptake (OAT1)

    2. Pars recta region (S_3)—glutamine synthase activity

H. Whole animal still preferred for kidney toxicity test but *in vitro* tests are whole kidney perfusion (direct effects), renal cortical slices (simple multicellular model for rapid species comparisons that can indicate cell viability through dye exclusion and can be sampled for synthesis of macromolecules, proliferation, certain carrier-mediated transport, endocytosis, barrier functions including plasma membrane, nuclear activity including expression and mutations, cytoplasmic evaluations, lysosomal assay, mitochondrial function, movement of compound through cells and metabolism all the way to targets, cell repair and cell death), renal epithelial cell lines, and biochemical endpoints

I. Model kidney toxicity compounds—biphenyl, CCl_4, and $HgCl_2$, which indicate the most sensitive kidney tests to involve kidney weight and *in vitro* renal cortical tissue's ability to accumulate organic ions and concentrate urine

CONCEPTUALIZING TOXICOLOGY 23-1 (*continued*)

As toxicants are excreted from the body, they may cause damage along the way. Even natural waste products produced by the body such as bilirubin or creatinine can be damaging. For example, muscle wasting (rhabdomyolysis) caused by a statin medication may lead to excess creatinine in the blood and renal failure. The symptoms of renal failure are usually based on the poor production of urine and less or no excretion of nitrogenous wastes leading to higher creatinine and blood urea nitrogen (BUN) as clinically relevant parameters. However, due to failure of the endocrine portion of the kidney (production of erythropoietin), an anemia may develop, and the effect of angiotensin I may lead to changes in blood pressure. Less developed markers include the amino acid content of urine indicating a specific damage of certain heavy metals such as Pb or Hg. The liver can also be the kidney's "worst enemy" by converting a toxic species via conjugation to something the kidney tries to reabsorb due to the conjugation product, thus it succumbs to the toxicity instead of the liver. The human kidney starts its young adult life with approximately 1 million nephrons (decreases with age, disease processes, and toxicity), or the physiological functional unit for filtration, reabsorption, and secretion that leads to urine formation and preservation of important physiological substance. The vasculature leading to the glomerulus or filter starts the process of filtration and regulates flow into this region based on the blood

pressure. The proximal tubule of the kidney does most of the "heavy lifting" of reabsorption (and some secretion of waste products such as nitrogenous compounds) for the kidney; it resembles the duodenum with a brush border and specific transporters linked to sodium reabsorption and may damage mostly the kidney cortical cells. Additionally, the loop of Henle is a countercurrent concentrator that may inadvertently concentrate a toxic chemical to the detriment of the medulla of the kidney.

This chapter begins with an examination of the prerenal or vascular perfusion of the kidney (takes ~20% of blood volume in the normal unstressed human), followed by vascular injury, moving on to glomerulus of the nephron (GFR or glomerular filtration rate is a key kidney parameter for function), and then proceeding through the proximal convoluted tubule, interstitium (between tubular cells and capillaries), the descending thin loop of Henle, the thick ascending loop of Henle, distal convoluted tubule, and finally the collecting duct to examine kidney toxicity by mechanism and section. The kidney anatomy and physiology play a distinct role in toxicity, because the proximal tubule may concentrate a compound more than threefold, while the distal convoluted tubule and the collecting duct may do so to > 2 log units (100-fold). This of course would increase the toxicity of an agent. The proximal tubule's transport systems for reabsorption make this tubule particularly sensitive to toxicant action. The loop of Henle is known for its countercurrent concentrating action, and the medulla where it is located is hypoxic. This combination may concentrate certain compounds that have increased oxygen metabolism and make the tubules susceptible to injury (Bonventre et al., 2010). As certain data may be more specific to a portion of a section, that will be included. More general data on kidney damage are included in a miscellaneous group of agents. First look at **Figure 23-1**. In this figure, medications that affect various regions of the kidney are noted, as are available biomarkers to assess damage to this region. Also examine **Table 23-1** that summarizes kidney toxicities from various compounds.

Site	Biomarker	Medications
Glomerulus	Total protein, cystatin C (urinary), β_2-microglobulin, α_1-microglobulin, albumin	Doxorubicin (Adriamycin), Puromycin, gold, pamidronate, penicilliamine
Proximal tubule	KIM-1, clusterin, NGAL, GST-α, β_2-microglobulin, α_1-microglobulin, NAG, osteopontin, cystatin C (urinary), netrin-1, RBP IL-18, HGF, cyr61, NHE-3, exosomal fetuin-A, L-FABP, albumin	Cyclosporine, tacrolimus, cisplatin, vancomycin, gentamicin, neomycin, tobramycin, amikacin, ibandronate, zoledronate, hydroxyethyl starch, contrast agents, foscarnet, cidofovir, adefovir, tenofovir, intravenous immunoglobulin
Loop of Henle	Osteopontin, NHE-3	Analgesics (chronic)
Distal tubule	Osteopontin, clusterin, GST-μ/π, NGAL, H-FABP, calbindin D28	Cyclosporine, tacrolmius, sulfadiazine, lithium (chronic), amphotericin B
Collecting duct	Calbindin D28	Amphotericin B, acyclovir, lithium (acute)

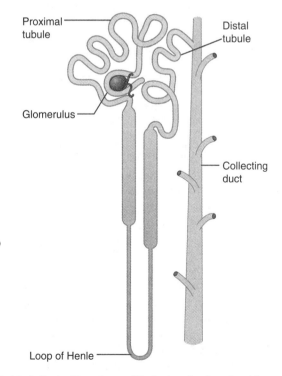

FIGURE 23-1 Sites of Kidney Toxicity Indicating Biomarkers and Medications that Cause Renal Damage

TABLE 23-1 Forensic Chart of Renal Toxicity	
Renal System Toxicity	**Toxic Agents**
Prerenal azotemia	Use of more than one diuretic class, ACE inhibitors, angiotensin receptor antagonists, COX inhibitors, agents causing rapid blood pressure drop (Choudhury and Ahmed, 2006)
Vascular damage	Cancer chemotherapy medications, immunosuppressants, antiplatelet agents, antivirals, anticoagulants, thrombolytics (Choudhury and Ahmed, 2006)
Glomerular damage	Aminoglycosides, fenoprofen, mefenamate, Au, Hg, penicillamine, ACE inhibitors, foscarnet, interferon-α (Choudhury and Ahmed, 2006), doxorubicin, puromycin, pamidronate (Bonventre et al., 2010)
Interstitium	Antibiotics, anti-gout, diuretics, H_2 antagonists, interferon, NSAIDs, proton pump inhibitors (Choudhury and Ahmed, 2006), Au, Hg (Bigazzi, 1999)
Proximal tubule damage	
Ischemia	Amphotericin B, immunosuppressants, radiocontrast agents (Choudhury and Ahmed, 2006)
Fanconi-type	Antiretroviral medications (Choudhury and Ahmed, 2006)
Toxic necrosis	Bisphosphonates (Choudhury and Ahmed, 2006)
Osmotic nephrosis	IV immunoglobulin + osmotic agents (Choudhury and Ahmed, 2006)
S_1, S_2 segments	Aminoglycosides (Choudhury and Ahmed, 2006; Karasawa and Steyger, 2011), cephaloridine (Cristofori et al., 2007), Cd, Cr, solvents, K_2CrO_7 (Cristofori et al., 2007)
S_3 segment	Cisplatin (Choudhury and Ahmed, 2006), Hg, HCBD (Cristofori et al., 2007), chlorinated anilines (Rankin et al., 2008)
Loop of Henle	NSAIDs, acetaminophen (Choudhury and Ahmed, 2006)
Distal convoluted tubule	Foscarnet, immunosuppressants, amphotericin B, gentamicin, carboplatin (Choudhury and Ahmed, 2006), sulfadiazine, chronic Li poisoning (Bonventre et al., 2010)
Collecting duct	Aminoglycosides, cisplatin (Choudhury and Ahmed, 2006), amphotericin B, acyclovir, acute Li poisoning (Bonventre et al., 2010), F (Cittanova et al., 1996)

Prerenal Azotemia

Azotemia is the increase in BUN as an indication of renal damage. Use of a combination of loop (inhibition of Na^+-K^+-$2Cl^-$ cotransport in the ascending thick loop of Henle) and thiazide (inhibition of Na^+-Cl^- symport in the distal convoluted tubule of the kidney) diuretics or large doses of osmotic diuretics such as mannitol (water loss into urine with relatively low rate of renal tubular reabsorption of these molecules) stimulates NaCl uptake and renal vasoconstriction. Osmotic contrast dye also can yield acute vasoconstriction with fractional excretion of Na^+ less than 1%. It is this combination that leads to tubular dysfunction and necrosis. Similarly, agents that cause a sudden or rapid

decrease in blood pressure (alpha$_1$-receptor blockers especially in combination with erectile dysfunction medications such as sildenafil citrate, nitroglycerin, Ca^{2+}-channel blockers, diazoxide, hydralazine, angiotensin-converting enzyme [ACE] inhibitors, and angiotensin receptor antagonists) yield similar results, especially in humans with compromised kidney autoregulation (lack vasodilatory response in the glomerular afferent arteriole and vasoconstriction of the efferent arteriole in a response to decreased renal perfusion). These problems are augmented in the elderly, especially in those with renal artery stenosis. Nonsteroidal anti-inflammatory drugs (NSAIDs; vasodilatory prostaglandin formation inhibitors due to COX enzymes inhibition), ACE inhibitors, or angiotensin receptor antagonists can also make human patients' kidneys less able to autoregulate and therefore subject to the toxic action of severe perfusion loss through vasoconstriction. Some of the toxicity of vasoconstriction from COX inhibitors may be reversible unless the effects are long term. ACE inhibitors also may cause transient increases in BUN and creatinine due to prevention of the efferent arteriole vasoconstriction, which is key to maintaining GFR in volume-contraction or low-perfusion conditions. However, taken together with diuretics, these agents alter renal function presenting with sodium avidity. Any agent that results in hypovolemia from loss of sodium may increase prerenal failure (Choudhury and Ahmed, 2006).

Vascular Damage

Damage to the endothelial cell lining of blood vessels in the kidney may result in the release of thromboxane by those vessels, which initiates platelet aggregation and clot formation. Thrombotic (clot) microangiopathy and renal vascular injury result. Cyclosporine, tacrolimus, and muromonab-CD3 are immunosuppressive agents that cause this type of injury. Interferon and valacyclovir are antiviral compounds that damage these vessels. Compounds that are especially damaging to these small vessels are gastrointestinal (GI) cancer chemotherapy agents mitomycin C in combination with cisplatin and bleomycin and gemcitabine or mitomycin C alone. Thrombotic thrombocytopenic purpura–hemolytic uremic syndrome is related to increased doses of these agents. Antiplatelet agents, such as ticlopidine and clopidogrel, and the antimalarial agent quinine more often produce this syndrome via immune-mediated reactions. Interferon is both dose and immune mediated in generation of thrombotic microangiopathy. Why would anticoagulant therapy or "clot-busters" be problematic for these vessels, since one would expect less clot formation? The problem lies elsewhere, because warfarin (interferes with vitamin K action in clotting), heparin (anti-thrombin physiological anticoagulant), streptokinase, or tissue-plasminogen activator (dissolve clots or "clot-busters") starts to reduce atherosclerotic plaques.

The cholesterol released from these plaques may occlude (block) small-diameter arcuate and interlobular arteries, terminal arterioles, and glomerular capillaries. Just as blocking a heart vessel causes an infarct of myocardium, this type of blockage in kidney vessels causes similar ischemic disease, necrosis, and infarction. Inflammation of the surrounding interstitium broadens the damage (Choudhury and Ahmed, 2006).

Glomerular Damage

Medications that affect the filtering cellular architecture of the glomerulus cause proteinuria (protein and blood should be prevented from finding their way into the tubular filtrate). The lymphokines (to be discussed later in the section on interstitial inflammatory damage) may mediate some of the damage to the glomerulus, as may leukotriene formation (increased by COX inhibitors such as the NSAIDs, with lesions present by mefenamate and fenoprofen). White blood cells may find their way into the filtrate due to hypersensitivity reactions. Lesions of the filtration membrane occur with older toxic rheumatoid arthritis medications (gold and penicillamine), ACE inhibitors (blood pressure medications), and foscarnet (see distal tubule toxicity for this medication; Choudhury and Ahmed, 2006). Some of the larger heavy metals are known to produce autoimmune reactions and damage the glomerulus, but not always in the human kidney. Ag, Au, Hg, and Li induce autoimmunity in various parts of the body. Some metals (Cd, Cr, Cu, Pb, Pt, Zn) only produce autoimmunity infrequently. Other metals are immunotoxic (As, Be, Fe, Ni, V) but do not appear to cause immune reactions. The reactions appear to be species dependent. For example, Cd induces autoimmunity in rodents, but the renal pathology does not appear to be autoimmune mediated in the human. Chronic gold therapy, on the other hand, yields autoimmune thrombocytopenia and immune-complex glomerulonephritis along with other autoimmune reactions. Hg similarly has clear evidence of autoimmune disease in human kidneys and elsewhere (Bigazzi, 1994; Suzuki et al., 2011). Mouse models appear to indicate that autoimmunity from Hg exposure leads to antibodies to nucleolar antigens with a general activation of the immune system, especially the Th2 subset. Glomerulonephritis is transient in these murine models but includes Ig deposits (Bagenstose et al., 1999). Immune reactions of the kidney glomerulus involve a number of disorders. The first is thickening of the glomerular basement membranes (GBM) leading to increased glomerular permeability to proteinuria and edema. It can be purely nephrotic (albumin but no red blood cells in the urine). No detectable immune deposits may be seen in this early phase, but podocyte foot processes are effaced accompanied by swelling of epithelial cells and perhaps some small subendothelial deposits. Membranous nephropathy/membranous glomerulonephritis (or glomerulonephropathy) is characterized by capillary wall thickening and no detectable inflammatory cells. Immunoglobulins (Igs) cause granular deposits that are seen in GBM. Thin argyrophilic projections or spikes are found in this condition in the lamina densa of GBM. Mixed nephrotoxic/nephritis form of nephrotic syndrome includes both blood and albumin in the urine. Mesangial cell and matrix increases plus capillary wall thickening are characteristic of mesangiocapillary glomerulonephritis. Lupus nephritis can occur with small mesangial immune deposits (class I), pure mesangial alterations (class II), focal proliferative glomerulonephritis (class III), diffuse proliferative glomerulonephritis (class IV), membranous glomerulonephritis (class V), and advanced sclerosing glomerulonephritis (class VI; Bigazzi, 1999). Interferon-α has yielded reversible focal segmental hyalinosis associated with visceral epithelial hyperplasia, crescentic glomerulonephritis, and membranous nephropathy. Biphosphonates (i.e., pamidronate) damage the tubules as discussed in the proximal tubular injury section, but also can similarly damage the podocytes of the glomerulus by a T cell–mediated reaction (production of interferon-γ and other cytokines). A late-stage effect of aminoglycoside toxicity (discussed more fully in the proximal tubule section due to the importance of this site for the toxicity of these antibiotics) is alteration of glomerular filtration. In this stage, the density and number

of glomerular fenestrae decrease along with tubular backleak. Tubular obstruction occurs, and mesangial platelet-activating factor is found at higher concentrations (Choudhury and Ahmed, 2006).

Proximal Convoluted Tubular (PCT) Injury

Damage to tubules includes toxic, ischemic, inflammatory, and obstructive injury. Because the vasoconstriction for prerenal azotemia has already been discussed, the examination of this tubule first involves the effects of vasoconstriction on tubular injury. Ischemic tubular injury is a consequence of acute vasoconstriction induced by immunosuppressive agents, radiocontrast agents, and antifungal amphotericin B. The immunosuppressant agents may have the toxicity mediated through or augmented by decreased prostaglandin production and increased vascular renin activity and endothelin. Basolateral transport by the $3Na^+,2K^+$-ATPase results in Na^+ reabsorption in the proximal convoluted tubule, driving other cotransport of reabsorbed nutrients from the luminal side of the cells. Improper insertion of that sodium and potassium pump into the apical membrane due to alterations in polarity leads to epithelium that has too high calcium levels. The signaling by increased calcium leads to altered ion homeostasis and cell death. Proximal tubule damage may result in Fanconi-type dysfunction seen as increased sodium and chloride excretion in the urine (saluresis), potassium excretion (kaliuresis), decreased ammonia in the urine, glucose in the urine (glucosuria which usually by itself would be a sign of diabetes mellitus), protein in the urine (proteinuria), the physiological buffer bicarbonate in the urine (bicarbonaturia), and higher phosphate in the urine (phosphaturia). The human organic anion transporter (hOAT) in the basolateral membrane is responsible for the uptake of anionic, charged metabolites and medications (and other toxicants of similar chemical nature). The medications that are concentrated into these cells by hOAT include the chemotherapy agent methotrexate, antiretroviral nucleoside analogs, NSAID salicylates, and urate. The medication probenecid, which is used to excrete more uric acid in gout or prevent penicillin excretion, blocks hOAT and thereby decreases the accumulation of these compounds. The Fanconi-type abnormality is mostly associated with antiretrovirals cidofovir and adefovir. Toxic tubular necrosis characterized by loss of brush border and apoptosis of cells is caused by biphosphonates used in the treatment of multiple myeloma and Paget's disease. Biphosphonates are only cleared by the energy-requiring mechanisms of active transport following filtrations. Then they are secreted by the tubular cells, unless the proximal tubule cells' internalization leads to incorporation into adenosine triphosphate (ATP) analogs. This will inhibit ATP-dependent pathways including the vital $3Na^+$, $2K^+$-ATPase. Actin ring assembly can also be blocked by this compound and lead to other alterations of cellular architecture. Intravenous administration of Igs for skin problems, immune-associated disease states, neurological disorders, or rheumatoid arthritis–associated pathologies (including those involving the kidney) may lead to osmotic nephrosis. In this context, the stabilizing agent for Ig administration can be a sugar such as sucrose (or other osmotic agents such as dextran, hydroxyethyl starch, or mannitol). Sucrose resists metabolism and causes swelling and proximal tubule damage.

The proximal tubule may be subdivided into S_1 and S_2 (pars convoluta or convoluted part) segments versus the S_3 segment (pars recta or straight part). The first two segments are likely damaged by overburdened lysosomes and toxic groups bound to proteins, while the S_3 segment usually is damaged by metabolic activation, accumulation of compounds by specific transporters, and hypoxia/reperfusion injury (Cristofori et al., 2007). The S_1 and S_2 segments are damaged by aminoglycosides (organic bases with cationic groups), which by the nature of the number of aminoglycoside linkages are transported from the luminal brush border of these proximal cells (likely via multi-ligand endocytic receptor megalin) into the lysosomal compartment. They stay there for an enormous $t_{1/2}$ of 100 hours (plasma $t_{1/2}$ of 3 hours) and inhibit lysosomal enzymes. Neomycin is most toxic and has the most aminoglycoside

linkages, and gentamycin, tobramycin, amikacin, and streptomycin proceed down the severity scale (Choudhury and Ahmed, 2006). Further research indicates that there are aminoglycoside-binding proteins (HSP73, calreticulin, CLIMP-53) that lead to stimulation of caspases and Bcl-2 signal transduction pathways that mediate aminoglycoside cytotoxicity (Karasawa and Steyger, 2011). Another antibiotic known as cephaloridine also targets the S_1 and S_2 segments. Certain metals, such as Cd and Cr(VI), and solvents damage the S_1 and S_2 segments (Cristofori et al., 2007). Acute Cd toxicity yields hepatotoxicity. Chronic Cd toxicity appears to involve metallothionein conjugation in the liver and transport to the kidney. In this chronic toxicity model, Cd stimulates *de novo* synthesis of metallothionein (MT). When the loading of Cd ions exceeds the chelation or "buffering" capacity of intracellular MTs, it reaches the kidneys via the circulation. In this case, the liver unintentionally sets up the kidney toxicity (this role of the liver is revisited later with glutathione (GSH) conjugation of hexachlorobutadiene and cisplatin). In the proximal tubule, the filtered CdMT is endocytosed and degraded by lysosomes. This frees the metal to do damage to various structures (Sabolić et al., 2010). Cr(VI) appears to achieve its toxicity through accumulation via the anion transport system followed by intracellular reduction. It can react with H_2O_2 and yield OH.. An industrial-use metallic oxide (potassium dichromate or K_2CrO_7) also specifically damages in this region, producing vacuolization 24 hours after introduction and diffuse necrosis after 48 hours (Cristofori et al., 2007).

Cisplatin, a chlorinated (2 groups + 2 amino groups) platinum cancer chemotherapy agent, is biotransformed to an aquated species that reacts on nucleophilic sites in DNA to treat cancers. In the kidney, this cytotoxic agent is most damaging to the S_3 segment of the proximal tubule. Oxidative stress and heat shock protein appear to be mechanisms of tubular cell depletion in the kidney. It is of interest that hydration and chloride stabilization of the cisplatin by saline (chloride diuresis) prior to treatment largely prevents the renal damage. Any medication or toxin that causes significant tubular injury can lead to acute renal failure due to induction of apoptosis and sloughing of tubular cells, active urinary sediment abnormalities, intratubular blockage, and less urine formation (Choudhury and Ahmed, 2006). Heavy metals can also damage the tubules (and interstitium) directly or via immune reactions. Immune reactions include acute tubulointerstitial nephritis including fever and hematuria accompanied by interstitial edema, leukocyte infiltration, and focal tubular necrosis. Polyuria, nocturia, and mild proteinuria characterize chronic tubulointerstitial nephritis with infiltration with monocytes, interstitial fibrosis, and tubular atrophy. The direct toxicity of Au and immune recognition thereof may be linked to the chelates between Au(I) and cysteine thiol groups (similarly Hg forms S-conjugates). This is also related to gold's immunosuppressive action on rheumatoid arthritis. Monocytes are capable of generating an active metabolite of gold known as Au(III). Wistar rats treated with aurothiomalate show thickened glomerular capillary walls and granular glomerular deposition of Igs and complement, but detectable Au is only found in the PCT. Inbred mice of the A.SW strain treated with gold sodium thiomalate give some indication that the autoantigen is fibrillarin (U3 RNP protein), similar to Hg-induced renal autoimmunity. Brown Norway rats appear to react to laminin 1 (GBM), which is a component of the extracellular matrix (Bigazzi, 1999). Direct mercury toxicity in the proximal tubule occurs via organic anion transporter OAT1/ Slc22a6 as mice Oat1 knockouts abolished the observed damage in wild-type mice (Torres et al., 2011). This direct damage due to Hg is also found in the S_3 segment, as are the toxic effects of hexachloro-1,3-butadiene (CBD) and Pd. Hexachlorobutadiene (HCBD) and cisplatin (cis-Pt) are observed to cause a diffuse necrosis in this pars recta section in the outer stripe of the outer medulla. This is a case where the liver unintentionally injures the kidney. Both cis-Pt and HCBD are conjugated by GSH in the liver to prevent hepatotoxicity and removal to the kidney. The GSH-conjugated halogenated alkane (HCBD) is further metabolized to S-(pentachlorobutadienyl)-L-cysteine. This molecule is acted upon by cysteine conjugate β-lyase to become the reactive thioketene that

ultimately does the kidney damage. In similar fashion, cis-Pt is conjugated in the liver and becomes toxic in the kidney. In the case of cis-Pt, γ-glutamyl transpeptidase appears to play a crucial role in the nephrotoxicity of cis-Pt, while it decreases the therapeutic value in causing toxicity to the carcinoma (Cristofori et al., 2007).

The chlorinated anilines are extremely nephrotoxic. One of the worst is 3,5-dichloroaniline, an intermediate of fungicide manufacture. Aminochlorophenols are also nephrotoxicants, and the role of parent compound and metabolites in this toxicity have been investigated. It is of interest that one of the metabolites of 3,5-dichloroaniline is likely 4-amino-2,6-dichlorophenol. These compounds cause proximal renal necrosis in the corticomedullary region (S_3). If this were the liver, cytochrome P450 (CYP) or flavin-containing monooxygenase (FMO) N-oxidation would be expected to metabolize to a toxic benzoquinoneimine, reminiscent of acetaminophen metabolism/activation to a toxic metabolite. However, neither CYP inhibitors of metyrapone or piperonyl butoxide or isoniazid nor FMO inhibitor (methimazole) or enhancer (N-octylamine) appeared to have any evidence for impacting the toxicity of the aminochlorophenol. Rather, an inhibitor of prostaglandin H synthase activity (indomethacin) appeared to partially reduce the toxicity of this compound. So oxidation by non-microsomal oxidative enzymes appears to be responsible for the toxicity of this compound in the kidney. Also, ascorbate (2 mM) and GSH (1 mM) appear to also diminish the toxicity of the compound if the concentration of the aminochlorophenol is not too high (0.05–0.1 mM). N-Acetylcysteine was less able to reduce the toxicity of the aminochlorophenol. Structure is important for the renal toxicity as 4-aminophenol toxicity is indeed more attenuated by ascorbic acid. This suggests that oxidative stress is the major mechanism for less complex aromatic hydrocarbons' renal damage, whereas the more complex chlorinated anilines appear to involve alkylation and oxidative stress mechanisms. Because GSH reduces the toxicity of the more complex aminochlorophenol but increases the toxicity of 4-aminophenol, this indicates a differing role for GSH-produced metabolites and their metabolism through γ-glutamyl transpeptidase. The aminochlorophenol appears not to follow the classic GSH conjugate/cysteine conjugate β-lyase nephrotoxicity (Rankin et al., 2008).

Interstitium

Immune responses by T cells predominate here and can form granulomas. Antibodies can form in the basement membrane for certain medications such as the antibiotic methicillin. Most antibiotics carry some risk of kidney toxicity. Tubulitis associated with proinflammatory and profibrotic cytokine formation are induced by antibiotics (cephalosporins, clarithromycin, penicillins, rifampin), diuretics (furosemide, thiazides), cimetidine or ranitidine (H_2 antagonists = antiacid), anti-gout medication (allopurinol), antiviral interferon, proton-pump inhibitors (e.g., omeprazole), and NSAIDs (Choudhury and Ahmed, 2006).

Loop of Henle

The loop of Henle is the region of the nephron closely associated with chronic renal damage from NSAIDs and acetaminophen (analgesic but not anti-inflammatory). Acetaminophen toxicity appears to be the classic case of the GSH depletion mechanism similar to the liver (but not the same metabolite). Acetaminophen-cysteine administration increases the toxicity of acetaminophen in the kidney while sparing hepatic thiols. Aromatic thiol ethers appear to be metabolized by cysteine conjugate β-lyase (as opposed to the chloroaniline). Once acted upon by this enzyme, they are able to covalently bind to macromolecules, deplete nonprotein sulfhydryls, and generate lipid peroxides. Pretreatment with aminooxyacetic acid (AOAA), a renal cysteine conjugate β-lyase inhibitor, does not affect acetaminophen's renal damage. However, acetaminophen toxicity is reduced by acivicin, a γ-glutamyl transpeptidase inhibitor. This appears to rule out the kidney's ability to take quinone thioethers and target them through the mercapturic acid pathway–coupled transport processes, which ultimately leads to macromolecule (DNA or protein) alkylation and lipid peroxidation.

Instead, it appears to support the hypothesis that acetaminophen-cysteine functions as a γ-glutamyl acceptor substrate. The GSH used for this reaction would not be available to conjugate/detoxify the reactive metabolite of acetaminophen, N-acetyl-p-benzoquinoneimine (Stern et al., 2005). This depletion/toxicity mechanism in the γ-glutamyl cycle starting by GSH conjugation in the renal proximal tubule cells is illustrated in **Figure 23-2**.

Other chronic damaging agents of the kidney are Li^+ (causes interstitial fibrosis and nephrogenic diabetes insipidus with dysregulation of aquaporins-2,3, but also damages the glomerulus and other tubules as part of is cortical toxicity with disruption of epithelial Na^+ channels and urea transporters UT-A1 and UT-b) and the immunosuppressant calcineurin inhibitors. The renal medulla as a countercurrent concentrator accumulates within the medullary gradient with more at the papillary tip. Lipid peroxidation produces the damage to this region. Chronic fibrosis creates shrinkage of the kidney size while a further association with obliterative arteriolopathy and tubular collapse leads to renal failure. Calcineurin inhibitors may achieve this end via enhanced release of endothelin-1, decreased nitric oxide, and increased transforming growth factor-β (Choudhury and Ahmed, 2006).

Distal Convoluted Tubule

The immunosuppressant calcineurin inhibitors mentioned earlier in the discussion of proximal tubule damage can also lead to distal magnesium wasting and tubular collapse, vacuolization, and nephrocalcinosis. Amphotericin B also causes direct distal tubular damage with nonoliguric renal failure accompanied by distal tubular acidosis. Concentrating problems and potassium wasting are also generated in this region as this antifungal agent (leading to acute tubular necrosis at high doses). It is of interest that lipid-based formulations of amphotericin B cause less kidney toxicity. Foscarnet is an acyclic nucleoside phosphonoformic acid (treats immunocompromised patients with cytomegalovirus retinitis and mucocutaneous acyclovir-resistant herpes simplex virus) that leads to

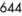

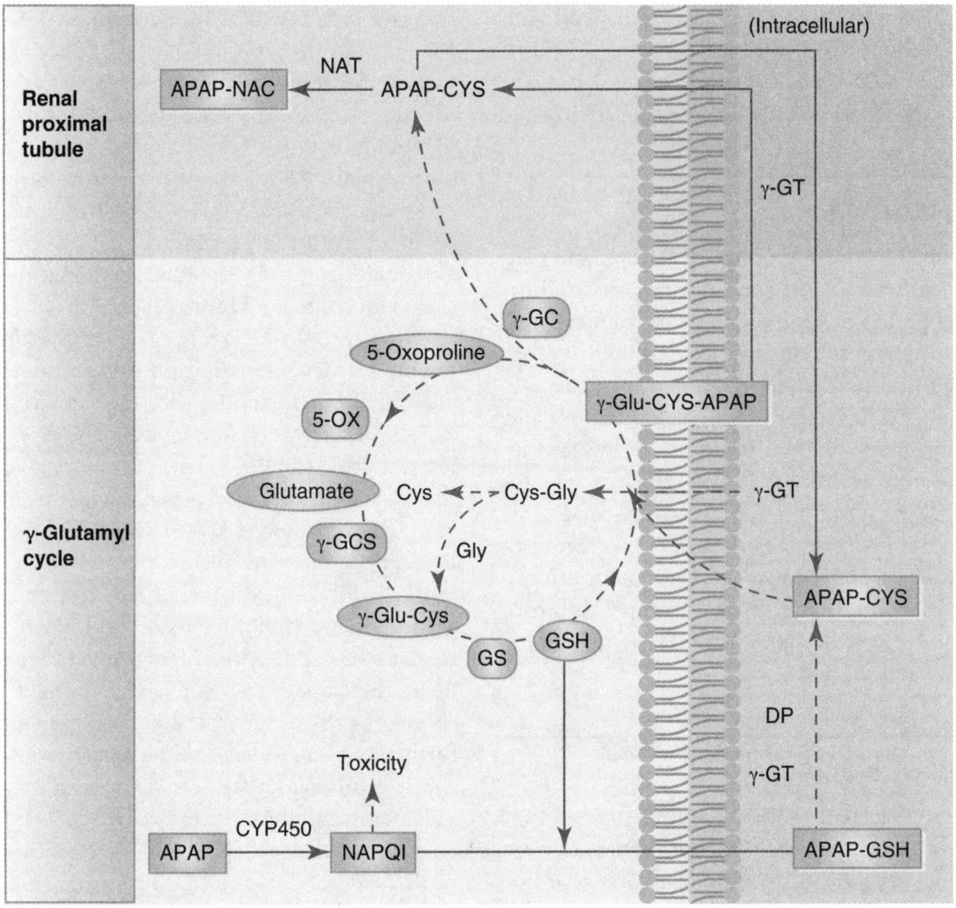

FIGURE 23-2 Participation of Acetaminophen in the γ-Glutamyl Cycle

Note: APAP (acetaminophen) is metabolized by cytochrome P450 (CYP450) to the reactive metabolite *N*-acetyl-*p*-benzoquinone (NAPQI) unless conjugated by glutathione (GSH). However, this conjugate (APAP-GSH) becomes acetaminophen cysteine (APAP-CYS) via enzymatic conversion to by g-glutamyltranspeptidase (g-GT) followed by dipeptidase (DP). This is the species that feeds into the g-glutamyl cycle and depletes GSH. g-glutamylcysteinylacetaminophen (g-GLUCYS-APAP) is acted upon in the cycle by g-glutamylcyclotransferase (g-GC). The APAP-CYS can be regenerated at this step and be acetylated via n-acetyl tranferase to acetaminophen-mercapturate (APAP-NAC). Other enzymes in the cycle are: oxoprolinase (5-OX), g-glutamylcysteine synthetase (g-GCS), and glutathione synthetase (GS finishing the pivotal sequence of GSH synthesis).

distal tubular acidosis and nephrogenic diabetes insipidus (dehydration due to lack of antidiuretic hormone [ADH] action). This compound is capable of chelating divalent metal ions such as Ca^{2+} and Mg^{2+}. Activated platinum (cisplatin) can also damage here as well (Choudhury and Ahmed, 2006).

Collecting Duct

Aminoglycosides result in urinary magnesium loss (hypomagnesemia) and resistance to ADH with nonoliguric (having good GFR but low tubular reabsorption rates) acute tubular necrosis. Cisplatin damages here similarly to its action on the distal tubule and damage, where lysosomal and tubular hyperplasia and necrosis can occur extending down into the renal papilla (Choudhury and Ahmed, 2006). Fluoride toxicity to the collecting duct may involve mitochondrial toxicity as exposure of immortalized human collecting duct cells decreased cell number and total protein content and increased lactate dehydrogenase release at a threshold concentration of 5.0 mM. $3Na^+$-$2K^+$ ATPase activity is also inhibited by more than half at this same concentration. At 1.0 mM, crystal formation and other morphological alterations of the mitochondria are noted. In patients this would turn into clinical Na^+ and water disturbances in response to fluoride toxicity (Cittanova et al., 1996).

Acid–Base Balance and Electrolyte Balance

Although this can just yield systemic problems, such as heart arrhythmias, certain toxic agents cause this type of problem. For example, most diuretics lead to low potassium (hypokalemia), but agents that damage the distal tubule (carboplatin, cisplatin, gentamicin) cause potassium loss from the kidney. The opposite, dangerous hyperkalemia (can stop the heart), can occur with spironolactone or other potassium-sparing diuretics (aldosterone antagonists at the distal convoluted tubule), especially in concert with K^+ supplementation. However, the use of agents that affect renin-angiotensin or aldosterone activity also may yield similar dangerous accumulation of potassium, such as ACE inhibitors and angiotensin receptor antagonists (COX-2 inhibitors may be considered a subset of NSAIDs). Blocking Na^+ channel activity via pentamidine, trimethoprim, or NSAIDs or decreased adrenergic activity via use of betablockers may also worsen hyperkalemia. Low sodium levels occur when sodium is excreted out of the body faster than water or water levels rise in the body faster than sodium. Thiazide diuretics dump sodium and elicit an increase in antidiuretic hormone (ADH) and aldosterone secondary to water loss, causing hyponatremia. Cyclophosphamide and vincristine (cancer chemotherapy) have an antidiuretic effect on free water excretion in the distal tubules yielding similar results. NSAIDs prevent the formation of prostaglandins potentiating the action of ADH and causing hyponatremia. Li^+ and demeclocycline yield nephrogenic diabetes insipidus. As water is eliminated too fast, the dehydration results (hypernatremia).

Proximal tubular acidosis results from carbonic anhydrase inhibition (used to treat altitude sickness, a variety of neurological and GI disorders, glaucoma, osteoporosis). It is caused by acetazolamide, dorzolamide, mafenide acetate, 6-mercaptopurine, and sulfanilamide. Aminoglycoside or cisplatin proximal tubule damage can also spur acidosis. Compounds that inhibit the distal tubular Na^+/H^+ exchange yield distal tubular acidosis (amphotericin B, cyclosporine, Li^+, and vitamin D [high dose]).

Species Specificity

Sustiva (efavirenz) was a medication that was abandoned due to renal epithelial cell necrosis in the rat. This toxicity does not appear in the human or the cynomolgus monkey, because neither produces the toxic GSH-conjugated metabolite (Bonventre et al., 2010).

Kidney Toxicity Tests

The clinical standards for toxicity testing are still serum creatinine and BUN. Creatinine synthesis rate alterations in individuals indicate comparable toxicity but may not cause similar changes in creatinine kinetics (creatinine clearance) or steady-state serum concentrations. It also may be a highly delayed signal following injury. Additionally, 50% of kidney function must be lost to observe elevations of serum creatinine (Dent et al., 2007). BUN is also problematic because many factors lead to its concentration variations. BUN may simply increase when plasma volume decreases, as in dehydration. If urea synthesis is increased, BUN will also rise, as in people who use protein supplements to build muscle tissue. Additionally, catabolic states causing muscle wasting or blood in the GI tract will cause protein loads and increased BUN.

Histopathology is the standard that appears to have the most influence on determining toxicity. In the clinic, the desirability of taking a biopsy is not favored unless a cancer is evident. Even in animal models, there are non-histopathology-associated kidney toxicities such as interference with proximal tubule transport (leading to aminoaciduria, glucosuria, or hyperuricosuria) or prevention of ADH activity in the collecting duct as observed earlier for agents producing apparent diabetes insipidus.

Changes in GFR are also problematic, because its threshold for determining toxicity in an organ with reserve functional capacity is too high by this method. **Table 23-2** reviews the toxicity tests by region, while this discussion augments the table and marks toxicity based on clinical models. The glomerulus and/or proximal tubule may leak protein (albumin), smaller proteins (microglobins, cysteine-rich proteins), and a lipoprotein involved in prevention of glomerular immune complexes (clusterin depletion in kidney leads to more immune complex formation at the glomerulus and proximal convoluted tubule; Ghiggeri et al., 2002). Preclinical or clinical studies suggest that the following biomarkers have use in these perturbations of normal kidney function. Nephrotoxic acute kidney injury is assessed by urinary albumin, α-GST, α_1-microglobulin, β_2-microglobulin, clusterin, cystatin-C, heart-type L-fatty acid–binding protein (signals hypoxia), hepatocyte growth factor (prevents fibrosis), IL-18 (signals tubule-interstitial damage and kidney disease progression to more fatal outcomes in intensive care units; Shi et al., 2012), KIM-1 (kidney injury protein-1 or transmembrane protein with Ig and mucin domains), liver-type fatty acid protein (involved in fatty acid transport to plasma membrane for β-oxidation, protects against oxidative stress, and marks injury), N-acetyl-β-glucosaminidase (elevated in chromium workers; Liu et al., 1998), netrin-1 (prevents inflammatory reactions due to ischemia followed by reperfusion injury; Wang et al., 2008), neutrophil gelatinase-associated lipocalin (expressed at low amounts normally but elevates dramatically in injured kidney cells; Dent et al., 2007), osteopontin (upregulated in ischemia/perfusion injury and macrophage chemoattractant; Persy et al., 2003), retinol-binding protein, and Na^+/H^+ exchanger isoform 3 (most prevalent apical Na^+ transporter differentiating prerenal azotemia, acute tubular necrosis, and intrinsic acute renal failure other than acute tubular necrosis; du Cheyron et al., 2003). Ischemic injury is assessed by urinary albumin, α-GST, α_1-microglobulin, β_2-microglobulin, clusterin, cysteine-rich protein, cystatin-C, exosomal fetuin-A, heart-type fatty acid–binding protein, hepatocyte growth

TABLE 23-2	Renal Toxicity Tests
Testing For	**Individual Assays**
Glomerular damage	Permeability changes may be reflected in albumin in urine (proteinuria, cystatin-C; Bonventre et al., 2010)
Proximal tubule damage	Decreased reabsorption mechanisms (proteinuria, α_1-microglobulin, β_2-microglobulin, cysteine-rich protein, cystatin-C, retinol-binding protein), damaged leaky cells (α-GST, exosomal fetuin-A, N-acetyl-β-glucosaminidase; Liu et al., 1998), netrin-1 (Wang et al., 2008), neutrophil gelatinase-associated lipocalin (Dent et al., 2007), Na^+/H^+ exchanger isoform 3 (du Cheyron et al., 2003), fibrosis (hepatocyte growth factor, KIM-1, liver-type fatty acid protein, osteopontin; Persy et al., 2003), immune complex (clusterin, IL-18; Bonventre et al., 2010; Ghiggeri et al., 2002; Shi et al., 2012)
S_1–S_2 segments	p-aminohippuric acid uptake (Cristofori et al., 2007)
S_3 segment	glutamine synthetase (Cristofori et al., 2007)
Loop of Henle	Fibrosis (osteopontin), leaky damaged loop cells (Na^+/H^+ exchanger isoform 3; Bonventre et al., 2010)
Distal convoluted tubule	Leaky damaged distal tubule cells (clusterin, neutrophil gelatinase-associated lipocalin), hypoxia (heart-type L-fatty-acid-binding protein), fibrosis (hepatocyte growth factor, osteopontin; Bonventre et al., 2010)
Collecting duct	Ability to respond to ADH (Choudhury and Ahmed, 2006), other toxicity tests based on organelle function (e.g., mitochondrial function; Cittanova et al., 1996)
In vitro tests	Perfused kidney, renal cortical slices, renal cortical cells in isolation (Hawksworth et al., 1995)

factor, IL-18, KIM-1, liver-type fatty acid protein, N-acetyl-β-glucosaminidase, netrin-1, neutrophil gelatinase–associated lipocalin, osteopontin, retinol-binding protein, and Na^+/H^+ exchanger isoform 3. Septic injury is marked by urinary albumin, α-GST, $α_1$-microglobulin, $β_2$-microglobulin, cystatin-C, exosomal fetuin-A, hepatocyte growth factor, IL-18, KIM-1, liver-type fatty acid protein, N-acetyl-β-glucosaminidase, netrin-1, neutrophil gelatinase–associated lipocalin, retinol-binding protein, and Na^+/H^+ exchanger isoform 3. Renal transplantation is marked by urinary α-GST, $α_1$-microglobulin, $β_2$-microglobulin, heart-type fatty acid–binding protein, hepatocyte growth factor, IL-18, KIM-1, liver-type fatty acid protein, N-acetyl-β-glucosaminidase, retinol-binding protein, and Na^+/H^+ exchanger isoform 3 (Bonventre et al., 2010).

When determining proximal tubule sections, the uptake of p-aminohippuric acid (pAH—not to be confused with polycyclic aromatic hydrocarbons) is indicative of nephrotoxicity to the pars convoluta region, while glutamine synthetase activity (mitochondrial enzyme crucial in nitrogen metabolism) denotes pars recta (proximal and distal portions of S_3) toxicity. The use of pAH uptake of a specific marker of one segment of the proximal tubule is complicated by its uptake mechanism in a variety of species. pAH transport appears to involve OAT1, one of three organic anion transporters of the basolateral membranes. As mentioned earlier, OAT4 appears to be associated with the apical membrane in rat proximal tubule cells. In the rabbit and mouse, OAT1 appears to be localized in the S_2 segment. In the rat, the site of this transport appears to have conflicting data. In a study using segment-specific nephrotoxicants such as HCBD, both the S_2 and S_3 segments appeared to be involved in pAH transport (Roch-Ramel and Weiner, 1980; Roch-Ramel et al., 1980) or just localized to the S3 segment (Hook et al., 1982). A study using similar techniques 20 years later suggested the S_1 and S_2 segments (Trevisan et al., 2001). In 2005 (Kwak et al., 2005), rat OAT1 mRNA was found to involve the cortex and outer medulla (Cristofori et al., 2007).

On the whole, it still appears that the intact animal (or human clinical findings) predominate as the renal toxicity tests. However, *in vitro* models involving whole kidney perfusion (single pass, recirculation of perfusate, and recirculation and dialysis of perfusate), renal cortical slices, use of renal epithelial cell lines, and biochemical endpoints indicate some possible alternatives. Isolated perfused kidney models are most appropriate for direct effects of toxicants, although they have a limited lifetime of use. These perfused kidneys also have higher renal vascular flow and lower GFRs and decreased filtration fractions than normal kidneys. They also lack the influence of the other organ systems in renal control and toxicity (such as the liver). Isolated perfused nephrons are not suitable toxicity models. Renal cortical slices may be used because they are simple, are multicellular, require no enzymatic tissue digestion, and are three-dimensional, plus cell–cell contacts exist, site specificity is intact, several functional parameters can be evaluated, renal-specific parameters are intact, and they can allow for rapid species comparisons. However, these slices also have a limited lifetime; have heterogenicity of morphology, function, and biochemistry; lack reproducibility of nephron segments; and may have collapsed lumen leading to lack of active transport of pAH; additionally, the surface of the slice is by definition damaged. Cell lines offer an ease of handling and rapid results, but do not exhibit complete proximal tubule function. These *in vitro* tests can test for cell viability by dye exclusion or enzyme or ion leakage. They can also look for synthesis of macromolecules (DNA, RNA, protein, matrix elements). They can assay rate of proliferation (clonogenic assays). Carrier-mediated transport can be assessed (glucose, organic ions, inorganic ions, low-molecular-weight proteins). Cultured cells of proximal tubule origin can be assayed for endocytosis of labeled proteins or carbohydrates. Barrier functions can also be assessed electrophysiologically or by diffusion of extracellular markers. Biochemically, they can assess damage to the plasma membrane via ion regulation, signal transduction, membrane leakage, and lipid peroxidation. Nuclear activity can be determined by gene expression, endonuclease activation, and mutations. Cytoplasm/cytoskeletal evaluations involve GSH depletion and protein processing. Degradative enzymes of the lysosomes indicate the function of this important organelle. Mitochondrial function can be determined via ATP synthesis, cellular respiration, and ion regulation. Along with these functions, the entry of the chemical or metabolite into cells, metabolism, and interactions at target sites (protein/DNA/lipid) may be evaluated along with the larger response of cell repair (no effect to proliferation toward becoming a cancer cell) to cell death (apoptosis to necrosis; Hawksworth et al., 1995). Model kidney toxicity compounds of biphenyl, CCl_4, and $HgCl_2$ indicate that standard urinalysis (urine specific gravity, pH, volume, glucosuria, proteinuria, urinary electrolytes), serum analyses (BUN, creatinine and creatinine clearance, electrolytes), quantitative enzymuria, and histopathological changes were inconsistent and less sensitive measures of subacute renal toxicity than were tests that quantified total functional renal capacity. The most sensitive tests interestingly enough appeared to involve kidney weight and *in vitro* renal cortical tissue's ability to accumulate organic ions and concentrate urine (Kluwe, 1981).

Questions

1. What mechanisms underlie the development of prerenal azotemia?
2. What are some agents that damage kidney vascular directly? What agents also require an immune reaction?
3. How is the severity of glomerulonephritis indicated by urine contents?
4. Why is cisplatin toxic to the S_3 segment of the kidney, while aminoglycoside antibiotics are toxic to the S_1 and S_2 segments?
5. How does chronic acetaminophen administration damage the loop of Henle?
6. What is different about the consequences of damage to the distal convoluted tubule by compounds that damage elsewhere (such as the PCT)?
7. What are the biomarkers of toxicity to the S_1 and S_2 segments versus S_3 segment of the proximal convoluted tubule?

References

Bagenstose LM, Salgame P, Monestier M. 1999. Murine mercury-induced autoimmunity: a model of chemically related autoimmunity in humans. *Immunol Res.* 20:67–78.

Bigazzi PE. 1994. Autoimmunity and heavy metals. *Lupus.* 3:449–453.

Bigazzi PE. 1999. Metals and kidney autoimmunity. *Environ Health Perspect.* 107(Suppl 5):753–765.

Bonventre JV, Vaidya VS, Schmouder R, Feig P, Dieterle F. 2010. Next-generation biomarkers for detecting kidney toxicity. *Nat Biotechnol.* 28:436–440.

Choudhury D, Ahmed Z. 2006. Drug-associated renal dysfunction and injury. *Nat Clin Pract Nephrol.* 2:80–91.

Cittanova ML, Lelongt B, Verpont MC, Geniteau-Legendre M, Wahbe F, Prie D, Coriat P, Ronco PM. 1996. Fluoride ion toxicity in human kidney collecting duct cells. *Anesthesiology.* 84:428–435.

Cristofori P, Zanetti E, Fregona D, Piaia A, Trevisan A. 2007. Renal proximal tubule segment-specific nephrotoxicity: an overview on biomarkers and histopathology. *Toxicol Pathol.* 35:270–275.

Dent CL, Ma Q, Dastrala S, Bennett M, Mitsnefes MM, Barasch J, Devarajan P. 2007. Plasma neutrophil gelatinase-associated lipocalin predicts acute kidney injury, morbidity and mortality after pediatric cardiac surgery: a prospective uncontrolled cohort study. *Crit Care.* 11:R127.

du Cheyron D, Daubin C, Poggioli J, Ramakers M, Houillier P, Charbonneau P, Paillard M. 2003. Urinary measurement of Na^+/H^+ exchanger isoform 3 (NHE3) protein as new marker of tubule injury in critically ill patients with ARF. *Am J Kidney Dis.* 42:497–506.

Ghiggeri GM, Bruschi M, Candiano G, Rastaldi MP, Scolari F, Passerini P, Musante L, Pertica N, Caridi G, Ferrario F, Perfumo F, Ponticelli C. 2002. Depletion of clusterin in renal diseases causing nephrotic syndrome. *Kidney Int.* 62:2184–2194. Erratum in: *Kidney Int.* 2003;63:1602.

Hawksworth GM, Bach PH, Nagelkerke JF, Decant W, Diezi JE, Harpur E, Lock EA, MacDonald C, Morin J-P, Pfaller W, Rutten FAJJL, Ryan MP, Toutain HJ, Trevisan A. 1995. Nephrotoxicity testing *in vitro*: the report and recommendations of ECVAM Workshop 10. *Altern Lab Anim.* 23:713–727.

Hook JB, Rose MS, Lock EA. 1982. The nephrotoxicity of hexachloro-1:3-butadiene in the rat: studies of organic anion and cation transport in renal slices and the effect of monooxygenase inducers. *Toxicol Appl Pharmacol.* 65:373–82.

Karasawa T, Steyger PS. 2011. Intracellular mechanisms of aminoglycoside-induced cytotoxicity. *Integr Biol (Camb)*. 3:879–886.

Kluwe WM. 1981. Renal function tests as indicators of kidney injury in subacute toxicity studies. *Toxicol Appl Pharmacol*. 57:414–424.

Kwak J-O, Kim H-W, Oh K-J, Kim DS, Han KO, Cha SH. 2005. Co-localization and interaction of organic anion transporter 1 with caveolin-2 in rat kidney. *Exp Mol Med*. 37:204–212.

Liu CS, Kuo HW, Lai JS, Lin TI. 1998. Urinary *N*-acetyl-beta-glucosaminidase as an indicator of renal dysfunction in electroplating workers. *Int Arch Occup Environ Health*. 71:348–352.

Persy VP, Verhulst A, Ysebaert DK, De Greef KE, De Broe ME. 2003. Reduced postischemic macrophage infiltration and interstitial fibrosis in osteopontin knockout mice. *Kidney Int*. 63:543–553.

Rankin GO, Hong SK, Anestis DK, Ball JG, Valentovic MA. 2008. Mechanistic aspects of 4-amino-2, 6-dichlorophenol-induced *in vitro* nephrotoxicity. *Toxicology*. 245:123–129.

Roch-Ramel F, Weiner IM. 1980. Renal excretion of urate: factors determining the actions of drugs. *Kidney Int*. 18:665–676.

Roch-Ramel F, White F, Vowles L, Simmonds HA, Cameron JS. 1980. Micropuncture study of tubular transport of urate and PAH in the pig kidney. *Am J Physiol Renal Physiol*. 239:F107–F112.

Sabolić I, Breljak D, Skarica M, Herak-Kramberger CM. 2010. Role of metallothionein in cadmium traffic and toxicity in kidneys and other mammalian organs. *Biometals*. 23:897–926.

Shi B, Ni Z, Cao L, Mou S, Wang Q, Zhang M, Fang W, Yan Y, Qian J. 2012. Serum IL-18 is closely associated with renal tubulorinterstitial injury and predicts renal prognosis in IgA nephropathy. *Mediators Inflamm*. 2012:728417.

Stern ST, Bruno MK, Horton RA, Hill DW, Roberts JC, Cohen SD. 2005. Contribution of acetaminophen-cysteine to acetaminophen nephrotoxicity II. Possible involvement of the gamma-glutamyl cycle. *Toxicol Appl Pharmacol*. 202:160–171.

Suzuki Y, Inoue T, Ra C. 2011. Autoimmunity-inducing metals (Hg, Au and Ag) modulate mast cell signaling, function and survival. *Curr Pharm Des*. 17:3805–3814.

Torres AM, Dnyanmote AV, Bush KT, Wu W, Nigam SK. 2011. Deletion of multispecific organic anion transporter Oat1/Slc22a6 protects against mercury-induced kidney injury. *J Biol Chem*. 286:26391–26395.

Trevisan A, Giraldo M, Borella M, Bottegal S, Fabrello A. 2001. Tubular segment-specific biomarkers of nephrotoxicity in the rat. *Toxicol Lett*. 124:113–20.

Wang W, Reeves WB, Ramesh G. 2008. Netrin-1 and kidney injury. I. Netrin-1 protects against ischemia-reperfusion injury of the kidney. *Am J Physiol Renal Physiol*. 294:F739–F747.

PART IV

Toxic Reactions of Ecosystems

Dispersion Modeling in Air, Water, and Soil: Likely Route of Exposure and Most Sensitive Organism Based on Dispersion and Concentration

This is a chapter outline intended to guide and familiarize you with the content to follow.

I. Ecotoxicology and environmental toxicity

    A. Comparison of environmental toxicology and ecotoxicology approaches

        1. Environmental toxicology examines the separate effects of toxicants on specific environmental species under controlled conditions in a laboratory. This information is coupled to estimated environmental concentrations under worst case scenarios to assess risk

        2. Ecotoxicology examines the effects of toxicant in the degraded current environment with species abundance and so forth monitored along with measured concentrations of the toxicant(s) at various selected sites. See USEtox program in Figure 24-2. Environmental species other than humans have a fate factor and an ecotox effect factor to assess impact, while humans have an intake fraction and a human effect factor to determine human disease

    B. Dispersion modeling to assess concentration and risk

        1. Simple modeling

            a. Exponential drop-off in three dimensions from a point source with an initial concentration $C_0 \rightarrow$ a simplistic first approximation:
C_d (concentration at distance d) = $C_0 e^{-d}$—see Figure 24-1

            b. AUC = area under curve = integral from 0 to d of $C_0 e^{-e}$ dx dy dz

        2. Radiation—falls off as inverse of the square of distance ($1/d^2$), not exponential

        3. More advanced initial models include moving to a dilution grid model based on height of the building and height of the stack to see if more advanced modeling is warranted

        4. Older models used similar topographies to estimate dispersions (e.g., EPA rolling hills model), but newer models employ advanced meteorological and topographical data now available via GIS (Geographic Information Systems). Then the worst case scenario is envisioned through the model to determine maximum exposure following regulations of application instructions

    C. Dispersion models

        1. K_{ow} (octanol/water partition coefficient) is an important factor in assessing transport and adsorption to particles of absorption into an organism of hydrophobic chemicals. Other chemical parameters also help with determining fate of chemicals (e.g., Hg is dense and tends to sink to the bottom of water)

        2. Air dispersion models—see Figure 24-3

            a. Box, plume, and puff of particles models predict different dispersion characteristics

            b. EPA screening models

                 (1) AERSCREEN (1-h worst-case scenario and estimate 3-h, 8-h, 24-h, and annual concentrations without meteorological data) composed of MAKEMET (site-specific matrix of meteorological conditions) and AERSCREEN command-prompt interface program.

CONCEPTUALIZING TOXICOLOGY 24-1

Uses source input entries then to determine emissions profile (e.g., emission rate, stack height, stack diameter). Despite its apparent complexity, it is still only a screening tool

(2) COMPLEX1 is a multiple point source model

(3) CTSCREEN assumes Gaussian plume dispersion into a complex terrain

(4) RTDM3.2 is a sequential Gaussian plume dispersion into a complex terrain

(5) SCREEN3 uses a single-source Gaussian model that generates maximum ground-level estimations for point, flare, and volume sources

(6) TSCREEN also employs Gaussian model for toxic emissions from a variety of release modes for superfund sites

(7) VALLEY incorporates up to 50 point sources into a steady-state, complex terrain, univariate Gaussian plume algorithm to estimate 24-h or annual concentrations

(8) VISCREEN provides a quantified estimate of the potential impact of a plume of a specified emission for a given set of transport and dispersion conditions

c. Recommended EPA air dispersion models

(1) AERMOD = steady-state plume model (as opposed to non-steady-state plume model of CALPUFF) employing planetary boundary layer turbulence structure and scaling concepts to calculate dispersion into simple or complex terrains. Composed of AERMET, a meteorological data preprocessor in three stages (assesses data quality → merges UPPERAIR, SURFACE, and ONSITE data for 24-h periods → reads merged data file and develops necessary boundary layer for dispersion calculations), and AERMAP, a terrain data preprocessor (user needs to define location, receptors including elevation, and other raw types of terrain data)

(2) CALPUFF = a multilayer, multi-species, non-steady-state puff dispersion model that simulates changing meteorological conditions. Instead of assuming a normally distributed plume model of which the Gaussian model is the oldest, this model follows a random walk of plume parcels or particles in a Lagrangian model as the statistics of their trajectories. The benefit of this model is that it does not assume particles stay together, but can have puff splitting due to complex wind fields. This air dispersion model can also determine wet and dry deposition/fallout

(3) BLP is a special case Gaussian plume dispersion model applicable to Al reduction plants and other industrial sources where plume rise and downwash effects from stationary line sources are critical to proper modeling

(4) CALINE3 employs a Gaussian plume dispersion model to model toxicant emissions downwind of highways in uncomplicated terrain

(5) CAL3QHC/CAL3QHCR is a CALINE-based carbon monoxide model queuing hotspot calculations and with a traffic model (emissions from vehicles that experience delays at signal lights, etc.)

(6) CTMPLUS uses a refined point source Gaussian air quality model in all stability conditions for terrains that are not easily modeled in simpler form

(7) OCD employs a straight-line Gaussian model to determine impacts of offshore emissions on air quality of coastal regions (as may occur from a burning oil spill such as occurred in the Gulf of Mexico in 2010)

d. Alternative air dispersion models

(1) ADAM—employs modified box and Gaussian dispersion model; AFTOX—Gaussian model for liquid gas releases; ASPEN—Gaussian model estimating annual average concentration for each census tract (population); DEGADIS—simulates deposition from dense gases or aerosol clouds in level terrain; HGSYSTEM—dispersion of accidental releases of denser-than-air compounds; HOTMAC/RAPTAD—3-D Eulerian model and Lagrangian random puff model for pollutant transport and diffusion; HYROAD—traffic emissions and dispersions; ISC3—steady-state Gaussian model for industrial complex emissions; ISC-PRIME—incorporates building downwash into ISCST3 model; OBODM—open burning and detonation of obsolete munitions and solid propellants; OZIPR—1-D photochemical box model alternative to

CONCEPTUALIZING TOXICOLOGY 24-1 (*continued*)

OZIP; Panache—Eulerian 3-D finite volume fluid mechanics model and Lagrangian model for particulate matter; PLUVUEII—estimates visual range reduction and atmospheric discoloration by particles in plumes on NO_x or SO_x gases; SCIPUFF—an alternative second-order closure integration puff model; SDM—determines ground-level concentrations from stationary point source emissions near a shoreline; SLM—denser-than-air release models using 1-D equations of momentum, conservation of mass, species and energy, and equation of state

(2) Pesticide models: AgDRIFT for aerial spray deposition patterns; AgDISP for sprays from aircraft; PERFUM for soil fumigants; SOFEA and FEMS for fumigant exposures to bystanders near treated fields

3. Soil and water movement models

a. Movement in fracture rock

(1) Diffusive exchange based on properties of rock matrix, permeability features, advection (fluid movement based on bulk flow), and dispersion all add the mean velocity which in fracture rock can vary over a number of orders of magnitude. In porous media, the void space length and width are similar dimensions, while in fractured rock a few preferential paths may control the majority of flow. Models focusing on regional water balance are more successful in modeling these flows, while stochastic methods are able to account for extreme variability in velocity

b. Movement in soils

(1) Soil vapor extraction model indicates parameters that need including in a soil model such as permeability of the soil to the toxics or water based on soil texture and type, soil structure and stratification, soil moisture, and depth to groundwater. Specific changes are based on pollutant chemistry, the slope of the topography, rainfall events, and other factors that make the models more specific to the ecology of the area and how the chemicals move (as in applications on land) or are likely to move (predicted effects of spills) in that environment

c. Modeling of watershed systems

(1) PRMS simulates the hydrologic cycle at a watershed scale based on climate, biota, geology, and human activities. The four objectives are simulation of hydrologic processes, simulation of water budgets at watershed scale, integration of PRMS with other natural resource management models, and providing modular design for selection of hydrologic-process algorithms

d. Modeling of surface waters

(1) USGS has the most developed surface water models for a variety of conditions. The NRCS has a number of hydrology models based on their involvement in soils and agriculture (AGNPS model utilizes an "annualized" science and technology loading model for agriculture-related watersheds). EPA has pesticide movement models (GENEEC and SWAMP for exposure of and risk to aquatic organisms; FIRST FQPA Index Reservoir Screening Tool for drinking water impacts; KABAM bioaccumulation of hydrophobic pesticides in aquatic food webs; PRZM simulates hydrophobic movement of pesticides in soils within and immediately below plant root zone to surface waters; EXAMS models fate, transport, and exposure to pesticides; EXPRESS assesses aquatic pesticide exposure; SWIMODEL for pesticides used in pools)

e. Solute transfer in ground water

(1) PRZM also follows the pesticide in soil to ground water as well as surface waters. SCIGROW specializes in estimating pesticide concentrations in ground water. USGS is interested in solute transport into ground water and has programs to simulate various parameters as they affect that transport (HST3D, HYDROTHERM, PHAST)

D. Route of exposure

1. Respiratory routes—rapid peaks through lung or gill and respiratory damage, immune reactions, and cancer of the respiratory tract. Pesticides have STIR (Screening Tool for Respiratory Risk) for human exposures

CONCEPTUALIZING TOXICOLOGY 24-1 (*continued*)

2. Oral—slower and shorter but possibly extended peak if drinking water for humans (SIP, or Screening Imbibition Program). Avian and mammalian food items can be modeled for pesticide concentration estimates (T-REX, or Terrestrial Residue Exposure). Terrestrial organisms are more thoroughly investigated for their risk of pesticide exposure through TIM (Terrestrial Investigation Model)

3. Non-target plant pesticide exposures from a single application can be estimated through TerrPlant. T-HERPS simulates pesticide exposure to terrestrial reptiles and amphibians

E. Health effects

1. Human lung—asthma, emphysema, chronic obstructive pulmonary disease, lung cancer

2. Human heart—organ directly after the lung

3. Human brain—organ directly after the heart

4. Human GI tract—food and drinking water contamination

5. Modeling best done through PBPK/PD (Physiological-Based Pharmacokinetic/Pharmacodynamic) but also expensive to gather exact human data

6. Fish—FGETS models food and gill exchange of toxic substances—lethality based on narcotic mode of action. The whole body concentration of C_f then is represented by the following equations: $C_f = B_f/W = (P_a + P_l K_l = P_s K_s)C_a$, where P_a = the aqueous fraction of the whole fish, P_l = the lipid fraction of the whole fish, K_l = partition coefficient between lipid and water (e.g., K_{ow}), P_s = the structural organic fraction of the whole fish, and K_s = partition coefficient between lipid and structural organic matter (e.g., $K_{oc} = 0.4K_{ow}$)

7. Most sensitive organism/biomarkers—direct toxicity measurement of fish miss tertiary effects that occur to algae, which impact zooplankton and therefore fish populations. This is only modeled well by microcosm (tank containing various organisms) or mesocosm (artificial lakes or streams) studies. As these studies are expensive, reproductive success and flow-through exposure of fish yield increased sensitivity to compounds in aquatic systems that may be closer to true environmental impacts excluding habitat issues, climate change, and so forth

8. Ecotoxicology studies indicate no current ecosystem is free from impacts of air pollution. Acidity, eutrophication of and toxic cyanobacterial blooms in estuaries and lakes by excess nutrients (nitrogen, phosphorus), and mercury in benthic organisms are a few of the major concerns of the role of excess compounds having impacts on the environment. Macroinvertebrate sampling can indicate local effects of pollution on streams, and other ecotoxicology indices are also important measures to compare with the simulated models mentioned earlier. The uncertainties in ecotoxicology testing involve the selection of the test species and endpoint (species representative of the ecosystem or other species and endpoints could be varied or incomparable), the validity of a theoretical distribution function (species sensitivity distribution may not fit that function), biological variability within and between species, comparability of laboratory-derived data to field data (bioavailability of toxicant in lab versus field setting and exposure time), variation of scientific data (in a particular researcher's own studies and between researchers both in the lab and the field), and the ever-present problem in field work of other compounds exerting antagonistic, additive, or synergistic effects (less problematic in environmental toxicology laboratory testing under controlled conditions but perhaps less applicable to field results)

CONCEPTUALIZING TOXICOLOGY 24-1 (*continued*)

Ecotoxicology and Environmental Toxicology

This chapter first examines the differences between environmental toxicology and eco-toxicology. Environmental toxicology uses data derived from selected organisms in isolation exposed to pollutants found in the environment and characterizes the hazard. It is similar to taking selected cells out of the body and making them the biomarker for the whole physiology of the body. Ecotoxicology takes into account that the ecosystem has been impacted by human agriculture, industry, and so forth. It is unwise to talk of the Great Plains region when there is the great agricultural region instead. Agricultural regions have drained swamps that have acted as natural holding ponds and filters for pollutants, retarding water flow into rivers. Making tile drains and affecting water flow rapidity into rivers have led to run-off of soil causing erosion and streams or rivers rising too fast and cutting away at their banks. For example, the Minnesota River and its impact on Lake Pepin in the upper Mississippi basin (filling it in with eroded soil and riverbank soil) is part of the legacy of changing the ecosystem. Cities have been placed on waterways, influencing their flows and contents. Streets, storm sewers, and the like have affected stream flows as well. Ecotoxicology recognizes that these systems are already degraded and further examines influences such as global climate change, dead zones, toxic algal blooms, aquifer pollution by toxic plumes, endocrine disruption of wildlife (and humans), and other manifestations of toxic inputs that have large effects on the ecosystem. In U.S. law, ecotoxicology is defined at the company line, farm line, property line, or other border. Thus, within the scope of property rights, a person or a company (which can now been also viewed as a person by the U.S. Supreme Court decision called the Citizens United decision) may store toxic substances on their property, but once they cross the property line in the air/water or form a plume down into the soil toward an aquifer, then ecotoxicity is considered. This requires modeling for dispersion, because no country can afford to put monitors on all property lines.

Dispersion indicates that the highest concentration is likely at the source, which may be a point source such as a discharge pipe from a sewage treatment plant. Nonpoint source pollution refers to inputs from every farm field or every lawn that cannot be reasonably assessed individually, but must be considered as a whole. This does not mean that extreme overuse of a pesticide or pumping a septic tank or manure lagoon directly into a county ditch or river will not be detected as a point source requiring law enforcement and regulatory authorities to come into play, but rather that acceptable practices still have profound impacts as the "price of doing business (public or private)." The topics covered in this chapter are introduced by some simple modeling considerations. As shown in **Figure 24-1**, the point source starts with the highest concentration or C_0 (concentration

at time 0 and distance 0 from source). This does not mean that certain organisms can't bioaccumulate the toxic substance, as was found for dichlorodiphenyltrichloroethane (DDT) and the California condor. The key here is to find the concentration in the air, water, or soil once it gets past the private part and becomes part of the public domain or larger ecosystem.

The initial concentration from a source should decrease rapidly in all three dimensions equally if no wind or current or slope exists—dx, dy, dz (calculus terms meaning that it SLOPES down from a higher concentration). For example, being downwind, downstream, or downhill from a source will dramatically increase this calculation (as indicated in the book *Living Downstream* [Steingraber, 2010], a resident of New Orleans may feel the effects from Minneapolis resident who fouls their river, or people downwind from the Bhopal, India or Chernobyl, Ukraine disasters will be greatly affected), while being upwind, upstream, or uphill will dramatically decrease the calculated concentration. As a first approximation in three-dimensional (3-D) space, the first assumption may be an exponential drop-off. Therefore, each line in the figure represents an exponential decline of an equation e^{-d}, where d is the distance from C_0 in any direction. Solving for concentration yields:

$$C_0 e^{-d} = C_d, \text{ or the concentration at distance } d$$

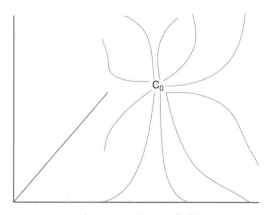

FIGURE 24-1 The Exponential Drop-Off of the Initial Concentration or C_0 of a Point Source in Three Dimensions *dx, dy,* and *dz*

To solve for this equation using a given distance, the natural logarithm or ln would be taken of both sides. A rearrangement yields ln $C_0/C_d = -d$ or ln $C_d/C_0 = d$. From this simple model, it is relatively easy (but not necessarily very accurate) to find how far a living organism would have to be from a source to achieve a certain concentration as long as the dimensions of d are in mm, m, km, or other measure of distance. In radiation, the square of the distance determines radiation dose, so a person 1 m from a radioactive source receives 100 times the radiation than someone 10 m from a source receives. This is important for toxicity. For example, during the making of the atomic bomb during the Manhattan Project era of the 1940s, a person close to two sources that were brought too close together died that week after calculating the dose he received; his colleagues behind him received doses that were not acutely toxic. Back to the former example, the area under the curve would be:

$$\int_0^d C_0 e^{-d}\, dx\, dy\, dz$$

This is not a bad first approximation; however, density of the chemical (lighter or heavier than water or air), hydrophobicity (adsorption), charge (ion exchange), viscosity, vapor pressure, and so forth will interact with the ambient conditions (temperature, humidity, sun intensity, etc.). The direction will greatly be affected by the wind, rain, soil properties (impermeable to highly permeable or cracked), and other factors.

To solve for the air concentration, for instance, at a given distance d, a dilution grid that was determined in the 1981 by the Michigan short-term model air pollution model (specifies building height, stack height, emission concentrations, and a dilution grid based on distance from stack on the ground) may be used as an initial test to see if more advanced modeling should be used (Su and Wurzel, 1981). More advanced topographical modeling for air in a river valley using the U.S. Environmental Protection Agency (EPA) rolling hills model (similar topography for a given terrain modeled in the past) of air pollution was the next innovation in dispersion modeling. Newer models discussed later in the dispersion section use more advanced meteorological and topographical data available in this computer information age for the specific local conditions rather than a simplified similar modeled topography. Once the concentration at a given distance is known to a reasonable degree, the worst case scenario is determined. The reasoning here is that someone can stand 24 hours a day in the plume of a smokestack blown to the ground or their lofty apartment building, but the EPA or similar agency doesn't have the money to actually measure everyone's true exposure. The worst case scenario conveys a sense of maximum exposure. Then, the toxicity indicated in the organ systems part of this text predicts the hazard. Putting that together yields the risk. Now this is environmental toxicology, as a model system is employed using laboratory data instead of a degraded ecosystem with meager habitat and other stressors.

Only ecotoxicologists may truly determine risk by proper design and sampling of impact in the ecosystem of species such as may be done by macroinvertebrate counts, fish abundance, and so forth. Also, the sexes of the species, their malformations, pathologies, and so on may be determined. In humans, epidemiology comes into play to determine whether a cancer cluster or other problem exists in the plume of the pollutant. Scientists then look for the most sensitive species to warn humans of effects that may impact them or the food web of other species that humans wish to conserve or consume in their diet. If a mine "ecosystem" is examined, the human is one of the few species in that mine unless bats reside there, or fungi or bacteria are considered. The miners of the historic past brought a canary as a sensitive organism to signal the presence of mine gas at levels that would not yet affect the miner. The canary's high heart rate, respiration rate, and metabolic rate would make it more susceptible to toxic gases' effects on its central nervous system (CNS). Because the canary would not normally use a working mine as a habitat, the miners were really engaging in environmental toxicology—employing a sensitive model species as an indicator/biomarker of danger.

Before examining dispersion into the environment, route of entry, and health effects (most sensitive species) to characterize exposure and hazard, consider the following sophisticated ecotoxicity model. The USEtox program is an effort of the United Nations Environmental Program (UNEP) and the Society of Environmental Toxicology and Chemistry (SETAC; Rosenbaum et al., 2008). As shown in **Figure 24-2**, this integrated approach looks at the environmental fate of the emissions, the intake fraction into the human/ecosystem, and the human disease outcomes or damage to ecosystems. This figure covers all the aspects of the following sections of this chapter. A deep examination of this international ecotoxicity model requires that fate (FF) is expressed in days, the exposure (XF) in day^{-1} for human toxicity, and effects (EF) in $cases/kg_{intake}$ for human toxicity or potential affected fraction of species (PAF) m^3/kg for ecotoxicity. Another approach for ecotoxicity

assessment is using the potential disappeared fraction (PDF) that has uses in climate change, ozone layer, and acidification (Sharaai et al., 2009). This leads to a set of scale-specific characterization factors (CF) where $CF = EF \times XF \times FF = EF \times iF$ (intake fraction from the figure). The human exposure matrix XF includes inhalation of rural or urban air, ingestion of untreated surface drinking water, and ingestion of exposed produce (leaf crops), unexposed produce (root crops), meat, milk, and fish from freshwater and marine compartments for the entire human population studied. The intake fraction matrix includes the fraction of the emission that is taken by the whole population. The risk to that human population is based on data for cancer and non-cancer effects based on laboratory studies. The toxicity takes on a linear dose–response

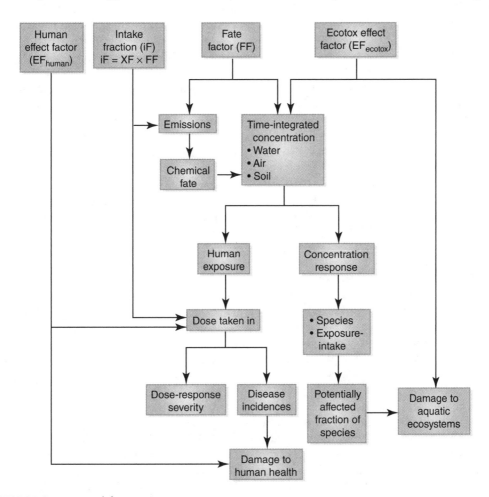

FIGURE 24-2 A Framework for Comparative Toxicity Assessment

function where the human effect is calculated to be $0.5/ED_{50}$, where ED_{50} represents the lifetime daily dose that results in a probability effect of 0.5. This model does not take into account differences in metabolic activation between animals and humans. For freshwater ecosystems the effect factor is calculated using a similar linear concentration–response behavior that results in a slope of $0.5/HC_{50}$. The designation of HC_{50} represents the hazardous concentration at which 50% of the species are above the ED_{50} (e.g., > 50% may be sick or dead depending on how the hazard is defined). Aquatic ecotoxicological effect factors have the dimensions of m^3 kg^{-1}. Once the scale-specific factors, exposure factors, and effect factors are inputted into the model, the final characterization factor for human toxicity and aquatic ecotoxicity result. Summation of characterization factors from continental- and global-scale assessments completes the analysis. Carcinogenic and non-carcinogenic effects are also summed, unless these effects are not equally weighted. The human toxicity potential is expressed in comparative toxic units (CTU_h) by calculating the estimated increase in morbidity (note sickness is the threshold for humans—not as far as deaths) in the total human population per unit of mass of a chemical emitted (clinical cases per kilogram emission). Aquatic ecotoxicity is also expressed in CTU_e, providing an estimate of PAF integrated over time and volume per unit mass of a chemical emitted (PAF m^3 day kg^{-1}, and this time may involve deaths rather than more subtle morbidity or reproductive outcomes). Even this modeling does not include all environments. Freshwater is the aquatic system modeled by USEtox. In contrast, the ocean is viewed as so vast that it represents a sink rather than an impacted location, although human activity has clearly affected coral reefs and produced dead zones in the ocean close to shore. The pH of the ocean is also altered/reduced by increasing CO_2 levels in the atmosphere, and humans are warned that ocean-caught tuna, swordfish, and other species have high mercury levels. This will impact sea fish at the top of the food chain such as sharks, sea mammals such as dolphins or seals, and birds feeding off of marine fish.

Dispersion

Although the EPA uses dispersion specifically to define movement of a toxicant in the air, the idea that a pollutant moves or disperses into its environment is still a valuable concept for all transport of a toxicant into the ecosystem. The lipophilic (as determined by log K_{OW} or similar partition coefficient) and charged molecules affect their ability to adsorb to soil or air particles (or soil in air as in dust storms). The pH of the water or soil may also affect its movement or stability. The density of the compound may drive it to the soil at the bottom of a lake or river or stream (benthic zone), which may then adsorb the compound or allow anaerobic organisms to modify the compound (as in the case of Hg becoming an organic form of mercury that is more easily absorbed and accumulated up the food web). Air, soil, and water are not separate compartments but are interlinked. Wind can erode soil and lift compounds associated with soil into the air, or microorganisms can take applied nitrates to the soil and denitrify the nitrogen into a gaseous form that enters the atmosphere. A volcano or large explosion such as occurs from nuclear fission or fusion may send particles high into the atmosphere and affect climate as well as put heavy metals and other toxic substances into the air from which they settle as "fallout." Water takes particles out of the lower troposphere in the form of snow and rain. The melting snow or rain can cause compounds to move through the soil at various levels depending on the soil texture and its water infiltration rate. Clay soils will resist water entering the soil and have more runoff from the surface, while sand will have deeper penetration and threaten aquifers. This is especially important for the highest peak of pesticide found in nearby ditches or streams following the first heavy rain after application. A heavy rainstorm or a large snowmelt will erode the soil and associated toxicants.

Air Dispersion Models

Three models are used as a reference for how dispersions are treated: box, plume, and puff. The three models are simplified in **Figure 24-3**. One looks at a "box" a certain distance from

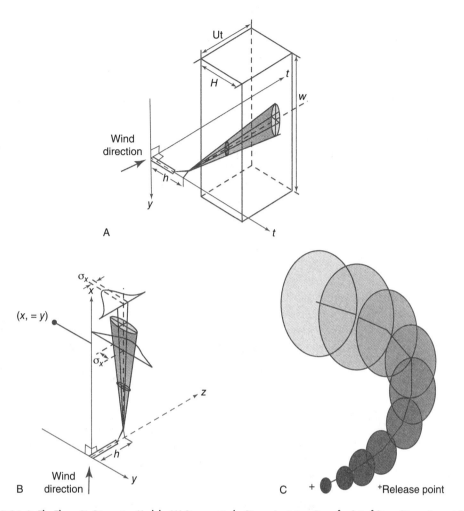

FIGURE 24-3 The Three Air Dispersion Models: (A) Represents the Dispersion into a Box of a Set of Given Dimensions at Certain Distances from the Source; (B) Represents the Formation of a Plume Which is Evaluated at a Certain Distances from the Source as Indicated by the Ellipse; and (C) Looks at Particle Dispersions at Various Distances from a Source Generating Elliptical "Puffs."

a source, while the other two treat a plume at a distance or discrete puffs of particles at a distance. More complicated application of these models is applied by the EPA in screening models followed by more complete models. The Technology Transfer Network Support Center for Regulatory Atmospheric Modeling is available at the EPA (2010) website and includes mathematical equations utilizing emission and meteorological data.

Screening Models

Prior to using a refined, expensive model with intensive data requirements, it is useful to use a screen to see if further modeling is necessary

to protect humans or the organisms in the ecosystem they occupy. Also, it can be important to consider the fragility or unique wilderness classification of a protected area.

AERSCREEN

AERSCREEN is a recommended screening model based on AERMOD. It performs a 1-hour worst case scenario from a single source without meteorological data and then similarly estimates 3-hour, 8-hour, 24-hour, and annual concentrations. AERSCREEN has two major components: MAKEMET (site-specific matrix of meteorological conditions for input in AERMOD model) and AERSCREEN command-prompt interface program. MAKEMET interfaces with AERMAP for terrain information and BPIPPRM to automate processing building information.

Inputs or options in AERSCREEN involve source parameters (point, rectangular area, circular area, volume, capped stack, horizontal stack, or flare sources), building downwash information (point, capped stack, horizontal stack, or flare sources), ability to model nitrogen oxide conversions (NO_x to NO_2, plume volume molar ratio [PVMRM]), ozone-limiting method (OLM), input of representative O_3 background concentration; can adjust to terrain heights for source (stack) and receptors through AERMAP; specify minimum and maximum temperatures for MAKEMET, minimum wind speed and anemometer height for MAKEMET, surface characteristics for MAKEMET input (user-defined single values for albedo, Bowen ration, and surface roughness, AERMET seasonal tables, or values listed in an external file such as an AERSURFACE output file or surface characteristics listed in AERMET), and probe or maximum downwind distance of receptors; employ flagpole receptors and flagpole height, urban and urban population or rural source (important in consideration of farm ecosystems versus urban ecosystems that have been created), and minimum ambient distance for ambient air receptors; allow up to 10 discrete receptor distances; perform error checks on AERSCREEN inputs or AERMOD and/or AERMAP outputs; and use a search routine to find the maximum 1-hour concentration as a worst case scenario. To determine other periods of time, the averaging period ratios are 1.0, 0.9, 0.6, and 0.1 for 3-hour, 8-hour, 24-hour, and annual "worst cases."

MAKEMET inputs generate a matrix of meteorological conditions based on looping through a range of wind speeds, cloud covers, ambient temperatures, solar elevation angles, and convective velocity scales. Once these data are gathered, source input entries such as emission rate (lb/h or g/s), stack height (ft or m), stack diameter (in or m), stack temp (°F or K), and stack velocity (ft/s or m/s) or flow rate (actual cubic feet per minute) are considered. The point, capped stack, horizontal stack, or flare must be specified. Flare requires not only the emission rate and stack height, but also the total heat release rate (cal/sec) and radiative heat loss fraction. In this setup, the effective stack diameter or $D = 9.88 \times 10^{-4} \times (HR \times -HL)^{1/2}$, where HR = heat release rate and HL is the heat loss fraction. The effective stack height or $H_{eff} = H_s + 4.56 \times 10^{-3} \times HR^{0.478}$ where H_s is the stack height. Volume sources require emission rate, release height at center of volume, and initial lateral and vertical dimensions of that volume. Rectangular area sources also require emission rate and release height above ground, but also need long and short dimensions of the area and the initial vertical dimension of the plume. Circular area sources have the first two parameters and the fourth one (of rectangular area) along with radius of circle. Downwash uses building and stack height/location and dimensions to calculate the effect of the building on dilution to the ground. It is of interest that the meteorological and surface data not only determine temperatures, but also define the surface as water, forest type (deciduous, coniferous), swamp, cultivated land (farm), grassland, urban, desert shrub land, or other criteria that better describe the surface with average moisture or dry conditions. This description may appear intensive, but still simplifies the parameters used for a recommended screening tool rather than a much more complex air model. Note that the parameters are interested in the emission, the stack, the building, the ecological setting, and the meteorological data. This is consistent with many models of air pollution (EPA, 2011).

COMPLEX1

COMPLEX1 is a multiple point source model that utilizes terrain adjustment in combination with the plume impaction algorithm of the VALLEY model (discussed later).

CTSCREEN

CTSCREEN supposes a Gaussian plume dispersion into a complex terrain. It is a screening version of the CTMPLUS model.

RTDM3.2

RTDM3.2 of Rough Terrain Diffusion Model utilizes a sequential Gaussian plume model that estimates ground-level concentration in rough or flat terrain in the locale of at least one co-located point source.

SCREEN3

SCREEN3, a screening version of ISC3, uses a single-source Gaussian plume model that yields maximum ground-level estimated concentrations for point, flare, and volume sources. It also provides cavity zone concentrations due to inversion breakup and shoreline fumigation.

TSCREEN

TSCREEN is a Toxics Screening Model that also uses a Gaussian model for toxic emissions and subsequent dispersion from a variety of release modes for superfund sites. This model is a compilation of SCREEN3, PUFF, and Relief Valve Discharge (RVD).

VALLEY

VALLEY uses a steady-state, complex terrain, univariate Gaussian plume algorithm to estimate 24-hour or annual concentrations that result from emissions from as many as 50 total point sources and area sources.

VISCREEN

VISCREEN provides a quantified estimate of the potential impact of a plume of specified emission for a given set of transport and dispersion conditions.

Recommended EPA Dispersion Models

EPA recommends AERMOD and CALPUFF. It also has BLP, CALINE3, CAL3QHC/ CAL3QHCR, CTDMPLUS, and OCD models.

AERMOD

AERMOD is a steady-state plume model as opposed to the non-steady-state puff model of CALPUFF. AERMOD uses planetary boundary layer turbulence structure and scaling concepts to determine the treatment of surface and elevated sources to calculate dispersion into simple and complex terrains. The two regulatory components of AERMOD are AERMET, a meteorological data preprocessor that encompasses the air dispersion portion based on planetary boundary layer turbulence structure and scaling concepts, and AERMAP, which performs preprocessing of terrain data using U.S. Geological Survey (USGS) Digital Elevation Data.

AERMET is run in three stages. Three basic data types are used generated by the National Oceanic and Atmospheric Administration's (NOAA) National Weather Service (NWS), Federal Aviation Administration (FAA) or other hourly surface observations, NWS upper air sounds twice a day, and data collected from an on-site measurement program such as an instrument tower. The first stage of AERMET retrieves data from the raw data files and assesses data quality. The second stage merges the UPPERAIR, SURFACE, and ONSITE data for 24-hour periods and creates an intermediate file. The final stage reads that merged data file, develops the necessary boundary layer parameters for dispersion calculations by AERMOD, and sends a meteorological data output that is AERMOD-ready.

AERMAP uses a variety of terrain information as a preprocessor of that information. Horizontal datum refers to the model or method used to identify locations on the Earth with different geographical coordinates depending on the reference datum. This also models the size and shape of the Earth or reference ellipsoid used to project geographic coordinates to other coordinate systems (e.g., Universal Transverse Mercator or UTM using Cartesian/rectangular X and Y coordinates). The USGS Digital Elevation Model data serve as reference ellipsoids. The domain must then be defined for all receptors and sources. The user may define the user-specified coordinate system for source and receptor locations to the UTM coordinate system using east–west (X) and north–south (Y) Cartesian grid system directions. Defining where the receptors are in this system is considered the anchor point specifications. There is then a need to specify elevation by the USGS Digital Elevation Model (DEM) or National Elevation Dataset (NED). The raw type of terrain data specified in either of these systems must be specified. The elevation of the receptors and handling of gaps in the DEM files due to conversion of the data to the norm of the North American Datum of 1983 (NAD83) must be specified. A FILLGAPS option can be used to help generate data for those areas; otherwise, the gaps are assigned a missing code (-9999.0). Users are encouraged to check whether the results for gap receptors relative to the topographical map are accurately accounted for in the program. Using the NED elevation data solves these problems. AERMAP then uses a two-dimensional bilinear interpolation method for calculating receptor elevations. Once both of these preprocessors (AERMET and AERMAP) have been debugged and validated by the user, then AERMOD is run to assess the concentrations for steady-state data. However, some emissions are pulsed into the environment as stochastic functions (pesticide runoff is similarly pulsed at rain or snowmelt intervals) as the emissions are not constant. Other modeling needs to be run in these cases.

CALPUFF

As indicated earlier, CALPUFF is a multilayer, multi-species, non-steady-state puff dispersion model that simulates changing meteorological conditions (time- and space-varying) that affect transport, transformation, and removal of toxicants in the air. It has algorithms that model effects of terrain (subgrid scale effects). It can also estimate effects of fallout (dry and wet deposition), chemical transformation, or particulate visibility (three factors in longer range effects). CALPUFF can simulate atmospheric deposition from tens of meters to hundreds of kilometers.

CALPUFF/CALMET integrates mesoscale meteorological models such as MM4/5 and CSUMM with a diagnostic, mass-consistent wind model. It is able to integrate local effects such as slope flow, kinematic terrain effects, terrain blocking, and sea breeze circulations. Instead of assuming a normally distributed plume model (oldest model is the Gaussian model), this dispersion model follows the random walk of plume parcels or particles (Lagrangian model) as the statistics of their trajectories. There are other models that assume a box model, Eulerian model (following particles in a 3-D Cartesian grid), and dense (heavier than air) gas model. This model does not assume that the particles stay together, but can have puff splitting occur due to complex wind fields. The steps in CALMET are to specify domain and

coordinate systems, prepare geophysical data, prepare meteorological data, prepare user control file, run CALMET and produce outputs, and post-process outputs. The reason CALMET is indicated first here is that there is a requirement to do near-field (building downwash, subgrid scale complex terrain) and far-field (puff splitting, deposition) applications. Far-field applications need two input files, CALMET. DAT and CALPUFF.INP for sources with constant release rates (not stochastic). Similar to CALMET, the domain and coordinate system must be specified. There can be a user-defined Cartesian coordinate system (not limited to just UTM or Lambert Conformal). The geophysical data may come from CALMET, but may be specified separately. Meteorological data may come from CALMET or other meteorological files. Sources, species, and emissions data should be included and species specified. Chemistry and deposition data should be included next into the model. Receptor coverage is again specified as in other models. Run conditions should also be specified and then run CALPUFF and produce outputs. The post-processing is again important here as in CALMET.

BLP

BLP is a special case Gaussian plume dispersion model associated with the complexity of aluminum reduction plants and other industrial sources where plume rise and downwash effects from stationary line sources are critical to the analyses.

CALINE3

CALINE3 is another steady-state Gaussian dispersion model meant to model toxicant emissions to concentrations at receptor locations downwind of highways in uncomplicated terrain.

CAL3QHC/CAL3QHCR

CAL3QHC/CAL3QHCR is a CALINE-based carbon monoxide (CO) model with queuing hotspot calculations and with a traffic model to calculate delays and queues that are likely at intersections with signal lights. The CAL3QHCR uses local meteorological data and is therefore considered more refined.

CTMPLUS

CTMPLUS is the Complex Terrain Dispersion Model Plus Algorithms for Unstable Situations. This model uses a refined point source Gaussian air quality model in all stability conditions for terrains that are not easily modeled in simpler form.

OCD

OCD is the Offshore and Coastal Dispersion Model 5. It uses a straight-line Gaussian model to determine the impacts of offshore emissions from point, area, or line sources on the air quality of coastal regions. This model could be used to determine if a burning oil spill may affect the respiratory health of coastal residents.

Alternative Air Dispersion Models

Alternative models are:

- ADAM—Air Force Assessment Model using a modified box and Gaussian dispersion model
- AFTOX—Gaussian model for continuous or instantaneous liquid gas from elevated or surface releases
- ASPEN—Assessment System for Population Exposure Nationwide using a Gaussian formulation for dispersion based on ISCST3 or Industrial Source Complex Short Term Model estimating annual average concentrations and a mapping module that produces a concentration at each census tract
- DEGADIS—Simulates atmospheric deposition at ground levels of area dense gas or aerosol clouds released with zero momentum into the atmospheric boundary layer over flat, level terrain
- HGSYSTEM—Collection of computer programs predicting the source-term and subsequent dispersion of accidental chemical releases emphasizing denser-than-air behavior
- HOTMAC/RAPTAD-3-D—Eulerian model for weather forecasting and Lagrangian random puff model for pollutant transport and diffusion, respectively
- HYROAD—Hybrid Roadway Model integrates three historically individual

models that simulate traffic, emissions, and dispersion
- ISC3-steady-state—Gaussian plume model that can assess pollutant concentrations from an industrial complex
- ISC-PRIME—Plume Rise Model Enhancements incorporates building downwash into ISCST3 model
- OBODM—Determines air quality effects of open burning and detonation of obsolete munitions and solid propellants
- OZIPR—One-dimensional photochemical box model alternative to OZIP
- Panache—Eulerian, 3-D finite volume fluid mechanics model and Lagrangian model for particulate matter simulating continuous and short-term pollutant dispersions
- PLUVUEII—Estimates visual range reduction and atmospheric discoloration caused by plumes resulting from emitted particles, NO_x gases, and SO_x gases from a single source
- SCIPUFF—Second-order Closure Integration PUFF model using Lagrangian puff dispersion model employing a collection of Gaussian puffs to predict 3-D, time-dependent pollutant concentrations
- SDM—Shore Dispersion Model using a multiple-point dispersion model to determine ground-level concentrations from tall stationary point source emissions near a shoreline
- SLM—Denser-than-air releases treated by solving one-dimensional equations of momentum, conservation of mass, species, and energy, and equation of state
- Pesticides have a number of atmospheric models from the EPA such as:
  - AgDRIFT—Aerial spray deposition patterns
  - AgDISP—Sprays from aircraft
  - PERFUM—Probabilistic Exposure and Risk Model for [soil] Fumigants
  - SOFEA—Soil Fumigant Exposure Assessment to bystanders in proximity to treated fields
  - FEMS—Fumigant Emissions Modeling System to bystanders in proximity to treated fields

Movement in Soil and Water

It seems that movement into soil and water and the creation of a plume should involve just soil or just water. That is a rare event, because hydrology plays a huge role depending on the hydrophilic or hydrophobic nature of the toxic substance. The soils have been characterized by the former U.S. Soil Conservation Service, now known as the Natural Resources Conservation Service (NRCS) under the authority of the U.S. Department of Agriculture. The USGS also studies and models the movement of toxicant into soils and waters through its Toxic Substances Hydrology Program. One would think that a clean lake or river would not involve soil, but that would negate soil particles suspended in those systems, the benthic or bottom layer, aquatic plants, and anything else that may add to the organic matter in the water. Soil is a complex system and its integrity is critical to movement of substances. Sand is porous, while clay is fairly difficult to permeate with water. However, cracks, fractures, wells, and so forth can make movement of toxicants easier deeper into the soil and into underground aquifers (shallow and deep) that are used for drinking water and agricultural irrigation. A drought may produce more cracks or harden soil, depending on the situation. A flood may wash a toxicant adsorbed to soil such as hydrophobic pesticides, or a high water table may increase the runoff of water-soluble pollutants such as nitrates and phosphates. The USGS is concerned with subsurface point source contamination, larger considerations of watershed and regional scale contamination (nonpoint and distributed point source contamination from hard-rock mining, pesticide use/contamination, mercury, "emerging" contaminants such as hormone medications, priority ecosystem studies such as the Gulf of Mexico hypoxic zone or the Everglades in Florida, and amphibian research as impacted by pesticides, fungi, and parasites), and methods development (microbial geochemistry, geochemistry, hydrology, contaminant geophysics, and modeling). Listed under point source contamination (USGS, 2015a) modeling is contamination in fractured-rock aquifers,

petroleum-related contamination (from spills or above ground or below ground storage tanks), chlorinated solvent contamination (as occurs from dry-cleaning facilities and industrial chemical sites), and contamination from mixed sources (landfills and wastewater discharge).

Movement in Fractured Rock

Of greatest concern are areas of fractured-rock aquifers for subsurface point source contamination as opposed to sand and gravel aquifers (although both are of interest and importance). More uncertainties arise in these fractured systems with respect to direction and rate of contaminant migration and chemical and microbial transformations that occur while in transit. This is mainly a concern of hydraulic properties such as fractures, joints, conduits, and bugs that provide principal pathways for flow, but vary by orders of magnitude (large errors for local effects if only considering larger scales). For example, crystalline rocks have matrix porosity as great as 3%, while sedimentary rocks that used to be under water have larger matrix porosity. In these geological formations, diffusive (based on the properties of the rock matrix) exchange from or to permeable features changes environmental tracers trying to model the movement of the pollutant. Advection (fluid movement based on bulk flow) or dispersion equations may underestimate the groundwater velocity by orders of magnitude. The usual assumption is that the mean velocity of chemical transport controls chemical advection, and the variability about the mean velocity is incorporated into the dispersion. In fractured rock, velocities usually vary over a number of orders of magnitude, and variability is significantly higher than in porous media, meaning that behavior in porous media cannot be used to model fractured rock chemical dispersion. In porous media, the void space length and width are similar dimensions, while in fracture rock a few preferential paths may control the majority of groundwater flow. Models that focus on regional water balance (spatially distributed bulk properties estimated from recharge, discharge, and measurements of hydraulic head but do not consider individual preferential flow paths) over meters to kilometers may have greater success with these flows in these geological formations. Stochastic methods that take into account the extreme variability of the velocity show promise, but need to evaluate complexities of recharge and regional geologic features that constrain flow (Shapiro, 2011).

Movement in Soils

The EPA a number of soil movement models for toxics and pesticides. An example of this modeling is the soil vapor extraction model (EPA, 2012). This model is used as an example for it includes the permeability of the soil to the toxics or water based on soil texture and type, soil structure and stratification, soil moisture, and depth to groundwater. These are essential components with specific changes based on the pollutant chemistry, the slope of the topography, rainfall events, and other factors that make the models more specific to the ecology of the area and how the chemicals move (as in applications on land) or are likely to move (predicted effects of spills) in that environment. The Ground Water and Ecosystems Research of the EPA (Chen et al., 2002; using radionuclide fate and transport—similar to NRCS's tracing methodology) tries to assess uncertainties of peak contaminant concentrations and time to peak concentrations at the water table. This group analyzed CHAIN, MULTIMED-DP 1.0, FECTUZ, CHAIN 2D, and HYDRUS. Important properties of these models are soil structure and texture, bulk density, water content, and hydraulic conductivity. Chemical properties such as distribution coefficient, degradation half-life, dispersion coefficient, and molecular diffusion were analyzed. Other properties of the soil and site were equilibrium/nonequilibrium sorption sites, rooting depth, recharge rate, hysteretic effects, and precipitation/evapotranspiration.

Modeling of Watershed Systems (MOWS)

USGS modeling includes normal to extreme climatic conditions (USGS, 2015b). The Precipitation Runoff Modeling System (PRMS) helps to simulate the hydrologic cycle at a watershed scale based on climate, biota, geology, and human activities. Its four primary objectives are simulation of hydrologic processes (evaporation, transpiration, runoff, infiltration, and interflow taking into account energy and water budgets of plant canopy, snowpack, and soil zone), simulation of water budgets at watershed scale for temporal scales (days to centuries), integration of PRMS with other natural resource management models, and provision of a modular design for proper selection of hydrologic process algorithms. This model may be part of a way of determining runoff for water-soluble pollutants such as nitrates and phosphates, and less so for hydrophobic pesticides.

Surface Waters

The USGS has ANNIE, BRANCH, BSDMS, CAP, CGAP, DR3M, FEQ, FESWMS-2DH, FourPt, GCLAS, GenScn, GLSNet, GSFLOW, HSexp, HSPF, HYSEP, INFIL3.0, IOWDM, KTRLine, LOADEST, MEASERR, MODEIN, NCALC, NFF, NSS, OTEQ, OTIS, PeakFQ, PRMS, SAC, SEDDISCH, SEDSIZE, StreamStats, SWSTAT, WREG, and WSPRO as surface water programs for a variety of conditions (from rainfall to culverts to watersheds to types of sediments). The NRCS has AGNPS (Agricultural Non-Point Source Pollution model), HecRas (water surface profiles), hydraulic formulas (hydraulics calculator), cross-section analyzer (hydraulic parameters with uniform flow), SITES (rainfall/runoff for dam and spillway analysis and design), WinDAM (estimates erosion or earthen embankments and auxiliary spillways of dams), TR-19 (reservoir storage requirements analysis), WinTR-20, NRCS Geo-Hydro (ArcView interface to Win TR-20), WinTR-55 (Windows version of TR-55), frequency curves, EFH2 (peak discharge determination), and other hydrology models they no longer support.

The AGNPS is a model worth examining, because the Midwest farm region has significant erosion, fertilizer (nitrates and phosphates), and pesticide inputs into ditches, streams, and rivers, ultimately coming together in the Mississippi River and the Gulf of Mexico. The smaller ditches and streams have high short peak concentrations after the first heavy rainfall following application, while larger rivers have lower but more sustained pollutant concentrations. The AGNPS model uses an "annualized" science and technology loading model for agricultural-related watersheds. This is a more reliable stable number but is less predictive of peak concentrations and the impact of those concentrations on the crucial spring oxygen formation (via beneficial algal populations) versus oxygen demand of bacteria in warmer months. The model looks at stream network processes, stream corridor modeling (accounting for erosion of banks during high spring flows or summer floods), an instream water temperature model, and several related salmonid models. This produces an approximation of an ecological picture of the impact of farm-related activities on surface waters and an important fish family.

The EPA (2015) has programs to model pesticide movements specifically as they represent a large landmass in the country (agriculture, lawns, golf courses) with impacts on soils and waters of the area. GENEEC models surface water for exposures to aquatic organisms/environment. FIRST (FQPA [Food Quality Protection Act] Index Reservoir Screening Tool) is also a surface water model but is more applicable to drinking water. KABAM estimates bioaccumulation of hydrophobic pesticides in aquatic food webs and higher level risks to mammals and birds consuming those aquatic species. PRZM (Pesticide Root Zone Model) is also a surface water model, but simulates movement of hydrophobic pesticides in soil within and immediately below the plant root zone to surface waters via tile drains or through stream banks, or other areas. This model has a long history and has exposures refined by EXAMS (Exposure Analysis Modeling System evaluating fate, transport, and exposure to pesticides as a surface water model). EXPRESS (EXAMS–PRZM Exposure Simulation Shell) provides a rapid and consistent assessment of aquatic pesticide exposure on a variety of crops. SWAMP estimates the probability, magnitude, and certainty of risk to aquatic organisms from exposure to pesticides. If a farmer is raising rice in a paddy, then the movement in the surface water of the paddy into the environment is estimated by the Tier I Rice

Model. A swimming pool may be considered a surface water that can be assessed using the SWIMODEL (Swimmer Exposure Assessment Model) to evaluate expose to pesticides used in indoor swimming pools and spas.

Solute Transport in Groundwater

Continuing the EPA discussion of pesticides, it is important to note that PRZM has a soil movement property as well. In addition, SCIGROW (Screening Concentration in Ground Water) estimates pesticide concentrations in groundwater from land or air applications to fields. USGS has a variety of software to ascertain movement of solutes in groundwater (Kipp, 2008). These include HST3D (simulation of heat and solute in 3-D groundwater flow systems), HYDROTHERM (simulation of two-phase groundwater flow and heat transport from 0–1,000°C), and PHAST (simulation of multi-component geochemical reactions and transport in 3-D groundwater flow systems).

Route of Exposure

Pesticide programs provide some of the ways that exposure can develop into toxicity. Respiratory routes may provide rapid peaks and affect the lung (or gill) of the respiring organism, leading to respiratory damage (fibrosis, emphysema, etc.), immune system reactions (allergy, asthma, pneumonitis), and cancer of various parts of the respiratory tract (lung cancer, mesothelioma). For pesticides, STIR (Screening Tool for Inhalation Risk) estimates the exposure due to inhalation. If drinking water is considered, SIP (Screening Imbibition Program) estimates pesticide exposure from drinking water alone to birds and mammals. Estimates of pesticide concentration on avian and mammalian food items can be made via T-REX (Terrestrial Residue Exposure). Terrestrial organisms can be evaluated more thoroughly for probability, magnitude, and certainty of risk from pesticide exposure through TIM (Terrestrial Investigation Model). Plants (non-target plants that may represent crops or are not considered weeds in the local ecology) may have their pesticide exposure from single application through TerrPlant (Tier I). T-HERPS simulates exposure to terrestrial reptiles and amphibians such as occurred in Lake Apopka alligators.

Health Effects

Air pollutants come into the system via respiration and affect the lung (asthma, emphysema, chronic obstructive pulmonary disease, lung cancer), then the heart (via the pulmonary circulation), followed by the brain (off the aortic arch toward the head). Food and drinking water contamination impacts the absorption (gastrointestinal tract) and processing centers (such as the liver and kidney) or target organs such as the CNS. Humans are usually given the highest consideration followed by biomarker species, fish kills, and so forth depending on the severity of the contamination. Health effects models for humans exposed to pesticides include DEEM (Dietary Exposure Evaluation Model), CAL-ENDEX™-FCID (aggregated exposure across multiple pathways), CARES (Cumulative and Aggregate Risk Evaluation System), LifeLine™ Version 2.0 (diet, tap water, and in residential environments) or Version 4.3 (dietary, aggregate, and cumulative risks), OPHED (Occupational Pesticide Handler Exposure Data—these workers get the highest exposure via mixing, loading, and application), OPPED (Occupational Pesticide Post-application Exposure Data such a harvesting, weeding, and other post-application exposures), Rex (Residential Exposure Assessment), SHEDS (Stochastic Human Exposure and Dose Simulation Model, a physically based stochastic model to quantify exposure and dose via multimedia and multi-pathways), PBPK/PD (Physiologically Based Pharmacokinetic/Pharmacodynamic, the most accurate model but expensive to gather the exact human data), and Residential SOPs (Standard Operating Procedures for Residential Pesticide Exposure from lawn/garden care, foggers, and pet treatments).

For fish, the routes of exposure via gill and food can be modeled using the EPA's (1994) Food and Gill Exchange of Toxic Substances (FGETS), which can model water only (acute exposure similar to respiratory in human) or water and food (chronic exposures). These can be modeled for exposure to nonionic, non-metabolized, organic chemicals that bioaccumulate in this organism. The lethality is based on a narcotic mode of action. FGETS considers the biological attributes of the fish (body weight, fractional aqueous, lipid and structural organic composition, feeding, and metabolic demands of that species of fish) and the physic-chemical properties of the toxicant (aqueous diffusivity, molar volume/aqueous diffusivity, n-octanol water partition coefficient or log P/bioconcentration factor; together melting point and log P estimate chemical's activity in fish) that determine diffusive exchange across the gill membranes (gill morphometry) and the intestinal mucosa (morphometry). It is worthwhile to examine this model more carefully to see how the respiratory (gill) route has the greater impact. The fish's whole body concentration of C_f (ppm = μg chemical/g live weight fish) is calculated via the total body burden B_f (μg chemical/fish)/W (live weight). Fish growth is modeled via:

$$dW/dt = F \times E \times R \times SDA$$

where F = fish's feeding fluxes (g/day), E = fish's egestive fluxes (g/day), R = fish's respiratory fluxes (g/day, which is based on how active the gill is), and SDA = fish's specific dynamic action (g/day). The total body burden is expressed as:

$$dB_f/dt = S_g J_g + J_i = S_q k_w (C_w - C_a)$$

where S_g = the fish's total gill area (cm^2), J_g = the net diffusive flux across the gills (μg/cm^2/day), J_i = the net mass exchange across the fish's intestine from food (μg/day), k_w = the chemical's mass conductance through the inter-lamellar water of the gills (cm/day), C_w = the chemical's concentration in the environmental water (ppm), and C_a = the chemical's concentration in the fish's aqueous blood (ppm). The gill exchange represents a direct application of Fick's first law of diffusion. FGETS can have three formulations for chemical exchange of food—it can be assumed that a constant toxicant assimilation efficiency occurs (thermodynamic equilibrium of fish's feces and whole body)—or kinetic uses of Fick's first law of diffusion. Fish are conceptualized as a three-phase solvent consisting of water, lipid, and structural organic matter. The exchange in these three phases is considered relatively rapid compared with exchange across the gill and intestine. The whole body concentration of C_f thus is represented by the following equations:

$$C_f = B_f/W = (P_a = P_1K_1 + P_sK_s)C_a$$

where P_a = the aqueous fraction of the whole fish, P_1 = the lipid fraction of the whole fish, K_1 = partition coefficient between lipid and water (e.g., K_{ow}), P_s = the structural organic fraction of the whole fish, and K_s = partition coefficient between lipid and structural organic matter (e.g., $K_{OC} = 0.4K_{OW}$). If only the gill is considered, then the bioconcentration factor or $BCF = C_f/C_w = P_a + P_1K_1 + P_aK_a$ and can generate the body burden as:

$$dB/dt = S_gK_w(C_w - C_fBCF) + J_i$$

which allows substitution of B_f/W for C_f leading to:

$$dB/dt = S_gKw(C_w - B_f/W\,BCF) = J_i$$

or a simple juxtaposition of the initial equations. It this model, the species data generate necessary aqueous and structural organ fractions for fish. The user then specifies an adjustment factor ($0.33 <$ active gill < 1) for active gill, which is crucial in calibrating the fish's predicted mass exchange of the chemical across the gill based on the difference between the fish's physiological and anatomical surface area (Barber et al., 1988).

Other later versions of this program have been modified, but have many of the same underlying assumptions. There are many papers and a whole journal devoted to ecological modeling, which cannot be adequately addressed in a single chapter. However, modeling is important to try to predict impacts by computer when testing in the environment is expensive and does not prevent sensitive organisms from succumbing to effects of emissions prior to the completion of an assessment.

Most Sensitive Organism/Biomarkers

The most sensitive organism is usually ascertained by exposing organisms to a logarithmic series of toxicity concentrations in the lab.

There are some problems with this approach ecologically. A sensitive fish such as the trout may appear resistant to an herbicide compared to algae. Many Midwestern rivers depend on the algae that produce oxygen at the beginning of the spring season, because they do not have a significant elevation drop to oxygenate by that method. At that point, herbicide runoff into the stream may not support trout. On top of that are secondary and tertiary toxicities as indicated by toxicity to an algal species that affects the zooplankton followed by a reduction in a fish population. Mesocosm studies (using artificial lakes) indicated those secondary to tertiary effects (Kettle et al., 1987). However, one does not have to go that far. If reproductive success in terms of egg production, success of larvae, and so forth is measured, then a far lower concentration is found to cause damage to the following generations by influencing reproduction. In addition, the use of a flow-through system allows higher toxicities associated with the flow of a stream instead of a static tank exposure. At that point, even a highly pesticide-resistant fish such as the fathead minnow exhibits reproductive abnormalities (lower egg production and gonad abnormalities in male and female fish exposed for one-half to a full month at 0.5–50 µg/L) at low concentrations once thought to be relatively harmless to adult fish (Tillitt et al., 2010). Thus, it is not so easy to assess the most sensitive organisms, because the direct toxicity and secondary and tertiary outcomes to future generations must be assessed as well. It depends where society wants to regulate activities that clearly affect fish populations at parts per billion (ppb). Scientists can now find effects at concentrations that would either preclude the use of a product or produce an unachievable reduction with reasonable costs in runoff from an agricultural field. The same could be said for endocrine disruptors causing reproductive abnormalities from sewage effluent that may need to be as clean as drinking water (or better at ppb). For areas with highly sloping soils or climate change that results in more heavy rain events than predicted from past climatic data, the impacts would be expected to increase. In another example, if a cold-water fish becomes exposed to warmer water from the effluent of a nuclear electrical generation facility or climate change, the species would either have to adapt or suffer high toxicities from compounds and concentrations formerly thought to be tolerable.

The kind of study that shows more ecotoxicity is hopefully similar to those reported by The Nature Conservancy and similar groups. For example, one study (Lovett and Tear, 2007) investigated the effects of atmospheric deposition on biological diversity in the eastern United States. The summary of the report indicated that none of the ecosystems examined were free from the effects of air pollution. The industrialization of economies worldwide has generated pollutants that affect aquatic ecosystems (acidity, eutrophication of estuaries and lakes—nitrogen, mercury) and biogeological cycling in terrestrial systems. There is also evidence of effects of nitrogen deposition on grasslands, alpine areas, bogs, and forest mycorrhizae. Soil acidification from SO_x also impacts entire forests, as does climate change. Ozone also reduces photosynthesis in many terrestrial plant species. These pollutants represent chronic exposure that is usually only realized during other stressors such as drought, freezing, or increased pathogen action. Acid/aluminum effects are exceptional in that they can be lethal to aquatic organisms in short order.

For water pollution aquatic macroinvertebrate analyses from Hester-Dendy samplers or similar devices test these very sensitive organisms to assess stream toxicity, because they are affected by the physical, chemical, and biological changes that occur in the stream and can't travel long distances to avoid local impacts. Macroinvertebrates may also register cumulative toxicity and habitat loss. As a critical part of the food web of this aquatic system (stream, river, or interlocking lakes found at the headwaters of the Mississippi River, for instance), they are sensitive to and represent impacts on other species that depend on them as a food source. Speciation and abundance of algae and dissolved oxygen readings that are seasonally relevant (during early spring planting) may indicate the impacts of agricultural applications. Effluents from cities have more unusual compounds such as hormones and other medications that make fish studies important for endocrine disruption,

heart effects, and so forth. *Daphnia magna* also show effects of cardiovascular medications and have been used in environmental toxicity testing for years (as opposed to ecotoxicity analysis of existing species diversity and abundance).

For terrestrial toxicity, one of the least resistant organisms to effects of insecticides is the honeybee. Pollination of many plants is dependent on this species. The long-distance flying behavior of the bees and the multiple plants they sample make them good carriers of pesticide residues in the pollen or susceptible to toxicity of compounds such as methyl parathion formerly used to control pest insect species (Chauzat et al., 2006). Some raptors representing the high end of the food chain are sensitive to bioaccumulative effects, such as the often cited California condor's sensitivity to DDT. Certain non-target plant species are also sensitive to broadleaf weed pesticides such as 2,4-D. It would be nice to protect the most sensitive species of an ecosystem and its community integrity. However, using the most sensitive organism as the measure of ecotoxicity may reflect the uniqueness of that organism and certainly this species cannot predict the realm of toxicities to other organisms. Additionally, the most sensitive assay or species may overregulate the use of a product with excellent pesticide control that in reality has less acute toxicity concerns in the ecosystem than another less effective product. That is why rodents or fathead minnows and other hearty species are used in comparison to toxicity to bees or green algae. Also the toxicant itself may not be as complex as DDT and its reproductive toxicity to raptors. For example, heavy metal toxicity appears relatively straightforward on first glance (Forbes and Forbes, 1993; DeVries and Bakker, 1998). The uncertainties inherent in environmental toxicity or ecotoxicity testing and regulation involve the selection of the test species and endpoint (species representative of the ecosystem or other species and endpoints could be varied or incomparable), the validity of a theoretical distribution function (species sensitivity distribution may not fit that function), biological variability within and between species, comparability of laboratory-derived data to field data (bioavailability of toxicant in lab versus field setting and exposure time), variation of scientific data (in a particular researcher's own studies and between researchers both in the lab and the field), and the ever-present problem in field work of other compounds exerting antagonistic, additive, or synergistic effects (less problematic in environmental toxicology laboratory testing under controlled conditions but perhaps less applicable to field results).

Questions

1. What is the difference between environmental toxicology and ecotoxicology?
2. Why is K_{OW} an important factor in fate of a chemical in the environment or absorption into an organism?
3. Why is it necessary to have a variety of screening models for air dispersion?
4. Why is it important to have both the AERMOD and CALPUFF modeling available for air dispersion modeling?
5. What are essential differences in modeling movement of compounds in fractured rock, soils, and watershed systems?
6. Why can the EPA PRZM model be used as a tool for surface water and water movement in groundwater?
7. Why are many environmental models including route of exposure based on pesticides?
8. How are the FGETS program assumptions for assessing fish toxicity different from human modeling?
9. How can sensitivity be built into environmental toxicity testing without resorting to expensive mesocosm studies?

References

Barber MC, Suarez LA, Lassiter RR. 1988. FGETS (Food and Gill Exchange of Toxic Substances): a simulation model for predicting bioaccumulation of nonpolar organic pollutants by fish. Athens, GA: U.S. Environmental Protection Agency.

Chauzat M-P, Faucon J-P, Martel A-C, Lachaize J, Cougoule N, Aubert M. 2006. A survey of pesticide residues in pollen loads collected by honey bees in France. *J Econ Entomol.* 99:253–262.

Chen J-S, Drake, RL, Lin, Z., Jewett DG, Burden DS. 2002. Simulating radionuclide fate and transport in the unsaturated zone: evaluation and sensitivity analyses of select computer models. U.S. Environmental Protection Agency document EPA/600/R-02/082.

DeVries W, Bakker DJ. 1998. *Manual for calculating critical loads of heavy metals for terrestrial ecosystems. Guideline for critical limits, calculation methods and input data.* Report 166. Wageningen, the Netherlands: DLO Winand Staring Centre.

Forbes TL, Forbes VE. 1993. A critique of the use of distribution-based models in ecotoxicology. *Funct Ecol.* 7:249–254.

Kettle WD, DeNoyelles F Jr, Heacock BD, Kadoum AM. 1987. Diet and reproductive success of bluegill recovered from experimental ponds treated with atrazine. *Bull Environ Contam Toxicol.* 8:345–353.

Kipp KL. 2008. Solute transport simulation in groundwater systems. http://wwwbrr.cr.usgs.gov/projects/GW_Solute

Lovett GM, Tear TH. 2007. Effects of atmospheric deposition on biological diversity in the eastern United States. http://www.ecostudies.org/reprints/Effects_of_atmospheric_deposition_on_biodiversity.pdf.

Rosenbaum RK, Bachmann TM, Gold LS, Huijbregts MAJ, Joliet O, Juraske R, Koehler A, Larsen HR, MacLeod M, Margni N, McKone TE, Payet J, Schuhmacher M, van de Meent D, Hauschild MZ. 2008. USEtox—the UNEP-SETAC toxicity model: recommended characterization factors for human toxicity and freshwater ecotoxicity in life cycle impact assessment. *Int J Life Cycle Assess.* 13:532–546.

Sharaai AH, Mahmood NZ, Sulaiman AH. 2009. Life cycle impact assessment (LCIA) of potable water treatment process in Malaysia: comparison between dissolved air flotation (DAF) and ultrafiltration (UF) technology. *Aust J Basic Appl Sci.* 3:3625–3632.

Shapiro AM. 2011. The challenge of interpreting environmental tracer concentrations in fractured rock and carbonate aquifers. *Hydrogeol J.* 19:9–12.

Steingraber S. 2010. *Living downstream: An ecologist's personal investigation of cancer and the environment.* 2nd ed. Cambridge, MA: De Capo Press.

Su G, Wurzel KA. 1981. A regulatory framework for setting air emission limits for noncriteria pollutants. *J Air Pollut Control Assoc.* 31:160–162.

Tillitt DE, Papoulias DM, Whyte JJ, Richter CA. 2010. Atrazine reduces reproduction in fathead minnow (*Pimephales promelas*). *Aquat Toxicol.* 99:149–159. U.S. Environmental Protection

Agency. 1994. FGETS. http://www2.epa.gov/exposure-assessment-models/fgets.

U.S. Environmental Protection Agency. 2010. Dispersion modeling. http://www.epa.gov/scram001/dispersionindex.htm.

U.S. Environmental Protection Agency. 2011. AERSCREEN user's guide. EPA-454/B-11-001. http://www.epa.gov/scram001/models/screen/aerscreen_userguide.pdf

U.S. Environmental Protection Agency. 2012. Soil vapor extraction (SVE). http://www.epa.gov/oust/cat/sve1.htm

U.S. Environmental Protection Agency. 2015. Pesticides: Science and policy: Models. http://www.epa.gov/pesticides/science/models_pg.htm

U.S. Geological Survey. 2015a. Environmental health – toxic substances: Contaminated site management and remediation investigations. http://toxics.usgs.gov/investigations/subsurface_point_index.html

U.S. Geological Survey. 2015b. Watershed Modeling: Modeling of watershed systems (MOWS). http://wwwbrr.cr.usgs.gov/projects/SW_MoWS/

CHAPTER 25

Agricultural Chemicals (Pesticides and Fertilizers): Exposure and Impacts

This is a chapter outline intended to guide and familiarize you with the content to follow.

I. Agricultural chemicals

    A. Fertilizers/nutrients—see Figure 25-1 for NH_4^+, NO_2^-, NO_3^-, and PO_4^{3-} in the Mississippi River for 1991–1992

        1. Ammonia nitrogen

            a. Human toxicity—applied as a gas (anhydrous ammonia) and becomes NH_4^+. Ammonia is also emitted from manure (prevented by inhibiting microbial uricase). Ammonia gas contacts respiratory tract → chemical burns and pneumonia (NH_3 in combination with H_2O → alkaline NH_4OH). Passes into blood → neurotoxicity = synthesis of glutamine by glutamine synthase → astrocytes and transport glutamine to mitochondria → conversion back to NH_3 → generates ROS and mitochondrial permeability transition. "Trojan Horse" hypothesis = interference of glutamine with activation of NMDA/NO/cGMP pathway by NH_3. NH_3 depolarizes neurons directly, substituting for K^+, or causes ↑ Ca^{2+} → cell death via stimulation of NMDA receptor

            b. Fish toxicity—NH_4^+ does not pass well through biological membranes, but NH_3 does. As pH ↑, so does NH_3/NH_4 reaction (pK = 9.5). NH_3 toxicity is ranked as diatom > barnacle > fish and amphipod > shrimp—see Figure 25-2. Exercise augments NH_3 in fish, and therefore NH_3 toxicity (rainbow trout at rest LC_{50} = ~200 mg/L N at rest; exercising ~30 mg/L N). Resistant weather loaches volatilize NH_3 and the mudskipper actively pumps NH_4^+ out of its system. Elasmobranchs and some teleosts convert NH_3 → urea, similar to human liver

        2. Nitrite/Nitrate

            a. In humans, especially fetuses and babies with limited NADH and methemoglobin (metHb) reductase (diaphorase I) activity, the oxidation (via H_2O_2 formation) of the oxygen-binding Fe^{3+} form of Hb to the Fe^{2+} metHb makes an unsuitable binding site for oxygen, but can now bind CN. Can happen to cattle given high nitrate silage (not given enough time to denitrify by bacteria)

            b. In normoxic fish (more than hypoxic benthic fish), NO_3^- uptake → ↑ S-nitroso, N-nitroso, and Fe-nitrosyl compounds → nitrosative stress

            c. Nitrogenous compounds and wastes plus bacterial action in stratified waters at river mouths into the ocean have created dead or hypoxic zones

        3. Orthophosphate

            a. Excess PO_4^{3-} in humans → vascular calcification as it combines with Ca^{2+}. Can lead to secondary hyperparathyroidism as plasma free Ca^{2+} ↓ in the blood. Excess phosphate in foods → ↑ Akt-mediated signal transduction pathway → growth of lung tumors

CONCEPTUALIZING TOXICOLOGY 25-1

b. Mice respond to excess phosphate by experiencing premature aging

c. In agricultural lakes, $\uparrow PO_4^{3-} \rightarrow$ cyanobacterial blooms $\rightarrow$ direct liver toxicity to pets who drink from the lake and $\uparrow$ risk of ALS for humans living by lake

B. Pesticides

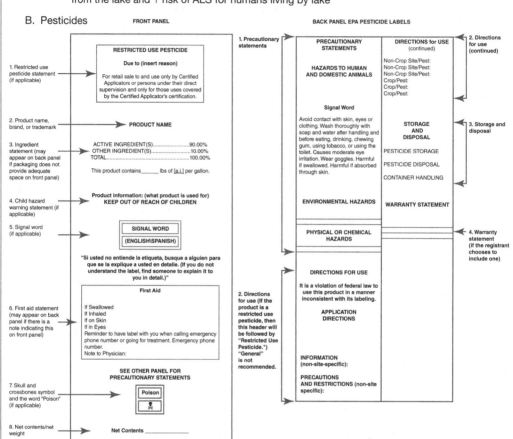

Data from Environmental Protection Agency. Retrieved from: http://www.epa.gov/pesticides/regulating/labels/pest-label-training/module2

1. Herbicides target plant pests (weed is a plant growing where it is not wanted)—see Table 25-1

   a. ACCase (acetylCoA carboxylase) inhibitors include arylphenoxypropionates (clodinafop-propargyl appears to be a peroxisome proliferator [cancer] and is cytotoxic through propargyl alcohol generation), cyclohexanones (tralkoxydim causes Leydig cell tumors in rat testes), and phenyl pyrazoline (major concern for birds and mammals relying on monocots and nonflowering plants for food)

   b. Acetolactate synthase/acetohydroxyacid synthase (ALS/AHAS) inhibitors include sulfonylureas (liver target organ in all test species), imidazolinones (imazapyr $\rightarrow$ irreversible eye damage), triazolopyrimidines (mainly a concern to applicators), pyrimidinyl(thio)benzoates (bispyribac-Na high half-life in environment = concern for groundwater contamination), and sulfonylaminocarbonyl triazolinones (affect dog's thyroid function, so endocrine disruption a possibility)

   c. Triazines move into the arena of disrupting photosynthesis (PSII) and represent many formerly primary herbicides (e.g., atrazine) used in the United States and still have use in formulations. Triazines act at Q_B site by binding adjacent positions on D-1 quinone protein (see Figure 25-3). This diverts electrons into production of free radicals and the thylakoid membrane for photosynthesis. Sunlight then is only toxic and cannot generate energy in these plants. Corals are very sensitive to PSII inhibition. Mainly used on corn because it has an effective detoxification

CONCEPTUALIZING TOXICOLOGY 25-1 (*continued*)

system employing GSH. Atrazine is an endocrine disruptor (via suppression of LH in rat reproductive function). It is also a persistent chlorinated compound, whose metabolites contaminate water supplies. Ultralow levels of atrazine cause malformations if exposed at early stages of amphibian metamorphosis

d. Other PSII disruptors: Triazinone inhibits all Hill-reactions (H_2O + electron acceptor + light in chloroplasts → electron acceptor-H_2 + $\frac{1}{2}O_2$) by interrupting electron flow between the primary (Q) and secondary (plastoquinone) electron acceptor of photosystem II. Metribuzin (triazinone) is an irritant and ↑ rat liver and thyroid (endocrine disruption). Triazolinone is similar to triazines and triazinones in binding to Q_B. Amicarbazone (triazolinone) → thyroid vacuolization in dog (EPA does not consider this an endocrine disruptor because liver metabolism may play a large role in thyroid effects). Uracil herbicides (bromacil and terbacil) inhibit D1 protein of PSII. Bromacil → inhibit thyroid peroxidase → thyroid tumors in male rats. Other uracil compounds inhibit iodine uptake. Pyridazinones (pyrazon/chloridazon) bind to same site as triazines, but with different binding behavior. Phenyl-carbamates (betanal, phenmedipham) bind to Q_B on one of five niches. Betanal may have some embryotoxic action based on one article (Medved, 1984) and also cause allergic contact dermatitis (Nater and Grosfeld, 1979). Phenmedipham + Cu → inhibit cholinesterase activity (important as carbamate insecticides are AChE inhibitors) in white worm. Ureas (linuron) → interferes with transmission of male hormones (endocrine disruption) with similar toxicity profile to plasticizer dibutyl phthalate → testicular tumors in mice (Group C carcinogen). Amides (propanil) = primary eye irritant. Propanil = novel endocrine disruptor active through enhanced immune response in C57BL/6 mice, which requires steroid synthesis (GnRH antagonist antide prevented immune response). Nitriles (bromoxynil, ioxynil) ↓ redox potential or Em thereby ↑ sensitivity of PSII to light damage. Bromoxynil butyrate caused developmental toxicity (canceled by manufacturer) while phenol = Group C carcinogen. Bromoxynil and ioxynil both uncouple oxidative phosphorylation. Benzothiadiazinones (bentazon) also have similar action to triazines and ureas with PSII electron transport, but in extreme human poisoning lead to hepatorenal dysfunction, ↑ perspiration, breathing difficulties, and heart failure. Phenylpyridazine (pyridate) = canceled, but is of interest to endocrine disruption due to competing with estrogen for ERα binding

e. Bipyridylium (Paraquat and diquat) herbicides are toxic oxidation-reduction indicators that produce $O_2^{\cdot-}$ following reduction and presence of O_2. These herbicides interfere with electron transfer in PSI and cause triplet chlorophyll by PSII inhibition. Paraquat's lung half-life is very long due to the polyamine uptake system (P_5-ATPase ATP13A2), and it does lung damage regardless of route of administration. Diquat usually causes kidney damage unless inhaled

f. Inhibition of protoporphyrinogen oxidase (PPO): All inhibitors of PPO are developmentally suspect due to interference with heme synthetic pathway. Diphenyl ethers inhibit PPO in plants (causing light absorption and peroxidative degradation of membrane lipids) and humans (leading to porphyria and porphyria variegate). These compounds, depending on their structure, also generate ROS and activate mast cells (nitrofen) and have strong antiandrogenic activities (chlornitrofen and chlormethoxyfen). Phenylpyrazoles (pyraflufen-ethyl) also inhibit PPO, may cause irreversible eye damage, and are considered to be likely human carcinogens (mouse liver tumor induction). N-phenylphthalimides (flumioxazin) inhibit PPO (especially formulated product) as well, and its phototoxic mode may occur in plants and fish. They cause heart septal defects in developing rats, possibly related to ↓ heme biosynthesis, and are endocrine disruptors based on atrophied and hypoplastic testes and/or epididymides in male rats. Thiadiazoles' (fluthiacet-methyl) GSH metabolite inhibits PPO, is clastogenic (micronuclei induced in rat liver cells), and ↑ trend toward exocrine and pancreatic islet cell adenomas in male rats and liver tumors in mice (likely human carcinogens). Oxadiazoles (oxadiazon) inhibit PPO, are peroxisome proliferators, ↑ aromatase activity, and likely induce liver cancer in humans (endocrine disruptors and carcinogens). Triazolinones (azafenidin) inhibit PPO and cause liver toxicity and anemia. Oxazolidinediones (pentoxazone), pyrimidinediones (butafenacil), and pyridazinones (flufenpyr-ethyl) also are used to inhibit PPO for their herbicidal activity

g. Bleaching: Pyridazinones (norflurazon) inhibit phytoene desaturase step of carotenoid biosynthesis/bleaching and affect thyroid of dogs at high-dose (endocrine disruption) and non-quantifiable Group C carcinogen. Pyridine carboxamides (diflufenican) also inhibit this step and high doses affect testes and thymus weights, but only when body weight is affected as

CONCEPTUALIZING TOXICOLOGY 25-1 (*continued*)

well. Another herbicide that inhibits this step is fluridone, whose N-methyl formamide metabolite is more toxic than parent compound. The formulation of this agent is 60-fold more toxic to water mites than the active ingredient and has been listed by the U.S. Fish and Wildlife Service as a threat to all listed U.S. freshwater aquatic species

h. Bleaching/4-hydroxyphenylpyruvate dioxygenase (4-HPPD) inhibitors lead to high blood tyrosine levels in dog causing eye lesions and liver and kidney effects. Isoxaflutole is a toxic 4-HPPD inhibitor $\rightarrow$ developmental toxicity, Group B_2 human carcinogen (liver tumors), and endocrine disruption (thyroid $\downarrow T_4$) and is extremely phytotoxic. Pyrazoles (pyrazoxyfen) are 4-HPPD inhibitors used in rice paddies with mainly aquatic species concerns. Benzobicyclons fit the "other" category of 4-HPPD inhibitors used on rice fields of Japan with concerns for carp and other aquatic species

i. Bleaching/inhibition of carotenoid biosynthesis: Triazoles (amitrol = lycopene cyclase inhibitor) are thyroid disruptors ($\downarrow$ TSH receptor on surface of rat thyroid follicle cells) and cause thyroid, pituitary, and liver tumors (Group B_2 carcinogen). Isoxazolidinone (clomazone) inhibits carotenoid biosynthesis via metabolites (5-ketoclomazone) and causes oxidative stress in human RBCs, and ROS also inhibit AChE. Diphenyl ether (aclonifen) is highly persistent and very toxic to aquatic organisms

j. Glycine: Glyphosate is a widely used pesticide known as Roundup. This herbicide inhibits 5-enolpyruvylshikimate 3-phosphate synthase (EC 2.5.1.19), the sixth enzyme in the shikimate pathway that leads to the formation of aromatic amino acids in algae, higher plants, bacteria, fungi, and apicomplexan parasites, but is an enzyme not present in mammals. Rat testicular toxicity/necrosis appears to indicate that glyphosate is a potent endocrine disruptor. Parkinson's disease in accidental spills on humans and damage to GABAergic and dopaminergic neurons in a worm species points to neurotoxicity of this herbicide. Additionally, cytotoxicity linked to dose-dependent DNA breaks in frog neonates sprayed with glyphosate formulations indicates ecotoxicological risks to anuran species

k. Phosphinic acid (glufosinate-ammonium) inhibits glutamine synthetase and neurotoxicity in rats linked to inhibition of the same enzyme found in plants

l. Carbamate (asulam) inhibits dihydropteroate synthase (an enzyme found in plants and microbes) involved in folic acid synthesis. A second activity of this herbicide is prevention of microtubule assembly (mitosis inhibition by chlorpropham, propham, and carbetamide). Thyroid and adrenal tumors in male rats indicate Group C carcinogen

m. Microtubule assembly inhibitors: Dinitroaniline (benefin) is a microtubule assembly inhibitor (plants) and skin sensitizer, and high doses yield liver and thyroid tumors. Developmental toxicity was also evident with benefin (dead pups and progressive neuropathy and liver and kidney enlargement in survivors). Also very highly toxic to freshwater fish. Phosphoramidate (amiprophos-methyl) higher specificity for tubulin than colchicine, a natural antimitotic agent, makes it an oral poison (and eye irritant) based on that property alone. Pyridine (dithiopyr) is highly toxic to freshwater fish and aquatic invertebrates. Benzamide (propyzamide) causes hepatic, thyroid, and pituitary toxicity (endocrine). Group B_2 carcinogen due to liver cancer in male mice and testicular and thyroid tumors in rats (organochlorine compound). Benzoic acid (DCPA) had manufacturing impurities on 2,3,7,8-TCDD and HCB = oncogenic, developmental toxicity, and immunotoxicity

n. Inhibitors of cell division, protein synthesis, and very long chain fatty acids (VLCFAs): Chloroacetamide (acetochlor) probable human carcinogen based on high-dose hepatocarcinomas and thyroid cell adenomas (endocrine) in male rat, lung tumors in females at all dose levels, and other growths in nasal tract, femur, and stomach. Acetamide (napropamide) also disrupts cell division and inhibits VLCFAs 7. Its toxicity is related to diarrhea, excessive tearing and urination, depression, salivation, rapid weight loss, respiratory changes, $\downarrow$ blood pressure, and fluid in body cavities. Oxyacetamide (flufenacet) also inhibits VLCFAs and induces changes in gait, convulsions, etc. Tetrazolinone (fentrazamide) inhibits VLDFAs $\rightarrow$ $\downarrow$ cell division. Another VLDFA synthesis inhibitor is the organophosphate anilofos (also therefore inhibits AChE)

o. Inhibitors of cellulose/cell wall synthesis: Nitrile (dichlobenil) has high phytotoxicity for emerging crops and is a class C carcinogen ($\uparrow$ rat tumors). Triazolocarboxamide (flupoxam) = obsolete

CONCEPTUALIZING TOXICOLOGY 25-1 (*continued*)

herbicide of this category. Quinone carboxylic acid (quinclorac) has activities of ↓ cellulose synthesis and mimics growth hormone auxin. Quinclorac is a dermal sensitizer and chronic toxicity = kidney, liver, and pancreatic acinar alterations

p. Uncouplers of oxidative phosphorylation: Dinitrophenol (DNOC), based on mechanism, is toxic to a variety of cells and organisms

q. Inhibition of lipid synthesis by route other than ACC inhibition: Thiocarbamate (butylate) is a strong eye irritation agent with ↑ risk of prostate cancer and non-Hodgkin lymphoma, is highly toxic to freshwater fish, and has historically had fatal injuries among farmers along with four other famous herbicides (banned 2,4,5-T, Paraquat, alachlor, metribuzin). Phosphorodithioate (bensulide) also prevents lipid synthesis and has neurotoxicity based on cholinesterase inhibition. Benzofuran (benfuresate) is another example of this class of agents, as is chloro-carbonic-acid (dalapon), which also is a growth regulator

r. Auxin-like activity: Phenoxy-carboxylic acid (2,4-D) is a famous dandelion (broadleaf) control agent for lawns—acid and salt forms are severe irritants. Dogs are most sensitive to 2.4-D's effects due to limited capacity to excrete organic acids. Once renal clearance reaches saturation 2,4-D → eye, thyroid, kidney, and ovary toxicity (endocrine). Pyridine carboxylic acid (clopyralid) = synthetic auxin mainly concerned with eye irritation. Benazolin-ethyl is another synthetic auxin with moderate toxicity to fish

s. Inhibitors of auxin transport: Phthalamate (naptalam) is an eye irritant in a granular formulation (Alanap, technical) as is semicarbazole (diflufenzopyr-sodium)

t. Anti-microtubule mechanism involving spindle formation: arylaminopropionic acid (flamprop-M-methyl). Mainly nontarget plant, algae, and *Daphnia* concerns

u. Destruction of cell membranes: pyrazolium (difenzoquat) canceled due to moderate toxicity to mammals, bees, etc.

v. Organic arsenicals: Inhibition of plant growth by uncoupling oxidative phosphorylation → chlorosis (loss of chlorophyll). Inorganic As = carcinogen but organic arsenicals less toxic than inorganic form (opposite of Hg). Target organs for DSMA and MSMA = large intestine and kidney. DMA targets urinary bladder and thyroid (endocrine). Higher exposures target CNS. Circulatory or renal failure → death

w. Bromobutide may be amide herbicide or organic bromide or 4-HPPD inhibitor. This compound loses bromine on metabolism and ecological significance uncertain at this point

x. Cinmethylin = monoterpene inhibits tyrosine aminotransferase

y. Cumyluron = urea analog—liver as target from centrilobular hepatocellular swelling → hepatocellular adenomas. Dymron substituted urea, preventing germination of target plants and elongation of roots

z. Soil fumigant (herbicidal, fungicidal, nematocidal): Dazomet degrades in methyl isothiocyanate (eye, systemic, and respiratory toxicity)

aa. Biopesticide: Pelargonic acid (nonanoic acid) blossom thinner in apple and pear trees—skin and eye irritation

bb. Plant growth regulators—see Table 25-2

(1) Gibberellic acid synthesis inhibitors: Pyrimidine (ancymidol) produces little toxicity unless spilled to nontarget organisms. Quaternary ammonium (chlormequat chloride)—mouthful of this agent made worker die of cholinergic crisis. Triazole (paclobutrazol)—implications for steroid synthesis (inhibits CYP51 family) affecting endocrine, reproduction, and development

(2) Pinchers (↓ growth of suckers): Cyclohexaketone (dikegulac sodium) is a DNA synthesis inhibitor and has mainly ocular concerns. Methyl esters of fatty acids are also pinchers, and inhalation can lead to chemical pneumonia for greenhouse workers

(3) Growth promoters: Gibberellin/cytokinin produce endocrine disruption (oxidative stress → ↓ thyroid function) and reproductive toxicity (↓ spermatogenesis and derangement of germ cells), and cytokinins also block cAMP-dependent microfilament organization (endocrine). Acid (ethephon) is an organophosphate that stimulates ethylene (ripening) generation = severe

CONCEPTUALIZING TOXICOLOGY 25-1 (*continued*)

eye risk. Rooting hormones (IBA) = native auxin accelerates cell elongation in stem cuttings. IBA affects glucose tolerance, antioxidant defense, and cholinesterase (neurotoxicity) and myeloperoxidase (immunotoxicity) inhibition

2. Insecticides/miticides—see Table 25-3

   a. AChE inhibitors

      (1) Carbamates—reversible AChE inhibitors (neurotoxic especially to honeybees that don't develop resistance), likely human carcinogen due to vascular tumors in mice and inhibits steroidogenesis

      (2) Organophosphates—stronger AChE inhibitors; malathion and parathion metabolism to oxon = active form of these organophosphates (more in insects than in mammalian metabolism due to hydrolysis deactivation in mammal); hepatic tumors in rats suggests carcinogenicity

   b. Cyclodiene organochlorines

      (1) DDT—held Na^+ channel open (action potential)

      (2) Endosulfan—interfered with presynaptic GABA receptors

   c. Pyrethroids/botanical pyrethrins

      (1) Prolong Na^+ permeability (action potential)—Bifenthrin is highly toxic to honeybees, possible human carcinogen and endocrine disruptor ($\downarrow$ secretion of progesterone and PGE^2); pyrethrin $\rightarrow$ neurobehavioral toxicity, chronic thyroid toxicity (endocrine), and liver damage

      (2) Synergists that prevent metabolism of these agents are MGK-264 and piperonyl butoxide (possible human carcinogen due to ileocecal ulcers and adenomas and carcinomas of the liver in rats)

   d. Neonicotinoids/nicotine

      (1) Agonists or antagonists of cholinergic nicotinic receptors disrupt nerve transmission—nicotine is a powerful neurotoxin

      (2) Neonicotinoids have $\downarrow$ bumblebee colony growth and queen production

   e. Spinosyns disrupt nicotinic/GABA-gated chloride channels and affect reproduction and thyroid (endocrine)

   f. Glycosides—avermectin B1 = GABA receptor antagonist = extreme mammalian and aquatic invertebrate toxicity (but not birds) and also affects male rat fertility (reproduction and endocrine)

   g. Juvenile hormone mimics—mainly influences *Daphnia* as nontarget species

   h. Selective feeding blockers—pyridine azomethines and carboxamides (neurotoxic in rats = $\downarrow$ body temperature and motor activity, function, and observation of battery changes and cancer = liver tumors)

   i. Mite growth inhibitors—tetrazines/thiazolidinones/oxazolines—clofentezine $\uparrow$ liver metabolism and excretion of thyroid hormone; etoxazole $\uparrow$ formation of superoxide radicals

   j. Bioinsecticides—BT is a soil bacterium toxic to insects but not humans

   k. Organotins—inhibition of oxidative phosphorylation in mites and severe eye irritant in rabbits

   l. Pyrroles—chlorfenapyr uncouples oxidative phosphorylation via disruption of H^+ gradient

   m. Benzoyl urea insect growth regulators—low toxicity but affects Hb in animals

   n. Chitin synthesis inhibitor—buprofezin had some thyroid effects (endocrine); triazine cyromazine affects molting and estuarine/marine invertebrates

   o. Growth regulators—ecdysone = steroidal prohormone promoting premature molting

   p. Coupling site II electron transport inhibitors at cyt bc_1 complex—only toxic to rats at near lethal doses, but some are possible human carcinogens (hydramethylnon and acequinocyl)

   q. Pyridazinones and phenoxypyrazoles—pyridaben = site I mitochondrial electron transport inhibitor that is acute toxic to mice; methylpyrazoles are genotoxic to SH-SY5Y neuroblastoma line

CONCEPTUALIZING TOXICOLOGY 25-1 (*continued*)

    r. Inhibitors of acetyl CoA carboxylase—spiromesifen = contact sensitizer, endocrine disruptor (thyroid), liver and immune (spleen) toxicant; spirotetramat targets thyroid and thymus (endocrine and immune)

    s. Unknown action—bifenazate targets liver, spleen, and adrenal cortex (endocrine); azadirachtin from neem tree at high doses inhibits AChE; pyridalyl activated by CYP in mites → ROS → damage cellular macromolecules and ↑ proteasome activity

    t. Miscellaneous—biopesticide *Beauveria bassiana* strain HF23 = eye irritant, strain ATCC 74040 = dermal sensitizer

3. Fungicides—see Table 25-4

    a. Thiophanates, methyl benzimidazole, and carbamates inhibit tubulin in mitosis and thiophanate-methyl is both a skin sensitizer and affects liver and thyroid (endocrine and cancer)

    b. Dicarboximides—inhibits DNA/RNA synthesis and metabolism = likely human carcinogen based on liver tumors in mice and Leydig cells of rats (reproductive and endocrine)

    c. Demethylation inhibitors of sterol synthesis (imidazole, pyrimidine, triazole) destabilize fungal cell walls—triflumizole metabolized to 4-chloro-2-trifluoromethyl aniline targeting liver but also chronic exposure to rats → hyperplastic lesions of endocrine glands and lymph nodes—also some neurotoxicity on oral exposure; fenarimol can cause hydronephrosis and ↓ fertility and dystocia in rats along with hepatic adenomas and hyperplastic nodules; propiconazole → dermal sensitization, developmental toxicity (malformations), acute neurotoxicity, and chronic liver toxicity including cancer; 1,2,5-triazole has mainly endocrine effects, but 1,2,4-triazole as a compound or metabolite of triadimefon = neurotoxin and thyroid adenomas

    d. Acrylamine affects RNA synthesis in fungi but also causes bradycardia → cardiac arrest at high doses

    e. Piperidines inhibit isomerase of ergosterol synthesis = skin irritant

    f. Phenyl-benzamines affect mitochondrial electron transport with reproductive and developmental toxicities

    g. Strobilurins, imidazolinones—quinone outside inhibitors (cytochrome bc_1 at Q_o site of complex III)—compounds toxic to fish or mysid shrimp, but relatively nontoxic to mammals or birds

    h. Phenylpyrrole (fludioxonil) alter MAP kinase in osmotic signal transduction—again more aquatic organism toxicity

    i. Aromatic hydrocarbon and thiadiazole—produce lipid peroxidation products; PCNB chronic exposure = liver and thyroid hyperplasia (toxicity and cancer with a threshold effect and is persistent due to high chlorination) and very acutely toxic to estuarine/marine fish and invertebrates

    j. Hydroxyanalide—fenhexamid affects the 3-keto reductase during C4 demethylation in ergosterol biosynthesis—adrenal (endocrine) toxicity

    k. Polyoxins—biopesticides inhibiting chitin synthase

    l. Cyano-imidazole—quinone inside inhibitor

    m. Carbamate—propamocarb hydrochloride affects cell wall permeability, but causes brain lesions in rats

    n. Ethyl phosphonates and phosphite (phosphorus acid directly inhibits oxidative phosphorylation in oomycetes)—acidic content = human concern

    o. Cinnamic acid amides—inhibits fungal ergosterol synthesis and affects prostate (endocrine) weights in high-dosed male dogs

    p. Copper—broad-spectrum fungicide, bactericide, aquatic herbicide, algaecide, and molluscicide

    q. Dithiocarbamates affect fungi at multiple sites of action—mancozeb is thiol-reactive and affects thyroid (endocrine and cancer) and causes peripheral nerve damage in rat

    r. Phthalimides—captan has nonspecific thiol reactivity and inhibition of cellular respiration in fungi (thiophosgene degradation product)—severe eye irritant, affects thyroid (endocrine) and

CONCEPTUALIZING TOXICOLOGY 25-1 (*continued*)

other key organ weights such as heart and brain, and is a probable human carcinogen due to intestinal, liver, and kidney alterations. THPI metabolite is also a risk factor. Highly toxic to fish

    s. Chloronitriles—chlorothalonil is a polychlorinated aromatic that causes severe eye irritation and based on its ability to cause cell proliferation = probable human carcinogen (renal tumors in rats)

    t. Biopesticides—organisms such as bacteria with antifungal properties/components such as rhizocticin antifungal phosphono-oligopeptide produced by *Bacillus subtilis* ATCC 6633

    u. Bicarbonate—disrupts K^+ balance of cells and causes fungal cell wall collapse

    v. Neem oil—long-chain fatty acids and glycerides

    w. Plant extracts—especially toxic to fungi are antifungal isoquinoline alkaloids from plume poppy used in Chinese medicine for anti-inflammatory and antibacterial properties

4. Rodenticides/fumigants—see Table 25-5

    a. One of the most toxic categories, because rodenticides are targeting mammalian species and fumigants generate gases toxic to many species of organisms

    b. Organic fumigants

        (1) Acrylonitrile—former fumigant in food industry—high acute respiratory and extreme oral and dermal toxicity, which are indicated in humans by limb weakness, labored and irregular breathing, dizziness and impaired judgment, cyanosis, nausea, collapse, and convulsions; also causes lung cancer

        (2) Calcium cyanide, cyanogen bromide, cyanogen chloride (all degrade or are metabolized to CN gas)—insect fumigants (inhibits cyt a_3 = cellular respiration in mitochondria)

        (3) CS_2—psychosis and at increased exposure nausea, vomiting, dizziness, fatigue, headache, mood changes, lethargy, blurred vision, delirium, and convulsions—also affects sperm count and menstrual disturbances

        (4) CCl_4—former fumigant that causes CNS (as original compound), liver (CYP metabolism to trichloromethyl radical species), and kidney toxicity—also a probable human carcinogen

        (5) Chloropicrin = soil fumigant (fungicidal, herbicidal, insecticidal, and nematocidal properties) that is highly toxic to mammals and is very highly toxic to fish and aquatic invertebrates

        (6) Dazomet = nonselective soil fumigant that degrades to methyl isothiocyanate (MITC) that caused the Bhopal disaster (pulmonary edema); metam sodium/potassium also generates MITC

        (7) 1,2-Dibromo-3-chloropropane = former soil fumigant → pulmonary congestion, moderate CNS depression and probable human carcinogen; 11,3-dichloropropene = component of soil fumigants causing respiratory difficulties and is a carcinogen in male mice and to workers accidentally exposed to vapors of a tank truck spill (lymphoma and leukemia); propylene dichloride was a soil fumigant with human lung, GI tract, blood, liver, kidney, CNS, and eye toxicity; probable human carcinogen

        (8) *p*-Dichlorobenzene = fumigant insecticide and moth repellant (clothes); also used for ticks and lice control around bird cages—main concern eye or dermal irritation because it does not generate overwhelming gas or vapor as classic fumigants do—tumor promoter but not directly carcinogenic (mitogenic)

        (9) Ethylene dibromide = fumigant that is extremely toxic to humans (liver, kidney, and testes regardless of route—also a severe skin irritant) and on inhalation causes depression and collapse (or bronchitis if not fatal) and probable human carcinogen

        (10) Ethylene dichloride = former fumigant that caused CNS, liver, kidney, and respiratory toxicity along with cardiac arrhythmias and probable human carcinogen (gavage study in rodents yielded forestomach squamous cell carcinomas, circulatory system hemangiosarcomas, mammary adenocarcinoma, alveolar/bronchiolar adenomas, endometrial stromal polyps and sarcomas, and hepatocellular carcinomas)

        (11) Ethylene oxide used only in small amounts as fumigant due to depression of CNS, irritation to eyes and mucous membranes, and increased incidence of cancers (leukemia, stomach cancer, pancreatic cancer, and Hodgkin's disease); propylene oxide = fumigant

CONCEPTUALIZING TOXICOLOGY 25-1 (*continued*)

of foodstuffs and plastic medical instruments that is an irritant (eye, skin necrosis, and respiratory tract) and has neurological effects, and tumors develop in animals (nasal and forestomach)

(12) Methyl bromide (heavier than air fumigant)—neurotoxicity (especially dogs) is most common effect including human deaths due to accidental exposure. Stratospheric ozone depletion is a major environmental concern ($\uparrow$ UV); bromide ion = concern to aquatic organisms; trichloroethane discontinued due to Montreal Protocol (stratospheric ozone depletion agent)

(13) Iodomethane = newer pre-plant soil fumigant viewed as alternative to methyl bromide, which has toxicity concerns—iodomethane has thyroid toxicity (contains iodide), alkylating properties (cancer potential), irreversible neurological toxicity, and fetal toxicity

(14) Naphthalene used in mothballs → hemolytic anemia, liver damage, and neurological damage. Chronic human exposure → cataracts and damage to the retina. Possible human carcinogen based on female mice alveolar/bronchiolar adenomas

c. Inorganic fumigants

(1) Al and Mg phosphide → form highly toxic phosphine gas when exposed to moisture—rats develop coagulative necrosis of kidney and pulmonary congestion—shown to be clastogen *in vitro* and in applicators

(2) SO_2—low toxicity except for humans with sulfite sensitivity (asthma)

(3) Sulfuryl fluoride—fluoride toxicity caused this to be withdrawn as fumigant

d. Anticoagulant rodenticides

(1) Warfarin (anticoagulant medication in humans)—interferes with vitamin K and has developmental effects in humans

(2) Most agents EPA classifies as Category I (highest toxicity) are rodenticides. Only one is a neurotoxin (bromethalin)

e. Neurotoxic rodenticides

(1) Strychnine—interferes with glycine's postsynaptic inhibition at motoneurons and interneurons

(2) Red squill, zinc phosphide, and bromethalin = other neurotoxins

f. Circulatory collapse—cholecalciferol (vitamin D) given in extreme excess → calcification → occlusion of circulatory system and death

References

Medved IL. 1984. [Potential hazardousness of the embryotoxic action of the herbicide Betanal (experimental data)]. *Gig Sanit.* Apr (4):16-18.

Nater JP, Grosfeld JC. 1979. Allergic contact dermatitis from Betanal (phenmedipham). *Contact Dermatitis.* 5:59-60.

CONCEPTUALIZING TOXICOLOGY 25-1 (*continued*)

Since Europeans settled in the United States, the forests, plains, and other existing ecosystems have been transformed by clear-cutting and planting as well as development of cities on water routes. The current landscapes are rural (farm crop rows or grazing pastures) and urban (cities with large water usage and sewage effluents as well as congested industrial and automobile emission areas). Both impact the air, soil, and water, although there appears to be a lot of finger pointing and denial from both city dwellers and farm communities. This chapter focuses on agricultural chemicals and their impacts. Of greatest interest are the fertilizers that now are mainly of chemical origin instead of human or animal waste. It is probably a good thing that human waste is not used due to parasites and diseases that result from crops raised using human waste as fertilizer in other countries and in the United States up to the

1920s. The animal waste for large-scale animal facilities has become a problem that has led to anaerobic hydrogen sulfide- and ammonia-producing manure lagoons and similar storage or disposal sites. In this chapter, it is of greatest interest to investigate the nitrogen and phosphorus inputs that have led to eutrophication/dead zones of U.S. waters and toxic cyanobacterial blooms in agricultural lakes, respectively. Additionally, pesticide use since the 1950s has led to a number of problems that have resulted in bans of certain compounds and restricted use of others. Thus, it is necessary to determine the composition of chemical fertilizers (liquid, solid) and their impacts and the ingredients and formulations of pesticides (liquid, solid, fumigants). Pesticides by definition usually encompass herbicides and insecticides (fumigants may fall under insecticides). Fungicides, which are used to treat mold "pests" that grow on crops and foods, also fall into this category. Because they can be applied from the air, on the ground, or into the ground, pesticides affect air quality, water contamination, and soil residues based on their application technique. Wind, precipitation of various sorts, slopes, and proximity to residential communities and delicate ecologies or apiaries (as with methyl parathion and honeybee sensitivity) make application restrictions important and put the farmer in a difficult situation because effects may spread for miles. Additionally, because rural areas drain into larger rivers such as the Mississippi, large loads of eroded soil, fertilizer runoff, and fertilizer contents add to enormous loads reflected at the mouths of these rivers (in the water and deposited sediments).

Fertilizers/Nutrients

Nutrients in river water come from natural sources and anthropogenic sources. Agricultural contaminants are mainly fertilizers and animal wastes (including waste from slaughterhouses), while urban/industrial areas produce human sewage, lawn fertilizers, household products, and industrial wastes (fertilizer manufacturing, petrochemical byproducts, and agrochemical byproducts). As shown in **Figure 25-1**, the Mississippi River's 1991–1992 season shows which nutrients generally result from agricultural activities.

The situation has become worse than what is depicted in the figure, especially for nitrates because corn prices and use of corn for energy and animal feed have resulted in more acres planted in corn, which requires high nutrient inputs. However, Figure 25- is still useful for providing an illustration of the important nutrients and their impacts. Nitrogen sources are NH_4^+ (more localized impacts involving application and air drift of anhydrous ammonia to farm fields exceeding water quality criteria for this compound set by the EPA; EPA, 1998a), NO_2^-, and NO_3^- (with longer range effects of nitrates to create dead zones in the stratified Mississippi River mouth/Gulf of Mexico—freshwater/saltwater layering and bacteria action to create a hypoxic area). The orthophosphate loading parallels the nitrate picture due to its presence in fertilizer and the water solubility of this nutrient. Here, toxic cyanobacterial blooms in rural lakes are of major concern and how these blooms may have some linkage to amyotrophic lateral sclerosis (or Lou Gehrig's disease—a progressive, usually fatal neurodegenerative disorder now associated with cyanobacterial toxin β-N-methylamino-L-alanine; Banack et al., 2010). This chapter does not cover the salts that arise from use of irrigation or agricultural products, because road salt use in the northern United States appears to be a greater potential impact on the waters of this area.

Ammonia Nitrogen

Ammonia is applied as a gas, and, when it comes rapidly into contact with water, it becomes ammonium ion. Another source of ammonia gas is ammonia emission from manure. The manure emission may be controllable via supplementing with dietary zinc and other minerals to inhibit the action of the microbial uricase (Hunde et al., 2012). The ammonia gas is most problematic to the farm worker or producer of the anhydrous ammonia. The first concern is the contact in the respiratory tract, including chemical burns and pneumonia. NH_3 rapidly contacts water to become the alkaline NH_4OH Once it passes into the blood, it is a major neurotoxin and may cause encephalopathy. The neurotoxicity appears to be mediated through glutamine synthesized from the excess

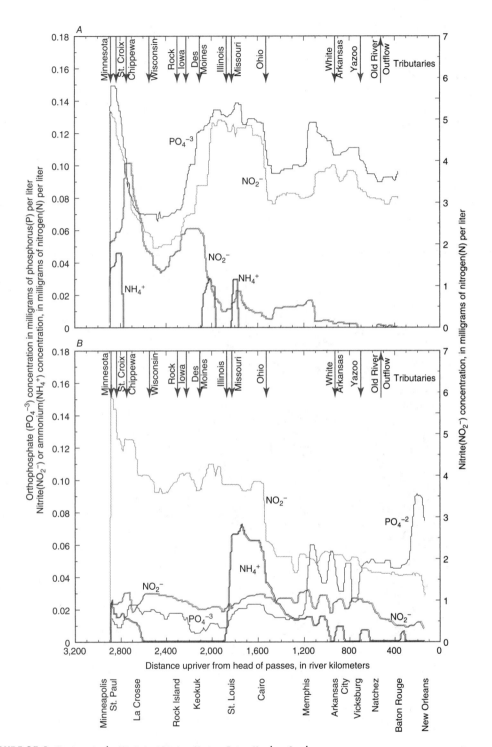

FIGURE 25-1 Nutrients in the Mississippi River at Various Points North to South

A) When taken as a snapshot for June and July 1991, nitrates (NO_3^-, pale green line) and orthophosphate (PO_4^{3-}, brown line) parallel each other in the corn belt of Minnesota/Northern Iowa (Minnesota River) and then increase from the corn regions of Iowa and northern Illinois. Ammonium ion (NH_4^+, purple line) shows distinct peaks on inputs from this region then is assimilated by bacteria (converted to NO_3^- or NO_2^-) of adsorbed to sediment. NO_2^- (aquamarine line) is similar to NH_4^+ in its conversion by bacteria and algae (to NO_3^-) but not as rapidly as NH_4^+ conversion. B) March and April 1992 show seasonal variations in nutrient loading/transport.

Data from Antweiler RC, Goolsby DA, Taylor HE. 1995. Nutrients in the Mississippi River. In: *Contaminants in the Mississippi River.* RH Meade, ed., USGS Circular 1133.

ammonia by the astrocyte enzyme glutamine synthase (glutamate + ammonia → glutamine). Astrocytes subsequently swell on transport of the glutamine to the mitochondria and convert back into ammonia. This ammonia generates reactive oxygen species (ROS) and the mitochondrial permeability transition. There is also a "Trojan Horse" hypothesis connected with these phenomena including the interference of glutamine with the activation of the NMDA/NO/cGMP pathway by ammonia (Albrecht et al., 2010). Some researchers suggest that ammonia either depolarizes neurons directly, substituting for K^+, or causes excess Ca^{2+}, leading to cell death in central nervous system (CNS) cells

of all vertebrates via stimulation of the NMDA receptor (Binstock and Lecar, 1969; Beaumont et al., 2000; Randall and Tsui, 2002). Toxicity to fish involves mainly ammonia, because ammonium ion does not pass well through biological membranes. As the pH of the water increases, the amount of ammonia rather than ammonium increases, and the pK for the NH_3/NH_4^+ reaction is 9.5. This increases ammonia toxicity in fish, pushing the lethal concentration (LC_{50}) down between pH 7.5 and 8.5. The diatom > barnacle > fish and amphipod > shrimp, as ranked in terms of susceptibility to ammonia in **Figure 25-2** (lower LC_{50}s for most susceptible species). Exercise also exacerbates ammonia

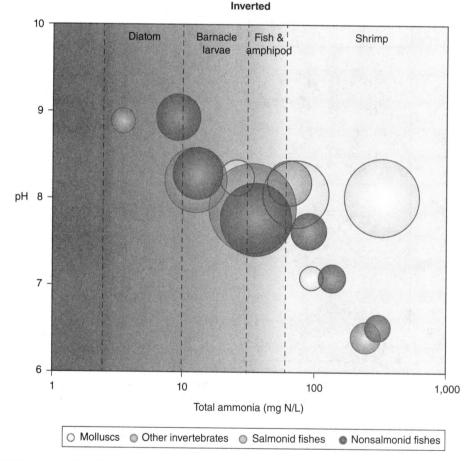

FIGURE 25-2 Acute LC_{50}s (U.S. Environmental Protection Agency, 1998) Used to Derive Final Acute Values (FAV) and Criterion Maximum Concentrations (CMCs) for Ammonia. (Wu, 2001; from Randall and Tsui, 2002)

Note: The labels at the top from Hong Kong species are not meant to imply that these species are affected at all pH values or at the range of the dotted lines. Rather at pH values of 7.5-8.3 the diatoms are most affected (~4 mg N/L), followed by barnacle larvae (~10 mg N/L), fish & amphipod (~40 mg N/L), and shrimp most resistant (~80 mg N/L).

toxicity. For example, it is generated in fish during exercise: The rainbow trout at rest has an ammonium LC_{50} of ~200 mg/L N, while it is ~30 mg/L N in exercising fish. Some of the least sensitive species have developed methods to eliminate ammonia from their systems or detoxify ammonia by metabolic conversion. Weather loaches (*Misqurnus anquillicaudatus*) volatilize ammonia (reemits into the environment), and the mudskipper (*Periophthalmodon schlosseri*) has an active pump to remove ammonium ion out of its system. Elasmobranchs and some teleosts convert ammonia into urea similar to the mechanism of the human liver. Some species resort to less proteolysis and amino acid catabolism to reduce ammonia production (Randall and Tsui, 2002).

Nitrite/Nitrate

Two oxidative nitrogen compounds lead to the formation of methemoglobin (metHB), which is the oxidized (Fe^{3+}) state of hemoglobin that does not bind to oxygen. It needs to be reduced by methemoglobin reductase to continue normal function. It appears that oxyhemoglobin may indeed react with nitrite anion to form hydrogen peroxide and nitrogen dioxide. It appears that H_2O_2 is the initiator species, and NO_2 is the autocatalytic propagatory species for metHb formation (Keszler et al., 2008). Deaths in children due to metHb formation occur in rural areas with high nitrate and nitrite levels in well water because the children have less ability to convert metHb to the reduced oxygen-carryring form (Nițuc et al., 2010). Pregnant women run the risk of metHb formation if they consume contaminated well water, which will be a negative outcome for the developing organism within them. Ruminants make NO_2 in their rumens when consuming silage or grasses high in nitrite/nitrate (fresh, high nitrogen–containing grasses or corn stalks that have not been allowed bacterial action and time to denitrify). The NO_2 transfers to plasma and also leads to metHb formation (McKenzie et al., 2004). Even fish can succumb to nitrite poisoning but are less sensitive to nitrate (Jensen and Hansen, 2011). Nitrite is taken up by normoxic fish more than hypoxic fish and

results in elevated S-nitroso (thiols), N-nitroso (amines), and Fe-nitrosyl (metHb and nitrosylHb) compounds or nitrosative stress. However, even adult humans can show an increase in metHb, with complaints of stomach/intestinal difficulties (such as gastroesophageal reflux) and bone and nerve pain (e.g., osteoarthritis). Bone and joint disorders have also been associated with an increase in *ex vivo* production of tumor necrosis factor beta (TNFβ) or Th2/T_{reg} cytokine IL-10 (Zeman et al., 2011). Nitrates can be reduced by bacteria to nitrite ions, even in aqueous media. This may lead further to nitrous anhydride, which then generates nitrosonium ions. Secondary amines then can react with nitrosium ions to yield carcinogenic nitrosoamines. Even urea—excreted from humans and animals alike—can proceed down this bacterial transformation pathway to become a cancer-causing agent (Hamon, 2007). Clearly, the worldwide hypoxic zones are created by microbial action induced by nitrogenous wastes and chemical fertilizers in stratified freshwater/seawater and represent indirect action of nitrates and nitrites on a variety of organisms. Eutrophication also has far-reaching effects on the biota of the world and is also an indirect effect of nitrogen compound loading into aquatic ecosystems (marshes, lakes).

Orthophosphate

In humans excess phosphates (usually from enemas but can come from drinking water because phosphate is readily absorbed in the gastrointestinal [GI] tract) result in vascular calcification as they combine with Ca^{2+} in the blood. This can lead to secondary hyperparathyroidism as calcium levels drop in the blood. Tetany, dehydration, hypotension, tachycardia, hyperpyrexia, cardiac arrest, and coma can result in severe cases. Some of these complications are a result of ion/electrolyte imbalance due to increased anion gaps. In a young girl, phosphate toxicity resulted in a generalized seizure that only responded to intravenous $CaCl_2$ (Marraffa et al., 2004). Animals given 30–50 mL/kg of a phosphate-containing enema die (100%; Martin et al., 1987). Mice (*klotho*-null) with phosphate toxicity experience premature aging (loss of body weight, kyphosis, hypogonadism, infertility, generalized tissue atrophy, and reduced lifespan). High phosphate levels in foods (meats, cheeses, soft drinks, and bakery items) may also simulate the growth of lung tumors (increases Akt-mediated signal transduction pathway), but are capable of dysregulating parathyroid hormone and vitamin D (decreasing bone mineralization) and hypocalcemia, especially in postmenopausal women (Razzaque, 2011). Phosphate in the water and/or kidney damage from sewage effluents or agricultural runoff may increase plasma phosphate in fish (Gunnarsson et al., 2009). Indirect exposure to phosphates appears to be greater in species drinking or swimming in surface waters. Phosphate detergents had to be reduced based on their negative impact on waterways. Now, agricultural runoff of phosphates into rural lakes can result in the growth of toxic cyanobacteria and the emerging possibility that not only do direct toxicities and deaths result to aquatic life, pets (dogs that drink from the lakes), other domestic animals used for meat, and humans, but there is an increased possibility of developing chronic neurodegenerative disease (amyotrophic lateral sclerosis) associated with living by these cyanobacterial toxin-contaminated lakes.

Pesticides

The Office of Chemical Safety and Pollution Prevention at the U.S. Environmental Protection Agency (EPA) regulates pesticides under the authority of the Federal Insecticide, Fungicide, and Rodenticide Act (FIFRA). It also regulates toxic substances (Toxic Subtances Control Act), foods, drugs, and cosmetics (Federal Food, Drug, and Cosmetic Act) and is also empowered by the Pollution Prevention Act. Under the auspices of the EPA's Pesticide Program, regulation of pesticide applications, registration (Pesticide Registration Improvement Renewal Act), and manufacture are subject to these acts and also the Food Quality Protection Act and the Endangered Species Act. These acts provide an excellent source of information on pesticides, as does EXTOXNET (*Extension Toxicology Network*), which is maintained at Oregon State University.

Herbicides

Herbicides target plant pests or weeds. A weed is a plant growing in a field of crops where it does not belong. By this definition, a soybean growing in a field of corn represents a weed. Usually, the term is reserved for grasses and other plants that no one ever wants in their crops, lawns, or gardens. This discussion focuses on the target and then the toxicity as shown in **Table 25-1**. The nontarget plant species for pesticide testing by Environment Canada have included phytoplanktonic algae and cyanobacteria. Among these are non-nitrogen-fixing diatoms (*Cyclotella meneghiama*, *Nitzchia* sp.), green algae (*Scenedesmus quadicauda* and *S. capricornutum*), unicellular cyanobateria (*Microcystis aeruginosa*), and filamentous cyanobacteria (*Oscillatoria* sp. and *Pseudoanabaena* sp.). Nitrogen-fixing filamentous cyanobacteria are represented by *Aphanizomenon flos-aquae* and *Anabaena inequalis*). Duckweed (*Lemna minor*) represents a floating vascular plant. Depending on the herbicide, sometimes the eukaryotes (green algae, diatoms, and duckweed) were more sensitive (to the broad-spectrum contact herbicide hexazinone) than were cyanobacteria. Another broad-spectrum contact herbicide (diquat) was most toxic to diatoms followed by cyanobacteria, while green algae were comparatively tolerant (Peterson et al., 1997). That is why individual classes of herbicides may have differential effects on plants and animals and must be viewed separately. The actions of herbicides that affect photosynthesis usually are grouped into electron transport inhibitors, uncouplers, energy transfer inhibitors, inhibitory uncouplers, or electron acceptors (Fuerst and Norman, 1991).

Arylphenoxypropionate

These compounds target grasses via inhibition of acetyl coenzyme A (CoA) carboxylase (ACCase). Two gramineous weeds, *Lolium rigidum* Gaud and *Alopecurus myosuroides* Huds, develop resistance to this chemical class of pesticides and cyclohexanedione herbicide cycloxydim by a leucine allele in the ACCase gene (Délye et al., 2002). Arylalkanoate dioxygenase enzymes (AADs) can degrade

TABLE 25-1   Herbicide Listing by Mechanism of Action and Toxicity

Target of Herbicidal Action	Chemical Family of Herbicide	Active Ingredient	Toxicity
Inhibition of acetyl CoA carboxylase	Arylphenoxypropionate "FOPs"	Clodinafop-propargyl Cyhalofop-butyl Diclofop-methyl Fenoxaprop-P-ethyl Fluazifop-P-butyl Haloxyfop-R-methyl Propaquizafop Quizalofop-P-ethyl	Peroxisome proliferator so some cancer potential, skin irritant and sensitizer in formulated pesticide (EPA pesticide fact sheet), and zebrafish developmental toxicity for ventrally derived gastrula ectoderm cells (Gui et al., 2011).
	Cyclohexanedione "DIMs"	Alloxydim Butroxydim Clethodim Cycloxydim Profoxydim Tepraloxydim Tralkoxydim	Mainly danger to applier (inhalation, dermal) and likely male carcinogen (Leydig cell tumors in rats). Also danger to nontarget plants such as tomatoes that may occur via drift or granular formulation.
	Phenylpyrazoline "DENs"*	Pinoxaden	Nontarget plants and animals that rely on them for food.
Inhibition of acetolactate synthase (ALS; acetohydroxyacid synthase [AHAS])	Sulfonylurea	Amidosulfuron Aximsulfuron Bensulfuron-methyl Chlorimuron-ethyl Chlorsulfuron Cinosulfuron Cyclosulfamuron Ethametsulfuron-methyl Ethoxysulfuron Flazasulfuron Flupyrsulfuron-methyl-Na Formasulfuron Halosulfuron-methyl Imazosulfuron Iodosulfuron Mesosulfuron Metsulfuron-methyl Nicosulfuron Oxasulfuron Primisulfuron-methyl Pyraxosulfuron-ethyl Rimsulfuron Sulfometuron-methyl Sulfosulfuron Thifensulfuron-methyl Triasulfuron Tribenuron-methyl Trifloxysulfuron Triflusulfuon-methyl Tritosulfuron	Main toxicity to nontarget plants, especially duckweed (Peterson et al., 1994). Low mammalian toxicity although high-dose chronic eye damage is noted in rats and liver toxicity to all 1test species. Some thyroid effects in the dog may be evident. As usual respiratory concentrations reflect some concern for application personnel.

(*continues*)

TABLE 25-1 Herbicide Listing by Mechanism of Action and Toxicity (*continued*)

Target of Herbicidal Action	Chemical Family of Herbicide	Active Ingredient	Toxicity
Inhibition of acetolactate synthase (ALS; acetohydroxyacid synthase [AHAS]) (cont'd)	Imidazolinone	Imazapic Imazamethabenz-methyl Imazamox Imazapyr Imazaquin Imazethapyr	Inhalation and irreversible eye damage concerns. Ecotoxicity to nontarget monocots and dicots and especially the aquatic vascular plant duckweed.
	Triazolopyrimidine	Cloramsulam-methyl Diclosulam Florasulam Flumetsulam Metosulam Penoxsulam	There appear to be high-dose concerns for liver and kidney toxicity. Main concerns are for nontarget plant species such as duckweed and green algae.
	Pyrimidinyl(thio) benzoate	Bispyribac-Na Pyrbenzoxim Pyriftalid Pyrithiobac-Na Pyriminobac-methyl	These compounds appear to be more irritating, but present little problem beyond applicator. Again, native, nontarget plants (Sago pondweed) = concern.
	Sulfonrylaminocarbonyltriazolinone	Flucarbazone-Na Propoxycarbazone-Na	The thyroid disruption in the dog is unlike the other compounds that affect ALS in plants. However, it is relatively nontoxic to many species and has similar applicator inhalation warnings. In this case, the duckweed appears more affected than nonvascular nontarget plants.
Inhibition of photosystem II	Triazine	Ametryne Atrazine Cyanazine Desmetryne Dimethametryne Prometon Prometryne Propazine Simetryne Terbumeton Terbuthylazine Terbutryne Trietazine	Beyond the usual nontarget species, atrazine shows low-concentration endocrine disruption in fish and amphibian reproductive or toxicity in early development. That in combination with indirect effects on fish via habitat disturbances (phytoplankton and zooplankton effects), heavy use, and persistence make this group a strong risk concern.
	Triazinone	Hexazinone Metamitron Metribuzin	Nontarget plants, birds, and possible thyroid disruption at high doses in rats.
	Triazolinone	Amicarbazone	Highest concern for nontarget plants (especially algae) due to potency. Persistence leads to chronic neurotoxicity and growth risk in mammals and growth and reproductive risk in birds and estuarine/marine invertebrates.
	Uracil	Bromacil Lenacil Terbacil	Bromacil appears to be both a possible human carcinogen and thyroid disruptor. It is also very toxic to nontarget algae (ppb).

TABLE 25-1   Herbicide Listing by Mechanism of Action and Toxicity (*continued*)

Target of Herbicidal Action	Chemical Family of Herbicide	Active Ingredient	Toxicity
Inhibition of photosystem I	Pyridazinone	Pyrazon = Chloridazon	Relatively nontoxic except at high levels to dogs (renal damage) and macrophytes in states with high application rates (CA, MN).
	Phenyl-carbamate	Desmedipham Phenmedipham	While the EPA is mainly concerned about phemedipham's eye irritation properties, these herbicides may interact with CNS medications (Vincent et al., 2009), inhibit cholinesterases (Howcroft et al., 2011), cause allergic contact dermatitis (Nater and Grosfeld, 1979) and embryotoxicity (Medved, 1984).
Inhibition of photosystem II	Urea	Chlorobomuron Chlorotoluron Chloroxuron Dimefuron Diuron Ethidimuron Fenuron Flumeturon Isoproturon Isouron Linuron Methabenzthiazuron Metobromuron Metoxuron Monolinuron Neburon Siduron Tebuthiuron	Linuron has chronic toxicity to wildlife (including mammals) and is highly toxic to estuarine/marine species and aquatic invertebrates. It is also an endocrine disruptor as an antiandrogen and other possible mechanisms similar in action to a plasticizer, dibutyl phthalate (Gray et al., 1999).
	Amide	Propanil Pentanochlor	Propanil may pose a risk to plants, birds, fish, invertebrates, and estuarine/marine species. It is also an endocrine disruptor that increases associated antibody-secreting cells by a mechanism requiring steroid synthesis.
Inhibition of photosystem II	Nitrile	Bromofenoxim Bromoxynil Ioxynil	Developmentally toxic, uncoupler of oxidative phosphorylation (mitochondria), and interacts with transthyretin in rats (thyroid disruption).
	Benzothiadiazinone	Bentazon	Its reproductive effects in rabbits and its positive result in a yeast assay for anti-reproductive hormones indicate an endocrine and reproductive toxicant with high-dose blood clotting alterations and organ damage.
	Phenyl-pyridazine	Pyridate Pyridafol	Although pyridate has been voluntarily withdrawn in the United States, it was neurotoxic to the rat and was an endocrine disruptor (ERα and AR binding; Okubo et al., 2004).

(continues)

TABLE 25-1 Herbicide Listing by Mechanism of Action and Toxicity (*continued*)

Target of Herbicidal Action	Chemical Family of Herbicide	Active Ingredient	Toxicity
Photosystem I electron diversion	Bipyridylium	Diquat Paraquat	Redox cycling leads to $O_2^{\cdot-}$, cellular damage, genotoxicity, and reproductive and endocrine organ damage.
Inhibition of protoporphyrinogen oxidase (PPO)	Diphenylether	Acifluorfen-Na Bifenox Chlomethoxyfen Chlornitrofen Fluoroglycofen-ethyl Fomesafen Halosafen Lactofen Nitrofen Oxyfluorfen	The nitrogenous compounds seem the most toxic, changing redox states of cells and mast cell activation. These same compounds also are antiandrogenic and estrogenic or endocrine disruptors. The others may cause some damage to crops or induce fish kills, especially with post-emergence application.
	Phenylpyrazole	Fluzaolate Pyraflufen-ethyl	The long-term carcinogenicity to mice leads all concerns.
	N-Phenylphthalimide	Cindon-ethyl Flumioxazin Flumiclorac-pentyl	The ventricular septal thinning during development in rats may be due to the loss of embryonic blood cells. Male reproductive organ abnormalities may indicate endocrine disruption. High toxicity to mysid shrimp, lettuce, and cucumber.
	Thiadiazole	Fluthiacet-methyl Thidiazimin	Leading the list of toxicities are pancreatic and liver cancers followed by very high toxicity to fish and moderate toxicity to freshwater invertebrates.
Inhibition of the phytoene desaturase step of carotenoid biosynthesis/ bleaching	Pyrazdinone	Oxadiazon Oxadiargyl	The liver cancer, nontarget plant toxicity, and chronic toxicity including possible endocrine disruption top the list for oxadiazon.
		Azafenidin Carfentrazone-ethyl Sulfentrazone	Reproductive toxicity and nontarget plant toxicity mirror many PPO inhibitors.
		Pentoxazone	High algal toxicity and moderate toxicity to fish, aquatic invertebrates, honeybees, and earthworms.
		Benzfendizone Butafenacil	Mice most sensitive mammalian enzyme to PPO inhibition by butafenacil. Nontarget plants, invertebrates, and shrimp are highly sensitive.
		Pyraclonil Profluazol Flufenpyr-ethyl	Chronic liver toxicity and hematologic changes evident with some thymus enlargement.
Inhibition of phytoene desaturase step of carotenoid biosynthesis/ bleaching	Pyrazinone	Norflurazon	Desaturase enzyme inhibition leads to abnormal fatty acid metabolism in the liver and thyroid disruption. Inflammation in the kidney may be a precursor to cancer.

TABLE 25-1	Herbicide Listing by Mechanism of Action and Toxicity (*continued*)		
Target of Herbicidal Action	**Chemical Family of Herbicide**	**Active Ingredient**	**Toxicity**
Inhibition of phytoene desaturase step of carotenoid biosynthesis/ bleaching (cont'd)	Pyridinecarboxamide	Diflufenican Picolinafen	May have limited aquatic or nontarget toxicity but no clear evidence of endocrine disruption.
	Other	Benflubutamid Fluridone Flurochloridone Flurtamone	Fluridone appears to decrease cells in the G2 phase of the cell cycle in a mammalian cytotoxicity assay, but main concern in aquatic toxicity viewed as a major threat by U.S. Fish and Wildlife Service.
Inhibition of 4-hydroxyphenyl-pyruvate-dioxygenase/ bleaching (4-HPPD)	Triketone	Mesotrione Sulcotrione	4-HPPD inhibition increases tyrosine leading to eye, liver, and kidney toxicity. Delayed fetal ossification and nontarget plants/algae mark other effects.
	Isoxazole	Isoxachlortole Isoxaflutole	Liver cancer, thyroid disruption and tumors, and high phytotoxicity and toxicity to shrimp + eye damage.
Inhibition of 4-hydroxyphenyl-pyruvate-dioxygenase/ bleaching (4-HPPD)	Pyrazole	Benzofenap (obsolete) Pyrazolynate (obsolete) Pyrazoxyfen (not U.S.)	Fits the slightly hazardous category with some aquatic toxicity especially to trout.
Inhibition of carotenoid biosynthesis/bleaching (target unknown)	Other	Benzobicyclon	Moderately toxic to aquatic invertebrates, carp, and algae.
	Triazole	Amitrole (*in vivo* lycopene cyclase inhibitor)	Thyroid (disruption), pituitary, and liver cancers lead the list. Also nontarget plants may be extremely sensitive.
	Isoxazolidinone	Clomazone	Mostly toxic to nontarget plants and aquatic invertebrates, but does generate ROS and inhibit AChE in human RBCs.
	Urea	Fluometuron	This compound was covered under urea (PSII inhibition).
	Diphenylether	Aclonifen	High toxicity to aquatic plants make it a concern for all aquatic organisms. Moderate toxicity to honeybees, earthworms, fish, sediment-dwelling organisms and algae.
Inhibition of 5-enolpyruvylshikimate 3-phosphate (EPSP) synthase	Glycine	Glyphosate Sulfosate	Potent toxicity to nontarget plants, testicular toxicity (mammals), and dopaminergic and GABAergic neurodegeneration (worms and possibly humans).
Inhibition of glutamine synthetase	Phosphinic acid	Glufosinate-ammonium Bialaphos—Bilanaphos	Mainly neurotoxic/behavioral alterations via glutamine synthetase inhibition or NMDA receptor activation.
Inhibition of dihydropteroate (DHP) synthase	Carbamate	Asulam	Appears to cause thyroid and adrenal tumors and exceed the LOC for nontarget plants.
Microtubule assembly inhibition	Dinitroanaline	Benefin = Benfluralin Butralin Dinitramine	These pesticides are known to cause kidney, liver, hematological, and thyroid toxicity. Concerns for avian reproduction and very high toxicity noted

(*continues*)

TABLE 25-1   Herbicide Listing by Mechanism of Action and Toxicity (*continued*)

Target of Herbicidal Action	Chemical Family of Herbicide	Active Ingredient	Toxicity
Microtubule assembly inhibition (cont'd)		Ethalfluralin Orylzalin Pendimethalin Trifluralin	for freshwater fish and estuarine/marine invertebrates.
	Phosphoroamidate	Amiprophos-methyl Butamiphos	Because microtubules are potently inhibited = oral poison at high doses and induces polyploidy in surviving plant cells.
Inhibition of mitosis/ microtubule organisation	Pyridine	Dithiopyr Thiazopyr	Main concern is freshwater fish and aquatic invertebrate toxicity.
	Benzamide	Propyzamide = Pronamide Tebutam	Cancer, endocrine disruption, and green algae concerns.
	Benzoic acid	DCPA = chlorthal-dimethyl	Main concerns arise from impurities of TCDD and HCB in manufacture process.
	Carbamate	Chlorpropham Propham Carbetamide	Not of major concern acutely if used properly; some chronic concern for algae and earthworms.
Inhibition of cell division/ very long chain fatty acids (VLCFAs)	Chloroacetamide	Acetochlor Alachlor Butachlor Dimethachlor Dimethanamid Metazachlor Metolochlor Pethoxamid Pretilachlor Propachlor Propisochlor Thenylchlor	Mutagenic action, clastogenesis, cancer formation, and endocrine disruption lead the list of effects of high doses. Environmental toxicity to fish and honeybees are also of concern.
Inhibition of cell division/ very long chain fatty acids (VLCFAs)	Acetamide	Diphenamid Napropamide Naproanilide	Napropamide appears to be a concern for fish, certain marine organisms, and chronically to mammals ingesting treated pastures or foods.
	Oxyacetamide	Flufenacet Mefenacet	The main toxicity appears to be nontarget plants.
	Tetrazolinone	Fentrazamide	Chronic ingestion and algae.
	Other	Anilofos Cafenstrole Piperophos	Anilofos' organophosphate structure makes it more like a neurotoxic insecticide.
Inhibition of cellulose synthesis (cell wall)	Nitrile	Dichlobenil Chlorthiamid	Mainly toxic to aquatic insects and sowed or emerging plants.
	Benzamide	Isoxaben	Cancer and inhalation concerns.
	Triazolocarboxamide	Flupoxam	Obsolete.
	Quinoline carboxylic acid	Quinclorac (for monocots)	Liver, kidney, and pancreatic damage and nontarget plants.

TABLE 25-1	Herbicide Listing by Mechanism of Action and Toxicity (*continued*)		
Target of Herbicidal Action	**Chemical Family of Herbicide**	**Active Ingredient**	**Toxicity**
Uncoupling oxidative phosphorylation— membrane disruption	Dinitrophenol	DNOC (4,6-dinitro-*o*-cresol) Dinoseb Dinotert	Their mechanism of action makes them toxic to all mitochondrial activity.
Inhibition of lipid synthesis—not acetyl-CoA carboxylase (ACCase) inhibition	Thiocarbamate	Butylate Cycloate Dimepiperate EPTC (5-ethyl dipropylthiocarbamate) Esprocarb Molinate Orbencarb Pebulate Prosulfocarb Thiobencarb = Benthiocarb Tiocarbazil Trialate Vernolate	Primary eye irritant, with concerns for human cancer and fatal exposures not observed in animal studies.
	Phosphorodithioate	Bensulide	AChE inhibition = neurotoxic
	Benzofuran	Benfuresate Ethofumesate	Main concern aquatic toxicity.
	Chloro-carbonic-acid	TCA Dalapon	Main concern = irritant but not used in United States.
Synthetic auxins (plant hormones that act like indole acetic acid)	Phenoxy-carboxylic-acid	Clomeprop 2,4-D 2,4-DB Dichlorprop = 2,4-DP MCPA MCPB Mecoprop = MCPP = CMPP	Main concerns are to the liver, kidney, and endocrine organs especially in the dog and can even have neurotoxicity at high doses. Vascular plants and certain marine invertebrates may also be at risk.
	Benzoic acid	Chloramben Dicamba TBA	Major concern as irritant and nonvascular aquatic plants except at high doses in goat.
	Pyridine carboxylic acid	Clopyralid Fluroxypyr Picloram Triclopyr	Main acute concern = eye irritation, but at high doses may affect barrier function of GI tract (endocrine).
	Quinoline carboxylic acid	Quinclorac Quimerac	Liver, kidney, and pancreatic damage and nontarget plants.
	Other	Benazolin-ethyl	Some moderate toxicity to aquatic species and earthworms.
Inhibition of auxin transport	Phthalamate	Naptalam	Eye irritation + nontarget plants
	Semicarbazole	Diflufenzopyr-Na	Eye irritation + nontarget plants

(*continues*)

TABLE 25-1   Herbicide Listing by Mechanism of Action and Toxicity (*continued*)

Target of Herbicidal Action	Chemical Family of Herbicide	Active Ingredient	Toxicity
Unknown or controversial (developing concepts of action)	Arylaminopropionic acid	Flamprop-M-methyl/-isopropyl	Major concern for nontarget plants (e.g., algae) + *Daphnia*.
	Pyrazolium	Difenzoquat	Quaternary ammonium structure key to action + toxicity to a variety of species.
	Organoarsenical	DSMA MSMA	GI and renal toxicity and neurotoxicity at high doses.
	Other	Bromobutide (chloro)-flurenol	A 4-HPPD inhibitor causing skin and eye irritation with uncertain environmental effects.
		Cinmethylin	Moderate oral and dermal toxicity.
		Cumyluron	Moderate toxicity and liver alterations—possible carcinogen/chromosome alterations.
		Dazomet	Methyl isothiocyanate degradation product acute toxic.
		Dymron—Daimuron Methyl-dimuron Methyl-dymron Etobenzanid Fosamine Indanofan Metam Oxazicolmefone Oleic acid	Toxicity to mammals not a major concern, but environmental influences are being studied in Asia.
		Pelargonic acid Pyributicarb	Biopesticide that has eye and skin irritation properties + nontarget plant concerns.

* FOPs, DIMs, and DENS refer to chemical classes based on suffix on most of the active ingredients given to arylphenoxypropionates, cyclohexanediones, and phenylpyrazolines, respectively.

Data from http://pested.okstate.edu/pdf/herbicide%20moa.pdf

the widely used broadleaf herbicide 2,4-dichlorophenoxyacetic acid (2,4-D), the aryloxyphenoxypropionate grass-active herbicides, and pyridyloxyacetate herbicides such as triclopyr and fluroxypyr. This confers resistance to plants such as Arabidopsis (of the family Brassicaceae and related to the cabbage and mustard), maize (corn), and transgenic soybean plants (Wright et al., 2010). This indicates that as more plants become pesticide resistant (such as Roundup Ready® crops), this will find its way into other plants (pollination and other gene-transfer mechanisms). The pesticide fact sheet from the EPA (2000a) indicates a high oral lethal dose (LD_{50}) in rats (> 1,000 mg/kg) and greater dermal LD_{50} indicating low toxicity for clodinafop-propargyl (technical grade) used extensively to control annual grasses. This specific pesticide is only a slight eye irritant in the rabbit test and is a nonirritant for primary skin irritation in the rabbit (it is a severe irritant as part of the pesticide Discover); however, it is a skin sensitizer in the rat. The 28-day oral gavage comes with a no-observed-adverse-effect-level (NOAEL) < 5 mg/kg, which is not that toxic. The 90-day oral toxicity in dogs gives a NOAEL of 0.346 mg/kg/day. This may be true, because dogs generally have a difficult time clearing certain pesticides (such as 2,4-D) and can have more chronic effects (such as leukemia). At 750 ppm in rats, prostate and ovarian tumors are increased by clodinafop-propargyl, so the NOAEL for these effects is 10-fold lower at 0.03 mg/kg/day. However, this pesticide does not come up positive in a mutagenicity test. Its carcinogenicity may be linked to its action as a peroxisome proliferator in the rat liver similar to hypolipidemic compounds and phenoxyacetic acid derivatives. In hepatocytes, clodinafop-propargyl can induce cytoxicity through propargyl alcohol. The acute reference dose (R_fD) for this compound in females 13–50 years of age is calculated to be 0.05 mg/kg/day. Developmental toxicity in rats was calculated as LOAEL of 40 mg/kg/day based on bilateral distension and torsion of the ureters, unilateral 14th ribs, and incomplete ossification of metacarpals and various cranial bones. More sensitive environmental toxicity testing indicates that the zebrafish (*Danio rerio*) exposed to 0.2–5.0 μM clodinafop-propargyl showed a minimum teratogenic concentration of 0.6 μM. When exposed at 2 hours postfertilization (2 hpf), the zebrafish exhibited various embryonic phenotypes such as fin gap in ventral tail and coiled tail. Exposure 10 hpf resulted in failed detachment of tail. This indicated posterior and ventral gene expression changes that were found to show reduced expression of the ventral ectoderm marker gata-3 (ventrally derived gastrula ectoderm cells; Gui et al., 2011). These aquatic organism larvae/embryo studies are the kind that feed the notion that pesticides always cause some level of ecotoxicity at levels used in the environment, especially in developing fish and amphibians. Also, herbicides may impact beneficial algae as nontarget plant species.

Cyclohexanedione

The cyclohexanedione herbicides affect the same target (ACCase) as the arylphenoxypropionate derivatives. This is why, as mentioned earlier, certain weeds are resistant to both chemical classes of herbicides (and more). Again, these herbicides target grasses. However, some of them also impact rice crops in submerged or paddy conditions (e.g., tralkoxydim). A differently formulated version (EK-2612) appears to inhibit ACCase, but more so in target grasses such as barnyardgrass (*Ehcinochloa crus-galli*) than in rice crops (*Oryza sativa*; Kim et al., 2004). The EPA (1998b) pesticide fact sheet indicates that tralkoxydim is used to control wild oats, green foxtail, yellow foxtail, annual ryegrass, and Persian darnel in wheat and barley fields. The NOAEL for tralkoxydim is 30 mg/kg/day in the rat and 200 mg/kg/day for the rabbit for maternal and developmental toxicity. There is no developmental toxicity below doses associated with maternal toxicity. Again, the 90-day or 1-year dog chronic feeding study reported in the EPA fact sheet calculates the lowest NOAEL at 0.5 mg/kg/day. The appearance of Leydig cell tumors in rat testes rates a positive/likely carcinogenic response for this pesticide. Systemic toxicity occurred in male rats fed ~188 mg/kg/day and female rats fed ~163 mg/kg/day (high) and caused decreased body weight gain, reduced food consumption, and higher liver weights with clear cell areas and higher alanine aminotransferase (ALT) levels in exposed females. The R_fD = 0.005 mg/kg/day based on the dog and a 100-fold safety factor (10 × for interspecies extrapolation and 10 × for intraspecies variability). The drinking water level of comparison (DWLOC) for cancer is extrapolated to be 1 part per billion (ppb). The EEC (estimated environmental concentration) in surface water and groundwater is 0.528 ppb and 0.016 ppb, respectively, based on PRZM-EXAMS and SCI-GROW2 computer models. The acute dermal LD_{50} > 2,000 mg/kg is high but still a source of some concern. Cyclohexanedione is a moderate eye irritant (rabbit), slight skin irritant (rabbit), and the LC_{50} > 3.71 mg/L makes it a respiratory concern when applying the granular herbicide without proper protection (toxicity to liver and adrenals, and can lead to fatality if inhaled or significant amounts are absorbed through the skin). It is not considered a problem to aquatic birds (mallard duck > 150 ppm) or honeybees (> 50 μg/bee for formulated product) based on their LD_{50}s. A nontarget species that may be a sensitive plant is the tomato (most sensitive dicot), while ryegrass and corn are sensitive monocots. Green algae are the most sensitive nonvascular plant species. This pesticide has yet to generate sufficient data on endocrine disruption to clearly state any danger except to nontarget plants or to application personnel.

Phenylpyrazoline

Pinoxaden is a newer ACCase inhibitor used on wheat and barley for post-emergence control of grass weeds. This herbicide is not an acute toxin (oral, dermal, and inhalation Categories III and IV), but is irritating to the eye. Its major concern is for birds and mammals that rely on monocots and nonflowering, nontarget plants.

Sulfonylureas

Sulfonourea herbicides inhibit acetolactate synthase (ALS), otherwise known as acetyhydroxyacid synthase (AHAS). This action prevents the synthesis of branch-chain amino acids such as valine, leucine, and isoleucine, which are key to the formation of new cells. Imazosulfuron is a systemic sulfonylurea that is absorbed by the roots and foliage. From this point, the sulfonourea is translocated to the xylem and phloem of vascular plants (pre- and post-emergence control of sedges and broadleaf weeds). The sulfonylureas are acutely toxic to duckweed (Peterson et al., 1994), but are relatively nontoxic to adult mammals (rat oral and dermal LD_{50} > 5,000 mg/kg and > 2,000 mg/kg, respectively; not a dermal or eye irritant in rabbit assays) based on the EPA (2010a) pesticide fact sheet for imazosulfuron. Inhalation LC_{50} > 2.12 mg/L should carry the usual caution for application personnel. The EPA fact sheet data indicate that the liver appears be the target organ in repeated-dose studies in all test species. Some thyroid effects were only apparent in the dog (again the organism that has a difficult time clearing pesticides). Rats fed > 1,000 mg/kg/day (high dose) are observed to have retinal degeneration, lens vascularization, cataracts, and corneal scarring.

Imidazolinone

Imidazolinones target ALS/AHAS, as do the sulfonylureas. These herbicides are applied at low rates due to their high potency. Imazapyr was the only one of this class that was considered for reregistration by the EPA. It is a systemic, non-selective pre- and post-emergent herbicide used to control a variety of terrestrial and aquatic weed species that may come in the form of a liquid, wettable powder, or granule. It has low potential for oral or dermal toxicity. However, it exceeds the sulfonylureas to be considered an acute Toxicity Category II (Category I is highly toxic and severely irritating; Category II is moderately toxic and moderately irritating; Category III is slightly toxic and slightly irritating; Category IV is practically nontoxic and not an irritant) inhalation hazard to appliers. It is not considered a skin irritant or dermal sensitizer. Because it does irreversible eye damage, it is considered the highest Toxicity Category (I) by the EPA. Although maternal toxicity to the rabbit (salivation) was noted at 300 mg/kg/day, imazapyr did not cause increased susceptibility to the fetus. The dog did not show any toxicity over the tested doses and this chemical is not considered a carcinogen. The chronic R_fD = 2.5 mg/kg/day (EPA, 2006a). This compound is also not considered toxic to fish, invertebrates, and nonvascular aquatic plants. There are ecotoxicological risks to nontarget terrestrial plants and aquatic vascular plants (monocots such as wheat and dicots such as sugar beets and cucumbers), especially seedling emergence (EC_{25} < 0.005 lb [acid equivalent [ae]/acre) and vegetative vigor (EC_{25} < 0.015 lb ae/acre). Again, duckweed appears to be a sensitive aquatic vascular plant (EC_{50} = 0.018 mg ae/L). No endocrine disruption has been demonstrated so far with the imidazolinones.

Triazolopyrimidine

Triazolopyrimidine herbicides also have the same target (ALS/AHAS) as the previous herbicides. A representative of this group, cloransulam-methyl, is applied to the soil surface to control broadleaf weeds pre-emergence or post-emergence. It is defined as (Toxicity Category III—caution) toxic for acute dermal or inhalation toxicity and eye irritation studies. No carcinogenicity assays yielded significant problems and the chronic feeding NOAEL = 75 mg/kg/day and LOAEL = 325 mg/kg/day in the rat based on significant increases in hemoglobin, hematocrit, red blood cell (RBC) count, relative liver and testes weights, and collecting duct hypertrophy with decreases in liver enzymes (aspirate and alanine aminotransferases) in male rats and decreases in cholesterol, urine specific gravity, and increased kidney vacuolation in female rats. The R_fD = 0.1 mg/kg/day for cloransulam-methyl. Because this compound's half-life in aerobic versus anaerobic (deeper) soils is 9–13 days versus 16 days, respectively, a groundwater advisory/monitoring is a condition of EPA registration. Fish (96-h LC_{50} > 86 ppm in rainbow trout), small mammals, birds (5-day LC_{50} > 520 ppm in bobwhite quail or mallard duck), and bees (LD_{50} > 25 µg active ingredient [ai]/bee) have little toxicity associated with this product's use, but nontarget plants are again of greatest concern. The onion (monocot) has an EC_{25}/EC_{05} = 0.0054 (lb ai/acre), while the tomato has an EC_{25}/EC_{05} = 0.0076 (lb ai/acre) based on phytotoxicity and an EC_{25} of 0.0006 (lb ai/acre) based on vegetative vigor. Again, the duckweed (EC_{50}/EC_{05} = 0.00312 ppm) and green algae (EC_{50}/EC_{05} = 0.00346 ppm) seem most sensitive as nontarget vascular and nonvascular plants, respectively. The acute oral and dermal LD_{50} > 5,000 mg/kg and >2,000 mg/kg, respectively (rat). The acute inhalation LC_{50} > 3.77 mg/L is of concern for application purposes. Endocrine disruption studies have yet to find problem in this category of herbicides (EPA, 1997).

Pyrmidinyl(thio)benzoate

ALS/AHAS is again the target of this chemical family of herbicide. One of these chemicals, bispyribac-Na, is used to treat invasive Eurasian watermilfoil (*Myriophyllum spicatum*) and hydrilla *(Hydrilla verticillata)*, but as usual may also affect native aquatic species of plants such as Sago pondweed (*Stuckinea pectinata*). These herbicides are systemic and must be maintained for 60–90 days to control the invasive plant species. A half-life of 42–115 days makes bispyribac-Na a concern for groundwater contamination. This compound does not bind to soil. As with other herbicides with the same target, it is relatively nontoxic to trout, bluegill, minnows, oysters, shrimp, and water fleas (*Daphnia* sp.). Birds and mammals are similarly resistant to its toxic effects at levels used in the environment, and it does not bioaccumulate. As usual, applicators might experience minor eye and

skin irritation and respiratory irritation at high concentrations. Again, endocrine disruption or reproductive effects have not as yet been found.

Sulfonylaminocarbonyltriazolinone

This is the final chemical family that targets ALS/AHAS. The EPA (2010b) puts this group into the sulfonylureas for application onto wheat fields. Their oral (rat) and dermal (rat, rabbit) LD_{50} > 5,000, so this chemical family represents little toxicity. It is a slight irritant to the rabbit eye (Category III). Again, the applicator must guard against inhalation as the acute inhalation LC_{50} > 5.113 mg/L. The NOAEL = 33.8 mg/kg/day based on the 90-day oral toxicity to (sensitive) dogs. Maternal toxicity (decreased food consumption and increased clinical signs) sets an LOAEL = 300 mg/kg/day, which is the NOAEL level that would ensure that fetal weights and delayed fetal ossification would not occur. Reproductive concerns at high levels (LOAEL = 800 mg/kg/day for males and 991 mg/kg/day for females) are based on decreased male liver weights and decreased uterine weights and increased severe cecal enlargement in females. These are the same levels that reduce pup weights in rats, decrease liver weight in male pups, cause marbled liver, and fill the stomach with air. Chronic toxicity in dogs caused body weight gain reductions and increased N-demethylase in both sexes, with females additionally showing decreased T4 levels (thyroid) and marginally increased liver weight. The EPA fact sheet noted no evidence for these compounds causing cancer. However, the fact sheet data reported decreased body weight and thickening mucosa of the glandular stomach in a 2-year feeding study in rats. Females increased food consumption and experienced vacuolation of the squamous epithelium in the forestomach. Males experienced immunological alterations. High doses caused some neurotoxicity in males by increased incidence of perianal staining (males) and decreased motor and locomotor activity as wells as open field activity (both sexes). The R_fD = 3.0 mg/kg/day for females 13–50 years of age and a chronic R_fD = 0.36 mg/kg/day for all populations based on dog body weight and thyroid disruption. Again, birds (LD_{50} > 2,000 mg/kg; LC_{50} > 4,621 ppm), mammals ($LD_{50} > 5,000$ mg/kg), and honeybees ($LD_{50} > 200$ µg/bee) are relatively unaffected. However, the onion appears again to be a sensitive nontarget species of all monocots or dicots tested at an $EC_{35} = 0.00034$ lb ai/acre. For flucarbazone-Na, it is of interest that duckweed appears sensitive to its action ($EC_{50} = 12.3$ ppb), while nonvascular plants (algae or diatom) are much less sensitive ($EC_{50} = 2,510$). Clearly, if the dog's thyroid is affected, endocrine disruption cannot be ruled out for this family of chemicals.

Triazine

As the discussion moves into the inhibition of photosynthesis via disrupting photosystem II (PSII), a wider scope of toxicity to plants and animals is found in these herbicides. Corals are very sensitive to all PSII inhibitors at low concentrations (ng/L; Jones, 2005). The *s*-triazines appear to interfere with electron transport in photosystem II to inhibit O_2 evolution in plants such as spinach (*Spionacia oleracea*). PSII herbicides appear to act at second electron acceptor B

by decreasing the oxidation/reduction potential of B, thereby making the primary acceptor Q unable to reduce B (Allen et al., 1983). It is important to examine photosynthesis more closely and the action of herbicides that interfere with the two photosystems (PSII and PSI in that order), as shown in **Figure 25-3**. Note that the mechanism of triazine action is specifically related to the Q_B site by binding adjacent positions on the D-1 quinone protein. This diverts electrons into the production of free radicals, which ultimately destroy cells' macromolecules and the cell membrane. The chloroplast chloroplast's thylakoid membrane is important for photosynthesis (site of PSI and PSII). Damaging this membrane essentially makes the plant only susceptible to the toxic influences of sunlight instead of the benefits of photosynthesis, although some herbicides (phenols) appear to be more damaging in this regard. Why can the triazines be used on any crop if they interfere with photosynthesis? The reason is that corn has an effective detoxification system using a reaction with glutathione, a protective tripeptide, and transport to the plant cell's vacuole.

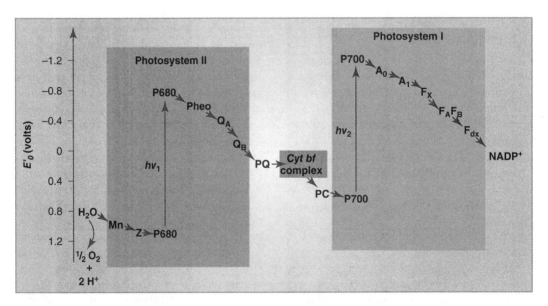

FIGURE 25-3 Electron Flow in Photosynthesis Through Photosystem II Followed by Photosystem I

Note: The Q_B site is where triazines act diverting electron energy into and damaging the cell and its membranes. The bipyridillium herbicides inhibit at ferrodoxin (Fdx), accepting electrons from photosystem I and donating them to oxygen creating O_2^-.

If there are effects, they appear to be noted at the leaf's periphery (as seen in a target weed such as velvetleaf).

Of the triazines, atrazine has topped the list of herbicides for years as the most used herbicide. It has an extensive literature due to its use, and because endocrine disruption is a manifested action. It is also persistent (anaerobic aquatic study determined overall, water, and sediment half-lives of 608, 578, and 330 days, respectively), carrying over into the next year's growing season and contamination of well water (Ballantine et al., 1998). It appears to be more persistent in the soil in cold climates (20-fold different for a northern state, Minnnesota, versus a southern state, Georgia). This brings a sharper focus to its effects. Atrazine has been used to control broadleaf and some grassy weeds in crops such as corn (the biggest use in Iowa, Illinois, Indiana, Ohio, Nebraska, and Delaware; ~75% of field corn acreage), sorghum, sugarcane, wheat (stubble), guava, macadamia nuts, hay, pasture, summer fallow, forestry or woodlands, conifer, woody ornamentals, Christmas trees, sod, and residential (mainly Florida and Southeast) and recreational turf (parks and golf courses). Glyphosate use is starting to overtake atrazine's use for clearing an area for planting or in crops with an introduced gene discussed earlier resistant to the action of glyphosate. Glyphosate is investigated later in the herbicide section where its mechanism is discussed.

Atrazine was the subject of a controversy of the rat breast cancer model, because atrazine increased breast cancers in these animals. However, increased cancer risk even among applicators cannot be confirmed with any degree of certainty. This does not mean that atrazine poses no mechanisms that may increase cancer risk. It appears that atrazine-responsive adrenal carcinoma cells (H295R) express 54 times more steroidogenic factor 1 than nonresponsive granulosa KGN cells. Atrazine is viewed here as a possible cancer-causing agent (prostate cancer in rats and correlations of reproductive cancers in humans to atrazine exposure) that increases aromatase expression in some human cancer lines by inhibition of phosphodiesterase and subsequent increase in cAMP (Fan et al., 2007).

As a result, the female Sprague Dawley (SD) rat became the focus of endocrine disruption instead. Because atrazine caused disruption of the hypothalamic-pituitary with an attenuation of the luteinizing hormone (LH) surge in the female rats, this suppression of LH and its possible developmental and reproductive effects cannot be overlooked by the EPA. Its neuroendocrine mode of action and the possibility of development of the young have currently not been accounted for in the toxicity endpoints and traditional uncertainty factors employed in risk assessment. Complicating the picture is the finding that atrazine disrupts the mitochondrial membrane potential ($\Delta\psi_m$), increases intracellular Ca^{2+}, generates ROS, and depletes adenosine triphosphate (ATP) in a dose- and time-dependent manner, inducing apoptosis in grass carp (*Ctenopharyngodon idellus*) cell line XC7901 (Liu et al., 2006).

Additionally, atrazine and its persistent chlorinated metabolites appear to be a chronic risk in contaminated drinking water supplies. The NOAEL is 10 mg/kg/day for acute dietary intake for females 13–50 years old (delayed ossification of certain cranial bones in fetuses and decreased weight gain in adult). The Hayes laboratory has weighed in with very low atrazine concentrations causing malformations in amphibians (Hayes et al., 2006). Sometimes the effects require clever experimentation, because direct toxicity is not noted. For example, Atlantic croaker (*Micropogonias undulatus*) sperm exposed to 0.01–10 µM atrazine (or estrogenic or nonestrogenic organic compounds of which atrazine is currently classified) showed no effects on motility. Atrazine did block the nongenomic action of the progestin 17,20β,21-trihydroxy-4-pregnen-3-one's ability to upregulate sperm motility at concentrations < 0.1 µM. This indicates the inadequacy of standard assays in detecting physiological actions in a whole organism that may be disrupted by antagonizing important (hormonal) signals (Thomas and Doughty, 2004). These effects and atrazine's persistence warrant the low chronic R_fD of 0.018 mg/kg/day and the chronic population adjusted dose (PAD) of 0.0018 mg/kg/day. The biggest concern was community water systems that were > 100% of the infant PAD (some > 500%) in the United States (especially in the Midwestern corn belt of Illinois followed by a number states—Indiana, Kentucky, Louisiana, Missouri, Ohio). The EPA made note of certain studies that reinforced its calculation of NOAELs and LOELs including delayed pubertal separation in male offspring after 30 dosing days (oral, dermal, and inhalation, short-term) and attenuating LH surge in SD rats (oral, dermal, and inhalation, intermediate-term). This is despite acute rat oral LD_{50} > 1,869 mg/kg (> 2,000 mg/kg dermal). This looks similar to the other classes of herbicides, but low-level effects and persistence drive a more cautious view of the triazines. It is not an irritant nor a sensitizer, so the effects on children LC_{50} > 5.8 mg/L is the usual caution to applicators. But now, concern for children playing on treated lawns is a chronic concern to a sensitive population. It is not an irritant nor a sensitizer, so the effects on children would not likely be picked up in this fashion.

In regard to other creatures, atrazine is either nontoxic or slightly toxic in adult birds and mammals and relatively nontoxic to honeybees. Cucumber is the most sensitive dicot, and oats are the most sensitive monocot for germination. Seedling emergence places the carrot as the most sensitive dicot and oats and ryegrass as the most sensitive monocots. Vegetative vigor still has the cucumber as the most sensitive dicot, while the most sensitive monocot is the onion. The duckweed is still sensitive to atrazine for < 10-day exposure (170 ppb set as 50% affected) and > 10-day exposure concentration (NOAEC < 3.4 ppb). The *Chlorophyceae* have only a < 10-day exposure (49 ppb set as 50% reduction in cell growth). A refined aquatic assessment was based on a number of parameters; examples include the following: fish population and invertebrate reductions at > 62 µg/L, food and habitat effects that reduce fish populations indirectly > 20 µg/L, likely reduction in invertebrate populations > 10 µg/L, reduction in primary (nonvascular plant) production > 1 µg/L, acute effects phytoplankton > 32 µg/L, acute effects in macrophytes > 18 µg/L, reductions in macrophytes or primary production > 2.3 µg/L, fish mortality > 5,300 µg/L, reduced fish growth > 88 µg/L, reduction fish population > 62 µg/L. Thus, atrazine has a wide-ranging toxicity profile (as do other triazines) that makes registration and regulation more difficult (EPA, 2012a).

Triazinone

An herbicide of this family of chemicals, metribuzin, also inhibits all Hill-reactions when water is the electron donor by interrupting electron flow between the primary (Q) and secondary (plastoquinone) electron acceptor of photosystem II (Trebst and Wietoska, 1975). As shown in Figure 25-3, the photosystem II herbicides usually bind to a polypeptide on Q_B, leaving Q_A in a reduced state (that is how nondestructive fluorescence detects the herbicidal action; Ahrens, 1989). Triazone herbicides are used to control annual grasses and numerous broadleaf weeds in field and vegetative crops. The crops' resistance has to do with metabolism of the herbicide similar to the triazines. Metribuzin is slightly to moderately toxic in humans by oral, skin, or inhalation. Sedation (toxic CNS depression) and labored breathing were symptoms of poisoning in rats given high doses. Acute inhalation can result in irritation of the mucous membranes of the upper respiratory tract. The acute oral LD_{50} is 1,090–2,300, 700, and 245–274 mg/kg for technical grade metribuzin in rats, mice, and guinea pigs, respectively. Its 4-hour LC_{50} for inhalation in rats is 885 mg/m³. This herbicide does not show eye or skin irritation to rabbits or human volunteers. Dogs show reduced weight gain, deaths, blood chemistry alterations, and hepatic and renal damage after 2 years of 37.5 mg metribuzin/kg/day. Rats given 25 and 75 mg/kg/day exhibited enlarged livers and thyroid glands after 3 months. The enlargement of the thyroid suggests that this compound should be considered as a thyroid endocrine disruptor. The EPA has a drinking water standard of 200 ppb. Animal studies indicate the risk of chronic kidney damage at high concentrations. Metribuzin is moderately acutely toxic to birds that consume it (LD_{50} > 100 mg/kg) and slightly toxic to fish (96-h LC_{60} > 10 mg/L in goldfish). This herbicide is moderately toxic to freshwater invertebrates (96-h LC_{60} > 48.3 mg/L in marine/estuarine shrimp) and nontoxic to bees. The half-lives of metribuzin are 7 days and 28 weeks in pond water and distilled water (hydrolysis), respectively (EPA, 1998c).

Triazolinone

Amicarbazone is a triazolinone herbicide that also works at photosystem II. It binds to the Q_B domain of photosystem II similarly to triazines and triazinones. It has a broad spectrum of weed control (velvetleaf, common lambsquarters, pigweed species, common cocklebur, and morning glory species) when planting corn or sugar cane, and causes chlorosis, stunted growth, tissue necrosis, and death of target plants. This herbicide is more potent than atrazine and can be applied on the leaves or roots (Dayan et al., 2009). The EPA fact sheet reported the acute $R_fD = 0.10$ mg/kg/day based on acute rat neurotoxicity. The fact sheet data also reported a chronic $R_fD = 0.023$ mg/kg/day based on a chronic rat study (increased relative liver weights, minimal hepatocytomegaly, minimal spleen pigmentation, decreased body weight and RBC (red blood cell) indices, increased cholesterol, T4 and T3 thyroid hormones in male, CYP demethylase activities) and hepatic alterations in a chronic dog study. The fact sheet also reported a NOAEL = 6.28 mg/kg/day in 90-day oral toxicity to the beagle dog based on thyroid vacuolization; decreased food consumption and glucose in females; increased platelets, phosphate, bile acids, and absolute and relative liver weights; lymphoid hyperplasia of the gall bladders in males; and decreased albumin and increased triglycerides and CYP demethylase activity in both sexes. Despite the thyroid effects, this compound is not currently considered an endocrine disruptor by EPA, because the liver alterations and metabolism of the thyroid hormones may play some role in thyroid hormone alterations. This is another persistent compound similar to the triazines with biotransformation requiring 87 days to reduce to half its concentration ($t_{1/2}$). It is practically nontoxic to honeybees, slightly toxic to mammals (90-day oral rat NOAEL =33/38 mg/kg/day), and slightly toxic to practically nontoxic to birds. The fact sheet indicates this pesticide is an eye irritant that caused corneal opacity in the New Zealand white rabbit, but cleared by day 7.

However, chronic exposure indicates growth and reproductive effects in birds (decreased viable embryos per eggs set, number of hatchlings per egg set, and eggshell thickness in bobwhite quail and mallard ducks) and toxicity to parents and offspring (both exhibiting decreased body weight gain and incomplete ossification of bones in portions of developing Himalayan rabbits) in mammals. Nontarget dicots are more sensitive to this herbicide's toxic action, but monocots are also affected. Amicarbazone is practically acutely nontoxic to freshwater fish and estuarine/marine fish, slightly toxic to freshwater invertebrates, and slightly toxic to practically nontoxic to estuarine/marine invertebrates. However, aquatic animals have decreased growth (freshwater fish) and growth and reproductive parameters (freshwater and estuarine/marine invertebrates) upon longer-term exposure. This herbicide is particularly toxic to algae, but also affects vascular plants (EPA, 2005a).

Uracil

Uracil herbicides also bind and inhibit the D1 protein as do the other photosystem II herbicides mentioned earlier. Bromacil and terbacil are used to control a broad spectrum of weeds (broadleaves and grasses). Bromacil is particularly used in citrus and pineapple fields. The EPA's analysis of bromacil showed decreased body weight, focal atrophy of seminiferous tubules (testicular abnormalities), hydronephrosis, histological evidence for antithyroid activity (cystic follicle in thyroid and enlargement of centrilobular cells of the liver), and a positive trend in thyroid tumors (C-cell adenomas and follicular cell adenomas and/or carcinomas) in male rats (C classification or possible human carcinogen for carcinogenicity). These troubling findings make this compound suspect both as a carcinogen and a thyroid (endocrine) disruptor. Bromacil is a mild eye irritant to the rabbit. How does bromacil disrupt thyroid function and produce thyroid tumors? Amitrole, ethylene thiourea, and mancozeb do so by inhibiting thyroid peroxidase, causing a high thyroid tumor incidence. Amitrole, ethylene thiourea, mancozeb, ethiozin, and pentachloronitrobenzene inhibit iodine uptake into the thyroid (first three may reduce uptake via alterations of thyroid peroxidase activity). Five pesticides actually increase iodine uptake by the thyroid. Liver damage is another mechanism that affects thyroid function as with amicarbazone. Bromacil is an odd one, in that it is the only one of 19 pesticides that induce thyroid tumors that does not exhibit cellular hypertrophy, hyperplasia, increase in thyroid weight, decrease in thyroid hormone, or increase in thyroid-stimulating hormone (TSH; Hurley et al., 1998). Developmental testing again showed some retarded or partial ossification of the axial and appendicular skeleton. The EPA fact sheet reported an $R_fD =$ 0.1 mg/kg/day based on the no observed effect level (NOEL) of 9.82 mg/kg/day in the chronic rat study. Bromacil is practically nontoxic to avian and reptilian species (acute and subacute). It is relatively nontoxic to bees, estuarine species, and aquatic invertebrates as well. This herbicide does exhibit slight toxicity to fish and amphibians in 96-hour acute toxicity tests. The half-life of this compound in soil is ~2 months. Rape (canola) is the most sensitive dicot and wheat is the most sensitive monocot to the herbicidal action of this compound. It is considered very highly toxic to *Selenastrum capricornutum* (EC_{50} = 6.8 ppb; EPA, 1996a).

Pyridazinone

Pyrazon/chloridazon binds to the same sites as triazine herbicides, but with different binding behavior. This herbicide is used to grow beets (and on bulb crops and roses) by inhibiting the growth of various weeds pre-plant, pre-emergence, and early post-emergence. This is a relatively low-toxicity chemical via oral, dermal, and inhalation routes of exposure and is not viewed as an irritant or sensitizer. At high doses over a longer term, the only effect on animals appears to be reduced food consumption and body weight. Dogs develop renal distal tubule vacuolation and lymphoreticular hyperplasia of the gastric mucosa at higher chronic doses. Developmental and reproductive effects are negligible, and pyrazon is not likely to be a carcinogen in humans. Neurobehavioral toxicity is also not apparent. An acute R_fD has not been established for this compound, but based on body weight effects warrants a chronic $R_fD =$ 0.18 mg/kg/day. The risk to aquatic organisms is considered low, and this herbicide is also practically acutely nontoxic to birds or mammals by the oral route. The risk to macrophytes (aquatic plants) was only exceeded in California and Minnesota, where application rates were assumed to be 7.3 lb ai/acre and 3.5 lb ai/acre were assumed by the EPA (EPA, 2005b).

Phenyl-carbamate

These herbicides work on annual broadleaf weeds, but they are weak on grasses in sugar beet crops. Most of the photosystem II inhibitors, of which phenyl-carbamates are one chemical family, bind to quinone Q_B on one of five binding niches. This quinone is on the chloroplast D1 thylakoid membrane protein. Desmedipham is a post-emergence herbicide used in both table beets and Swiss chard seed production in the state of Washington. Desmedipham is practically nontoxic for acute oral toxicity, inhalation toxicity, and dermal irritation (Category IV). It is slightly toxic via the dermal route (Category III). It is moderately toxic for eye irritation (Category II). This herbicide is also not considered a developmental toxicant or mutagen (Group E). Minimal effects are expected to aquatic plants and animals or acutely to insects, birds, or mammals (as is the chronic risk to mammals). In a pesticide mix (Betanal Expert), phenmedipham was most toxic to *Vibrio fischeri* (bacterium) and *Lemna minor* (macrophyte). Desmedipham was most toxic to *Pseudokirchneriella subcapitata* (microalgae), *Daphnia magna*, and *Daphnia longispina* (cladocerans; Vidal et al., 2011). One Russian article indicates that perhaps Betanal may have some embryotoxic action (Medved, 1984), while an article from the late 1970s indicates an allergic contact dermatitis from the same herbicide blend (Nater and Grosfeld, 1979). The white worm (*Enchytraeus albidus*) is an important soil organism and has cholinesterases similar to mammalian enzymes. The cholinesterase activity was inhibited by phenmedipham and copper (Howcroft et al., 2011). This might signal an important toxicity (carbamate insecticides are known to be cholinesterase inhibitors). Phenmedipham (and amperozide) also has possible pharmaceutical properties for pain, anxiety, depression, and other CNS activities as an inhibitor of fatty acid amide hydrolase (Vincent et al., 2009). Because this may interact with other medications from sewage and would certainly not be a regularly tested toxic interaction, this may pose an unknown risk to humans and animals consuming the water.

Urea

Although most of the phenylureas are inhibitors of photosystem II, siduron inhibits cell division and is a root growth inhibitor used to control warm-season grass instead of cool-season grass in lawns, golf courses, and sod farms. It is important to examine the more common action of the phenylureas, because nontarget species are most likely affected by mechanisms associated with these herbicides. Linuron, for example, is used to control germinating and newly emerging grasses and broadleaf weeds. Most of the linuron used in the United States is for growth of soybeans. Linuron acts on photosystem II and stresses freshwater plants (macrophytes and algae) due to this action (Snel et al., 1998). Linuron has relatively low acute toxicity to animals. It is slightly toxic (Category III) via oral, dermal, and inhalation routes. It causes slight eye irritation to rabbits and causes some skin irritation or sensitization. Subchronic testing yielded high-dose alteration in blood cell counts and retarded growth. Chronic toxicity and carcinogenicity testing in beagle dogs yielded RBC destruction and liver weight changes. Rats developed testicular tumors (male) and RBC destruction. Mice developed liver tumors, decreased body weight gain, increased liver weights, and other liver alterations in response to chronic linuron dosing. These tests suggest that linuron may be an unquantifiable Group C carcinogen (possible human carcinogen with limited animal evidence). Some developmental toxicity in rats (fetal resorptions) and rabbits (more abortions, fewer fetuses/litter, decreased fetal body weight, increased incidence of fetal skeletal skull variations) was evident at levels that caused maternal toxic effects. A two-generation reproductive toxicity study caused eye and testes abnormalities in rats. Linuron appeared to interfere with the transmission of male hormones. In this respect and others, it must be considered an endocrine disruptor. Linuron treatment results in male offspring with reduced anogenital distance, retained nipples, and a low incidence of hypospadias due to its low affinity for the androgen receptor. It also causes malformed epididymides and testes atrophy. Linuron's profile of effects appears similar to that of the plasticizer dibutyl phthalate, indicating that this herbicide may have several mechanisms of endocrine toxicity (Gray et al., 1999). Linuron is moderately persistent ($t_{1/2}$ = 57–100 days in aerobic soil) and relatively immobile except in the case of coarse textured soils and soils with little organic matter. This herbicide is practically acutely nontoxic to mammals or honeybees, but likely poses chronic risk to wild mammals. It is slightly acutely toxic to birds, but does cause reproductive alterations in birds. Linuron is moderately toxic to cold- and warm-water fish (affected fish length at lowest dose level). It is highly toxic to aquatic invertebrates and moderately toxic to freshwater aquatic invertebrates. This EPA fact sheet indicates that this herbicide shows high toxicity toward the sheepshead minnow and moderate toxicity toward the eastern oyster and mysid shrimp (estuarine/marine acute toxicity studies). Aquatic plants are at risk from linuron exposure, and risk to terrestrial plants cannot be ruled out (EPA, 1995a). The urea herbicide fluometuron fits both the PSII inhibitor and inhibition of carotenoid biosynthesis by bleaching. Carotenoids are essential components of photosynthetic membranes (plastic organization and function), aid in light harvesting, and stabilize the lipidic phase of thylakoid membranes. The bleaching done by herbicides that prevent carotenoid biosynthesis eliminates the photo-oxidation protection offered by carotenoids as quenching agents against triplet chlorophyll and single oxygen (Vecchia et al., 2001). Fluometuron, the last herbicide mentioned so far, is used either pre- or post-emergence to control susceptible weeds in cotton fields. Fluometuron is moderately toxic to humans (especially inhaled or absorbed through skin causing toxicity to liver, kidneys, and intestinal tract) and is a mild inhibitor of acetylcholinesterase. It has been found to increase white blood cell counts in agricultural workers and can also lead to abnormalities of RBCs accompanied by increased spleen weight. It is a skin sensitizer and creates corneal opacity as well. Chronic exposure can lead to conjunctivitis. Resorptions in pregnant rabbits occurred on exposure to fluometuron. This herbicide also appears to interfere with mouse testes DNA synthesis, so it must be considered an endocrine disruptor on this evidence alone (EPA, 2005c).

Amide

Propanil is an amide herbicide used to control broadleaf and grass weeds in rice crops. This herbicide binding site is again in the electron transport chain of PSII. Is has low acute toxicity (Category III) to practically no toxicity by other acute tests (dermal, inhalation, and primary skin irritation). It is considered a primary eye irritant based on rabbit testing. Chronic risks exist for small mammals, freshwater fish, and invertebrates. Its maximum application rate also poses a threat to nontarget aquatic vascular/nonvascular plants and terrestrial plants in semi-aquatic areas, and acute risks to birds, small mammals, freshwater fish and invertebrates, and estuarine/marine fish and invertebrates. Propanil is a novel type of endocrine disruptor that enhances humoral (antibody) immune responses in C57BL/6 mice. It does so through the increase in phosphorylcholine-specific IgG2b, IgG3, and IgM antibody-secreting cells in the spleen four- to sixfold 1 week after vaccination of the female mice with heat-killed *Streptococcus pneumonia*. Propanil neither binds to the estrogen receptors (α or β) nor do estrogen or progesterone receptor antagonists prevent the increase in antibody-secreting cells. Male mice have similar responses to propanil, and orchiectomy (removal of testes = source of testosterone) did not prevent the increased humoral immune response. Complete inhibition of steroid synthesis with gonadotropin-releasing hormone antagonist antide did prevent the increased immune response. Thus, it appears that steroid synthesis is required for the endocrine-disrupting effect of propanil (Salazar et al., 2006). Clearly, this type of endocrine disruption is not part of any standard assay for pesticide toxicity.

Nitrile

The urea herbicides such as 3-(3,4-dichlorophenyl)-1,1-dimethylurea bind and protect the D1 protein from photodamage as they block PSII electron flow (raise redox potential or Em of the Q_A/Q_A^- redox couple by 50 mV). The phenolic nitriles such as bromoxynil lower the Em by approximately 45 mV and increase the sensitivity of PSII to light damage (Krieger-Liszkay and Rutherford, 1998). These nitrile herbicides are used as selective contact foliage applied chemicals to control grasses and broadleaf weeds. Bromoxynil was originally available in phenol, butyrate, heptanoate, and octanoate, but due to developmental toxicity bromoxynil butyrate was voluntarily canceled by the manufacturer. Bromoxynil phenol is a Category II acute oral or inhalation toxicant and Category III for acute dermal effects. The octanoate form is Category II for acute inhalation effects. The phenol form is a possible human carcinogen (Group C). Bromoxynil is a developmental toxicant and a skin irritant at high doses (100 mg/kg/day). Bromoxynil and ioxynil may be very important in another important fashion—uncoupling of oxidative phosphorylation in mitochondria. People who were poisoned by this agent show excessive perspiration, thirst, fever, emesis, myalgia, and weight loss that usually accompanies mitochondrial uncoupling of ATP synthesis. The effect of bromoxynil can be observed in mitochondria of mouse liver (Guan et al., 2009; articles back to the 1960s indicate these effects at μM concentrations) or higher plants (Zottini et al., 1994). Bromoxynil is a strong competitor for the thyroxine binding site of transthyretin and reduces level of both T4 and T3 in rat plasma (Van den Berg et al., 1991). Although human risk may not be clinically significant due to differences in transporter binding and thyroxine levels, the rat has indicated endocrine disruption. The $R_fD = 0.015$ mg/kg/day based on 1-year oral toxicity in dogs. The risk to birds and insects is low, while it is medium to high for mammals based on developmental effects. The risk is also medium for freshwater invertebrates.

Benzothiadiazinone

Bentazon is applied as a post-emergent herbicide used to control broadleaf weeds and yellow nutsedge (*Cyperus esculentus*) in alfalfa, soybean, sorghum, rice, corn, peanut, and certain vegetable crops such as navy beans and lima beans. This herbicide also interferes with PSII electron transport similar to the triazine and urea herbicides (Baltazar and Monaco, 1984). However, in algae it produced an increase of pigment (chlorophylls a and c and carotenoids) content, ATP synthesis, rates of photosynthesis and respiration, and thiobarbituric acid reactive substances (TBARS; as one measure of lipid peroxidation). Because it caused toxicity to a marine diatom, pigments cannot be used as biomarkers of toxicity for this herbicide (Hourmant et al., 2009). Bentazon is slightly acutely toxic via oral, dermal and inhalation routes (Category III). Guinea pigs show skin sensitization with this compound. At the highest dose tested, bentazon caused reductions in body weight gain, increased blood clotting times, and increased renal and hepatic weights in rats. In beagle dogs, the two highest doses of bentazon resulted in anemia-like changes in blood, reduced body weight gains, intestinal inflammation, and congestion of the small intestine and the spleen. In chronic toxicity and carcinogenicity studies in rats reported in the EPA (1994a) fact sheet, it was not found to increase tumors but did cause alterations in blood clotting and alterations of the testes, pancreas, and liver at the highest dose tested. Changes in kidney, thyroid, and pituitary weights were also noted at this highest dose, as were reduced body weight gain and hemorrhage in the liver and heart. In poisoning of rabbits and pheasants, respiratory symptoms were noted with increased body temperatures, and ultimately rapid and high-intensity rigor mortis (Neuschl and Kacmár, 1993). In extreme human poisoning, acute hepatorenal dysfunction leading to death is noted (Wu et al., 2008), but has also yielded increased perspiration, breathing difficulties, and heart failure along with extreme general muscle rigidity (Turcant et al., 2003). Maternal and developmental toxicities were mostly observed in rabbits. Low-dose exposure to male mice caused cell association to the 12 stages of the seminiferous epithelium of adults (frequency of stages VII, IX, and XII), while male mice exposed *in utero* and sampled 100 days following birth (frequency of stages I, III, and VII) were significantly different from controls (Garagna et al., 2005). This may indicate endocrine disruption as possibly confirmed by a positive recombinant yeast screen (for anti-estrogenic/antiandrogenic activity) and inhibition of ovulation *in vivo* due to decreased testosterone production (Orton et al., 2009). The $R_fD = 0.03$ mg/kg bwt/day based on the dog feeding study reported in the EPA fact sheet. Bentazon is a concern for leaching into ground and surface waters. This herbicide is slightly toxic to birds (acute oral and subacute dietary) and exceeds level of concern for chronic avian exposure (reproductive risk). It is slightly acutely toxic to small mammals and practically nontoxic to honeybees, fish (warm or cold water), aquatic invertebrates, and estuarine/marine organisms. Aquatic plant risk is low, but may be hazardous to nontarget terrestrial and semiaquatic plants.

Phenylpyridazine

Pyridate was a terrestrial post-emergent herbicide for broadleaf weeds used in chickpeas (cancelled by registrant in 2004 and final remaining products in 2007) that is a slightly acute toxicant orally or dermally (Category III). It caused some slight skin irritation, but not to the eye. It showed sensitizing activity in the Maximization test and the Buehler test. Pyridate was not a concern for acute inhalation exposure (Category IV). According to the EPA (2000b) fact sheet, dogs given the highest dose of this pesticide experienced severe emesis, ataxia, opisthotonos, nystagmus, and mydriasis were noted 3 hours after dosing (neurotoxicity). Developmental toxicity data from that same fact sheet indicated some maternal toxicity (mortality, decreased body weight, food consumption, ventral body position alterations, dyspnea, sedation, and loss of reaction to external stimuli) and the usual unossified and/or missing bones caused by a number of herbicides. The $R_fD = 0.11$ mg/kg/day. The European Union's NOEC (21 days) = 0.08 mg/L in rainbow trout and 0.01 mg/L for *Daphnia magna*. Pyridate's acute toxicity to algae indicated an $EC_{50} > 2.0$ mg/L for *Anabaena flos-aquae*. It was practically nontoxic to honeybees (> 100 µg/bee). Pyridate appeared to be an endocrine disruptor in an estrogen receptor (ER)–dependent MDF-7 cell proliferation assay. This herbicide bound to both ERα and the androgen receptor (AR). It was more effective in competing with estrogen for the ERα binding than androgen binding to AR (Okubo et al., 2004).

Bipyridylium

Paraquat has been used to control weeds and grasses in agricultural (pre-emergence on vegetables, grains, cotton, grasses, sugar cane, peanuts, potatoes, and tree plantation and post-emergence on fruit crops, vegetable, trees, vines, grains, soybeans, and sugar cane) and nonagricultural areas. Diquat has been used in lakes to eliminate or control invasive aquatic plants, but has major concerns for algal and faunal community dynamics. Paraquat and diquat are quite toxic compounds in their own right. They are oxidation-reduction indicators that can form superoxide in the test tube just by shaking the tube following chemical reduction. In the body, the cytochrome P450 oxidoreductase reduces these compounds and initiates the generation of superoxide radical in the presence of oxygen (variants of this enzyme Tyr181Asp, Ala287Pro, Arg457His, Val492Glu, and Val608Phe reduce Paraquat toxicity and indicate possible resistance in the human population to Paraquat poisoning; Han et al., 2006). These herbicides interfere with electron transfer in photosystem I. Photosystem II inhibition results in production of triplet chlorophyll and singlet oxygen, which peroxidizes membrane lipids. PSI electron acceptors such as bipyridylium herbicides on the other hand accept their electrons from iron-sulfur protein $F_A F_B$. The free radical form of the herbicide then results in lipid peroxidation (Fuerst and Norman, 1991). These herbicides do not hydrolyze rapidly except in highly alkaline conditions, so may be considered persistent in water and are highly dangerous to applicators and wildlife right after application (raptors that may consume voles and become intoxicated via accumulation). Paraquat is far more dangerous because the half-life in the lung is longer due to the polyamine uptake system (cells expressing the human P_5-ATPase ATP13A2, membrane transporters energized by ATP), and it causes lung damage regardless of route

of administration to animals. This polyamine uptake is likely started by a plasma membrane carrier and subsequent sequestration into acidic vesicles of ATP13A2 found in lysosomes and late endosomes (Pinto Fde et al., 2012). Diquat causes lung toxicity if inhaled, but is more likely to cause renal damage if consumed. These factors have rated Paraquat as highly acutely toxic (Category I) via the inhalation route and moderately toxic (Category II) orally. It is only considered slightly toxic dermally due to its hydrophilicity (poor skin absorption). It is a moderate to severe eye irritant but a minimal dermal irritant. Any developmental toxicity with Paraquat appears to be related to maternal toxicity. The $R_f D = 0.45$ mg/kg/day based on chronic pneumonitis. One would think that such a water-soluble compound would leach easily into water; however, it appears that the charge has it bound tightly to soil (especially clay). The major concern for nontarget plants is drift, so applications should be made to reduce this possibility (low wind and application close to the soil surface). Paraquat at lower concentrations in female fish (Nile tilapia, or *Oreochromis niloticus*) appears to affect CYP activity (ethoxyresorufin O-deethylase activity) and liver histology (parenchymal vacuolization, necrosis, and increase in macrophage aggregates and eosinophilic granular cells) and increase the late vitellogenic and mature percentage of oocytes. This indicates at least some reproductive toxicity associated with metabolic alterations and cellular damage (Figueiredo-Fernandes et al., 2006). Dermal application decreased sperm counts in rats (D'Souza et al., 2006). Damage to the zebra mussel (*Dreissena polymorpha*) was found in sub-mg/L exposures causing cellular vacuolation, lysis, and thinness of the germinative epithelia of the digestive gland and the testes. Increased granulocytes also indicated inflammatory capacity of from 0.125–0.5 mg Paraquat/L. Genotoxicity was found with increased micronucleus formation in these mussels (Mantecca et al., 2006). It appears that from its damage to endocrine organs, changes in xenobiotic metabolism, and genotoxicity, low concentrations of Paraquat are suspect in endocrine disruption, reproductive toxicity, and destruction of genetic material that could aid in the formation of cancer or at least cellular dysfunction.

Diphenyl Ether

Inhibition of protoporphyrinogen oxidase (PPO) appears to be the target for diphenyl ether herbicides allowing the accumulation of protoporphyrin IX (porphyrins strongly generate singlet oxygen) in plant tissues. It inhibits this enzyme in plants (corn etioplast IC_{50} = 4 nM), mouse mitochondria, or yeast mitochondrial membranes. The toxicity is exerted by light absorption and peroxidative degradation of membrane lipids (and other cellular entities). These herbicides have been used to control annual grasses and dicotyledonous weeds (pre-emergence or post-emergence) in soybeans, peanuts, cotton, rice, and other crops. Accumulation of protoporphyrin in humans leads to porphyria and porphyria variegate (Matringe et al., 1989). Experimental hepatic uroporphyria was induced in male DBA/2 mice by fomesafen (Krijt et al., 2003). Nitrofen is one of the more toxic members of this group, inducing changes in the cellular redox states of P19 teratocarcinoma cells, generating ROS, and increasing apoptosis via TUNEL-positivity and caspase-3 cleavage (Kling et al., 2005). Nitrofen and another nitrogenous diphenyl ether herbicide, chlornitrofen, induced mast cell activation (increased degranulation and proinflammatory cytokine-production; Teshima et al., 2004). Fomesafen is persistent and mobile in water, so it poses some risk to aquatic plants (although below level of concern based on estimated environmental concentrations) but is of most concern for nontarget terrestrial plants. This herbicide applied post-emergence causes 0–40% damage for monocots and 40–80% range for dicots. Ecotoxicity was tested in planktonic communities in mesocosms over a 9-month period. Chlorophyceae (green algae) were the most sensitive algal community to fomesafen, while no effects were seen in zooplankton (with the exception of fomesafen plus Agral 90 adjuvant; Caquet et al., 2005). At least two of these herbicides, chlornitrofen and chlormethoxyfen, have antiandrogenic activities (chlornitrofen or chlornitrofen-amino has

ER agonist activities as well) higher than those of known AR antagonists vinclozolin and p,p-dichlorodiphenyldichloroethylene as indicated using *in vitro* Chinese hamster ovary cells (Kojima et al., 2004). This makes some of the compounds suspect endocrine disruptors (some strongly). Ecotoxicity testing would indicate no direct action of acifluorfen on *Daphnia magna* Strauss; however, 36 hours of UV exposure produced photoproducts that were toxic to this organism (Scrano et al., 2002). Small mammals exceed the LOCs for acute exposure to endangered species for fomesafen. Although fish show little direct effects of fomesafen, there was a fish kill (~200 fish) that occurred after a legal application (this was marked as possible by the EPA).

Phenylpyrazole

Pyraflufen-ethyl is potent inhibitor of PPO. It is mainly used to control broadleaf weeds in cereal crops, in cotton or potato as a harvest aid/defoliant, and as a burn-down/pre-plant application for cotton, soybeans, and corn (Scroggs et al., 2006). It is listed as high toxicity (Category I) for irreversible eye damage. Otherwise, it has low toxicity on the skin and very low toxicity for oral or inhalation routes. Rats given this herbicide orally for 104 weeks had liver and kidney abnormalities. Rabbit reproductive/developmental toxicity tests revealed maternal mortality at moderate doses and increased abortion at high doses. Pyraflufen-ethyl is considered to be a likely human carcinogen based on a 78-week mouse study that indicated higher liver tumor incidence (EPA, 2002). This herbicide is considered practically acutely nontoxic to mammals and birds via the oral route. It is considered highly toxic to rainbow trout but has lower toxicity to bluegill sunfish. The aquatic insect tests were highly variable (from practically nontoxic to highly toxic), but indicate only direct contact as a problem (Washington State Department of Transportation, 2006).

N-Phenylphthalimide

Flumioxazin is another PPO inhibitor used on soybeans and peanuts to provide pre- and post-emergent control of annual and perennial weeds. The phototoxic mode of action may occur in plants and in fish. It is of interest that the formulated product inhibits this enzyme more than the active ingredient (Daugrois et al., 2005). Flumioxazin is a Category III toxicant for acute dermal exposure (rat) or eye irritation (rabbit). Decreases in mean corpuscular volume in both sexes and an increase in platelets in female rats with 90-day oral dosing established the NOEAEL as low as 65 mg/kg/day. The dog had a lower 90-day exposure NOAEL (10 mg/kg/day) based on dose-dependent increases in cholesterol, phospholipid, and alkaline phosphatase. The mouse 90-day NOAEL was higher (429 mg/kg/day) based on liver weight increases. On exposure to pregnant females, flumioxazin induced ventricular septal defects in the developing rat heart. The critical time for developmental toxicity appeared to be day 12, because dosing at this time yielded the highest embryonic death incidence, lowest fetal body weight, and most frequent induction of ventricular septal defects plus wavy ribs. The thin ventricular septal defects may result from compensation for loss of embryonic blood cells, although mitochondrial lesions were apparent as a result of abnormal iron deposits from lack of heme biosynthesis in erythrocytes derived from the yolk sac (Kawamura et al., 1996). Maternal effects were also noted such as red substance found in the vagina, decreased body weight/body weight gain (and food consumption), and increased female mortality. Flumioxazin may be an endocrine disruptor in mammals as it increased the incidence of atrophied and hypoplastic testes and/or epididymides in male rats at an LOAEL of 200 ppm. This herbicide was not found to be carcinogenic, but at high concentrations (500 M) induced chromatid breaks and exchanges in Chinese hamster ovary cells. Bobwhite quail and the mallard duck are practically unaffected by this herbicide (nontoxic due to $LD_{50} > 2,250$ mg/kg and 5-day $LC_{50} > 5,620$ ppm). Flumioxazin is similarly nontoxic to small mammals and honeybees. Bluegill sunfish show slight toxicity (96-h $LC_{50} > 21$ ppm), while rainbow trout (96-h $LC_{50} = 2.3$ ppm), sheepshead minnow (96-h $LC_{50} > 4.7$ ppm), eastern oyster (96-h $LC_{50}/EC_{50} = 2.4$ ppm), and *Daphnia pulex* (96-h $LC_{50} = 5.5$ ppm) exhibit moderate toxicity to this compound. Mysid shrimp are very sensitive to

flumioxazin (96-h $LC_{50}/EC_{50} = 0.23$ ppm or highly toxic). Terrestrial plants also fall into the highly toxic category for this herbicide, especially lettuce for seedling emergence ($EC_{25} = 0.0008$ lb ai/acre) and cucumber for vegetative vigor ($EC_{25} = 0.00008$ lb ai/acre).

Thiadiazole

Fluthiacet-methyl is first converted to its urazole by glutathione S-transferase and inhibits PPO in velvetleaf (and other broadleaf weeds) and cotton at I_{50}s ranging from 10–12 nM (Shmizu et al., 1995) in soybean fields. Acute dermal toxicity puts this herbicide in Category III (caution), but it is not a sensitizer. Fluthiacet-methyl is not considered mutagenic in a number of bacterial and mammalian cell assays, but was clastogenic with and without S9 activation in two different mammalian cell lines. Micronuclei were induced in rat liver cells exposed *in vivo* to this compound. There was some decrease in mean litter body weights at high doses (313 and 388 mg fluthiacet-methyl/kg/day in male and female rats, respectively) given to rats in a reproductive study. As expected, potent inhibition of heme synthesis had effects on the rat erythropoietic system and the liver over a 90-day feeding study. The systemic toxicity from a rat chronic feeding/carcinogenicity study was observed as decreased body weights, liver damage, pancreatic toxicity, and microcytic anemia in males and liver toxicity, uterine toxicity, and slight microcytic anemia in females. In male rats there was also an increasing trend toward exocrine and pancreatic islet cell adenomas. In the mouse carcinogenicity study, males had increasing hepatocellular adenomas, carcinomas, and/or adenomas/carcinomas, thus fluthiacet-methyl is categorized as a likely human carcinogen (pancreas in male rats and liver tumors in mice). The R_fD is set at 0.001 mg/kg/day based on the mouse carcinogenicity study. This herbicide was practically nontoxic to birds, small mammals, bees, and other beneficial insects. However, it was very highly toxic to fish (96-h $LC_{50} = 140$ ppb and 43 ppb for bluegill sunfish and rainbow trout, respectively; LOAEC = 6 ppb for fathead minnow based on weight and length) and moderately toxic to freshwater invertebrates (*Daphnia magna* lifecycle toxicity LOAEC =

70 ppb based on length; the 48-h EC_{50} exceeded the solubility limit for this compound at 2.3 ppm), so it carries an environmental hazard precautionary statement. The monocot most sensitive to fluthiacet-methyl is the onion with an $EC_{25} = 0.01$ lb ai/acre for seedling emergence and vegetative vigor. The cucumber is the most sensitive dicot with an $EC_{25} = 0.0006$ lb ai/acre (vegetative vigor). Duckweed, green algae, and diatoms are sensitive with an $EC_{50}s = 2.2$ ppb, 2.51 ppb, and 5.13 (marine) and 7.22 (freshwater) ppb, respectively (EPA, 1999a).

Oxadiazole

Oxadiazon is a pre-emergent and early post-emergent inhibitor of PPO (light-dependent peroxidizing compound) that is used on turf or sod farms to control grassy weeds such as goosegrass and crabgrass and broadleaf weeds. It causes skin, eye, and mucous membrane irritation in humans and due to consistent hepatic effects across a variety of species is considered a likely inducer of liver cancer in humans. This herbicide binds to organic matter, thus it persists in the environment. The NOAEC = 0.01275 μg/L for lack of peroxidation and necrotic leaves for the aquatic macrophyte *Callitriche obtusangula* (Iriti et al., 2009). Oxadiazon induced aromatase activity in human choriocarcinoma JEG-3 cells after 24 hours of exposure (Laville et al., 2006). Oxadiazon oxiconazole also activates the human pregnane receptor in a stable reporter cell system (Lemaire et al., 2006). This herbicide and oxadiazon are also peroxisome proliferators (Krijt and Vokurka, 1997). These features may mark it as an endocrine disruptor and confirm its carcinogenic potential. Significant fetal toxicity occurs in both rats and rabbits (resorptions, post-implantation loss, decreased fetal weight, skeletal variations) at a dose at which slight maternal toxicity was observed (weight loss/decreased weight gain). Oxadiazon appears to present no acute risk to birds, but may pose a chronic risk that may be more important for endangered species. Chronic risk also exists for mammalian herbivores and insectivores. There appears to be a low risk of acute fish toxicity to this herbicide, but in shallow waters with significant solar radiation (which may also degrade the compound), the toxicity of recently applied compound may have enhanced risk to aquatic organisms. Chronic risk does exist for freshwater and estuarine/marine fish and aquatic invertebrates. Because this compound does bind to sediment, benthic organisms may be at increased risk of exposure and toxicity. Acute plant risk levels are exceeded for oxadiazon for both vascular and nonvascular plants.

Triazolinone

Azafenidin is another PPO inhibitor used for pre- and post-emergent control of broadleaf weeds and grasses. Humans contacting high doses of this compound can expect liver toxicity and anemia, and lower external exposure may yield mild, temporary skin irritation to moderate eye irritation. This herbicide will be lethal to nontarget bushy/woody plants. It is considered practically nontoxic to honeybees or to terrestrial animals on acute exposure and slightly toxic to fish or aquatic invertebrates. Evaluation of azafenidin for the European Union indicated repeated dosing of pregnant rats (subchronic) caused *in utero* deaths and low NOAELs indicated adverse effects on fertility and/or early developmental toxicity by mechanisms that do not require interaction with steroid receptors. All the inhibitors of protoporphyrinogen oxidase are developmentally suspect as interfering with the heme biosynthetic pathway (common to other toxicants such as hexachlorobenzene, griseofulvin, diazinon, phenobarbital, and lead) would be expected to affect the intricate, interwoven pathways leading to fertilization/conception and implantation (Dent, 2007).

Oxazolidinedione

Yet another PPO inhibitor is pentoxazone. Pentoxazone should be considered as toxic based on this activity alone. It has moderate acute fish, aquatic invertebrate, earthworm, and honeybee toxicity. This herbicide has low acute mammalian and avian toxicity as with most other PPO inhibitors. In its use for control of weeds in rice paddy agriculture, it has algicidal effects only (versus algistatic) on *Pseudokirchneriella subcapitata*, so is highly toxic to nontarget plants (EU data from University of Herfordshire Pesticide Properties Database, 2014).

Pyrimidinedione

Butafenacil is also a PPO inhibitor. It is used to control broadleaf and annual grasses in Argentina, Brazil, Japan, Switzerland, and Thailand in cotton, citrus, non-cropland, pome fruit, stone fruit, grapes, garlic, and onions (Australian data from Davies, 2002). This herbicide has low acute oral, dermal, and inhalation toxicity. It is a slight eye irritant, but is not a skin irritant or sensitizer. The PPO inhibition (especially for the mouse enzyme = 16-fold lower IC_{50} than in human) leads to reduction of red cell number and liver enlargement in mice, rats, and dogs. The NOEL for the mouse is 0.36 mg/kg bw/day in males due to hematologic effects and liver toxicity in both sexes. Butafenacil is practically nontoxic to mallard ducks and bobwhite quail; moderately toxic to rainbow trout, bluegill sunfish, sheepshead minnow, and the eastern oyster; and highly toxic to *Daphnia magna*, marine mysid shrimp, and algae. Additionally, chronic exposure made daphnids highly sensitive compared to only slightly toxic acutely (high acute to chronic ratio). Nontarget plants are also of concern close to the area of application.

Other PPO Inhibitors

Flufenpyr-ethyl (pyridazinone herbicide) is used on corn, soybeans, and sugarcane to control velvetleaf and morning glory (*Ipomoea violacea*). As usual for PPO inhibitors, acute mammalian toxicity is low, but chronic liver toxicity (hepatocellular fatty vacuolation and necrosis) and hematologic changes are evident. The EPA (2003a) memorandum indicates that a one-generation reproduction study on this herbicide indicated kidney lesions (interstitial fibrosis of cortex NOAEL = 100 ppm). The memorandum data also indicate that thymus weights were also increased on a 13-week feeding study. Clearly, nontarget plants must again be considered at risk.

Pyridazinone

The mechanism of the pyridazinone class of herbicides involves inhibition of the phytoene desaturase step of carotenoid biosynthesis/bleaching. Norflurazon is a selective pre-emergent herbicide used in the control of germinating annual grasses and broadleaf weeds that may grow in fruit, vegetable, nut, cotton, peanut, and soybean fields. It has low acute toxicity. Subchronic toxicity studies indicate liver and thyroid weight changes, increased cholesterol levels, and decreased RBC counts (dog). Because the thyroid is an endocrine organ, this must be considered at least a high-dose endocrine disruptor. The EPA (1996b) fact sheet indicated that a 2-year carcinogenicity study in mice also observed increased liver weight and nodular enlargement of the liver, enlarged spleen, and nephritis. In rat liver cells, norflurazon has been shown to affect delta-6 fatty acid desaturation more efficiently than delta-5 or delta-4 (Hagve et al., 1985). This herbicide is listed as a non-quantifiable (Group C) possible human carcinogen. It has also been linked to an allergic contact dermatitis (Leow and Maibach, 1996). Norflurazon is practically nontoxic acutely to avian species, mammals, and honeybees, but does yield reproductive alterations in birds. It is slightly toxic to fish (cold or warm water) and aquatic invertebrates. This herbicide is also moderately toxic to selected estuarine/marine organisms. It is highly toxic to aquatic plants and can damage terrestrial plants.

Pyridinecarboxamide

Diflufenican also exerts its herbicidal activity through bleaching/inhibition of carotenoid biosynthesis at the phytoene desaturase step. Although this compound may cause irritation to mucous membranes and the skin, it is not considered acutely toxic. It is not toxic to birds or bees and has listed LC_{50}s of 56–100 mg/L for rainbow trout, 105 mg/L for carp, and > 20 mg/L for *Daphnia*. There appears to be some effect of high doses on testes and thymus weights, but only at levels that affect body weight as well. This is not clear evidence of endocrine disruption, but perhaps a result of systemic toxicity.

Other Agents That Inhibit Carotenoid Biosynthesis at the Phytoene Desaturase Step

Fluridone is a systemic aquatic herbicide used to control aquatic weeds in various surface waters ranging from ponds to rivers. This herbicide is practically acutely nontoxic to birds, mammals, and terrestrial invertebrates. However, it is a moderate eye irritant and causes increased abortions in rats (developmental toxicity). Furidone was found to be more cytotoxic in a mammalian *in vitro* cell cytotoxicity assay than the herbicide atrazine but less than herbicides diquat and acetochlor. It shares the ability of atrazine to decrease the number of cells in the G2 phase of the cell cycle (Freeman and Rayburn, 2006). A metabolite, N-methyl formamide, is more acutely toxic than the parent compound to mammals. Aquatic organisms are more sensitive to its effects, varying from slightly to moderately toxic to aquatic vertebrates and invertebrates. In the fluridone summary document of the EPA (2009a), The U.S. Fish and Wildlife Service is mentioned as having issued an opinion in 1984 that registration of this product could provide a threat to the viability of all listed U.S. freshwater aquatic species with impacts including untoward habitat changes. The formulated herbicide is 60-fold more toxic to water mites than the active ingredient and reinforces the documentation of aquatic impacts of this herbicide (Yi et al., 2011).

Triketone

Mesotrione starts the inhibitors of 4-hydroxyphenylpyruvate dioxygenase (4-HPPD) leading to bleaching of broadleaf weeds (pre- and post-emergent). Inhibition of this enzyme in the rat, mouse, and dog leads to high blood tyrosine levels that cause eye (lesions), liver, and kidney effects. Delayed ossification in fetuses treated with mesotrione occurs at doses below those yielding maternal toxicity (decreased body weight gain in rat; decreased food consumption, abortions, and GI effects in rabbit). This herbicide is a mild eye irritant but is practically nontoxic to avian species, small mammals, and aquatic species. Microalgae, especially *Ankistrodesmus fusiformis* of the Chlorophyceae class, had a low IC_{50} (0.05 mg/L) for mesotrione (Moro et al., 2012).

Isoxazole

Isoxaflutole appears to be more toxic as a 4-HPPD inhibitor causing developmental toxicity, classed as a probable human carcinogen (Group B_2) and extremely phytotoxic (EC_{25} = 10^{-5} lb ai/acre). The EPA (2010c) summary document on this pesticide indicated that isoxaflutole increased liver weights in a 21-day rat dermal toxicity test and hemolysis in dogs in a chronic study. Chronic exposure leads to liver tumors (adenomas and carcinomas). Thyroid hyperplasia with reductions in thyroxine (T_4) production also marks this herbicide as a chronic endocrine disruptor in rats (and causes thyroid tumors via the lack of negative feedback on the thyroid-pituitary axis). Eye lesions were also observed similar to mesotrione. There also may be some high-dose subchronic neurotoxicity in rats (reduced mean hind limb grip strength in male rats). However, isoxaflutole is practically nontoxic to the mallard duck and acutely but slightly toxic subacutely to the bobwhite quail. Honeybees and rats have little to fear from this compound in the wild. Rainbow trout, *Daphnia magna*, the sheepshead minnow, and the eastern oyster respond with moderate toxicity to this herbicide, but isoxaflutole is highly toxic to mysid shrimp.

Pyrazole

Pyrazole herbicides such as pyrazoxyfen are also inhibitors of 4-HPPD used in paddy rice to control annual and perennial weeds (not in the United States). The chief concern is to *Daphnia*, killifish, carp, and especially rainbow trout with LC_{50}s = 127, 2.7, 2.5, and 0.79 mg/L, respectively. Otherwise pyrazoxyfen fits the slightly hazardous category.

Benzobicyclon

Benzobicyclon fits the "other" category for 4-HPPD inhibitors. This is another herbicide not used in the United States but used on rice fields of Japan. This herbicide is moderately toxic to carp (acute 96-h LC_{50} = 10.0 mg/L), *Daphnia* (acute 48-h LC_{50} = 1.0 mg/L), and algae (acute 72-h LC_{50} = 1.0 mg/L to *Pseudokirchneriella subcapitata*), but has a low toxicity to honeybees.

Triazole

With this class of agents, bleaching is still a mechanism of herbicide action with inhibition of carotenoid biosynthesis. Amitrole, an *in vivo* inhibitor of lycopene cyclase and chlorophyll formation and limited regrowth of buds, is used primarily on nonagricultural areas to control weeds in industrial areas, fencerows, shade trees, and ornamental shrubs and vines. Due to this herbicide's ability to have antithyroid effects, it must be considered an endocrine disruptor. It also causes thyroid, pituitary (also endocrine), and liver tumors (Group B_2—probable human carcinogen), so it has special handling instructions for applicators. The mechanism for the thyroid disruption may involve reduction of TSH receptor on the surface of rat thyroid follicle cells and therefore decreases thyroid hormone synthesis as shown in other studies (Pan and Zhang, 2011). Otherwise, amitrole is practically nontoxic acutely or causes dermal irritation and is slightly toxic for dermal exposure and primary eye irritation. Ecological assessment indicates that this herbicide is practically nontoxic to avian species on an acute oral and subacute basis and to freshwater fish. Mammals similarly have little to fear on an acute oral basis. Mammalian reproduction may be affected locally as the two-generation rat reproduction study indicated untoward effects. Moderate toxicity may be expected to marine invertebrates and slightly toxic to freshwater invertebrates. Nontarget monocots (especially wheat) and dicots (most sensitive is pepper) are affected at very low levels (< 0.1 lb ai/acre) and may be of concern.

Isoxazolidinone

Clomazone is another bleaching agent that inhibits carotenoid biosynthesis caused by a plant metabolite, 5-ketoclomazone. This herbicide is used typically pre-plant or pre-emergent or plant incorporated on cotton, tobacco, soybeans, rice, and sugarcane to control annual grasses and broadleaf weeds. Clomazone has been shown to cause oxidative stress in human RBCs *in vitro* and also appears to inhibit acetylcholinesterase (AChE) in these cells via ROS generation (Santi et al., 2011). There may some acute risk to nonlisted freshwater and estuarine/marine invertebrates, terrestrial plants, and aquatic nonvascular plants and chronic risk exceeding the LOC for nonlisted mammals. Clomazone is slightly toxic to freshwater or estuarine/marine fish, moderately toxic to freshwater invertebrates, and highly to moderately

toxic to estuarine/marine invertebrates. Nontarget plants have experienced whitening under field application conditions (lettuce most sensitive dicot; oat most sensitive monocot).

Diphenyl Ether

Aclonifen is used outside the United States (Europe, South America) to control broadleaf weeds and grass weeds in fields of corn, legumes, potatoes, sunflowers, and vegetables via bleaching/inhibition of carotenoid biosynthesis. It has low mammalian acute toxicity and is slightly irritating to the eye of the rabbit. However, it is highly persistent in the environment and is considered very toxic to aquatic organisms. Moderate toxicity is noted with an acute 96-h $LC_{50} = 0.005$ in *Oncorhynchus mykiss* to high toxicity indicated by a 21-day chronic $LC_{50} = 0.67$ in *Pimephales promelas*. Moderate toxicity is also noted in sediment-dwelling organisms (*Chironomus riparius*) with 28-day chronic NOECs of 0.472 mg/L water and 32.0 mg/kg sediment. High toxicity for aquatic plants (acute 7-day $EC_{50} = 0.006$ mg/L for *Lemna gibba*) makes aclonifen a concern for all aquatic organisms. Moderate toxicities are noted for algae, honeybees, and earthworms.

Glycine

Glyphosate is an active ingredient in an herbicide that has crops designed to be resistant to its action (Roundup Ready®). It works via inhibition of 5-enolpyruvylshikimate 3-phosphate synthase (EC 2.5.1.19), the sixth enzyme in the shikimate pathway that leads to the formation of aromatic amino acids in algae, higher plants, bacteria, fungi, and apicomplexan parasites, but is an enzyme not present in mammals. Glyphosate appears to bind to the phosphoenolpyruvate (second) site of the enzyme, thereby providing herbicidal or antiparasitic (*Plasmodium falciparum* [malaria], *Toxoplasma gondii*, and *Cryptosporidium parvum*) action (Schönbrunn et al., 2001). This herbicide is nonselective and at lower rates represents a plant growth regulator. It appears to affect all plant life that is not resistant based on genetics, but has a short half-life in soil (2–197 days). It has low oral and dermal acute toxicity (Category III) to mammals. The EPA (2009b) registration review document indicated that a subchronic rat feeding study indicated some blood and pancreatic effects. Developmental studies of pregnant rats indicated that glyphosate treatment led to diarrhea, decreased body weight gain, nasal discharge, and death in the high-dose group. The main ecological concern for the use of glyphosate is the possibility of fish kills if aquatic weeds die, decompose, and result in oxygen loss or the loss of endangered or nontarget plants and animals that feed off those plants such as the Houston toad. These data produce overconfidence in the low toxicity of this compound. In more recent studies, evidence of lowered testosterone production in rat testicular cells at very low environmental doses and acute rat testicular toxicity/necrosis at high doses indicate a potent endocrine disruptor (Clair et al., 2012). There also appears to be concern for either accidental high exposure to glyphosate and Parkinson's disease in the human or chronic exposure and dopaminergic (affecting movement such as Parkinson's disease) and GABAergic (affecting sleep and inhibitory neural pathways) neuron degeneration as indicated in the worm *Caenorhabditis elegans* (Negga et al., 2012). Spraying glyphosate formulations on the direct-developing frog *Eleutherodactylus johnstonei* neonates led to clear cytotoxicity and DNA breaks in a dose-dependent manner (Meza-Joya et al., 2013).

Phosphinic Acid

Glufosinate-ammonium works as an herbicide via inhibition of glutamine synthetase, an enzyme found in plants and animals. This herbicide has low acute oral toxicity and has a LOAEL and NOAEL or 64–90 and 6.2–8.8 mg/kg/day for 90 days of oral exposure in male rats based on glutamine synthetase inhibition in the brains of male rats (neurotoxicity). There may even be direct convulsant action of glufosinate-ammonium as indicated in mice injected intraperitoneally with 80 mg/kg, which is partially antagonized by NMDA receptor antagonists. Clinical chemistries and liver weights marked toxicity to male mice at doses exceeding 192 mg/kg/day for 90 days. Dermal toxicity in rats was observed as increases in aggressive behavior, piloerection, and high startle response. Maternal effects in rats were based on vaginal bleeding and hyperactivity while developmental responses included dilated renal pelvis. Prenatal toxicity in the rabbit was manifested as decreased body weights and fetal deaths. Reproductive and fertility effects in the rat included decreased numbers of viable pups. Dog toxicity was observed as changes in the electrocardiogram at 6 months of treatment. The EPA (2008a) fact sheet reported no carcinogenicity in rats, but did find increased incidence of retinal atrophy. Similarly, a lack of carcinogenic responses was found in the mouse, but in this animal this herbicide caused increase in glucose levels, changes in glutathione (GSH) levels, and decreased albumin and total proteins.

Carbamate

Asulam is a selective post-emergent systemic carbamate herbicide effective against annual grasses and broadleaf weeds that may grow in areas for plantings such as sugarcane (major use), Christmas trees, ornamentals, St. Augustine grass, Bermuda grass, and non-cropland uses. Its mode of action is via inhibition of dihydropteroate synthase, an enzyme involved in folic acid synthesis. A secondary activity of this herbicide appears to involve prevention of microtubule assembly/mitosis inhibition. Asulam is practically nontoxic via acute oral and inhalation routes and is not a skin sensitizer. It is slightly toxic via the dermal route and causes slight eye irritation in rabbits. Thyroid and adrenal tumors have been discovered in male rats exposed to high doses (Group C or possible human carcinogen). The EPA (2010d) summary document reported chronically exposed dogs had decreased body weight gain, decreased food consumption, vomiting, diarrhea, and RBC reductions. Also, the dogs given the highest doses had increased thyroid and kidney weights and decreased testicular weights. The same EPA document indicated that a mouse cancer study yielded higher spleen weights in males and decreased brain weights and survival in females. This herbicide does exceed the LOC for endangered and nonendangered terrestrial and semiaquatic plants. Other carbamates are considered primary in disrupting microtubule organization such as chlorpropham, propham, and carbetamide. Carbetamide is a pre- and post-emergence herbicide used on a variety of field crops in Europe to control annual grasses and some broadleaf weeds. It is considered of moderate acute toxicity (rat oral LD_{50} = 1718 mg/kg, bird—*Colinus virginianus* LD_{50} > 2000 mg/kg, fish—*Oncorhynchus mykiss* 96-h LC_{50} > 100 mg/L, *Daphnia magna* 48-h EC_{50} = 81 mg/L). This herbicide has low toxicity to aquatic plants or acute toxicity to algae or honeybees, but has moderate toxicity to algae based on the 96-h NOEC (0.14 mg/L) and earthworms based on 14-day LC_{50} (660 mg/kg soil).

Dinitroaniline

Asulam breached the subject of microtubule assembly inhibition. The dinitroaniline compounds have that as their primary herbicidal activity, as do a number of other chemical classes of herbicides to follow. Benefin is a dinitroaniline pre-emergent herbicide used to control annual grasses and broadleaf weeds in direct-seeded lettuce, established turf, seeded alfalfa, red clover, birdsfoot trefoil, and ladino clover. This herbicide has low acute toxicity via oral and dermal routes (Category IV) and is listed as Category III for primary eye and skin irritation. It is listed as a skin sensitizer in the Buehler test (7/12 guinea pigs tested positive). However, if dermal exposure is continued, severe dermal effects are seen at high doses of benfluralin. This compound is toxic to the kidneys and liver in longer-term studies (20 mg/kg/day in female rats) and is toxic to the thyroid at high doses (136.3 mg/kg/day in male rats) as indicated in the EPA (2004a) reregistration document. Dinitroaniline pesticides usually cause toxicity to the kidney, liver, blood, and thyroid. Because the two highest doses of benefin cause an increase in liver and thyroid tumors, it is classified as having suggestive evidence of carcinogenicity. Birds show no mortality as adults to acute or subacute doses of benfluralin. However, avian reproductive toxicity was noted in the EPA document in tests using the northern bobwhite quail (decrease in number of surviving hatchlings, egg set, and 14-day hatchling survivor weight) or mallard duck (% eggs that cracked). The EPA also noted a mammalian two-generation rat reproductive study that produced

animals with decreased body weight, body weight gains, and food consumption. More importantly, there were dead pups and survivors with progressive chronic neuropathy and liver and kidney enlargement. Benefin is also acutely very highly toxic to freshwater fish (*Lepomis macrochirus* or bluegill sunfish) and estuarine/marine invertebrates (*Americamysis bahia*).

Phosphoramidate

Amiprophos-methyl has greater specificity for tubulin (low concentrations are needed to inhibit microtubule proliferation) *in vitro* than colchicine, a natural antimitotic agent. It is used throughout the world to control weeds, because it is quickly degraded and leaves little residue (Rodrigues et al., 2011). Due to its effect on dividing cells, it is considered an oral poison and is an eye irritant.

Pyridine

Dithiopyr is used on terrestrial non-food sites as a pre-emergent and post-emergent herbicide to control crabgrass and other susceptible annual grasses and broadleaf weeds in turf. Although this herbicide has low acute toxicity, it is a Category II dermal and eye irritant in rabbits and was positive for dermal sensitization by the Buehler method as part of Dimension Turf Herbicide, MON-15151. It is also highly toxic to freshwater fish and aquatic invertebrates.

Benzamide

Propyzamide (pronamide) is a selective, systemic, pre- and post-emergence herbicide that also inhibits microtubule assembly/plant cell division. It controls grasses and broadleaf weeds in lettuce (highest use), endive, alfalfa, rhubarb, pome and stone fruits, artichokes, berries, grapes, and legumes (also used on woody ornamentals, Christmas trees, turf, and fallow land). It is practically nontoxic (acute oral) to slightly toxic (dermal and inhalation). The EPA (1994b) fact sheet reported subchronic tests with rats that indicated hepatic, thyroid, and pituitary toxicity (endocrine toxicity = thyroid, pituitary, and testes). Propyzamide is a Group B_2 probable human carcinogen based on liver cancer in male mice (chronic feeding) and benign testicular and thyroid tumors in rats (related to organochlorine compounds). Ecological toxicity is based on effects on green algae. Isoxaben is a different kind of benzamide that inhibits the conversion of glucose to cellulose thereby preventing cell wall synthesis in its pre-emergent action against broadleaf weeds for use in noncrop areas and non-fruit-bearing fruit and nut crops. This herbicide has low toxicity orally or dermally (Category III and IV), but is more toxic if inhaled (Category II and III). In rats, live hypertrophy occurs at high doses while mice develop benign liver adenomas. This makes it a cancer concern consistent with other benzamides that have a different mechanism of herbicidal action. Isoxaben is moderately toxic to freshwater fish and invertebrates, estuarine/marine fish and invertebrates, and green algae.

Benzoic Acid

Dimethyl tetrachloroterephthalate (DCPA) is the last of the category of microtubule assembly inhibitors. DCPA and its metabolites have low acute and chronic toxicity, but manufacturing impurities in the past have contained 2,3,7,8-TCDD and hexachlorobenzene (HCB), which are oncogenic (probable human carcinogens), developmentally toxic, and cause adverse effects on the immune response. Benzoic acid analogs can also act as plant hormones (auxins—see phenoxy-carboxylic-acid for this mechanism later in this chapter). Dicamba is an herbicide used pre-plant, pre-emergence, and post-emergence in control of broadleaf weeds in right-of-way areas, asparagus, barley, corn, grasses grown in pasture and rangeland, oats, proso millet, rye, sorghum, soybeans, sugarcane, wheat, residential lawns, and golf courses. Its major acute concerns are as irritation to the eye and skin (Category II). At high doses in goats the dimethyl amine salt of this herbicide dicamba produced cellular changes in the lungs, liver, kidney, adrenal gland (endocrine), and spleen. Aquatic nonvascular plants were considered at risk in the environmental risk analysis.

Chloroacetamide

Acetochlor is one of a long list of herbicides that inhibit cell division (also protein synthesis inhibition noted) and affect very long chain fatty acids (VLCFAs). This herbicide is used pre-emergence to control annual grasses, certain broadleaf weeds, and yellow nutsedge on a wide range of crops. It is considered moderately acutely toxic orally. This herbicide is considered Category II for eye irritation; Category III for acute toxicity via oral, dermal, and inhalation routes; and Category IV for skin irritation, but is considered a skin sensitizer. Positive (weak) mutagenicity findings for acetochlor were found in the CHO/HGPRT gene mutation assay, a strain of *Salmonella typhimurium* reversion assay requiring metabolic activation, clastogenic with cultured human lymphocytes, and in a structural chromosome aberration study using fertility/pregnancy outcomes (EPA, 2005d). These findings were reinforced by cancer studies indicating high-dose hepatocarcinomas in males, lung tumors in females at all dose levels, and total benign ovarian tumors in mid-dose females. In a chronic feeding study, additional thyroid cell adenomas in males were noted along with high-dose papillary edema of the mucosa of the nose and nasal epithelial adenomas. Rare tumors of the benign chondroma of the femur and basal cell tumor of the stomach were also seen with chronic high doses in the rat. These results gave acetochlor a probable human carcinogen classification, which was reexamined by EPA (2007a) to insure that the chronic RfD (cRfD) of 0.02 mg/kg/day was indeed protective of both non-cancer and cancer effects. Repeated doses also increased liver, kidney, and testicular weights. Environmentally, acetochlor is considered moderately toxic to honeybees and is toxic to rainbow trout and bluegill sunfish (fish 96-h LC_{50}s = 0.45 and 1.30 mg/L, respectively). Acetochlor is also an endocrine disruptor (Hinther et al., 2010; Rollerova et al., 2011).

Acetamide

Napropamide takes the discussion of the herbicides further into the disruption of cell division and inhibition of VLCFAs. This compound is a selective systemic amide herbicide that controls annual grasses and broadleaf weeds on vegetables, fruit trees and bushes, vines, strawberries, sunflowers, tobacco, olives, and mint. Napropamide is not very toxic dermally (Category III), orally, or via inhalation (Category IV). Its toxicity is observed via diarrhea, excessive tearing and urination, depression, salivation, rapid weight loss, respiratory changes, decreased blood pressure, and fluid in body cavities. Conflicting studies suggest that incomplete bone formation may occur during development on exposure to this compound. It is also a moderate eye irritant in the rabbit (Category II). Environmentally, this herbicide is moderately toxic to freshwater fish species and marine organisms such as the pink shrimp and eastern oyster. It also exceeds the LOC for mammals that feed on all treated food types. Napropamide is also a risk to aquatic vascular plants and terrestrial and semi-aquatic plants.

Oxyacetamide

Again, the inhibition of cell division in the roots and shoots of germinating seeds via inhibition of VLCFAs (required for cell plate formation; Bach et al., 2011) is the mechanism of flufenacet's action. Flufenacet is a selective pre- or post-emergence herbicide used to control annual grasses and broadleaf weeds in corn, soybeans, triticale, wheat, and forests. The slight acute toxicity to mammals was indicated by uncoordinated gait and decreased activity, hot-to-touch bodies, urine stains, increased reactivity, convulsions, ungroomed appearance, salivation, lacrimation, and various stains about the head and forepaws (rats). It is moderately toxic to freshwater and estuarine/marine fish and some studies of freshwater and estuarine/marine invertebrates. This herbicide is highly toxic to vascular and nonvascular aquatic plants. The tomato is the most sensitive dicot and sorghum is the most sensitive monocot (seedling emergence), yet for vegetative vigor the cucumber is the dicot most sensitive to flufenacet's action. Flufenacet is not an endocrine disruptor per se, but can reduce serum thyroxine levels by increased biotransformation of the hormone in the liver (Christenson et al., 1996).

Tetrazolinone

Fentrazamide also inhibits VLCFA synthesis and subsequently cell division. Again broadleaf weeds and grasses are the focus of this herbicide in rice, cereals, and corn. Acute oral toxicity for fentrazamide is low in the rat, but switches to high for the short-term dietary NOEL and to green algae. This herbicide is moderately toxic to birds, fish, *Daphnia*, and earthworms. At extremely high doses (3,000–4,000 ppm) given to rats over their lifespan, there was axonal degeneration of the sciatic nerve due to interference with glucose utilization, an effect not considered relevant to usual human exposures (Schmuck et al., 2003).

Other VLCFA Synthesis Inhibitors

Anilofos is one of three other pre- and post-emergence application herbicides that inhibit cell division via blocking the synthesis of VLCFAs and are used to control sedges, annual grasses, and some broadleaf weeds in rice fields. It has moderate acute toxicity in the rat (LD_{50} = 472 mg/kg), fish (96-h LC_{50} = 2.8 mg/L in *Oncorhynchus mykiss*), and *Daphnia*. Since it is an organophosphate in structure it is also and acetylcholinesterase inhibitor (neurotoxic similar to many insecticides of the same class). Anilofos inhibits total ATPase and the $3Na^+,2K^+$-ATPase and may also affect ion transport into neurons (neurotoxicity) and other cells (Hazarika and Sarkar, 2001). This herbicide is also a respiratory tract irritant. The World Health Organization gives it overall a Category II classification, while the EPA is less concerned based on its formulation and use (Category III).

Nitrile

Dichlobenil represents a group of herbicides based on interfering with cellulose/cell wall synthesis that are used for selective weed control in cranberry bogs, ornamentals, nurseries, fruit orchards, vineyards, forestry plantations, public green areas, and along industrial or railway property. This herbicide should not be applied between sowing and emergence of crop as prohibitive phytotoxicity is noted. It has low oral or inhalation toxicity but is of moderate toxicity via the dermal route. The EPA (1998d) fact sheet mentions liver changes in the rat and dog following 2-year feeding studies. The same fact sheet data indicate skeletal changes at high doses in a developmental study employing pregnant rats. Dichlobenil is classified as a possible human carcinogen (Class C) based on an observed increase in tumors in rats at the highest dose. This compound is slightly to moderately toxic to fish and moderately to highly toxic to aquatic insects.

Triazolocarboxamide

Flupoxam is an obsolete herbicide used to control broadleaf weeds in winter cereals by interfering with cellulose synthesis.

Quinoline Carboxylic Acid

Quinclorac is the last agent examined that interferes with cellulose synthesis, yet can also mimic the plant growth hormone auxin. It is a systemic pre- and post-emergent herbicide used in the control of broadleaf weeds and grass on rice, sorghum, wheat, residential lawns, ornamentals, and turf grass. This herbicide is classified as Category III for acute oral, dermal, and inhalation toxicity and is only a mild eye irritant. It is a dermal sensitizer. Subchronic toxicity included lower body weight and gain, increased water intake, increased liver enzymes, and focal chronic interstitial nephritis. Chronic toxicity also adds pancreatic acinar cell hyperplasia to the kidney and liver alterations. It appears that the major environmental concerns are for nontarget terrestrial and aquatic plants.

Dinitrophenol

As these compounds uncouple oxidative phosphorylation in mitochondria by membrane disruption, they must all be considered toxic to a variety of cells and organisms. They may be used as herbicides, insecticides, and fungicides. DNOC (4,6-dinitro-o-cresol), sodium salt fits all these activities and toxicities. Diaphoresis, thirst, fever (hyperthermia), tachycardia, tachypnea, headache, confusion, malaise, and restlessness mark the signs of dinitrophenol exposure, as do yellowing of the skin and hair with dermal exposure. Cataracts and glaucoma may result from chronic exposure. DNOC was used primarily as a blossom-thinning agent on fruit trees and as an insecticide, miticide, and fungicide. Terrestrial vertebrate toxicity is based on 90-day rat dietary exposure with the geometric mean of the LOEL (2.5 mg/kg/day) and NOEL (0.25 mg/kg/day) = 0.8 mg/kg/day, a very low value. Aquatic species are also affected, with the

rainbow trout having LC$_{50}$s ranging from 0.066–0.45 mg/L dependent on the study.

Thiocarbamate

Butylate introduces the inhibition of lipid synthesis via routes other than ACC inhibition that cause weed seeds in the germination stage of development to slow shoot growth and leaves to become twisted. It is usually used in combination with a triazine herbicide. Butylate is used on corn fields just prior to planting to control grassy weeds (e.g., nutgrass, millet grass) and some broadleaf weeds. Butylate and other thiocarbamates are known to cause irritation of the skin, eyes (Category I), and mucous membranes of the respiratory tract. Otherwise, it is characterized as Class III, or slightly toxic. The chronic toxicity of this herbicide causes liver and testicular lesions and affects blood clotting. Beagle dogs also experience increased thyroid weight from chronic exposure to this herbicide. Although animal studies failed to find increased cancer risk, butylate use was associated with increased risk of prostate cancer and non-Hodgkin's lymphoma (Lynch et al., 2009). It has also been historically linked with 4 other herbicides (2,4,5-T, Paraquat, alachlor, metribuzin) resulting in fatal injuries among farmers (Waggoner et al., 2012). Butylate is highly toxic to freshwater fish.

Phosphorodithioate

Bensulide also prevents lipid synthesis and is used to control grasses and other weeds in food crops such as vegetables and melons. It has the property of a cholinesterase inhibitor, acting like an insecticide, so neurotoxicity is of major concern. Chronic risks to birds and mammals are expected from this activity alone.

Benzofuran

Benfuresate is another lipid synthesis inhibitor used for post-emergence control of grass and broadleaf weeds. This herbicide does not pose an acute risk to mammals but is moderately toxic to fish, earthworms, *Daphnia*, and algae.

Chloro-Carbonic Acid

Dalapon finishes the lipid synthesis inhibitors and is also classified as a growth regulator. This herbicide is used for grass weeds, cattails, and rush control in non-cropland and crops such as alfalfa, asparagus, flax, potatoes, rapeseed, and sugar beets. Is a moderate skin and eye irritant and can also irritate the upper respiratory tract especially upon repeated prolonged contact. Poisoning symptoms are lassitude, vomiting, diarrhea, slowing pulse, and loss of appetite (general). It is not used in the United States.

Phenoxy-Carboxylic Acid

Most people in the United States have sprayed or been exposed to spray of dandelions (post-emergence) and other broadleaf weeds on lawns with 2,4-dichlorophenoxyacetic acid (2,4-D). It was so widely used in North Dakota that box elder trees (a sensitive tree species) were no longer carried by nurseries. This is the introduction of the first chemical family acting like plant growth hormones (auxins) based on synthetic forms of indole acetic acid. 2,4-D has use as an herbicide, a plant growth regulator, and as a fungicide. The EPA (2005e) in a reregistration eligibility decision mentioned a pre-Special Review status since 1986 based on epidemiological links of 2,4-D exposure (occupational or residential) to non-Hodgkin's lymphoma. Despite this association, the same EPA document noted that the Scientific Advisory Board/Scientific Advisory Panel Special Joint Committee of the EPA did not see a cause-and-effect relationship and has classified 2,4-D as Group D (not classifiable as to human carcinogenicity). 2,4-D appears to increase cell-wall plasticity, biosynthesis of proteins, and the production of ethylene causing uncontrolled cell division and growth and subsequent damage to vascular tissue. This herbicide has low acute toxicity by oral, dermal, or inhalation routes (Categories III or IV). The acid and salt forms of 2,4-D are severe irritants. 2,4-D is actively secreted by the proximal tubules of the kidney. Because the dog has a limited capacity to excrete organic acids, the usual mammalian model of the rat is less sensitive than the dog to the chronic effects of this herbicide. Once the renal clearance saturation threshold is reached, toxicity is observed in the eye, thyroid (endocrine), kidney, adrenals (endocrine), and ovaries/testes (endocrine). Exceeding this threshold in pregnant rats led to skeletal abnormalities in the developing pups. In pregnant rabbits, high-dose levels also cause neurotoxicity (ataxia, decreased motor activity, myotonia, prostration, lateral recumbency, impaired/loss of the righting reflex, and skin cold to the touch). Birds show a range of toxicity to this herbicide from practically nontoxic to moderately toxic. Marine invertebrate LC_{50}s range from > 0.092 (highly toxic) to > 66 mg ae/L (practically nontoxic) for 2,4-D esters. Nontarget vascular plants are two orders of magnitude more sensitive to 2,4-D than nonvascular plants.

Pyridine Carboxylic Acid

Clopyralid, similar to 2,4-D, is a synthetic auxin and is used for selective post-emergence control of broadleaf weeds along roadsides or crops. Its acute concern is mainly eye irritation. Chronic exposure to rats at moderate to high doses caused slight changes in body, liver, and kidney weights and some stomach tissue structural alterations (may involve endocrine cells of the GI tract involved in the barrier functions of this region; Iaglov and Ptashekas, 1989). Environmental concerns center on contact with nontarget plants.

Other Synthetic Auxins

Benazolin-ethyl is used to control annual broadleaf weeds, especially black bindweed and cleavers. This herbicide has low acute toxicity in the rat, birds, and algae but moderate toxicity to fish, *Daphnia*, and earthworms. Benazolin-ethyl is moderately toxic to algae following 96-hour chronic exposure.

Phthalamate

Naptalam inhibits auxin transport and so serves as a pre-emergent herbicide for control of broadleaf weeds in cucurbits and wood nursery stock. This herbicide is Category IV for acute dermal irritation and inhalation exposure and Category III for oral and dermal toxicity to the rat. However, a granular formulation (Alanap, technical) was a Category I eye irritant that led to corneal opacity. The target organ for naptalam sodium is the liver. Nontarget plants are the main environmental concern.

Semicarbazole

Diflufenzopyr-sodium is also an inhibitor of auxin transport and is used in combination with dicamba to be a post-emergence herbicide for broadleaf weed control in corn. Irritation responses (mammal) and nontarget plants lead the list of toxicity concerns.

Arylaminopropionic Acid

Flamprop-M-methyl is a selective, post-emergent, systemic herbicide whose mode of action depends on being absorbed by the leaves, hydrolyzed to the active flamprop-M, and transported to the meristems. It appears to act via a new anti-microtubule mechanism of action involving spindle organization (Tresch et al., 2008). This compound is used to control wild oats (*Avena* spp.) in barley and wheat, but can also control *Alopecurus myosuroides* and *Arrhenatherum elatius*. *Daphnia* and algae/nontarget plants appear to be the major concerns.

Pyrazolium

Difenzoquat was a selective post-emergence quaternary ammonium herbicide used on wheat and barley to control wild oats (voluntarily canceled registration with EPA). It acts by rapid destruction of cell membranes. It has moderate acute toxicity in the rat/mammal, honeybees, earthworms, *Daphnia*, and algae due to its chemical nature. It is also an eye irritant.

Organic Arsenicals

Disodium methanearsonate (DSMA) and monosodium methanearsonate (MSMA) are registered herbicides that the EPA would like to have voluntarily discontinued or phased out based on their toxicity and the availability of less toxic alternatives. These herbicides are used for weed control on cotton, on turf/lawns, and under trees, vines, and shrubs. Their mode of action appears to be inhibition of plant growth by uncoupling phosphorylation with plants exhibiting chlorosis caused by loss of chlorophyll. Because arsenic is ubiquitous, one must consider background inorganic versus synthetic organic arsenic compounds. Where methyl mercury is more toxic than mercury based on percent absorption, the opposite is true for

arsenic. Despite the presence of arsenic in the compounds, organic arsenical herbicides have low to moderate acute toxicity via oral, dermal, and inhalation routes. The target organs for exposure to DSMA and MSMA are the large intestine (GI tract) and the kidney. DMA (cacodylic acid) appears to target the urinary bladder and the thyroid. CNS effects can occur at higher exposures including muscle weakness, spasms, coma, and convulsions. Circulatory failure can then result in death, as may renal failure. Inorganic arsenic is a human carcinogen, so compounds containing arsenic must have cancer risk assessed. Inorganic arsenic via high levels in drinking water results in liver, kidney, lung, bladder, and skin cancer. Based on the "worst case scenario" DSMA or MSMA does not exceed the LOC for cancer by exposure from registered uses or by animal testing. However, terrestrial mammals have chronic concerns many times exceeding the LOCs (arsenic compounds biotransform but never lose their arsenic). The same can be said for endangered and nonendangered plants.

Bromobutide

This may fit into the chemical class of amide herbicides, but also fits into organic bromide. It is used on rice paddy fields outside of the United States or Europe (Asia). Mechanistically, bromobutide may fit into the 4-hydroxyphenylpyruvate dioxygenase inhibitors, bleaching compounds. It has low acute rat toxicity, but is a skin and eye irritant. Other than this compound losing its bromine on metabolism, its ecological significance is still being studied by researchers in Japan (Tsuda et al., 2011).

Cinmethylin

This oxybicycloheptane compound is structurally similar to natural monoterpene 1,4-cineole that is used in the control of grass weeds preplant or pre-emergence. It was thought that this compound or the natural monoterpene prevents the plant from synthesizing the amino acid asparagine and that the metabolite of this herbicide (1,4-cineole) derivative was the true inhibitor asparagine synthetase (Romagni et al., 2000); however, that research article was retracted 5 years later. Another researcher discovered that cinmethylin inhibits plant tyrosine aminotransferase (conversion of tyrosine to 4-hydroxyphenylpyruvate; Grossman et al., 2012). Cinmethylin has moderate toxicity via the oral and dermal routes.

Cumyluron

Cumyluron is a urea analog. It has moderate acute oral toxicity in the rat and moderate acute toxicity to fish. In a summary of toxicology data by the California EPA (2009) on cumyluron, centrilobular hepatocellular swelling marks the liver as a target in chronic studies with the dog. Increased hepatocellular adenomas of the liver were found in the mouse. This compound also was slightly positive for mutagenicity by the bacterial reverse mutation assay. The activated method treated cells in the mammalian chromosome aberration test found chromosome aberration and polyploid cells. Subacute toxicity to rats indicated liver, kidney, and blood alterations.

Dazomet

Dazomet is a nonselective soil fumigant with herbicidal, fungicidal, and nematicidal properties. When applied, this compound rapidly degrades into the toxic methyl isothiocyanate (MITC) that is a volatile fumigant. MITC is a major concern, because levels exceeding 22 ppb causes eye irritation and systemic or respiratory effects, as expected from the Bhopal, India incident and other cyanide compounds' effects.

Dymron

Dymron (daimuron) is a novel substituted urea herbicide that is strongly inhibitory to the germination of sensitive plant species (Cyperaceae weeds) and prevents the elongation of the roots and underground stems (works efficiently late in the process) used in rice, cotton, corn, soybeans, and other crops. It is only slightly toxic via ingestion and subcutaneous routes. Similarly to bromobutide, it has use in rice paddy agriculture, and its environmental influences are being studied by Japanese researchers (Vu et al., 2006).

Pelargonic Acid

Nonanoic acid is another name of this chemical naturally found in almost all species of animals and plants. This biopesticide is an herbicide use to prevent growth of weeds indoors and outdoors and is a blossom thinner for apple and pear trees. This chemical is a skin and eye irritant but otherwise is not considered overtly toxic. Environmentally, nontarget plants are the only concern for herbicidal concentrations of pelargonic acid.

Plant Growth Regulators

Plant growth regulators are used to alter plant growth but not to kill them (dose-dependent). **Table 25-2** lists plant growth regulators, their action, and toxicity. The use of plant growth regulators can only be understood with the realization of factors controlling germination and growth. Water activates the germ plasm and protein synthesis resumes as protein formed during seed development reactivate. Control of the germination process occurs with four plant hormones. Abscisic acid blocks germination. Auxins control root formation and growth. Gibberellins regulate protein synthesis and stem elongation. Finally, cytokinins control organ differentiation. Ethylene gas is used for ripening of fruits and appears to have some regulatory role in certain plants.

Pyrimidine

Ancymidol initiates the discussion of gibberellic acid synthesis inhibitors of plant growth regulation use in treating container-grown herbaceous plants, ornamental woody shrubs, and bedding plants. Ancymidol has low acute oral, inhalation (Category III), and dermal (Category IV) toxicities and causes mild eye (Category III) and skin (Category IV) irritation. Clearly, the way it is used presents little human concern or ecological concern. However, an accidental spill may have ecological consequences at least to nontarget plants, but the data still need to be developed.

Ammonium

Chlormequat chloride is a quaternary ammonium compound that also inhibits gibberellic acid synthesis. The growth regulator is applied onto ornamental plants grown in greenhouses, nurseries, and shade houses. Although no human concerns of use are expressed by

TABLE 25-2   Plant Growth Regulator Listing by Mechanism of Action and Toxicity

Target of Regulator Action	Chemical Family of Regulator	Active Ingredient	Toxicity
Gibberellic acid synthesis inhibition	Pyrimidine	Ancymidol Flurprimidol	Nontarget plants possibly affected—unintended exposure
	Ammonium	Chlormequat chloride Daminozide	Can cause cholinergic crisis on high exposure but main concern is avian reproduction
	Triazole	Paclobutrazol Uniconazole-p	CYP51 inhibition = steroid synthesis inhibition + resulting endocrine, developmental, and reproductive toxicities
DNA synthesis inhibition	Cyclohexaketone	Dikegulac sodium	Only other fruiting trees nearby
Chemical pincher	Fatty acid	Methyl esters of fatty acids	Inhalation and chemical pneumonia
Growth promoter	Gibberellin	Gibberellic acid	Slight eye irritation + endocrine disruption + reproductive toxicity
	Synthetic cytokinin/gibberellin	Cytokinin/gibberellic acid	Cytokinin = thyroid microtubules inhibited
Ethylene generator	Acid	Ethephon	Severe eye irritant + blood cholinesterase inhibitor + danger to terrestrial plants
Rooting hormones	Rooting hormones Synthetic auxin	IBA IBA + NAA	Neurotoxic, immunotoxic, affects glucose tolerance, increases cGMP (IBA)

Based on Chemical Class Chart volume XI http://www.ohp.com/Labels_MSDS/PDF/CCC_XI.pdf

the EPA (although a worker who consumed a mouthful of this agent died of ventricular fibrillation to asystole typical of cholinergic crisis; Winek et al., 1990), the NOAEC could not be established for avian reproduction as the lowest dose yielded effects. Chlormequat chloride poses only a slight toxic risk to adult birds, reptile, and terrestrial amphibians. Based on how the compound is used, the application methods were defined by the EPA to prevent environmental drift and nontarget plant and animal exposures.

Triazole

Paclobutrazol is the final plant growth regulator examined that inhibits gibberellin synthesis. This chemical is used in nurseries, greenhouses, shade houses, and interior landscapes but can also be applied to turf with fertilizers. Applied in the latter way outside, it is classified as a nonselective post-emergent herbicide for control of annual grasses and broadleaf weeds (reduces need for lawn mowing and increases turf density) The EPA (2007b) did not have chronic data on this specific compound for ecological analysis, so it looked through triazole herbicides that were structurally similar and shared mechanisms in common of being demethylation inhibitor (DMI) fungicides that inhibited the CYP51 family (lanosterol 14-α-demethylase which is a critical enzyme in the synthesis of cholesterol from lanosterol). This CYP enzyme is conserved in plants, fungi, bacteria, and animals and may be the ancestor to all eukaryotic

CYPs. This has implications for steroid synthesis, endocrine disruption, and reproductive and developmental toxicity.

Cyclohexaketone

Dikegulac sodium is a DNA synthesis inhibitor (interferes with terminal growth areas) that is structurally similar to natural products involved in the biosynthesis of L-ascorbic acid and structurally similar to other plant cell wall components. This allows lateral shoots to be enhanced over the usual apical dominance (growth points). This agent is used as a chemical pincher (inhibits growth of suckers—a method for chemical pruning) for greenhouse and nursery ornamentals, growth control of landscape ornamentals, growth retardant for broadleaf trees, and suppression of flower and fruit formation in fruiting landscape trees and shrubs. This chemical carries a Category IV toxicity rating for acute oral, dermal, and inhalation exposure. Ocular irritation, iridial, and conjunctival changes that subsided after 10 days gave dikegulac sodium a Category II toxicity rating. Freshwater fish and invertebrates are little impacted by this chemical. Similarly, aquatic plants are not considered at risk from this plant growth regulator. Potentially, multiple applications and drift may affect fruiting trees adjacent to the sprayed area, but the overall impact is not considered problematic.

Fatty Acid

Methyl esters of fatty acids (aliphatic ester category of EPA) serve as chemical pinchers preventing sucker growth and also fall under plant growth regulators. These chemicals are methyl esters of hexanoic, octanoic, decanoic, and dodecanoic acid. They are slight skin and eye irritants and are not toxic orally. Acute inhalation analysis concerned the EPA regarding the development of chemical pneumonia by greenhouse handlers. However, based on their usage and structure, the environmental impact was considered to be minimal.

Gibberellin/Cytokinin

Shifting the focus to gibberellic acid or synthetic variants and cytokinin leads to the area of growth promoters (stimulate cell division

and elongation). They are applied to growing crops, ornamental and shade trees, shrubs, and vines and are considered nontoxic/natural. They do cause slight eye irritation (Category III), but otherwise are not a concern to humans, animals, or nontarget organisms. However, endocrine disruption (oxidative stress and decreased thyroid function; Troudi et al., 2011) and reproductive toxicity (inhibition of spermatogenesis and derangement of germ cells; Ravikumar and Srikumar, 2005) have occurred in rats. Cytokinin is not orally toxic, but causes slight toxicity (Category III) via the dermal route (acute or irritation—rabbit) and eye irritation (rabbit). Again, cytokinin's natural origin swayed EPA to a nontoxic classification including nontarget environmental species. However, plant cytokinins are derivatives of adenosine and interfere with thyroid function (dog follicular cells; Fernandez-Pol et al., 1977) via blocking cAMP-dependent microfilament organization (endocrine disruption; Laezza et al., 1997).

Acid

Ethephon is an organophosphonate plant growth regulator that works via stimulating ethylene generation. Ethylene is a ripening agent in fruit. It also aids in abscission (plant drops one or more parts as in fruit), flower induction, and breaking of apical dominance. This chemical poses a severe risk of eye irritation (Category I). There is some chronic risk to mammals (decreased growth); acute risk to birds, terrestrial-phase amphibians, and reptiles (mortality); and phytotoxicity to terrestrial plants. The animal effects may relate to ethephon's blood but not brain cholinesterase inhibition.

Rooting Hormones

IBA (indole-3-butyric acid) is a native auxin that is considered a rooting hormone because it promotes and accelerates cell elongation within stem cuttings. This process leads to the plant increasing its roots. As a common metabolite of tryptophan in humans, this substance is considered negligible in terms of toxicity by EPA. One study outlined possible effects of IBA on glucose tolerance in normal rats (Losert and Kraaz, 1975). A more recent study indicated deleterious effects of IBA on the antioxidant defense system of rat cells (Topalca et al., 2009). Another study indicated cholinesterase inhibition (neurotoxicity) and increased myeloperoxidase activity (immunotoxicity) in rats (Yilmaz and Celik, 2009). A mechanistic study of interest indicated that IBA increased rat guanylyl cyclase activity in the lung, small intestine, liver, and renal cortex (not just a plant effector; Vesely et al., 1985). Naphthalene acetic acid (NAA) is a potent synthetic auxin that increases root formation (number, length/dry weight root hairs, small and large) and is registered for use on fruit crops. The EPA suggests little risk to humans, other mammals, or nontarget environmental species. This is difficult to reconcile with naphthalene as a PAH that is known to have toxic effects on the neuroendocrine systems of species such as the teleost fish (e.g., rainbow trout; Gesto et al., 2009). However, making the compound more water soluble does allow conjugation prior to attaching the ring structures via oxidation and is mentioned prominently as safe glycine and glucuronide conjugates of the acid form by EPA.

Insecticides/Miticides

Insecticides are usually more toxic to humans as mechanisms are chosen that may compromise neurological function or by other action. Also, nontarget populations of insects such as bees are of concern, because it is generally not desirable to eliminate pollinators in crop production. **Table 25-3** lists insecticides/miticides, their action, and toxicity.

Carbamates

Carbaryl is one of the most widely used broad-spectrum insecticides for treating pets for fleas, in agricultural insect pest management, in professional turf management, and in garden markets. The concerns regarding this pesticide also extend to its manufacture after Bhopal, India experienced many deaths from methyl isothiocyanate used in the synthesizing carbaryl. Carbaryl use in the home is of concern as the reversible AChE inhibition (unless a lethal dose is administered without antidote of atropine) is higher in young rats that older ones. Handlers may suffer neurotoxicity from carbaryl's action. Carbaryl is also classified as a

likely human carcinogen, because it produces vascular tumors in mice. Unfortunately, bees cannot develop resistance to this type of insecticide, so carbaryl is considered very highly toxic to honeybees, estuarine/marine invertebrates, and other aquatic species such as the Atlantic salmon. Carbaryl is also an endocrine disruptor that appears to inhibit steroidogenesis in primary human granulosa-lutein cells at least in part by preventing the delivery of cholesterol over mitochondrial membranes and decreasing cAMP formation (Cheng et al., 2006).

Organophosphates

Organophosphates are usually stronger AChE inhibitors. Methyl parathion used to be one of these agents. Parathion had to be converted to paraoxon as the active form of this insecticide. It is so strong that it should not be sprayed within 1-2 miles of an apiary (bee facility). Some unlicensed users sprayed this substance into houses, which made the pets and people living inside ill as it was never meant to be used inside structures. It was voluntarily withdrawn from the United States in 2010. Malathion is a similar broad-spectrum insecticide and miticide in that it requires conversion to malaoxon to be active. This is done by oxidation of the $P = S$ moiety to $P = O$ via fast microsomal enzymes found in the insect or mammal to the active product. The reason the insect is more susceptible to AChE inhibition is that the mammal can convert malathion to inactive products via hydrolysis and binding, which is slow in the insect but fast in the mammal. Also, the malaoxon is rapidly hydrolyzed by A-esterases in the mammal to inactive products, while this process is slow in the insect. However, malaoxon can be an environmental breakdown product of malathion, making it readily available for neurotoxicity. Malathion has been used in agriculture, home use, and eradication programs for the boll weevil (southern United States), medfly (California), and mosquito control. It is also used as a pharmaceutical agent (pediculicide to treat head lice and their eggs). The acute toxicity by any route is considered low in rats, but young animals exhibit adverse effects more readily. There is suggestive evidence of carcinogenicity due to occurrence of hepatic tumors in rats at

TABLE 25-3　Insecticides/Miticides Listing by Mechanism of Action and Toxicity

Target of Insecticidal Action	Chemical Family	Active Ingredient	Toxicity
GABA-gated chloride channel antagonists	Cyclodiene organochlorines	Endosulfan	Banned based on persistence, neurotoxicity and organ toxicity including male reproductive organs.
Sodium channel modulators	Botanical	Pyrethrins	Neurotoxic, thyroid, cancer.
	Pyrethroids	Bifenthrin Cyfluthrin Fenpropathrin Fluvalinate Lambda-Cyhalothrin Permethrin	Neurotoxicity, possible carcinogen, and endocrine disruptor with chiral specificity of action.
Acetylcholinesterase Inhibitors	Carbamates	Carbaryl	AChE inhibition + vascular cancer + endocrine disruption.
	Organophosphates	Acephate Chlorpyrifos Dichlorvos Dimethoate Malathion Methidathion Oxydemeton-methyl Phosmet	AChE inhibition, parathyroid hyperplasias (both sexes), thyroid adenomas and carcinomas (male). Very high dose cytotoxic actions on liver, lung, disruption of adrenal medulla.
Nicotinic acetylcholine receptor agonists/antagonists (group 4)	Botanicals	Nicotine	Being phased out due to its high neurotoxicity.
	Neonicotinoids	Acetamiprid Dinotefuran Imidacloprid Thiamethoxam	Moderate oral toxicity, hepatic damage, developmental toxicity, and environmental concentrations & bee toxicity.
Nicotine acetylcholine receptor agonists (not group 4)	Spinosyns	Spinosad Spinetoram	Neurotoxic, reproductive toxin, thyroid disruption.
Chloride channel activators by interfering with GABA receptors in insects	Glycosides	Avermectin B1/Abamectin Milbemectin	Neurotoxicity, developmental and reproductive toxin + endocrine disruption (male rat).
Juvenile insect hormone mimics (growth regulator)	O-ethyl carbamate Pyridine	Fenoxycarb Pyriproxyfen s-Kinoprene	Clearly endocrine disruption in a limited species group based on activity + liver + kidney toxicity for pyriproxyfen.
Feeding blockers	Pyridine carboxyamides Pyridine azomethines	Flonicamid Pymetrozine	Neurotoxicity/liver cancer. Endocrine, liver, spleen, kidney, bone marrow changes.
Mite growth inhibitors	2,4-Diphenyloxazoline derivatives Tetrazines Thiazolidinones	Etoxazole Clofentezine Hexythiazox	Toxic degradation products. Freshwater species effects. ROS & genotoxicity in human lymphocyte assays.

TABLE 25-3 Insecticides/Miticides Listing by Mechanism of Action and Toxicity (*continued*)

Target of Insecticidal Action	Chemical Family	Active Ingredient	Toxicity
Site I electron transport inhibitor (METI acaracides/insecticides)	Pyridazinones	Pyridaben	Acute neurotoxicity & Parkinson's disease pathway.
	Phenoxypyrazoles	Fenpyroximate	Heart block + *in vitro* genotoxicity.
Inhibitors of acetyl CoA carboxylase	Tetronic acids	Spiromesifen	Liver, spleen, thyroid, adrenal.
	Tetramic acids	Spirotetramat	Thyroid & thymus (dog), testes epididymides (rat), bee brood disruption.
Inhibit microsomal metabolism (not insecticidal on their own)	Synergizing agents	MGK-264 Piperonyl butoxide	Liver damage + aquatic organisms sensitivity.
Unknown or uncertain action	Carbazates	Bifenazate	Liver, spleen, adrenal cortex.
	Biopesticide insect growth regulators	Azadirachtin	Some dermal sensitization. High human dose neurotoxicity
		Pyridalyl	Toxic to target insect cells but not mammalian in cell culture.
Miscellaneous	Oils	Clarified hydrophobic extract of neem oil Paraffinic oil Petroleum oil	Generally considered low toxicity but should avoid application to sensitive plants or on water surfaces. Dermal, eye (NH_4^+), aquatic invertebrates
	Soaps	Potassium salts of fatty acids	(K^+).
	Biopesticides	*Beauveria bassiana*	Eye irritation, dermal sensitizer, honeybees.
Microbial disruption of insect midgut membranes	Bioinsecticides	*Bacillus Thuringiensis* (BT) Karstaki or Israelensis	Butterfly species lethality (controversial).
Disrupt oxidative phosphorylation	Organotins	Fenbutatin-oxide	Persistent aquatic organism toxicity/bioaccumulation.
Uncouple oxidative phosphorylation	Pyrroles	Chlorfenapyr	Highly toxic to birds — EPA rejected registration request.
Inhibit chitin biosynthesis — type 0/Lepidopteran	Benzoyl urea insect growth regulators	Diflubenzuron Novaluron	Aquatic invertebrates + marine/estuarine crustaceans, carcinogenic metabolite
Inhibit chitin biosynthesis — type 1, Homopteran		Buprofezin	Liver and thyroid (endocrine).
Molting disruptor, Dipteran	Triazine insect growth regulators	Cyromazine	Estuarine/marine invertebrates? Birds, fish, mammals- not acute
Ecdysone agonist/molting disruptors	Growth regulators	Tebufenozide	Reproduction in quail.
Coupling site II electron transport inhibitors (Complex III)	Amidinohydrazone	Hydramethylnon	Mitochondrial poison, male reproduction, cancer, aquatic.
	Napthoquinone derivates	Acequinocyl	Vitamin K antagonism & hemorrhaging.

Modified from Chemical Class Chart volume XI http://www.ohp.com/Labels_MSDS/PDF/CCC_XI.pdf

high doses and the presence of few rate tumors of rats. Chronic studies reported in the EPA (2009c) summary document indicated parathyroid hyperplasia in male and female rats and a significant trend in male rats of thyroid follicular cell adenomas and carcinomas and thyroid c-cell carcinomas (endocrine disruption and cancer—but not a major concern according to EPA). Very high doses (33,051 mg/kg/day) to Wistar rats for 40 days caused regular arrangement of hepatocytes with dilated sinusoidal spaces, thickened lung epithelium, regression of adrenal medulla with congestion and disruption of the germ line as cytotoxic actions of malathion (Saadi et al., 2008).

Cyclodiene Organochlorines

DDT was a neurotoxic persistent organochlorine insecticide that was found to accumulate in species and decimated the California condor population, eagles, and other raptors at the top of the food chain. There were also concerns for DDT and DDE (breakdown product) in human females and breast cancer. Similar organochlorines have been banned by the EPA. Endosulfan can now be added to the banned compounds. It was used as a contact insecticide and acaricide for agricultural (crops) and ornamental plants. Endosulfan interfered with inhibitory presynaptic GABA (γ-aminobutyric acid) receptors on insect neurons leading to repetitive nervous discharges. Unfortunately, GABA is the most prevalent inhibitory CNS neurotransmitter in mammals and other organisms as well. The organochlorine nature of this compound made it more persistent than the EPA thought in 2002 and a suit by farm workers convinced the agency to reassess the exposure data. Workers' health risks (high acute oral and inhalation toxicity) were assessed to be greater than already known (even to those using personal protective equipment), and increased risk to fish and birds was also found (bioaccumulation in fish and up the food chain = persistence issues). Endosulfan is neurotoxic and damages the kidneys, liver, and male reproductive organs (endocrine disruption) in lab animal testing.

Pyrethroids/Botanical Pyrethrins

Pyrethroids and synthetic and pyrethrins are naturally obtained neurotoxic sodium channel modulators. They poison the axon by interfering with sodium channels (prolonging Na^+ permeability during the excitatory phase of the action potential) in both the central and peripheral nervous systems, causing paralysis via repetitive nervous discharges. One of the synthetic pyrethroids used to mimic natural substances from chrysanthemums found in Australia and Africa was sprayed in 2012 over Dallas and similar communities to kill mosquito vectors of West Nile virus. Bifenthrin is an example of a Type I pyrethroid insecticide used to control aphids, worms, ants (including southern fire ants), gnats, moths, beetles, grasshoppers, mites, midges, spiders, ticks, yellow jackets, maggots, thrips, caterpillars, flies, fleas, and other pests in domestic, public health, agricultural, and industrial settings. Bifenthrin is highly toxic to terrestrial invertebrates including honeybees. This insecticide is categorized as a possible human carcinogen and is an endocrine disruptor. Specifically, this chiral pesticide, the 1S-cis isomer of bifenthrin (but not the 1R-cis isomer), significantly reduced the secretion of progesterone and prostaglandin E$_2$, decreased expression of genes regulating rate-limiting steps in progesterone biosynthesis (P450$_{scc}$, StAR, PBR, DBI, COX-2), disrupted transcription activation of StAR and COX-2 promoter, and inhibited protein kinase C (PKC; signaling mediator of progesterone and PGE$_2$ synthesis) by forming a hydrogen bond between PKC and the 1S-cis isomer of bifenthrin in rat ovarian granulosa cells (Liu et al., 2011). As might be expected, aquatic organisms such as fish are highly sensitive to the action of these compounds. Pyrethrins are botanical insecticides containing six naturally active ingredients: pyrethrin 1, pyrethrin 2, cinerin 1, cinerin 2, jasmolin 1, and jasmolin 2. The critical toxicological effects of pyrethrins according to the EPA (2006b) are neurobehavioral toxicity, chronic thyroid toxicity (changes in serum thyroid hormones = endocrine disruption), and liver damage. Inhalation can also cause lesions in the respiratory tract. There is also suggestive evidence of carcinogenicity (benign liver tumors in female rats). Synergists that inhibit the metabolism of pyrethroids or pyrethrins are MGK-264 and piperonyl butoxide (inhibits microsomal enzymes). Piperonyl butoxide

(PBO) has been around since the 1950s and has been used as a synergizing agent with pyrethrins, pyrethroids, and organophosphates. This synergizing agent has low acute toxicity by all three routes but is a dermal sensitizer. The main target organ of PBO is the liver, increasing liver weight and liver histopathology (enlarged hepatocytes with glassy cytoplasm, oval cell proliferation, bile duct hyperplasia, and focal necrosis in rats). Because PBO works effectively as a synergist in insects (inhibits microsomal enzymes at effective doses) but not in mammals (inhibits microsomal enzymes transiently only at high doses), the EPA saw no reason to assess human health risks of mixtures of PBO with other insecticide ingredients. PBO is a possible human carcinogen (high ileocecal ulcers, liver adenomas and carcinomas with Fisher 344 rats at very high doses or in CD-1 mice, slight increase in thyroid follicular cell tumors in Sprague Dawley rats). PBO is moderately acutely toxic to freshwater and estuarine/marine fish, moderately to highly acutely toxic to freshwater invertebrates, and highly acutely toxic to estuarine invertebrates and amphibians.

Neonicotinoids/Nicotine

These bind to nicotinic acetylcholine receptors, disrupting nerve transmission (agonists or antagonists) and causing paralysis and death of the target insects. Acetamiprid is not very acutely toxic dermally or inhaled, but was moderately toxic on oral dosing to lab animals. High doses of this insecticide appear to cause hepatic vacuolation in rats. Some rib abnormality was noted in rat developmental studies. The neonicotinoid insecticides have come under recent scrutiny due to studies indicating reduced bumblebee colony growth and queen production (especially the most utilized agent imidacloprid; Whitehorn et al., 2012) and questions of the role of these agents in the noted collapse of certain colonies in the United States and Europe. Foraging efficiency of worker bees may play some role in this effect (Mommaerts et al., 2010). The EPA is reassessing the benefit of this class of insecticides based on these findings. Nicotine (from tobacco) can be used on ornamental plants (poinsettias popular in December) in greenhouses only but not on violets. Some of the benefit of nicotine is that white flies

have not been reported to develop resistance to this agent. Unfortunately, nicotine is a powerful neurotoxic (and active at neuromuscular junctions) agent categorized as highly acutely toxic (Category I) by all routes of exposure (1–4 mg in adult humans may yield toxicity). This is clearly an insecticide that is being phased out as other agents are less toxic and yield similar benefit.

Spinosyns

Spinosad (and spinetoram) is used on a variety of crops, ornamentals, poultry, pet kennels, domestic dwellings, aquatic sites, food-handling establishments, refuse sites, ant mounds, and seed treatment, and as a mosquitocide and fruit fly bait. It works and is neurotoxic to nontarget species due to disruption of the nicotinic/GABA-gated chloride channels. There is an acute risk to freshwater, free-swimming invertebrates; risk to mammals; and potential risk to terrestrial invertebrates. Only spinetoram is a dermal sensitizer, but not spinosad. High doses ($\geq$ 0.05% in feed) of spinosad damage the adrenal glands, liver, lymphoid cells, reproductive tissues, kidney, thyroid, stomach, lung, and skeletal muscles of rats. Chronic toxicity was observed at $\geq$ 0.05% spinosad in feed in rats with vacuolation and inflammation of the thyroid, which extends into the lymphoid tissue and lung if given over a 2-year period. This makes this compound a neurotoxin, a reproductive toxin, and an endocrine disruptor.

Glycosides

Avermectin B1 (Abamectin) is a natural macrocyclic lactone (from *Streptomyces avermitilis*) used as an anthelmintic (treats parasitic worms), insecticide, and miticide due to its GABA receptor antagonism in the insect, parasite, or mite. This compound has extreme mammalian and aquatic invertebrate acute toxicity and is highly toxic to fish and bees. Interestingly, avermectin is relatively nontoxic to birds. This insecticide is also a developmental toxicant as it induces cleft palate in the CF1 mouse. Avermectin also causes testicular infiltration of blood vessels with marked hemorrhage and a significant accumulation of connective tissue surrounding the seminiferous tubules (affects male rat fertility—reproductive toxicant and endocrine disruptor; Elbetieha and Da'as, 2003).

Juvenile Hormone Mimics

Juvenile hormone-mimicking agents (s-Kinoprene, fenoxycarb, and the pyridine compound pyriproxyfen) prevent molting from the larval stage to the adult stage. Overall, kinoprene appears to have low acute toxicity except to *Daphnia* (moderate toxicity based on 48-h EC_{50}) and honeybees (moderate based on 48-h LD_{50}). However, this chemical is irritating to the eyes and the skin. It is of interest that *Daphnia* were also used to screen juvenoid activity of kinoprene and found to potentiate the activity of methyl farnesoate, a chemical that determines male sex hormone regulation in this species, so at least for a certain grouping of species this qualifies under endocrine disruption (relatively obvious from its insecticidal activity; Wang et al., 2005). s-Kinoprene and fenoxycarb are not really in use, but the growth regulator pyriproxyfen does target metamorphosis in insects and is used on various vegetable crops, vine-climbing fruits, and watercress. In subchronic and chronic analyses, pyriproxyfen affects the liver and kidneys. It also appears to affect genes in *Daphnia* (inducing Hb; Gorr et al., 2006; or increasing number of males; Oda et al., 2006). Again, this is clearly a case of endocrine disruption in a limited group of species.

Pyridine Azomethines and Carboxamides

These agents are selective feeding blockers with unknown or nonspecific mode of action. Pymetrozine (azomethine) is used to control certain aphids on cucurbit vegetables, fruiting vegetables, potatoes (tubers), and tobacco. This insecticide yields only slight dermal sensitization and is not acutely toxic. The EPA (2000c) fact sheet mentioned neurotoxicity in an acute neurotoxicity study (reduced body temperature, function observation battery changes, and decreased motor activity in male rats at lowest dose tested). Subchronic neurotoxicity was noted by stereotypy in males and tiptoe gait in females). In chronic feeding studies, hepatocellular hypertrophy was noted (and hemosiderosis in mice) and liver tumors (female rats positive for hepatomas and/or carcinomas = likely human carcinogen). Flonicamid (carboxamide but can also be considered a nicotinoid insecticide) also

affects feeding behavior. This insecticide causes hyaline deposits in kidneys and liver centrilobular hypertrophy in rats on a subchronic feeding study in rats. Mice given this compound over a 90-day period showed liver, spleen, and bone marrow histopathologic changes. Dogs given flonicamid also had increased adrenal and decreased thymus weights (endocrine/immune). Mice over a chronic exposure had increased alveolar/bronchiolar adenomas.

Tetrazines/Thiazolidinones/2,4-Diphenyloxazoline Derivatives

All these agents are mite growth inhibitors that work via unknown or nonspecific mode of action. Clofentezine is a tetrazine miticide that acts as an ovicide used on fruits, walnuts, and ornamental plants. This compound is not necessarily a cause for concern, but its abiotic hydrolysis product 2-chlorobenzoic acid hydrazide and direct photolysis product 2-chlorobenzonitrile may indeed be of concern. However, it does appear that one bivalve mollusk finds this type of insecticide problematic for its antioxidant defense systems (thiols, GSH, metallothioneins; Falfushinska et al., 2012). Additionally, clofentezine appears to increase liver metabolism and excretion of thyroid hormone (Hurley, 1998). Hexythiazox is an ovicide of the thiazolidinone chemical class (kills mite eggs at early stages of development by an unknown mechanism) used on a variety of fruit crops. Although mammals and honeybees are not very affected by this compound, hexythiazox is acutely highly toxic to freshwater fish and invertebrates (bluegill and *Daphnia* $LC_{50}s$ = 0.53 and 0.74 ppm, respectively). Etoxazole is a 2,4-diphenyloxzoline derivative acaricide (mites), but has low toxicity to beneficial non-mite arthropods such as pirate bugs and does not pose a threat to honeybees. It is used on fruit crops and walnuts and appears to act via chitin biosynthesis inhibition (Nauen and Smagghe, 2006). Fish have been tested for oxidative stress with various pesticides, and etoxazole exposure was associated with generation of superoxide radicals that decreased catalase activity and increased phagocytic activity of splenocytes (Slaninova et al., 2009). In human lymphocytes, this insecticide had troubling aspects of positive results in the chromosome aberration test, sister chromatid exchange, and micronucleus test (three genotoxic assays). This compound also decreased the mitotic index while not affecting the replication index at all tested concentrations. All three of the miticides discussed in this section have to be rotated along with integrated pest management because mites can develop resistance to any of these agents.

Bioinsecticides

Bacillus thuringiensis is a soil bacterium famous as Bt corn and other products (Bt cotton). This engineered crop is controversial with natural food advocates, but has the advantage of being an organism with toxicity to insects but not to people. The major concern for EPA is resistance and overuse of the product. However, despite the National Academy of Science's analysis with regard to the monarch butterfly (Hellmich et al., 2001), articles still appear indicating lethal effects of Bt products on certain butterfly species such as Bt176 maize/corn pollen on the European Peacock butterfly (Felke et al., 2010).

Organotins

Inhibition of oxidative phosphorylation/ATP biosynthesis at the site of dinitrophenol uncoupling is the mechanism affected by organotins such as fenbutatin oxide that work as an acaricide (mite control). This insecticide is a severe eye irritant in rabbits (Category I). This miticide is persistent (Sn) and is highly toxic to aquatic organisms and can bioaccumulate in these species. Reductions in spermatogenesis and steroidogenesis were observed in mice treated with fentin and fenbutatin, so there may be some reproductive and endocrine effects at least in certain mixtures (Reddy et al., 2006).

Pyrroles

Chlorfenapyr uncouples oxidative phosphorylation via disruption of the H^+ gradient (chemiosmotic coupling). This pesticide did not meet the requirements for EPA registration because it had severe effects on bird reproduction and high to very high oral toxicity in adult birds (risks outweigh benefits and Spinosad and Tebufenozide

are suggested alternatives to control beet armyworms). This insecticide is also persistent ($t_{1/2} = 9$ months). Mallard ducks receiving 10 ppm experienced neurotoxicity, and half of the ducks died (LD_{50}). Emaciation and elevated organ weight/body weight are indicators of chlorfenapyr exposure, with the liver as the preferred tissue for chemical confirmation (Albers et al., 2006).

Benzoyl Urea Insect Growth Regulators

Diflubenzuron inhibits chitin biosynthesis in lepidopterans. It does affect molting hormone source in its control of insect growth in development of *Tenebrio molitor* (darkling beetle; Soltani et al., 1989). This insecticide is usually of low acute toxicity but does affect Hb of animals. A metabolite of diflubenzuron is *p*-chloroaniline, a probable human carcinogen (as is likely also true for another metabolite *p*-chlorphenylurea). Environmentally, freshwater aquatic invertebrates and marine/estuarine crustaceans experience high toxicity to this insecticide, which affects reproduction, growth, and survival in these aquatic species.

Buprofezin

Buprofezin is a chitin synthesis inhibitor in Homopterans. It disrupts molting, suppresses oviposition, and reduces egg viability in planthoppers, leafhoppers, whiteflies, and scales. This insecticide has little acute impact. The EPA (2003b) reports that subchronic studies in the rat resulted in microscopic lesions in the liver and thyroid weight increases in males. Chronic male rat studies yielded follicular cell hyperplasia and hypertrophy. Chronic mouse studies were more likely to produce hepatocellular adenomas and carcinomas in females (suggestive but weak evidence for cancer).

Triazine Insect Growth Regulators

Molting disruption in dipterans is the mechanism of action of cyromazine. This insecticide reduces fathead minnow growth at 36 mg/L and daphnid growth and reproduction at 0.64 mg/L. As cyromazine inhibits chitin synthesis, it may have chronic effects in estuarine/marine invertebrates (survivorship, growth, and reproduction). The EPA (2007c) cyromazine summary document listed chronic studies with the mallard duck that indicated significant reductions in hatchlings at 300 ppm (reproduction). Slight treatment-related increase in the number of male bobwhite quails with regressed testes was also noted at 300 ppm of cyromazine. The EPA suggests a presumptive risk for mammals and birds (surrogate for reptiles and terrestrial-phase amphibians).

Growth Regulators—Ecdysone

Ecdysone is a steroidal prohormone secreted by the prothoracic gland that promotes molting (premature molting). Tebufenozide is an ecdysone agonist that targets molting in lepidopterans, classifying it as an insect endocrine disruptor. Human concerns are small because acute toxicity assays have not indicated toxicity. The EPA (2008b) tebufenozide summary document described the results a quail study (no mallard duck study) suggesting reproductive effects on birds. Reproductive effects in fish had not been addressed by chronic exposures, so this was noted by the EPA.

Coupling Site II Electron Transport Inhibitors

Hydramethylnon and the naphthoquinone derivative acequinocyl fit the profile of inhibition of mitochondrial electron transport at the cytochrome bc_1 complex. Acutely this insecticide is not considered very toxic, but at near lethal oral doses in rats it caused excess salivation, decreased activity, anorexia, bloody nose, and difficulty with coordination/balance. Male rats showed less inclination to mate and testicular degeneration, prostate atrophy, and germ cell damage (reproduction and endocrine). Calves (Holsteins) given 113.5 g hydramethylnon developed leucopenia, lymphopenia, and eosinopenia. Mice given 50–100 ppm in their diet chronically developed lung adenomas and carcinomas (possible human carcinogen). There is also moderate to very high toxicity in freshwater fish (can bioaccumulate due to high K_{OW}) and moderate toxicity to freshwater invertebrates. Acequinocyl is a miticide but is also a vitamin K antagonist. This latter activity disrupts blood coagulation, which was observed as internal hemorrhages in a subchronic rat study as listed in the EPA (2003c) acequinocyl fact sheet.

Bulging eyeballs were also noted. The mouse also experiences liver damage (histopathology and liver enzymes in the plasma) with chronic exposure to this insecticide.

Pyridazinones and Phenoxypyrazoles

Pyridaben is a pyridazinone miticide/insecticide that works via inhibition of site I mitochondrial electron transport. Orally it is acutely toxic to the mouse (Category II), but produces slight eye irritation or other acute toxicity. However, acute neurotoxicity in rats may be of consequence especially considering that this insecticide, the herbicide Paraquat, and the fungicide maneb share some troubling disruption of concordant signaling pathways of idiopathic Parkinson's disease (axonal guidance signaling, Wnt/β-catenin signaling, IL-6 signaling, ephrin receptor signaling, TGF-β signaling, PPAR signaling, and G-protein coupled receptor signaling; Gollamudi et al., 2012). Developmental toxicity was illustrated by incomplete ossification of some bones. The phenoxypyrazole fenpyroximate shares the same insecticidal mode of action, but is more toxic (moderate acute oral and inhalation toxicity and is a slight to moderate skin sensitizer). The NY State Department of Environmental Conservation (2003) lists a number of animal studies showing toxicity of this insecticide especially in dogs and rats. Fenpyroximate caused first- and second-degree heart block (bradycardia) at high doses in dogs in a subchronic study. Liver damage (hepatocellular necrosis) was observed in a subchronic oral rat study in females. Although carcinogenesis was not observed with this compound, it appears that many methylpyrazoles share genotoxic activity in the SH-SY5Y neuroblastoma line (Graillot et al., 2012).

Tetronic and Tetramic Acids

This category is characterized by insecticidal inhibitors of acetyl CoA carboxylase. Spiromesifen is a tetronic acid that overall has low acute toxicity potential except as a contact sensitizer (moderate toxicity). Short- and long-term animal toxicity tests yielded loss of body weight adrenal effects (endocrine—discoloration, increase in fine vesiculation, and presence of cytoplasmic eosinophilia in zona fasciculate cells), thyroid effects (endocrine—decreased T_3 and T_4, increased TSH, increased thyroxine binding capacity, colloidal alteration, follicular cell hypertrophy), liver effects (increased alkaline phosphatase, ATL and decreased cholesterol, triglycerides), and spleen effects (atrophy, decreased spleen cell count, and increased macrophages). Spirotetramat is a tetramic acid that exhibits low to moderate acute toxicity via oral, dermal, and inhalation routes. This insecticide is an eye irritant and shows skin-sensitization potential in animals and humans. Spirotetramat targets the thyroid and thymus (endocrine and immune) in oral subchronic exposure to dogs. The testes-epididymides were the target organs for the subchronic oral rat study (EPA, 2013). The Australian Pesticides and Veterinary Medicines Authority (2007) indicated that adult honeybees do not experience harm from this insecticide, but that brood disruption was observed in field feeding studies (recovered following spirotetramat dissipation).

Unknown or Uncertain Action

Carbazates (bifenazate) and the biopesticide insect growth regulators azadirachtin and pyridalyl fit into this category. It appears that bifenazate has an allosteric modulator effect on spider mite GABA receptors (site distinct from GABA binding site) that currently is not conclusively related to its miticide activity (Hiragaki et al., 2012). Bifenazate appears to target the liver, spleen, and adrenal cortex (endocrine). Azadirachtin is a mixture of limonoid compounds extracted from seeds of the neem tree, *Azadirachta indica* A. Juss native to India. It interferes with feeding, molting, mating, and egg laying and at high doses causes mortality an inhibition of AChE (Senthil Nathan et al., 2008). It is a Category III or IV acute toxicant but is a dermal sensitizer. It can produce reversible neurotoxicity if consumed in high doses in humans (Iyyadurai et al., 2010). Pyridalyl is a newer agent that affects cells from Lepidoptera or Thysanoptera without mammalian cell activity. It requires CYP activation resulting in the production of ROS that damage cellular macromolecules and enhance proteasome activity. Protein degradation and necrotic cell death result. This mechanism was discovered by introducing sublethal doses of pyridalyl and noting upregulation of thiol peroxiredoxin in resistant cells and is prevented by CYP inhibitors. Additionally, three proteasome subunits were upregulated in susceptible cells along with Hsp70 stress protein and glyceraldehyde 3-phosphate dehydrogenases (Powell, 2011).

Miscellaneous

The biopesticide *Beauveria bassiana* strains 447, ATCC 74040, GHA, and HF23 are based on ubiquitous soil fungi and control insects by germination and growth on the exoskeletons of target pests and secretion of enzymes into their soft tissue. It is mainly a Category III (eye irritation or acute inhalation) to Category IV toxicity indicating small effects at worst acutely. However, strain HF23 was a Category II eye irritant. Strain ATCC 74040 is a dermal sensitizer. There may be some effects on beneficial insects such as honeybees at temperatures below 37°C as this microbe does not survive above this temperature. Cold-pressed neem oil is now approved by the EPA as the need to control bed bugs has become a problem seeking a solution (other than heating the infested house to 120°F). This mixture of several C_{26} terpenoids has yielded only a Category III for acute dermal exposure. The terpenoids are likely the insecticidal nature of neem oil. Other oils may work via preventing respiration/gas exchange in insects as well as prevent feeding on sprayed surfaces. Oils are also fungistatic, preventing further mold growth. Highly refined stylet oils may also control insects from spreading plant viruses as well as insect, mite, and fungal pathogens by preventing the retention in the stylets of aphid mouthparts. These nonspecific oils (petroleum for instance) may have to be used carefully if used in the environment because an oil layer on top of water may affect a variety of beneficial insects and aquatic organisms. Additionally, unsaturated hydrocarbons are unstable and may form toxic substances when sprayed on plants. This can be avoided by selecting oils with high-percentage unsulfonated residue (degree of oil refinement). Also, oils with low viscosity (expressed in Saybolt seconds) are less likely to produce plant injury. Soap salts (potassium or ammonium salts of fatty acids) are also used to control insects. Potassium salts of fatty acids are used as insecticides/acaricides, herbicides, and algaecides. Ammonium salts of fatty acids are used as rabbit and deer repellents. Soap salts overall have low toxicity but can yield moderate dermal irritation with repeated exposure. Ammonium salts can also permanently damage the eye. Potassium salts are highly toxic to aquatic invertebrates.

Fungicides

Fungicides are used to eliminate mold (rust, mildew, rot, scab, blight, spot) growth on seeds, crops, or harvested produce. Their occasional antimicrobial action is used in preserving wood, paints, and so forth. **Table 25-4** lists fungicides, their action, and toxicity.

Thiophanates, Methylbenzimidazole, Carbamates

These compounds have antifungal activity via inhibition of tubulin formation in mitosis. Acute toxicity was low for thiophanate-methyl

(EPA, 2005f) but was a skin sensitizer (Magnusson guinea pig maximization test). Other studies listed by the EPA included chronic feeding studies yielded liver and thyroid gland hypertrophy and thyroid hyperplasia (endocrine) in rats. Developmental toxicity was observed as increased incidence of supernumerary ribs and decreased fetal weights in rabbits. Chronically exposed mice were found to have statistically significant dose-dependent increases in hepatocellular adenomas (and carcinomas in males) and thyroid cell adenomas in males at the highest tested dose (likely to be carcinogenic in humans).

Dicarboximides

Iprodione is a contact and/or locally systemic fungicide registered for a variety of crops, lawns, and ornamental plants acting by inhibiting cell division (DNA/RNA synthesis and metabolism). It is a Category III acute toxicant by most routes and is not a dermal sensitizer. This fungicide is not mutagenic but is a likely human carcinogen based on evidence of liver

---

TABLE 25-4   Fungicides Listing by Mechanism of Action and Toxicity

Target of Fungicidal Action	Chemical Family	Active Ingredient	Toxicity
Affect cell division, DNA/RNA synthesis and metabolism	Dicarboximides	Iprodione Thiophanate-methyl	Cancer, developmental, reproductive, fish and marine/estuarine invertebrates.
Inhibition of tubulin formation in mitosis	Carbamates (MBC fungicides) Thiophanates Methyl benzimidazole		Cancer, liver, thyroid, development.
Demethylation (DMI) inhibition of sterol synthesis	Demethylation Inhibitors	Triadimefon Myclobutanil	Neurotoxicity, possible cancer, freshwater fish & invertebrates.
	Imidazole	Triflumizole Imazalil	Liver, lymph, endocrine, neurotoxicity.
	Triazole Pyrimidine	Propiconazole Fenarimol	Reproductive, fish, green algae. Developmental, neurotoxicity, possible cancer, liver, endocrine.
Affect RNA synthesis	Phenylamides/Acylamine	Metalaxyl-M	Cardiac toxicity.
Inhibition of isomerase in sterol synthesis	Piperadines Morpholine	Piperalin	Skin irritation, aquatic organisms (not plant).
Affect mitochondrial transport chain	Phenyl-benzamides	Flutolanil	Liver, developmental, reproductive.

TABLE 25-4   Fungicides Listing by Mechanism of Action and Toxicity (*continued*)

Target of Fungicidal Action	Chemical Family	Active Ingredient	Toxicity
Quinone inside inhibitors	Cyano-imidazole	Cyazofamid	Weak allergic reactions in mice, kidney, endocrine, development.
Quinone outside inhibitors	Srobilurins	Azoxystrobin Kresoxim-methyl Trifloxystrobin Pyraclostrobin	Fish and aquatic invertebrates.
	Imidazolinones	Fenamidone	Shrimp, fish, aquatic invertebrates.
MAP protein kinase in osmotic signal transduction	Phenylpyrrole (PP fungicides)	Fludioxonil	Liver, kidney, aquatic organisms, endocrine
Lipid peroxidation (proposed)	Thiadiazole	Etridiazole	Cancer, liver, endocrine, reproductive.
	Aromatic Hydrocarbon	Pentachloronitrobenzene (PCNB)	Cancer, aquatic organisms, bioaccumulation + volatile long-range air pollutant.
3-Keto reductase during C4 demethylation in sterol biosynthesis	Hydroxyanilide	Fenhexamid	Blood, adrenal.
Chitin synthase inhibition in cell wall development	Polyoxins (biopesticides)		Trout, *Daphnia*.
Affect cell membrane permeability (proposed)	Carbamate	Propamocarb	Neurotoxic, oxidative, GI, endocrine
Mode of action unknown or cannot be place in any grouping	Phosphite Ethyl phosphonates	Phosphorus acid	Harmful as acid via all routes and moderate eye irritant.
Phospholipid biosynthesis and cell wall deposition (proposed)	Cinnamic acid amides	Dimethomorph	Prostate, liver, arteritis, trout, estuarine invertebrates.
Multisite activity (M1)	Copper, fixed Copper, complex	Copper hydroxide Copper sulfate	Liver, neurological, possible cancer, aquatic organisms.
(M3)	Dithiocarbamates & relatives	Mancozeb	ETU metabolite — thyroid cancer, neurotoxicity.
(M4)	Phthalimides	Captan	Endocrine, cancer, eye irritant, fish, crab, *Daphnia* reproduction, algae growth
(M5)	Chloronitriles	Chlorothalonil	GI, kidney, cancer, eye irritant.
Not classified	Botanic extract	*Macheaya* extract	May have medicinal properties.
		Raynoutria sachalinesis	Antioxidant but may be slightly harmful to egg parasitoid.
	Oil	Clarified hydrophobic extract of neem oil	Low dermal toxicity, eye irritation, and mild sensitizer.
	Biopesticide	*Bacillus subtilis* GB03 *Bacillus subtilis* QST713	Some plant diseases may be possible but is not likely to lead to human toxicity/disease.
		Trichoderma harzianum T22 *Trichoderma virens* GL21	No mammalian toxicity. Unlikely with registered use to have aquatic toxicity.
		Streptomyces lydicus WYEC108	No plant or mammalian toxicity noted.

(*continues*)

Target of Fungicidal Action	Chemical Family	Active Ingredient	Toxicity
TABLE 25-4 Fungicides Listing by Mechanism of Action and Toxicity (*continued*)			
Not classified (cont'd)	Bicarbonate	Potassium bicarbonate	Considered relatively non-toxic with cautionary statement for child access to pure chemical.
	Hydrogen dioxide	Hydrogen peroxide	Natural oxidizing agent with limited toxicity.
Not classified	Biopesticide	*Trichoderma harzianum* T22 *Trichoderma virens* GL21	No mammalian toxicity. Unlikely with registered use to have aquatic toxicity.
		Bacillus subtilis GB03 *Bacillus subtilis* QST713	Some plant diseases may be possible but is not likely to lead to human toxicity/disease.
		Streptomyces lydicus WYEC108	No plant or mammalian toxicity noted.
	Bicarbonate	Potassium bicarbonate	Considered relatively non-toxic with cautionary statement for child access to pure chemical.
	Hydrogen dioxide	Hydrogen peroxide	Natural oxidizing agent with limited toxicity.
	Oil	Clarified hydrophobic extract of neem oil	Low dermal toxicity, eye irritation, and mild sensitizer.
	Botanic extract	*Macheaya* extract	May have medicinal properties.
		Raynoutria sachalinesis	Antioxidant but may be slightly harmful to egg parasitoid.

Modified from Chemical Class Chart volume XI http://www.ohp.com/Labels_MSDS/PDF/CCC_XI.pdf

tumors in mice and Leydig cells of the male rat (reproductive or endocrine as well). Developmental toxicity is noted by decreased anogenital distance. This compound can also be metabolized to 3,5-dichloroanaline (3,5-DCA) and its estimate of cumulative risk assessment from consumption of food and water is based on the 3,5-DCA content. Environmentally, iprodione represents little risk to birds, small mammals, and honeybees, but is moderately toxic to fish (freshwater or estuarine/marine), and is moderately to highly toxic to estuarine/marine invertebrates.

Imidazole, Pyrimidine, Triazole, Demethylation Inhibitors

These compounds have antifungal activity via inhibition of demethylation inhibition (DMI) of sterol (ergosterol is fungal sterol) synthesis, thereby destabilizing fungal cell walls.

Triflumizole (imidazole) is a broad-spectrum foliar fungicide. Toxicological concern extends to the 4-chloro-2-trifluoromethyl aniline metabolite. The EPA (2007d) triflumizole summary document lists this fungicide's primary target as the liver in subchronic studies on rodents, which appear more sensitive than the dog (unusual) for this compound. At high doses, microsomal induction was noted. The same EPA document lists the results of chronic rat exposure that resulted in cystic or hyperplastic lesions of endocrine glands and lymph nodes. Acute oral and inhalation in rats and mice indicated signs of neurotoxicity. Fenarimol (pyrimidine) is a systemic foliar fungicide. Acutely, fenarimol is Category III and is not a skin sensitizer (but can cause hydronephrosis). This fungicide causes reduced fertility and dystocia (abnormal labor or childbirth) in rats as low as 1.2 mg/kg/day. In a chronic rat feeding study

(EPA, 2007e) this compound increased hepatic adenomas and hyperplastic nodules. Fenarimol is moderately toxic to freshwater invertebrates and highly toxic to freshwater fish and most toxic to green algae (*Selenastrum capricornutum*). Propiconazole (triazole) is both a fungicide and an antimicrobial compound targeting fungi, bacteria, and plant viruses. This fungicide is an acute Category III (oral, dermal, eye irritation) or Category IV (inhalation, skin irritation) toxicant. Propiconazole caused dermal sensitization (guinea pigs). Developmental toxicity in rats was marked by increased incidence of rudimentary ribs, cleft palate, unossified sternebrae, and increased incidence of shortened and absent renal papillae. Acute neurotoxicity was noted by piloerection, diarrhea, and tiptoe gait. The 2-year mouse study (EPA, 2006c) indicated this fungicide caused liver toxicity (increased weight). Increased hepatocellular adenomas/carcinomas in male rats also rate this compound as a possible human carcinogen (Group C—not genotoxic but threshold mechanism). 1,2,5-Triazole showed potential estrogen, androgen, and/or thyroid-mediated toxicity including testicular changes and sperm abnormalities, ovarian changes, delays in sexual maturation, and dose-related decreases in TSH (thyroid). Triadimefon (DMI) is a broad-spectrum fungicide. Triadimenol is a primary metabolite of this fungicide and is registered under its own active ingredient number. The toxicity of either of these compounds extends to a common metabolite, 1,2,4-triazole. Neurotoxicity (in rats, mice, and rabbits) is the key concern for this compound. However, a chronic concern as a possible human carcinogen developed from increases in thyroid adenomas in male Wistar rats (endocrine) and hepatocellular adenomas in both sexes of the NMRI mouse. This fungicide is moderately acutely toxic to freshwater fish and invertebrates.

Acylamine

Metalaxyl-M works as a fungicide by affecting RNA synthesis by soil- and airborne Peronosporales. It has moderate acute toxicity in the rat (but high short-term when considering the NOEL). Some of these effects may be explained by a metalaxyl-induced bradycardia, which at high doses leads to cardiac arrest (Naidu and Radhakrishnamurty, 1988). This fungicide also had moderate acute toxicity in birds, fish, aquatic invertebrates, and earthworms but low toxicity in honeybees, aquatic plants, and algae. It is also a skin and eye irritant.

Piperadines

Piperalin functions as a fungicide (controls powdery mildew) due to inhibition of isomerase in ergosterol synthesis. Although acutely it has low toxicity overall, it causes moderate to severe skin irritation. In feeding pregnant rats, the dams experienced excess salivation, soiled fur, decreased body weight, and decreased food consumption. This compound is not toxic to birds but is highly toxic to fish and moderately toxic to aquatic invertebrates.

Phenylbenzamides

Flutolanil functions as a fungicide via affecting the mitochondrial transport chain. The EPA (2008c) flutolanil summary document listed increased liver weights in 90-day feeding studies in the rat or dog. The same document indicated opposite effects in two-year feeding studies in rats—decreased liver (also liver-to-body) and body weights. Reproductive and development toxicities were marked by decreased pup weight and body weight gain and fetal mortality in the high-dose group of rats fed over three generations. Enlargement of the renal pelvis was also found in the high-dose group.

Strobilurins, Imidazolinones

These compounds have fungicidal activity due to the action as quinone outside inhibitors (inhibit electron transport by binding to the outer binding site of the cytochrome bc_1 at Q_o site of complex III). Azoxystrobin (strobilurin or β-methoxyacrylate) has uses as a fungicide and as an antimicrobial. It is highly acutely toxic to freshwater fish and invertebrates amd estuarine/marine invertebrates. Fenamidone (imidazolinone) is a broad-spectrum foliar fungicide that is Category IV for acute oral and dermal exposure or primary dermal irritation and Category III for acute inhalation and eye irritation. It is extremely toxic to mysid shrimp, highly toxic to fish (bluegill sunfish and rainbow trout), oysters, and *Daphnia*, and moderately toxic to sheepshead minnow. This fungicide is relatively nontoxic on an acute basis to mammals (rats) or birds (mallard duck and bobwhite quail).

Phenylpyrrole (PP Fungicides)

Fludioxonil is a fungicide and an antimicrobial via its ability to alter mitogen-activated protein (MAP) kinase in osmotic signal transduction. This fungicide is highly toxic to aquatic organisms but is practically nontoxic to terrestrial organisms. The primary target organs are the liver and kidney (microscopic pathology—centrilobular hypertrophy and nephropathy in exposed mice). Although this compound is not considered a cancer-causing agent by the EPA (2011), some increases in liver tumors (combined adenomas and carcinomas) in female rats were noted in a lifetime exposure. That same EPA document indicated that female mice lymphomas found in one study failed to replicate in a second murine study. This compound (and dimethomorph, fenhexamid, quinoxyfen, cyprodinil, λ-cyhalothrin, pyrimethanil, azinphosmethyl, pirimiphos-methyl) was shown to have antiandrogenic activity in an *in vitro* AR receptor assay (Orton et al., 2011)

Aromatic Hydrocarbon and Thiadiazole

These chemicals are proposed to work via production of lipid peroxidation products. *Pentachloronitrobenzene* (PCNB) is an aromatic nonsystemic fungicide applied to soil, mainly turf, and seeds to control plant diseases. Acutely, PCNB is only slightly toxic (Category III for inhalation and primary eye irritant and dermal for one formulation) to practically nontoxic (Category IV for oral or dermal from one formulation and dermal sensitization). Chronic dietary exposure to the rat caused hepatocellular hypertrophy and hyperplasia and thyroid (endocrine) hypertrophy. This fungicide also is considered a Group C (possible human) carcinogen with a threshold effect. Because this compound is highly chlorinated, its persistence, bioaccumulation potential, and potential for long-range transport (found in Saskatchewan, Canada where it is not used) are high and of concern to the EPA. Its concern to aquatic species is the bioaccumulation factor > 5,000 and

a K_{OW} > 5. PCNB is highly toxic to freshwater fish and invertebrates and very highly toxic to estuarine/marine fish and invertebrates acutely. Chronically, it is toxic to aquatic and terrestrial animals (meets adverse criterion of Stockholm Convention as indicated by the EPA, 2006d). Its ability to volatilize makes it an addition to the list established by the Convention on Long-range Transboundary Air Pollution in the same EPA document. Etridiazole is a soil fungicide. Chronic rat toxicity data reported by the EPA (2000d) suggest that the liver is the target organ, increasing liver weight, hepatocytomegaly in males; spongiosis hepatis in males; clear, basophilic, and eosinophilic hepatocellular alterations in both sexes; hepatic centrilobular pigmentation in females; cholangiectasis in females; renal tubule karyomegaly in males and females; and testicular hyperplasia (reproductive/endocrine) in males. This fungicide is a probable human carcinogen based on multiple tumor types in male and female rats (liver, bile duct, mammary gland, thyroid, and testes) including a rare bile duct tumor known as cholangiocarcinoma, non-neoplastic lesions mentioned earlier for chronic organ toxicity, and positive mutagenicity data (*Salmonella typhimurium*, *in vitro* cytogenetics assay in Chinese hamster ovary cells, and two *in vitro* sister chromatid exchange assays listed in same EPA document).

Hydroxyanalide

Fenhexamid works as a fungicide via affecting the 3-keto reductase during C4 demethylation in ergosterol biosynthesis. Acute exposures do not seem to indicate significant toxicity. A 1-year dog feeding study (EPA, 1999b) indicated that this fungicide causes decreased RBC count, hemoglobin, and hematocrit and increased Heinz bodies in males and females. Also, increased adrenal weight (endocrine) and intracytoplasmic vacuoles in adrenal cortex in female dogs were noted.

Polyoxins

Polyoxins are biopesticides with systemic fungicidal activity related to inhibition of chitin synthase inhibition in fungal cell wall development (prevents elongation of growing mycelia and causes cell wall rupture). Polyoxin-D is practically nontoxic (Category IV) for acute oral and inhalation exposure and causes dermal irritation or sensitization. It is slightly toxic (Category II) for acute dermal exposure or eye irritation. Although this compound is relatively nontoxic in the rat and mallard duck, it is moderately toxic to rainbow trout or *Daphnia magna*.

Cyano-imidazole

Cyazofamid has fungicidal activity as a quinone inside inhibitor (Q,I). This fungicide has low-order acute toxicity via the oral, dermal, and inhalation routes. Minimal reversible eye irritation can occur; similarly, it is a slight dermal irritant and a weak sensitizer. The EPA (2012b) lists a variety of animal studies including the following data. Subchronic toxicity studies in that rat indicated mild to low renal effects (basophilic kidney tubules) as the primary organ toxicity. A 1-year dog study indicated parathyroid and pituitary (endocrine) cysts in the high-dose groups. An 18-month mouse carcinogenicity study indicated possible allergic effects of the sulfonamide moiety of this cyazofamid as indicated by skin lesions and at the high dose hair loss due to scratching. The high dose in developmental toxicity studies employing the rat indicated increased incidence of bent ribs in the absence of maternal toxicity.

Carbamate

Propamocarb hydrochloride functions as a fungicide by a proposed mechanism of affecting cell membrane permeability. This fungicide has low acute toxicity by oral, dermal, or inhalation routes. It causes slight eye irritation but is not a dermal irritant or sensitizer. The EPA (1995b) reregistration eligibility decision list a number of animal studies including the following. Subchronic and chronic rat studies indicate neurotoxicity with decreased motor activity, brain lesions, and ocular effects. In a dog study, GI toxicity and lesions in the trachea and lungs were noted upon oral exposure. Some developmental qualitative effects were noted in rat offspring (post-implantation losses, minor skeletal abnormalities, and minor lesions of the ears, heart, and upper GI tract). It

poses a potential chronic risk to birds but not to other terrestrial or aquatic organisms. However, frogs sampled from a site polluted with TATTU fungicide (mixture of propamocarb and mancozeb) had oxidative damage as illustrated by decreased Mn-SOD activity and oxidative destruction of lipids and proteins, neurotoxicity as evidenced by depletion of AChE activity and endocrine disruption as increased vitellogenin-like proteins (estrogenic effects; Falfushinska et al., 2008).

Ethyl Phosphonates and Phosphite

Phosphorus acid is used to control plant pathogens from the Oomycota phylum. This is not truly a fungus but often grouped with fungi due to filament structures that these organisms make that are similar to fungi. The oomycetes differ from true fungi by containing cellulosic compounds and glycan rather than chitin in their cell walls and are diploid rather than haploid for their genetic information. Phosphorous acid directly inhibits oxidative phosphorylation in oomycetes and stimulates the plant's natural defense response against pathogen attack (Brunings et al., 2012). This compound is organic but is an acid, which makes it harmful if swallowed, inhaled, or absorbed through the skin. It also causes moderate eye irritation. Phosphorus acid is not considered a dermal irritant or sensitizer.

Cinnamic Acid Amides

Dimethomorph is a systemic morpholine fungicide that inhibits ergosterol synthesis (proposed mechanism of affecting phospholipid biosynthesis and cell wall deposition). This fungicide is classified as Category III (conjunctiva of the eye, dermal) or IV (eye irritation cleared in 48 hours, oral, another dermal exposure test, skin irritation) for acute toxicity indicating little to no practical toxicity and is not a dermal sensitizer. The EPA (1998e) fact sheet reports that the highest dose given in a 90-day dog feeding study produced prostate fibrosis in four of the males. The critical toxic effect was characterized as a significant decrease in prostate weights of high-dose male dogs (endocrine). There were also possible threshold liver effects (increased alkaline phosphatase activity). Chronic rat exposure to dimethomorph yielded "ground glass" foci in liver and arteritis in male rats at doses higher than those that caused liver toxicity. Although dimethomorph is practically nontoxic to birds, mammals, and honeybees, it is slightly toxic to estuarine fish and moderately toxic to rainbow trout and estuarine invertebrates. Used in combination with mancozeb, dimethomorph is very highly toxic to freshwater fish and invertebrates. Dimethomorph fits the "pure" androgen receptor antagonism model (Orton et al., 2012) and must be considered an endocrine disruptor (hinted already from prostate results).

Copper — Complex or Fixed

Copper sulfate is the complex form of copper; the copper hydroxide fixed form of these fungicides dissociates into cupric ion (Cu^{2+}), which is an active broad-spectrum fungicide, bactericide, aquatic herbicide, algaecide, and molluscicide. Because copper is a naturally occurring element, its concentration is the key element (plus oxidation state). Low nutritional levels of copper maintain copper-binding proteins involved in blood (hemoglobin formation), blood vessel development, growth, immune function, and connective tissue composition. Copper toxicity occurs for microbial heterotrophic metabolism as low as 10 µg/L, while phytoplankton community photosynthesis is reduced significantly by concentrations as low as 25 µg/L (Jonas, 1989). Some humans with abnormal copper metabolism causing excess retention or who are incapable of absorption might have Wilson's disease (starts with liver and spills into neurological toxicity of excess copper and accumulations in the kidneys and eyes), occipital horn syndrome (defective biliary excretion of copper causing a lysyl oxidase deficiency and skin and joint laxity), Tyrolean infantile cirrhosis, Indian childhood cirrhosis, idiopathic copper toxicosis (three forms of hepatic copper toxicosis), or aceruloplasminemia (lack of ceruloplasmin in the blood lacks binding of copper and leads to iron deposits that account for the neurodegeneration, diabetes mellitus due to pancreatic damage, and liver damage). Menkes syndrome is another deficiency in copper/ceruloplasmin that causes neurodegeneration in infants, poor growth, and

"kinky" hair. The main toxicological concern is the effect of excesses of copper that lead to liver damage and neurotoxicity. As sensitive human populations already have been characterized, animal models are not as informative. Copper hydroxide acutely is a Category I eye irritant causing corneal opacity, iris irritation, chemosis, and invasion of corneal blood vessels. Otherwise, it is mainly Category III or IV. Similarly, copper sulfate pentahydrate causes Category I severe eye irritation and is also Category II for acute oral exposure in the rat. This may be due to the gastric irritation and corrosion caused by excess copper ingestion. The EPA (2009d) in its reregistration eligibility decision lists that some vineyard workers exposed to copper sulfate and hydrated lime mixtures (Bordeaux mixture) had increased cancer rates, but this finding is not definite as it lacks any chemical contact information . However, it is not known what else they were exposed to and does not present a definitive case to indicate copper's role in their disease. However, high concentrations of copper (≥ 400 ppm) are mutagenic in two types of microorganisms and caused endocrine tumors in chickens injected (intravenously or intramuscularly) with 10 mg/kg copper sulfate. Its uses also indicate an environmental toxicity danger to a variety of aquatic organisms. Copper paints used on boats negatively affected reef systems, and effects of sublethal concentrations of copper on the mussel *Mytilus coruscus* were observed by the following biomarkers: increased catalase activity; decreased SOD, glutamic-oxaloacetic transaminase, glutamic-pyruvic transaminase, and acid phosphatase activities in digestive gland; and decreased catalase and acid phosphatase activity in the gill. Other tissues showed differing effects based on copper concentration (Li et al., 2012).

Dithiocarbamates and Relatives

Mancozeb, an ethylene bis-dithiocarbamate (EBDC), has been mentioned previously as used in toxic combinations with other fungicides. It is a contact (not systemic) fungicide that disrupts cell metabolism at several sites in the target fungus. Ethylene thiourea (ETU) is a metabolite, environmental degradation product, and cooking byproduct of EBCD fungicides, which is also a concern along with the fungicide itself. The yeast *Saccharomyces cerevisiae* reveals how this fungicide has multiple sites of action. Altogether 286 genes confer protection against mancozeb, including those associated with transcriptional machinery, vacuolar organization and biogenesis, intracellular trafficking, and cellular pH regulation. Also, oxidative stress response, protein degradation, and carbohydrate/energy metabolism were involved with tolerance to this fungicide. Mancozeb is not a free-radical generator but is thiol reactive (genes involved in GSH biosynthesis also confer protection; Dias et al., 2010). The thyroid is the target organ (mainly thyroid follicular hyperplasia and tumors—endocrine and cancer). The EPA (2005g) lists a number of animal studies for mancozeb including the following. A rat subchronic study indicated microscopic neuropathology (peripheral nerve damage). Developmental neurotoxicity of mancozeb (hydrocephaly and other malformations) and ETU are of concern to the EPA. Acutely, no route (oral, dermal, inhalation) is considered toxic, although eye irritation was noted. Skin sensitization may occur in humans with end-use products. The metabolite ETU is the main culprit for these effects and has also been found to cause overt liver toxicity in a chronic dog study. A toxic effect not ascribed to ETU is a significant decrease in lipopolysaccharide-induced TNF-α production in leukocytes of agricultural workers exposed to mancozeb (Corsini et al., 2006).

Phthalimides

Captan is a familiar chloroalkylthio (dicarboximide) fungicide used on a variety of fruits such as the strawberry to prevent fungal growth. It appears to have nonspecific thiol reactivity and inhibition of cellular respiration as its antifungal action. A short-lived thiophosgene degradation product may be the reason this fungicide reacts with thiols and other functional groups. This fungicide listed by EPA (2004b) amendment to the reregistration eligibility decision as causing a number of the following toxicities including severe eye irritation (Category I due to corneal opacity in a rabbit study) and moderate skin sensitization (guinea pigs). Signs of captan

exposure in animals are hypothermia, listlessness, depression, diarrhea, weight loss, anorexia, and increased water consumption. It is also a probable human carcinogen (intestinal tumors in rodents, male rat hepatocellular hypertrophy, and adenomas and carcinomas in male rat kidney). Exposed rats of both sexes exhibited increased kidney weights and males had increased heart, brain, liver, and thyroid/parathyroid weights (endocrine). A metabolite THPI is also considered a risk factor. Captan is highly toxic to very highly toxic to bluegill sunfish, fathead minnows, brook trout, coho salmon, harlequin fish, and brown trout and is moderately toxic to Dungeness crab. It also affects *Daphnia magna* reproduction at 0.56 to 1.0 mg/L. Algae growth inhibition occurs for several species at captan concentrations < 1.0 mg/L.

Chloronitriles

Chlorothalonil (polychlorinated aromatic) is a broad-spectrum, nonsystemic protectant pesticide used as a fungicide to control fungal foliar diseases. This fungicide causes severe (Category I due to corneal opacity) eye irritation in the rabbit and moderate toxicity for inhalation exposure in the rat (Category II). Otherwise, it is Category IV in other routes (oral and dermal) and is not a dermal sensitizer. On subchronic exposure, it caused hyperplasia, hyperkeratosis of the epithelium of the forestomach of the mouse, dilated renal tubules and similar toxicity (hyperplasia/hyperkeratosis) of the stomach in the rat, and reduced alanine aminotransferase and body weight gain in the beagle. Chronic toxicity yielded renal and stomach tumors in the mouse and renal adenomas/carcinomas and stomach papillomas in the rat. Cell proliferation appears to be the mode of development of renal tumors in rats. Chlorothalonil is rated as a Group B or probable human carcinogen.

Biopesticides

Trichoderma harzianum strain T22G or F-Stop (KRL-AG2) is a rapidly growing common soil, litter, and wood fungus that is not toxic to rats or avian species. Its other effects were waived by the EPA based on the usage (seed treatment) and unlikelihood of this fungicide entering the environment (it is a natural organism). This fungus grows tropically toward hyphae of other fungi, coils about them in a lectin-mediated reaction, and degrades the cell walls of target plant pathogenic fungi (Harman, n.d.). *Trichoderma virens* GL21 is another of the rapidly growing common soil hyphomycetes found in all climate zones that is not toxic to rats but has fungicidal activity similar to *Trichoderma virens*. *Bacillus subtilis* (strains GB03 and QST713) is a ubiquitous, rod-shaped, Gram-positive (in early stages of growth) bacterium that produces an endospore that allows it to endure extreme conditions and produces a variety of proteases and other enzymes that allows it to contribute to nutrient cycling. It does not have attachment abilities or toxins that might cause pathogenesis in humans. It will infect and cause mortality of the second instar larvae of the malarial mosquito, *Anopheles culicifacies*. This organism is not considered a plant pathogen, but may be associated with certain plant diseases. This organism does produce antibacterial and antifungal compounds that are the basis for its use as a fungicide. Difficidin and oxydifficidin have antibiotic activity on a broad spectrum of aerobic and anaerobic bacteria. Rhizocticin was an antifungal phosphono-oligopeptide produced by *Bacillus subtilis* ATCC 6633. Peptidases may split rhizocticin into inactive L-arginine and toxic L-2-amino-5-phosphono-3-cis-pentenoic acid (L-APPA). L-APPA appears to interfere with the threonine or threonine-related metabolism (Kugler et al., 1990). Other antifungal antibiotics are produced by *Bacillus subtilis* (e.g., bacillomycin D, iturin, bacillomycin L), some of which are volatiles. *Streptomyces lydicus* (WYEC108) is a ubiquitous, free-living saprophytic soil bacterium used as a soluble powder fungicide for controlling root rot and damping off fungi. By colonizing the roots system, this bacterium protects it from harmful fungi. *Streptomyces lydicus* is absent of toxicological or pathogenic effects. Some effective human antibiotics such as streptomycin and neomycin have come from *Streptomyces* species. Antifungal metabolites are clearly produced by this organism and some are used based on their ability to colonize the protected plant roots. For example, *S. lydicus* WYEC is a good colonizer of certain plants, but is a poor colonizer of sagebrush root (*Streptomyces* sp. stain RG colonizes sagebrush roots well). Only two of the 500 known species of this bacterium are plant pathogens (*S. scabies* and *S. ipomoea*).

Bicarbonate

Potassium bicarbonate is effective against powdery mildew diseases. Baking soda was credited to a Russian plant pathologist as a fungicide. This disrupts the potassium balance of the cells (the sodium form in baking soda would disrupt the sodium balance) and cause the fungal cell wall to collapse (EPA, 2004c). Since potassium bicarbonate is a natural substance and exposure under normal conditions would not be expected to prove harmful, this compound has received an EPA exemption from determination of tolerance for residues. The pure substance should be kept away from young children as many similar agents in a kitchen used in foods or cleaning supplies would similarly be labeled with cautionary statements regarding storage. Hydrogen peroxide is a natural oxidizer found in many homes as an antiseptic agent, and it has antifungal properties. Used at ≤ 1% it is not a danger to mammals and even gargling with such an agent might provide beneficial rather than toxic reactions in an infection. An EPA exemption from determination of tolerance for residues was clearly appropriate for this antifungal chemical.

Neem Oil

Clarified hydrophobic extract of neem oil (long chain fatty acids and glycerides) is considered a biochemical pesticide and nontoxic with the exception of eye irritation and acute dermal exposure (Category III). This extract is also a mild contact sensitizer.

Plant Extracts

Extracts of *Macleaya cordata* (plume poppy) contain potent (IC$_{50}$s ranging from 0.47 to 6.13 µg/mL) antifungal isoquinoline alkaloids (sanguinarine, chelerythrine, protopine, α-allocryptopine; Liu et al., 2009). This plant is an herbal traditional Chinese medicine used for its anti-inflammatory and antibacterial properties. One of these alkaloids, sanguinarine, used in µM nontoxic concentrations elevated antioxidant defense systems via elevating heme oxygenase-1 and thioredoxin 1 via activation of the p38 MAPK/Nrf2 pathway in primary culture of human hepatocytes (Vrba et al., 2012). Similarly, the extract of the *Reynoutria sachalinensis* (giant knotweed) flower has three flavonoids (quercetin-3-O-alpha-L-arabinofuranoside, quercetin-3-O-beta-D-galactopyranoside, quercetin-3-O-beta-D-glucuronopyranoside) that are potent scavengers of superoxide radical (antioxidant) and three anthraquinones (emodin, emodin-8-O-beta-D-glucopyranoside, physcion-8-O-beta-D-glucopyranoside) in methanol extracts (Zhang et al., 2005). This extract has antifungal properties against powdery mildew. Although this extract may be somewhat harmful to the egg parasitoid *Trichogramma cacoeciae* Marchal, it is far less harmful than conventional fungicides (Hafez et al., 1999).

Rodenticides/Fumigants

Animal pests are sometimes eliminated by chemicals that are more toxic to species that cannot vomit but that also have toxicity to humans and other mammals. Both rodents and insects get into grain bins and must be controlled, typically with the use of fumigants. They are liquids/gases that are generally neurotoxic in nature and have been known to cause human toxicity and deaths if not well sealed in and separated from workers or people living close to the treated material (e.g., a factory turned into residential complex in Minneapolis lead to methyl bromide deaths because the pipes were not well sealed between the grain storage area and the former factory). The EPA lists fumigants as pesticides that form gases and vapors toxic to plants, animals, and microorganisms. **Table 25-5** lists rodenticides/ fumigants, their action, and toxicity. The list of grain fumigants comes from the U.S. Department of Labor (OSHA, 2015).

Organic Fumigants

In the past, acrylonitrile was used as a fumigant in the food industry. It has high acute inhalation toxicity in rodent testing and high to extreme toxicity via oral and dermal exposures. Human workers with exposures < 1 hour experienced mucous membrane irritation, headaches, nausea, feelings of apprehension, nervous irritability, low-grade anemia, leukocytosis, kidney irritation, and mild jaundice. Acrylonitrile poisoning is characterized by limb weakness, labored and irregular breathing, dizziness and impaired judgment, cyanosis, nausea, collapse, and convulsions. Lung cancer has also been seen with this chemical, which has been discontinued due to its overall toxicity (no reason to use it except in manufacturing of acrylic and modacrylic fibers, plastics, surface coatings, nitrile elastomers, barrier resins, and adhesives.

Calcium cyanide has been used as an insect fumigant in enclosed spaces. Because cyanide inhibits cytochrome a_3 in mitochondrial oxidative phosphorylation, it is a toxicant of cellular respiration. Its CNS toxicity marks its action and its extreme toxicity to humans. People can experience symptoms from headaches to dizziness to numbness, tremor, and loss of visual acuity as well as cardiovascular and respiratory effects that lead to rapid death. Lower levels over a longer period affect the thyroid gland, result in myelin degeneration, and cause irritation to the eyes and skin. Cyanogen bromide rapidly gives off hydrogen bromide gas in acids and decomposes or is ingested and breaks down to hydrogen cyanide. Cyanogen chloride is used as a fumigant, in tear gas, and in industrial synthesis; it was also used as an antipersonnel agent in World War I. An early 1950s study indicated metabolism to cyanide ion in rat blood by hemoglobin and GSH and the use of thiosulfate therapy in cyanide poisoning (Chen and Rose, 1952).

Carbon disulfide has been used as a fumigant for insects in stored grain and removes botfly infestations from the stomachs of horses and ectoparasites from pigs. Humans experience breathing and chest pains from inhalation as well as nausea, vomiting, dizziness, fatigue, headache, mood changes, lethargy, blurred vision, delirium, and convulsions. Psychosis is a marked feature of this strange solvent. CS_2 also affects sperm count and causes menstrual disturbances in males and females, respectively, if exposed via inhalation.

Carbon tetrachloride was a discontinued fumigant that had toxicity for the CNS, liver, and kidneys. The solvent itself at high concentrations was CNS toxic, but the liver toxicity is

TABLE 25-5   Fumigants and Rodenticides Listing by Mechanism of Action and Toxicity

Target of Fumigant/ Rodenticide Action	Chemical Family	Active Ingredient	Toxicity
Respiratory (especially fumigants) and possible neurotoxicity based on agent	Organic fumigants	Acrylonitrile	CNS, respiratory, cancer (discontinued)
		Calcium cyanide/cyanogen bromide/cyanogen chloride/ hydrogen cyanide	CNS, cellular respiration
		Carbon disulfide	Neurobehavioral
		Carbon tetrachloride/chloroform	CNS, liver, kidney, cancer (both discontinued)
		Chloropicrin	Eye, respiratory tract, CNS
		Dazomet	Respiratory, neurobehavioral
		1,2-Dibromo-3-chloropropane	Respiratory, CNS, cancer (discontinued)
		1,3-Dichloropropene	Respiratory, bladder, cancer
		p-Dichlorobenzene	Liver, kidney, tumor promoter
		Ethylene dibromide	Liver, kidney, bronchitis, cancer (discontinued)
		Ethylene dichloride	Respiratory, heart, liver, kidneys, CNS, cancer (discontinued)
		Ethylene oxide	Respiratory, CNS, eyes, cancer
		Iodomethane	Cancer, neurological, thyroid, developmental
		Metam sodium/potassium	Respiratory, neurobehavioral
		Methyl bromide	Neurotoxicity + stratospheric ozone depletion (phasing out)
		Methylene chloride Naphthalene	Hemolytic anemia, liver, neurological, eye, cancer
		Propylene dichloride	Lung, GI, blood, liver, kidney, CNS, eye, development, cancer (discontinued)
		Propylene oxide	Irritant, respiratory, neurological, cancer
		1,1,1-Trichloroethane	CNS, liver, stratospheric ozone depletion (discontinued)
	Inorganic fumigants	Aluminum/magnesium phosphide/Phosphine	Respiratory, clastogen, kidney
		Sulfur dioxide	Migraines, asthma attacks
		Sulfuryl fluoride	Kidney, respiratory, CNS, dental fluorosis (phased-down withdrawal)
Anticoagulant rodenticides		Warfarin Fumarin Pival PMP Diphacinone Chlorophacinone Brodifacoum Bromadiolone Difethialone	High acute toxicity and developmental at clinical doses
Neurotoxic rodenticides		Strychnine Bromethalin	Motoneurons and interneurons
Circulatory system rodenticide		Cholecalciferol	Hypercalcification

due to biotransformation by CYP and reductive dehalogenation to a trichloromethyl radical species ($Cl_3C\cdot$) as indicated by ESR (Connor et al., 1986). It also is considered a probable human carcinogen (Group B) based on liver cancer. Chloroform was similarly used (discontinued) to affect the CNS and caused liver and kidney toxicity and tumors due to reductive dehalogenation forming a radical.

Chloropicrin is a soil fumigant that the EPA compares with other soil fumigants (dazomet, methyl bromide, metam sodium/potassium, iodomethane, 1,3-dichloropropene) to be consistent and assess risk tradeoffs and economic outcomes. Chloropicrin is considered to be nonselective with fungicidal, herbicidal, insecticidal, and nematicidal properties. It is sometimes used as a warning agent prior to sulfuryl fluoride residential structure fumigations. As with most volatile fumigants, inhalation is the greatest concern as it causes eye, nose, throat, and upper respiratory irritation. Chloropicrin is highly toxic to mammals and is very highly toxic to fish and aquatic invertebrates.

Dazomet is a nonselective soil fumigant that is fungicidal, herbicidal, and nematicidal. Its major toxic degradation gas product is methyl isothiocyanate (MITC), which is the agent that caused the Bhopal disaster with severe and lethal respiratory damage (pulmonary edema). At lower concentrations, it is still highly irritating to the skin, eyes, and mucous membranes and may result in headache, vomiting (GI irritation), abdominal pain, insomnia, and anxiety neurosis with depression or paranoid tendencies. This product, of course, is acutely toxic to mammals and birds by inhalation of the MITC gas or oral granule ingestion. Fish and aquatic invertebrates are also affected by MITC deposition into water bodies.

1,2-Dibromo-3-chloropropane was used as a soil fumigant and nematicide, but is currently only an intermediate in chemical synthesis. Humans experience pulmonary congestion and moderate CNS depression on inhalation or GI disturbances and pulmonary edema from ingestion. Chronic exposure decreases sperm counts in humans (testicular effects noted in animals = reproductive + endocrine). This chemical was also listed as a probable human carcinogen (Group B2) due to high incidence of tumors of the nasal tract, tongue, adrenal cortex, and lungs of rodents upon inhalation exposure. 1,3-Dichloropropene is a component of soil fumigants. It causes mucous membrane irritation, chest pain, and breathing difficulties (human exposed to spill). Humans also exhibit skin sensitization upon chronic exposure. 1,3-Dichloropropene causes nasal mucosal tissue and urinary bladder damage in rodents exposed via inhalation. This agent is both a carcinogen in male mice (bronchoalveolar adenomas upon chronic inhalation) and in humans accidentally exposed to vapors during cleanup of a tank truck spill (histiocytic lymphoma and leukemia). This classifies 1,3-dichloropropene as a Group B carcinogen.

p-Dichlorobenzene is a fumigant insecticide used as a moth repellant (garments), and it controls lice and ticks around bird cages. No outdoor use means that ecological risk was not assessed but can be assumed in a spill. This compound has moderate toxicity orally or primary eye or dermal irritation. Low toxicity was found for inhalation or dermal routes as it is not a classic fumigant in the sense of overwhelming gases/vapors formed in its use (it is a solid and volatilizes from that state). Rodents given p-dichlorobenzene orally have mainly suffered liver and kidney damage. The EPA indicates that cancer caused in rodents was due to a mitogenic/cell proliferation effect, not a mutagenic one. Because the effect was not long lasting, if not resulting in overt liver damage, then it was not carcinogenic by EPA's standards. However, p-dichlorobenzene is still viewed as a tumor promoter (Hernández et al., 2009).

Ethylene dibromide (dibromoethane) was used as a fumigant but is extremely toxic to humans. Liver, kidney, and testes (endocrine/reproductive and dose damage sperm cells) damage occur regardless of route. It is a severe skin irritant, and acute inhalation results in depression and collapse (inhalation results in bronchitis if the effects are not lethal). This compound proved to be a probable human carcinogen (Group B) as a variety of tumors developed in both sexes of rodents. Similarly, ethylene dichloride (dichloroethane) was discontinued as a fumigant due to CNS, liver, kidney, and respiratory toxicity. It also caused cardiac arrhythmias, nausea, and vomiting. Animal studies (rodents) indicated that dichloroethane (by gavage administration) is a probable human carcinogen (Group B2) based on increased incidences of forestomach squamous cell carcinomas, circulatory system hemangiosarcomas, mammary adenocarcinoma, alveolar/bronchiolar adenomas, endometrial stromal polyps and sarcomas, and hepatocellular carcinomas (EPA, 2000e).

Ethylene oxide is used in small amounts as a fumigant as it depresses the human CNS and irritates eyes and mucous membranes (including bronchitis, pulmonary edema, and emphysema), and exposed human workers have higher incidences of leukemia, stomach cancer, pancreatic cancer, and Hodgkin's disease. These data are limited, so animal studies (EPA, 2008d) led to focus on lung, gland, and uterine tumors as a probable human carcinogen (Group B1). Iodomethane is a newer pre-plant soil fumigant viewed as an alternative to methyl bromide (toxicity concerns and protection of stratospheric ozone) to control plant pathogens, nematodes, insects, and weeds. Some 54 scientists have been puzzled about the methyl iodide substitution as the EPA (2007f) data indicate cancer potential (alkylating agent was the major thrust of the scientists letter to EPA and methyl iodide's volatility and water solubility), thyroid toxicity (this endocrine disruption is not surprising as it is an iodide), permanent neurological damage, and fetal toxicity (EPA, 2007g).

Metam sodium/potassium (methyldithiocarbamate salts) again is similar to dazomet as the major degradation product is MITC. Both salts of metam are broad-spectrum fumigants that treat for fungal, bacterial, algal, weed, insect, and nematode pests. Of course, the irritation of the respiratory tract and other exposed regions are the major concerns, because they lead to death and neurobehavioral damage for the survivors.

Methyl bromide is a broad-spectrum fumigant (acaricide, antimicrobial, fungicidal, herbicidal, insecticide, nematicide, and vertebrate/rodent and snake control agent). Its main use that is being phased out is as a soil fumigant.

Neurotoxicity is the most common effect of exposure (decreased activity, tremors, ataxia, and paralysis). Chronic exposure in rodents indicated degenerative changes in the cerebellum. Dogs were the most sensitive species of mammal tested to the neurotoxicity of this compound. Its environmental damage extends to the atmosphere—decreasing the UV-protective influences of the stratospheric ozone and indirectly leading to increased skin cancers and other mutagenic pressures on all biota subjected to sunlight. Nontarget mammals and birds would be exposed to this volatile chemical (as all fumigants pose this kind of risk) and respond with moderate toxicity similar to the other tested animals. Similarly, concerns for aquatic invertebrates also are raised. Fish show also low to moderate toxicity to methyl bromide. Bromide ion has to be considered in all aquatic risk assessments. Naphthalene may be something that older people are aware of, because it was used extensively in homes as mothballs in the past. Acute exposure results in hemolytic anemia, liver damage, and neurological damage. Cataracts and damage to the retina have been reported in human chronic exposure. Due to limited human reports without proper controls, laryngeal carcinomas or neoplasms of the pylorus and the cecum (GI tract) in humans are inconclusive. However, alveolar/bronchiolar adenomas in exposed female mice classify naphthalene as a possible human carcinogen (Group C).

Propylene dichloride (1,2-dichloropropane) was used as a soil fumigant, but had human toxicity (lung, GI tract, blood, liver, kidney, CNS, and eye toxicity). The EPA (2000f) reported animal studies resulting in respiratory and blood effects from inhalation exposure (expected route of entry and order of adverse effects). Developmental toxicity was noted in animals exposed by gavage. Propylene dichloride was classified as a probable human carcinogen (Group B2) due to increased mammary gland tumors in female rats and liver tumors in both sexes of mice (gavage exposure). Propylene oxide is used as a fumigant of foodstuffs and plastic medical instruments. It is an irritant (eye, skin necrosis, and respiratory tract). Inflammatory lesions of the nasal cavity, trachea, and lungs, and neurological effects are noted in chronic animal studies (EPA, 2000g). Tumors have been found in the cells lining the nasal cavity (inhalation) or forestomach (gavage) of exposed animals, so propylene oxide classified as a probable human carcinogen (Group B2). Trichloroethane is similar to methyl bromide except that it has been discontinued based on toxicity and the Montreal Protocol (EPA, 2012 advisories on the 25th anniversary of the Montreal Protocol [UNEP, 1987]) —risk to the potential ozone depletion caused by small halogenated compounds. Humans exposed to this compound exhibited mainly CNS (and possibly cardiac) depression and other neurological effects such as memory. Animal studies focus on the liver as the target organ.

Inorganic Fumigants

Aluminum phosphide and magnesium phosphide are formulated as tablets and pellets to control burrowing rodents and form highly toxic phosphine gas when exposed to moisture. This gas is highly toxic with an $LC_{50} > 11$ ppm. Rats exposed to this compound had coagulative necrosis in the tubules of the kidney and pulmonary congestion. Although phosphine does not appear to cause cancer in rat studies (EPA, 1999c), pesticide applicators exposed to this compound had chromosomal damage and increased chromosomal damage in bone marrow of exposed Sprague Dawley male rats (not mutagenic but is a clastogen *in vitro*). Sulfur dioxide has very low acute oral toxicity, does not irritate the skin, and has been recognized as a GRAS (generally recognized as safe) food preservative that has been used in wines and for a while in salads at restaurants. Due to some people's sensitivity to sulfites (people with migraine headaches with sulfite concentration > 10 ppm), some of this has been discontinued, especially at salad bars. However, some people respond with nausea and diarrhea, and it may precipitate a dangerous asthma attack (bronchospasm). Sulfuryl fluoride was a hopeful replacement for methyl bromide (ozone depletion); however, the reevaluation of fluoride toxicology has prompted a phased-down withdrawal of this compound as a fumigant (insect control

in grain storage). The human consequence of water contamination is severe dental fluorosis (enamel of tooth compromised by excess fluoride with sensitivity in first 8 years of life). Fatal human exposures have occurred with this compound. Sulfuryl fluoride causes respiratory irritation, pulmonary edema, nausea, abdominal pain, CNS depression, and numbness of the extremities. In rats, chronic inhalation exposure resulted in renal failure and death. Other treatment-related effects in rats were vacuolation of the cerebrum and thalamus/hypothalamus, and reactive hyperplasia and inflammation of the respiratory epithelium of the nasal turbinates, lung congestion, and aggregates of alveolar macrophages.

Anticoagulant Rodenticides

Warfarin was developed from a mycotoxin found on moldy sweet clover and its first use was not for medical purposes as an anticoagulant but rather as a rodenticide (kills mice and rats). The rats and mice cannot vomit, and this synthetic derivative of dicoumarol has toxic anticoagulant action by interfering with the role of vitamin K (from green leafy vegetables such as spinach) in the platelet clotting cascade. Due to its high acute toxicity orally to rodents, it is listed for humans as toxicity Category I (the most toxic category EPA has developed). It is also a developmental toxicant and causes birth defects in women taking clinical doses during any trimester of pregnancy. Six to 9 weeks' gestation yield the most commonly reported defect of chondrodysplasia punctata (shortened bones, punctuated or dot-like calcification in the cartilage, and abnormal peroxisomes). CNS effects, eye disorders, and developmental delays are also part of the human reactions during gestation. However, the amount used in many traditional rat bait products was very low (unlikely to cause teratogenic effects). The U.S. Department of Agriculture used to regulate vertebrate control agents, under which category rodenticides fall. EPA (1998f) Reregistration for Eligibility Decision (RED) Rodenticide Cluster covered 243 of the 406 products used and the remaining 182 products used to eliminate small vertebrate pests. Brodifacoum, bromadiolone, bromethalin, chlorophacinone, and diphacinone and its sodium salt were identified by the EPA as the Rodenticide Cluster and are all Category I (highly acutely toxic) for all three routes except that bromethalin is Category II for dermal exposure. It appears that all rodenticides, as expected, are potentially dangerous to all mammals/vertebrates. It is of interest that only one of the cluster is a neurotoxin (bromethalin). The rest are anticoagulants.

Neurotoxic Rodenticides

Strychnine has been a popular poison for rodents and other pests, and it was occasionally used in murders. It was hard to detect. In the mid-1990s its only registered use by EPA was for control of pocket gophers as a grain-based bait or paste. In old medicine kits from the United States, small amounts of strychnine were used as a nonspecific CNS stimulant. That use disappeared many years ago. Strychnine makes all muscle groups contract at the same time as the antagonist muscle is stimulated along with the agonist. This may break bones and send the poisoned person or animal hurling across a room. Strychnine accomplishes this action via interfering with postsynaptic inhibition by glycine at motoneurons and interneurons. As a potent neurotoxin, it is classified as toxicity Category I. Of course, birds and small mammals are at high risk of toxicity if exposed. Similarly, fish respond either with moderate or high toxicity. Red squill and zinc phosphide were other single-dose neurotoxic agents, as is bromethalin—the sole neurotoxin among EPA's rodenticide cluster.

Cholecalciferol

Vitamin D has many good properties as a nutrient involving calcium and phosphorus absorption and balance. However, in excess calcium will rise to levels that exceed the ability of hormones to control calcium homeostasis. The calcification can occur over a few days in dosed rodents resulting in calcification diseases, which include occlusion (block) of the circulatory system and death. The pure technical form of this compound is quite toxic to humans, but the bait itself contains only 740 ppm cholecalciferol, resulting in waving of acute-hazard evaluation studies by the EPA.

Questions

1. Why does ammonia gas damage on the way down the respiratory tract of the human as ammonium hydroxide, but actually damage mitochondria in the brain as ammonia gas?

2. Why is drinking untreated well water from corn-growing farms an issue, especially for pregnant women?

3. Why have triazine herbicides received more attention tha, other herbicides that may be more directly toxic to humans (such as Paraquat)?

4. Why is bromacil of the uracil herbicides important for endocrine disruption?

5. Why are the nitriles important for mitochondrial action if their primary herbicidal effects are on chloroplasts?

6. Why is the bipyridylium herbicide Paraquat always a lung toxicant? Why is diquat usually a kidney toxicant unless inhaled?

7. What do bleaching agents share in common?

8. Glyphosate is widely used on driveways to kill all plant life that comes up though concrete and is used in agriculture to clear fields of unwanted plant life prior to planting. Why can it be used that way and what are the risks related to application?

9. Why would an organochlorine mitosis-inhibiting herbicide be an oral poison and a possible human carcinogen?

10. Why is the dog more sensitive to dandelion control agent 2,4-D than other mammals?

11. What appears to be a common theme for many insecticides/miticides in common use such as carbamates and organophosphates?

12. Some fungicides act on ergosterol synthesis mechanisms, but the strobilurins/imidazolinones and phenylpyrrole compounds affect electron transport and MAP kinase signal transduction, respectively. Which ones have more concerns for humans versus aquatic species?

13. Why are fumigants very toxic?

14. Which rodenticide category has the most toxic chemicals according to EPA's classification system?

References

Ahrens WH. 1989. Uptake and action of metribuzin in soybeans (*Glycine max*) and two weed species as monitored by chlorophyll fluorescence. *Weed Sci.* 37:631–638.

Albers PH, Klein PN, Green DE, Melancon MJ, Bradley BP, Noguchi G. 2006. Chlorfenapyr and mallard ducks: overview, study design, macroscopic effects, and analytical chemistry. *Environ Toxicol Chem.* 25(2):438–445.

Albrecht J, Zielińska M, Norenberg MD. 2010. Glutamine as a mediator of ammonia neurotoxicity: a critical appraisal. *Biochem Pharmacol.* 80:1303–1308.

Allen MM, Turnburke AC, Legace EA, Steinback KE. 1983. Effects of photosystem II herbicides on the photosynthetic membranes of the cyanobacterium *Aphanocapsa* 6308. *Plant Physiol.* 71:388–392.

Antweiler RC, Goolsby DA, Taylor HE. 1995. Nutrients in the Mississippi River. In: RH Meade, ed. *Contaminants in the Mississippi River.* Reston, VA: U.S. Geological Survey Circular 1133.

Australian Pesticide and Veterinary Medicines Authority. 2007. Advice Summary. Application for Variation of a Registered Chemical Product. Product name: Movento 240 SC Insecticide. Applicant: Bayer Cropscience Pty Ltd. Product number: 61864. Application number: 46145. Purpose of Application and Description of Use: Variation of registration and label approval to include specified pests in onions, citrus and mangoes.Active Constituent(s): Spiroteramat. http://archive.apvma.gov.au/advice_summaries/46145.rtf

Bach L, Gissot L, Marion J, Tellier F, Moreau P, Satiat-Jeunemaître B, Palauqui JC, Napier JA, Faure JD. 2011. Very-long-chain fatty acids are required for cell plate formation during cytokinesis in *Arabidopsis thaliana. J Cell Sci.* 124(Pt 19):3223–3234.

Ballantine LG., McFarland JE, Hackett DS, eds. 1998. *Triazine Herbicides Risk Assessment.* Washington, DC: American Chemical Society.

Baltazar AM, Monaco TJ. 1984. Uptake, translocation, and metabolism of bentazon by two pepper species (*Capsicum annum* and *Capsicum chinense*). *Weed Sci.* 32:258–263.

Banack SA, Caller TA, Stommel EW. 2010. The cyanobacteria derived toxin Beta-N-methylamino-L-alanine and amyotrophic lateral sclerosis. *Toxins (Basel).* 2:2837–2850.

Beaumont MW, Taylor EW, Butler PJ. 2000. The resting membrane potential of white muscle from brown trout (*Salmo trutta*) exposed to copper in soft, acidic water. *J. Exp. Biol.* 203:2229–2236.

Binstock L, Lecar H. 1969. Ammonium ion currents in the squid giant axon. *J. Gen. Physiol.* 53:342–361.

Brunings AM, Liu G. Simonne EH, Zhang S, Li Y, Datnoff LE. 2012. *Are the phosphorous and phosphoric acids equal phosphorus sources for plant growth?* HS1010, Horticultural Sciences Department, Florida Cooperative Extension Service, Institute of Food and Agricultural Sciences, University of Florida.

California Environmental Protection Agency. 2009. Summary of Toxicology Data. Cumyluron. Medical Toxicology Branch. Chemical Code #: 5986. Tolerance #: 53067. SB 950 # NA. http://www.cdpr.ca.gov/docs/risk/toxsums/pdfs/5986.pdf

Caquet T, Deydier-Stephan L, Lacroix G, Le Rouzic B, Lescher-Moutoué F. 2005. Effects of fomesafen, alone and in combination with an adjuvant, on plankton communities in freshwater outdoor pond mesocosms. *Environ Toxicol Chem.* 24:1116–1124.

Chen KK, Rose CL. 1952. Nitrite and thiosulfate therapy in cyanide poisoning. *JAMA.* 149:113–115.

Cheng S, Chen J, Qiu Y, Hong X, Xia Y, Feng T, Liu J, Song L, Zhang Z, Wang X. 2006. Carbaryl inhibits basal and FSH-induced progesterone biosynthesis of primary human granulosa-lutein cells. *Toxicology.* 220:37–45.

Christenson WR, Becker BD, Wahle BS, Moore KD, Dass PD, Lake SG, Van Goethem DL, Stuart BP, Sangha GK, Thyssen JH. 1996. Evidence of chemical stimulation of hepatic metabolism by an experimental acetanilide (FOE 5043) indirectly mediating reductions in circulating thyroid hormone levels in the male rat. *Fundam Appl Toxicol.* 29:251–259.

Clair E, Mesnage R, Travert C, Séralini GÉ. 2012. A glyphosate-based herbicide induces necrosis and apoptosis in mature rat testicular cells *in vitro*, and testosterone decrease at lower levels. *Toxicol In Vitro.* 26:269–279.

Connor HD, Thurman RG, Galizi MD, Mason RP. 1986. The formation of a novel free radical metabolite from CCl_4 in the perfused rat liver and *in vivo.* *J Biol Chem.* 261:4542–4548.

Corsini E, Viviani B, Birindelli S, Gilardi F, Torri A, Codecà I, Lucchi L, Bartesaghi S, Galli CL, Marinovich M, Colosio C. 2006. Molecular mechanisms underlying mancozeb-induced inhibition of TNF-alpha production. *Toxicol Appl Pharmacol.* 212:89–98.

Daugrois JH, Hoy JW, Griffin JL. 2005. Protoporphyrinogen oxidase inhibitor herbicide effects on pythium root rot of sugarcane, pythium species, and the soil microbial community. *Phytopathology.* 95:220–226.

Davies, BA. 2002 Butafenacil – a new complimentary premix partner for triasulfuron or glyphosate for the enhanced knockdown and residual control of weeds in broadacre cropping situations.

In: Jacob HS, Dodd J, Moore JH, eds. *Thirteen Australian Weeds Conference Papers and Proceedings.* Plant Protection Society of Western Australia, Victoria Park, pp. 311–314.

Dayan FE, Trindade MLB, Velini ED. 2009. Amicarbazone, a new photosystem II inhibitor. *Weed Sci.* 57:579–583.

Délye C, Matéjicek A, Gasquez J. 2002. PCR-based detection of resistance to acetyl-CoA carboxylase-inhibiting herbicides in black-grass (*Alopecurus myosuroides* Huds) and ryegrass (*Lolium rigidum* Gaud). *Pest Manag Sci.* 58:474–478.

Dent MP. 2007. Strengths and limitations of using repeat-dose toxicity studies to predict effects on fertility. *Regul Toxicol Pharmacol.* 48:241–258.

Dias PJ, Teixeira MC, Telo JP, Sá-Correia I. 2010. Insights into the mechanisms of toxicity and tolerance to the agricultural fungicide mancozeb in yeast, as suggested by a chemogenomic approach. *OMICS.* 14:211–227.

D'Souza UJ, Narayana K, Zain A, Raju S, Nizam HM, Noriah O. 2006. Dermal exposure to the herbicide-paraquat results in genotoxic and cytotoxic damage to germ cells in the male rat. *Folia Morphol (Warsz).* 65:6–10.

Elbetieha A, Da'as SI. 2003. Assessment of antifertility activities of abamectin pesticide in male rats. *Ecotoxicol Environ Saf.* 55:307–313.

Falfushinska HI, Romanchuk LD, Stolyar OB. 2008. Different responses of biochemical markers in frogs (*Rana ridibunda*) from urban and rural wetlands to the effect of carbamate fungicide. *Comp Biochem Physiol C Toxicol Pharmacol.* 148:223–229.

Falfushinska HI, Hnatyshyna LL, Stoliar OB. 2012. [Population-related peculiarities of molecular stress-responsive systems of bivalve mollusk under the effect of tetrazine pesticide]. *Ukr Biokhim Zh.* 84:90–97.

Fan W, Yanase T, Morinaga H, Gondo S, Okabe T, Nomura M, Komatsu T, Morohashi K, Hayes TB, Takayanagi R, Nawata H. 2007. Atrazine-induced aromatase expression is SF-1 dependent: implications for endocrine disruption in wildlife and reproductive cancers in humans. *Environ Health Perspect.* 115:720–727.

Felke M, Langenbruch GA, Feiertag S, Kassa A. 2010. Effect of Bt-176 maize pollen on first instar larvae of the Peacock butterfly (Inachis io) (Lepidoptera; Nymphalidae). *Environ Biosafety Res.* 9:5–12.

Fernandez-Pol JA, Hays MT, Binette JP. 1977. Actions of plant cytokinins on dog thyroid follicular cells *in vitro. Exp Mol Pathol.* 26:251–259.

Figueiredo-Fernandes A, Fontaínhas-Fernandes A, Rocha E, Reis-Henriques MA. 2006. The effect of paraquat on hepatic EROD activity, liver, and gonadal histology in males and females of Nile tilapia, *Oreochromis niloticus*, exposed at different temperatures. *Arch Environ Contam Toxicol.* 51:626–632.

Freeman JL, Rayburn AL. 2006. Aquatic herbicides and herbicide contaminants: *in vitro* cytotoxicity and cell-cycle analysis. *Environ Toxicol.* 21:256–263.

Fuerst EP, Norman MA. 1991. Interactions of herbicides with photosynthetic electron transport. *Weed Sci.* 39:458–464.

Garagna S, Vasco C, Merico V, Esposito A, Zuccotti M, Redi CA. 2005. Effects of a low dose of bentazon on spermatogenesis of mice exposed during foetal, postnatal and adult life. *Toxicology.* 212:165–174.

Gesto M, Tintos A, Rodríguez-Illamola A, Soengas JL, Míguez JM. 2009. Effects of naphthalene, beta-naphthoflavone and benzo(a)pyrene on the diurnal and nocturnal indoleamine metabolism and melatonin content in the pineal organ of rainbow trout, *Oncorhynchus mykiss. Aquat Toxicol.* 92(1):1–8.

Gollamudi S, Johri A, Calingasan NY, Yang L, Elemento O, Beal MF. 2012. Concordant signaling pathways produced by pesticide exposure in mice correspond to pathways identified in human Parkinson's disease. *PLoS One.* 7:e36191.

Gorr TA, Rider CV, Wang HY, Olmstead AW, LeBlanc GA. 2006. A candidate juvenoid hormone receptor cis-element in the *Daphnia magna* hb2 hemoglobin gene promoter. *Mol Cell Endocrinol.* 247:91–102.

Graillot V, Tomasetig F, Cravedi JP, Audebert M. 2012. Evidence of the *in vitro* genotoxicity of methyl-pyrazole pesticides in human cells. *Mutat Res.* 748:8–16.

Gray LE Jr, Wolf C, Lambright C, Mann P, Price M, Cooper RL, Ostby J. 1999. Administration of potentially antiandrogenic pesticides (procymi-done, linuron, iprodione, chlozolinate, p,p'-DDE, and ketoconazole) and toxic substances (dibutyl- and diethylhexyl phthalate, PCB 169, and ethane dimethane sulphonate) during sexual differentiation produces diverse profiles of reproductive malformations in the male rat. *Toxicol Ind Health.* 15:94–118.

Grossmann K, Hutzler J, Tresch S, Christiansen N, Looser R, Ehrhardt T. 2012. On the mode of action of the herbicides cinmethylin and 5-benzy-loxymethyl-1, 2-isoxazolines: putative inhibitors of plant tyrosine aminotransferase. *Pest Manag Sci.* 68:482–492.

Guan XF, Zhao GJ, Cai QQ, Wang ZY, Lu ZQ, Qiu QM, Hong GL, Liang H. 2009. [Effect of bromoxynil on membrane potential and respiratory control rate in isolated mitochondria from mice liver and intervention effect of NAC]. *Zhonghua Lao Dong Wei Sheng Zhi Ye Bing Za Zhi.* 27:472–475.

Gui W, Dong Q, Zhou S, Wang X, Liu S, Zhu G. 2011. Waterborne exposure to clodinafop-propargyl disrupts the posterior and ventral development of zebrafish embryos. *Environ Toxicol Chem*. 30:1576–1581.

Gunnarsson L, Kristiansson E, Rutgersson C, Sturve J, Fick J, Förlin L, Larsson DG. 2009. Pharmaceutical industry effluent diluted 1:500 affects global gene expression, cytochrome P450 1A activity, and plasma phosphate in fish. *Environ Toxicol Chem*. 28:2639–2647.

Hafez MB, Schmitt A, Hassan SA. 1999. The side-effects of plant extracts and metabolites of *Reynoutria sachalinensis* (F. Schmidt) Nakai and conventional fungicides on the beneficial organism *Trichogramma cacoeciae* Marchal (Hym., Trichogrammatidae). *J Appl Entomol*. 123:363–368.

Hagve TA, Christophersen BO, Böger P. 1985. Norflurazon—an inhibitor of essential fatty acid desaturation in isolated liver cells. *Lipids*. 20:719–722.

Hamon M. 2007. [Can nitrates lead to indirect toxicity?]. *Ann Pharm Fr*. 65:347–355.

Han JF, Wang SL, He XY, Liu CY, Hong JY. 2006. Effect of genetic variation on human cytochrome p450 reductase-mediated paraquat cytotoxicity. *Toxicol Sci*. 91:42–48.

Harman GE. n.d. *Trichoderma* for biocontrol of plant pathogens: from basic research to commercialized products. http://web.entomology.cornell.edu/shelton/cornell-biocontrol-conf/talks/harman.html

Hayes TB, Stuart AA, Mendoza M, Collins A, Noriega N, Vonk A, Johnston G, Liu R, Kpodzo D. 2006. Characterization of atrazine-induced gonadal malformations in African clawed frogs (*Xenopus laevis*) and comparisons with effects of an androgen antagonist (cyproterone acetate) and exogenous estrogen (17beta-estradiol): Support for the demasculinization/feminization hypothesis. *Environ Health Perspect*. 114(Suppl 1):134–141.

Hazarika A, Sarkar SN. 2001. Effect of isoproturon pretreatment on the biochemical toxicodynamics of anilofos in male rats. *Toxicology*. 165:87–95.

Hellmich RL, Siegfried BD, Sears MK, Stanley-Horn DE, Daniels MJ, Mattila HR, Spencer T, Bidne KG, Lewis LC. 2001. Monarch larvae sensitivity to Bacillus thuringiensis- purified proteins and pollen. *Proc Natl Acad Sci USA*. 98:11925–11930.

Hernández LG, van Steeg H, Luijten M, van Benthem J. 2009. Mechanisms of non-genotoxic carcinogens and importance of a weight of evidence approach. *Mutat Res*. 682:94–109.

Hinther A, Domanski D, Vawda S, Helbing CC. 2010. C-fin: a cultured frog tadpole tail fin biopsy approach for detection of thyroid hormone-disrupting chemicals. *Environ Toxicol Chem*. 29:380–388.

Hiragaki S, Kobayashi T, Ochiai N, Toshima K, Dekeyser MA, Matsuda K, Takeda M. 2012. A novel action of highly specific acaricide; bifenazate as a synergist for a GABA-gated chloride channel of *Tetranychus urticae* [Acari: Tetranychidae]. *Neurotoxicology*. 33:307–313.

Hourmant A, Amara A, Pouline P, Durand G, Arzul G, Quiniou F. 2009. Effect of bentazon on growth and physiological responses of marine diatom: *Chaetoceros gracilis*. *Toxicol Mech Methods*. 19:109–115.

Howcroft CF, Gravato C, Amorim MJ, Novais SC, Soares AM, Guilhermino L. 2011. Biochemical characterization of cholinesterases in *Enchytraeus albidus* and assessment of *in vivo* and *in vitro* effects of different soil properties, copper and phenmedipham. *Ecotoxicology*. 20:119–130.

Hunde A, Patterson P, Ricke S, Kim WK. 2012. Supplementation of poultry feeds with dietary zinc and other minerals and compounds to mitigate nitrogen emissions-a review. *Biol Trace Elem Res*. 147(1–3):386–394.

Hurley PM. 1998. Mode of carcinogenic action of pesticides inducing thyroid follicular cell tumors in rodents. *Environ Health Perspect*. 106:437–445.

Hurley PM, Hill RN, Whiting RJ. 1998. Mode of carcinogenic action of pesticides inducing thyroid follicular cell tumors in rodents. *Environ Health Perspect*. 106:437–445.

Iaglov VV, Ptashekas IuR. 1989. [The reaction of the endocrine cells of the gastrointestinal tract in response to exposure to 3,6-dichloropicolinic acid]. *Biull Eksp Biol Med*. 107:758–761.

Iriti M, Castorina G, Picchi V, Faoro F, Gomarasca S. 2009. Acute exposure of the aquatic macrophyte *Callitriche obtusangula* to the herbicide oxadiazon: the protective role of N-acetylcysteine. *Chemosphere*. 74:1231–1237.

Iyyadurai R, Surekha V, Sathyendra S, Paul Wilson B, Gopinath KG. 2010. Azadirachtin poisoning: a case report. *Clin Toxicol (Phila)*. 48:857–858.

Jensen FB, Hansen MN. 2011. Differential uptake and metabolism of nitrite in normoxic and hypoxic goldfish. *Aquat Toxicol*. 101:318–325.

Jonas RB. 1989. Acute copper and cupric ion toxicity in an estuarine microbial community. *Appl Environ Microbiol*. 55:43–49.

Jones R. 2005. The ecotoxicological effects of photosystem II herbicide3s on corals. *Mar Pollut Bull*. 51:495–506.

Kawamura S, Yoshioka T, Kato T, Matsuo M, Yasuda M. 1996. Histological changes in rat embryonic blood cells as a possible mechanism for ventricular septal defects produced by an N-phenylimide herbicide. *Teratology*. 54:237–244.

Keszler A, Piknova B, Schechter AN, Hogg N. 2008. The reaction between nitrite and oxyhemoglobin: a mechanistic study. *J Biol Chem*. 283:9615–9622.

Kim TJ, Kim JS, Hong KS, Hwang IT, Kim KM, Kim HR, Cho KY. 2004. EK-2612, a new cyclohexane-1,3-dione possessing selectivity between rice (*Oryza sativa*) and barnyardgrass (*Echinochloa crus-galli*). *Pest Manag Sci.* 60:909–913.

Kling DE, Aidlen JT, Fisher JC, Kinane TB, Donahoe PK, Schnitzer JJ. 2005. Nitrofen induces a redox-dependent apoptosis associated with increased p38 activity in P19 teratocarcinoma cells. *Toxicol In Vitro.* 19:1–10.

Kojima H, Katsura E, Takeuchi S, Niiyama K, Kobayashi K. 2004. Screening for estrogen and androgen receptor activities in 200 pesticides by *in vitro* reporter gene assays using Chinese hamster ovary cells. *Environ Health Perspect.* 112:524–531.

Krieger-Liszkay A, Rutherford. 1998. Influence of herbicide binding on the redox potential of the quinone acceptor in photosystem II: relevance to photodamage and phytotoxicity. *Biochemistry.* 37:17339–17334.

Krijt J, Psenák O, Vokurka M, Chlumská A, Fakan F. 2003. Experimental hepatic uroporphyria induced by the diphenyl-ether herbicide fomesafen in male DBA/2 mice. *Toxicol Appl Pharmacol.* 189:28–38.

Krijt J, Vokurka M. 1997. Herbicide oxadiazon induces peroxisome proliferation. *Toxicol Appl Pharmacol.* 146:170–171.

Kugler M, Loeffler W, Rapp C, Kern A, Jung G. 1990. Rhizocticin A, an antifungal phosphono-oligopeptide of *Bacillus subtilis* ATCC 6633: biological properties. *Arch Microbiol.* 153:276–281.

Laezza C, Migliaro A, Cerbone R, Tedesco I, Santillo M, Garbi C, Bifulco M. 1997. N6-isopentenyl-adenosine affects cAMP-dependent microfilament organization in FRTL-5 thyroid cells. *Exp Cell Res.* 234:178–182.

Laville N, Balaguer P, Brion F, Hinfray N, Casellas C, Porcher JM, Aït-Aïssa S. 2006. Modulation of aromatase activity and mRNA by various selected pesticides in the human choriocarcinoma JEG-3 cell line. *Toxicology.* 228:98–108.

Lemaire G, Mnif W, Pascussi JM, Pillon A, Rabenoelina F, Fenet H, Gomez E, Casellas C, Nicolas JC, Cavaillès V, Duchesne MJ, Balaguer P. 2006. Identification of new human pregnane X receptor ligands among pesticides using a stable reporter cell system. *Toxicol Sci.* 91:501–509.

Leow YH, Maibach HL. 1996. Allergic contact dermatitis from norflurazon (Predict). *Contact Dermatitis.* 35:369–370.

Li Y, Gu Z, Liu H, Shen H, Yang J. 2012. Biochemical response of the mussel *Mytilus coruscus* (Mytiloida: Mytilidae) exposed to *in vivo* sub-lethal copper concentrations. *Chinese J Oceanol Limnol.* 30:738–745.

Liu H, Wang J, Zhao J, Lu S, Wang J, Jiang W, Ma Z, Zhou L. 2009. Isoquinoline alkaloids from *Macleaya cordata* active against plant microbial pathogens. *Nat Prod Commun.* 4:1557–1560.

Liu J, Yang Y, Zhuang S, Yang Y, Li F, Liu W. 2011. Enantioselective endocrine-disrupting effects of bifenthrin on hormone synthesis in rat ovarian cells. *Toxicology.* 290:42–49.

Liu XM, Shao JZ, Xiang LX, Chen XY. 2006. Cytotoxic effects and apoptosis induction of atrazine in a grass carp (*Ctenopharyngodon idellus*) cell line. *Environ Toxicol.* 21:80–89.

Losert W, Kraaz W. 1975. [Influence of indole-3-alkanecarboxylic acids on glucose utilization in rats]. *Arzneimittelforschung.* 25:880–887.

Lynch SM, Mahajan R, Beane Freeman LE, Hoppin JA, Alavanja MC. 2009. Cancer incidence among pesticide applicators exposed to butylate in the Agricultural Health Study (AHS). *Environ Res.* 109:860–868.

Mantecca P, Vailati G, Bacchetta R. 2006. Histological changes and micronucleus induction in the zebra mussel *Dreissena polymorpha* after paraquat exposure. *Histol Histopathol.* 21:829–840.

Marraffa JM, Hui A, Stork CM. 2004. Severe hyperphosphatemia and hypocalcemia following the rectal administration of a phosphate-containing Fleet pediatric enema. *Pediatr Emerg Care.* 20:453–456.

Martin RR, Lisehora GR, Braxton M Jr, Barcia PJ. 1987. Fatal poisoning from sodium phosphate enema. Case report and experimental study. *JAMA.* 257:2190–2192.

Matringe M, Camadro JM, Labbe P, Scalla R. 1989. Protoporphyrinogen oxidase as a molecular target for diphenyl ether herbicides. *Biochem J.* 260:231–235.

McKenzie RA, Rayner AC, Thompson GK, Pidgeon GF, Burren BR. 2004. Nitrate-nitrite toxicity in cattle and sheep grazing *Dactyloctenium radulans* (button grass) in stockyards. *Aust Vet J.* 82:630–634.

Medved IL. 1984. [Potential hazardousness of the embryotoxic action of the herbicide betanal (experimental data)]. *Gig Sanit.* Apr (4):16–18.

Meza-Joya FL, Ramírez-Pinilla MP, Fuentes-Lorenzo JL. 2013. Toxic, cytotoxic, and genotoxic effects of a glyphosate formulation (Roundup® SL-Cosmoflux®411F) in the direct-developing frog *Eleutherodactylus johnstonei*. *Environ Mol Mutagen.* 54:362–373.

Mommaerts V, Reynders S, Boulet J, Besard L, Sterk G, Smagghe G. 2010. Risk assessment for side-effects of neonicotinoids against bumblebees with and without impairing foraging behavior. *Ecotoxicology.* 19:207–215.

Moro CV, Bricheux G, Portelli C, Bohatier J. 2012. Comparative effects of the herbicides chlortoluron and mesotrione on freshwater microalgae. *Environ Toxicol Chem*. 31:778–786.

Naidu KA, Radhakrishnamurty R. 1988. Metalaxyl-induced bradycardia in rats: mediated by alpha-adrenoreceptors. *J Toxicol Environ Health*. 23:495–498.

Nater JP, Grosfeld JC. 1979. Allergic contact dermatitis from Betanal (phenmedipham). *Contact Dermatitis*. 5:59–60.

Nauen R, Smagghe G. 2006. Mode of action of etoxazole. *Pest Manag Sci*. 62:379–382.

Negga R, Stuart JA, Machen ML, Salva J, Lizek AJ, Richardson SJ, Osborne AS, Mirallas O, McVey KA, Fitsanakis VA. 2012. Exposure to glyphosate-and/or Mn/Zn-ethylene-bis-dithiocarbamate-containing pesticides leads to degeneration of γ-aminobutyric acid and dopamine neurons in *Caenorhabditis elegans*. *Neurotox Res*. 21:281–290.

Neuschl J, Kacmár P. 1993. [Acute oral toxicity of bentazon, an herbicide developed in Czechoslovakia, in pheasants and rabbits and the clinical symptoms of poisoning]. *Vet Med (Praha)*. 38:115–121.

New York State Department of Environmental Conservation. 2003. Fenpyroximate (AkariTM 5SC) NYS DEC Letter - Registration of Active Ingredient 5/03. Division of Solid and Hazardous Materials. http://pmep.cce.cornell.edu/profiles/insect-mite/fenitrothion-methylpara/fenpyroximate/fenpyrox_reg_0503.html

Nițuc E, Năstase V, Mihăilescu G, Chioveanu D. 2010. Researches of the nitrates and nitrites in some well waters from rural area in correlation with methoglobinemia morbidity. *Rev Med Chir Soc Med Nat Iasi*. 114:580–586.

Occupational Safety and Health Administration. 2015. Chemical Grain Fumigant. SHIP 01-06-2015. https://www.osha.gov/dts/shib/shib010615.html

Oda S, Tatarazako N, Watanabe H, Morita M, Iguchi T. 2006. Genetic differences in the production of male neonates in *Daphnia magna* exposed to juvenile hormone analogs. *Chemosphere*. 63:1477–1484.

Okubo T, Yokoyama Y, Kano K, Soya Y, Kano I. 2004. Estimation of estrogenic and antiestrogenic activities of selected pesticides by MCF-7 cell proliferation assay. *Arch Environ Contam Toxicol*. 46:445–453.

Orton F, Lutz I, Kloas W, Routledge EJ. 2009. Endocrine disrupting effects of herbicides and pentachlorophenol: *in vitro* and *in vivo* evidence. *Environ Sci Technol*. 43:2144–2150.

Orton F, Rosivatz E, Scholze M, Kortenkamp A. 2011. Widely used pesticides with previously unknown endocrine activity revealed as *in vitro* antiandrogens. *Environ Health Perspect*. 119:794–800.

Orton F, Rosivatz E, Scholze M, Kortenkamp A. 2012. Competitive androgen receptor antagonism as a factor determining the predictability of cumulative antiandrogenic effects of widely used pesticides. *Environ Health Perspect*. 120(11):1578–1584.

Pan H, Zhang L. 2011. [Mechanism of the effects of amitrole on the thyroglobulin in Fischer rat thyroid follicle-5 cell]. *Wei Sheng Yan Jiu*. 40:434–436, 440.

Peterson HA, Boutin C, Martin PA, Freemark KE, Ruecker NJ, Moody MJ. 1994. Aquatic phytotoxicity of 23 pesticides applied at expected environmental concentrations. *Aquat Toxicol*. 28:275–292.

Peterson HA, Boutin C, Freemark KE, Martin PA. 1997. Toxicity of hexazinone and diquat to green algae, diatoms, cyanobacteria and duckweed. *Aquat Toxicol*. 39:111–134.

Pinto Fde T, Corradi GR, Hera DP, Adamo HP. 2012. CHO cells expressing the human P_5-ATPase ATP13A2 are more sensitive to the toxic effects of herbicide paraquat. *Neurochem Int*. 60:243–248.

Powell GF, Ward DA, Prescott MC, Spiller DG, White MR, Turner PC, Earley FG, Phillips J, Rees HH. 2011. The molecular action of the novel insecticide, Pyridalyl. *Insect Biochem Mol Biol*. 41:459–469.

Randall DJ, Tsui TKN. 2002. Ammonia toxicity to fish. *Mar Pollut Bull*. 45:17–23.

Ravikumar S, Srikumar K. 2005. Metabolic dysregulation and inhibition of spermatogenesis by gibberellic acid in rat testicular cells. *J Environ Biol*. 26:567–569.

Razzaque MS. 2011. Phosphate toxicity: new insights into an old problem. *Clin Sci (Lond)*. 120:91–97.

Reddy PS, Pushpalatha T, Reddy PS. 2006. Reduction of spermatogenesis and steroidogenesis in mice after fentin and fenbutatin administration. *Toxicol Lett*. 166:53–59.

Rodrigues FA, Soares JDR, Santos RRS, Pasqual M, Silva SO. 2011. Colchicine and amiprophos-methyl in polyploidy induction in banana plant. *Afr J Biotechnol*. 10:13476–13481.

Rollerova E, Wsolova L, Urbancikova M. 2011. Neonatal exposure to herbicide acetochlor alters pubertal development in female wistar rats. *Toxicol Mech Methods*. 21:406–417.

Romagni JG, Duke SO, Dayan FE. 2000. Inhibition of plant asparagine synthetase by monoterpene cineoles. *Plant Physiol*. 123:725–732. Retraction in: Romagni JG, Duke SO, Dayan FE. 2005. *Plant Physiol*. 137:1487.

Saadi L, Lebaili N, Benyoussi M. 2008. Exploration of cytotoxic effect of malathion on some rat organs structure. *Commun Agric Appl Biol Sci*. 73:875–881.

Salazar KD, Miller MR, Barnett JB, Schafer R. 2006. Evidence for a novel endocrine disruptor: the pesticide propanil requires the ovaries and steroid synthesis to enhance humoral immunity. *Toxicol Sci.* 93:62–74.

Santi A, Menezes C, Duarte MM, Leitemperger J, Lópes T, Loro VL. 2011. Oxidative stress biomarkers and acetylcholinesterase activity in human erythrocytes exposed to clomazone (*in vitro*). *Interdiscip Toxicol.* 4:149–153.

Schmuck G, Freyberger A, Ahr HJ, Stahl B, Kayser M. 2003. Effects of the new herbicide fentrazamide on the glucose utilization in neurons and erythrocytes *in vitro*. *Neurotoxicology*. 24:55–64.

Schönbrunn E, Eschenburg S, Shuttleworth WA, Schloss JV, Amrhein N, Evans JN, Kabsch W. 2001. Interaction of the herbicide glyphosate with its target enzyme 5-enolpyruvylshikimate 3-phosphate synthase in atomic detail. *Proc Natl Acad Sci USA*. 98:1376–1380.

Scrano L, Bufo SA, D'Auria M, Meallier P, Behechti A, Shramm KW. 2002. Photochemistry and photo-induced toxicity of acifluorfen, a diphenyl-ether herbicide. *J Environ Qual.* 31:268–274.

Scroggs DM, Miller DK, Vidrine PR, Downer RG. 2006. Evaluation of weed control and crop tolerance with co-application of glyphosate and pyraflufen-ethyl in glyphosate-resistant soybean (*Glycine max*). *Weed Technol.* 20:1035–1039.

Senthil Nathan S, Young Choi M, Yul Seo H, Hoon Paik C, Kalaivani K, Duk Kim J. 2008. Effect of azadirachtin on acetylcholinesterase (AChE) activity and histology of the brown planthopper *Nilaparvata lugens* (Stål). *Ecotoxicol Environ Saf.* 70:244–250.

Shmizu T, Hashimoto N, Nakayama I, Nakao T, Mizutani H, Unai T, Yamaguchi M, Abe H. 1995. A novel isourazole herbicide, fluthiacet-methyl, is a potent inhibitor of protoporphyrinogen oxidase after isomerization by glutathione S-transferase. *Plant Cell Physiol.* 36:625–632.

Slaninova A, Smutna M, Modra H, Svobodova Z. 2009. A review: oxidative stress in fish induced by pesticides. *Neuro Endocrinol Lett.* 30(Suppl 1): 2–12.

Snel JFH, Vos JH, Gylstra R, Brock TCM, 1998. Inhibition of photosystem II (PSII) electron transport as a convenient endpoint to assess stress of the herbicide linuron on freshwater plants. *Aquat Ecol.* 32:113–123.

Soltani N, Delachambre J, Delbecque JP. 1989. Stagespecific effects of diflubenzuron on ecdysteroid titers during the development of *Tenebrio molitor*: evidence for a change in hormonal source. *Gen Comp Endocrinol.* 76:350–356.

Teshima R, Nakamura R, Nakajima O, Hachisuka A, Sawada J. 2004. Effect of two nitrogenous diphenyl ether pesticides on mast cell activation. *Toxicol Lett.* 150:277–283.

Thomas P, Doughty K. 2004. Disruption of rapid, nongenomic steroid actions by environmental chemicals: interference with progestin stimulation of sperm motility in Atlantic croaker. *Environ Sci Technol.* 38:6328–6332.

Topalca N, Yegin E, Celik I. 2009. Influence of indole-3-butyric acid on antioxidant defense systems in various tissues of rats at subacute and subchronic exposure. *Food Chem Toxicol.* 47:2441–2444.

Trebst A, Wietoska H. 1975. [Mode of action and structure-activity-relationships of the amino-triazinone herbicide Metribuzin. Inhibition of photosynthetic electron transport in chloroplasts by Metribuzin (author's transl)]. *Z Naturforsch C*. 30:499–504.

Tresch S, Niggeweg R, Grossmann K. 2008. The herbicide flamprop-M-methyl has a new antimicrotubule mechanism of action. *Pest Manag Sci.* 64:1195–1203.

Troudi A, Amara IB, Samet AM, Fetoui H, Soudani N, Guermazi F, Boudawara T, Zeghal N. 2011. Oxidative stress and thyroid impairment after gibberellic acid treatment in pregnant and lactating rats and their offspring. *Biofactors.* 37:429–438.

Tsuda T, Igawa T, Tanaka K, Hirota D. 2011. Changes of concentrations, shipment amounts and ecological risk of pesticides in river water flowing into Lake Biwa. *Bull Environ Contam Toxicol.* 87:307–311.

Turcant A, Harry P, Cailleux A, Puech M, Bruhat C, Vicq N, Le Bouil A, Allain P. 2003. Fatal acute poisoning by bentazon. *J Anal Toxicol.* 27:113–117.

United Nations Environment Programme (UNEP). 1987. The Montreal Protocol on Substances that Deplete the Ozone Layer. Treaty. http://ozone .unep.org/en/handbook-montreal-protocol-substances-deplete-ozone-layer/5

U.S. Environmental Protection Agency (EPA). 1994a. R.E.D FACTS: Bentazon. EPA-738-F-94-026. http://www.epa.gov/pesticides/reregistration/REDs/factsheets/0182fact.pdf

U.S. Environmental Protection Agency. 1994b. R.E.D FACTS: Pronamide. EPA-738-F-94-007. http://www.epa.gov/opp00001/chem_search/reg_actions/reregistration/fs_PC-101701_1-May-94.pdf

U.S. Environmental Protection Agency. 1995a. R.E.D FACTS: Linuron. EPA-738-F-95-003. http://www.epa.gov/pesticides/reregistration/REDs/factsheets/0047fact.pdf

U.S. Environmental Protection Agency. 1995b. Reregistration Eligibility Decision (RED) Propamocarb. EPA-738-F-95-036. http://nepis.epa.gov/Exe/ZyNET.exe/20000ILL.TXT?ZyActionD=ZyDocument&Client=EPA&Index=1995+Thru+1999 &Docs=&Query=&Time=&EndTime=&Se archMethod=1&TocRestrict=n&Toc=&TocEn try=&QField=&QFieldYear=&QFieldMonth= &QFieldDay=&IntQFieldOp=0&ExtQFieldOp

=0&XmlQuery=&File=D%3A\zyfiles\Index%20
Data\95thru99\Txt\00000001\20000ILL.txt&U
ser=ANONYMOUS&Password=anonymous&
SortMethod=h|-&MaximumDocuments=1&
FuzzyDegree=0&ImageQuality=r75g8/r75g8/
x150y150g16/i425&Display=p|f&DefSeekPage
=x&SearchBack=ZyActionL&Back=ZyActionS
&BackDesc=Results%20page&MaximumPages=
1&ZyEntry=1&SeekPage=x&ZyPURL

U.S. Environmental Protection Agency. 1996a. R.E.D
FACTS: Bromacil. EPA-738-F-96-013. http://nepis
.epa.gov/Exe/ZyNET.exe/200006AX.TXT?ZyActio
nD=ZyDocument&Client=EPA&Index=1995+
Thru+1999&Docs=&Query=&Time=&EndTim
e=&SearchMethod=1&TocRestrict=n&Toc=&T
ocEntry=&QField=&QFieldYear=&QFieldMont
h=&QFieldDay=&IntQFieldOp=0&ExtQFieldO
p=0&XmlQuery=&File=D%3A\zyfiles\Index%20
Data\95thru99\Txt\00000005\200006AX.txt&
User=ANONYMOUS&Password=anonymous
&SortMethod=h|-&MaximumDocuments=1&
FuzzyDegree=0&ImageQuality=r75g8/r75g8/
x150y150g16/i425&Display=p|f&DefSeekPage=
x&SearchBack=ZyActionL&Back=ZyActionS&Ba
ckDesc=Results%20page&MaximumPages=1&Zy
Entry=1&SeekPage=x&ZyPURL

U.S. Environmental Protection Agency. 1996b. R.E.D
FACTS: Nonflurzon. EPA-738-F-96-012. http://
www.epa.gov/opp00001/chem_search/reg_
actions/reregistration/fs_PC-105801_1-Jul-96.pdf

U.S. Environmental Protection Agency. 1997. Pesticide
Fact Sheet: Cloransulam-methyl. http://www.epa
.gov/pesticides/chem_search/reg_actions/
registration/fs_PC-129116_29-Oct-97.pdf

U.S. Environmental Protection Agency. 1998a.
Addendum to "Ambient water quality criteria for
ammonia--1984." Springfield, VA: National
Technical Information Service.

U.S. Environmental Protection Agency. 1998b.
Pesticide Fact Sheet: Tralkoxydim. http://www.epa
.gov/pesticides/chem_search/reg_actions/
registration/fs_PC-121000_04-Dec-98.pdf.

U.S. Environmental Protection Agency. 1998c. R.E.D
FACTS: Metribuzin. EPA-738-F-98-006. http://
nepis.epa.gov/Adobe/PDF/200006DV.PDF

U.S. Environmental Protection Agency. 1998d.
R.E.D FACTS: Dichlobenil. EPA-738-F-98-005.
http://www.epa.gov/opp00001/chem_
search/reg_actions/reregistration/fs_PC-
027401_1-Oct-98.pdf

U.S. Environmental Protection Agency. 1998e.
Pesticide Fact Sheet: Dimethomorph. http://
nepis.epa.gov/Exe/ZyNET.exe/P100BNIM.TXT?
ZyActionD=ZyDocument&Client=EPA&Index
=1995+Thru+1999&Docs=&Query=&Time=
&EndTime=&SearchMethod=1&TocRestrict=
n&Toc=&TocEntry=&QField=&QFieldYear=

&QFieldMonth=&QFieldDay=&IntQFieldOp=
0&ExtQFieldOp=0&XmlQuery=&File=D%3A\
zyfiles\Index%20Data\95thru99\Txt\00000031\
P100BNIM.txt&User=ANONYMOUS&Passwo
rd=anonymous&SortMethod=h|-&Maximum
Documents=1&FuzzyDegree=0&ImageQualit
y=r75g8/r75g8/x150y150g16/i425&Display=p
|f&DefSeekPage=x&SearchBack=ZyActionL&
Back=ZyActionS&BackDesc=Results%20pag
e&MaximumPages=1&ZyEntry=1&SeekPage
=x&ZyPURL

U.S. Environmental Protection Agency. 1998f.
R.E.D. Facts: Rodenticide Cluster. http://
www.epa.gov/pesticides/reregistration/REDs/
factsheets/2100fact.pdf

U.S. Environmental Protection Agency. 1999a.
Pesticide Fact Sheet: Fluthiacet-methyl. http://
www.epa.gov/pesticides/chem_search/reg_actions/
registration/fs_PC-108803_01-Apr-99.pdf

U.S. Environmental Protection Agency. 2000a.
Pesticide Fact Sheet: Clodinafop-propargyl.

U.S. Environmental Protection Agency. 1999b.
Pesticide Fact Sheet: Fenhexamid. http://www.epa
.gov/pesticides/chem_search/reg_actions/
registration/fs_PC-090209_20-May-99.pdf

U.S. Environmental Protection Agency. 1999c. Pesti-
cide Fact Sheet: Phosphine. http://nepis.epa.gov/
Exe/ZyNET.exe/P100BIXW.TXT?ZyActionD=Zy
Document&Client=EPA&Index=1995+Thru+
1999&Docs=&Query=&Time=&EndTime=&S
earchMethod=1&TocRestrict=n&Toc=&TocEn
try=&QField=&QFieldYear=&QFieldMonth=
&QFieldDay=&IntQFieldOp=0&ExtQFieldOp
=0&XmlQuery=&File=D%3A\zyfiles\Index%20
Data\95thru99\Txt\00000031\P100BIXW.txt&
User=ANONYMOUS&Password=anonymous
&SortMethod=h|-&MaximumDocuments=1&
FuzzyDegree=0&ImageQuality=r75g8/r75g8/
x150y150g16/i425&Display=p|f&DefSeekPage=
x&SearchBack=ZyActionL&Back=ZyActionS&Ba
ckDesc=Results%20page&MaximumPages=1&Zy
Entry=1&SeekPage=x&ZyPURL

U.S. Environmental Protection Agency. 2000b.
Pyridate (Lentagram, Tough) Pesticide Tolerance
4/00. Fed. Reg. 65:25647-25652.

U.S. Environmental Protection Agency. 2000c.
Pesticide Fact Sheet: Pymetrozine. http://nepis
.epa.gov/Exe/ZyNET.exe/P100BIBS.txt?ZyAction
D=ZyDocument&Client=EPA&Index=2000%20
Thru%202005&Docs=&Query=&Time=&End
Time=&SearchMethod=1&TocRestrict=n&To
c=&TocEntry=&QField=&QFieldYear=&QFiel
dMonth=&QFieldDay=&UseQField=&IntQFie
ldOp=0&ExtQFieldOp=0&XmlQuery=&File=
D%3A\ZYFILES\INDEX%20DATA\00THRU05\
TXT\00000028\P100BIBS.txt&User=ANON
YMOUS&Password=anonymous&SortMetho

d=h|-&MaximumDocuments=1&FuzzyDegree
=0&ImageQuality=r75g8/r75g8/x150y150g16/
i425&Display=p|f&DefSeekPage=x&SearchBack
=ZyActionL&Back=ZyActionS&BackDesc=Resu
lts%20page&MaximumPages=1&ZyEntry=1

U.S. Environmental Protection Agency. 2000d. Reregistration Eligibility Decision (RED) Etridiazole (Terrazole®). EPA-738-R-00-019. http://www.epa.gov/pesticides/reregistration/REDs/0009red.pdf

U.S. Environmental Protection Agency. 2000e. Ethylene Dichloride (1,2-Dichloroethane) 107-06-2. Hazard Summary-Created in April 1992; Revised in January 2000. http://www.epa.gov/ttnatw01/hlthef/di-ethan.html

U.S. Environmental Protection Agency. 2000f. Propylene Dichloride (1,2-Dichloropropane) 78-87-5. Hazard Summary-Created in April 1992; Revised in January 2000. http://www.epa.gov/ttn/atw/hlthef/di-propa.html

U.S. Environmental Protection Agency. 2000g. Propylene Oxide 75-56-9. Hazard Summary-Created in April 1992; Revised in January 2000. http://www.epa.gov/ttn/atw/hlthef/prop-oxi.html

U.S. Environmental Protection Agency. 2002. Cancer Assessment Document. *Evaluation of the carcinogenic potential of pyraflufen-ethyl*, PC Code 030090. Memorandum. *Pyraflufen-Ethyl – Report of the Cancer Assessment Review Committee* Health Effects Division, Office of Pesticide Programs.

U.S. Environmental Protection Agency. 2003a. Memorandum PP#: OF06164. Flufenpyr-Ethyl in/on field corn, soybeans and sugarcane. Health Effects Division (HED) Risk 1 Assessment. PC Code: 108853. DP Barcode: D270403. Case: 293057. Submission: S582174. http://www.epa.gov/pesticides/chem_search/hhbp/R064999.pdf

U.S. Environmental Protection Agency. 2003b. Buprofezin, Pesticide Tolerance 6/03. Fed. Reg. 68:37765-37772.

U.S. Environmental Protection Agency. 2003c. Acequinocyl Pesticide Fact Sheet. http://nepis.epa.gov/Exe/ZyNET.exe/P100BICM.TXT?ZyActionD=ZyDocument&Client=EPA&Index=2000+Thru+2005&Docs=&Query=&Time=&EndTime=&SearchMethod=1&TocRestrict=n&Toc=&TocEntry=&QField=&QFieldYear=&QFieldMonth=&QFieldDay=&IntQFieldOp=0&ExtQFieldOp=0&XmlQuery=&File=D%3A\zyfiles\Index%20Data\00thru05\Txt\00000028\P100BICM.txt&User=ANONYMOUS&Password=anonymous&SortMethod=h|-&MaximumDocuments=1&FuzzyDegree=0&ImageQuality=r75g8/r75g8/x150y150g16/i425&Display=p|f&DefSeekPage=x&SearchBack=ZyActionL&Back=ZyActionS&BackDesc=Results%20page&MaximumPages=1&ZyEntry=1&SeekPage=x&ZyPURL

U.S. Environmental Protection Agency. 2004a. Reregistration Eligibility Decision (RED) for Benfluralin. EPA-738-R-04-012. http://www.epa.gov/opp00001/chem_search/reg_actions/reregistration/red_PC-084301_22-Jul-04.pdf

U.S. Environmental Protection Agency. 2004b. Ammendment to the 1999 Captan RED. http://www.epa.gov/oppsrrd1/reregistration/REDs/0120red.pdf

U.S. Environmental Protection Agency. 2004c. Kaligreen® (fungicide label). http://www.epa.gov/pesticides/chem_search/ppls/070231-00001-20040617.pdf

U.S. Environmental Protection Agency. 2005a. Pesticide Fact Sheet: Amicarbazone. http://www.epa.gov/pesticides/chem_search/reg_actions/registration/fs_PC-114004_04-Oct-05.pdf

U.S. Environmental Protection Agency. 2005b. R.E.D FACTS: Pyrazon. EPA-738-F-05-012. http://www.epa.gov/pesticides/reregistration/REDs/factsheets/pyrazon_factsheet.pdf

U.S. Environmental Protection Agency. 2005c. Reregistration Eligibility Decision (RED) for Fluometuron. http://www.epa.gov/oppsrrd1/reregistration/REDs/fluometuron_red.pdf

U.S. Environmental Protection Agency. 2005d. Acetochlor Docket. EPA-HQ-OPP-2005-0227. http://www.regulations.gov/fdmspublic/component/main?main=DocketDetail&d=EPA-HQ-OPP-2005-0227

U.S. Environmental Protection Agency. 2005e. Reregistration Eligibility Decision for 2,4-D. EPA-738-R-05-002. http://www.epa.gov/oppsrrd1/reregistration/REDs/24d_red.pdf

U.S. Environmental Protection Agency. 2005f. Reregistration Eligibility Decision Thiophane-Methyl. http://www.epa.gov/oppsrrd1/reregistration/REDs/tm_red.pdf

U.S. Environmental Protection Agency. 2005g. Reregistration Eligibility Decision Mancozeb. http://www.epa.gov/pesticides/reregistration/REDs/mancozeb_red.pdf

U.S. Environmental Protection Agency. 2006a. Reregistration Eligibility Decision for Imazapyr. EPA-738-R-06-007. http://www.epa.gov/pesticides/reregistration/REDs/imazapyr_red.pdfhttp://www.epa.gov/pesticides/reregistration/REDs/imazapyr_red.pdf

U.S. Environmental Protection Agency. 2006b. Reregistration Eligibility Decision for Pyrethrins. EPA-738-R-06-004. http://www.epa.gov/oppsrrd1/reregistration/REDs/pyrethrins_red.pdf

U.S. Environmental Protection Agency. 2006c. Reregistration Eligibility Decision (RED) for Propiconazole. EPA-738-R-06-027. http://www.epa.gov/pesticides/reregistration/REDs/propiconazole_red.pdf

U.S. Environmental Protection Agency. 2006d. Reregistration Eligibility Decision (RED) for Pentachloronitrobenzne. List A. Case No. 0128. http://www.epa.gov/pesticides/reregistration/REDs/pcnb_red.pdf

U.S. Environmental Protection Agency. 2007a. Memorandum. Acetochlor: Fifth Report of the Cancer Assessment Review Committee. PC Code: 121601.

U.S. Environmental Protection Agency. 2007b. Paclobutrazol Summary Document. Registration Review: Initial Docket March 2007. In Docket Number: EPA-HQ-EPA-2006-0109. http://www.epa.gov/oppsrrd1/registration_review/paclobutrazol/paclobutrazol_summary.pdf

U.S. Environmental Protection Agency. 2007c. Cyromazine Summary Document. Registration Review: Initial Docket March 2007. In Docket Number: EPA-HQ-EPA-2006-0108. http://www.regulations.gov/fdmspublic/component/main?main=DocumentDetail&d=EPA-HQ-OPP-2006-0108-0003

U.S. Environmental Protection Agency. 2007d. Triflumizole Summary Document. Reregistration Review Docket March 2007. In Docket. EPA-HQ-OPP-2006-0115. http://www.regulations.gov/fdmspublic/component/main?main=DocumentDetail&d=EPA-HQ-OPP-2006-0115-0003

U.S. Environmental Protection Agency. 2007e. Fenarimol Summary Document. Registration Review: Initial Docket March 23, 2007. In Docket. EPA-HQ-OPP-2006-0241. http://www.regulations.gov/fdmspublic/component/main?main=DocumentDetail&d=EPA-HQ-OPP-2006-0241-0003

U.S. Environmental Protection Agency. 2007f. Pesticide Fact Sheet: Iodomethane. http://www.epa.gov/pesticides/chem_search/reg_actions/registration/fs_PC-000011_01-Jan-07.pdf

U.S. Environmental Protection Agency. 2007g. September 24, 2007 Letter to Mr. Stephen Johnson, Administrator, United States Environmental Protection Agency. Signatures Bergman RG, Hoffmann R., Fenn JB, Knowles WS, Ernst RR, Grubbs RH, Moore CB, Berson JA, Herschback D, Hoffman BM, DePuy CH, Saykally RJ, Heathcock C, Bercaw JE, Silbey RJ, Berne BJ, Stang PJ, Waugh JS, Murray RW, Corbett JD, Bruice TC, Roberts JD, Parmenter CS, Nicolauo KC, Lippard SJ, Kiessling L, Caruthers MH, Barry RS, Saunders M, Brookhart MS, Dye JL, Duilio A, Saveant J-M, Chisholm MH, Bigeleisen J, Zare RN, Casey CP, Bard AJ, Seyferth D, Gray HB, McLafferty FW, Bax A, Yates JTJr, Wibery KB, Letsinger RL, Meinwald J, Scheraga HA, Wolynes PG, Leone SR, Solomon EI, Schettler T,

McConnell RS, Orris P, Ervan PB. http://www.epa.gov/opp00001/factsheets/iodomethane_letter.pdf

U.S. Environmental Protection Agency. 2008a. Glufosinate Summary Document. EPA-HQ-OPP-2008-0190. http://www.regulations.gov/fdmspublic/component/main?main=DocumentDetail&d=EPA-HQ-OPP-2008-0190-0003

U.S. Environmental Protection Agency. 2008b. Tebufenozide Summary Document. Registration Review Initial Docket. Case 7417. December 2008. EPA-HQ-OPP-2008-0824. http://www.regulations.gov/fdmspublic/component/main?main=DocumentDetail&d=EPA-HQ-OPP-2008-0824-0003

U.S. Environmental Protection Agency. 2008c. Flutolanil Summary Document. Registration Review Initial Docket. Case 7410. September 2008. EPA-HQ-OPP-2008-0148. http://www.regulations.gov/fdmspublic/component/main?main=DocumentDetail&d=EPA-HQ-OPP-2008-0148-0008

U.S. Environmental Protection Agency. 2008d. Reregistration Eligibility Decision for Ethylene Oxide. EPA-738-R-08-003. http://www.epa.gov/pesticides/reregistration/REDs/ethylene-oxide-red.pdf

U.S. Environmental Protection Agency. 2009a. Fluridone Summary Document. EPA-HQ-OP-2009-0160. http://www.regulations.gov/fdmspublic/component/main?main=DocumentDetail&d=EPA-HQ-OPP-2009-0160-0002

U.S. Environmental Protection Agency. 2009b. Registration Review Document for Glyphosate. Case Number: 0178. EPA-HQ-OPP-2009-0361. http://www.regulations.gov/fdmspublic/component/main?main=DocumentDetail&d=EPA-HQ-OPP-2009-0361-0003

U.S. Environmental Protection Agency. 2009c. Malathion Summary Document. Registration Review: Initial Docket June 2009. EPA-HQ-OPP-2009-0317. http://www.regulations.gov/fdmspublic/component/main?main=DocumentDetail&d=EPA-HQ-OPP-2009-0317-0006

U.S. Environmental Protection Agency. 2009d. Reregistration Eligibility Decision (RED) for Coppers. EPA-738-R-09-304. http://www.epa.gov/opp00001/reregistration/REDs/copper_red_amend.pdf

U.S. Environmental Protection Agency. 2010a. Pesticide Fact Sheet: Imazosulfuron. http://www.epa.gov/pesticides/chem_search/reg_actions/registration/fs_PC-118602_14-Dec-10.pdf

U.S. Environmental Protection Agency. 2010b. Pesticide Fact Sheet: Flucarbazone-sodium. http://www.epa.gov/opp00001/

chem_search/reg_actions/registration/fs_PC-114009_29-Sep-00.pdf

U.S. Environmental Protection Agency. 2010c. Isoxaflutole Summary Document. EPA-HQ-OPP-2010-0979. http://www.regulations.gov/#!documentDetail;D=EPA-HQ-OPP-2010-0979-0008

U.S. Environmental Protection Agency. 2010d. Summary Document for Sodium Asulam Registration Review: Initial Docket. EPA-HQ-OPP-2010-0783. http://www.regulations.gov/#!documentDetail;D=EPA-HQ-OPP-2010-0783-0002

U.S. Environmental Protection Agency. 2011. Fludioxonil Summary Document Registration Review: Initial Docket June 2011. In Docket EPA-HQ-OPP-2010-1067. http://www.regulations.gov/#!documentDetail;D=EPA-HQ-OPP-2010-1067-0002

U.S. Environmental Protection Agency. 2012a. Problem formulation for the reassessment of ecological risks from the use of atrazine. EPA-HQ-OPP-2012-0230. http://www.epa.gov/oppsrrd1/reregistration/atrazine/

U.S. Environmental Protection Agency. 2012b. Cyazofamid; Pesticide Tolerances. *Fed. Reg.* 77:59114-59120.

U.S. Environmental Protection Agency. 2012c. Ozone Depleting Substances. http://www.epa.ie/air/airenforcement/ozone/#.Vd4FL5dLoUo

U.S. Environmental Protection Agency. 2013. Spirotetramat; Pesticide Tolerances. Fed. Reg. 78: 28507-28513.

University of Herfordshire Pesticide Properties Database. 2014. Pentoxazone (Ref:KPP314). http://sitem.herts.ac.uk/aeru/ppdb/en/Reports/1162.htm

Van den Berg KJ, van Raaij JA, Bragt PC, Notten WR. 1991. Interactions of halogenated industrial chemicals with transthyretin and effects on thyroid hormone levels *in vivo*. *Arch Toxicol.* 65:15-19.

Vecchia FD, Barbato R, La Rocca N, Moro I, Rascio N. 2001. Responses to bleaching herbicides by leaf chloroplasts of maize plants grown at different temperatures. *J Exp Bot.* 52:811-820.

Vesely DL, Hudson JL, Pipkin JL Jr, Pack LD, Meiners SE. 1985. Plant growth-promoting hormones activate mammalian guanylate cyclase activity. *Endocrinology.* 116:1887-1892.

Vidal T, Abrantes N, Gonçalves AM, Gonçalves F. 2011. Acute and chronic toxicity of Betanal®Expert and its active ingredients on nontarget aquatic organisms from different trophic levels. *Environ Toxicol.* 27(9):537-548.

Vincent F, Nguyen MT, Emerling DE, Kelly MG, Duncton MA. 2009. Mining biologically-active molecules for inhibitors of fatty acid amide hydrolase (FAAH): identification of phenmedipham and amperozide as FAAH inhibitors. *Bioorg Med Chem Lett.* 19:6793-6796.

Vrba J, Orolinova E, Ulrichova J. 2012. Induction of heme oxygenase-1 by *Macleaya cordata* extract and its constituent sanguinarine in RAW264.7 cells. *Fitoterapia.* 83:329-335.

Vu SH, Ishihara S, Watanabe H. 2006. Exposure risk assessment and evaluation of the best management practice for controlling pesticide runoff from paddy fields. Part 1: Paddy watershed monitoring. *Pest Manag Sci.* 62:1193-1206.

Waggoner JK, Henneberger PK, Kullman GJ, Umbach DM, Kamel F, Beane Freeman LE, Alavanja MC, Sandler DP, Hoppin JA. 2012. Pesticide use and fatal injury among farmers in the Agricultural Health Study. *Int Arch Occup Environ Health.* 86(2):177-187.

Wang HY, Olmstead AW, Li H, Leblanc GA. 2005. The screening of chemicals for juvenoid-related endocrine activity using the water flea *Daphnia magna*. *Aquat Toxicol.* 74:193-204.

Washington State Department of Transportation. 2006. Pyraflufen roadside vegetation management herbidice fact sheet. http://www.wsdot.wa.gov/NR/rdonlyres/2514F1B8-C9FA-4BF9-AB38-71AC04EA189F/0/Pyraflufen.pdf

Whitehorn PR, O'Connor S, Wackers FL, Goulson D. 2012. Neonicotinoid pesticide reduces bumble bee colony growth and queen production. *Science.* 336:351-352.

Winek CL, Wahba WW, Edelstein JM. 1990. Sudden death following accidental ingestion of chlormequat. *J Anal Toxicol.* 14:257-258.

Wright TR, Shan G, Walsh TA, Lira JM, Cui C, Song P, Zhuang M, Arnold NL, Lin G, Yau K, Russell SM, Cicchillo RM, Peterson MA, Simpson DM, Zhou N, Ponsamuel J, Zhang Z. 2010. Robust crop resistance to broadleaf and grass herbicides provided by aryloxyalkanoate dioxygenase transgenes. *Proc Natl Acad Sci U S A.* 107:20240-20245.

Wu IW, Wu MS, Lin JL. 2008. Acute renal failure induced by bentazone: 2 case reports and a comprehensive review. *J Nephrol.* 21:256-260.

Wu RSS. 2001. *Consultancy studies on Fisheries and Marine Ecological Criteria for Impact Assessment, Final Report.* Hong Kong Government, SAR, People's Republic of China: Environmental Protection Department.

Yi SA, Francis BM, Jarrell WM, Soucek DJ. 2011. Toxicological effects of the aquatic herbicide, fluridone, on male water mites (Hydrachnidiae: Arrenurus: Megaluracarus). *Ecotoxicology.* 20:81–87.

Yilmaz Z, Celik I. 2009. Neurotoxic and immunotoxic effects of indole-3-butyric acid on rats at sub-acute and subchronic exposure. *Neurotoxicology.* 30:382–385.

Zeman C, Beltz L, Linda M, Maddux J, Depken D, Orr J, Theran P. 2011. New questions and insights into nitrate/nitrite and human health effects: a retrospective cohort study of private well users'

immunological and wellness status. *J Environ Health.* 74:8–18.

Zhang X, Thuong PT, Jin W, Su ND, Sok DE, Bae K, Kang SS. 2005. Antioxidant activity of anthraquinones and flavonoids from flower of *Reynoutria sachalinensis. Arch Pharm Res.* 28:22–27.

Zottini M, Scoccianti V, Zannoni D. 1994. Effects of 3,5-dibromo-4-hydroxybenzonitrile (bromoxynil) on bioenergetics of higher plant mitochondria (*Pisum sativum*). *Plant Physiol.* 106:1483–1488.

CHAPTER 26

Industrial Chemicals That Biodegrade: Organic Chemical Exposures and Impacts

This is a chapter outline intended to guide and familiarize you with the content to follow.

I. Organic chemical toxicity (chemicals that biodegrade)

    A. Nonspecific CNS effects from Type I (fatigue, memory impairment, irritability, difficulty concentrating, mild mood disturbance) → moderate severity characterized as mild chronic toxic encephalopathy or Types 2A (sustained personality/mood changes—emotional instability, diminished impulse control, motivation) or 2B (affected intellect—diminished concentration, memory, and learning capacity) → pronounced or severe chronic toxic encephalopathy or Type 3 (global deterioration in intellect and memory = dementia)

        1. Toxic metabolites (e.g., formaldehyde → formate crystals in brain) ↑ toxicity (neurotoxicity of n-hexane related to formation of 2,5,-hexanedione) and possibly lead to cancer (benzene, CCl_4, trichloroethylene, 1,1,2,2-tetrachloroethane) or reproductive toxicity (2-methoxyethanol, 2-ethoxyethanol, and methyl chloride)

    B. Solvents—see Table 26-1

        1. Nonspecific, high-ppm effects → chronic solvent-induced encephalopathy (CSE) also known as "painters' syndrome," "organic solvent syndrome," or "psycho-organic syndrome"

        2. Psychosis and CS_2

        3. Peripheral nerve damage—CS_2, n-hexane, methyl n-butyl ketone and bromopropane substitutes for ozone-depleting CFCs

        4. Sensorineural hearing loss—toluene and styrene

        5. Long-chain alkanes (petroleum distillates)

            a. Secondary ketone metabolites (2nd position) induce CYP2E1 activity → ↑ toxic metabolites of CCl_4 and $HCCl_3$ especially in the liver

            b. PETROTOX model attempts to determine the toxic effects of mixtures of petroleum distillates on aquatic organisms—see Figure 26-1 for use of hydrocarbon block method (additivity) along with Raoult's Law and Henry's Law (solubility of partitioning of hydrocarbons to headspace complex mixtures in water-accommodating fractions). This model works for algae but overestimates toxicity to fish because it does not account for biotransformation or loss via volatilization. Underestimates of toxicity to *Daphnia* or repeated exposures to green algae, which appears to lie with high-molecular-weight, less water-soluble aromatic constituents of kerosene, naphtha, and gas oils (minor changes in solubility have large impacts on the model)

            c. Oil spills of water-soluble fraction of light Arabian crude oil, dispersed oil, or dispersant → liver toxicity; the dispersant mediated a T cell response that was confirmed by ↑ IFNγ. The dispersant (Corexit EC9500A) may be neurotoxic as indicated by rats' loss of olfactory marker protein (inhalation), ↓ tyrosine hydroxylase in striatum, alterations in synaptic and neuronal intermediate filament proteins, and astrogliosis of hippocampus and frontal cortex

CONCEPTUALIZING TOXICOLOGY 26-1

d. Gasoline can be lethal at high concentrations as indicated by Australian deaths. Additives to gasoline usually more toxic than the petroleum distillates themselves. Gas used to contain lead. Now it contains MTBE (oxygenate), which causes cancer in animals (cytotoxic, hormonal mechanisms and/or promoter) such as hepatocellular adenomas in female mice (antiestrogen effects) and renal tubular cell tumors in male rats ($\uparrow$ α2u-globin nephropathy). Other additives with toxic implications are ethanol, methanol, *t*-butyl alcohol, TAME, ethyl *t*-butyl ether, ethylene dibromide, ethylene dichloride (mutagenic metabolite = chloroacetaldehyde), MMT (Canadian additive contains toxic Mn damaging CNS, lung, reproductive and immune systems), benzene (forms phenoxy radical → leukemia or aplastic anemia, alkyl benzenes (CNS, liver, kidney and heart)

e. Jet fuels—older JP-4 less toxic than current JP-8 (weak dermal sensitizer but is a greater irritant of respiratory tract). Both jet fuels can cause hearing loss by mechanisms similar to components of gasoline

6. Alcohols

a. Ethanol—formation of acetaldehyde = toxic species in addition to direct action of ethanol on the CNS—see Figure 26-2. Ethanol also affects immune responses via alteration of LPS-induced TLR4 signaling in macrophages

b. Methanol—formation of formate = toxic species in addition to direct action of methanol on CNS; ethanol can be used to compete with methanol for alcohol dehydrogenase to prevent methanol → formate. Methanol and isopropanol affect immune response via creating transcriptional interference that decreases lymphocyte activation

c. Figure 26-3 indicates that ethanol leads human poisoning cases followed by isopropanol, glycols, and then methanol. Other alcohols have few cases

7. Amines

a. Easily protonated compounds with cyclohexylamine causing developmental toxicity, mutations, and cancer. N-hydroxylation of amines via CYP → toxic hydroxylamines → oximes. The alkaline pH of aliphatic amines and formation of active metabolites → toxicity beyond their lipophilicity. Linear amines appear to have the highest toxicity. Some structures containing amines also generate quinones, polynitroaromatic compounds, and imidazoles, which are highly reactive (higher toxicity as electrophiles reacting with nucleophilic groups). Polynitroaromatics uncouple oxidative phosphorylation (especially acidic phenolic compounds)

8. Ketones/aldehydes

a. Formaldehyde and acetaldehyde → cancer ± ROS formation. Formaldehyde and glutaraldehyde = fixatives (formalin causes clastogenesis via chromosome pieces sticking together). Glutaraldehyde = irritant, skin sensitizer, and damages a variety of key organs and is toxic to fetus including inducing malformations

b. Ecotoxicity can be modeled for α,β-unsaturated aldehydes and ketones using quantum calculations to indicate their reactivity with GSH or methanethiol. Most toxic compound using this method along with water as a possible catalytic pathway was acrolein (had lowest activation energy)

c. Methyl *n*-butyl ketone inhaled → $\uparrow$ neurofilaments in large myelinated nerve fibers → axonal swelling with secondary thinning of myelin sheath. 2,5-hexanedione mentioned earlier as metabolite of *n*-hexane or methyl *n*-butyl ketone → axonal degeneration in mammillary body and visual nuclei of cats

9. Halogenated hydrocarbons

a. Reductive dehalogenation and radical formation via CYP2E1 makes highly halogenated compounds toxic (electron-withdrawing properties of halogens increase the carbon atom radical formation probability); CCl$_4$ as model compound activation → steatosis and hepatic cancer/necrosis (TNFα signals apoptosis, while TGFα and TGFβ formation → cell self-destruction and fibrosis)

b. Perchloroethylene (dry cleaning solvent) and trichloroethylene (degreaser) have similar metabolites such as trichloroacetic acid (from trichloroethylene) → liver and kidney damage/cancer

CONCEPTUALIZING TOXICOLOGY 26-1 (*continued*)

    c. Chloroform causes kidney damage based on metabolites made there (liver CYP reductase gene deletion = liver-Cpr-null mice), not necessarily from liver metabolites. However, halogenated alkanes ↑ toxicity by GSH conjugation (GSH conjugates and forming episulfonium ions)

10. Aromatics

    a. Benzene and its derivatives are very toxic, especially if there is no side group to conjugate. Benzene via CYP → phenol or hydroquinone via PHS myeloperoxidase → phenoxy radical → leukemia or bone marrow destruction depending on dose and duration of exposure. Important that animal models do not develop same type of cancer (Zymbal's gland tumors and mammary glands, oral tissues, lung, nasal cavities, lymphoma, liver, forestomach, skin, uterus, ovary, Harderian, and preputial gland tumors)

    b. 1,3-Butadiene → different tumors based on dose

    c. Catechol → tumors of tongue, esophagus, forestomach, and stomach (not liver, urinary bladder, or thyroid), while hydroquinone → renal tubule cell adenomas at high doses and leukemia

    d. Toluene mainly a neurotoxin → low dose causes a deficit in spatial learning and memory; prolonged exposure → ↑ expression of NMDA receptor subunit NR2B, as do other volatile organic chemicals (VOCs). T cells recruited in attempts to clear toluene from the brain, but as toluene concentrations ↑, T cell deficiencies → dysregulation of neuroimmune crosstalk. See Figure 26-4. Toluene metabolized to hippuric acid for excretion

    e. Xylenes similar to toluene (lipophilicity = CNS depression and disruption of lipid environment of membrane proteins) and cleared as methyl hippuric acid. The reactive aldehyde (methyl benzaldehyde) may be key toxic metabolite. In the rodent, CYP2F metabolites coumarin, naphthalene, and styrene drive cytotoxicity and nasal and lung tumors (mouse rich in CYP2F2 in nasal tissue, while rat nasal tissue rich in CYP2F4). Mice do not respond to ethylbenzene metabolite, but their terminal bronchioles develop tumors to coumarin, naphthalene, styrene, ethylbenzene, cumene, α-methylstyrene, divinylbenzene, and benzofuran. Rats do not respond similarly nor do they respond to styrene or divinylbenzene induction of lung tumors

11. Halogenated aromatics' toxicity related to metabolic activation as seen in Figure 26-5 for bromobenzene. Primary metabolites of bromobenzene damage the liver (bromohydroquinone) while secondary metabolites damage the kidneys (GSH metabolite → kidney where it becomes a cysteine → lowers the redox potential → ↑ conversion to quinone species)

12. Hexachlorobenzene fits in better with persistent polychlorinated dibenzo-p-dioxins/furans, DDT, and β-hexachlorocyclohexane → less involved in displacement of halogens and more action on nuclear receptors (estrogen, androgen, progesterone, glucocorticoid, constitutive androstane, rodent prename X, mineralocorticoid/aldosterone, thyroid hormone) and AhR

13. Sulfur-containing organic chemical solvents

    a. Mercaptans (mercury capturer) = odiferous toxic compounds; methyl mercaptan gas → irritation to pain, depresses CNS, and similar to H_2S can cause death by respiratory paralysis; as ↑ alkyl chain length, mercaptans are less toxic as liquids

    b. DMSO = solvent associated with breaching skin barrier for other chemicals, but has systemic toxicity at high concentrations including producing acute respiratory distress

    c. CS_2 → coronary heart disease, coronary risk factors (hypercholesterolemia), retinal angiopathy, problems with color discrimination, effects on peripheral nerves, psychophysiological effects, morphological and other CNS effects (psychosis), and changes in fertility and other hormonal effects have been reported in workers in viscose fiber manufacture. Retinal microaneurysms, EGG changes, altered peripheral nerve conduction velocities, MRI hyperintensive spots, and hearing alterations in Japanese workers

14. Glycols

    a. Ethylene glycol (antifreeze component) via alcohol dehydrogenase → glycolate → metabolic acidosis

15. Glycol ethers

CONCEPTUALIZING TOXICOLOGY 26-1 (*continued*)

C. Polycyclic aromatic hydrocarbons (PAHs)
   1. Burn products activated by CYP → epoxides especially critical in bay region of their structure. PAHs also generate ROS. PAHs also absorb light energy → photo-excited states. DNA adducts → cancer

D. Polychlorinated biphenyls (PCBs)
   1. Persistent based on number of Cl molecules—coplanar congeners act similar to dioxins and toxicity based on AhR cell proliferation potential (TEQ)

E. Dibenzodioxins and dibenzofurans
   1. Most potent AhR agonists → chloracne, birth defects (very potent reproductive toxicant), neurotoxicity, immunotoxicity, and cell proliferation that promotes cancer growth

---

CONCEPTUALIZING TOXICOLOGY 26-1 (*continued*)

Many people, especially in the chemical industry or petroleum refining, come into contact with organic solvents. Organic solvents are a heterogeneous classification of compounds that are usually liquid between 0–250°C and include alcohols, aldehydes, aliphatic hydrocarbons, amines, aromatic hydrocarbons, cyclic hydrocarbons, esters, ethers, halogenated hydrocarbons, and ketones. They are used for dissolving certain hydrophobic industrial chemicals, chemical synthesis, extraction of various products, and refining of oil to products used in pharmaceuticals, plastics, automotive industry, personal care products, and so forth. Because many of these solvents are also volatile (such as paint thinner fumes), many people are exposed chronically to high concentrations. Even those that are considered consumable (ethanol) have deleterious effects over time to the brain, liver, heart, and other organs. At the highest concentrations found in large storage containers (> 5,000 ppm), they are immediately toxic or lethal via inhalation.

Nonspecific neurotoxicity may come about as can be seen in persons consuming alcohol, for example. First they may seem euphoric as inhibitions to certain behaviors are removed, then ataxic (uncoordinated) as the cerebellum becomes involved. At higher concentrations, speech becomes slurred. Then, people become unconscious and drift into coma as alcohol toxemia is achieved. Some have seizures prior to coma and death. The National Institute for Occupational Safety and Health (NIOSH)

indicates that the worker or animal exposed to organic solvents proceeds from narcosis, anesthesia, central nervous system (CNS) depression, respiratory arrest, and unconsciousness to death. Reaction time, manual dexterity, coordination, and balance are affected and can be quantitatively examined in exposed people or animals. Peripheral neuropathies (sensory and motor conduction velocities and electromyogram/muscle abnormalities) and mild toxic encephalopathy have been found in animal studies and in workers. Changes in behavior such as reversible subjective symptoms (e.g., fatigability, irritability, and memory impairment) have been noted, as have alterations in personality or mood including emotional instability and diminished impulse control and motivation. Diminished intellectual function was reflected in reduced ability to concentrate, memory, and ability to learn new tasks. More severe irreversible damage is marked by structural changes in the CNS and dementia and an increase in brain protein levels.

A scale developed in 1985 indicated more reversible (minimal) organic affective syndrome as Type I (fatigue, memory impairment, irritability, difficulty in concentrating, mild mood disturbance) proceeding to moderate severity characterized as mild chronic toxic encephalopathy or Types 2A (sustained personality/mood changes—emotional instability, diminished impulse control, motivation) or 2B (affected intellect—diminished concentration, memory, and learning capacity), and finally graduating to pronounced or severe chronic toxic encephalopathy or Type 3 (global deterioration in intellect and memory—dementia). More toxic solvents have effects at lower concentrations due to their toxicity or that of their metabolite(s), such as methanol becoming formaldehyde via alcohol dehydrogenase (then to formate crystals in brain) or *n*-hexane and methyl *n*-butyl ketone becoming 2,5-hexanedione via cytochrome P450 (CYP). There is some thought that acute reversible effects may be due to the parent compound, while chronic effects are more applicable to activation to reactive intermediates via biotransformation (NIOSH, 1987). However, very little is known about many of these agents except those that have had an extensive history of exposure to human workers such as benzene, *n*-butyl ketone, carbon disulfide, *n*-hexane, or methanol. It is believed that regional blood flow coupled to the lipophilicity of these compounds make the brain and nerves likely targets for accumulation following inhalation (Kulig, 1990).

Many organic solvents are recognized by NIOSH as carcinogens (benzene, carbon tetrachloride, trichloroethylene, and 1,1,2, 2-tetrachloroethane) and/or reproductive toxicants (2-methoxyethanol, 2-ethoxyethanol, and methyl chloride) in workplaces, but neurotoxicity appears to be more of a generalized risk of exposure. In 1987, it was estimated that ~10 million workers were exposed to products containing these solvents in paints, adhesives, glues, coatings, and degreasing/cleaning agents and in the manufacture/synthesis of dyes, polymers, plastics, textiles, printing inks, agricultural products, and pharmaceuticals (NIOSH, 1987). Chronic exposure has clearly been linked to benzene-induced leukemia, scleroderma with mixed solvents, and kidney cancer in those workers exposed to chlorinated hydrocarbons. As indicated earlier, metabolites may be more responsible for these diseases and for chronic neurotoxicity. Some chronic diseases such as Parkinson's may be exacerbated by solvent exposure (develop disease 3 years younger and less responsive to L-DOPA treatment). Solvent exposure may increase risk of essential tremor, but currently the data are not very compelling. Alzheimer's disease does not appear to be caused by solvents. However, chronic solvent exposure is a marker for premorbid intelligence (risk factor

for dementia). Amyotrophic lateral sclerosis (ALS) appears to be more linked to toxic cyanobacteria than to solvents. Similarly, multiple sclerosis (MS) has not had a clear link to solvent exposure. The strongest links are still the peripheral neuropathies caused by the 2,5-hexanedione metabolite of *n*-hexane and a general mild cognitive impairment with most organic solvents, the subclinical color vision loss with particular agents, and some hearing loss possible (Dick, 2006). Qualitative structure–activity relationship (QSAR) studies indicate that log P or the *n*-octanol/water partition explains much of the general toxicity (anesthesia) or ecotoxicity of organic solvents such as acrylates, alcohols, alkanes, amines, anilines, chlorophenols, ethers, ketones, methacrylates, nitriles, and phenols. Their penetration into skin was also based on their hydrophobicity. For inhalation and respiratory tract toxicity, the gas/liquid partition into organic bases such as tricresyl phosphate appeared most important. The haloalkanes appear to be subject to QSAR analysis for mutagenicity as well (Tanii, 1994).

Solvents

The effects of organic solvents on specific organs are summarized in **Table 26-1**.

Nonspecific High-ppm Effects

Chronic exposure to organic solvents leads to chronic solvent-induced encephalopathy (CSE). Human patients with CSE had an increase in electroencephalogram (EEG) total power, which resembles slight metabolic encephalopathy. CSE also is marked by an increased latency to doing certain tasks such as increased P300 latency in an odd-ball counting or odd-ball reaction time task. Patients with CSE also had lower cerebral blood flow as a major prognostic factor. There appear to be age differences in response as younger people had a greater increase on electroneuromyography (ENMG) amplitude of the sural electrode and a greater decrease in conduction velocity of the median IIIN and median IN electrodes compared to the older workers with CSE. Even following treatment, CSE was complicated or its recovery less successful in those humans using

TABLE 26-1　Organic Solvent and Persistent Organic Chemical Toxicity

Toxicity	Compound Key Examples	Toxic Mechanism
Chronic solvent-induced encephalopathy	All organic solvents	CNS depression—respiratory arrest
Peripheral neuropathy	n-Hexane Methyl n-butyl ketone	2,5-hexanedione toxicity to peripheral nerves
Blindness	Methanol	Formate crystal formation
Color discrimination changes	CS_2	Receptiveness of ganglion cells of demyelination of optic nerve fibers
Hearing loss	Gasoline, jet fuel, solvents	CNS brain region damage
Giant axonal neuropathy	Methyl n-butyl ketone	Increased neurofilaments
Neuroimmune dysfunction	Toluene	Decreased T cell recruitment
Immunotoxicity	Naphthalene, ethanol, persistent organochlorines	Active metabolites' effect on cell signaling
Hematological toxicity	Glycol ethers	Via aldehyde or alkoxyacetic acids
Tongue/forestomach/stomach/esophagus	Ethanol, benzene	Active metabolites
Liver damage	Methanol/formaldehyde CCl_4, $HCCl_3$ Gasoline	Formate and ROS formation Carbene-centered radical Female rat induction of estrogen metabolism
Kidney damage	Ethylene dibromide Gasoline	Oxide reactive adduct Male rat–specific $\alpha2u$-globin
Coronary heart disease	CS_2	Increased cholesterol
Testes	Ethylene dibromide, glycol ethers	Oxide reactive adduct
Ovarian tumors	Benzene	Active metabolites
Adrenal cortex	Ethylene dibromide	Oxide reactive adduct
Leukemia	Benzene	Phenoxy radical
Yolk sac edema	Amines	Alkyl amines
Developmental abnormalities	Xylenes, 2,4-DNP, 4-AP, hydroquinone	Toxic metabolites interfere with developmental stages
Asthma/respiratory damage	Ketone/aldehydes Benzene derivatives Xylene	Irritation Toluene affects neutrophils Pulmonary edema—severe irritation and toxicity
Mouse-specific lung cancers	Styrene	CYP2F metabolites
Skin	Most organic solvents such as xylene	Dissolves skin-protective oils and can blister or burn
Cell proliferation	Dibenzodioxins, dibenzofurans, HCB	Src activation (HCB), AhR activation (dioxins and furans)
DNA adducts	PAHs	CYP epoxide formation
Skin cancer	PAHs	Photoreaction

medications affecting the CNS. Thus, solvents interact with medications that may treat mental health issues. Neuropsychological function impairments were also noted with CSE (van Valen et al., 2009). Some solvents are more apt to affect neuropsychiatric analysis (e.g., carbon disulfide and psychosis), so this can be an important feature at lower concentrations as well. This CSE has originally been linked to Danish painters and therefore was known as "painters' syndrome," "organic solvent syndrome," "psycho-organic syndrome," or CSE. At lower chronic occupational exposure limits, there is no "symptomatic" neurological dysfunction. Carbon disulfide, n-hexane, and methyl n-butyl ketone affect the CNS and peripheral nervous system (PNS) specifically. 2-Bromopropane and 1-bromopropane substitutes for the ozone-depleting chlorofluorocarbons (CFCs) caused peripheral nerve toxicity in animal studies (similar to p-bromophenylacetyl urea causing dying-back axonopathies while chlorophenylacetyl urea has anti-seizure properties), but was subsequently found to cause CNS and PNS dysfunction in workers in the United States and China. Toluene and styrene cause sensorineural hearing loss and acquired color vision disturbances in workers. Toluene abusers suffer toluene leukoencephalopathy marked in magnetic resonance imaging (MRI) studies as cerebral atrophy, patchy periventricular hyperintensities, and hypointensities of the basal ganglia (Matsuoka, 2007).

Alkanes, Long-Chain Hydrocarbons, Crude Oil to Diesel Fuel to Gasoline to Jet Fuel From Petroleum Distillation

Small alkanes are very volatile and formed easily by bacteria as evidenced by methane emissions from landfills and thawed permafrost soils. They are toxic in high concentrations, so people need to "air out" enclosed disposal sites including animal wastes prior to entry. Methane in high concentrations is also apparently an ozone-depletion agent. Ethane is similarly volatile, and liquid propane has been used as fuel for years. Longer alkanes may be toxic if the second position is converted into a ketone as with n-hexane. These ketones also potentiate the toxicity of haloalkanes such as CCl_4.

The potentiation in the liver was thought to occur via similar alterations of plasma membrane enzymes and basal canalicular membrane fluidity, but only acetone appears to have that effect of the solvents acetone, methyl ethyl ketone, and methyl isobutyl ketone (Raymond and Plaa, 1996). Ketones induce CYP activity that appears to play a key role in the activation of CCl_4 or $HCCl_3$ in this potentiation, especially in the liver (Raymond and Plaa, 1995).

Petroleum distillation has taken thick oil and distilled it into various weights of refined fuel—from diesel fuel to gasoline to jet fuel. These are mixtures that contain long-chain hydrocarbons and aromatics that may be more toxic such as benzene, toluene, and xylenes. The PETROTOX model (Redman et al., 2012) attempts to deal with these complex mixtures of petroleum distillates and their impact on aquatic organisms. The assumptions of the model are that there is additivity of effects for similar modes of action, toxicity of blocks, and the petroleum compounds chemistry. This is known as the hydrocarbon block method based on the physicochemical and degradation properties essential to understanding and modeling the distribution and fate of the components of complex mixtures of hydrocarbons. The lethal loading approach standardizes testing and assessment of aquatic toxicity of complex mixtures of hydrophobic compounds in water media. Following equilibration of the loaded concentration of the petroleum mixture with the solvent (defined water media), test organisms are added to quantify and note adverse response. The acute LL_{50} or the EL_{50} is a 50% population response to the lethal (L) or effect (E) loading—similar to the lethal concentration (LC_{50}) and the effective concentration (EC_{50}). The chronic responses are reported as the no-observed-effect-level (NOEL) of EL_{10} values, similar to the no-observed-adverse-effect-level (NOAEL) and the lowest-observed-adverse-effect-level (LOAEL). Boiling-point intervals subdivide the petroleum mixtures into seven fractions and can accommodate distinguishing between aliphatic and the more toxic aromatic hydrocarbon classes via two-dimensional gas chromatography.

The target lipid model is a quantitative method for prediction of toxicity of hydrocarbons individually or in mixtures. The model in

Figure 26-1 employs a three-phase partitioning based on a combination of Raoult's law and Henry's law based on solubility of partitioning of hydrocarbons to the headspace complex mixtures in water-accommodating fractions (WAFs—validated parts of model use gasoline and crude oil). The equation for partitioning is $f_{d,I} = (1 + POC \cdot K_{OC,i})$, where $f_{d,I}$ = dissolved fraction for each structure, i; POC = particulate organic carbon content (kg/L); K_{OC} = organic carbon-water partition coefficient. The target lipid model or modified TLM is the basis for calculating the toxicity of these hydrocarbons dissolved in a water medium to aquatic organisms. This narcosis model is similar to high concentrations causing anesthetic to lethal depression of the CNS in mammals. The TLM employs critical target lipid body burdens (CTLBGB) to model sensitivity of different organisms to narcosis. Experimental results provide acute to chronic ratios (ACR) that are used to predict chronic effects irrespective of true molecular or physiological mechanisms. One of the assumptions of the modification to the TLM is that high log K_{OW} hydrocarbons are less bioavailable. The toxic units or T_{UW} = C_W/C^*_W, where C_W = estimated concentration based on partitioning model divided by the C^*_W or critical acute or chronic (depending on what duration of effect is desired) aqueous concentration such as the median lethal concentration LC_{50} or the NOEC. Individual TUs are then added together to estimate the mixture's effects acutely or chronically on aquatic organisms. When estimates were compared with actual concentrations, the dissolved hydrocarbon concentrations were consistent over four orders of magnitude for gasoline, kerosene, gas oil, heavy fuel oil, and crude oil. There were some outliers for lower kerosene and naphtha loadings that were well below predicted dissolved concentrations, while heavier polycyclic aromatic hydrocarbons (PAHs), weathered crude oil, kerosene, heavy fuel oil, and gas oil preparations were enriched when compared with the model estimates. The algal toxicity was consistent with that found in experiments when the additional POC phase was included. However, it appears that the model overestimated the toxicity in fish. The

assumptions of no losses via volatilization and biotransformation were clearly too conservative and harder to assess in large complex organisms with longer exposure periods. The model still was a good estimate for certain chemical mixtures as 49 observations of toxicity indicated that 21 of the model predictions were within a factor of 2, while 34 predictions were within a factor of 4. Only three observations showed greater toxicity than predicted. Two cases were distillate aromatics (biotransformation may yield toxic metabolites) in which *Daphnia magna* (aquatic invertebrate) experienced an LL_{50} of 36 mg/L, while the model indicates that the chemical mixture was nontoxic. Another aromatic caused an EL_{50} in *Pseudokirchneriella subcapitata* (green algae) of 19 mg/L with a predicted value of 230 mg/L. It gets worse on repeated exposure, because a third exposure of algae to heavy fuel oil yielded an EL_{50} of 0.75 mg/L with a prediction of 140 mg/L. The problem appears to lie with the presence of high-molecular-weight, less water-soluble aromatic constituents of kerosene, naphtha, and gas oils. Minor changes in solubility really impact the model (Redman et al., 2012).

In a metaphase chromosome analysis of rats chronically exposed to volatile petroleum fractions (may be especially problematic for aromatics), chromosomal aberrations and genomic changes (aneuploidy, polyploidy) were noted in bone marrow ("Study of the mutagenic activity of petroleum," 2012). For the heavier fuels such as diesel oil, the mixtures become more complex. Heavier fuels include PAHs, which are cytotoxic and include compounds such as naphthalene, acenaphthylene, acenaphthene, fluorene, and phenanthrene. The PAHs chemically quantified in specified extracts of biodiesel contain these compounds and have been found to be cytotoxic via CYP activation. The genotoxicity/weak mutagenicity of diesel fuel or biodiesel may be related to the presence of fatty acid methyl esters associated with the fuel itself or impurities from feedstock used to produce biodiesel. Biodiesel has the added potential of soybean constituents including phytoestrogens and phytosterols that may oxidized during preparation of the biofuel. Together these components may be responsible for chromosome aberrations and base-pair

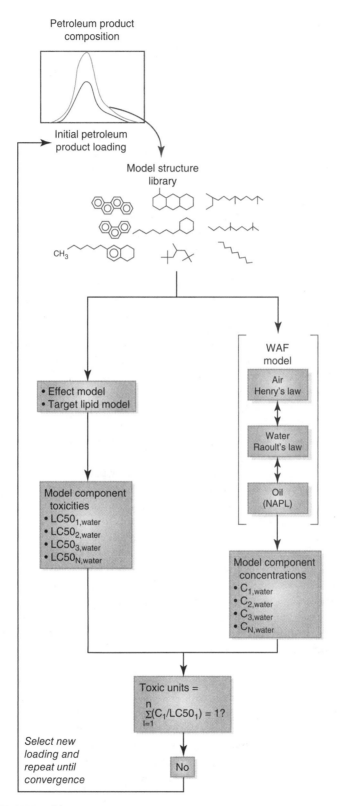

FIGURE 26-1 The PETROTOX Model

substitution mutations (Leme et al., 2012). The layperson does not need to read peer-reviewed articles to know the effects of crude oil on the aquatic ecosystem. News organizations have reported on ongoing unplanned experiments due to large spills in Alaska (Prince William Sound in 1989) and the Gulf of Mexico (3-month spill in 2010). People saw pictures of birds coated in oil getting washed in dish soap to restore their thermal barrier and prevent other toxicity from the oil (killed birds, fish, increased erosion of wetlands of Louisiana, killed shrimp and other life on the sea floor, and enormous impacts on the fishing industry). Medical personnel are concerned about the effects of inhalation of the volatile components of the crude oil (benzene, toluene, naphthalene, xylene, and hydrogen sulfide) on the cleanup crews' long-term health (Solomon and Janssen, 2010). The other issue that has arisen out of the Gulf of Mexico spill is the use of dispersants. The dispersant Corexit 9500 was used to enhance microbial degradation of the crude oil spill. The combination of 50:1 or 10:1 weathered crude oil and Corexit 9500 was applied to mallard duck eggs. Median lethal applications for 50:1 and 10:1 mixtures of the oil and dispersant were ~21 mg/egg (~322 µg/g egg) and ~33 mg/egg (517 µg/g egg), respectively. Spleen masses of the hatchlings exposed to the 50:1 mixture were the only physiological measures that were different from controls. Toxicity to mallard embryos was reduced by decreasing ratios of dispersant to weathered crude (Finch et al., 2012). The liver of the juvenile rabbit fish (*Siganus canaliculatus*) showed similar toxicity to the water-soluble fraction of light Arabian crude oil, dispersed oil, or dispersant with hepatocyte swelling and cytoplasmic vacuolization, megalocytosis, coagulative dispersed necrosis, lymphocytic infiltration, melano-macrophage aggregates, spongiosis hepatis, pericholangitis, and bile stagnosis. The total liver index resulting from circulatory, degenerative, proliferative, and inflammatory changes indicated that dispersed oil is no more toxic to this fish species' liver than crude oil or dispersant (Agamy, 2012).

The workers involved in the cleanup had acute pulmonary and dermatological adverse reactions that might have come from the cleanup. The dispersant Corexit 9500A was considered the possible culprit. This dispersant has dioctyl sodium sulfosuccinate (DSS) as an active ingredient. In mouse models for hypersensitivity and immune suppression (local lymph node assay, phenotypic analysis of draining lymph node cells, mouse ear swelling rest, total serum IgE, and the plaque-forming cell assay), dermal application resulted in skin irritation and lymphocyte proliferation. EC_3 values for Corexit 9500A and DSS were 0.4% (potent sensitizer) and 3.9% (moderate sensitizer), respectively. A T lymphocyte–mediated mechanism was the cause of the local lymph node assay that yielded mouse ear swelling tests for both the dispersant and its active ingredient. The lack of an IgE response in any assay (serum of node cell) eliminates the possibility of immediate hypersensitivity or allergic reaction. Increased IFN-γ but not IL-4 protein in stimulated node cells confirmed a T cell response. Neither the dispersant nor its active ingredient was immunosuppressive (Anderson et al., 2011).

The model oil dispersant Corexit EC9500A may be neurotoxic and was sprayed onto oil slicks possibly resulting in inhalation. When rats were exposed via inhalation to this dispersant, they had a partial loss of olfactory marker protein in the olfactory bulb. Tyrosine hydroxylase protein content in the striatum was decreased. Synaptic and neuronal intermediate filament proteins in specific brain areas were changed. In the hippocampus and frontal cortex, exposure to this dispersant yielded reactive astrogliosis (increased expression of fibrillary acidic protein). The events taken together indicate perturbed olfactory signal transduction, axonal function, and synaptic vesicle fusion presaging an imbalance in neurotransmitter signaling (Sriram et al., 2011). Other than the immune, pulmonary, and nervous system toxicity of the major dispersants used during the Gulf oil spill (mainly Corexit 9527 and 9500), the lack of knowledge of 35 different chemical dispersants, many of which have proprietary ingredients, is reflected in the 38 peer-reviewed articles on their toxicity in 2011. As dispersants will likely continue to be used as oil drilling becomes more difficult and accidental spills continue to occur, the toxicity of these substances to the ecosystem and cleanup personnel will become more important to assess and identify for clinical treatment or environmental remediation (Wise and Wise, 2011).

It takes high concentrations of gasoline to be lethal, but in Australia some have inhaled gasoline with lethal effects (Byard et al., 2003). Lead now has had been removed from gasoline and is replaced by oxygenate. First, consider the additives, which are often more toxic than gasoline itself. Methyl tert-butyl ether (MTBE) is the most widely used oxygenate, while ethanol is the next. MTBE causes cancer in animals and is considered a "nontraditional" genotoxicant because it is cytotoxic (as differentiated from mitogenic), using hormonal mechanisms or acting as a promoter. It is possible that because formaldehyde and tributanol are reactive carcinogens, MTBE causes cancer in animals and occupationally exposed individuals. This gasoline additive causes female mice to develop hepatocellular adenoma (via nongenotoxic anti-estrogen effects, mentioned in the discussion later in this chapter, on unleaded gasoline) and male rats to increase renal tubular cell tumors and interstitial cell tumors (via α2u-globin nephropathy unique to male rats, also discussed in the unleaded gasoline section). MTBE may increase its own metabolism via CYP induction. Many people consider ethanol to be a safer alternative, but they are not considering that ethanol extends gasoline plumes through the groundwater, leading to increased exposure of humans and other organisms in the soil or who rely on groundwater. Also, acetaldehyde is a reactive metabolite that at high concentrations certainly does liver damage and may cause liver cancer and is related to the CNS toxicity of ethanol as discussed under alcohols. Ethanol also is subject to reaction in the atmosphere to create peroxyacylnitrate, which is the respiratory irritant in smog (Ahmed, 2001). Methanol is another possible gasoline additive that has powerful neurotoxicity associated with its metabolism (see alcohols). It is also a dysmorphogenic agent (deaths of rat and mouse embryos following exposure or yielding craniofacial abnormalities). Methanol can also accelerate the degeneration of the testes in male rats. t-Butyl alcohol is another possible additive that targets the urinary tract of rodents (nephropathy in male rats with increased hyaline protein). Another possible gasoline additive is t-amyl methyl ether (TAME), which causes CNS depression as other volatiles do, while also appearing to increase the incidence of cleft palate in developing mice. TAME-exposed Chinese hamster ovary cells in vitro showed a positive concentration-dependent response for chromosome alterations. Ethyl t-butyl ether is another possible antiknock additive that is not predicted to be genotoxic or carcinogenic on a structure–activity relationship analysis. Ethylene dibromide (EDB; probable carcinogen—Group 2A) and ethylene dichloride (EDC; possible human carcinogen—Group 2B) are used to remove lead from engines (Pb scavengers) and are similar to fumigants (former chapter on agricultural chemicals covered the properties of fumigants). Their metabolites exert their toxicity. Ethylene dibromide damages the liver, stomach, adrenal cortex, and the testes. Urinary metabolites in rats and mice following oral or intraperitoneal (IP) administration of EDB were S-(2-hydroxyethyl)cysteine, N-acetyl-S-(2-hydroxyethyl)cysteine, and N-acetyl-S-(2-hydroxyethyl)cysteine-S-oxide (reactive adduct formation from metabolites noted on human albumin). Chloroacetaldehyde is a mutagen and possible metabolite of EDC. An octane enhancer used in Canada is methyl-cyclopentadienyl manganese tricarbonyl (MMT); its combustion makes toxic Mn available causing lung and immune system damage (coughs, colds, dyspnea during exercise, bronchitis, altered ventilatory volumes), reproductive problems (decreased fertility, impotence), and toxicity to the primary target of the CNS (headache, insomnia, disorientation, anxiety, lethargy, memory loss progressing to motor disturbances, tremors, difficulty walking mimicking Parkinsonism; Francis and Forsyth, 1995). Benzene is sometimes added even though it would already be present in gasoline as a blending agent; it forms the phenoxy radical in the bone marrow that causes leukemia or aplastic anemia depending on the severity of bone marrow damage. Alkyl benzenes of toluene and xylene are found in gasoline blends. Dermal exposure results in defatting of the keratin layer, vasodilation, erythema, and dry, scaly dermatitis (xylenes are potent skin irritants as well). CNS is the principle organ for toxicity, although the liver, kidney, and heart may be affected as well. Toluene acts to cause Parkinson's disease–like damage to the rat's dopaminergic nigrostriatal system and progressive hearing loss with cochlear cell damage demonstrated for *in vitro* exposure of cochlear cells. Xylenes cause an increase in pre-implantation losses, skeletal anomalies, reduced fetal body weight, and delayed development, while toluene is only fetotoxic (does not induce malformations).

Now that the additives have been examined, consider the mixture known as gasoline. Associations have been made between gasoline exposure and kidney (Enterline, 1993) and liver (Standeven et al., 1993) cancer, acute myeloid leukemia (Jakobsson et al., 1993), myeloma (Wong and Raabe, 1997), heart disease (Kranjcec et al., 2007), CNS alterations (Ritchie et al., 2001), skin changes including malignant melanoma (Infante, 1993), and mucous membrane changes (Baraniuk, 2009). These studies have included smokers and exclusion removes renal cell cancer. Melanomas could come from sunlight exposure, benzene, and gasoline as well as a combination of these, so the true role of gasoline is not easily dissected out of these studies. Nordic countries have also reported increases in service station workers and pharyngeal, laryngeal, and lung cancers. Exhaust fumes must also be considered in these exposures. Benzene is the agent that may be potentiated by other gasoline components to cause leukemia. Animal studies indicate that exposed female mice exhibit liver tumors, while renal tumors are found in male rats (exposure + hormone action). Female rats only have mild proximal tubule dysfunction when exposed to gasoline. Hyaline droplets or an increase in $\alpha 2u$-globin were found in renal tubules of male rats, possibly due to the higher component of branched hydrocarbons. Renal tubule cell death from $\alpha 2u$-globin nephropathy would be followed by a proliferative sequence leading to renal cancer in male rats. However, this $\alpha 2u$-globin protein is unique to the male rat and has questionable human implications. The female mice that developed liver tumors were found to have an induction of estrogen metabolism in isolated hepatocytes explaining the anti-estrogen activity of unleaded

gasoline (and induction of CYP2B). The cancer may develop as a result of altered cell turnover or altered cell growth. Gas fumes exceeding 200 ppm irritate the eyes. Skin exposure decreased glutathione (GSH) and GSH *S*-transferase activity, and increased lipid peroxidation in the brain and liver. Heart disease is not confirmed in refinery workers whose exposure may be quite high. Psychomotor and visual motor functions, immediate and delayed memory, and decreased intellectual capacity mark long-term neurotoxic findings in exposed workers. Ataxia, tremor, and acute or subacute encephalopathic syndrome result from intentional gas sniffers such as mentioned earlier regarding a subset of the Australian population (Caprino and Togna, 1998).

Jet fuel depends on its mix, as expected. The first jet fuel produced for the U.S. Air Force in 1951 was JP-4. JP-4 had low acute toxicity with slight dermal irritation. The current jet fuel, JP-8, is similar to JP-4 in its acute toxicity but adds a weak dermal sensitization. JP-8 is also a greater irritant of the respiratory tract than the older jet fuel mix. Both jet fuels may contribute to hearing loss similar to some of the components of gasoline. The male rat–specific nephropathy that was found in gasoline-exposed animals is similarly generated by the jet fuels. JP-8 has also caused immunosuppression. JP-8 has limited neurobehavioral toxicity, developmental toxicity, and reproductive toxicity. JP-4 is too old to have immune, neurobehavioral, or reproductive tests performed to assess its impacts. Neither jet fuels show mutagenicity, but JP-4 increased unscheduled DNA synthesis. The naphthalene content of the current and alternative or future fuels is an issue along with the immunotoxicity and inhalation exposure (Mattie and Sterner, 2011).

Alcohols

Ethanol is a good starting point, because people appear to voluntarily achieve toxicity. Certain populations genetically have more alcohol dehydrogenase and never experience the more "enjoyable" effects of ethanol, such as relaxation, release from behavioral inhibitions, and euphoria (despite these substances being CNS depressants), because more rapid formation of the toxic acetaldehyde makes them feel sickened instead (Stamatoyannopoulos et al., 1975). How alcohol affects the body can be determined by blood alcohol percentage as indicated in **Figure 26-2**. Methanol or "wood alcohol" is known to cause blindness and has caused deaths due to teenagers drinking fluids they thought contained Everclear, or strong ethanol (Davis et al., 2002). The slow formation of formaldehyde via alcohol dehydrogenase (ADH) and then rapid conversion to formate is the basis of early metabolic acidosis in primates. Lactate may accumulate due to formate inhibition of the respiratory chain/oxidative phosphorylation. Formate-induced tissue hypoxia may underlie the visual damage and general toxicity (Jacobsen and McMartin, 1986). The liver is less of a concern for acute toxicity due to the prominent neurotoxicity. However, acute hepatotoxicity is possible.

It is of interest that at 95% O_2, methanol has little toxicity to isolated rat hepatocytes, but is toxic to the centrilobular region at 50 mM in 1% O_2 (hypoxic) due to increased NADH levels. NADH is increased by methanol metabolism by ADH1. Reductive stress yields released forms of Fe^{2+} iron from ferritin causing reactive oxygen species (ROS) formation. Similar mechanisms exist for ethanol-induced liver damage. Iron chelators of various sorts including deferoxamine, NADH oxidizers, and ATP generators such as fructose protected hepatocytes and reduced the formation and toxicity of ROS. Formaldehyde formation via a Fenton reaction using Fe^{2+}/H_2O_2 at 1% O_2 is still a toxic issue in hepatocytes because there is increased protein carbonylation. This ferrous iron/hydrogen peroxide catalysis oxidizes methanol/formaldehyde to pro-oxidant radicals (oxidative stress through protein carbonylation

Number of Alcoholic Drinks Consumed by 70 kg Person	Blood Ethanol Content	Neurological Effects
1	0.02–0.03%	Slight euphoria, loss of shyness, no ataxia or apparent depressive effects.
2	0.04–0.06%	Feeling of well-being; relaxed, lowered inhibitions; warm sensation; euphoria. Minor impairment of reasoning, memory; less cautious in behavior.
3	0.07–0.09%	Euphoria; slightly impaired balance, speech, vision, reaction time, and hearing. Reduced self-control and judgment with impaired caution, reason, and memory.
4	0.10–0.125%	Euphoria; significantly ataxia and loss of judgment; slurred speech and affected balance, vision, reaction time, and hearing. Most states have this level as definitely illegal to operate motor vehicles.
5	0.13–0.15%	Gross ataxia–loss of physical control, blurred vision, major loss of balance. Euphoria reduced and dysphoria (anxiety, restlessness) appears.
6	0.16–0.20%	Dysphoria predominates, nausea possible ("sloppy drunk" appearance).
7	0.25%	Needs assistance in walking, total mental confusion. Dysphoria, nausea, and some vomiting.
>7	Over 0.30%	Loss of consciousness unless a chronic alcoholic with no clinical indications of liver damage. Over 0.40% blood ethanol content is the onset of coma and death due to respiratory arrest.

FIGURE 26-2 Percent Ethanol and Neurological Effects

Data from http://chavesdwiprogram.us/pdf/Effects%20of%20Alcohol%20Intoxication.pdf.

and ROS formation) yielding cell death (MacAllister et al., 2011).

The exposure to other alcohols based on the number of poison control center cases per year is shown in **Figure 26-3**. Note that ethanol dramatically leads the list, followed by isopropanol/isopropyl alcohol, glycols, and then methanol or methanol mixtures, with glycols and other alcohols representing a very small percentage. This means that allyl alcohol may be a good way of modeling the oxidative toxicity in zone one, but allyl alcohol does not approach the others in its uses or effects on the human population and ecosystem as a whole. Ethanol consumption through alcoholic beverages does not even have to be included to still be the cause of the majority of alcohol poisonings—just the amounts used in mouthwash, hand sanitizer, and cleaning products lead to ethanol toxicosis. Many households use isopropanol, which comes next on the list, whereas glycols are mainly associated with automotive products. Methanol appears to be low on the list in occurrences but has one of the highest mortality rates (15–36%) due to the delayed formation of its toxic metabolites. Immunomodulatory properties of ethanol have led to correct hypotheses that other short-chain alcohols similarly inhibit the inflammatory response via preventing leukocyte/endothelial cell interactions and affecting monocytes through the NFAT family of transcription factors with or without the involvement of AP-1.

When looking at the effects of alcohols, it helps to think of them in terms of their former use in the "old West" as an anesthetic agent, which obeys the Meyer-Overton rule that potency is more able to dissolve in olive oil than in water. This makes longer chain hydrocarbons more anesthetic, but their diffusion rate is based on the square root of their molecular weight favoring smaller molecules. As with luciferase, the hydrophobic binding pocket of proteins may indeed be linked to the size of the hydrocarbon chain. This would make very long hydrocarbons (longer than two *n*-hexanol molecules or one *n*-dodecanol molecule) "stick out" into the solvent and favor hydrophobic compounds of a certain length. The targets proteins are mainly neuromodulatory, although the field of psychoneuroimmunology indicates that systems are interrelated in their functions. Biochemical and mutation analyses identify target proteins as pentameric ligand-gated ion channels (GABA$_A$ receptor, glycine receptor, nicotinic acetylcholine receptor, N-methyl-D-aspartate (NMDA)–type glutamate receptors, bacterial homologue

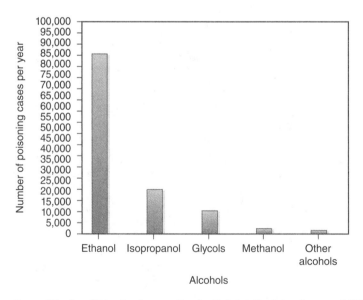

FIGURE 26-3 Acute Reported Number of Poisoning Cases per Year for Alcohols in North America up until 2010

Note: 188 Cases of methanol and glycol mixtures were also part of the methanol portion of the pie chart.

of pLGIC or GLIC), potassium channels (Shaw2, G protein–gated inwardly rectifying potassium channel 2, IRK1), adhesion molecules (L1), odorant-binding proteins (LUSH), and enzymes (luciferase alcohol dehydrogenase of ADH, adenylyl cyclase). The molecules that co-crystallized with these proteins were the anesthetic agents propofol (GLIC), 2-methyl,2,4,-pentanediol (IRK1), ethanol, 1-propanol, and 1-butanol (LUSH); bromoform (luciferase); and pentafluorobenzyl alcohol and trifluoroethanol (ADH). This hydrophobic action at the site of ion channels and adhesion molecules may explain the neurotoxicity of these compounds, yet it is known that these substances affect many signal transduction pathways leading to immunotoxicity as well. The most is known about ethanol, which appears to affect lipopolysaccharide-induced TLR4 signaling in macrophages at the membrane level. Methanol and isopropanol work more downstream to cause transcriptional problems that mark the immunotoxicity (decreased lymphocyte activation) of these compounds. It appears that isopropanol decreases cytokine release *in vitro* from T cells, natural killer cells, monocytes (with exception of increased IL-6), and macrophages (again excepting IL-6), while methanol appears to augment cytokine production. Thus, it appears that the complexity of the toxicity of alcohols depends on their hydrophobicity and interactions with signal transduction through membrane proteins and transcription factors. The neurotoxicity, immunotoxicity, and so forth may be more amenable to analysis by weighing the dysregulation that occurs with these compounds at relevant doses/concentrations (Désy et al., 2012).

Amines

Amines by their chemical nature are bases, because they can easily be protonated. Aliphatic amines used in medications, cosmetics, dyes, and pesticide synthesis, and as synthetic intermediates are likewise strong organic bases. Primary aliphatic amines C_8 to C_{18} are mainly used in the synthesis of ethoxylated fatty amines widely employed as cationic, surface-active compounds (textile industry, mineral oil, antistatic compounds in plastics). The remaining aliphatic amines are flotation agents, dispersing agents for pigments (bear some relationship to oil dispersants), and agents that prevent corrosion (cyclohexylamine in steam lines and boiler systems in the United States). Cyclohexylamine is thought to be developmentally toxic (no teratogenic effects for this amine in zebrafish embryos), mutagenic, and carcinogenic. In any hydrophobic compound, the generalized narcosis must still be considered (aliphatic moiety), but the polar amine and its metabolism must also be considered. The N-oxidation via CYPs in humans and animals yields the toxic hydroxylamines then oximes from primary amines:

$$R-CH_2-NH_2 \rightarrow R-CH_2-NH-OH \rightarrow R-CH=N-OH$$

Hydroxylamines and possible nitrones from secondary amines in the alpha carbon have an available hydrogen:

$$R^1(R^2)-CH-NH-R^s \rightarrow R^1(R^2)-CH-NOH-R^3$$
$$R^1(R^2)-C=NO-R^3 \leftrightarrow R^1(R^2)-C-NO-R^3$$

Tertiary amines can be metabolized to *N*-oxides that can be desalkylated and/or reduced:

$$R^1(R^2)(R^3)-N \rightarrow R^1(R^2)(R^3)-N-O$$

The alkaline pH these aliphatic amines in aquatic media and the formation of active metabolites mark their toxicity beyond their lipophilicity. A pH of 11.2 with zebrafish embryos was lethal (pKa values range from 8.49 [morpholine] to 11.3 [piperidine], but degree of ionization was also very important ranging from 2% [morpholine] to 90% [piperidine] or even 99% tributylamine). Of the amines tested on zebrafish embryos, *n*-decylamine had the lowest LC_{50} (20 μmol/L), while isopropylamine had the highest LC_{50} for a primary amine (2,531 μmol/L), indicating linear amines were the most toxic. Not surprisingly based on its chemistry, morpholine had the highest LC_{50} for a secondary amine (6,901 μmol/L), while dicyclohexylamine had the lowest LC_{50} value (172 μmol/L). Tertiary amine toxicity was led by N,N-dimethylcyclohexylamine (417 μmol/L), while tributylamine was the least toxic (LC_{50} = 1,625 μmol/L). For the tertiary amines, chain length exceeding six carbon atoms appeared to decrease toxicity rather than increase toxicity with dimethylcyclohexylamine as the notable exception (8 carbons). Lethal effects for these embryos involve mechanisms such as cardiac arrest (no heart beat), while sublethal effects are characterized by hypopigmentation (all amines tested excepting cyclohexylamine and dimethylbutylamine), yolk sac edema (all amines tested and usually is coupled to lethal results) or edema of the pericard/pericardium (lack of circulation), and deformed tail region. Missing otoliths or sacculi (part of hearing system) were also observed in affected embryos. Primary amines did not affect the sacculus, while secondary and tertiary amines have this effect. Granulated otoliths were observed in embryos treated with primary or secondary amines or only 1-ethylpiperidine, triethylamine, and tripropylamine of the tertiary amines. No otoliths occurred with all three classes of amines tested. Some spina bifida (unclosed spinal column due to incomplete closure of embryonic neural tube) was also caused by hexylamine, diisobutylamine, dibutylamine, and dimethylbutylamine. Apart from their lipophilicity, some notable outliers are 4-aminophenol (4-AP), 2,4-dinitrophenol (DNP), 4-nitrophenol (4-NP), and 3,4-dichloroaniline (3,4-DCA). This is where their mechanisms of action may come more into play. 2,4-DNP, 4-AP, and hydroquinone led to a lack of completion of the gastrula stage of embryonic development. 4-NP formed a hyperblastula (gastrula stage not even reached). Quinones, polynitroaromatic compounds, and imidazoles are highly reactive chemical species. These electrophiles react with nucleophilic groups such as amines, hydroxyls, or sulfhydryls found on proteins and DNA bases. Uncoupling oxidative phosphorylation is associated with polynitroaromatics such as 2,4-DNP. Increasing the acidity of a phenol group also increases their toxicity (e.g., 2,4-DNP pKa = 4.1, compared with 4-NP pKa = 7.21; Burst, 2001).

Ketones/Aldehydes

Small aldehydes such as formaldehyde (Mathison et al., 1997) and acetaldehyde are known for their toxicity to a variety of cells leading to cancer using metabolites with or without ROS. Formaldehyde and glutaraldehyde are commonly used as fixatives, and formaldehyde can cause chromosome pieces to stick together resulting in clastogenesis. Glutaraldehyde is an irritant and skin sensitizer, occasionally produces asthma, and is found to damage the heart, kidneys, and liver. If inhaled, glutaraldehyde also produces lung damage. Fetal toxicity and malformations have resulted from this aldehyde. It is not surprising that this compound is found to be mutagenic in the Ames test, but has failed to produce animal results (cancer) consistent with this finding (Takigawa and Endo, 2006). In ecotoxicity, it is easier to start by considering fish. 11 α,β-unsaturated aldehydes and ketones can be modeled using quantum calculations to explore their Michael reactions with methanethiol or glutathione. Water presence or absence also may be important in the catalytic pathway, so modeling must try both schemes (although aquatic systems should have plenty of water available). The most toxic compound was acrolein, which had the lowest activation energy and used water to calculate its activation energy of the reaction (Furuhama et al., 2012).

One must not only consider the most offending ketone or aldehyde, but also its synergism with other close chemical species. Methyl n-butyl ketone (MBK) following inhalation increased the number of neurofilaments in large myelinated nerve fibers resulting in axonal swelling with secondary thinning of the myelin sheath ("giant axonal" neuropathy). Additionally, inpouchings of the myelin sheath were observed. This pathology extended itself to abnormalities of the neuromuscular junction including main nerve trunk, nerve roots, and intramuscular nerves. Although methyl ethyl ketone (MEK) did not show this type of neurotoxicity, MEK potentiated the effects of MBK in a ratio of 1:5; MBK:MEK (Saida et al., 1976). As mentioned earlier in the organic solvents section, the toxic species of n-hexane or methyl n-butyl ketone is 2,5-hexanedione as seen in the axonal degeneration in the mammillary body and visual nuclei of cats (Schaumburg and Spencer, 1978). This same sort of problem developed in Berlin solvent sniffers with a hexane/MEK mixture (1:9 mixture; Altenkirch et al., 1978). Part of the synergistic toxicity of secondary ketones with increasing carbon chain length of highly chlorinated methane derivatives such as carbon tetrachloride and chloroform appears to occur due to an induction of CYP2E1 (inhibited this interaction by monoclonal antibody to this isoenzyme or other substrates for CYP2E1). Acetone-treated rats had a three-fold induction of this monooxygenase and increased metabolism of chloroform as measured by headspace gas chromatography (Brady et al., 1989).

Halogenated Hydrocarbons

Halogenated hydrocarbons such as alkanes, alkenes, and alkynes are not only anesthetizing, but are subject to reductive dehalogenation and radical formation based on CYP2E1, which is induced by ethanol and other compounds that become ketones/aldehydes. Some have remained as anesthetic agents such as halothane or enflurane, while others such as CCl_4, $HCCl_3$, trichloroethylene, and vinylidene chloride have remained as solvents (Raucy et al., 1993). Carbon tetrachloride, due to its complete electron withdrawal by halogens from its sole carbon, serves as the model of halogenated alkane reductive hepatic toxicity damage. The generation and stabilization of the trichloromethyl radical ($Cl_3C.$) by CYP2E1, CYP2B1, CYP2B2, and possibly CYP3A is the essential event leading to binding of the radical to nucleic acids, protein, and lipid, interfering with essential processes of lipid metabolism. This may lead to steatosis (fatty liver), while the radical binding to DNA leads to hepatic cancer. This radical can also react with oxygen, forming the $Cl_3COO.$ radical that initiates lipid peroxidation, especially with polyunsaturated fatty acids. The lipid peroxidation leads to increased permeability of the plasma membrane, mitochondrial membrane, and endoplasmic reticulum. One lipid peroxide product is 4-hydroxynonenal, a reactive aldehyde that binds to proteins/enzymes. Ca homeostasis becomes disrupted and leads to apoptosis and necrosis depending on the severity of the damage (whether an inexorable series of events has occurred or whether repair is still possible). The formation of tumor

necrosis factor alpha (TNFα) signals for apoptosis (counteracted by IL-10), while transforming growth factor alpha (TGFα) and beta (TGFβ) formation cause cell self-destruction and fibrosis. Carbon tetrachloride poisoning also results in hypomethylation of cellular components. In the case of RNA hypomethylation, this is thought to inhibit protein synthesis. For phospholipids, hypomethylation prevents the export of phospholipids via prevention of lipoprotein secretion (Weber et al., 2003). Perchloroethylene has also been used as a "dry" cleaning solvent. The solvent trichloroethylene (TCE)—used for degreasing of metal parts—and its ability to cause liver and kidney cancer via its metabolites, including trichloroacetic acid and dichloroacetic acid, may appear straightforward on first examination. Perchloroethylene has similar metabolites and may add to the toxicity of TCE and similar halogenated hydrocarbons. Ethanol and other chemicals that induce CYP2E1 may also prove to enhance the toxicity of these compounds, and generation of ROS may also accompany the metabolism of chemicals toxic to the lung, nervous system, heart, liver, kidney, cervix, and lymphatic system. This may give a more complete picture of actions of TCE that lead to cancer (lung, liver, kidney, and testicular tumors along with lymphoma). However, coexposures of mixtures of solvents, haloacetates, and ethanol with TCE involve both pharmacodynamic and pharmacokinetic considerations (Caldwell et al., 2008). One has to consider tissue repair in the toxicity observed for these and other chemicals, because cell-signaling mechanisms involve chemokines, cytokines, growth factors, and nuclear receptors lead to promitogenic gene expression and cell division. The regeneration of hepatic extracellular matrix and angiogenesis also relate to liver toxicity. Tissue repair increases up to the threshold dose that delays or impairs cell signaling for repair resulting in unchecked secondary effects of tissue destruction, organ failure, and mortality (Mehendale, 2005).

Chloroform has one less chlorine than carbon tetrachloride and was an anesthetic agent that was discontinued due to its carcinogenicity and liver toxicity. It appears that CYP2E1 plays a role in the liver toxicity and the kidney toxicity in male mice, as CYP2E1-null mice are resistant to the hepatic and renal toxicity of this solvent. The liver biotransformation plays no role in the renal toxicity to these susceptible male mice based on their CYP2E1 content, because deletion of the liver CYP reductase gene (liver-Cpr-null) left more chloroform to become toxic in the kidney. The liver-Cpr-null mice exposed to chloroform had raised blood urea nitrogen (BUN) levels (a clinical measure of how well the kidney is working to rid the body of nitrogenous wastes) that were five times higher than that of unexposed (vehicle-treated) mice and had severe kidney lesions, while BUN was only slightly elevated with mild kidney lesions in wild-type mice with the same 150 mg/kg chloroform dose. At 300 mg/kg, chloroform caused severe kidney lesions in liver-Cpr-null and wild-type mice, but the BUN levels were still higher in the liver-Cpr-null mice than in the HCCl$_3$-exposed wild-type mice (Fang et al., 2008). Halogenated alkanes can also be made more toxic by GSH conjugation. This seems to be the opposite of what happens with acetaminophen. These conjugates can be unstable and form an aldehyde or be toxic in their own right. Ethane with two halogens can also form GSH conjugates and then episulfonium ions that are both toxic to the proximal tubule of the kidney and mutagenic as well. Highly halogenated alkanes also may be conjugated by GSH and ultimately be taken up by kidney tubules. The renal mitochondrial enzyme responsible for the conversion to various toxic thiol species is cysteine-conjugate β-lyase.

Aromatics (Arenes → Benzene Derivatives)

Benzene has a long history of human exposure and animal testing. It is fully capable of neurotoxic consequences, but its metabolism to a species that is damaging to the bone marrow is the most important (benzene → phenol → hydroquinone via CYPs in liver and the phenol or hydroquinone metabolites are converted to the phenoxy radical by the prostaglandin H synthase (PHS) myeloperoxidase in the bone marrow). Depending on exposure duration and concentrations, the bone marrow can be severely damaged yielding aplastic anemia/pancytopenia or leukemia with lower, more chronic insults. The first animal cancer models indicated

Zymbal's gland carcinomas in rats given benzene orally or by inhalation (Maltoni and Scarnato, 1979; Maltoni et al., 1982a). Because the Zymbal's gland was regarded as a vestigial organ in the ear of the rat not found in humans, this gave industrial producers grounds to dispute benzene's carcinogenicity. However, inhalation exposure yielded anemia, lymphocytopenia, and bone marrow hyperplasia with an increase in lymphoid tumors in male mice. Although humans exhibit leukemia on exposure, rats and mice did not exhibit this type of cancer. Lung adenomas in male mice were observed by IP injection of benzene (Stoner et al., 1986), and rat inhalation studies yielded mainly carcinomas in various sites (Maltoni et al., 1982a,b; Maltoni et al., 1983; Maltoni et al., 1985; Snyder et al., 1984). Epidemiological evidence has added multiple myeloma, lung cancer, and non-Hodgkin's lymphoma to leukemia as cancers caused by benzene exposure in humans. The history of this discrepancy between animal models and humans is fascinating and important. Professor Cesare Maltoni attempted to identify occupational carcinogens and had early models of croton oil on rabbit skin (Parmeggiani et al., 1957), 9,10-dimethyl-1,2-benzanthracene on hamster skin (Maltoni and Prodi, 1957), and other bioassays for vinyl chloride (Maltoni and Lefemine, 1974), gasoline products (benzene part of the mix with toluene, xylenes, and naphthalene; Maltoni et al., 1997), and ethanol (Soffritti et al., 2002) as the starting points. David Rall (Huff et al., 1984) followed up with the National Toxicology Program to elucidate the nature of toxicants in animals and humans. For both researchers, benzene was an enigma to be solved. In addition to Zymbal's gland tumors, three strains of mice and three strains of rats exhibited tumors in mammary glands, oral tissues, lungs, nasal cavities, lymph nodes, liver, forestomach, skin, uterus, ovaries, and Harderian and preputial glands. Malignancies were found in both species and all strains. Human exposure to benzene was more frequently associated with leukemia due to its relatively fast onset and diagnosis.

Other cancers may take more time to develop. 1,3-Butadiene is a potent carcinogen whose concentration–response indicates some important findings about cancer development: At lower concentrations different tumor patterns become evident. Different exposure patterns for humans to benzene may indeed yield different tumor origins. Also, the most abundant and highest half-life metabolites—catechol, hydroquinone, and phenol—should be examined more closely. Catechol is a strong promoter of cancer and by itself causes forestomach hyperplasia, a few nonglandular papillomas of the forestomach in mice, and adenocarcinomas of the glandular stomach in nearly all rats. Catechol appears to increase the initiator-target tumors in the tongue, esophagus, forestomach, and stomach (benzene only increases forestomach tumors but not stomach tumors) but not in the liver, urinary bladder, or thyroid of mice. Hydroquinone appears to cause nephropathy in rats with hyperplasia of the renal pelvic transitional epithelium and renal cortical cysts in male rats leading to renal tubular cell hyperplasia and renal tubule cell adenomas at high doses. This same chemical in mice caused thyroid follicular cell hyperplasia and in females increased mononuclear cell leukemia. Livers of male mice with hydroquinone exposure increased anisokaryosis, multinucleated hepatocytes, and basophilic foci and possible progression to liver tumors. Phenol given for 2 years (lifetime) in rats and mice caused only leukemia as a cancer. Other low-dose tumors in male rats included C cell tumors of the thyroid, adrenal gland pheochromocytomas, and interstitial cell tumors of the testes. Hydroquinone and to a lesser degree phenol are associated with leukemia in animal models (Huff, 2007).

Toluene is mainly known for its neurotoxicity, although it can irritate the respiratory tract on inhalation or eye irritation from the fumes. It also can be absorbed through the skin and gastrointestinal tract. It is similar to alcohol and benzodiazepines in its CNS effects (sleep, headaches, memory impairment). Depression, dizziness, and fatigue have occurred in paint workers who have inhaled too much of this solvent. Toluene is marked by a low-dose deficit in spatial learning and memory. "Fetal solvent syndrome" is associated with embryopathy (growth retardation and microencephaly). Toluene affects a variety of neurotransmitters in its CNS effects. As expected from a CNS depressant, it inhibits excitatory NMDA receptors and nicotinic acetylcholine (ACh) receptors, while enhancing $GABA_A$ and glycine receptors. IP toluene injection decreases ACh in the striatum and hippocampus in a dose-dependent manner in freely moving rats. However, the neurotransmitter picture is more complicated than just these findings. Abusive levels of toluene exposure to rodents caused an upregulation of the expression of NMDA in rat hippocampal neurons. NMDA-glutamate receptors, responsible for visual-evoked potentials in rodents, appear to be a likely target of toluene toxicity. Exposure of adult mice to 50 ppm toluene over a prolonged period resulted in upregulation of NMDA receptor subunit NR2B expression with simultaneous induction of CaMKIV, CREB1, and GosB/ΔFosB in the hippocampus. As opposed to a decrease in NMDA receptor activity suggested by early experiments in this area of study, it appears that volatile organic chemicals (VOCs) may increase NMDA receptor activity via increasing NO (stimulate NMDA receptors) and peroxynitrite (increase NMDA receptor sensitivity) levels. Glutamate (a stimulatory neurotransmitter that can lead to toxicity when abusively stimulated) and taurine but not GABA and glycine were rapidly and reversibly increased in a dose-dependent manner 30 minutes after toluene administration. Toluene inhalation by rats caused an increase in prefrontal cortex extracellular dopamine concentration (an excitatory neurotransmitter involved in manic behavior), but not in the nucleus accumbens. Xenopus oocyte exposure to benzene potentiated serotonin-activated currents as indicated by serotonin-3A receptor responses. It is also of interest how the immune system may play a role in neurobehavioral function. T cell presence in the hippocampus as a result of very low levels of toluene result in upregulation of memory function–related gene expression as the immune system attempts to clear to toxicant from the brain (recruitment of peripheral T cells activate microglia that induce secretion of cytokines). However, as toluene concentration increases, T cell deficiencies result in dysregulation of neuroimmune crosstalk. Additionally, neurotrophins involved in the survival, differentiation, and maintenance of neuronal populations are upregulated along with their accompanying related receptors by low levels of toluene exposure. This expression of neurotrophins can also aggravate airway inflammatory responses in asthmatic populations, leading to a link between immune, neuronal, and respiratory system toxicities. The stress hormones also play a role in toxicity, as toluene exposure appears to induce adrenocortical hypertrophy via the hypothalamic-pituitary-adrenal axis. The stress response involves catecholamines as well and appears to explain the increased heart rate and respiratory sinus arrhythmia associated with toluene (and other mixed organic solvents) exposure (Win-Shwe and Fujimaki, 2010). The link of key systems for toluene toxicity and possibly for other solvents is indicated in **Figure 26-4**.

Xylene is similar to toluene as it has one more methyl group in a meta- (40–60% of laboratory-grade xylene), para- (20%), and ortho-position (20%), and is usually also contaminated with ethyl benzene (6–20%), toluene, trimethylbenzene, phenol, thiophene, pyridine, and hydrogen sulfide. It is similarly converted to the methyl hippuric acid (hippuric acid for toluene) and excreted. The CNS depression effects are obvious based the lipophilicity of xylenes and disruption of the lipid environment of the membrane proteins or direct binding to hydrophobic pockets. Again, the reactive aldehyde (methyl benzaldehyde) may be the key toxic metabolite. Xylene is an irritant of the nose, throat, and the lungs (yielding pulmonary edema) and can damage the surface of the eye if splashed into it. Xylenes can damage the liver and kidneys, but this is extremely unlikely without prominent CNS effects, which may also appear as a neurologically caused muscle weakness. Contamination with benzene is the only reason xylenes may affect blood cell numbers and formation. Xylenes, as they are also representative of other organic solvents, dissolve the skin's protective oils and at high concentrations in continued contact yield burns and blistering. The fetal toxicity, delayed skeletal ossification, and behavioral effects of xylenes have already been mentioned earlier (Kandyala et al., 2010). It appears that in the mouse and rat that, the CYP2F metabolites of compounds such as coumarin, naphthalene, and

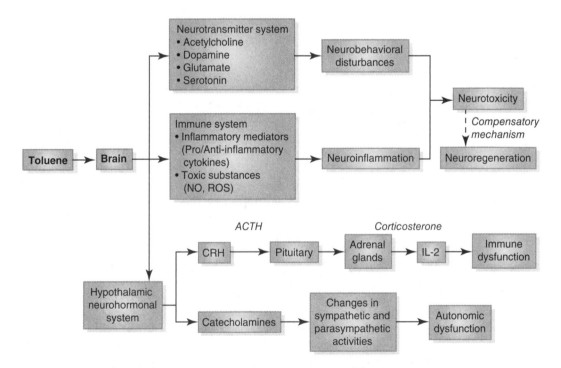

FIGURE 26-4 The Effects of Toluene on Neurotransmission, Immune Function, and the Stress Response

styrene drive the cytotoxicity and nasal and lung tumors in the mouse (rich in CYP2F2) and nasal tissue of rats (rich in CYP2F4). Rat CYP2F4 is fully capable of metabolizing these compounds, however CYP2F4 occurs at amounts lower than in the mouse and not in sufficient activity to cause rat lung cytotoxicity. Human lungs have far fewer Clara cells, and human lung microsomes either do not create the cytotoxic metabolites or only in biologically insignificant quantities. The morphology of the human lung's Clara cells also makes human lung tissue less sensitive to toxic metabolites compared with the rodent (especially mice). CYP2E1 (primarily alkyl oxidation) played little role in the toxicity of these compounds in mice. Additionally, the primary metabolite of ethylbenzene lacks lung toxicity in the mouse. This explains why coumarin, naphthalene, styrene, ethylbenzene, cumene, α-methylstyrene, divinylbenzene, and benzofuran cause toxicity to the terminal bronchioles leading to late-developing bronchoalveolar tumors in the lungs of mice but not rats. Additionally, this indicates the reason for styrene- or divinylbenzene-induced lung tumors in mice but not rats. Some of these are carcinogens in their own right, but not at these specific sites such as naphthalene and nasal cancers (via epoxide formation by CYPs). Because human workers have uncontrolled exposure to mixtures of chemicals, it has become clear that the methylbenzenes are mainly neurotoxic and that styrene has an uncertain association with cancers, chromosomal aberrations, sister chromatid exchanges, and micronuclei formation in some studies and not in others. The presence of 1,3-butadiene also complicates the issue as this alone could explain clastogenic effects (Cruzan et al., 2009).

Halogenated Aromatics

Algae respond to halogenated benzenes as a result of their K_{ow} (Zeng et al., 2011). The halogenated benzene derivatives are found to cause hepatic necrosis in a variety of species. They do so via metabolic activation, as shown in **Figure 26-5** For example, primary metabolites of bromobenzene potently damage the liver, while secondary metabolites cause severe damage to the kidney. As with benzene, the reactive

3,4 epoxide catalyzed by CYP starts the toxic process by binding to proteins. Again, the epoxides are converted to phenols, which are given a secondary oxidation reaction to hydroquinones, which are oxidized to electrophilic quinones (bind to sulfhydryl groups of protein or GSH). Bromobenzene is toxic to the liver until as a bromohydroquinone it is conjugated to GSH and sent off to the kidney. Via processing in the proximal tubular cells by γ-glutamyl transferase and membrane alanyl aminopeptidase, it becomes a cysteine similar to other aromatic compounds such as naphthalene. Unfortunately, the cysteine lowers the redox potential of this compound making it more subject to conversion to a reactive quinone species.

Now that the metabolic activation of halogenated aromatic compounds has been illustrated, how is this modeled? Considering high doses as toxic to the liver, the hydrophobicity (log P), ease of oxidation (EHOMO or energy of the highest molecular orbital), and the dipole moment (μ; asymmetric charge distribution of halogen substituents) correlate with human or rat hepatocyte toxicity. However, in phenobarbital-treated rats that have increased expression of CYP2B/3A, hydrophobicity and dipole moment predominate—not the ease of oxidation. This finding confirms that the initial activation of bromobenzene by CYP is the rate-limiting step proceeding to damage in the liver (and consequently to what it might do to the kidney; Chan et al., 2007). At the other end of the spectrum is hexachlorobenzene, which fits in more with the polychlorinated dibenzo-p-dioxins/furans, dichlorodiphenyltrichloroethane (DDT), and β-hexachlorohexacyclohexane under the category of persistent organic pollutants, as their chlorine atoms do not yield easily to nucleophilic displacement and elimination reactions. The major focus of these compounds is their action on nuclear receptors such as the estrogen receptor, androgen receptor, progesterone receptor, glucocorticoid receptor, constitutive androstane receptor, rodent prename X receptor, mineralocorticoid/aldosterone receptor, and thyroid hormone receptors. The aryl/aromatic hydrocarbon receptor (AhR) is clearly of interest here as too. Binding to these receptors causes translocation of the nuclear receptors and/or

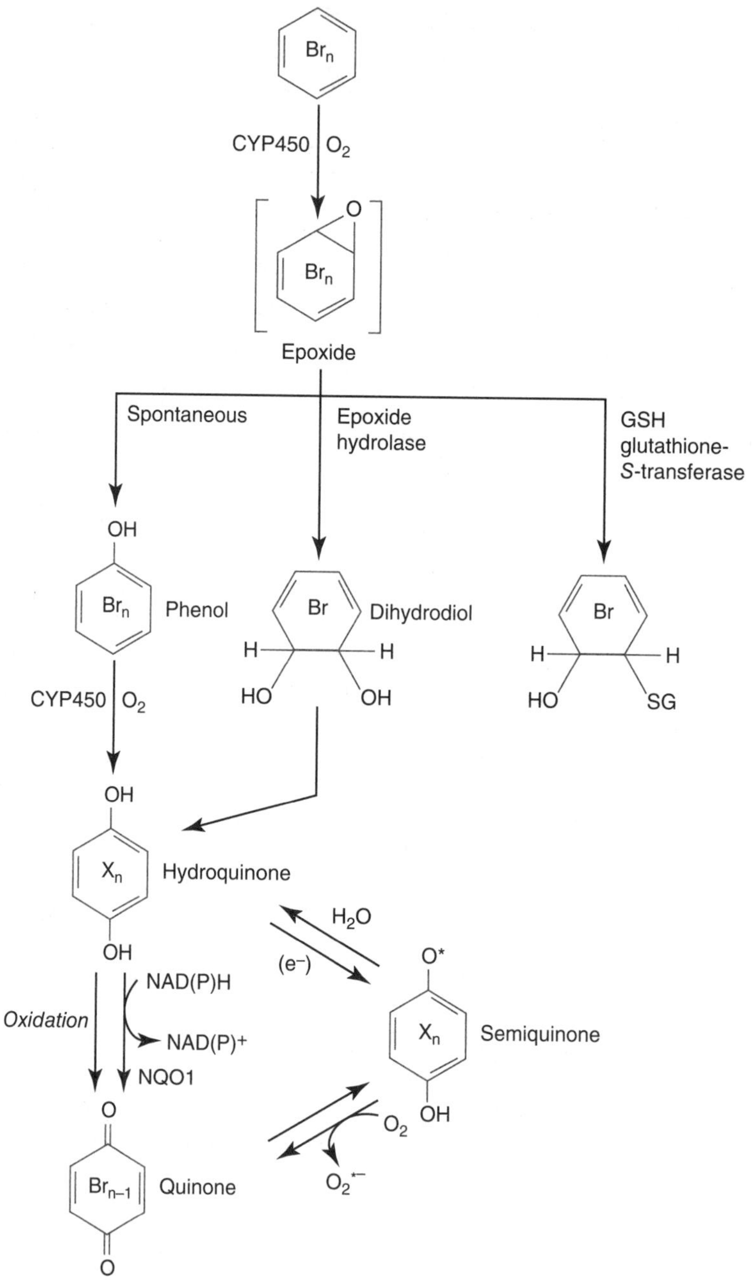

FIGURE 26-5 Metabolic Activation of Halogenated Benzenes as Represented by Bromobenzene

Note: The binding of bromines to the ring at n positions on outside of the benzene is indicated by the Br$_n$ inside the ring rather than outside the ring. Other n moieties are indicated by X$_n$. The formation of the reactive electrophilic epoxide is seen at the top of the figure. Isomerization to phenols, conversion to dihydrodiols (epoxide hydrolase) or GSH conjugation (via glutathione S-transferase) to prevent adduct formation of cellular macromolecules (proteins and DNA) is the second tier down. Formation of the hydroquinone to a quinone by CYP is displayed on the left just below the second tier. Electrophilic quinines (conjugated by GSH, forming adducts, or generating ROS as a result of redox cycling) are found in the triangular reaction sequence on the bottom of the figure.

the AhR to the nucleus. Hexachlorobenzene (HCB) actually would be regarded as a fungicide and not a solvent per se. It has a half-life of 6 years in the human, so it is capable of causing long-term effects even after an acute dose. HCB mainly targets the liver, ovary, and the CNS (as expected of any volatile chemical). It also generates free radicals (reactive tetrachloro-1,4-benzoquinone) on metabolism that leads to porphyria (can present as skin or neurological problem based on accelerated heme production). HCB does not have affinity for the estrogen receptor and is a weak agonist of the AhR protein. Those properties clearly separate this compound from the potent cell proliferation agents of TCDD or highly chlorinated dibenzofurans. To elicit mammary tumors, HCB requires the strong mutagen N-nitroso-N-methylurea, so HCB has some cancer-promoting activity. The way HCB accomplishes cell proliferation is complicated. It appears to involve Src activation (pro-oncogene tyrosine-protein kinase), which is not AhR dependent. It also appears to involve insulin receptor substrate 1 (IRS-1) phosphorylation, therefore activating the insulin-like growth factor-insulin receptor pathway involved in the development of breast cancer (Mrema et al., 2012).

Sulfur-Containing Organic Chemical Solvents

Mercaptans are toxic odiferous compounds used to scent natural gas or as mercury chelators (a contraction of mercury capturer is how this group of compounds obtained their name). Methyl mercaptan is a gas employed in the manufacture of methionine, plastics, pesticides, and jet fuel. It causes eye irritation, redness, and pain. Methyl mercaptan also leads to respiratory tract irritation. This compound also depresses the CNS including the respiratory center similar to hydrogen sulfide and produces death by respiratory paralysis. As the alkyl chain is increased, the mercaptans become liquid and therefore can be used as solvents. They tend to be less toxic but can still be slightly irritating to the eyes of rabbits (n-butyl mercaptan is used as an animal repellant). Dimethylsulfoxide (DMSO) is a well known solvent whose major problem with dermal administration is

altering the skin as a barrier to other compounds. However, it appears to have systemic toxicity with dismal prognoses for human patients for which it was used as part of cord blood stem cell transplant (Ruiz-Delgado et al., 2009) and appears to play some role in acute respiratory distress syndrome, despite its nature as a radical scavenger (Tawil et al., 2011). DMSO is also a pharmacologic agent that helps with circulatory problems in the heart and CNS and can attenuate the cytotoxicity associated with excess glutamate release (CNS; Jacob and de la Torre, 2009). A small compound that has industrial solvent applications and a distinct set of toxicities is carbon disulfide.

Carbon Disulfide

Many of the toxic effects of CS_2 have already been discussed, but the workers in the viscose fiber industry are key examples of human toxicity. They have experienced coronary heart disease, coronary risk factors, retinal angiopathy, problems with color discrimination, effects on peripheral nerves, psychophysiological effects, morphological and other CNS effects, and changes in fertility and other hormonal effects. Japanese workers have been reported to have retinal microaneurysms plus electrocardiogram changes, altered peripheral nerve conduction velocities, MRI hyperintensive spots, and changes in hearing that are currently unclear as to their distinct linkage to CS_2 exposure (Gelbke et al., 2009). The coronary heart disease may be related to hypercholesterolemia (Kotseva, 2001). The changes in color discrimination involve either receptiveness alterations in ganglion cells or demyelination of optic nerve fibers (Raitta et al., 1981).

Glycols

Ethylene glycol as the basis of antifreeze solutions used in automobile radiator cooling systems is metabolized more rapidly than methanol via alcohol dehydrogenase to glycolate (or glyoxylic acid) resulting in metabolic acidosis. The toxin oxalate may be formed from here and rapidly precipitates calcium in various tissues and the urine (Jacobsen and McMartin, 1986).

Glycol Ethers

Compounds such as ethyl ether represent older solvents that were also used as anesthetic agents. Their toxicity is similar in nature to that of other organic solvents in the CNS. Ethylene glycol alkyl ethers such as 2-methoxyethanol, 2-ethoxyethanol, 2-isopropoxyethanol, and 2-butoxyethanol, however, have toxicity that spans a variety of organ systems. These compounds are found in many products of industrial or home use including paints, varnishes, engine fuels, hydraulic fluids, floor polishes, and cleaners of glass, leather, and upholstery. Their ether composition makes them easily absorbed via inhalation, dermally, or by ingestion, and their oxidation into aldehydes and alkoxyacetic acids yields their toxic species. Along with CNS toxicity, hematopoietic organs and reproductive organs also succumb to the toxic influences of these compounds both acutely and chronically (Starek and Szabla, 2008).

PAHs (Arenes — Multiple Rings)

These chemicals have been around for millions of years; they represent burn products. An evaluation of diesel exhaust found a variety of PAHs, such as 3-nitrobenzanthrone (Hallberg et al., 2012). This compound has been identified in urban air and has been linked to micronucleus formation in DNA of human hepatoma cells. Diesel exhaust has been shown to increase mutagenicity of *Salmonella typhimurium* and mammalian cells. ICR mice respond to diesel exhaust with an increase in the incidence of tumors and induction of 8-hydroxy-deoxyguanosine adducts (Hallberg et al., 2012). Most PAHs are activated by CYPs to epoxides, especially critical in the bay region. Less examined is the effect of sunlight radiation in the presence of oxygen on the formation of oxygenated PAHs, PAH quinones, nitro-PAHs, and halogenated PAHs. PAHs and PAH photoreaction products appear to absorb light energy to achieve photo-excited states. Together with molecular oxygen, medium, and coexisting chemicals, ROS are formed along with other reactive intermediates (oxygenated PAHs and free radicals). These reactive intermediates, which include ROS, produce lipid peroxidation, DNA strand breaks, oxidation of certain sensitive DNA bases (to 8-oxo-2′-deoxyguanosine), and DNA adducts. This photoreaction can occur on human skin and therefore should be of concern regarding skin cancer (Fu et al., 2012).

Polychlorinated Biphenyls (PCBs)

These are persistent chemicals, especially as the number of chlorines increases. PCBs were used as a coolant for electrical transformers. The less chlorinated species (one to two chlorines) are less of a concern due to their metabolism, but the hexachlorobiphenyl congeners are very persistent and have chronic cancer potential. Coplanar congeners act very similarly to dioxins and may be viewed in dioxin-equivalent toxicity (TEQ based on AhR activation) units. PCBs have hormone-like properties and exhibit neuro- and immunotoxicity (immune system suppression is a common mechanism for organochlorines). They have been associated with liver/biliary cancer, breast cancer, and skin cancer. They have recently been linked to the increased risk of non-Hodgkin's lymphoma (Freeman and Kohles, 2012).

Dibenzodioxins and Dibenzofurans

As a result of the burning of plastics and heavy fuels such as diesel oil or synthesized chlorinated pesticides such as 2,4,5-T, 2,3,7, 7-tetrachlorodibenzo-*p*-dioxin (TCDD) is generated. TCDD is the most potent dibenzodioxin as indicated by TEQ analysis. The manufacture of pesticides had these as important contaminants, especially of Agent Orange defoliant used in the Vietnam War in the 1960s. This exposure to dioxin has been linked to birth defects including spina bifida (Ngo et al., 2010). Polyhalogenated aromatic hydrocarbons such as the organochlorine pesticides, PCBs, and polychlorinated dibenzodioxins (PCDDs) and dibenzofurans (PCDFs) are fetotoxic, neurotoxic, and immunotoxic. They are especially toxic to guinea pigs, but are more chronically toxic to humans. They promote carcinogens and/or interfere with hormonal receptors. They pass the placenta and also equilibrate with lipid compartments of the body including breastmilk lipids. The exposure via breastmilk in industrialized countries is 10–100 times (1–2 log units) higher than the tolerable daily intake (TDI) of 1–4 toxic equivalents (WHO-TEQ) pg/kg/day established in 1998 by the World Health Organization for dioxins and dioxin-like PCBs, but is a potentially "late" exposure in development lasting 0.6% of the expected lifespan (Przyrembel et al., 2000). This pg/kg/day may seem low, but is three orders of magnitude higher than the 1.0 ng/kg/day NOAEL set for rat carcinogenicity and reproductive toxicity for TCDD. However, it appears that for humans 600 g TCDD TEQs can be taken in daily for a 60-kg average body weight without deleterious effects. The only sustained toxic consequence in humans exposed to PCDD/PCDF is chloracne and other skin conditions (Feeley and Grant, 1993).

Questions

1. What chemical parameter is a good indication of the anesthesia potential of organic solvents? Why does it miss the chronic toxicity of n-hexane or formaldehyde?
2. Why does the PETROTOX model overestimate the toxicity of petroleum distillates to fish?
3. Why are gasoline additives usually more toxic than the long-chain hydrocarbons that predominate in gasoline?
4. Why is ethanol an antidote to methanol toxicity?
5. Why are aliphatic amines more toxic than their log P would indicate?
6. What is the link between the synergism between ketones and halogenated hydrocarbon toxicity?
7. What do catechol, phenol, and hydroquinone indicate about animal models of benzene-induced cancers?
8. Why is hexachlorobenzene sometimes viewed as more similar to TCDD and DDT than to bromobenzene in its activation and

effects, yet is actually distinct from those larger compounds in its toxicity?
9. What are the unusual features of CS_2 poisoning?
10. Ethylene glycol is toxic on ingestion (from drinking antifreeze) due to the formation of glycolate resulting in metabolic acidosis. Why are the glycol ethers more toxic and have a variety of systemic effects?
11. Why are PAHs viewed as mutagenic, while highly toxic TCDDs (especially to guinea pig) are cancer-promotion agents?

References

Agamy E. 2012. Histopathological liver alterations in juvenile rabbit fish (*Siganus canaliculatus*) exposed to light Arabian crude oil, dispersed oil and dispersant. *Ecotoxicol Environ Saf.* 75:171–179.

Ahmed FE. 2001. Toxicology and human health effects following exposure to oxygenated or reformulated gasoline. *Toxicol Lett.* 123:89–113.

Altenkirch H, Stoltenburg G, Wagner HM. 1978. Experimental studies on hydrocarbon neuropathies induced by methyl-ethyl-ketone (MEK). *J Neurol.* 219:159–170.

Anderson SE, Franko J, Lukomska E, Meade BJ. 2011. Potential immunotoxicological health effects following exposure to COREXIT 9500A during cleanup of the Deepwater Horizon oil spill. *J Toxicol Environ Health A.* 74:1419–1430.

Baraniuk JN. 2009. Pathogenic mechanisms of idiopathic nonallergic rhinitis. *World Allergy Organ J.* 2:106–114.

Brady JF, Li D, Ishizaki H, Lee M, Ning SM, Xiao F, Yang CS. 1989. Induction of cytochromes P450IIE1 and P450IIB1 by secondary ketones and the role of P450IIE1 in chloroform metabolism. *Toxicol Appl Pharmacol.* 100:342–349.

Burst, K. 2001. Toxicity of aliphatic amines on the embryos of zebrafish *Danio rerio*—experimental studies and QSAR [Dissertation]. Dresden, Technical University, Germany.

Byard RW, Chivell WC, Gilbert JD. 2003. Unusual facial markings and lethal mechanisms in a series of gasoline inhalation deaths. *Am J Forensic Med Pathol.* 24:298–302.

Caldwell JC, Keshava N, Evans MV. 2008. Difficulty of mode of action determination for trichloroethylene: an example of complex interactions of metabolites and other chemical exposures. *Environ Mol Mutagen.* 49:142–154.

Caprino L, Togna GI. 1998. Potential health effects of gasoline and its constituents: a review of current literature (1990-1997) on toxicological data. *Environ Health Perspect.* 106:115-125.

Chan K, Jensen NS, Silber PM, O'Brien PJ. 2007. Structure-activity relationships for halobenzene induced cytotoxicity in rat and human hepatocytes. *Chem Biol Interact.* 165:165-174.

Cruzan G, Bus J, Banton M, Gingell R, Carlson G. 2009. Mouse specific lung tumors from CYP2F2-mediated cytotoxic metabolism: an endpoint/toxic response where data from multiple chemicals converge to support a mode of action. *Regul Toxicol Pharmacol.* 55:205-218.

Davis LE, Hudson D, Benson BE, Jones Easom LA, Coleman JK. 2002. Methanol poisoning exposures in the United States: 1993-1998. *J Toxicol Clin Toxicol.* 40:499-505.

Désy O, Carignan D, de Campos-Lima PO. 2012. Short-term immunological effects of non-ethanolic short-chain alcohols. *Toxicol Lett.* 210:44-52.

Dick FD. 2006. Solvent neurotoxicity. *Occup Environ Med.* 63:221-226, 179.

Enterline PE. Review of new evidence regarding the relationship of gasoline exposure to kidney cancer and leukemia. *Environ Health Perspect.* 101 (Suppl 6):101-103.

Fang C, Behr M, Xie F, Lu S, Doret M, Luo H, Yang W, Aldous K, Ding X, Gu J. 2008. Mechanism of chloroform-induced renal toxicity: non-involvement of hepatic cytochrome P450-dependent metabolism. *Toxicol Appl Pharmacol.* 227:48-55.

Feeley MM, Grant DL. 1993. Approach to risk assessment of PCDDs and PCDFs in Canada. *Regul Toxicol Pharmacol.* 18:428-437.

Finch BE, Wooten KJ, Faust DR, Smith PN. 2012. Embryotoxicity of mixtures of weathered crude oil collected from the Gulf of Mexico and Corexit 9500 in mallard ducks (*Anas platyrhynchos*). *Sci Total Environ.* 426:155-159.

Francis AA, Forsyth C. 1995. Toxicity profiles. The Risk Assessment Information System. http://rais .ornl.gov/tox/profiles/mn.html

Freeman MD, Kohles SS. 2012. Plasma levels of polychlorinated biphenyls, non-Hodgkin lymphoma, and causation. *J Environ Public Health.* 2012:258981. doi: 10.1155/2012/258981.

Fu PP, Xia Q, Sun X, Yu H. 2012. Phototoxicity and environmental transformation of polycyclic aromatic hydrocarbons (PAHs)-light-induced reactive oxygen species, lipid peroxidation, and DNA damage. *J Environ Sci Health C Environ Carcinog Ecotoxicol Rev.* 30:1-41.

Furuhama A, Aoki Y, Shiraishi H. 2012. Consideration of reactivity to acute fish toxicity of α,β-unsaturated carbonyl ketones and aldehydes. *SAR QSAR Environ Res.* 23:169-184.

Gelbke HP, Göen T, Mäurer M, Sulsky SI. 2009. A review of health effects of carbon disulfide in viscose industry and a proposal for an occupational exposure limit. *Crit Rev Toxicol.* 39(Suppl 2):1-126.

Hallberg LM, Ward JB, Hernandez C, Ameredes BT, Wickliffe JK; HEI Health Review Committee. 2012. Part 3. Assessment of genotoxicity and oxidative stress after exposure to diesel exhaust from U.S. 2007-compliant diesel engines: report on 1- and 3-month exposures in the ACES bioassay. *Res Rep Health Eff Inst.* Sep;(166):163-184.

Huff J, Moore J, Rall D. 1984. The National Toxicology Program and preventive oncology. In: Estrin N, Estrin N, editors. *The Cosmetic Industry: Scientific and Regulatory Foundations.* (pp. 647-676). New York: Marcel Dekker.

Huff J. 2007. Benzene-induced cancers: abridged history and occupational health impact. *Int J Occup Environ Health.* 13:213-221.

Infante PF. 1993. State of the science on the carcinogenicity of gasoline with particular reference to cohort mortality study results. *Environ Health Perspect.* 101(Suppl 6): 105-109.

Jacob SW, de la Torre JC. 2009. Pharmacology of dimethyl sulfoxide in cardiac and CNS damage. *Pharmacol Rep.* 61:225-235.

Jacobsen D, McMartin KE. 1986. Methanol and ethylene glycol poisonings. Mechanism of toxicity, clinical course, diagnosis and treatment. *Med Toxicol.* 1:309-334.

Jakobsson R, Ahlbom A, Bellander T, Lundberg I. 1993. Acute myeloid leukemia among petrol station attendants. *Arch Environ Health.* 48:255-259.

Kandyala R, Raghavendra SP, Rajasekharan ST. 2010. Xylene: an overview of its health hazards and preventive measures. *J Oral Maxillofac Pathol.* 14:1-5.

Kotseva K. 2001. Occupational exposure to low concentrations of carbon disulfide as a risk factor for hypercholesterolaemia. *Int Arch Occup Environ Health.* 74:38-42.

Kranjcec D, Bergovec M, Rougier JS, Raguz M, Pavlovic S, Jespersen T, Castella V, Keller DI, Abriel H. 2007. Brugada syndrome unmasked by accidental inhalation of gasoline vapors. *Pacing Clin Electrophysiol.* 30:1294-1298.

Kulig BM. 1990. Neurotoxic effects of organic solvents. In: Russell RW, Flattau PE, Pope AM, eds., *Behavioral Measures of Neurotoxicity.* Washington, DC: National Academies Press.

Leme DM, Grummt T, Heinze R, Sehr A, Renz S, Reinel S, de Oliveira DP, Ferraz ER, de Marchi MR, Machado MC, Zocolo GJ, Marin-Morales MA. 2012. An overview of biodiesel soil pollution: data based on cytotoxicity and genotoxicity assessments. *J Hazard Mater.* 199-200:343-349.

MacAllister SL, Choi J, Dedina L, O'Brien PJ. 2011. Metabolic mechanisms of methanol/formaldehyde in isolated rat hepatocytes: carbonyl-metabolizing enzymes versus oxidative stress. *Chem Biol Interact.* 191:308–314.

Maltoni C, Ciliberti A, Pinto C, Soffritti M, Belpoggi F, Menarini L. 1997. Results of long-term experimental carcinogenicity studies of the effects of gasoline, correlated fuels, and major gasoline aromatics on rats. *Ann NY Acad Sci.* 837:15–52.

Maltoni C, Conti B, Cotti G. 1983. Benzene: a multipotential carcinogen. Results of long-term bioassays performed at the Bologna Institute of Oncology. *Am J Ind Med.* 4:589–630.

Maltoni C, Conti B, Cotti G, Belpoggi F. 1985. Experimental studies on benzene carcinogenicity at the Bologna Institute of Oncology: current results and ongoing research. *Am J Ind Med.* 7:415–446.

Maltoni C, Cotti G, Valgimigli L, Mandrioli A. 1982a. Zymbal gland carcinomas in rats following exposure to benzene by inhalation. *Am J Ind Med.* 3:11–16.

Maltoni C, Cotti G, Valgimigli L, Mandrioli A. 1982b. Hepatocarcinomas in Sprague-Dawley rats, following exposure to benzene by inhalation. First experimental demonstration. *Med Lav.* 4:446–450.

Maltoni C, Lefemine G. 1974. Carcinogenicity bioassays of vinyl chloride. I. Research plan and early results. *Environ Res.* 7:387:405.

Maltoni C, Prodi G. 1957. [Cutaneous oncogenesis in *Cricetus auratus* (hamster) by 9,10-dimethyl-1,2-benzanthracene.] *Boll Soc Ital Biol Sper.* 33:506–507.

Maltoni C, Scarnato C. 1979. First experimental demonstration of the carcinogenic effects of benzene; long-term bioassays on Sprague-Dawley rats by oral administration. *Med Lav.* 70:352–357.

Mathison BH, Harman AE, Bogdanffy MS. 1997. DNA damage in the nasal passageway: a literature review. *Mutat Res.* 380:77–96.

Matsuoka M. 2007. [Neurotoxicity of organic solvents-recent findings]. *Brain Nerve.* 59:591–596.

Mattie DR, Sterner TR. 2011. Past, present and emerging toxicity issues for jet fuel. *Toxicol Appl Pharmacol.* 254:127–132.

Mehendale HM. 2005. Tissue repair: an important determinant of final outcome of toxicant-induced injury. *Toxicol Pathol.* 33:41–51.

Mrema EJ, Rubino FM, Brambilla G, Moretto A, Tsatsakis AM, Colosio C. 2012. Persistent organochlorinated pesticides and mechanisms of their toxicity. *Toxicology.* 307:74–88.

National Institute for Occupational Safety and Health. 1987. Organic solvent neurotoxicity. *Current Intelligence Bulletin.* 48(87–104). http://www.cdc.gov/niosh/docs/87-104/.

Ngo AD, Taylor R, Roberts CL. 2010. Paternal exposure to Agent Orange and spina bifida: a meta-analysis. *Eur J Epidemiol.* 25:37–44.

Parmeggiani A, Prodi G, Maltoni C. 1957. [Incorporation of radioactive sulfate in sulfurated polysaccharides of rabbit skin during treatment with cocarcinogenic substance (Croton oil)] Boll Soc Ital Biol Sper. 33:496–499.Przyrembel H, Heinrich-Hirsch B, Vieth B. 2000. Exposition to and health effects of residues in human milk. *Adv Exp Med Biol.* 478:307–325.

Raitta C, Teir H, Tolonen M, Nurminen M, Helpiö E, Malmström S. 1981. Impaired color discrimination among viscose rayon workers exposed to carbon disulfide. *J Occup Med.* 23:189–192.

Raucy JL, Kraner JC, Lasker JM. 1993. Bioactivation of halogenated hydrocarbons by cytochrome P4502E1. *Crit Rev Toxicol.* 23:1–20.

Raymond P, Plaa GL. 1995. Ketone potentiation of haloalkane-induced hepato- and nephrotoxicity. II. Implication of monooxygenases. *J Toxicol Environ Health.* 46:317–328.

Raymond P, Plaa GL. 1996. Ketone potentiation of haloalkane-induced hepatotoxicity: CCl_4 and ketone treatment on hepatic membrane integrity. *J Toxicol Environ Health.* 49:285–300.

Redman AD, Parkerton TF, McGrath JA, Di Toro DM. 2012. PETROTOX: An aquatic toxicity model for petroleum substances. *Environ Toxicol Chem.* 31:2498–2506.

Ritchie GD, Still KR, Alexander WK, Nordholm AF, Wilson CL, Rossi J 3rd, Mattie DR. 2001. A review of the neurotoxicity risk of selected hydrocarbon fuels. *J Toxicol Environ Health B Crit Rev.* 4:223–312.

Ruiz-Delgado GJ, Mancías-Guerra C, Tamez-Gómez EL, Rodríguez-Romo LN, López-Otero A, Hernández-Arizpe A, Gómez-Almaguer D, Ruiz-Argüelles GJ. 2009. Dimethyl sulfoxide-induced toxicity in cord blood stem cell transplantation: report of three cases and review of the literature. *Acta Haematol.* 122:1–5.

Saida K, Mendell JR, Weiss HS. 1976. Peripheral nerve changes induced by methyl *n*-butyl ketone and potentiation by methyl ethyl ketone. *J Neuropathol Exp Neurol.* 35:207–225.

Schaumburg HH, Spencer PS. 1978. Environmental hydrocarbons produce degeneration in cat hypothalamus and optic tract. *Science.* 199:199–200.

Snyder CA, Goldstein BD, Sellakumar AR, Albert RE. 1984. Evidence for hematotoxicity and tumorigenesis in rats exposed to 100 ppm benzene. *Am J Ind Med.* 5:429–434.

Solomon GM, Janssen S. 2010. Health effects of the Gulf oil spill. *JAMA.* 304:1118–1119.

Soffritti M, Belpoggi F, Cevolani D, Guarino M, Padovani M, Maltoni C. 2002. Results of long-term experimental studies on the carcinogenicity of methyl alcohol and ethyl alcohol in rats. *Ann NY Acad Sci.* 982:46–69.

Sriram K, Lin GX, Jefferson AM, Goldsmith WT, Jackson M, McKinney W, Frazer DG, Robinson VA, Castranova V. 2011. Neurotoxicity following acute inhalation exposure to the oil dispersant COREXIT EC9500A. *J Toxicol Environ Health A.* 74:1405–1418.

Stamatoyannopoulos G, Chen SH, Fukui M. 1975. Liver alcohol dehydrogenase in Japanese: high population frequency of atypical form and its possible role in alcohol sensitivity. *Am J Hum Genet.* 27:789–796.

Standeven AM, Goldsworthy TL. 1993. Promotion of preneoplastic lesions and induction of CYP2B by unleaded gasoline vapor in female B6C3F1 mouse liver. *Carcinogenesis.* 14:2137–2141.

Starek A, Szabla J. 2008. [Ethylene glycol alkyl ethers-the substances noxious to health]. *Med Pr.* 59:179–185.

Stoner GD, Conran PB, Greisiger EA, Stober J, Morgan M, Pereira MA. 1986. Comparison of two routes of chemical administration on the lung adenoma response in strain A/J mice. *Toxicol Appl Pharmacol.* 82: 19–31.

[Study of the mutagenic activity of petroleum upon chronic exposure in laboratory animals]. 2012. *Gig Sanit.* Jul-Aug:69–73.

Takigawa T, Endo Y. 2006. Effects of glutaraldehyde exposure on human health. *J Occup Health.* 48:75–87.

Tanii H. 1994. [Structure-activity relationships of organic solvents and related chemicals]. *Sangyo Igaku.* 36:299–313.

Tawil I, Carlson AP, Taylor CL. 2011. Acute respiratory distress syndrome after onyx embolization of arteriovenous malformation. *Crit Care Res Pract.* 2011:918185.

van Valen E, Wekking E, van der Laan G, Sprangers M, van Dijk F. 2009. The course of chronic solvent induced encephalopathy: a systematic review. *Neurotoxicology.* 30:1172–1186.

Weber LW, Boll M, Stampfl A. 2003. Hepatotoxicity and mechanism of action of haloalkanes: carbon tetrachloride as a toxicological model. *Crit Rev Toxicol.* 33:105–136.

Win-Shwe TT, Fujimaki H. 2010. Neurotoxicity of toluene. *Toxicol Lett.* 198:93–99.

Wise J, Wise JP Sr. 2011. A review of the toxicity of chemical dispersants. *Rev Environ Health.* 26:281–300.

Wong O, Raabe GK. 1997. Multiple myeloma and benzene exposure in a multinational cohort of more than 250,000 petroleum workers. *Regul Toxicol Pharmacol.* 26:188–199.

Zeng M, Lin Z, Yin D, Zhang Y, Kong D. 2011. A K(ow)-based QSAR model for predicting toxicity of halogenated benzenes to all algae regardless of species. *Bull Environ Contam Toxicol.* 86:565–570.

CHAPTER 27

Industrial Chemicals That Change Lipophilicity But Do Not Biodegrade: Metal Impacts

This is a chapter outline intended to guide and familiarize you with the content to follow.

I. Metals

    A. Change hydrophobicity but do not biodegrade = higher toxicity and pass through skin more easily (e.g., Hg^0 vs. dimethylmercury)

    B. Se and Hg are volatile if heated (the rest are particle associated)

    C. Some metals are nutrients but lead to liver damage (accumulates metals in diet) and other toxicity if ingested in toxic amounts (e.g., Fe, Se)

    D. Toxic metals—see Table 27-1

        1. Arsenic (As)—skin lesions (pigmentation and keratosis), weakness, conjunctival congestion, hepatomegaly, portal hypertension, lung disease, polyneuropathy, solid edema of limbs, ischemic heart disease, peripheral vascular disease, hypertension, and anemia; methylation reactions used to help remove As from body. First methylation reaction and As^{3+} state (arsenite) important to As toxicity such as cancer, diabetes mellitus, cardiovascular toxicity, neurotoxicity, and nephrotoxicity. The ϖ isoform of GSH S-transferase and purine nucleoside phosphorylase catalyze the reduction of As(V) to the more toxic As(III). Polynucleotide phosphorylase and mitochondrial ATP synthase also do this reduction in the presence of GSH. As non-conjugated arsenicals are highly reactive with thiols and easily converted to less toxic pentavalent arsenicals, the As(III)-GSH conjugate may be a key factor in As toxicity. The methylation of As(III) requires S-adenosylmethionine (catalyzed by rat cytosolic enzyme arsenite methyltransferase) and leads both to ↑ toxicity and excretion ("double-edged sword"). As is not a mutagen but a clastogen that leads to cancer of various organs via mechanisms such as cell-cycle checkpoint dysregulation, DNA damage response, abnormal chromosomal segregation, defects in cell-cycle checkpoints, disabled apoptosis, telomere dysfunction, altered chromatin structure, and other toxic mechanisms including inhibition or loss of the expression of tumor suppressor gene and activation of oncogenes. DNA repair is also inhibited (skin lesions)

        2. Cadmium (Cd)—especially known for renal proximal tubule damage to S_1 and S_2 segments (apoptosis). This is caused by endoplasmic reticulum (ER) stress → ER stress transducers (RNA-dependent protein kinase-like ER kinase [PERK]), activating transcription factor 6 (ATF6), and inositol-requiring ER-to-nucleus signal kinase 1 (IRE1) → ATF6 activates apoptosis through induction of CCAAT/enhancer-binding protein-homologous protein (CHOP), while IRE1 produces apoptosis by stimulation of X-box binding protein 1 (XBP1) and subsequent phosphorylation of c-jun N-terminal kinase (JNK). ER stress also leads to Ca^{2+} release and induction of apoptosis (calpain-caspase signal transduction pathway). Cd also acts directly on kidney mitochondria → mitochondrial swelling → cyt c release. Cd also affects Ub-proteasome system responsible for degradation of damaged proteins. At high concentrations, Cd causes a painful deterioration of bones (Itai-Itai disease). Chronic exposure can lead to liver or kidney tumors and diabetes mellitus

CONCEPTUALIZING TOXICOLOGY 27-1

3. Lead (Pb) causes neurodegeneration including increased incidence of Parkinson's disease, activation of astroglial, and inflammatory processes. Pb blocks long-term potentiation (brain acquiring new skills) via blocking NMDA receptors channel. Also ↓ number of synapses where nR2A subunit of NMDA receptor is expressed. This ↓ brain-derived neurotrophic factor → activation of Trk receptors. At high doses, Pb → encephalopathy. Lead also inhibits the formation of myelin, which affects white matter in the brain and peripheral nerves and additionally disrupts the formation of the blood–brain barrier. Pb, Ga, Cu, Hg, and Al also affect heme synthesis. Pb toxicity is especially marked by inhibition of δ-aminolevulinic acid dehydratase (ALAD inhibition = clinical measure), although other enzymes of heme synthesis are affected. Kidney also affected by Pb (and other heavy metals) with impaired tubular transport mechanisms and appearance of degenerative changes in tubular epithelium and nuclear inclusion bodies containing Pb-protein complexes. Fanconi syndrome = Pb-induced ↑ glucose, phosphates, and amino acids but not protein in the urine. Pb is also a reproductive and developmental toxicant. Generation of ROS and substitution for divalent cations such as Ca^{2+}, Mg^{2+}, and Fe^2 are other mechanisms of Pb toxicity

4. Mercury (Hg)—truly heavy metal (> 13 g/mL) that is volatile if heated. Hg^0 not dangerous unless injected or inhaled. Hg^0 oxidized by RBCs → Hg^+ or Hg^{2+} → kidney toxicity or inhaled gas in CNS → Hg^{2+}, which interacts with –SH → ↓ clearance of glutamine → excitotoxicity via NMDA receptors → "mad hatter's" disease = triad of gingivitis (gum disease), tremor, and erethism (behavior change). Hg is methylated to MeHg by anaerobic bacteria, is highly absorbed by all routes including skin, is transported to CNS via MeHg-L-cysteine (l-type neutral amino acid transporter), and reacts with selenols similar to Hg^{2+} → Minamata disease → cortical atrophy, neuronal loss and gliosis marked by cortical blindness, decreased hand proprioception, choreoathetosis, and attention deficits. Hg → ↑ expression of amyloid precursor protein → insoluble β-amyloid of Alzheimer's disease. CH_3Hg^+ = monocation electrophile → oxidizes nucleophilic groups (–SH) → disrupts homeostasis of neuronal and glial cells affecting a variety of sulfhydryl-containing enzymes. GSH depletion and H_2O_2 generation also add to MeHg's toxicity. Thus, a combination of glutamate and Ca^{2+} homeostasis disruption and oxidative stress → MeHg neurotoxicity. See Figure 27-1

5. Uranium (U)—mainly known for its radioactivity—is mainly a very heavy metal that has found toxicity as depleted uranium used in antitank shells. On explosion of these shells, inhalation of the uranium dust → leukemia, congenital abnormalities, and Kaposi sarcoma. U can also affect the brain, reproduction (including estrogenic effects), gene expression, and uranium metabolism in areas surrounding uranium mining (chronic exposure). As a heavy metal, U kidney toxicity affects rodents and dogs (transport mechanisms altered, ROS generated, altered oxidative phosphorylation, and disrupted metabolism of AChE and monoamines)

E. Essential metals

1. Calcium (Ca)—deficiency = osteoporosis; hypercalcemia (90% due to primary hyperparathyroidism and malignancy) → given mnemonic of (kidney) stones, bones, groans, thrones, and psychiatric overtones toxicities (and abnormal ECG rhythms)

2. Chromium (Cr)—maintains normal glucose balance due to Cr(III); Cr(VI) excess = strong oxidizing agent (even low intake) → moves from low-dose immunostimulation to high-dose immunosuppression, mutagenicity, genotoxicity (SCE and chromosome aberrations + enhances damage by inhibiting nucleotide excision repair), carcinogenicity, neurotoxicity, and reproductive toxicity

3. Cobalt (Co)—part of vitamin B$_{12}$, but inorganic form not necessary in diet and had been used clinically to stimulate erythropoietin production by the kidney to treat anemias and protect against hypoxia via inducing HIF, heme oxygenase, and metallothionein (also prevents oxidative damage following hypoxia); Co excess → goiter via inhibition of tyrosine iodonase, Co-asthma and hard metal disease (lung damage), allergic contact dermatitis (skin exposure), immune alterations, and possibly cancer. Co in beer → cardiomyopathy. Like other heavy metals, Co has affinity for –SH groups and thereby inhibits mitochondrial respiration. Co also generates ROS via Fenton-like reactions. Induction of HIF most likely associated with cancer. At high concentrations, Co ions and nanoparticles → cytotoxicity → apoptosis or necrosis

4. Copper (Cu)—involved in mitochondrial respiration, antioxidant defense, neurotransmitter synthesis, formation of connective tissue, pigmentation, and iron metabolism. Hard to develop

CONCEPTUALIZING TOXICOLOGY 27-1 (*continued*)

deficiency, but molybdenum can generate unabsorbable Cu-thiomolybdate complexes even in humans (human swayback). Wilson's disease = excess copper due to mutation in $ATP_{7B} \rightarrow$ liver, brain, and cornea accumulation. Hepatic cirrhosis (such as found in Indian childhood cirrhosis or Wilson's disease) and neurological dysfunctions (in Wilson's disease) develop in copper toxicosis. Liver damage starts in zone 3 (centrilobular) as opposed to Fe in zone 1 (periportal). Progressive inflammation $\rightarrow$ necrosis bridging fibrosis between centrilobular areas $\rightarrow$ irreversible liver cirrhosis

5. Iron (Fe)—deficiency $\rightarrow$ microcytic hypochromic anemia; excess $\rightarrow$ ROS via Fenton and Haber-Weiss reactions as shown in Figure 27-2. Fe deposition in basal ganglia = mediating factor in neurodegeneration (Parkinson's and Alzheimer's diseases). Children taking too many Fe supplements $\rightarrow$ liver damage and death (periportal damage)

6. Magnesium (Mg)—deficiency difficult to find except in pregnancy $\rightarrow$ profound effects on parturition, post-uterine involution, and fetal growth and development. Deficiency can also contribute to sudden infant death syndrome (SIDS) since there will be less control of brown adipose tissue thermoregulation in the fetus. Mg deficiency brought on by chemotherapeutic medication anti-EGFR monoclonal antibodies $\rightarrow$ serious cardiac arrhythmias and convulsions. Mg excess of greatest danger to fetus as fetal kidney does not excrete Mg as efficiently as mature kidney $\rightarrow$ hyporeflexia, poor suckling, and occasional respiratory depression. $MgSO_4$ may be more toxic than $MgCl_2$ because it may interact with paracellular components and not be as efficacious as a pharmaceutical agent. Mg^{2+} enters the cell via the Ca^{2+} TRPM7 channel. Excess intracellular Mg^{2+} $\rightarrow$ NMDA channel hyperactivity $\rightarrow$ neuronal cell death due to effects of Mg^{2+} on mitochondrial activities. Mg^{2+} reduces ACh and NE levels $\rightarrow \downarrow$ neuromuscular transmission. As $\uparrow Mg^{2+} \rightarrow \uparrow$ ATP utilization, facilitates nerve conduction, skin flushing (physiological) $\rightarrow$ depression of CNS and uterine smooth muscle (therapeutic) $\rightarrow$ arrest of deep reflexes to respiratory depression to respiratory arrest to cardiac arrest (toxic)

7. Manganese (Mn)—deficiency $\rightarrow \downarrow$ MnSOD in mitochondria (oxidant defense), skeletal abnormalities, and $\downarrow$ collagen formation in wound healing. Excess Mn $\rightarrow$ manganism (extrapyramidal syndrome similar to idiopathic Parkinson's disease) due to autoxidation of dopamine as shown in Figure 27-3

8. Molybdenum (Mo)—deficiency difficult to find in humans (parenteral nutrition) but in goats had $\downarrow$ weight gain, food consumption, and reproduction. Mo = part of important oxidases. Molybdenum trioxide = most toxic compound. Mo can cause kidney failure, but lesser toxicity results in a wasting disease resulting from disruptions of Cu metabolism

9. Potassium (K)—Hypokalemia affects muscles and renal tubule cells and can lead to arrhythmias. Cardiac signs = most associated with hyperkalemia $\rightarrow$ cardiac arrest and death. Acidosis $\uparrow$ hyperkalemia as it $\uparrow K^+$ efflux from cells

10. Selenium (Se)—component of important SeGSHpx antioxidant enzyme whole deficiency $\rightarrow$ cardiomyopathy (Keshan disease). If accompanied by vitamin E deficiency in chickens $\rightarrow$ exudative diathesis. Selenosis $\rightarrow$ hair and nail loss/brittleness, garlic breath, skin rash, GI disturbances, and nervous system disruptions. As a nutrient Se is an antioxidant, while in excess the mineral is a prooxidant forming selenodiglutathione and other metabolites

11. Sodium (Na)—deficiency = low blood volume and affects membrane potentials. Excess $\rightarrow$ hypertension or dehydration

12. Vanadium (V)—Insulin mimic and is cardioprotective. Deficiency = $\downarrow$ growth rate, infancy survival, hematocrit, and thyroid function. Excess $\rightarrow$ green tongue, diarrhea, abdominal cramping, and mental function changes. V $\rightarrow$ oxidative stress via interference with ferritin's ability to deliver Fe to oligodendrocyte progenitor cells during development $\rightarrow$ apoptosis and hypomyelination. V_2O_5 toxic to miners as does not transport well out of lung, affects cardiac function and generates inflammatory cytokines and chemokines on hepatocyte exposure, and impairs mitochondrial function. Renal toxicity may be due to $\downarrow$ citrate uptake and $3Na^+, 2K^+$-ATPase activity in brush border membrane vesicles. Male infertility results from necrosis of spermatogonium, spermatocytes, and Sertoli cells

13. Zinc (Zn)—essential for ribonucleic polymerases, alcohol dehydrogenase, carbonic anhydrase, and alkaline phosphatase activity. Deficiency $\rightarrow \downarrow$ appetite, slowing growth, skin alterations, and immunological abnormalities. Zn excess $\rightarrow$ GI irritation and vomiting, and immune system function is reduced

CONCEPTUALIZING TOXICOLOGY 27-1 (*continued*)

F. Biological interest

1. Nickel (Ni)—Neuroendocrine and gonadal influences on HPG axis. Ni substitution in metal-dependent enzymes disrupts protein function. Ni enters via Ca channel and competes with Ca for receptors. Ni cross-links DNA and amino acids, forms ROS, and mimics hypoxia. Ni targets histone-modifying enzymes → toxicity and cancer

G Medical

1. Aluminum (Al)—Medically used for OTC medical products as phosphate-binding agents, antiperspirants, adjuvant for immunizations, renal dialysis, and bladder irrigation. Neurotoxicity linked to action of ATP production/mitochondrial function. Al causes oxidative stress in brain. Chelation of Al slows progression of Alzheimer's disease. Osteomalacia is a bone deformity caused by Al. Al either suppresses immune function via ↓ CD4+ T lymphocytes or ↑ allergy via chronic fatigue syndrome and macrophagic myofasciitis

2. Bismuth (Bi)—Medically used OTC to treat digestive disorders (antipepsin and coating properties). Bismuth subcitrate → nausea, vomiting, and facial paresthesia. Chronic Bi administration → encephalopathy. Bi also shows toxicity to liver, bladder, joints, gums, stomach, and colon

3. Gallium (Ga)—Medically used as a diagnostic and therapeutic agent in cancer and bone metabolism with anti-inflammatory and immunosuppressant activity. Some gallium compounds are also antimicrobial. Ga especially interferes with Fe metabolism → microcytic anemia without ↓ platelet or WBC counts. It also disrupts Ca homeostasis and has been used to treat hypercalcemia, however Ga's renal toxicity limits its usefulness

4. Gold (Au)—One of oldest treatments for rheumatoid arthritis. Au → dermatitis, stomatitis, transient hematuria, and mild proteinuria (renal). Vasomotor toxicity may develop. One of three metals (Ag, Au, Hg) that produce autoimmunity. Au also affects mast cell survival, protein kinase activation, and ROS and NO generation along with Ca^{2+} influx. Au is taken up by choroid plexus, which is central to brain development and function. Au may lead to neurodegeneration. Gold salts also can cause pulmonary injury. Au(I) salts → uptake by lysosomes → myeloperoxidase and other lysosomal enzymes oxidize gold to Au(III)Cl_3, a stronger producer of prooxidants by lysosomal oxidative bursts that yields pharmaceutical and toxic reactivity. Conversely, $AuCl_3$ is also a scavenger of ROS such as hypochlorous acid. Anti-inflammatory activity may be due to denaturation of proteins including lysosomal enzymes. ROS scavenging, protein denaturation, and antigen processing interference → reduced production of arthritogenic peptides, but denaturing self-proteins → autoimmunity (recognition)

5. Lithium (Li)—Used to treat bipolar disorders. Li toxicity mainly involved in pyramidal tract, but can also affect brain stem and peripheral nerves. Thyroid disruption occurs by ↓ thyroid hormone synthesis and release and ↑ risk of thyroid autoimmunity (↑ B cell activity). Li also ↓ GFR (renal) and urinary concentration ability due to nephrogenic diabetes insipidus. Li's therapeutic to neurotoxic effects are due to glutamatergic/NDMAR signaling alterations or indirectly via GABAergic transmission of brain-derived neurotrophic factor. Li also affects the GI tract via L-arginine/NO pathway. Impotence may develop as altering NO levels → lack of erectile response

6. Silver (Ag)—Used for wound treatment and deodorant powders. Ag nanoparticles (g NPs) = industrial antimicrobial agents (photocatalytic properties → oxidative damage), but also damage algae more than Ag^+. Ag NPs are cytotoxic and genotoxic to rodent cells, but human cells have more resistance. Still, toxicity exists in rat liver and neuronal cells, human lung epithelial cells, and mouse stem cells. Silver deposits in eye and skin → reactions. Ag → autoimmunity. Major toxicity of ionic silver = mitochondrial damage to most cells via the permeability transition pathway (Ag-induced formation of proteinaceous pores). Ag NPs use "Trojan Horse" mechanism as Ag NPs permeate cell membranes ↑ intracellular Ag^+ and cause cytotoxicity and genotoxicity via interference with cell transport and local GSH depletion (protective mechanism along with metallothionein and cysteine) → ROS via interference with ion and electron flow across mitochondrial membrane and damage DNA via ROS or ↓ ATP production/DNA repair mechanisms. High doses of Ag NPs → ↑ NO and cell proliferation and damage circulatory, respiratory, CNS, and hepatic systems. Ag NPs also affect development of zebrafish

CONCEPTUALIZING TOXICOLOGY 27-1 (*continued*)

Metals are elements found in the periodic table with multiple oxidation states that never biodegrade, but can be biotransformed to more lipophilic compounds. This is not necessarily positive; for example, methylation by anaerobic bacteria of mercury leads to methyl or dimethyl mercury, both of which have been known to pass through certain types of gloves, making contact with the skin and killing humans. Metals also concentrate up the food chain more readily in hydrophobic forms. Two of the metals, mercury and selenium, are volatile and easily escape most pollution control equipment. Others associate with particles and are more readily captured. However, small particles containing heavy metals (such as occurs in pica or sanded-off lead paint instead of a wet removal of old lead-based paints) may be inhaled or ingested and cause heavy metal poisoning. Mining operations make these compounds available, and some operations use acids or metals (mercury recovery of gold) that yield more hazardous conditions for workers in these industries. Mining operations have always been hazardous and heavy metal poisoning was a common occurrence in Roman times when mining operations were performed by captured slave populations. Additionally, in the past food and water was handled with lead pipes, plates, and vessels, leading to lead poisoning in well-to-do parts of the population. Lead acetate may also have been the first "artificial sweetener" as old wine in lead containers leached lead when the wine became vinegar (acetic acid). Metals' developmental effects on the central nervous system (CNS) are most problematic during development in the womb or in childhood potentially hindering learning.

Some metals are nutritive, so their biphasic toxicity curve proceeds from deficiency to health to pharmacological doses to poisons. Inclusion in the correct storage form of a nutrient metal such as Fe in ferritin or function in hemoglobin or CYPs would be advantageous, while hemosiderin would lead to oxidative damage and liver toxicity. Some metals have very small ranges where they are nutritive, such as selenium; for example, the sodium selenate form has much higher toxicity than selenocysteine. Selenite and the formation of the toxic selenodiglutathione in cells may damage the liver but also provide some protection against certain forms of cancer. This complicates the toxicity profiles depending on the use of some toxic metals as possible chemotherapy or chemoprevention agents. Gold compounds have been used in the past to treat rheumatoid arthritis. Other metals have also been used in dentistry, such as the gold fillings and silver amalgams (mainly mercury) that were used in the past. Because mercury is volatile, uncapped mercury-containing amalgams can be a source of inhaled mercury body burdens.

Some metals are referred to as heavy metals, which may be characterized by atomic weight and density (e.g., > 4 or 5), and may or may not include the actinides. Medical personnel rarely encounter heavy metal poisoning in their practice. Lead, mercury, and cadmium may be considered toxic metals with no benefits to human physiology. Iron, zinc, cobalt, copper, manganese, selenium, chromium, and molybdenum are trace elements that have beneficial nutritional roles but can be problematic at higher intakes. Aluminum, bismuth, gold, gallium, lithium, and silver are important in medical treatment and diagnostic procedures. Developmental categories exist for metals as well, because the developing organism is more susceptible to absorption and the plasticity of the brain. Of greatest toxicity concerns here are arsenic, cadmium, lead, mercury, and uranium as they are widespread in the environment. Essential trace metals include chromium, cobalt, manganese, selenium, and zinc. Those of biological "interest" are nickel and vanadium. Aluminum, gallium, and lithium are most important as pharmacologic versus toxic agents (Domingo, 1994).

Toxic Metals

The toxic effects of metals are summarized in **Table 27-1**

Arsenic

Arsenic has been a problem in water supplies for years especially in certain areas of the world where As levels are high such as Chile, Thailand, Bangladesh, and India. It is also known in literature/movies as a poison of choice (e.g., in the 1944 dark comedy *Arsenic and Old Lace).*

TABLE 27-1   Metal Toxicity

Toxicity	Key Examples	Toxic Mechanism
Neurodegeneration	Fe, Hg, Mn, Pb, Cr(VI), Cu, Se, V, Ni (vapor), Al, Bi, Au, Li, Ag	ROS generation
Visual/auditory alone	Ga	
Neurotransmission	Mg, Ni (neuroendocrine), Al	Decreased ACh and NE
Cancer	As, U, Cr (VI), Co, Se, Ni	Genomic instability induction, estrogen receptor upregulation (chronic exposure), for Co activation of HIF
Pain/bone	Cd, Al (osteomalacia)	Joint and spine pain associated with deformities
Hyporeflexia	Mg	Decreased ACh and NE
Renal toxicity S_1 and S_2 segments	Cd	Apoptosis
Acute and chronic nephropathy	Pb, U (nitrate damages S_2, S_3 segments), V, Li	Damage to tubular transport deteriorating to renal breakdown
Glomerulonephritis	Au	
Kidney failure	Mo, Bi, Ga	Diuresis and proteinuria
Diabetes mellitus	Cd	Liver and kidney damage and gluconeogenesis inhibition
Hematopoietic	Pb, Ga, Cu, Hg, Al, Co, Ga, Au	Iron transport and heme synthesis pathway inhibition
Reproductive/developmental	Pb, U, Cr(VI), Mg, Ni, Li (Ebstein's anomaly may not be significant for Li but sexual function affected), Ag	Inhibited spermatogenesis and/or chromosome damage in men and infertility or spontaneous abortion in women
Respiratory	Cr(VI), Co	ROS leads to cancer or other severe pulmonary conditions, Co asthma and hard-metal disease
	Mg, V_2O_5, Ni_3S_2, Au, Ag	Respiratory depression via decreased ACh
Immune reaction/immunotoxicity	Cr(VI), Co, Zn, Ni, Al, Ga, Au, Li, Ag	Haptenization of proteins and/or immunosuppression at high doses
Thyroid toxicity	Co, Li	Inhibition of tyrosine iodonase, other thyroid enzymes
Cardiac/cardiovascular damage	Co	Cardiomyopathy
	Ag (nanoparticles)	NO production and cell proliferation
Cardiac arrhythmia	Mg, K, V	Depression to arrest
Hypertension	Na	Increased blood volume
Hepatic and/or mitochondrial	Cu, Fe, V, Ni (vapor), Al, Ag	Inflammatory → apoptosis or necrosis
Dehydration	Mg (citrate)	Osmotic diuretic
	Na	Increased osmotic pressure

TABLE 27-1   Metal Toxicity (*continued*)

Toxicity	Key Examples	Toxic Mechanism
GI disturbances	Se, Zn, and high levels of many metals such as V	From irritation and vomiting to loss of cells/linking
Gout-like symptoms	Mo	
Hair and fingernail loss to DNA damage	Se	Oxidative toxicity
Skin and eye reactions	As, Ag	
Metabolic acidosis	K	Ion exchange
Mimics hypoxia	Co, Ni	Signal transduction pathway
Parathyroid/Ca	Li	Increased both

It is well known to cause skin lesions marked by pigmentation and keratosis 5 to 10 years after exposure starts. In adults arsenic poisoning is marked by weakness, conjunctival congestion, hepatomegaly, portal hypertension, lung disease, polyneuropathy, solid edema of limbs, ischemic heart disease, peripheral vascular disease, hypertension, and anemia. Children appear affected but are identified by pigmentation and/or keratosis, pulmonary interstitial fibrosis with mild bronchiectasis, and reduced intellectual function.

It is important to note the methylation of arsenic, for this is used to remove As from the system. It appears that the second methylation step may be higher in certain children, indicating that As spends less time in the body and may have less skin reactions as a result (Majumdar and Guha Mazumder, 2012). However, the first methylation reaction may be important for arsenic's toxicity. The +3 oxidation state appears in the most toxic species of arsenic leading to hyperkeratosis, cancer, diabetes mellitus, cardiovascular toxicity, neurotoxicity, kidney damage, and other organ damage at high, acute, or chronic exposures. Inorganic arsenate (As[V]) is reduced to arsenite (As[III]) and methylated to mono- (MMA) and dimethylated forms (DMA) that are found in the urine. The ϖ isoform of glutathione (GSH) S-transferase and purine nucleoside phosphorylase catalyze the

reduction of As(V) to the more toxic As(III). Polynucleotide phosphorylase and mitochondrial adenosine triphosphate (ATP) synthase also do this reduction in the presence of GSH. The methylation of As(III) requires S-adenosylmethionine as the methyl donor and produces MMA(V), MMA(III), and DMA(III). As(III) methyltransferase (As3MT) appeared to be the rat liver cytosolic enzyme responsible for arsenic methylation.

Two pathways have been proposed for methylation. The classic one employs As3MT to convert As(III) to MMA(V) and from MMA(III) to DMA(V). The other novel pathway uses GSH conjugation of As(III), then the methylation of GSH-conjugate of As(III) (Sumi and Himeno, 2012). Newer evidence from *in vitro* studies suggests that the oxidative methylation route is not the one that occurs in mammals. Arsenic is only methylated in the presence of GSH of other thiols, which indicates that As is methylated in the trivalent oxidation state. Because nonconjugated arsenicals are highly reactive with thiols and are easily converted to less toxic corresponding pentavalent arsenicals, the As(III)-GSH conjugate may be the key factor in As toxicity (Watanabe and Hirano, 2013). The methylation of As(III) is a "double-edged sword" as the methylation to MMA(III) or DMA(III) leads to excretion and higher toxicity. Lastly, the long-term ingestion of arsenic must be considered as it leads to cancer of the skin, lung, liver, urinary bladder, kidney, and other organs. As(III) is not a point mutagen but is a potent clastogen. The most carcinogenic species is the trivalent methylated form, while the pentavalent methylated form is least toxic. Thioarsenicals formed during As metabolism are extremely genotoxic and cytotoxic.

Arsenic in these various toxic forms disrupt the genomic integrity via cell-cycle checkpoint dysregulation, DNA damage response, abnormal chromosomal segregation, defects in cell-cycle checkpoints, disabled apoptosis, telomere dysfunction, altered chromatin structure, and other toxic mechanisms including inhibition or loss of the expression of tumor suppressor gene and activation of oncogenes. Schematically, As converts a normal cell with DNA repair and chromosome segregation that has genomic integrity to one that has persistent DNA damage, inefficient DNA repair, telomere dysfunction, mitotic arrest, apoptosis, and epigenetic dysregulation. These mechanisms lead to an unstable genome that can proceed further with replication errors with defects in repair machineries (microsatellite instability associated with small insertion/deletion of bases within short clusters of nucleotide repeats associated with cancers such as colorectal cancer and sporadic renal cell carcinoma) or defects in spindle assembly leading to chromosome rearrangements (chromosome instability). Chronic arsenic exposure leads to gross structural changes such as end-to-end fusion, abnormal sister chromatid separation, aberrant chromosome separation, and numerical chromosome changes (aneuploidy and polyploidy).

Hungarian children with high chronic As exposure exhibited aberrant cells with chromatid type deletions, acentric fragments, and dicentric chromosomes and rings (Paldy et al., 1991). Chromatid breaks and gaps were found by a Finnish group (Mäki-Paakkanen et al., 1998). These types of alterations lead to activation of proto-oncogenes and therefore move directly into malignancy. This poisoning is malicious as the clastogenic and aneugenic properties persist to keep the genome unstable and propagate beyond the exposure period. The formation of micronuclei As confirms the genomic instability at the nuclear level. Micronuclei form when reactive oxygen species (ROS) generated by As exposure inhibit nucleotide mismatch repair and generate microsatellite instability. Arsenic and methylated metabolites cause single-strand and double-strand breaks via ROS and also reactive nitrogen species (RNS). Even the least toxic DMA(V) is capable of lung and skin tumor production via dimethylated arsenic peroxide formation (an ROS).

Arsenite can induce 8-OHdG and promote genomic instability (DNA damage), inducing oncogene expression. The formamidopyrimidine–DNA glycosylase (Fpg) modified comet assay has shown the oxidative nature of As-induced DNA adducts via a Ca^{2+}-mediated production or peroxynitrite, hypochlorous acid, and hydroxyl radicals. Because the mitochondria are large sources of intracellular ROS and As induces apoptosis through mitochondrial dysfunction, these two processes synergistically enhance the mutagenic potential of As. DNA repair through strand break rejoining is inhibited by As. ROS may cause single- or double-strand breaks, with the double-strand breaks persisting and less repaired. Even DMA(V) affects repair and replication mechanisms in human alveolar cells, increasing the persistence of DNA damage. Usually small amounts of damage would be sensed by poly(ADP-ribose) polymerase (PARP) and DNA-dependent protein kinase (DNA-PK), which through signal transduction via ATM/ATR activates effectors CHK1, CHK2, and p53. PARP has a high affinity for single- and double-strand DNA breaks. The lack of PARP-1 enhances sensitivity to As(III). Bladder cancer may be induced by a 12-week exposure of human urothelial cells to MMA(III) through the generation of ROS (producing ssDNA breaks) and inhibition of PARP-1 activity. Skin cells exposed to arsenite show the co-mutagenic and co-carcinogenic effects as the p53-dependent increase in p21 expression is deficient. This pathway normally would block the cell-cycle progression following DNA damage. Additionally, arsenite causes poly(ADP-ribosyl)ation of P53 protein and PARP-1 protein. Nucleotide bond damage induced by ROS can also be repaired by base excision repair (DNA polymerase β, DNA ligase I, and apurinic endonuclease 1) and nucleotide excision repair (for bulky distortion in DNA double helix via ligases), both of which are inhibited by arsenite. Inefficient DNA repair capacity is a key mechanism in the development of skin lesions from As.

Telomere instability is another feature of As poisoning and carcinogenesis. It is of interest that human cells have shorter telomeres than rodent cells and are more sensitive to arsenite. Telomeres play a key role in aging and cancer and are also crucial in genomic integrity. At low doses of arsenic, telomerase activity and telomere length are not affected to any great extent, while high As doses lead to loss of telomerase activity and telomeric DNA attrition and apoptosis. It is the change in the state of the telomere that appears to be more important than the reduction of telomerase activity of As-induced senescence. Some mechanisms that might be important here are upregulation of heat shock proteins, oncogenes, and cell growth factors. Arsenic also induces mitotic arrest, and MMA(III), DMA(III), MMA(V), and DMA(V) are all strong spindle disruptors. This feature has also been used to develop arsenic trioxide as a chemotherapeutic agent in the treatment of leukemia, because this compound along with the chemotherapeutic mitosis disruptor paclitaxel causes mitotic arrest followed by apoptosis at low concentrations. Arsenic appears to induce apoptosis through induction of mitochondrial instability in lymphocytes of exposed humans. However, chronic As exposure results in an increase in the stability of nuclear protein kinase B, an antiapoptotic molecule, and activates transcription factor Nrf2 constitutively. These processes lead to apoptosis resistance and increase the risk of skin cancer development.

Arsenic has epigenetic effects as well, leading to DNA hypomethylation. This increases the genome susceptibility to movement toward malignancy, as cancer cells are characterized by global DNA hypomethylation. *S*-adenosyl methionine is used to methylate As and becomes depleted leading to less of this methyl donor for DNA transcription regulation via methylation. Rodents exposed over a lifetime to As levels similar to the high concentrations in drinking water humans have been exposed to developed many cancers (e.g., lung adenocarcinoma, hepatocellular carcinoma, adrenal tumors, gall bladder tumor, ovarian tumors), which were more aggressive in nature and had higher incidence compared to *in utero* exposure only. Some upregulation of the estrogen receptor is also found with As exposure along with associated genes NF-κB, COX-2, and cyclin D1 (Bhattacharjee et al., 2013).

Cadmium

Cadmium is a ubiquitous pollutant that affects multiple organs such as the kidneys, the lungs, and the liver. It is especially known in occupational exposure for renal proximal tubule damage to S_1 and S_2 segments. Apoptosis appears to be a mechanism for cadmium's renal toxicity as well as to mouse liver, rat testes, human T cell line (CEM-C12 cells), lymphoma U937 cells, hepatocytes and liver L-02 cells, fetal lung fibroblast MRC-5 cells, prostate epithelial cells, mouse mesangial cells, rat lung epithelial cells, and cortical neurons. In pig renal proximal tubular epithelial LLC-PK$_1$ cells, apoptosis is induced through stress on the endoplasmic reticulum (ER). ER stress transducers are RNA-dependent protein kinase-like ER kinase (PERK), activating transcription factor 6 (ATF6), and inositol-requiring ER-to-nucleus signal kinase 1 (IRE1). ATF6 activates apoptosis through induction of CCAAT/enhancer-binding protein-homologous protein (CHOP), while IRE1 produces apoptosis by stimulation of X-box binding protein 1 (XBP1) and subsequent phosphorylation of c-jun N-terminal kinase (JNK). Cd also elevates cytosolic Ca^{2+} by release from an intracellular storage site such as the ER and to calcium uptake. This rise in cytosolic Ca^{2+} starts apoptosis by the familiar calpain-caspase signal transduction pathway. Cd may cause calcium release from the ER by the phospholipase C (PLC) pathway that produces inositol-1,4,5-triphosphate (IP_3) that subsequently binds to IP_3 receptors that regulate calcium release. This was suggested by experiments employing human embryonic kidneys (Lawal and Ellis, 2012). A PLC-specific inhibitor, U73122, prevented the Cd-dependent increase in cytosolic Ca^{2+} levels and the activation of calpain and caspase-3. Cd can also activate a G-protein coupled receptor, which is followed by PLC activation leading to increased cytosolic calcium in renal distal epithelial A6 cells. Cd-induced synthesis of ceramide is a second messenger that leads to renal tubule epithelial cell apoptosis through the calpain-caspases. Use of a ceramide synthesis inhibitor prevents calpain activation and apoptotic cell death due to acute Cd exposure.

Chronic Cd exposure may produce oxidative stress via ROS generation in porcine kidney LLC-PK$_1$ cells. Antioxidants or stable overexpression of superoxide dismutase (SOD) reduce Cd-induced ER stress and proapoptotic unfolded protein response signaling cascades. Mitochondrial effects of Cd may also play a role in apoptotic mechanisms, such as the induction of caspase-9 and -3 in kidney proximal tubule cells. Rat proximal tubule WKPT-0293 Cl.2 cells and mouse renal mesangial cells have an alternative approach to apoptosis through the release of endonuclease apoptosis-inducing factor from the mitochondria (caspase-dependent and -independent pathways activated). Cd can also act directly on isolated kidney mitochondria, as indicated by mitochondrial swelling followed by cyt c release. DNA microarray technology indicates that Cd affects normal rat kidney epithelial cells (NRK-52E cells) by increasing the expression of 73 genes and decreasing the expression of 42 genes (Tokumoto et al., 2011).

The Ub-proteasome gene is a focus for cadmium toxicity, because the expression of Ubc4 in yeast alters the sensitivity of yeast cells to Cd (Hwang et al., 2008). In the exposed kidney cells, *Ube2d4* (a family homolog to the yeast Ubc4) was downregulated. This is of concern as this Ub-proteasome system is an ATP-dependent degradation unit for damaged (or short-lived) proteins (ubiquitinates the protein which then proceeds to proteasome degradation). Other members of the *Ubde2d* gene family with decreased gene expression due to Cd exposure in kidney cells were *Ube2d1*, *Ube2d2*, and *Ube2d3*. This is important, for in human breast carcinoma MCF7 cells, Ubde2d2 and Ubde2d3 are responsible for ubiquitination of the tumor suppressor p53. The regulation of p53 appears to be via the rate of degradation. In the NRK-52E cells, Cd substantially increased p53 intracellular accumulation, which is then phosphorylated. The p53 pathway leads to apoptosis along with

the other pathways affected by Cd (Fujiwara et al., 2012). At high levels, Cd causes painful deterioration of the bones as indicated by the itai-itai or "ouch-ouch" disease. It also has been linked to pre-diabetes mellitus, diabetes mellitus, and overall cancer mortality with sex differences in the types of cancer. The liver and kidneys have been mentioned before as target organs for Cd poisoning, but their link to maintenance of blood glucose may be related to the diabetogenic effect of Cd. Heme is known to inhibit gluconeogenesis, so Cd poisoning may mimic heme oxygenase-2 (HO-2) deficiency. Two of the key co-regulators of glucose may be HO-2 and the key regulator of glycolysis, 6-phospho-fructo-2-kinase/fructose-2,6-bisphosphatase 4 (PFKFB4). Cd-caused cancer may be related to HO-2 activity, as cancer-prone cells require PFKFB4 and glycolysis for cell proliferation and resistance to apoptosis. Thus, depending on the dose and duration of exposure and sex of the Cd-exposed individual, cells may be damaged and proceed to apoptosis or to diabetes mellitus and cancer (Satarug and Moore, 2012).

Lead

Lead is one the oldest known toxicants that chiefly affects the nervous system. The CNS effects are more pronounced in children (more Pb gets into the brain, and the developing brain is more sensitive), while peripheral effects are more evident in adults. Adults are not completely resistant to the CNS effects of lead as neurodegeneration can occur along with activation of astroglia and inflammatory processes similar to what occurs in Alzheimer's disease. Also, lead levels appear to correlate with increased incidence of Parkinson's disease.

Some synaptic effects for Pb exposure may be the N-methyl-D-aspartate (NMDA) receptors. Long-term potentiation is how the brain acquires new skills. Lead appears to affect this long-term potentiation via blocking the NMDA receptor channel, and that blockage depends on the structure of the NMDA receptor's subunits. In the case of the NR2A subunit, which increases gradually through maturation of the brain, Pb binding occurs only partly at the Zn binding site and in the case of NR2B only partly overlaps with the binding site for Zn. This phenomenon points to a particular sensitivity to Pb of this subunit that controls excitatory neurotransmission via glutamine and the concentration of calcium in neural cells. Pb also inhibits the expression of the nR2A subunit, and in the hippocampus (the site of short-term memory) it reduces the number of synapses where the NR2A subunit of the NMDA receptor is expressed. This also decreases the secretion of brain-derived neurotrophic factor (BDNF). This leads to a decrease in activation of presynaptic Trk receptors. Positive reverse signaling is reduced and results in a decrease in the incorporation of the synaptic vesicle proteins synaptobrevin and syntaxin. Pb also impairs vesicular release. Ultimately, Pb disturbs neuronal signaling pathways (Baranowska-Bosiacka et al., 2012). Encephalopathy is a progressive degeneration of certain brain areas that can occur with lead poisoning and is marked by dullness, irritability, poor attention span, headache, muscular tremor, loss of memory, and hallucinations. At very high Pb exposures, the CNS effects can deteriorate further into delirium, lack of coordination, ataxia, convulsions, paralysis, and coma. Children show inattentiveness, hyperactivity, and irritability even at low Pb exposures. At higher levels, permanent brain damage and death may occur. Peripheral neuropathy and reduced motor activity due to loss of the myelination around the nerve mark the peripheral nervous system effects (Flora et al., 2012).

Another problem with metals such as Pb, Ga, Cu, Hg, and Al is that they affect heme synthesis. Pb and other metals compete with iron on transporters, reduce the iron pool, and bind to proteins causing physical and mental disruptions. These metals may affect gene expression, enzymatic activity, and iron integration into protoporphyrin IX and therefore decrease heme synthesis (Schauder et al., 2010). Enzymes affected by Pb are δ-aminolevulinic acid dehydratase (ALAD = cytosolic enzyme catalyzing δ-aminolevulinic acid [ALA] → porphobilinogen), aminolevulinic acid synthase (ALAS = mitochondrial enzyme catalyzing formation of ALA), and ferrochelatase (catalyzing insertion of iron into protoporphyrin to form heme; inhibition yields coproporphyrin in urine,

accumulation of protoporphyrin in red blood cells [RBCs], and substitution of Zn in porphyrin ring). As can be seen, heme synthesis starts in the mitochondria and intermediate steps follow in the cytoplasm. ALAD activity appears most sensitive to Pb inhibition (accumulation of aminolevulinic acid in the plasma) and is used as a clinical measure of Pb poisoning. Heme synthesis is not significantly altered until ALAD inhibition reaches 80−90%. Lead also increases the fragility of RBCs leading to hemolytic anemia with high lead levels and the degradation of ribonucleic acid in RBCs as indicated by basophilic stippling. Frank anemia occurs with an extended period of lead exposure.

As with most heavy metals, the kidney is a target organ with acute nephropathy. This acute renal toxicity is marked by impaired tubular transport mechanisms and appearance of degenerative changes in tubular epithelium and nuclear inclusion bodies containing lead-protein complexes. The increase of glucose, phosphates, and amino acids, but not protein, in the urine induced by Pb is known as Fanconi's syndrome. Chronic nephropathy is characterized by glomerular and tubulointerstitial changes with resulting renal breakdown, hypertension, and hyperuricemia. The hypertension from kidney effects also translates into cardiovascular disease and other disorders such as ischemic heart disease (myocardial infarction [MI]), cerebrovascular accidents (stroke), and peripheral vascular disease.

Reproductive damage happens in men (reduced libido, reduced sperm motility and number, chromosomal damage, infertility, abnormal prostatic function, and changes in serum testosterone) and women (infertility, miscarriage, premature membrane rupture, pre-eclampsia, pregnancy hypertension, and premature delivery). Developmental toxicity to the fetus occurs as well. Bone is a storage place for Pb and accounts for 40−70% of Pb released into the blood in adults. Oxidative stress results from lead forming ROS and antioxidant reserve depletion (binds to sulfhydryl groups including GSH and the sensitive enzymes such as ALAD, glutathione reductase, glutathione peroxidase, and glutathione-S-transferase). SOD and catalase are antioxidant enzymes inhibited by Pb.

Pb can do so by replacing binding to sulfhydryl moieties or replacing Zn in the enzyme. Pb causes lipid peroxidation and hemoglobin oxidation, which is the direct cause of hemolysis.

Pb also may substitute for divalent cations, such as Ca^{2+}, Mg^{2+} and Fe^{2+}, and monovalent cations like Na^+. These ionic effects disrupt intra- and intercellular signaling, cell adhesion, protein folding and maturation, apoptosis, ionic transport, enzyme regulation, and release of neurotransmitters. Ionic mechanisms of action of Pb mainly are related to neurological impairments, with lead accumulating in astroglial cells and blocking the formation of myelin responsible for white matter and peripheral nerve insulation and conduction velocities. This also disrupts the formation of the blood–brain barrier. The replacement of calcium can affect protein kinase C activity thereby affecting long-term neural excitation and memory storage. The effects on sodium ion concentration will affect the action potential, uptake of neurotransmitters, and regulation and uptake of calcium by synaptosomes. Antioxidants can prevent Pb toxicity via preventing ROS formation (primary antioxidants such as flavonoids, tocopherol, and ascorbic acid), chelating Pb ion, or chelating lead and maintaining its redox state and not having it reduce O_2. Secondary antioxidants such as low-molecular-weight polyphenols slow down the rate of oxidation but do not convert free radicals into stable molecules (Flora et al., 2012).

Mercury

Mercury is truly a "heavy" metal as its density is > 13 g/mL. In aquatic systems, mercury descends to the bottom of the water that it enters. Mercury is a volatile transition metal that comes from natural processes such as evaporation and volcanic activity and human activities such as the burning of coal and incinerators. Elemental Hg^0 is not dangerous on the skin as long as no cracks in the skin surface exist. It is most dangerous if exposed to heat (such as breaking an old thermometer over a hot plate) and vaporizes and is $> 90\%$ absorbed via inhalation. Hg^0 becomes a vapor from tooth fillings that are not crowned, from industrial production of caustic soda and chlorine, and from artisanal miners burning off mercury used to amalgamate gold. Hg^0 vapor causes neurotoxicity (as well as damage to other organs) characterized by decreased strength and coordination and increased tremor. Hg^0 is oxidized by erythrocyte catalase to mercurous (Hg^+) and mercuric (Hg^{2+}) ions that are mainly toxic to the kidney, but also damage other organs (e.g., the lung and gastrointestinal [GI] tract). This Hg^{2+} is also formed from the vapor in the CNS interacting with sulfhydryl groups and leads to inhibition of clearance of extracellular glutamate and excitotoxicity (this is discussed more fully later for similar dysregulation by methylmercury). Also similar to methylmercury, Hg^{2+} has a high affinity to selenols and inhibits the selenoprotein thioredoxin reductase, which may be the major molecular mechanism of the toxicity of Hg^{2+}. Inorganic forms (Hg^+ and Hg^{+2}) are more mobile in aqueous media and are known to cause the classic "mad hatters" disease (from spraying mercuric nitrate), comprising the triad of gingivitis, tremor, and erethism (irritability, low self-confidence, depression, apathy, shyness, and timidity leading in prolonged exposure to delirium, personality change, and memory loss).

Methylmercury (MeHg) is most dangerous, because it can be easily absorbed via ingestion (~95% absorbed), inhalation, dermally, and easily crosses the blood–brain barrier. MeHg is as high as 1 ppm in predatory fish. Minamata disease occurred in Minamata Bay due to mercury dumping by a Japanese industry that lead to the contamination of seafood with MeHg due to bacterial methylation of the inorganic mercury. After absorption, $> 90\%$ of MeHg in the blood is bound to erythrocyte hemoglobin (intracellular). Only 6% remains in the blood after equilibration with the tissues and excretion. Inorganic mercury is an important excretory metabolite of MeHg, with 73% found in the urine, 39% in breastmilk, and 7% in the blood. CH_3Hg-SG is the biliary product (GSH mercaptide). The CNS is the main target for MeHg transported as a MeHg-L-cysteine complex by L-type neutral amino acid transporter. It similarly transports across the placenta and affects differentiation, migration, and synaptogenesis of the developing fetal brain at concentrations that are lower than would damage the adult brain. A human exposed to MeHg at 8 years of age, showed evidence of cortical atrophy, neuronal loss, and gliosis—most evident in the paracentral and parietooccipital regions 22 years later. Before this person died, the neurological signs were cortical blindness, decreased hand proprioception, choreoathetosis, and attention deficits. Hg likely persists in the brain as inorganic mercury bound to sulfhydryl groups of proteins. Mercury shares the mechanisms of oxidative stress and neurodegeneration as part of its overall toxicity with an overabundance of Fe and Mn.

Mercury lead and aluminum are related to the development of neuropathological conditions. Hg induces glial cell reactivity/inflammation, and upregulates the expression of amyloid precursor protein increasing the formation of insoluble β-amyloid (Alzheimer's disease pathogenic factors). MeHg is a monoalkylmercurial and its Hg atom is a CH_3-Hg^+, a monocation, which has electrophilic properties. This electrophilic property allows MeHg to oxidize nucleophilic groups such as sulfhydryls. This disrupts the homeostasis provided to neuronal and glial cells by sulfhydryl-containing proteins. Some enzymes affected are Ca^{2+}-ATPase, choline acetyltransferase, creatine kinase, enolase, GSH reductase, and thioredoxin reductase.

Selenols are more nucleophilic than thiols; so selenoproteins such as GSH peroxidase (GSH peroxidase-1 inhibited by nM concentrations of MeHg in cultured neurons) and thioredoxin reductase are critical and primary targets of MeHg and resulting neurotoxicity. Other selenoproteins such as selenoprotein W and 5′-deiodinase are also found to downregulate their activity in the presence of MeHg. Nonprotein thiols such as GSH are targets that allow deposition of MeHg in tissues. This leads to GSH depletion (concentrations dropping from mM to low μM range in the cerebrum and cerebellum) and adds to MeHg's neurotoxicity. MeHg does cause the generation of H_2O_2, which downregulates the activity of glutamate transporters. This leads to abusive stimulation of NMDA subtype glutamate receptors/excitotoxicity (increasing Na^+ and Ca^{2+} influx leading to oxidative stress and neurotoxicity). The Ca^{2+} influx alone increases NO production due to

activation of neuronal NO synthase and leads to mitochondrial collapse. The events of ROS generation, and glutamate and calcium dyshomeostasis leading to neurotoxicity are summarized in **Figure 27-1**. It appears that the neurotoxicity of the adults exposed to high MeHg levels at Minamata Bay, Japan had cerebellar ataxia, concentric constriction of their visual fields, and sensory disturbances indicating selective neurodegeneration of the calcarine, temporal, pre-, and postcentral cortices, as well as the cerebellar hemispheres. Various chelation therapies have been tried including penicillamine, dimercaprol, 2,3-dimercaptopropane-1-sulphonate, meso-2,3-dimercaptocsuccinic acid, and a thiolated resin. It appears that although some mercury may be removed from the system, the CNS damage persists (Farina et al., 2013).

Uranium

When most laypeople think of uranium, radioactivity comes to mind in the manufacture of nuclear fuel or weapons. Radon gas evolution from uranium and its radioactive impact as a gas that gives off alpha particles is also a concern to uranium miners and homeowners in areas rich in uranium. However, it is a very heavy metal, and most of its toxicity is based on that aspect. It is so heavy or dense that depleted uranium (DU) is used to coat antitank shells. In places where these shells have been used and uranium dust has been violently created via explosions, there have been increases in leukemia (Balkans), congenital abnormalities, and Kaposi sarcoma (Iraq; Shelleh, 2012). As a heavy metal, it damages the kidneys, causes development effects, and leads to genotoxicity. More recent findings suggest that U can affect the brain, reproduction (including estrogenic effects), gene expression, and uranium metabolism. These effects appear to be manifested not at high radiation areas like mines but rather in surrounding residential areas, where the heavy metal effects predominate due to lower chronic exposure (Brugge and Buchner, 2011). The sensitivity to U has the following order: rabbit > rat > guinea pig > pig > mouse > dog > cat > human. Doses of ≥ 5 mg U/kg are overtly toxic to the kidneys of rodents and dogs.

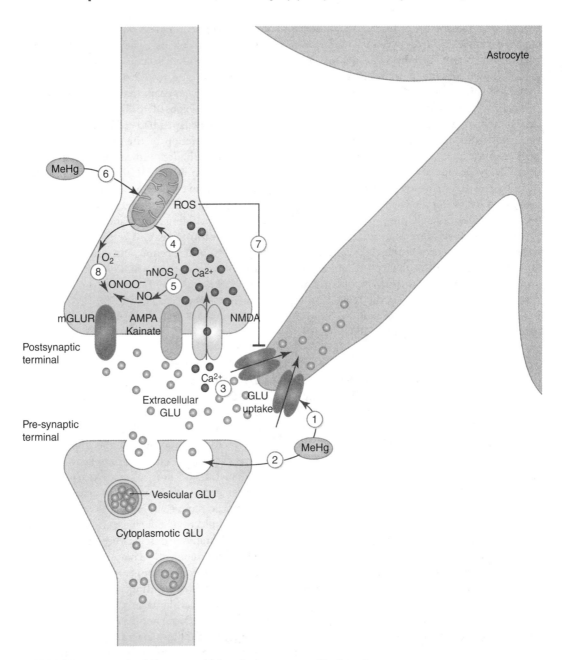

FIGURE 27-1 MeHg-Induced Glutamate and Calcium Dyshomeostasis and Oxidative Stress

Note: MeHg causes increased extracellular glutamate (GLU) levels via the inhibition of astrocytic glutamate uptake (event 1) and the stimulation of glutamate release from pre-synaptic terminals (event 2). Increased extracellular glutamate levels overactivate *N*-methyl D-aspartate (NMDA)-type glutamate receptors, increasing calcium influx into neurons (event 3). Increased levels of intracellular calcium, which can lead to mitochondrial collapse (event 4), activate neuronal nitric oxide synthase (nNOS) (event 5), thus increasing nitric oxide (NO) formation. MeHg affects the mitochondrial electron transfer chain (mainly at the level of complexes II–III) (event 6), leading to increased formation of reactive oxygen species [ROS; superoxide anion ($O_2^{\cdot-}$) and hydrogen peroxide (H_2O_2)]. H_2O_2 can inhibit astrocyte glutamate transporters (event 7), contributing to the excitotoxic cycle. reacts with NO (event 8), generating peroxynitrite ($ONOO^-$), a highly oxidative molecule.

The low specific radioactivity of U effects cannot explain the production of cancer, so an examination of U and its mechanisms of damage as another heavy metal become important. The acute effects of U decrease the glomerular filtration rate (GFR) in the kidney due to a combination of glomerular effects and tubuloglomerular feedback as a result of tubular insult (by increasing electrolytes, β-2-microglobin, proteins, and glucose excretion). As a heavy metal, U causes kidney damage by altered transport mechanisms or oxidative stress via ROS generation or changing oxidative phosphorylation along with disruptions of acetylcholinesterase and monoamine metabolism. The alterations of Na/K ATPase or Na ATPase affect Na transport, which is responsible for most tubular reabsorption processes via secondary active transport. This leads to tubular reuptake dysfunction. The interference with Na/P_i II transporter affects P_i reabsorption, and reduction of sodium-glucose transporters affects glucose reabsorption. Together, they reduce the ability of the renal cells to support cellular respiration and can lead to apoptosis. Direct action on the mitochondria also produces ROS (including oxidized glutathione) that lead to lipid peroxidation and the activation of proapoptotic mechanisms through caspases. There is also physical loss of villi in the proximal tubules increasing alkaline phosphatase activity in the urine. Uranyl nitrate intraperitoneal injection specifically damages the S_2 and S_3 segments of the proximal tubule with cell vacuolization, loss of brush border membrane, and increase in the lysosomal and vacuolar mass of the S_1 segment. Tissue lesions in the kidney lead to increases in urinary activities of N-acetyl glucosaminidase, γ-glutamyl transpeptidase, lactate dehydrogenase, and acid phosphatase. Except for lactate dehydrogenase (nonspecific marker of tissue damage), the other enzymes are indications of proximal tubule damage. Uranium also affects various enzymes in glycolysis, the Krebs cycle, and gluconeogenesis; increases the activity of SOD (disrupts oxidative balance); and raises blood pressure via plasma renin levels. High levels can lead to necrosis of the proximal tubules and adherences and congestion in the glomerular epithelium with loss of glomerular surface. In chronic, exposure the species

sensitivity changes—with the rat more sensitive than the rabbit. Chronic exposure to diabetes mellitus increases the susceptibility to metal nephrotoxicity, so human patients in the past treated for diabetes with U might have exhibited chronic nephrotoxicity if current diagnostic techniques were available in the 19th century. However, it has been difficult in current human exposures to find a relationship between exposure level, duration of exposure, and observed kidney alterations. Chronic exposure leads to variable degrees of renal damage from no detectable alterations to mild injury of tubular function. However, undetermined comorbidity factors may play a role in the final influence of long-term exposure to U (Vicente-Vicente et al., 2010).

Essential Metals

In the discussion of essential metals, deficiency and toxicity due to overnutrition (both are malnutrition) should be examined.

Calcium

Calcium is necessary for a variety of cell-signaling functions; release of neurotransmitters; contraction of the heart, skeletal muscle, and smooth muscle; and the formation of bone. A deficiency of calcium is usually marked by osteoporosis, because bones will be subject to calcium release by osteoclasts stimulated by parathyroid hormone in low free-plasma calcium states. Hypercalcemia, which humans have been aware of for a very long time, can originate from excess intake, hypervitaminosis D, administration of dihydrotachysterol, parathyroid poisoning (90% of hypercalcemic cases in humans are due to primary hyperparathyroidism and malignancy), milk-alkali syndrome, primary and secondary skeletal neoplasms, immobilization, multiple myeloma, Paget's disease, Boeck's sarcoidosis, administration of anterior pituitary extracts, and administration of gonadotrophic hormones and estrogens, and it occasionally occurs in advanced nephritis with uremia (Hollinger and Pattee, 1956). Signs of hypercalcemia are easily memorized as "stones, bones, groans, thrones, and psychiatric overtones."

Renal or biliary stones; bone pain; abdominal pain and vomiting; polyuria; and depression, anxiety, cognitive dysfunction, insomnia and, in extreme cases, coma may result. Abnormal electrocardiogram (ECG) rhythms include a short QT interval and widening of the T wave. In more extreme cases, the ECG can mimic an acute MI or hypothermia (Osborn wave). Excess vitamin D (cholecalciferol) can be used as a rodenticide causing excess calcium and phosphate absorption and has devastating effects on the cardiovascular system with other impacts on the CNS, muscles, the GI tract (oral administration), and the kidneys.

Chromium

Chromium appears to maintain normal glucose tolerance as demonstrated in rats (Striffler et al., 1998). Humans also benefit from chromium supplementation in mildly impaired glucose tolerance. Chromium deficiency appears to enhance the progression of impairment of glucose tolerance with advanced age and appears to increase the risk of diabetes mellitus. The interaction of chromium and glucose metabolism is complex. A glucose tolerance test yields acute increments of plasma Cr in normal subjects, which does not appear to occur in certain patients with diabetes mellitus. Chromium supplementation causes the reappearance of that increment in those same people with diabetes mellitus. Some studies have shown an increase in Cr (Glinsmann et al., 1966) and others a decrease in the presence of a glucose challenge (Davidson and Burt, 1973). It appears to have something to do with insulin. Those normal-weight people who showed a low, normal insulin response to a glucose challenge showed a 98% increase in plasma Cr concentration, while those heavier body weight people with high insulin response also had a 24% decline in their plasma Cr concentration.

Cr appears to be incorporated into a 70-kDa protein containing 5–6 atoms of Cr per molecule and induced in regenerating liver. This form of chromium appears to bind to nucleolar chromatin and yields a substantial increase in RNA synthesis. This contrasts with the uncontrolled reaction of Cr(VI) with genetic material.

Another protein that binds Cr is ~1.5 kDa and is composed of aspartic acid, glutamic acid, glycine, and cysteine. It appears to be a detoxication mechanism, while it also has some physiological activity on glucose oxidation by isolated fat cells similar to glucose tolerance factor preparations (Mertz, 1993). The oxidation state of Cr is important as +3 yields a nutrient in moderate intake, while +6 is considered a toxicant even at low intake. Cr(VI) is an irritant of the nasal mucosa with concentrations as low as 2 µg/m³ and is also a skin irritant and sensitizer. Cr(VI) is reduced to Cr(III) in the body and then haptenizes by binding to proteins (immune reactions then occur). At higher doses, a biphasic curve is generated as immunosuppression occurs rather than immunostimulation (T and B cell proliferation by lipopolysaccharide-stimulated B cells inhibited by Cr(VI) particles).

Cr(VI) is a strong oxidizing agent (generates ROS), yielding mutagenicity, gene mutations/genotoxicity (sister-chromatid exchanges and chromosome aberrations), carcinogenicity (lung cancer in miners or in poorly ventilated plating facilities especially in combination with cigarette smoking) or other tumors, immunotoxicity, neurotoxicity, and reproductive toxicity. Cr(VI) to Cr(III) reduction appears to result in oxidative DNA damage including strand breaks, Cr-DAN adducts, DNA–DNA interstrand cross-links (most responsible for blocking DNA replication), and DNA–protein cross-links. Low levels of damage from ROS generation yield genomic instability and cancer, while high-level damage leads to cell-cycle arrest and apoptosis. The generation of lung cancer appears to be via Cr(VI) deposits that persist at bronchial bifurcations. These particles dissolve outside of the cell and then enter the cell as their respective ions. Chromate ion reduction to Cr(III) yields Cr(V), Cr(IV), and free radicals as intermediates. Cr(VI), one of the intermediates, or some combination of both appears to cause the chromosomal aberrations, adducts, cross-links, and strand breaks. In the lung, DNA-phosphate-based adducts yield various types of damage to genetic material and activate the p53 signaling pathway (cell-cycle arrest or apoptosis via expression of BH3 domain-containing proteins PUMA and NOXA, which work via the multidomain

Bcl-2 family member BAX). The activation of cyclin-dependent kinase inhibitor CDKN1A then arrests growth, and the induction of mitochondrial membrane permeabilization releases apoptogenic factors from the mitochondrial intermembrane space. Cr(VI) additionally causes ataxia-telangiectasia mutated-dependent DNA damage response pathway, which serves dichotomous roles of apoptosis and cell survival. Cd(VI) also inhibits nucleotide excision repair, which disables the principle route for eliminating Cr(VI)-DNA adducts in human cells. This enhances the mutagenicity, carcinogenicity, and cytotoxicity of Cr(VI). Occupational exposure usually is through inhalation (shortness of breath, coughing, wheezing, perforations and ulcerations of the septum, bronchitis, decreased pulmonary function, pneumonia, and asthma), and nonoccupational exposure is usually from contaminated food and/or water (Das and Singh, 2011).

Cobalt

Cobalt is an essential micronutrient as part of vitamin B_{12} (hydroxocobalamin), but inorganic Co is not considered necessary in the diet. Several bacterial metalloenzymes have been described that are Co-dependent for activation. A Co^{2+}-activated enzyme in humans is methionine aminopeptidase, which achieves cotranslational proteolytic excision of the initiator methionine from the N-terminus of nascent polypeptide chains. Co also stimulates erythropoietin production by the kidney and was used in clinical practice to treat anemias secondary to chronic renal failure and malignancies without much evident toxicity. Cobalt may stimulate erythropoietin by inhibition of the oxygen-dependent hydroxylases, hypoxia-inducible factor (HIF)-α prolyl hydroxylase and HIF-α asparaginyl hydroxylase, that are the hypothesized oxygen sensors that induce erythropoietin in hypoxia. Cobalt's induction of erythropoietin is also enhanced by hypoxia. This hypoxic production of erythropoietin gives low levels of cobalt as a preconditioning agent the possibility of being protective against cardiac ischemia, renal damage, and neural damage during low oxygen states similar to

hypoxic preconditioning. Low levels of cobalt by inducing HIF, heme oxygenase, and metallothionein also prevent oxidative damage following hypoxia. Indeed, low cobalt levels appeared to protect rat skeletal muscles from oxidative damage and improved endurance during training under hypoxic conditions.

Excessive exposure to Co results in inhibition of tyrosine iodonase (goiter and myxedema of the thyroid), Co-asthma and hard-metal disease (inhalation and lung damage), allergic contact dermatitis (skin exposure), immune system function alterations, and possibly cancer. Co (as chloride or sulfate) also used to be present in beer in the 1960s to keep the "head" stable. Heavy beer drinkers suffered cardiomyopathy as a result of Co accumulation in the myocardium, possibly exacerbated by nutritional deficiencies. At lower exposure, alterations in ventricular diastolic function were noted by echocardiography without accompanying major cardiac dysfunction. Co, like many other heavy metals, has affinity for sulfhydryl groups and can thereby inhibit mitochondrial respiration. Co^{2+} can also replace other divalent ions off the ion center of metal-activated enzymes (including intracellular Ca^{2+}-binding proteins). This divalent ion property also allows Co to interfere with Ca^{2+} entry and signaling. Heme synthesis is also impaired by Co similar to other metals via inhibition of δ-aminolevulinic acid synthase and porphobilinogen synthase (or δ-aminolevulinic acid dehydratase), which appears to be dichotomous from its stimulation of erythropoietin. Like other metals, Co can also lead to the formation of damaging ROS via Fenton-like reactions. This leads to lipid and DNA damage (in animals oxidative DNA damage and possible inhibition of DNA repair are sufficient evidence for carcinogenicity, but inadequate for characterization as a human carcinogen). Cobalt's stimulation of the metal-induced HIF is most likely associated with tumor development and growth in the living organism through activation of angiogenic growth factors and angiogenesis genes, glucose transporters, glycolytic enzymes, and affecting genes responsible for apoptosis/cell proliferation. At high concentrations, Co ions and Co metal nanoparticles are cytotoxic, induce apoptosis, or lead to necrosis with inflammation.

Long-term exposure to cobalt appears to accumulate this metal in the liver and kidneys. However, it may also be sequestered in RBCs due to oxidation from Co^{2+} to Co^{3+}, which will tightly bind to hemoglobin. Cobalt in either oxidation state is also not subject to calcium pump removal from the RBC (Simonsen et al., 2012).

Copper

Copper is an important nutrient involved in mitochondrial respiration, antioxidant defense, neurotransmitter synthesis, formation of connective tissue, pigmentation, and iron metabolism (leading to heme formation; Fieten et al., 2012). It is difficult to find copper deficiency in the population. It is easier to find copper deficiency in ruminants as the rumen bacteria produce hydrogen sulfide reducing Cu availability from forage and creating swayback in lambs. Molybdenum-rich pasturelands increase thiomolybdate (TM) synthesis and unabsorbable complexes of Cu-TM. Human swayback has been discovered and the use of TM to treat abnormalities related to Cu metabolism (e.g., Wilson's diseases) or states where copper plays a role (tumor growth, inflammatory diseases, and Alzheimer's disease) results in long-term copper depletion (Suttle, 2012). The neurodegeneration of Alzheimer's disease may be due to ROS/RNS generation. Cu, Fe, and heme can bind to amyloid-β and generate oxidative stress (Chassaing et al., 2012). Most of what is known about human copper toxicity comes from the literature on Menkes disease and Wilson's disease, which are due to mutations in the genes coding for the homologous Cu-transporting ATPases (ATP7A [Kaler, 2014] and ATP 7B [Lutsenko et al., 2002], respectively).

Copper is taken up in the diet by CTR1 (and possibly CTR2) into enterocytes and transported by serum proteins to the liver where the same transporter stores Cu in hepatocytes via metallothionein and GSH in the cytosol followed by copper chaperones (such as COX_{17} copper chaperone for cytochrome c oxidase in the mitochondrial inner membrane). For Cu export into the plasma, the copper chaperone $ATOX_1$ delivers copper to ATP_{7B} in the trans-Golgi compartment and forms holo-ceruloplasmin for secretion. Wilson's disease, which is an autosomal recessive disorder due to a mutation in ATP_{7B}, accumulates Cu in the liver, brain, and cornea. Hepatic and neurologic or psychiatric dysfunctions are noted in the person's 20s or 30s. Other forms of copper toxicosis are Indian childhood cirrhosis, endemic Tyrolean infantile cirrhosis, and idiopathic copper toxicosis. Those diseases of early childhood appear to involve only the hepatic damage and none of the neurological toxicity of Wilson's disease, and only consanguinity and high dietary copper appear to be related to their onset. Certain dog breeds have Cu toxicosis as well, with the mutation in the $COMMD_1$ (copper metabolism gene MURR1 containing Domain 1) gene associated with Bedlington terriers. These dogs have a huge accumulation of Cu in hepatic lysosomes, indicating not only a Cu transport role, but a degranulation of lysosomal content into the bile for this gene product. This gene product may also play a role in maturation of SOD, and RNAi-mediated knockout of $COMMD_1$ expression results in significant induction of SOD_1 activity. In dogs of various breeds, Cu toxicosis appears to start in the liver by inflammatory changes in the centrilobular regions of the liver (zone 3). This is opposite that of Fe, where high oxygen levels result in damage in the periportal (zone 1) region. The hepatocytes progress to apoptosis and are phagocytized, concentrating Cu in the Kupffer cells. The progressive inflammation leads to necrosis, bridging fibrosis between centrilobular areas, and ultimately leading to irreversible liver cirrhosis. The liver enzyme that indicates copper toxicosis is alanine-aminotransferase rather than alkaline phosphatase, which is consonant with hepatocellular damage rather than cholestasis (Fieten et al., 2012).

Iron

Iron is one of the most plentiful elements in the Earth's crust. It has oxidation states from −2 to +6, but is mainly found in organisms bound to specific metalloproteins in the +2 and +3 oxidation states (although there may be a transient Fe[IV] oxo state for CYPs). Fe plays important roles in energy/oxidative metabolism. Deficiency is usually marked by microcytic hypochromic anemia. Due to the ferric (Fe^{3+}) and ferrous (Fe^{2+}) oxidation states, Fe is an inherent generator of ROS such as indicated by the Fenton reaction and Haber-Weiss reaction that appears to be critical in developing mitochondrial damage and central in neurodegeneration as displayed in **Figure 27-2.** Fe can be a mediating factor in neurodegenerative processes such as Parkinson's disease and Alzheimer's disease. The basal ganglia appear to be the preferred site of iron deposition in the neurodegenerative

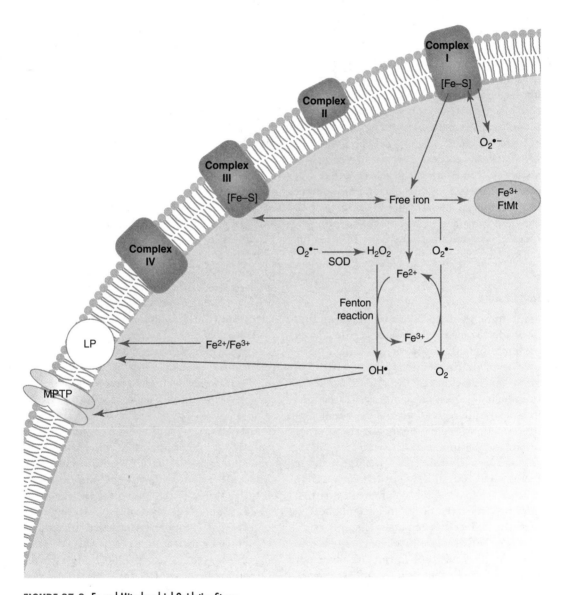

FIGURE 27-2 Fe and Mitochondrial Oxidative Stress

Note: Fe can start mitochondrial oxidative stress via interaction with different ROS. Free Fe can be released from mitochondrial Fe–sulfur clusters in complexes I and III upon interaction with ROS (in the figure it is shown the release of superoxide anion by these complexes and the potential oxidation of Fe–S cluster by ; the oxidation of the Fe–sulfur clusters can increase the free Fe in the mitochondrial matrix. This can facilitate the operation of the toxic Haber–Weiss and Fenton reactions, feeding a general pro-oxidant cycle). The redox pair Fe^{2+}–Fe^{3+} can also directly stimulate lipid peroxidation, which can intensify the oxidative stress and contribute to mitochondrial and cellular demise via mPTP formation. Free cationic Fe (regardless of the redox state) is the critical element for neurotoxicity and it can be buffered by intramitochondrial ferritin (FtMt), which acts as an antioxidant protein in the mitochondrial matrix.

diseases. Fe overload as caused by hemorrhage into the brain appears to indicate more heme uptake by the neurons than glial cells. Iron-induced cell death, known as ferroptosis, is morphologically, biochemically, and genetically distinct from apoptosis, necrosis, or autophagy and can be activated by glutamate. Three types of Fe absorption involvethe uptake of heme-Fe by proton-coupled folate transport (PCFT/HCP1); absorption of mineralized Fe^{3+} in ferritin present in legume seeds via clathrin-dependent, receptor-mediated endocytosis; and non-heme Fe^{2+} uptake from salts or chelators that may be part of iron supplements (Farina et al., 2013). Children taking too many iron supplements at one sitting can develop liver damage that leads to death. Hemochromatosis is a state of iron overload of genetic origin but can be modeled by uptake of Fe-fumarate into periportal hepatocytes leading to ROS and lipid peroxidation (as opposed to intraperitoneal Fe-dextran injections that affect mainly the Kupffer cells; Younes et al., 1989).

Magnesium

Magnesium deficiency is again difficult to find normally, except in pregnancy. Mg deficiency has profound effects on parturition and post-uterine involution and interferes with fetal growth and development. Morbidity may result from hematological alterations, perturbations in temperature regulation, and developmental malformations. Mg deficiency can also contribute to sudden infant death syndrome (SIDS) through less control of brown adipose tissue thermoregulation in the fetus (Durlach, 2004). A cancer chemotherapy agent, anti-epidermal growth factor receptor monoclonal antibodies, may also induce hypomagnesemia and hypocalcemia. Early symptoms of magnesium deficiency are difficult to discern clinically if not monitored closely, but serious cardiac arrhythmias and convulsions may result in longer term Mg depletion (Costa et al., 2011).

At other times, Mg and Ca have been used in prophylaxis of neurotoxicity caused by the colorectal cancer chemotherapeutic agent oxaliplatin, a Pt compound (Khattak, 2011). Magnesium sulfate has been used for a variety

of disorders including pre-eclampsia and eclampsia (danger of magnesium toxicity to the neonate; Drinkwater, 2011) and asthma (Song and Chang, 2012), among others (vaso- and neuroprotective properties after spinal cord injury, postnatal treatment of severe birth asphyxia, antithrombotic, antiarrhythmic, treats cardioplegia, improved mitochondrial respiratory function following traumatic brain injury, smooth muscle relaxation, anesthetic adjunct medication, improves pulmonary hypertension in newborn, cerebral palsy treatment, improves insulin sensitivity in type 2 diabetes mellitus; Durlach et al., 2005). The danger to the fetus is of concern, because the fetal kidney does not excrete Mg as efficiently as the mature kidney. Neonatal hypermagnesemia can result in hyporeflexia, poor suckling, and on occasion respiratory depression. Hypermagnesemia can also affect intracardial and peripheral circulation, APGAR score at birth, and Ca metabolism, and it can induce meconial discharge. In animal models, fetal mortality was related to $MgSO_4$ dose (Durlach, 2004). Magnesium citrate has been used as a purgative (osmotic laxative) prior to colonoscopy, but can cause dehydration, electrolyte shift, and magnesium retention (Adamcewicz et al., 2011).

Magnesium may also have some efficacy in other metal poisoning (e.g., Cd; Matović et al., 2010). However, the form of Mg may be important even in clinical practice. $MgCl_2$ crystals are dianions with Mg coordinated with six water molecules $[Mg(H_2O)_6]^{2+}$ and two independent chloride atoms, while $MgSO_4$ is also a hexa-aqueous molecule with an additional water molecule associated with the sulfate anion $[Mg(H_2O)_6]^{2+}[SO_4 \cdot H_2O]$. This gives the magnesium sulfate the possibility of reacting with paracellular components rather than cellular components, increasing toxicity while decreasing efficacy (Durlach et al., 2005). Mg excess is important because Mg^{2+} inhibits various species of ionic channels either extracellularly or intracellularly. The Ca^{2+} TRPM7 is the channel through which Mg^{2+} enters the intracellular space. An excess of intracellular Mg^{2+} induces hyperactivity of the NMDA channels and can cause neuronal cell death due to inhibitory effects of this ion on mitochondrial activities

(Sato and Fukuda, 2004). Mg also decreases the levels of acetylcholine and norepinephrine. Neuromuscular transmission is reduced and muscles relax. Depression of acetylcholine in the heart and lung fortunately occurs at higher concentrations than the concentrations that relax the uterus (tocolytic activity). In the physiological range of 1.3–2.1 mEq/L, Mg couples with ATP to increase utilization of ATP and activates many enzyme systems, facilitates nerve conduction, and promotes K^+ transport. At 3–5 mEq/L (pharmacological loading dose), peripheral vasodilation occurs (skin flushing and feeling warmth, nausea, and vomiting if overly rapid administration occurs). At 4–6 mEq/L therapeutic concentrations, depression of CNS and uterine smooth muscle occurs. Depression of deep reflexes (7–8 mEq/L), arrest of deep reflexes (9–12 mEq/L), respiratory depression (12–15 mEq/L), respiratory arrest (15–18 mEq/L), arrhythmia, bradycardia, heart block (18–24 mEq/L), and cardiac arrest (25–35 mEq/L) occur at higher Mg concentrations in ascending order (Nick, 2004).

Manganese

Mn is another plentiful element in the Earth's crust, but is mainly found as carbonates, oxides, and silicates. Oxidation states for Mn are 2+, 3+, 4+, 6+, and 7+ in salts such as sulfate, chloride, and gluconate and chelates such as aspartate, fumarate, and succinate. Manganese deficiency results in a variety of diseases, as it is part of the MnSOD, a key enzyme for antioxidant protection in mitochondria. Skeletal abnormalities are found in animals that are Mn-deficient, and wound healing is compromised as collagen production is inhibited. Uptake of Mn can come from infant formula (higher amounts found than in breast milk) or other dietary supplements, fumes, aerosols, or suspended particulate matter. Intestinal absorption is tightly regulated at 3–5%, with Mn ions binding to the same location as Fe^{3+} ions on mucin (large glycoprotein). Iron and Mn also find to the intercellular metal binding protein mobilferrin. The absorption of reduced iron (via ascorbate or surface ferrireductases) and Mn^{2+} occurs via the divalent metal transporter 1 (DMT1)

into enterocytes from the proximal small bowel. As the number of transporters increase in iron deficiency, more Mn may be absorbed in this condition. Nasal inhalation results in particulate transport through the olfactory bulb with deposition in the striatum and cerebellum. Also, methcathinone hydrochloride in drug-addicted humans in Eastern Europe and the Baltic states results in Mn poisoning due to the use of potassium permanganate as the oxidant for pseudoephedrine hydrochloride. Mn overload causes manganism, an extrapyramidal syndrome appearing similar to idiopathic Parkinson's disease. This disease appears to occur due to the autoxidation of dopamine via generation of ROS and dopamine-o-quinone. These events are shown in **Figure 27-3.** Other accompanying problems of this redox cycling are NADH/NADPH depletion and inactivation of enzymes by oxidizing thiol groups or essential amino acids in addition to the generation of ROS and lipid peroxidation (Farina et al., 2013).

Molybdenum

Molybdenum is essential for the function of important oxidases (aldehyde oxidase, xanthine oxidase, and sulfite oxidase). Although molybdenum deficiency has not been observed in humans except in cases of long-term parenteral nutrition, goats fed a diet with < 0.00007 mg Mo/g had reduced weight gain, decreased food consumption, and affected reproduction. Mo toxicity has been observed in the former Soviet Union, where gout-like syndrome with elevated blood Mo levels, uric acid, and xanthine oxidase were noted. Rats given 80 mg Mo/kg/day had kidney failure (Goldhaber, 2003). Mo(VI) chemical species is part of the molybdate anion, $[MoO_4]^{2-}$, that enters animal and plant cells. However, it appears that molybdenum trioxide is a more toxic compared to other chemical forms of molybdenum (De Schamphelaere et al., 2010). As noted earlier, Mo interferes with Cu absorption and may have some pharmacological and toxicological applications based on this interaction. Molybdenosis and Mo disruptions of Cu metabolism appear to cause a wasting disease in the Swedish moose (*Alces alces* L.) with a multitude of severe lesions, disturbed glucose metabolism,

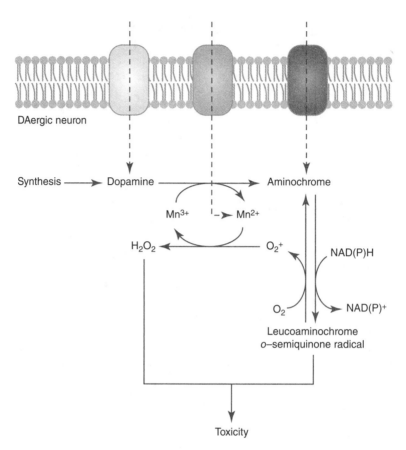

FIGURE 27-3 Mn-Induced Dopamine (DA) Oxidation: Primary Reactions Involved in Reactive Oxygen Species (ROS) and o-Quinones Radical Generation

Note: Mn-catalyzes the autoxidation of DA, involving the redox cycling of Mn^{2+} and Mn^{3+} in a reaction that generates ROS and DA-o-quinone or catalyzes the production of H_2O_2 inside the neurons, thereby leading to oxidative damage in DAergic neurons.

and decreased activity of Cu-containing enzymes (ceruloplasmin, SOD in blood, myocardial cytochrome *c* oxidase; Frank, 2004).

Potassium

Hypokalemia and hyperkalemia are familiar clinical states. Because K^+ is the major intracellular cation, many electrophysiological functions depend on its intake (50 mEq/kg body weight in humans). Because the kidneys excrete 80% of potassium intake, use of diuretics leads to hypokalemia (as do alcoholism, GI disturbances, renal tubular acidosis types I and II, primary and secondary hyperaldosteronism, Bartter's syndrome, Liddle syndrome, certain antibiotics, Mg depletion, trauma, albuterol, theophylline, and certain leukemias or ACTH-producing tumor). Potassium balance depends on acid–base status, plasma insulin concentration, plasma catecholamine levels, and to a small degree aldosterone levels. Muscles (skeletal more so than cardiac) and renal tubule cells are most affected by hypokalemia. Effects include muscle weakness, paralytic ileus, ECG changes (flat or inverted T waves, prominent U waves, ST segment depression), and cardiac arrhythmias (atrial tachycardia with or without block, AV dissociation, ventricular tachycardia, and ventricular fibrillation, which can lead to rapid death). Renal effects of hypokalemia include reduced creatinine clearance, inhibition of Cl⁻ fractional absorption by diluting segments, and depression of diuretic response to a water load.

Hyperkalemia can come from an excess of K intake or pseudohyperkalemia (extravascular hemolysis, severe leukocytosis, or thrombocytosis). Extracellular acidosis also produces hyperkalemia (efflux of potassium from inside of cells as a result of cellular buffering of H^+ ions while alkalosis produces hypokalemia due to potassium influx). True hyperkalemia (serum $K^+ >$ 5.5 mEq/L) is accompanied by low CO_2 content, and elevated blood urea nitrogen and serum creatinine. Kidney failure (complications arising from chronic kidney failure) could be a cause of hyperkalemia. Additonally, a variety of medications can lead to hyperkalemia, including potassium-sparing diuretics, angiotensin-converting enzyme (ACE) inhibitors, certain non-steroidal anti-inflammatory drugs (NSAIDs), anti-infectives, anticoagulants, digitalis, and antihypertensives. Cardiac signs are the most telling toxicity of hyperkalemia (progression of ECG problems start with tall, peaked T waves, widening of QRS, smaller P wave amplitude, QRS-T fusion, proceeding to AV dissociation, ventricular tachycardia, ventricular fibrillation, cardiac arrest, and death). Potassium intake also leads to azotemia (high nitrogen-containing compounds in plasma/serum) and metabolic acidosis (H^+/K^+ exchange). The metabolic acidosis aggravates hyperkalemia as it leads to potassium efflux from cells (Mandal, 1997).

Selenium

Selenium is an important component of the antioxidant enzyme selenium-dependent glutathione peroxidase, other antioxidant selenoproteins, and Se-containing proteins regulating redox states of important molecules such as ascorbic acid. It is also found in enzymes regulating thyroid hormone metabolism. Se deficiency was found in China as Keshan disease, a cardiomyopathy due to oxidative stress that must originate from an accompanying infection or chemical exposure. Exudative diathesis occurs in chickens low in vitamin E and Se, as oxidative damage is magnified in animals by this combination of antioxidant deficiency states. Selenosis is the excess Se toxicity state that includes hair and nail loss and brittleness, garlic breath (from dimethylselenide), skin rash, GI disturbances, and nervous

system disruptions (Goldhaber, 2003). However, selenium may be important as a cancer chemoprevention agent or to prevent the toxicity of As or Cd (Zwolak and Zaporowska, 2012). The anticancer action of Se is both as an antioxidant and prooxidant. Se metabolites inhibit tumor cell growth, modulate the cell cycle, and cause apoptosis. At low dietary concentrations, Se is part of antioxidant enzymes, while sodium selenite is prooxidant at high concentrations, forming selenodiglutathione and other metabolites. This apoptosis-induced prooxidant form of selenium is also highly toxic and can induce DNA damage (Brozmanová et al., 2010).

Sodium

Lack of sodium leads to low blood volume and blood pressure and has effects on membrane potentials and the balance of other ions as well if low enough. Excess sodium clearly leads to hypertension or dehydration depending on the level consumed. Sodium excess is a problem in processed foods, and drinking seawater has dehydrated many a victim without water rescued from a shipwreck at sea.

Vanadium

Vanadium is an essential micronutrient that is satisfied by 10–25 μg in the diet (from cereals, fruit juices, fish, shellfish, mushrooms, parsley, spinach, wine, and beer). It appears to be an insulin mimic and is anti-diabetes mellitus and cardioprotective (antihypertensive; Verma et al., 1998). V deficiency may reduce growth rate, infancy survival, hematocrit, and thyroid function (utilization of iodine). However, it is clear that V is toxic at low ($>$ 10 mg daily) intakes. Green tongue, diarrhea, abdominal cramping, and mental function changes are signs of vanadium toxicity. Vanadium appears to generate oxidative stress via interfering with ferritin's ability to deliver iron to oligodendrocyte progenitor cells during development. This leads to apoptosis and hypomyelination (Todorich et al., 2011). Vanadium pentoxide is a toxic species that is toxic by inhalation exposure (miners). It does not transport well out of the lung and may cause acute chemical pneumonitis, pulmonary edema, and/or acute tracheobronchitis. This compound also appears to negatively affect cardiac autonomic function. Cytokine and chemokine secretion by hepatocytes exposed to vanadium pentoxide leads to inflammation. This compound also impairs mitochondrial function. V_2O_5 also changes the permeability of epithelium, promoting inflammatory mediators and resulting in underlying neuronal tissue damage and death. Citrate uptake and $3Na^+$, $2K^+$-ATPase are inhibited by vanadium pentoxide in renal brush border membrane vesicles that may be a contributing cause of nephrotoxicity. Male infertility also results from vanadium pentoxide administration via necrosis of the spermatogonium, spermatocytes, and Sertoli cells (Cooper, 2007).

Zinc

Zinc is essential for ribonucleic polymerases, alcohol dehydrogenase, carbonic anhydrase, and alkaline phosphatase activity. Zinc deficiency in humans appears as decreased appetite, slowing growth, skin alterations, and immunological abnormalities. During pregnancy Zn deficiency yields developmental disorders. Zn oxide has been used pharmacologically as a healing agent (part of diaper rash cream). High levels of Zn (≥ 2 g zinc sulfate) result in GI irritation and vomiting. Copper status is reduced (decrease in erythrocyte SOD in adult females). Immune system function is reduced (biphasic for immune function; Goldhaber, 2003).

Biological Interest: Nickel

Nickel's toxicity as a carcinogen may indeed be its reproductive toxicity as well. It has neuroendocrine and gonadal influences on the hypothalamic-pituitary-gonadal (HPG) axis. Substitution of Ni into metal-dependent enzymes disrupts protein function. Ni crosses the cell membrane via Ca channel and competes with Ca for receptors that bind that ion. Ni cross-links DNA and amino acids, forms ROS, and mimics hypoxia (Forgacs et al., 2012). Histone-modifying enzymes (e.g., iron- and 2-oxoglutarate-dependent dioxygenase family enzymes) appear to be targets that lead to the toxicity/carcinogenicity of Ni (Chervona et al.,

2012). Respiratory cancers (and lung irritation, lung inflammation/pneumonia, emphysema, fibrosis, pneumoconiosis, allergic asthma) would be associated with inhalation of Ni species, with key Ni species of less soluble oxidic and particularly sulfidic nickel (Ni_3S_2). Skin contact is more associated with allergic contact dermatitis (Schaumlöffel, 2012). Other symptoms associated with exposure to nickel include nausea, vomiting, diarrhea, headache, chest pain, weakness, and coughing. Nickel vapor may cause irritation to eyes, nose, and throat, and on systemic distribution swelling of the brain and liver, liver degeneration, and various types of cancer.

Medical

Aluminum

Aluminum is abundant in over-the-counter (OTC) medical products such as phosphate-binding agents (aluminum hydroxide), in adjuvant for immunizations, via dialysate for patients on renal dialysis or total parenteral nutrition contamination, through bladder irrigation, and transdermal use of antiperspirants. One of the possible outcomes of overuse of this and similar products is neurotoxicity. The inhibitory actions of Al on ATP production/mitochondrial function cause the formation of globular astrocytes that generate fat. This appears to be a root cause of brain disorders that some used to think mirrored Alzheimer's-like behavior in animals exposed to Al (Lemire and Appanna, 2011). It is of interest that chelation of Fe and/or Al with desferrioxamine slows the progression of Alzheimer's disease (possibly by reducing ROS formation; Percy et al., 2011). Al does cause oxidative stress in the brain. Other diseases associated with Al toxicity are Parkinson's disease–like effects (decreased dopamine content of striatum), dialysis encephalopathy, and osteomalacia. In isolate cultured hepatoblastoma cells (HepG2) Al seems to interfere with iron-dependent and redox-sensitive enzymes in the Krebs cycle and oxidative phosphorylation. As a compensatory mechanism, HIF-1α (the same factor mentioned in cobalt's carcinogenic action) is stabilized to increase

ATP synthesis in the cytosol by glycolysis. Lipid is also accumulated in these hepatic origin cells via increased lipid synthesis and reduced β-oxidation of fatty acids. Oxidative stress that accompanies Al toxicity is battled by α-ketoglutarate quenching and succinate accumulation, which stabilizes HIF-1α. The use of α-ketoglutarate in this manner decreases L-carnitine biosynthesis and fatty acid oxidation (Mailloux et al., 2011).

Aluminum has been reported to cause either suppression of immune function (chronic high Al exposure and decreased CD4+ T lymphocytes) or increased reactivity via allergy and autoimmunity (chronic fatigue syndrome and macrophagic myofasciitis due to Al in adjuvant for immunization). Al can increase IgE levels and therefore induce immediate hypersensitivity. Limited data suggest that Al can affect Type II hypersensitivity (as occurs with aluminum-containing adjuvants involving IL-1β, IL-18 and especially IL-33; Li et al., 2007; Schmitz et al., 2005) to cell surface or matrix antigens and can also trigger Type III hypersensitivity to soluble antigens generating tissue damage by prevention of removal of circulatory immune complex. Sometimes both results occur, as high Al doses first decrease CD8[+] T lymphocytes in exposed rats and then the organism adapts over a longer time of exposure to increase these cytotoxic T cells. Al also increases oral tolerance to foreign antigens by inducing the expression of the suppressive cytokine IL-4 (Zhu et al., 2012). An aluminum-related bone disease is osteomalacia, in which excessive deposits at the site of osteoid mineralization occur instead of Ca. Hematopoiesis (proposed interference with Fe absorption and utilization and hemolysis) is also inhibited by Al excess, yielding microcytic anemia (similar to Pb poisoning).

Bismuth

Bismuth has been part of medicinal products for years (digestive disorders). Although its toxicity is not considered relevant at usual pharmacological doses in healthy people, inadvertent or intentional (suicidal) ingestion of bismuth subcitrate has resulted in nausea, vomiting, and facial paresthesia. Acute renal failure as a result of bismuth toxicity has occurred in a human patient even though supportive treatment and dialysis were required. Chronic administration causes encephalopathy (Cengiz et al., 2005). It is of interest that Bi salts are less toxic than water-soluble organic complexes of this metal. The water-soluble organic complexes yield much higher Bi levels than ionic Bi (Serfontein and Mekel, 1979). Bismuth also affects the liver, bladder, joints, gums, stomach, and colon. The kidney usually has the highest concentration, and Bi is specifically bound to protein there. The prodromal phase of Bi toxicity starts as problems with walking, standing, writing, memory, behavior (psychiatric symptoms), insomnia, and muscle cramps. The manifest phase is an abrupt appearance of alterations in awareness, myoclonia, astasia (lack of motor coordination) and/or abasia (inability to walk as a result of coordination problems) and dysarthria. The encephalopathy that might result is due to neuronal dysfunction caused by this metal (Slikkerveer and de Wolff, 1989). Bi can also cause skin and respiratory irritation if exposed via external routes/dusts.

Gallium

Gallium has been a diagnostic and therapeutic agent in cancer and Ca/bone metabolism (radioactive, ^{67}Ga citrate scan/uptake for lymphoma malignancy determination, and gallium nitrate's antineoplastic activity). Ga also has anti-inflammatory and immunosuppressive activity (gallium nitrate inhibits carp Ig production, phagocyte killing ability, and blood leukocytes). Some gallium compounds may be antimicrobial as well. This discussion will not include the use of gallium arsenide used in the semiconductor industry, as the toxicity manifested appears to lie with the arsenic moiety. Gallium interacts with a variety of cellular processes, especially involving iron metabolism. Gallium interferes with calcium and has been used to treat hypercalcemia, but causes renal toxicity that makes this compound dose limiting. Microcytic anemia may result from gallium's interference with Fe metabolism, but does not result in reductions of thrombocyte or leukocyte counts.

Ga can in a few people lead to visual and auditory toxicities (Chitambar, 2010).

Gold

Gold is one of the older medications for treatment of rheumatoid arthritis. Patients receiving Au therapy may have dermatitis, stomatitis, transient hematuria, and mild proteinuria. Some diarrhea may also occur. Patients with rheumatoid arthritis and HLA-DR3 also are more likely to develop proteinuria (nephropathy) and thrombocytopenia. Post-injection of gold compounds, nitritoid (vasomotor) reactions can occur including weakness, dizziness, nausea, vomiting, perspiration, and facial flushing. Slower, non-vasomotor reactions may also appear following injection of Au compounds characterized by arthralgia (joint pain), joint swelling, easily becoming fatigued, and malaise. Gold is one of three heavy metals (Ag, Au, Hg) that can lead to autoimmunity, increases in serum IgG and IgE, polyclonal activation of B and T lymphocytes, and renal immune complex deposition and glomerulonephritis. Mast cells represent an important target for metals that result in autoimmunity as these metals cause mast cell degranulation and secretion of arachidonic acid metabolites and cytokines such as IL-4. Mast cell survival is also influenced by Au. Mitogen-activated protein kinase activation, ROS, and NO generation along with Ca^{2+} influx are altered by metals such as Au (Suzuki et al., 2011).

Gold also appears to be taken up by the choroid plexus (as are Hg and Cd). Plexus regulatory pathways that are central to brain development and function are then affected. This metal accumulation may lead to neurodegeneration (Zheng, 2001). Pulmonary injury from gold salts are associated with bronchiolitis obliterans organizing pneumonia, characterized on radiography and on radiographs as hetero- and homogeneous peripheral opacities (upper and lower lobes) and on CT scans as poorly defined nodular consolidation, centrilobular nodules, and bronchial dilatation (Rossi et al., 2000). The odd portion of the use of Au is that it was mistaken for an immunosuppressant agent in its ability to treat rheumatoid arthritis, but it actually can

stimulate immune reactivity as indicated by skin and mucous membrane reactions (pruritus, rash, cheilitis [lips], eosinophilia, chronic papular eruptions, contact sensitivity, erythema nodosum, allergic contact purpura, pityriasis rosea, lichenoid and exfoliative dermatitis), blood dyscrasias, pulmonitis, nephrotoxicity, and nephrotic syndrome.

Mechanisms of action of Au(I) salts begin with uptake by lysosomes. Once there, myeloperoxidase and other lysosomal enzymes oxidize gold in aurothiomalate to Au(III; auric) chloride. $AuCl_3$ is a better oxidant than Au(I) and is the predominant species for its pharmaceutical anti-inflammatory action and toxic reactivity. A rapid oxidative burst by the lysosome may be responsible for the oxidation of gold and the Au(III) can diffuse away from its site of oxidation to react with protein reductants. This could generate immunological reactions responsible both for its therapeutic action and adverse effects. The production of Au(III) is interestingly an oxidant former and a scavenger of ROS such as hypochlorous acid. Au(III) irreversibly denatures protein including lysosomal enzymes and may be responsible for its anti-inflammatory activity. Additionally, Au(III) may interfere with antigen processing of may alter major histocompatibility complex (MHC) molecules in the lysosomal-endosomal pathway. The three mechanisms just enumerated (ROS scavenging, protein denaturation, and antigen-processing interference) may account for reduced production of arthritogenic (self) peptides. However, denaturation of self-proteins may instead induce autoimmunity if now recognized in that state as "foreign" protein (Merchant, 1998).

Lithium

Lithium is a medication used in the treatment of bipolar disorders. Based on its action, at high levels over a substantial period of time (> 2 months) reversible (mainly problems of pyramidal tract in acute Li neurotoxicity—tremor, ataxia, gait problems, myoclonus, hyperreflexia, dysarthria, convulsions, incontinence) or irreversible (cerebellar impairment, dementia, Parkinsonian syndromes, choreoathetosis, brain stem syndromes, peripheral neuropathies) lithium neurotoxicity may result (Netto amd Phutane, 2012). It is a thyroid disruptor by decreasing thyroid hormone synthesis and release, reducing peripheral iodination of T4 by inhibiting 5′ deiodinase, and increasing the risk of thyroid autoimmunity by augmenting B lymphocyte activity and reducing the ratio of circulating cytotoxic T cells (Kibirige et al., 2013). Other symptoms of Li toxicity are decreased GFR and reduced urinary concentration ability (polyuria and polydipsia due to nephrogenic diabetes insipidus) and weight gain. End-stage renal failure risk from Li therapy is low (0.5% in a Swedish population treated with Li). Congenital abnormalities (Ebstein's anomaly) are increased 400-fold by Li treatment but represent still a low number of events (may not be statistically; McKnight et al., 2012). Lithium's therapeutic action was first thought to result from inhibition of signal transduction through G-protein-couple receptor pathways or inositol monophosphatase and glycogen synthase kinase-2. There is more recent evidence suggesting that Li may act via N-methyl-D-aspartate receptor (NDAR) nitric oxide signaling. This pathway appears to regulate monoaminergic neurotransmission in a bidirectional manner. However, Li appears to also affect the monoaminergic system, GSK-3β, adenylyl cyclase, and key proteins involved in neuroprotection (e.g., p53, BAX, Bcl-2, caspase, and cytochrome c). The therapeutic to neurotoxic effects of Li appear to result from changes in glutamatergic/NDMAR signaling (disturbing glutamate uptake, regulation of NMDAR phosphorylation, NMDAR mRNA level), or indirectly via GABAergic transmission of brain-derived neurotrophic factor (BDNF) in the CNS.

Lithium's renal effects may be due to decreased formation of cAMP in renal tubules. However, Li also has some neuroendocrine effects that may bear on this system, such as upregulation of nNOS (neuronal nitric oxide synthase) gene expression, decreased NOS activity, and elevation of arginine vasopressin. Li affects GI motility and gastric function mostly during early phases of treatment via reduction in NO-mediated non-adrenergic, non-cholinergic neurogenic relaxation of the gastric fundus (in the rat *in vitro*), which is augmented by L-NAME (precursor to NOS inhibitor L-NNA) and is ameliorated by L-arginine. This indicates the role of Li in its disruption of the L-arginine/NO pathway. This same action of Li on the GI tract has an interesting protective action on the rat model of irritable bowel syndrome by increasing the threshold for pain (nociception) and reducing defecation frequency. Li pretreatment also reduced ethanol-induced gastric damage. Affecting NO levels may lead to impotence as erection is not possible without relaxation of the corpus cavernosum (Ghasemi and Dehpour, 2011).

Silver

Silver has been used for wound treatment and deodorant powders as an antibacterial (used even in Roman times to treat potable water). Silver nanoparticles have been used industrially as antimicrobial agents and may have some interesting cancer chemotherapeutic action (Ong et al., 2013). The antimicrobial action of silver nanoparticles is increased due to its surface and photocatalytic properties that generate oxidative damage (Stensberg et al., 2011). Argyria and argyrosis are skin and eye reactions to silver deposits in the dermis and cornea/conjunctiva. Silver binds to metallothionein I and II, which chelate and therefore reduce the toxicity to many heavy metals such as Ag (Miyayama et al., 2012). As mentioned for Au and Hg, silver is also a metal that causes the formation of autoantibodies/autoimmunity (Suzuki et al., 2011).

Ag nanoparticles are of particular interest due to their size and developing information on their toxicity as an emerging product. Algal species are more sensitive to silver nanoparticles than to free Ag^+. The addition of the sulfhydryl-containing amino acid cysteine (similar moieties in GSH and metallothionein) decreases toxic effects of ionic or nanoparticle silver (Stensberg et al., 2011). Silver nanoparticles are quite ubiquitous now due to industrial usage and are cytotoxic and genotoxic to mammalian (rodents) cells with more resistance of human cells (de Lima et al., 2012). Rat liver (BRL3A) and neuronal cells, human lung epithelial cells, and mouse stem cells all exhibit the toxic effects of Ag nanoparticles. Aquatic invertebrates and vertebrates also demonstrate Ag nanoparticle toxicity and that microorganisms and plants can accumulate silver nanoparticles in the food chain. The major toxicity of ionic silver is via the mitochondrial damage to most cells via the permeability transition pathway. In rat liver, mitochondria swelling, disrupted metabolism, and subsequent apoptosis occur due to the Ag-induced formation of proteinaceous pores in the mitochondrial membranes. However, silver nanoparticles (Ag NPs) appear to take the "Trojan Horse" mechanism. The Ag NPs permeate cell membranes (< 5 nm passively; > 5 nm by endosomal mechanisms) increasing intracellular Ag^+. This ionic form of silver then causes cytotoxic and genotoxic effects via interference with cell transport and local GSH depletion along with other antioxidants. ROS are generated (via interference with ion and electron flow across the mitochondrial membrane), as occurs with other heavy metals along with the familiar accompanying DNA damage (via ROS or decreased ATP production/ATP-dependent DNA repair mechanisms) and effects on cytokine production (alveolar macrophages increased NF-α, MIP-2 and IL-1β; human epidermal cells IL-1β, IL-6, IL-8, and TNF-α; human mesenchymal cells increased IL-8 at < 5 µg/mL Ag NPs and decreased IL-6 and IL-8 at higher concentrations). The degree of damage determines whether apoptosis or necrosis occurs. The mean Ag NP size that appears to induce the most loss of mitochondrial activity appears to be 15 nm. Rat coronary endothelial cells exposed to high doses of Ag NP increase NO and cell proliferation. Ag NPs appear to affect multiple systems including circulatory (decreased platelet aggregation), respiratory (inflammatory), CNS (neuronal degeneration and necrosis), and hepatic (accumulation results in vacuolization, hepatic focal necrosis, hyperplasia of bile ducts, more inflammatory cell infiltration, and dilation of central veins) systems. Topical exposure to Ag NPs causes pigs at the highest doses to experience edema, epidermal hyperplasia, and focal inflammation. Ag NPs also affected zebrafish (developmental model organism) including mortality, heart rate, and hatching rates as well as morphological alterations, edema, and retarded development (Stensberg et al., 2011).

Questions

1. Why are GSH S-transferase and purine nucleoside phosphorylase considered activating enzymes and S-adenosylmethionine considered an activator for As toxicity?
2. What organelle is primarily responsible for renal proximal tubule damage?
3. What receptor does lead affect in the CNS and what is the clinical measure of Pb poisoning?
4. What mechanisms lead to MeHg neurotoxicity?
5. Histologically, how has copper excess been differentiated from iron excess in the liver?
6. Why does Mo toxicity look like a deficiency of another metal?
7. Why is Ni considered a metal of biological interest instead of a toxic metal?
8. Why is Ag NP toxicity different from Ag^+ exposure?

References

Adamcewicz M, Bearelly D, Porat G, Friedenberg FK. 2011. Mechanism of action and toxicities of purgatives used for colonoscopy preparation. *Expert Opin Drug Metab Toxicol.* 7:89–101.

Baranowska-Bosiacka I, Gutowska I, Rybicka M, Nowacki P, Chlubek D. 2012. Neurotoxicity of lead. Hypothetical molecular mechanisms of synaptic function disorders. *Neurol Neurochir Pol.* 46:569–578.

Bhattacharjee P, Banerjee M, Giri AK. 2013. Role of genomic instability in arsenic-induced carcinogenicity. A review. *Environ Int.* 53C:29–40.

Brozmanová J, Mániková D, Vlcková V, Chovanec M. 2010. Selenium: a double-edged sword for defense and offence in cancer. *Arch Toxicol.* 84:919–938.

Brugge D, Buchner V. 2011. Health effects of uranium: new research findings. *Rev Environ Health.* 26:231–249.

Cengiz N, Uslu Y, Gök F, Anarat A. 2005. Acute renal failure after overdose of colloidal bismuth subcitrate. *Pediatr Nephrol.* 20:1355–1358.

Chassaing S, Collin F, Dorlet P, Gout J, Hureau C, Faller P. 2012. Copper and heme-mediated Abeta toxicity: redox chemistry, Abeta oxidations and anti-ROS compounds. *Curr Top Med Chem.* 12:2473–2595.

Chervona Y, Arita A, Costa M. 2012. Carcinogenic metals and the epigenome: understanding the effect of nickel, arsenic, and chromium. *Metallomics.* 4:619–627.

Chitambar CR. 2010. Medical applications and toxicities of gallium compounds. *Int J Environ Res Public Health.* 7:2337–2361.

Cooper RG. 2007. Vanadium pentoxide inhalation. *Indian J Occup Environ Med.* 11:97–102.

Costa A, Tejpar S, Prenen H, Van Cutsem E. 2011. Hypomagnesaemia and targeted anti-epidermal growth factor receptor (EGFR) agents. *Target Oncol.* 6:227–233.

Das AP, Singh S. 2011. Occupational health assessment of chromite toxicity among Indian miners. *Indian J Occup Environ Med.* 15:6–13.

Davidson IWF, Burt RL. 1973. Physiological changes in plasma chromium of normal and pregnant women: effect of glucose load. *Am J Obstet Gynecol.* 116:601–608.

de Lima R, Seabra AB, Durán N. 2012. Silver nanoparticles: a brief review of cytotoxicity and genotoxicity of chemically and biogenically synthesized nanoparticles. *J Appl Toxicol.* 32:867–879.

De Schamphelaere KA, Stubblefield W, Rodriguez P, Vleminckx K, Janssen CR. 2010. The chronic toxicity of molybdate to freshwater organisms. I. Generating reliable effects data. *Sci Total Environ.* 408:5362–5371.

Domingo JL. 1994. Metal-induced developmental toxicity in mammals: a review. *J Toxicol Environ Health.* 42:123–141.

Drinkwater J. 2011. Magnesium sulphate for pre-eclampsia: care of the neonate. *Pract Midwife.* 14:17–19.

Durlach J. 2004. New data on the importance of gestational Mg deficiency. *J Am Coll Nutr.* 23:694S–700S.

Durlach J, Guiet-Bara A, Pagès N, Bac P, Bara M. 2005. Magnesium chloride or magnesium sulfate: a genuine question. *Magnes Res.* 18:187–192.

Farina M, Avila DS, da Rocha JB, Aschner M. 2013. Metals, oxidative stress and neurodegeneration: a focus on iron, manganese and mercury. *Neurochem Int.* 62:575–594.

Fieten H, Leegwater PA, Watson AL, Rothuizen J. 2012. Canine models of copper toxicosis for understanding mammalian copper metabolism. *Mamm Genome.* 23:62–75.

Flora G, Gupta D, Tiwari A. 2012. Toxicity of lead: a review with recent updates. *Interdiscip Toxicol.* 5:47–58.

Forgacs Z, Massányi P, Lukac N, Somosy Z. 2012. Reproductive toxicology of nickel—review. *J Environ Sci Health A Tox Hazard Subst Environ Eng.* 47:1249–1260.

Frank A. 2004. A review of the "mysterious" wasting disease in Swedish moose (*Alces alces* L.) related to molybdenosis and disturbances in copper metabolism. *Biol Trace Elem Res.* 102:143–159.

Fujiwara Y, Lee JY, Tokumoto M, Satoh M. 2012. Cadmium renal toxicity via apoptotic pathways. *Biol Pharm Bull.* 35:1892–1897.

Ghasemi M, Dehpour AR. 2011. The NMDA receptor/nitric oxide pathway: a target for the therapeutic and toxic effects of lithium. *Trends Pharmacol Sci.* 32:420–434.

Glinsmann WH, Feldman FJ, Mertz W. 1966. Plasma chromium after glucose administration. *Science.* 152:1243–1245.

Goldhaber SB. 2003. Trace element risk assessment: essentiality vs. toxicity. *Regul Toxicol Pharmacol.* 38:232–242.

Hollinger HZ, Pattee CJ. 1956. A review of abnormal calcium and phosphorus metabolism. I. Hypercalcaemia. *Can Med Assoc J.* 75:941–948.

Hwang GW, Furuchi T, Naganuma A. 2008. The ubiquitin-conjugating enzymes, Ubc4 and Cdc34, mediate cadmium resistance in budding yeast through different mechanisms. *Life Sci.* 82:1182–1185.

Kaler SG. 2014. Translational research investigations on ATP7A: an important human copper ATPase. *Ann NY Acad Sci.* 1314:64–8.

Khattak MA. 2011. Calcium and magnesium prophylaxis for oxaliplatin-related neurotoxicity: is it a trade-off between drug efficacy and toxicity? *Oncologist.* 16:1780–1783.

Kibirige D, Luzinda K, Ssekitoleko R. 2013. Spectrum of lithium induced thyroid abnormalities: a current perspective. *Thyroid Res.* 6:3.

Lawal AO, Ellis EM. 2012. Phospholipase C mediates cadmium-dependent apoptosis in HEK 293 cells. *Basic Clin Pharmacol Toxicol.* 110:510–517.

Lemire J, Appanna VD. 2011. Aluminum toxicity and astrocyte dysfunction: a metabolic link to neurological disorders. *J Inorg Biochem.* 105:1513–1517.

Li H, Nookala S, Re F. 2007. Aluminum hydroxide adjuvants activate caspase-1 and induce IL-1beta and IL-18 release. *J Immunol.* 178:5271–5276.

Lutsenko S, Efremov RG, Tsivkovskii R, Walker JM. 2002. Human copper-transporting ATPase ATP7B (the Wilson's disease protein): biochemical properties and regulation. *J Bioenerg Biomembr.* 34:351–362.

Mailloux RJ, Lemire J, Appanna VD. 2011. Hepatic response to aluminum toxicity: dyslipidemia and liver diseases. *Exp Cell Res.* 317:2231–2238.

Mäki-Paakkanen J, Kurttio P, Paldy A, Pekkanen J. 1998. Association between the clastogenic effect of peripheral lymphocytes and human exposure to arsenic through drinking water. *Environ Mol Mutagen.* 32:301–313.

Majumdar KK, Guha Mazumder DN. 2012. Effect of drinking arsenic-contaminated water in children. *Indian J Public Health.* 56:223–226.

Mandal AK. 1997. Hypokalemia and hyperkalemia. *Med Clin North Am.* 81:611–639.

Matović V, Plamenac Bulat Z, Djukić-Cosić D, Soldatović D. 2010. Antagonism between cadmium and magnesium: a possible role of magnesium in therapy of cadmium intoxication. *Magnes Res.* 23:19–26.

McKnight RF, Adida M, Budge K, Stockton S, Goodwin GM, Geddes JR. 2012. Lithium toxicity profile: a systematic review and meta-analysis. *Lancet.* 379:721–728.

Merchant B. 1998. Gold, the noble metal and the paradoxes of its toxicology. *Biologicals.* 26:49–59.

Mertz W. 1993. Chromium in human nutrition: a review. *J Nutr.* 123:626–633.

Miyayama T, Arai Y, Hirano S. 2012. [Environmental exposure to silver and its health effects]. *Nihon Eiseigaku Zasshi.* 67:383–389.

Netto I, Phutane VH. 2012. Reversible lithium neurotoxicity: review of the literature. *Prim Care Companion CNS Disord.* 14:PCC.11r01197.

Nick JM. 2004. Deep tendon reflexes, magnesium, and calcium: assessments and implications. *J Obstet Gynecol Neonatal Nurs.* 33:221–230.

Ong C, Lim JZ, Ng CT, Li JJ, Yung LY, Bay BH. 2013. Silver nanoparticles in cancer: therapeutic efficacy and toxicity. *Curr Med Chem.* 20:772–781.

Paldy A. Farkas I, Markus B, Gundy S. 1991. Chromosomal aberrations in children exposed to high concentrations of arsenic in drinking water. 21st Annual Meeting of the European Mutagen Society (EEMS) on Environmental Mutagens-Carcinogens.

Percy ME, Kruck TP, Pogue AI, Lukiw WJ. 2011. Towards the prevention of potential aluminum toxic effects and an effective treatment for Alzheimer's disease. *J Inorg Biochem.* 105:1505–1512.

Rossi SE, Erasmus JJ, McAdams HP, Sporn TA, Goodman PC. 2000. Pulmonary drug toxicity: radiologic and pathologic manifestations. *Radiographics.* 20:1245–1259.

Satarug S, Moore MR. 2012. Emerging roles of cadmium and heme oxygenase in type-2 diabetes and cancer susceptibility. *Tohoku J Exp Med.* 228:267–288.

Sato Y, Fukuda J. 2004. [Physiological role of Mg2+ in neurons]. *Clin Calcium.* 14:50–57.

Schauder A, Avital A, Malik Z. 2010. Regulation and gene expression of heme synthesis under heavy metal exposure—review. *J Environ Pathol Toxicol Oncol.* 29:137–158.

Schaumlöffel D. 2012. Nickel species: analysis and toxic effects. *J Trace Elem Med Biol.* 26:1–6.

Schmitz J, Owyang A, Oldham E, Song Y, Murphy E, McClanahan TK, Zurawski G, Moshrefi M, Qin J, Li X, Gorman DM, Bazan JF, Kastelein RA. 2005. IL-33, an interleukin-1-like cytokine that signals via the IL-1 receptor-related protein ST2 and induces T helper type 2-associated cytokines. *Immunity.* 23:479–490.

Serfontein WJ, Mekel R. 1979. Bismuth toxicity in man II. Review of bismuth blood and urine levels in patients after administration of therapeutic bismuth formulations in relation to the problem of bismuth toxicity in man. *Res Commun Chem Pathol Pharmacol.* 26:391–411.

Shelleh HH. 2012. Depleted uranium. Is it potentially involved in the recent upsurge of malignancies in populations exposed to war dust? *Saudi Med J.* 33:483–488.

Slikkerveer A, de Wolff FA. 1989. Pharmacokinetics and toxicity of bismuth compounds. *Med Toxicol Adverse Drug Exp.* 4:303–323.

Simonsen LO, Harbak H, Bennekou P. 2012. Cobalt metabolism and toxicology—a brief update. *Sci Total Environ.* 432:210–215.

Song WJ, Chang YS. 2012. Magnesium sulfate for acute asthma in adults: a systematic literature review. *Asia Pac Allergy.* 2:76–85.

Stensberg MC, Wei Q, McLamore ES, Porterfield DM, Wei A, Sepúlveda MS. 2011. Toxicological studies on silver nanoparticles: challenges and opportunities in assessment, monitoring and imaging. *Nanomedicine (Lond).* 6:879–898.

Striffler JS, Polansky MM, Anderson RA. 1998. Dietary chromium decreases insulin resistance in rats fed a high-fat, mineral-imbalanced diet. *Metabolism.* 47:396–400.

Sumi D, Himeno S. 2012. Role of arsenic (+3 oxidation state) methyltransferase in arsenic metabolism and toxicity. *Biol Pharm Bull.* 35:1870–1875.

Suttle NF. 2012. Copper imbalances in ruminants and humans: unexpected common ground. *Adv Nutr.* 3:666–674.

Suzuki Y, Inoue T, Ra C. 2011. Autoimmunity-inducing metals (Hg, Au and Ag) modulate mast cell signaling, function and survival. *Curr Pharm Des.* 17:3805–3814.

Todorich B, Olopade JO, Surguladze N, Zhang X, Neely E, Connor JR. 2011. The mechanism of vanadium-mediated developmental hypomyelination is related to destruction of oligodendrocyte progenitors through a relationship with ferritin and iron. *Neurotox Res.* 19:361–373.

Tokumoto M, Ohtsu T, Honda A, Fujiwara Y, Nagase H, Satoh M. 2011. DNA microarray analysis of normal rat kidney epithelial cells treated with cadmium. *J Toxicol Sci.* 36:127–129.

Verma S, Cam MC, McNeill JH. 1998. Nutritional factors that can favorably influence the glucose/insulin system: vanadium. *J Am Coll Nutr.* 17:11–18.

Vicente-Vicente L, Quiros Y, Pérez-Barriocanal F, López-Novoa JM, López-Hernández FJ, Morales AI. 2010. Nephrotoxicity of uranium: pathophysiological, diagnostic and therapeutic perspectives. *Toxicol Sci.* 118:324–347.

Watanabe T, Hirano S. 2013. Metabolism of arsenic and its toxicological relevance. *Arch Toxicol.* 87:969–979.

Younes M, Eberhardt I, Lemoine R. 1989. Effect of iron overload on spontaneous and xenobiotic-induced lipid peroxidation *in vivo. J Appl Toxicol.* 9:103–108.

Zheng W. 2001. Toxicology of choroid plexus: special reference to metal-induced neurotoxicities. *Microsc Res Tech.* 52:89–103.

Zhu YZ, Liu DW, Liu ZY, Li YF. 2013. Impact of aluminum exposure on the immune system: a mini review. *Environ Toxicol Pharmacol.* 35:82–87.

Zwolak I, Zaporowska H. 2012. Selenium interactions and toxicity: a review. Selenium interactions and toxicity. *Cell Biol Toxicol.* 28:31–46.

CHAPTER 28

Industrial Chemicals That Cause Atmospheric Changes and Direct Versus Indirect Toxicity: Gases, Vapors, Aerosols, and Radiation

This is a chapter outline intended to guide and familiarize you with the content to follow.

I. Atmospheric chemicals

   A. Dispersion of gas—see Figure 28-1 for sulfur particles over Namibia

   B. Gases and vapors

      1. Direct effects—see Table 28-1

         a. Based on toxic gas accidents in the EU, the gases are CO, F_2, NH_3, H_2S, SO_2, $COCl_2$, HF, and NO_2/N_2O_4 —see Figure 28-2

         b. Gases = formless fluids that expand to fill any enclosure and obey gas laws

         c. Vapors = evaporated liquids or solids that are in a gaseous phase and obey gas laws

         d. Henry's Law for gases and vapors: Henry's Law Constant = C_{liquid}/C_{gas}; with 200 ppm $< LC_{50} \leq$ 2,000 ppm by volume for gas or vapor for 1 hour = toxic, while $LC_{50} <$ 200 ppm = highly toxic

         e. For dusts, mists, and fumes 2 mg/L $< LC_{50} \leq$ 20 mg/L for 1 hour = toxic and $<$ 2 mg/L = highly toxic. For gas mixtures $LC_{50m} = 1/[C_i/LC_{50i}]$, where $LC_{50m} = LC_{50}$ of the mixture, $C_i =$ concentration of the component i in decimal %, and $LC_{50i} = LC_{50}$ of component i. Normalization factors adjust exposure to 1 hour if not tested for that time period. For gases with $LC_{50} \leq$ 100 ppm, 500 ppm, 2,500 ppm, and 20,000 ppm by volume = categories 1–4, respectively. Vapors are done by mg/L with $LC_{50} \leq$ 0.5 mg/L, 2.0 mg/L, 10 mg/L, and 20 mg/L = categories 1–4, respectively. Dust and fumes are also determined by mg/L with $LC_{50} \leq$ 0.05 mg/L, 0.5 mg/L, 1.0 mg/L, and 5 mg/L as categories 1–4, respectively

         f. The National Fire Protection Agency has colors (blue = health hazard, yellow = instability of compound, red = flammable, white = special) and categories of 0 (no risk such as water), 1 (irritation and minor residual injury such a acetone), 2 (temporary incapacitation or some residual injury such as diethyl ether), 3 (serious temporary or moderate residual injury such as chlorine gas), and 4 (neurotoxins such an HCN gas)

         g. Certain gases target the mucosal tissue (formaldehyde); others may be scrubbed out of the respiratory tract by the nose for short durations of exposure (isopropyl alcohol, NH_3, HF, SO_2), while other less water-soluble compounds target the conducting airways (phosgene, NO_2, O_3). Water-soluble compounds can enter all cells along the tract to do damage, while gases pass through the conductive airways to the blood and on to target organs. Type I pneumocytes are most likely affected in the conducting airway as they line the alveolar wall surface. If pulmonary surfactant production is affected, then atelectasis results. Inflammation → pulmonary edema,

---

CONCEPTUALIZING TOXICOLOGY 28-1

which can be fatal. Irritants are NH_3, NO_x, SO_x, F_2, PH_3 (phosphine), and acrolein, which affect the area of lung based on their water solubility and reactivity. Sensitizations, allergy, and asthma are associated with isocyanates and amines. CO and H_2S are insoluble gases that affect mitochondria/neurons. Fuming gases (HCl, HBr, HF) corrode the respiratory tract CO, NO_x, SO_x, and O_3 damage directly or form peroxyacyl nitrates (smog) by photochemical reactions in mixtures. VOCs form from combustion or evaporation of fuels and solvents

   h. Dog is best human model due to branching of airway and responsiveness/presence of bronchiole constriction

2. Indirect effects

   a. CFCs depleting atmospheric O_3 ($Cl + O_3 \rightarrow ClO + O_2$ and $ClO + O_3 \rightarrow Cl + 2\,O_2$) $\rightarrow \uparrow$ UV irradiation $\rightarrow$ cataracts, malignant melanoma, basal cell carcinoma, and squamous cell carcinoma

   b. Smog (peroxyacyl nitrates) formed from NO + hydrocarbons + O_2 + O_3, which damage and irritate the lung and damage plants (generate ROS and Ca^{2+}-mediated cell death)

   c. CO_2 is changing temperature and pH of oceans along with UV $\uparrow$ already mentioned $\rightarrow$ coral bleaching affecting a variety of sea life in those communities

C. Aerosols (100 nm - 100 μm) are small particles composed of solids or liquids such as fumes, dusts, smoke, fogs, and mists suspending in air long enough to be dispersed

1. Direct effects

   a. Aerosols' toxicity depends on size of particle, size distribution, and concentration. Vaporizers produce large droplets that don't find their way far into the respiratory tract, while ultrasonic humidifiers may experience the toxicity of metals in the tap water as small aerosols are created. Inertia and sedimentation velocity (affected by mass and aerodynamic drag as determined by aerodynamic diameter, $D_{AE} = D(QC)^{1/2}/(Q_0 C_{AE})^{1/2}$; Q_0 = unit density; C and C_{AE} = slip correction factors applied when the diameter of the particle is close to the mean free path of gas molecules) and diffusion rate determine deposition. Particle size 0.1 μm $< D_{AE} <$ 3 μm $\rightarrow$ tracheobronchial deposition nearly constant. Small geometric standard deviation, σ_g, in particle size is considered a monodisperse group of particles, and toxicity is based on tidal volume of breathing and breathing rate. Large particles deposit in upper respiratory tract and are cleared by cilia (unless paralyzed by nicotine), while small particles are deposited farther down. The retained dose = $\alpha \cdot$ (VT·f) C·t (α = deposition fraction; VT = tidal volume; f = respiratory frequency; C = [toxicant]$_{atmosphere}$; t = exposure time). Particles' composition may yield lung cancer ($>$ 10 μm fibers), mesothelioma (~5 μm fibers), and fibrosis (~2 μm fibers) for insoluble agents such as asbestos that cause oxidative toxicity via macrophage activation. The smallest particle ($<$ 1 μm) will access the alveoli and sediment or diffuse ($<$ 0.5 μm) into the circulation. Nanosized particles should be assessed by their diffusion into the circulation and into target organs. Mineral dusts $\rightarrow$ pneumoconiosis (Fe, Sn, Ba). Collagenous pneumoconiosis $\rightarrow$ irreversible fibrosis (asbestos, silica, coal dust). As, Be, Cd, Ni, or silica fiber dusts $\rightarrow$ lung cancer

2. Indirect effects

   a. Atmospheric aerosol formation (growing molecular clusters) usually involves organic compounds. Sulfuric acid is a driver of smaller clusters, while amines are part of the next order of clusters. Organic vapors represent a portion of the third size of clusters, especially highly oxidized organic molecules. Nitrate or nitric acid can also be part of these larger clusters. These aerosols are influenced by and affect the biosphere, clouds, and climate

D. Radiation

1. Unstable isotopes give off particles of various sizes, charges, and velocities, which determine toxicity based on absorbed energy (Gy or Sv depending on whether the linear energy transfer is considered such as the mass of the particle) per depth of tissue and formation of ROS by

CONCEPTUALIZING TOXICOLOGY 28-1 (*continued*)

interaction with water. Ionizing radiation + $H_2O \rightarrow HOH^+ + e^-$ (tissue gains 34 ev); $e^- + H_2O \rightarrow$ HOH^-; $HOH^+ \rightarrow H^+ + OH^{\cdot}$ (hydroxyl radical); $HOH^- \rightarrow HO^- + H^{\cdot}$ (hydrogen radical)

2. Exposure was first measured by roentgen or r with ~83 erg/g air from the measurement of a Geiger counter. Correction for α or β radiation generated the equivalent roentgen (e.r.). This developed into rep/day = $60 \times E_m \times C$ (C = [isotope] in μc/g or mc/kg; E_m = mean energy of the radiation in million electron volts). This further developed into rads, where 500 rad = lethal human dose for X-rays or γ-rays. In this model ^{24}Na would give a whole body irradiation, while ^{89}Sr would involve bone and bone marrow. X-rays or γ-irradiation would also involve the bone (absorbed there) and soft tissue in that region. However, rads do not consider the energy impact of large particles like high-energy neutrons or α particles. The rem replaced the rad to indicate energy transfer. Now, 100 rad = 1 Gray (Gy), and 100 rems = 1 Sievert (Sv). This now takes into account relative biological effectiveness (RBE) where H = DQN (D = absorbed dose; Q = quality factor or RBE; N = additional modifying factors). Note α particles are most dangerous (Q = 20) over a short distance as they have a He nucleus mass and double charge. Neutrons have half the mass of α particles, but lack charge (more penetrating) and have Q = 10 along with protons. β particles are quenched over short distances even by water, but share the same Q = 1 with penetrating X-rays and g-rays. Tissues reactions are accounted by $H_E = \Sigma w_T H_T$ (w = weighting factor for organ or tissue; T and H_T = mean dose equivalent to organ or tissue T (w_T = 0.25 for gonads, 0.15 for breast, 0.12 for red marrow and lungs, 0.06 for five remaining organs or tissues receiving highest radiation dose, and 0.03 for thyroid, bone surface, remainder of organs). ^{222}Rn is a short-lived but dangerous α-emitting decay product that is characterized as working level (WL). Exposure is considered to have no threshold for toxicity, so the longer exposed over a lifetime, the higher the risk of cancer and other diseases as shown in Figure 28-4. Limits are set for exposure in most countries to 20 mSv/year for radiation workers (not pregnant) with a maximum of 50 mSv in any 1 year above background radiation. Fukushima workers were allowed 250 mSv due to the severity of the problem with radiation containment in a tsunami-breached nuclear power plant. The 570 PBq of ^{131}I released from the Fukushima plant is of concern for thyroid cancer

3. γ-rays or X-rays $\rightarrow$ photoelectric effects, Compton scattering, and pair production on entering matter. α particles have two neutrons and two protons, so their large size prevents their penetration, but their double positive charge has high ionizing potential. β particles have lower ionizing potential, but higher penetrating capability. Neutrons produce ionizations directly and have no charge so penetrate well. Neutrons are very toxic as they have high kinetic energy. Distance from a radiation source helps tremendously as does dense material shielding such as lead due to the 1/distance^2 rule of radiation dose

4. Half-life and radioactivity (based on dps as 1 dps = Bq) indicate the possible exposure to radioactive sources. See Table 28-2 for Bq from various common sources. Short-lived isotopes, such as ^{24}Na, ^{42}K, ^{131}I, and possibly ^{32}P were considered less dangerous β and γ emitters, while long-lived isotopes ^{22}Na and ^{36}Cl were used with more caution

5. Must consider $t_{1/2}$ and equivalent doses between particles to understand their toxicity

6. Radiation use in society is shown in Figure 28-3 and indicates relative radiation hazards of industry or atmospheric exposure

7. Radionuclides—toxicity based on organ (Table 28-3) and particles emitted (Table 28-4)

   a. Lung—inhaled soluble ^{238}Pu, ^{222}Rn, ^{241}Am, ^{144}CeO$_2$, ^{244}CmO$_2$, ^{243}EsCl$_3$, ^{210}Po—α particles and γ-rays $\rightarrow$ more associated with single- or double-strand breaks in DNA than β particles

   b. Thyroid—^{131}I

   c. Bone—^{90}Sr is of concern but more likely is an α emiiter ^{226}Ra (bone sarcomas). ^{239}Pu, ^{235}U, ^{90}Y, ^{140}Ba, ^{140}La, and the rare earth metals have strong affinity for bone

   d. Fast-growing tissues such as skin, GI tract, bone marrow, lymphatic tissues, and reproductive organs depend on radionuclide and intake (e.g., oral)

CONCEPTUALIZING TOXICOLOGY 28-1 (*continued*)

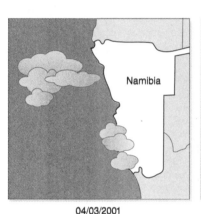 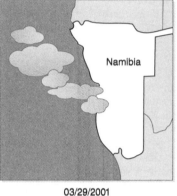 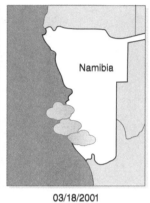

| 04/03/2001 | 03/29/2001 | 03/18/2001 |

FIGURE 28-1 Reversed Dispersion Diagram of Suspended Sulphur Granules (represented by light blue clouds) off the Namibian Coast

Modified from Weeks SJ, Currie B, Bakun A. 2002. Satellite imaging: massive emissions of toxic gas in the Atlantic. *Nature* 415: 493–494.

The examination of environmental toxicology now moves into the arena of inhalation toxicology, which covers gases, vapors, and aerosols, including radioactive gases such as radon. Note the dispersion of gas in **Figure 28-1**. High concentrations follow the wind patterns from the source and can affect organs near the source and downwind (Weeks et al., 2002). Lethal concentrations (LC_{50}s)/radioactivity and time spent in the presence of these agents are most important for toxicity (Hayes and Bakand, 2010). Although one can make a good case for skin and eye toxicity from exposure to oxidants that generate reactive oxygen species (ROS) such as certain low-wavelength UV radiation, diesel fuel exhaust, cigarette smoke, halogenated hydrocarbons, heavy metals, and ozone (Valacchi et al., 2012), this chapter focuses on air pollutants that can diffuse through the alveoli into circulation based on lipid solubility, molecular weight/volume, aerodynamic diameter, and other factors. Direct effects are due to reaction of the cells lining the airway to irritants resulting in systemic effects. Indirect effects are those that form smog (peroxyacyl nitrates) or other products in the atmosphere (not the original compound) and changes in the UV protection offered by stratospheric O_3 or similar changes (for fish that might be changing the pH and temperature of the water by increased CO_2 in the atmosphere).

Gases and Vapors—Direct Effects

Note the toxicities of gases, vapors, and aerosols in **Table 28-1**. Juxtapose those toxicities with the compounds that have generated the most toxicity reports for chemical accidents by the European Union shown in **Figure 28-2**. Toxic

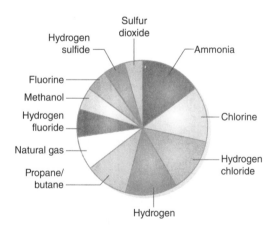

FIGURE 28-2 Relativistic Scale of Chemicals Involved in Accidents, Reported in Descending Order from Major Accident Reporting System (MARS) Database 1984–2004 of the European Union

TABLE 28-1   Gases, Vapors, and Aerosols Toxicity

Gases and Vapors Toxicity	Key Examples	Toxic Mechanism
Nasal tissue	O_3 vs. HCHO	Transitional epithelium vs. Respiratory mucosal damage
Pneumonitis/bronchitis → pulmonary edema → acute respiratory distress	Irritants such as NH_3, SO_2, phosgene, O_3	Inflammatory mediators: Start with upper airway Start at conducting airways
Sensitization, allergy, asthma	Isocyanates, amines	Hyper-responsiveness of airway and/or immune stimulation
Reactive airways dysfunction syndrome	Irritants	
Destruction of alveolar cells, capillary endothelium → acute respiratory failure → death	Overwhelming chlorine	Damages cells along entire respiratory tract
Affect internal organs/neurotoxicity	Anesthetics, CO	Insoluble and non-reactive gases pass through alveolar wall and systemic circulation to CNS and other organs
Corrosion of the respiratory tract	Strong acid fumes, caustic mists	Cellular damage followed by inflammation
Simple asphyxiants	N_2, H_2, CH_4, noble gases excluding radon, C_2H_5, C_2H_6	Dilution
Chemical asphyxiants	CO, HCN, H_2S	Disrupt cellular respiration
Cancer of the respiratory tract	HCHO (nose), isopropyl alcohol	Genotoxicity
Other organ systems cancer	Benzene	Reactive metabolites/genotoxic

Aerosol/Particulate Toxicity	Key Examples	Toxic Mechanism
Irritation	V	Airway reactivity to inflammation and asthma depending on dose and exposure duration
Bronchitis	Cr(VI), V	Inflammation
Pneumonia	Be, Cd oxide, Mn pneumonia	Too low oxygen into circulation, cough
Emphysema	Cd oxide	Lymphocyte infiltration, damage to alveoli, FEV_1 decreased
Tuberculosis	Silicotuberculosis	Yields blood on cough, extensive damage to lung
Cor pulmonale (enlargement of right ventricle due to increased resistance/pulmonary hypertension)	Be, Cd oxide	Resistance builds as lung toxicity prevents good perfusion of lung
Granulomatosis	Be	Immune reaction to particles
Pneumoconiosis (lung disease caused by chronic inhaled mineral or metallic dust)/metal/fiber/particle disease	Aluminosis, asbestosis, berylliosis, byssinosis (cotton), coal miner's pneumoconiosis, kaolinosis, manganism, siderosis (Fe oxides), silicosis, talcosis, stenosis (tin), hard metal disease (tungsten carbide)	From benign symptoms to collagenous irreversible fibrosis and other structural changes
Fibrosis of the respiratory tract	Asbestos (small), Al, coal dust, iron oxides, kaolin, silica, talc, tungsten carbide	

(continues)

TABLE 28-1 Gases, Vapors, and Aerosols Toxicity (*continued*)

Aerosol/Particulate Toxicity	Key Examples	Toxic Mechanism
Edema	Al (alveolar), Be, and Ni (pulmonary)	Leaky capillaries
Pleural plaques	Asbestos	Macrophage-induced ROS
Cancer of the respiratory tract	Asbestos (fiber size: lung cancer > mesothelioma), Ni (nose, lung), wood dusts, leather work (nose), As or Be or Cd (lung cancer)	Genotoxicity
Hyperplasia of bronchial epithelium	Tungsten carbide	

Data from Hayes A, Bakand S. 2010. Inhalation toxicology. EXS. 100: 461–488.

gases are CO, F_2 (9th most accidents), NO, HCl (3rd most accidents), H_2S (10th most accidents), HBr, Cl_2 (2nd most accidents), NH_3 (most accidents), SO_2 (11th most accidents, $COCl_2$ (phosgene), HF (7th most accidents), and NO_2/N_2O_4. Those starting with hydrogen in their chemical formula may also be volatilized acid that has not condensed into fumes (that is why people are supposed to use hoods when opening a bottle of acid)—except H_2S, which becomes a weak acid known as sulfhydric or hydrosulfuric acid. Remaining chemicals on the list of 11 most identified chemical accidents in the European Union (EU) result from flammable gases such as propane/butane or natural gas (which can be narcotizing/toxic at high concentrations) and a toxic solvent's vapor (methanol). From 1979 to September 2011, the EU reported through electronic medication administration records (eMARs) that chemical accidents that occurred with ≥ 10 events involved oxidizers (10 events), extremely flammable and toxic for an identified agent (11 events), highly flammable (13 events), explosive (18 events), dangerous for the environment as well as flammable and toxic (20 events), flammable and toxic (20 events), very toxic and flammable and toxic (25 events), toxic for a named substance (27 events), highly flammable (29 events), named substance (30 events), flammable (37 events), extremely flammable for a named substance (49 events), toxic (60 events),

extremely flammable (68 events), and not provided information (111 events). (Joint Research Centre, n.d.)

Gases are formless fluids that expand to fill any enclosure and observe universal gas laws. Vapors result from evaporation from a liquid state and are not considered different from gases except that a vapor is the gaseous phase of a compound that normally would be found as a solid or liquid at room temperature and atmospheric pressures similar to sea level (clearly, a very hot day in Denver, Colorado may yield more boiling solvents). They may be volatile organic compounds (VOCs) or other vapors from liquids such as HCN, C_3H_6O (propylene oxide), CS_2, C_3H_4O (acrolein), Br_2, CH_3OH, C_2H_5OH (from an ethanol plant), C_3H_3N (acrylonitrile), C_6H_6, off-gassing solutions such as HCN, ammonium hydroxide solution, formalin, acetyl chlorine (HCl released), HCl, carbonic acid (CO_2 released), HF, nitric acid, phosphoric acid, sulfuric acid, SO_3 (oleum), or off-gassing of other solid materials such as formaldehyde from composite cabinets or synthetic carpet fibers (Hayes and Bakand, 2010).

Because gas concentrations are reached faster with deeper breaths, ventilation is the first factor to be considered. This is followed by perfusion (heart rate and volume). Animals with high heart rates (canary in the mine) have faster rates of equilibration with the body. Diffusion is the final measure as the gas exposure area is high in the human (140 m²). This is a little more than half the intestinal area but 80 times the skin surface area. Because gases do not normally permeate the skin well, the lung is the entrance point. Then one has to consider a gas versus other forms such as aerosol or vapors. Gases and vapors are considered in the same toxicity category as they obey Henry's Law:

$$\text{Henry's Law Constant} = C_{\text{liquid}}/C_{\text{gas}}$$

Toxicity is defined as 200 ppm < LC_{50} ≤ 2,000 ppm by volume of gas or vapor continuous inhalation for 1 hour (or < 1 hour if death occurs), and LC_{50} ≤ 200 ppm is highly toxic. Note that for dusts, mists, or fumes, 2 mg/L < LC_{50} ≤ 20 mg/L for the same breathing interval is characterized as toxic and < 2 mg/L as highly toxic. For gas mixtures, binary mixture = hazardous component + nonhazardous gases comprising the remainder of the mixture = $LC_{50m} = 1/[C_i/LC_{50i}]$, where $LC_{50m} = LC_{50}$ of the mixture, C_i = concentration of the component i in decimal %, and $LC_{50i} = LC_{50}$ of component i. Normalization factors must adjust LC_{50} results to exposures of 1 hour (0.5 hour exposure multiply by 0.7; 1.5 hour multiply by 1.2; 2 hours multiply by 1.4; 3 hours multiply by 1.7; 4 hours multiply by 2; 5 hours multiply by 2.2; 6 hours multiply by 2.4; 7 hours multiply by 2.6; 8 hours multiply by 2.8). Another way of categorizing respiratory toxicity led to the following (United Nations, 2007): For gases LC_{50} ≤ 100 ppm, 500 ppm, 2,500 ppm, and 20,000 ppm by volume = categories 1–4, respectively. Vapors are done by mg/L with LC_{50} ≤ 0.5 mg/L, 2.0 mg/L, 10 mg/L, and 20 mg/L = categories 1–4, respectively. Dust and fumes are also determined by mg/L with LC_{50} ≤ 0.05 mg/L, 0.5 mg/L, 1.0 mg/L, and 5 mg/L as categories 1–4, respectively.

The National Fire Protection Association (NFPA) 704 (most current edition; NFPA, 2012): Standard System for Identification of the Hazards of Materials for Emergency Response of 1960 recognizes categories within a color as blue (health hazard), yellow (instability/reactivity), red (flammability), and white (special). Under blue, category 0 chemicals pose no health hazard (e.g., water), category 1 agents yield irritation with minor residual injury (e.g., acetone), category 2 chemicals cause either temporary incapacitation or possible residual injury (e.g., diethyl ether), category 3 chemicals such as chlorine may cause serious temporary or moderate residual injury, and category 4 chemicals are usually neurotoxic compounds (e.g., HCN, phosphine, CO, and sarin) to which very limited exposure may cause mortalities or major residual injury. Under yellow, category 0 gases' stability is good (e.g., He), category 1 includes gases that may become unstable at elevated temperatures and pressures such as propene, category 2 involves violent chemical changes at elevated temperatures and pressures or violent or explosive reactions with water (e.g., white phosphorus, K metal, Na metal), category 3 encompasses those chemicals that detonate or undergo explosive decomposition with a strong initiating source or initiate with heating under confinement or reacts explosively with water or detonate if severely shocked (e.g., ammonium nitrate, chlorine trifluoride), and category 4 compounds readily detonate or undergo explosive decomposition at normal temperatures and pressures (e.g., nitroglycerin, chlorine azide, and chlorine dioxide). Under red, category 0 gases will not burn under typical fire conditions (such as CO_2) or are solids such as concrete, stone, or sand; category 1 compounds require considerable preheating to combust such as mineral oil (flash point ≥ 93.4°C); category 2 chemicals only require moderate heating or high ambient temperature (flash point 38–93°C) to ignite (diesel fuel); category 3 includes liquids and solids that can be ignited at almost all ambient temperatures (flash point 23–38°C) such as gasoline; and category 4 will rapidly or completely vaporize at normal temperatures and pressures (flash point < 23°C) and will burn readily such as acetylene and diethylzinc (pyrophoric substances). White includes OX (oxidizers such as potassium perchlorate, ammonium nitrate, hydrogen peroxide), W (reacts with water in an unusual or dangerous manner such as cesium, sodium, sulfuric acid), and SA (simple asphyxiant gases limited to nitrogen, helium, neon, argon, krypton, and xenon). Methane, hydrogen, ethylene, and ethane may also cause dilution asphyxiation, but are not officially in the SA category. Chemical asphyxiants such as

CO, HCN, and H_2S disrupt mitochondrial oxidative phosphorylation/cellular respiration. Now, clearly the NFPA standards involve more than just gases, but the toxicity and chemical reactivity for those that are gases fall under these categories.

It is important to keep in mind the NFPA categories, because irritant gases may damage all areas of the respiratory tract from nasopharyngeal to tracheobronchial to pulmonary (respiratory bronchioles and alveoli) regions. Structure-activity of irritant compounds may be related to sensory irritants (RD_{50}) that for nonreactive volatile organics are simply related to vapor pressure and gas–liquid partition coefficients, while chemically reactive $-CH_2$-halogen compounds K_{OW} and a chemical reactivity factor describe their action (Greenwood, 2006). The nasal passages themselves have transitional epithelium damage from O_3, while formaldehyde targets the respiratory mucosal tissue. However, at low concentrations over short time periods, gases such as HCHO and isopropyl alcohol (too efficient scrubbing by the nose yielding nasal cancer), NH_3, HF, and SO_2 may be "scrubbed" by the upper airway leading to the types of irritation that make an animal move from the area. Phosgene, NO_2, and O_3 are not very water soluble and produce their toxic actions in conducting airways such as the bronchioles and alveoli (Hayes and Bakand, 2010). Longer exposure or higher concentrations may affect the entire airway and lead to more severe consequences. For short durations of exposure, physiological reflexes limit exposure via stimulation of the trigeminal nerve/burning sensations of the nasopharynx, oropharynx, and eyes. Rhinorrhea, profuse tearing (lacrimation), coughing, and sneezing occur. With respiratory distress comes inflammation of the glottis, excessive secretions, and laryngospasm. Small rodents used as inhalation models also have a reduction in respiratory rate from sensory irritation as a consequence of a distinctive delay in the exhalation phase (one reason the beagle dog is a better human model of respired toxicants). In humans bronchoconstriction can also occur due to parasympathetic nerve innervations or localized inflammatory chemical mediator release (histamine and similar agents).

High concentrations of irritants can lead to reactive airways dysfunction syndrome (RADS), which causes asthma with a 24-hour latency period. However, gases, vapors, particulates, and allergens can lead to hyper-responsiveness of the airway known as asthma. Workers exposed to agents such as benzene-1,2,4-tricarboxylicacid-1,2-anhydride, chlorine, platinum salt, isocyanates, cement dust, grain dust, animal farming, environmental tobacco smoke, welding fumes, or construction work were most likely to experience asthma due to chronic inflammation of the airway (along with coughing, wheezing, chest tightness, dyspnea, shortness of breath at rest, and reversible airway flow limitations) or chronic obstructive pulmonary disease (COPD; associated with chronic productive cough, not fully reversible airflow limitation, and a progressive, abnormal inflammatory response of lungs with increased neutrophils and alveolar macrophages due to chronic smoking or exposure to noxious gases or particles). There was a moderate association between work with phthalic anhydride, glutaraldehyde, sulfur dioxide, cotton dust, cleaning agents, potrooms, farming (various), and foundries and these two pulmonary disorders.

Asthma has a clear mechanism from exposure to occupational allergens, as the IgE-mediated release of histamine leads to bronchoconstriction and inflammatory responses. Respiratory irritants that cause asthma are usually low-molecular-weight chemicals ($< 5,000$ Daltons) such as Cl_2, acids, welding fumes, and isocyanates that also yield COPD. COPD is related to chronic bronchitis, bronchiolitis, and asthma and may have sites of emphysema, which indicate that lymphocyte accumulation is starting to reduce the forced expiratory volume at 1.0 second (FEV1). A third ground of agents induce asthma via unknown toxic/pathophysiologic mechanisms. Irritants that cause asthma have permissible exposure limits (PELs) such as pig confinement facilities (possibly high in NH_3, H_2S), cleaning agents (again NH_3, acids, chlorine compounds, solvents), ozone, endotoxin, HCHO, quaternary ammonium compounds, Cl_2, bisulfate or SO_2, acid mist, diesel exhaust, fumigant residues, dusts in textile paper, mineral fiber or construction industries or mines, potrooms, and meatwrappers or even cold weather athletes (Baur et al., 2012). Gases toxic to other organs would only concern the concentration of the gas as it enters the blood stream via the respiratory bronchioles and alveoli and attains a specified concentration at target organs. Water-soluble toxins may enter via all cells along the tract. However, toxicants that affect respiratory cells are more likely to damage type I pneumocytes, as they cover ~90% of the alveolar wall surface. If the pulmonary surfactant layer is damaged, then inflammation of the pulmonary parenchyma can result in atelectasis. If the inflammatory substances are substantial, pulmonary capillaries will leak protein-rich exudates that will result in dangerous or fatal pulmonary edema. The activation of neutrophils appears to be responsible for acute lung injury as elimination of neutrophils reduces lung injury and capillary permeability from hemorrhagic or endotoxin exposure.

Acute injury appears with characteristic shortness of breath, cough, and hypoxemia. As indicated in NFPA category blue, irritants of the respiratory tract such as phosgene gas may lead to pneumonitis progressing to pulmonary edema and respiratory distress syndrome over time. However, a high concentration of chlorine is worse as it immediately damages alveolar epithelial cells, capillary endothelial cells, and results in death as a consequence of acute respiratory failure (Greenwood, 2006). Other irritants such as ammonia, NO_x, SO, F_2, PH_3 (phosphine), and acrolein irritate in the area of the lung based on their water solubility and reactivity and can lead to bronchitis. Sensitization, allergy, and asthma usually come from isocyanates and amines. CO and H_2S are very insoluble gases and exert their mitochondrial/neurotoxicity (and toxicity to other organs) via the pulmonary veins and then systemically (first heart then brain; Hayes and Bakand, 2010). A list of toxic gases would involve fuming acids (e.g., HCl, HBr, HF) leading to corrosion of the respiratory tract. The mode of action of Cl_2 may be comparable in some respects to F_2, another reactive halogen gas that has toxic properties. Air pollutants, such as CO, NO_x, SO_x, and O_3, damage directly individually in high concentrations or indirectly via photochemical formation of peroxyacyl nitrates (smog). VOCs form from combustion of fuels or from evaporation from solvents (such as occurs during painting in confined spaces).

Aerosols — Direct Effects

Aerosols (100 nm to over 100 μm) are small particles composed of solids or liquids such as fumes (solid particles condensed from a gaseous state), dusts (solid particles temporarily suspended in air—usually largest), smoke (dry and liquid particles suspended in the gases resulting from combustion of organic material from 0.01–1.0 μm but can aggregate into soot), fogs (liquid water droplets or ice crystals suspended in air), and mists (liquid finely divided from few to over 100 μm) that are suspended in air sufficiently long to remain dispersed. Clearly, concentration is as important for aerosols and vapors as it is for gases. In the case of aerosols, it is first important to note the size of the particle. For example, if people use a vaporizer to help with sinus drainage, they generally don't have to worry much about the quality of the tap water as the droplet size is large. Ultrasonic humidifiers may have to have cleaner water as metals in that water may now be available due to the aerosols created.

Particles deposited depend on particle size and particle size distribution in the aerosol. Inertia, sedimentation velocity, and diffusion rate determine this deposition. Mass and aerodynamic drag affect the particle's inertia and sedimentation rate (gravitational sedimentation velocity). The aerodynamic diameter helps determine these functions with the diameter of a spherical particle D, density Q, and the aerodynamic diameter $D_{AE} = D(QC)^{1/2}/(Q_0 C_{AE})^{1/2}$, where Q_0 represents the unit density and C and C_{AE} are slip correction factors that must be applied when the diameter of the particle is close to the mean free path of gas molecules. Small changes (~4%) occur with temperature changes in the lung air as the mean free path varies with pressure and sedimentation rate. If the aerosol is dense (> 1) and small, then deposition would exceed that calculated by aerodynamic diameter. However, this aerodynamic diameter function does not determine diffusional deposition, because particle density does not impact diffusion (diffusional collection calculated by total deposition – extrapolated inertial deposition curve). In 0.1 μm $< D_{AE} <$ 3 μm, tracheobronchial deposition is nearly constant. With variable-sized particles of interval $x \pm (dx/2)$, the distribution of the relative frequency of particle is represented by:

$$f(x) \, dx = 1/\sigma(2\pi)^{\frac{1}{2}} \exp\{-(x - \mu)^2/2 \, \sigma^2\} \, dx$$

where $x = \ln D$ (still represents particle diameter) and $\sigma = \ln \sigma_g$ where σ_g is the geometric standard deviation, CMD is count median diameter, and $\mu = -\ln$ CMD. The values m and s give estimates of μ and σ_g as determined by sampling the aerosol. For N particles, m is equal to the summation from $i = 1$ to N of $\ln D_i/N$ and s is the square root of the summation from $i = 1$ to N of $(\ln D_i - \ln \text{CMD})^2/(N - 1)$. Aerosols with small σ_g values (< 1.22) are classed as monodisperse. At this point, the tidal volume and breathing rate become important. Particle size also matters for clearance, because large particles (high aerodynamic diameter) deposited in the upper respiratory tract are rapidly cleared by ciliary movement of the mucus layer (unless it contains nicotine or similar toxicants that paralyze the cilia; Tillery et al., 1976). The dose is described as:

$$\text{Retained dose} = \alpha \cdot (\text{VT} \cdot f) \, C \cdot t$$

where α is the deposition fraction, VT is the tidal volume, f is the respiratory frequency, C is the concentration of the toxicant in the atmosphere, and t is the exposure time. In the determination of gases such as inhalation anesthetics and CO, α is not determined as retention is not an issue as long as the subject remains in the gas concentration (will equilibrate or die at some point during exposure depending on the depth of the initial breaths and tidal volume and rate of biotransformation).

As indicated earlier, particle retention depends on size, shape, density, electrostatic charge, and hygroscopicity (Greenwood, 2006). In this arena, lung cancer (> 10 μm fibers), mesothelioma (~5 μm fibers) and fibrotic (~2 μm fibers) agent asbestos (and macrophage recruitment and activation; Choe et al., 1997), cigarette smoke, and various other agents can be considered. Particles

will affect the area where they are impacting (inertial), intercepted, sediment (settling), electrostatically precipitated, or diffuse (move by Brownian motion; Greenwood, 2006). Larger particles or fibers (5–30 μm) sill lodge in the nasopharyngeal region, while aerosols of 1–5 μm will find their way to be deposited in the tracheobronchial region, but may still be cleared by cilia. The smallest (< 1 μm) will access the alveolar region and sediment and/or diffuse (for particle < 0.5 μm) into the circulation. Diffusion is especially important for determining the toxicity of new nanosized particles, which penetrate easily into the circulation and target organs. Insoluble particles at this level that do not diffuse may remain in the lung essentially for the lifetime of the exposed individual.

Chronic exposure to mineral dusts and associated tissue reactions characterize pneumoconiosis. In the benign form, pneumoconiosis from iron (siderosis), tin (stannosis), and baritosis (barium) does not involve alveolar changes or increased collagenous fibrosis. Collagenous pneumoconiosis in comparison is characterized by structural alterations in lung tissue and irreversible fibrosis from exposure to asbestos fibers (asbestosis), silica not in fiber form (silicosis), and coal miner's pneumoconiosis. Particles containing metals such as As, Be, Cd, Ni, or silica fibers (asbestos and macrophage activation to form damaging ROS) are associated with the development of lung cancer (as is the radioactive gas Rn to be discussed later under radiation). Silica (not fibers), other synthetic fibers, and welding fumes are suspected carcinogens. Cigarette smoke clearly leads to lung cancer based on the particles and the content of polycyclic aromatic hydrocarbons that are biotransformed/activated into genotoxic compounds. Larger particles appear to cause nasal cancer (wood dusts or leather workers) or upper respiratory irritation (Hayes and Bakand, 2010).

Gases and Vapors — Indirect Effects

Gases also affect the composition of the atmosphere, generate other chemicals via photochemical reactions, change the climate, and change the protection of the atmosphere to certain types of radiation. All these factors must be taken into account. Chlorofluorocarbons (CFCs) were banned in the United States because they were found to decrease stratospheric ozone and increase UV irradiation. CFC-11, CFC-12, and CFC-13 last 74, 111, and 90 years, respectively, in the atmosphere. Every CFC molecule leads to thousands of stratospheric O_3 molecules' destruction, as do CCl_4, halons, and trichloroethane. They do so by electromagnetic radiation exciting those compounds, releasing Cl or Br atoms. For example, $Cl + O_3 \rightarrow ClO + O_2$ and $ClO + O_3 \rightarrow Cl + 2 O_2$, which destroys two ozone molecules and regenerates the original Cl atom. The Montreal Protocol sought the ban of these ozone-depleting chemicals after observing increases in UVB radiation (280–315 nm UV light increased impacts on or reduced plankton populations in ocean's photic zone, damaged other plant life, and increased malignant melanomas and other skin cancers), snow blindness, cataracts, and immune suppression in human. Based on epidemiological information, a 1% decrease in stratospheric ozone produces a 0.3–0.6% increase in cataracts, 0.6% increase in malignant melanoma, 2.7% increase in basal cell carcinoma, and 4.6 % increase in squamous cell carcinoma. There may also be elevated cases and severity of infection due to immune system suppression. This sets the stage for radiation toxicity, as UVB is in the upper wavelengths, which define ionizing radiation (exciting water to ultimately becoming hydroxyl radical; Ando, 1990). Note that emitted gases may react together to form peroxyacyl nitrate (PAN) via NO + hydrocarbons + O_2 + $O_3 \rightarrow$ peroxyacyl nitrates + oxygen products. This not only damages/irritates the lung but also damages plants along with ozone found in the lower troposphere. When smog-sensitive tobacco variety cell suspensions (ironic—because tobacco yields a toxic smoke) were exposed to PAN, ROS were generated (indicated by increased intracellular H_2O_2 and protection by ROS scavengers and related inhibitors) and Ca^{2+}-mediated cell death occurred (decreased by Ca^{2+} chelator; Yukihiro et al., 2012).

Another effect of gases is well modeled by the one with the most diverse impact—CO_2. Carbon dioxide at high levels can cause narcotizing effects on flies or asphyxiation in mammals. At lower concentrations, it stimulates respiration in mammals resulting in the feeling of being hot, and it causes vasodilation in the skin and vasoconstriction internally yielding hypertensive activity. At the levels it is being emitted now and over the industrial period, it has dramatically affected the global climate and the pH of aquatic bodies including the ocean. The combination is toxic to aquatic species (Pandolfi et al., 2011). Consequences include coral bleaching as sea surface temperatures rise, CO_2 increases in seawater, rising sea levels, potentially shifting ocean currents, increasing UV concentrations, and intensifying storms over the ocean (hurricanes and cyclones). Other gases such as methane (which is explosive at high concentrations and can lead to asphyxiation) may be more influential in the future leading to climate change.

Particles — Indirect Effects

Particles that have seen massive increases in the past (such as the Dust Bowl era of the 1930s) have yielded respiratory toxicity, as has volcanic activity. High atmospheric emissions of particles such as occurs through volcanic activity, nuclear explosions, and similar explosive activity have actually changed the climate for as much as a year due to less sunlight and radiation making it to the Earth's surface. Atmospheric aerosol formation (molecular clusters growing to larger sizes) via nucleation starting at the < 2 nanometer size range have physical, chemical, and dynamic parameters that guide their formation via neural pathways. Especially important are organic compounds in aerosol formation, growth, radiative forcing and associated feedbacks between biogenic emissions, clouds, and climate. Sulfuric acid is a main gaseous driver of daytime aerosol formation and the smallest clusters (very slowly growing clusters derived from gas-phase reactions, cluster formation/ evaporation). Amines also appear to be part of the second size regime of clusters (slowly growing clusters involving sulfuric acid–amine clusters, stabilizing organic compounds; determines the formation rate at 1.5 nm range or $J_{1.5}$).

Organic vapors are the candidates for the third size clusters (rapidly growing sub-3 nm following Nano-Köhler theory of neural clusters forming by condensable vapors similar to a cloud and determining formation rate at 3.0-nm range or J_3), especially highly oxidized organic molecules. These clusters can also involve nitrate or nitric acid as well in compounds such as $C_{10}H_{15}N_2O_{11}$. These clusters are influenced by and affect the biosphere, clouds, and climate (Kulmala et al., 2013).

Radiation

Radiation involves the formation of particles from an unstable nucleus at a certain rate of decay. Unstable isotopes are indicated as follows:

$$_{\text{atomic number}}^{\text{mass number}}X$$

(X is the symbol for the element.) Radioactive decay is given as NRC (2012): Human Resources Training and Development. [H-201 – Health Physics Technology] Health Physics Fundamentals http://pbadupws.nrc.gov/docs/ML1126/ML11262A154.pdf.

$$_{95}^{241}Am \rightarrow \,_{93}^{237}Am \,+\, _{2}^{4}He^{++}$$

[241]Americium (atomic number 95) decays to [237]Neptunium and an α particle. Carbon-14 (atomic number 6) is a β emitter as it has more neutrons than protons. The neutrons divide into a proton and an electron. The electrons are represented by the negatively charged e that is emitted:

$$_{6}^{14}C \rightarrow \,_{7}^{14}N \,+\, _{-1}^{0}e$$

When an excited nucleus gives off a photon (no mass and no charge) in the gamma range of the electromagnetic spectrum (close in wavelength to X-rays), it is represented as the penetrating and ionizing γ irradiation and usually follows the β particle emission of that unstable nucleus. An X-ray comes from a machine-produced electron field (not from the nucleus). [137]Cs (atomic number 55) decays by one of its neutrons becoming a proton and a beta particle; however, the additional proton changes the atom to [137]Ba. The nucleus ejects the beta particle, but is still

too unstable. That is when it ejects a gamma photon to become more stable. A positron has the same mass as an electron but has a positive charge and is released from an artificially created unstable nucleus as represented by:

$$_{1}^{0}e$$

Similarly, an unstable nucleus may be created that takes an electron from its inner shell to help stabilize the nucleus. This is called electron capture and is represented by:

$$_{19}^{40}K + \,_{-1}^{0}e \rightarrow \,_{18}^{40}Ar$$

Sometimes in physics experiments, large accelerators are used to bombard a nucleus yielding particles such as alpha particles and neutrons or an entire nucleus to create other particles such as looking for the Higgs boson. Not only do scientists need to know which particles are given off, but the half-life determines how fast a nucleus may decay. Fast-decaying nuclei may be dangerous because they give off their radiation in a relatively short half-life (when half the source or isotope is decayed giving off half the radiation). However, for highly radioactive materials, fast decay is easier to store such as radioactive iodine and then safely dispose of, while plutonium lasts many generations. The half-life is given by the equation:

$$A_E = A_0 \times 0.5^{t/t_{1/2}}$$

where A_E is the amount of radioactive material left, A_0 is the initial amount of the radioactive material, t is the time since the material had its initial radioactivity, and $t_{1/2}$ is the half-life. Other equations using log functions are also used to determine half-life such as $t = \log[(A_E/A_0)/\log 0.5] \times t_{1/2}$ or this same equation solved for $t_{1/2}$ instead.

The units used to describe decay are disintegrations per second (dps), or formerly disintegrations per minute (dpms—used more in radiation counting as in a gamma counter or scintillation counter for beta emitters). William Conrad Röntgen's discovery of X-rays in 1895 started the unit named after him for radiation, which persisted beyond WWII and the development of the atomic bomb in the Manhattan Project. Henri Becquerel was a French physicist and Nobel laureate who in 1896 described rays from radioactive uranium salts that appeared to act similarly to X-rays. Radioactive thorium was discovered and Becquerel's doctoral student Marie Skłodowska-Curie and her husband Pierre Curie discovered radioactive polonium and radium and shared the Nobel Prize with Becquerel. The Curie couple also performed biological experiments with rodents indicating the toxic nature of this radiation. From this history, 1 disintegration per second was relatively recently taken as the unit of radioactivity as the Becquerel or Bq. This is a useful number in physics, but has no biological meaning—similar to a molecule having little toxicity to a cell. A mole of an ion such as Na or compound is certainly toxic to a single cell. Similarly, the former designation of a gram of Ra as the unit of radioactivity known as the Curie or Ci has a unit of 3.7×10^{10} disintegrations per second or Bqs. As strange as this unit may appear, it has definite biological meaning/toxicity as opposed to the Bq. As confirmed in **Table 28-2**, humans have 65 Bq/kg or for an average weight human 4,500 Bq of natural radiation. Some have jokingly suggested the banana as a standard as it has 15 Bq of radioactivity. It stops being a joking matter when radon in homes is considered. This is due to radon's emission of very toxic alpha particles that damage nearby tissue by delivering all their energy due to their high mass for a particle and velocity, which can occur at

TABLE 28-2 Radioactivity of Common Materials	
1 Adult Human (65 Bq/kg)	**4,500 Bq**
1 kg of coffee	1,000 Bq
1 kg of brazil nuts	400 Bq
1 banana	15 Bq
The air in a 100-m² Australian home (radon)	3,000 Bq
The air in many 100-m² European homes (radon)	up to 30,000 Bq
1 household smoke detector (with americium)	30,000 Bq
Radioisotope for medical diagnosis	70 million Bq
Radioisotope source for medical therapy	100,000,000 million Bq (100 TBq)
1 kg 50-year-old vitrified high-level nuclear waste	10,000,000 million Bq (10 TBq)
1 luminous exit sign (1970s)	1,000,000 million Bq (1 TBq)
1 kg uranium	25 million Bq
1 kg uranium ore (Canadian, 15%)	25 million Bq
1 kg uranium ore (Australian, 0.3%)	500,000 Bq
1 kg low-level radioactive waste	1 million Bq
1 kg of coal ash	2,000 Bq
1 kg of granite	1,000 Bq
1 kg of superphosphate fertilizer	5,000 Bq

Though the intrinsic radioactivity is the same, the radiation dose received by someone handling a kilogram of high-grade uranium ore will be much greater than for the same exposure to a kilogram of separated uranium, because the ore contains a number of short-lived decay products (indicating decay rate as important) while the uranium has a very long half-life (which makes it more dangerous for chronic or multigeneration exposure).

Reproduced from http://www.world-nuclear.org/info/inf05.html.

low-level concentrations in a one-story house, for example. Thus, radiation toxicologists/ health physicists must consider the half-life and the equivalent doses between particles just to determine dose.

Because radioisotopes may also distribute into and concentrate in various parts of the body, the distribution of isotopes must be considered as well. Sources of radiation are noted in **Figure 28-3**. This account indicates that the "average" person is not an appropriate measure, because exposure may depend on global location, medical procedures, profession (uranium miner), and other factors. The average dose from background radiation is determined by absorbed radiation dose. Back in the 1940s, the roentgen (r) had the physical meaning based on the measurement of ion concentration in the air and was the basis of Geiger counters. Roentgen had the dimensions of energy per unit of mass and was considered to be ~83 erg/g air. Correction for alpha or beta radiation gave the equivalent roentgen, and the energy release in tissue was considered similar to air (but not exactly the same) on a mass basis.

H.M. Parker came up with the rem to indicate the equivalence of the roentgen unit in terms of mammalian toxicity. In those days, the alpha particle was considered 5–10 times as effective as beta rays yielding equivalent energy. This has been altered since, as experimental results even in the 1940s indicated that ^{239}Pu was 50 times more effective than radium in producing acute radiation disease, presumed at that time to be due to its heterogeneous tissue distribution.

The tissue dosage was given by rep/day = 60 × E_m × C, where C = concentration of the isotope in μc/g or mc/kg, and E_m = mean energy of the radiation in million electron volts. The surface of a mass of tissue was assumed to be a plane with the dosage at the surface equal to one half of the calculation by the rep/day equation. This situation was meant to apply to beta radiation from radioactive iodine. Other beta dosage sources would be defined by simple geometry as long as the beta ray spectrum was defined for that source. The impact on mitotic changes around a point source in tissue was the model used. 500 r or 500 rad was considered the absorbed dose that is lethal for a human exposed once to X-rays or gamma radiation. This supposition becomes more complicated as one notes the presence of radio-sensitive cells such as the hematopoietic tissue of the bone marrow.

Ionic isotopes such as ^{24}Na (^{24} is the isotope) would be assumed to give whole body irradiation, while ^{89}Sr would involve bone and bone marrow as it distributes to bone. Similarly, intermittent or continuous X- or γ-irradiation would damage the bone marrow as the particle penetrates soft tissue to the dense bone and is absorbed there. This is where the reactions occur that lead to aplastic anemia. Elements such as radiocesium lead to hypertrophy at the edges of the liver, where cesium levels are relatively low and radiation dosage is small, and necrosis in the bulk of the liver, where the damage is extensive. Radium used to be painted by hand (dipping the brush on the tongue to moisten the brush between applications)

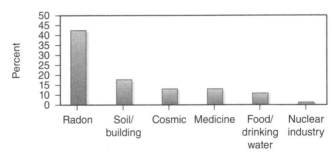

FIGURE 28-3 Sources of Radiation

onto watches before electric watch dials. This element went to the bone and caused bone sarcoma (1 μg of retained dose). Colloidal thorium dioxide resulted in liver sarcoma. Skin and subcutaneous malignant tumors can be achieved by high-dose external beta radiation. Feeding radioyttrium to rats instead caused colon carcinomas. The distribution of ^{32}P would resemble the pattern expected of acute radiation syndrome. There was reasoning back in the 1940s that ^{24}Na, ^{42}K, ^{131}I, and possibly ^{32}P were beta and gamma emitters and could be tolerated between 1 and 10 rep to the critical tissue, since they had a short half-life (such as the thyroid for radioiodine). Bone-seeking isotopes were excluded from this category, especially ^{14}C. ^{55}Fe, ^{59}Fe, ^{45}Ca, and long-lived isotopes ^{22}Na and ^{36}Cl were viewed as borderline or used with more caution (Brues, 1949).

The understanding of radiation has changed since the late 1940s and more is known of the mechanisms involved in radiation damage and carcinogenesis. The units have changed as scientists have come to understand that rads (1 rad = 100 erg/gram), which correspond to the roentgens for X-rays or gamma irradiation, do not contain the full linear energy impact of larger particles. Therefore, 100 rad now equals 1 Gy (Gray) or the absorbed dose of 1 joule/kg; this unit is toxic, but not necessarily lethal except for neutrons and alpha particles. The rem takes into account the weighting factor by using an equation generated by the International Commission on Radiological Protection Publication 26 (ICRP, 1977). The IRCP started to relate release to human doses (ICRP, 1979). IRCP published material is used by the U.S. Environmental Protection Agency (EPA, 2012).

The rem = the rad for beta and gamma radiation, but not for alpha particles and neutrons. The rem has been replaced by the Sievert (Sv), which is 100 rems and is likely toxic, but now equivalent for all radiation energy. As the Sv takes into account various types of radiation, it is important to standardize the equivalence of those radiation particle energies absorbed for radiation protection regulations. The absorbed dose of the radiation that the subject is exposed to is divided by the absorbed dose of traditionally 250 kVp X-rays as the reference

that produces the *same biological endpoint* (the biological effects not the radiation itself are the basis of this comparison) and is referred to as the relative biological effectiveness or RBE. An arbitrary consensus RBE estimate known as the quality factor (Q) is usually employed. This is similar to the effective dose equivalent, H, which has been used to normalize the tissue absorption/impact of different particles' energies. The equation for H is:

$$H = DQN$$

where D = absorbed dose, Q = quality factor (RBE), and N is the product of additional modifying factors. Note that alpha particles are the most dangerous (Q = 20), but only over a short distance as they have a helium nucleus composition (large mass compared to beta or gamma radiation) and a double charge (EPA, 2012). Neutrons (half the mass of alpha but more penetrating as they are uncharged) and protons (same mass as neutrons but have a single charge that limits their penetrating capacity) are half the Q value (10). The speed and penetration ability of other particles vary for beta radiation (particles are quenched or absorbed by water molecules over relatively short distances), positrons, X-rays (absorbed by bone surface and soft tissue inside and outside of bone,) and gamma rays (similar to X-rays), but all have the same Q (an order of magnitude down from the alpha, neutrons, and positrons with a Q = 1). H_E, which is a weighted sum of dose equivalents to all organs and tissues, is defined as:

$$H_E = \sum_T w_T H_T$$

where w is the weighting factor for organ or tissue T and H_T is the mean dose equivalent to organ or tissue T (EPA, 2012). The factor w_T is normalized so that the summation of all organ weighting factors is equal to 1. This w_T factor also takes into account the fractional contribution of organ or tissue T to the total risk of stochastic health effects when the body is uniformly irradiated. Additionally, the committed effective dose equivalent, $H_{E,50}$, incorporates into its calculation of absorbed dose the weighted sum of committed dose equivalents to all irradiated organs and tissues and is expressed as:

$$H_{E,50} = \Sigma\, w_T\, H_{T,50}$$
$$T$$

H_E and $H_{E,50}$ (the $_{50}$ reflects the tissue for 50 years following intake as cancer may be a slow process at lower doses for long half-life isotopes) thus reflect both the distribution of isotopes to tissues and the absorbed nature of the particles they emit (EPA, 2012). The organ and tissue weighting factors for $w_T = 0.25$ (gonads), 0.15 (breast), 0.12 (red marrow, lungs), 0.06 (five remaining organs or tissues receiving the highest dose of radiation), and 0.03 (thyroid, bone surface, remainder of organs).

Working level (WL) is used to characterize the short-lived radioactive decay products of radon (^{222}Rn). The WL is any mixture of short-lived radon decay products per liter of air that emit 1.3×10^5 MeV of alpha particle energy (EPA, 2012). That is why plastic is used in homes to detect Rn as alpha delivers enough energy to streak that material. The working level month (WLM) is defined as exposure to 1 WL over 170 hours (1 working month). Gamma rays and X-rays involve photoelectric effects, Compton scattering, and pair production on entering matter. It is important to note here that particles can damage not only by direct damage by absorbed radiation, but more importantly ionize water (water constitutes much of the composition of tissues) to radicals that mediate their damage as indicated by the following equations:

Ionizing radiation + $H_2O \rightarrow HOH^+$ + e^- (tissue gains 34 ev); $e^- + H_2O \rightarrow HOH^-$; $HOH^+ \rightarrow H^+ + OH^{\cdot}$(hydroxyl radical); $HOH^- \rightarrow HO^- + H^{\cdot}$ (hydrogen radical)

Alpha particles have two neutrons and two protons, so their large size prevents their penetration, but their double-positive charge has high ionizing potential. Beta particles have lower ionizing potential, but higher penetrating capability. Neutrons produce ionizations directly and have no charge so penetrate well. They also have high kinetic energy and are quite toxic.

With this information in place, how does radiation protection fit into the calculation of

radiation dose over a lifetime? The answer is given simplistically in **Figure 28-4**. The assumption is that increased exposure increases the risk of genetic and other cellular damage. There is a belief in hormesis that small amounts of toxicants including radiation may be beneficial as they stimulate repair mechanisms. This assumption does not take into account that the biphasic approach is the basis of radiation protection regulations. However, it is naïve to assume that humans are not subject to background radiation all the time. Cosmic radiation comes from directly ionizing to photon component (E = $h\upsilon$, where $h = 6.26 \times 10^{-34}$ J s, or Planck's constant, and υ = the frequency of the photon or gamma or X-rays) at 0.28 mSv, neutron component (particulate or corpuscular energy comes from alpha, beta, positrons, electrons, protons, and neutrons with E = ½mV^2) at 0.10 mSv, and cosmogenic radionuclides at 0.01 mSv for a total of 0.39 (0.3–1.0 mSv range) depending mainly on altitude and protection of atmosphere (more at the poles due to the magnetic forces of the Earth causing the aurorae). External terrestrial radiation outdoors is 0.07 mSv to 0.41 mSv indoors for a total of 0.48 mSv (0.3–1.0 mSv range). Inhalation of U and Th leads to 0.006 mSv of absorbed radiation dose (excepting miners or

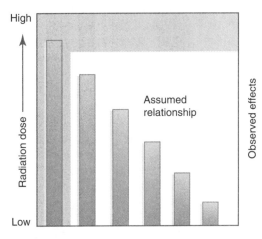

The linear hypothesis (inverted)

FIGURE 28-4 The Assumption of Radiation's Effects That Indicate That No Radiation Exposure Is Safe

those who live close to a U mine—those living close should be limited to 1 mSv/yr above background), ^{222}Rn gives 1.15 mSv, and thoron (^{220}Rn) gives 0.1 mSv for a total of 1.26 mSv (0.2–10 mSv range). Clearly, Rn exposure is of greatest concern and variability (alpha particles and E = 0.511 + [5.11/(1 − u^2/c^2)$^{1/2}$], where 1 eV = 1.6 × 10^{-19} J and energy absorption is fast in tissue with a falloff of dE/dx = 3.8 × 10^{-25} C NZ/E ln{549E/I} MeV μm^{-1}, where N = number of atoms/cm^3 in medium; Z = atomic number of medium; I = ionization of medium; E = energy of α particle; C = charge correction for α particles with energy < 1.6 MeV with a simple estimation of I = 10(Z); for an α particle of 5 MeV such as Ra → Rn, the equation becomes dE/dx = [0.126C/E] ln{7.99 E} MeV μm^{-1} or with proper values becomes dE/dx = 0.126(1.0)/5.0 ln{7.99 × 5} = 0.093 μm^{-1} tissue) worldwide, and indoor exposure can be similar to smoking cigarettes even in the United States. The importance of this rapid energy absorption indicates that α emitters such as Rn may impart their radiation to a single cell, which may lead to cell death, significant irreparable damage, and the development of cancer at low doses and higher doses to radiation poisoning. Ingestion of ^{40}K leads to 0.17 mSv, while U and Th lead to 0.12 mSv (0.2 − 1.0 mSv range). Total background radiation amounts to 2.4 mSv/yr (1.0–13 mSv range) for the average person, while nuclear submarines have the least exposure at 0.3 mSv/yr in a well shielded environment. Radiation assumes the linear no-threshold model of Figure 28-4 despite lack of evidence for toxicity at < 1 Sv/yr, but radiation effects are based mostly on atomic bomb survivors in Hiroshima and Nagasaki, Japan.

For more ordinary conditions, exposure must be justified (net benefit), optimized (as low as reasonably achievable, or ALARA), and limited for individuals. Most countries set a limit of 20 mSv/year over 5 years for radiation workers with a maximum of 50 mSv in any 1 year above background radiation and excludes medical exposure (ICRP, 1977) with a proviso that attempts to keep exposure ALARA based on social and economic factors. Medical procedures now involve dosimetry, benefit–risk assessment, and total lifetime dose calculations. However, in the past X-ray machines were available to people to

see how a foot fit into a shoe or used to treat diseases such as ankylosing spondylitis (along with a possible second treatment with X-rays or thorium) with excess cancers noted in the population (leukemia, lung, and esophageal, although the spine received the highest radiation dose; UNSCEAR, 2000).

How much radiation is toxic? Average background radiation is 2.4 mSv/yr, with 1.5 mSv/yr in Australia and 3 mSv/yr in North America. An additional 1.5–2.5 mSv/year can be experienced on average as an Australian or U.S. uranium miner or nuclear industry worker above background and medical procedures (including diagnostic X-rays). Aircrews due to flying at middle latitudes and radiation scanning devices may have up to 5 mSv/yr. Polar route aircrews (New York to Tokyo) experience 9 mSv/yr. Australian miners' maximum radiation dose is 10 mSv/yr. An abdominal and pelvis CT scan will rate an additional 10 mSv/scan. The current average limit for U miners and nuclear industry employees is 20 mSv/yr but was 50 mSv/yr as a former (longer-term older employees might have experienced this in the past) standard and for nations with high background radiation levels (parts of Iran, India, and Europe). Emergency workers can experience 50 mSv for one occurrence (International Atomic Energy Agency [IAEA, 2014] regulations). 100 mSv is the lowest radiation level that accompanies a higher cancer risk (UNSCEAR, 2000) and is allowed for vital remediation work by emergency personnel (IAEA, 2014). Higher than this absorption dose is expected to increase the risk but not necessarily the severity of neoplastic diseases.

Other than nuclear bomb victims in Japan in 1945, nuclear reactor accidents have added more recent human risk data of exposure to radiation. After the Fukushima Daiichi nuclear disaster in 2011, workers were allowed a short-term dose of 250 mSv despite the increased possible risk of future cancers. Of special concern at Fukushima was the inhalation of the 570 PBq (petabecquerels) of ^{131}I released (more than the nuclear accident at Three Mile Island near Harrisburg, Pennsylvania in 1979, but much less than Chernobyl). The 167 workers exposed to possible thyroid damage from radioactive iodine inhalation had doses of 100–150 mSv

(135 workers), 150–200 mSv (23 workers), 200–250 mSv (3 workers), and > 250 mSv (6 workers; UNSCEAR, 2013). Ramsar, Iran has a background level of 250 mSv/yr with no reported increase in health problems over the general population. However, the 1986 Chernobyl accident exposed 24,000 people within 15 km of the nuclear plant explosion to 0.45 Sv before evacuation. The World Health Organization (WHO, 2006) set a limit of 0.35 Sv/lifetime based on this experience as a dose warranting evacuation. Of the 134 most heavily exposed firefighters and workers at Chernobyl, 28 died from acute radiation poisoning within 3 months of the accident (20 received > 6.5 Gy, 7 received 4.2–6.4 Gy, and one received 2.2–4.1 Gy). Nineteen others died from other causes between the years of 1987 and 2004. Exposure to lower doses caused 4.6% of the Russian emergency workers to die of radiation-induced diseases (average external dose = 1.07 Sv for solid neoplasms, circulatory disorders, and leukemias). The extreme dose of 500 mSv is allowed for life-saving purposes only by emergency workers. A 5% increase in the fatal cancer rate is expected for someone exposed to 1,000 mSv short term with the person experiencing temporary radiation sickness of nausea and decreased white blood cell count, but not death. However, above this level, the severity of the illness increases with dose. An LD_{50} in humans over a 1-month period would occur with 5,000 mSv short term. Guaranteed fatality within

a few weeks occurs with 10,000 mSv short term (World Nuclear Association, 2015).

Radiation protection consists of limiting time and distance to protect people handling highly radioactive material at fatal or disease-inducing doses. Radiation falls off by distance squared. For example, a person died in less than 1 week as a result of a flash of radiation when bringing two highly radioactive sources just under the critical mass/source together too fast during the Manhattan Project died, but this incident did not have acute effects on colleagues not far behind him. Another form of protection is dense shielding such as lead or plexiglass-coated lead to prevent X-ray formation from a highly radioactive source bombarding metal directly. Other shielding is provided by storing highly radioactive materials under water or concrete or lead-lined rooms and handling using remove controls. Containment is the fourth protection, with closed systems and multiple barriers within closed systems.

Radionuclides

The radionuclides and their isotopes determine the types of particles emitted, half-lives, and distribution to organs depending on route of administration. **Table 28-3** indicates the target organ for each set of radionuclides, their emitted particles, and their half-lives. These factors taken together form the picture of radiation damage in the body. **Table 28-4** will help

TABLE 28-3	Radionuclides' Toxicity	
Target Organ	**Toxicity**	**Radionuclide Examples, Particles Emitted, and Half-Lives**
Lung (inhalation)	Radiation pneumonitis → fibrosis → lung tumors (adenocarcinomas at lower doses)	Transuranics ($^{238 \text{ or } 239}PuO_2$): Alpha: $t_{1/2}$ = 24,100 years, ^{222}Rn: $t_{1/2}$ = 3 days
	Squamous cell carcinomas	Beta and gamma emitters or high-dose insoluble transuranics
	Pulmonary edema	High fatal radiation dose
Thyroid	Thyroid dysfunction → cancer	^{131}I
Bone	Sarcomas and affecting blood flow	^{226}Ra and possibly ^{90}Sr; strong affinity for bone; ^{239}Pu, ^{235}U, ^{90}Y, ^{140}Ba, ^{140}La, and the rare earth metals
Fast-growing cells	Skin, GI tract, bone marrow, lymphatic tissues, reproductive organs	Dependent on distribution/intake (e.g., oral)
Clearance tissues	Kidney and urinary bladder	Most radionuclides

TABLE 28-4   Radiological Characteristics of Selected Radionuclides Found at Superfund Sites

Nuclide	Half-Life	Mean α Energy, MeV/decay	Mean β Energy, MeV/decay	Mean γ Energy, MeV/decay
α, β, γ Emitters				
^{241}Am	4.32×10^2 y	5.57×10^0	5.21×10^{-2}	3.25×10^{-2}
^{243}Am	7.38×10^3 y	5.36×10^0	2.17×10^{-2}	5.61×10^{-2}
^{243}Cm	2.85×10^1 y	5.89×10^0	1.38×10^{-1}	1.35×10^{-1}
^{244}Cm	1.81×10^1 y	5.89×10^0	8.59×10^{-3}	1.70×10^{-3}
^{237}Np	2.14×10^6 y	4.85×10^0	7.01×10^{-2}	3.46×10^{-2}
^{210}Po	1.38×10^2 y	5.40×10^0	8.19×10^{-2}	8.51×10^{-6}
^{238}Pu	8.77×10^1 y	5.59×10^0	1.06×10^{-2}	1.81×10^{-3}
^{239}Pu	2.41×10^4 y	5.24×10^0	6.74×10^{-3}	8.07×10^{-4}
^{240}Pu	6.54×10^3 y	5.24×10^0	1.06×10^{-2}	1.73×10^{-3}
^{241}Pu	1.44×10^1 y	1.22×10^{-4}	5.25×10^{-3}	2.55×10^{-6}
^{242}Pu	3.76×10^5 y	4.97×10^0	8.73×10^{-3}	1.44×10^{-3}
^{226}Ra	1.60×10^3 y	4.86×10^0	3.59×10^{-3}	6.75×10^{-3}
^{230}Th	7.70×10^4 y	4.75×10^0	1.42×10^{-2}	1.55×10^{-3}
^{232}Th	1.41×10^{10} y	4.07×10^0	1.25×10^{-2}	1.33×10^{-3}
^{234}U	2.44×10^5 y	4.84×10^0	1.32×10^{-2}	1.73×10^{-3}
^{235}U	7.04×10^8 y	4.47×10^0	4.92×10^{-2}	1.56×10^{-1}
^{238}U	4.47×10^9 y	4.26×10^0	1.00×10^{-2}	1.36×10^{-3}
β, γ Emitters				
^{137m}Ba	2.25×10^0 h	—	6.37×10^{-2}	5.98×10^{-1}
^{144}Ce	2.84×10^2 d	—	9.22×10^{-2}	2.07×10^{-2}
^{60}Co	5.27×10^0 y	—	9.65×10^{-2}	2.50×10^0
^{51}Cr	2.77×10^1 d	—	31.56×10^{-1}	3.26×10^{-2}
^{134}Cs	2.06×10^0 y	—	1.64×10^{-1}	1.55×10^0
^{59}Fe	4.45×10^1 d	—	1.17×10^{-1}	1.19×10^0
^{129}I	1.57×10^7 y	—	6.38×10^{-2}	2.46×10^{-2}
^{131}I	8.04×10^0 d	—	1.92×10^{-1}	3.81×10^{-1}
^{40}K	1.28×10^9 y	—	5.23×10^{-1}	1.56×10^{-1}
^{54}Mn	3.13×10^2 d	—	4.22×10^{-3}	8.36×10^{-1}
^{99}Mo	6.60×10^1 h	—	3.93×10^{-1}	1.50×10^{-1}
^{94}Nb	2.03×10^4 y	—	1.68×10^{-1}	1.57×10^0
^{210}Pb	2.23×10^1 y	—	3.80×10^{-2}	4.81×10^{-3}
^{228}Ra	5.75×10^0 y	—	1.69×10^{-2}	4.14×10^{-9}
^{89}Sr	5.05×10^1 d	—	5.83×10^{-1}	8.45×10^{-5}
^{99m}Tc	6.02×10^0 h	—	1.62×10^{-2}	1.26×10^{-1}

(continues)

TABLE 28-4   Radiological Characteristics of Selected Radionuclides Found at Superfund Sites (*continued*)

Nuclide	Half-Life	Mean α Energy, MeV/decay	Mean β Energy, MeV/decay	Mean γ Energy, MeV/decay
β Emitters				
^{14}C	5.73×10^3 y	—	4.95×10^{-2}	—
^{135}Cs	2.30×10^6 y	—	6.73×10^{-2}	—
^{137}Cs	3.00×10^1 y	—	1.87×10^{-1}	—
^3H	1.23×10^1 y	—	5.68×10^{-3}	—
^{32}P	1.43×10^1 d	—	6.95×10^{-1}	—
^{106}Ru	3.68×10^2 d	—	1.00×10^{-2}	—
^{35}S	8.74×10^1 d	—	4.88×10^{-2}	—
^{90}Sr	2.91×10^1 y	—	1.96×10^{-1}	—
^{99}Tc	2.13×10^5 y	—	1.01×10^{-1}	—

Data from EPA. Retrieved from: http://www.epa.gov/oswer/riskassessment/ragsa/pdf/rags_ch10.pdf

understand alpha emitters, beta emitters, and gamma emitters. There is a reason alpha emissions are the focus of the radiation danger from those sources that emit alpha radiation along with other radioactive particles. It is based on the energy the alpha particles emit. Beta and gamma emitters may affect surrounding tissue (beta) and more dense tissue such as bone as well (gamma) unless the element distributes to bone, then all forms of radiation affect the bone (as does radium used to make luminous dial watches).

Lung Damage

Because this chapter started with inhalation and the emergencies such as Fukushima and Chernobyl generated radioactive gases and other radionuclides that should not be inhaled (therefore the importance of respirator use), this examination of radionuclides begins with lung toxicity. Similar to other particles, radionuclide deposition can occur in nasopharyngeal, tracheobronchial, pulmonary (alveolar), and thoracic lymph node compartments. Retention of inhaled radionuclides is dependent on the chemical form of the compound (solubility, ability to be engulfed and cleared by macrophages and cilia, and transport

to extrapulmonary tissues). The ICRP (1994) proposes that compounds of D, W, and Y classes have average clearance times in the lung of 0.5, 50, or 500 days (orders of magnitude separating them). Oxides of plutonium, americium, and curium have pulmonary clearance times from 50–1,000 days (high-temperature oxidation forms more insoluble compounds). More soluble compounds such as actinide nitrates have more rapid clearance from the lung.

Particle size and specific activity (amount of energy released per unit of mass of the radionuclide and faster decay leading to higher specific energies) also influence retention. Macrophages are damaged (cytotoxicity) with increased particle size, higher specific activities, and increased quantity of material deposited in the lung. Macrophage cytotoxicity increases the development of fibrosis and longer retention times ("double-edged sword"). If the specific activity is high enough, it can also cause "dissolution" and increased solubility and consequently shorter retention times. The damage associated with its particles is determined by Gy absorbed and the linear energy transfer as determined by Sv. For example, the alpha particle has a track length of the width of many cells (~40 μm). Distribution to the whole lung is more toxic than concentration in one part, because the "wasted" energy released to an area of few cells could have less overall biological effect, or a tumor or damage there could be removed surgically. Lung cell movements, particle movements, solubility, and particle size appear over time to average the dose-distribution pattern from initially a nonhomogeneous pattern to increased homogeneity. The nonhomogeneity is increased for insoluble, alpha particle–emitting transuranic oxides than for more soluble transuranics or beta and gamma emitters. No matter the particle emitted, the early deaths of cells result in radiation pneumonitis or fibrosis as repair is attempted at high radiation doses. If other cells survive, hyperplasia of pulmonary epithelium can lead to lung tumors. Because dividing cells are more susceptible to cancer formation, it is important to note that alveoli multiply throughout a lifetime and bronchiolar and alveolar epithelial cells have a 30-day or less turnover rate. Mechanical irritation; chemical, physical, and infectious agents; and vitamin A deficiency can lead to squamous and adenomatous metaplasia, which can augment radiation-induced cancer formation, while constant irritation stimulates lung tumor formation. Progressing toward a malignant focus appears to involve a multiplication of the number of ionizing events/cell × number of cells irradiated. Rats rarely develop spontaneous lung tumors, but are models of epithelial cell tumors such as adenocarcinoma, bronchoalveolar carcinoma, undifferentiated carcinoma, or squamous cell carcinoma. Transuranic compounds usually cause well differentiated adenocarcinomas and squamous cell carcinomas and less frequently form hemangiosarcoma, fibrosarcoma, and mesothelioma.

Rat lungs exposed to 6–20 µCi/g of plutonium-238 (half-life 87.74 years) or plutonium-239 ($t_{1/2}$ = 24,100 years) dioxide died 6–7 days later (the longest-lived isotope of plutonium is ^{244}Pu with a half-life of 80.8 million years). This plutonium-239 isotope is formed as follows: ^{238}U (atomic number 92) is bombarded with neutrons forming ^{239}U (atomic number 92). The ^{239}U loses a beta particle in 23.5 minutes becoming ^{239}Np (atomic number 93), which also loses a beta particle over 2.36 days

becoming ^{239}Pu (atomic number 94), causing the toxic alpha emitter to become ^{235}U. ^{238}Pu is formed by bombarding ^{238}U with deuterons (heavy hydrogen) to become ^{238}Np plus two neutrons. This ^{238}Np isotope loses a beta particle over 2.12 days to become the alpha-emitting ^{238}Pu that becomes ^{234}U. Thus, the radiation level and the particles emitted from the plutonium isotopes caused equivalent damage as the half-lives were irrelevant at this high-dose level. At ~0.2 µCi/g rats survived longer (less edema), but deposited fibrin and displayed early proliferation of bronchiolar and alveolar epithelium. Rats inhaling ^{239}PuO$_2$ developed a progressive radiation pneumonitis with a characteristic accumulation of collagen (maximal at 200 days after exposure) and elastin in damaged pulmonary epithelium and thickened septal walls. Alpha emitters such as ^{239}PuO$_2$ or ^{222}Rn (half-life 3.8 days) are of most concern. Short-lived ^{219}Rn or ^{220}Rn isotopes have $t_{1/2}$ = 4 and 55.3 seconds respectively, so they do not last long enough to be inhaled at a high, sustained dose. Adenomatous metaplasia (irregular proliferation of cuboidal epithelial cells forming papillary patterns) and adenomas precede the development of malignant adenocarcinomas (invasion of the pleura, blood, or lymphatic vessels), the most frequent lung cancer associated with rat exposure to alpha emitters. Epidermoid carcinomas in rats (irregular proliferation of stratified squamous keratinizing epithelium, which may replace entire lobes) appear in conjunction with radiation-induced fibrosis and are more likely to metastasize to other regions such as the kidney. The isotope is important when considering hemangiosarcomas (originating from central regions of the lung). ^{239}PuO$_2$ with the much longer half-life is more likely to produce this form of cancer than ^{238}PuO$_2$. ^{239}PuO$_2$, however, appears to develop malignant mesotheliomas similarly to intraperitoneal injections of chrysotile asbestos. These tumors are also produced by inhalation of ^{241}Am (alpha emitter used in smoke detectors), ^{144}CeO$_2$, ^{244}CmO$_2$, ^{243}EsCl$_3$, ^{210}Po, soluble Pu, and ^{222}Rn. Radiation dose and dose distribution alter the cancer produced. High doses of insoluble ^{238}PuO$_2$ or ^{239}PuO$_2$ particles result in more squamous cell cancers, as do beta- and gamma-emitting radionuclides

(^{90}Y or ^{91}Y, ^{144}Ce, and ^{90}Sr fused to aluminum silicate as these metals may not stay in the lung without this fusion—for, example ^{90}Sr is a "bone-seeker"), while adenocarcinomas occur more often at lower doses and for soluble transuranics such as ^{244}CmO$_2$ and soluble ^{238}Pu (Dagle and Sanders, 1984). The large airways usually exhibit the squamous cell carcinoma and small-cell carcinoma, while bronchiolar epithelium and alveolar-interstitial tissue cancers arise from respective progenitor cells with preferential formation of adenocarcinoma. Alpha particles and gamma rays produce single- or double-stand breaks, while beta particles appear to affect the connections between bases (Sturm, 2011).

Thyroid

Radioactive iodine has resulted in exposure from nuclear explosions, nuclear reactor accidents, misuse of radioimmunoassay (accidents by mouth pipette use or gamma radiation exposure from source of radioactive iodine–labeled materials), and from medical uses. As the thyroid accumulates the iodine, the ^{131}I is the usual isotope, which fortunately has a short half-life for time of exposure, but unfortunately gives off more energy than ^{129}I in that time if it is already in the thyroid. People exposed to high levels of radioactive iodine are subject to thyroid dysfunction and cancer. As the thyroid is damaged, part of the problem is the lack of negative feedback from T$_4$ and T$_3$ to the hypothalamus and the pituitary, resulting in high thyroid-stimulating hormone release and promotion of hyperplasia of thyroid follicles that already are have mutagenic injury if they have not already died.

Bone

^{90}Sr was a concern to baby boomers because they were potentially exposed to this radionuclide via atmospheric testing of atomic and hydrogen bombs during the 1950s. It acts very much like calcium in its distribution to bone. ^{226}Ra is the most stable form and glows a faint blue. Those who used this compound to make watches were subject to bone sarcomas as a result of the relocation from the digestive tract into the blood circulation and the bone. As an alpha emitter, it is a very toxic material. Because

it is also a gamma emitter, its uses in Denver, Colorado warranted concern. Ra had been processed from mining operations, which led to the Denver Radium Superfund site. Development of this area was watched closely by the EPA and environmental groups. Other radionuclides, including ^{239}Pu, ^{235}U, ^{90}Y, ^{140}Ba, ^{140}La, and the rare earth metals, also have strong affinity for bone (Loutit et al., 1976). The bone-seeking radionuclides appear to be directed by blood flow rather than the rate of osteogenesis as indicated by rat studies (Genant et al., 1974). Bone-seeking radionuclides lead to osteosarcomata, primitive mesenchymal (angio-) sarcomata, and fibrosarcomata in mice (Loutit et al., 1976).

Fast-Growing Cells

Skin, gastrointestinal tract (including associated glands and organs such as the salivary glands, regenerative liver, and the pancreas), bone marrow (leukemia), lymphatic tissues, and reproductive organs are highly susceptible to cancers. Mitotic index may be a presupposing factor in radiation-induced cancers (whole body radiation poisoning causes severe damage to many of these tissues as seen from nuclear facility accidents and atomic bomb survivors).

Clearance Tissues

Kidney and urinary bladder cancers may result from clearance of radionuclides.

Questions

1. Why is a short duration of exposure to isopropyl alcohol, ammonia, hydrogen fluoride, or sulfur dioxide of less concern for the entire respiratory tract than ozone, phosgene, or nitrogen dioxide?

2. What factor is different in determining the impact of aerosols versus gases and vapors?

3. What are the famous ways that gases and vapors can lead to problems in the stratosphere and troposphere?

4. Why are the emissions of sulfuric acid, amines, organic vapors, and nitrate or nitric acid so important in the indirect effects of these particles?

5. Why are Sv more indicative of radiation damage than Gy?

6. Inhalation of radiation may lead to lung cancer, but what other tissues are susceptible to various types of radioactive particles?

References

Ando M. 1990. [Risk evaluation of stratospheric ozone depletion resulting from chlorofluorocarbons (CFC) on human health]. *Nihon Eiseigaku Zasshi.* 45:947–953.

Baur X, Bakehe P, Vellguth H. 2012. Bronchial asthma and COPD due to irritants in the workplace—an evidence-based approach. *J Occup Med Toxicol.* 7:19.

Brues AM. 1949. Biological hazards and toxicity of radioactive isotopes. *J Clin Invest.* 28:1286–1296.

Choe N, Tanaka S, Xia W, Hemenway DR, Roggli VL, Kagan E. 1997. Pleural macrophage recruitment and activation in asbestos-induced pleural injury. *Environ Health Perspect.* 105(Suppl 5):1257–1260.

Dagle GE, Sanders CL. 1984. Radionuclide injury to the lung. *Environ Health Perspect.* 55:129–137.

Genant HK, Bautovich GJ, Singh M, Lathrop KA, Harper PV. 1974. Bone-seeking radionuclides: an *in vivo* study of factors affecting skeletal uptake. *Radiology.* 113:373–382.

Greenwood MA. 2006. A brief review of inhalation toxicology and the development of a research proposal to demonstrate the relevance of an established mouse bioassay to biodefense objectives [Masters Thesis]. University of Pittsburgh.

Hayes A, Bakand S. 2010. Inhalation toxicology. *EXS.* 100:461–488.

International Atomic Energy Agency. 2014. Radiation Protection and Safety of Radiation Sources: International Basic Safety Standards General Safety Requirements Series No. GSR Part 3, Vienna, Austria.

International Commission on Radiological Protection (IRCP). 1977. Recommendations of the IRCP. Publication 26. *Ann ICRP.* 1(3).

International Commission on Radiological Protection (IRCP). 1979. Radionuclide Release into the Environment - Assessment of Doses to Man. Publication 29. *Ann ICRP.* 2(2).

International Commission on Radiological Protection (IRCP). 1994. Human Respiratory Tract Model for Radiological Protection. Oxford: Pergamon Press, ICRP Publication 66, Part 1; *Ann. ICRP.* 24(1-3).

Joint Research Centre. n.d. The EU Major Accident Reporting System—eMARS. European Commission. http://www.unece.org/fileadmin/DAM/env/teia/doc/COP-7/10.5_EMARS.pdf

Kulmala M, Kontkanen J, Junninen H, Lehtipalo K, Manninen HE, Nieminen T, Petäjä T, Sipilä M, Schobesberger S, Rantala P, Franchin A, Jokinen T, Järvinen E, Äijälä M, Kangasluoma J, Hakala J, Aalto PP, Paasonen P, Mikkilä J, Vanhanen J, Aalto J, Hakola H, Makkonen U, Ruuskanen T, Mauldin RL 3rd, Duplissy J, Vehkamäki H, Bäck J, Kortelainen A, Riipinen I, Kurtén T, Johnston MV, Smith JN, Ehn M, Mentel TF, Lehtinen KE, Laaksonen A, Kerminen VM, Worsnop DR. 2013. Direct observations of atmospheric aerosol nucleation. *Science.* 339:943–946.

Loutit JF, Corp MJ, Ardran GM. 1976. Radiographic features of bone in several strains of laboratory mice and of their tumours induced by bone-seeking radionuclides. *J Anat.* 122:357–375.

National Fire Protection Association (NFPA). 2012. *Standards System for the Identification of Hazards of Materials for Emergency Response, 2012 Edition.* Quincy, MA: NFPA.

Nuclear Regulatory Commission (NRC). 2012. Human Resources Training and Development. [H-201 – Health Physics Technology] Health Physics Fundamentals, pg 5. http://pbadupws.nrc.gov/docs/ML1126/ML11262A154.pdf

Pandolfi JM, Connolly SR, Marshall DJ, Cohen AL. 2011. Projecting coral reef futures under global warming and ocean acidification. *Science.* 333:418–422.

Sturm R. 2011. Radioactivity and lung cancer-mathematical models of radionuclide deposition in the human lungs. *J Thorac Dis.* 3:231–243.

Tillery MI, Wood GO, Ettinger HJ. 1976. Generation and characterization of aerosols and vapors for inhalation experiments. *Environ Health Perspect.* 16:25–40.

United Nations. 2007. Globally Harmonized System of Classification and Labeling of Chemicals, Part 3. http://www.unece.org/fileadmin/DAM/trans/danger/publi/ghs/ghs_rev02/English/03e_part3.pdf

U.S. Environmental Protection Agency. 2012. Radiation Risk Assessment Guidance. http://www.epa.gov/oswer/riskassessment/ragsa/pdf/rags_ch10.pdf

UNSCEAR. 2000. *Sources and effects of ionizing radiation. Report of the United Nations Scientific Committee on the Effects of Atomic Radiation.* New York: UNSCEAR.

UNSCEAR. 2013. *Report of the United Nations Scientific Committee on the Effects of Ionizing Radiation. A/68/46.* New York: UNSCEAR.

Valacchi G, Sticozzi C, Pecorelli A, Cervellati F, Cervellati C, Maioli E. 2012. Cutaneous responses to environmental stressors. *Ann NY Acad Sci.* 1271:75–81.

Weeks SJ, Currie B, Bakun A. 2002. Satellite imaging: massive emissions of toxic gas in the Atlantic. *Nature*. 415:493–494.

WHO. 2006. WHO Expert Group report. *Health Effects of the Chernobyl Accident and Special Health Care Programmes: Report of the UN Chernobyl Forum Health Expert Group*. Burton B, Repacholi M, Zhanat Carr C, eds. Geneva, Switzerland: World Health Organization.

World Nuclear Association. 2015. Nuclear Radiation and Health Effects. http://www.world-nuclear.org/info/inf05.html

Yukihiro M, Hiramatsu T, Bouteau F, Kadono T, Kawano T. 2012. Peroxyacetyl nitrate-induced oxidative and calcium signaling events leading to cell death in ozone-sensitive tobacco cell-line. *Plant Signal Behav*. 7:113–120.

CHAPTER 29

Toxicity of Pharmaceuticals and Personal Care Products (PPCPs) into Water

This is a chapter outline intended to guide and familiarize you with the content to follow.

I. Pharmaceutical and personal care products

    A. Emerging field based on human use of pharmaceuticals and the improper disposal of those medications and urinary metabolites. Also consists of personal care products such as musks (fragrances), cosmetics, sunscreen agents, and nutraceuticals. See Figure 29-1

    B. Species effects modeled by Interspecies Correlation Estimate (ICE), which uses surrogate species Model II least squares regression analysis and Acute to Chronic Estimation (ACE) Model (NOAEL or LOAEL predictions from linear regression analysis of was acute toxicity testing). Both models account for mode of action, chemical class, and taxonomic distance

        1. Fathead minnow = model fish species and vitellogenin gene expression indicates estrogenic endocrine disruption in males

        2. Modeling by EPA concerned with hydrolytic transformation of emerging contaminants, the same protein expression chip data used for human estimation of effects of PPCPs, development of a Tier II two-generation guideline for the sheepshead minnow, linkage of exposure and effects using genomics, proteomics, and metabolomics in small fish, use of an amphibian model of lack of morphogenesis from tadpole to adult frog to characterize and predict thyroid disruptors, emission of natural substances and medications from concentrated animal feeding operations and their effects on endocrine functions, development and evaluation of long-term testing protocols for endocrine-disrupting chemicals (EDCs) and reproductive toxicants in small fish, analytical methods for detection of 65 ecologically relevant metabolites from pharmaceuticals, development of molecular indicators of exposure to pharmaceuticals and EDCs, an informatics approach to estimating ecological risks posed by pharmaceuticals, identifying ecological and molecular indicator responses to pharmaceuticals under simulated field conditions at an EPA experimental stream facility, national screening for EDCs including medications in municipal sewage effluents, development of receptor-to population-level analytical tools for assessing EDC exposure to wastewater-impacted estuaries, rapid assessment tool development for biological effects of complex and biologically active chemical mixtures, and alkylphenols and alkylphenol ethoxylates plus metabolites as potential key agents in endocrine disruption into Great Lakes tributaries

    C. Environmental Effects of PPCPs

        1. Exposure concentrations = 0–10 µg/L acetaminophen (liver), 0–22 µg/L for the NSAID ibuprofen, 0–0.65 µg/L for the anti-seizure and mood-stabilizing drug carbamazepine, and 0–0.73 µg/L for the veterinary antibiotic lincomycin. Caffeine is another substance found in an Indiana stream (mean concentration = 0.044 µg/L). The maximum concentrations of other PPCPs in that same stream were 0.45 µg/L for acetaminophen, the antiseptic soap ingredient triclosan at 0.23 µg/L, the insect repellant DEET at 0.18 µg/L, caffeine at 0.14 µg/L, and the stimulant paraxanthine at 0.12 µg/L. The frequency of detection for these substances in that stream was also important, with the highest for human PPCP DEET (70%), followed by the human PPCP paraxanthine (64%),

the veterinary sulfamethazine (59%), the human PPCP triclosan and veterinary lincomycin (both at 57%), then by human PPCP acetaminòphen (56%), human PPCP caffeine (52%), followed by the human nicotine metabolite cotinine (43%), human sulfamethoxazole (30%), human NSAID naproxen (28%), human PPCP carbamazepine (12%), human PPCP ibuprofen, human fibrate used to lower cholesterol and triglycerides gemfibrozil (10%), the veterinary coccidiostat tylosin (6%), human antibiotic trimethoprim (2%), and the human disinfectant and soap antifungal triclocarban (1%). Calculated pharmaceutical loads for that stream were higher for human medications (378.2, 360.1, 189.5, 97.7, and 49.8 µg/s for triclosan, paraxanthine, caffeine, acetaminophen, and DEET, respectively) than medications used in veterinary practice (35.6 and 27.6 µg/s for lincomycin and sulfamethazine, respectively)

2. Uptake of PPCPs into plants appears to involve the dissolved organic matter in the planting matrix

3. Effects of organisms—see Table 29-1

   a. Cytogenetic effects on zebra mussel for human PPCPs rank soap antiseptic ingredient triclosan > antibiotic trimethoprim > NSAID ibuprofen > diclofenac (NSAID) = analgesic acetaminophen measured as a biomarker response index

   b. Wastewater treatment plant mixtures induced CYP (EROD activity in rainbow trout cell line RTG-2) and inhibited β-galactosidase (6/7 mixtures)

   c. Whole Japanese medaka fish indicated that exposure to carbamazepine and diclofenac ↓ feeding behavior, while carbamazepine triclosan ↓ swimming speed

   d. Freshwater crustacean (*Thamnocephalus platyurus*) also indicated the triclosan and the musk mefenamic acid had the lowest 24-h LC_{50}s (most toxic), while anti-seizure carbamazepine had the highest LC_{50} (> 2 orders of magnitude). A whole fish (*Oryzias latipes*) showed a similar pattern, with the 96-h LC_{50} for triclosan and mefenamic acid still the lowest values, but now the antibiotic clarithromycin was least toxic (> 2 orders of magnitude). Some medications had no observable effects at the concentrations tested (> 100 mg/L) such as the cardiac beta-blocker atenolol, antiarrhythmic disopyramide, H_2 antihistamine famotidine, or antibiotics erythromycin or levofloxacin. Mixtures of medications naproxen, gemfibrozil, diclofenac, ibuprofen, triclosan (antiseptic), salicylic acid (NSAID), and acetaminophen from 10–1,000 ng/L nominal concentration had little effect on the lifecycle of fathead minnows, although larval deformities ↑ ~5% from controls. Triclosan in particular was toxic to marine phytoplankton (*Dunaliella tertiolecta*), with medications being at least 50-fold or much less toxic in a 96-h static algal bioassay (EC_{50}). However, additivity was noted for mixtures of simvastatin-clofibric acid and fluoxetine-triclosan. Hormones, as expected, are very potent endocrine-disrupting agents on juvenile zebrafish with dose-dependent ↑ vitellogenin and complete sex reversal at 2 ng/L 17α-ethynylestradiol (EE2) with significant sex ratios at 1 ng/L. The androgen 17α-methyltestosterone (MT) caused complete sex reversal at all concentrations tested between 26 and 1,000 ng/L

   e. Human effects—see Table 29-2

      (1) Triclosan is not problematic unless environmental regulations are lax. It is a persistent chlorinated product with byproducts such as methyltriclosan and other chlorinated phenols. Despite this possible lack of proven effects, triclosan is measurable in human breast milk, urine, and plasma. In animals, triclosan disrupts the thyroid and possibly the reproductive axis

      (2) Musks' estrogenicity → breast cancer concerns (E-screen assay → significantly ↑ growth rate of human MCF-7 breast cancer cells exposed to musk xylene or musk ketone, which is inhibited by tamoxifen), but far less potent than 17β-estradiol

      (3) Fathead minnows exposed to a mixture of 3 psychoactive agents 10 µg/L fluoxetine, 50 µg/L venlafaxine, and 100 µg/L carbamazepine → enrichment of genes similar to human idiopathic autism

      (4) Human cases of toxicity may result from China's production of pharmaceuticals and used in farming and aquaculture facilities at levels not allowed in U.S. facilities. One major global concern of these compounds in the rivers is the development of bacteria highly resistant to antibiotics

CONCEPTUALIZING TOXICOLOGY 29-1 (*continued*)

There is now a whole lab in Las Vegas of the U.S. Environmental Protection Agency (EPA) devoted to pharmaceuticals and personal care products (EPA, 2012). PPCPs include prescription, over-the-counter (OTC), and veterinary medications; fragrances; cosmetics; sunscreen products; diagnostic agents; and nutraceuticals (dietary supplements such as vitamins and minerals). Sources of this material come from human waste (mainly metabolites) and disposal of expired or unused medication, regulated residues from drug manufacture, illicit drug use and manufacture (uncontrolled), residues from hospitals, veterinary drug use with focus on antibiotics and steroids, and agribusiness. **Figure 29-1** refers to the origins of PPCPs in the environment. The active metabolites of medications (especially slow-dissolving drugs), including those flushed down toilets that leak from sewage systems and from medicated animal carcasses, serve to provide a mixture of low-level pharmaceuticals in scavengers, drinking water for humans, and aquatic species.

Endocrine disruption as a result of PPCPs adds to the concern that they will end up downstream from sewage effluents. Pharmacies, physicians, humanitarian medication surpluses, and hospital wastes especially from cancer chemotherapeutic agents that do not biodegrade (such as cisplatin) may also find their way into sewage systems. Septic systems and other uses of sewage (land application, illegal direct discharge into water bodies, and manure lagoons provide these products into agriculture or waters (surface and/or ground water especially if old wells are not capped off). People evacuating wastes during use of surface waters or dumping their wash water into surface waters are another source of contamination. Manufacturers' waste streams and illegal drug operations add to the contamination, making many a locality unfit for habitation. Landfill and cemetery leakage provide other avenues for these products to make their way into the ecosystem. Certain medications have dual use for control of birds (4-aminopyridine), rodents (azacholesterol, warfarin), snakes (acetaminophen), plant pathogens (selected antibiotics), and amphibians (caffeine). Usually waters are at risk, but some medicated

animal feeds are dusty and may be respired, while others volatilize and may react with ultraviolet (UV) light (Daughton, 2007).

The EPA is modeling human health effects by toxicity pathway–specific protein chip array analysis for chemical screening and prioritization of PPCPs (EPA, 2010). Figure 29-1 Illustrates the EPA's approach to PPCPs. Note the sources and fates of pharmaceuticals, personal care products, and their biological metabolites and photochemical degradation products. Two software products are used to evaluate the impact and the possible impact of chemicals (including those having relevant toxicity data) to a variety of species including threatened and endangered species. One is the Interspecies Correlation Estimate (ICE) model using surrogate species Model II least squares regression, which should now be expanded into wildlife and other aquatic species. The other Acute to Chronic Estimation (ACE) model is used to predict the no-observed-adverse-effect-level (NOAEL) or lowest-observed-adverse-effect-level (LOAEL) concentrations for chronic mortality from raw acute toxicity data employing accelerated life testing and linear regression analysis. Both are subject to rigorous quality assurance/quality control, bootstrap validation, and the scrutiny of peer-reviewed publications. These models are also meant to take into account mode of action, chemical class, and taxonomic distance. The fathead minnow (*Pimephales promelas*) is the lab rat of the aquatic world (including sequenced genome), and vitellogenin gene expression yields important information about estrogenic endocrine disruption effects of chemicals or mixtures found in sewage effluents. The fathead minnow and pearl dace (*Margariscus margarita*) were exposed in an experimental lake in northwestern Ontario to 17α-ethynylestradiol at ~4–6 ng/L for 3 years starting in 2001 (Kidd et al., 2007). Comparing these data with the same species in reference lakes gives a more long-term understanding of the impacts of low levels of potent estrogenic compounds on aquatic species.

Additionally, the EPA has considered the persistence of many agents from wastewater effluents in the treatment of, removal from, and

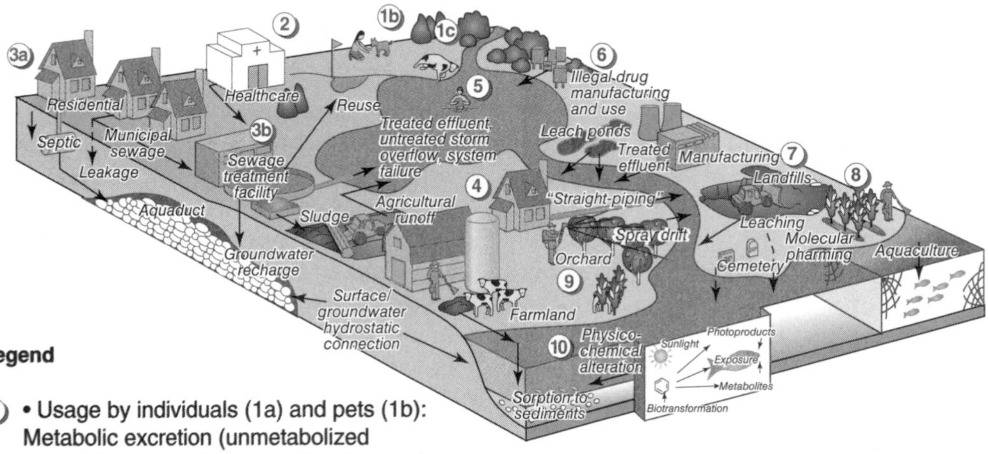

Legend

① • Usage by individuals (1a) and pets (1b): Metabolic excretion (unmetabolized parent drug, parent-drug conjugates, and bioactive metabolites); sweat and vomitus. Excretion exacerbated by disease and slow-dissolving medications
  • Disposal of unused/outdated medication to sewage systems
  • Underground leakage from sewage system infrastructure
  • Disposal of euthanized/medicated animal carcasses serving as food for scavengers (1c)

② • Release of treated/untreated hospital wastes to domestic sewage systems (weighted toward acutely toxic drugs and diagnostic agents, as opposed to long-term medications); also disposal by pharmacies, physicians, humanitarian drug surplus

③ • Release to private septic/leach fields (3a)
  • Treated effluent from domestic sewage treatment plants discharged to surface waters, re-injected into aquifers (recharge), recycled/reused (irrigation or domestic uses) (3b)
  • Overflow of untreated sewage from storm events and system failures directly to surface waters (3b)

④ • Transfer of sewage solids ("biosolids") to land (e.g., soil amendment/fertilization)
  • "Straight-piping" from homes (untreated sewage discharged directly to surface waters)
  • Release from agriculture: spray drift from tree crops (e.g., antibiotics)
  • Dung from medicated domestic animals (e.g., feed) - CAFOs (confined animal feeding operations)

⑤ • Direct release to open waters via washing/bathing/swimming

⑥ • Discharge of regulated/controlled industrial manufacturing waste streams
  • Disposal/release from clandestine drug labs and illicit drug usage

⑦ • Disposal to landfills via domestic refuse, medical wastes, and other hazardous wastes
  • Leaching from defective (poorly engineered) landfills and cemeteries

⑧ • Release to open waters from aquaculture (medicated feed and resulting excreta)
  • Future potential for release from molecular pharming (production of therapeutics in crops)

⑨ • Release of drugs that serve double duty as pest control agents: examples: 4-aminopyridine, experimental multiple sclerosis drug → used as avicide; warfarin, anticoagulant → rat poison; azacholesterol, antilipidemics → avian/rodent reproductive inhibitors; certain antibiotics → used for orchard pathogens; acetaminophen, analgesic → brown tree snake control; caffeine, stimulant → *coqui* frog control

⑩ Ultimate environmental transport/fate:
  • Most PPCPs eventually transported from terrestrial domain to aqueous domain
  • Phototransformation (both direct and indirect reactions via UV light)
  • Physicochemical alteration, degradation, and ultimate mineralization
  • Volatilization (mainly certain anesthetics, fragrances)
  • Some uptake by plants
  • Respirable particulates containing sorbed drugs (e.g., medicated-feed dusts)

FIGURE 29-1 PPCP Origins

Repropduced from Environmental Protection Agency. Retrieved from: https://uwphi.pophealth.wisc.edu/programs/health-policy/ebhpp/events/20140313/ppcps-in-the-environment.pdf

potential human exposure to drinking water. Ecological concerns of the EPA include:

- Hydrolytic transformation of emerging contaminants
- Protein expression chip data used for human estimation of effects of PPCPs
- Development of a Tier II two-generation guideline for the sheepshead minnow
- Linkage of exposure and effects using genomics, proteomics, and metabolomics in small fish
- Use of an amphibian model of lack of morphogenesis from tadpole to adult frog to characterize and predict thyroid disruptors
- Emission of natural substances and medications from concentrated animal feeding operations and their effects on endocrine functions; development and evaluation of long-term testing protocols for endocrine-disrupting chemicals (EDCs) and reproductive toxicants in small fish
- Analytical methods for detection of 65 ecologically relevant metabolites from pharmaceuticals; development of molecular indicators of exposure to pharmaceuticals and EDCs
- An informatics approach to estimating ecological risks posed by pharmaceuticals; identifying ecological and molecular indicator responses to pharmaceuticals under simulated field conditions at an EPA experimental stream facility; national screening for EDCs including medications in municipal sewage effluents; development of receptor- to population-level analytical tools for assessing EDC exposure to wastewater-impacted estuaries
- Rapid assessment tool development for biological effects of complex and biologically active chemical mixtures; and alkylphenols and alkylphenolethoxylates plus metabolites as potential key agents in endocrine disruption into Great Lakes tributaries.

This is quite a wish list that EPA hopes to have successful research outcomes for analysis. This chapter examines the known effects that are of primary concern based on published accounts.

Environmental Effects of PPCPs

To understand the effects of PPCPs, exposure concentrations must be known or estimated. Concentrations for human PPCPs range from 0–10 µg/L for the hepatotoxic analgesic agent acetaminophen, 0–22 µg/L for the nonsteroidal anti-inflammatory drug (NSAID) ibuprofen, 0–0.65 µg/L for the anti-seizure and mood-stabilizing drug carbamazepine, and 0–0.73 µg/L for the veterinary antibiotic lincomycin. Pharmaceutical mean concentrations in a rural Indiana stream were 0.17 µg/L for acetaminophen and 0.044 µg/L for the stimulant caffeine, which were an order of magnitude higher than veterinary antibiotics lincomycin or sulfamethazine at 0.006 µg/L (Bernot et al., 2013). Maximum concentrations in that same stream were also highest for human medications with acetaminophen reaching 0.45 µg/L, the antiseptic soap ingredient triclosan at 0.23 µg/L, the insect repellant DEET at 0.18 µg/L, caffeine at 0.14 µg/L, and the stimulant paraxanthine at 0.12 µg/L. The frequency for detection of PPCPs in those Indiana stream samples were highest for human PPCP DEET (70%), followed by the human PPCP paraxanthine (64%), the veterinary sulfamethazine (59%), the human PPCP triclosan and veterinary lincomycin (both at 57%), then by human PPCP acetaminophen (56%), human PPCP caffeine (52%), followed by the human nicotine metabolite cotinine (43%), human sulfamethoxazole (30%), human NSAID naproxen (28%), human PPCP carbamazepine (12%), human PPCP ibuprofen, human fibrate used to lower cholesterol and triglycerides gemfibrozil (10%), the veterinary coccidiostat tylosin (6%), human antibiotic trimethoprim (2%), and the human disinfectant and soap antifungal triclocarban (1%). The pharmaceutical load calculated as µg/s (µg/L times the discharge rate of L/s) in that stream were higher for human medications (378.2, 360.1, 189.5, 97.7, and 49.8 µg/s for triclosan, paraxanthine, caffeine, acetaminophen, and DEET, respectively) than medications used in veterinary practice (35.6 and 27.6 µg/s for lincomycin and sulfamethazine, respectively). There are of course seasonal variations in the concentrations of these compounds and net retention of the reach input in µg/m/d (highest for paraxanthine in March at 1,667 µg/m/d; Bernot et al., 2013).

PPCPs can be taken up into plants such as the Chinese cabbage (*Brassica campestris*). Soil was contaminated with 2.6 ng/g carbamazepine, 3.1 ng/g sulfamethoxazole, 5.4 ng/g salbutamol (β_2 agonist antiasthma agent), or 0.5 ng/g trimethoprim and in a second experiment exposed to biosolids from a wastewater treatment plant containing 93.1 mg/g carbamazepine, 67.4 ng/g sulfamethoxazole, 30.3 ng/g salbutamol, 433.7 ng/g triclosam, and 24.7 ng/g trimethoprim (Holling et al., 2012). Aerials and roots of the cabbage plant were analyzed separately. In the first experiment, all four pharmaceuticals were detected with median concentrations of 255.4 ng/g aerials and 272.9 ng/g roots carbamazepine, 222.8 ng/g aerials and 260.3 ng/g roots sulfamethoxazole,108.3 ng/g aerials and 140.6 ng/g roots salbutamol, and 20.6 ng/g aerials and 53.7 ng/g (-1) roots trimethoprim. For those cabbages exposed to biosolids, pharmaceuticals detected in the aerials were carbamazepine (317.6 ng/g aerials and 416.2 ng/g roots), salbutamol (21.2 ng/g aerials and 187.6 ng/g roots), and triclosan (22.9 ng/g aerials and 1220.1 ng/g roots). Sulfamethoxazole was detected only in the roots of one the plants exposed to biosolid-amended soil. The study suggested that the rhizosphere

conditions such as dissolved organic matter in the planting matrix appear to be key factors in predicting mobilization and bioavailability of these PPCPs (Holling et al., 2012).

Fish in a German study were analyzed for the presence of 15 pharmaceuticals, 2 pharmaceutical metabolites, and 12 personal care products (Subedi et al., 2012). Researchers found only two pharmaceuticals, diphenhydramine (antihistamine) at four sites with concentrations of 0.04–0.07 ng/g wet weight (ww) and desmethylsertraline (metabolite of the antidepressant selective serotonin reuptake inhibitor [SSRI] sertraline) at two sites with concentrations of 1.65–3.28 ng/g ww. Galaxolide (polycyclic musk used in perfumes) was found at 0.69–0.89 ng/g ww with a maximum concentration of 447 ng/g ww at the Rehlingen sampling site in the Saar River. Tonalide (a macrocyclic musk) was similarly found at 0.89–0.97 ng/g ww with a maximum concentration of 15 ng/g ww in fish tissue at that same contaminated site. These concentrations for galaxolide and tonalide in fish tissue have decreased from 1995–2008 and are 19 and 28 times, respectively, lower than those concentrations found in the United States. **Table 29-1** summarizes some of the studies

TABLE 29-1 Environmental Toxicity from PPCPs		
Toxicity	**Compound Key Examples**	**Toxic Mechanism**
96-hour toxicity to zebra mussel	Acetaminophen, diclofenac, ibuprofen, triclosan, trimethoprim	Cytogenetic disruption by eight different assays merged into a biomarker response index
RTG-2 rainbow trout cell line	WWTP effluent mixtures	CYP1A, EROD activity, ROS, β-galactosidase, cellular senescence, cell viability
Japanese medaka fish behavior	Carbamazepine, diclofenac, triclosan	Feeding behavior and swimming speed
Freshwater fish vs. crustacean	Triclosan, mefenamic acid, ifenprodil, propranolol, indomethacin, ibuprofen, clarithromycin, carbamazepine	LC_{50}s indicate highest toxicity for triclosan or mefenamic acid otherwise order of toxicity different for different aquatic species
Fathead minnows lifecycle	Naproxen, gemfibrozil, diclofenac, ibuprofen, triclosan, salicylic acid, acetaminophen	Larval deformities increased by 5–6% over controls
Phytoplankton	Triclosan, fluoxetine, simvastatin, diclofenac, clofibric acid, carbamazepine	EC_{50} problematic especially for triclosan, but additivity of others in a mixture problematic
Juvenile zebrafish sex changes	17α-ethynylestradiol, 17α-methyltestosterone	Complete sex reversal by either agent in ng/L or 10s of ng/L range

indicating effects of PPCPs on aquatic species. Note that sometimes these reflect the additive effects of mixtures, the potency of hormones, or the sensitivity of a given species to physiological disruption.

The freshwater bivalve *Dreissena polymorpha* (zebra mussel) was employed to measure the biomarker response index (BRI) using eight cytogenetic effects induced by a 96-hour exposure to 1 nM of various human PPCPs. This BRI found that the cytogenetic toxicity ranked triclosan > trimethoprim > ibuprofen > diclofenac (NSAID) = acetaminophen (paracetamol; Parolini et al., 2013). A rainbow trout cell line (RTG-2) was first used to assess the lowest observable adverse effect concentration (LOAEC) and half maximal effective concentration (EC_{50}) within the range of 0.15–784.47 μg/L. Four out of the seven tested wastewater treatment plant (WWTP) mixtures induced 7-ethoxyresorufin-*O*-deethylase (EROD) CYP activity. Reactive oxygen species (ROS) presence was detected following exposure to two of the mixtures. Six of seven of the mixtures inhibited β-galactosidase at concentrations higher than those that induced EROD activity or ROS production. The evaluation of toxicity of PPCPs to rainbow trout cells also evaluated cellular senescence and cell viability (Fernández et al., 2013).

Whole fish (Japanese medaka; *Oryzias latipes*) were evaluated for the effects of 6.15 mg/L carbamazepine, 1.0 mg/L diclofenac, and 0.17 mg/L triclosan (all concentrations represent 10% of the 96-hour LC_{50} calculated for medaka for these compounds) on feeding behavior and swimming speed 5 to 9 days (especially effective on days 8 and 9) into the exposure. Feeding behavior (time it took to eat midge larvae) was negatively impacted by carbamazepine and diclofenac, while swimming speed was decreased by exposure to carbamazepine and triclosan (Nassef et al., 2010).

Selected PPCPs were tested on two aquatic species, a freshwater crustacean (*Thamnocephalus platyurus*) and a fish species (*Oryzias latipes*). The 24-hour median LC_{50}s were (from most to least toxic) 0.47, 3.95, 4.43, 10.31, 16.14, 19.59, 94.23, and > 100 mg/L for *Thamnocephalus platyurus* exposed to triclosan, mefenamic acid (NSAID), ifenprodil (NMDA receptor antagonist for

vasodilation), propranolol (antiarrhythmic), indomethacin (NSAID), ibuprofen, clarithromycin (antibiotic), and carbamazepine, respectively. The fish *O. latipes* showed a different sensitivity with 96-hour LC_{50}s of 0.60, 8.04, 8.71, 11.40, 45.87, 81.92, and > 100 mg/L for exposure to triclosan, mefenamic acid, ifenprodil, propranolol, carbamazepine, indomethacin, and ibuprofen or clarithromycin, respectively. Note that except for the antiseptic triclosan and the musk agent mefenamic acid, the aquatic organisms were differentially sensitive to these agents (different hierarchical order of toxicities). However, atenolol (β_1 antagonist), disopyramide (antiarrhythmic), famotidine (H$_2$ antihistamine = stomach acid inhibitor), fluconazole (antifungal), erythromycin (antibiotic), and levofloxacin (antibiotic) yielded no acute toxicity (> 100 mg/L; Kim et al., 2009).

A mixture of PPCPs at nominal concentrations of 10, 30, 100, 300, and 1000 ng/L for naproxen, gemfibrozil, diclofenac, ibuprofen, triclosan, salicylic acid (NSAID), and acetaminophen had little effects on the lifecycle of fathead minnows (growth and development) including length, weights, condition factors, liver weights, gonad weights, external sex characteristics, or egg production of females. The percentage of larval deformities was increased in the F1 generation at 100 and 300 ng/L nominal concentrations from a control of 4.7% for water controls and 3.4% for solvent controls to 9.3% and 9.2% deformities for 100 ng/L and 300 ng/L PPCP mixture, respectively (Parrott and Bennie, 2009).

Marine phytoplankton species, which are important for nutrient cycling and food availability for higher trophic levels, are also responsive to PPCPs. *Dunaliella tertiolecta* in a 96-hour static algal bioassay protocol exhibited 96-hour EC_{50} values of 3.55 μg/L for triclosan (also most toxic for other aquatic species listed earlier), 169.81 μg/L for the SSRI fluoxetine, 22,800 μg/L for the cholesterol synthesis inhibitor simvastatin, 195,690 μg/L for diclofenac, and 224,180 μg/L for the fibrate clofibric acid. An EC_{50} value could not be determined for carbamazepine, but the highest concentration tested of 80,000 μg/L reduced cell density of this phytoplankton species by 42%. Only triclosan was lethal at usual environmental concentrations found in WWTP effluents or surface waters associated with discharge of effluents. However, it is important to note that mixtures of simvastatin-clofibric acid and fluoxetine-triclosan yielded additive toxicity (DeLorenzo and Fleming, 2008).

There are also very sensitive species that are very labile to sex change as noted by fisheries for years. One such model species is the juvenile zebrafish (*Danio rerio*), which exhibited a dose-dependent increase in vitellogenin production and complete sex reversal at 2 ng/L 17α-ethynylestradiol (EE2) with significant sex ratios at 1 ng/L. The androgen 17α-methyltestosterone (MT) caused complete sex reversal at all concentrations tested between 26 and 1,000 ng/L. Intersex fish were noted at the highest concentration of 1,000 ng/L EE2. Although EE2 was clearly more potent, the ng/L potencies of both hormones indicate a strong ability to influence sex by hormones in effluent or estrogenic or androgenic compounds discharged into surface waters (Orn et al., 2003).

Possible Human Effects of PPCPs

Table 29-2 summarizes the possible human effects of PPCPs. Note that it is difficult except for the antiseptic triclosan to find levels that humans are exposed to that might be problematic except in countries where environmental regulations are lax and production of pharmaceuticals and personal care products are high. Triclosan (5-chloro-2-[2,4-dichloro-2'-hydroxy-diphenoxy]phenol, TCS) is a chemical that is currently allowed by the U.S. Food and Drug Administration and EPA in antiseptic soaps, but is now banned for government agencies in Minnesota. However, its structure should give pause as highly chlorinated products tend to be persistent and this one is found in surface waters. It is of concern that its byproducts such as methyltriclosan and other chlorinated phenols appear to be more resistant to degradation and are more toxic than the parent compound (photooxidation to strong Ah-receptor agonists chlorinated dibenzodioxins). TCS has been found in human breast milk, urine, and plasma. Although the usual rodent data do not indicate systemic toxicity, it has been found in animals to disrupt thyroid hormone homeostasis and possibly the reproductive axis. Algae (high toxicity), invertebrates, and selective fish (including reproductive and developmental toxicity in fish) are considerably more sensitive to the toxic action of TCS than mammalian species (Dann and Hontela, 2011).

Estrogenicity and breast cancer are concerns for certain metabolites of musks prevalent in fragrances. An E-screen assay indicated a statistically significant elevation of the growth rate of human MCF-7 breast cancer cells when exposed to musk xylene or musk ketone (nitro musks), p-amino-musk xylene metabolite, and polycyclic musk fragrance 7-acetyl-1,1,3,4,4,6-hexamethyl-tetrahydronaphthalene (AHTN). Their estrogenicity was confirmed by tamoxifen inhibition of these effects. However, all these compounds are far less estrogenic than 17β-estradiol (Bitsch et al., 2002).

One interesting study suggested that idiopathic autism is a genetic disease with unknown environmental triggers (Thomas and Klaper,

TABLE 29-2	Possible Human Toxicity from PPCPs	
Toxicity	**Compound Key Examples**	**Toxic Mechanism**
Thyroid disruption and possibly reproductive axis	Triclosan	Toxic metabolite methyltriclosan
Idiopathic autism	Fluoxetine, venlafaxine, carbamazepine	Enhanced expression of a pattern of autism-like genes at high concentrations
Increased cancer incidence, decreased fertility, increased antibiotic resistance	Antibiotics, soaps, musks, other pharmaceutical compounds such as potent synthetic estrogen (ethynylestradiol)	Variety of toxic mechanisms such as endocrine disruption and include additivity with other persistent organic chemicals

2012). The use of antidepressants by women is associated with autism in their offspring. Environmental concentrations of fluoxetine (SSRI), venlafaxine (serotonin-norepinephrine reuptake inhibitor), and carbamazepine varied from as little as 0.14 µg/L, no data reported, and 0.25 µg/L in drinking water, respectively, to 0.841 µg/L (from a WWTP effluent), 2.19 µg/L (from raw sewage), to 22.0 µg/L (from a WWTP), respectively. Fathead minnows treated with a mixture of three psychoactive pharmaceuticals—fluoxetine at 10 µg/L, venlafaxine at 50 µg/L, and carbamazepine at 100 µg/L (concentrations intended to be similar to the highest expected environmental estimates)—exhibited unambiguous enrichment only of a pattern of genes similar to human idiopathic autism (Thomas and Klaper, 2012).

These experimental values appeared rather high, and it is difficult to see how humans could be exposed to sustained concentrations of 10s to 100s of micrograms without taking the medications. That is the difficulty with many studies of PPCPs: Do the concentrations that exist in nature really have effects on humans or do they disrupt only aquatic species from WWTP effluents? Because there are ~3,000 different substances used as medications for the treatment of humans and animals and thousands of personal care products including skin care products, dental care products, soaps, sunscreens, and hair care products, the discharge into the aquatic environment is problematic as annual production exceeds 10^6 metric tons (one metric ton = 10^3 kilograms) worldwide. China and Southeast Asia have found alkylated musks in WWTP in Guangdong, China and antibiotics from aquaculture in Vietnam. At a pharmaceutical plant in Taizhou, China, chemical runoff from the factory into an open creek was so high that it led to deaths and illnesses of workers (not PPCPs per se). China's medications are 70% prescribed as antibiotics for bacterial infections and used in farming and in aquaculture facilities. In 2003, China led the world in annual production of penicillin (28,000 metric tons = 60% of world's production), oxytetracycline (10,000 metric tons = 6% of world's production), and is ranked high for production of doxycycline and cephalosporins. Concerns

for Hong Kong and the Pearl River Delta for human and environmental exposures are manifested by these astounding numbers. Concerns for human exposure are endocrine disruption or other abnormal physiological responses, reproductive dysfunction, increased cancer incidence, development of "super" bacteria with multiple antibiotic resistance, and potentiating the toxicity of other more persistent highly chlorinated organic compounds and metals in drinking water and estuaries (endocrine disruption from ethynylestradiol and 4-alkylphenols, amphipod population effects of ethynylestradiol, inhibition of CYP1A and other gizzard shad liver cells, and spotted sea trout estrogen receptor antagonism by tamoxifen). Because PPCPs are considered "emerging" toxicants of interest, increases in cancer rates, reductions in human fertility, more resistant bacterial infections, and forth were not generally associated with PPCP exposure (Richardson et al., 2005).

Treatment of Effluents to Prevent Exposure to PPCPs

Bacteria are being selected that remove PPCPs to ng/L concentrations such as triclosan, bisphenol A (endocrine disruptor from plastic baby bottles), ibuprofen (commonly used analgesic), 17β-estradiol (from humans and other forms from synthetic birth control pills and medications to treat menopausal symptoms), and gemfibrozil (fibrate used to lower cholesterol and triglycerides in people with pancreatitis; Zhou et al., 2013).

Questions

1. There is a controversy between rural and urban areas about who produces the most water pollution. In the arena of PPCPs, do animal/veterinary products or human medications, soaps, and other products predominate?
2. What is considered the most toxic PPCPs based on data from crustaceans or fish?
3. Which are the most potent PPCP endocrine disruptors?

References

Bernot MJ, Smith L, Frey J. 2013. Human and veterinary pharmaceutical abundance and transport in a rural central Indiana stream influenced by confined animal feeding operations (CAFOs). *Sci Total Environ.* 445–446:219–230.

Bitsch N, Dudas C, Körner W, Failing K, Biselli S, Rimkus G, Brunn H. 2002. Estrogenic activity of musk fragrances detected by the E-screen assay using human mcf-7 cells. *Arch Environ Contam Toxicol.* 43:257–264.

Dann AB, Hontela A. 2011. Triclosan: environmental exposure, toxicity and mechanisms of action. *J Appl Toxicol.* 31:285–311.

Daughton CG. 2007. Pharmaceuticals in the environment: sources and their management. In: M. Petrovic and D. Barcelo, Eds., *Analysis, Fate and Removal of Pharmaceuticals in the Water Cycle* (Vol. 50). Amsterdam, The Netherlands: Elsevier Science; 1–58.

DeLorenzo ME, Fleming J. 2008. Individual and mixture effects of selected pharmaceuticals and personal care products on the marine phytoplankton species *Dunaliella tertiolecta. Arch Environ Contam Toxicol.* 54:203–210.

Fernández C, Carbonell G, Babín M. 2013. Effects of individual and a mixture of pharmaceuticals and personal-care products on cytotoxicity, EROD activity and ROS production in a rainbow trout gonadal cell line (RTG-2). *J Appl Toxicol.* 33:1203–1212.

Holling CS, Bailey JL, Vanden Heuvel B, Kinney CA. 2012. Uptake of human pharmaceuticals and personal care products by cabbage (*Brassica campestris*) from fortified and biosolids-amended soils. *J Environ Monit.* 14:3029–3036.

Kidd KA, Blanchfield PJ, Mills KH, Palace VP, Evans RE, Lazorchak JM, Flick RW. 2007. Collapse of a fish population after exposure to a synthetic estrogen. *Proc Natl Acad Sci USA.* 104:8897–8901.

Kim JW, Ishibashi H, Yamauchi R, Ichikawa N, Takao Y, Hirano M, Koga M, Arizono K. 2009. Acute toxicity of pharmaceutical and personal care products on freshwater crustacean (*Thamnocephalus platyurus*) and fish (*Oryzias latipes*). *J Toxicol Sci.* 34:227–232.

Nassef M, Matsumoto S, Seki M, Khalil F, Kang IJ, Shimasaki Y, Oshima Y, Honjo T. 2010. Acute effects of triclosan, diclofenac and carbamazepine on feeding performance of Japanese medaka fish (*Oryzias latipes*). *Chemosphere.* 80:1095–1100.

Orn S, Holbech H, Madsen TH, Norrgren L, Petersen GI. 2003. Gonad development and vitellogenin production in zebrafish (*Danio rerio*) exposed to ethinylestradiol and methyltestosterone. *Aquat Toxicol.* 65:397–411.

Parolini M, Pedriali A, Binelli A. 2013. Application of a biomarker response index for ranking the toxicity of five pharmaceutical and personal care products (PPCPs) to the bivalve *Dreissena polymorpha. Arch Environ Contam Toxicol.* 64:439–447.

Parrott JL, Bennie DT. 2009. Life-cycle exposure of fathead minnows to a mixture of six common pharmaceuticals and triclosan. *J Toxicol Environ Health A.* 72:633–641.

Richardson BJ, Lam PK, Martin M. 2005. Emerging chemicals of concern: pharmaceuticals and personal care products (PPCPs) in Asia, with particular reference to Southern China. *Mar Pollut Bull.* 50:913–920.

Subedi B, Du B, Chambliss CK, Koschorreck J, Rüdel H, Quack M, Brooks BW, Usenko S. 2012. Occurrence of pharmaceuticals and personal care products in German fish tissue: a national study. *Environ Sci Technol.* 46:9047–9054.

Thomas MA, Klaper RD. 2012. Psychoactive pharmaceuticals induce fish gene expression profiles associated with human idiopathic autism. *PLoS One.* 7:e32917.

U.S. Environmental Protection Agency. 2010. Toxicity pathway-specific protein expression models for chemical screening and prioritization. http://www.epa.gov/ppcp/projects/toxicity.html

U.S. Environmental Protection Agency. 2012. Pharmaceuticals and Personal Care Products as Pollutants (PPCPs). http://www.epa.gov/ppcp/

Zhou NA, Lutovsky AC, Andaker GL, Gough HL, Ferguson JF. 2013. Cultivation and characterization of bacterial isolates capable of degrading pharmaceutical and personal care products for improved removal in activated sludge wastewater treatment. *Biodegradation.* 24:813–827.

Biological Toxicants

Venoms and Injection Toxicity Versus Poisonous Animals or Cells and Ingestion or Contact Toxicity

This is a chapter outline intended to guide and familiarize you with the content to follow.

I. Animal venoms and poisons

    A. Venoms—Injection route and composition, depending on snake and need to digest tissue for spread of toxin, cause hemorrhage or aid digestion of prey (crotalids) versus neurotoxins of sea snakes and spitting cobras. Other venoms change composition in certain other organisms such as scorpions based on perceived need for protection. Defensive toxins from bees and venomous fishes based on need to inflict pain. See Figure 30-1. See Table 30-1

        1. Hemotoxic venoms →

            a. Hypotension from vasodilation by kinin-releasing activity of blarina toxin and kallikrein from short-tailed shrews or peptidase S1 toxins from toxicoferan reptiles; vasodilation by kinin-like activity of tachykinin-like peptide(s) from cephalopods and hymenopteran insects

            b. Hemorrhage from inhibition of epinephrine-induced platelet aggregation by Type III (anguimorph lizards) or Type IB (snakes) phospholipase A_2; inhibition of ADP-induced platelet aggregation by snake venom metalloproteinases and Type IB or Type IIA phospholipase A_2 or by hymenopteran insects' apyrase; inhibition of collagen-induced platelet aggregation by snake venom C-type lectins and metalloproteinases; inhibition of platelet aggregation by GPIIb/IIIa receptor antagonism by snake venom disintegrins and mambin/dendroaspin; thrombin inhibition by snake venom C-type lectins, textilinins, and Type IIA phospholipase A_2

            c. Clot formation from prothrombin activation via mechanisms such as formation of meizothrombin, promoting phospholipid and Factor Va, or just promoting phospholipid action by snake venom Factor V, Factor X, or metalloproteinases

        2. Neurotoxic venoms through nerve or neuromuscular action → paralysis, pain and/or death:

            a. Modulate the Na^+ channel (block by cone snails channel (block by cone snails μ- or μ-O-conotoxins, scorpions Cn-11, and spider hainantoxin-1 or protoxin-II); activation at site 4 by scorpion β-toxins and spider δ-palutoxins or μ-agatoxins; prolongation by cone snail δ-conotoxins (site 6 on Na^+ channel), Irukandji syndrome jellyfish uncharacterized toxin, scorpion α-toxins, sea anemone Na^+ channel inhibitory toxins, and spider δ-atracotoxins) and/or:

            b. Block the K^+ channel (cone snail κ-conotoxin, hymenopteran insect apamin, short scorpion toxins, Cnidaria Kunitz-type proteinase inhibitors, sea anemone type 3 (BDS) K^+ channel toxins, snake venom dendrotoxins, spider κ-atracotoxins, and toxicoferan reptile CRISP toxins) and/or:

            c. Block the Ca^{2+} channel (cone snail ω-conotoxins, snake venom calcicludine and calciseptine/FS2, spider ω-neurotoxins, and toxicoferan reptile CRISP toxins), antagonism of nicotinic cholinergic receptors (snake venom α-neurotoxins and cone snail α-conotoxins) and/or:

            d. Antagonize nicotinic cholinergic receptors (snake venom α-neurotoxins and cone snail α-conotoxins) and/or:

CONCEPTUALIZING TOXICOLOGY 30-1

e. Antagonize the muscarinic cholinergic receptors (scorpion uncharacterized toxin[s], and snake venom phospholipase A_2 toxins and type-A and type-B muscarinic toxins)

3. Evolutionary development

a. Cysteine-rich secretory (glycol)-proteins (CRISP) genes are positively selected in snakes more than in lizards. Mammalian CRISP genes were strongly negatively selected. CRISPs in Elapidae (venomous snakes in tropical and subtropical regions) have undergone less selection pressure compared with colubrids (most snake species that are nonvenomous or whose venom produces little harm in humans with notable exceptions such as genus *Boiga* or *Rhabdophis*) that may use grip or constriction to kill their prey. Viperidae also have similar high positive selection pressure on molecular evolution of CRISPs, employing hemotoxins to kill or disable prey. Anguimorph lizards have low positive pressure on CRISPs as they use pace and powerful jaws rather than metabolically costly venom to attack prey

4. Venom based on biological classification

a. Chordata: Amniota: Reptilia: Squamata (lizards and snakes)

(1) Serpentes (snakes)

(a) Crotalids (and Mayan pit viper with its thrombin-like enzymes = hemorrhagins which are generally metalloproteinases and cleave collagenous basement membrane → weakening blood vessel walls) are known for hemotoxic effects while elapids are known for their neurotoxicity. Peptides → toxicity and are also insecticidal. Enzymatic proteins metalloproteinase, hyaluronidase, and myotoxic phospholipase A_2 → tissue necrosis. Nonenzymatic snake venoms proteins = three-finger toxins, proteinase inhibitors, snaclecs (C-type lectins and related proteins), nerve growth factors, bradykinin-potentiating peptides, natriuretic peptides, cysteine-rich secretory proteins (CRISPs) or helveprins, sarafotoxins, cobra venom factors, vascular endothelial growth factors, waprins, vespryns, and veficolins. Neurotoxins can be subdivided also for their action: For example, long-chain α-neurotoxins bind to N_M and N_N receptors, causing neuromuscular toxicity and CNS neurotoxicity, respectively. Short-chain α-neurotoxins bind to N_M receptors only, causing only muscle paralysis. Cholinergic toxicity is a property of cobra venom due to polypeptides of ~7K molecular weight that bind to postsynaptic cholinergic receptors. Cardiotoxicity is also a property of cobra venoms due to irreversible depolarization of cell membrane by similarly sized polypeptides. Some enzymes have multiple toxicities such as the phospholipase A_2 of sea snakes that causes presynaptic neuromuscular block, but also has hemolytic, anticoagulant, myonecrotic, and hemorrhaging activities. Mambas have α-dendrotoxin that blocks a group of of voltage-gated K^+ channels, while producing convulsions by increasing glutamate release in the brain. Some of these same venoms also have pharmacologically relevant compounds. Mamba venom contains a three-fingered peptide producing analgesia via inhibiting acid-sensing ion channels in the peripheral nervous system and CNS without respiratory depression, which may be helpful in treating diabetic neuropathy. L-amino acid oxidase is found in all snake venoms and has antibacterial, antifungal, antiprotozoal, and antiviral activities along with an uncertain action on platelet aggregation

(b) Venom hierarchy based on volume and toxicity: cobra (↑ volume and ↑ toxicity) similar to lethality of Mojave rattlesnakes > Eastern diamondback rattlesnake (↑ volume but one to two orders of magnitude less toxic than those indicated as ↑ toxicity) > tiger snake (↑ volume and ↑ toxicity) sea snake (↑ toxicity) = Indian krait or Eastern coral snake or Australian brown snake (↑ toxicity) > puff adder and Gaboon viper and timber rattler (volumes enough to kill but lower toxicity than mamba by an order of magnitude) > mamba (not a lethal dose depending on attack and number of bites, but still quite toxic) > cottonmouth moccasin = American copperhead

(2) Lacertilia (lizards)

(a) Gila monster and beaded lizard make helokinestatins 1–6 (bradykinin antagonist peptides) which cause hypotension (led to development of angiotensin-converting enzyme inhibitors)

CONCEPTUALIZING TOXICOLOGY 30-1 (*continued*)

b. Eumetazoa: Bilateria: Ecdysozoa: Arthropod

(1) Spiders and scorpions (Arachnida)

(a) Brown recluse spiders cause extensive skin necrosis through activity of sphingomyelinase D (phospholipases-D) + other venom constituents which are neurotoxic, metalloproteinases, serine-proteases, lectin-like molecules, translationally controlled tumor protein, etc.

(b) Scorpions release tityustoxin, hemicalcin, and a complex mixture of basic proteins → skin necrosis, bullae, and multisystem failure (↑ venom). The *Buthidae* produce the most toxic venom containing hyaluronidase (neurotoxic). Presence of disulfide bonds and lysine residues in the small basic protein are central to the toxin's biologic activity → ↑ Na^+ permeability and potentiates ACh release from motoneurons and postganglionic autonomic neurons

(c) Brazilian tarantula releases diverse low MW compounds, acylpolyamines, linear peptides, cysteine-knotted mini-proteins, neurotoxic proteins, and enzymes

(d) Most African and South American spiders cause phases of reaction: activate primary sensory neurons followed by afferent input and central sensitization of the dorsal horn via transient receptor potential ankyrin-1 receptors and inflammatory cytokines, eicosanoids and NO

(e) Tarantula spiders work via activating tetrodotoxin-resistant Na^+ channels → cardiac arrest. Conversely, dialyzed *P. nigriventer* (wandering spider) venom → ↑ heart rate, while whole venom of this species had the opposite effect (neurotoxins alter Na^+ activity = sympathetic, while biogenic amines have parasympathetic effects)

(f) Black widow spider produces a 5 K MW protein → explosive release of neurotransmitter (ACh), which then depletes nerve terminal and swelling ensues → failure of neuromuscular transmission

(g) Ticks and mites activate IgE-driven T_H2 skin reactions

(2) Millipedes and centipedes (*Myriapoda*)

(a) Centipede bites are myotoxic, cardiotoxic, and neurotoxic due to metalloproteinases

(b) Millipedes cause erythema and hyperpigmentation due to cyanide and quinones

(3) Insecta

(a) Caterpillars—toxic and painful venom delivered by setae from puss slug caterpillars and giant silkworm moth caterpillars

(b) True bugs—stylets deliver toxic and painful venom from assassin bugs

(c) Bees and wasps—sting = most toxic venoms of insects. Harvester ants (leads toxic list), velvet ants, bees, yellowjackets, and hornets deliver toxic and painful venoms. Key honeybee toxin = melittin, a cationic polypeptide, that is hemolytic, cardiotoxic, and myotoxic. Membrane damage accounts for majority of bee venom's effects other than anaphylaxis in sensitized individuals

(d) Activities of insect venoms (neurotoxic, hemolytic, digestive, hemorrhagic, and pain-producing) due to components including alkaloids, biogenic amines, polysaccharides, organic acids (formic), amino acids, and peptides and proteins similar to other venomous species

c. Chordata: Craniata

(1) Scorpionfish is most toxic of the Scorpaenidae—venom delivery through 1–17 dorsal, 3 anal, and 2 pelvic fin spines that causes hemorrhaging, hemolysis, and proteolysis and ↓ blood pressure via Sp-CTx protein (cytolytic/hemolytic and vasodilatory). Fresh venom also affects mean arterial pressure (coronary vasoconstriction) and heart rate (positive chronotropic, lusitropic [conduction system], and inotropic effects). Stonefish (*Synanceiidae*) antivenom prevents inflammation and ↓ cardiovascular effects to scorpionfish

CONCEPTUALIZING TOXICOLOGY 30-1 (*continued*)

    d. Lophotrochozoa: Mollusca

      (1) Cone snails use small peptides (ω-conotoxins) squeezed through barbed radula to paralyze their prey. α-Conotoxins antagonize N_M and N_N (nicotinic muscle- and neuronal-type acetylcholine) receptors. μ-Conotoxins inhibit Na^+ channels on the sarcolemma at site 1 (same site for tetrodotoxin and saxitoxin). Interestingly, the ω-conotoxins may have medical application in neuropathic pain management. The target of these toxins is the voltage-gated Ca^{2+} channels. The targeting of $Ca_v2.2$ channels that is responsible for neurotransmitter release is shared by peptides from spiders, snakes, assassin bugs, centipedes, and scorpions

    e. Eumetazoa: Cnidaria

      (1) Nematocyst venoms of jellyfish, sea anemones, corals, and sea pens contain 250 peptides, proteins, enzymes, and proteinase inhibitors as well as purines, quaternary ammonium compounds, biogenic amines, and betaines. Sea anemone toxins are primarily cytolytic (cytolysins) or neurotoxic peptides and proteins targeting voltage-gated Na^+ (preventing inactivation), K^+, and acid-sensing ion channels

      (2) A coral, *Palythoa toxica*, produces highly toxic venom displayed in Figure 30-2. Jellyfish, especially the Portuguese man-of-war, are known for toxic stings. The key hemolysin is known as physalitoxin. Another toxin found in the venom produces cardiac toxicity. It causes Ca^{2+} influx (not related to L-type or T-type Ca^{2+} channels), but is not sensitive to ouabain, vanadate, or organic Ca^{2+} channel blocker. This toxin's action is blocked by transition metals La^{2+} or Zn^{2+}. The loss of membrane integrity is reminiscent of black widow spider venom α-latrotoxin in the development of nonclosing ionic channels permeable to K^+, Na^+, and Ca^{2+}, which are not blocked by the usual Na^+ or Ca^{2+} channel blockers. Cell lysis also occurs due to the change in ion permeability. The difference between man-of-war venom and α-latrotoxin is the order of potency of block by divalent cations—$Co^{2+} > Ni^{2+} > Zn^{2+}$ for spider venom and $Zn^{2+} > Ni^{2+} = Co^{2+}$ for the man-of-war venom (note reversed order). The man-of-war toxin is also similar to the dinoflagellate *Gambierdiscus toxicus* maitotoxin as both toxins cause Ca^{2+} uptake, K^+ efflux, and Na^+ influx, with the Ca^{2+} and Na^+ movements not altered by conventional organic blocking agents. Maitotoxin also has Zn^{2+} as the most potent divalent ion in blocking the ion permeability caused by the toxin with an IC_{50} of 41 versus 34 μM for man-of-war venom. Miatoxin also lyses BC_3H_1 cells

    f. Echinodermata: Holothuroidea

      (1) Sea cucumbers will expel their viscera and Cuvierian organ containing saponins or holothurin (a lanosteroid-type triterpene glycoside that is hemolytic and cytolytic and causes contraction then relaxation of mammalian phrenic nerve preparation) when disturbed. Long, sticky, white threads adhere to offending species, weakening muscles of the enemy and potentially causing permanent blindness

    g. Chordata: Mammalia: Eutheria: Soricomorpha: Soricidae

      (1) Northern short-tailed shrew produces venom from submaxillary and sublingual glands containing lethal blarina toxin (N-linked microheterogeneous glycoprotein with tissue kallikrein-like activity). Toxin converts kininogens to kinins

  5. Venom economy

    a. Venom optimization hypothesis based on frugality of venom use. Protein-rich venom has a high metabolic cost. The larger the prey, the more resistant the prey to venom, difficult to handle prey, and repletion of venom glad will ↑ venom dose. There is also some redundancy in venom components (in the scorpion 17 different toxins target Na_v channels). Certain scorpions, spiders, or the red spitting cobra change venom composition based on number of venom releases. First venom may be far less toxic than subsequent releases

B. Poisonous animals

  1. Rely on oily substances that produce hallucinations or neurotoxic action that might be released on skin or feathers or in ovaries to insure that death will occur to prevent that prey species from consuming reproductive ability/survival of the poisonous species

CONCEPTUALIZING TOXICOLOGY 30-1 (*continued*)

2. See Table 30-2 for activity of various animal poisons

3. Toads and frogs are a good starting point as they secrete oily poisons onto their skin (aromatic amines acting as vasoconstrictors, convulsants, hallucinogens, and cholinergic agents). Some of the mass spectra of important indolealkylamines of toads are displayed in Figure 30-3. These compounds are 3Na$^+$, 2K$^+$-ATPase inhibitors, affect Na$^+$/ Ca^{2+} exchange in cardiac myocytes causing ↑ intracellular Ca2+, and cause heart failure at high concentrations. Lately, these substances have also been noted for their antitumor activities as they inhibit cell proliferation, induce differentiation, and promote apoptosis cancer cells by G$_2$/M arrest with cyclin A and B1 downregulation and decreased CDK1 protein level. Upstream regulators of CDK/cyclin such as cell division cycle (CDC)25A, CDC25B, and CDC25C all were inhibited by toad toxin bufotalin. Bufadienolides displayed in Figure 30-4 activate caspases, alter the mitochondrial membrane potential (extreme swelling of mitochondria), increase intracellular Ca^{2+}, decrease anti-apoptotic protein bcl-2, and increase pro-apoptotic protein bax expression. Akt, a factor key to cell growth and survival by phosphorylating and thereby inhibiting pro-apoptotic molecules, was also dramatically reduced by bufotalin treatment. ROS expression appears increased as well in response to this class of toad poisons

   Frogs have a variety of toxins reflecting diversity of origins. Non-lens βγ-crystallins and trefoil factor hemolyze human RBCs via membrane pore formation. Frogs also have steroid alkaloid poisons (keeping Na$^+$ channels open) with variants found in toads such as batrachotoxin displayed in Figure 30-5. This toxin's actions are reversed by tetrodotoxin or saxitoxin (from dinoflagellate). Interestingly, the Panamanian golden frog produces a guanidinium alkaloid zetekitoxin similar to saxitoxin affecting Na+ channels. Neotropical poison frogs share a lipophilic alkaloid, pumiliotoxin, which targets the voltage-sensitive Na+ channels, causing them to prolong opening similar to the effects of batrachotoxins. Many of these venoms originate from ant venoms and trail-marking alkaloids consumed by dendrobatid frogs (histrionicotoxin). Some frogs (Harlequin poison dart frog or Ecuadorean tree frog) have compounds that are strong noncompetitive antagonists to nicotinic cholinergic receptor channel complexes. Other alkaloids isolated from frog skin are monocyclic pyrrolidines and piperidines; bicyclic decahydroquinolines, pyrrolizidines, indolizidines, and quinolizidines; and tricyclic gephyrotoxins, pyrrolizidine oximes, pseudophrynamines, and coccinellines that affect ion channels. These alkaloids stored in skin glands again appear to originate from dietary consumption of small arthropods

4. Salamanders and newts have a poison also found in the infamous pufferfish. Fish and especially shellfish may consume protistans that confer toxicity to themselves

5. Origins of these poisons: Marine organisms → polyethers, macrolides, terpenes, unusual amino acids/peptides, and alkaloids. Nonmarine organisms → similar chemical classes of agents, but with notable structural differences. However, tetrodotoxin and its congeners, which include chiriquitoxin and the similarity between saxitoxin and zetekitoxin, show some similarities between marine and amphibian species. Tetrodotoxin (TTX) is found in frogs, the blue-ringed octopus, mollusks, salamanders, newts, and of course the pufferfish from which it was first isolated. TTX selectively blocks voltage-gated Na$^+$ channels. This toxin may be the result of synthesis by symbiotic microorganisms in higher taxa, rather than a marine or amphibian animal. This makes the biological classification of a toxicant difficult at best to be true to its biological origins

6. Fish poisons: Pufferfish = historic discovery of the guanidinium alkaloid tetrodotoxin in the liver, gonads, and skin, which varies based on reproductive cycle—see Figure 30-6 for structures. Toxicity by consuming fish flesh varies from Group 1 GI symptoms (slime of lampreys and hagfish, etc.); Group 2 GI and neurological symptoms (pufferfish *Tetraodon*, hypervitaminosis A from shark liver, saxitoxin from paralytic shellfish poisoning actually resulting from dinoflagellate or cyanobacteria, etc.); Group 3 GI and cardiac symptoms (Clupeotoxin from anchovies, sardines, and herring); Group 4 assorted GI, neurological, cardiac, joint, and other organ system toxicities (such as Ciguatera from a variety of fish species that really are from a photosynthetic dinoflagellate or Gymnothorax toxin from Moray eel); Group 5 anaphylactoid reactions (high histamine concentrations resulting from microbial action on poorly cooled Scombroid fish); and Group 6 hallucinations (Chimaera from ratfish, indole from surgeon fish, mullet hallucinogenic fish poisoning)

CONCEPTUALIZING TOXICOLOGY 30-1 (*continued*)

7. Poisonous bird—*Pitohui dichrous* of New Guinea has homobatrachotoxin, an amphibian toxin, in its feathers, which may be sequestered in uropygial gland through diet of Choresine beetles. *Ifrita kowaldi* contains batrachotoxinin-A *cis*-crotonate

8. Evolution of poisons and proper attribution: Botulism toxin actually is the result of a phage gene, so is not a bacterial poison per se. The toxicity of pertussis and cholera toxin involves ADP-ribosylation of different proteins, yielding different toxicities. Anthrax toxin has structure of A_s-B with the B fragment as the protective antigen and A (Zn^{2+}-dependent metalloproteinase, seen in tetanus toxin and snake venoms) representing the lethal or edema factor. Thus, the structure of toxins and their activities may be charted across organisms to discover similarities that may lead to understanding of their origins and differing modes of action that may have evolved into different toxins from an earlier form of a toxin. Cyanobacteria, one of the oldest species of organisms, produces toxins including hepatotoxins (OAT protein access to liver cells → inhibit eukaryotic protein phosphatases), neurotoxins (became the snail/dinoflagellate saxitoxin), cytotoxins, and irritant or dermatoxins

9. Dinoflagellates (photosynthetic eukaryotes) co-evolved saxitoxin ($binds to Na^+$ channel at site 1 where blocks pore, modifies K^+ channel which appears to be the original target and partially blocks Ca^{2+} channel) with cyanobacteria. Saxitoxin was designed as a grazing deterrent for zooplankton, fish, and macroinvertebrates. Brevetoxins A and B work in the Na^+ channel at site 5 to keep always activated. Ciguatoxin works at the same site to shift activation gating. Maitotoxin allows nonselective ion passage through cation channels. Azaspiracid blocks K^+ pore. Palytoxin inhibits the Na^+, K^+-ATPase. Yessotoxin affects cytoskeleton (paralysis). Ostreotoxin 3 = inactivation gating modifier. Cooliatoxin = neurotoxin associated with paralytic shellfish poisoning. See marine toxin structures in Figure 30-7

10. Diatoms (algae) are plants but are associated with amnesic shellfish poisoning via domoic acid, which works at glutamate receptors (↑ duration of influx of Na^+ and Ca^{2+})

11. Fungal poisons—see structures in Figure 30-8. Aflatoxins are mycotoxins activated by CYPs to cause liver damage and cancer (synergize with hepatitis B). Ipomeanol, a furan derivative, produces lung edema in cattle due to CYPs found in the lung (forms epoxide). Ochratoxin A → oxidative stress and DNA damage and ↓ intracellular Zn (Zn supplementation ↓ DNA strand breaks but does not help with mitochondrial membrane potential). Trichothecenes were probably developed as bactericidal and also fungicidal and insecticidal. A *Penicillium* strain produces a tubulin-binding compound that inhibits mitosis. Another fungal compound, α-amanitin, selectively inhibits eukaryotic RNA polymerase II. Another fungal compound, coprine, inhibits the low K_m form of liver acetaldehyde dehydrogenase by active metabolite cyclopropanone hydrate. Ergots affect the nervous system (hallucinations) and are vasoconstrictive and contract uterine smooth muscle continuously. Psilocybin was used by Aztecs to generate spiritual hallucinations. Zearalenone is estrogenic and produces hyperestrogenic effects, especially in pigs that eat moldy (*Fusarium*) feed

12. Bacterial poisons—see botulism, cyanobacterial, cholera, and pertussis in previous sections. Botulism heavy chain is the transport mechanism to neuronal cytoplasm by acting with luminal domain of synaptobrevin, while the light chain produces the lysis preventing ACh release. As mentioned earlier, lysogenic phage genes play a large role in the development of toxins for botulism, anthrax, tetanus, diphtheria, toxic shock, scarlet fever, exfoliative dermatitis, food poisoning, traveler's diarrhea, *Shigella* dysentery, necrotizing pneumonia, and cholera. However, *Clostridium perfringens* α-toxin is encoded by a standard chromosomal gene and can cause fatal gangrene. *Staphylococcus* pathogenicity islands encode for superantigens (15–20 kb) in toxicogenic strains; some important toxins are toxic shock syndrome toxin-1, Sags, SEK, SEL, and enterotoxins. Lipopolysaccharide is an important non-protein toxin and endotoxin that is part of the cell wall of gram-negative (double-walled) bacteria. As indicated earlier, protein toxins from bacteria have an A-B structure (A = enzyme and B = receptor-binding polypeptide). They are activated in bacteria via nicking by proteases when synthesized by bacteria or attached to membrane receptors. ↑ cAMP results due to enzymatic ADP-ribosylation of adenylyl cyclase regulatory proteins (e.g., cholera affecting GTP-regulatory protein → extreme and painful diarrhea). Diphtheria toxin inhibits protein synthesis by ADP-ribosylation of elongation factor-2 (EF-2). Most bacteria affect target cells where they bind with the exceptions of botulism and especially tetanus toxin (Zn^{2+}-dependent metalloproteinase cleaves VAMP in GABAergic and glycinergic neurons →

CONCEPTUALIZING TOXICOLOGY 30-1 (*continued*)

> muscle rigidity and spasms or "lockjaw") that move up axons and inhibit more distant structures. Cells can be resistant to incorporation of the toxin as is the case for mouse or rat cells L-929 and 3T3 and diphtheria toxin. *Shigella* toxin works through a protein exotoxin that inactivates the 60S eukaryotic ribosomal subunit → cytotoxicity, neurotoxicity, and enterotoxicity. *E. coli* toxin prevalent in the news due to meat contamination has two enterotoxins. The heat-labile enterotoxin is similar to cholera and binds to the same G_{M1}-containing receptor activating adenylyl cyclase (blocked by cholera toxin antibody), but has less activity (less violent diarrhea). The heat-stable enterotoxin stimulates guanylyl cyclase. The *Bordetella pertussis* toxin is unusual in that the B oligomer blocks the biological activity of the A-B toxin by competing for receptor occupancy. The B oligomer by itself induces mitogenic responses. The A portion by itself is not toxic, but pretreatment of the cells with the B oligomer and washing them allows the A promoter to deliver its enzymatic activity/toxicity. The pertussis toxin causes ADP-ribosylation of the G_i or N_i protein distinct from the G protein action of cholera or heat-labile *E. coli* enterotoxins

CONCEPTUALIZING TOXICOLOGY 30-1 (*continued*)

Venoms are one of the few toxicants for which injection is the normal route of administration. They are composed of a mixture that reflects the environment of the animal. For instance, rattlesnakes and copperheads (crotalids) are likely to be stepped on by an animal with a hoof and thick furry skin on its legs. This makes penetrability of the venom an issue and is reflected in the composition. Digestion may also be a quality of venoms for consumption of prey. Also, quick changes in blood pressure by polypeptides in the venom may cause immune reactions and therefore confer resistance to large animals such as humans (also the basis of production of antivenoms). Sea snakes and spitting cobras may rely more on the neurotoxicity of their venoms.

Venoms serve as a foraging adaptation in venomous groups of organisms (mammals, snakes, selected lizards, spiders, scorpions, centipedes, some insects, cephalopods). In others such as Helodermatidae lizards, the majority of venomous fishes, echinoderms, lepidopteran larvae, and other insects, venoms serve a protective adaptation. Intraspecific conflict seems to be reserved for organisms such as the platypus. Defensive venoms usually involve inflicting severe localized pain, such as occurs from bee stings and venomous fishes. Predatory venoms are far more complex. The composition of the venoms may also vary based on the degree of threat perceived by the venomous organism. A low treat for a scorpion produces a low metabolically challenging pain-inducing pre-venom, while a high threat yields a proteinaceous main venom. The actions of venoms are based on their hemotoxic versus neurotoxic properties (see **Figure 30-1**).

The hemotoxic venoms include those that cause hypotension (vasodilation by kinin-releasing activity of blarina toxin and kallikrein from short-tailed shrews or peptidase S1 toxins from toxicoferan reptiles; vasodilation by kinin-like activity of tachykinin-like peptide[s] from cephalopods and hymenopteran insects), hemorrhage (inhibition of epinephrine-induced platelet aggregation by Type III [anguimorph lizards] or Type IB [snakes] phospholipase A_2; inhibition of adenosine diphosphate [ADP]-induced platelet aggregation by snake venom metalloproteinases and Type IB or Type IIA phospholipase A_2 or by hymenopteran insects' apyrase; inhibition of collagen-induced platelet aggregation by snake venom C-type lectins and metalloproteinases; inhibition of platelet aggregation by GPIIb/IIIa receptor antagonism by snake venom disintegrins and mambin/dendroaspin; thrombin inhibition by snake venom C-type lectins, textilinins, and Type IIA phospholipase A_2), and clot formation (prothrombin activation via mechanisms such as formation of meizothrombin, promoting phospholipid and Factor Va, or just promoting phospholipid action by snake venom Factor V, Factor X, or metalloproteinases; Speijer et al., 1986).

Neurotoxins (toxins that result in nerve or neuromuscular action that causes paralysis, pain, and/or death) modulate the Na^+ channel (block by cone snails μ- or μ-O-conotoxins,

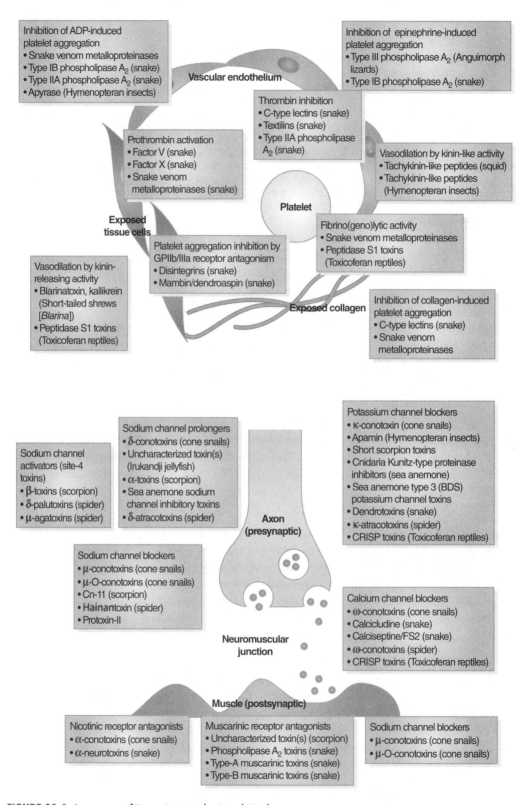

FIGURE 30-1 Convergence of Venom Action in the Animal Kingdom

scorpions Cn-11, and spider hainantoxin-1 or protoxin-II; activation at site 4 by scorpion β-toxins and spider δ-palutoxins or μ-agatoxins; prolongation by cone snail δ-conotoxins (site 6 on Na^+ channel), Irukandji syndrome jellyfish uncharacterized toxin, scorpion α-toxins, sea anemone Na^+ channel inhibitory toxins, and spider δ-atracotoxins), block the K^+ channel (cone snail κ-conotoxin, hymenopteran insect apamin, short scorpion toxins, Cnidaria Kunitz-type proteinase inhibitors, sea anemone type 3 [BDS] K^+ channel toxins, snake venom dendrotoxins, spider κ-atracotoxins, and toxicoferan reptile CRISP toxins), block the Ca^{2+} channel (cone snail ù-conotoxins, snake venom calcicludine and calciseptine/FS2, spider ω-neurotoxins, and toxicoferan reptile toxins), antagonize nicotinic cholinergic receptors (snake venom α-neurotoxins and cone snail α-conotoxins), and/or antagonize muscarinic cholinergic receptors (scorpion uncharacterized toxin[s], snake venom phospholipase A_2 toxins, and type-A and type-B muscarinic toxins; Casewell et al., 2013).

Analysis of the molecular evolution of cysteine-rich secretory (glyco)proteins (CRISPs— exclusive vertebrate protein with activities in mammalian reproduction and reptilian venom) compared nonvenomous mammalian CRISPs with those found in toxicoferan reptiles. The CRISP gene in reptiles was significantly influenced by positive selection in snakes ($\omega = 3.84$) more than in lizards ($\omega = 2.33$). Mammalian CRISPs were oppositely selected (strong negative selection; CRISP1 = 0.55, CRISP2 = 0.40, and CRISP3 = 0.68). The most pertinent of portion of this study (Sunagar et al., 2012) to this discussion is how the evolution of the toxicoferan reptiles differed by specific predatory mechanism employed by the venomous organism. CRISPs in Elapidae have undergone less selection pressure ($\omega = 2.86$) compared with the colubrids ($\omega = 4.10$). This may reflect the use of neurotoxins by the elapids versus grip and constriction to kill their prey. The Viperidae have similar high positive selection pressure on the molecular evolution of their CRISPS ($\omega = 4.19$), as they rely on their hemotoxins to disable and capture their prey. Anguimorph lizards have lower positive pressure to modify their CRISPs ($\omega = 2.33$) than snakes ($\omega = 3.84$), which may indicate their use

of pace and powerful jaws rather than relying on metabolically costly venom to attack their prey (Sunagar et al., 2012).

Poisonous animals such as amphibians and birds rely on oily substances that may quickly tell an animal via hallucinations or neurotoxic action in the oral cavity that this animal should not be eaten but spit out. Otherwise, poisons may reside in the ovaries to insure that the predatory animal will not consume more of the species trying to protect itself with the poison, or other animals may note the toxicity experienced by another predator and avoid eating the poisonous animal. This chapter also examine poisonous Protista up to complex organisms and the chemical structures of the poisons to indicate how these toxins are synthesized by biological organisms that have resistance to their own venoms or poisons.

Chordata: Amniota: Reptilia: Squamata Venoms

Reptiles are often the first class of animals that laypersons consider as being venomous. Much is known of reptile venoms, as they have been the source of human concern even in literature and in recent history the development of antivenoms. Venomous lizards and snakes (suborder Serpentes) fall under the order Squamata.

Serpentes (Snake) Venoms

Table 30-1 lists the venoms by toxicity while the descriptions in this chapter list by species. Snake venoms are the usual toxic mixture people would think of first as having toxic or lethal consequences depending on the snake such as the mamba, cobra, or rattlesnake. The Crotalids (rattlesnakes, copperheads) are usually known for their hemotoxic effects, while the Elapids such as the coral snakes (*Micrurus*), cobras (*Naja*), kraits (*Bungarus*), and mambas are known for the neurotoxicity of their venoms. Even if a person survives the systemic action of the snake venom, permanent tissue damage is associated with the site of the bite. Snake venom metalloproteinase, hyaluronidase, and myotoxic phospholipase A_2 are the key factors

TABLE 30-1　Toxicity of Venoms

Toxicity	Venom Toxins	Toxic Mechanism
Neuromuscular	Saponins—sea cucumber	Muscles less responsive
	Cone snail μ-conotoxins, scorpion Cn-11, spider haniantoxin-1 and protoxin-II	Na$^+$ channel block
	Scorpion β-toxins, spider δ-palutoxins or μ-agatoxins	Na$^+$ channel activation
	Cone snail δ-conotoxins, Irukandji syndrome jellyfish uncharacterized toxin, scorpion α-toxins, sea anemone Na$^+$ channel inhibitory toxins, spider δ-atracotoxins	Na$^+$ channel prolongation
	Cone snail κ-conotoxins, hymenopteran insects apamin, short scorpion toxins, Cnidaria Kunitz-type proteinase inhibitors, sea anemone type 3 (BDS) K$^+$ channel toxins, snake venom dendrotoxins, spider κ-atracotoxins, toxicoferan reptile CRISP toxins	K$^+$ channel block
	Cone snail ω-conotoxins, snake venom calcicludine and calciseptine/FS2, spider ω-neurotoxins, toxicoferan reptile CRISP toxins	Inhibit Ca^{2+} channel
	Snake venom α-neurotoxins, cone snail α-conotoxins	Antagonism of nicotinic (N$_M$ and N$_N$) receptors
	Scorpion uncharacterized toxin(s), snake venom phospholipase A$_2$ toxins and type-A and type-B muscarinic toxins	Antagonism of muscarinic (M) receptors
Neurotoxicity/cellular potentials	Coral palytoxin	Potent inhibitor of 3Na$^+$, 2K$^+$-ATPase
Neurotoxicity— neurotransmitter release	Black widow spider—latrotoxin	Presynaptic action causing explosive neurotransmitter release
Tissue necrosis and extracellular matrix degradation	Snake venom metalloproteinase (and centipede), hyaluronidase, and myotoxic phospholipase A$_2$, brown recluse spider phospholipases-D	Tissue digestion/degradation—can also be myotoxic, cardiotoxic, and neurotoxic Necrosis and edema → renal failure + hematological reactions
Apoptosis and necrosis	L-amino acid oxidase from all snake venoms, some fungi, and marine species	ROS formation
Physical damage and pain	Spider venoms (selected)	Transient receptor potential ankyrin-1 receptors
Inflammation	Spider venoms	Cytokines, eicosanoids, NO release
Cardiac toxicity	Spider venoms (selected)—parasympathomimetic	TTX-resistant Na$^+$ channel changes and/or ACh release and/or direct cholinergic activity (biogenic amines) leading to bradycardia and less contraction force
	Spider venoms (selected)—sympathomimetic	Fraction left after dialysis alters Na$^+$ channel in opposite way to increase heart rate and contraction force

TABLE 30-1   Toxicity of Venoms (*continued*)

Toxicity	Venom Toxins	Toxic Mechanism
Cardiac toxicity (*continued*)	Jellyfish	Na$^+$ channel effects yield high catecholamine release and cardiovascular stress — hypertension and cardiomyopathy
	Snake (elapid)	Irreversible depolarization
Changes in blood pressure	Jellyfish	Hypertension from Na$^+$ channel alterations
	Short-tailed shrews — blarina toxin, kallikrein Toxicoferan reptiles — peptidase S1 toxins	Hypotension from kinin-releasing activity
	Hymenopteran insects and cephalopods — tachykinin-like peptides	Hypotension from kinin-like activity
	Scorpionfish and stone fish	Cardiovascular Sp-CTx
	Stiletto snake venom endothelin-like sarafotoxins	Severe vasoconstriction of coronary arteries
	Green mamba (*Dendroaspis*) natriuretic peptide	Activates guanylate cyclase
	Viperid snakes VEGF-F	Hypotension and proliferation of vascular endothelial cells
Hemorrhage	Anguimorph lizards — Type III phospholipase A$_2$ Snakes — Type IB phospholipase A$_2$	Inhibition of epinephrine-induced platelet aggregation
	Snake venom — metalloproteinases and Type IB or Type IIA phospholipase A$_2$	Inhibition of ADP-induced platelet aggregation
	Hymenopteran insects — apyrase	
	Snake venom — C-type lectins, metalloproteinases	Inhibition of collagen-induced platelet aggregation
	Snake venom — disintegrins, mambin/ dendroaspin	Inhibition of platelet aggregation by GPIIb/IIIa antagonism
	Snake venom — C-type lectins, textilinins, Type IIA phospholipase A$_2$	Thrombin inhibition
	Snake venom — metalloproteinases and peptidase S1 toxins	Fibrino(geno)lytic activity
	Japanese pit viper	Binds factor IX/factor X-binding protein
Hemolytic anemia	Brown recluse spider	Venom "lytic" enzymes
	Scorpionfish and stone fish	Cytolytic Sp-CTx
	Holothurians/saponins from sea cucumber	Cytolytic
Blood clot formation	Snake venom — Factor V and X and metalloproteinases	Prothrombin activation
	Neotropical snake venom convulxin	Collagen receptor binding causing platelet aggregation
Renal failure	Snake venom crotoxin	Acute tubular necrosis
Membrane ion channels and cytolysis	Man-of-war jellyfish, black widow spider, and bee venoms	Changes in membrane permeability to ions by forming channels and cytolysis that may be by same (jellyfish) or different mechanisms (bee)

for inducing tissue necrosis and extracellular matrix degradation. Even though antivenoms may prevent mortality, tissue necrosis and extracellular matrix degradation continue despite the antidote. Plant secondary metabolites of snake venoms with anti-ophidian (anti-snake) properties are being used to elicit antibodies (Santhosh et al., 2013).

Peptides of snake venom are not only toxic to humans but also have insecticidal activity that may make for a promising new class of pesticide (Smith et al., 2013). The categories of non-enzymatic snake venom proteins are three-finger toxins, proteinase inhibitors, snaclecs (snake C-type lectins and related proteins), nerve growth factors, bradykinin-potentiating peptides, natriuretic peptides, cysteine-rich secretory proteins (CRISPs) or helveprins, sarafotoxins, cobra venom factors, vascular endothelial growth factors (VEGFs), waprins, vespryns, and veficolins. These compounds are not only toxic, but also have pharmaceutical and physiological research activities shedding light on the mechanism involved in ion channel function (green mamba venom dendrotoxin–blocking specific voltage-gated K^+ channels and prolonged release of acetylcholine [ACh]; Australian elapid *Pseudechis australis* produces pseudechetoxin, which is a member of CRISPs and blocks cyclic nucleotide-gated channels, high conductance Ca^{2+}-activated channels, and possibly L-type Ca^{2+}-channels, which appear to be involved in smooth muscle contraction and inflammation), vasoconstriction (stiletto snake sarafotoxins = strong vasoconstriction coronary vessels and similar to endothelins), blood vessel growth (VEGFs from *Vipera ammodytes ammodytes* and *Daboia russelli* venoms), complement system activity (cobra venom factor activates complement cascade similar to human C3b), platelet aggregation, blood coagulation (coagulation due to Neotropical rattlesnake binding to collagen receptor; detection of the absence of von Willebrand factor in a hereditary blood coagulation abnormality by botrocetin, a South American snake snaclec coagglutinin; anticoagulant effects of Japanese pit viper, *Protobothrops flavoviridis*, and binding to/inhibition of factor IX/factor X-binding protein), signal transduction (nerve growth factor in cottonmouth

snake venom), and blood pressure regulation (extreme vasodilation due to activation of guanylate cyclase by green mamba natriuretic peptide; bradykinin-potentiation peptides first recognized in Brazilian pit viper venom made possible antihypertensive medications ramipril, captopril, enalapril, lisinopril, and perindopril; hypotension and vascular endothelial cell proliferation by VEGF-F from viperid snakes; McCleary and Kini, 2013).

Neurotoxic venoms were isolated from snake venom in the early 1960s and classified as peptides by zone electrophoresis as α-, β-, and γ-bungarotoxin from the many-braided krait. Because these agents are really d-tubocurarine/curare-mimicking agents (postsynaptic block of acetylcholine at the motor end plate), they have been reclassified as α-neurotoxins (classic neurotoxic venomous snakes such as the elapid, hydrophid, and "harmless" colubrid). The alpha refers to the antagonism at the nicotinic subclass of cholinergic receptors. There is a suggestion that the family of snake then be included in the naming of the toxin such as elapitoxin for Elapidae family followed by two letters such as Aa for *Acanthophis antarcticus*. Then a number system should be employed to note short chain α-neurotoxin (number 1) of a long-chain α-neurotoxin (number 2) or a κ-neurotoxin (number 3). The chick biventer cervicis nerve-muscle preparation screens well between presynaptic β-neurotoxins and postsynaptic α-neurotoxins. Elapids have three-fingered toxins (flat molecules with small hydrophobic core with four disulfide bridges/bonds with three adjacent loops of "fingers" that are crossed by five anti-parallel β-strands creating a large β-pleated sheet) that characterize their α-neurotoxins in their venoms. The short-chain α-neurotoxins have a molecular weight (MW) of 6–7 kDa and usually inhibit nerve-mediated twitch responses in the chick biventer preparation with 30 min at 1 µM with high variability in reversibility of this effect. Long-chain neurotoxins consist of 66–75 amino acids with an MW of 7–9 kDa and contain five disulfide bridges. ACh must be able to bind to two portions (between subunits δ–α and α–ε) of its receptor ($[\alpha_1]_2\beta1\delta\varepsilon$ stoichiometry for the adult receptor) for activating the nicotinic receptor (nAChR). Prior to binding to the nAChR, α-neurotoxins' positively charged "head" region binds with the lipid bilayer close to the receptor. Hydrogen bonds form between polar head groups of the phospholipid bilayer and the hydrophilic, positively charged side chains of the head region residues of the short-chain α-neurotoxin II from *Naja oxiana*. This results in a positioning of loop II of the neurotoxin by the nAChR binding site. Both short- and long-chain neurotoxins bind to the N_M receptor, while only long-chain α-neurotoxins bind with high affinity for the N_N receptor (Barber et al., 2013).

Cobra venoms are neurotoxic also due to the irreversible binding of the small (7,000 molecular weight) basic polypeptide to postsynaptic cholinergic receptors (slow-acting neuromuscular blocking agent leading to drooping of eyelids, flaccid paralysis, and neck flexor weakness progressing to respiratory failure; Hodgson, 2012). Cardiotoxins are also present in the cobra with nonenzymatic polypeptides with 6,000–7,000 MW that produce their effects by causing irreversible depolarization of the cell membrane. Sea snakes and kraits have neurotoxic peptides of ~11,000 MW that work presynaptically as phospholipase A_2 to produce a neuromuscular block. This same enzyme activity also has direct hemolytic, anticoagulant, myonecrotic, or hemorrhaging activities. Venoms also contain arginine ester hydrolases that are thrombin-like enzymes that lead to defibrination syndrome *in vivo* or induce release of bradykinin. Hyaluronidase helps the venom spread after the bite. Protease activity may yield hemorrhage or edema. Other enzymes such as acetylcholinesterase, phosphodiesterase, and 5′-nucleotidase also add to the venom's overall toxicity (Tan, 2005). Mambas produce one of the most toxic venoms with α-dendrotoxin being a specific blocking agent of a group of voltage-gated K^+ channels, while producing convulsions by increasing glutamate release in the brain. *Dendroaspis* venom additionally has a natural peptide inhibitor of acetylcholinesterase known as fasciculin and protein toxins that agonize the muscarinic cholinergic receptors (Hodgson, 2012). In contrast, the three-finger peptide in mamba venom produces analgesia by inhibiting the acid-sensing ion channels in the peripheral and central

nervous systems without respiratory depression and may have pharmacologic potential in treating diabetic neuropathy, which appears to result from post-translational (methylglyoxal-induced) alterations in Nav1.8, a voltage-gated Na^+ channel expressed only in pain fibers (Woolf, 2013).

One component found in all snake venoms and also in microscopic fungi and certain marine species is L-amino acid oxidase (LAAO). LAAO has antibacterial, antifungal, antiprotozoal, and antiviral activities along with an uncertain action on platelet aggregation. As its name suggests, LAAO reduces all L-amino acid content of exposed animals and forms H_2O_2. Reactive oxygen species (ROS) generated from the hydrogen peroxide stimulate apoptotic and necrotic signaling pathways. Local hydrogen peroxide concentrations are high as LAAO has carbohydrate moieties that attach to the cell's surface (Lukasheva et al., 2012).

Moving away from the more neurotoxic venoms, the Malayan pit viper (*Calloselasma rhodostoma*) is closer to the rattlesnake in that it is known for its hemorrhagic properties (potent thrombin-like enzyme and moderate hemorrhagic activities). This viper has thrombin-like enzymes, hemorrhagins (the major one is rhodostoxin in this species; hemorrhagins are generally metalloproteinases that cleave collagenous basement membrane thereby weakening blood vessel walls), platelet aggregation inducers (aggretin = nonenzymatic protein producing thrombocytopenic syndrome), platelet aggregation inhibitors/disintegrins, fibrinogenase, LAAO, proteases, phospholipase A_2 enzymes, and arginine esterases. The systemic bleeding occurring from this viper's venom is probably due to the thrombocytopenia enhanced by defibrination syndrome. The swelling, hemorrhage, and necrosis may be a result of the actions of the hemorrhagins and edema-producing elements including the autopharmacologic (have pharmacologic activities in the body such as occurs with autacoids or hormones) actions of the venom. The drop in blood pressure leads to shock due to loss of blood (hypovolemia) and bradykinin release (autopharmacologic action; Tan, 2005).

Rattlesnake venom targets the lung via numerous agents that increase vascular permeability (pulmonary congestion and hemorrhage) and hemolysis. Localized bleeding, intense pain, edema that is superficial but quickly develops, and development of hemorrhagic blistering are noted symptoms of Crotalidae bites (fang marks obvious to the eye; Hodgson, 2012). Although the rattlesnake is usually considered hemorrhagic, crotoxin and crotamine (myonecrotic toxin targeting voltage-sensitive Na$^+$ channels; Marcussi et al., 2011) are neurotoxic components of the Neotropical rattlesnake, *Crotalus durissus terrificus*. However, the venom of this rattlesnake produced convulsions and changes in breathing patterns not explained by its neurotoxic components. Convulxin isolated from this venom caused vocalizations in dogs and changes in breathing patterns. It is a C-type lectin and causes platelet aggregation in mammalian prey by binding and clustering to p62/GPVI collagen receptor (McCleary and Kini, 2013). Crotoxin (composed of a nonenzymatic acidic component A and a basic phospholipase A$_2$ activity component B has presynaptic β-neurotoxicity along with myalgic symptoms, coagulation disturbances, and often kidney failure with acute tubular necrosis; Calvete et al., 2010) and crotapotin also cause significant DNA damage as indicated by micronucleus and comet assays. Crotoxin alone is cytotoxic to several human and murine tumor cell lines. Crotoxin and crotamine also have bactericidal, anti-HIV, analgesic, and antitumor activities (Marcussi et al., 2011).

To compare snake venom toxicity, it is necessary to consider both the venom amount delivered per bite (and number of bites) and the lethal human dose. The cobra delivers about 3–19 times the amount of venom needed to kill a human (15–350 mg venom; 18–45 mg lethal human dose). Sea snake venom is more toxic, but less venom is delivered (1–15 mg venom; 2–4 mg lethal human dose). The Indian krait is similar to the sea snake (8–20 mg venom, 3 mg lethal human dose), as is the Eastern coral snake (3–5 mg venom, 4 mg lethal human dose) or the Australian brown snake (5–10 mg venom, 3 mg lethal human dose). The tiger snake delivers much more venom than it needs to kill a person similar to the cobra, but is similar in lethal dose to the sea snake or the Indian krait (35–65 mg

venom, 3 mg human lethal dose). Mambas may not deliver enough to kill a human or may exceed the dose significantly, so are dependent on species and severity of the attack (6–100 mg venom, 12–15 mg human lethal dose). The puff adder needs to deliver much more venom to be lethal, but just exceeds the dose for humans (160–200 mg venom, 95 mg human lethal dose). The Gaboon viper is similarly grouped as requiring an order of magnitude higher venom than the more neurotoxic species of snakes (450–600 mg venom, human lethal dose may be ~180 mg). The American copperhead also has to deliver ~100 mg to be lethal to humans, but rarely achieves that in the first bite (40–70 mg venom). The cottonmouth moccasin similarly is close to the lethal dose depending on the size of its victim and the severity of the attack (100–150 mg venom, 125 mg human lethal dose). The rattlesnakes have the Mojave as the most toxic based on lethal human dose (50–90 mg venom, 15 mg human lethal dose); however, the Eastern diamondback significantly delivers the most venom (400–700 mg venom, human lethal dose 100 mg). The Western diamondback rattlesnake (200–300 mg venom, 100 mg human lethal dose) and the timber rattler (100–150 mg venom, 75 mg human lethal dose) are in between. It does appear, however, that the hemotoxic species must deliver more venom to achieve lethality than the neurotoxic snakes (Cobra Master, 1994).

Lacertilia (Lizards) Venoms

The Gila monster (*Heloderma suspectum*) and the beaded lizard (*Heloderma horridum*) make helokinestatins 1–6, which are a family of bradykinin antagonist peptides from venoms of the Gila monster and the Mexican beaded lizard. They are classed into bradykinin-potentiating peptides similar to that of the venom of the snake known as the South American arrowhead viper (*Bothrops jararaca*) and were lead agents in the development of angiotensin-converting enzyme (ACE) inhibitors used in the treatment of hypertension. Two novel tridecapeptides have been isolated from the Gila monster's venom: helokinestatin-7S (FDDDSTELILEPR—1550 Da) and helokinestatin-7H (FDDDSRKLILEPR—1604 Da). A synthetic replicate of helokinestatin-7H had no physiological activity on rat arterial smooth muscle by itself, but did antagonize the vasodilatory effects of bradykinin. However, a synthetic replicate of helokinestatin-7S had the opposite vasoconstrictive action (Ma et al., 2012).

Eumetazoa: Bilateria: Ecdysozoa: Arthropod Venoms

These organisms have an exoskeleton. The subphylum Chelicerata covers the Arachnida (spiders, scorpions), Merostomata, and Pycnogonoda. Myriapoda involves the centipedes and millipedes, Crustacea the shrimp, and Hexapoda the insects including wingless organisms. Spiders (eight legs vs. insects that have six legs) are usually the next species people consider when they think of venomous creatures. However, centipedes (Chilopoda), millipedes (Diplopoda), and Arachnida (spiders and scorpions) cause tissue injury at the very least at the dermatological level through bites, stings, and the release of toxins. Ticks and mites are more known for being vectors of disease such as Lyme disease. Centipede bites elicit pain and erythema through release of metalloproteinases. These metalloproteinases are myotoxic, cardiotoxic, and neurotoxic. Tarantulas use the capsaicin receptor to cause pain. Dermatitis and conjunctivitis may result from allergic reactions to tarantula contact with body bristles. Cyanide and quinones of millipedes cause erythema and hyperpigmentation. Loxoscelism (extensive skin necrosis) through the activity of sphingomyelinase D is characteristic of the brown recluse spider bite. Scorpions via release of tityustoxin, hemicalcin, and a complex mixture of basic proteins can cause skin necrosis, bullae, and in severe envenomation can result in multisystem failure. Tick bites or burrowing mites activate IgE-driven T_H2 skin reactions (erythema, edema, papules, pruritus; Haddad et al., 2012).

The Brazilian tarantula *Acanthoscurria paulensis* has a diverse mixture of low-molecular-weight mass compounds (16% of venom compounds), acylpolyamines (11%), linear peptides (6%), cysteine-knotted mini-proteins (60%), neurotoxic proteins (1%), and enzymes (6%). Different assays were used to assess nociception (pain; mouse model; Le Bars et al., 2001), edema (rat hindpaw intradermal injection; Mortari et al., 2012), and cardiotoxicity (*in situ* frog heart; Schwartz et al., 1999; and isolated ventricle strip; Mourão et al., 2013). Chromatographic analysis yielded 97 distinct components of the venom with molecular masses between 601.4 and 21,932.3 Da (Mourão et al., 2013). This tarantula venom did not show a pain response but did yield a dose-dependent edematous activity in the rat hind-paw. The effects of the venom overall were hypoactivity, anuria, constipation, dyspnea, and prostration and ultimately death. The interesting part was the diastolic arrest caused by the venom on the *in situ* frog heart preparation. This arrest was similar to a high dose of acetylcholine in the same preparation. Atropine (a muscarinic cholinergic receptor antagonist) blocked the arrest (negative chronotropic effect) and the negative inotropic effect (decreased contraction strength) of the venom on the heart. Only the low-molecular-mass fraction had these cardiotoxic effects that were antagonized by atropine, but not the proteinaceous portion of that fraction. For this spider, it was not clear whether the low-molecular-weight fraction caused ACh to be released or worked as a cholinergic agent. Other spiders may induce mild to severe pain, itching, and increased sensitivity including possible muscle spasms. The pain from other spiders appears to be due to a combined effect of mechanical damage due to large chelicerae, low pH of the venom (~5), and the presence of the biogenic amines serotonin and histamine in the venom along with adenosine and adenosine triphosphate (ATP). Deaths in mice from 55 spider venoms seemed to vary between 3 minutes and 2 hours including rigid or flaccid paralysis, piloerection, lacrimation, excessive salivation, hyperextension of the tail, and seizure. Asian and African spider species appear to be more toxic, as are arboreal species such as *Heteroscodra*, *Poecilotheria*, and *Stromatopelma*. Twelve of the South American species such as *Acanthoscurria* species and *Grammostola spatulata* led to mouse deaths in < 30 minutes. Most of the Theraphosidae spider bites involve severe pain. The first phase involves direct activation of the primary sensory neurons. The second phase combines afferent input and central sensitization of the dorsal horn. Both of these phases involve the transient receptor potential ankyrin-1 receptors. The second phase also involves inflammatory cytokines such as IL-1β, IL-6, IL-8, and TNF-α as well as eicosanoids and NO. The *Lasiodora* species of tarantula spiders appears to work via activating tetrodotoxin (TTX; see pufferfish under poisonous fish)-resistant Na$^+$ channels as indicated by (1) dose-dependent bradycardia (slowing of the heart), transient cardiac arrest, and arrhythmia enhanced by anticholinesterase medications and ameliorated by atropine; (2) inhibition of these heart disturbances by an inhibitor of ACh transport; and (3) cardiotoxic effects unchanged by tetrodotoxin (see pufferfish under poisonous fish). Conversely, dialyzed *P. nigriventer* (wandering spider) venom increased heart rate (positive chronotropic effect) and contraction strength and was inhibited by β-adrenergic antagonists and synergized by atropine. Whole venom by this species had the opposite effect. The sympathetic effects are likely the product of neurotoxins that alter Na$^+$ channel activity, while the parasympathetic effects eliminated by dialysis were likely biogenic amines (Mourão et al., 2013).

The brown recluse spider or *Loxosceles reclusa* is part of the brown spider genus. This spider is known for its necrosis-inducing factors rather than neurotoxins. Phospholipases-D (sphingomyelinase D) causes dermonecrosis, lipid hydrolysis, hemolysis, *in vitro* platelet aggregation, infiltration of inflammatory cells, edema, renal disturbances, cytokine activation, *in vitro* cytotoxicity, and lethality. This factor alone describes the bite proceeding from a cutaneous lesion to a necrotizing wound that appears dark, blue-violet in color and becomes indurated (hardened by increase in fibrous elements). Scar tissue forms as a result of these factors. There is also erythema and edema surrounding the lesion. When the venom reaches the systemic circulation, fever, weakness, vomiting, pruritic reactions, kidney failure, thrombocytopenia, disseminating intravascular coagulation, and hemolytic anemia may occur. Insecticidal peptides from LiTx family members and Magi

3-related peptides may cause flaccid paralysis to *S. frugiperda*, and affect Na$^+$ channels. Astacin-like metalloproteinases act on gelatin, fibronectin, fibrinogen, and entactin. Hyaluronidases (endo-beta-N-acetyl-d-hexosaminidases hydrolases) act on hyaluronic acid and chondroitin sulfate. Serine-proteases have gelatinolytic activity and are activated by trypsin *in vitro*. Serine/cysteine protease inhibitors appear to be related to coagulation processes, fibrinolysis, and inflammation. Translationally controlled tumor protein may promote histamine release in the extracellular environment and affect embryonic development, cell proliferation, and stabilization of microtubules. Lectin-like molecules bind carbohydrates, alter extracellular matrix organization, promote endocytosis, and activate complement. Alkaline phosphatase is a venom enzyme that mimics the activity of a liver enzyme. ATPase causes ATP hydrolysis. Neurotoxic and non-neurotoxic peptides, polyamines, and other components of brown recluse spider venom have not been studied sufficiently to characterize their effects (Chaim et al., 2011).

The black widow spider or *Lactrodectus mactans* produces a 5 K molecular weight protein that accumulates in the central and peripheral nervous systems and results in explosive release of neurotransmitter (ACh) followed by depletion of vesicles and swelling of nerve terminal with failure of neuromuscular transmission. Small animals and children may experience a life-threatening reaction. However, for adult humans the symptoms and severe pain, restlessness, irritability, tremors, superficial breathing, tachycardia, and hypertension usually occur.

The Scorpionidae have painful stings, and the most toxic are the family Buthidae. This family of scorpions has complex venom containing hyaluronidase components that are neurotoxic. The presence of disulfide bonds and lysine residues in the small basic protein are central to the toxin's biologic activity. This scorpion toxin increases axonal Na$^+$ permeability and potentiates acetylcholine release from motor neurons and postganglionic autonomic neurons. Toxicity is characterized by local inflammation, pain, restlessness, malaise, sympathetic discharge, cardiac arrhythmias, and respiratory arrest/death in severe cases (Hodgson, 2012).

Insecta Venoms

Most people are aware of allergies to bee stings, but do not normally think of insects as having venom. Venomous insects can be of the orders Lepidoptera (caterpillars), Hemiptera (true bugs), and Hymenoptera (bees and wasps). Bees and wasps deliver venom via a sting apparatus, Hemiptera via stylets, and passively via modified setae in Lepidoptera that break and pierce the surface of the receiving organism (in this case caterpillars are the example). Other orders such as Diptera (true flies), Neuroptera (net-winged insects), and Coleoptera (beetles) have also been classified in the past as having oral venoms, but these insects may not have true venoms as they just might be ejecting digestive fluid. Classification of venoms is based on their biologic activities such neurotoxic, hemolytic, digestive, hemorrhagic, and allogeneic or pain-producing similar to snakes or other venomous animals. The chemical composition of alkaloids, biogenic amines, polysaccharides, organic acids such as formic acid, amino acids, and mainly peptides and proteins is also similar to other venomous species. The death of King Menes of Egypt in the 26th century BCE is the earliest account of a toxic (lethal) response to envenomation by a wasp or hornet.

Some of the most toxic or painful venoms come from harvester ants (*Pogonomyrmex*; Hymenoptera: Formicidae), bees (Hymenoptera: Apidae), yellowjackets and hornets (*Vespula*, *Dolichovespula*; Hymenoptera: Vespidae), velvet ants (Hymenoptera: Mutillidae*)*, puss caterpillars (*Megalopyge opercularis*; Lepidoptera: Megalopygidae), slug caterpillars (*Acharia stimulea*; Lepidoptera: Limacodidae), giant silkworm moth caterpillars (*Lonomia* sp. and *Automeris io*; Lepidoptera: Saturniidae), and assassin bugs (*Rasahus* sp.; Hemiptera: Reduviidae). However, based on the lethal dose (LD_{50}), the Hymenopteran insects have the most toxic venoms. Of those, the harvester ant, *Pogonomyrmex maricopa*, leads the list with the lowest LD_{50} (0.12 mg/kg) in a mouse (6 stings for a 1-kg animal = LD_{50}). A predator of this insect species, the lizard *Phrynosoma cornutum* has a much higher LD_{50} of 162 mg/kg, so one must be careful when talking about relative toxicity of venoms or susceptibility by species to venoms (Meyer, 1996). The honeybee (European or Africanized honey bee; *Apis mellifera*) venom is a mixture of melittin, phospholipase A_2, apamin, and hyaluronidase. Melittin is the key component and as a cationic polypeptide exhibits cytotoxic effects such as hemolysis, cardiotoxicity, and myotoxicity. This agent synergizes with phospholipase A_2 to lyse biological membranes composed of phospholipids. Suramin, a polyanion polysulfonated naphthylurea derivative prevented the lethality of the bee venom and protected all membranes, which eliminated the edema, vascular permeability, cultured endothelial cell lesion, and myotoxicity (sarcolemma protected indicated by rate of creatine kinase release), and inhibited the activity of venom phospholipase A_2. This indicates that membrane damage can account for the majority of bee venom's effects other than anaphylactic/allergic reactions that may occur in sensitized individuals (El-Kik et al., 2013).

Chordata: Craniata Venoms

Fish include all gill-bearing craniate animals that lack limbs with digits. The classes of fish are Agnatha (jawless fish including hagfish and lampreys), Chondrichthyes (cartilaginous fish such as the sharks and rays), Placodermi (armored fish), Acanthodii (so-called spiny sharks), Osteichthyes (ray-finned fishes, fleshy finned fishes ancestral to tetrapods). Within this classification, tetrapods such as mammals, birds, and amphibians do not belong to this grouping despite the fact that lungfish and coelacanths are closer relatives to the tetrapods.

Scorpaenidae and Synanceiidae (stonefish) are venomous fish of which the genus *Synanceia* (scorpionfish) is the most toxic of the Scorpaenidae (lionfish and scorpion fish). The venom delivery system involves 11–17 dorsal, 3 anal, and 2 pelvic fin spines with glandular tissue of different cellular structure found in grooves along opposite sides of the spines. The venom of *Scaevola plumieri* has an LD_{50} of 0.28 mg/kg intravenously in mice. The venom has activities that can generate hemorrhaging, hemolysis, and proteolysis. Fresh venom also affects mean arterial pressure (coronary vasoconstriction) and heart rate (positive chronotropic, lusitropic [conduction system], and inotropic effects). A cytolytic/hemolytic toxin with vasoactive (vasorelaxation) properties, Sp-CTx is a protein. The adult human usually does not die, but may have symptoms of severe pain with irradiation of the pain, edema, erythema, sometimes skin necrosis, adenopathy, nausea, vomiting, agitation, malaise, diaphoresis, diarrhea, tachycardia, and other arrhythmias. Stonefish antivenom appears to prevent or ameliorate the inflammation and lower the cardiovascular effects of the venom of the scorpionfish. This indicates some sequence similarity between proteinaceous toxins in fish venoms (Gomes et al., 2011).

Lophotrochozoa: Mollusca Venoms

Cone snails of the *Conus* species are gastropod mollusks that use small peptides known as ω-conotoxins synthesized in their tubular ducts and squeezed through a barbed radula to paralyze their prey. Their venoms consist of 100–200 peptides of 9–100 amino acids in length. These peptides target the neuromuscular system via ion channels, membrane receptors, and transporters. α-Conotoxins antagonize N_M and N_N (nicotinic muscle- and neuronal-type acetylcholine) receptors. μ-Conotoxins inhibit Na^+ channels on the sarcolemma at site 1 (same site for tetrodotoxin and saxitoxin). Interestingly, the ω-conotoxins may have medical application in neuropathic pain management. The target of these toxins is the voltage-gated Ca^{2+} channels, composed of heteromeric proteins comprising five subunits. These calcium channels have a pore-forming $α_1$ subunit and smaller auxiliary β, $α_2$, δ, and γ subunits. There are two distinct classes of these voltage-gated calcium channels—high voltage-activated (L-type found in skeletal muscle, neurons, cardiac myocytes, endocrine cells, pancreatic β cells, and retinal cells; P/Q- and N-type found on neurons and pancreatic β cells; and R-type found in neurons and endocrine cells) and low voltage-activated (T-type found on neurons, cardiac myocytes, smooth muscle, endocrine cells, and kidney

cells) channels. By inhibiting these channels the ω-conotoxins also block neurotransmitter release in mammalian systems *in vitro* (Hannon and Atchison, 2013). Not only do cone snails produce peptides in their venom that affect $Ca_v2.2$ channels, but spiders, snakes, assassin bugs, centipedes, and scorpions are sources high in potent selective inhibitors of this channel responsible for neurotransmitter release (Sousa et al., 2013).

Eumetazoa: Cnidaria Venoms

This phylum consists of some of the most unrecognized but most venomous animals, including jellyfish, sea anemones, corals (hard and soft), and sea pens. Approximately 250 peptides, proteins, enzymes, and proteinase inhibitors have been identified along with purines, quaternary ammonium compounds, biogenic amines, and betaines. Prey acquisition, predator deterrents, and territory defense involve neurotoxic and cardiotoxic effects of the nematocyst venoms located on the tentacles, acrorhagi, and acontia and in the mucous coat that covers the body of the animal. Sea anemone toxins are fundamentally cytolytic or neurotoxic peptides and proteins. These toxins target voltage-gated Na^+ (at site 3 = S3-S4 loop of domain IV binding keeping that segment in the inward position and preventing channel inactivation), K^+, and acid-sensing ion channels. There are also cytolysins, Kunitz-type protease inhibitors, and phosphodiesterase A_2 activity (Frazão et al., 2012).

A coral, *Palythoa toxica*, produces one of the most toxic venoms as displayed in **Figure 30-2**. Palytoxin has also been found in the dinoflagellate genus *Ostreopsis*. It has an LD_{50} of 300 ng/kg in mice due to its potent inhibition of the $3Na^+,2K^+$-ATPase that is critical to maintain membrane potentials in all cells (Ramos and Vasconcelos, 2010).

Jellyfish, especially the Portuguese man-of-war (*Physalia physalis*), are known for toxic stings. The key protein in the venom is a hemolysin known as physalitoxin. However, this jellyfish's nematocyst venom also has dramatic cardiac toxicity as noted by arrhythmias and positive inotropy (based on external Ca^{2+} concentration but not related to L-type of T-type Ca^{2+}

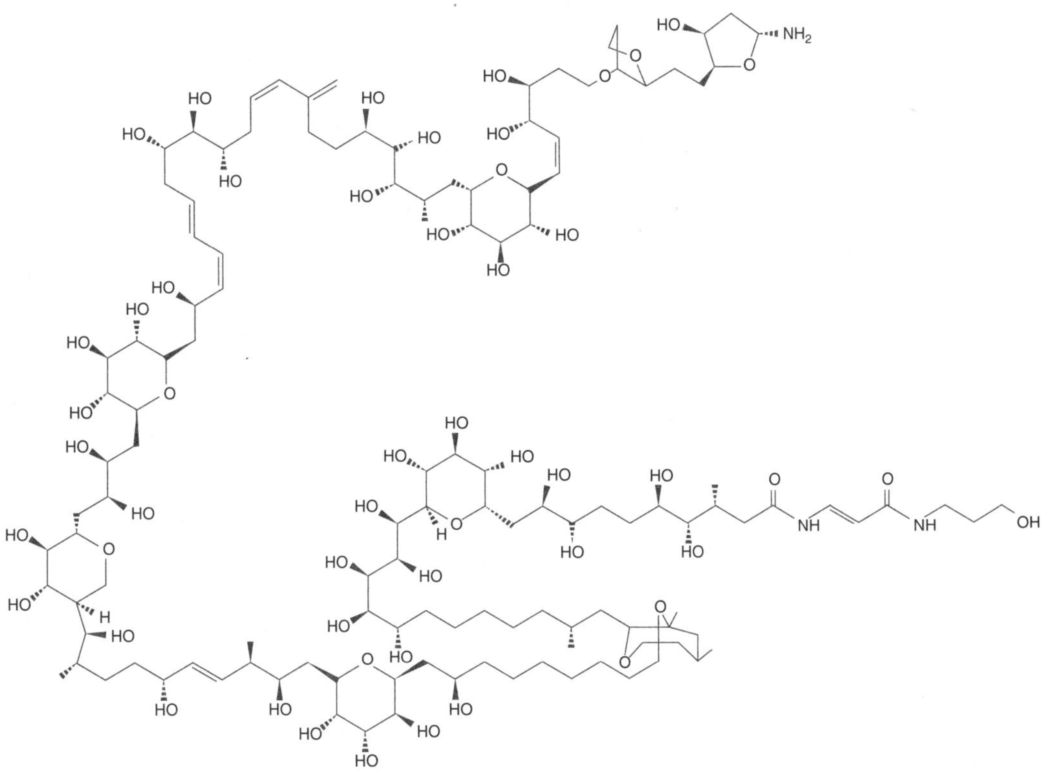

FIGURE 30-2 Structure of Palytoxin

channels). This component of the venom, which causes calcium influx into L-929, GH_4C_1, FRL, in embryonic chick cells, is not sensitive to ouabain, vanadate, or organic Ca^{2+} channel blocker. However, it is blocked by transition metals La^{2+} and Zn^{2+}. This venom component also causes a loss of membrane integrity as noted by the release of intracellular lactate dehydrogenase. In this regard, this toxin may be similar to α-latrotoxin, maitotoxin, and mellitin. Black widow spider venom's α-latrotoxin develops nonclosing ionic channels permeable to K^+, Na^+, and Ca^{2+}, which are not blocked by the usual Na^+ of Ca^{2+} channel blockers. Cell lysis also occurs due to the change in ion permeability. The difference between man-of-war venom and α-latrotoxin is the order of potency of block by divalent cations—$Co^{2+} > Ni^{2+} > Zn^{2+}$ for spider venom and $Zn^{2+} > Ni^{2+} = Co^{2+}$ for the man-of-war venom (note reversed order). Man-of-war venom is also similar to maitotoxin

produced by the dinoflagellate *Gambierdiscus toxicus* as both toxins cause Ca^{2+} uptake, K^+ efflux, and Na^+ influx, with the calcium and sodium movements not altered by conventional organic blocking agents. Maitotoxin also has Zn^{2+} as the most potent divalent ion in blocking the ion permeability caused by the toxin with an IC_{50} of 41 versus 34 μM for man-of-war venom. Maitotoxin also lyses BC_3H_1 cells. Bee venom mellitin is also a cytolytic agent, but appears to cause half-maximal cytolysis (EC_{50} for LDH release = 1 μg/mL) at ~1/9 of the concentration, which causes half-maximal Ca^{2+} influx (EC_{50} = 91 μg/mL). This means that, at least for the bee venom, the cytolytic effects are apparently not related to the change in Ca^{2+} permeability. Lanthanum's block of the Ca^{2+} uptake and cytolytic activity of the man-of-war venom at the target cell plasma membrane level does not, however, neutralize the overall cytolytic nature of the venom. The effect of La^{2+}

and Zn^{2+} may influence membrane fluidity and not allow the toxin(s) in the venom to oligomerize in the target membrane (Edwards and Hessinger, 2000).

The Australian Carybdea jellyfish appear to be associated with Irukandji syndrome, starting with severe muscle pains with primary symptoms involving the lower back. Muscle cramps appear to progress to vomiting, diaphoresis, agitation, vasoconstriction/hypertension, and prostration. In extreme cases of envenomation, acute heart failure appears to result from affecting neuronal sodium channels. This sodium channel effect causes a huge release of endogenous catecholamines by jellyfish of species *Carukia barnesi*, *Alatina mordens*, and *Malo maxima*. This high venom-induced release of stress-linked neurotransmitters may be responsible for cardiomyopathy. Jellyfish venom from *C. xaymacana* may also cause pore formation in myocardial cellular membranes. Leakage of troponin from cardiac membranes is associated with extreme cases of envenomation in humans. In the clinic, parenteral analgesia, antihypertensive therapy, oxygen, and mechanical ventilation are used to try to manage the venom toxicity, but no antidotal first-aid has yet been developed (Tibballs et al., 2012).

Echinodermata: Holothuroidea Venom

Sea cucumbers (*Pearsonothuria graeffei*) will expel their viscera and the Cuvierian organ containing saponins or holothurin when disturbed. Long, white, sticky threads adhere to the offending species and the venom weakens the muscles of the enemy and can cause permanent blindness. Holothurin is a lanosteroid-type triterpene glycoside. Holothurin is hemolytic, cytolytic, and can first cause contracture then relaxation of the mammalian phrenic nerve-diaphragm preparation. The triterpene glycosides are secondary metabolites of holothurians and have anti-tumor and anti-angiogenic properties through actions on receptor tyrosine kinases or VEGF-induced kinase insert domain receptor signaling pathways (Zhao et al., 2011).

Chordata: Mammalia: Eutheria: Soricomorpha: Soricidae Venoms

It is unusual to have a venomous mammal. However, the northern short-tailed shrew (*Blarina brevicauda*) venom arising from the submaxillary and sublingual glands contains a lethal blarina toxin that possesses an N-linked microheterogeneous glycoprotein with tissue kallikrein-like activity. The isolated 253 amino acid protein contains three serine proteases and a very close identity to tissue kallikreins. This toxin converts kininogens to kinins, is vasodilatory, and is proteolytic. Toxicity is manifested by irregular respiration, paralysis, and convulsions prior to death, and is inhibited by aprotinin, a kallikrein inhibitor (Kita et al., 2004). A pharmacologic peptide soricidin used in treating ovarian cancer is also a component of the toxin.

Venom Economy

There exists a venom optimization hypothesis based on the frugality of venom use. The reason for using other methods for prey capture and ingestion or predator deterrence is due to the high metabolic cost of producing the protein-rich venom. If possible due to small prey, competitor, or predator size, adult scorpions of the *Pandinus* genera use massive pedipalps and avoid venom use while juveniles frequently envenomate. The Arizona Desert hairy scorpion, *Hadrurus arizonensis*, on the other hand, uses its venom at least once per encounter with prey despite its large physical size. Some venomous snakes use a combination of constriction and venom to economize on use. However, the larger the prey, the more resistant the prey to venom, the handling difficulty of the prey, and repletion of the venom gland will increase the venom dose. Another reason certain venomous animals use venom frugally is the functional redundancy of the animal venom components. In the scorpion *Leiurus quinquestriatus hebraeus* there are 17 different toxins that target site 3 of the insect Na_V channel. Certain scorpions or spiders or the red spitting cobra also change the composition of their venom based on number of venom releases. The first venom may be far less toxic than subsequent releases based on observation of milking certain spiders (Morgenstern and King, 2013).

Chordata: Tetrapoda: Amphibia Poisons

Table 30-2 lists the animal poisons by toxic compounds, while this section focuses on species as the organizing principle. This portion of the chapter considers poisons rather than venoms. Toads and frogs (Anura) are a good starting point, as their products represent that the secretions onto the skin that will hopefully prevent consumption and protect the organism. Salamanders and newts (Urodela)

also introduce a poison that is found in the infamous pufferfish. Fish occasionally have to be consumed first and may have the toxic property inside that protects others of their species but not that individual if consumed. Fish and especially shellfish may also consume a toxin from aquatic protistans that confer toxicity to those that eat that fish such as humans. Aromatic amines are secreted onto amphibian skin of three chemical classes of agents: indolealkylamines (5-HT or serotonin and N-methylated derivatives), imidazole alkylamines and histamine, and monohydroxy phenylalkylamines and catecholamines. These agents act as vasoconstrictors, convulsants, hallucinogens, and cholinergic agents. Indolealkylamines are the key biogenic amines of amphibian skin secretions. The evolutionary basis of these secretions have been evaluated in anurans

TABLE 30-2   Toxicity of Animal Poisons

Toxicity	Animal Poisons	Toxic Mechanism
Vasoconstriction	Indolealkylamines from toads, fungal ergot alkaloids	Pharmacologic action on biogenic amine receptors
Cardiac strength and heart rate	Bufadienolides from toads	$3Na^+,2K^+$-ATPase inhibitors
Cardiotoxins, neurotoxicity, and neuromuscular junction	Histrionicotoxin alkaloids from frog *Oophaga histrionica*	Non-competitive nicotinic receptor antagonists
Convulsants, hallucinogens, cholinergic neurotoxicity	Indolealkylamines from toads, fungal ergot alkaloids, psilocybin	Pharmacologic action on biogenic amine receptors
Membrane depolarizations— neurotoxic and cardiotoxic	Batrachotoxin(s) from frog *Phyllobates aurotaenia*	Na^+ channel modulation (Open)
	Pumiliotoxins from Dendrobatidae frogs	
	Frog zetekitoxin, frog + newts + salamander + octopus + puffer fish tetrodotoxin	(Inhibit)
	Dinoflagellates and cyanobacteria saxitoxin	(Site 1 pore blocker)
	Dinoflagellates brevetoxins	(Site 5 activation)
	Dinoflagellates ciguatoxin	(Site 5 shift activation gating)
	Dinoflagellates ostreotoxin 3	Inactivation gating modifier
	Dinoflagellates maitotoxin	Nonselective cation entry
	Dinoflagellates azaspiracid	K^+ channel pore blocker

(continues)

TABLE 30-2   Toxicity of Animal Poisons (*continued*)

Toxicity	Animal Poisons	Toxic Mechanism
Amnesia	Diatom domoic acid	Glutamate receptor-linked Na^+ and Ca^{2+} influx
Neurotoxicity at high-affinity and low-affinity binding sites	*Epipedobates tricolor* frog epibatidine	Very potent nicotinic receptor agonist
Preventing neurotransmitter release—flaccid paralysis	Bacteria *Clostridium botulinum* + phage toxin	$Zn2^+$ metalloproteinase lysis of membrane fusion proteins (SNAP-25)
Preventing inhibitory neurotransmitter release—flaccid paralysis $\rightarrow$ rigidity and spasm	Bacteria *Clostridium tetani*	$Zn2^+$ metalloproteinase lysis of VAMP 1st at motor nerve terminals $\rightarrow$ $\downarrow$ GABAergic and $\downarrow$ glycinergic
Other paralysis	Dinoflagellates yessotoxin	Cytoskeletal interactions
Fungal microtubule function	Fungal griseofulvin	Tubulin binding = $\downarrow$ mitosis
Hemolysis	$\beta\gamma$-Crystallin and trefoil factor from *Bombina maxima* frog	Membrane pore formation
Cell-cycle arrest	Bufadienolides from toads	Effects on cell-cycle regulation
DNA damage	Fungal ochratoxins	ROS generation and zinc depletion
Mitochondrial	Bufadienolides from toads, fungal ochratoxin	Apoptosis generation via caspases, Ca^{2+}, mitochondrial membrane potential
Apoptosis of immune cells	Bacterial anthrax lethal factor	Zn^{2+}- dependent metalloproteinase action on MAPKK
Protein synthesis inhibition	Bacterial diphtheria toxin and *Pseudomonas* exotoxin A	ADP-ribose transfer to elongation factor-2 but cell sensitivity first due to surface-binding receptors
	Pseudomonas exoenzyme S (not an effective toxin)	ADP ribosylates different eukaryotic proteins
	Shigella toxin (neurotoxic, cytotoxic and enterotoxic)	Inactivates 60S ribosomal subunit of eukaryotic cells
	Bacillus anthracis toxin edema factor	Edema factor = calmodulin-dependent adenylyl cyclase
mRNA synthesis inhibition	Fungal α-amanitin	Eukaryote RNA polymerase II inhibition
Increased cAMP	Bacterial cholera toxin, *E. coli* heat-labile enterotoxin, pertussis toxin	Changes ion fluxes via ADP-ribosylation of adenylyl cyclase regulation
Increased cGMP	Bacterial *E. coli* heat-stable enterotoxin	Stimulates guanylyl cyclase
Uterine motility	Fungal ergot alkaloids	Pharmacologic action on biogenic amine receptors
Hepatic damage and cancer	Fungal aflatoxins	CYP forms epoxide
	Cyanobacteria microcystins and nodularins	Protein phosphatase inhibition $\rightarrow$ liver hemorrhage
Hepatotoxicity/cytotoxicity/ neurotoxicity	Cyanobacterial cylindrospermopsin	GSH, protein synthesis, CYP inhibition
Lung damage	Fungal ipomeanol	CYP activation to epoxide
Reproduction deficit	Fungal aflatoxins	CYP forms epoxide
Steroid-like action	Fungal zearalenone	Estrogenic
Enhanced ethanol toxicity	Fungal coprine	Low Km liver acetaldehyde dehydrogenase inhibition

such as leptodactylid frogs, *Litoria rubella*, and Bufonidae, of which the last group is the most striking example of indolealkylamine synthesis and secretion.

Figure 30-3 examines the structures and mass spectra of three important indolealkylamines from toads. There were differences in the composition of serotonin (5-HT), bufotenin (BTN), dehydrobufotenine (DHB), and bufotenidine (BTD) between species of toads and the cutaneous versus parotid gland secretions within a species. For example, indolealkylamine composition of skin secretions is similar between *Bufo rubescens* (DHB and DHB-S), *Bufo ictericus*, and *Bufo arenarum*, while parotid gland secretions are close for *B. rubescens* (DHB, DHB-S, and 5-HT), *Bufo crucifer*, and *Bufo marinus*. In the same species, *B. arenarum* has BTD, DHB, DHB-S, 5-HT, and BTN in its parotid gland, but excludes BTD from its skin secretions. *B. crucifer*, on the other hand, has DHB, DHB-S,

5-HT, and a small amount of BTN in the parotid gland secretion, while including more indolealkylamines in its skin secretions (BTD, DHB, DHB-S, 5-HT, and BTN). Similarly, *Bufo granulosus* has fewer compounds in its parotid secretion (DHB, DHB-S, 5-HT, and BTN) and more in its skin secretions (BTD, DHB, DHB-S, T-HT, and BTN). Other species such as *Brachycephalus ephippium* present no indoleamines in their skin secretions and do not have parotid glands (Maciel et al., 2003). Powerful bufadienolides such as bufalin, cinobufotalin, resibufogenin, and cinobufagin have been isolated in traditional Chinese medicine from the auricular and skin glands of *Bufo bufo gargarizans* Cantor or *Bufo melanostictus* Schneider.

Note the structures in **Figure 30-4** are more akin to cholesterol than resembling biogenic amines of other toad skin poisons. These compounds are $3Na^+$, $2K^+$-ATPase inhibitors (similar to the plant poison and medication

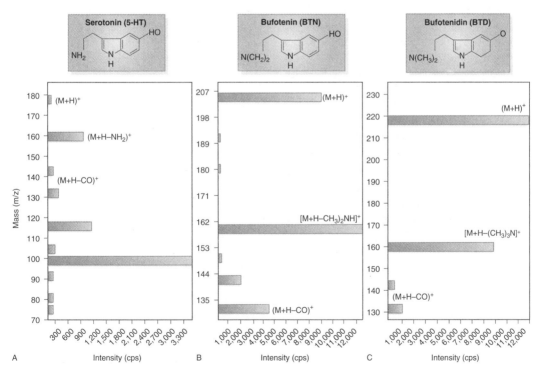

FIGURE 30-3 Mass Spectra and Structures of Three Important Indolealkylamines: (A) Serotonin, (B) Bufotenin, (C) Bufotenidine from Standards to Characterize Bufonid Skin Secretions

	Bufalin	Bufotalin	Cinobufagin	Telocinobufagin
R_1	H	H	H	OH
R_2	OH	OH	-O-	OH
R_3	H	H	-O-	H
R_4	H	OAc	OAc	H

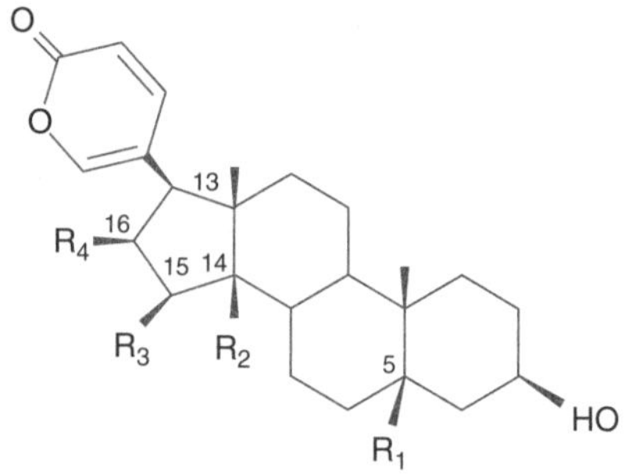

FIGURE 30-4 The Structures of the Bufadienolides

digitalis), affect Na^+/Ca^{2+} exchange in cardiac myocytes causing an increase in intracellular Ca^{2+}, and thereby have a positive inotropic effect. Higher concentrations can cause heart failure. Lately, these substances have also been noted for their antitumor activities as they inhibit cell proliferation, induce differentiation, and promote apoptosis in U973, LNCaP, PC-3, THP-1, HL-60, and BEL-7402 cancer cells. They do so by G_2/M arrest with cyclin A and B1 downregulation and decreased CDK1 protein level. Upstream regulators of CDK/cyclin such as cell division cycle (CDC)25A, CDC25B, and CDC25C all were inhibited by bufotalin. Aurora A (involved in multiple mitotic events such as centrosome cycle, spindle assembly, microtubule-kinetochore attachment, a spindle checkpoint) was also highly downregulated. CDK inhibitors p21 and p53 were found to be elevated. The mitochondrial effects of these bufadienolides activate caspases, alter the mitochondrial membrane potential (extreme swelling of mitochondria), increase intracellular Ca^{2+}, decrease anti-apoptotic protein bcl-2, and increase pro-apoptotic protein bax expression. Akt, a factor key to cell growth and survival by phosphorylating and thereby inhibiting pro-apoptotic molecules, was also dramatically reduced by bufotalin treatment. ROS expression also appears increased in response to this class of toad poisons (Zhang et al., 2012).

Returning to the variety of poisons found in frogs, their diversity probably reflects their manifold origins. Hemolytic compounds were found in certain snake species, and the protein non-lens $\beta\gamma$-crystallins (structural proteins in vertebrates) and trefoil factor complex of the Chinese red belly frog (*Bombina maxima* found in the mountainous region of southwestern China) hemolyzes mammalian red blood cells via membrane pore formation. This frog toxin has pharmaceutical properties as it stimulates cell migration and wound healing. Depending on the dose, it also is capable of causing cell detachment and apoptosis using human umbilical endothelial cells as the assay (Liu et al., 2008).

As the toad discussion ended with steroidal alkaloid poisons, examinations of the frog versions are warranted. Batrachotoxin (BTX; 3′,9′-epoxy-14a, *18a*-[epoxyethano-*N*-methylimino]-5β-pregna-7,16-diene-3β, 11α, 20α (2,4-dimethyl-1*H*-pyrrole-3-carboxylate]) and its variants (batrachotoxin A, homo-batrachotoxin, dihydrobatrachotoxin, and 3-*O*-methylbatrachotoxin) are extremely toxic in mice (BTX's LD_{50} = 2.0 µg/kg intravenously) and are found in the skin secretions of the Columbian arrow poison frog, *Phyllobates aurotaenia*. Note the steroid structure as illustrated in **Figure 30-5**. BTX causes the Na^+ channels to remain open by binding to the receptor similar to other neurotoxins such as veratridine, aconitine, and grayanotoxin. This leads to peripheral and central neurotoxicity and cardiac arrest. Tetrodotoxin and saxitoxin

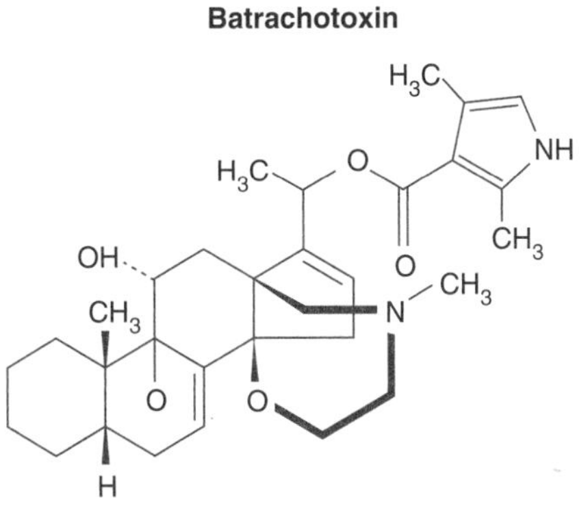

Batrachotoxin

FIGURE 30-5 The Structure of the Frog Steroid Alkaloid Batrachotoxin

prevent or reverse the depolarization caused by batrachotoxin, but do not bind at the same site as BTX (Hodgson, 2012). Neotropical poison frogs, Dendrobatidae, share a lipophilic alkaloid known as pumiliotoxins or allopumiliotoxins (7-hydroxypumiliotoxins). 8-Hydroxy-8-methyl-6-(2′-methylhexylidene)-1-azabicyclo[4.3.0]nonane of pumiliotoxin 251D [PTX (+)-251D], a skin alkaloid shared among all genera of dendrobatids and other anurans. A 10-mg/kg dose of PTX (+)-251D administered via subcutaneous injection caused convulsions, hyperalgesia (increased pain), and death, while the (–) enantiomer had not effect. Pumiliotoxins target the voltage-sensitive sodium channels, causing them to prolong opening similar to the effects of batrachotoxins. This causes cardiac stimulation and at high doses convulsions and death, and pumiliotoxins are potent insecticides for mosquitoes (Weldon et al., 2006).

How did the frogs develop or obtain their toxic alkaloids? It is likely that ant venoms and trail-marking alkaloids are consumed by dendrobatid frogs. For example, histrionicotoxin alkaloids have been recently isolated from ants (Jones et al., 2012). They are found in frogs such as *Oophaga histrionic* or Harlequin poison dart frogs and are strong noncompetitive antagonists and ligands for nicotinic cholinergic receptor channel complexes (δ subunit). Epibatidine is another alkaloid isolated from the Ecuadorean tree frog, *Epipedobates tricolor*, with strong nicotinic receptor agonist activity

in the mammalian brain and antinociceptive (reduces pain) activity. Other alkaloids from frog skin are monocyclic pyrrolidines and piperidines; bicyclic decahydroquinolines, pyrrolizidines, indolizidines, and quinolizidines; and tricyclic gephyrotoxins, pyrrolizidine oximes, pseudophrynamines, and coccinellines that affect ion channels. Frog skin alkaloids appear to be dietary from small arthropods that are then stored in the skin glands. Ants in the diet are sources of pyrrolidines, piperidines, 3,5-disubstituted pyrrolizidines, and 3,5-disubstituted indolizidines in frogs (Daly, 1995). A guanidinium alkaloid, zetekitoxin AB from the Panamanian golden frog, *Atelopus zeteki*, appears close to saxitoxin, a paralytic poison from a dinoflagellate found in shellfish and is in the same chemical class as tetrodotoxin, a toxin from the pufferfish. While the steroidal bufadienolides inhibit the sodium-potassium ATPase, the guanidinium alkaloids block the voltage-gated sodium channels (Yotsu-Yamashita et al., 2004).

The evolution of these toxins starts with marine organisms' polyethers, macrolides, terpenes, unusual amino acids/peptides, and alkaloids. Nonmarine organisms yield similar chemical classes of agents, but with notable structural differences. However, tetrodotoxin and its congeners, which include chiriquitoxin, and the similarity between saxitoxin and zetekitoxin show some similarities between marine and amphibian species (Daly, 2004). Tetrodotoxin (TTX) is found in frogs, the blue-ringed octopus, mollusks, salamanders, newts, and of course the pufferfish from which it was first isolated. TTX selectively blocks voltage-gated sodium channels. This toxin may be the result of synthesis by symbiotic microorganisms in higher taxa rather than a marine or amphibian animal. This makes the biological classification of a toxicant difficult at best to be true to its biological origins (Chau et al., 2011).

Fish Poisons

The historic discovery of tetrodotoxin was found in the pufferfish (Animalia: Chordata: Vertebrata: Actinopterygii: Neopterygii:

Teleostei: Tetraodontidae). The complex ring structure of TTX, a guanidinium alkaloid, is displayed in **Figure 30-6**. However, the suspected microbial origins of TTX confound the classification. TTX concentrates in the liver, gonads, and skin, but can be found in other parts of the viscera. Symbiosis appears to be at work in the development of these "animal" toxins. However, it is also dependent on the fish as well. For instance, pufferfish or tetraodontoid fish toxicity follows closely with their reproductive cycle, with highest levels during late spring and early summer (Halstead, 1958).

It cannot always be assumed that a seasonal variation in toxin level reflects the ingestion by the marine organism of another toxic species such as the organism that produces the red tide. As opposed to fish venoms, the poisons appear relatively stable. Marine organisms can have a variety of size compounds and chemical classes similar to the amphibians as well as activities that may be single, such as vasoconstriction, or complex. The pufferfish produce what are

known as ichthyosarcotoxins (poisoning by fish flesh). The clinical designations are the reason for the classifications, with Group 1 causing mild gastrointestinal (GI) symptoms only (Cyclostome from slime of lampreys and hagfish, Elasmobranch usually from Greenland sleeper shark, and Gempylid yielding strong purgative reactions from ingesting snake mackerel, castor oil fish, and skilfish). Group 2 involves GI and neurological symptoms (*Tetraodon* from pufferfish and porcupine fish, Elasmobranch shark liver-caused hypervitaminosis A, and ichthyotoxism from roe and caviar poisoning and may be related to saxitoxin or paralytic shellfish poisoning resulting from the *Gonyaulax catenella* dinoflagellate or cyanobacteria). Group 3 is determined by GI and cardiac symptoms (clupeotoxin from episodic exposures to anchovies, sardine, and herring). Group 4 has a complex assortment of GI, neurological, cardiac, joint, and other organ system problems (ciguatera from a variety of fish species, and *Gymnothorax* from Moray eel and is likely a severe form

	TTX	6-*epi*TTX	11-deoxyTTX	11-*nor*TTX -6(S)-ol	11-*nor*TTX- 6(R)-ol	11-*nor*TTX-6, 6-diol
R$_1$	OH	CH$_2$OH	OH	OH	H	OH
R$_2$	CH$_2$OH	OH	CH$_3$	H	OH	OH

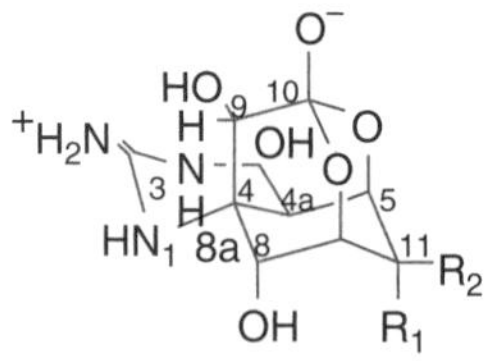

	5-deoxyTTX	5,6,11-trideoxyTTX	1-hydroxy-5,11-dideoxyTTX
R$_1$	H	H	H
R$_2$	OH	H	OH
R$_3$	CH$_2$OH	CH$_3$	CH$_3$
R$_4$	H	H	OH

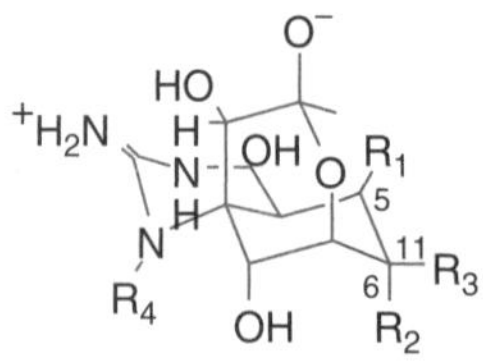

	4,9-anhydroTTX	6-*epi*-4,9-anhydroTTX
R$_1$	OH	CH$_2$OH
R$_2$	CH$_2$OH	OH

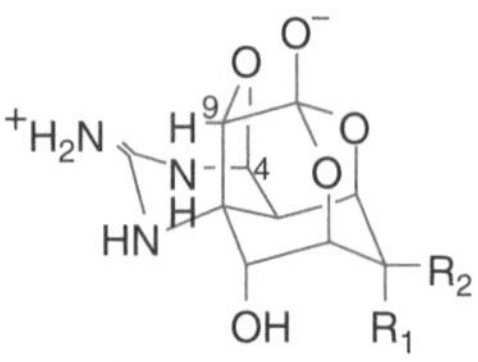

FIGURE 30-6 The Structures of Tetrodotoxin and its Analogs

of ciguatera). Group 5 involves anaphylactoid reactions (Scombroid). Group 6 involves hallucinogens (Chimaera from ratfish and elephant fish, hallucinogenic fish poisoning from mullet, and surgeonfish possibly related to maitotoxin, a ciguateric toxin, but more likely an indole as is found on amphibian skin; Grant, 1997).

The ciguateric fish poisonings (GI and neurological) are really caused by a photosynthetic benthic dinoflagellate known as *Gambierdiscus toxicus*, so again the diet rather than the fish is responsible for this type of poisoning. Scombroid fish poisoning is really of microbial origin even though it falls under the same classification as an ichthyosarcotoxin, which calls into question the classification system. Tuna and mackerel (Scombridae) of even dark-fleshed fish such as the sardine and anchovy need to be quickly cooled. Otherwise, the enteric gram-negative bacteria such as *Morganella morganii*, *Escherichia coli*, *Klebsiella* species, and *Pseudomonas aeruginosa* of the fish's cutis and intestine will decarboxylate the amino acid histidine found in the muscle of the fish into histamine, giving an apparent allergic-type reaction with flushing, rash, urticaria (usually extensive erythema without wheals), palpitations, headache, dizziness, sweating, burning of the mouth and throat, abdominal cramps, nausea, vomiting, and diarrhea. This, this type of fish poisoning is actually that of "spoiled" fish and is not truly an intrinsic fish toxin (Stratta and Badino, 2012).

Chordata: Avialae: Aves Poisons

Pitohui dichrous birds from New Guinea have homobatrachotoxin, an amphibian toxin, in their feathers. This bird is polyphyletic and represents several lineages among the corvoid families of passerine birds. This indicates that other corvoid birds indeed may harbor this toxin after consuming the toxin through their diet of insects (Choresine beetles of the Melyridae family) and secrete it through the uropygial gland (Jønsson et al., 2008). A second toxic bird genus that lives at higher altitudes than the *Pitohui*, *Ifrita kowaldi*, was discovered to contain batrachotoxinin-A *cis*-crotonate (Dumbacher et al., 2000).

Discussion of Poisons' Evolution and Proper Attribution/Biological Classification

The animal poisons and some of their origins indicate numerous cases of poisons coming from consumption of venomous insects, symbiosis with other organisms, and bacterial spoilage. In a text about biological toxicology, it is important to ferret out the evolutionary or dietary origins of these toxins. Earlier papers may give the false illusion that scientists had solid evidence of the origins of toxins. For instance, laypeople know that *Clostridium botulinum* produces the most potent toxins, a Zn^{2+} metalloproteinase that cleaves the membrane fusion proteins (synaptobrevin, synaptosomal-associated protein or SNAP-25, and syntaxin) and prevents neurotransmitter release for 6 months in mammals (Ahnert-Hilger et al., 2013). A number of cultures of strains of *C. botulinum* with specific toxicities exist. Group I appear to be proteolytic and produce toxin type A, B, or F. The non-proteolytic strains are designated as group II and produce toxin type B, E, or F. Group III are weakly proteolytic or non-proteolytic strains that contain toxin C_1, C_2, or D. Non-saccharolytic but proteolytic strains are in Group IV and produce type C toxin. There are also strains that produce type E toxin. Analysis of botulinum-neurotoxin carrying prophage indicates that group III of this toxin should also include *C. novyi* and *C. haemolyticum*. Is this genetic material transfer by plasmids or does this call into question the true origin of this toxin (Skarin et al., 2011)? Actually, lysogenic association between phage and bacteria produced the most toxigenic type C strain of *Clostridium botulinum* (Hariharan and Mitchell, 1976). From experiments also done decades ago, it appears that bacteriophages control production of C_1 and D toxins (Sugiyama, 1980). If bacteria, bacteriophages, fungi, dinoflagellates, and so forth are at the core of many poisons, scientists are really examining many kingdoms of biological classification and can only refer to the animal "host" of the toxin as animal-associated toxicity such as paralytic shellfish poisoning or plant-associated toxicity such as aflatoxin B_1 poisoning.

Bacteria are prokaryotes, and protists are unicellular eukaryotes. The protists could be labeled as their own taxon, but that would be inaccurate. Protists are in all five kingdoms and polyphyletic. The most problematic of the protists are the Myxozoa. They are plasmodial in the trophic state. Myxozoa are derived from bilateral animal ancestors through the loss of gastrointestinal and nervous systems. It also appears that this protest has anaerobic microsporidia that evolved from the aerobic filamentous zygomatic fungi. Even if the higher classification of kingdom Protozoa is revised, 11 phyla still need to be used under this classification. Complementary gene fusion indicates that there were two clades of eukaryotes. One is the ancestral uniciliate or unicentriolar unikonts. The other originates from ancestral biciliate bikonts, which go through ciliary transformation (younger anterior cilium → dissimilar older posterior cilium). Amoebozoa and the opisthokonts (Animalia: Choanozoa and Fungi) are unikonts, which have triple-gene fusion in common and are not in bikonts. Plants and all other protists include protozoan infrakingdoms Rhizaria (phyla Cercozoa and Retaria [Radiozoa, Foraminifera]), Excavata (phyla Loukozoa, Metamonada, Euglenozoa, Percolozoa), kingdom Plantae (Viridiplantae, Rhodophyta [sisters]; Glaucophyta), the chromalveolate clade, and the protozoan phylum Apusozoa (Thecomonadea, Diphylleida). Further classification of the chromalveolates involve members of the kingdom Chromista (Cryptista, Heterokonta, Haptophyta) and the protozoan infrakingdom Alveolata (phyla Ciliophora and Miozoa [= Protalveolata, Dinozoa, Apicomplexa]), which deviated from a common ancestor that enslaved a red alga and through evolution developed unique plastid protein-targeting mechanisms through the host rough (ribosome-containing) endoplasmic reticulum and an enslaved algal plasma/periplastid membrane. Branching order for the five bikont groups is unclear, although Plantae may be sisters or ancestors of chromalveolates (designated corticates as they both possess cortical alveoli). Rhizaria and Excavata, together known as cabozoa, are likely sisters supposing that there was an enslavement of formerly green algal plastic

or euglenoids and chlorarachneans (*Cercozoa*) in a single event in the ancestor they share in common. It is also possible that the pairings of Apusozoa and Excavata, or centrohelid heliozoa and Haptophyta are sisters (Cavalier-Smith, 2003). Because it is not possible to give every classification in a single chapter as might be warranted from a purist point of view, it is more expeditious to separate into animal and plant those poisons belonging to cells "closest" to that grouping despite its clear problems.

Eukarya: Chromalveolata: Alveolata: Dinoflagellata Poisons

The dinoflagellates are photosynthetic eukaryotes, but a large number are mixotrophic in that they ingest prey as well. The trouble is that as paralytic shellfish poisoning by saxitoxin is examined more closely, *Gonyaulax catenella* may not be the origin of saxitoxin. A shellfish, a dinoflagellate, and ultimately prokaryotic cyanobacteria (domain Bacteria and phylum Cyanobacteria) share the toxin attributed to the dinoflagellate. Both the dinoflagellates and cyanobacteria (*Cylindrospermopsis raciborskii* T3, *Anabaena circinalis*, *Aphanizomenon* sp., and *Lyngbya wollei*) have genes that cause the biosynthesis of saxitoxin. In examining this toxin more closely, the phytoplankton (more like plant cells, but are prokaryotes) species' eco-evolution becomes apparent. Saxitoxin is part of the marine neurotoxins produced by phytoplankton, select invertebrates, and fish, thus evolutionary patterns can be realized for protection of a variety or marine life. It does appear from critical saxitoxin-related genes that the biosynthesis pathway was developed independently in dinoflagellates and cyanobacteria even though there are some evolutionary-related proteins. These marine toxins interact with voltage-gated Na^+, K^+, and Ca^{2+} channels. The structures of these marine toxins are displayed in **Figure 30-7**. Saxitoxin is an alkaloid that appears to work via blocking nerve impulses by binding to the Na^+ channel (site 1 where pore-blocking toxin prevents ion conductance through affinity for outer mouth), but also targets the other two ion channels (modifying the K^+ channel and partially

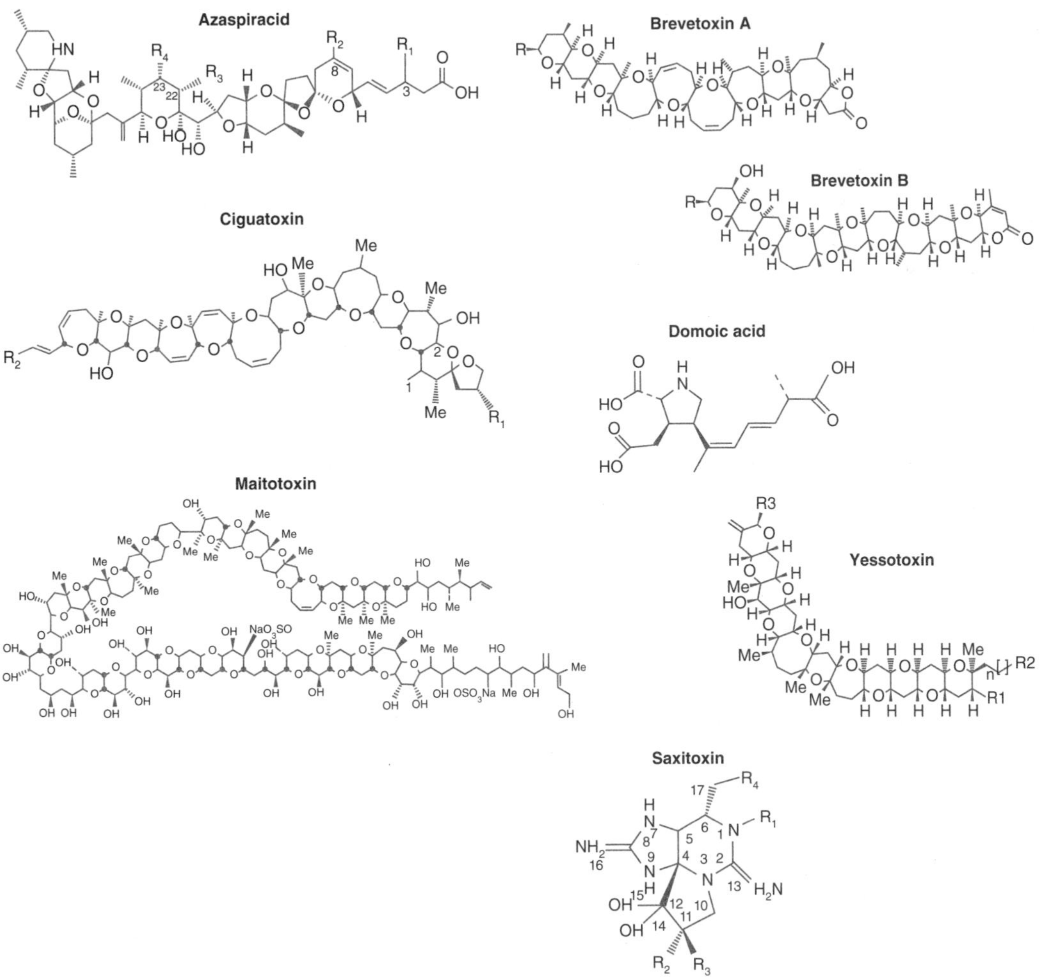

FIGURE 30-7 Structures of Marine Toxins

blocking the Ca²⁺ channel extracellularly) and has been associated with dinoflagellates *Pyrodinium bahamense*, *Alexandrium* spp., and *Gymnodinium catenatum*. The 7,8,9-guanidinium moiety acts as a cationic substitute for Na⁺ and works best at neutral pH. Saxitoxin gene cluster antiquity indicates that the potassium channel may have been the original target prior to evolution of this toxin to its present form and may serve as a grazing deterrent for zooplankton, fish, and macroinvertebrates that prey on dinoflagellates.

Brevetoxin A and B are polyketides that are found in dinoflagellates and work to enhance activation and inactivation block on Na⁺ channel site 5 (sites 2 and 5 binding

to intramembrane allosteric receptors changes voltage gating when channel is in its active state = always activated). The polyketide ciguatoxin also works at site 5 to shift activation gating. Dinoflagellate polyketide maitotoxin appears to allow nonselective ion passage through cation channels. Azaspiracid is a polyketide from dinoflagellates that blocks the K⁺ pore. Palytoxin's (polyketide) inhibition of the sodium-potassium ATPase has already been discussed for coral venom, but also represents a dinoflagellate poison. Dinoflagellate yessotoxin is also a polyketide that may possibly paralyze via cytoskeletal interactions. Ostreotoxin 3 is a polyketide from dinoflagellates that is an inactivation-gating modifier. Cooliatoxin is another dinoflagellate polyketide with neurotoxic properties of paralytic shellfish poisoning (Cusick and Sayler, 2013).

Eukaryota: Chromalveolata: Heterokontophyta: Bacillariophyceae Poisons

Diatoms are a major group of algae, which should normally put them with plants. However, their close association with amnesic shellfish poisoning deserves mention. Domoic acid is an amino acid from diatoms that works at glutamate receptors to cause depolarization via increased duration of influx of Ca^{2+} and Na^+ (Cusick and Sayler, 2013).

Eukaryota: Opisthokonta: Fungi Poisons

Another group of toxins comes from the molds that grow on animal and plant material and in the soil, where they have to develop mechanisms to combat bacteria. Mycotoxins have a variety of activities. Note the structures of some key mycotoxins in **Figure 30-8**. Aflatoxins' metabolism by CYPs is emphasized, because aflatoxin activation to an extremely reactive epoxide leads to liver damage and cancer in the dietary ppb range. Hepatitis B virus appears to synergize with aflatoxin to produce liver cancer in Africa and Asia. The genus *Aspergillus* produces aflatoxin B_1, the most toxic form, in moldy grain, maize, peanuts (peanut butter contains small amounts of these compounds), and other crops. It was first noted

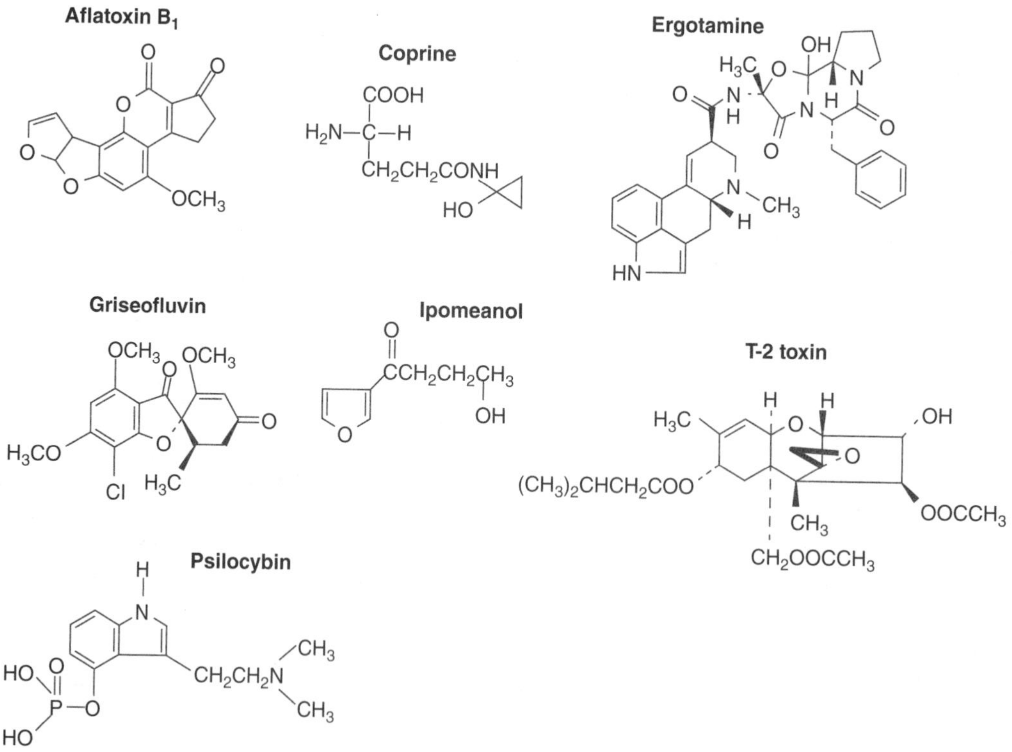

FIGURE 30-8 Structures of Mycotoxins

as a disease of poultry (Turkey-X disease) and affects reproduction and growth rate of birds. Ipomeanol (the "LE factor") produces lung edema in cattle given a sweet potato diet that has the fungus *Fusarium solani* growing on it. In this case, the liver is not the activating organ, but rather the CYPs commonly found in the lung with activity toward activating this furan derivative (1-(3-furyl)-4-hydroxypentanone) through epoxide formation (Hodgson, 2012).

Oxidative stress and DNA damage are caused by the ochratoxin A that is the key toxic agent produced by *Aspergillus ochraceus* and *Penicillium viridicatum*. This fungal toxin reduces intracellular zinc concentration, generates ROS, decreases superoxide dismutase (SOD), and decreases the mitochondrial membrane potential ($\Delta\psi$m). Zinc supplementation helps with ROS, SOD, and ochratoxin-induced DNA strand breaks, but does not help with the effects on the mitochondrial membrane potential (Zheng et al., 2013).

Trichothecenes are sesquiterpenoid *Fusarium* and *Trichoderma* genera fungal metabolites such as the T-2 toxin displayed in Figure 30-8. They are bactericidal (probably reflecting their original intent), fungicidal (competition), and insecticidal. Diarrhea, anorexia, and ataxia are mammalian signs of toxicity yielding Abakabi disease in Japan and stachybotryotoxicosis in Russia. A purer fungicidal compound comes from *Penicillium griseofulvum* strain that produces a tubulin-binding compound (griseofulvin = 2S-7-chloro-2,4,6-trimethoxy-6-methylspiro[benzofuran-2(3H),1′[2] cyclohexene-3,4-dione) that alters microtubule function and inhibits mitosis. A much more toxic fungus is the *Amanita phalloides* or death cap producing α-amanitin, a cyclic octapeptide with selective inhibition of RNA polymerase II in eukaryotes. This effectively eliminates mRNA synthesis at concentrations below 1.0 μg/mL. Edible fungi known as the death cap or ink cap also come from the genus *Coprinopsis*. The toxin coprine is a cyclopropanol glutamine derivative as shown in Figure 30-8. Coprine inhibits the low K_m form of liver acetaldehyde dehydrogenase due the active metabolite cyclopropanone hydrate, thereby increasing the toxicity of ethanol via halting the further metabolism of the acetaldehyde metabolite of alcohol dehydrogenase.

Ergot alkaloids from *Claviceps purpurea*–contaminated grain lead to ergotism, known previously as St. Anthony's fire in animals. These compounds affect the nervous system and are also vasoconstrictive. They are similar agents to the hallucinogen LSD as they are amides of lysergic acid and can be amine alkaloids such as lysergic acid and amino acid alkaloids such as ergotamine. The effects of these agents involve their agonist, partial agonist, and/or antagonistic effects at biogenic amine receptors, which lead to nausea, vomiting, decreased circulation, rapid and weak pulse, stimulated uterine motility in females, and coma. The 1960s saw many humans taking a variety of psychoactive agents including synthetic and natural hallucinogens. The Aztecs used "magic" mushrooms (genera *Psilocybe*, *Stropharia*, and *Conocybe*) to generate a spiritual state via the hallucinogen psilocybin (O-phosphoryl-4-hydroxy-N,N-dimethyltryptamine). Psilocybin can also cause psychosis in people likely to develop that condition without the action of this serotonin analogue (most likely works at biogenic amine/serotonin receptors). One of the most interesting toxins produced by the *Fusarium* fungus growing in corn, barley, wheat, hay, and oats is zearalenone, a natural endocrine disruptor. This mycotoxin is estrogenic and produces hyperestrogenic effects affecting reproduction, especially in pigs (Hodgson, 2012).

Bacteria Poisons

Moving into the prokaryotes, the bacteria include gram-negative (double-walled and do not stain) and positive (single wall and do stain) bacteria and photosynthetic cyanobacteria. The discussion of cyanobacteria could be reserved for the beginning of the plant section (similar or part of cycad poisoning); however, it has already been mentioned how cyanobacteria may have poisons similar to that found in dinoflagellates and plants (cycad poisoning). *Clostridium botulinum* toxin has already been discussed. The heavy chain of botulism toxin is the mechanism of transport to the intracellular (neuronal cytoplasm) compartment by interacting with the luminal domain of synaptobrevin (Ahnert-Hilger et al., 2013), while the light chain actually produces the lysis involved in preventing acetylcholine release. This process leads to muscle fatigue, ptosis, dysarthria, and death as a result of respiratory paralysis (Hodgson, 2012). Phage genes appeared to play a large role in the development of the botulinum toxin. The same is true for anthrax, tetanus, diphtheria, toxic shock, scarlet fever, exfoliative dermatitis, food poisoning, traveler's diarrhea, *Shigella* dysentery, necrotizing pneumonia, and cholera (although others also include mobile genetic elements). A family of related staphylococcal pathogenicity islands encoding superantigens is characterized by 15–20 kb elements that occupy constant positions in toxigenic strains. This region encodes integrases, helicases, and terminases with flanking direct repeats. The prototype is SaPI1 of *Staphylococcus aureus*, which encodes TSST-1 (toxic shock syndrome toxin-1) plus Sags, SEK, and SEL. Other family members encode enterotoxins B (SaPI3) and C (SaPI4) with the minimum of two more Sags each. SaPI1 and SaPI2 also encode TSST-1 and are excised and induced to replicate by specific staphylococcal phages. The way these toxins are transferred indicates that they come from other species other than bacilli (*Bacillus cereus*), staphylococci (*Staphylococcus aureus*), and clostridia (*Clostridium perfringens* and *Clostridium botulinum*). *Clostridium perfringens* α-toxin is an exception, as it is encoded by a standard chromosomal gene and can cause fatal gangrene on its own (Novick, 2003).

It is of evolutionary interest how the phage obtained these genes and the advantage conferred to the bacterium by the introduction of a gene that encodes for toxins. Lysogenic phages are part of the chromosomes of toxigenic bacteria. Toxins are generally released by lysis, but some are released with outer-membrane proteins in outer-membrane vesicles. Lipopolysaccharide represents an important non-protein toxin and endotoxin, which is part of the cell wall of gram-negative bacteria. Toxins can alter the eukaryotic cell membrane by changing a structural component and/or its function. Some toxins bind to specific glycoprotein or ganglioside receptors on the surface membrane. The toxin is then incorporated via

absorptive endocytosis. Protein toxins have two components: A, an enzyme, and B, a polypeptide that binds to the receptor. A majority of these toxins may be activated via nicking by proteases when synthesized by the bacterium or attached to the membrane receptor. Intracellular cAMP increases in cells affected by many of these toxins due to the enzymatic ADP-ribosylation of the adenylyl cyclase regulatory proteins as occurs with cholera toxin (*Vibrio cholera* causes extreme and painful diarrhea and dehydration via affecting the GTP-regulatory protein). Protein synthesis inhibition occurs with diphtheria toxin via the transfer of ADP-ribose to elongation factor-2 (EF-2). The majority of bacterial toxins also target cells where they bind, but tetanus toxin and to a lesser extent botulinum toxin move up axons and inhibit more distant structures (Lubran, 1988).

Approximately 50 toxins appear to be at least partially to fully responsible for the pathological manifestations and/or mortality that are caused by host infection or contamination of food (intoxication). These toxins may travel in the bloodstream and affect internal organs or destroy host tissue and kill phagocytes in the vicinity of the infection leading to bacterial growth and spread (Alouf, 1998). *Pseudomonas* exotoxin A works similarly to diphtheria toxin by ADP-ribosylation of EF-2, but has no immunological cross-reactivity and exhibits extremely different cell-line specificities. Both toxins bind to different cell surface receptors and have different internalization pathways. While the Vero cell line is a good test for sensitivity to diphtheria toxin, there is no such cell line for *Pseudomonas* exotoxin A. The mouse or rat cells L-929 and 3T3 that respond with a lethal dose value of 0.10 and 0.15 ng/mL, respectively, are totally resistant to diphtheria toxin. Thus, the internal toxicity mechanism can be similar, but the cell surface protein must first make the cell sensitive to binding and incorporation of the toxin. *Pseudomonas* exoenzyme S also causes ADP-ribosylation of eukaryotic proteins, but is not correlated to morbidity in cells or animals.

Shigella toxin causes extreme diarrhea and dysenteric syndrome though a protein exotoxin, which is cytotoxic, neurotoxic, and enterotoxic. Its primary toxicity is inhibition of protein synthesis via inactivation of the 60S eukaryotic ribosomal subunit. *Escherichia coli* enterotoxins have two distinct types. The heat-labile enterotoxin is similar to cholera toxin in that it binds to the same G_{M1}-containing receptor and has similar but usually less dramatic internal activity producing "traveler's diarrhea." This enterotoxin's activity is so close to cholera toxin that the cholera toxin antibody inhibits enterotoxin's activation of adenylyl cyclase. The heat-stable enterotoxin stimulates guanylyl cyclase.

Bordetella pertussis toxin similarly to the cholera toxin or heat-labile *E. coli* heat-labile enterotoxin has an A portion that causes ADP-ribosylation and increased cAMP formation. However, the B oligomer blocks the biological action of the entire toxin likely by competing for receptor occupancy. Alone, the B oligomer induces insulin-like or mitogenic responses from other cells, possible by cross-linking or aggregation of cell surface proteins similar to concanavalin A or anti-receptor antibodies. However, the A promoter added alone lacked its toxic activity, but pretreatment of cells with the B oligomer and washing them allowed the A promoter to deliver its enzymatic activity/toxicity. The mode of action of this pertussis toxin is different from cholera toxin. The pertussis toxin results in ADP-ribosylation of a 41,000-MW membrane protein with an affinity for guanine nucleotides, while the cholera toxin ADP-ribosylates a 45,000-MW G protein. Thus, it appears that cholera or *E. coli* heat-labile enterotoxin acts on the G protein, while pertussis toxin causes ADP-ribosylation of the G_i or N_i protein.

Anthrax toxin from *Bacillus anthracis* is familiar to veterinarians for its occasional outbreaks, but recently has been used as a bioterrorism toxin. This toxin has a protective antigen, edema factor, and a lethal factor, each of which is a protein. None of the components alone are active. In this case the A_s-B structure has the B fragment as the protective antigen and A representing the lethal factor or edema factor. The B fragment binds to the tumor endothelium marker-8 and capillary morphogenesis protein 2. After membrane endoproteases from the furan family cleave a fragment off the B protein, a pre-pore oligomer can bind to the lethal factor or the edema factor. It is of interest

that the edema factor itself is an adenylyl cyclase that raises cAMP in conjunction with a cellular cofactor that is calmodulin (Middlebrook and Dorland, 1984). The lethal factor of bacillus anthracis acts as a Zn^{2+}-dependent metalloproteinase that cleaves the N-terminus of mitogen-activated protein kinase kinases (MAPKK) disrupting signal transduction and causes apoptotic pathways to be activated, especially problematic for immune cells responding to the infection (Chauncey et al., 2012).

Tetanus toxin (tetanospasmin) is produced by the anaerobic bacterium *Clostridium tetani* where spores infect contaminated wounds. Tetanus and botulinum toxin are taken up similarly into nerve terminals of lower motor neurons. The tetanus toxin is a Zn^{2+}-dependent metalloproteinase that cleaves synaptobrevin/vesicle-associated membrane protein (VAMP) that is required for release of neurotransmitter from nerve endings via fusion of synaptic vesicles with neuronal plasma membrane. The initial symptom of flaccid paralysis due to decreased release of ACh is similar to botulism. Unlike botulism toxin, tetanus toxin is transported retrograde up the axons of motor neurons until it reaches the spinal cord or brainstem. It crosses synapses and is taken up by the GABAergic neurons (presynaptic inhibitory neurotransmitter) or glycinergic neurons (postsynaptic inhibitory neurotransmitter of motor neurons). Cleaving VAMP prevents release of GABA and glycine leading to a partial, functional denervation of lower motor neurons progressing to hyperactivity and increased muscle activity including rigidity and spasms ("lockjaw"). Because botulinum toxin A prevents ACh at the same neuromuscular junctions by cleaving a different protein (SNAP-25) rather than synaptobrevin, which is cleaved both by tetanus and botulinum toxins B, D, F, and G, this may be used to treat the rigidity and spasms caused by tetanus toxin (Hassel, 2013).

Toxins from cyanobacteria or "blue-green algae" of species *Anabaena*, *Aphanizomenon*, *Microcystis*, *Nodularia*, and *Oscillatoria* are found in eutrophic freshwater rivers, lakes, and streams (usually associated with fertilizer runoff). There are four major classes of cyanotoxins including hepatotoxins, neurotoxins, cytotoxins, and irritant or dermatoxins. *Microcystis aeruginosa* releases heptapeptides (cyclo-D-Ala-L-X-erythro-β-methyl-D-iso-Asp-L-Y-[3-amino-9-methoxy-2,6,8-trimethyldehydroAla]-D-isoGlu-N-methyldehydroAla; where X and Y are variable amino acids for the 90 microcystin isoforms) known as microcystins, which are hepatotoxic. The microcystins are biosynthesized non-ribosomally by the thiotemplate function of a large multifunctional enzyme complex including a non-ribosomal peptide synthetase and polyketide synthase (familiar polyketides in dinoflagellate poisons) domains. They may be released into the water or be taken up with the cyanobacterium into fish, dogs, or even humans. The organic anion transport (OAT) proteins allow the microcystins access to hepatocytes where they inhibit eukaryotic protein phosphatases 1 and 2A. This leads to increased phosphorylation of structural filaments followed by cytoskeletal degradation and the destruction of the acinar structural of the liver. Hepatocytes then retract from surrounding tissue and sinusoidal capillaries allow blood pooling in the liver. Death results from local tissue damage proceeding to liver failure and hemorrhagic shock. Nonlethal exposures in humans may lead to development of cancer via protein phosphatase inhibition. The cyclic pentapeptide nodularin is produced by *Nodularia spumigena*. Nodularins and microcystins usually produce similar action and so are usually lumped together even in testing kits. The potent neurotoxin saxitoxin is a cyanobacterial neurotoxin (its mechanism of action was examined in the section on snails followed by dinoflagellates earlier in this chapter). The cyanobacteria species that produce saxitoxin are *Anabaena circinalis*, *Aphanizomenon* species, *Aphanizomenon gracile*, *Cylindrospermopsis raciborskii*, and *Lyngbya wollei*, while the dinoflagellate species producing saxitoxins are *Alexandrium*, *Pyrodinium*, and *Gymnodinium*. This trialkyl tetrahydropurine is the parent compound of more than 30 naturally occurring derivatives due to different moieties at four positions due to hydroxylation, sulfation, or carbamoylation. The carbamate toxins are 10–10,00 times more potent than the *N*-sulfo-carbamoyl derivatives. The guanidinium groups and the carbon-12 hydroxyls in saxitoxin are crucial to binding to sodium channel α subunit. The carbamoyl

side chain aids in the binding process. A single mutation in that Na^+ channel subunit can confer complete insensitivity to saxitoxin by sacrificing speed of that channel. Cylindrospermopsin is a polyketide-derived alkaloid toxin with a central functional guanidine portion and a hydroxymethyluracil linked to a tricyclic carbon backbone produced by *Cylindrospermopsis raciborskii* (major toxin producer), *Aphanizomenon ovalisporum*, *Aphanizomenon flosaquae*, *Umezakia natans*, *Raphidiopsis curvata*, *Anabaena bergii*, *Anabaena lapponica*, and *Lyngbya wollei*. This toxin is hepatotoxic, cytotoxic, and neurotoxic as well, with its toxicity linked to its uracil and C7 hydroxyl interfering with GSH, protein synthesis, and CYPs (Pearson et al., 2010).

Questions

1. What is the difference between animal venoms and poisons?
2. How can CRISPs give an accounting of evolution of venoms?
3. What is the difference between the activities of short- and long-chain α-neurotoxins?
4. What are the toxicity dimensions of the enzyme phospholipase A_2?
5. What toxins do Gila monsters and beaded lizards produce, and what is their physiological action?
6. Botulism toxin prevents ACh release. How does black widow spider venom accomplish a similar endpoint by a substantially different mechanism?
7. Why are the fish of Synanceiidae (stonefish) and Scorpaenidae (scorpionfish) considered arising from similar molecular evolutionary origins?
8. What property do some conotoxins share with other venomous species, including spiders, snakes, assassin bugs, and scorpions?
9. What are the similarities and differences between Portuguese man-of-war jellyfish nematocyst toxin and α-latrotoxin from the black widow spider?
10. What are the origins of frog poisons?
11. What do the trichothecenes indicate about the original purpose of the fungal toxins α-amanitins?

12. Why is it important to find the origins of bacterial or shellfish toxins?
13. Why is the A-B structure so important for bacterial toxin activity?

References

Ahnert-Hilger G, Münster-Wandowski A, Höltje M. 2013. Synaptic vesicle proteins: targets and routes for botulinum neurotoxins. *Curr Top Microbiol Immunol*. 364:159–177.

Alouf J. 1998. [Implications of bacterial protein toxins in infectious and food-borne diseases]. *C R Seances Soc Biol Fil*. 192:485–502.

Barber CM, Isbister GK, Hodgson WC. 2013. Alpha neurotoxins. *Toxicon*. 66:47–58.

Calvete JJ, Sanz L, Cid P, de la Torre P, Flores-Díaz M, Dos Santos MC, Borges A, Bremo A, Angulo Y, Lomonte B, Alape-Girón A, Gutiérrez JM. 2010. Snake venomics of the Central American rattlesnake *Crotalus simus* and the South American *Crotalus durissus* complex points to neurotoxicity as an adaptive paedomorphic trend along *Crotalus* dispersal in South America. *J Proteome Res*. 9:528–544.

Casewell NR, Wüster W, Vonk FJ, Harrison RA, Fry BG. 2013. Complex cocktails: the evolutionary novelty of venoms. *Trends Ecol Evol*. 28:219–229.

Cavalier-Smith T. 2003. Protist phylogeny and the high-level classification of Protozoa. *Europ J Protistol*. 39:338–348.

Chaim OM, Trevisan-Silva D, Chaves-Moreira D, Wille ACM, Ferrer VP, Matsubara FH, Mangili OC, da Silveira RB, Gremski LH, Gremski W, Senff-Ribeiro A, Veiga SS. 2011. Brown spider (*Loxosceles* genus) venom toxins: tools for biological purposes. *Toxins (Basel)*. 3:309–344.

Chau R, Kalaitzis JA, Neilan BA. 2011. On the origins and biosynthesis of tetrodotoxin. *Aquat Toxicol*. 104:61–72.

Chauncey KM, Lopez MC, Sidhu G, Szarowicz SE, Baker HV, Quinn C, Southwick FS. 2012. *Bacillus anthracis'* lethal toxin induces broad transcriptional responses in human peripheral monocytes. *BMC Immunol*. 13:33.

Cobra Master. 1994. Cobra venom vs other snakes: case study. http://cobras.org/cobra-venom/

Cusick KD, Sayler GS. 2013. An overview on the marine neurotoxin, saxitoxin: genetics, molecular targets, methods of detection and ecological functions. *Mar Drugs*. 11:991–1018.

Daly JW. 1995. Alkaloids from frog skins: selective probes for ion channels and nicotinic receptors. *Braz J Med Biol Res*. 28:1033–1042.

Daly JW. 2004. Marine toxins and nonmarine toxins: convergence or symbiotic organisms? *J Nat Prod*. 67:1211–1215.

Dumbacher JP, Spande TF, Daly JW. 2000. Batrachotoxin alkaloids from passerine birds: a second toxic bird genus (*Ifrita kowaldi*) from New Guinea. *Proc Natl Acad Sci USA*. 97:12970–12975.

Edwards L, Hessinger DA. 2000. Portuguese Man-of-war (*Physalia physalis*) venom induces calcium influx into cells by permeabilizing plasma membranes. *Toxicon*. 38:1015–1028.

El-Kik CZ, Fernandes FF, Tomaz MA, Gaban GA, Fonseca TF, Calil-Elias S, Oliveira SD, Silva CL, Martinez AM, Melo PA. 2013. Neutralization of *Apis mellifera* bee venom activities by suramin. *Toxicon*. 67C:55–62.

Frazão B, Vasconcelos V, Antunes A. 2012. Sea anemone (*Cnidaria, Anthozoa, Actiniaria*) toxins: an overview. *Mar Drugs*. 10(8):1812–1851.

Gomes HL, Menezes TN, Carnielli JB, Andrich F, Evangelista KS, Chávez-Olórtegui C, Vassallo DV, Figueiredo SG. 2011. Stonefish antivenom neutralises the inflammatory and cardiovascular effects induced by scorpionfish *Scorpaena plumieri* venom. *Toxicon*. 57:992–999.

Grant IC. 1997. Ichthyosarcotoxism: poisoning by edible fish. *J Accid Emerg Med*. 14:246–251.

Haddad V Jr, Cardoso JL, Lupi O, Tyring SK. 2012. Tropical dermatology: venomous arthropods and human skin: part II. *Diplopoda, Chilopoda*, and *Arachnida. J Am Acad Dermatol*. 67:347.e1–9; quiz 355.

Halstead, BW. 1958. Poisonous fishes. *Public Health Rep*. 73:302–312.

Hannon HE, Atchison WD. 2013. Omega-conotoxins as experimental tools and therapeutics in pain management. *Mar Drugs*. 11:680–699.

Hariharan H, Mitchell WR. 1976. Observations on bacteriophages of *Clostridium botulinum* type C isolates from different sources and the role of certain phages in toxigenicity. *Appl Environ Microbiol*. 32:145–158.

Hassel B. 2013. Tetanus: pathophysiology, treatment, and the possibility of using botulinum toxin against tetanus-induced rigidity and spasms. *Toxins (Basel)*. 5:73–83.

Hodgson E. 2012. Toxins and venoms. *Prog Mol Biol Transl Sci*. 112:373–415.

Jones TH, Adams RM, Spande TF, Garraffo HM, Kaneko T, Schultz TR. 2012. Histrionicotoxin alkaloids finally detected in an ant. *J Nat Prod*. 75:1930–1936.

Jønsson KA, Bowie RCK, Norman JA, Christidis L, Fjeldså J. 2008. Polyphyletic origin of toxic *Pitohui* birds suggests widespread occurrence of toxicity in corvoid birds. *Biol Lett*. 4:71–74.

Kita M, Nakamura Y, Okumura Y, Ohdachi SD, Oba Y, Yoshikuni M, Kido H, Uemura D. 2004.

Blarina toxin, a mammalian lethal venom from the short-tailed shrew *Blarina brevicauda*: isolation and characterization. *Proc Natl Acad Sci USA.* 101:7542-7547.

Le Bars D, Gozariu M, Cadden SW. 2001. Animal models of nociception. *Pharmacol. Rev.* 53:597-652.

Liu S-B, He Y-Y, Zhang Y, Lee W-H, Qian J-Q, Lai R, Jin Y. 2008. A novel non-lens βγ–crystallin and trefoil factor complex from amphibian skin and its functional implications. *PLoS ONE.* 3:e1770.

Lubran MM. 1988. Bacterial toxins. *Ann Clin Lab Sci.* 18:58-71.

Lukasheva EV, Efremova AA, Treshchalina EM, Arinbasarova AIu, Medentsev AG, Berezov TT. 2012. [L-amino acid oxidases: properties and molecular mechanisms of action]. *Biomed Khim.* 58:372-384.

Ma C, Wang H, Wu Y, Zhou M, Lowe G, Wang L, Zhang Y, Chen T, Shaw C. 2012. Helokinestatin-7 peptides from the venoms of *Heloderma* lizards. *Peptides.* 35:300-305.

Maciel NM, Schwartz CA, Rodrigues Pires Júnior O, Sebben A, Castro MS, Sousa MV, Fontes W, Ferroni Schwartz EN. 2003. Composition of indolealkylamines of *Bufo rubescens* cutaneous secretions compared to six other Brazilian bufonids with phylogenetic implications. *Comp Biochem Physiol B Biochem Mol Biol.* 134:641-649.

Marcussi S, Santos PR, Menaldo DL, Silveira LB, Santos-Filho NA, Mazzi MV, da Silva SL, Stábeli RG, Antunes LM, Soares AM. 2011. Evaluation of the genotoxicity of *Crotalus durissus terrificus* snake venom and its isolated toxins on human lymphocytes. *Mutat Res.* 724:59-63.

McCleary RJ, Kini RM. 2013. Non-enzymatic proteins from snake venoms: a gold mine of pharmacological tools and drug leads. *Toxicon.* 62:56-74.

Meyer WL. 1996. Most toxic insect venom. In: *Book of Insect Records.* Gainesville, FL: University of Florida. http://entnemdept.ufl.edu/walker/ufbir/chapters/chapter_23.shtml

Middlebrook JL, Dorland RB. 1984. Bacterial toxins: cellular mechanisms of action. *Microbiol Rev.* 48:199-221.

Morgenstern D, King GF. 2013. The venom optimization hypothesis revisited. *Toxicon.* 63:120-128.

Mortari MR, do Couto LL, dos Anjos LC, Mourão CBF, Camargos TS, Vargas JA, Oliveira FN, Gati Cdel C, Schwartz CA, Schwartz EF. 2012. Pharmacological characterization of *Synoeca cyanea* venom: an aggressive social wasp widely distributed in the Neotropical region. *Toxicon.* 59:163-170.

Mourão CB, Oliveira FN, e Carvalho AC, Arenas CJ, Duque HM, Gonçalves JC, Macêdo JK, Galante P, Schwartz CA, Mortari MR, Almeida Santos Mde F, Schwartz EF. 2013. Venomic and pharmacological activity of *Acanthoscurria paulensis* (Theraphosidae) spider venom. *Toxicon.* 61:129-138.

Novick RP. 2003. Mobile genetic elements and bacterial toxinoses: the superantigen-encoding pathogenicity islands of *Staphylococcus aureus.* *Plasmid.* 49:93-105.

Pearson L, Mihali T, Moffitt M, Kellmann R, Neilan B. 2010. On the chemistry, toxicology and genetics of the cyanobacterial toxins, microcystin, nodularin, saxitoxin and cylindrospermopsin. *Mar Drugs.* 8:1650-1680.

Ramos B, Vasconcelos V. 2010. Palytoxin and analogs: biological and ecological effects. *Mar Drugs.* 8:2021-2037.

Santhosh MS, Hemshekhar M, Sunitha K, Thushara RM, Jnaneshwari S, Kemparaju K, Girish KS. 2013. Snake venom induced local toxicities: plant secondary metabolites as an auxiliary therapy. *Mini Rev Med Chem.* 13:106-123.

Schwartz EN, Schwartz CA, Sebben A, Largura SW, Mendes EG. 1999. Indirect cardiotoxic activity of the caecilian *Siphonops paulensis* (Gymnophiona, Amphibia) skin secretion. *Toxicon.* 37:47-54.

Skarin H, Håfström T, Westerberg J, Segerman B. 2011. *Clostridium botulinum* group III: a group with dual identity shaped by plasmids, phages and mobile elements. *BMC Genomics.* 12:185.

Smith JJ, Herzig V, King GF, Alewood PF. 2013. The insecticidal potential of venom peptides. *Cell Mol Life Sci.* 70:3665-3693.

Sousa SR, Vetter I, Lewis RJ. 2013. Venom peptides as a rich source of cav2.2 channel blockers. *Toxins (Basel).* 5:286-314.

Speijer H, Govers-Riemslag JW, Zwaal RF, Rosing J. 1986. Prothrombin activation by an activator from the venom of *Oxyuranus scutellatus* (Taipan snake). *J Biol Chem.* 261:13258-13267.

Stratta P, Badino G. 2012. Scombroid poisoning. *CMAJ.* 184:674.

Sugiyama H. 1980. *Clostridium botulinum* neurotoxin. *Microbiol Rev.* 44:419-448.

Sunagar K, Johnson WE, O'Brien SJ, Vasconcelos V, Antunes A. 2012. Evolution of CRISPs associated with toxicoferan-reptilian venom and mammalian reproduction. *Mol Biol Evol.* 29:1807-1822.

Tan NH. 2005. Toxins from venoms of poisonous snakes indigenous to Malaysia: a review. http://www.tanngethong.com/toxins_from_venoms_of_poisonous_.htm

Tibballs J, Li R, Tibballs HA, Gershwin LA, Winkel KD. 2012. Australian carybdeid jellyfish causing "Irukandji syndrome". *Toxicon.* 59:617-625.

Weldon PJ, Kramer M, Gordon S, Spande TF, Daly JW. 2006. A common pumiliotoxin from poison frogs exhibits enantioselective toxicity against mosquitoes. *Proc Natl Acad Sci USA.* 103:17818-17821.

Woolf CJ. 2013. Pain: morphine, metabolites, mambas, and mutations. *Lancet Neurol.* 12:18-20.

Yotsu-Yamashita M, Kim YH, Dudley SC Jr, Choudhary G, Pfahnl A, Oshima Y, Daly JW. 2004. The structure of zetekitoxin AB, a saxitoxin analog from the Panamanian golden frog *Atelopus zeteki*: a potent sodium-channel blocker. *Proc Natl Acad Sci USA*. 101:4346–4351.

Zhang DM, Liu JS, Tang MK, Yiu A, Cao HH, Jiang L, Chan JY, Tian HY, Fung KP, Ye WC. 2012. Bufotalin from Venenum Bufonis inhibits growth of multidrug resistant HepG2 cells through G2/M cell cycle arrest and apoptosis. *Eur J Pharmacol*. 692:19–28.

Zhao Q, Liu ZD, Xue Y, Wang JF, Li H, Tang QJ, Wang YM, Dong P, Xue CH. 2011. Ds-echinoside A, a new triterpene glycoside derived from sea cucumber, exhibits antimetastatic activity via the inhibition of NF-κB-dependent MMP-9 and VEGF expressions. *J Zhejiang Univ Sci B*. 12:534–544.

Zheng J, Zhang Y, Xu W, Luo Y, Hao J, Shen XL, Yang X, Li X, Huang K. 2013. Zinc protects HepG2 cells against the oxidative damage and DNA damage induced by ochratoxin A. *Toxicol Appl Pharmacol*. 268:123–131.

CHAPTER 31

Poisonous Plants or Plant Cells and Ingestion or Contact Toxicity

This is a chapter outline intended to guide and familiarize you with the content to follow.

I. Poisonous plants or plant cells—see Figure 31-1, Table 31-1

  A. Protection of plant from herbivores, bacteria, and fungi

  B. Seed poisons

   1. Castor bean's ricin lectin has N-glycosidase activity for 28S rRNA of mammalian 60S subunit → cytotoxic and neurotoxic properties + has hemagglutinin property as well and ricinine → GI poisoning, liver and kidney damage, and in extreme CNS poisoning potentiates glutamate release. Small-seeded castor bean plant produces more ricinine, which also has antibacterial activity

   2. Rosary pea's abrin lectin's two polypeptide chains → GI toxin (A-B structure similar to many bacterial toxins with B gaining access for other chain [RNA-N-glycosidase]) → ribosomal protein synthesis inhibition and is part of the ribosomal-inactivating proteins represented by ricin, abrin (type II ribosomal inactivating protein), gelonin, momordin, and mistletoe lectin. Intraperitoneally injected abrin → toxicity to MAPK pathway, cytokine-cytokine receptor interaction, calcium signaling pathway, Jak-STAT signaling pathway, and natural killer cells

   3. Bouncing bet's saponins → CNS and cardiac depression and GI complications via membranolytic effects and toxic effects (as well as fungitoxic effect)

   4. Strychnine alkaloid → antagonism of inhibitory glycine receptors

   5. Grasspea's toxic amino acid β-N-oxalyl-α, β-L-diaminoproprionic acid (ODAP) → neurolathyrism (motoneuron dysfunction) depleting thiols through oxidative stress and mitochondrial dysfunction. As ODAP is transported intracellularly via system xc-glutamate/cysteine transporter, presence of cysteine may inhibit uptake and toxicity of ODAP

   6. Soybean's trypsin/protease inhibitors → pancreatic hypertrophy → death

   7. Chickpeas, mung beans, lentils, and broad beans also have protease inhibitors that are eliminated by requisite soaking in water for 24 hours at room temperature

   8. Cyanogenic glycosides are found in stone fruits → cyanide by gut bacteria exocellulase β-glucosidase or via exposure to heat, mineral acids, or megadoses of ascorbic acid

   9. Cycad poisoning → Guamanian form of amyotrophic lateral sclerosis/parkinsonism dementia complex. Neurotoxic properties are due to toxic cyanobacterial amino acid β-methylaminoalanine (BMAA which is found in brain tissue of some patients from Guam and North America with Alzheimer's disease) and cycasin, a developmental neurotoxin and alkylating agent (hepatotoxic, developmentally toxic, and carcinogenic)

   10. Cottonseeds' gossypol (terpenoid aldehyde of polyphenolic compound) → apoptosis via inhibition of calcineurin. Temporary paralysis due to ↓ K+ levels. Hemolysis → anemia. Gossypol's toxicity partially due to ROS production in reproductive system (antifertility agent in male mammals), heart,

CONCEPTUALIZING TOXICOLOGY 31-1

liver, and biological membranes in general and its constituent electron transfer functionalities and those of gossypol's metabolites

11. Solanine (glycoalkaloid) from green potato eyes, skin, stem, and sprouts → reversible inhibitors of human plasma butyrylcholinesterase, but toxicity related to cytotoxicity, GI, and neurological effects

C. Root poisons

1. Monkshood synthesizes alkaloids aconitine, mesaconitine, and jesaconitine → bind to Na^+ channels prolonging their open state similar to frog batrachotoxins and pumiliotoxins. In the heart ↑ Na^+ → ↑ Ca^{2+} and fatal arrhythmias (torsades de pointes)

2. Large liana of South America produces d-tubocurarine → nonspecific cholinergic nicotinic cholinergic antagonist that acts to paralyze muscles (does not cross BBB)

3. Licorice roots triterpenoid glycyrrhizin inhibits 11β-hydroxysteroid dehydrogenase, which is responsible for inactivating cortisol → state resembling ↑ aldosterone levels with Na^+ retention and hypertension. Triterpenoids also have immunomodulatory and antitumor activities related to ↑ apoptosis and inhibition of oncogenic and anti-apoptotic signaling pathways and suppression or nuclear translocation of transcription factors such as NF-κB

4. Umbelliferae toxin 7-hydroxycoumarins interfere with vitamin K → bloody diarrhea (fungal contamination as fungi produce coumarin)

D. Fruit poisons

1. Buckthorn toxins coyotillo and tullidora produce segmental demyelination of peripheral nerves due to alterations of Schwann cell metabolism

2. Berries of *Amrita cocculus* and bicuculline of Dutchman's breeches → $GABA_A$ antagonism and epileptic seizures as opposed to the agonistic sedative-hypnotic actions of medicinal plant *Loeselia mexicana* compound daphnoretin or fungal chemicals muscimol and ibotenic acid at the same receptor

E. Plant leaves and flowers

1. Tobacco plant's nicotine is famous for its addictive properties due to binding to nicotinic cholinergic receptors. Nicotine has developmental effects on zebrafish (neural differentiation and axon path-finding errors)

2. Coca leaves produce cocaine → blocks Na^+ channel (local anesthetic) and prevents reuptake of dopamine (stimulant), serotonin, norepinephrine and epinephrine

3. Opium poppy produces a paste that contains a powerful addictive analgesic, respiratory center depression agent, and constipating chemical leading to the discovery of the opioid receptors (especially μ). Papaverine in the opium plant inhibits cyclic nucleotide phosphodiesterase → smooth muscle relaxation

4. Marijuana plant produces Δ^9-tetrahydrocannabinol that produces CNS depression and physical dependence, acute anxiety, and psychosis on heavy use

5. Toxicodendrons are known for urushiol, a mixture of catechols that help develop allergic reactions known as poison ivy, poison oak, or poison sumac reactions

6. Bracken or coarse ferns or aquatic ferns have thiaminase in rhizomes and young fronds that are protective against insects. In monogastrics such as humans or especially horses, demyelination of peripheral nerves is the sign of thiamine deficiency. In this same plant, ptaquiloside → bone marrow depression and acute hemorrhagic syndrome

7. *Prosopis juliflora* plant produces cara-torta or pie face due to cranial nerve dysfunction if used as a grazing food source for long periods. This plant also contains piperidine alkaloid juliprosopine → uncoupling oxidative phosphorylation in neurons due to arrangement of inner mitochondrial membrane

8. Pyrrolizidine alkaloids produced by > 6,000 plants mostly in the Boraginaceae, Asteraceae, Orchidaceae, and Leguminosae families are CYP-activated hepatotoxins that cause veno-occlusive

CONCEPTUALIZING TOXICOLOGY 31-1 (*continued*)

disease and cancer. Other CYP-activated compounds are teucrin A from germander (liver damage due to reactive epoxide that inactivates CYP3A and epoxide hydrolase) and safrole from black pepper (DNA adducts formed following 1-hydroxylation and sulfation). Aristolochic acids from *Aristolochia* species form a reduction of a nitro group by CYP1A1/2 or peroxidases to reactive cyclic nitrenium ions. Furanocoumarins from grapefruit juice irreversibly inhibit CYP3A causing medication overdoses such as the statins used to control cholesterol. Other suicide substrates for CYPs come from capsaicin in chili peppers, diallyl sulfone in garlic, methysticin and dihydromethysticin in kava, oleuropein in olive oil, and resveratrol found in grape seeds. GSH depletion can result from catnip's pulegone and kava's quinone

9. Lupines contain piperidine alkaloids and quinolizidine alkaloids → muscle weakness and ataxia (incoordination) and fetal contracture-type skeletal defects and cleft palate. Poison hemlock's coniine results in similar effects in pigs and sheep (birds not similarly affected)

10. Plants of the Ericaceae family contain diterpene grayanotoxins or andromedotoxin, acetylandromedol, or rhodotoxin in the leaves, twigs, and flowers → "mad honey disease" due to binding to the group II receptor site in voltage-gated Na^+ channels ($Na_v1·x$), probably on the internal surface of the membrane so that they cannot be inactivated

11. Pokeweed antiviral protein is an N-glycosidase similar to ricin or abrin

12. Belladonna or "beautiful women" refers to the atropine in this plant that dilates the pupil (and causes CNS toxicity and bradycardia) due to its muscarinic cholinergic receptor antagonism. Scopolamine is a similarly acting agent from the nightshades

13. The chrysanthemum produces pyrethrins with action on Na^+ channel (retard opening and closing) → neurotoxicity and used as a natural insecticide

14. Other CNS-active compounds are arecoline, (nicotinic receptor antagonist from *Areca catechu* L.), caffeine (increased norepinephrine secretion by competitive antagonism at adenosine receptors from *Coffea* spp., *Cola* spp., etc.), cathinone (stimulant that leads to release and inhibits reuptake of dopamine from *Catha edulis*), codeine (another μ- and κ-opioid receptor agonist similar to morphine from *Papaver somniferum*), dimethyltryptamine (causes hallucinations via serotonin receptor agonism from *Anadenanthera peregrina* and *Virola theiodora*), ephedrine (stimulant from *Ephedra nevadensis*), ginkgolides and bilobalide (interferes with platelet function but is not really neurological despite ads stating benefits of *Ginkgo biloba*), harmine and harmaline (hallucinogen, serotonin syndrome, and hypertension via MAO inhibition and sedation from *Banisteriopsis* spp., etc.), hyoscyamine (muscarinic receptor antagonist similar to atropine from *Atropa belladonna*, etc.), ibogaine (hallucinations via α3β4 nicotinic receptor antagonism from *Tabernanthe iboga*), lysergic acid amide/ergine (hallucinogen via serotonin receptor agonism from *Argyreia nervosa*, etc.), mescaline (hallucinations via serotonin receptor agonism from *Lophophora williamsii* and *Trichocereus pachanoi*), methysticin, dihydromethysticin, yangonin, desmethoxyyangonin, kavain, dihydro-kavain (all sedative products of rhizomes of *Piper methysticum* with actions of inhibition of norepinephrine reuptake [kavain], reversible MAO B inhibition [desmethoxyyangonin], and some analgesic activities), mitragynine (opioid receptor agonism from *Mitragyna speciosa*), muscarine (dysphoria produced through muscarinic agonism from *Amanita muscaria*), muscimol (sedation through GABA agonism also from *Amanita muscaria*), physostigmine (reversible AChE inhibitor from *Physostigma venenosum*), pilocarpine (muscarinic receptor agonist from *Pilocarpus microphyllus*), psilocybin metabolizes to active psilocin (hallucinogen via 5-HT1A and 5-HT2A/2C agonism from *Psilocybe* spp.), reserpine (depressant, antipsychotic via depletion of vesicular stored monoamines from *Rauvolfia serpentine*), salicin and salicylic acid (NSAIDs/analgesic and antipyretic that can also disturb acid/base balance via nonselective COX inhibition from *Salix alba* and *Spiraea* spp.), salvinorin-A (hallucinations through κ-opioid receptor agonism from *Salvia divinorum*), and scopolamine (depression and euphoria via muscarinic receptor antagonism from *Atropa belladonna*, etc.)

15. Yellow star thistle produces sesquiterpene → depletes GSH → ↑ ROS → cell membrane damage and nigropallidal encephalomalacia in horses (high MAO activity = susceptible to oxidative injury)

16. *N*-Methylphenethylamine = alkaloid from *Acacia* plants is a pressor (↑ blood pressure) and produces "limberleg" (locomotor ataxia)

CONCEPTUALIZING TOXICOLOGY 31-1 *(continued)*

17. Low larkspurs produce *N*-methylsuccinimidoanthranoyllycoctonine = alkaloid that causes antagonism at N_M receptors → muscle weakness, respiratory depression, death

18. Quinine alkaloid poisoning → cinchonism (bark of *Cinchona officinalis*) = ↓ hearing, GI problems, vasodilation, diaphoresis, headache → blindness and cardiac and neurological toxicity with possibilities of thrombocytopenia (and purpura). Malarial patients receiving pure quinine also experience anemia, intravascular hemolysis, and renal failure. This same plant also produces quinidine = antiarrhythmic medication that blocks Na^+ current and multiple cardiac K^+ currents with marked Q-T prolongation. Quinidine and cinchonine are alkaloids that also potentiate the cytotoxicity and apoptosis induced by cancer chemotherapeutic medication paclitaxel by accumulation of P-glycoprotein-positive (P-gp) substrate rhodamine and cleaved the poly (ADP-ribose) polymerase, activated caspase 3 and downregulated P-gp expression

19. Paclitaxel (taxane) is from yew bark and needles (see Figure 31-2 for structures) → at high concentrations cardiotoxic due to action on myocardium (↑ Ca^{2+} by affecting Na^+ and Ca^{2+} conductance → ↑ A-V conduction and QRS duration) and used at therapeutic concentrations for cancer due to binding to β-tubulin → prevents the disassembly of this critical cytoskeletal protein → mitotic arrest

20. The tropolone alkaloid colchicine from *Gloriosa superba* causes mitotic arrest by interfering with microtubule and spindle formation, but also lowers body temperature, ↑ sensitivity to CNS depressants, depresses respiratory center, ↑ activity of sympathomimetic compounds, constricts blood vessels (hypertension), induces seizures, and ↑ GI motility. The vinca alkaloids from the Madagascar periwinkle plant also interfere with microtubule via binding to β-tubulin and prevent polymerization with α-tubulin

21. Other cancer chemotherapeutic agents arising from Chinese medicinal plants are more toxic such as etoposide (derivative of podophyllotoxin of the mandrake plant) → forms ternary complexes with topoisomerase II and DNA preventing resealing of breaks following topoisomerase binding to DNA. Topotecan (derivative of cytotoxic quinone alkaloid camptothecin from *Camptotheca acuminate* Decne) inhibits topoisomerase I → DNA damage and apoptosis. Gambogic acid from *Garcinia* spp. = cytotoxic compound → G0/G1 cell-cycle arrest in chronic myeloid leukemia through interference with steroid receptor coactivator-3 and has proapoptotic activities via binding to the transferrin receptor and inhibition of Bcl-2 family proteins and topoisomerase IIα. Gambogic acid also inhibits activation of VEGFR2 and downstream protein kinases → prevent angiogenesis (microvessels). The "thunder god vine" contains terpenoids (and alkaloids) such a triptolide → induces overexpression of cytomembrane death receptor in cholangiocarcinoma cells and uses mitochondrial-mediated pathways to induce apoptosis in leukemia cells. Tripterine from the same plant celastrol uses NF-κB, caspase family proteins, VEGF receptors, heat shock proteins, K^+ and Ca^{2+} channels, and Ig Fc ε receptor 1 to affect apoptosis, cell cycle arrest, and decreased angiogenesis and metastasis. Other Chinese medicinal plants vary in toxicity from dehydration or GI problems (slightly toxic such as *Evodia rutaecarpa*, *Prunus armeniaca*, *Melia toosendan*); to cough, dyspnea, vomiting, goiter, urticaria or similar symptoms (toxic such as *Pinellia ternate*, *Xanthium sibricum*); to toxic or deadly (*Strychnos nux-vomica* containing strychnine)

22. Cardiac active compounds are digitalis from foxglove plant → inhibition of $3Na^+$, $2K^+$-ATPase → ↑ Ca^{2+}

23. Accumulation of Cu in people with Wilson's disease = copper-accumulating *Trifolium* spp. Accumulation of nitrates → metHb formation (forage sorghum, sudangrass, sudan-sorghum hybrids). Nitrate accumulation from protein concentrate–amended corn silage or free-choice hay also ↓ progesterone via inhibition of CYP. Lush pasture grazing → Mg deficiency in ruminants. Brown and red seaweed diet to sheep → Cu deficiency. Cyanosis induced by sorghums (contain prussic acid). Calcium oxalate crystals in dumbcane or *Halogeton glomeratus* → irritation of lips, GI tract, and possibly respiratory irritation. Irritation is also caused by a sanguinarine alkaloid from *Sanguinaria canadensis*. Irritation can also be caused by diterpene or triterpene in spurge. Emesis caused by lycorine alkaloid from Amaryllidaceae on neurokinin-1 receptor and serotonin 3 receptor. The terpenoid glycoside ligustrin from the privet also causes vomiting and diarrhea, but can also lead to convulsions and death. Tannins from tree leaves ↓ vertebrate protein digestion but not in insects. Insects' high pH intestinal tract → formation of semiquinone radicals, quinones, and ROS from tannins. Acorns high in tannins cause kidney damage in cattle. Hypericin from

CONCEPTUALIZING TOXICOLOGY 31-1 (*continued*)

St. John's wort → photosensitization via yield of singlet oxygen and ROS and also ↑ diarrhea, heart and respiration rate, and fever. Eating too many carrots (β-carotene) or furocoumarins from wild parsnip also causes photosensitization. Cattle can be photosensitized by phylloerythrin, a chlorophyll degradation product formed in the rumen. *Tetradymia* spp. yield phototoxic syndrome especially problematic in sheep (big head and loss of lips). Hemolytic anemias develop in ruminants fed high amounts of rape forage. *Brassica oleracea* contain glucosinolates → hydrolyze to isothiocyanates → goitrogens (inhibition I uptake by thyroid). Tansy mustard → blindness by unknown mechanism. Walnut tree bark contains naphthoquinones → laminitis and fish toxicity (especially juglone) and ROS generation accompanied by GSH depletion → apoptosis

CONCEPTUALIZING TOXICOLOGY 31-1 (*continued*)

This chapter covers mainly macrophyte/aquatic plants and vascular terrestrial plants or tracheophytes. These are definitely of the kingdom Plantae. The first focus is the seed of the plant and why a seed needs to develop a toxin. Plants such as the sunflower or the pumpkin produce enough seeds to waste many of them without concern, while a peach only has one "pit" and will protect it with a cyanide-containing toxin. However, does it matter which herbivore this toxin is affecting the most? For example, the insect may be highly affected based on its size. Mammals also have to be separated based on size (small mouse intestine versus extensive transit time in an elephant's intestinal tract) and whether they are monogastrics or ruminants. Some toxins, if they are further metabolized by the bacteria in the rumen, will release more of the toxic compound. Ruminants can also be sensitive to rumen stasis. Others will be ineffective in ruminants such as a thiaminase, as the rumen bacteria make abundant thiamine. Certain birds are not sensitive to the coniine in hemlock, while a human eating that contaminated bird would succumb to the toxin. Certain birds of South America eat toxic seeds and then eat clay so they can adsorb the toxic component(s) of the seed onto the clay and retain the nutrients for absorption.

Ecotoxicologists need to consider whether a precious seed is also producing the toxin to prevent germination under improper conditions such as low moisture and low activity of soil bacteria, which are needed to promote hydrolysis of certain compounds. Or, is the toxin antibacterial and protecting the seed from bacterial degradation that may interfere with germination and growth? The fruit, leaf, or root of the plant may also be toxic. However, certain omnivores or herbivores have developed systems that are resistant to toxicity. For example, the golden bamboo (*Cephalostachyum* cf. *viguieri* contains 0.015% cyanide in the plant) lemur (*Hapalemur aureus*) eats 12 times the lethal dose of cyanide compared with other mammals. It is not yet known how they avoid cyanide poisoning.

In this chapter, plant toxins are examined starting with the seeds and working from there to other parts of the plant. Plant poisons can involve a variety of compounds such as alkaloids (organic hydroxyl acids such as hydroxybutanedioic acid, 2-hydroxy-1,2,3,-propanetricarboxylic acid, tannic, and quinic acids from dicotyledonous plants), glycosides, lipids (neutral fats, phospholipids, and sterols), phenols, sulfur compounds, lipids, and phenols. Some have been used in bioterrorism and others as medicines (cocaine, opiates), illegal and legal drugs of abuse (cannabinoids from marijuana, opium from poppies, nicotine from tobacco), and legal stimulants (caffeine). Human diets have carcinogens in them as represented by safrole in black pepper and cholinesterase inhibitors such as solanine and glycoalkaloid α-chaconine found in the green portions of improperly stored potatoes (left out in the light; Hodgson, 2012). Representative structures of plant poisons are displayed in **Figure 31-1**. Toxicity of plant poisons are summarized in **Table 31-1**.

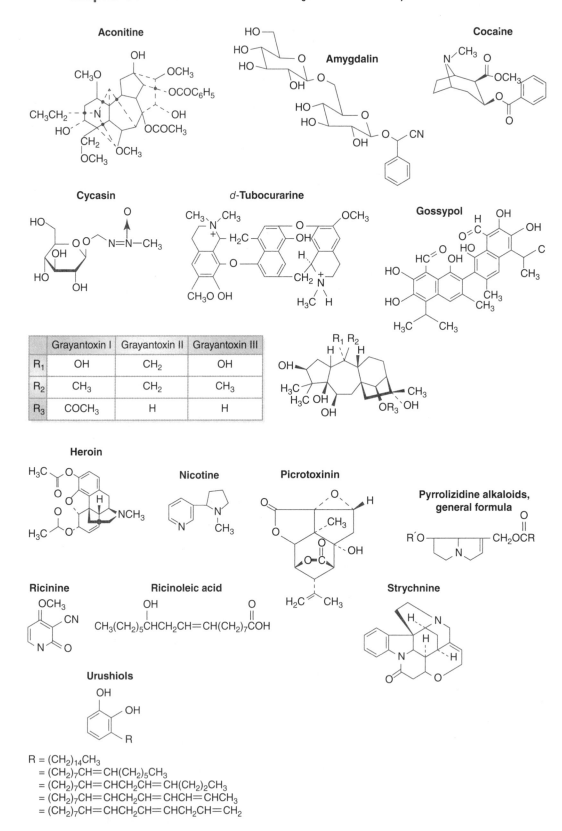

FIGURE 31-1 Structures of Plant Poisons

TABLE 31-1   Toxicity of Plants

Toxicity	Plant toxins	Toxic Mechanism
Neurotoxicity	Ricinine	Increased glutamate release
	Buckthorn toxin, fern thiaminase	Peripheral demyelination & possible autism development
Lathyrism	β-N-oxalyl-α, β-L-diaminoproprionic acid	Mitochondrial dysfunction + thiol ↓ in motor neurons
Neurotoxicity → bradycardia & respiratory depression	Grayanotoxins	Prevents voltage-gated Na^+ channel inactivation
Hyperexcitability	Pyrethrum/pyrethrins	Na^+ channel ↓ response
Drugs of abuse toxicities	Cocaine	Na^+ channel and reuptake of monoamine blocks
	Morphine, codeine, mitragynine	Depress respiratory center, μ
Sedation	$Δ^9$-tetrahydrocannabinol methysticin, dihydromethy-sticin, yangonin, desmethoxy-yangonin, kavain, dihydro-kavain	Cannabinoid receptor type 1 Various mechanisms including MAO B inhibition, NE reuptake inhibition, analgesic activity
Stimulants	Cathionine, ephedrine	Adrenergic-like effects
Hallucinations	Dimethyltryptamine, lysergic acid amide, mescaline, psilocin	Serotonin receptor agonist
	Ibogaine	$α3β4$ nicotinic receptor antagonism
	Salvinorin-A	κ-opioid receptor agonist
Serotonin syndrome	Harmine, harmaline	MAO inhibition
(+ heart and muscle)	Nicotine, arecoline	nAChR binding
Dysphoria	Muscarine, pilocarpine	Muscarinic receptor agonism
Neurotoxicity → respiratory depression	Atropine, scopolamine, hyoscyamine	Muscarinic antagonism
Seizures	Picrotoxin, bicuculline	$GABA_A$ antagonism
Sedation/hypnosis	Daphnoretin, muscimol	$GABA_A$ agonism
Hypersensitivity to sensory inputs + convulsions	Strychnine	Glycine receptor antagonism
Neurodegeneration	Cycasin, β-methylamionalanine	ALS/parkinsonism & possible Alzheimer's tangles
Neurotoxicity + G.I. symptoms	Solanine	Cytotoxic + inhibit butyrylcholinesterase
	Physostigmine	AChE inhibition
Nigropallidal encephalomalacia	Repin	ROS, cell membrane damage
Antipsychotic/depressant	Reserpine	Depletion of vesicular stored monoamines
Neurotoxicity	Amygdalin, other cyanogenic glycosides, prussic acid	CN inhibits cytochrome a_3
	Juliprosopine	Uncouples oxidative phosphorylation
	Saponins	CNS depression
Blindness, tinnitus, cardiac effects, G.I., drop in blood pressure, platelet effects.	Quinine	Direct effects on neurons — curare-like action on neuromuscular junctions
Blindness	Tansy mustard	Unknown
Emesis	Lycorine	Neurokinin-1 & $5-HT_3$ receptors

(continues)

TABLE 31-1　Toxicity of Plants (*continued*)

Toxicity	Plant toxins	Toxic Mechanism
NSAID analgesia/antipyretic	Salicin, salicylic acid	COX inhibition
Fatal cardiac ventricular arrhythmias	Aconitine	Prolonged opening Na^+ channel $\rightarrow Ca^{2+}$ triggering
Arrhythmias + b.p. changes + CNS stimulation	Caffeine (for susceptible individuals)	$\uparrow$NE secretion via competitive antagonism adenosine receptors
Torsades de pointes	Quinidine	Blocking Na^+ and multiple K^+ cardiac current
Heart block & cardiac arrest	Taxine B	Block Ca^{2+} (& Na^+) channels
Heart block & hyperkalemia	Digoxin	$3Na^+$, $2K^+$-ATPase inhibition
Heart arrest	Saponins	Cardiac depression
Neuromuscular	d-Tubocurarine, MSAL-type alkaloids	N_M antagonist
Tetany $\rightarrow$ death	Low Mg, high K, high nitrogen (NH_3-producing) forage	Mg deficiency
Muscle weakness/ataxia	Quinolizidine & piperidine alkaloids, NMPEA	Inhibition of muscle movement
Hemagglutinin	Ricin	RCA120 action
Hemorrhage	Fern ptaquiloside	Bone marrow damage
	Gikgolides, hydrangin	Platelet function interference
Hemolytic anemia	Forage brassicas	Metabolic disorders $\rightarrow$ Hb oxidation
Aneurysm (dissecting extra-aortic)	*Lathryus odoratus* seeds	Alterations of elastic fibers in arteries & membranes
Cyanosis & CYP inhibition leading to $\downarrow$ progresterone at lower concentrations	High nitrate (nitrite)	Methemoglobin formation
Blood pressure changes	Papaverine	Smooth muscle relaxation
	Glycerrhizin	Inhibits 11b-hydroxysteroid dehydrogenase
Mitosis arrest	Paclitaxel vs. colchicine and vinca alkaloids	Increasing vs. decreasing microtubule formation
Kidney cancer	Aristolochic acids	CYP1A1/2 or peroxidase activation
Pancreas damage	Soybean trypsin inhibitors	Protease inhibition hypertrophies pancreas as need for production increases
Goiter	Glucosinolates/isothiocyanates	$\downarrow$ I uptake by thyroid
G.I., hepatic, kidney toxicity	Ricinine	Alkaloid toxicity
Liver damage/cancer/hemo-occlusive disease	Pyrrolizidine alkaloids	CYP activation
Liver damage	Teucrin A, teuchamaedryn A	CYP3A4 activation – inactivation of CYP3A and epoxide hydrolase
G.I. tract effects + kidney damage	Tannins	ROS (insects) + $\downarrow$protein digestion (vertebrates)
Serosal edema of stomachs	Allylisothiocyanate	Irritation & cytotoxicity
Make medications such as the liver toxic acetaminophen or statins more toxic due to lack of proper metabolism	Pulegone, kava (quinone) Sulfone, methysticin, dihydromethysticin, oleuropein, resveratrol, furanocoumarins	GSH depletion CYP suicide substrates
Liver damage	*Trifolium* spp.	Cu accumulation

TABLE 31-1   Toxicity of Plants (*continued*)

Toxicity	Plant toxins	Toxic Mechanism
Reproductive followed by liver, heart, lung, RBC (hemolysis)	Gossypol	ROS, electron transfer, apoptosis
Developmental (cleft palate + "crooked calf disease")	Quinolizidine & piperidine alkaloids	Inhibit muscle movement
DNA adducts with possible cancer formation	Safrole, methyleugenol, estragole, quercitin	1-Hydroxylation & sulfation
	Cycasin	
DNA strand breaks → cell death	Podophyllotoxin	Inhibition topoisomerase II
	Camptothecin	Inhibition topoisomerase I
Apoptosis	Plumgagin, juglone	ROS + GSH-depletion
Irritation	Urushiols	Allergic contact dermatitis
	Calcium oxalate, sanguinarine alkaloids, diterpene /triterpene esters	Edema/erythema
Photosensitization	β-carotene, furocoumarins, hypericin, phylloerythrin	Coloration/skin reactions
Vomiting, diarrhea, convulsions → death	Glycoside ligustrin	Unknown action
G.I.problems, slowed respiration, dizziness, weakness	Githagenein	

Seed Poisons

The most infamous seed toxin is the ricin (toxic lectin protein) or alkaloid ricinine (1,2,-dihydro-4-methoxy-1-methyl-2-oxo-3-pyridinecarbonitrile) produced by the castor bean (*Ricinus communis*). This white compound in its crude state has easily been removed from the castor bean and has been mailed as a bioterrorism tool. The ricin toxin A chain is the cytotoxic component of the dimeric protein and depurinates the α-sarcin/ricin loop following retrograde trafficking to the cytosol (B chain = sugar binding). Ricin has an N-glycosidase activity, which cleaves a single N-glycosidic bond at position A-4324 of the 28S rRNA of the mammalian 60S subunit and thereby confers its cytotoxic and neurotoxic properties (Tong et al., 2012). Ricin (RCA60) is an antitumor agent at lower doses and a hemagglutinin (2 proteins = RCA120) and toxin (2 proteins). Ricin E has a hybrid B-chain of ricin and *R. communis* agglutinin (Worbs

et al., 2011). Ricinine causes gastrointestinal (GI) poisoning symptoms, liver and kidney damage, and in extreme poisoning convulsions, coma, hypotension and death due to increased glutamate release in the central nervous system (CNS; Ferraz et al., 2002). It is of interest that the small-seeded variety of the castor bean plant produced more ricinine, which has antibacterial activity. So the plant seed is protecting itself against herbivores and bacteria that may affect germination and growth (Khafagi, 2007).

Abrin (toxalbumin) is another lectin (glycoprotein) and biological warfare agent similar to ricin that is composed of two polypeptide chains with a disulfide bond connecting them produced by *Abrus precatorius*, the rosary pea or jequirity bean. It is a GI toxin, with one polypeptide chain (polypeptide B chain as a galactose-specific lectin) binding to the intestinal cell membrane which facilitates the entrance of the other chain (A-chain portion) into the cytoplasm. Ribosomal protein synthesis is inhibited causing cell death and loss of intestinal function (secondarily causing plasma composition changes that progress to cerebral edema and cardiac arrhythmia). Ricin, abrin, gelonin (from Himalayan plant *Gelonium multiflorum*), momordin (a saponin derived from the bitter melon, *Momordica charantia*, and the balsam apple, *Momordica balsamina*), mistletoe lectin (fermented preparations of *Viscum album* or common mistletoe a hemi-parasitic shrub that grows on stems of white fir, *Abies pectinata*), and other plant proteins are known as ribosomal-inactivating proteins (ironically known as RIPs). Abrin and ricin are two of the most toxic substances known to exist, only exceeded by botulinum toxin. Abrin is a member of the family of type II ribosomal inactivating proteins composed of A and B subunits (appears similar to many bacterial toxins). The A chain has enzymatic function as an RNA-N-glycosidase, resulting in depurination of adenine at 4325 in the 28S rRNA. This activity abolishes all mammalian cellular translation. Similar to ricin, the modification of the ribosomal subunit prevents elongation factor 2 binding (note that diphtheria toxin did another method of interfering with EL-2 by ADP-ribosylation), thereby preventing protein synthesis. When abrin is injected intraperitoneally into the mouse, the brain effects start with rapid induction of the immune and inflammatory response, progressing to severe damage. Organ damage throughout the organism was indicated by increases in serum lactate dehydrogenase, aspartate aminotransferase, urea, and creatinine. Microarray analysis of the brain tissue indicated toxicity to a remarkable array of regulators of signaling pathways including the mitogen-activated protein kinase (MAPK) pathway, cytokine-cytokine receptor interaction, calcium signaling pathway, Jak-STAT signaling pathway, and natural killer cells (Bhaskar et al., 2012).

Saponins from the bouncing bet (*Saponaria officinalis*) and corn cockle (*Agrostemma githago*) lead to CNS and cardiac depression as well as GI complications. Saponins have membranolytic effects, toxic and fungitoxic effects, adverse effects on animal growth and performance, and hypocholesterolemic effects (Price et al., 1987).

Strychnine is a familiar alkaloid seed poison originating from *Strychnos nux-vomica*. This compound works by antagonism of inhibitory glycine receptors (postsynaptic control of motoneurons, interneurons as in antagonistic muscle group, afferent sensory neurons including pain fibers, and visual and auditory processing). Not surprisingly, strychnine makes the animal or human hypersensitive to sensory stimuli, induces convulsions, and the resulting respiratory deficits may lead to rapid death after very few convulsions (Dutertre et al., 2012).

Another seed poison depends on the species of animal and the diet of humans (undernutrition combined with high seed ingestion). A toxic amino acid β-N-oxalyl-α, β-L-diaminopropionic acid (ODAP) from the grasspea and its metabolism and distribution to tissue underlie the development of neurolathyrism, a spastic paraparesis that originates from an upper motoneuron dysfunction. However, *Lathyrus sativus* has a high quantity of protease inhibitors that complicates the picture, especially in feeds of poultry and pigs. Similarly, soybean (*Glycine max*) trypsin/protease inhibitors (heat labile so cooked soybeans are not toxic) caused pancreatic hypertrophy and death, if the pancreas was sufficiently inhibited. These proteinaceous and polyphenolic enzyme (protease) inhibitors cause fecal loss of sulfur amino acids through formation of enzyme-inhibitor complexes (chickpea, mung bean, lentil, and broad bean also have protease inhibitors that are mainly eliminated by soaking the beans in water for 24 hours at room temperature). ODAP further depletes reduced thiols through oxidative stress and mitochondrial dysfunction in the motor cortex and lumbar spinal cord of mice. ODAP also inhibits tyrosine amino transferase, which leads to elevated levels of l-3,4-dihydroxyphenylalanine (L-DOPA). L-DOPA is O-methylated requiring S-adenosylmethionine, which further stresses sulfur amino acids by drawing on methionine. ODAP additionally inhibits cystathionine-γ-lyase. Because ODAP or homocystic acid sensitize CA1 pyramidal neurons in hippocampal neurons to cysteine toxicity and ODAP is transported intracellularly by system xc-glutamate/cysteine transporter, the presence of cysteine may inhibit the uptake and toxicity of ODAP. Thus, it appears that a species has to have a reduced amount of thiols that sensitizes them to ODAP and the development of lathyrism (Enneking, 2011).

Seeds from *Lathyrus odoratus* alter elastic cartilage in arteries and membranes causing extra-aortic dissecting aneurysms (Walker, 1957). Pits from the *Prunus* genus found in stone fruits such apricots, bitter almonds, peaches, black or wild cherries, and the chokecherry have amygdalin, a cyanogenic glycoside. Other plants (e.g., macadamia nuts and almonds) have this chemically bonded cyanide, aldehyde or ketone, and sugar. This is the form in which most cyanide is formed in plants. It has been used as a fraudulent ineffective and toxic medication, laetrile, to treat cancer. The cyanide is released as hydrogen cyanide (prussic acid) in the gut by the bacterial exocellulase β-glucosidase or via exposure to heat, mineral acids, or megadoses of ascorbic acid (vitamin C). This makes the amygdalin more toxic in ruminants as more complete digestion may occur in the rumen with crude pit ingestion. Humans usually need to eat the seed contents. The poisoning is clearly cyanosis (inhibition of cellular respiration by inhibition of cytochrome a_3; Herbert, 1979).

Another plant toxin may have some origins in cyanobacteria. The development of the neurodegenerative disease known initially as cycad (division Cycadophyta) poisoning or Lytico-Bodig disease is actually a Guamanian form of amyotrophic lateral sclerosis/parkinsonism dementia complex. The indigenous Chamorro people of the Mariana Islands use cycad seeds that have neurotoxic properties due to the toxic cyanobacterial amino acid β-methylaminoalanine (BMAA) and cycasin, a developmental neurotoxin and alkylating agent (methylazoxymethanol-β-D-glucoside). Cycasin is hepatotoxic, carcinogenic (digestive tract, liver, and kidney tumors when fed to rats), and a developmental toxin in addition to its neurotoxicity. It is of ecotoxicologic interest that fruit bats feed on cycad seeds and bioaccumulate BMAA. BMAA is found in brain tissue of Guam patients and some North American patients dying of Alzheimer's disease. The biochemical evidence suggests Alzheimer's disease-like combined 3R and 4R tau species resulting in neuropathologic tangles and neurodegeneration. This may be a cyanobacterial link to at least to part of the neurodegeneration that is caused by plants, herbivores, and animals that feed off those herbivores (food chain biomagnification; Ince and Codd, 2005).

Gossypol is a terpenoid aldehyde of the polyphenolic compound (six phenolic hydroxyl groups and two reactive aldehyde moieties, formula $C_{30}H_{30}O_8$) found in cotton (genus *Gossypium*, family Malvaceae) seeds (Wang et al., 2009). If given too high in an animal diet, it can have effects on milk production in cows, despite the rumen bacterial ability to metabolize gossypol at a low percentage of the diet. Gossypol is an effective antifertility agent in male mammals, as it appears to substantially lower testosterone levels in long-term (12–20 week) feeding studies in male rabbits and reduce testosterone release from the rat testes. However, feeding levels of about 20 mg/kg/day into Dutch-belted male rabbits caused loss of appetite, hind limb paralysis, and breathing difficulties with liver and lung congestion and intestinal gases (Saksena et al., 1981). Gossypol causes apoptosis via regulation of Bax and Bcl2, reversibly inhibits calcineurin, and binds to calmodulin. The temporary paralysis is likely due to reduced K^+ levels caused by this agent. Gossypol is also hemolytic and can cause anemia through this activity (Zbidah et al., 2012). Part of gossypol's toxicity may be related to generating reactive oxygen species (ROS) in the reproductive system, heart, liver, and biological membranes in general and its constituent electron transfer functionalities and those of gossypol's metabolites (conjugated dicarbonyl—a quinone derivative; Kovacic, 2003).

The potato is a tuberous (tubers are botanically separate from the "true seed") plant of the family Solanaceae (the deadly nightshades). That biological classification defines the toxin, the alkaloid solanine, which is rich in areas of high metabolic activity such as eyes, skin, stem, and sprouts. These plants have natural plant glycoalkaloids, which include nitrogen in a steroid structure, and hexacyclic alkaloid aglycones that are biosynthesized from cholesterol. Glycoalkaloids are α-solanine (tri-glycoside containing galactose, glucose, and rhamnose) and α-chaconine (glucose + two rhamnose groups) from the potato, α-tomatine and dehydrotomatine from the tomato, and solasonine and solamargine from the eggplant. These glycoalkaloids are found in tubers, roots, sprouts, and leaves of the potato plant and are α compounds. Both α-solanine and α-chaconine are reversible inhibitors of human plasma cholinesterase (butyrylcholinesterase). This is of interest, but solanine toxicity appears not to be related to cholinergic syndrome. Instead, the toxicity observed in animals is characterized by GI and neurologic symptoms including vomiting, headache, and flushing. These compounds are also cytotoxic (Barceloux, 2009). The glycoside githagenin from *Agrostemma githago* (corn cockle) causes GI problems and a "cheesy" discharge from the mouths of birds, slow breathing, dizziness, and weakness (Hebestreit and Melzig, 2003). Acute mustard seed toxicosis in beef cattle was reported in 1988 in Saskatchewan related to allyl isothiocyanate content causing extensive serosal edema of the stomach and reduction of brain cholinesterase activity (Kernaleguen, 1989).

Root Poisons

Aconitine, mesaconitine, and jesaconitine are alkaloids from the roots of the family Ranunculaceae, including *Aconitum* genus with the name of Monkshood, including medicines and poisons such as monkshood, wolf's bane (used historically to kill wolves), leopard's bane, women's banc, devil's helmet, blue rocket, or queen of the poisons. Aconitine itself may be isolated from *Aconitum napellus* and binds to the Na^+ channels prolonging their open state (remember batrachotoxins or pumiliotoxins from frogs). The increase in cytosolic Na^+ is accompanied in heart cells by excess Ca^{2+} due to the activation of the Na^+/Ca^{2+} exchange system or L-type Ca^{2+} channels and proceeds to triggered activity. The repeated discharges of the focal myocardial area induce arrhythmias. The development of torsades de pointes (rare variety of polymorphic ventricular tachycardia characterized by the apparent "twisting" of the QRS about the isoelectric baseline which may be brought about by long QT syndrome) and ventricular fibrillation via reentry and breakup of wave propagation

can be deadly unless immediately reversed (Jung et al., 2011).

A historic toxic plant compound is curare (used as a weapon against invading Spanish Conquistadors), which is made from the roots and stems of a large liana or vine of the South American rainforest, *Chondrodendron tomentosum*. Its active ingredient, d-tubocurarine, was isolated in 1935 and is a nonspecific nicotinic cholinergic receptor antagonist. As little of this compound crosses the blood–brain barrier (BBB), its major action is muscle relaxation to the point of respiratory paralysis as occurs in those subject to the arrow poisons of indigenous peoples of that region (Heier, 2010).

Licorice roots produce the triterpenoid glycyrrhizin, which inhibits 11β-hydroxysteroid dehydrogenase, which is responsible for inactivating cortisol. As a result, a state resembling high aldosterone levels leads to increased sodium retention and hypertension in those humans or animals consuming natural licorice at high levels in their daily diet. Glycyrrhizin has some therapeutic actions such as for treatment of ulcers, viral infections, and offering liver protection (Isbrucker and Burdock, 2006).

Glycyrrhizic acid and other triterpenoids such as ursolic acid, oleanolic acid, and nomlin; diterpenoids such as andrographolide; and monoterpenoids such as limonene and perillic acid also have immunomodulatory and antitumor activities by inducing apoptosis and inhibiting oncogenic and anti-apoptotic signaling pathways and suppression or nuclear translocation of diverse transcription factors such as NF-κB (Kuttan et al., 2011). Bloody diarrhea can result from consuming roots and rhizomes of the Umbelliferae toxin 7-hydroxycoumarins or hydrangin, which blocks multiple sites of the coagulation cascade but is mainly thought to work via interference with vitamin K (Toohey, 1952).

Fruit Poisons

Buckthorn toxins, such as coyotillo and tullidora, are likely defenses for a desert shrub *Karwinskia humboldtiana* of the Southwestern United States and Northern Mexico. Four key anthracenones (T-544, T-496, T-516, and T-514) produced in the endocarp of the coyotillo fruit yield segmental demyelination of peripheral nerves/peripheral neuropathy such as the sciatic nerve and progressive paralysis similar to Guillain-Barré syndrome in a Wistar rat model and humans (Salazar-Leal et al., 2006). Primary action of these compounds appears to be on Schwann cell metabolism (Mitchell et al., 1978). Berries of a plant native to Southeast Asia, *Amrita cocculus*, produce an agent that affects/antagonizes GABA$_A$ receptors (inhibitory presynaptic GABAergic neurotransmission). By doing so it causes seizures and convulsions and is medicinal in that it can be used to treat overdoses of sedative/hypnotic agents that work via agonism at that receptor. Another agent that has the epileptic GABA$_A$-inhibiting properties is a plant alkaloid, bicuculline, produced by Dutchman's breeches (*Dicentra cucullaria*). Similar but opposite-acting agents that act as agonists of the GABA$_A$ receptor are muscimol and ibotenic acid, the prodrug to muscimol, both produced by the fungus *Amanita muscaria*. Sedative-hypnotic activity and dissociation and synesthesia can occur that are more like psychedelic drugs. This opposite activity of a plant compound versus a fungal compound at the same receptor demonstrates diverging actions of toxins from organisms from different kingdoms. However, plant compounds can also yield sedation via similar mechanisms to the fungal compound. The medicinal plant *Loeselia mexicana* (Polemoniaceae) produces compounds that are used to treat fever, dysentery, stomach pain, swelling, diarrhea, vomiting, headache, dandruff, hair fall, and shock. The compounds consist of flavonols, including quercetin, kaempferol, and glycoflavones, a pentacyclic triterpene, and three coumarins—daphnoretin and its precursors scopoletin and umbelliferone. It is the daphnoretin that has the anti-anxiety activity as would be expected from a GABA$_A$ agonist (Herrera-Ruiz et al., 2011).

Plant Leaves and Flowers

Addictive Neurotoxic Products

The most famous leaf comes from the tobacco plant (*Nicotiana tabacum*). Nicotine is an addiction (tolerance and dependence)-producing alkaloid in the plant. Nicotine binds to the nicotinic acetylcholine (ACh) receptors (nAChRs) and can stimulate some receptors while desensitizing other receptors. Nicotine can increase sympathetic nervous system activation including increases in heart rate via excitation of sympathetic ganglia and causes a discharge of epinephrine from the adrenal medulla or paralysis of parasympathetic ganglia. It can also do the exact opposite (slow heart rate via sympathetic ganglia paralysis and activation of parasympathetic ganglia), depending on dose. Small nicotine doses directly simulate ganglion cells, which is followed by blockade of transmission at high doses. Nicotine also alters the nAChR sensitivity to itself on chronic administration as well as GABAergic systems in nicotine reward reinforcement and increased physiological activity (addiction model). Zebrafish show this biphasic response with rhythmic muscular bending followed by paralysis. Neurological changes in these adult fish occur with 15 and 25 μM nicotine as indicated by an increase in startle response. Embryonic zebrafish exposed to nicotine have alterations in neural differentiation and axon path-finding errors. Adolescent rats exposed to acute nicotine followed by withdrawal exhibited changes in the serotonin receptor response, while prenatal exposure increased locomotive activity in adolescent male rats. Increased dopaminergic activity is also observed in nicotine-enhanced learning pathways (Klee et al., 2011).

Coca leaves produce local anesthesia by blocking the sodium channel and acting centrally as a stimulant via prevention of reuptake of dopamine (most important), serotonin, norepinephrine, and epinephrine (monoamines). Administration of a monoclonal catalytic antibody (1510), mutant butyrylcholinesterase, and mutant cocaine esterase derivative may be an approach to decreasing cocaine dependence and toxicity (Schindler and Goldberg, 2012).

Opium is known by all who have watched *The Wizard of Oz*, in which the poppy was "attractive to the eye but has poison in it." The opium poppy (*Papaver somniferum*) produces opium as a paste. It contains ~12% morphine, an alkaloid, which decreases nociception (opiates produce analgesia via μ, κ, and δ receptors, but morphine is mainly μ with a little κ activity) and produces sedation (via μ and κ receptors). The acetylated version is heroin, which is extremely addictive (induces tolerance and dependence). The μ receptors decreases ACh and μ and δ receptors decrease dopamine neurotransmitter release. Both μ and κ receptors induce constipation, but the real danger of overdose is the depression of central nervous system control of respiration by μ (Pasternak, 1993).

Another less well known or active compound found in opium is the alkaloid papaverine, which appears to involve smooth muscle relaxation via inhibition of cyclic nucleotide phosphodiesterase. However, clinically this compound administered intracisternally to treat aneurysmal subarachnoid hemorrhage caused hypertension and tachycardia in a human patient (Srivastava et al., 2011).

An additional famous drug of abuse and recently medically-prescribed agent, marijuana, comes from the genus *Cannabis* as in the hemp plant *Cannabis sativa*. Cannabinoids, terpenoids, and other compounds are secreted by the glandular trichomes of floral calyxes and bracts of female plants. Marijuana is a product of the flower buds and hashish of the resin. Only the Δ^9-tetrahydrocannabinol (THC) is neurologically active at the cannabinoid receptor type 1. Some heavy users develop a cannabis use disorder and physical dependence (withdrawal induced by abstinence). Also, acute anxiety, psychosis, and other brain deterioration may result from chronic use (Gunderson et al., 2012).

Other Neurotoxic and Neuromuscular Toxicity Agents

The bracken or coarse ferns (genus *Pteridium*) or aquatic ferns (genus *Marsilea*) have a toxin in the rhizomes and young fronds with thiaminase activity that offers these plants protection from insects. In monogastrics such as the horse, the thiamine deficiency leads to demyelination of peripheral nerves that is first noticed by scruffy appearance, weight loss without loss of appetite, and uncoordinated movements. Untreated, this will progress to a crouching stance and loss of muscular control including twitches and tremors. In ruminants, such as cattle, the

chemical ptaquiloside bone marrow depression and following thrombocytopenia lead to an acute hemorrhagic syndrome (Bracken fern poisoning, 2005). It is of interest that the daughter of a woman who drank alcohol and took a thiaminase in the form of an herbal remedy of 1,200 mg/day of *Equisetum arvense* (horsetail) had autism spectrum disorder (Ortega García et al., 2011).

Another neurotoxic plant is *Prosopis juliflora*, which produces cara-torta or pie face due to cranial nerve dysfunction if used as a grazing food source for long periods. One of the piperidine alkaloids in this plant is juliprosopine that causes uncoupling of oxidative phosphorylation in mitochondria in neurons due to arrangement of the inner mitochondrial membrane (increased fluorescent responses of mitochondria labeled with 1-aniline-8-naphthalene sulfonate and 1,6-diphenyl-1,3,5,-hexatriene; Maioli et al., 2012).

The lupines contain piperidine alkaloids and quinolizidine alkaloids. They similarly induce muscle weakness and ataxia as well as fetal contracture-type skeletal defects and cleft palate. Similar malformations are caused in goats and cattle with the lupines, which include the piperidine alkaloids ammodendrine, N-methyl ammodendrine, and N-acetyl hystrine. If pigs and sheep are included with the affected species, then poison hemlock's coniine or γ-coniceine and *Nicotiana glauca*'s anabasine result in similar toxic and developmental effects (Panter et al., 1999). It is of interest that certain bird species, such as the skylark, chaffinch, and robin, are not subject to poisoning by coniine (Vetter, 2004).

Honey is not only toxic to infants due to presence of *Clostridium botulinum* and the lack of immunity in infants, but also to adults if the bees had been in contact with the plants of the Ericaceae family such as the *Rhododendron*, *Pieris*, *Agarista*, and *Kalmia*. These plants contain diterpene (25 isoforms of polyhydroxylated cyclic hydrocarbon with a 5/7/6/5 structure and no nitrogen) grayanotoxin or andromedotoxin, acetylandromedol, or rhodotoxin in the leaves, twigs, and flowers. The first symptoms of "mad honey disease" are due to binding to the group II receptor site in voltage-gated Na^+ channels ($Na_v1\cdot x$), probably on the internal surface of the membrane (only active as hydrophobic binding on the cytoplasmic side). This binding keeps the channels' configuration such that it cannot be inactivated. The neurons are the key target for this action. The increase in vagal tone leads to bradycardia, which is prevented by bilateral vagotomy in rats. Atropine as an acetylcholine antagonist prevented the vagal stimulation that induced the bradycardia and the respiratory depression (Jansen et al., 2012).

Belladonna means "pretty woman" and is a sexist term for toxicity women were subjected to by administration of a toxic alkaloid to dilate their eyes (and cause more glaucoma or blindness from increased light exposure of the retina). The plant *Atropa belladonna* indicates an atropine (muscarinic antagonist) and its use in women. This compound was also a dangerous herbal medicine used as an anti-rheumatic and anti-arthritic agent in Abruzzo, Italy (Leporatti and Impieri, 2007).

Scopolamine is another organic ester of tropic acid from the deadly nightshade plants that blocks acetylcholine at muscarinic receptors. As would be expected from blocking ACh action at these receptors, dry mouth, blurred vision, increased temperature, memory disturbance/amnesia, hallucinations, depression, circulatory collapse, and death due to respiratory failure may result (Hodgson, 2012).

A famous class of neurotoxic agents used commonly as a natural insecticide is pyrethrum (or pyrethrins) isolated from *Chrysanthemum cinerariaefolium*. By action on the nerve membrane Na^+ channels (retarding opening and closing), Na^+ permeability is increased and hyperexcitability results (Katsuda, 2012).

These neuroactive muscarinic antagonists (which can also come from *Brugmansia aurea* L., *Datura stramonium* L., and *Mandragora officinalis* L.) point to the origins of some Western medicines as having been taken from herbal medicine. Other CNS-active compounds are arecoline (nicotinic receptor antagonist from *Areca catechu* L.), caffeine (increased norepinephrine secretion by competitive antagonism at adenosine receptors from *Camellia sinensi*, *Coffea* spp., *Cola* spp., *Ilex* spp., two *Paullina* spp., and *Theobroma cacao*), cathinone (stimulant that leads to release and inhibits reuptake of dopamine from *Catha edulis*), codeine (another μ- and κ-opioid receptor agonist similar to morphine from *Papaver somniferum*), dimethyltryptamine (causes hallucinations via serotonin receptor agonism from *Anadenanthera peregrina* and *Virola theiodora*), ephedrine (stimulant from *Ephedra nevadensis*), ginkgolides and bilobalide (interferes with platelet function but is not really neurological despite common advertising claims for *Ginkgo biloba*), harmine and harmaline (hallucinogen, serotonin syndrome, and hypertension via monoamine oxidase [MAO] inhibition and sedation from *Banisteriopsis caapi*, *Banisteriopsis inebrians*, *Peganum harmala*, and *Passiflora incarnata*), hyoscyamine (muscarinic receptor antagonist similar to atropine from *Atropa belladonna*, *Hyoscyamus niger*, and *Mandragora officinalis*), ibogaine (hallucinations via α3β4 nicotinic receptor antagonism from *Tabernanthe iboga*), lysergic acid amide/ergine (hallucinogen via serotonin receptor agonism from *Argyreia nervosa*, *Ipomoea violacea*, and *Turbina corymbosa*), mescaline (hallucinations via serotonin receptor agonism from *Lophophora williamsii* and *Trichocereus pachanoi*), methysticin, dihydromethysticin, yangonin, desmethoxyyangonin, kavain, dihydro-kavain (all sedative products of rhizomes of *Piper methysticum* with actions of inhibition of norepinephrine reuptake [kavain], reversible MAO B inhibition [desmethoxyyangonin], and some analgesic activities), mitragynine (opioid receptor agonism from *Mitragyna speciosa*), muscarine (dysphoria produced through muscarinic agonism from *Amanita muscaria*), muscimol (sedation through GABA agonism also from *Amanita muscaria*), physostigmine (reversible AChE inhibitor from *Physostigma venenosum*), pilocarpine (muscarinic receptor agonist from *Pilocarpus microphyllus*), psilocybin which metabolizes to active psilocin (hallucinogen via 5-HT1A and 5-HT2A/2C agonism from *Psilocybe* spp.), reserpine (depressant, antipsychotic via depletion of vesicular stored monoamines from *Rauvolfia serpentina*), salicin and salicylic acid (nonsteroidal anti-inflammatory drugs [NSAIDs]/analgesics and antipyretics that can also disturb acid–base balance via nonselective COX inhibition from *Salix alba* and *Spiraea* spp.), salvinorin-A (hallucinations through κ-opioid receptor agonism from *Salvia divinorum*), and scopolamine (depression and euphoria via muscarinic receptor antagonism from *Atropa belladonna*, *Brugmansia aurea*, *Datura metal*, *Datura stramonium*, *Hyoscyamus niger*, and *Mandragora officinalis*; McClatchey et al., 2009).

The yellow star thistle (*Centaurea solstitialis*) and Russian knapweed (*Centaurea repens*) produce a sesquiterpene lactone that depletes GSH, increases ROS, and causes cell membrane damage in cell cultures and ultimately leads to nigropallidal encephalomalacia in horses likely due to susceptibility of this brain region to oxidation due to high activity of MAO (Chang et al., 2012).

N-Methylphenethylamine (NMPEA) is an alkaloid isolated from *Acacia* plants such as *rigidula* or *berlandieri*. NMPEA is a pressor that can increase blood pressure, but it is more known for "limberleg" or "guajillo wobbles." This locomotor ataxia is found in sheep and goats grazing on this plant during droughts (Pemberton et al., 1993).

Achnatherum robustum (also known as *Stipa* spp.) is commonly called sleepy grass, but its activity is actually due to ergine, a product of a fungus growing on the plant. Low larkspurs of the genus *Delphinium* produce toxic alkaloids of the *N*-methylsuccinimidoanthranoyllycoctonine (MSAL) type and less toxic methylenedioxylycoctonine (MDL) type. The toxicity of MSAL-type alkaloids is due to antagonism of the nicotinic ACh receptors at the neuromuscular junction (N_M) causing muscle weakness, tachycardia, failure of voluntary muscular coordination, sternal recumbency, lateral recumbency, respiratory depression, and death. The order of MSAL-type toxicity is nudicauline > 14-deacetylnudicauline > methyllycaconitine >> geyerline (Green et al., 2013).

Quinine alkaloid poisoning is known by the term *cinchonism*, indicating its plant origin (*Cinchona officinalis* bark). Symptoms involve changes in hearing, GI problems, vasodilation, diaphoresis, and headache turning to blindness and cardiac and neurological toxicity, including effects on the chemoreceptor trigger zone. Thrombocytopenia and purpura are possible. Malarial patients may also experience anemia, acute intravascular hemolysis, and renal failure (Bateman and Dyson, 1986). Some reproductive effects have also been examined (Farombi

et al., 2012). This same plant also produces other alkaloids such as the cardioactive/toxic quinidine (blocks Na^+ current and multiple cardiac K^+ currents with marked Q-T prolongation; Grace and Camm, 1998) and cinchonine. It is of interest that these two alkaloids potentiate the cytotoxicity and apoptosis induced by the cancer chemotherapeutic medication paclitaxel in multidrug resistance. They do so by accumulation of P-glycoprotein-positive (P-gp) substrate rhodamine and cleaving the poly (ADP-ribose) polymerase, activating caspase 3, and downregulating P-gp expression (and increasing sub-GI apoptotic portion; Lee et al., 2011). The chemotherapeutic medication paclitaxel also is of plant origin: The yew (*Taxus* spp.) bark and needles contains the highest amount of this toxic therapeutic medication.

The taxine alkaloids were first isolated as taxine with a chemical formula of $C_{37}H_{52}NO_{10}$, but are now represented by two major types: taxine A and taxine B. The structures of these two types of compounds are exhibited in **Figure 31-2**. Taxanes A and B are cardiotoxic with direct action on depressing the myocardium leading to hypotension and cardiac arrest. However, taxine B is more potent in this regard, increasing A-V conduction and QRS duration. These toxic actions lead to second-degree and complete heart block and diastolic cardiac arrest. Taxines yield these effects via an increase in cytosolic Ca^{2+} by affecting Na^+ and Ca^{2+} channel conductance. Paclitaxel, the diterpenoid cancer medication, also inhibits the calcium pump at high concentrations. Its therapeutic concentrations are more specific to the mitotic spindle. Paclitaxel binds to the β-tubulin subunit of microtubules and prevents the disassembly of this critical cytoskeletal protein. Bundles of excess microtubules with aberrant structures develop, causing mitotic arrest (Wilson et al., 2001). Mitotic arrest can also be obtained by blocking microtubule formation. *Gloriosa superba* is known as the glory lily and is used as an industrial medicinal crop in South India due to its high colchicine alkaloid content. The tuber of the plant is highly toxic and has been used to commit suicide or murder, while the leaves have pharmacologic properties. All the tropolone alkaloids isolated from this plant have

	3a	3b	3c	3d
R_1	OH	OH	H	H
R_2	Ac	H	Ac	H
R_3	H	Ac	H	H
R_4	H	H	Ac	H
Taxine alkaloids	Taxine B	Isotaxine B	I-Deoxytaxine B	I-Deoxyisotaxine B

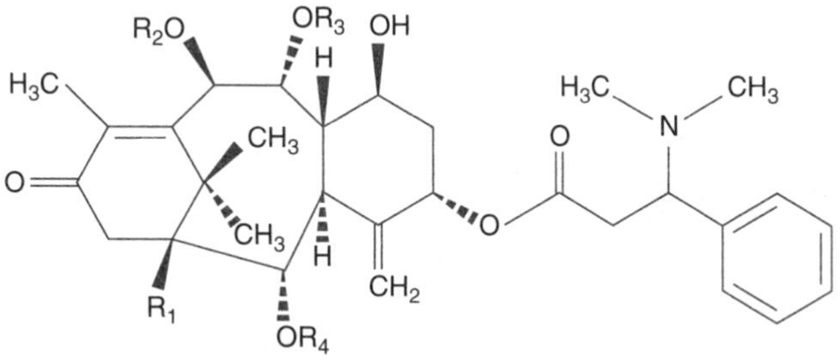

	2a	2b
R_1	Ac	H
Taxine alkaloids	Taxine A	2-Deacetyltaxine A

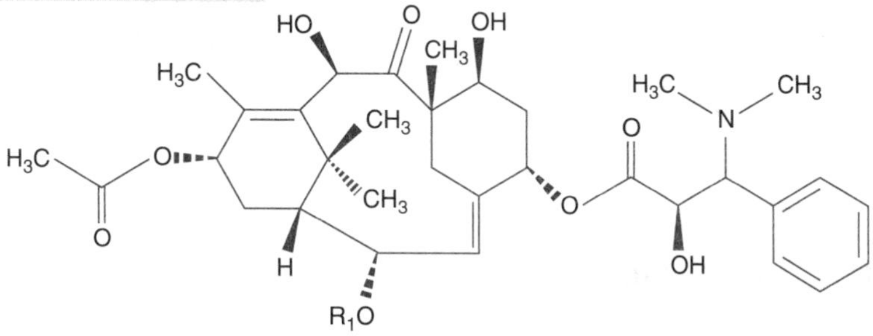

FIGURE 31-2 Structures of the Taxine Alkaloids from the Yew

been identified as colchicine, lumicolchicine, 3-demethyl-N-deformyl-N-deacetyl colchicines, and 3-demethylcholchicine. The leaves also contain superbine, gloriosine, gloriosol, phytosterols, and stigmasterin. Colchicine causes metaphase arrest as its key activity by interfering with microtubule and spindle formation but can also lower body temperature, increase sensitivity to CNS depressants, depress the respiratory center, increase activity of sympathomimetic compounds, constrict blood vessels, yield hypertension via central vasomotor stimulation, induce seizures, and increase GI motility via its action on the nervous system (Jana and Shekhawat, 2011).

Contact Dermal Toxicity/Sensitization or Phototoxicity

Another infamous species of plants, the *Toxicodendron*, is part of the Anacardiaceae family including poison ivy (*Toxicodendron radicans*), western poison oak (*Toxicodendron diversilobum*), eastern poison oak (*Toxicodendron quercifolium*), and poison sumac (*Toxicodendron vernix*). The allergic compound found in the sap/oils of this plant (leaves, stems, and roots) is urushiol, a mixture of catechols. Somewhere between 50 and 70% of the population is sensitized to these compounds and can develop allergic contact dermatitis (Lee and Arriola, 1999).

Hypericin from St. John's wort can lead to photosensitization via a high yield of singlet oxygen and other ROS (Olivo et al., 2006), but also increases heart and respiration rate, induce fever, and lead to diarrhea. Eating too many carrots (β-carotene) can photosensitize the skin. A European weed that is now invasive in the U.S. is the wild parsnip, *Pastinaca sativa*. This plant's dermal (blisters) toxicity from furanocoumarins is elicited under light classifying it as phototoxic. It is of interest that attempts to use insect herbivores to control this weed only increased the toxic furoanocoumarin content of resistant plants (Zangerl and Berenbaum, 2005). Photosensitization in livestock is a problem that results from a primary phototoxic agent that reaches the skin unchanged by metabolism following ingestion or porphyrin phylloerythrin as a degradation product of chlorophyll produced in the rumen. *Tetradymia* species and phototoxic syndrome (including big head production and possible loss of lips and ability to eat) is especially problematic for sheep (Johnson, 1982).

Oral, GI and Liver Toxicity

Pyrrolizidine alkaloids (> 600 pyrrolizidine alkaloids and N-oxides) are produced by > 6,000 plants, mostly in the Boraginaceae, Asteraceae, Orchidaceae, and Leguminosae families, which are used in traditional medicine practices such as the popular Ayurveda. These hepatotoxins activated by CYPs are found in honey, grains, milk, offal, and eggs. They cause hepatic venoocclusive disease and liver cancer (Roeder and Wiedenfeld, 2013).

Other plant/herbal preparations are bioactivated. Liver damage results from CYP3A4 activation of teucrin A and teuchamaedryn, two diterpenoids from germander (*Teucrium chamaedrys*), to a reactive epoxide that inactivates CYP3A and epoxide hydrolase. Some compounds such as safrole from black pepper (or methyl eugenol or estragole from plants) are alkenylbenzenes and others are flavonoids such as quercetin that form DNA adducts via 1-hydroxylation and sulfation and possible cancer after prolonged heavy use in susceptible individuals. Glutathione (GSH) can be depleted by pulegone (from catnip or *Nepeta cataria*) or by the reactive quinone formed from kava (Chen et al., 2011). Other compounds such as the furanocoumarins in grapefruit juice (Hanley et al., 2011) irreversibly inhibit CYP3A and other suicide substrates for various CYPs such as capsaicin from chili peppers, diallyl sulfone in garlic, methysticin and dihydromethysticin in kava, oleuropein in olive oil, and resveratrol found in grape seeds. Some of these last compounds are also viewed favorably for their other activities. These agents are not so much toxic in their own right but may increase the toxicity of liver-toxic agents such as acetaminophen if GSH is lacking or statins (which also cause rhabdomyolysis or muscle wasting and high creatinine release leading to kidney failure) if CYPs are inhibited. Kidney cancer results from activation of aristolochic acids from *Aristolochia* species via a reduction of a nitro group by CYP1A1/2 or peroxidases to reactive cyclic nitrenium ions (DNA and protein → H-ras and myc oncogene activation and gene mutation in renal cells; Chen et al., 2011).

Calcium oxalate crystals known as raphides in the *Dieffenbachia* spp. (dumbcane) or *Arisaema triphyllum* (Jack-in-the-pulpit) cause irritation to the lips and GI tract, and may extend irritation into the respiratory tract depending on the how the animal reacts to the intense irritation (Pedaci et al., 1999). Another plant containing high oxalates, *Halogeton glomeratus*, affects sheep if large amounts are consumed acutely (James and Butcher, 1972). *Sanguinaria canadensis* contains a sanguinarine alkaloid that is also a severe irritant.

Some plants cause severe emesis. For example, the lycorine alkaloid from the Amaryllidaceae causes severe emesis, but it is completely blocked by the neurokinin-1 receptor antagonist maropitant, which significantly decreases the severity of nausea and prolongs the lag time until the start of emesis by the 5-HT$_3$ receptor antagonist ondansetron. It appears that the key factors in producing emesis are neurokinin-1 and to some degree the serotonin 3 receptor (Kretzing et al., 2011).

Tannins are defensive secondary metabolite deterrents or toxins of tree leaves, representing 5–10% dry weight. They reduce vertebrate herbivore protein digestion, but not that of insects. Instead, insect digestive tracts have a high pH, leading to formation of semiquinone radicals and quinones along with other ROS. They can also cause kidney damage (renal tubules) as indicated in cattle eating acorns. Insects protect themselves from tannins by high pH, surfactants, antioxidants, and a protective peritrophic envelope midgut lining (Barbehenn and Peter Constabel, 2011). Irritation can also be due to *Euphorbia esula* (spurge—named so for its use as a purgative), which contain diterpene or triterpene esters in the sap that are severe irritants and herbivore deterrents and can lead to temporary changes in vision prior to treatment upon eye contact (Eke et al., 2000). The terpenoid glycoside ligustrin from the privet or *Ligustrum vulgare* also causes vomiting, diarrhea, convulsions, and death if enough is consumed (Gao et al., 2013).

Cytotoxic Agents

Pokeweed antiviral protein is an N-glycosidase that is similar to ricin and abrin, for example, in that it is a ribosome-inactivating protein that acts when the A-site of the ribosomal peptidyl-transferase center is unoccupied. All these proteins are known for their ability to depurinate the highly conserved sarcin/ricin loop of large ribosomal RNA, therefore not allowing EL-2 binding and preventing translation (Mansouri et al., 2006). Colchine and other microtubule affecting agents such a paclitaxel mentioned in the neurotoxicity and neuromuscular toxicity section could also fit in this category.

Herbal Anticancer Agents

The vinca alkaloids isolated from the Madagascar periwinkle (*Catharanthus roseus*, also historically referred to as *Vinca rosea*) also inhibit microtubule formation via binding to β-tubulin and prevent polymerization with α-tubulin. Other plant products used in the treatment of cancer besides vinca alkaloids or taxanes in order to "fight fire with fire (toxic plant compounds)" are epipodophyllotoxin derivatives and camptothecin derivatives. Etoposide is a derivative of podophyllotoxin of the mandrake plant or mayapple (*Podophyllum peltatum*) that forms a ternary complex with topoisomerase II and DNA, preventing resealing a break that usually follows topoisomerase binding to DNA. This increases DNA strand breaks and cell death. Topotecan (derivative of cytotoxic quinone alkaloid camptothecin from *Camptotheca acuminate* Decne) inhibits topoisomerase I by intercalation in DNA and similarly leads to DNA damage and apoptosis. A number of poisonous Chinese herbal medicines also hold the promise of anti-tumor activity. Gambogic acid comes from a resin of the *Garcinia* species and has cytotoxic properties causing growth inhibition and G0/G1 cell-cycle arrest in chronic myeloid leukemia cells through interference of steroid receptor coactivator-3. This compound also binds to the transferrin receptor and inhibits Bcl-2 family proteins and topoisomerase IIα as part of its proapoptotic activities. Gambogic acid also inhibits activation of VEGFR2 and downstream protein kinases, preventing proliferation, migration, invasion, tube formation, and microvessel growth. *Tripterygium wilfordii*, the "thunder god vine," contains diterpenes, triterpenes, sesquiterpenoids, and alkaloids. The principal terpenoids triptolide and tripterine have anti-tumor activity. Triptolide appears to induce apoptosis through different pathways in a diversity of cell lines. This compound induces overexpression of cytomembrane death receptor in cholangiocarcinoma cells, but uses mitochondrial-mediated pathways to induce apoptosis in leukemic cells. Tripterine or celastrol uses NF-κB, caspase family proteins, VEGF receptors, heat shock proteins, K$^+$ and Ca^{2+} channels, and Ig Fc ε receptor 1 to affect apoptosis, cell-cycle arrest, and decreased angiogenesis and metastasis. Other plants have been used in Chinese medicine that vary from the slightly toxic—such as those that might involve GI problems or dehydration (*Evodia rutaecarpa, Prunus armeniaca* discussed previously, *Melia toosendan*)—to toxic as indicated by cough, dyspnea, vomiting, goiter, urticaria, or similar symptoms (*Pinellia ternate*, *Xanthium sibricum*) to highly toxic (*Strychnos nux-vomica* containing strychnine as discussed earlier; Wang et al., 2012).

Pharmaceutical Cardioactive Compounds

Another class of pharmaceutical agents that have been derived from plant poisons is cardioactive agents such as digitalis or digoxin, a secondary glycoside isolated from the foxglove plant *Digitalis purpurea* that acts via inhibition of the $3Na^+$, $2K^+$-ATPase. This drug at therapeutic concentrations can increase heart contractility via elevated intracellular Ca^{2+}, but at toxic concentrations can lead to arrhythmias of various sorts including AV node block and hyperkalemia. Interestingly, digoxin and its analogs are also potential cancer therapeutic medications (Elbaz et al., 2012).

Conditionally Toxic Compounds

Some plants are not toxic on their own, but can be toxic to organisms with certain conditions. For example, a person with Wilson's disease or similar inability to deal with Cu accumulation should avoid eating animals grazing on *Trifolium* spp. because these plants are Cu accumulators and can lead to liver degeneration (Barry et al., 1983). Accumulation of nitrates in plants such as forage sorghum, sudangrass, sudan-sorghum hybrids, and pearl millet lead to high levels in cattle and horses due to their consumption rate (not in sheep and swine as they do not consume enough of this forage to be a problem). Normally, the bacteria of the rumen convert the nitrate to the toxic form nitrite, but then proceed to use the nitrite as a nitrogen source by the same bacteria. However, when nitrate is > 6,000 ppm in the feed, it is potentially toxic to cattle and at > 9,000 ppm lethal due to rapid absorption of nitrite into the blood and oxidation of hemoglobin to methemoglobin (metHb), which leads to cyanosis (metHb cannot carry oxygen as Fe^{3+} must first must be reduced by metHb reductase to Fe^{2+}). Red maple (*Acer rubrum*) also cause metHb formation in addition

to depression, anorexia, hemolytic anemia, and dehydration. Sorghums contain prussic acid (HCN) and also can yield lethal cyanosis at > 1,000 ppm in cattle feed via inhibition of cytochrome a_3 (Fjell et al., 1991). In an 8-week study, nitrate poisoning at 1,600 ppm in protein concentrate-amended corn silage and 4,000 ppm in free-choice hay indicate depressed serum progesterone concentrations through inhibition of CYP (Page et al., 1990). Similarly, grazing on lush, cool-season pastures can lead to incoordination, salivation, aggressive behavior, tetany, convulsions, and death due to magnesium deficiency. Older cows cannot mobilize magnesium stores from their older bones and are susceptible to low Mg content of the forage, high K levels that reduce Mg absorption, high nitrogen fertilizing (buildup of ammonia in rumen that reacts with Mg and makes it less absorbable), and certain organic acids in the forage (Rasby, 2013). Similarly, giving an exclusive brown and red seaweed (*Rhodymenia palmate*) diet to sheep over a 6- to 8-week period in Iceland led to a fatal demyelination disorder in newborn lambs that appears to have resulted from a copper deficiency (Hallsson, 1961).

Ruminants are sensitive to grazing on forage consisting of plants such as *Brassica napus* (rapeseed), developing hemolytic anemias via a variety of metabolic disorders. Hemoglobin oxidation and precipitation as Heinz-Ehrlich bodies are the key events leading to hemolysis (Prache, 1994). *Brassica oleracea* contain glucosinolates that hydrolyze to isothiocyanates, which are goitrogens due to inhibition of iodine uptake by the thyroid (Stoewsand, 1995). The tansy mustard *(Descurainia pinnata)* of the Brassicaceae produces blindness (blind staggers) in cattle that consume this plant in the Southern and Western United States by an unknown mechanism or toxic agent (Department of Ecosystem Science and Management Texas A&M University, 2015). Juglone and plumbagin are naphthoquinones from the Plumbaginaceae and Droseraceae families and the *Juglans* spp. (walnut tree bark), respectively. Juglone ingestion can lead to laminitis and is toxic to fish. These naphthoquinones also involve ROS generation and GSH depletion in causing apoptosis (Seshadri et al., 2011).

Questions

1. What is the mechanism of the lectin ricin's extremely poisonous activities?
2. Why might cysteine inhibit ODAP motoneuron toxicity?
3. Why is gossypol a dangerous antifertility agent?
4. How does aconitine lead to dangerous heart arrhythmias?
5. Spanish Conquistadors were surprised when poison darts stopped the breathing of their soldiers. What caused this and why?
6. Why would certain plant or fungal compounds produce sedative-hypnotic action yet another plant compound would cause epileptic seizures via action at the same receptor of a human who ate that plant or fungus?
7. List some famous toxins that come from the leaves and flowers of plants. What do they do?
8. How does paclitaxel from the yew plant help treat metastatic cancers? Why do quinidine and cinchonine from the bark of the *Cinchona officinalis* plant aid in the chemotherapeutic action of paclitaxel?

References

Barbehenn RV, Peter Constabel C. 2011. Tannins in plant-herbivore interactions. *Phytochemistry.* 72:1551–1565.

Barceloux DG. 2009. Potatoes, tomatoes, and solanine toxicity (*Solanum tuberosum* L., *Solanum lycopersicum* L.). *Dis Mon.* 55:391–402.

Barry TN, Millar KR, Bond G, Duncan SJ. 1983. Copper metabolism in growing sheep given kale (*Brassica oleracea*) and ryegrass (*Lolium perenne*)-clover (*Trifolium repens*) fresh forage diets. *Br J Nutr.* 50:281–289.

Bateman DN, Dyson EH. 1986. Quinine toxicity. *Adverse Drug React Acute Poisoning Rev.* 5:215–233.

Bhaskar AS, Gupta N, Rao PV. 2012. Transcriptomic profile of host response in mouse brain after exposure to plant toxin abrin. *Toxicology.* 299:33–43.

Bracken fern poisoning: Introduction. In: *The Merck Veterinary Manual,* 9th ed. Whitehouse Station, NJ: Merck & Co., Inc. and Merial Ltd., 2005.

Chang HT, Rumbeiha WK, Patterson JS, Puschner B, Knight AP. 2012. Toxic equine parkinsonism: an immunohistochemical study of 10 horses with nigropallidal encephalomalacia. *Vet Pathol.* 49:398–402.

Chen XW, Serag ES, Sneed KB, Zhou SF. 2011. Herbal bioactivation, molecular targets and the toxicity relevance. *Chem Biol Interact.* 192:161–176.

Department of Ecosystem Science and Management Texas A&M University. 2015. Plant of the Texas Rangeland Virtual Herbarium: Tansy Mustard *Descurainia pinnata.* http://essmextension.tamu .edu/plants/plant/tansy-mustard/

Dutertre S, Becker CM, Betz H. 2012. Inhibitory glycine receptors: an update. *J Biol Chem.* 287: 40216–40223.

Eke T, Al-Husainy S, Raynor MK. 2000. The spectrum of ocular inflammation caused by euphorbia plant sap. *Arch Ophthalmol.* 118:13–16.

Elbaz HA, Stueckle TA, Tse W, Rojanasakul Y, Dinu CZ. 2012. Digitoxin and its analogs as novel cancer therapeutics. *Exp Hematol Oncol.* 1:4.

Enneking D. 2011. The nutritive value of grasspea (*Lathyrus sativus*) and allied species, their toxicity to animals and the role of malnutrition in neurolathyrism. *Food Chem Toxicol.* 49:694–709.

Farombi EO, Ekor M, Adedara IA, Tonwe KE, Ojujoh TO, Oyeyemi MO. 2012. Quercetin protects against testicular toxicity induced by chronic administration of therapeutic dose of quinine sulfate in rats. *J Basic Clin Physiol Pharmacol.* 23:39–44.

Ferraz AC, Anselmo-Franci JA, Perosa SR, de Castro-Neto EF, Bellissimo MI, de Oliveira BH, Cavalheiro EA, Naffah-Mazzacoratti Mda G, Da Cunha C. 2002. Amino acid and monoamine alterations in the cerebral cortex and hippocampus of mice submitted to ricinine-induced seizures. *Pharmacol Biochem Behav.* 72:779–786.

Fjell D, Blasi D, Towne G. 1991. *Nitrate and prussic acid toxicity in forage: causes, prevention, and feeding management.* MF-1018. Manhattan, KS: Departments of Agronomy & Animal Sciences, Kansas State University.

Gao BB, She GM, She DM. 2013. Chemical constituents and biological activities of plants from the genus *Ligustrum. Chem Biodivers.* 10:96–128.

Grace AA, Camm J. 1998. Quinidine. *N Engl J Med.* 322:35–45.

Green BT, Welch KD, Gardner DR, Stegelmeier BL, Lee ST. 2013. A toxicokinetic comparison of two species of low larkspur (*Delphinium* spp.) in cattle. *Res Vet Sci.* 95:612–615.

Gunderson EW, Haughey HM, Ait-Daoud N, Joshi AS, Hart CL. 2012. "Spice" and "K2" herbal highs: a case series and systematic review of the clinical effects and biopsychosocial implications of synthetic cannabinoid use in humans. *Am J Addict.* 21:320–326.

Hallsson SV. 1961. The uses of seaweed in Iceland. *Fourth International Seaweed Symposium.* Biarritz, France. http://www.noamkelp.com/technical/iceland.html

Hanley MJ, Cancalon P, Widmer WW, Greenblatt DJ. 2011. The effect of grapefruit juice on drug disposition. *Expert Opin Drug Metab Toxicol. Expert Opin Drug Metab Toxicol.* 7:267–286.

Hebestreit P, Melzig MF. 2003. Cyctotoxic activity of the seeds from *Agrostemma githago* var. githago. *Planta Med.* 69:921–925.

Heier T. 2010. [Muscle relaxants]. *Tidsskr Nor Laegeforen.* 130:398–401.

Herrera-Ruiz M, González-Carranza A, Zamilpa A, Jiménez-Ferrer E, Huerta-Reyes M, Navarro-García VM. 2011. The standardized extract of *Loeselia mexicana* possesses anxiolytic activity through the γ-amino butyric acid mechanism. *J Ethnopharmacol.* 138:261–267.

Herbert V. 1979. Laetrile: the cult of cyanide. Promoting poison for profit. *Am J Clin Nutr.* 32:1121–1158.

Hodgson E. 2012. Toxins and venoms. *Prog Mol Biol Transl Sci.* 112:373–415.

Ince PG, Codd GA. 2005. Return of the cycad hypothesis—does the amyotrophic lateral sclerosis/parkinsonism dementia complex (ALS/PDC) of Guam have new implications for global health? *Neuropathol Appl Neurobiol.* 31:345–353.

Isbrucker RA, Burdock GA. 2006. Risk and safety assessment on the consumption of Licorice root (*Glycyrrhiza* sp.), its extract and powder as a food ingredient, with emphasis on the pharmacology and toxicology of glycyrrhizin. *Regul Toxicol Pharmacol.* 46:167–192.

James LF, Butcher JE. 1972. Halogeton poisoning of sheep: effect of high level oxalate intake. *J Anim Sci.* 35:1233–1238.

Jana S, Shekhawat GS. 2011. Critical review on medicinally potent plant species: *Gloriosa superba. Fitoterapia.* 82:293–301.

Jansen SA, Kleerekooper I, Hofman ZLM, Kappen IFPM, Stary-Weinzinger A, van der Heyden MAG. 2012. Grayanotoxin poisoning: 'mad honey disease' and beyond. *Cardiovasc Toxicol.* 12:208–215.

Johnson AE. 1982. Toxicologic aspects of photosensitization in livestock. *J Natl Cancer Inst.* 69:253–258.

Jung B-C, Lee S-H, Cho Y-K, Park H-S, Kim Y-N, Lee Y-S, Shin D-G. 2011. Role of the alternans of action potential duration and aconitine-induced arrhythmias in isolated rabbit hearts. *J Korean Med Sci.* 26:1576–1581.

Katsuda Y. 2012. Progress and future of pyrethroids. *Top Curr Chem.* 314:1–30.

Kernaleguen A. 1989. Satkatchewan: acute mustard seed toxicosis in cattle. *Can Vet J.* 30:324.

Khafagi IK. 2007. Variation of callus induction and active metabolite accumulation in callus cultures of two varieties of *Ricinus communis* L. *Biotechnology.* 6:193–201.

Klee EW, Ebbert JO, Schneider H, Hurt RD, Ekker SC. 2011. Zebrafish for the study of the biological effects of nicotine. *Nicotine Tob Res.* 13:301–312.

Kovacic P. 2003. Mechanism of drug and toxic actions of gossypol: focus on reactive oxygen species and electron transfer. *Curr Med Chem.* 10:2711–2718.

Kretzing S, Abraham G, Seiwert B, Ungemach FR, Krügel U, Teichert J, Regenthal R. 2011. *In vivo* assessment of antiemetic drugs and mechanism of lycorine-induced nausea and emesis. *Arch Toxicol.* 85:1565–1573.

Kuttan G, Pratheeshkumar P, Manu KA, Kuttan R. 2011. Inhibition of tumor progression by naturally occurring terpenoids. *Pharm Biol.* 49:995–1007.

Lee SY, Rhee YH, Jeong SJ, Lee HJ, Lee HJ, Jung MH, Kim SH, Lee EO, Ahn KS, Ahn KS, Kim SH. 2011. Hydrocinchonine, cinchonine, and quinidine potentiate paclitaxel-induced cytotoxicity and apoptosis via multidrug resistance reversal in MES-SA/DX5 uterine sarcoma cells. *Environ Toxicol.* 26:424–431.

Lee NP, Arriola ER. 1999. Poison ivy, oak, and sumac dermatitis. *West J Med.* 171:354–355.

Leporatti ML, Impieri M. 2007. Ethnobotanical notes about some uses of medicinal plants in Alto Tirreno Cosentino area (Calabria, Southern Italy). *J Ethnobiol Ethnomed.* 3:34.

Mansouri S, Nourollahzadeh E, Hudak KA. 2006. Pokeweed antiviral protein depurinates the sarcin/ricin loop of the rRNA prior to binding of aminoacyl-tRNA to the ribosomal A-site. *RNA.* 12:1683–1692.

Maioli MA, Lemos DE, Guelfi M, Medeiros HC, Riet-Correa F, Medeiros RM, Barbosa-Filho JM, Mingatto FE. 2012. Mechanism for the uncoupling of oxidative phosphorylation by juliprosopine on rat brain mitochondria. *Toxicon.* 60:1355–1362.

McClatchey WC, Mahady GB, Bennett BC, Shiels L, Savo V. 2009. Ethnobotany as a pharmacological research tool and recent developments in CNS-active natural products from ethnobotanical sources. *Pharmacol Ther.* 123:239–254.

Mitchell J, Wellerr RO, Evans H, Arai I, Daves GD jr. 1978. Buckthorn neuropathy: effects of intraneural injection of *Karwinskia hummoldtiana* toxin. *Neuropath Appl Neurobiol.* 4:85–97.

Olivo M, Du HY, Bay BH. 2006. Hypericin lights up the way for the potential treatment of nasopharyngeal cancer by photodynamic therapy. *Curr Clin Pharmacol.* 1:217–222.

Ortega García JA, Angulo MG, Sobrino-Najul EJ, Soldin OP, Mira AP, Martínez-Salcedo E, Claudio L. 2011. Prenatal exposure of a girl with autism spectrum disorder to 'horsetail' (*Equisetum arvense*) herbal remedy and alcohol: a case report. *J Med Case Rep.* 5:129.

Page RD, Gilson WD, Guthrie LD, Mertens DR, Hatch RC. 1990. Serum progesterone and milk production and composition in dairy cows fed two concentrations of nitrate. *Vet Hum Toxicol.* 32:27–31.

Panter KE, James LF, Gardner DR. 1999. Lupines, poison-hemlock and *Nicotiana* spp: toxicity and teratogenicity in livestock. *J Nat Toxins.* 8:117–134.

Pasternak GW. 1993. Pharmacological mechanisms of opioid analgesics. *Clin Neuropharmacol.* 16:1–18.

Pedaci L, Krenzelok EP, Jacobsen TD, Aronis J. 1999. *Dieffenbachia* species exposures: an evidence-based assessment of symptom presentation. *Vet Hum Toxicol.* 41:335–338.

Pemberton IJ, Smith GR, Forbes TD, Hensarling CM. 1993. Technical note: an improved method for extraction and quantification of toxic phenethylamines from *Acacia berlandieri. J Anim Sci.* 71:467–470.

Prache S. 1994. Haemolytic anaemia in ruminants fed forage brassicas: a review. *Vet Res.* 25:497–520.

Price KR, Johnson IT, Fenwick GR. 1987. The chemistry and biological significance of saponins in foods and feedingstuffs. *Crit Rev Food Sci Nutr.* 26:27–135.

Rasby R. 2013. Grass tetany management for cattle grazing lush, cool season pastures. University of Nebraska-Lincoln. http://beef.unl.edu/web/cattleproduction/grasstetanymanagement

Roeder E, Wiedenfeld H. 2013. Plants containing pyrrolizidine alkaloids used in the traditional Indian medicine—including Ayurveda. *Pharmazie.* 68:83–92.

Saksena SK, Salmonsen R, Lau IF, Chang MC. 1981. Gossypol: its toxicological and endocrinological effects in male rabbits. *Contraception.* 24:203–214.

Salazar-Leal ME, Flores MS, Sepulveda-Saavedra J, Romero-Diaz VJ, Becerra-Verdin EM, Tamez-Rodriguez VA, Martinez HR, Piñeyro-Lopez A, Bermudez MV. 2006. An experimental model of peripheral neuropathy induced in rats by *Karwinskia humboldtiana* (buckthorn) fruit. *J Peripher Nerv Syst.* 11:253–261.

Schindler CW, Goldberg SR. 2012. Accelerating cocaine metabolism as an approach to the treatment of cocaine abuse and toxicity. *Future Med Chem.* 4:163–175.

Seshadri P, Rajaram A, Rajaram R. 2011. Plumbagin and juglone induce caspase-3-dependent apoptosis involving the mitochondria through ROS generation in human peripheral blood lymphocytes. *Free Radic Biol Med.* 51:2090–2107.

Srivastava VK, Agrawal S, Sahu S. 2011. Association of acute onset hypertension and tachycardia following intracisternal papaverine administration during intracranial aneurysm surgery: a case report and review of the literature. *J Clin Anesth.* 23:224–226.

Stoewsand GS. 1995. Bioactive organosulfur phytochemicals in *Brassica oleracea* vegetables—a review. *Food Chem Toxicol.* 33:537–543.

Tong WM, Sha O, Ng TB, Cho EY, Kwong WH. 2012. Different *in vitro* toxicity of ribosome-inactivating proteins (RIPs) on sensory neurons and Schwann cells. *Neurosci Lett.* 524:89–94.

Toohey M. 1952. Antagonism of anticoagulants dicoumarol, tromexan, and phenylindandione by vitamin K. *Br Med J.* 2:687–690.

Vetter J. 2004. Poison hemlock (*Conium maculatum* L.). *Food Chem Toxicol.* 42:1373–1382.

Walker DG. 1957. Elastic fiber alterations in rats treated with *Lathyrus odoratus*; histopathologic study of elastic cartilage and of elastic fibers in arteries and membranes, with special reference to the occurrence of extra-aortic dissecting aneurysms. *AMA Arch Pathol.* 64:434–445.

Wang S, Wu X, Tan M, Gong J, Tan W, Bian B, Chen M, Wang Y. 2012. Fighting fire with fire: poisonous Chinese herbal medicine for cancer therapy. *J Ethnopharmacol.* 140:33–45.

Wang X, Howell CP, Chen F, Yin J, Jiang Y. 2009. Gossypol—a polyphenolic compound from cotton plant. *Adv Food Nutr Res.* 58:215–263.

Wilson CR, Sauer J, Hooser SB. 2001. Taxines: a review of the mechanism and toxicity of yew (*Taxus* spp.) alkaloids. *Toxicon.* 39:175–185.

Worbs S, Köhler K, Pauly D, Avondet MA, Schaer M, Dorner MB, Dorner BG. 2011. *Ricinus communis* intoxications in human and veterinary medicine-a summary of real cases. *Toxins (Basel).* 3:1332–1372.

Zangerl AR, Berenbaum MR. 2005. Increase in toxicity of an invasive weed after reassociation with its coevolved herbivore. *Proc Natl Acad Sci USA.* 102:15529–15532.

Zbidah M, Lupescu, A, Shaik N, Lang F. 2012. Gossypol-induced suicidal erythrocyte death. *Toxicology.* 302:101.

Index

Note: Page numbers followed by *f* and *t* refer to figures and tables respectively

About the Author

Herbert Schildt is a leading authority on C#, C++, C, and Java. His programming books have sold more than 3.5 million copies worldwide and have been translated into all major foreign languages. He is the author of numerous bestsellers, including *Java: The Complete Reference*, *C++: The Complete Reference*, *C: The Complete Reference*, and *C#: A Beginner's Guide*. Although interested in all facets of computing, his primary focus is computer languages, including compilers, interpreters, and robotic control languages. He also has an active interest in the standardization of languages. Schildt holds both graduate and undergraduate degrees from the University of Illinois. He can be reached at his consulting office at (217) 586-4683. His web site is **www.HerbSchildt.com**.

About the Technical Editor

Michael Howard (Austin, Texas) is a principal security program manager on the Trustworthy Computing (TwC) Group's Security Engineering team at Microsoft, where he is responsible for managing secure design, programming, and testing techniques across the company. Howard is an architect of the Security Development Lifecycle (SDL), a process for improving the security of Microsoft's software. Howard speaks regularly on the topic of securing code for Microsoft and at conferences worldwide. He regularly publishes articles on security design and is the co-author of six security books, including the award-winning *Writing Secure Code*, *19 Deadly Sins of Software Security*, *The Security Development Lifecycle*, and his most recent release, *Writing Secure Code for Windows Vista*.

C# 3.0:
The Complete Reference

Herbert Schildt

New York Chicago San Francisco
Lisbon London Madrid Mexico City
Milan New Delhi San Juan
Seoul Singapore Sydney Toronto

The McGraw·Hill Companies

Cataloging-in-Publication Data is on file with the Library of Congress

McGraw-Hill books are available at special quantity discounts to use as premiums and sales promotions, or for use in corporate training programs. To contact a special sales representative, please visit the Contact Us page at www.mhprofessional.com.

C# 3.0: The Complete Reference

1234567890 DOC DOC 0198

ISBN 978-0-07-158841-6
MHID   0-07-158841-8

Sponsoring Editor	**Proofreader**
Jane K. Brownlow	Paul Tyler
Editorial Supervisor	**Indexer**
Patty Mon	Sheryl Schildt
Project Editor	**Production Supervisor**
LeeAnn Pickrell	Jean Bodeaux
Acquisitions Coordinator	**Composition**
Carly Stapleton	Apollo Publishing Service
Technical Editor	**Illustration**
Michael Howard	Apollo Publishing Service
Copy Editor	**Art Director, Cover**
LeeAnn Pickrell	Jeff Weeks

Contents at a Glance

Contents

Special Thanks

Special thanks go to Michael Howard for his excellent technical edit of this book. His expertise, insights, suggestions, and advice were of great value.

Preface

We programmers are a demanding bunch, always looking for ways to improve the performance, efficiency, and portability of our programs. We also demand much from the tools we use, especially when it comes to programming languages. There are many programming languages, but only a few are great. A great programming language must be powerful, yet flexible. Its syntax must be terse, but clear. It must facilitate the creation of correct code while not getting in our way. It must support state-of-the-art features, but not trendy dead ends. Finally, a great programming language must have one more, almost intangible quality: It must feel right when we use it. C# is such a language.

Created by Microsoft to support its .NET Framework, C# builds on a rich programming heritage. Its chief architect was long-time programming guru Anders Hejlsberg. C# is directly descended from two of the world's most successful computer languages: C and C++. From C, it derives its syntax, many of its keywords, and its operators. It builds upon and improves the object model defined by C++. C# is also closely related to another very successful language: Java.

Sharing a common ancestry, but differing in many important ways, C# and Java are more like cousins. Both support distributed programming and both use intermediate code to achieve safety and portability, but the details differ. They both also provide a significant amount of runtime error checking, security, and managed execution, but again, the details differ. However, unlike Java, C# also gives you access to pointers—a feature supported by C++. Thus, C# combines the raw power of C++ with the type safety of Java. Furthermore, the trade-offs between power and safety are carefully balanced and are nearly transparent.

Throughout the history of computing, programming languages have evolved to accommodate changes in the computing environment, advances in computer language theory, and new ways of thinking about and approaching the job of programming. C# is no exception. In the ongoing process of refinement, adaptation, and innovation, C# has demonstrated its ability to respond rapidly to the changing needs of the programmer. This fact is testified to by the many new features added to C# since its initial 1.0 release in 2000.

Consider the first major revision, C# 2.0. It added several features that made it easier for programmers to write more resilient, reliable, and nimble code. Without question, the most important 2.0 addition was generics. Through the use of generics, it became possible to create type-safe, reusable code in C#. Thus, the addition of generics fundamentally expanded the power and scope of the language.

Now consider the second major revision, C# 3.0. This is the latest version of C# and is the version described in this book. It is not an exaggeration to say that C# 3.0 has added features that have redefined the very core of C#, raising the bar in computer language development in the process. Of its many innovative features, two stand out: LINQ and lambda expressions. LINQ, which stands for Language Integrated Query, enables you to create database-style queries by using elements of the C# language. Lambda expressions implement a functional-style syntax that uses the => lambda operator, and lambda expressions are frequently used in LINQ expressions.

As you will see in the course of this book, the combination of LINQ and lambda expressions represents a radically powerful subset of C#. Furthermore, they are revolutionary features that

are redefining how solutions are crafted for many different types of programming tasks, not just database queries. In essence, they let you approach old problems in new ways. Their use not only streamlines a solution, but also helps you conceptualize a problem from a different point of view. Simply put, the addition of LINQ and lambda expressions is both significant and far reaching. They are changing the way we think about the job of programming.

Because of its ability to adapt rapidly to the changing demands of the programming landscape, C# has remained a vibrant and innovative language. As a result, it defines one of the most powerful, feature-rich languages in modern computing. It is also a language that no programmer can afford to ignore. This book is designed to help you master it.

What's Inside

This book describes C# 3.0. It is divided into two parts. Part I provides a comprehensive discussion of the C# language, including the new features added by version 3.0. This is the largest part in the book, and it describes the keywords, syntax, and features that define the language. I/O, file handling, reflection, and the preprocessor are also discussed in Part I.

Part II explores the C# class library, which is the .NET Framework class library. This library is huge! Because of space limitations, it is not possible to cover the entire .NET Framework class library in one book. Instead, Part II focuses on the core library, which is contained in the **System** namespace. Also covered are collections, multithreading, networking, and Windows Forms. These are the parts of the library that nearly every C# programmer will use.

A Book for All Programmers

This book does not require any previous programming experience. If you already know C++ or Java, you will be able to advance quite rapidly because C# has much in common with those languages. If you don't have any previous programming experience, you will still be able to learn C# from this book, but you will need to work carefully through the examples in each chapter.

Required Software

To compile and run C# 3.0 programs, you must use Visual Studio 2008 or later.

Don't Forget: Code on the Web

Remember, the source code for all of the programs in this book is available free-of-charge on the Web at **www.mhprofessional.com**.

For Further Study

C# 3.0: The Complete Reference is your gateway to the Herb Schildt series of programming books. Here are some others that you will find of interest.

For a carefully paced introduction to C#, try

C# 3.0: A Beginner's Guide

To learn about Java programming, we recommend the following:

Java: The Complete Reference

Java: A Beginner's Guide

Swing: A Beginner's Guide

The Art of Java

Herb Schildt's Java Programming Cookbook

To learn about C++, you will find these books especially helpful:

C++: The Complete Reference

C++: A Beginner's Guide

C++ From the Ground Up

STL Programming From the Ground Up

The Art of C++

Herb Schildt's C++ Programming Cookbook

If you want to learn about the C language, the foundation of all modern programming, the following title will be of interest:

C: The Complete Reference

When you need solid answers, fast, turn to Herbert Schildt, the recognized authority on programming.

PART I

The C# Language

Part I discusses the elements of the C# language, including its keywords, syntax, and operators. Also described are several foundational C# techniques, such as using I/O and reflection, which are tightly linked with the C# language.

The Creation of C#

C# is Microsoft's premier language for .NET development. It leverages time-tested features with cutting-edge innovations and provides a highly usable, efficient way to write programs for the modern enterprise computing environment. It is, by any measure, one of the most important languages of the 21st century.

The purpose of this chapter is to place C# into its historical context, including the forces that drove its creation, its design philosophy, and how it was influenced by other computer languages. This chapter also explains how C# relates to the .NET Framework. As you will see, C# and the .NET Framework work together to create a highly refined programming environment.

C#'s Family Tree

Computer languages do not exist in a void. Rather, they relate to one another, with each new language influenced in one form or another by the ones that came before. In a process akin to cross-pollination, features from one language are adapted by another, a new innovation is integrated into an existing context, or an older construct is removed. In this way, languages evolve and the art of programming advances. C# is no exception.

C# inherits a rich programming legacy. It is directly descended from two of the world's most successful computer languages: C and C++. It is closely related to another: Java. Understanding the nature of these relationships is crucial to understanding C#. Thus, we begin our examination of C# by placing it in the historical context of these three languages.

C: The Beginning of the Modern Age of Programming

The creation of C marks the beginning of the modern age of programming. C was invented by Dennis Ritchie in the 1970s on a DEC PDP-11 that used the UNIX operating system. While some earlier languages, most notably Pascal, had achieved significant success, C established the paradigm that still charts the course of programming today.

C grew out of the *structured programming* revolution of the 1960s. Prior to structured programming, large programs were difficult to write because the program logic tended to degenerate into what is known as "spaghetti code," a tangled mass of jumps, calls, and returns that is difficult to follow. Structured languages addressed this problem by adding well-defined control statements, subroutines with local variables, and other improvements. Through the use of structured techniques programs became better organized, more reliable, and easier to manage.

Although there were other structured languages at the time, C was the first to successfully combine power, elegance, and expressiveness. Its terse, yet easy-to-use syntax coupled with its philosophy that the programmer (not the language) was in charge quickly won many converts. It can be a bit hard to understand from today's perspective, but C was a breath of fresh air that programmers had long awaited. As a result, C became the most widely used structured programming language of the 1980s.

However, even the venerable C language had its limits. One of the most troublesome was its inability to handle large programs. The C language hits a barrier once a project reaches a certain size, and after that point, C programs are difficult to understand and maintain. Precisely where this limit is reached depends upon the program, the programmer, and the tools at hand, but there is always a threshold beyond which a C program becomes unmanageable.

The Creation of OOP and C++

By the late 1970s, the size of many projects was near or at the limits of what structured programming methodologies and the C language could handle. To solve this problem, a new way to program began to emerge. This method is called *object-oriented programming* (OOP). Using OOP, a programmer could handle much larger programs. The trouble was that C, the most popular language at the time, did not support object-oriented programming. The desire for an object-oriented version of C ultimately led to the creation of C++.

C++ was invented by Bjarne Stroustrup beginning in 1979 at Bell Laboratories in Murray Hill, New Jersey. He initially called the new language "C with Classes." However, in 1983 the name was changed to C++. C++ contains the entire C language. Thus, C is the foundation upon which C++ is built. Most of the additions that Stroustrup made to C were designed to support object-oriented programming. In essence, C++ is the object-oriented version of C. By building upon the foundation of C, Stroustrup provided a smooth migration path to OOP. Instead of having to learn an entirely new language, a C programmer needed to learn only a few new features before reaping the benefits of the object-oriented methodology.

C++ simmered in the background during much of the 1980s, undergoing extensive development. By the beginning of the 1990s, C++ was ready for mainstream use, and its popularity exploded. By the end of the decade, it had become the most widely used programming language. Today, C++ is still the preeminent language for the development of high-performance system code.

It is critical to understand that the invention of C++ was not an attempt to create an entirely new programming language. Instead, it was an enhancement to an already highly successful language. This approach to language development—beginning with an existing language and moving it forward—established a trend that continues today.

The Internet and Java Emerge

The next major advance in programming languages is Java. Work on Java, which was originally called Oak, began in 1991 at Sun Microsystems. The main driving force behind Java's design was James Gosling. Patrick Naughton, Chris Warth, Ed Frank, and Mike Sheridan also played a role.

Java is a structured, object-oriented language with a syntax and philosophy derived from C++. The innovative aspects of Java were driven not so much by advances in the art of programming (although some certainly were), but rather by changes in the computing environment. Prior to the mainstreaming of the Internet, most programs were written,

compiled, and targeted for a specific CPU and a specific operating system. While it has always been true that programmers like to reuse their code, the ability to port a program easily from one environment to another took a backseat to more pressing problems. However, with the rise of the Internet, in which many different types of CPUs and operating systems are connected, the old problem of portability reemerged with a vengeance. To solve the problem of portability, a new language was needed, and this new language was Java.

Although the single most important aspect of Java (and the reason for its rapid acceptance) is its ability to create cross-platform, portable code, it is interesting to note that the original impetus for Java was not the Internet, but rather the need for a platform-independent language that could be used to create software for embedded controllers. In 1993, it became clear that the issues of cross-platform portability found when creating code for embedded controllers are also encountered when attempting to create code for the Internet. Remember: the Internet is a vast, distributed computing universe in which many different types of computers live. The same techniques that solved the portability problem on a small scale could be applied to the Internet on a large scale.

Java achieved portability by translating a program's source code into an intermediate language called *bytecode*. This bytecode was then executed by the Java Virtual Machine (JVM). Therefore, a Java program could run in any environment for which a JVM was available. Also, since the JVM is relatively easy to implement, it was readily available for a large number of environments.

Java's use of bytecode differed radically from both C and C++, which were nearly always compiled to executable machine code. Machine code is tied to a specific CPU and operating system. Thus, if you wanted to run a C/C++ program on a different system, it needed to be recompiled to machine code specifically for that environment. Therefore, to create a C/C++ program that would run in a variety of environments, several different executable versions of the program would be needed. Not only was this impractical, it was expensive. Java's use of an intermediate language was an elegant, cost-effective solution. It is also a solution that C# would adapt for its own purposes.

As mentioned, Java is descended from C and C++. Its syntax is based on C, and its object model is evolved from C++. Although Java code is neither upwardly nor downwardly compatible with C or C++, its syntax is sufficiently similar that the large pool of existing C/C++ programmers could move to Java with very little effort. Furthermore, because Java built upon and improved an existing paradigm, Gosling, et al., were free to focus their attention on the new and innovative features. Just as Stroustrup did not need to "reinvent the wheel" when creating C++, Gosling did not need to create an entirely new language when developing Java. Moreover, with the creation of Java, C and C++ became an accepted substrata upon which to base a new computer language.

The Creation of C#

While Java has successfully addressed many of the issues surrounding portability in the Internet environment, there are still features that it lacks. One is *cross-language interoperability*, also called *mixed-language programming*. This is the ability for the code produced by one language to work easily with the code produced by another. Cross-language interoperability is needed for the creation of large, distributed software systems. It is also desirable for programming software components because the most valuable component is one that can be used by the widest variety of computer languages, in the greatest number of operating environments.

Another feature lacking in Java is full integration with the Windows platform. Although Java programs can be executed in a Windows environment (assuming that the Java Virtual Machine has been installed), Java and Windows are not closely coupled. Since Windows is the most widely used operating system in the world, lack of direct support for Windows is a drawback to Java.

To answer these and other needs, Microsoft developed C#. C# was created at Microsoft late in the 1990s and was part of Microsoft's overall .NET strategy. It was first released in its alpha version in the middle of 2000. C#'s chief architect was Anders Hejlsberg. Hejlsberg is one of the world's leading language experts, with several notable accomplishments to his credit. For example, in the 1980s he was the original author of the highly successful and influential Turbo Pascal, whose streamlined implementation set the standard for all future compilers.

C# is directly related to C, C++, and Java. This is not by accident. These are three of the most widely used—and most widely liked—programming languages in the world. Furthermore, at the time of C#'s creation, nearly all professional programmers knew C, C++, and/or Java. By building C# upon a solid, well-understood foundation, C# offered an easy migration path from these languages. Since it was neither necessary nor desirable for Hejlsberg to "reinvent the wheel," he was free to focus on specific improvements and innovations.

The family tree for C# is shown in Figure 1-1. The grandfather of C# is C. From C, C# derives its syntax, many of its keywords, and its operators. C# builds upon and improves the object model defined by C++. If you know C or C++, then you will feel at home with C#.

C# and Java have a bit more complicated relationship. As explained, Java is also descended from C and C++. It too shares the C/C++ syntax and object model. Like Java, C# is designed to produce portable code. However, C# is not descended from Java. Instead, C# and Java are more like cousins, sharing a common ancestry, but differing in many important ways. The good news, though, is that if you know Java, then many C# concepts will be familiar. Conversely, if in the future you need to learn Java, then many of the things you learn about C# will carry over.

C# contains many innovative features that we will examine at length throughout the course of this book, but some of its most important relate to its built-in support for software components. In fact, C# has been characterized as being a component-oriented language because it contains integral support for the writing of software components. For example,

FIGURE 1-1
The C# family tree

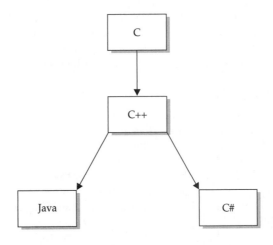

C# includes features that directly support the constituents of components, such as properties, methods, and events. However, C#'s ability to work in a secure, mixed-language environment is perhaps its most important component-oriented feature.

The Evolution of C#

Since its original 1.0 release, C# has been evolving at a rapid pace. Not long after C# 1.0, Microsoft released version 1.1. It contained many minor tweaks but added no major features. However, the situation was much different with the release of C# 2.0.

C# 2.0 was a watershed event in the lifecycle of C# because it added many new features, such as generics, partial types, and anonymous methods, that fundamentally expanded the scope, power, and range of the language. Version 2.0 firmly put C# at the forefront of computer language development. It also demonstrated Microsoft's long-term commitment to the language.

The next major release of C# was 3.0, and this is the version of C# described by this book. Because of the many new features added by C# 2.0, one might have expected the development of C# to slow a bit, just to let programmers catch up, but this was not the case. With the release of C# 3.0, Microsoft once again put C# on the cutting edge of language design, this time adding a set of innovative features that redefined the programming landscape. Here is a list of what 3.0 has added to the language:

- Anonymous types
- Auto-implemented properties
- Extension methods
- Implicitly typed variables
- Lambda expressions
- Language-integrated query (LINQ)
- Object and collection initializers
- Partial methods

Although all of these features are important and have significant impact on the language, the two that are the most exciting are language-integrated query (LINQ) and lambda expressions. LINQ enables you to write database-style queries using C# programming elements. However, the LINQ syntax is not limited to only databases. It can also be used with arrays and collections. Thus, LINQ offers a new way to approach several common programming tasks. Lambda expressions are often used in LINQ expressions, but can also be used elsewhere. They implement a functional-style syntax that uses the lambda operator =>. Together, LINQ and lambda expressions add an entirely new dimension to C# programming. Throughout the course of this book, you will see how these features are revolutionizing the way that C# code is written.

How C# Relates to the .NET Framework

Although C# is a computer language that can be studied on its own, it has a special relationship to its runtime environment, the .NET Framework. The reason for this is twofold. First, C# was initially designed by Microsoft to create code for the .NET

Framework. Second, the libraries used by C# are the ones defined by the .NET Framework. Thus, even though it is theoretically possible to separate C# the language from the .NET environment, in practice the two are closely linked. Because of this, it is important to have a general understanding of the .NET Framework and why it is important to C#.

What Is the .NET Framework?

The .NET Framework defines an environment that supports the development and execution of highly distributed, component-based applications. It enables differing computer languages to work together and provides for security, program portability, and a common programming model for the Windows platform. As it relates to C#, the .NET Framework defines two very important entities. The first is the *Common Language Runtime* (CLR). This is the system that manages the execution of your program. Along with other benefits, the Common Language Runtime is the part of the .NET Framework that enables programs to be portable, supports mixed-language programming, and provides for secure execution.

The second entity is the .NET *class library*. This library gives your program access to the runtime environment. For example, if you want to perform I/O, such as displaying something on the screen, you will use the .NET class library to do it. If you are new to programming, then the term *class* may be new. Although it is explained in detail later in this book, for now a brief definition will suffice: a class is an object-oriented construct that helps organize programs. As long as your program restricts itself to the features defined by the .NET class library, your programs can run anywhere that the .NET runtime system is supported. Since C# automatically uses the .NET Framework class library, C# programs are automatically portable to all .NET environments.

How the Common Language Runtime Works

The Common Language Runtime manages the execution of .NET code. Here is how it works: When you compile a C# program, the output of the compiler is not executable code. Instead, it is a file that contains a special type of pseudocode called *Microsoft Intermediate Language* (MSIL). MSIL defines a set of portable instructions that are independent of any specific CPU. In essence, MSIL defines a portable assembly language. One other point: although MSIL is similar in concept to Java's bytecode, the two are not the same.

It is the job of the CLR to translate the intermediate code into executable code when a program is run. Thus, any program compiled to MSIL can be run in any environment for which the CLR is implemented. This is part of how the .NET Framework achieves portability.

Microsoft Intermediate Language is turned into executable code using a *JIT compiler*. "JIT" stands for "Just-In-Time." The process works like this: When a .NET program is executed, the CLR activates the JIT compiler. The JIT compiler converts MSIL into native code on demand as each part of your program is needed. Thus, your C# program actually executes as native code even though it is initially compiled into MSIL. This means that your program runs nearly as fast as it would if it had been compiled to native code in the first place, but it gains the portability benefits of MSIL.

In addition to MSIL, one other thing is output when you compile a C# program: *metadata*. Metadata describes the data used by your program and enables your code to interact easily with other code. The metadata is contained in the same file as the MSIL.

Managed vs. Unmanaged Code

In general, when you write a C# program, you are creating what is called *managed code*. Managed code is executed under the control of the Common Language Runtime as just described. Because it is running under the control of the CLR, managed code is subject to certain constraints—and derives several benefits. The constraints are easily described and met: the compiler must produce an MSIL file targeted for the CLR (which C# does) and use the .NET class library (which C# does). The benefits of managed code are many, including modern memory management, the ability to mix languages, better security, support for version control, and a clean way for software components to interact.

The opposite of managed code is unmanaged code. Unmanaged code does not execute under the Common Language Runtime. Thus, all Windows programs prior to the creation of the .NET Framework use unmanaged code. It is possible for managed code and unmanaged code to work together, so the fact that C# generates managed code does not restrict its ability to operate in conjunction with preexisting programs.

The Common Language Specification

Although all managed code gains the benefits provided by the CLR, if your code will be used by other programs written in different languages, then for maximum usability, it should adhere to the Common Language Specification (CLS). The CLS describes a set of features that different .NET-compatible languages have in common. CLS compliance is especially important when creating software components that will be used by other languages. The CLS includes a subset of the *Common Type System* (CTS). The CTS defines the rules concerning data types. Of course, C# supports both the CLS and the CTS.

An Overview of C#

By far, the hardest thing about learning a programming language is the fact that no element exists in isolation. Instead, the components of the language work together. This interrelatedness makes it difficult to discuss one aspect of C# without involving another. To help overcome this problem, this chapter provides a brief overview of several C# features, including the general form of a C# program, some basic control statements, and operators. It does not go into too many details, but rather concentrates on the general concepts common to any C# program. Most of the topics discussed here are examined in greater detail in the remaining chapters of Part I.

Object-Oriented Programming

At the center of C# is *object-oriented programming* (OOP). The object-oriented methodology is inseparable from C#, and all C# programs are to at least some extent object oriented. Because of its importance to C#, it is useful to understand OOP's basic principles before you write even a simple C# program.

OOP is a powerful way to approach the job of programming. Programming methodologies have changed dramatically since the invention of the computer, primarily to accommodate the increasing complexity of programs. For example, when computers were first invented, programming was done by toggling in the binary machine instructions using the computer's front panel. As long as programs were just a few hundred instructions long, this approach worked. As programs grew, assembly language was invented so that a programmer could deal with larger, increasingly complex programs, using symbolic representations of the machine instructions. As programs continued to grow, high-level languages such as FORTRAN and COBOL were introduced that gave the programmer more tools with which to handle complexity. When these early languages began to reach their breaking point, structured programming languages, such as C, were invented.

At each milestone in the history of programming, techniques and tools were created to allow the programmer to deal with increasingly greater complexity. Each step of the way, the new approach took the best elements of the previous methods and moved forward. The same is true of object-oriented programming. Prior to OOP, many projects were nearing (or exceeding) the point where the structured approach no longer worked. A better way to handle complexity was needed, and object-oriented programming was the solution.

Object-oriented programming took the best ideas of structured programming and combined them with several new concepts. The result was a different and better way of organizing a program. In the most general sense, a program can be organized in one of two ways: around its code (what is happening) or around its data (what is being affected). Using only structured programming techniques, programs are typically organized around code. This approach can be thought of as "code acting on data."

Object-oriented programs work the other way around. They are organized around data, with the key principle being "data controlling access to code." In an object-oriented language, you define the data and the code that is permitted to act on that data. Thus, a data type defines precisely the operations that can be applied to that data.

To support the principles of object-oriented programming, all OOP languages, including C#, have three traits in common: encapsulation, polymorphism, and inheritance. Let's examine each.

Encapsulation

Encapsulation is a programming mechanism that binds together code and the data it manipulates, and that keeps both safe from outside interference and misuse. In an object-oriented language, code and data can be bound together in such a way that a self-contained *black box* is created. Within the box are all necessary data and code. When code and data are linked together in this fashion, an *object* is created. In other words, an object is the device that supports encapsulation.

Within an object, the code, data, or both may be *private* to that object or *public*. Private code or data is known to and accessible by only another part of the object. That is, private code or data cannot be accessed by a piece of the program that exists outside the object. When code or data is public, other parts of your program can access it even though it is defined within an object. Typically, the public parts of an object are used to provide a controlled interface to the private elements.

C#'s basic unit of encapsulation is the *class*. A class defines the form of an object. It specifies both the data and the code that will operate on that data. C# uses a class specification to construct *objects*. Objects are instances of a class. Thus, a class is essentially a set of plans that specify how to build an object.

Collectively, the code and data that constitute a class are called its *members*. The data defined by the class is referred to as *fields*. The terms *member variables* and *instance variables* also are used. The code that operates on that data is contained within *function members,* of which the most common is the *method*. Method is C#'s term for a subroutine. (Other function members include properties, events, and constructors.) Thus, the methods of a class contain code that acts on the fields defined by that class.

Polymorphism

Polymorphism (from Greek, meaning "many forms") is the quality that allows one interface to access a general class of actions. A simple example of polymorphism is found in the steering wheel of an automobile. The steering wheel (the interface) is the same no matter what type of actual steering mechanism is used. That is, the steering wheel works the same whether your car has manual steering, power steering, or rack-and-pinion steering. Thus, turning the steering wheel left causes the car to go left no matter what type of steering is used. The benefit of the uniform interface is, of course, that once you know how to operate the steering wheel, you can drive any type of car.

The same principle can also apply to programming. For example, consider a *stack* (which is a first-in, last-out list). You might have a program that requires three different types of stacks. One stack is used for integer values, one for floating-point values, and one for characters. In this case, the algorithm that implements each stack is the same, even though the data being stored differs. In a non-object-oriented language, you would be required to create three different sets of stack routines, with each set using different names. However, because of polymorphism, in C# you can create one general set of stack routines that works for all three specific situations. This way, once you know how to use one stack, you can use them all.

More generally, the concept of polymorphism is often expressed by the phrase "one interface, multiple methods." This means that it is possible to design a generic interface to a group of related activities. Polymorphism helps reduce complexity by allowing the same interface to be used to specify a *general class of action.* It is the compiler's job to select the *specific action* (that is, method) as it applies to each situation. You, the programmer, don't need to do this selection manually. You need only remember and utilize the general interface.

Inheritance

Inheritance is the process by which one object can acquire the properties of another object. This is important because it supports the concept of hierarchical classification. If you think about it, most knowledge is made manageable by hierarchical (that is, top-down) classifications. For example, a Red Delicious apple is part of the classification *apple,* which in turn is part of the *fruit* class, which is under the larger class *food.* That is, the *food* class possesses certain qualities (edible, nutritious, and so on) which also, logically, apply to its subclass, *fruit.* In addition to these qualities, the *fruit* class has specific characteristics (juicy, sweet, and so on) that distinguish it from other food. The *apple* class defines those qualities specific to an apple (grows on trees, not tropical, and so on). A Red Delicious apple would, in turn, inherit all the qualities of all preceding classes and would define only those qualities that make it unique.

Without the use of hierarchies, each object would have to explicitly define all of its characteristics. Using inheritance, an object need only define those qualities that make it unique within its class. It can inherit its general attributes from its parent. Thus, the inheritance mechanism makes it possible for one object to be a specific instance of a more general case.

A First Simple Program

It is now time to look at an actual C# program. We will begin by compiling and running the short program shown here:

```
/*
   This is a simple C# program.

   Call this program Example.cs.
*/

using System;

class Example {
```

```
// A C# program begins with a call to Main().
static void Main() {
  Console.WriteLine("A simple C# program.");
}
}
```

The primary development environment for C# is Microsoft's Visual Studio. To compile all of the programs in this book, including those that use the new C# 3.0 features, you will need to use a version of Visual Studio 2008 (or later) that supports C#. A good choice for learning C# 3.0 is Visual C# 2008 Express Edition because (at the time of this writing) it is available free of charge from Microsoft. Visual C# 2008 Express Edition contains a full-featured compiler that supports all of C# 3.0 and is, therefore, able to compile all of the code in this book. It also includes Visual Studio, which is Microsoft's integrated programming environment (IDE). Although the Express Edition does not supply all of the tools that a commercial developer will want, it is perfect for learning C#. At the time of this writing, Visual C# 2008 Express Edition can be downloaded from **microsoft.com/express/**. All of the code in this book has been tested against this compiler.

Using Visual C#, there are two general approaches that you can take to creating, compiling, and running a C# program. First, you can use the Visual Studio IDE. Second, you can use the command-line compiler, **csc.exe**. Both methods are described here.

Using csc.exe, the C# Command-Line Compiler

Although the Visual Studio IDE is what you will probably be using for your commercial projects, some readers will find the C# command-line compiler more convenient, especially for compiling and running the sample programs shown in this book. The reason is that you don't have to create a project for the program. You can simply create the program and then compile it and run it—all from the command line. Therefore, if you know how to use the Command Prompt window and its command-line interface, using the command-line compiler will be faster and easier than using the IDE.

CAUTION *If you are not familiar with the Command Prompt window, then it is probably better to use the Visual Studio IDE. Although its commands are not difficult to learn, trying to learn both the Command Prompt and C# at the same time will be a challenging experience.*

To create and run programs using the C# command-line compiler, follow these three steps:

1. Enter the program using a text editor.
2. Compile the program using **csc.exe**.
3. Run the program.

Entering the Program

The source code for programs shown in this book are available at **www.mhprofessional.com**. However, if you want to enter the programs by hand, you are free to do so. In this case, you must enter the program into your computer using a text editor, such as Notepad. Remember,

you must create text-only files, not formatted word-processor files, because the format information in a word processor file will confuse the C# compiler. When entering the program, call the file **Example.cs**.

Compiling the Program

To compile the program, execute the C# compiler, **csc.exe**, specifying the name of the source file on the command line, as shown here:

```
C:\>csc Example.cs
```

The **csc** compiler creates a file called **Example.exe** that contains the MSIL version of the program. Although MSIL is not executable code, it is still contained in an **exe** file. The Common Language Runtime automatically invokes the JIT compiler when you attempt to execute **Example.exe**. Be aware, however, that if you try to execute **Example.exe** (or any other **exe** file that contains MSIL) on a computer for which the .NET Framework is not installed, the program will not execute because the CLR will be missing.

NOTE *Prior to running* **csc.exe** *you will need to open a Command Prompt window that is configured for Visual Studio. The easiest way to do this is to select Visual Studio 2008 Command Prompt under Visual Studio Tools in the Start menu. Alternatively, you can start an unconfigured Command Prompt window and then run the batch file* **vsvars32.bat**, *which is provided by Visual Studio. You may, however, encounter a problem with the command-line approach. At the time of this writing, Visual C# 2008 Express Edition does not provide the Visual Studio Tools menu or the* **vsvars32.bat** *file. Therefore, if you are using Visual C# 2008 Express, you may not be able to configure a command prompt window automatically. In this case, use the Visual Studio IDE instead. However, Visual C++ 2008 Express Edition does supply both* **vsvars32.bat** *and the Visual Studio 2008 Command Prompt menu selection. Therefore, if you also install Visual C++ 2008 Express Edition, you will be able to start a properly configured command prompt window that will also work for C#.*

Running the Program

To actually run the program, just type its name on the command line, as shown here:

```
C:\>Example
```

When the program is run, the following output is displayed:

```
A simple C# program.
```

Using the Visual Studio IDE

Visual Studio is Microsoft's integrated programming environment. It lets you edit, compile, run, and debug a C# program, all without leaving its well-thought-out environment. Visual Studio offers convenience and helps manage your programs. It is most effective for larger projects, but it can be used to great success with smaller programs, such as those that constitute the examples in this book.

The steps required to edit, compile, and run a C# program using the Visual Studio 2008 IDE are shown here. These steps assume the IDE provided by Visual C# 2008 Express Edition. Slight differences may exist with other versions of Visual Studio 2008.

1. Create a new, empty C# project by selecting File | New Project. Next, select Empty Project:

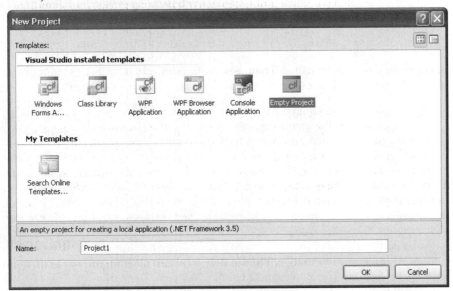

Then, press OK to create the project.

2. Once the new project is created, the Visual Studio IDE will look like this:

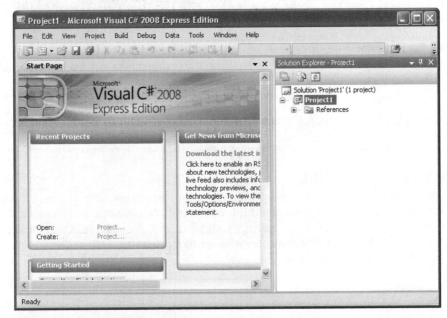

This is the second type of comment supported by C#. A single-line comment begins with a // and ends at the end of the line. Although styles vary, it is not uncommon for programmers to use multiline comments for longer remarks and single-line comments for brief, line-by-line descriptions. (The third type of comment supported by C# aids in the creation of documentation and is described in Appendix A.)

The next line of code is shown here:

```
static void Main() {
```

This line begins the **Main()** method. As mentioned earlier, in C#, a subroutine is called a method. As the comment preceding it suggests, this is the line at which the program will begin executing. All C# applications begin execution by calling **Main()**. The complete meaning of each part of this line cannot be given now, since it involves a detailed understanding of several other C# features. However, since many of the examples in this book will use this line of code, we will take a brief look at it here.

The line begins with the keyword **static**. A method that is modified by **static** can be called before an object of its class has been created. This is necessary because **Main()** is called at program startup. The keyword **void** indicates that **Main()** does not return a value. As you will see, methods can also return values. The empty parentheses that follow **Main** indicate that no information is passed to **Main()**. Although it is possible to pass information into **Main()**, none is passed in this example. The last character on the line is the {. This signals the start of **Main()**'s body. All of the code that comprises a method will occur between the method's opening curly brace and its closing curly brace.

The next line of code is shown here. Notice that it occurs inside **Main()**.

```
Console.WriteLine("A simple C# program.");
```

This line outputs the string "A simple C# program." followed by a new line on the screen. Output is actually accomplished by the built-in method **WriteLine()**. In this case, **WriteLine()** displays the string that is passed to it. Information that is passed to a method is called an *argument*. In addition to strings, **WriteLine()** can be used to display other types of information. The line begins with **Console**, which is the name of a predefined class that supports console I/O. By connecting **Console** with **WriteLine()**, you are telling the compiler that **WriteLine()** is a member of the **Console** class. The fact that C# uses an object to define console output is further evidence of its object-oriented nature.

Notice that the **WriteLine()** statement ends with a semicolon, as does the **using System** statement earlier in the program. In general, statements in C# end with a semicolon. The exception to this rule are *blocks*, which begin with a { and end with a }. This is why those lines in the program don't end with a semicolon. Blocks provide a mechanism for grouping statements and are discussed later in this chapter.

The first } in the program ends **Main()**, and the last } ends the **Example** class definition.

One last point: C# is case-sensitive. Forgetting this can cause serious problems. For example, if you accidentally type **main** instead of **Main**, or **writeline** instead of **WriteLine**, the preceding program will be incorrect. Furthermore, although the C# compiler *will* compile classes that do not contain a **Main()** method, it has no way to execute them. So, had you mistyped **Main**, you would see an error message that states that **Example.exe** does not have an entry point defined.

Handling Syntax Errors

If you are new to programming, it is important to learn how to interpret and respond to errors that may occur when you try to compile a program. Most compilation errors are caused by typing mistakes. As all programmers soon find out, accidentally typing something incorrectly is quite easy. Fortunately, if you type something wrong, the compiler will report a *syntax error* message when it tries to compile your program. This message gives you the line number at which the error is found and a description of the error itself.

Although the syntax errors reported by the compiler are, obviously, helpful, they sometimes can also be misleading. The C# compiler attempts to make sense out of your source code no matter what you have written. For this reason, the error that is reported may not always reflect the actual cause of the problem. In the preceding program, for example, an accidental omission of the opening curly brace after the **Main( )** method generates the following sequence of errors when compiled by the **csc** command-line compiler. (Similar errors are generated when compiling using the IDE.)

```
EX1.CS(12,21): error CS1002: ; expected
EX1.CS(13,22): error CS1519: Invalid token '(' in class, struct, or
interface member declaration
EX1.CS(15,1): error CS1022: Type or namespace definition, or
end-of-file expected
```

Clearly, the first error message is completely wrong, because what is missing is not a semicolon, but a curly brace. The second two messages are equally confusing.

The point of this discussion is that when your program contains a syntax error, don't necessarily take the compiler's messages at face value. They may be misleading. You may need to "second guess" an error message in order to find the problem. Also, look at the last few lines of code immediately preceding the one in which the error was reported. Sometimes an error will not be reported until several lines after the point at which the error really occurred.

A Small Variation

Although all of the programs in this book will use it, the line

```
using System;
```

at the start of the first example program is not technically needed. It is, however, a valuable convenience. The reason it's not necessary is that in C# you can always *fully qualify* a name with the namespace to which it belongs. For example, the line

```
Console.WriteLine("A simple C# program.");
```

can be rewritten as

```
System.Console.WriteLine("A simple C# program.");
```

Thus, the first example could be recoded as shown here:

```
// This version does not include "using System;".

class Example {
```

```
  // A C# program begins with a call to Main().
  static void Main() {

    // Here, Console.WriteLine is fully qualified.
    System.Console.WriteLine("A simple C# program.");
  }
}
```

Since it is quite tedious to always specify the **System** namespace whenever a member of that namespace is used, most C# programmers include **using System** at the top of their programs, as will all of the programs in this book. It is important to understand, however, that you can explicitly qualify a name with its namespace if needed.

A Second Simple Program

Perhaps no other construct is as important to a programming language as the variable. A *variable* is a named memory location that can be assigned a value. It is called a variable because its value can be changed during the execution of a program. In other words, the content of a variable is changeable, not fixed.

The following program creates two variables called **x** and **y**.

```
// This program demonstrates variables.

using System;

class Example2 {
  static void Main() {
    int x; // this declares a variable
    int y; // this declares another variable

    x = 100; // this assigns 100 to x

    Console.WriteLine("x contains " + x);

    y = x / 2;

    Console.Write("y contains x / 2: ");
    Console.WriteLine(y);
  }
}
```

When you run this program, you will see the following output:

```
x contains 100
y contains x / 2: 50
```

This program introduces several new concepts. First, the statement

```
int x; // this declares a variable
```

declares a variable called **x** of type integer. In C#, all variables must be declared before they are used. Further, the kind of values that the variable can hold must also be specified. This is called the *type* of the variable. In this case, **x** can hold integer values. These are whole

numbers. In C#, to declare a variable to be of type integer, precede its name with the keyword **int**. Thus, the preceding statement declares a variable called **x** of type **int**.

The next line declares a second variable called **y**.

```
int y; // this declares another variable
```

Notice that it uses the same format as the first except that the name of the variable is different.

In general, to declare a variable, you will use a statement like this:

type var-name;

Here, *type* specifies the type of variable being declared, and *var-name* is the name of the variable. In addition to **int**, C# supports several other data types.

The following line of code assigns **x** the value **100**:

```
x = 100; // this assigns 100 to x
```

In C#, the assignment operator is the single equal sign. It copies the value on its right side into the variable on its left.

The next line of code outputs the value of **x** preceded by the string "x contains ".

```
Console.WriteLine("x contains " + x);
```

In this statement, the plus sign causes the value of **x** to be displayed after the string that precedes it. This approach can be generalized. Using the **+** operator, you can chain together as many items as you want within a single **WriteLine( )** statement.

The next line of code assigns **y** the value of **x** divided by **2**:

```
y = x / 2;
```

This line divides the value in **x** by 2 and then stores that result in **y**. Thus, after the line executes, **y** will contain the value 50. The value of **x** will be unchanged. Like most other computer languages, C# supports a full range of arithmetic operators, including those shown here:

+	Addition
–	Subtraction
*	Multiplication
/	Division

Here are the next two lines in the program:

```
Console.Write("y contains x / 2: ");
Console.WriteLine(y);
```

Two new things are occurring here. First, the built-in method **Write( )** is used to display the string "y contains x / 2: ". This string is *not* followed by a new line. This means that when the next output is generated, it will start on the same line. The **Write( )** method is just like **WriteLine( )**, except that it does not output a new line after each call. Second, in the call

to **WriteLine()**, notice that **y** is used by itself. Both **Write()** and **WriteLine()** can be used to output values of any of C#'s built-in types.

One more point about declaring variables before we move on: It is possible to declare two or more variables using the same declaration statement. Just separate their names by commas. For example, **x** and **y** could have been declared like this:

```
int x, y; // both declared using one statement
```

NOTE   *C# 3.0 includes a new feature called an* implicitly typed variable. *Implicitly typed variables are variables whose type is automatically determined by the compiler. Implicitly typed variables are discussed in Chapter 3.*

Another Data Type

In the preceding program, a variable of type **int** was used. However, an **int** variable can hold only whole numbers. It cannot be used when a fractional component is required. For example, an **int** variable can hold the value 18, but not the value 18.3. Fortunately, **int** is only one of several data types defined by C#. To allow numbers with fractional components, C# defines two floating-point types: **float** and **double**, which represent single- and double-precision values, respectively. Of the two, **double** is the most commonly used.

To declare a variable of type **double**, use a statement similar to that shown here:

```
double result;
```

Here, **result** is the name of the variable, which is of type **double**. Because **result** has a floating-point type, it can hold values such as 122.23, 0.034, or –19.0.

To better understand the difference between **int** and **double**, try the following program:

```
/*
   This program illustrates the differences
   between int and double.
*/

using System;

class Example3 {
  static void Main() {
    int ivar;     // this declares an int variable
    double dvar;  // this declares a floating-point variable

    ivar = 100;    // assign ivar the value 100

    dvar = 100.0; // assign dvar the value 100.0

    Console.WriteLine("Original value of ivar: " + ivar);
    Console.WriteLine("Original value of dvar: " + dvar);

    Console.WriteLine(); // print a blank line

    // Now, divide both by 3.
    ivar = ivar / 3;
    dvar = dvar / 3.0;
```

```
Console.WriteLine("ivar after division: " + ivar);
Console.WriteLine("dvar after division: " + dvar);
  }
}
```

The output from this program is shown here:

```
Original value of ivar: 100
Original value of dvar: 100

ivar after division: 33
dvar after division: 33.3333333333333
```

As you can see, when **ivar** (an **int** variable) is divided by 3, a whole-number division is performed, and the outcome is 33—the fractional component is lost. However, when **dvar** (a **double** variable) is divided by 3, the fractional component is preserved.

As the program shows, when you want to specify a floating-point value in a program, you must include a decimal point. If you don't, it will be interpreted as an integer. For example, in C#, the value 100 is an integer, but the value 100.0 is a floating-point value.

There is one other new thing to notice in the program. To print a blank line, simply call **WriteLine()** without any arguments.

The floating-point data types are often used when working with real-world quantities where fractional components are commonly needed. For example, this program computes the area of a circle. It uses the value 3.1416 for pi.

```
// Compute the area of a circle.

using System;

class Circle {
  static void Main() {
    double radius;
    double area;

    radius = 10.0;
    area = radius * radius * 3.1416;

    Console.WriteLine("Area is " + area);
  }
}
```

The output from the program is shown here:

```
Area is 314.16
```

Clearly, the computation of a circle's area could not be satisfactorily achieved without the use of floating-point data.

Two Control Statements

Inside a method, execution proceeds from one statement to the next, top to bottom. It is possible to alter this flow through the use of the various program control statements supported by C#. Although we will look closely at control statements later, two are briefly introduced here because we will be using them to write sample programs.

The if Statement

You can selectively execute part of a program through the use of C#'s conditional statement: the **if**. The **if** statement works in C# much like the IF statement in any other language. For example, it is syntactically identical to the **if** statements in C, C++, and Java. Its simplest form is shown here:

if(*condition*) *statement*;

Here, *condition* is a Boolean (that is, true or false) expression. If *condition* is true, then the statement is executed. If *condition* is false, then the statement is bypassed. Here is an example:

```
if(10 < 11) Console.WriteLine("10 is less than 11");
```

In this case, since 10 is less than 11, the conditional expression is true, and **WriteLine()** will execute. However, consider the following:

```
if(10 < 9) Console.WriteLine("this won't be displayed");
```

In this case, 10 is not less than 9. Thus, the call to **WriteLine()** will not take place.

C# defines a full complement of relational operators that can be used in a conditional expression. They are shown here:

Operator	Meaning
<	Less than
<=	Less than or equal to
>	Greater than
>=	Greater than or equal to
==	Equal to
!=	Not equal

Here is a program that illustrates the **if** statement:

```
// Demonstrate the if.

using System;

class IfDemo {
  static void Main() {
    int a, b, c;

    a = 2;
    b = 3;

    if(a < b) Console.WriteLine("a is less than b");

    // This won't display anything.
    if(a == b) Console.WriteLine("you won't see this");

    Console.WriteLine();
```

```
    c = a - b; // c contains -1

    Console.WriteLine("c contains -1");
    if(c >= 0) Console.WriteLine("c is non-negative");
    if(c < 0) Console.WriteLine("c is negative");

    Console.WriteLine();

    c = b - a; // c now contains 1
    Console.WriteLine("c contains 1");
    if(c >= 0) Console.WriteLine("c is non-negative");
    if(c < 0) Console.WriteLine("c is negative");
  }
}
```

The output generated by this program is shown here:

```
a is less than b

c contains -1
c is negative

c contains 1
c is non-negative
```

Notice one other thing in this program. The line

```
int a, b, c;
```

declares three variables, **a**, **b**, and **c**, by use of a comma-separated list. As mentioned earlier, when you need two or more variables of the same type, they can be declared in one statement. Just separate the variable names with commas.

The for Loop

You can repeatedly execute a sequence of code by creating a *loop*. C# supplies a powerful assortment of loop constructs. The one we will look at here is the **for** loop. Like the **if** statement, the C# **for** loop is similar to its counterpart in C, C++, and Java. The simplest form of the **for** loop is shown here:

for(*initialization*; *condition*; *iteration*) *statement*;

In its most common form, the *initialization* portion of the loop sets a loop control variable to an initial value. The *condition* is a Boolean expression that tests the loop control variable. If the outcome of that test is true, the **for** loop continues to iterate. If it is false, the loop terminates. The *iteration* expression determines how the loop control variable is changed each time the loop iterates. Here is a short program that illustrates the **for** loop:

```
// Demonstrate the for loop.

using System;

class ForDemo {
  static void Main() {
    int count;
```

```
    for(count = 0; count < 5; count = count+1)
      Console.WriteLine("This is count: " + count);

    Console.WriteLine("Done!");
  }
}
```

The output generated by the program is shown here:

```
This is count: 0
This is count: 1
This is count: 2
This is count: 3
This is count: 4
Done!
```

In this example, **count** is the loop control variable. It is set to zero in the initialization portion of the **for**. At the start of each iteration (including the first one), the conditional test **count < 5** is performed. If the outcome of this test is true, the **WriteLine()** statement is executed. Next, the iteration portion of the loop is executed, which adds 1 to **count**. This process continues until **count** reaches 5. At this point, the conditional test becomes false, causing the loop to terminate. Execution picks up at the bottom of the loop.

As a point of interest, in professionally written C# programs you will almost never see the iteration portion of the loop written as shown in the preceding program. That is, you will seldom see statements like this:

```
count = count + 1;
```

The reason is that C# includes a special increment operator that performs this operation. The increment operator is **++** (that is, two consecutive plus signs). The increment operator increases its operand by one. By use of the increment operator, the preceding statement can be written like this:

```
count++;
```

Thus, the **for** in the preceding program will usually be written like this:

```
for(count = 0; count < 5; count++)
```

You might want to try this. As you will see, the loop still runs exactly the same as it did before.

C# also provides a decrement operator, which is specified as **– –**. This operator decreases its operand by one.

Using Code Blocks

Another key element of C# is the *code block*. A code block is a grouping of statements. This is done by enclosing the statements between opening and closing curly braces. Once a block of code has been created, it becomes a logical unit that can be used any place a single statement can. For example, a block can be a target for **if** and **for** statements. Consider this **if** statement:

```
if(w < h) {
  v = w * h;
```

```
    w = 0;
  }
```

Here, if **w** is less than **h**, then both statements inside the block will be executed. Thus, the two statements inside the block form a logical unit, and one statement cannot execute without the other also executing. The key point here is that whenever you need to logically link two or more statements, you do so by creating a block. Code blocks allow many algorithms to be implemented with greater clarity and efficiency.

Here is a program that uses a code block to prevent a division by zero:

```
// Demonstrate a block of code.

using System;

class BlockDemo {
  static void Main() {
    int i, j, d;

    i = 5;
    j = 10;

    // The target of this if is a block.
    if(i != 0) {
      Console.WriteLine("i does not equal zero");
      d = j / i;
      Console.WriteLine("j / i is " + d);
    }
  }
}
```

The output generated by this program is shown here:

```
i does not equal zero
j / i is 2
```

In this case, the target of the **if** statement is a block of code and not just a single statement. If the condition controlling the **if** is true (as it is in this case), the three statements inside the block will be executed. Try setting **i** to zero and observe the result.

Here is another example. It uses a code block to compute the sum and the product of the numbers from 1 to 10.

```
// Compute the sum and product of the numbers from 1 to 10.

using System;

class ProdSum {
  static void Main() {
    int prod;
    int sum;
    int i;

    sum = 0;
    prod = 1;
```

```
   for(i=1; i <= 10; i++) {
     sum = sum + i;
     prod = prod * i;
   }
   Console.WriteLine("Sum is " + sum);
   Console.WriteLine("Product is " + prod);

  }
}
```

The output is shown here:

```
Sum is 55
Product is 3628800
```

Here, the block enables one loop to compute both the sum and the product. Without the use of the block, two separate **for** loops would have been required.

One last point: Code blocks do not introduce any runtime inefficiencies. In other words, the { and } do not consume any extra time during the execution of a program. In fact, because of their ability to simplify (and clarify) the coding of certain algorithms, the use of code blocks generally results in increased speed and efficiency.

Semicolons, Positioning, and Indentation

In C#, the semicolon signals the end of a statement. That is, each individual statement must end with a semicolon.

As you know, a block is a set of logically connected statements that are surrounded by opening and closing braces. A block is *not* terminated with a semicolon. Since a block is a group of statements, it makes sense that a block is not terminated by a semicolon; instead, the end of the block is indicated by the closing brace.

C# does not recognize the end of the line as the end of a statement—only a semicolon terminates a statement. For this reason, it does not matter where on a line you put a statement. For example, to C#,

```
x = y;
y = y + 1;
Console.WriteLine(x + " " + y);
```

is the same as

```
x = y;   y = y + 1;   Console.WriteLine(x + " " + y);
```

Furthermore, the individual elements of a statement can also be put on separate lines. For example, the following is perfectly acceptable:

```
Console.WriteLine("This is a long line of output" +
                  x + y + z +
                  "more output");
```

Breaking long lines in this fashion is often used to make programs more readable. It can also help prevent excessively long lines from wrapping.

You may have noticed in the previous examples that certain statements were indented. C# is a free-form language, meaning that it does not matter where you place statements relative to each other on a line. However, over the years, a common and accepted indentation style has developed that allows for very readable programs. This book follows that style, and it is recommended that you do so as well. Using this style, you indent one level after each opening brace and move back out one level after each closing brace. There are certain statements that encourage some additional indenting; these will be covered later.

The C# Keywords

At its foundation, a computer language is defined by its keywords because they determine the features built into the language. C# defines two general types of keywords: *reserved* and *contextual*. The reserved keywords cannot be used as names for variables, classes, or methods. They can be used only as keywords. This is why they are called *reserved*. The terms *reserved words* or *reserved identifiers* are also sometimes used. There are currently 77 reserved keywords defined by version 3.0 of the C# language. They are shown in Table 2-1.

C# 3.0 defines 13 contextual keywords that have a special meaning in certain contexts. In those contexts, they act as keywords. Outside those contexts, they can be used as names for other program elements, such as variable names. Thus, they are not technically reserved. As a general rule, however, you should consider the contextual keywords reserved and avoid using them for any other purpose. Using a contextual keyword as a name for some other program element can be confusing and is considered bad practice by many programmers. The contextual keywords are shown in Table 2-2.

abstract	as	base	bool	break
byte	case	catch	char	checked
class	const	continue	decimal	default
delegate	do	double	else	enum
event	explicit	extern	false	finally
fixed	float	for	foreach	goto
if	implicit	in	int	interface
internal	is	lock	long	namespace
new	null	object	operator	out
override	params	private	protected	public
readonly	ref	return	sbyte	sealed
short	sizeof	stackalloc	static	string
struct	switch	this	throw	true
try	typeof	uint	ulong	unchecked
unsafe	ushort	using	virtual	volatile
void	while			

TABLE 2-1 The C# Reserved Keywords

from	get	group	into	join
let	orderby	partial	select	set
value	where	yield		

TABLE 2-2   The C# Contextual Keywords

Identifiers

In C#, an identifier is a name assigned to a method, a variable, or any other user-defined item. Identifiers can be one or more characters long. Variable names may start with any letter of the alphabet or an underscore. Next may be a letter, a digit, or an underscore. The underscore can be used to enhance the readability of a variable name, as in **line_count**. However, identifers containing two consecutive underscores, such as **max_ _value**, are reserved for use by the compiler. Uppercase and lowercase are different; that is, to C#, **myvar** and **MyVar** are separate names. Here are some examples of acceptable identifiers:

Test	x	y2	MaxLoad
up	_top	my_var	sample23

Remember, you can't start an identifier with a digit. Thus, **12x** is invalid, for example. Good programming practice dictates that you choose identifiers that reflect the meaning or usage of the items being named.

Although you cannot use any of the reserved C# keywords as identifiers, C# does allow you to precede a keyword with an @, allowing it to be a legal identifier. For example, **@for** is a valid identifier. In this case, the identifier is actually **for** and the @ is ignored. Here is a program that illustrates the use of an @ identifier:

```
// Demonstrate an @ identifier.

using System;

class IdTest {
  static void Main() {
    int @if; // use if as an identifier

    for(@if = 0; @if < 10; @if++)
      Console.WriteLine("@if is " + @if);
  }
}
```

The output shown here proves the **@if** is properly interpreted as an identifier:

```
@if is 0
@if is 1
@if is 2
@if is 3
@if is 4
```

```
@if is 5
@if is 6
@if is 7
@if is 8
@if is 9
```

Frankly, using @-qualified keywords for identifiers is not recommended, except for special purposes. Also, the @ can precede any identifier, but this is considered bad practice.

The .NET Framework Class Library

The sample programs shown in this chapter make use of two built-in methods: **WriteLine()** and **Write()**. As mentioned, these methods are members of the **Console** class, which is part of the **System** namespace, which is defined by the .NET Framework's class library. As explained earlier in this chapter, the C# environment relies on the .NET Framework class library to provide support for such things as I/O, string handling, networking, and GUIs. Thus, C# as a totality is a combination of the C# language itself, plus the .NET standard classes. As you will see, the class library provides much of the functionality that is part of any C# program. Indeed, part of becoming a C# programmer is learning to use these standard classes. Throughout Part I, various elements of the .NET library classes and methods are described. Part II examines portions of the .NET library in detail.

Data Types, Literals, and Variables

This chapter examines three fundamental elements of C#: data types, literals, and variables. In general, the types of data that a language provides define the kinds of problems to which the language can be applied. As you might expect, C# offers a rich set of built-in data types, which makes C# suitable for a wide range of applications. You can create variables of any of these types, and you can specify constants of each type, which in the language of C# are called *literals*.

Why Data Types Are Important

Data types are especially important in C# because it is a strongly typed language. This means that all operations are type-checked by the compiler for type compatibility. Illegal operations will not be compiled. Thus, strong type-checking helps prevent errors and enhances reliability. To enable strong type-checking, all variables, expressions, and values have a type. There is no concept of a "typeless" variable, for example. Furthermore, a value's type determines what operations are allowed on it. An operation allowed on one type might not be allowed on another.

C#'s Value Types

C# contains two general categories of built-in data types: *value types* and *reference types*. The difference between the two types is what a variable contains. For a value type, a variable holds an actual value, such 3.1416 or 212. For a reference type, a variable holds a reference to the value. The most commonly used reference type is the class, and a discussion of classes and reference types is deferred until later in this book. The value types are described here.

At the core of C# are the 13 value types shown in Table 3-1. Collectively, these are referred to as the *simple types*. They are called simple types because they consist of a single value. (In other words, they are not a composite of two or more values.) They form the foundation of C#'s type system, providing the basic, low-level data elements upon which a program operates. The simple types are also sometimes referred to as *primitive types*.

Type	Meaning
bool	Represents true/false values
byte	8-bit unsigned integer
char	Character
decimal	Numeric type for financial calculations
double	Double-precision floating point
float	Single-precision floating point
int	Integer
long	Long integer
sbyte	8-bit signed integer
short	Short integer
uint	An unsigned integer
ulong	An unsigned long integer
ushort	An unsigned short integer

TABLE 3-1   The C# Value Types

C# strictly specifies a range and behavior for each value type. Because of portability requirements, C# is uncompromising on this account. For example, an **int** is the same in all execution environments. There is no need to rewrite code to fit a specific platform. Although strictly specifying the size of the value types may cause a small loss of performance in some environments, it is necessary in order to achieve portability.

NOTE *In addition to the simple types, C# defines three other categories of value types. These are enumerations, structures, and nullable types, all of which are described later in this book.*

Integers

C# defines nine integer types: **char**, **byte**, **sbyte**, **short**, **ushort**, **int**, **uint**, **long**, and **ulong**. However, the **char** type is primarily used for representing characters, and it is discussed later in this chapter. The remaining eight integer types are used for numeric calculations. Their bit-width and ranges are shown here:

Type	Width in Bits	Range
byte	8	0 to 255
sbyte	8	–128 to 127
short	16	–32,768 to 32,767
ushort	16	0 to 65,535
int	32	–2,147,483,648 to 2,147,483,647
uint	32	0 to 4,294,967,295
long	64	–9,223,372,036,854,775,808 to 9,223,372,036,854,775,807
ulong	64	0 to 18,446,744,073,709,551,615

As the table shows, C# defines both signed and unsigned versions of the various integer types. The difference between signed and unsigned integers is in the way the high-order bit of the integer is interpreted. If a signed integer is specified, then the C# compiler will generate code that assumes the high-order bit of an integer is to be used as a *sign flag*. If the sign flag is 0, then the number is positive; if it is 1, then the number is negative. Negative numbers are almost always represented using the *two's complement* approach. In this method, all bits in the negative number are reversed, and then 1 is added to this number.

Signed integers are important for a great many algorithms, but they have only half the absolute magnitude of their unsigned relatives. For example, as a **short**, here is 32,767:

    0 1 1 1 1 1 1 1 1 1 1 1 1 1 1 1

For a signed value, if the high-order bit were set to 1, the number would then be interpreted as –1 (assuming the two's complement format). However, if you declared this to be a **ushort**, then when the high-order bit was set to 1, the number would become 65,535.

Probably the most commonly used integer type is **int**. Variables of type **int** are often employed to control loops, to index arrays, and for general-purpose integer math. When you need an integer that has a range greater than **int**, you have many options. If the value you want to store is unsigned, you can use **uint**. For large signed values, use **long**. For large unsigned values, use **ulong**. For example, here is a program that computes the distance from the Earth to the sun, in inches. Because this value is so large, the program uses a **long** variable to hold it.

```
// Compute the distance from the Earth to the sun, in inches.

using System;

class Inches {
  static void Main() {
    long inches;
    long miles;

    miles = 93000000; // 93,000,000 miles to the sun

    // 5,280 feet in a mile, 12 inches in a foot.
    inches = miles * 5280 * 12;

    Console.WriteLine("Distance to the sun: " +
                      inches + " inches.");

  }
}
```

Here is the output from the program:

```
Distance to the sun: 5892480000000 inches.
```

Clearly, the result could not have been held in an **int** or **uint** variable.

The smallest integer types are **byte** and **sbyte**. The **byte** type is an unsigned value between 0 and 255. Variables of type **byte** are especially useful when working with raw binary data, such as a byte stream produced by some device. For small signed integers, use **sbyte**. Here is an example that uses a variable of type **byte** to control a **for** loop that produces the summation of the number 100:

```
// Use byte.
```

```
using System;

class Use_byte {
  static void Main() {
    byte x;
    int sum;

    sum = 0;
    for(x = 1; x <= 100; x++)
      sum = sum + x;

    Console.WriteLine("Summation of 100 is " + sum);
  }
}
```

The output from the program is shown here:

```
Summation of 100 is 5050
```

Since the **for** loop runs only from 0 to 100, which is well within the range of a **byte**, there is no need to use a larger type variable to control it.

When you need an integer that is larger than a **byte** or **sbyte**, but smaller than an **int** or **uint**, use **short** or **ushort**.

Floating-Point Types

The floating-point types can represent numbers that have fractional components. There are two kinds of floating-point types, **float** and **double**, which represent single- and double-precision numbers, respectively. The type **float** is 32 bits wide and has an approximate range of 1.5E–45 to 3.4E+38. The **double** type is 64 bits wide and has an approximate range of 5E–324 to 1.7E+308.

Of the two, **double** is the most commonly used. One reason for this is that many of the math functions in C#'s class library (which is the .NET Framework library) use **double** values. For example, the **Sqrt( )** method (which is defined by the library class **System.Math**) returns a **double** value that is the square root of its **double** argument. Here, **Sqrt( )** is used to compute the radius of a circle given the circle's area:

```
// Find the radius of a circle given its area.

using System;

class FindRadius {
  static void Main() {
    Double r;
    Double area;

    area = 10.0;

    r = Math.Sqrt(area / 3.1416);
```

```
    Console.WriteLine("Radius is " + r);
  }
}
```

The output from the program is shown here:

```
Radius is 1.78412203012729
```

One other point about the preceding example. As mentioned, **Sqrt( )** is a member of the **Math** class. Notice how **Sqrt( )** is called; it is preceded by the name **Math**. This is similar to the way **Console** precedes **WriteLine( )**. Although not all standard methods are called by specifying their class name first, several are, as the next example shows.

The following program demonstrates several of C#'s trigonometric functions, which are also part of C#'s math library. They also operate on **double** data. The program displays the sine, cosine, and tangent for the angles (measured in radians) from 0.1 to 1.0.

```
//  Demonstrate Math.Sin(), Math.Cos(), and Math.Tan().

using System;

class Trigonometry {
  static void Main() {
    Double theta; // angle in radians

    for(theta = 0.1; theta <= 1.0; theta = theta + 0.1) {
      Console.WriteLine("Sine of " + theta + "  is " +
                    Math.Sin(theta));
      Console.WriteLine("Cosine of " + theta + "  is " +
                    Math.Cos(theta));
      Console.WriteLine("Tangent of " + theta + "  is " +
                    Math.Tan(theta));
      Console.WriteLine();
    }
  }
}
```

Here is a portion of the program's output:

```
Sine of 0.1  is 0.0998334166468282
Cosine of 0.1  is 0.995004165278026
Tangent of 0.1  is 0.100334672085451

Sine of 0.2  is 0.198669330795061
Cosine of 0.2  is 0.980066577841242
Tangent of 0.2  is 0.202710035508673

Sine of 0.3  is 0.29552020666134
Cosine of 0.3  is 0.955336489125606
Tangent of 0.3  is 0.309336249609623
```

To compute the sine, cosine, and tangent, the standard library methods **Math.Sin( )**, **Math.Cos( )**, and **Math.Tan( )** are used. Like **Math.Sqrt( )**, the trigonometric methods are called with a **double** argument, and they return a **double** result. The angles must be specified in radians.

The decimal Type

Perhaps the most interesting C# numeric type is **decimal**, which is intended for use in monetary calculations. The **decimal** type utilizes 128 bits to represent values within the range 1E–28 to 7.9E+28. As you may know, normal floating-point arithmetic is subject to a variety of rounding errors when it is applied to decimal values. The **decimal** type eliminates these errors and can accurately represent up to 28 decimal places (or 29 places in some cases). This ability to represent decimal values without rounding errors makes it especially useful for computations that involve money.

Here is a program that uses a **decimal** type in a financial calculation. The program computes the discounted price given the original price and a discount percentage.

```
// Use the decimal type to compute a discount.

using System;

class UseDecimal {
  static void Main() {
    decimal price;
    decimal discount;
    decimal discounted_price;

    // Compute discounted price.
    price = 19.95m;
    discount = 0.15m; // discount rate is 15%

    discounted_price = price - ( price * discount);

    Console.WriteLine("Discounted price: $" + discounted_price);
  }
}
```

The output from this program is shown here:

```
Discounted price: $16.9575
```

In the program, notice that the decimal constants are followed by the *m* suffix. This is necessary because without the suffix, these values would be interpreted as standard floating-point constants, which are not compatible with the **decimal** data type. You can assign an integer value, such as 10, to a **decimal** variable without the use of the *m* suffix, though. (A detailed discussion of numeric constants is found later in this chapter.)

Here is another example that uses the **decimal** type. It computes the future value of an investment that has a fixed rate of return over a period of years.

```
/*
   Use the decimal type to compute the future value
   of an investment.
*/

using System;

class FutVal {
```

```
static void Main() {
  decimal amount;
  decimal rate_of_return;
  int years, i;

  amount = 1000.0M;
  rate_of_return = 0.07M;
  years = 10;

  Console.WriteLine("Original investment: $" + amount);
  Console.WriteLine("Rate of return: " + rate_of_return);
  Console.WriteLine("Over " + years + " years");

  for(i = 0; i < years; i++)
    amount = amount + (amount * rate_of_return);

  Console.WriteLine("Future value is $" + amount);
  }
}
```

Here is the output:

```
Original investment: $1000
Rate of return: 0.07
Over 10 years
Future value is $1967.15135728956532249000
```

Notice that the result is accurate to several decimal places—more than you would probably want! Later in this chapter you will see how to format such output in a more appealing fashion.

Characters

In C#, characters are not 8-bit quantities like they are in many other computer languages, such as C++. Instead, C# uses a 16-bit character type called *Unicode*. Unicode defines a character set that is large enough to represent all of the characters found in all human languages. Although many languages, such as English, French, or German, use relatively small alphabets, some languages, such as Chinese, use very large character sets that cannot be represented using just 8 bits. To address this situation, in C#, **char** is an unsigned 16-bit type having a range of 0 to 65,535. The standard 8-bit ASCII character set is a subset of Unicode and ranges from 0 to 127. Thus, the ASCII characters are still valid C# characters.

A character variable can be assigned a value by enclosing the character inside single quotes. For example, this assigns X to the variable **ch**:

```
char ch;
ch = 'X';
```

You can output a **char** value using a **WriteLine( )** statement. For example, this line outputs the value in **ch**:

```
Console.WriteLine("This is ch: " + ch);
```

Although **char** is defined by C# as an integer type, it cannot be freely mixed with integers in all cases. This is because there are no automatic type conversions from integer to **char**. For example, the following fragment is invalid:

```
char ch;

ch = 88; // error, won't work
```

The reason the preceding code will not work is that 10 is an integer value, and it won't automatically convert to a **char**. If you attempt to compile this code, you will see an error message. To make the assignment legal, you would need to employ a cast, which is described later in this chapter.

The bool Type

The **bool** type represents true/false values. C# defines the values true and false using the reserved words **true** and **false**. Thus, a variable or expression of type **bool** will be one of these two values. Furthermore, there is no conversion defined between **bool** and integer values. For example, 1 does not convert to true, and 0 does not convert to false.

Here is a program that demonstrates the **bool** type:

```
// Demonstrate bool values.

using System;

class BoolDemo {
  static void Main() {
    bool b;

    b = false;
    Console.WriteLine("b is " + b);
    b = true;
    Console.WriteLine("b is " + b);

    // A bool value can control the if statement.
    if(b) Console.WriteLine("This is executed.");

    b = false;
    if(b) Console.WriteLine("This is not executed.");

    // Outcome of a relational operator is a bool value.
    Console.WriteLine("10 > 9 is " + (10 > 9));
  }
}
```

The output generated by this program is shown here:

```
b is False
b is True
This is executed.
10 > 9 is True
```

There are three interesting things to notice about this program. First, as you can see, when a **bool** value is output by **WriteLine( )**, "True" or "False" is displayed. Second, the value of a **bool** variable is sufficient, by itself, to control the **if** statement. There is no need to write an **if** statement like this:

```
if(b == true) ...
```

Third, the outcome of a relational operator, such as **<**, is a **bool** value. This is why the expression **10 > 9** displays the value "True." Further, the extra set of parentheses around **10 > 9** is necessary because the **+** operator has a higher precedence than the **>**.

Some Output Options

Up to this point, when data has been output using a **WriteLine( )** statement, it has been displayed using the default format. However, the .NET Framework defines a sophisticated formatting mechanism that gives you detailed control over how data is displayed. Although formatted I/O is covered in detail later in this book, it is useful to introduce some formatting options at this time. Using these options, you will be able to specify the way values look when output via a **WriteLine( )** statement. Doing so enables you to produce more appealing output. Keep in mind that the formatting mechanism supports many more features than described here.

When outputting lists of data, you have been separating each part of the list with a plus sign, as shown here:

```
Console.WriteLine("You ordered " + 2 + " items at $" + 3 + " each.");
```

While very convenient, outputting numeric information in this way does not give you any control over how that information appears. For example, for a floating-point value, you can't control the number of decimal places displayed. Consider the following statement:

```
Console.WriteLine("Here is 10/3: " + 10.0/3.0);
```

It generates this output:

```
Here is 10/3: 3.33333333333333
```

Although this might be fine for some purposes, displaying so many decimal places could be inappropriate for others. For example, in financial calculations, you will usually want to display two decimal places.

To control how numeric data is formatted, you will need to use a second form of **WriteLine( )**, shown here, which allows you to embed formatting information:

WriteLine(*"format string"*, *arg0*, *arg1*, ... , *argN*);

In this version, the arguments to **WriteLine( )** are separated by commas and not **+** signs. The *format string* contains two items: regular, printing characters that are displayed as-is, and format specifiers. Format specifiers take this general form:

{*argnum*, *width*: *fmt*}

Here, *argnum* specifies the number of the argument (starting from zero) to display. The minimum width of the field is specified by *width*, and the format is specified by *fmt*. The *width* and *fmt* are optional.

During execution, when a format specifier is encountered in the format string, the corresponding argument, as specified by *argnum*, is substituted and displayed. Thus, the position of a format specification within the format string determines where its matching data will be displayed. Both *width* and *fmt* are optional. Therefore, in its simplest form, a format specifier simply indicates which argument to display. For example, {0} indicates *arg0*, {1} specifies *arg1*, and so on.

Let's begin with a simple example. The statement

```
Console.WriteLine("February has {0} or {1} days.", 28, 29);
```

produces the following output:

```
February has 28 or 29 days.
```

As you can see, the value 28 is substituted for {0}, and 29 is substituted for {1}. Thus, the format specifiers identify the location at which the subsequent arguments, in this case 28 and 29, are displayed within the string. Furthermore, notice that the additional values are separated by commas, not + signs.

Here is a variation of the preceding statement that specifies minimum field widths:

```
Console.WriteLine("February has {0,10} or {1,5} days.", 28, 29);
```

It produces the following output:

```
February has         28 or    29 days.
```

As you can see, spaces have been added to fill out the unused portions of the fields. Remember, a minimum field width is just that: the *minimum* width. Output can exceed that width if needed.

Of course, the arguments associated with a format command need not be constants. For example, this program displays a table of squares and cubes. It uses format commands to output the values.

```
// Use format commands.

using System;

class DisplayOptions {
  static void Main() {
    int i;

    Console.WriteLine("Value\tSquared\tCubed");

    for(i = 1; i < 10; i++)
      Console.WriteLine("{0}\t{1}\t{2}", i, i*i, i*i*i);
  }
}
```

The output is shown here:

```
Value    Squared Cubed
1        1       1
2        4       8
3        9       27
4        16      64
5        25      125
6        36      216
7        49      343
8        64      512
9        81      729
```

In the preceding examples, no formatting was applied to the values themselves. Of course, the purpose of using format specifiers is to control the way the data looks. The types of data most commonly formatted are floating-point and decimal values. One of the easiest ways to specify a format is to describe a template that **WriteLine( )** will use. To do this, show an example of the format that you want, using **#**s to mark the digit positions. You can also specify the decimal point and commas. For example, here is a better way to display 10 divided by 3:

```
Console.WriteLine("Here is 10/3: {0:#.##}", 10.0/3.0);
```

The output from this statement is shown here:

```
Here is 10/3: 3.33
```

In this example, the template is **#.##**, which tells **WriteLine( )** to display two decimal places. It is important to understand, however, that **WriteLine( )** will display more than one digit to the left of the decimal point, if necessary, so as not to misrepresent the value.

Here is another example. This statement

```
Console.WriteLine("{0:###,###.##}", 123456.56);
```

generates this output:

```
123,456.56
```

If you want to display monetary values, use the **C** format specifier. For example:

```
decimal balance;

balance = 12323.09m;
Console.WriteLine("Current balance is {0:C}", balance);
```

The output from this sequence is shown here (in U.S. dollar format):

```
Current balance is $12,323.09
```

The **C** format can be used to improve the output from the price discount program shown earlier:

```
// Use the C format specifier to output dollars and cents.

using System;
```

```
class UseDecimal {
  static void Main() {
    decimal price;
    decimal discount;
    decimal discounted_price;

    // Compute discounted price.
    price = 19.95m;
    discount = 0.15m; // discount rate is 15%

    discounted_price = price - ( price * discount);

    Console.WriteLine("Discounted price: {0:C}", discounted_price);
  }
}
```

Here is the way the output now looks:

```
Discounted price: $16.96
```

Literals

In C#, *literals* refer to fixed values that are represented in their human-readable form. For example, the number 100 is a literal. For the most part, literals and their usage are so intuitive that they have been used in one form or another by all the preceding sample programs. Now the time has come to explain them formally.

C# literals can be of any simple type. The way each literal is represented depends upon its type. As explained earlier, character literals are enclosed between single quotes. For example, 'a' and '%' are both character literals.

Integer literals are specified as numbers without fractional components. For example, 10 and −100 are integer literals. Floating-point literals require the use of the decimal point followed by the number's fractional component. For example, 11.123 is a floating-point literal. C# also allows you to use scientific notation for floating-point numbers.

Since C# is a strongly typed language, literals, too, have a type. Naturally, this raises the following question: What is the type of a numeric literal? For example, what is the type of 12, 123987, or 0.23? Fortunately, C# specifies some easy-to-follow rules that answer these questions.

First, for integer literals, the type of the literal is the smallest integer type that will hold it, beginning with **int**. Thus, an integer literal is either of type **int**, **uint**, **long**, or **ulong**, depending upon its value. Second, floating-point literals are of type **double**.

If C#'s default type is not what you want for a literal, you can explicitly specify its type by including a suffix. To specify a **long** literal, append an *l* or an *L*. For example, 12 is an **int**, but 12L is a **long**. To specify an unsigned integer value, append a *u* or *U*. Thus, 100 is an **int**, but 100U is a **uint**. To specify an unsigned, long integer, use *ul* or *UL*. For example, 984375UL is of type **ulong**.

To specify a **float** literal, append an *F* or *f* to the constant. For example, 10.19F is of type **float**. Although redundant, you can specify a **double** literal by appending a *D* or *d*. (As just mentioned, floating-point literals are **double** by default.)

To specify a **decimal** literal, follow its value with an *m* or *M*. For example, 9.95M is a **decimal** literal.

Although integer literals create an **int**, **uint**, **long**, or **ulong** value by default, they can still be assigned to variables of type **byte**, **sbyte**, **short**, or **ushort** as long as the value being assigned can be represented by the target type.

Hexadecimal Literals

As you probably know, in programming it is sometimes easier to use a number system based on 16 instead of 10. The base 16 number system is called *hexadecimal* and uses the digits 0 through 9 plus the letters A through F, which stand for 10, 11, 12, 13, 14, and 15. For example, the hexadecimal number 10 is 16 in decimal. Because of the frequency with which hexadecimal numbers are used, C# allows you to specify integer literals in hexadecimal format. A hexadecimal literal must begin with **0x** (a 0 followed by an *x*). Here are some examples:

```
count = 0xFF; // 255 in decimal
incr = 0x1a;  // 26 in decimal
```

Character Escape Sequences

Enclosing character literals in single quotes works for most printing characters, but a few characters, such as the carriage return, pose a special problem when a text editor is used. In addition, certain other characters, such as the single and double quotes, have special meaning in C#, so you cannot use them directly. For these reasons, C# provides special *escape sequences*, sometimes referred to as *backslash character constants*, shown in Table 3-2. These sequences are used in place of the characters they represent.

For example, this assigns **ch** the tab character:

```
ch = '\t';
```

The next example assigns a single quote to **ch**:

```
ch = '\'';
```

Escape Sequence	Description
\a	Alert (bell)
\b	Backspace
\f	Form feed
\n	New line (linefeed)
\r	Carriage return
\t	Horizontal tab
\v	Vertical tab
\0	Null
\'	Single quote
\"	Double quote
\\	Backslash

TABLE 3-2   Character Escape Sequences

String Literals

C# supports one other type of literal: the *string*. A string literal is a set of characters enclosed by double quotes. For example,

```
"this is a test"
```

is a string. You have seen examples of strings in many of the **WriteLine( )** statements in the preceding sample programs.

In addition to normal characters, a string literal can also contain one or more of the escape sequences just described. For example, consider the following program. It uses the **\n** and **\t** escape sequences.

```
// Demonstrate escape sequences in strings.

using System;

class StrDemo {
  static void Main() {
    Console.WriteLine("Line One\nLine Two\nLine Three");
    Console.WriteLine("One\tTwo\tThree");
    Console.WriteLine("Four\tFive\tSix");

    // Embed quotes.
    Console.WriteLine("\"Why?\", he asked.");
  }
}
```

The output is shown here:

```
Line One
Line Two
Line Three
One      Two      Three
Four     Five     Six
"Why?", he asked.
```

Notice how the **\n** escape sequence is used to generate a new line. You don't need to use multiple **WriteLine( )** statements to get multiline output. Just embed **\n** within a longer string at the points where you want the new lines to occur. Also note how a quotation mark is generated inside a string.

In addition to the form of string literal just described, you can also specify a *verbatim string literal*. A verbatim string literal begins with an @, which is followed by a quoted string. The contents of the quoted string are accepted without modification and can span two or more lines. Thus, you can include newlines, tabs, and so on, but you don't need to use the escape sequences. The only exception is that to obtain a double quote ("), you must use two double quotes in a row (""). Here is a program that demonstrates verbatim string literals:

```
// Demonstrate verbatim literal strings.

using System;

class Verbatim {
```

```
    static void Main() {
      Console.WriteLine(@"This is a verbatim
string literal
that spans several lines.
");
      Console.WriteLine(@"Here is some tabbed output:
1      2      3      4
5      6      7      8
");
      Console.WriteLine(@"Programmers say, ""I like C#.""");
    }
}
```

The output from this program is shown here:

```
This is a verbatim
string literal
that spans several lines.

Here is some tabbed output:
1      2      3      4
5      6      7      8

Programmers say, "I like C#."
```

The important point to notice about the preceding program is that the verbatim string literals are displayed precisely as they are entered into the program.

The advantage of verbatim string literals is that you can specify output in your program exactly as it will appear on the screen. However, in the case of multiline strings, the wrapping will obscure the indentation of your program. For this reason, the programs in this book will make only limited use of verbatim string literals. That said, they are still a wonderful benefit for many formatting situations.

One last point: Don't confuse strings with characters. A character literal, such as 'X', represents a single letter of type **char**. A string containing only one letter, such as "X", is still a string.

A Closer Look at Variables

Variables are declared using this form of statement:

   type var-name;

where *type* is the data type of the variable and *var-name* is its name. You can declare a variable of any valid type, including the value types just described. It is important to understand that a variable's capabilities are determined by its type. For example, a variable of type **bool** cannot be used to store floating-point values. Furthermore, the type of a variable cannot change during its lifetime. An **int** variable cannot turn into a **char** variable, for example.

All variables in C# must be declared prior to their use. This is necessary because the compiler must know what type of data a variable contains before it can properly compile any statement that uses the variable. It also enables C# to perform strict type-checking.

C# defines several different kinds of variables. The kind that we have been using are called *local variables* because they are declared within a method.

Initializing a Variable

One way to give a variable a value is through an assignment statement, as you have already seen. Another way is by giving it an initial value when it is declared. To do this, follow the variable's name with an equal sign and the value being assigned. The general form of initialization is shown here:

type var-name = value;

Here, *value* is the value that is given to the variable when it is created. The value must be compatible with the specified type.

Here are some examples:

```
int count = 10; // give count an initial value of 10
char ch = 'X';  // initialize ch with the letter X
float f = 1.2F; // f is initialized with 1.2
```

When declaring two or more variables of the same type using a comma-separated list, you can give one or more of those variables an initial value. For example:

```
int a, b = 8, c = 19, d; // b and c have initializations
```

In this case, only **b** and **c** are initialized.

Dynamic Initialization

Although the preceding examples have used only constants as initializers, C# allows variables to be initialized dynamically, using any expression valid at the point at which the variable is declared. For example, here is a short program that computes the hypotenuse of a right triangle given the lengths of its two opposing sides.

```
// Demonstrate dynamic initialization.

using System;

class DynInit {
  static void Main() {
    // Length of sides.
    double s1 = 4.0;
    double s2 = 5.0;

    // Dynamically initialize hypot.
    double hypot = Math.Sqrt( (s1 * s1) + (s2 * s2) );

    Console.Write("Hypotenuse of triangle with sides " +
                  s1 + " by " + s2 + " is ");

    Console.WriteLine("{0:#.###}.", hypot);

  }
}
```

Here is the output:

```
Hypotenuse of triangle with sides 4 by 5 is 6.403.
```

Here, three local variables—**s1, s2,** and **hypot**—are declared. The first two, **s1** and **s2**, are initialized by constants. However, **hypot** is initialized dynamically to the length of the hypotenuse. Notice that the initialization involves calling **Math.Sqrt( )**. As explained, you can use any expression that is valid at the point of the initialization. Since a call to **Math.Sqrt( )** (or any other library method) is valid at this point, it can be used in the initialization of **hypot**. The key point here is that the initialization expression can use any element valid at the time of the initialization, including calls to methods, other variables, or literals.

Implicitly Typed Variables

As explained, in C# all variables must be declared. Normally, a declaration includes the type of the variable, such as **int** or **bool**, followed by the name of the variable. However, beginning with C# 3.0, it is possible to let the compiler determine the type of a local variable based on the value used to initialize it. This is called an *implicitly typed variable.*

An implicitly typed variable is declared using the keyword **var**, and it must be initialized. The compiler uses the type of the initializer to determine the type of the variable. Here is an example:

```
var e = 2.7183;
```

Because **e** is initialized with a floating-point literal (whose type is **double** by default), the type of **e** is **double**. Had **e** been declared like this:

```
var e = 2.7183F;
```

then **e** would have the type **float**, instead.

The following program demonstrates implicitly typed variables. It reworks the program shown in the preceding section so that all variables are implicitly typed.

```
//   Demonstrate implicitly typed variables.

using System;

class ImplicitlyTypedVar {
  static void Main() {

    // These are now implicitly typed variables. They
    // are of type double because their initializing
    // expressions are of type double.
    var s1 = 4.0;
    var s2 = 5.0;

    // Now, hypot is implicitly typed.  Its type is double
    // because the return type of Sqrt() is double.
    var hypot = Math.Sqrt( (s1 * s1) + (s2 * s2) );

    Console.Write("Hypotenuse of triangle with sides " +
                s1 + " by " + s2 + " is ");

    Console.WriteLine("{0:#.###}.", hypot);

    // The following statement will not compile because
    // s1 is a double and cannot be assigned a decimal value.
```

```
//     s1 = 12.2M;   // Error!
    }
}
```

The output is the same as before.

It is important to emphasize that an implicitly typed variable is still a strongly typed variable. Notice this commented-out line in the program:

```
//     s1 = 12.2M;   // Error!
```

This assignment is invalid because **s1** is of type **double**. Thus, it cannot be assigned a **decimal** value. The only difference between an implicitly typed variable and a "normal" explicitly typed variable is how the type is determined. Once that type has been determined, the variable has a type, and this type is fixed throughout the lifetime of the variable. Thus, the type of **s1** cannot be changed during execution of the program.

Implicitly typed variables were not added to C# to replace "normal" variable declarations. Instead, implicitly typed variables are designed to handle some special-case situations, the most important of which relate to Language-Integrated Query (LINQ), which is described in Chapter 19. Therefore, for most variable declarations, you should continue to use explicitly typed variables because they make your code easier to read and easier to understand.

One last point: Only one implicitly typed variable can be declared at any one time. Therefore, the following declaration,

```
var s1 = 4.0, s2 = 5.0; // Error!
```

is wrong and won't compile because it attempts to declare both **s1** and **s2** at the same time.

The Scope and Lifetime of Variables

So far, all of the variables that we have been using are declared at the start of the **Main()** method. However, C# allows a local variable to be declared within any block. As explained in Chapter 1, a block begins with an opening curly brace and ends with a closing curly brace. A block defines a *scope*. Thus, each time you start a new block, you are creating a new scope. A scope determines what names are visible to other parts of your program without qualification. It also determines the lifetime of local variables.

The most important scopes in C# are those defined by a class and those defined by a method. A discussion of class scope (and variables declared within it) is deferred until later in this book, when classes are described. For now, we will examine only the scopes defined by or within a method.

The scope defined by a method begins with its opening curly brace and ends with its closing curly brace. However, if that method has parameters, they too are included within the scope defined by the method.

As a general rule, local variables declared inside a scope are not visible to code that is defined outside that scope. Thus, when you declare a variable within a scope, you are protecting it from access or modification from outside the scope. Indeed, the scope rules provide the foundation for encapsulation.

Scopes can be nested. For example, each time you create a block of code, you are creating a new, nested scope. When this occurs, the outer scope encloses the inner scope. This means that local variables declared in the outer scope will be visible to code within the inner scope.

However, the reverse is not true. Local variables declared within the inner scope will not be visible outside it.

To understand the effect of nested scopes, consider the following program:

```
// Demonstrate block scope.

using System;

class ScopeDemo {
  static void Main() {
    int x; // known to all code within Main()

    x = 10;
    if(x == 10) { // start new scope
      int y = 20; // known only to this block

      // x and y both known here.
      Console.WriteLine("x and y: " + x + " " + y);
      x = y * 2;
    }
    // y = 100; // Error! y not known here.

    // x is still known here.
    Console.WriteLine("x is " + x);
  }
}
```

As the comments indicate, the variable **x** is declared at the start of **Main( )**'s scope and is accessible to all subsequent code within **Main( )**. Within the **if** block, **y** is declared. Since a block defines a scope, **y** is visible only to other code within its block. This is why outside of its block, the line **y = 100;** is commented out. If you remove the leading comment symbol, a compile-time error will occur because **y** is not visible outside of its block. Within the **if** block, **x** can be used because code within a block (that is, a nested scope) has access to variables declared by an enclosing scope.

Within a block, variables can be declared at any point, but are valid only after they are declared. Thus, if you define a variable at the start of a method, it is available to all of the code within that method. Conversely, if you declare a variable at the end of a block, it is effectively useless, because no code will have access to it.

If a variable declaration includes an initializer, then that variable will be reinitialized each time the block in which it is declared is entered. For example, consider this program:

```
// Demonstrate lifetime of a variable.

using System;

class VarInitDemo {
  static void Main() {
    int x;

    for(x = 0; x < 3; x++) {
      int y = -1; // y is initialized each time block is entered
      Console.WriteLine("y is: " + y); // this always prints -1
```

```
      y = 100;
      Console.WriteLine("y is now: " + y);
    }
  }
}
```

The output generated by this program is shown here:

```
y is: -1
y is now: 100
y is: -1
y is now: 100
y is: -1
y is now: 100
```

As you can see, **y** is always reinitialized to –1 each time the inner **for** loop is entered. Even though it is subsequently assigned the value 100, this value is lost.

There is one quirk to C#'s scope rules that may surprise you: Although blocks can be nested, no variable declared within an inner scope can have the same name as a variable declared by an enclosing scope. For example, the following program, which tries to declare two separate variables with the same name, will not compile.

```
/*
   This program attempts to declare a variable
   in an inner scope with the same name as one
   defined in an outer scope.

   *** This program will not compile. ***
*/

using System;

class NestVar {
  static void Main() {
    int count;

    for(count = 0; count < 10; count = count+1) {
      Console.WriteLine("This is count: " + count);

      int count; // illegal!!!
      for(count = 0; count < 2; count++)
        Console.WriteLine("This program is in error!");
    }
  }
}
```

If you come from a C/C++ background, then you know that there is no restriction on the names you give variables declared in an inner scope. Thus, in C/C++ the declaration of **count** within the block of the outer **for** loop is completely valid. However, in C/C++, such a declaration hides the outer variable. The designers of C# felt that this type of *name hiding* could easily lead to programming errors and disallowed it.

Type Conversion and Casting

In programming, it is common to assign one type of variable to another. For example, you might want to assign an **int** value to a **float** variable, as shown here:

```
int i;
float f;

i = 10;
f = i; // assign an int to a float
```

When compatible types are mixed in an assignment, the value of the right side is automatically converted to the type of the left side. Thus, in the preceding fragment, the value in **i** is converted into a **float** and then assigned to **f**. However, because of C#'s strict type-checking, not all types are compatible, and thus, not all type conversions are implicitly allowed. For example, **bool** and **int** are not compatible. Fortunately, it is still possible to obtain a conversion between incompatible types by using a *cast*. A cast performs an explicit type conversion. Both automatic type conversion and casting are examined here.

Automatic Conversions

When one type of data is assigned to another type of variable, an *implicit* type conversion will take place automatically if

- The two types are compatible.
- The destination type has a range that is greater than the source type.

When these two conditions are met, a *widening conversion* takes place. For example, the **int** type is always large enough to hold all valid **byte** values, and both **int** and **byte** are compatible integer types, so an implicit conversion can be applied.

For widening conversions, the numeric types, including integer and floating-point types, are compatible with each other. For example, the following program is perfectly valid since **long** to **double** is a widening conversion that is automatically performed.

```
// Demonstrate implicit conversion from long to double.

using System;

class LtoD {
  static void Main() {
    long L;
    double D;

    L = 100123285L;
    D = L;

    Console.WriteLine("L and D: " + L + " " + D);
  }
}
```

Although there is an implicit conversion from **long** to **double**, there is no implicit conversion from **double** to **long** since this is not a widening conversion. Thus, the following version of the preceding program is invalid:

```
// *** This program will not compile. ***

using System;

class LtoD {
  static void Main() {
    long L;
    double D;

    D = 100123285.0;
    L = D; // Illegal!!!

    Console.WriteLine("L and D: " + L + " " + D);

  }
}
```

In addition to the restrictions just described, there are no implicit conversions between **decimal** and **float** or **double**, or from the numeric types to **char** or **bool**. Also, **char** and **bool** are not compatible with each other.

Casting Incompatible Types

Although the implicit type conversions are helpful, they will not fulfill all programming needs because they apply only to widening conversions between compatible types. For all other cases you must employ a cast. A *cast* is an instruction to the compiler to convert the outcome of an expression into a specified type. Thus, it requests an explicit type conversion. A cast has this general form:

   (*target-type*) *expression*

Here, *target-type* specifies the desired type to convert the specified expression to. For example, given

```
double x, y;
```

if you want the type of the expression **x/y** to be **int**, you can write

```
(int) (x / y)
```

Here, even though **x** and **y** are of type **double**, the cast converts the outcome of the expression to **int**. The parentheses surrounding x / y are necessary. Otherwise, the cast to **int** would apply only to the **x** and not to the outcome of the division. The cast is necessary here because there is no implicit conversion from **double** to **int**.

When a cast involves a *narrowing conversion*, information might be lost. For example, when casting a **long** into an **int**, information will be lost if the **long**'s value is greater than the range of an **int** because its high-order bits are removed. When a floating-point value is cast to an integer type, the fractional component will also be lost due to truncation. For

example, if the value 1.23 is assigned to an integer, the resulting value will simply be 1. The 0.23 is lost.

The following program demonstrates some type conversions that require casts. It also shows some situations in which the casts cause data to be lost.

```
// Demonstrate casting.

using System;

class CastDemo {
  static void Main() {
    double x, y;
    byte b;
    int i;
    char ch;
    uint u;
    short s;
    long l;

    x = 10.0;
    y = 3.0;

    // Cast double to int, fractional component lost.
    i = (int) (x / y);
    Console.WriteLine("Integer outcome of x / y: " + i);
    Console.WriteLine();

    // Cast an int into a byte, no data lost.
    i = 255;
    b = (byte) i;
    Console.WriteLine("b after assigning 255: " + b +
                      " -- no data lost.");

    // Cast an int into a byte, data lost.
    i = 257;
    b = (byte) i;
    Console.WriteLine("b after assigning 257: " + b +
                      " -- data lost.");
    Console.WriteLine();

    // Cast a uint into a short, no data lost.
    u = 32000;
    s = (short) u;
    Console.WriteLine("s after assigning 32000: " + s +
                      " -- no data lost.");

    // Cast a uint into a short, data lost.
    u = 64000;
    s = (short) u;
    Console.WriteLine("s after assigning 64000: " + s +
                      " -- data lost.");
    Console.WriteLine();
```

```
    // Cast a long into a uint, no data lost.
    l = 64000;
    u = (uint) l;
    Console.WriteLine("u after assigning 64000: " + u +
                      " -- no data lost.");

    // Cast a long into a uint, data lost.
    l = -12;
    u = (uint) l;
    Console.WriteLine("u after assigning -12: " + u +
                      " -- data lost.");
    Console.WriteLine();

    // Cast an int into a char.
    b = 88; // ASCII code for X
    ch = (char) b;
    Console.WriteLine("ch after assigning 88: " + ch);
  }
}
```

The output from the program is shown here:

```
Integer outcome of x / y: 3

b after assigning 255: 255 -- no data lost.
b after assigning 257: 1 -- data lost.

s after assigning 32000: 32000 -- no data lost.
s after assigning 64000: -1536 -- data lost.

u after assigning 64000: 64000 -- no data lost.
u after assigning -12: 4294967284 -- data lost.

ch after assigning 88: X
```

Let's look at each assignment. The cast of (x / y) to int results in the truncation of the fractional component, and information is lost.

No loss of information occurs when b is assigned the value 255 because a byte can hold the value 255. However, when the attempt is made to assign b the value 257, information loss occurs because 257 exceeds a byte's range. In both cases the casts are needed because there is no implicit conversion from int to byte.

When the short variable s is assigned the value 32,000 through the uint variable u, no data is lost because a short can hold the value 32,000. However, in the next assignment, u has the value 64,000, which is outside the range of a short, and data is lost. In both cases the casts are needed because there is no implicit conversion from uint to short.

Next, u is assigned the value 64,000 through the long variable l. In this case, no data is lost because 64,000 is within the range of a uint. However, when the value –12 is assigned to u, data is lost because a uint cannot hold negative numbers. In both cases the casts are needed because there is no implicit conversion from long to uint.

Finally, no information is lost, but a cast is needed when assigning a byte value to a char.

Type Conversion in Expressions

In addition to occurring within an assignment, type conversions also take place within an expression. In an expression, you can freely mix two or more different types of data as long as they are compatible with each other. For example, you can mix **short** and **long** within an expression because they are both numeric types. When different types of data are mixed within an expression, they are converted to the same type, on an operation-by-operation basis.

The conversions are accomplished through the use of C#'s *type promotion rules*. Here is the algorithm that they define for binary operations:

IF one operand is a **decimal**, THEN the other operand is promoted to **decimal** (unless it is of type **float** or **double**, in which case an error results).

ELSE IF one operand is a **double**, the second is promoted to **double**.

ELSE IF one operand is a **float**, the second is promoted to **float**.

ELSE IF one operand is a **ulong**, the second is promoted to **ulong** (unless it is of type **sbyte**, **short**, **int**, or **long**, in which case an error results).

ELSE IF one operand is a **long**, the second is promoted to **long**.

ELSE IF one operand is a **uint** and the second is of type **sbyte**, **short**, or **int**, both are promoted to **long**.

ELSE IF one operand is a **uint**, the second is promoted to **uint**.

ELSE both operands are promoted to **int**.

There are a couple of important points to be made about the type promotion rules. First, not all types can be mixed in an expression. Specifically, there is no implicit conversion from **float** or **double** to **decimal**, and it is not possible to mix **ulong** with any signed integer type. To mix these types requires the use of an explicit cast.

Second, pay special attention to the last rule. It states that if none of the preceding rules applies, then all other operands are promoted to **int**. Therefore, in an expression, all **char**, **sbyte**, **byte**, **ushort**, and **short** values are promoted to **int** for the purposes of calculation. This is called *integer promotion*. It also means that the outcome of all arithmetic operations will be no smaller than **int**.

It is important to understand that type promotions only apply to the values operated upon when an expression is evaluated. For example, if the value of a **byte** variable is promoted to **int** inside an expression, outside the expression, the variable is still a **byte**. Type promotion only affects the evaluation of an expression.

Type promotion can, however, lead to somewhat unexpected results. For example, when an arithmetic operation involves two **byte** values, the following sequence occurs. First, the **byte** operands are promoted to **int**. Then the operation takes place, yielding an **int** result. Thus, the outcome of an operation involving two **byte** values will be an **int**. This is not what you might intuitively expect. Consider the following program.

```
// A promotion surprise!

using System;

class PromDemo {
  static void Main() {
    byte b;

    b = 10;
    b = (byte) (b * b); // cast needed!!

    Console.WriteLine("b: "+ b);
  }
}
```

Somewhat counterintuitively, a cast to **byte** is needed when assigning **b * b** back to **b**! The reason is because in **b * b**, the value of **b** is promoted to **int** when the expression is evaluated. Thus, **b * b** results in an **int** value, which cannot be assigned to a **byte** variable without a cast. Keep this in mind if you get unexpected type-incompatibility error messages on expressions that would otherwise seem perfectly correct.

This same sort of situation also occurs when performing operations on **char**s. For example, in the following fragment, the cast back to **char** is needed because of the promotion of **ch1** and **ch2** to **int** within the expression

```
char ch1 = 'a', ch2 = 'b';

ch1 = (char) (ch1 + ch2);
```

Without the cast, the result of adding **ch1** to **ch2** would be **int**, which can't be assigned to a **char**.

Type promotions also occur when a unary operation, such as the unary –, takes place. For the unary operations, operands smaller than **int** (**byte**, **sbyte**, **short**, and **ushort**) are promoted to **int**. Also, a **char** operand is converted to **int**. Furthermore, if a **uint** value is negated, it is promoted to **long**.

Using Casts in Expressions

A cast can be applied to a specific portion of a larger expression. This gives you fine-grained control over the way type conversions occur when an expression is evaluated. For example, consider the following program. It displays the square roots of the numbers from 1 to 10. It also displays the whole number portion and the fractional part of each result, separately. To do so, it uses a cast to convert the result of **Math.Sqrt( )** to **int**.

```
// Using casts in an expression.

using System;

class CastExpr {
  static void Main() {
    double n;

    for(n = 1.0; n <= 10; n++) {
```

```
      Console.WriteLine("The square root of {0} is {1}",
                        n, Math.Sqrt(n));

      Console.WriteLine("Whole number part: {0}" ,
                        (int) Math.Sqrt(n));

      Console.WriteLine("Fractional part: {0}",
                        Math.Sqrt(n) - (int) Math.Sqrt(n) );
      Console.WriteLine();
    }
  }
}
```

Here is the output from the program:

```
The square root of 1 is 1
Whole number part: 1
Fractional part: 0

The square root of 2 is 1.4142135623731
Whole number part: 1
Fractional part: 0.414213562373095

The square root of 3 is 1.73205080756888
Whole number part: 1
Fractional part: 0.732050807568877

The square root of 4 is 2
Whole number part: 2
Fractional part: 0

The square root of 5 is 2.23606797749979
Whole number part: 2
Fractional part: 0.23606797749979

The square root of 6 is 2.44948974278318
Whole number part: 2
Fractional part: 0.449489742783178

The square root of 7 is 2.64575131106459
Whole number part: 2
Fractional part: 0.645751311064591

The square root of 8 is 2.82842712474619
Whole number part: 2
Fractional part: 0.82842712474619

The square root of 9 is 3
Whole number part: 3
Fractional part: 0

The square root of 10 is 3.16227766016838
Whole number part: 3
Fractional part: 0.16227766016838
```

As the output shows, the cast of **Math.Sqrt( )** to **int** results in the whole number component of the value. In this expression

```
Math.Sqrt(n)  -  (int) Math.Sqrt(n)
```

the cast to **int** obtains the whole number component, which is then subtracted from the complete value, yielding the fractional component. Thus, the outcome of the expression is **double**. Only the value of the second call to **Math.Sqrt( )** is cast to **int**.

Operators

C# provides an extensive set of operators that give the programmer detailed control over the construction and evaluation of expressions. Most of C#'s operators fall into the following categories: *arithmetic, bitwise, relational,* and *logical.* These operators are examined in this chapter. Also discussed are the assignment operator and the **?** operator. C# also defines several other operators that handle specialized situations, such as array indexing, member access, and the lambda operator. These special operators are examined later in this book, when the features to which they apply are described.

Arithmetic Operators

C# defines the following arithmetic operators:

Operator	Meaning
+	Addition
–	Subtraction (also unary minus)
*	Multiplication
/	Division
%	Modulus
++	Increment
– –	Decrement

The operators **+**, **–**, *****, and **/** all work in the expected way. These can be applied to any built-in numeric data type.

Although the actions of arithmetic operators are well known to all readers, a few special situations warrant some explanation. First, remember that when **/** is applied to an integer, any remainder will be truncated; for example, 10/3 will equal 3 in integer division. You can obtain the remainder of this division by using the modulus operator, **%**. The **%** is also referred to as the *remainder operator.* It yields the remainder of an integer division. For example, 10 % 3 is 1. In C#, the **%** can be applied to both integer and floating-point types.

Thus, 10.0 % 3.0 is also 1. (This differs from C/C++, which allow modulus operations only on integer types.) The following program demonstrates the modulus operator:

```
// Demonstrate the % operator.

using System;

class ModDemo {
  static void Main() {
    int iresult, irem;
    double dresult, drem;

    iresult = 10 / 3;
    irem = 10 % 3;

    dresult = 10.0 / 3.0;
    drem = 10.0 % 3.0;

    Console.WriteLine("Result and remainder of 10 / 3: " +
                      iresult + " " + irem);
    Console.WriteLine("Result and remainder of 10.0 / 3.0: " +
                      dresult + " " + drem);
  }
}
```

The output from the program is shown here:

```
Result and remainder of 10 / 3: 3 1
Result and remainder of 10.0 / 3.0: 3.33333333333333 1
```

As you can see, the % yields a remainder of 1 for both integer and floating-point operations.

Increment and Decrement

Introduced in Chapter 2, the ++ and the − − are the increment and decrement operators. As you will see, they have some special properties that make them quite interesting. Let's begin by reviewing precisely what the increment and decrement operators do.

The increment operator adds 1 to its operand, and the decrement operator subtracts 1. Therefore,

```
x = x + 1;
```

is the same as

```
x++;
```

and

```
x = x - 1;
```

is the same as

```
x--;
```

Understand, however, that in the increment or decrement forms, **x** is evaluated only once, not twice. This can improve efficiency in some cases.

Both the increment and decrement operators can either precede (prefix) or follow (postfix) the operand. For example

```
x = x + 1;
```

can be written as

```
++x; // prefix form
```

or as

```
x++; // postfix form
```

In the foregoing example, there is no difference whether the increment is applied as a prefix or a postfix. However, when an increment or decrement is used as part of a larger expression, there is an important difference. When an increment or decrement operator *precedes* its operand, the result of the operation is the value of the operand *after* the increment. If the operator *follows* its operand, the result of the operation is the value of the operand *before* the increment. Consider the following:

```
x = 10;
y = ++x;
```

In this case, **y** will be set to 11. This is because **x** is first incremented and then its value is returned. However, if the code is written as

```
x = 10;
y = x++;
```

then **y** will be set to 10. In this case, the value of **x** is first obtained, **x** is incremented, and then the original value of **x** is returned. In both cases, **x** is still set to 11. The difference is what is returned by the operation.

There are significant advantages in being able to control when the increment or decrement operation takes place. Consider the following program, which generates a series of numbers:

```
// Demonstrate the difference between prefix and
// postfix forms of ++.

using System;

class PrePostDemo {
  static void Main() {
    int x, y;
    int i;

    x = 1;
    Console.WriteLine("Series generated using y = x + x++;");
    for(i = 0; i < 10; i++) {

      y = x + x++; // postfix ++
```

```
    Console.WriteLine(y + " ");
  }
  Console.WriteLine();

  x = 1;
  Console.WriteLine("Series generated using y = x + ++x;");
  for(i = 0; i < 10; i++) {

    y = x + ++x; // prefix ++

    Console.WriteLine(y + " ");
  }
  Console.WriteLine();

  }
}
```

The output is shown here:

```
Series generated using y = x + x++;
2
4
6
8
10
12
14
16
18
20

Series generated using y = x + ++x;
3
5
7
9
11
13
15
17
19
21
```

As the output confirms, the statement

```
y = x + x++;
```

adds the original value of **x** to **x** and assigns this result to **y**. The value of **x** is incremented after its value has been obtained. However, the statement

```
y = x + ++x;
```

obtains the value of **x**, increments **x**, and then adds that value to the original value of **x**. The result is assigned to **y**. As the output shows, simply changing **++x** to **x++** changes the number series from even to odd.

One other point about the preceding example: Don't let expressions like

```
x + ++x
```

intimidate you. Although having two operators back-to-back is a bit unsettling at first glance, the compiler keeps it all straight. Just remember, this expression simply adds the value of x to the value of x incremented.

Relational and Logical Operators

In the terms *relational operator* and *logical operator, relational* refers to the relationships that values can have with one another, and *logical* refers to the ways in which true and false values can be connected together. Since the relational operators produce true or false results, they often work with the logical operators. For this reason they will be discussed together here.

The relational operators are as follows:

Operator	Meaning
= =	Equal to
!=	Not equal to
>	Greater than
<	Less than
>=	Greater than or equal to
<=	Less than or equal to

The logical operators are shown next:

Operator	Meaning
&	AND
|	OR
^	XOR (exclusive OR)
||	Short-circuit OR
&&	Short-circuit AND
!	NOT

The outcome of the relational and logical operators is a **bool** value.

In general, objects can be compared for equality or inequality using == and !=. However, the comparison operators, <, >, <=, or >=, can be applied only to those types that support an ordering relationship. Therefore, all of the relational operators can be applied to all numeric types. However, values of type **bool** can only be compared for equality or inequality since the **true** and **false** values are not ordered. For example, **true > false** has no meaning in C#.

For the logical operators, the operands must be of type **bool**, and the result of a logical operation is of type **bool**. The logical operators, **&**, **|**, **^**, and **!**, support the basic logical operations AND, OR, XOR, and NOT, according to the following truth table:

p	q	p & q	p	q	p ^ q	!p
False	False	False	False	False	True
True	False	False	True	True	False
False	True	False	True	True	True
True	True	True	True	False	False

As the table shows, the outcome of an exclusive OR operation is true when one and only one operand is true.

Here is a program that demonstrates several of the relational and logical operators:

```
// Demonstrate the relational and logical operators.

using System;

class RelLogOps {
    static void Main() {
        int i, j;
        bool b1, b2;

        i = 10;
        j = 11;
        if(i < j) Console.WriteLine("i < j");
        if(i <= j) Console.WriteLine("i <= j");
        if(i != j) Console.WriteLine("i != j");
        if(i == j) Console.WriteLine("this won't execute");
        if(i >= j) Console.WriteLine("this won't execute");
        if(i > j) Console.WriteLine("this won't execute");

        b1 = true;
        b2 = false;
        if(b1 & b2) Console.WriteLine("this won't execute");
        if(!(b1 & b2)) Console.WriteLine("!(b1 & b2) is true");
        if(b1 | b2) Console.WriteLine("b1 | b2 is true");
        if(b1 ^ b2) Console.WriteLine("b1 ^ b2 is true");
    }
}
```

The output from the program is shown here:

```
i < j
i <= j
i != j
!(b1 & b2) is true
b1 | b2 is true
b1 ^ b2 is true
```

The logical operators provided by C# perform the most commonly used logical operations. However, several other operations are defined by the rules for formal logic. These other logical operations can be constructed using the logical operators supported by C#. Thus, C# supplies a set of logical operators sufficient to construct any other logical operation. For example, another logical operation is *implication*. Implication is a binary operation in which the outcome is false only when the left operand is true and the right operand is false. (The implication operation reflects the idea that true cannot imply false.) Thus, the truth table for the implication operator is shown here:

p	q	p implies q
True	True	True
True	False	False
False	False	True
False	True	True

The implication operation can be constructed using a combination of the ! and the | operator, as shown here:

!p | q

The following program demonstrates this implementation:

```
// Create an implication operator in C#.

using System;

class Implication {
  static void Main() {
    bool p=false, q=false;
    int i, j;

    for(i = 0; i < 2; i++) {
      for(j = 0; j < 2; j++) {
        if(i==0) p = true;
        if(i==1) p = false;
        if(j==0) q = true;
        if(j==1) q = false;

        Console.WriteLine("p is " + p + ", q is " + q);
        if(!p | q) Console.WriteLine(p + " implies " + q +
                    " is " + true);
        Console.WriteLine();
      }
    }
  }
}
```

The output is shown here:

```
p is True, q is True
True implies True is True

p is True, q is False
```

```
p is False, q is True
False implies True is True

p is False, q is False
False implies False is True
```

Short-Circuit Logical Operators

C# supplies special *short-circuit* versions of its AND and OR logical operators that can be used to produce more efficient code. To understand why, consider the following. In an AND operation, if the first operand is false, then the outcome is false no matter what value the second operand has. In an OR operation, if the first operand is true, then the outcome of the operation is true no matter what the value of the second operand. Thus, in these two cases there is no need to evaluate the second operand. By not evaluating the second operand, time is saved and more efficient code is produced.

The short-circuit AND operator is **&&** and the short-circuit OR operator is | |. As described earlier, their normal counterparts are **&** and |. The only difference between the normal and short-circuit versions is that the normal operands will always evaluate each operand, but short-circuit versions will evaluate the second operand only when necessary.

Here is a program that demonstrates the short-circuit AND operator. The program determines if the value in **d** is a factor of **n**. It does this by performing a modulus operation. If the remainder of **n** / **d** is zero, then **d** is a factor. However, since the modulus operation involves a division, the short-circuit form of the AND is used to prevent a divide-by-zero error.

```
// Demonstrate the short-circuit operators.

using System;

class SCops {
  static void Main() {
    int n, d;

    n = 10;
    d = 2;
    if(d != 0 && (n % d) == 0)
      Console.WriteLine(d + " is a factor of " + n);

    d = 0; // now, set d to zero

    // Since d is zero, the second operand is not evaluated.
    if(d != 0 && (n % d) == 0)
      Console.WriteLine(d + " is a factor of " + n);

    // Now, try the same thing without short-circuit operator.
    // This will cause a divide-by-zero error.
    if(d != 0 & (n % d) == 0)
      Console.WriteLine(d + " is a factor of " + n);
  }
}
```

To prevent a divide-by-zero error, the **if** statement first checks to see if **d** is equal to zero. If it is, then the short-circuit AND stops at that point and does not perform the modulus

division. Thus, in the first test, **d** is 2 and the modulus operation is performed. The second test fails because **d** is set to zero, and the modulus operation is skipped, avoiding a divide-by-zero error. Finally, the normal AND operator is tried. This causes both operands to be evaluated, which leads to a runtime error when the division-by-zero occurs.

Since the short-circuit operators are, in some cases, more efficient than their normal counterparts, you might be wondering why C# still offers the normal AND and OR operators. The answer is that in some cases you will want both operands of an AND or OR operation to be evaluated because of the side effects produced. Consider the following:

```
// Side effects can be important.

using System;

class SideEffects {
  static void Main() {
    int i;
    bool someCondition = false;

    i = 0;

    // Here, i is still incremented even though the if statement fails.
    if(someCondition & (++i < 100))
      Console.WriteLine("this won't be displayed");
    Console.WriteLine("if statement executed: " + i); // displays 1

    // In this case, i is not incremented because the short-circuit
    // operator skips the increment.
    if(someCondition && (++i < 100))
      Console.WriteLine("this won't be displayed");
    Console.WriteLine("if statement executed: " + i); // still 1 !!
  }
}
```

First, notice that the **bool** variable **someCondition** is initialized to **false**. Next, examine each **if** statement. As the comments indicate, in the first **if** statement, **i** is incremented despite the fact that **someCondition** is false. When the **&** is used, as it is in the first **if** statement, the expression on the right side of the **&** is evaluated no matter what value the expression on the left has. However, in the second **if** statement, the short-circuit operator is used. In this case, the variable **i** is not incremented because the left operand, **someCondition**, is false, which causes the expression on the right to be skipped. The lesson here is that if your code expects the right-hand operand of an AND or OR operation to be evaluated, then you must use C#'s non-short-circuit forms for these operations.

One other point: The short-circuit AND is also known as the *conditional AND*, and the short-circuit OR is also called the *conditional OR*.

The Assignment Operator

The *assignment operator* is the single equal sign, =. The assignment operator works in C# much as it does in other computer languages. It has this general form:

> *var-name* = *expression*;

Here, the type of *var-name* must be compatible with the type of *expression*.

The assignment operator does have one interesting attribute that you may not be familiar with: It allows you to create a chain of assignments. For example, consider this fragment:

```
int x, y, z;

x = y = z = 100; // set x, y, and z to 100
```

This fragment sets the variables **x**, **y**, and **z** to 100 using a single statement. This works because the = is an operator that yields the assigned value. Thus, the value of **z = 100** is 100, which is then assigned to **y**, which in turn is assigned to **x**. Using a "chain of assignment" is an easy way to set a group of variables to a common value.

Compound Assignments

C# provides special compound assignment operators that simplify the coding of certain assignment statements. Let's begin with an example. The assignment statement shown here:

```
x = x + 10;
```

can be written using a compound assignment as

```
x += 10;
```

The operator pair **+=** tells the compiler to assign to **x** the value of **x** plus 10.
    Here is another example. The statement

```
x = x - 100;
```

is the same as

```
x -= 100;
```

Both statements assign to **x** the value of **x** minus 100.
    There are compound assignment operators for many of the binary operators (that is, those that require two operands). The general form of the shorthand is

   var-name op = expression;

Thus, the arithmetic and logical assignment operators are

+=	-=	*=	/=
%=	&=	|=	^=

Because the compound assignment statements are shorter than their noncompound equivalents, the compound assignment operators are also sometimes called the *shorthand assignment* operators.
    The compound assignment operators provide two benefits. First, they are more compact than their "longhand" equivalents. Second, they can result in more efficient executable code (because the left-hand operand is evaluated only once). For these reasons, you will often see the compound assignment operators used in professionally written C# programs.

The Bitwise Operators

C# provides a set of *bitwise* operators that expand the types of problems to which C# can be applied. The bitwise operators act directly upon the bits of their operands. They are defined only for integer operands. They cannot be used on **bool**, **float**, or **double**.

They are called the *bitwise* operators because they are used to test, set, or shift the bits that comprise an integer value. Among other uses, bitwise operations are important to a wide variety of systems-level programming tasks, such as analyzing status information from a device. Table 4-1 lists the bitwise operators.

The Bitwise AND, OR, XOR, and NOT Operators

The bitwise operators AND, OR, XOR, and NOT are &, |, ^, and ~. They perform the same operations as their Boolean logic equivalents described earlier. The difference is that the bitwise operators work on a bit-by-bit basis. The following table shows the outcome of each operation using 1s and 0s:

p	q	p & q	p | q	p ^ q	~p
0	0	0	0	0	1
1	0	0	1	1	0
0	1	0	1	1	1
1	1	1	1	0	0

In terms of its most common usage, you can think of the bitwise AND as a way to turn bits off. That is, any bit that is 0 in either operand will cause the corresponding bit in the outcome to be set to 0. For example

```
     1101 0011
&  1010 1010
   --------------------
     1000 0010
```

Operator	Result
&	Bitwise AND
|	Bitwise OR
^	Bitwise exclusive OR (XOR)
>>	Shift right
<<	Shift left
~	One's complement (unary NOT)

TABLE 4-1 The Bitwise Operators

The following program demonstrates the **&** by using it to convert odd numbers into even numbers. It does this by turning off bit zero. For example, the low-order byte of the number 9 in binary is 0000 1001. When bit zero is turned off, this number becomes 8, or 0000 1000 in binary.

```
// Use bitwise AND to make a number even.

using System;

class MakeEven {
  static void Main() {
    ushort num;
    ushort i;

    for(i = 1; i <= 10; i++) {
      num = i;

      Console.WriteLine("num: " + num);

      num = (ushort) (num & 0xFFFE);

      Console.WriteLine("num after turning off bit zero: "
                          +  num + "\n");
    }
  }
}
```

The output from this program is shown here:

```
num: 1
num after turning off bit zero: 0

num: 2
num after turning off bit zero: 2

num: 3
num after turning off bit zero: 2

num: 4
num after turning off bit zero: 4

num: 5
num after turning off bit zero: 4

num: 6
num after turning off bit zero: 6

num: 7
num after turning off bit zero: 6

num: 8
num after turning off bit zero: 8

num: 9
num after turning off bit zero: 8
```

```
num: 10
num after turning off bit zero: 10
```

The value **0xFFFE** used in the AND statement is the hexadecimal representation of
1111 1111 1111 1110. Therefore, the AND operation leaves all bits in **num** unchanged except
for bit zero, which is set to zero. Thus, even numbers are unchanged, but odd numbers are
made even by reducing their value by 1.

The AND operator is also useful when you want to determine whether a bit is on or off.
For example, this program determines if a number is odd:

```
// Use bitwise AND to determine if a number is odd.

using System;

class IsOdd {
  static void Main() {
    ushort num;

    num = 10;

    if((num & 1) == 1)
      Console.WriteLine("This won't display.");

    num = 11;

    if((num & 1) == 1)
      Console.WriteLine(num + " is odd.");

  }
}
```

The output is shown here:

```
11 is odd.
```

In the **if** statements, the value of **num** is ANDed with 1. If bit zero in **num** is set, the result
of **num & 1** is 1; otherwise, the result is zero. Therefore, the **if** statement can succeed only
when the number is odd.

You can use the bit-testing capability of the bitwise **&** to create a program that uses the
bitwise **&** to show the bits of a **byte** value in binary format. Here is one approach:

```
// Display the bits within a byte.

using System;

class ShowBits {
  static void Main() {
    int t;
    byte val;

    val = 123;
    for(t=128; t > 0; t = t/2) {
      if((val & t) != 0) Console.Write("1 ");
```

```
   if((val & t) == 0) Console.Write("0 ");
  }
 }
}
```

The output is shown here:

```
0 1 1 1 1 0 1 1
```

The **for** loop successively tests each bit in **val**, using the bitwise AND, to determine if it is on or off. If the bit is on, the digit **1** is displayed; otherwise, **0** is displayed.

The bitwise OR can be used to turn bits on. Any bit that is set to 1 in either operand will cause the corresponding bit in the variable to be set to 1. For example

```
    1101 0011
|   1010 1010
    -------------------
    1111 1011
```

You can make use of the OR to change the make-even program shown earlier into a make-odd program, as shown here:

```
//  Use bitwise OR to make a number odd.

using System;

class MakeOdd {
  static void Main() {
    ushort num;
    ushort i;

    for(i = 1; i <= 10; i++) {
      num = i;

      Console.WriteLine("num: " + num);

      num = (ushort) (num | 1);

      Console.WriteLine("num after turning on bit zero: "
                        +  num + "\n");
    }
  }
}
```

The output from this program is shown here:

```
num: 1
num after turning on bit zero: 1

num: 2
num after turning on bit zero: 3

num: 3
num after turning on bit zero: 3
```

```
num: 4
num after turning on bit zero: 5

num: 5
num after turning on bit zero: 5

num: 6
num after turning on bit zero: 7

num: 7
num after turning on bit zero: 7

num: 8
num after turning on bit zero: 9

num: 9
num after turning on bit zero: 9

num: 10
num after turning on bit zero: 11
```

The program works by ORing each number with the value 1, because 1 is the value that produces a value in binary in which only bit zero is set. When this value is ORed with any other value, it produces a result in which the low-order bit is set and all other bits remain unchanged. Thus, a value that is even will be increased by 1, becoming odd.

An exclusive OR, usually abbreviated XOR, will set a bit on if, and only if, the bits being compared are different, as illustrated here:

```
    0 1 1 1 1 1 1 1
^   1 0 1 1 1 0 0 1
    -------------------------
    1 1 0 0 0 1 1 0
```

The XOR operator has an interesting property that is useful in a variety of situations. When some value X is XORed with another value Y, and then that result is XORed with Y again, X is produced. That is, given the sequence

    R1 = X ^ Y;
    R2 = R1 ^ Y;

R2 is the same value as X. Thus, the outcome of a sequence of two XORs using the same value produces the original value. This feature of the XOR can be put into action to create a simple cipher in which some integer is the key that is used to both encode and decode a message by XORing the characters in that message. To encode, the XOR operation is applied the first time, yielding the ciphertext. To decode, the XOR is applied a second time, yielding the plaintext. Of course, such a cipher has no practical value, being trivially easy to break. It does, however, provide an interesting way to demonstrate the effects of the XOR, as the following program shows:

```
// Demonstrate the XOR.

using System;
```

```
class Encode {
  static void Main() {
    char ch1 = 'H';
    char ch2 = 'i';
    char ch3 = '!';
    int key = 88;

    Console.WriteLine("Original message: " + ch1 + ch2 + ch3);

    // Encode the message.
    ch1 = (char) (ch1 ^ key);
    ch2 = (char) (ch2 ^ key);
    ch3 = (char) (ch3 ^ key);

    Console.WriteLine("Encoded message: " + ch1 + ch2 + ch3);

    // Decode the message.
    ch1 = (char) (ch1 ^ key);
    ch2 = (char) (ch2 ^ key);
    ch3 = (char) (ch3 ^ key);

    Console.WriteLine("Encoded message: " + ch1 + ch2 + ch3);
  }
}
```

Here is the output:

```
Original message: Hi!
Encoded message: ☐1y
Encoded message: Hi!
```

As you can see, the result of two XORs using the same key produces the decoded message. (Remember, this simple XOR cipher is not suitable for any real-world, practical use because it is inherently insecure.)

The unary one's complement (NOT) operator reverses the state of all the bits of the operand. For example, if some integer called **A** has the bit pattern 1001 0110, then ~**A** produces a result with the bit pattern 0110 1001.

The following program demonstrates the NOT operator by displaying a number and its complement in binary:

```
// Demonstrate the bitwise NOT.

using System;

class NotDemo {
  static void Main() {
    sbyte b = -34;

    for(int t=128; t > 0; t = t/2) {
      if((b & t) != 0) Console.Write("1 ");
      if((b & t) == 0) Console.Write("0 ");
    }
    Console.WriteLine();
```

```
   // reverse all bits
   b = (sbyte) ~b;

   for(int t=128; t > 0; t = t/2) {
      if((b & t) != 0) Console.Write("1 ");
      if((b & t) == 0) Console.Write("0 ");
   }
 }
}
```

Here is the output:

```
1 1 0 1 1 1 1 0
0 0 1 0 0 0 0 1
```

The Shift Operators

In C# it is possible to shift the bits that comprise an integer value to the left or to the right by a specified amount. C# defines the two bit-shift operators shown here:

<<	Left shift
>>	Right shift

The general forms for these operators are shown here:

value << num-bits
value >> num-bits

Here, *value* is the value being shifted by the number of bit positions specified by *num-bits*.

A left shift causes all bits within the specified value to be shifted left one position and a zero bit to be brought in on the right. A right shift causes all bits to be shifted right one position. In the case of a right shift on an unsigned value, a zero is brought in on the left. In the case of a right shift on a signed value, the sign bit is preserved. Recall that negative numbers are represented by setting the high-order bit of an integer value to 1. Thus, if the value being shifted is negative, each right shift brings in a 1 on the left. If the value is positive, each right shift brings in a 0 on the left.

For both left and right shifts, the bits shifted out are lost. Thus, a shift is not a rotate and there is no way to retrieve a bit that has been shifted out.

Here is a program that graphically illustrates the effect of a left and right shift. Here, an integer is given an initial value of 1, which means that its low-order bit is set. Then, eight shifts are performed on the integer. After each shift, the lower eight bits of the value are shown. The process is then repeated, except that a 1 is put in the eighth bit position, and right shifts are performed.

```
// Demonstrate the shift << and >> operators.

using System;

class ShiftDemo {
  static void Main() {
    int val = 1;
```

```
    for(int i = 0; i < 8; i++) {
      for(int t=128; t > 0; t = t/2) {
        if((val & t) != 0) Console.Write("1 ");
        if((val & t) == 0) Console.Write("0 ");
      }
      Console.WriteLine();
      val = val << 1; // left shift
    }
    Console.WriteLine();

    val = 128;
    for(int i = 0; i < 8; i++) {
      for(int t=128; t > 0; t = t/2) {
        if((val & t) != 0) Console.Write("1 ");
        if((val & t) == 0) Console.Write("0 ");
      }
      Console.WriteLine();
      val = val >> 1; // right shift
    }
  }
}
```

The output from the program is shown here:

```
0 0 0 0 0 0 0 1
0 0 0 0 0 0 1 0
0 0 0 0 0 1 0 0
0 0 0 0 1 0 0 0
0 0 0 1 0 0 0 0
0 0 1 0 0 0 0 0
0 1 0 0 0 0 0 0
1 0 0 0 0 0 0 0

1 0 0 0 0 0 0 0
0 1 0 0 0 0 0 0
0 0 1 0 0 0 0 0
0 0 0 1 0 0 0 0
0 0 0 0 1 0 0 0
0 0 0 0 0 1 0 0
0 0 0 0 0 0 1 0
0 0 0 0 0 0 0 1
```

Since binary is based on powers of 2, the shift operators can be used as a way to multiply or divide an integer by 2. A shift left doubles a value. A shift right halves it. Of course, this works only as long as you are not shifting bits off one end or the other. Here is an example:

```
// Use the shift operators to multiply and divide by 2.

using System;

class MultDiv {
  static void Main() {
    int n;

    n = 10;
```

```
        Console.WriteLine("Value of n: " + n);

        // Multiply by 2.
        n = n << 1;
        Console.WriteLine("Value of n after n = n * 2: " + n);

        // Multiply by 4.
        n = n << 2;
        Console.WriteLine("Value of n after n = n * 4: " + n);

        // Divide by 2.
        n = n >> 1;
        Console.WriteLine("Value of n after n = n / 2: " + n);

        // Divide by 4.
        n = n >> 2;
        Console.WriteLine("Value of n after n = n / 4: " + n);
        Console.WriteLine();

        // Reset n.
        n = 10;
        Console.WriteLine("Value of n: " + n);

        // Multiply by 2, 30 times.
        n = n << 30; // data is lost
        Console.WriteLine("Value of n after left-shifting 30 places: " + n);
    }
}
```

The output is shown here:

```
Value of n: 10
Value of n after n = n * 2: 20
Value of n after n = n * 4: 80
Value of n after n = n / 2: 40
Value of n after n = n / 4: 10

Value of n: 10
Value of n after left-shifting 30 places: -2147483648
```

Notice the last line in the output. When the value 10 is left-shifted 30 times, information is lost because bits are shifted out of the range of an **int**. In this case, the garbage value produced is negative because a 1 bit is shifted into the high-order bit, which is used as a sign bit, causing the number to be interpreted as negative. This illustrates why you must be careful when using the shift operators to multiply or divide a value by 2. (See Chapter 3 for an explanation of signed vs. unsigned data types.)

Bitwise Compound Assignments

All of the binary bitwise operators can be used in compound assignments. For example, the following two statements both assign to **x** the outcome of an XOR of **x** with the value 127:

```
x = x ^ 127;
x ^= 127;
```

The ? Operator

One of C#'s most fascinating operators is the **?**, which is C#'s conditional operator. The **?** operator is often used to replace certain types of if-then-else constructions. The **?** is called a *ternary operator* because it requires three operands. It takes the general form

Exp1 ? *Exp2* : *Exp3;*

where *Exp1* is a **bool** expression, and *Exp2* and *Exp3* are expressions. The type of *Exp2* and *Exp3* must be the same. Notice the use and placement of the colon.

The value of a **?** expression is determined like this: *Exp1* is evaluated. If it is true, then *Exp2* is evaluated and becomes the value of the entire **?** expression. If *Exp1* is false, then *Exp3* is evaluated, and its value becomes the value of the expression. Consider this example, which assigns **absval** the absolute value of **val**:

```
absval = val < 0 ? -val : val; // get absolute value of val
```

Here, **absval** will be assigned the value of **val** if **val** is zero or greater. If **val** is negative, then **absval** will be assigned the negative of that value (which yields a positive value).

Here is another example of the **?** operator. This program divides two numbers, but will not allow a division by zero.

```
// Prevent a division by zero using the ?.

using System;

class NoZeroDiv {
  static void Main() {
    int result;

    for(int i = -5; i < 6; i++) {
      result = i != 0 ? 100 / i : 0;
      if(i != 0)
        Console.WriteLine("100 / " + i + " is " + result);
    }
  }
}
```

The output from the program is shown here:

```
100 / -5 is -20
100 / -4 is -25
100 / -3 is -33
100 / -2 is -50
100 / -1 is -100
100 / 1 is 100
100 / 2 is 50
100 / 3 is 33
100 / 4 is 25
100 / 5 is 20
```

Pay special attention to this line from the program:

```
result = i != 0 ? 100 / i : 0;
```

Here, **result** is assigned the outcome of the division of 100 by **i**. However, this division takes place only if **i** is not 0. When **i** is 0, a placeholder value of 0 is assigned to **result**.

You don't actually have to assign the value produced by the **?** to some variable. For example, you could use the value as an argument in a call to a method. Or, if the expressions are all of type **bool**, the **?** can be used as the conditional expression in a loop or **if** statement. For example, the following program displays the results of dividing 100 by only even, non-zero values:

```
// Divide by only even, non-zero values.

using System;

class NoZeroDiv2 {
  static void Main() {

    for(int i = -5; i < 6; i++)
      if(i != 0 ? (i%2 == 0) : false)
        Console.WriteLine("100 / " + i + " is " + 100 / i);
  }
}
```

Notice the **if** statement. If **i** is zero, then the outcome of the **if** is false. Otherwise, if **i** is non-zero, then the outcome of the **if** is true if **i** is even and false if **i** is odd. Thus, only even, non-zero divisors are allowed. Although this example is somewhat contrived for the sake of illustration, such constructs are occasionally very useful.

Spacing and Parentheses

An expression in C# can have tabs and spaces in it to make it more readable. For example, the following two expressions are the same, but the second is easier to read:

```
x=10/y*(127+x);

x = 10 / y * (127 + x);
```

Parentheses can be used to group subexpressions, thereby effectively increasing the precedence of the operations contained within them, just like in algebra. Use of redundant or additional parentheses will not cause errors or slow down execution of the expression. You are encouraged to use parentheses to make clear the exact order of evaluation, both for yourself and for others who may have to figure out your program later. For example, which of the following two expressions is easier to read?

```
x = y/3-34*temp+127;

x = (y/3) - (34*temp) + 127;
```

Operator Precedence

Table 4-2 shows the order of precedence for all C# operators, from highest to lowest. This table includes several operators that will be discussed later in this book.

Highest									
()	[]	.	++ (postfix)	– – (postfix)	checked	new	sizeof	typeof	unchecked
!	~	(cast)	+ (unary)	– (unary)	++ (prefix)	– – (prefix)			
*	/	%							
+	–								
<<	>>								
<	>	<=	>=	is					
==	!=								
&									
^									
|									
&&									
||									
??									
?:									
=	op=	=>							
Lowest									

TABLE 4-2   The Precedence of the C# Operators

Program Control Statements

This chapter discusses C#'s program control statements. There are three categories of program control statements: *selection* statements, which are the **if** and the **switch**; *iteration* statements, which consist of the **for**, **while**, **do-while**, and **foreach** loops; and *jump* statements, which include **break**, **continue**, **goto**, **return**, and **throw**. Except for **throw**, which is part of C#'s exception-handling mechanism and is discussed in Chapter 13, the others are examined here.

The if Statement

Chapter 2 introduced the **if** statement. It is examined in detail here. The complete form of the **if** statement is

    if(*condition*) *statement*;
    else *statement*;

where the targets of the **if** and **else** are single statements. The **else** clause is optional. The targets of both the **if** and **else** can be blocks of statements. The general form of the **if** using blocks of statements is

    if(*condition*)
    {
      statement sequence
    }
    else
    {
      statement sequence
    }

If the conditional expression is true, the target of the **if** will be executed; otherwise, if it exists, the target of the **else** will be executed. At no time will both of them be executed. The conditional expression controlling the **if** must produce a **bool** result.

Here is a simple example that uses an **if** and **else** to report if a number is positive or negative:

```
// Determine if a value is positive or negative.

using System;
```

```
class PosNeg {
  static void Main() {
    int i;

    for(i=-5; i <= 5; i++) {
      Console.Write("Testing " + i + ": ");

      if(i < 0) Console.WriteLine("negative");
      else Console.WriteLine("positive");
    }
  }
}
```

The output is shown here:

```
Testing -5: negative
Testing -4: negative
Testing -3: negative
Testing -2: negative
Testing -1: negative
Testing 0: positive
Testing 1: positive
Testing 2: positive
Testing 3: positive
Testing 4: positive
Testing 5: positive
```

In this example, if **i** is less than zero, then the target of the **if** is executed. Otherwise, the target of the **else** is executed. In no case are both executed.

Nested ifs

A *nested if* is an **if** statement that is the target of another **if** or **else**. Nested **ifs** are very common in programming. The main thing to remember about nested **ifs** in C# is that an **else** clause always refers to the nearest **if** statement that is within the same block as the **else** and not already associated with an **else**. Here is an example:

```
if(i == 10) {
  if(j < 20) a = b;
  if(k > 100) c = d;
  else a = c; // this else refers to if(k > 100)
}
else a = d; // this else refers to if(i == 10)
```

As the comments indicate, the final **else** is not associated with **if(j < 20)** because it is not in the same block (even though it is the nearest **if** without an **else**). Rather, the final **else** is associated with **if(i == 10)**. The inner **else** refers to **if(k > 100)** because it is the closest **if** within the same block.

The following program demonstrates a nested **if**. In the positive/negative program shown earlier, zero is reported as positive. However, as a general rule, zero is considered signless. The following version of the program reports zero as being neither positive nor negative.

```
// Determine if a value is positive, negative, or zero.

using System;

class PosNegZero {
  static void Main() {
    int i;

    for(i=-5; i <= 5; i++) {

      Console.Write("Testing " + i + ": ");

      if(i < 0) Console.WriteLine("negative");
      else if(i == 0) Console.WriteLine("no sign");
        else Console.WriteLine("positive");
    }
  }
}
```

Here is the output:

```
Testing -5: negative
Testing -4: negative
Testing -3: negative
Testing -2: negative
Testing -1: negative
Testing 0: no sign
Testing 1: positive
Testing 2: positive
Testing 3: positive
Testing 4: positive
Testing 5: positive
```

The if-else-if Ladder

A common programming construct that is based upon the nested **if** is the *if-else-if* ladder. It looks like this:

> if(*condition*)
>   *statement*;
> else if(*condition*)
>   *statement*;
> else if(*condition*)
>   *statement*;
>   .
>   .
>   .
> else
>   *statement*;

The conditional expressions are evaluated from the top downward. As soon as a true condition is found, the statement associated with it is executed, and the rest of the ladder is bypassed.

If none of the conditions is true, then the final **else** clause will be executed. The final **else** often acts as a default condition. That is, if all other conditional tests fail, then the last **else** clause is executed. If there is no final **else** and all other conditions are false, then no action will take place.

The following program demonstrates the **if-else-if** ladder. It finds the smallest single-digit factor (other than 1) for a given value.

```
// Determine smallest single-digit factor.

using System;

class Ladder {
  static void Main() {
    int num;

    for(num = 2; num < 12; num++) {
      if((num % 2) == 0)
        Console.WriteLine("Smallest factor of " + num + " is 2.");
      else if((num % 3) == 0)
        Console.WriteLine("Smallest factor of " + num + " is 3.");
      else if((num % 5) == 0)
        Console.WriteLine("Smallest factor of " + num + " is 5.");
      else if((num % 7) == 0)
        Console.WriteLine("Smallest factor of " + num + " is 7.");
      else
        Console.WriteLine(num + " is not divisible by 2, 3, 5, or 7.");
    }
  }
}
```

The program produces the following output:

```
Smallest factor of 2 is 2.
Smallest factor of 3 is 3.
Smallest factor of 4 is 2.
Smallest factor of 5 is 5.
Smallest factor of 6 is 2.
Smallest factor of 7 is 7.
Smallest factor of 8 is 2.
Smallest factor of 9 is 3.
Smallest factor of 10 is 2.
11 is not divisible by 2, 3, 5, or 7.
```

As you can see, the **else** is executed only if none of the preceding **if** statements succeeds.

The switch Statement

The second of C#'s selection statements is **switch**. The **switch** provides for a multiway branch. Thus, it enables a program to select among several alternatives. Although a series of nested **if** statements can perform multiway tests, for many situations the **switch** is a more efficient approach. It works like this: The value of an expression is successively tested against a list of constants. When a match is found, the statement sequence associated with that match is executed. The general form of the **switch** statement is

```
switch(expression) {
  case constant1:
    statement sequence
    break;
  case constant2:
    statement sequence
    break;
  case constant3:
    statement sequence
    break;
    .
    .
    .
  default:
    statement sequence
    break;
}
```

The **switch** expression must be of an integer type, such as **char**, **byte**, **short**, or **int**, of an enumeration type, or of type **string**. (Enumerations and the **string** type are described later in this book.) Thus, floating-point expressions, for example, are not allowed. Frequently, the expression controlling the **switch** is simply a variable. The **case** constants must be of a type compatible with the expression. No two **case** constants in the same **switch** can have identical values.

The **default** sequence is executed if no **case** constant matches the expression. The **default** is optional; if it is not present, no action takes place if all matches fail. When a match is found, the statements associated with that **case** are executed until the **break** is encountered.

The following program demonstrates the **switch**:

```
// Demonstrate the switch.

using System;

class SwitchDemo {
  static void Main() {
    int i;

    for(i=0; i<10; i++)
      switch(i) {
        case 0:
          Console.WriteLine("i is zero");
          break;
        case 1:
          Console.WriteLine("i is one");
          break;
        case 2:
          Console.WriteLine("i is two");
          break;
        case 3:
          Console.WriteLine("i is three");
          break;
```

```
        case 4:
          Console.WriteLine("i is four");
          break;
        default:
          Console.WriteLine("i is five or more");
          break;
      }
  }
}
```

The output produced by this program is shown here:

```
i is zero
i is one
i is two
i is three
i is four
i is five or more
i is five or more
i is five or more
i is five or more
i is five or more
```

As you can see, each time through the loop, the statements associated with the **case** constant that matches **i** are executed. All others are bypassed. When **i** is five or greater, no **case** constants match, so the **default** is executed.

In the preceding example, the **switch** was controlled by an **int** variable. As explained, you can control a **switch** with any integer type, including **char**. Here is an example that uses a **char** expression and **char case** constants:

```
// Use a char to control the switch.

using System;

class SwitchDemo2 {
  static void Main() {
    char ch;

    for(ch='A'; ch<= 'E'; ch++)
      switch(ch) {
        case 'A':
          Console.WriteLine("ch is A");
          break;
        case 'B':
          Console.WriteLine("ch is B");
          break;
        case 'C':
          Console.WriteLine("ch is C");
          break;
        case 'D':
          Console.WriteLine("ch is D");
          break;
        case 'E':
          Console.WriteLine("ch is E");
```

```
        break;
      }
    }
}
```

The output from this program is shown here:

```
ch is A
ch is B
ch is C
ch is D
ch is E
```

Notice that this example does not include a **default** case. Remember, the **default** is optional. When not needed, it can be left out.

In C#, it is an error for the statement sequence associated with one **case** to continue on into the next **case**. This is called the "no fall-through" rule. This is why **case** sequences end with a **break** statement. (You can avoid fall-through in other ways, such as by using the **goto** discussed later in this chapter, but **break** is by far the most commonly used approach.) When encountered within the statement sequence of a **case**, the **break** statement causes program flow to exit from the entire **switch** statement and resume at the next statement outside the **switch**. The **default** sequence also must not "fall through," and it too usually ends with **break**.

The no fall-through rule is one point on which C# differs from C, C++, and Java. In those languages, one **case** may continue on (that is, fall through) into the next **case**. There are two reasons that C# instituted the no fall-through rule for **case**s: First, it allows the compiler to freely rearrange the order of the **case** sequences, perhaps for purposes of optimization. Such a rearrangement would not be possible if one **case** could flow into the next. Second, requiring each **case** to explicitly end prevents a programmer from accidentally allowing one **case** to flow into the next.

Although you cannot allow one **case** sequence to fall through into another, you can have two or more **case** labels refer to the same code sequence, as shown in this example:

```
// Empty cases can fall through.

using System;

class EmptyCasesCanFall {
  static void Main() {
    int i;

    for(i=1; i < 5; i++)
      switch(i) {
        case 1:
        case 2:
        case 3: Console.WriteLine("i is 1, 2 or 3");
          break;
        case 4: Console.WriteLine("i is 4");
          break;
      }

  }
}
```

The output is shown here:

```
i is 1, 2 or 3
i is 1, 2 or 3
i is 1, 2 or 3
i is 4
```

In this example, if **i** has the value 1, 2, or 3, then the first **WriteLine( )** statement executes. If **i** is 4, then the second **WriteLine( )** statement executes. The stacking of **case**s does not violate the no fall-through rule, because the **case** statements all use the same statement sequence.

Stacking **case** labels is a commonly employed technique when several **case**s share common code. This technique prevents the unnecessary duplication of code sequences.

Nested switch Statements

It is possible to have a **switch** as part of the statement sequence of an outer **switch**. This is called a *nested switch.* The **case** constants of the inner and outer **switch** can contain common values and no conflicts will arise. For example, the following code fragment is perfectly acceptable:

```
switch(ch1) {
  case 'A': Console.WriteLine("This A is part of outer switch.");
    switch(ch2) {
      case 'A':
        Console.WriteLine("This A is part of inner switch");
        break;
      case 'B': // ...
    } // end of inner switch
    break;
  case 'B': // ...
```

The for Loop

The **for** loop was introduced in Chapter 2. Here, it is examined in detail. You might be surprised at just how powerful and flexible the **for** loop is. Let's begin by reviewing the basics, starting with the most traditional forms of the **for**.

The general form of the **for** loop for repeating a single statement is

for(*initialization; condition; iteration*) *statement*;

For repeating a block, the general form is

for(*initialization; condition; iteration*)
{
    statement sequence
}

The *initialization* is usually an assignment statement that sets the initial value of the *loop control variable,* which acts as the counter that controls the loop. The *condition* is a Boolean expression that determines whether the loop will repeat. The *iteration* expression defines the amount by which the loop control variable will change each time the loop is repeated. Notice that these three major sections of the loop must be separated by semicolons. The **for** loop will

continue to execute as long as the condition tests true. Once the condition becomes false, the loop will exit, and program execution will resume on the statement following the **for**.

The **for** loop can proceed in a positive or negative fashion, and it can change the loop control variable by any amount. For example, the following program prints the numbers 100 to –100, in decrements of 5:

```
// A negatively running for loop.

using System;

class DecrFor {
  static void Main() {
    int x;

    for(x = 100; x > -100; x -= 5)
      Console.WriteLine(x);
  }
}
```

An important point about **for** loops is that the conditional expression is always tested at the top of the loop. This means that the code inside the loop may not be executed at all if the condition is false to begin with. Here is an example:

```
for(count=10; count < 5; count++)
  x += count; // this statement will not execute
```

This loop will never execute because its control variable, **count**, is greater than 5 when the loop is first entered. This makes the conditional expression, **count < 5**, false from the outset; thus, not even one iteration of the loop will occur.

The **for** loop is most useful when you will be iterating a known number of times. For example, the following program uses two **for** loops to find the prime numbers between 2 and 20. If the number is not prime, then its largest factor is displayed.

```
// Determine if a number is prime. If it is not, then
// display its largest factor.

using System;

class FindPrimes {
  static void Main() {
    int num;
    int i;
    int factor;
    bool isprime;

    for(num = 2; num < 20; num++) {
      isprime = true;
      factor = 0;

      // See if num is evenly divisible.
      for(i=2; i <= num/2; i++) {
        if((num % i) == 0) {
```

```
             // num is evenly divisible. Thus, it is not prime.
             isprime = false;
             factor = i;
           }
        }

      if(isprime)
         Console.WriteLine(num + " is prime.");
      else
         Console.WriteLine("Largest factor of " + num +
                           " is " + factor);
      }
   }
}
```

The output from the program is shown here:

```
2 is prime.
3 is prime.
Largest factor of 4 is 2
5 is prime.
Largest factor of 6 is 3
7 is prime.
Largest factor of 8 is 4
Largest factor of 9 is 3
Largest factor of 10 is 5
11 is prime.
Largest factor of 12 is 6
13 is prime.
Largest factor of 14 is 7
Largest factor of 15 is 5
Largest factor of 16 is 8
17 is prime.
Largest factor of 18 is 9
19 is prime.
```

Some Variations on the for Loop

The **for** is one of the most versatile statements in the C# language because it allows a wide range of variations. They are examined here.

Using Multiple Loop Control Variables

The **for** loop allows you to use two or more variables to control the loop. When using multiple loop control variables, the initialization and increments statements for each variable are separated by commas. Here is an example:

```
// Use commas in a for statement.

using System;

class Comma {
  static void Main() {
    int i, j;
```

```
  for(i=0, j=10; i < j; i++, j--)
     Console.WriteLine("i and j: " + i + " " + j);
   }
}
```

The output from the program is shown here:

```
i and j: 0 10
i and j: 1 9
i and j: 2 8
i and j: 3 7
i and j: 4 6
```

Here, commas separate the two initialization statements and the two iteration expressions. When the loop begins, both **i** and **j** are initialized. Each time the loop repeats, **i** is incremented and **j** is decremented. Multiple loop control variables are often convenient and can simplify certain algorithms. You can have any number of initialization and iteration statements, but in practice, more than two make the **for** loop unwieldy.

Here is a practical use of multiple loop control variables in a **for** statement. This program uses two loop control variables within a single **for** loop to find the largest and smallest factor of a number, in this case 100. Pay special attention to the termination condition. It relies on both loop control variables.

```
// Use commas in a for statement to find the largest and
// smallest factor of a number.

using System;

class Comma {
  static void Main() {
     int i, j;
     int smallest, largest;
     int num;

     num = 100;

     smallest = largest = 1;

     for(i=2, j=num/2; (i <= num/2) & (j >= 2); i++, j--) {

       if((smallest == 1) & ((num % i) == 0))
          smallest = i;

       if((largest == 1) & ((num % j) == 0))
          largest = j;

     }

     Console.WriteLine("Largest factor: " + largest);
     Console.WriteLine("Smallest factor: " + smallest);
   }
}
```

Here is the output from the program:

```
Largest factor: 50
Smallest factor: 2
```

Through the use of two loop control variables, a single **for** loop can find both the smallest and the largest factor of a number. The control variable **i** is used to search for the smallest factor. It is initially set to 2 and incremented until its value exceeds one half of **num**. The control variable **j** is used to search for the largest factor. Its value is initially set to one half the **num** and decremented until it is less than 2. The loop runs until both **i** and **j** are at their termination values. When the loop ends, both factors will have been found.

The Conditional Expression

The conditional expression controlling a **for** loop can be any valid expression that produces a **bool** result. It does not need to involve the loop control variable. For example, in the next program, the **for** loop is controlled by the value of **done**.

```
// Loop condition can be any bool expression.

using System;

class forDemo {
  static void Main() {
     int i, j;
     bool done = false;

     for(i=0, j=100; !done; i++, j--) {

       if(i*i >= j) done = true;

       Console.WriteLine("i, j: " + i + " " + j);
     }
   }
}
```

The output is shown here:

```
i, j: 0 100
i, j: 1 99
i, j: 2 98
i, j: 3 97
i, j: 4 96
i, j: 5 95
i, j: 6 94
i, j: 7 93
i, j: 8 92
i, j: 9 91
i, j: 10 90
```

In this example, the **for** loop iterates until the **bool** variable **done** is true. This variable is set to true inside the loop when **i** squared is greater than or equal to **j**.

Missing Pieces

Some interesting **for** loop variations are created by leaving pieces of the loop definition empty. In C#, it is possible for any or all of the initialization, condition, or iteration portions of the **for** loop to be empty. For example, consider the following program:

```
// Parts of the for can be empty.

using System;

class Empty {
  static void Main() {
    int i;

    for(i = 0; i < 10; ) {
      Console.WriteLine("Pass #" + i);
      i++; // increment loop control var
    }

  }
}
```

Here, the iteration expression of the **for** is empty. Instead, the loop control variable **i** is incremented inside the body of the loop. This means that each time the loop repeats, **i** is tested to see whether it equals 10, but no further action takes place. Of course, since **i** is incremented within the body of the loop, the loop runs normally, displaying the following output:

```
Pass #0
Pass #1
Pass #2
Pass #3
Pass #4
Pass #5
Pass #6
Pass #7
Pass #8
Pass #9
```

In the next example, the initialization portion is also moved out of the **for**:

```
// Move more out of the for loop.

using System;

class Empty2 {
  static void Main() {
    int i;

    i = 0; // move initialization out of loop
    for(; i < 10; ) {
      Console.WriteLine("Pass #" + i);
      i++; // increment loop control var
    }
  }
}
```

In this version, **i** is initialized before the loop begins, rather than as part of the **for**. Normally, you will want to initialize the loop control variable inside the **for**. Placing the initialization outside of the loop is generally done only when the initial value is derived through a complex process that does not lend itself to containment inside the **for** statement.

The Infinite Loop

You can create an *infinite loop* (a loop that never terminates) using the **for** by leaving the conditional expression empty. For example, the following fragment shows the way many C# programmers create an infinite loop:

```
for(;;) // intentionally infinite loop
{
  //...
}
```

This loop will run forever. Although there are some programming tasks, such as operating system command processors, that require an infinite loop, most "infinite loops" are really just loops with special termination requirements. (See "Using **break** to Exit a Loop," later in this chapter.)

Loops with No Body

In C#, the body associated with a **for** loop (or any other loop) can be empty. This is because a *empty statement* is syntactically valid. Bodyless loops are often useful. For example, the following program uses a bodyless loop to sum the numbers 1 through 5:

```
// The body of a loop can be empty.

using System;

class Empty3 {
  static void Main() {
    int i;
    int sum = 0;

    // Sum the numbers through 5.
    for(i = 1; i <= 5; sum += i++) ;

    Console.WriteLine("Sum is " + sum);
  }
}
```

The output from the program is shown here:

```
Sum is 15
```

Notice that the summation process is handled entirely within the **for** statement, and no body is needed. Pay special attention to the iteration expression:

```
sum += i++
```

Don't be intimidated by statements like this. They are common in professionally written C# programs and are easy to understand if you break them down into their parts. In words,

this statement says "add to **sum** the value of **sum** plus **i**, then increment **i**." Thus, it is the same as this sequence of statements:

```
sum = sum + i;
i++;
```

Declaring Loop Control Variables Inside the for Loop

Often the variable that controls a **for** loop is needed only for the purposes of the loop and is not used elsewhere. When this is the case, it is possible to declare the variable inside the initialization portion of the **for**. For example, the following program computes both the summation and the factorial of the numbers 1 through 5. It declares its loop control variable **i** inside the **for**:

```
// Declare loop control variable inside the for.

using System;

class ForVar {
  static void Main() {
    int sum = 0;
    int fact = 1;

    // Compute the factorial of the numbers 1 through 5.
    for(int i = 1; i <= 5; i++) {
      sum += i;  // i is known throughout the loop.
      fact *= i;
    }

    // But, i is not known here.

    Console.WriteLine("Sum is " + sum);
    Console.WriteLine("Factorial is " + fact);
  }
}
```

When you declare a variable inside a **for** loop, there is one important point to remember: The scope of that variable ends when the **for** statement does. (That is, the scope of the variable is limited to the **for** loop.) Outside the **for** loop, the variable will cease to exist. Thus, in the preceding example, **i** is not accessible outside the **for** loop. If you need to use the loop control variable elsewhere in your program, you will not be able to declare it inside the **for** loop.

Before moving on, you might want to experiment with your own variations on the **for** loop. As you will find, it is a fascinating loop.

The while Loop

Another of C#'s loops is the **while**. The general form of the **while** loop is

while(*condition*) *statement*;

where *statement* can be a single statement or a block of statements, and *condition* defines the condition that controls the loop and may be any valid Boolean expression. The statement is performed while the condition is true. When the condition becomes false, program control passes to the line immediately following the loop.

Here is a simple example in which a **while** is used to compute the order of magnitude of an integer:

```
// Compute the order of magnitude of an integer

using System;

class WhileDemo {
  static void Main() {
    int num;
    int mag;

    num = 435679;
    mag = 0;

    Console.WriteLine("Number: " + num);

    while(num > 0) {
      mag++;
      num = num / 10;
    };

    Console.WriteLine("Magnitude: " + mag);
  }
}
```

The output is shown here:

```
Number: 435679
Magnitude: 6
```

The **while** loop works like this: The value of **num** is tested. If **num** is greater than 0, the **mag** counter is incremented, and **num** is divided by 10. As long as the value in **num** is greater than 0, the loop repeats. When **num** is 0, the loop terminates and **mag** contains the order of magnitude of the original value.

As with the **for** loop, the **while** checks the conditional expression at the top of the loop, which means that the loop code may not execute at all. This eliminates the need for performing a separate test before the loop. The following program illustrates this characteristic of the **while** loop. It computes the integer powers of 2 from 0 to 9.

```
// Compute integer powers of 2.

using System;

class Power {
  static void Main() {
    int e;
    int result;

    for(int i=0; i < 10; i++) {
      result = 1;
      e = i;
```

```
      while(e > 0) {
        result *= 2;
        e--;
      }

      Console.WriteLine("2 to the " + i + " power is " + result);
    }
  }
}
```

The output from the program is shown here:

```
2 to the 0 power is 1
2 to the 1 power is 2
2 to the 2 power is 4
2 to the 3 power is 8
2 to the 4 power is 16
2 to the 5 power is 32
2 to the 6 power is 64
2 to the 7 power is 128
2 to the 8 power is 256
2 to the 9 power is 512
```

Notice that the **while** loop executes only when **e** is greater than 0. Thus, when **e** is 0, as it is in the first iteration of the **for** loop, the **while** loop is skipped.

The do-while Loop

The third C# loop is the **do-while**. Unlike the **for** and the **while** loops, in which the condition is tested at the top of the loop, the **do-while** loop checks its condition at the bottom of the loop. This means that a **do-while** loop will always execute at least once. The general form of the **do-while** loop is

> do {
>   *statements*;
> } while(*condition*);

Although the braces are not necessary when only one statement is present, they are often used to improve readability of the **do-while** construct, thus preventing confusion with the **while**. The **do-while** loop executes as long as the conditional expression is true.

The following program uses a **do-while** loop to display the digits of an integer in reverse order:

```
// Display the digits of an integer in reverse order.

using System;

class DoWhileDemo {
  static void Main() {
    int num;
    int nextdigit;

    num = 198;
```

```
    Console.WriteLine("Number: " + num);

    Console.Write("Number in reverse order: ");

    do {
      nextdigit = num % 10;
      Console.Write(nextdigit);
      num = num / 10;
    } while(num > 0);

    Console.WriteLine();
  }
}
```

The output is shown here:

```
Number: 198
Number in reverse order: 891
```

Here is how the loop works: With each iteration, the leftmost digit is obtained by computing the remainder of an integer division by 10. This digit is then displayed. Next, the value in **num** is divided by 10. Since this is an integer division, this results in the leftmost digit being removed. This process repeats until **num** is 0.

The foreach Loop

The **foreach** loop cycles through the elements of a *collection*. A collection is a group of objects. C# defines several types of collections, of which one is an array. The **foreach** loop is examined in Chapter 7, when arrays are discussed.

Using break to Exit a Loop

It is possible to force an immediate exit from a loop, bypassing any code remaining in the body of the loop and the loop's conditional test, by using the **break** statement. When a **break** statement is encountered inside a loop, the loop is terminated, and program control resumes at the next statement following the loop. Here is a simple example:

```
// Using break to exit a loop.

using System;

class BreakDemo {
  static void Main() {

    // Use break to exit this loop.
    for(int i=-10; i <= 10; i++) {
      if(i > 0) break; // terminate loop when i is positive
      Console.Write(i + " ");
    }
    Console.WriteLine("Done");
  }
}
```

This program generates the following output:

```
-10 -9 -8 -7 -6 -5 -4 -3 -2 -1 0 Done
```

As you can see, although the **for** loop is designed to run from –10 to 10, the **break** statement causes it to terminate early, when **i** becomes positive.

The **break** statement can be used with any of C#'s loops. For example, here is the previous program recoded to use a **do-while** loop:

```
// Using break to exit a do-while loop.

using System;

class BreakDemo2 {
  static void Main() {
    int i;

    i = -10;
    do {
      if(i > 0) break;
      Console.Write(i + " ");
      i++;
    } while(i <= 10);

    Console.WriteLine("Done");
  }
}
```

Here is a more practical example of **break**. This program finds the smallest factor of a number.

```
// Find the smallest factor of a value.

using System;

class FindSmallestFactor {
  static void Main() {
    int factor = 1;
    int num = 1000;

    for(int i=2; i <= num/i; i++) {
      if((num%i) == 0) {
        factor = i;
        break; // stop loop when factor is found
      }
    }
    Console.WriteLine("Smallest factor is " + factor);
  }
}
```

The output is shown here:

```
Smallest factor is 2
```

The **break** stops the **for** loop as soon as a factor is found. The use of **break** in this situation prevents the loop from trying any other values once a factor has been found, thus preventing inefficiency.

When used inside a set of nested loops, the **break** statement will break out of only the innermost loop. For example:

```
// Using break with nested loops.

using System;

class BreakNested {
  static void Main() {

    for(int i=0; i<3; i++) {
      Console.WriteLine("Outer loop count: " + i);
      Console.Write("    Inner loop count: ");

      int t = 0;
      while(t < 100) {
        if(t == 10) break; // terminate loop if t is 10
        Console.Write(t + " ");
        t++;
      }
      Console.WriteLine();
    }
    Console.WriteLine("Loops complete.");
  }
}
```

This program generates the following output:

```
Outer loop count: 0
    Inner loop count: 0 1 2 3 4 5 6 7 8 9
Outer loop count: 1
    Inner loop count: 0 1 2 3 4 5 6 7 8 9
Outer loop count: 2
    Inner loop count: 0 1 2 3 4 5 6 7 8 9
Loops complete.
```

As you can see, the **break** statement in the inner loop causes only the termination of that loop. The outer loop is unaffected.

Here are two other points to remember about **break**: First, more than one **break** statement may appear in a loop. However, be careful. Too many **break** statements have the tendency to destructure your code. Second, the **break** that exits a **switch** statement affects only that **switch** statement and not any enclosing loops.

Using continue

It is possible to force an early iteration of a loop, bypassing the loop's normal control structure. This is accomplished using **continue**. The **continue** statement forces the next iteration of the loop to take place, skipping any code in between. Thus, **continue** is essentially the complement of **break**. For example, the following program uses **continue** to help print the even numbers between 0 and 100.

```
// Use continue.

using System;

class ContDemo {
  static void Main() {

    // Print even numbers between 0 and 100.
    for(int i = 0; i <= 100; i++) {
      if((i%2) != 0) continue; // iterate
      Console.WriteLine(i);
    }
  }
}
```

Only even numbers are printed, because an odd number will cause the loop to iterate early, bypassing the call to **WriteLine( )**.

In **while** and **do-while** loops, a **continue** statement will cause control to go directly to the conditional expression and then continue the looping process. In the case of the **for**, the iteration expression of the loop is evaluated, then the conditional expression is executed, and then the loop continues.

Good uses of **continue** are rare. One reason is that C# provides a rich set of loop statements that fit most applications. However, for those special circumstances in which early iteration is needed, the **continue** statement provides a structured way to accomplish it.

return

The **return** statement causes a method to return. It can also be used to return a value. It is examined in Chapter 6.

The goto

The **goto** is C#'s unconditional jump statement. When encountered, program flow jumps to the location specified by the **goto**. The statement fell out of favor with programmers many years ago because it encouraged the creation of "spaghetti code." However, the **goto** is still occasionally—and sometimes effectively—used. This book will not make a judgment regarding its validity as a form of program control. It should be stated, however, that there are no programming situations that require the use of the **goto** statement—it is not necessary for making the language complete. Rather, **goto** is a convenience that, if used wisely, can be a benefit in certain programming situations. As such, the **goto** is not used in this book outside of this section. The chief concern most programmers have about the **goto** is its tendency to clutter a program and render it nearly unreadable. However, there are times when the use of the **goto** can clarify program flow rather than confuse it.

The **goto** requires a label for operation. A *label* is a valid C# identifier followed by a colon. The label must be in the same method as the **goto** that uses it and within scope. For example, a loop from 1 to 100 could be written using a **goto** and a label, as shown here:

```
x = 1;
loop1:
  x++;
  if(x < 100) goto loop1;
```

The **goto** can also be used to jump to a **case** or **default** statement within a **switch**. Technically, the **case** and **default** statements of a **switch** are labels. Thus, they can be targets of a **goto**. However, the **goto** statement must be executed from within the **switch**. That is, you cannot use the **goto** to jump into a **switch** statement. Here is an example that illustrates **goto** with a **switch**:

```
// Use goto with a switch.

using System;

class SwitchGoto {
  static void Main() {

    for(int i=1; i < 5; i++) {
      switch(i) {
        case 1:
          Console.WriteLine("In case 1");
          goto case 3;
        case 2:
          Console.WriteLine("In case 2");
          goto case 1;
        case 3:
          Console.WriteLine("In case 3");
          goto default;
        default:
          Console.WriteLine("In default");
          break;
      }

      Console.WriteLine();
    }

//    goto case 1; // Error! Can't jump into a switch.
  }
}
```

The output from the program is shown here:

```
In case 1
In case 3
In default

In case 2
In case 1
In case 3
In default

In case 3
In default

In default
```

Inside the **switch**, notice how the **goto** is used to jump to other **case** statements or the **default** statement. Furthermore, notice that the **case** statements do not end with a **break**. Since the **goto** prevents one **case** from falling through to the next, the no fall-through rule is not violated, and there is no need for a **break** statement. As explained, it is not possible to use the **goto** to jump into a **switch**. If you remove the comment symbols from the start of this line

```
//    goto case 1; // Error! Can't jump into a switch.
```

the program will not compile. Frankly, using a **goto** with a **switch** can be useful in some special-case situations, but it is not recommended style in general.

One good use for the **goto** is to exit from a deeply nested routine. Here is a simple example:

```
// Demonstrate the goto.

using System;

class Use_goto {
  static void Main() {
    int i=0, j=0, k=0;

    for(i=0; i < 10; i++) {
      for(j=0; j < 10; j++ ) {
        for(k=0; k < 10; k++) {
          Console.WriteLine("i, j, k: " + i + " " + j + " " + k);
          if(k == 3) goto stop;
        }
      }
    }

stop:
    Console.WriteLine("Stopped! i, j, k: " + i + ", " + j + " " + k);

  }
}
```

The output from the program is shown here:

```
i, j, k: 0 0 0
i, j, k: 0 0 1
i, j, k: 0 0 2
i, j, k: 0 0 3
Stopped! i, j, k: 0, 0 3
```

Eliminating the **goto** would force the use of three **if** and **break** statements. In this case, the **goto** simplifies the code. While this is a contrived example used for illustration, you can probably imagine situations in which a **goto** might be beneficial.

One last point: Although you can jump out of a block (as the preceding example shows), you can't use the **goto** to jump into a block.

6

Introducing Classes and Objects

This chapter introduces the class. The class is the foundation of C# because it defines the nature of an object. Furthermore, the class forms the basis for object-oriented programming. Within a class are defined both code and data. Because classes and objects are fundamental to C#, they constitute a large topic, which spans several chapters. This chapter begins the discussion by covering their main features.

Class Fundamentals

We have been using classes since the start of this book. Of course, only extremely simple classes have been used, and we have not taken advantage of the majority of their features. Classes are substantially more powerful than the limited ones presented so far.

Let's begin by reviewing the basics. A *class* is a template that defines the form of an object. It specifies both the data and the code that will operate on that data. C# uses a class specification to construct *objects*. Objects are *instances* of a class. Thus, a class is essentially a set of plans that specify how to build an object. It is important to be clear on one issue: A class is a logical abstraction. It is not until an object of that class has been created that a physical representation of that class exists in memory.

The General Form of a Class

When you define a class, you declare the data that it contains and the code that operates on it. While very simple classes might contain only code or only data, most real-world classes contain both.

In general terms, data is contained in *data members* defined by the class, and code is contained in *function members*. It is important to state at the outset that C# defines several specific flavors of data and function members. For example, data members (also called *fields*) include instance variables and static variables. Function members include methods, constructors, destructors, indexers, events, operators, and properties. For now, we will limit our discussion of the class to its essential elements: instance variables and methods. Later in this chapter constructors and destructors are discussed. The other types of members are described in later chapters.

109

A class is created by use of the keyword **class**. Here is the general form of a simple **class** definition that contains only instance variables and methods:

```
class classname {
    // declare instance variables
    access type var1;
    access type var2;
    // ...
    access type varN;

    // declare methods
    access ret-type method1(parameters) {
        // body of method
    }
    access ret-type method2(parameters) {
        // body of method
    }
    // ...
    access ret-type methodN(parameters) {
        // body of method
    }
}
```

Notice that each variable and method declaration is preceded with *access*. Here, *access* is an access specifier, such as **public**, which specifies how the member can be accessed. As mentioned in Chapter 2, class members can be private to a class or more accessible. The access specifier determines what type of access is allowed. The access specifier is optional, and if absent, then the member is private to the class. Members with private access can be used only by other members of their class. For the examples in this chapter, all members (except for the **Main( )** method) will be specified as **public**, which means that they can be used by all other code—even code defined outside the class. We will return to the topic of access specifiers in Chapter 8.

NOTE *In addition to an access specifier, the declaration of a class member can also contain one or more type modifiers. These modifiers are discussed later in this book.*

Although there is no syntactic rule that enforces it, a well-designed class should define one and only one logical entity. For example, a class that stores names and telephone numbers will not normally also store information about the stock market, average rainfall, sunspot cycles, or other unrelated information. The point here is that a well-designed class groups logically connected information. Putting unrelated information into the same class will quickly destructure your code.

Up to this point, the classes that we have been using have had only one method: **Main( )**. However, notice that the general form of a class does not specify a **Main( )** method. A **Main( )** method is required only if that class is the starting point for your program.

Define a Class

To illustrate classes, we will be evolving a class that encapsulates information about buildings, such as houses, stores, offices, and so on. This class is called **Building**, and it will store three

items of information about a building: the number of floors, the total area, and the number of occupants.

The first version of **Building** is shown here. It defines three instance variables: **Floors, Area**, and **Occupants**. Notice that **Building** does not contain any methods. Thus, it is currently a data-only class. (Subsequent sections will add methods to it.)

```
class Building {
  public int Floors;     // number of floors
  public int Area;       // total square footage of building
  public int Occupants;  // number of occupants
}
```

The instance variables defined by **Building** illustrate the way that instance variables are declared in general. The general form for declaring an instance variable is shown here:

access type var-name;

Here, *access* specifies the access; *type* specifies the type of variable; and *var-name* is the variable's name. Thus, aside from the access specifier, you declare an instance variable in the same way that you declare local variables. For **Building**, the variables are preceded by the **public** access modifier. As explained, this allows them to be accessed by code outside of **Building**.

A **class** definition creates a new data type. In this case, the new data type is called **Building**. You will use this name to declare objects of type **Building**. Remember that a **class** declaration is only a type description; it does not create an actual object. Thus, the preceding code does not cause any objects of type **Building** to come into existence.

To actually create a **Building** object, you will use a statement like the following:

```
Building house = new Building(); // create an object of type building
```

After this statement executes, **house** will be an instance of **Building**. Thus, it will have "physical" reality. For the moment, don't worry about the details of this statement.

Each time you create an instance of a class, you are creating an object that contains its own copy of each instance variable defined by the class. Thus, every **Building** object will contain its own copies of the instance variables **Floors, Area**, and **Occupants**. To access these variables, you will use the member access operator, which is a period. It is commonly referred to as the *dot operator*. The dot operator links the name of an object with the name of a member. The general form of the dot operator is shown here:

object.member

Thus, the *object* is specified on the left, and the *member* is put on the right. For example, to assign the **Floors** variable of **house** the value 2, use the following statement:

```
house.Floors = 2;
```

In general, you can use the dot operator to access both instance variables and methods.

Here is a complete program that uses the **Building** class:

```
// A program that uses the Building class.

using System;
```

```
class Building {
  public int Floors;     // number of floors
  public int Area;       // total square footage of building
  public int Occupants;  // number of occupants
}

// This class declares an object of type Building.
class BuildingDemo {
  static void Main() {
    Building house = new Building(); // create a Building object
    int areaPP; // area per person

    // Assign values to fields in house.
    house.Occupants = 4;
    house.Area = 2500;
    house.Floors = 2;

    // Compute the area per person.
    areaPP = house.Area / house.Occupants;

    Console.WriteLine("house has:\n   " +
                  house.Floors + " floors\n   " +
                  house.Occupants + " occupants\n   " +
                  house.Area + " total area\n   " +
                  areaPP + " area per person");
  }
}
```

This program consists of two classes: **Building** and **BuildingDemo**. Inside **BuildingDemo**, the **Main( )** method creates an instance of **Building** called **house**. Then the code within **Main( )** accesses the instance variables associated with **house**, assigning them values and using those values. It is important to understand that **Building** and **BuildingDemo** are two separate classes. The only relationship they have to each other is that one class creates an instance of the other. Although they are separate classes, code inside **BuildingDemo** can access the members of **Building** because they are declared **public**. If they had not been given the **public** access specifier, their access would have been limited to the **Building** class, and **BuildingDemo** would not have been able to use them.

Assume that you call the preceding file **UseBuilding.cs**. Compiling this program creates a file called **UseBuilding.exe**. Both the **Building** and **BuildingDemo** classes are automatically part of the executable file. The program displays the following output:

```
house has:
  2 floors
  4 occupants
  2500 total area
  625 area per person
```

It is not necessary for the **Building** and the **BuildingDemo** classes to actually be in the same source file. You could put each class in its own file, called **Building.cs** and **BuildingDemo.cs**, for example. Just tell the C# compiler to compile both files and link

them together. For example, you could use this command line to compile the program if you split it into two pieces as just described:

```
csc Building.cs BuildingDemo.cs
```

If you are using the Visual C++ IDE, you will need to add both files to your project and then build.

Before moving on, let's review a fundamental principle: Each object has its own copies of the instance variables defined by its class. Thus, the contents of the variables in one object can differ from the contents of the variables in another. There is no connection between the two objects except for the fact that they are both objects of the same type. For example, if you have two **Building** objects, each has its own copy of **Floors**, **Area**, and **Occupants**, and the contents of these can (and often will) differ between the two objects. The following program demonstrates this fact:

```csharp
// This program creates two Building objects.

using System;

class Building {
  public int Floors;    // number of floors
  public int Area;      // total square footage of building
  public int Occupants; // number of occupants
}

// This class declares two objects of type Building.
class BuildingDemo {
  static void Main() {
    Building house = new Building();
    Building office = new Building();

    int areaPP; // area per person

    // Assign values to fields in house.
    house.Occupants = 4;
    house.Area = 2500;
    house.Floors = 2;

    // Assign values to fields in office.
    office.Occupants = 25;
    office.Area = 4200;
    office.Floors = 3;

    // Compute the area per person in house.
    areaPP = house.Area / house.Occupants;

    Console.WriteLine("house has:\n  " +
                  house.Floors + " floors\n  " +
                  house.Occupants + " occupants\n  " +
                  house.Area + " total area\n  " +
                  areaPP + " area per person");
```

```
        Console.WriteLine();

        // Compute the area per person in office.
        areaPP = office.Area / office.Occupants;

        Console.WriteLine("office has:\n   " +
                          office.Floors + " floors\n   " +
                          office.Occupants + " occupants\n   " +
                          office.Area + " total area\n   " +
                          areaPP + " area per person");
    }
}
```

The output produced by this program is shown here:

```
house has:
  2 floors
  4 occupants
  2500 total area
  625 area per person

office has:
  3 floors
  25 occupants
  4200 total area
  168 area per person
```

As you can see, **house**'s data is completely separate from the data contained in **office**. Figure 6-1 depicts this situation.

How Objects Are Created

In the preceding programs, the following line was used to declare an object of type **Building**:

```
Building house = new Building();
```

This declaration performs three functions. First, it declares a variable called **house** of the class type **Building**. This variable is not, itself, an object. Instead, it is simply a variable that can *refer to* an object. Second, the declaration creates an actual, physical copy of the object.

FIGURE 6-1
One object's instance variables are separate from another's.

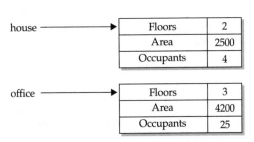

This is done by using the **new** operator. Finally, it assigns to **house** a reference to that object. Thus, after the line executes, **house** refers to an object of type **Building**.

The **new** operator dynamically allocates (that is, allocates at runtime) memory for an object and returns a reference to it. This reference is then stored in a variable. Thus, in C#, all class objects must be dynamically allocated.

As you might expect, it is possible to separate the declaration of **house** from the creation of the object to which it will refer, as shown here:

```
Building house; // declare reference to object
house = new Building(); // allocate a Building object
```

The first line declares **house** as a reference to an object of type **Building**. Thus, **house** is a variable that can refer to an object, but it is not an object, itself. The next line creates a new **Building** object and assigns a reference to it to **house**. Now, **house** is linked with an object.

The fact that class objects are accessed through a reference explains why classes are called *reference types*. The key difference between value types and reference types is what a variable of each type means. For a value type variable, the variable, itself, contains the value. For example, given

```
int x;
x = 10;
```

x contains the value 10 because **x** is a variable of type **int**, which is a value type. However, in the case of

```
Building house = new Building();
```

house does not, itself, contain the object. Instead, it contains a reference to the object.

Reference Variables and Assignment

In an assignment operation, reference variables act differently than do variables of a value type, such as **int**. When you assign one value type variable to another, the situation is straightforward. The variable on the left receives a *copy* of the *value* of the variable on the right. When you assign one object reference variable to another, the situation is a bit more complicated because the assignment causes the reference variable on the left to refer to the same object to which the reference variable on the right refers. The object, itself, is not copied. The effect of this difference can cause some counterintuitive results. For example, consider the following fragment:

```
Building house1 = new Building();
Building house2 = house1;
```

At first glance, it is easy to think that **house1** and **house2** refer to separate and distinct objects, but this is not the case. Instead, **house1** and **house2** will both refer to the *same* object. The assignment of **house1** to **house2** simply makes **house2** refer to the same object that **house1** does. Thus, the object can be acted upon by either **house1** or **house2**. For example, after the assignment

```
house1.Area = 2600;
```

executes, both of these **WriteLine( )** statements

```
Console.WriteLine(house1.Area);
Console.WriteLine(house2.Area);
```

display the same value: 2600.

Although **house1** and **house2** both refer to the same object, they are not linked in any other way. For example, a subsequent assignment to **house2** simply changes what object **house2** refers to. For example:

```
Building house1 = new Building();
Building house2 = house1;
Building house3 = new Building();

house2 = house3; // now house2 and house3 refer to the same object.
```

After this sequence executes, **house2** refers to the same object as **house3**. The object referred to by **house1** is unchanged.

Methods

As explained, instance variables and methods are two of the primary constituents of classes. So far, the **Building** class contains data, but no methods. Although data-only classes are perfectly valid, most classes will have methods. *Methods* are subroutines that manipulate the data defined by the class and, in many cases, provide access to that data. Typically, other parts of your program will interact with a class through its methods.

A method contains one or more statements. In well-written C# code, each method performs only one task. Each method has a name, and it is this name that is used to call the method. In general, you can name a method using any valid identifier that you please. However, remember that **Main( )** is reserved for the method that begins execution of your program. Also, don't use C#'s keywords for method names.

When denoting methods in text, this book has used and will continue to use a convention that has become common when writing about C#. A method will have parentheses after its name. For example, if a method's name is **GetVal**, then it will be written **GetVal( )** when its name is used in a sentence. This notation will help you distinguish variable names from method names in this book.

The general form of a method is shown here:

access ret-type name(parameter-list) {
    // body of method
}

Here, *access* is an access modifier that governs what other parts of your program can call the method. As explained earlier, the access modifier is optional. If not present, then the method is private to the class in which it is declared. For now, we will declare methods as **public** so that they can be called by any other code in the program. The *ret-type* specifies the type of data returned by the method. This can be any valid type, including class types that you create. If the method does not return a value, its return type must be **void**. The name of the method is specified by *name*. This can be any legal identifier other than those that would cause conflicts within the current declaration space. The *parameter-list* is a sequence of type

and identifier pairs separated by commas. Parameters are variables that receive the value of the *arguments* passed to the method when it is called. If the method has no parameters, then the parameter list will be empty.

Add a Method to the Building Class

As just explained, the methods of a class typically manipulate and provide access to the data of the class. With this in mind, recall that **Main( )** in the preceding examples computed the area-per-person by dividing the total area by the number of occupants. Although technically correct, this is not the best way to handle this computation. The calculation of area-per-person is something that is best handled by the **Building** class, itself. The reason for this conclusion is easy to understand: The area-per-person of a building is dependent upon the values in the **Area** and **Occupants** fields, which are encapsulated by **Building**. Thus, it is possible for the **Building** class to perform this calculation on its own. Furthermore, by adding this calculation to **Building**, you prevent each program that uses **Building** from having to perform this calculation manually. This prevents the unnecessary duplication of code. Finally, by adding a method to **Building** that computes the area-per-person, you are enhancing its object-oriented structure by encapsulating the quantities that relate directly to a building inside **Building**.

To add a method to **Building**, specify it within **Building**'s declaration. For example, the following version of **Building** contains a method called **AreaPerPerson( )** that displays the area-per-person for a building:

```
// Add a method to Building.

using System;

class Building {
  public int Floors;    // number of floors
  public int Area;      // total square footage of building
  public int Occupants; // number of occupants

  // Display the area per person.
  public void AreaPerPerson() {
    Console.WriteLine("  " + Area / Occupants + " area per person");
  }
}

// Use the AreaPerPerson() method.
class BuildingDemo {
  static void Main() {
    Building house = new Building();
    Building office = new Building();


    // Assign values to fields in house.
    house.Occupants = 4;
    house.Area = 2500;
    house.Floors = 2;

    // Assign values to fields in office.
    office.Occupants = 25;
```

```
    office.Area = 4200;
    office.Floors = 3;


    Console.WriteLine("house has:\n   " +
                      house.Floors + " floors\n   " +
                      house.Occupants + " occupants\n   " +
                      house.Area + " total area");
    house.AreaPerPerson();

    Console.WriteLine();

    Console.WriteLine("office has:\n   " +
                      office.Floors + " floors\n   " +
                      office.Occupants + " occupants\n   " +
                      office.Area + " total area");
    office.AreaPerPerson();
  }
}
```

This program generates the following output, which is the same as before:

```
house has:
  2 floors
  4 occupants
  2500 total area
  625 area per person

office has:
  3 floors
  25 occupants
  4200 total area
  168 area per person
```

Let's look at the key elements of this program, beginning with the **AreaPerPerson( )** method, itself. The first line of **AreaPerPerson( )** is

```
public void AreaPerPerson() {
```

This line declares a method called **AreaPerPerson** that has no parameters. It is specified as **public**, so it can be used by all other parts of the program. Its return type is **void**. Thus, **AreaPerPerson( )** does not return a value to the caller. The line ends with the opening curly brace of the method body.

The body of **AreaPerPerson( )** consists solely of this statement:

```
Console.WriteLine("   " + Area / Occupants + " area per person");
```

This statement displays the area-per-person of a building by dividing **Area** by **Occupants**. Since each object of type **Building** has its own copy of **Area** and **Occupants**, when **AreaPerPerson( )** is called, the computation uses the calling object's copies of those variables.

The **AreaPerPerson( )** method ends when its closing curly brace is encountered. This causes program control to transfer back to the caller.

Next, look closely at this line of code from inside **Main( )**:

```
house.AreaPerPerson();
```

This statement invokes the **AreaPerPerson( )** method on **house**. That is, it calls **AreaPerPerson( )** relative to the object referred to by **house**, by use of the dot operator. When a method is called, program control is transferred to the method. When the method terminates, control is transferred back to the caller, and execution resumes with the line of code following the call.

In this case, the call to **house.AreaPerPerson( )** displays the area-per-person of the building defined by **house**. In similar fashion, the call to **office.AreaPerPerson( )** displays the area-per-person of the building defined by **office**. Each time **AreaPerPerson( )** is invoked, it displays the area-per-person for the specified object.

There is something very important to notice inside the **AreaPerPerson( )** method: The instance variables **Area** and **Occupants** are referred to directly, without use of the dot operator. When a method uses an instance variable that is defined by its class, it does so directly, without explicit reference to an object and without use of the dot operator. This is easy to understand if you think about it. A method is always invoked relative to some object of its class. Once this invocation has occurred, the object is known. Thus, within a method, there is no need to specify the object a second time. This means that **Area** and **Occupants** inside **AreaPerPerson( )** implicitly refer to the copies of those variables found in the object that invokes **AreaPerPerson( )**.

NOTE *As a point of interest, in the* **AreaPerPerson()** *method,* **Occupants** *must not equal zero (which it won't for all of the examples in this chapter). If* **Occupants** *were zero, then a division-by-zero error would occur. In Chapter 13, you will learn about exceptions, which are C#'s approach to handling errors, and see how to watch for errors that can occur at runtime.*

Return from a Method

In general, there are two conditions that cause a method to return. The first, as the **AreaPerPerson( )** method in the preceding example shows, is when the method's closing curly brace is encountered. The second is when a **return** statement is executed. There are two forms of **return**: one for use in **void** methods (those that do not return a value) and one for returning values. The first form is examined here. The next section explains how to return values.

In a **void** method, you can cause the immediate termination of a method by using this form of **return**:

```
return ;
```

When this statement executes, program control returns to the caller, skipping any remaining code in the method. For example, consider this method:

```
public void MyMeth() {
  int i;

  for(i=0; i<10; i++) {
    if(i == 5) return; // stop at 5
    Console.WriteLine();
  }
}
```

Here, the **for** loop will only run from 0 to 5, because once **i** equals 5, the method returns.

It is permissible to have multiple **return** statements in a method, especially when there are two or more routes out of it. For example,

```
public void MyMeth() {
  // ...
  if(done) return;
  // ...
  if(error) return;
}
```

Here, the method returns if it is done or if an error occurs. Be careful, however. Having too many exit points in a method can destructure your code, so avoid using them casually.

To review: A **void** method can return in one of two ways—its closing curly brace is reached, or a **return** statement is executed.

Return a Value

Although methods with a return type of **void** are not rare, most methods will return a value. In fact, the ability to return a value is one of a method's most useful features. You have already seen an example of a return value when we used the **Math.Sqrt( )** function in Chapter 3 to obtain a square root.

Return values are used for a variety of purposes in programming. In some cases, such as with **Math.Sqrt( )**, the return value contains the outcome of some calculation. In other cases, the return value may simply indicate success or failure. In still others, it may contain a status code. Whatever the purpose, using method return values is an integral part of C# programming.

Methods return a value to the calling routine using this form of **return**:

return *value*;

Here, *value* is the value returned.

You can use a return value to improve the implementation of **AreaPerPerson( )**. Instead of displaying the area-per-person, a better approach is to have **AreaPerPerson( )** return this value. Among the advantages to this approach is that you can use the value for other calculations. The following example modifies **AreaPerPerson( )** to return the area-per-person rather than displaying it:

```
// Return a value from AreaPerPerson().

using System;

class Building {
  public int Floors;    // number of floors
  public int Area;      // total square footage of building
  public int Occupants; // number of occupants

  // Return the area per person.
  public int AreaPerPerson() {
    return Area / Occupants;
  }
}
```

```
// Use the return value from AreaPerPerson().
class BuildingDemo {
  static void Main() {
    Building house = new Building();
    Building office = new Building();
    int areaPP; // area per person

    // Assign values to fields in house.
    house.Occupants = 4;
    house.Area = 2500;
    house.Floors = 2;

    // Assign values to fields in office.
    office.Occupants = 25;
    office.Area = 4200;
    office.Floors = 3;

    // Obtain area per person for house.
    areaPP = house.AreaPerPerson();

    Console.WriteLine("house has:\n  " +
                house.Floors + " floors\n  " +
                house.Occupants + " occupants\n  " +
                house.Area + " total area\n  " +
                areaPP + " area per person");


    Console.WriteLine();

    // Obtain area per person for office.
    areaPP = office.AreaPerPerson();

    Console.WriteLine("office has:\n  " +
                office.Floors + " floors\n  " +
                office.Occupants + " occupants\n  " +
                office.Area + " total area\n  " +
                areaPP + " area per person");
  }
}
```

The output is the same as shown earlier.

In the program, notice that when **AreaPerPerson( )** is called, it is put on the right side of an assignment statement. On the left is a variable that will receive the value returned by **AreaPerPerson( )**. Thus, after

```
areaPP = house.AreaPerPerson();
```

executes, the area-per-person of the **house** object is stored in **areaPP**.

Notice that **AreaPerPerson( )** now has a return type of **int**. This means that it will return an integer value to the caller. The return type of a method is important because the type of data returned by a method must be compatible with the return type specified by the method. Thus, if you want a method to return data of type **double**, then its return type must be type **double**.

Although the preceding program is correct, it is not written as efficiently as it could be. Specifically, there is no need for the **areaPP** variable. A call to **AreaPerPerson( )** can be used in the **WriteLine( )** statement directly, as shown here:

```
Console.WriteLine("house has:\n   " +
                  house.Floors + " floors\n   " +
                  house.Occupants + " occupants\n   " +
                  house.Area + " total area\n   " +
                  house.AreaPerPerson() + " area per person");
```

In this case, when **WriteLine( )** is executed, **house.AreaPerPerson( )** is called automatically, and its value will be passed to **WriteLine( )**. Furthermore, you can use a call to **AreaPerPerson( )** whenever the area-per-person of a **Building** object is needed. For example, this statement compares the per-person areas of two buildings:

```
if(b1.AreaPerPerson() > b2.AreaPerPerson())
  Console.WriteLine("b1 has more space for each person");
```

Use Parameters

It is possible to pass one or more values to a method when the method is called. A value passed to a method is called an *argument.* Inside the method, the variable that receives the argument is called a *formal parameter,* or just *parameter,* for short. Parameters are declared inside the parentheses that follow the method's name. The parameter declaration syntax is the same as that used for variables. The scope of a parameter is the body of its method. Aside from its special task of receiving an argument, it acts like any other local variable.

Here is a simple example that uses a parameter. Inside the **ChkNum** class, the method **IsPrime( )** returns **true** if the value that it is passed is prime. It returns **false** otherwise. Therefore, **IsPrime( )** has a return type of **bool**.

```
// A simple example that uses a parameter.

using System;

class ChkNum {
  // Return true if x is prime.
  public bool IsPrime(int x) {
    if(x <= 1) return false;

    for(int i=2; i <= x/i; i++)
      if((x %i) == 0) return false;

    return true;
  }
}

class ParmDemo {
  static void Main() {
    ChkNum ob = new ChkNum();

    for(int i=2; i < 10; i++)
      if(ob.IsPrime(i)) Console.WriteLine(i + " is prime.");
```

```
   else Console.WriteLine(i + " is not prime.");
  }
}
```

Here is the output produced by the program:

```
2 is prime.
3 is prime.
4 is not prime.
5 is prime.
6 is not prime.
7 is prime.
8 is not prime.
9 is not prime.
```

In the program, **IsPrime( )** is called nine times, and each time a different value is passed. Let's look at this process closely. First, notice how **IsPrime( )** is called. The argument is specified between the parentheses. When **IsPrime( )** is called the first time, it is passed value 1. Thus, when **IsPrime( )** begins executing, the parameter **x** receives the value 1. In the second call, 2 is the argument, and **x** then has the value 2. In the third call, the argument is 3, which is the value that **x** receives, and so on. The point is that the value passed as an argument when **IsPrime( )** is called is the value received by its parameter, **x**.

A method can have more than one parameter. Simply declare each parameter, separating one from the next with a comma. For example, here the **ChkNum** class is expanded by adding a method called **LeastComFactor( )**, which returns the smallest factor that its two arguments have in common. In other words, it returns the smallest whole number value that can evenly divide both arguments.

```
// Add a method that takes two arguments.

using System;

class ChkNum {
  // Return true if x is prime.
  public bool IsPrime(int x) {
    if(x <= 1) return false;

    for(int i=2; i <= x/i; i++)
      if((x %i) == 0) return false;

    return true;
  }

  // Return the least common factor.
  public int LeastComFactor(int a, int b) {
    int max;

    if(IsPrime(a) || IsPrime(b)) return 1;

    max = a < b ? a : b;

    for(int i=2; i <= max/2; i++)
      if(((a%i) == 0) && ((b%i) == 0)) return i;
```

```
      return 1;
    }
  }

class ParmDemo {
  static void Main() {
    ChkNum ob = new ChkNum();
    int a, b;

    for(int i=2; i < 10; i++)
      if(ob.IsPrime(i)) Console.WriteLine(i + " is prime.");
      else Console.WriteLine(i + " is not prime.");

    a = 7;
    b = 8;
    Console.WriteLine("Least common factor for " +
                      a + " and " + b + " is " +
                      ob.LeastComFactor(a, b));

    a = 100;
    b = 8;
    Console.WriteLine("Least common factor for " +
                      a + " and " + b + " is " +
                      ob.LeastComFactor(a, b));

    a = 100;
    b = 75;
    Console.WriteLine("Least common factor for " +
                      a + " and " + b + " is " +
                      ob.LeastComFactor(a, b));

  }
}
```

Notice that when **LeastComFactor( )** is called, the arguments are also separated by commas. The output from the program is shown here:

```
2 is prime.
3 is prime.
4 is not prime.
5 is prime.
6 is not prime.
7 is prime.
8 is not prime.
9 is not prime.
Least common factor for 7 and 8 is 1
Least common factor for 100 and 8 is 2
Least common factor for 100 and 75 is 5
```

When using multiple parameters, each parameter specifies its own type, which can differ from the others. For example, this is perfectly valid:

```
int MyMeth(int a, double b, float c) {
  // ...
```

Add a Parameterized Method to Building

You can use a parameterized method to add a new feature to the **Building** class: the ability to compute the maximum number of occupants for a building assuming that each occupant must have a certain minimal space. This new method is called **MaxOccupant( )**. It is shown here:

```
// Return the maximum number of occupants if each
// is to have at least the specified minimum area.
public int MaxOccupant(int minArea) {
  return Area / minArea;
}
```

When **MaxOccupant( )** is called, the parameter **minArea** receives the minimum space needed for each occupant. The method divides the total area of the building by this value and returns the result.

The entire **Building** class that includes **MaxOccupant( )** is shown here:

```
/*
   Add a parameterized method that computes the
   maximum number of people that can occupy a
   building assuming each needs a specified
   minimum space.
*/

using System;

class Building {
  public int Floors;     // number of floors
  public int Area;       // total square footage of building
  public int Occupants; // number of occupants

  // Return the area per person.
  public int AreaPerPerson() {
    return Area / Occupants;
  }

  // Return the maximum number of occupants if each
  // is to have at least the specified minimum area.
  public int MaxOccupant(int minArea) {
    return Area / minArea;
  }
}

// Use MaxOccupant().
class BuildingDemo {
  static void Main() {
    Building house = new Building();
    Building office = new Building();

    // Assign values to fields in house.
    house.Occupants = 4;
    house.Area = 2500;
    house.Floors = 2;
```

```
// Assign values to fields in office.
office.Occupants = 25;
office.Area = 4200;
office.Floors = 3;

Console.WriteLine("Maximum occupants for house if each has " +
                  300 + " square feet: " +
                  house.MaxOccupant(300));

Console.WriteLine("Maximum occupants for office if each has " +
                  300 + " square feet: " +
                  office.MaxOccupant(300));
  }
}
```

The output from the program is shown here:

```
Maximum occupants for house if each has 300 square feet: 8
Maximum occupants for office if each has 300 square feet: 14
```

Avoiding Unreachable Code

When creating methods, you should avoid causing a situation in which a portion of code cannot, under any circumstances, be executed. This is called *unreachable code,* and it is considered incorrect in C#. The compiler will issue a warning message if you create a method that contains unreachable code. For example:

```
public void MyMeth() {
  char a, b;

  // ...

  if(a==b) {
    Console.WriteLine("equal");
    return;
  } else {
    Console.WriteLine("not equal");
    return;
  }
  Console.WriteLine("this is unreachable");
}
```

Here, the method **MyMeth( )** will always return before the final **WriteLine( )** statement is executed. If you try to compile this method, you will receive a warning. In general, unreachable code constitutes a mistake on your part, so it is a good idea to take unreachable code warnings seriously.

Constructors

In the preceding examples, the instance variables of each **Building** object had to be set manually using a sequence of statements, such as

```
house.Occupants = 4;
house.Area = 2500;
house.Floors = 2;
```

An approach like this would never be used in professionally written C# code. Aside from this approach being error prone (you might forget to set one of the fields), there is simply a better way to accomplish this task: the constructor.

A *constructor* initializes an object when it is created. It has the same name as its class and is syntactically similar to a method. However, constructors have no explicit return type. The general form of a constructor is shown here:

> *access class-name(param-list)* {
>   // constructor code
> }

Typically, you will use a constructor to give initial values to the instance variables defined by the class or to perform any other startup procedures required to create a fully formed object. Also, usually, *access* is **public** because constructors are normally called from outside their class. The *param-list* can be empty, or it can specify one or more parameters.

All classes have constructors, whether you define one or not, because C# automatically provides a default constructor that causes all member variables to be initialized to their default values. For most value types, the default value is zero. For **bool**, the default is **false**. For reference types, the default is null. However, once you define your own constructor, the default constructor is no longer used.

Here is a simple example that uses a constructor:

```
// A simple constructor.

using System;

class MyClass {
  public int x;

  public MyClass() {
    x = 10;
  }
}

class ConsDemo {
  static void Main() {
    MyClass t1 = new MyClass();
    MyClass t2 = new MyClass();

    Console.WriteLine(t1.x + " " + t2.x);
  }
}
```

In this example, the constructor for **MyClass** is

```
public MyClass() {
  x = 10;
}
```

Notice that the constructor is specified as **public**. This is because the constructor will be called from code defined outside of its class. This constructor assigns the instance variable **x** of **MyClass** the value 10. This constructor is called by **new** when an object is created. For example, in the line

```
MyClass t1 = new MyClass();
```

the constructor **MyClass( )** is called on the **t1** object, giving **t1.x** the value 10. The same is true for **t2**. After construction, **t2.x** has the value 10. Thus, the output from the program is

```
10 10
```

Parameterized Constructors

In the preceding example, a parameterless constructor was used. While this is fine for some situations, most often you will need a constructor that accepts one or more parameters. Parameters are added to a constructor in the same way they are added to a method: just declare them inside the parentheses after the constructor's name. For example, here **MyClass** is given a parameterized constructor:

```
// A parameterized constructor.

using System;

class MyClass {
  public int x;

  public MyClass(int i) {
    x = i;
  }
}

class ParmConsDemo {
  static void Main() {
    MyClass t1 = new MyClass(10);
    MyClass t2 = new MyClass(88);

    Console.WriteLine(t1.x + " " + t2.x);
  }
}
```

The output from this program is shown here:

```
10 88
```

In this version of the program, the **MyClass( )** constructor defines one parameter called **i**, which is used to initialize the instance variable, **x**. Thus, when the line

```
MyClass t1 = new MyClass(10);
```

executes, the value 10 is passed to **i**, which is then assigned to **x**.

Add a Constructor to the Building Class

We can improve the **Building** class by adding a constructor that automatically initializes the
Floors, Area, and **Occupants** fields when an object is constructed. Pay special attention to
how **Building** objects are created.

```
// Add a constructor to Building.

using System;

class Building {
  public int Floors;    // number of floors
  public int Area;      // total square footage of building
  public int Occupants; // number of occupants

  // A parameterized constructor for Building.
  public Building(int f, int a, int o) {
    Floors = f;
    Area = a;
    Occupants = o;
  }

  // Display the area per person.
  public int AreaPerPerson() {
    return Area / Occupants;
  }

  // Return the maximum number of occupants if each
  // is to have at least the specified minimum area.
  public int MaxOccupant(int minArea) {
    return Area / minArea;
  }
}

// Use the parameterized Building constructor.
class BuildingDemo {
  static void Main() {
    Building house = new Building(2, 2500, 4);
    Building office = new Building(3, 4200, 25);

    Console.WriteLine("Maximum occupants for house if each has " +
                      300 + " square feet: " +
                      house.MaxOccupant(300));

    Console.WriteLine("Maximum occupants for office if each has " +
                      300 + " square feet: " +
                      office.MaxOccupant(300));
  }
}
```

The output from this program is the same as for the previous version.

Both **house** and **office** were initialized by the **Building( )** constructor when they were created. Each object is initialized as specified in the parameters to its constructor. For example, in the following line,

```
Building house = new Building(2, 2500, 4);
```

the values 2, 2500, and 4 are passed to the **Building( )** constructor when **new** creates the object. Thus, **house**'s copy of **Floors**, **Area**, and **Occupants** will contain the values 2, 2500, and 4, respectively.

The new Operator Revisited

Now that you know more about classes and their constructors, let's take a closer look at the **new** operator. As it relates to classes, the **new** operator has this general form:

new *class-name*(*arg-list*)

Here, *class-name* is the name of the class that is being instantiated. The class name followed by parentheses specifies the constructor for the class. If a class does not define its own constructor, **new** will use the default constructor supplied by C#. Thus, **new** can be used to create an object of any class type.

Since memory is finite, it is possible that **new** will not be able to allocate memory for an object because insufficient memory exists. If this happens, a runtime exception will occur. (You will learn how to handle exceptions in Chapter 13.) For the sample programs in this book, you won't need to worry about running out of memory, but you may need to consider this possibility in real-world programs that you write.

Using new with Value Types

At this point, you might be asking why you don't need to use **new** for variables of the value types, such as **int** or **float**? In C#, a variable of a value type contains its own value. Memory to hold this value is automatically provided when the program is run. Thus, there is no need to explicitly allocate this memory using **new**. Conversely, a reference variable stores a reference to an object. The memory to hold this object must be allocated dynamically, during execution.

Not making the fundamental types, such **int** or **char**, into reference types greatly improves your program's performance. When using a reference type, there is a layer of indirection that adds overhead to each object access. This layer of indirection is avoided by a value type.

As a point of interest, it is permitted to use **new** with the value types, as shown here:

```
int i = new int();
```

Doing so invokes the default constructor for type **int**, which initializes **i** to zero. For example:

```
// Use new with a value type.

using System;

class newValue {
  static void Main() {
    int i = new int(); // initialize i to zero
```

```
      Console.WriteLine("The value of i is: " + i);
   }
}
```

The output from this program is

```
The value of i is: 0
```

As the output verifies, **i** is initialized to zero. Remember, without the use of **new**, **i** would be uninitialized, and it would cause an error to attempt to use it in the **WriteLine( )** statement without explicitly giving it a value first.

In general, invoking **new** for a value type invokes the default constructor for that type. It does not, however, dynamically allocate memory. Frankly, most programmers do not use **new** with the value types.

Garbage Collection and Destructors

As you have seen, objects are dynamically allocated from a pool of free memory by using the **new** operator. Of course, memory is not infinite, and the free memory can be exhausted. Thus, it is possible for **new** to fail because there is insufficient free memory to create the desired object. For this reason, one of the key components of any dynamic allocation scheme is the recovery of free memory from unused objects, making that memory available for subsequent reallocation. In many programming languages, the release of previously allocated memory is handled manually. For example, in C++, the **delete** operator is used to free memory that was allocated. However, C# uses a different, more trouble-free approach: *garbage collection.*

C#'s garbage collection system reclaims objects automatically—occurring transparently, behind the scenes, without any programmer intervention. It works like this: When no references to an object exist, that object is assumed to be no longer needed, and the memory occupied by the object is eventually released and collected. This recycled memory can then be used for a subsequent allocation.

Garbage collection occurs only sporadically during the execution of your program. It will not occur simply because one or more objects exist that are no longer used. Thus, you can't know, or make assumptions about, precisely when garbage collection will take place.

Destructors

It is possible to define a method that will be called just prior to an object's final destruction by the garbage collector. This method is called a *destructor*, and it can be used in some highly specialized situations to ensure that an object terminates cleanly. For example, you might use a destructor to ensure that a system resource owned by an object is released. It must be stated at the outset that destructors are a very advanced feature that are applicable only to certain rare cases. They are not normally needed. They are briefly described here for completeness.

Destructors have this general form:

~class-name( ) {
    // destruction code
}

Here, *class-name* is the name of the class. Thus, a destructor is declared like a constructor except that it is preceded with a ~ (tilde). Notice it has no return type and takes no arguments.

To add a destructor to a class, you simply include it as a member. It is called whenever an object of its class is about to be recycled. Inside the destructor, you will specify those actions that must be performed before an object is destroyed.

It is important to understand that the destructor is called just prior to garbage collection. It is not called when a variable containing a reference to an object goes out of scope, for example. (This differs from destructors in C++, which *are* called when an object goes out of scope.) This means that you cannot know precisely when a destructor will be executed. Furthermore, it is possible for your program to end before garbage collection occurs, so a destructor might not get called at all.

The following program demonstrates a destructor. It works by creating and destroying a large number of objects. During this process, at some point the garbage collector will be activated, and the destructors for the objects will be called.

```csharp
// Demonstrate a destructor.

using System;

class Destruct {
  public int x;

  public Destruct(int i) {
    x = i;
  }

  // Called when object is recycled.
  ~Destruct() {
    Console.WriteLine("Destructing " + x);
  }

  // Generates an object that is immediately destroyed.
  public void Generator(int i) {
    Destruct o = new Destruct(i);
  }

}

class DestructDemo {
  static void Main() {
    int count;

    Destruct ob = new Destruct(0);

    /* Now, generate a large number of objects. At
       some point, garbage collection will occur.
       Note: You might need to increase the number
       of objects generated in order to force
       garbage collection. */

    for(count=1; count < 100000; count++)
```

```
      ob.Generator(count);

    Console.WriteLine("Done");
  }
}
```

Here is how the program works. The constructor sets the instance variable **x** to a known value. In this example, **x** is used as an object ID. The destructor displays the value of **x** when an object is recycled. Of special interest is **Generator( )**. This method creates and then promptly destroys a **Destruct** object. The **DestructDemo** class creates an initial **Destruct** object called **ob**. Then using **ob**, it creates 100,000 objects by calling **Generator( )** on **ob**. This has the net effect of creating and destroying 100,000 objects. At various points in the middle of this process, garbage collection will take place. Precisely how often or when is dependent upon several factors, such as the initial amount of free memory, the operating system, and so on. However, at some point, you will start to see the messages generated by the destructor. If you don't see the messages prior to program termination (that is, before you see the "Done" message), try increasing the number of objects being generated by upping the count in the **for** loop.

One important point: The call to **WriteLine( )** inside **~Destruct( )** is purely for the sake of illustration in this rather contrived example. Normally, a destructor should act only on the instance variables defined by its class.

Because of the nondeterministic way in which destructors are called, they should not be used to perform actions that must occur at a specific point in your program. One other point: It is possible to request garbage collection. This is described in Part II, when C#'s class library is discussed. However, manually initiating garbage collection is not recommended for most circumstances, because it can lead to inefficiencies. Also, because of the way the garbage collector works, even if you explicitly request garbage collection, there is no way to know precisely when a specific object will be recycled.

The this Keyword

Before concluding this chapter, it is necessary to introduce **this**. When a method is called, it is automatically passed a reference to the invoking object (that is, the object on which the method is called). This reference is called **this**. Therefore, **this** refers to the object on which the method is acting. To understand **this**, first consider a program that creates a class called **Rect** that encapsulates the width and height of a rectangle and that includes a method called **Area( )** that returns its area.

```
using System;

class Rect {
  public int Width;
  public int Height;

  public Rect(int w, int h) {
    Width = w;
    Height = h;
  }

  public int Area() {
```

```
      return Width * Height;
   }
}

class UseRect {
  static void Main() {
    Rect r1 = new Rect(4, 5);
    Rect r2 = new Rect(7, 9);

    Console.WriteLine("Area of r1: " + r1.Area());

    Console.WriteLine("Area of r2: " + r2.Area());
  }
}
```

As you know, within a method, the other members of a class can be accessed directly, without any object or class qualification. Thus, inside **Area( )**, the statement

```
return Width * Height;
```

means that the copies of **Width** and **Height** associated with the invoking object will be multiplied together and the result returned. However, the same statement can also be written like this:

```
return this.Width * this.Height;
```

Here, **this** refers to the object on which **Area( )** was called. Thus, **this.Width** refers to that object's copy of **Width**, and **this.Height** refers to that object's copy of **Height**. For example, if **Area( )** had been invoked on an object called **x**, then **this** in the preceding statement would have been referring to **x**. Writing the statement without using **this** is really just shorthand.

It is also possible to use **this** inside a constructor. In this case, **this** refers to the object that is being constructed. For example, inside **Rect( )**, the statements

```
Width = w;
Height = h;
```

can be written like this:

```
this.Width = w;
this.Height = h;
```

Of course, there is no benefit in doing so in this case.

For the sake of illustration, here is the entire **Rect** class written using the **this** reference:

```
using System;

class Rect {
  public int Width;
  public int Height;

  public Rect(int w, int h) {
```

```
      this.Width = w;
      this.Height = h;
   }

   public int Area() {
     return this.Width * this.Height;
   }
}

class UseRect {
   static void Main() {
     Rect r1 = new Rect(4, 5);
     Rect r2 = new Rect(7, 9);

     Console.WriteLine("Area of r1: " + r1.Area());

     Console.WriteLine("Area of r2: " + r2.Area());

   }
}
```

Actually, no C# programmer would use **this** as just shown because nothing is gained and the standard form is easier. However, **this** has some important uses. For example, the C# syntax permits the name of a parameter or a local variable to be the same as the name of an instance variable. When this happens, the local name *hides* the instance variable. You can gain access to the hidden instance variable by referring to it through **this**. For example, the following is a syntactically valid way to write the **Rect( )** constructor:

```
public Rect(int Width, int Height) {
   this.Width = Width;
   this.Height = Height;
}
```

In this version, the names of the parameters are the same as the names of the instance variables, thus hiding them. However, **this** is used to "uncover" the instance variables.

Arrays and Strings

This chapter returns to the subject of C#'s data types. It discusses arrays and the **string** type. The **foreach** loop is also examined.

Arrays

An *array* is a collection of variables of the same type that are referred to by a common name. In C#, arrays can have one or more dimensions, although the one-dimensional array is the most common. Arrays are used for a variety of purposes because they offer a convenient means of grouping together related variables. For example, you might use an array to hold a record of the daily high temperature for a month, a list of stock prices, or your collection of programming books.

The principal advantage of an array is that it organizes data in such a way that it can be easily manipulated. For example, if you have an array containing the dividends for a selected group of stocks, it is easy to compute the average income by cycling through the array. Also, arrays organize data in such a way that it can be easily sorted.

Although arrays in C# can be used just like arrays in many other programming languages, they have one special attribute: They are implemented as objects. This fact is one reason that a discussion of arrays was deferred until objects had been introduced. By implementing arrays as objects, several important advantages are gained, not the least of which is that unused arrays can be garbage-collected.

One-Dimensional Arrays

A *one-dimensional array* is a list of related variables. Such lists are common in programming. For example, you might use a one-dimensional array to store the account numbers of the active users on a network. Another array might store the current batting averages for a baseball team.

Because arrays in C# are implemented as objects, two steps are needed to obtain an array for use in your program. First, you must declare a variable that can refer to an array. Second, you must create an instance of the array by use of **new**. Therefore, to declare a one-dimensional array, you will typically use this general form:

type[ ] *array-name* = new *type*[*size*];

Here, *type* declares the *element type* of the array. The element type determines the data type of each element that comprises the array. Notice the square brackets that follow *type*. They indicate that a one-dimensional array is being declared. The number of elements that the array will hold is determined by *size*.

NOTE *If you come from a C or C++ background, pay special attention to the way arrays are declared. Specifically, the square brackets follow the type name, not the array name.*

Here is an example. The following creates an **int** array of ten elements and links it to an array reference variable named **sample**.

```
int[] sample = new int[10];
```

The **sample** variable holds a reference to the memory allocated by **new**. This memory is large enough to hold ten elements of type **int**.

As is the case when creating an instance of a class, it is possible to break the preceding declaration in two. For example:

```
int[] sample;
sample = new int[10];
```

In this case, when **sample** is first created, it refers to no physical object. It is only after the second statement executes that **sample** refers to an array.

An individual element within an array is accessed by use of an index. An *index* describes the position of an element within an array. In C#, all arrays have 0 as the index of their first element. Because **sample** has 10 elements, it has index values of 0 through 9. To index an array, specify the number of the element you want, surrounded by square brackets. Thus, the first element in **sample** is **sample[0]**, and the last element is **sample[9]**. For example, the following program loads **sample** with the numbers 0 through 9:

```
// Demonstrate a one-dimensional array.

using System;

class ArrayDemo {
  static void Main() {
    int[] sample = new int[10];
    int i;

    for(i = 0; i < 10; i = i+1)
      sample[i] = i;

    for(i = 0; i < 10; i = i+1)
      Console.WriteLine("sample[" + i + "]: " + sample[i]);
  }
}
```

The output from the program is shown here:

```
sample[0]: 0
sample[1]: 1
sample[2]: 2
```

```
sample[3]:  3
sample[4]:  4
sample[5]:  5
sample[6]:  6
sample[7]:  7
sample[8]:  8
sample[9]:  9
```

Conceptually, the **sample** array looks like this:

0	1	2	3	4	5	6	7	8	9
sample [0]	sample [1]	sample [2]	sample [3]	sample [4]	sample [5]	sample [6]	sample [7]	sample [8]	sample [9]

Arrays are common in programming because they let you deal easily with large numbers of related variables. For example, the following program finds the average of the set of values stored in the **nums** array by cycling through the array using a **for** loop:

```
// Compute the average of a set of values.

using System;

class Average {
  static void Main() {
    int[] nums = new int[10];
    int avg = 0;

    nums[0] = 99;
    nums[1] = 10;
    nums[2] = 100;
    nums[3] = 18;
    nums[4] = 78;
    nums[5] = 23;
    nums[6] = 63;
    nums[7] = 9;
    nums[8] = 87;
    nums[9] = 49;

    for(int i=0; i < 10; i++)
      avg = avg + nums[i];

    avg = avg / 10;

    Console.WriteLine("Average: " + avg);
  }
}
```

The output from the program is shown here:

```
Average: 53
```

Initializing an Array

In the preceding program, the **nums** array was given values by hand, using ten separate assignment statements. While that is perfectly correct, there is an easier way to accomplish this. Arrays can be initialized when they are created. The general form for initializing a one-dimensional array is shown here:

type[ ] *array-name* = { *val1, val2, val3, ..., valN* };

Here, the initial values are specified by *val1* through *valN*. They are assigned in sequence, left to right, in index order. C# automatically allocates an array large enough to hold the initializers that you specify. There is no need to use the **new** operator explicitly. For example, here is a better way to write the **Average** program:

```
// Compute the average of a set of values.

using System;

class Average {
  static void Main() {
    int[] nums = { 99, 10, 100, 18, 78, 23,
                   63, 9, 87, 49 };
    int avg = 0;

    for(int i=0; i < 10; i++)
      avg = avg + nums[i];

    avg = avg / 10;

    Console.WriteLine("Average: " + avg);
  }
}
```

As a point of interest, although not needed, you can use **new** when initializing an array. For example, this is a proper, but redundant, way to initialize **nums** in the foregoing program:

```
int[] nums = new int[] { 99, 10, 100, 18, 78, 23,
                         63, 9, 87, 49 };
```

Although redundant here, the **new** form of array initialization is useful when you are assigning a new array to an already-existent array reference variable. For example:

```
int[] nums;
nums = new int[] { 99, 10, 100, 18, 78, 23,
                   63, 9, 87, 49 };
```

In this case, **nums** is declared in the first statement and initialized by the second.

One last point: It is permissible to specify the array size explicitly when initializing an array, but the size must agree with the number of initializers. For example, here is another way to initialize **nums**:

```
int[] nums = new int[10] { 99, 10, 100, 18, 78, 23,
                           63, 9, 87, 49 };
```

In this declaration, the size of **nums** is explicitly stated as 10.

Boundaries Are Enforced

Array boundaries are strictly enforced in C#; it is a runtime error to overrun or underrun the ends of an array. If you want to confirm this for yourself, try the following program that purposely overruns an array:

```
// Demonstrate an array overrun.

using System;

class ArrayErr {
  static void Main() {
    int[] sample = new int[10];
    int i;

    // Generate an array overrun.
    for(i = 0; i < 100; i = i+1)
      sample[i] = i;
  }
}
```

As soon as **i** reaches 10, an **IndexOutOfRangeException** is generated and the program is terminated. (See Chapter 13 for a discussion of exceptions and exception handling.)

Multidimensional Arrays

Although the one-dimensional array is the most commonly used array in programming, multidimensional arrays are certainly not rare. A *multidimensional array* is an array that has two or more dimensions, and an individual element is accessed through the combination of two or more indices.

Two-Dimensional Arrays

The simplest form of the multidimensional array is the two-dimensional array. In a two-dimensional array, the location of any specific element is specified by two indices. If you think of a two-dimensional array as a table of information, one index indicates the row, the other indicates the column.

To declare a two-dimensional integer array **table** of size 10, 20, you would write

```
int[,] table = new int[10, 20];
```

Pay careful attention to the declaration. Notice that the two dimensions are separated from each other by a comma. In the first part of the declaration, the syntax

```
[,]
```

indicates that a two-dimensional array reference variable is being created. When memory is actually allocated for the array using **new**, this syntax is used:

```
int[10, 20]
```

This creates a 10×20 array, and again, the comma separates the dimensions.

To access an element in a two-dimensional array, you must specify both indices, separating the two with a comma. For example, to assign the value 10 to location 3, 5 of array **table**, you would use

```
table[3, 5] = 10;
```

Here is a complete example. It loads a two-dimensional array with the numbers 1 through 12 and then displays the contents of the array.

```
// Demonstrate a two-dimensional array.

using System;

class TwoD {
  static void Main() {
    int t, i;
    int[,] table = new int[3, 4];

    for(t=0; t < 3; ++t) {
      for(i=0; i < 4; ++i) {
        table[t,i] = (t*4)+i+1;
        Console.Write(table[t,i] + " ");
      }
      Console.WriteLine();
    }
  }
}
```

In this example, **table[0, 0]** will have the value 1, **table[0, 1]** the value 2, **table[0, 2]** the value 3, and so on. The value of **table[2, 3]** will be 12. Conceptually, the array will look like the one shown in Figure 7-1.

NOTE *If you have previously programmed in C, C++, or Java, be careful when declaring or accessing multidimensional arrays in C#. In these other languages, array dimensions and indices are specified within their own set of brackets. C# separates dimensions using commas.*

Arrays of Three or More Dimensions

C# allows arrays with more than two dimensions. Here is the general form of a multidimensional array declaration:

type[, ...] *name* = new *type*[*size1*, *size2*, ..., *sizeN*];

FIGURE 7-1
A conceptual view of the **table** array created by the **TwoD** program

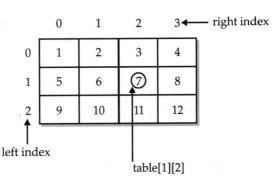

For example, the following declaration creates a 4×10×3 three-dimensional integer array:

```
int[,,] multidim = new int[4, 10, 3];
```

To assign element 2, 4, 1 of **multidim** the value 100, use this statement:

```
multidim[2, 4, 1] = 100;
```

Here is a program that uses a three-dimensional array that holds a 3×3×3 matrix of values. It then sums the value on one of the diagonals through the cube.

```
// Sum the values on a diagonal of a 3x3x3 matrix.

using System;

class ThreeDMatrix {
  static void Main() {
    int[,,] m = new int[3, 3, 3];
    int sum = 0;
    int n = 1;

    for(int x=0; x < 3; x++)
      for(int y=0; y < 3; y++)
        for(int z=0; z < 3; z++)
          m[x, y, z] = n++;

    sum = m[0, 0, 0] + m[1, 1, 1] + m[2, 2, 2];

    Console.WriteLine("Sum of first diagonal: " + sum);
  }
}
```

The output is shown here:

```
Sum of first diagonal: 42
```

Initializing Multidimensional Arrays

A multidimensional array can be initialized by enclosing each dimension's initializer list within its own set of curly braces. For example, the general form of array initialization for a two-dimensional array is shown here:

type[,] *array_name* = {
  { *val, val, val, ..., val* },
  { *val, val, val, ..., val* },

  .

  .

  .

  { *val, val, val, ..., val* }
};

Here, *val* indicates an initialization value. Each inner block designates a row. Within each row, the first value will be stored in the first position, the second value in the second position, and so on. Notice that commas separate the initializer blocks and that a semicolon follows the closing }.

For example, the following program initializes an array called **sqrs** with the numbers 1 through 10 and their squares.

```
// Initialize a two-dimensional array.

using System;

class Squares {
  static void Main() {
    int[,] sqrs = {
      { 1, 1 },
      { 2, 4 },
      { 3, 9 },
      { 4, 16 },
      { 5, 25 },
      { 6, 36 },
      { 7, 49 },
      { 8, 64 },
      { 9, 81 },
      { 10, 100 }
    };
    int i, j;

    for(i=0; i < 10; i++) {
      for(j=0; j < 2; j++)
        Console.Write(sqrs[i,j] + " ");
      Console.WriteLine();
    }
  }
}
```

Here is the output from the program:

```
1 1
2 4
3 9
4 16
5 25
6 36
7 49
8 64
9 81
10 100
```

Jagged Arrays

In the preceding examples, when you created a two-dimensional array, you were creating what C# calls a *rectangular array*. Thinking of two-dimensional arrays as tables, a rectangular array is a two-dimensional array in which the length of each row is the same for the entire array. However, C# also allows you to create a special type of two-dimensional array called a *jagged array*. A jagged array is an *array of arrays* in which the length of each array can differ. Thus, a jagged array can be used to create a table in which the lengths of the rows are not the same.

Jagged arrays are declared by using sets of square brackets to indicate each dimension. For example, to declare a two-dimensional jagged array, you will use this general form:

type[ ] [ ] *array-name* = new *type*[*size*][ ];

Here, *size* indicates the number of rows in the array. The rows, themselves, have not been allocated. Instead, the rows are allocated individually. This allows for the length of each row to vary. For example, the following code allocates memory for the first dimension of **jagged** when it is declared. It then allocates the second dimensions manually.

```
int[][] jagged = new int[3][];
jagged[0] = new int[4];
jagged[1] = new int[3];
jagged[2] = new int[5];
```

After this sequence executes, **jagged** looks like this:

jagged [0][0]	jagged [0][1]	jagged [0][2]	jagged [0][3]

jagged [1][0]	jagged [1][1]	jagged [1][2]

jagged [2][0]	jagged [2][1]	jagged [2][2]	jagged [2][3]	jagged [2][4]

It is easy to see how jagged arrays got their name!

Once a jagged array has been created, an element is accessed by specifying each index within its own set of brackets. For example, to assign the value 10 to element 2, 1 of **jagged**, you would use this statement:

```
jagged[2][1] = 10;
```

Note that this differs from the syntax that is used to access an element of a rectangular array.

The following program demonstrates the creation of a jagged two-dimensional array:

```
// Demonstrate jagged arrays.

using System;

class Jagged {
  static void Main() {
    int[][] jagged = new int[3][];
    jagged[0] = new int[4];
    jagged[1] = new int[3];
    jagged[2] = new int[5];

    int i;

    // Store values in first array.
    for(i=0; i < 4; i++)
      jagged[0][i] = i;

    // Store values in second array.
    for(i=0; i < 3; i++)
      jagged[1][i] = i;
```

```
    // Store values in third array.
    for(i=0; i < 5; i++)
      jagged[2][i] = i;

    // Display values in first array.
    for(i=0; i < 4; i++)
      Console.Write(jagged[0][i] + " ");

    Console.WriteLine();

    // Display values in second array.
    for(i=0; i < 3; i++)
      Console.Write(jagged[1][i] + " ");

    Console.WriteLine();

    // Display values in third array.
    for(i=0; i < 5; i++)
      Console.Write(jagged[2][i] + " ");

    Console.WriteLine();
  }
}
```

The output is shown here:

```
0 1 2 3
0 1 2
0 1 2 3 4
```

Jagged arrays are not used by all applications, but they can be effective in some situations. For example, if you need a very large two-dimensional array that is sparsely populated (that is, one in which not all of the elements will be used), then a jagged array might be a perfect solution.

One last point: Because jagged arrays are arrays of arrays, there is no restriction that requires that the arrays be one-dimensional. For example, the following creates an array of two-dimensional arrays:

```
int[][,] jagged = new int[3][,];
```

The next statement assigns **jagged[0]** a reference to a 4×2 array:

```
jagged[0] = new int[4, 2];
```

The following statement assigns a value to **jagged[0][1,0]**:

```
jagged[0][1,0] = i;
```

Assigning Array References

As with other objects, when you assign one array reference variable to another, you are simply making both variables refer to the same array. You are neither causing a copy of the

array to be created, nor are you causing the contents of one array to be copied to the other. For example, consider this program:

```
// Assigning array reference variables.

using System;

class AssignARef {
  static void Main() {
    int i;

    int[] nums1 = new int[10];
    int[] nums2 = new int[10];

    for(i=0; i < 10; i++) nums1[i] = i;

    for(i=0; i < 10; i++) nums2[i] = -i;

    Console.Write("Here is nums1: ");
    for(i=0; i < 10; i++)
      Console.Write(nums1[i] + " ");
    Console.WriteLine();

    Console.Write("Here is nums2: ");
    for(i=0; i < 10; i++)
      Console.Write(nums2[i] + " ");
    Console.WriteLine();

    nums2 = nums1; // now nums2 refers to nums1

    Console.Write("Here is nums2 after assignment: ");
    for(i=0; i < 10; i++)
      Console.Write(nums2[i] + " ");
    Console.WriteLine();

    // Next, operate on nums1 array through nums2.
    nums2[3] = 99;

    Console.Write("Here is nums1 after change through nums2: ");
    for(i=0; i < 10; i++)
      Console.Write(nums1[i] + " ");
    Console.WriteLine();
  }
}
```

The output from the program is shown here:

```
Here is nums1: 0 1 2 3 4 5 6 7 8 9
Here is nums2: 0 -1 -2 -3 -4 -5 -6 -7 -8 -9
Here is nums2 after assignment: 0 1 2 3 4 5 6 7 8 9
Here is nums1 after change through nums2: 0 1 2 99 4 5 6 7 8 9
```

As the output shows, after the assignment of **nums1** to **nums2**, both array reference variables refer to the same object.

Using the Length Property

A number of benefits result because C# implements arrays as objects. One comes from the fact that each array has associated with it a **Length** property that contains the number of elements that an array can hold. Thus, each array provides a means by which its length can be determined. Here is a program that demonstrates this property:

```
// Use the Length array property.

using System;

class LengthDemo {
  static void Main() {
    int[] nums = new int[10];

    Console.WriteLine("Length of nums is " + nums.Length);

    // Use Length to initialize nums.
    for(int i=0; i < nums.Length; i++)
      nums[i] = i * i;

    // Now use Length to display nums.
    Console.Write("Here is nums: ");
    for(int i=0; i < nums.Length; i++)
      Console.Write(nums[i] + " ");

    Console.WriteLine();
  }
}
```

This program displays the following output:

```
Length of nums is 10
Here is nums: 0 1 4 9 16 25 36 49 64 81
```

In **LengthDemo** notice the way that **nums.Length** is used by the **for** loops to govern the number of iterations that take place. Since each array carries with it its own length, you can use this information rather than manually keeping track of an array's size. Keep in mind that the value of **Length** has nothing to do with the number of elements that are actually in use. **Length** contains the number of elements that the array is capable of holding.

When the length of a multidimensional array is obtained, the total number of elements that can be held by the array is returned. For example:

```
// Use the Length array property on a 3D array.

using System;

class LengthDemo3D {
  static void Main() {
    int[,,] nums = new int[10, 5, 6];

    Console.WriteLine("Length of nums is " + nums.Length);
  }
}
```

The output is shown here:

```
Length of nums is 300
```

As the output verifies, **Length** obtains the number of elements that **nums** can hold, which is 300 (10×5×6) in this case. It is not possible to use **Length** to obtain the length of a specific dimension.

The inclusion of the **Length** property simplifies many algorithms by making certain types of array operations easier—and safer—to perform. For example, the following program uses **Length** to reverse the contents of an array by copying it back-to-front into another array:

```
// Reverse an array.

using System;

class RevCopy {
  static void Main() {
    int i,j;
    int[] nums1 = new int[10];
    int[] nums2 = new int[10];

    for(i=0; i < nums1.Length; i++) nums1[i] = i;

    Console.Write("Original contents: ");
    for(i=0; i < nums2.Length; i++)
      Console.Write(nums1[i] + " ");

    Console.WriteLine();

    // Reverse copy nums1 to nums2.
    if(nums2.Length >= nums1.Length) // make sure nums2 is long enough
      for(i=0, j=nums1.Length-1; i < nums1.Length; i++, j--)
        nums2[j] = nums1[i];

    Console.Write("Reversed contents: ");
    for(i=0; i < nums2.Length; i++)
      Console.Write(nums2[i] + " ");

    Console.WriteLine();
  }
}
```

Here is the output:

```
Original contents: 0 1 2 3 4 5 6 7 8 9
Reversed contents: 9 8 7 6 5 4 3 2 1 0
```

Here, **Length** helps perform two important functions. First, it is used to confirm that the target array is large enough to hold the contents of the source array. Second, it provides the termination condition of the **for** loop that performs the reverse copy. Of course, in this simple example, the size of the arrays is easily known, but this same approach can be applied to a wide range of more challenging situations.

Using Length with Jagged Arrays

A special case occurs when **Length** is used with jagged arrays. In this situation, it is possible to obtain the length of each individual array. For example, consider the following program, which simulates the CPU activity on a network with four nodes:

```
// Demonstrate Length with jagged arrays.

using System;

class Jagged {
  static void Main() {
    int[][] network_nodes = new int[4][];
    network_nodes[0] = new int[3];
    network_nodes[1] = new int[7];
    network_nodes[2] = new int[2];
    network_nodes[3] = new int[5];


    int i, j;

    // Fabricate some fake CPU usage data.
    for(i=0; i < network_nodes.Length; i++)
      for(j=0; j < network_nodes[i].Length; j++)
        network_nodes[i][j] = i * j + 70;


    Console.WriteLine("Total number of network nodes: " +
                      network_nodes.Length + "\n");

    for(i=0; i < network_nodes.Length; i++) {
      for(j=0; j < network_nodes[i].Length; j++) {
        Console.Write("CPU usage at node " + i +
                      " CPU " + j + ": ");
        Console.Write(network_nodes[i][j] + "% ");
        Console.WriteLine();
      }
      Console.WriteLine();
    }
  }
}
```

The output is shown here:

```
Total number of network nodes: 4

CPU usage at node 0 CPU 0: 70%
CPU usage at node 0 CPU 1: 70%
CPU usage at node 0 CPU 2: 70%

CPU usage at node 1 CPU 0: 70%
CPU usage at node 1 CPU 1: 71%
CPU usage at node 1 CPU 2: 72%
CPU usage at node 1 CPU 3: 73%
CPU usage at node 1 CPU 4: 74%
```

```
CPU usage at node 1 CPU 5: 75%
CPU usage at node 1 CPU 6: 76%

CPU usage at node 2 CPU 0: 70%
CPU usage at node 2 CPU 1: 72%

CPU usage at node 3 CPU 0: 70%
CPU usage at node 3 CPU 1: 73%
CPU usage at node 3 CPU 2: 76%
CPU usage at node 3 CPU 3: 79%
CPU usage at node 3 CPU 4: 82%
```

Pay special attention to the way **Length** is used on the jagged array **network_nodes**. Recall, a two-dimensional jagged array is an array of arrays. Thus, when the expression

```
network_nodes.Length
```

is used, it obtains the number of *arrays* stored in **network_nodes**, which is four in this case. To obtain the length of any individual array in the jagged array, you will use an expression such as this:

```
network_nodes[0].Length
```

which, in this case, obtains the length of the first array.

Implicitly Typed Arrays

As explained in Chapter 3, C# 3.0 adds the ability to declare implicitly typed variables by using the **var** keyword. These are variables whose type is determined by the compiler, based on the type of the initializing expression. Thus, all implicitly typed variables must be initialized. Using the same mechanism, it is also possible to create an implicitly typed array. As a general rule, implicitly typed arrays are for use in certain types of queries involving LINQ, which is described in Chapter 19. In most other cases, you will use the "normal" array declaration approach. Implicitly typed arrays are introduced here for completeness.

An implicitly typed array is declared using the keyword **var**, but you *do not* follow **var** with [ ]. Furthermore, the array must be initialized because it is the type of the initializers that determine the element type of the array. All of the initializers must be of the same or compatible type. Here is an example of an implicitly typed array:

```
var vals = new[] { 1, 2, 3, 4, 5 };
```

This creates an array of **int** that is five elements long. A reference to that array is assigned to **vals**. Thus, the type of **vals** is "array of **int**" and it has five elements. Again, notice that **var** is not followed by [ ]. Also, even though the array is being initialized, you must include **new[ ]**. It's not optional in this context.

Here is another example. It creates a two-dimensional array of **double**:

```
var vals = new[,] { {1.1, 2.2}, {3.3, 4.4},{ 5.5, 6.6} };
```

In this case, **vals** has the dimensions 2×3.

You can also declare implicitly typed jagged arrays. For example, consider the following program:

```
// Demonstrate an implicitly typed jagged array.

using System;

class Jagged {
  static void Main() {

    var jagged = new[] {
       new[] { 1, 2, 3, 4 },
       new[] { 9, 8, 7 },
       new[] { 11, 12, 13, 14, 15 }
    };

    for(int j = 0; j < jagged.Length; j++) {
      for(int i=0; i < jagged[j].Length; i++)
        Console.Write(jagged[j][i] + " ");

      Console.WriteLine();
    }
  }
}
```

The program produces the following output:

```
1 2 3 4
9 8 7
11 12 13 14 15
```

Pay special attention to the declaration of **jagged**:

```
var jagged = new[] {
   new[] { 1, 2, 3, 4 },
   new[] { 9, 8, 7 },
   new[] { 11, 12, 13, 14, 15 }
};
```

Notice how **new[ ]** is used in two ways. First, it creates the array of arrays. Second, it creates each individual array, based on the number and type of initializers. As you would expect, all of the initializers in the individual arrays must be of the same type. The same general approach used to declare **jagged** can be used to declare any implicitly typed jagged array.

As mentioned, implicitly typed arrays are most applicable to LINQ-based queries. They are not meant for general use. In most cases, you should use explicitly typed arrays.

The foreach Loop

In Chapter 5, it was mentioned that C# defines a loop called **foreach**, but a discussion of that statement was deferred until later. The time for that discussion has now come.

The **foreach** loop is used to cycle through the elements of a *collection*. A collection is a group of objects. C# defines several types of collections, of which one is an array. The general form of **foreach** is shown here:

foreach(*type loopvar* in *collection*) *statement*;

Here, *type loopvar* specifies the type and name of an *iteration variable*. The iteration variable receives the value of the next element in the collection each time the **foreach** loop iterates. The collection being cycled through is specified by *collection*, which, for the rest of this discussion, is an array. Thus, *type* must be the same as (or compatible with) the element type of the array. Beginning with C# 3.0, *type* can also be **var**, in which case the compiler determines the type based on the element type of the array. This can be useful when working with certain queries, as described later in this book. Normally, you will explicitly specify the type.

Here is how **foreach** works. When the loop begins, the first element in the array is obtained and assigned to *loopvar*. Each subsequent iteration obtains the next element from the array and stores it in *loopvar*. The loop ends when there are no more elements to obtain. Thus, the **foreach** cycles through the array one element at a time, from start to finish.

One important point to remember about **foreach** is that the iteration variable *loopvar* is read-only. This means you can't change the contents of an array by assigning the iteration variable a new value.

Here is a simple example that uses **foreach**. It creates an array of integers and gives it some initial values. It then displays those values, computing the summation in the process.

```
// Use the foreach loop.

using System;

class ForeachDemo {
  static void Main() {
    int sum = 0;
    int[] nums = new int[10];

    // Give nums some values.
    for(int i = 0; i < 10; i++)
      nums[i] = i;

    // Use foreach to display and sum the values.
    foreach(int x in nums) {
      Console.WriteLine("Value is: " + x);
      sum += x;
    }
    Console.WriteLine("Summation: " + sum);
  }
}
```

The output from the program is shown here:

```
Value is: 0
Value is: 1
Value is: 2
Value is: 3
Value is: 4
Value is: 5
Value is: 6
Value is: 7
```

```
Value is: 8
Value is: 9
Summation: 45
```

As this output shows, **foreach** cycles through an array in sequence from the lowest index to the highest.

Although the **foreach** loop iterates until all elements in an array have been examined, it is possible to terminate a **foreach** loop early by using a **break** statement. For example, this program sums only the first five elements of **nums**:

```
// Use break with a foreach.

using System;

class ForeachDemo {
  static void Main() {
    int sum = 0;
    int[] nums = new int[10];

    // Give nums some values.
    for(int i = 0; i < 10; i++)
      nums[i] = i;

    // Use foreach to display and sum the values.
    foreach(int x in nums) {
      Console.WriteLine("Value is: " + x);
      sum += x;
      if(x == 4) break; // stop the loop when 4 is obtained
    }
    Console.WriteLine("Summation of first 5 elements: " + sum);
  }
}
```

This is the output produced:

```
Value is: 0
Value is: 1
Value is: 2
Value is: 3
Value is: 4
Summation of first 5 elements: 10
```

As is evident, the **foreach** loop stops after the fifth element has been obtained.

The **foreach** loop also works on multidimensional arrays. It returns those elements in row order, from first to last.

```
// Use foreach on a two-dimensional array.

using System;

class ForeachDemo2 {
  static void Main() {
    int sum = 0;
    int[,] nums = new int[3,5];
```

```
    // Give nums some values.
    for(int i = 0; i < 3; i++)
      for(int j=0; j < 5; j++)
        nums[i,j] = (i+1)*(j+1);

    // Use foreach to display and sum the values.
    foreach(int x in nums) {
      Console.WriteLine("Value is: " + x);
      sum += x;
    }
    Console.WriteLine("Summation: " + sum);
  }
}
```

The output from this program is shown here:

```
Value is: 1
Value is: 2
Value is: 3
Value is: 4
Value is: 5
Value is: 2
Value is: 4
Value is: 6
Value is: 8
Value is: 10
Value is: 3
Value is: 6
Value is: 9
Value is: 12
Value is: 15
Summation: 90
```

Since the **foreach** loop can only cycle through an array sequentially, from start to finish, you might think that its use is limited. However, this is not true. A large number of algorithms require exactly this mechanism, of which one of the most common is searching. For example, the following program uses a **foreach** loop to search an array for a value. It stops if the value is found.

```
// Search an array using foreach.

using System;

class Search {
  static void Main() {
    int[] nums = new int[10];
    int val;
    bool found = false;

    // Give nums some values.
    for(int i = 0; i < 10; i++)
      nums[i] = i;

    val = 5;
```

```
    // Use foreach to search nums for key.
    foreach(int x in nums) {
      if(x == val) {
        found = true;
        break;
      }
    }

    if(found)
      Console.WriteLine("Value found!");
  }
}
```

The output is shown here:

```
Value found!
```

The **foreach** loop is an excellent choice in this application because searching an array involves examining each element. Other types of **foreach** applications include such things as computing an average, finding the minimum or maximum of a set, looking for duplicates, and so on. As you will see later in this book, **foreach** is especially useful when operating on other types of collections.

Strings

From a day-to-day programming standpoint, one of the most important of C#'s data types is **string**. **string** defines and supports character strings. In many other programming languages, a string is an array of characters. This is not the case with C#. In C#, strings are objects. Thus, **string** is a reference type. Although **string** is a built-in data type in C#, a discussion of **string** needed to wait until classes and objects had been introduced.

Actually, you have been using the **string** class since Chapter 2, but you did not know it. When you create a string literal, you are actually creating a **string** object. For example, in the statement

```
Console.WriteLine("In C#, strings are objects.");
```

the string "In C#, strings are objects." is automatically made into a **string** object by C#. Thus, the use of the **string** class has been "below the surface" in the preceding programs. In this section, you will learn to handle them explicitly.

Constructing Strings

The easiest way to construct a **string** is to use a string literal. For example, here **str** is a **string** reference variable that is assigned a reference to a string literal:

```
string str = "C# strings are powerful.";
```

In this case, **str** is initialized to the character sequence "C# strings are powerful."
You can also create a **string** from a **char** array. For example:

```
char[] charray = {'t', 'e', 's', 't'};
string str = new string(charray);
```

Once you have created a **string** object, you can use it nearly anywhere that a quoted string is allowed. For example, you can use a **string** object as an argument to **WriteLine( )**, as shown in this example:

```
// Introduce string.

using System;

class StringDemo {
  static void Main() {

    char[] charray = {'A', ' ', 's', 't', 'r', 'i', 'n', 'g', '.' };
    string str1 = new string(charray);
    string str2 = "Another string.";

    Console.WriteLine(str1);
    Console.WriteLine(str2);
  }
}
```

The output from the program is shown here:

```
A string.
Another string.
```

Operating on Strings

The **string** class contains several methods that operate on strings. Table 7-1 shows a few. The **string** type also includes the **Length** property, which contains the length of the string.

To obtain the value of an individual character of a string, you simply use an index. For example:

```
string str = "test";
Console.WriteLine(str[0]);
```

This displays "t", the first character of "test". Like arrays, string indexes begin at zero. One important point, however, is that you cannot assign a new value to a character within a string using an index. An index can only be used to obtain a character.

Method	Description
static string Copy(string *str*)	Returns a copy of *str*.
int CompareTo(string *str*)	Returns less than zero if the invoking string is less than *str*, greater than zero if the invoking string is greater than *str*, and zero if the strings are equal.
int IndexOf(string *str*)	Searches the invoking string for the substring specified by *str*. Returns the index of the first match, or –1 on failure.
int LastIndexOf(string *str*)	Searches the invoking string for the substring specified by *str*. Returns the index of the last match, or –1 on failure.
string ToLower( )	Returns a lowercase version of the invoking string.
string ToUpper( )	Returns an uppercase version of the invoking string.

TABLE 7-1 Some Common String Handling Methods

To test two strings for equality, you can use the = = operator. Normally, when the = = operator is applied to object references, it determines if both references refer to the same object. This differs for objects of type **string**. When the = = is applied to two **string** references, the contents of the strings, themselves, are compared for equality. The same is true for the != operator: When comparing **string** objects, the contents of the strings are compared. For other types of string comparisons, you will need to use the **CompareTo()** method.

Here is a program that demonstrates several string operations:

```
// Some string operations.

using System;

class StrOps {
  static void Main() {
    string str1 =
      "When it comes to .NET programming, C# is #1.";
    string str2 = string.Copy(str1);
    string str3 = "C# strings are powerful.";
    string strUp, strLow;
    int result, idx;

    Console.WriteLine("str1: " + str1);

    Console.WriteLine("Length of str1: " +
                      str1.Length);

    // Create upper- and lowercase versions of str1.
    strLow = str1.ToLower();
    strUp =  str1.ToUpper();
    Console.WriteLine("Lowercase version of str1:\n     " +
                      strLow);
    Console.WriteLine("Uppercase version of str1:\n     " +
                      strUp);

    Console.WriteLine();

    // Display str1, one char at a time.
    Console.WriteLine("Display str1, one char at a time.");
    for(int i=0; i < str1.Length; i++)
      Console.Write(str1[i]);
    Console.WriteLine("\n");

    // Compare strings.
    if(str1 == str2)
      Console.WriteLine("str1 == str2");
    else
      Console.WriteLine("str1 != str2");

    if(str1 == str3)
      Console.WriteLine("str1 == str3");
    else
      Console.WriteLine("str1 != str3");
```

```
  result = str1.CompareTo(str3);
  if(result == 0)
    Console.WriteLine("str1 and str3 are equal");
  else if(result < 0)
    Console.WriteLine("str1 is less than str3");
  else
    Console.WriteLine("str1 is greater than str3");

  Console.WriteLine();

  // Assign a new string to str2.
  str2 = "One Two Three One";

  // Search a string.
  idx = str2.IndexOf("One");
  Console.WriteLine("Index of first occurrence of One: " + idx);
  idx = str2.LastIndexOf("One");
  Console.WriteLine("Index of last occurrence of One: " + idx);

  }
}
```

This program generates the following output:

```
str1: When it comes to .NET programming, C# is #1.
Length of str1: 44
Lowercase version of str1:
    when it comes to .net programming, c# is #1.
Uppercase version of str1:
    WHEN IT COMES TO .NET PROGRAMMING, C# IS #1.

Display str1, one char at a time.
When it comes to .NET programming, C# is #1.

str1 == str2
str1 != str3
str1 is greater than str3

Index of first occurrence of One: 0
Index of last occurrence of One: 14
```

You can concatenate (join together) two strings using the **+** operator. For example, this statement:

```
string str1 = "One";
string str2 = "Two";
string str3 = "Three";
string str4 = str1 + str2 + str3;
```

initializes **str4** with the string "OneTwoThree".

One other point: The **string** keyword is an *alias* for (that is, maps directly to) the **System.String** class defined by the .NET Framework class library. Thus, the fields and methods defined by **string** are those of the **System.String** class, which includes more than the sampling described here. **System.String** is examined in detail in Part II.

Arrays of Strings

Like any other data type, strings can be assembled into arrays. For example:

```
// Demonstrate string arrays.
using System;

class StringArrays {
  static void Main() {
    string[] str = { "This", "is", "a", "test." };

    Console.WriteLine("Original array: ");
    for(int i=0; i < str.Length; i++)
      Console.Write(str[i] + " ");
    Console.WriteLine("\n");

    // Change a string.
    str[1] = "was";
    str[3] = "test, too!";

    Console.WriteLine("Modified array: ");
    for(int i=0; i < str.Length; i++)
      Console.Write(str[i] + " ");
  }
}
```

Here is the output from this program:

```
Original array:
This is a test.

Modified array:
This was a test, too!
```

Here is a more interesting example. The following program displays an integer value using words. For example, the value 19 will display as "one nine".

```
// Display the digits of an integer using words.

using System;

class ConvertDigitsToWords {
  static void Main() {
    int num;
    int nextdigit;
    int numdigits;
    int[] n = new int[20];

    string[] digits = { "zero", "one", "two",
                        "three", "four", "five",
                        "six", "seven", "eight",
                        "nine" };

    num = 1908;
```

```
   Console.WriteLine("Number: " + num);

   Console.Write("Number in words: ");

   nextdigit = 0;
   numdigits = 0;

   // Get individual digits and store in n.
   // These digits are stored in reverse order.
   do {
     nextdigit = num % 10;
     n[numdigits] = nextdigit;
     numdigits++;
     num = num / 10;
   } while(num > 0);
   numdigits--;

   // Display the words.
   for( ; numdigits >= 0; numdigits--)
     Console.Write(digits[n[numdigits]] + " ");

   Console.WriteLine();
  }
}
```

The output is shown here:

```
Number: 1908
Number in words: one nine zero eight
```

In the program, the **string** array **digits** holds in order the word equivalents of the digits from zero to nine. The program converts an integer into words by first obtaining each digit of the value and then storing those digits, in reverse order, in the **int** array called **n**. Then, this array is cycled through from back to front. In the process, each integer value in **n** is used as an index into **digits**, with the corresponding string being displayed.

Strings Are Immutable

Here is something that might surprise you: The contents of a **string** object are immutable. That is, once created, the character sequence comprising that string cannot be altered. This restriction allows strings to be implemented more efficiently. Even though this probably sounds like a serious drawback, it isn't. When you need a string that is a variation on one that already exists, simply create a new string that contains the desired changes. Since unused string objects are automatically garbage-collected, you don't even need to worry about what happens to the discarded strings.

It must be made clear, however, that **string** reference variables may, of course, change which object they refer to. It is just that the contents of a specific **string** object cannot be changed after it is created.

To fully understand why immutable strings are not a hindrance, we will use another of **string**'s methods: **Substring( )**. The **Substring( )** method returns a new string that contains a specified portion of the invoking string. Because a new **string** object is manufactured that

contains the substring, the original string is unaltered, and the rule of immutability is still intact. The form of **Substring( )** that we will be using is shown here:

string Substring(int *start*, int *len*)

Here, *start* specifies the beginning index, and *len* specifies the length of the substring.

Here is a program that demonstrates **Substring( )** and the principle of immutable strings:

```
// Use Substring().

using System;

class SubStr {
  static void Main() {
    string orgstr = "C# makes strings easy.";

    // construct a substring
    string substr = orgstr.Substring(5, 12);

    Console.WriteLine("orgstr: " + orgstr);
    Console.WriteLine("substr: " + substr);
  }
}
```

Here is the output from the program:

```
orgstr: C# makes strings easy.
substr: kes strings
```

As you can see, the original string **orgstr** is unchanged and **substr** contains the substring.

One more point: Although the immutability of **string** objects is not usually a restriction or hindrance, there may be times when it would be beneficial to modify a string. To allow this, C# offers a class called **StringBuilder**, which is in the **System.Text** namespace. It creates string objects that can be changed. For most purposes, however, you will want to use **string**, not **StringBuilder**.

Strings Can Be Used in switch Statements

A **string** can be used to control a **switch** statement. It is the only non-integer type that can be used in the **switch**. The fact that strings can be used in **switch** statements makes it possible to handle some otherwise challenging situations more easily than you might expect. For example, the following program displays the digit equivalent of the words "one," "two," and "three":

```
// A string can control a switch statement.

using System;

class StringSwitch {
  static void Main() {
    string[] strs = { "one", "two", "three", "two", "one" };
```

```
    foreach(string s in strs) {
      switch(s) {
        case "one":
          Console.Write(1);
          break;
        case "two":
          Console.Write(2);
          break;
        case "three":
          Console.Write(3);
          break;
      }
    }
    Console.WriteLine();
  }
}
```

The output is shown here:

```
12321
```

CHAPTER 8

A Closer Look at Methods and Classes

This chapter resumes the examination of classes and methods. It begins by explaining how to control access to the members of a class. It then discusses the passing and returning of objects, method overloading, the various forms of **Main()**, recursion, and the use of the keyword **static**.

Controlling Access to Class Members

In its support for encapsulation, the class provides two major benefits. First, it links data with code. You have been taking advantage of this aspect of the class since Chapter 6. Second, it provides the means by which access to members can be controlled. It is this second feature that is examined here.

Although C#'s approach is a bit more sophisticated, in essence, there are two basic types of class members: public and private. A public member can be freely accessed by code defined outside of its class. This is the type of class member that we have been using up to this point. A private member can be accessed only by methods defined by its class. It is through the use of private members that access is controlled.

Restricting access to a class' members is a fundamental part of object-oriented programming because it helps prevent the misuse of an object. By allowing access to private data only through a well-defined set of methods, you can prevent improper values from being assigned to that data—by performing a range check, for example. It is not possible for code outside the class to set the value of a private member directly. You can also control precisely how and when the data within an object is used. Thus, when correctly implemented, a class creates a "black box" that can be used, but the inner workings of which are not open to tampering.

C#'s Access Modifiers

Member access control is achieved through the use of four *access modifiers*: **public**, **private**, **protected**, and **internal**. In this chapter, we will be concerned with **public** and **private**. The **protected** modifier applies only when inheritance is involved and is described in Chapter 11.

The **internal** modifier applies mostly to the use of an *assembly*, which for C# loosely means a deployable program or library. The **internal** modifier is examined in Chapter 16.

When a member of a class is modified by the **public** specifier, that member can be accessed by any other code in your program. This includes methods defined inside other classes.

When a member of a class is specified as **private**, then that member can be accessed only by other members of its class. Thus, methods in other classes are not able to access a **private** member of another class. As explained in Chapter 6, if no access specifier is used, a class member is private to its class by default. Thus, the **private** specifier is optional when creating private class members.

An access specifier precedes the rest of a member's type specification. That is, it must begin a member's declaration statement. Here are some examples:

```
public string errMsg;
private double bal;
private bool isError(byte status) { // ...
```

To understand the difference between **public** and **private**, consider the following program:

```
// Public vs. private access.

using System;

class MyClass {
  private int alpha; // private access explicitly specified
  int beta;          // private access by default
  public int gamma;  // public access

  // Methods to access alpha and beta. It is OK for a member
  // of a class to access a private member of the same class.

  public void SetAlpha(int a) {
    alpha = a;
  }

  public int GetAlpha() {
    return alpha;
  }

  public void SetBeta(int a) {
    beta = a;
  }

  public int GetBeta() {
    return beta;
  }
}

class AccessDemo {
  static void Main() {
    MyClass ob = new MyClass();
```

```
      // Access to alpha and beta is allowed only through methods.
      ob.SetAlpha(-99);
      ob.SetBeta(19);
      Console.WriteLine("ob.alpha is " + ob.GetAlpha());
      Console.WriteLine("ob.beta is " + ob.GetBeta());

      // You cannot access alpha or beta like this:
//    ob.alpha = 10; // Wrong! alpha is private!
//    ob.beta = 9;   // Wrong! beta is private!

      // It is OK to directly access gamma because it is public.
      ob.gamma = 99;
    }
}
```

As you can see, inside the **MyClass** class, **alpha** is specified as **private**, **beta** is private by default, and **gamma** is specified as **public**. Because **alpha** and **beta** are private, they cannot be accessed by code outside of their class. Therefore, inside the **AccessDemo** class, neither can be used directly. Each must be accessed through public methods, such as **SetAlpha()** and **GetAlpha()**. For example, if you were to remove the comment symbol from the beginning of the following line

```
//   ob.alpha = 10; // Wrong! alpha is private!
```

you would not be able to compile this program because of the access violation. Although access to **alpha** by code outside of **MyClass** is not allowed, methods defined within **MyClass** can freely access it, as the **SetAlpha()** and **GetAlpha()** methods show. The same is true for **beta**.

The key point is this: A private member can be used freely by other members of its class, but it cannot be accessed by code outside its class.

Applying Public and Private Access

The proper use of public and private access is a key component of successful object-oriented programming. Although there are no hard and fast rules, here are some general principles that serve as guidelines:

- Members of a class that are used only within the class itself should be private.
- Instance data that must be within a specific range should be private, with access provided through public methods that can perform range checks.
- If changing a member can cause an effect that extends beyond the member itself (that is, affects other aspects of the object), that member should be private, and access to it should be controlled.
- Members that can cause harm to an object when improperly used should be private. Access to these members should be through public methods that prevent improper usage.
- Methods that get and set the values of private data must be public.
- Public instance variables are permissible when there is no reason for them to be private.

Of course, there are many nuances that the preceding rules do not address, and special cases cause one or more rules to be violated. But, in general, if you follow these rules, you will be creating resilient objects that are not easily misused.

Controlling Access: A Case Study

To better understand the "how and why" behind access control, a case study is useful. One of the quintessential examples of object-oriented programming is a class that implements a stack. As you probably know, a *stack* is a data structure that implements a last-in, first-out list. Its name comes from the analogy of a stack of plates on a table. The first plate on the table is the last one to be used.

A stack is a classic example of object-oriented programming because it combines storage for information along with the methods that access that information. Thus, a stack is a *data engine* that enforces the last-in, first-out usage. Such a combination is an excellent choice for a class in which the members that provide storage for the stack are private, and public methods provide access. By encapsulating the underlying storage, it is not possible for code that uses the stack to access the elements out of order.

A stack defines two basic operations: *push* and *pop.* A push puts a value onto the top of the stack. A pop removes a value from the top of the stack. Thus, a pop is consumptive; once a value has been popped off the stack, it has been removed and cannot be accessed again.

The example shown here creates a class called **Stack** that implements a stack. The underlying storage for the stack is provided by a private array. The push and pop operations are available through the public methods of the **Stack** class. Thus, the public methods enforce the last-in, first-out mechanism. As shown here, the **Stack** class stores characters, but the same mechanism could be used to store any type of data:

```
// A stack class for characters.

using System;

class Stack {
  // These members are private.
  char[] stck; // holds the stack
  int tos;     // index of the top of the stack

  // Construct an empty Stack given its size.
  public Stack(int size) {
    stck = new char[size]; // allocate memory for stack
    tos = 0;
  }

  // Push characters onto the stack.
  public void Push(char ch) {
    if(tos==stck.Length) {
      Console.WriteLine(" -- Stack is full.");
      return;
    }

    stck[tos] = ch;
    tos++;
  }

  // Pop a character from the stack.
```

```
public char Pop() {
  if(tos==0) {
    Console.WriteLine(" -- Stack is empty.");
    return (char) 0;
  }

  tos--;
  return stck[tos];
}

// Return true if the stack is full.
public bool IsFull() {
  return tos==stck.Length;
}

// Return true if the stack is empty.
public bool IsEmpty() {
  return tos==0;
}

// Return total capacity of the stack.
public int Capacity() {
  return stck.Length;
}

// Return number of objects currently on the stack.
public int GetNum() {
  return tos;
}
}
```

Let's examine this class closely. The **Stack** class begins by declaring these two instance variables:

```
// These members are private.
char[] stck; // holds the stack
int tos;     // index of the top of the stack
```

The **stck** array provides the underlying storage for the stack, which in this case holds characters. Notice that no array is allocated. The allocation of the actual array is handled by the **Stack** constructor. The **tos** member holds the index of the top of the stack.

Both the **tos** and **stck** members are private. This enforces the last-in, first-out stack mechanism. If public access to **stck** were allowed, then the elements on the stack could be accessed out of order. Also, since **tos** holds the index of the top element in the stack, manipulations of **tos** by code outside the **Stack** class must be prevented in order to avoid corruption of the stack. Access to **stck** and **tos** is available, indirectly, to the user of **Stack** through the various public methods described shortly.

The stack constructor is shown next:

```
// Construct an empty Stack given its size.
public Stack(int size) {
  stck = new char[size]; // allocate memory for stack
  tos = 0;
}
```

The constructor is passed the desired size of the stack. It allocates the underlying array and sets **tos** to zero. Thus, a zero value in **tos** indicates that the stack is empty.

The public **Push()** method puts an element onto the stack. It is shown here:

```
// Push characters onto the stack.
public void Push(char ch) {
  if(tos==stck.Length) {
    Console.WriteLine(" -- Stack is full.");
    return;
  }

  stck[tos] = ch;
  tos++;
}
```

The element to be pushed onto the stack is passed in **ch**. Before the element is added to the stack, a check is made to ensure that there is still room in the underlying array. This is done by making sure that **tos** does not exceed the length of **stck**. If there is still room, the element is stored in **stck** at the index specified by **tos**, and then **tos** is incremented. Thus, **tos** always contains the index of the next free element in **stck**.

To remove an element from the stack, call the public method **Pop()**. It is shown here:

```
// Pop a character from the stack.
public char Pop() {
  if(tos==0) {
    Console.WriteLine(" -- Stack is empty.");
    return (char) 0;
  }

  tos--;
  return stck[tos];
}
```

Here, the value of **tos** is checked. If it is zero, the stack is empty. Otherwise, **tos** is decremented, and the element at that index is returned.

Although **Push()** and **Pop()** are the only methods needed to implement a stack, some others are quite useful, and the **Stack** class defines four more. These are **IsFull()**, **IsEmpty()**, **Capacity()**, and **GetNum()**, and they provide information about the state of the stack. They are shown here:

```
// Return true if the stack is full.
public bool IsFull() {
  return tos==stck.Length;
}

// Return true if the stack is empty.
public bool IsEmpty() {
  return tos==0;
}

// Return total capacity of the stack.
```

```
public int Capacity() {
  return stck.Length;
}

// Return number of objects currently on the stack.
public int GetNum() {
  return tos;
}
```

The **IsFull()** method returns **true** when the stack is full and **false** otherwise. The **IsEmpty()** method returns **true** when the stack is empty and **false** otherwise. To obtain the total capacity of the stack (that is, the total number of elements it can hold), call **Capacity()**. To obtain the number of elements currently stored on the stack, call **GetNum()**. These methods are useful because the information they provide requires access to **tos**, which is private. They are also examples of how public methods can provide safe access to private members.

The following program demonstrates the stack:

```
// Demonstrate the Stack class.

using System;

class StackDemo {
  static void Main() {
    Stack stk1 = new Stack(10);
    Stack stk2 = new Stack(10);
    Stack stk3 = new Stack(10);
    char ch;
    int i;

    // Put some characters into stk1.
    Console.WriteLine("Push A through J onto stk1.");
    for(i=0; !stk1.IsFull(); i++)
      stk1.Push((char) ('A' + i));

    if(stk1.IsFull()) Console.WriteLine("stk1 is full.");

    // Display the contents of stk1.
    Console.Write("Contents of stk1: ");
    while( !stk1.IsEmpty() ) {
      ch = stk1.Pop();
      Console.Write(ch);
    }

    Console.WriteLine();

    if(stk1.IsEmpty()) Console.WriteLine("stk1 is empty.\n");

    // Put more characters into stk1.
    Console.WriteLine("Again push A through J onto stk1.");
    for(i=0; !stk1.IsFull(); i++)
      stk1.Push((char) ('A' + i));

    // Now, pop from stk1 and push the element in stk2.
```

```
    // This causes stk2 to hold the elements in reverse order.
    Console.WriteLine("Now, pop chars from stk1 and push " +
                      "them onto stk2.");
    while( !stk1.IsEmpty() ) {
      ch = stk1.Pop();
      stk2.Push(ch);
    }

    Console.Write("Contents of stk2: ");
    while( !stk2.IsEmpty() ) {
      ch = stk2.Pop();
      Console.Write(ch);
    }

    Console.WriteLine("\n");

    // Put 5 characters into stack.
    Console.WriteLine("Put 5 characters on stk3.");
    for(i=0; i < 5; i++)
      stk3.Push((char) ('A' + i));

    Console.WriteLine("Capacity of stk3: " + stk3.Capacity());
    Console.WriteLine("Number of objects in stk3: " +
                      stk3.GetNum());
  }
}
```

The output from the program is shown here:

```
Push A through J onto stk1.
stk1 is full.
Contents of stk1: JIHGFEDCBA
stk1 is empty.

Again push A through J onto stk1.
Now, pop chars from stk1 and push them onto stk2.
Contents of stk2: ABCDEFGHIJ

Put 5 characters on stk3.
Capacity of stk3: 10
Number of objects in stk3: 5
```

Pass References to Methods

Up to this point, the examples in this book have been using value types, such as **int** or **double**, as parameters to methods. However, it is both correct and common to use a reference type as a parameter. Doing so allows an object to be passed to a method. For example, consider the following program:

```
// References can be passed to methods.

using System;

class MyClass {
  int alpha, beta;
```

```
  public MyClass(int i, int j) {
    alpha = i;
    beta = j;
  }

  // Return true if ob contains the same values as the invoking object.
  public bool SameAs(MyClass ob) {
    if((ob.alpha == alpha) & (ob.beta == beta))
       return true;
    else return false;
  }

  // Make a copy of ob.
  public void Copy(MyClass ob) {
    alpha = ob.alpha;
    beta  = ob.beta;
  }

  public void Show() {
    Console.WriteLine("alpha: {0}, beta: {1}",
                      alpha, beta);
  }
}

class PassOb {
  static void Main() {
    MyClass ob1 = new MyClass(4, 5);
    MyClass ob2 = new MyClass(6, 7);

    Console.Write("ob1: ");
    ob1.Show();

    Console.Write("ob2: ");
    ob2.Show();

    if(ob1.SameAs(ob2))
      Console.WriteLine("ob1 and ob2 have the same values.");
    else
      Console.WriteLine("ob1 and ob2 have different values.");

    Console.WriteLine();

    // Now, make ob1 a copy of ob2.
    ob1.Copy(ob2);

    Console.Write("ob1 after copy: ");
    ob1.Show();

    if(ob1.SameAs(ob2))
      Console.WriteLine("ob1 and ob2 have the same values.");
    else
      Console.WriteLine("ob1 and ob2 have different values.");
  }
}
```

This program generates the following output:

```
ob1: alpha: 4, beta: 5
ob2: alpha: 6, beta: 7
ob1 and ob2 have different values.

ob1 after copy: alpha: 6, beta: 7
ob1 and ob2 have the same values.
```

The **SameAs()** and **Copy()** methods each take a reference of type **MyClass** as an argument. The **SameAs()** method compares the values of **alpha** and **beta** in the invoking object with the values of **alpha** and **beta** in the object passed via **ob**. The method returns **true** only if the two objects contain the same values for these instance variables. The **Copy()** method assigns the values of **alpha** and **beta** in the object referred to by **ob** to **alpha** and **beta** in the invoking object. As this example shows, syntactically, reference types are passed to methods in the same way as are value types.

How Arguments Are Passed

As the preceding example demonstrated, passing an object reference to a method is a straightforward task. However, there are some nuances that the example did not show. In certain cases, the effects of passing a reference type will be different than those experienced when passing a value type. To see why, let's review the two ways in which an argument can be passed to a subroutine.

The first way is *call-by-value.* This method *copies* the *value* of an argument into the formal parameter of the subroutine. Therefore, changes made to the parameter of the subroutine have no effect on the argument used in the call. The second way an argument can be passed is *call-by-reference.* In this method, a *reference* to an argument (not the value of the argument) is passed to the parameter. Inside the subroutine, this reference is used to access the actual argument specified in the call. This means that changes made to the parameter will affect the argument used to call the subroutine.

By default, C# uses call-by-value, which means that a copy of the argument is made and given to the receiving parameter. Thus, when you pass a value type, such as **int** or **double**, what occurs to the parameter that receives the argument has no effect outside the method. For example, consider the following program:

```
// Value types are passed by value.

using System;

class Test {
  /* This method causes no change to the arguments
     used in the call. */
  public void NoChange(int i, int j) {
    i = i + j;
    j = -j;
  }
}

class CallByValue {
  static void Main() {
    Test ob = new Test();
```

```
int a = 15, b = 20;

Console.WriteLine("a and b before call: " +
                  a + " " + b);

ob.NoChange(a, b);

Console.WriteLine("a and b after call: " +
                  a + " " + b);
  }
}
```

The output from this program is shown here:

```
a and b before call: 15 20
a and b after call: 15 20
```

As you can see, the operations that occur inside **NoChange()** have no effect on the values of **a** and **b** used in the call. Again, this is because *copies* of the *value* of **a** and **b** have been given to parameters **i** and **j**, but **a** and **b** are otherwise completely independent of **i** and **j**. Thus, assigning **i** a new value will not affect **a**.

When you pass a reference to a method, the situation is a bit more complicated. In this case, the reference, itself, is still passed by value. Thus, a copy of the reference is made and changes to the parameter will not affect the argument. (For example, making the parameter refer to a new object will not change the object to which the argument refers.) However—and this is a big however—changes *made to the object* being referred to by the parameter *will* affect the object referred to by the argument. Let's see why.

Recall that when you create a variable of a class type, you are only creating a reference to an object. Thus, when you pass this reference to a method, the parameter that receives it will refer to the same object as that referred to by the argument. Therefore, the argument and the parameter will both refer to the same object. This means that objects are passed to methods by what is effectively call-by-reference. Thus, changes to the object inside the method *do* affect the object used as an argument. For example, consider the following program:

```
// Objects are passed by reference.

using System;

class Test {
  public int a, b;

  public Test(int i, int j) {
    a = i;
    b = j;
  }

  /* Pass an object. Now, ob.a and ob.b in object
     used in the call will be changed. */
  public void Change(Test ob) {
    ob.a = ob.a + ob.b;
    ob.b = -ob.b;
  }
}
```

```
class CallByRef {
  static void Main() {
    Test ob = new Test(15, 20);

    Console.WriteLine("ob.a and ob.b before call: " +
                      ob.a + " " + ob.b);

    ob.Change(ob);

    Console.WriteLine("ob.a and ob.b after call: " +
                      ob.a + " " + ob.b);
  }
}
```

This program generates the following output:

```
ob.a and ob.b before call: 15 20
ob.a and ob.b after call: 35 -20
```

As you can see, in this case, the actions inside **Change()** have affected the object used as an argument.

To review: When a reference is passed to a method, the reference itself is passed by use of call-by-value. Thus, a copy of that reference is made. However, the copy of that reference will still refer to the same object as its corresponding argument. This means that objects are implicitly passed using call-by-reference.

Use ref and out Parameters

As just explained, value types, such as **int** or **char**, are passed by value to a method. This means that changes to the parameter that receives a value type will not affect the actual argument used in the call. You can, however, alter this behavior. Through the use of the **ref** and **out** keywords, it is possible to pass any of the value types by reference. Doing so allows a method to alter the argument used in the call.

Before going into the mechanics of using **ref** and **out**, it is useful to understand why you might want to pass a value type by reference. In general, there are two reasons: to allow a method to alter the contents of its arguments or to allow a method to return more than one value. Let's look at each reason in detail.

Often you will want a method to be able to operate on the actual arguments that are passed to it. The quintessential example of this is a **Swap()** method that exchanges the values of its two arguments. Since value types are passed by value, it is not possible to write a method that swaps the value of two **int**s, for example, using C#'s default call-by-value parameter passing mechanism. The **ref** modifier solves this problem.

As you know, a **return** statement enables a method to return a value to its caller. However, a method can return *only one* value each time it is called. What if you need to return two or more pieces of information? For example, what if you want to create a method that decomposes a floating-point number into its integer and fractional parts? To do this requires that two pieces of information be returned: the integer portion and the fractional component. This method cannot be written using only a single return value. The **out** modifier solves this problem.

Use ref

The **ref** parameter modifier causes C# to create a call-by-reference, rather than a call-by-value. The **ref** modifier is specified when the method is declared and when it is called. Let's begin with a simple example. The following program creates a method called **Sqr()** that returns in-place the square of its integer argument. Notice the use and placement of **ref**.

```
// Use ref to pass a value type by reference.

using System;

class RefTest {
  // This method changes its argument. Notice the use of ref.
  public void Sqr(ref int i) {
    i = i * i;
  }
}

class RefDemo {
  static void Main() {
    RefTest ob = new RefTest();

    int a = 10;

    Console.WriteLine("a before call: " + a);

    ob.Sqr(ref a); // notice the use of ref

    Console.WriteLine("a after call: " + a);
  }
}
```

Notice that **ref** precedes the entire parameter declaration in the method and that it precedes the argument when the method is called. The output from this program, shown here, confirms that the value of the argument, **a**, was indeed modified by **Sqr()**:

```
a before call: 10
a after call: 100
```

Using **ref**, it is now possible to write a method that exchanges the values of its two value-type arguments. For example, here is a program that contains a method called **Swap()** that exchanges the values of the two integer arguments with which it is called:

```
// Swap two values.

using System;

class ValueSwap {
  // This method now changes its arguments.
  public void Swap(ref int a, ref int b) {
    int t;
```

```
      t = a;
      a = b;
      b = t;
    }
}

class ValueSwapDemo {
  static void Main() {
    ValueSwap ob = new ValueSwap();

    int x = 10, y = 20;

    Console.WriteLine("x and y before call: " + x + " " + y);

    ob.Swap(ref x, ref y);

    Console.WriteLine("x and y after call: " + x + " " + y);
  }
}
```

The output from this program is shown here:

```
x and y before call: 10 20
x and y after call: 20 10
```

Here is one important point to understand about **ref**: An argument passed by **ref** must be assigned a value prior to the call. The reason is that the method that receives such an argument assumes that the parameter refers to a valid value. Thus, using **ref**, you cannot use a method to give an argument an initial value.

Use out

Sometimes you will want to use a reference parameter to receive a value from a method, but not pass in a value. For example, you might have a method that performs some function, such as opening a network socket, that returns a success/fail code in a reference parameter. In this case, there is no information to pass into the method, but there is information to pass back out. The problem with this scenario is that a **ref** parameter must be initialized to a value prior to the call. Thus, to use a **ref** parameter would require giving the argument a dummy value just to satisfy this constraint. Fortunately, C# provides a better alternative: the **out** parameter.

An **out** parameter is similar to a **ref** parameter with this one exception: It can only be used to pass a value out of a method. It is not necessary (or useful) to give the variable used as an **out** parameter an initial value prior to calling the method. The method will give the variable a value. Furthermore, inside the method, an **out** parameter is considered *unassigned*; that is, it is assumed to have no initial value. This implies that the method *must* assign the parameter a value prior to the method's termination. Thus, after the call to the method, an **out** parameter will contain a value.

Here is an example that uses an **out** parameter. In the class **Decompose**, the **GetParts()** method decomposes a floating-point number into its integer and fractional parts. Notice how each component is returned to the caller.

```
// Use out.

using System;

class Decompose {

  /* Decompose a floating-point value into its
     integer and fractional parts. */
  public int GetParts(double n, out double frac) {
    int whole;

    whole = (int) n;
    frac = n - whole; // pass fractional part back through frac
    return whole; // return integer portion
  }
}

class UseOut {
  static void Main() {
   Decompose ob = new Decompose();
    int i;
    double f;

    i = ob.GetParts(10.125, out f);

    Console.WriteLine("Integer portion is " + i);
    Console.WriteLine("Fractional part is " + f);
  }
}
```

The output from the program is shown here:

```
Integer portion is 10
Fractional part is 0.125
```

The **GetParts()** method returns two pieces of information. First, the integer portion of **n** is returned as **GetParts()**'s return value. Second, the fractional portion of **n** is passed back to the caller through the **out** parameter **frac**. As this example shows, by using **out**, it is possible for one method to return two values.

Of course, you are not limited to only one **out** parameter. A method can return as many pieces of information as necessary through **out** parameters. Here is an example that uses two **out** parameters. The method **HasComFactor()** performs two functions. First, it determines if two integers have a common factor (other than 1). It returns **true** if they do and **false** otherwise. Second, if they do have a common factor, **HasComFactor()** returns the least and greatest common factors in **out** parameters.

```
// Use two out parameters.

using System;

class Num {
  /* Determine if x and v have a common divisor.
```

```
       If so, return least and greatest common factors in
       the out parameters. */
   public bool HasComFactor(int x, int y,
                             out int least, out int greatest) {
     int i;
     int max = x < y ? x : y;
     bool first = true;

     least = 1;
     greatest = 1;

     // Find least and greatest common factors.
     for(i=2; i <= max/2 + 1; i++) {
       if( ((y%i)==0) & ((x%i)==0) ) {
         if(first) {
           least = i;
           first = false;
         }
         greatest = i;
       }
     }

     if(least != 1) return true;
     else return false;
   }
 }

 class DemoOut {
   static void Main() {
     Num ob = new Num();
     int lcf, gcf;

     if(ob.HasComFactor(231, 105, out lcf, out gcf)) {
       Console.WriteLine("Lcf of 231 and 105 is " + lcf);
       Console.WriteLine("Gcf of 231 and 105 is " + gcf);
     }
     else
       Console.WriteLine("No common factor for 35 and 49.");

     if(ob.HasComFactor(35, 51, out lcf, out gcf)) {
       Console.WriteLine("Lcf of 35 and 51 " + lcf);
       Console.WriteLine("Gcf of 35 and 51 is " + gcf);
     }
     else
       Console.WriteLine("No common factor for 35 and 51.");
   }
 }
```

In **Main()**, notice that **lcf** and **gcf** are not assigned values prior to the call to **HasComFactor()**. This would be an error if the parameters had been **ref** rather than **out**. The method returns either **true** or **false**, depending upon whether the two integers have a common factor. If they do, the least and greatest common factors are returned in the **out** parameters. The output from this program is shown here:

```
Lcf of 231 and 105 is 3
Gcf of 231 and 105 is 21
No common factor for 35 and 51.
```

Use ref and out on References

The use of **ref** and **out** is not limited to the passing of value types. They can also be used when a reference is passed. When **ref** or **out** modifies a reference, it causes the reference, itself, to be passed by reference. This allows a method to change the object to which the reference refers. Consider the following program, which uses **ref** reference parameters to exchange the objects to which two references are referring:

```
// Swap two references.

using System;

class RefSwap {
  int a, b;

  public RefSwap(int i, int j) {
    a = i;
    b = j;
  }

  public void Show() {
    Console.WriteLine("a: {0}, b: {1}", a, b);
  }

  // This method changes its arguments.
  public void Swap(ref RefSwap ob1, ref RefSwap ob2) {
    RefSwap t;

    t = ob1;
    ob1 = ob2;
    ob2 = t;
  }
}

class RefSwapDemo {
  static void Main() {
    RefSwap x = new RefSwap(1, 2);
    RefSwap y = new RefSwap(3, 4);

    Console.Write("x before call: ");
    x.Show();

    Console.Write("y before call: ");
    y.Show();

    Console.WriteLine();

    // Exchange the objects to which x and y refer.
    x.Swap(ref x, ref y);
```

```
    Console.Write("x after call: ");
    x.Show();

    Console.Write("y after call: ");
    y.Show();

  }
}
```

The output from this program is shown here:

```
x before call: a: 1, b: 2
y before call: a: 3, b: 4

x after call: a: 3, b: 4
y after call: a: 1, b: 2
```

In this example, the method **Swap()** exchanges the objects to which the two arguments to **Swap()** refer. Before calling **Swap()**, **x** refers to an object that contains the values 1 and 2, and **y** refers to an object that contains the values 3 and 4. After the call to **Swap()**, **x** refers to the object that contains the values 3 and 4, and **y** refers to the object that contains the values 1 and 2. If **ref** parameters had not been used, then the exchange inside **Swap()** would have had no effect outside **Swap()**. You might want to prove this by removing **ref** from **Swap()**.

Use a Variable Number of Arguments

When you create a method, you usually know in advance the number of arguments that you will be passing to it, but this is not always the case. Sometimes you will want to create a method that can be passed an arbitrary number of arguments. For example, consider a method that finds the smallest of a set of values. Such a method might be passed as few as two values, or three, or four, and so on. In all cases, you want that method to return the smallest value. Such a method cannot be created using normal parameters. Instead, you must use a special type of parameter that stands for an arbitrary number of parameters. This is done by creating a **params** parameter.

The **params** modifier is used to declare an array parameter that will be able to receive zero or more arguments. The number of elements in the array will be equal to the number of arguments passed to the method. Your program then accesses the array to obtain the arguments.

Here is an example that uses **params** to create a method called **MinVal()**, which returns the minimum value from a set of values:

```
// Demonstrate params.

using System;

class Min {
  public int MinVal(params int[] nums) {
    int m;

    if(nums.Length == 0) {
```

```
        Console.WriteLine("Error: no arguments.");
        return 0;
      }

    m = nums[0];
    for(int i=1; i < nums.Length; i++)
      if(nums[i] < m) m = nums[i];

    return m;
  }
}

class ParamsDemo {
  static void Main() {
    Min ob = new Min();
    int min;
    int a = 10, b = 20;

    // Call with 2 values.
    min = ob.MinVal(a, b);
    Console.WriteLine("Minimum is " + min);

    // Call with 3 values.
    min = ob.MinVal(a, b, -1);
    Console.WriteLine("Minimum is " + min);

    // Call with 5 values.
    min = ob.MinVal(18, 23, 3, 14, 25);
    Console.WriteLine("Minimum is " + min);

    // Can call with an int array, too.
    int[] args = { 45, 67, 34, 9, 112, 8 };
    min = ob.MinVal(args);
    Console.WriteLine("Minimum is " + min);
  }
}
```

The output from the program is shown here:

```
Minimum is 10
Minimum is -1
Minimum is 3
Minimum is 8
```

Each time **MinVal()** is called, the arguments are passed to it via the **nums** array. The length of the array equals the number of elements. Thus, you can use **MinVal()** to find the minimum of any number of values.

Notice the last call to **MinVal()**. Rather than being passed the values individually, it is passed an array containing the values. This is perfectly legal. When a **params** parameter is created, it will accept either a variable-length list of arguments or an array containing the arguments.

Although you can pass a **params** parameter any number of arguments, they all must be of a type compatible with the array type specified by the parameter. For example, calling **MinVal()** like this:

```
min = ob.MinVal(1, 2.2); // Wrong!
```

is illegal because there is no automatic conversion from **double** (2.2) to **int**, which is the type of **nums** in **MinVal()**.

When using **params**, you need to be careful about boundary conditions because a **params** parameter can accept any number of arguments—*even zero!* For example, it is syntactically valid to call **MinVal()** as shown here:

```
min = ob.MinVal(); // no arguments
min = ob.MinVal(3); // 1 argument
```

This is why there is a check in **MinVal()** to confirm that at least one element is in the **nums** array before there is an attempt to access that element. If the check were not there, then a runtime exception would result if **MinVal()** were called with no arguments. (Exceptions are described in Chapter 13.) Furthermore, the code in **MinVal()** was written in such a way as to permit calling **MinVal()** with one argument. In that situation, the lone argument is returned.

A method can have normal parameters and a variable-length parameter. For example, in the following program, the method **ShowArgs()** takes one **string** parameter and then a **params** integer array:

```
// Use regular parameter with a params parameter.

using System;

class MyClass {
  public void ShowArgs(string msg, params int[] nums) {
    Console.Write(msg + ": ");

    foreach(int i in nums)
      Console.Write(i + " ");

    Console.WriteLine();
  }
}

class ParamsDemo2 {
  static void Main() {
    MyClass ob = new MyClass();

    ob.ShowArgs("Here are some integers",
                1, 2, 3, 4, 5);

    ob.ShowArgs("Here are two more",
                17, 20);
  }
}
```

This program displays the following output:

```
Here are some integers: 1 2 3 4 5
Here are two more: 17 20
```

In cases where a method has regular parameters and a **params** parameter, the **params** parameter must be the last one in the parameter list. Furthermore, in all situations, there must be only one **params** parameter.

Return Objects

A method can return any type of data, including class types. For example, the following version of the **Rect** class includes a method called **Enlarge()** that creates a rectangle that is proportionally the same as the invoking rectangle, but larger by a specified factor:

```
// Return an object.

using System;

class Rect {
  int width;
  int height;

  public Rect(int w, int h) {
    width = w;
    height = h;
  }

  public int Area() {
    return width * height;
  }

  public void Show() {
    Console.WriteLine(width + " " + height);
  }

  /* Return a rectangle that is a specified
     factor larger than the invoking rectangle. */
  public Rect Enlarge(int factor) {
    return new Rect(width * factor, height * factor);
  }
}

class RetObj {
  static void Main() {
    Rect r1 = new Rect(4, 5);

    Console.Write("Dimensions of r1: ");
    r1.Show();
    Console.WriteLine("Area of r1: " + r1.Area());

    Console.WriteLine();

    // Create a rectangle that is twice as big as r1.
    Rect r2 = r1.Enlarge(2);
```

```
      Console.Write("Dimensions of r2: ");
      r2.Show();
      Console.WriteLine("Area of r2: " + r2.Area());
   }
}
```

The output is shown here:

```
Dimensions of r1: 4 5
Area of r1: 20

Dimensions of r2: 8 10
Area of r2: 80
```

When an object is returned by a method, it remains in existence until there are no more references to it. At that point, it is subject to garbage collection. Thus, an object won't be destroyed just because the method that created it terminates.

One application of object return types is the *class factory*. A class factory is a method that is used to construct objects of its class. In some situations, you may not want to give users of a class access to the class' constructor because of security concerns or because object construction depends upon certain external factors. In such cases, a class factory is used to construct objects. Here is a simple example:

```
// Use a class factory.

using System;

class MyClass {
  int a, b; // private

  // Create a class factory for MyClass.
  public MyClass Factory(int i, int j) {
    MyClass t = new MyClass();

    t.a = i;
    t.b = j;

    return t; // return an object
  }

  public void Show() {
    Console.WriteLine("a and b: " + a + " " + b);
  }

}

class MakeObjects {
  static void Main() {
    MyClass ob = new MyClass();
    int i, j;

    // Generate objects using the factory.
    for(i=0, j=10; i < 10; i++, j--) {
```

```
        MyClass anotherOb = ob.Factory(i, j); // make an object
        anotherOb.Show();
    }

    Console.WriteLine();
  }
}
```

The output is shown here:

```
a and b: 0 10
a and b: 1 9
a and b: 2 8
a and b: 3 7
a and b: 4 6
a and b: 5 5
a and b: 6 4
a and b: 7 3
a and b: 8 2
a and b: 9 1
```

Let's look closely at this example. **MyClass** does not define a constructor, so only the default constructor is available. Thus, it is not possible to set the values of **a** and **b** using a constructor. However, the class factory **Factory()** can create objects in which **a** and **b** are given values. Moreover, since **a** and **b** are private, using **Factory()** is the only way to set these values.

In **Main()**, a **MyClass** object is instantiated, and its factory method is used inside the **for** loop to create ten other objects. The line of code that creates objects is shown here:

```
MyClass anotherOb = ob.Factory(i, j); // get an object
```

With each iteration, an object reference called **anotherOb** is created, and it is assigned a reference to the object constructed by the factory. At the end of each iteration of the loop, **anotherOb** goes out of scope, and the object to which it refers is recycled.

Return an Array

Since in C# arrays are implemented as objects, a method can also return an array. (This differs from C++ in which arrays are not valid as return types.) For example, in the following program, the method **FindFactors()** returns an array that holds the factors of the argument that it is passed:

```
// Return an array.

using System;

class Factor {
  /* Return an array containing the factors of num.
     On return, numfactors will contain the number of
     factors found. */
  public int[] FindFactors(int num, out int numfactors) {
    int[] facts = new int[80]; // size of 80 is arbitrary
    int i, j;
```

```
// Find factors and put them in the facts array.
for(i=2, j=0; i < num/2 + 1; i++)
  if( (num%i)==0 ) {
    facts[j] = i;
    j++;
  }

numfactors = j;
return facts;
  }
}

class FindFactors {
  static void Main() {
    Factor f = new Factor();
    int numfactors;
    int[] factors;

    factors = f.FindFactors(1000, out numfactors);

    Console.WriteLine("Factors for 1000 are: ");
    for(int i=0; i < numfactors; i++)
      Console.Write(factors[i] + " ");

    Console.WriteLine();
  }
}
```

The output is shown here:

```
Factors for 1000 are:
2 4 5 8 10 20 25 40 50 100 125 200 250 500
```

In **Factor**, **FindFactors( )** is declared like this:

```
public int[] FindFactors(int num, out int numfactors) {
```

Notice how the **int** array return type is specified. This syntax can be generalized. Whenever a method returns an array, specify it in a similar fashion, adjusting the type and dimensions as needed. For example, the following declares a method called **someMeth( )** that returns a two-dimensional array of **double**:

```
public double[,] someMeth() { // ...
```

Method Overloading

In C#, two or more methods within the same class can share the same name, as long as their parameter declarations are different. When this is the case, the methods are said to be *overloaded,* and the process is referred to as *method overloading.* Method overloading is one of the ways that C# implements polymorphism.

In general, to overload a method, simply declare different versions of it. The compiler takes care of the rest. You must observe one important restriction: The type and/or number of the parameters of each overloaded method must differ. It is not sufficient for two methods to differ only in their return types. They must differ in the types or number of their parameters.

(Return types do not provide sufficient information in all cases for C# to decide which method to use.) Of course, overloaded methods *may* differ in their return types, too. When an overloaded method is called, the version of the method executed is the one whose parameters match the arguments.

Here is a simple example that illustrates method overloading:

```
// Demonstrate method overloading.

using System;

class Overload {
  public void OvlDemo() {
    Console.WriteLine("No parameters");
  }

  // Overload OvlDemo for one integer parameter.
  public void OvlDemo(int a) {
    Console.WriteLine("One parameter: " + a);
  }

  // Overload OvlDemo for two integer parameters.
  public int OvlDemo(int a, int b) {
    Console.WriteLine("Two parameters: " + a + " " + b);
    return a + b;
  }

  // Overload OvlDemo for two double parameters.
  public double OvlDemo(double a, double b) {
    Console.WriteLine("Two double parameters: " +
                        a + " "+ b);
    return a + b;
  }
}

class OverloadDemo {
  static void Main() {
    Overload ob = new Overload();
    int resI;
    double resD;

    // Call all versions of OvlDemo().
    ob.OvlDemo();
    Console.WriteLine();

    ob.OvlDemo(2);
    Console.WriteLine();

    resI = ob.OvlDemo(4, 6);
    Console.WriteLine("Result of ob.OvlDemo(4, 6): " + resI);
    Console.WriteLine();

    resD = ob.OvlDemo(1.1, 2.32);
    Console.WriteLine("Result of ob.OvlDemo(1.1, 2.32): " + resD);
  }
}
```

This program generates the following output:

```
No parameters

One parameter: 2

Two parameters: 4 6
Result of ob.OvlDemo(4, 6): 10

Two double parameters: 1.1 2.32
Result of ob.OvlDemo(1.1, 2.32): 3.42
```

As you can see, **OvlDemo()** is overloaded four times. The first version takes no parameters; the second takes one integer parameter; the third takes two integer parameters; and the fourth takes two **double** parameters. Notice that the first two versions of **OvlDemo()** return **void** and the second two return a value. This is perfectly valid, but as explained, overloading is not affected one way or the other by the return type of a method. Thus, attempting to use these two versions of **OvlDemo()** will cause an error:

```
// One OvlDemo(int) is OK.
public void OvlDemo(int a) {
  Console.WriteLine("One parameter: " + a);
}

/* Error! Two OvlDemo(int)s are not OK even though
    return types differ. */
public int OvlDemo(int a) {
  Console.WriteLine("One parameter: " + a);
  return a * a;
}
```

As the comments suggest, the difference in their return types is an insufficient difference for the purposes of overloading.

As you will recall from Chapter 3, C# provides certain implicit (i.e., automatic) type conversions. These conversions also apply to parameters of overloaded methods. For example, consider the following:

```
// Implicit type conversions can affect overloaded method resolution.

using System;

class Overload2 {
  public void MyMeth(int x) {
    Console.WriteLine("Inside MyMeth(int): " + x);
  }

  public void MyMeth(double x) {
    Console.WriteLine("Inside MyMeth(double): " + x);
  }
}

class TypeConv {
  static void Main() {
```

```
    Overload2 ob = new Overload2();

    int i = 10;
    double d = 10.1;

    byte b = 99;
    short s = 10;
    float f = 11.5F;


    ob.MyMeth(i); // calls ob.MyMeth(int)
    ob.MyMeth(d); // calls ob.MyMeth(double)

    ob.MyMeth(b); // calls ob.MyMeth(int) -- type conversion
    ob.MyMeth(s); // calls ob.MyMeth(int) -- type conversion
    ob.MyMeth(f); // calls ob.MyMeth(double) -- type conversion
  }
}
```

The output from the program is shown here:

```
Inside MyMeth(int): 10
Inside MyMeth(double): 10.1
Inside MyMeth(int): 99
Inside MyMeth(int): 10
Inside MyMeth(double): 11.5
```

In this example, only two versions of **MyMeth()** are defined: one that has an **int** parameter and one that has a **double** parameter. However, it is possible to pass **MyMeth()** a **byte**, **short**, or **float** value. In the case of **byte** and **short**, C# automatically converts them to **int**. Thus, **MyMeth(int)** is invoked. In the case of **float**, the value is converted to **double** and **MyMeth(double)** is called.

It is important to understand, however, that the implicit conversions apply only if there is no exact type match between a parameter and an argument. For example, here is the preceding program with the addition of a version of **MyMeth()** that specifies a **byte** parameter:

```
// Add MyMeth(byte).

using System;

class Overload2 {
  public void MyMeth(byte x) {
    Console.WriteLine("Inside MyMeth(byte): " + x);
  }

  public void MyMeth(int x) {
    Console.WriteLine("Inside MyMeth(int): " + x);
  }

  public void MyMeth(double x) {
    Console.WriteLine("Inside MyMeth(double): " + x);
  }
}
```

```
class TypeConv {
  static void Main() {
    Overload2 ob = new Overload2();

    int i = 10;
    double d = 10.1;

    byte b = 99;
    short s = 10;
    float f = 11.5F;


    ob.MyMeth(i); // calls ob.MyMeth(int)
    ob.MyMeth(d); // calls ob.MyMeth(double)

    ob.MyMeth(b); // calls ob.MyMeth(byte) -- now, no type conversion

    ob.MyMeth(s); // calls ob.MyMeth(int) -- type conversion
    ob.MyMeth(f); // calls ob.MyMeth(double) -- type conversion
  }
}
```

Now when the program is run, the following output is produced:

```
Inside MyMeth(int): 10
Inside MyMeth(double): 10.1
Inside MyMeth(byte): 99
Inside MyMeth(int): 10
Inside MyMeth(double): 11.5
```

In this version, since there is a version of **MyMeth()** that takes a **byte** argument, when **MyMeth()** is called with a **byte** argument, **MyMeth(byte)** is invoked and the automatic conversion to **int** does not occur.

Both **ref** and **out** participate in overload resolution. For example, the following defines two distinct and separate methods:

```
public void MyMeth(int x) {
  Console.WriteLine("Inside MyMeth(int): " + x);
}

public void MyMeth(ref int x) {
  Console.WriteLine("Inside MyMeth(ref int): " + x);
}
```

Thus,

```
ob.MyMeth(i)
```

invokes **MyMeth(int x)**, but

```
ob.MyMeth(ref i)
```

invokes **MyMeth(ref int x)**.

Although **ref** and **out** participate in overload resolution, the difference between the two alone is not sufficient. For example, these two versions of **MyMeth()** are invalid:

```
// Wrong!
public void MyMeth(out int x) { // ...
public void MyMeth(ref int x) { // ...
```

In this case, the compiler cannot differentiate between the two version of **MyMeth()** simply because one uses an **out int** parameter and the other uses a **ref int** parameter.

Method overloading supports polymorphism because it is one way that C# implements the "one interface, multiple methods" paradigm. To understand how, consider the following. In languages that do not support method overloading, each method must be given a unique name. However, frequently you will want to implement essentially the same method for different types of data. Consider the absolute value function. In languages that do not support overloading, there are usually three or more versions of this function, each with a slightly different name. For instance, in C, the function **abs()** returns the absolute value of an integer, **labs()** returns the absolute value of a long integer, and **fabs()** returns the absolute value of a floating-point value.

Since C does not support overloading, each function must have its own unique name, even though all three functions do essentially the same thing. This makes the situation more complex, conceptually, than it actually is. Although the underlying concept of each function is the same, you still have three names to remember. This situation does not occur in C# because each absolute value method can use the same name. Indeed, the .NET Framework class library includes an absolute value method called **Abs()**. This method is overloaded by the **System.Math** class to handle the numeric types. C# determines which version of **Abs()** to call based upon the type of argument.

A principal value of overloading is that it allows related methods to be accessed by use of a common name. Thus, the name **Abs** represents the *general action* that is being performed. It is left to the compiler to choose the right *specific* version for a particular circumstance. You, the programmer, need only remember the general operation being performed. Through the application of polymorphism, several names have been reduced to one. Although this example is fairly simple, if you expand the concept, you can see how overloading can help manage greater complexity.

When you overload a method, each version of that method can perform any activity you desire. There is no rule stating that overloaded methods must relate to one another. However, from a stylistic point of view, method overloading implies a relationship. Thus, while you can use the same name to overload unrelated methods, you should not. For example, you could use the name **Sqr** to create methods that return the *square* of an integer and the *square root* of a floating-point value. But these two operations are fundamentally different. Applying method overloading in this manner defeats its original purpose. In practice, you should only overload closely related operations.

C# defines the term *signature*, which is the name of a method plus its parameter list. Thus, for the purposes of overloading, no two methods within the same class can have the same signature. Notice that a signature does not include the return type since it is not used by C# for overload resolution. Also, the **params** modifier is not part of the signature.

Overload Constructors

Like methods, constructors can also be overloaded. Doing so allows you to construct objects in a variety of ways. For example, consider the following program:

```
// Demonstrate an overloaded constructor.

using System;

class MyClass {
  public int x;

  public MyClass() {
    Console.WriteLine("Inside MyClass().");
    x = 0;
  }

  public MyClass(int i) {
    Console.WriteLine("Inside MyClass(int).");
    x = i;
  }

  public MyClass(double d) {
    Console.WriteLine("Inside MyClass(double).");
    x = (int) d;
  }

  public MyClass(int i, int j) {
    Console.WriteLine("Inside MyClass(int, int).");
    x = i * j;
  }
}

class OverloadConsDemo {
  static void Main() {
    MyClass t1 = new MyClass();
    MyClass t2 = new MyClass(88);
    MyClass t3 = new MyClass(17.23);
    MyClass t4 = new MyClass(2, 4);

    Console.WriteLine("t1.x: " + t1.x);
    Console.WriteLine("t2.x: " + t2.x);
    Console.WriteLine("t3.x: " + t3.x);
    Console.WriteLine("t4.x: " + t4.x);
  }
}
```

The output from the program is shown here:

```
Inside MyClass().
Inside MyClass(int).
Inside MyClass(double).
Inside MyClass(int, int).
```

```
t1.x: 0
t2.x: 88
t3.x: 17
t4.x: 8
```

MyClass( ) is overloaded four ways, each constructing an object differently. The proper constructor is called based upon the arguments specified when **new** is executed. By overloading a class' constructor, you give the user of your class flexibility in the way objects are constructed.

One of the most common reasons that constructors are overloaded is to allow one object to initialize another. For example, here is an enhanced version of the **Stack** class developed earlier that allows one stack to be constructed from another:

```
// A stack class for characters.

using System;

class Stack {
  // These members are private.
  char[] stck; // holds the stack
  int tos;       // index of the top of the stack

  // Construct an empty Stack given its size.
  public Stack(int size) {
    stck = new char[size]; // allocate memory for stack
    tos = 0;
  }

  // Construct a Stack from a stack.
  public Stack(Stack ob) {
    // Allocate memory for stack.
    stck = new char[ob.stck.Length];

    // Copy elements to new stack.
    for(int i=0; i < ob.tos; i++)
      stck[i] = ob.stck[i];

    // Set tos for new stack.
    tos = ob.tos;
  }

  // Push characters onto the stack.
  public void Push(char ch) {
    if(tos==stck.Length) {
      Console.WriteLine(" -- Stack is full.");
      return;
    }

    stck[tos] = ch;
    tos++;
  }

  // Pop a character from the stack.
```

```
  public char Pop() {
    if(tos==0) {
      Console.WriteLine(" -- Stack is empty.");
      return (char) 0;
    }

    tos--;
    return stck[tos];
  }

  // Return true if the stack is full.
  public bool IsFull() {
    return tos==stck.Length;
  }

  // Return true if the stack is empty.
  public bool IsEmpty() {
    return tos==0;
  }

  // Return total capacity of the stack.
  public int Capacity() {
    return stck.Length;
  }

  // Return number of objects currently on the stack.
  public int GetNum() {
    return tos;
  }
}

// Demonstrate the Stack class.
class StackDemo {
  static void Main() {
    Stack stk1 = new Stack(10);
    char ch;
    int i;

    // Put some characters into stk1.
    Console.WriteLine("Push A through J onto stk1.");
    for(i=0; !stk1.IsFull(); i++)
      stk1.Push((char) ('A' + i));

    // Create a copy of stck1.
    Stack stk2 = new Stack(stk1);

    // Display the contents of stk1.
    Console.Write("Contents of stk1: ");
    while( !stk1.IsEmpty() ) {
      ch = stk1.Pop();
      Console.Write(ch);
    }
```

```
    Console.WriteLine();

    Console.Write("Contents of stk2: ");
    while ( !stk2.IsEmpty() ) {
      ch = stk2.Pop();
      Console.Write(ch);
    }

    Console.WriteLine("\n");

  }
}
```

The output is shown here:

```
Push A through J onto stk1.
Contents of stk1: JIHGFEDCBA
Contents of stk2: JIHGFEDCBA
```

In **StackDemo**, the first stack, **stk1**, is constructed and filled with characters. This stack is then used to construct the second stack, **stk2**. This causes the following **Stack** constructor to be executed:

```
// Construct a Stack from a stack.
public Stack(Stack ob) {
  // Allocate memory for stack.
  stck = new char[ob.stck.Length];

  // Copy elements to new stack.
  for(int i=0; i < ob.tos; i++)
    stck[i] = ob.stck[i];

  // Set tos for new stack.
  tos = ob.tos;
}
```

Inside this constructor, an array is allocated that is long enough to hold the elements contained in the stack passed in **ob**. Then, the contents of **ob**'s array are copied to the new array, and **tos** is set appropriately. After the constructor finishes, the new stack and the original stack are separate, but identical.

Invoke an Overloaded Constructor Through this

When working with overloaded constructors, it is sometimes useful for one constructor to invoke another. In C#, this is accomplished by using another form of the **this** keyword. The general form is shown here:

constructor-name(*parameter-list1*) : this(*parameter-list2*) {
   // ... body of constructor, which may be empty
}

When the constructor is executed, the overloaded constructor that matches the parameter list specified by *parameter-list2* is first executed. Then, if there are any statements inside the original constructor, they are executed. Here is an example:

```
// Demonstrate invoking a constructor through this.

using System;

class XYCoord {
  public int x, y;

  public XYCoord() : this(0, 0) {
    Console.WriteLine("Inside XYCoord()");
  }

  public XYCoord(XYCoord obj) : this(obj.x, obj.y) {
    Console.WriteLine("Inside XYCoord(obj)");
  }

  public XYCoord(int i, int j) {
    Console.WriteLine("Inside XYCoord(int, int)");
    x = i;
    y = j;
  }
}

class OverloadConsDemo {
  static void Main() {
    XYCoord t1 = new XYCoord();
    XYCoord t2 = new XYCoord(8, 9);
    XYCoord t3 = new XYCoord(t2);

    Console.WriteLine("t1.x, t1.y: " + t1.x + ", " + t1.y);
    Console.WriteLine("t2.x, t2.y: " + t2.x + ", " + t2.y);
    Console.WriteLine("t3.x, t3.y: " + t3.x + ", " + t3.y);
  }
}
```

The output from the program is shown here:

```
Inside XYCoord(int, int)
Inside XYCoord()
Inside XYCoord(int, int)
Inside XYCoord(int, int)
Inside XYCoord(obj)
t1.x, t1.y: 0, 0
t2.x, t2.y: 8, 9
t3.x, t3.y: 8, 9
```

Here is how the program works. In the **XYCoord** class, the only constructor that actually initializes the **x** and **y** fields is **XYCoord(int, int)**. The other two constructors simply invoke **XYCoord(int, int)** through **this**. For example, when object **t1** is created, its constructor, **XYCoord()**, is called. This causes **this(0, 0)** to be executed, which in this case translates into a call to **XYCoord(0, 0)**. The creation of **t2** works in similar fashion.

One reason why invoking overloaded constructors through **this** can be useful is that it can prevent the unnecessary duplication of code. In the foregoing example, there is no reason for all three constructors to duplicate the same initialization sequence, which the use of **this** avoids. Another advantage is that you can create constructors with implied "default arguments" that are used when these arguments are not explicitly specified. For example, you could create another **XYCoord** constructor as shown here:

```
public XYCoord(int x) : this(x, x) { }
```

This constructor automatically defaults the **y** coordinate to the same value as the **x** coordinate. Of course, it is wise to use such "default arguments" carefully because their misuse could easily confuse users of your classes.

Object Initializers

C# 3.0 added a new feature called *object initializers* that provides another way to create an object and initialize its fields and properties. (See Chapter 10 for a discussion of properties.) Using object initializers, you do not call a class' constructor in the normal way. Rather, you specify the names of the fields and/or properties to be initialized, giving each an initial value. Thus, the object initializer syntax provides an alternative to explicitly invoking a class' constructor. The primary use of the object initializer syntax is with anonymous types created in a LINQ expression. (Anonymous types and LINQ are described in Chapter 19.) However, because the object initializers can be used (and occasionally are used) with a named class, the fundamentals of object initialization are introduced here.

Let's begin with a simple example:

```
// A simple demonstration that uses object initializers.

using System;

class MyClass {
  public int Count;
  public string Str;
}

class ObjInitDemo {
  static void Main() {
    // Construct a MyClass object by using object initializers.
    MyClass obj = new MyClass { Count = 100, Str = "Testing" };

    Console.WriteLine(obj.Count + " " + obj.Str);
  }
}
```

This produces the following output:

```
100 Testing
```

As the output shows, the value of **obj.Count** has been initialized to 100 and the value of **obj.Str** has been initialized to "Testing". Notice, however, that **MyClass** does not define any explicit constructors, and that the normal constructor syntax has not been used. Rather, **obj** is created using the following line:

```
MyClass obj = new MyClass { Count = 100, Str = "Testing" };
```

Here, the names of the fields are explicitly specified along with their initial values. This results in a default instance of **MyClass** being constructed (by use of the implicit default constructor) and then **Count** and **Str** are given the specified initial values.

It is important to understand that the order of the initializers is not important. For example, **obj** could have been initialized as shown here:

```
MyClass obj = new MyClass { Str = "Testing", Count = 100 };
```

In this statement, the initialization of **Str** precedes the initialization of **Count**. In the program, it was the other way around. However, in either case, the end result is the same.

Here is the general form of object initialization syntax:

new *class-name* { *name* = *expr*, *name* = *expr*, *name* = *expr*, ... }

Here, *name* specifies the name of a field or property that is an accessible member of *class-name*. Of course, the type of the initializing expression specified by *expr* must be compatible with the type of field or property.

Although you can use object initializers with a named class (such as **MyClass** in the example), you usually won't. In general, you will use the normal constructor call syntax when working with named classes. As mentioned, object initializers are most applicable to anonymous types generated by a LINQ expression.

The Main( ) Method

Up to this point, you have been using one form of **Main()**. However, it has several overloaded forms. Some can be used to return a value, and some can receive arguments. Each is examined here.

Return Values from Main( )

When a program ends, you can return a value to the calling process (often the operating system) by returning a value from **Main()**. To do so, you can use this form of **Main()**:

static int Main()

Notice that instead of being declared **void**, this version of **Main()** has a return type of **int**.

Usually, the return value from **Main()** indicates whether the program ended normally or due to some abnormal condition. By convention, a return value of zero usually indicates normal termination. All other values indicate some type of error occurred.

Pass Arguments to Main( )

Many programs accept what are called *command-line* arguments. A command-line argument is the information that directly follows the program's name on the command line when it is executed. For C# programs, these arguments are then passed to the **Main()** method. To receive the arguments, you must use one of these forms of **Main()**:

static void Main(string[ ] *args*)
static int Main(string[ ] *args*)

The first form returns **void**; the second can be used to return an integer value, as described in the preceding section. For both, the command-line arguments are stored as strings in the

string array passed to **Main()**. The length of the *args* array will be equal to the number of command-line arguments, which might be zero.

For example, the following program displays all of the command-line arguments that it is called with:

```
// Display all command-line information.

using System;

class CLDemo {
  static void Main(string[] args) {
    Console.WriteLine("There are " + args.Length +
                      " command-line arguments.");

    Console.WriteLine("They are: ");
    for(int i=0; i < args.Length; i++)
      Console.WriteLine(args[i]);
  }
}
```

If **CLDemo** is executed like this:

```
CLDemo one two three
```

you will see the following output:

```
There are 3 command-line arguments.
They are:
one
two
three
```

To understand the way that command-line arguments can be used, consider the next program. It uses a simple substitution cipher to encode or decode messages. The message to be encoded or decoded is specified on the command line. The cipher is very simple: To encode a word, each letter is incremented by 1. Thus, A becomes B, and so on. To decode, each letter is decremented. Of course, such a cipher is of no practical value, being trivially easy to break. But it does provide an enjoyable pastime for children.

```
// Encode or decode a message using a simple substitution cipher.

using System;

class Cipher {
  static int Main(string[] args) {

    // See if arguments are present.
    if(args.Length < 2) {
      Console.WriteLine("Usage: encode/decode word1 [word2...wordN]");
      return 1; // return failure code
    }

    // If args present, first arg must be encode or decode.
```

```
    if(args[0] != "encode" & args[0] != "decode") {
      Console.WriteLine("First arg must be encode or decode.");
      return 1; // return failure code
    }

    // Encode or decode message.
    for(int n=1; n < args.Length; n++) {
      for(int i=0; i < args[n].Length; i++) {
        if(args[0] == "encode")
          Console.Write((char) (args[n][i] + 1) );
        else
          Console.Write((char) (args[n][i] - 1) );
      }
      Console.Write(" ");
    }

    Console.WriteLine();

    return 0;
  }
}
```

To use the program, specify either the "encode" or "decode" command followed by the phrase that you want to encrypt or decrypt. Assuming the program is called Cipher, here are two sample runs:

```
C:>Cipher encode one two
pof uxp

C:>Cipher decode pof uxp
one two
```

There are two interesting things in this program. First, notice how the program checks that a command-line argument is present before it continues executing. This is very important and can be generalized. When a program relies on there being one or more command-line arguments, it must always confirm that the proper arguments have been supplied. Failure to do this can lead to program malfunctions. Also, since the first command-line argument must be either "encode" or "decode," the program also checks this before proceeding.

Second, notice how the program returns a termination code. If the required command line is not present, then 1 is returned, indicating abnormal termination. Otherwise, 0 is returned when the program ends.

Recursion

In C#, a method can call itself. This process is called *recursion,* and a method that calls itself is said to be *recursive.* In general, recursion is the process of defining something in terms of itself and is somewhat similar to a circular definition. The key component of a recursive method is that it contains a statement that executes a call to itself. Recursion is a powerful control mechanism.

The classic example of recursion is the computation of the factorial of a number. The factorial of a number *N* is the product of all the whole numbers between 1 and *N*. For example, 3 factorial is 1×2×3, or 6. The following program shows a recursive way to

compute the factorial of a number. For comparison purposes, a nonrecursive equivalent is also included.

```
// A simple example of recursion.

using System;

class Factorial {
  // This is a recursive method.
  public int FactR(int n) {
    int result;

    if(n==1) return 1;
    result = FactR(n-1) * n;
    return result;
  }

  // This is an iterative equivalent.
  public int FactI(int n) {
    int t, result;

    result = 1;
    for(t=1; t <= n; t++) result *= t;
    return result;
  }
}

class Recursion {
  static void Main() {
    Factorial f = new Factorial();

    Console.WriteLine("Factorials using recursive method.");
    Console.WriteLine("Factorial of 3 is " + f.FactR(3));
    Console.WriteLine("Factorial of 4 is " + f.FactR(4));
    Console.WriteLine("Factorial of 5 is " + f.FactR(5));
    Console.WriteLine();

    Console.WriteLine("Factorials using iterative method.");
    Console.WriteLine("Factorial of 3 is " + f.FactI(3));
    Console.WriteLine("Factorial of 4 is " + f.FactI(4));
    Console.WriteLine("Factorial of 5 is " + f.FactI(5));
  }
}
```

The output from this program is shown here:

```
Factorials using recursive method.
Factorial of 3 is 6
Factorial of 4 is 24
Factorial of 5 is 120

Factorials using iterative method.
Factorial of 3 is 6
Factorial of 4 is 24
Factorial of 5 is 120
```

The operation of the nonrecursive method **FactI()** should be clear. It uses a loop starting at 1 and progressively multiplies each number by the moving product.

The operation of the recursive **FactR()** is a bit more complex. When **FactR()** is called with an argument of 1, the method returns 1; otherwise, it returns the product of **FactR(n–1)*n**. To evaluate this expression, **FactR()** is called with **n–1**. This process repeats until **n** equals 1 and the calls to the method begin returning. For example, when the factorial of 2 is calculated, the first call to **FactR()** will cause a second call to be made with an argument of 1. This call will return 1, which is then multiplied by 2 (the original value of **n**). The answer is then 2. You might find it interesting to insert **WriteLine()** statements into **FactR()** that show the level of recursion of each call and what the intermediate results are.

When a method calls itself, new local variables and parameters are allocated storage on the system stack, and the method code is executed with these new variables from the start. A recursive call does not make a new copy of the method. Only the arguments are new. As each recursive call returns, the old local variables and parameters are removed from the stack, and execution resumes at the point of the call inside the method. Recursive methods could be said to "telescope" out and back.

Here is another example of recursion. The **DisplayRev()** method uses recursion to display its string argument backward.

```
// Display a string in reverse by using recursion.

using System;

class RevStr {

  // Display a string backward.
  public void DisplayRev(string str) {
    if(str.Length > 0)
      DisplayRev(str.Substring(1, str.Length-1));
    else
      return;

    Console.Write(str[0]);
  }
}

class RevStrDemo {
  static void Main() {
    string s = "this is a test";
    RevStr rsOb = new RevStr();

    Console.WriteLine("Original string: " + s);

    Console.Write("Reversed string: ");
    rsOb.DisplayRev(s);

    Console.WriteLine();
  }
}
```

Here is the output:

```
Original string: this is a test
Reversed string: tset a si siht
```

Each time **DisplayRev( )** is called, it first checks to see if **str** has a length greater than zero. If it does, it recursively calls **DisplayRev( )** with a new string that consists of **str** minus its first character. This process repeats until a zero-length string is passed. This causes the recursive calls to start unraveling. As they do, the first character of **str** in each call is displayed. This results in the string being displayed in reverse order.

Recursive versions of many routines may execute a bit more slowly than the iterative equivalent because of the added overhead of the additional method calls. Too many recursive calls to a method could cause a stack overrun. Because storage for parameters and local variables is on the system stack, and each new call creates a new copy of these variables, it is possible that the stack could be exhausted. If this occurs, the CLR will throw an exception. However, you probably will not have to worry about this unless a recursive routine runs wild.

The main advantage to recursion is that some types of algorithms can be more clearly and simply implemented recursively than iteratively. For example, the quicksort sorting algorithm is quite difficult to implement in an iterative way. Also, some problems, especially AI-related ones, seem to lend themselves to recursive solutions.

When writing recursive methods, you must have a conditional statement, such as an **if**, somewhere to force the method to return without the recursive call being executed. If you don't do this, once you call the method, it will never return. This type of error is very common when working with recursion. Use **WriteLine( )** statements liberally so that you can watch what is going on and abort execution if you see that you have made a mistake.

Understanding static

There will be times when you will want to define a class member that will be used independently of any object of that class. Normally, a class member must be accessed through an object of its class, but it is possible to create a member that can be used by itself, without reference to a specific instance. To create such a member, precede its declaration with the keyword **static**. When a member is declared **static**, it can be accessed before any objects of its class are created and without reference to any object. You can declare both methods and variables to be **static**. The most common example of a **static** member is **Main( )**, which is declared **static** because it must be called by the operating system when your program begins.

Outside the class, to use a **static** member, you must specify the name of its class followed by the dot operator. No object needs to be created. In fact, a **static** member cannot be accessed through an object reference. It must be accessed through its class name. For example, if you want to assign the value 10 to a **static** variable called **count** that is part of a class called **Timer**, use this line:

```
Timer.count = 10;
```

This format is similar to that used to access normal instance variables through an object, except that the class name is used. A **static** method can be called in the same way—by use of the dot operator on the name of the class.

Variables declared as **static** are, essentially, global variables. When objects of its class are declared, no copy of a **static** variable is made. Instead, all instances of the class share the same

static variable. A **static** variable is initialized before its class is used. If no explicit initializer is specified, it is initialized to zero for numeric types, null in the case of reference types, or **false** for variables of type **bool**. Thus, a **static** variable always has a value.

The difference between a **static** method and a normal method is that the **static** method can be called through its class name, without any instance of that class being created. You have seen an example of this already: the **Sqrt()** method, which is a **static** method within C#'s **System.Math** class.

Here is an example that declares a **static** variable and a **static** method:

```
// Use static.

using System;

class StaticDemo {
  // A static variable.
  public static int Val = 100;

  // A static method.
  public static int ValDiv2() {
    return Val/2;
  }
}

class SDemo {
  static void Main() {

    Console.WriteLine("Initial value of StaticDemo.Val is "
                      + StaticDemo.Val);

    StaticDemo.Val = 8;
    Console.WriteLine("StaticDemo.Val is " + StaticDemo.Val);
    Console.WriteLine("StaticDemo.ValDiv2(): " +
                      StaticDemo.ValDiv2());

  }
}
```

The output is shown here:

```
Initial value of StaticDemo.Val is 100
StaticDemo.Val is 8
StaticDemo.ValDiv2(): 4
```

As the output shows, a **static** variable is initialized before any object of its class is created. There are several restrictions that apply to **static** methods:

- A **static** method does not have a **this** reference. This is because a **static** method does not execute relative to any object.

- A **static** method can directly call only other **static** methods of its class. It cannot directly call an instance method of its class. The reason is that instance methods operate on specific objects, but a **static** method is not called on an object. Thus, on what object would the **static** method operate?

- A similar restriction applies to **static** data. A **static** method can directly access only other **static** data defined by its class. It cannot operate on an instance variable of its class because there is no object to operate on.

For example, in the following class, the **static** method **ValDivDenom()** is illegal:

```
class StaticError {
  public int Denom = 3; // a normal instance variable
  public static int Val = 1024; // a static variable

  /* Error! Can't directly access a non-static variable
     from within a static method. */
  static int ValDivDenom() {
    return Val/Denom; // won't compile!
  }
}
```

Here, **Denom** is a normal instance variable that cannot be accessed within a **static** method. However, the use of **Val** is okay since it is a **static** variable.

The same problem occurs when trying to call a non-**static** method from within a **static** method of the same class. For example:

```
using System;

class AnotherStaticError {
  // A non-static method.
  void NonStaticMeth() {
    Console.WriteLine("Inside NonStaticMeth().");
  }

  /* Error! Can't directly call a non-static method
     from within a static method. */
  static void staticMeth() {
    NonStaticMeth(); // won't compile
  }
}
```

In this case, the attempt to call a non-**static** (that is, instance method) from a **static** method causes a compile-time error.

It is important to understand that a **static** method *can* call instance methods and access instance variables of its class if it does so through an object of that class. It is just that it cannot use an instance variable or method without an object qualification. For example, this fragment is perfectly valid:

```
class MyClass {
  // A non-static method.
  void NonStaticMeth() {
    Console.WriteLine("Inside NonStaticMeth().");
  }

  /* Can call a non-static method through an
     object reference from within a static method. */
```

```
public static void staticMeth(MyClass ob) {
  ob.NonStaticMeth(); // this is OK
  }
}
```

Here, **NonStaticMeth( )** is called by **staticMeth( )** through **ob**, which is an object of type **MyClass**.

Because **static** fields are independent of any specific object, they are useful when you need to maintain information that is applicable to an entire class. Here is an example of such a situation. It uses a **static** field to maintain a count of the number of objects that are in existence.

```
// Use a static field to count instances.

using System;

class CountInst {
  static int count = 0;

  // Increment count when object is created.
  public CountInst() {
    count++;
  }

  // Decrement count when object is destroyed.
  ~CountInst() {
    count--;
  }

  public static int GetCount() {
    return count;
  }
}

class CountDemo {
  static void Main() {
    CountInst ob;


    for(int i=0; i < 10; i++) {
      ob = new CountInst();
      Console.WriteLine("Current count: " + CountInst.GetCount());
    }
  }
}
```

The output is shown here:

```
Current count: 1
Current count: 2
Current count: 3
Current count: 4
Current count: 5
Current count: 6
```

```
Current count: 7
Current count: 8
Current count: 9
Current count: 10
```

Each time that an object of type **CountInst** is created, the **static** field **count** is incremented. Each time an object is recycled, **count** is decremented. Thus, **count** always contains a count of the number of objects currently in existence. This is possible only through the use of a **static** field. There is no way for an instance variable to maintain the count because the count relates to the class as a whole, not to a specific instance.

Here is one more example that uses **static**. Earlier in this chapter, you saw how a class factory could be used to create objects. In that example, the class factory was a non-**static** method, which meant that it could be called only through an object reference. This meant that a default object of the class needed to be created so that the factory method could be called. However, a better way to implement a class factory is as a **static** method, which allows the class factory to be called without creating an unnecessary object. Here is the class factory example rewritten to reflect this improvement:

```
// Use a static class factory.

using System;

class MyClass {
  int a, b;

  // Create a class factory for MyClass.
  static public MyClass Factory(int i, int j) {
    MyClass t = new MyClass();

    t.a = i;
    t.b = j;

    return t; // return an object
  }

  public void Show() {
    Console.WriteLine("a and b: " + a + " " + b);
  }
}

class MakeObjects {
  static void Main() {
    int i, j;

    // Generate objects using the factory.
    for(i=0, j=10; i < 10; i++, j--) {
      MyClass ob = MyClass.Factory(i, j); // get an object
      ob.Show();
    }

    Console.WriteLine();
  }
}
```

In this version, **Factory()** is invoked through its class name in this line of code:

```
MyClass ob = MyClass.Factory(i, j); // get an object
```

There is no need to create a **MyClass** object prior to using the factory.

Static Constructors

A constructor can also be specified as **static**. A **static** constructor is typically used to initialize features that apply to a class rather than an instance. Thus, it is used to initialize aspects of a class before any objects of the class are created. Here is a simple example:

```
// Use a static constructor.

using System;

class Cons {
  public static int alpha;
  public int beta;

  // A static constructor.
  static Cons() {
    alpha = 99;
    Console.WriteLine("Inside static constructor.");
  }

  // An instance constructor.
  public Cons() {
    beta = 100;
    Console.WriteLine("Inside instance constructor.");
  }
}

class ConsDemo {
  static void Main() {
    Cons ob = new Cons();

    Console.WriteLine("Cons.alpha: " + Cons.alpha);
    Console.WriteLine("ob.beta: " + ob.beta);
  }
}
```

Here is the output:

```
Inside static constructor.
Inside instance constructor.
Cons.alpha: 99
ob.beta: 100
```

Notice that the **static** constructor is called automatically (when the class is first loaded) and before the instance constructor. This can be generalized. In all cases, the **static** constructor will be executed before any instance constructor. Furthermore, **static** constructors cannot have access modifiers (thus, they use default access) and cannot be called by your program.

Static Classes

Beginning with C# 2.0, you can declare a class **static**. There are two key features of a **static** class. First, no object of a **static** class can be created. Second, a **static** class must contain only **static** members. A **static** class is created by modifying a class declaration with the keyword **static**, shown here.

     static class *class-name* { // ...

Within the cla ss, all members must be explicitly specified as **static**. Making a class **static** does not automatically make its members **static**.

    static classes have two primary uses. First, a **static** class is required when creating an *extension method*, which is a new feature added by C# 3.0. Extension methods relate mostly to LINQ, and a discussion of extensions methods is found in Chapter 19. Second, a **static** class is used to contain a collection of related **static** methods. This second use is demonstrated here.

    The following example uses a **static** class called **NumericFn** to hold a set of **static** methods that operate on a numeric value. Because all of the members of **NumericFn** are declared **static**, the class can also be declared **static**, which prevents it from being instantiated. Thus, **NumericFn** serves an organization role, providing a good way to logically group related methods.

```
// Demonstrate a static class.

using System;

static class NumericFn {
  // Return the reciprocal of a value.
  static public double Reciprocal(double num) {
    return 1/num;
  }

  // Return the fractional part of a value.
  static public double FracPart(double num) {
    return num - (int) num;
  }

  // Return true if num is even.
  static public bool IsEven(double num) {
    return (num % 2) == 0 ? true : false;
  }

  // Return true if num is odd.
  static public bool IsOdd(double num) {
    return !IsEven(num);
  }

}

class StaticClassDemo {
  static void Main() {
    Console.WriteLine("Reciprocal of 5 is " +
                      NumericFn.Reciprocal(5.0));
```

```
    Console.WriteLine("Fractional part of 4.234 is " +
                        NumericFn.FracPart(4.234));

    if(NumericFn.IsEven(10))
      Console.WriteLine("10 is even.");

    if(NumericFn.IsOdd(5))
      Console.WriteLine("5 is odd.");

    // The following attempt to create an instance of
    // NumericFn will cause an error.
//  NumericFn ob = new NumericFn(); // Wrong!
  }
}
```

The output from the program is shown here.

```
Reciprocal of 5 is 0.2
Fractional part of 4.234 is 0.234
10 is even.
5 is odd.
```

Notice that the last line in the program is commented-out. Because **NumericFn** is a **static** class, any attempt to create an object will result in a compile-time error. It would also be an error to attempt to give **NumericFn** a non-**static** member.

One last point: Although a **static** class cannot have an instance constructor, it can have a **static** constructor.

Operator Overloading

C# allows you to define the meaning of an operator relative to a class that you create. This process is called *operator overloading*. By overloading an operator, you expand its usage to your class. The effects of the operator are completely under your control and may differ from class to class. For example, a class that defines a linked list might use the + operator to add an object to the list. A class that implements a stack might use the + to push an object onto the stack. Another class might use the + operator in an entirely different way.

When an operator is overloaded, none of its original meaning is lost. It is simply that a new operation, relative to a specific class, is added. Therefore, overloading the + to handle a linked list, for example, does not cause its meaning relative to integers (that is, addition) to be changed.

A principal advantage of operator overloading is that it allows you to seamlessly integrate a new class type into your programming environment. This *type extensibility* is an important part of the power of an object-oriented language such as C#. Once operators are defined for a class, you can operate on objects of that class using the normal C# expression syntax. You can even use an object in expressions involving other types of data. Operator overloading is one of C#'s most powerful features.

Operator Overloading Fundamentals

Operator overloading is closely related to method overloading. To overload an operator, use the **operator** keyword to define an *operator method,* which defines the action of the operator relative to its class.

There are two forms of **operator** methods: one for unary operators and one for binary operators. The general form for each is shown here:

```
// General form for overloading a unary operator
public static ret-type operator op(param-type operand)
{
  // operations
}
```

```
// General form for overloading a binary operator
public static ret-type operator op(param-type1 operand1, param-type1 operand2)
{
  // operations
}
```

Here, the operator that you are overloading, such as + or /, is substituted for *op*. The *ret-type* specifies the type of value returned by the specified operation. Although it can be any type you choose, the return value is often of the same type as the class for which the operator is being overloaded. This correlation facilitates the use of the overloaded operator in expressions. For unary operators, the operand is passed in *operand*. For binary operators, the operands are passed in *operand1* and *operand2*. Notice that **operator** methods must be both **public** and **static**.

For unary operators, the operand must be of the same type as the class for which the operator is being defined. For binary operators, at least one of the operands must be of the same type as its class. Thus, you cannot overload any C# operators for objects that you have not created. For example, you can't redefine + for **int** or **string**.

One other point: Operator parameters must not use the **ref** or **out** modifier.

Overloading Binary Operators

To see how operator overloading works, let's start with an example that overloads two binary operators, the + and the −. The following program creates a class called **ThreeD**, which maintains the coordinates of an object in three-dimensional space. The overloaded + adds the individual coordinates of one **ThreeD** object to another. The overloaded − subtracts the coordinates of one object from the other.

```
// An example of operator overloading.

using System;

// A three-dimensional coordinate class.
class ThreeD {
  int x, y, z; // 3-D coordinates

  public ThreeD() { x = y = z = 0; }
  public ThreeD(int i, int j, int k) { x = i; y = j; z = k; }

  // Overload binary +.
  public static ThreeD operator +(ThreeD op1, ThreeD op2)
  {
    ThreeD result = new ThreeD();

    /* This adds together the coordinates of the two points
       and returns the result. */
    result.x = op1.x + op2.x; // These are integer additions
    result.y = op1.y + op2.y; // and the + retains its original
    result.z = op1.z + op2.z; // meaning relative to them.

    return result;
  }

  // Overload binary -.
  public static ThreeD operator -(ThreeD op1, ThreeD op2)
  {
    ThreeD result = new ThreeD();

    /* Notice the order of the operands. op1 is the left
       operand and op2 is the right. */
```

```
    result.x = op1.x - op2.x; // these are integer subtractions
    result.y = op1.y - op2.y;
    result.z = op1.z - op2.z;

    return result;
  }

  // Show X, Y, Z coordinates.
  public void Show()
  {
    Console.WriteLine(x + ", " + y + ", " + z);
  }
}

class ThreeDDemo {
  static void Main() {
    ThreeD a = new ThreeD(1, 2, 3);
    ThreeD b = new ThreeD(10, 10, 10);
    ThreeD c;

    Console.Write("Here is a: ");
    a.Show();
    Console.WriteLine();
    Console.Write("Here is b: ");
    b.Show();
    Console.WriteLine();

    c = a + b; // add a and b together
    Console.Write("Result of a + b: ");
    c.Show();
    Console.WriteLine();

    c = a + b + c; // add a, b, and c together
    Console.Write("Result of a + b + c: ");
    c.Show();
    Console.WriteLine();

    c = c - a; // subtract a
    Console.Write("Result of c - a: ");
    c.Show();
    Console.WriteLine();

    c = c - b; // subtract b
    Console.Write("Result of c - b: ");
    c.Show();
    Console.WriteLine();
  }
}
```

This program produces the following output:

```
Here is a: 1, 2, 3

Here is b: 10, 10, 10
```

```
Result of a + b: 11, 12, 13

Result of a + b + c: 22, 24, 26

Result of c - a: 21, 22, 23

Result of c - b: 11, 12, 13
```

Let's examine the preceding program carefully, beginning with the overloaded operator +. When two objects of type **ThreeD** are operated on by the + operator, the magnitudes of their respective coordinates are added together, as shown in **operator+( )**. Notice, however, that this method does not modify the value of either operand. Instead, a new object of type **ThreeD**, which contains the result of the operation, is returned by the method. To understand why the + operation does not change the contents of either object, think about the standard arithmetic + operation as applied like this: 10 + 12. The outcome of this operation is 22, but neither 10 nor 12 is changed by it. Although no rule prevents an overloaded operator from altering the value of one of its operands, it is best for the actions of an overloaded operator to be consistent with its usual meaning.

Notice that **operator+( )** returns an object of type **ThreeD**. Although the method could have returned any valid C# type, the fact that it returns a **ThreeD** object allows the + operator to be used in compound expressions, such as **a+b+c**. Here, **a+b** generates a result that is of type **ThreeD**. This value can then be added to **c**. Had any other type of value been generated by **a+b**, such an expression would not work.

Here is another important point: When the coordinates are added together inside **operator+( )**, the addition of the individual coordinates results in an integer addition. This is because the individual coordinates, **x**, **y**, and **z**, are integer quantities. The fact that the + operator is overloaded for objects of type **ThreeD** has no effect on the + as it is applied to integer values.

Now, look at **operator–( )**. The – operator works just like the + operator except that the order of the parameters is important. Recall that addition is commutative, but subtraction is not. (That is, A – B is not the same as B – A!) For all binary operators, the first parameter to an operator method will contain the left operand. The second parameter will contain the one on the right. When implementing overloaded versions of the noncommutative operators, you must remember which operand is on the left and which is on the right.

Overloading Unary Operators

The unary operators are overloaded just like the binary operators. The main difference, of course, is that there is only one operand. For example, here is a method that overloads the unary minus for the **ThreeD** class:

```
// Overload unary -.
public static ThreeD operator -(ThreeD op)
{
  ThreeD result = new ThreeD();

  result.x = -op.x;
  result.y = -op.y;
  result.z = -op.z;

  return result;
}
```

Here, a new object is created that contains the negated fields of the operand. This object is then returned. Notice that the operand is unchanged. Again, this is in keeping with the usual meaning of the unary minus. For example, in an expression such as this,

```
a = -b
```

a receives the negation of **b**, but **b** is not changed.

In C#, overloading **++** and **−−** is quite easy; simply return the incremented or decremented value, but don't change the invoking object. C# will automatically handle that for you, taking into account the difference between the prefix and postfix forms. For example, here is an **operator++()** method for the **ThreeD** class:

```
// Overload unary ++.
public static ThreeD operator ++(ThreeD op)
{
  ThreeD result = new ThreeD();

  // Return the incremented result.
  result.x = op.x + 1;
  result.y = op.y + 1;
  result.z = op.z + 1;

  return result;
}
```

Here is an expanded version of the previous example program that demonstrates the unary **−** and the **++** operator:

```
// More operator overloading.

using System;

// A three-dimensional coordinate class.
class ThreeD {
  int x, y, z; // 3-D coordinates

  public ThreeD() { x = y = z = 0; }
  public ThreeD(int i, int j, int k) { x = i; y = j; z = k; }

  // Overload binary +.
  public static ThreeD operator +(ThreeD op1, ThreeD op2)
  {
    ThreeD result = new ThreeD();

    /* This adds together the coordinates of the two points
       and returns the result. */
    result.x = op1.x + op2.x;
    result.y = op1.y + op2.y;
    result.z = op1.z + op2.z;

    return result;
  }

  // Overload binary -.
```

```csharp
    public static ThreeD operator -(ThreeD op1, ThreeD op2)
    {
      ThreeD result = new ThreeD();

      /* Notice the order of the operands. op1 is the left
         operand and op2 is the right. */
      result.x = op1.x - op2.x;
      result.y = op1.y - op2.y;
      result.z = op1.z - op2.z;

      return result;
    }

    // Overload unary -.
    public static ThreeD operator -(ThreeD op)
    {
      ThreeD result = new ThreeD();

      result.x = -op.x;
      result.y = -op.y;
      result.z = -op.z;

      return result;
    }

    // Overload unary ++.
    public static ThreeD operator ++(ThreeD op)
    {
      ThreeD result = new ThreeD();

      // Return the incremented result.
      result.x = op.x + 1;
      result.y = op.y + 1;
      result.z = op.z + 1;

      return result;
    }
    // Show X, Y, Z coordinates.
    public void Show()
    {
      Console.WriteLine(x + ", " + y + ", " + z);
    }
}

class ThreeDDemo {
  static void Main() {
    ThreeD a = new ThreeD(1, 2, 3);
    ThreeD b = new ThreeD(10, 10, 10);
    ThreeD c = new ThreeD();

    Console.Write("Here is a: ");
    a.Show();
    Console.WriteLine();
```

```
    Console.Write("Here is b: ");
    b.Show();
    Console.WriteLine();

    c = a + b; // add a and b together
    Console.Write("Result of a + b: ");
    c.Show();
    Console.WriteLine();

    c = a + b + c; // add a, b, and c together
    Console.Write("Result of a + b + c: ");
    c.Show();
    Console.WriteLine();

    c = c - a; // subtract a
    Console.Write("Result of c - a: ");
    c.Show();
    Console.WriteLine();

    c = c - b; // subtract b
    Console.Write("Result of c - b: ");
    c.Show();
    Console.WriteLine();

    c = -a; // assign -a to c
    Console.Write("Result of -a: ");
    c.Show();
    Console.WriteLine();

    c = a++; // post-increment a
    Console.WriteLine("Given c = a++");
    Console.Write("c is ");
    c.Show();
    Console.Write("a is ");
    a.Show();

    // Reset a to 1, 2, 3
    a = new ThreeD(1, 2, 3);
    Console.Write("\nResetting a to ");
    a.Show();

    c = ++a; // pre-increment a
    Console.WriteLine("\nGiven c = ++a");
    Console.Write("c is ");
    c.Show();
    Console.Write("a is ");
    a.Show();
  }
}
```

The output from the program is shown here:

```
Here is a: 1, 2, 3
```

```
Here is b: 10, 10, 10

Result of a + b: 11, 12, 13

Result of a + b + c: 22, 24, 26

Result of c - a: 21, 22, 23

Result of c - b: 11, 12, 13

Result of -a: -1, -2, -3

Given c = a++
c is 1, 2, 3
a is 2, 3, 4

Resetting a to 1, 2, 3

Given c = ++a
c is 2, 3, 4
a is 2, 3, 4
```

Handling Operations on C# Built-in Types

For any given class and operator, an operator method can, itself, be overloaded. One of the most common reasons for this is to allow operations between a class type and other types of data, such as a built-in type. For example, once again consider the **ThreeD** class. To this point, you have seen how to overload the + so that it adds the coordinates of one **ThreeD** object to another. However, this is not the only way in which you might want to define addition for **ThreeD**. For example, it might be useful to add an integer value to each coordinate of a **ThreeD** object. Such an operation could be used to translate axes. To perform such an operation, you will need to overload + a second time, as shown here:

```
// Overload binary + for ThreeD + int.
public static ThreeD operator +(ThreeD op1, int op2)
{
  ThreeD result = new ThreeD();

  result.x = op1.x + op2;
  result.y = op1.y + op2;
  result.z = op1.z + op2;

  return result;
}
```

Notice that the second parameter is of type **int**. Thus, the preceding method allows an integer value to be added to each field of a **ThreeD** object. This is permissible because, as explained earlier, when overloading a binary operator, one of the operands must be of the same type as the class for which the operator is being overloaded. However, the other operand can be of any other type.

Here is a version of **ThreeD** that has two overloaded + methods:

```
// Overload addition for ThreeD + ThreeD, and for ThreeD + int.

using System;

// A three-dimensional coordinate class.
class ThreeD {
  int x, y, z; // 3-D coordinates

  public ThreeD() { x = y = z = 0; }
  public ThreeD(int i, int j, int k) { x = i; y = j; z = k; }

  // Overload binary + for ThreeD + ThreeD.
  public static ThreeD operator +(ThreeD op1, ThreeD op2)
  {
    ThreeD result = new ThreeD();

    /* This adds together the coordinates of the two points
       and returns the result. */
    result.x = op1.x + op2.x;
    result.y = op1.y + op2.y;
    result.z = op1.z + op2.z;

    return result;
  }

  // Overload binary + for object + int.
  public static ThreeD operator +(ThreeD op1, int op2)
  {
    ThreeD result = new ThreeD();

    result.x = op1.x + op2;
    result.y = op1.y + op2;
    result.z = op1.z + op2;

    return result;
  }

  // Show X, Y, Z coordinates.
  public void Show()
  {
    Console.WriteLine(x + ", " + y + ", " + z);
  }
}

class ThreeDDemo {
  static void Main() {
    ThreeD a = new ThreeD(1, 2, 3);
    ThreeD b = new ThreeD(10, 10, 10);
    ThreeD c = new ThreeD();

    Console.Write("Here is a: ");
    a.Show();
    Console.WriteLine();
    Console.Write("Here is b: ");
```

```
    b.Show();
    Console.WriteLine();

    c = a + b; // ThreeD + ThreeD
    Console.Write("Result of a + b: ");
    c.Show();
    Console.WriteLine();

    c = b + 10; // ThreeD + int
    Console.Write("Result of b + 10: ");
    c.Show();
  }
}
```

The output from this program is shown here:

```
Here is a: 1, 2, 3

Here is b: 10, 10, 10

Result of a + b: 11, 12, 13

Result of b + 10: 20, 20, 20
```

As the output confirms, when the **+** is applied to two **ThreeD** objects, their coordinates are added together. When the **+** is applied to a **ThreeD** object and an integer, the coordinates are increased by the integer value.

While the overloading of **+** just shown certainly adds a useful capability to the **ThreeD** class, it does not quite finish the job. Here is why. The **operator+(ThreeD, int)** method allows statements like this:

   ob1 = ob2 + 10;

It does not, unfortunately, allow ones like this:

   ob1 = 10 + ob2;

The reason is that the integer argument is the second argument, which is the right-hand operand, but the preceding statement puts the integer argument on the left. To allow both forms of statements, you will need to overload the **+** yet another time. This version must have its first parameter as type **int** and its second parameter as type **ThreeD**. One version of the **operator+( )** method handles **ThreeD** + integer, and the other handles integer + **ThreeD**. Overloading the **+** (or any other binary operator) this way allows a built-in type to occur on the left or right side of the operator. Here is a version **ThreeD** that overloads the **+** operator as just described:

```
// Overload the + for ThreeD + ThreeD, ThreeD + int, and int + ThreeD.

using System;

// A three-dimensional coordinate class.
class ThreeD {
  int x, y, z; // 3-D coordinates
```

```
    public ThreeD() { x = y = z = 0; }
    public ThreeD(int i, int j, int k) { x = i; y = j; z = k; }

    // Overload binary + for ThreeD + ThreeD.
    public static ThreeD operator +(ThreeD op1, ThreeD op2)
    {
      ThreeD result = new ThreeD();

      /* This adds together the coordinates of the two points
         and returns the result. */
      result.x = op1.x + op2.x;
      result.y = op1.y + op2.y;
      result.z = op1.z + op2.z;

      return result;
    }

    // Overload binary + for ThreeD + int.
    public static ThreeD operator +(ThreeD op1, int op2)
    {
      ThreeD result = new ThreeD();

      result.x = op1.x + op2;
      result.y = op1.y + op2;
      result.z = op1.z + op2;

      return result;
    }

    // Overload binary + for int + ThreeD.
    public static ThreeD operator +(int op1, ThreeD op2)
    {
      ThreeD result = new ThreeD();

      result.x = op2.x + op1;
      result.y = op2.y + op1;
      result.z = op2.z + op1;

      return result;
    }

    // Show X, Y, Z coordinates.
    public void Show()
    {
      Console.WriteLine(x + ", " + y + ", " + z);
    }
}

class ThreeDDemo {
  static void Main() {
    ThreeD a = new ThreeD(1, 2, 3);
    ThreeD b = new ThreeD(10, 10, 10);
    ThreeD c = new ThreeD();
```

```
      Console.Write("Here is a: ");
      a.Show();
      Console.WriteLine();
      Console.Write("Here is b: ");
      b.Show();
      Console.WriteLine();

      c = a + b; // ThreeD + ThreeD
      Console.Write("Result of a + b: ");
      c.Show();
      Console.WriteLine();

      c = b + 10; // ThreeD + int
      Console.Write("Result of b + 10: ");
      c.Show();
      Console.WriteLine();

      c = 15 + b; // int + ThreeD
      Console.Write("Result of 15 + b: ");
      c.Show();
    }
}
```

The output from this program is shown here:

```
Here is a: 1, 2, 3

Here is b: 10, 10, 10

Result of a + b: 11, 12, 13

Result of b + 10: 20, 20, 20

Result of 15 + b: 25, 25, 25
```

Overloading the Relational Operators

The relational operators, such as = = or <, can also be overloaded and the process is straightforward. Usually, an overloaded relational operator returns a **true** or **false** value. This is in keeping with the normal usage of these operators and allows the overloaded relational operators to be used in conditional expressions. If you return a different type result, then you are greatly restricting the operator's utility.

Here is a version of the **ThreeD** class that overloads the < and > operators. In this example, these operators compare **ThreeD** objects based on their distance from the origin. One object is greater than another if its distance from the origin is greater. One object is less than another if its distance from the origin is less than the other. Given two points, such an implementation could be used to determine which point lies on the larger sphere. If neither operator returns true, then the two points lie on the same sphere. Of course, other ordering schemes are possible.

```
// Overload < and >.

using System;

// A three-dimensional coordinate class.
class ThreeD {
  int x, y, z; // 3-D coordinates

  public ThreeD() { x = y = z = 0; }
  public ThreeD(int i, int j, int k) { x = i; y = j; z = k; }

  // Overload <.
  public static bool operator <(ThreeD op1, ThreeD op2)
  {
    if(Math.Sqrt(op1.x * op1.x + op1.y * op1.y + op1.z * op1.z) <
       Math.Sqrt(op2.x * op2.x + op2.y * op2.y + op2.z * op2.z))
      return true;
    else
      return false;
  }

  // Overload >.
  public static bool operator >(ThreeD op1, ThreeD op2)
  {
    if(Math.Sqrt(op1.x * op1.x + op1.y * op1.y + op1.z * op1.z) >
       Math.Sqrt(op2.x * op2.x + op2.y * op2.y + op2.z * op2.z))
      return true;
    else
      return false;
  }

  // Show X, Y, Z coordinates.
  public void Show()
  {
    Console.WriteLine(x + ", " + y + ", " + z);
  }
}

class ThreeDDemo {
  static void Main() {
    ThreeD a = new ThreeD(5, 6, 7);
    ThreeD b = new ThreeD(10, 10, 10);
    ThreeD c = new ThreeD(1, 2, 3);
    ThreeD d = new ThreeD(6, 7, 5);

    Console.Write("Here is a: ");
    a.Show();
    Console.Write("Here is b: ");
    b.Show();
    Console.Write("Here is c: ");
    c.Show();
    Console.Write("Here is d: ");
    d.Show();
```

```
   Console.WriteLine();

   if(a > c) Console.WriteLine("a > c is true");
   if(a < c) Console.WriteLine("a < c is true");
   if(a > b) Console.WriteLine("a > b is true");
   if(a < b) Console.WriteLine("a < b is true");

   if(a > d) Console.WriteLine("a > d is true");
   else if(a < d) Console.WriteLine("a < d is true");
   else Console.WriteLine("a and d are same distance from origin");
  }
}
```

The output from this program is shown here:

```
Here is a: 5, 6, 7
Here is b: 10, 10, 10
Here is c: 1, 2, 3
Here is d: 6, 7, 5

a > c is true
a < b is true
a and d are same distance from origin
```

An important restriction applies to overloading the relational operators: You must overload them in pairs. For example, if you overload <, you must also overload >, and vice versa. The operator pairs are

= =	!=
<	>
<=	>=

One other point: If you overload the = = and != operators, then you will usually need to override **Object.Equals( )** and **Object.GetHashCode( )**. These methods and the technique of overriding are discussed in Chapter 11.

Overloading true and false

The keywords **true** and **false** can also be used as unary operators for the purposes of overloading. Overloaded versions of these operators provide custom determinations of true and false relative to classes that you create. Once true and false are overloaded for a class, you can use objects of that class to control the **if**, **while**, **for**, and **do-while** statements, or in a **?** expression.

The **true** and **false** operators must be overloaded as a pair. You cannot overload just one. Both are unary operators and they have this general form:

public static bool operator true(*param-type operand*)
{
   // return true or false
}

```
public static bool operator false(param-type operand)
{
    // return true or false
}
```

Notice that each returns a **bool** result.

The following example shows how **true** and **false** can be implemented for the **ThreeD** class. Each assumes that a **ThreeD** object is true if at least one coordinate is non-zero. If all three coordinates are zero, then the object is false. The decrement operator is also implemented for the purpose of illustration.

```
// Overload true and false for ThreeD.

using System;

// A three-dimensional coordinate class.
class ThreeD {
  int x, y, z; // 3-D coordinates

  public ThreeD() { x = y = z = 0; }
  public ThreeD(int i, int j, int k) { x = i; y = j; z = k; }

  // Overload true.
  public static bool operator true(ThreeD op) {
    if((op.x != 0) || (op.y != 0) || (op.z != 0))
      return true; // at least one coordinate is non-zero
    else
      return false;
  }

  // Overload false.
  public static bool operator false(ThreeD op) {
    if((op.x == 0) && (op.y == 0) && (op.z == 0))
      return true; // all coordinates are zero
    else
      return false;
  }

  // Overload unary --.
  public static ThreeD operator --(ThreeD op)
  {
    ThreeD result = new ThreeD();

    // Return the decremented result.
    result.x = op.x - 1;
    result.y = op.y - 1;
    result.z = op.z - 1;

    return result;
  }

  // Show X, Y, Z coordinates.
  public void Show()
  {
```

```
      Console.WriteLine(x + ", " + y + ", " + z);
   }
}

class TrueFalseDemo {
  static void Main() {
    ThreeD a = new ThreeD(5, 6, 7);
    ThreeD b = new ThreeD(10, 10, 10);
    ThreeD c = new ThreeD(0, 0, 0);

    Console.Write("Here is a: ");
    a.Show();
    Console.Write("Here is b: ");
    b.Show();
    Console.Write("Here is c: ");
    c.Show();
    Console.WriteLine();

    if(a) Console.WriteLine("a is true.");
    else Console.WriteLine("a is false.");

    if(b) Console.WriteLine("b is true.");
    else Console.WriteLine("b is false.");

    if(c) Console.WriteLine("c is true.");
    else Console.WriteLine("c is false.");

    Console.WriteLine();

    Console.WriteLine("Control a loop using a ThreeD object.");
    do {
      b.Show();
      b--;
    } while(b);
  }
}
```

The output is shown here:

```
Here is a: 5, 6, 7
Here is b: 10, 10, 10
Here is c: 0, 0, 0

a is true.
b is true.
c is false.

Control a loop using a ThreeD object.
10, 10, 10
9, 9, 9
8, 8, 8
7, 7, 7
6, 6, 6
5, 5, 5
```

```
4, 4, 4
3, 3, 3
2, 2, 2
1, 1, 1
```

Notice how the **ThreeD** objects are used to control **if** statements and a **while** loop. In the case of the **if** statements, the **ThreeD** object is evaluated using **true**. If the result of this operation is true, then the **if** statement succeeds. In the case of the **do-while** loop, each iteration of the loop decrements **b**. The loop repeats as long as **b** evaluates as true (that is, it contains at least one non-zero coordinate). When **b** contains all zero coordinates, it evaluates as false when the **true** operator is applied and the loop stops.

Overloading the Logical Operators

As you know, C# defines the following logical operators: **&**, **|**, **!**, **&&**, and **||**. Of these, only the **&**, **|**, and **!** can be overloaded. By following certain rules, however, the benefits of the short-circuit **&&** and **||** can still be obtained. Each situation is examined here.

A Simple Approach to Overloading the Logical Operators

Let's begin with the simplest situation. If you will not be making use of the short-circuit logical operators, then you can overload **&** and **|** as you would intuitively think, with each returning a **bool** result. An overloaded **!** will also usually return a **bool** result.

Here is an example that overloads the **!**, **&**, and **|** logical operators for objects of type **ThreeD**. As before, each assumes that a **ThreeD** object is true if at least one coordinate is non-zero. If all three coordinates are zero, then the object is false.

```
// A simple way to overload !, |, and & for ThreeD.

using System;

// A three-dimensional coordinate class.
class ThreeD {
  int x, y, z; // 3-D coordinates

  public ThreeD() { x = y = z = 0; }
  public ThreeD(int i, int j, int k) { x = i; y = j; z = k; }


  // Overload |.
  public static bool operator |(ThreeD op1, ThreeD op2)
  {
    if( ((op1.x != 0) || (op1.y != 0) || (op1.z != 0)) |
        ((op2.x != 0) || (op2.y != 0) || (op2.z != 0)) )
      return true;
    else
      return false;
  }

  // Overload &.
  public static bool operator &(ThreeD op1, ThreeD op2)
  {
```

```
        if( ((op1.x != 0) && (op1.y != 0) && (op1.z != 0)) &
            ((op2.x != 0) && (op2.y != 0) && (op2.z != 0)) )
          return true;
        else
          return false;
      }

      // Overload !.
      public static bool operator !(ThreeD op)
      {
        if((op.x != 0) || (op.y != 0) || (op.z != 0))
          return false;
        else return true;
      }

      // Show X, Y, Z coordinates.
      public void Show()
      {
        Console.WriteLine(x + ", " + y + ", " + z);
      }
    }

    class TrueFalseDemo {
      static void Main() {
        ThreeD a = new ThreeD(5, 6, 7);
        ThreeD b = new ThreeD(10, 10, 10);
        ThreeD c = new ThreeD(0, 0, 0);

        Console.Write("Here is a: ");
        a.Show();
        Console.Write("Here is b: ");
        b.Show();
        Console.Write("Here is c: ");
        c.Show();
        Console.WriteLine();

        if(!a) Console.WriteLine("a is false.");
        if(!b) Console.WriteLine("b is false.");
        if(!c) Console.WriteLine("c is false.");

        Console.WriteLine();

        if(a & b) Console.WriteLine("a & b is true.");
        else Console.WriteLine("a & b is false.");

        if(a & c) Console.WriteLine("a & c is true.");
        else Console.WriteLine("a & c is false.");

        if(a | b) Console.WriteLine("a | b is true.");
        else Console.WriteLine("a | b is false.");

        if(a | c) Console.WriteLine("a | c is true.");
        else Console.WriteLine("a | c is false.");
      }
    }
```

The output from the program is shown here:

```
Here is a: 5, 6, 7
Here is b: 10, 10, 10
Here is c: 0, 0, 0

c is false.

a & b is true.
a & c is false.
a | b is true.
a | c is true.
```

In this approach, the **&**, **|**, and **!** operator methods each return a **bool** result. This is necessary if the operators are to be used in their normal manner (that is, in places that expect a **bool** result). Recall that for all built-in types, the outcome of a logical operation is a value of type **bool**. Thus, having the overloaded versions of these operators return type **bool** is a rational approach. Unfortunately, this approach works only if you will not be needing the short-circuit operators.

Enabling the Short-Circuit Operators

To enable the use of the **&&** and **||** short-circuit operators, you must follow four rules. First, the class must overload **&** and **|**. Second, the return type of the overloaded **&** and **|** methods must be the same as the class for which the operators are being overloaded. Third, each parameter must be a reference to an object of the class for which the operator is being overloaded. Fourth, the **true** and **false** operators must be overloaded for the class. When these conditions have been met, the short-circuit operators automatically become available for use.

The following program shows how to properly implement the **&** and **|** for the **ThreeD** class so that the short-circuit operators **&&** and **||** are available.

```
/* A better way to overload !, |, and & for ThreeD.
   This version automatically enables the && and || operators. */

using System;

// A three-dimensional coordinate class.
class ThreeD {
  int x, y, z; // 3-D coordinates

  public ThreeD() { x = y = z = 0; }
  public ThreeD(int i, int j, int k) { x = i; y = j; z = k; }

  // Overload | for short-circuit evaluation.
  public static ThreeD operator |(ThreeD op1, ThreeD op2)
  {
    if( ((op1.x != 0) || (op1.y != 0) || (op1.z != 0)) |
        ((op2.x != 0) || (op2.y != 0) || (op2.z != 0)) )
      return new ThreeD(1, 1, 1);
    else
      return new ThreeD(0, 0, 0);
  }
```

```
    // Overload & for short-circuit evaluation.
    public static ThreeD operator &(ThreeD op1, ThreeD op2)
    {
      if( ((op1.x != 0) && (op1.y != 0) && (op1.z != 0)) &
          ((op2.x != 0) && (op2.y != 0) && (op2.z != 0)) )
        return new ThreeD(1, 1, 1);
      else
        return new ThreeD(0, 0, 0);
    }

    // Overload !.
    public static bool operator !(ThreeD op)
    {
      if(op) return false;
      else return true;
    }

    // Overload true.
    public static bool operator true(ThreeD op) {
      if((op.x != 0) || (op.y != 0) || (op.z != 0))
        return true; // at least one coordinate is non-zero
      else
        return false;
    }

    // Overload false.
    public static bool operator false(ThreeD op) {
      if((op.x == 0) && (op.y == 0) && (op.z == 0))
        return true; // all coordinates are zero
      else
        return false;
    }

    // Show X, Y, Z coordinates.
    public void Show()
    {
      Console.WriteLine(x + ", " + y + ", " + z);
    }
}

class TrueFalseDemo {
  static void Main() {
    ThreeD a = new ThreeD(5, 6, 7);
    ThreeD b = new ThreeD(10, 10, 10);
    ThreeD c = new ThreeD(0, 0, 0);

    Console.Write("Here is a: ");
    a.Show();
    Console.Write("Here is b: ");
    b.Show();
    Console.Write("Here is c: ");
    c.Show();
    Console.WriteLine();
```

```
      if(a) Console.WriteLine("a is true.");
      if(b) Console.WriteLine("b is true.");
      if(c) Console.WriteLine("c is true.");

      if(!a) Console.WriteLine("a is false.");
      if(!b) Console.WriteLine("b is false.");
      if(!c) Console.WriteLine("c is false.");

      Console.WriteLine();

      Console.WriteLine("Use & and |");
      if(a & b) Console.WriteLine("a & b is true.");
      else Console.WriteLine("a & b is false.");

      if(a & c) Console.WriteLine("a & c is true.");
      else Console.WriteLine("a & c is false.");

      if(a | b) Console.WriteLine("a | b is true.");
      else Console.WriteLine("a | b is false.");

      if(a | c) Console.WriteLine("a | c is true.");
      else Console.WriteLine("a | c is false.");

      Console.WriteLine();

      // Now use short-circuit ops.
      Console.WriteLine("Use short-circuit && and ||");
      if(a && b) Console.WriteLine("a && b is true.");
      else Console.WriteLine("a && b is false.");

      if(a && c) Console.WriteLine("a && c is true.");
      else Console.WriteLine("a && c is false.");

      if(a || b) Console.WriteLine("a || b is true.");
      else Console.WriteLine("a || b is false.");

      if(a || c) Console.WriteLine("a || c is true.");
      else Console.WriteLine("a || c is false.");
   }
}
```

The output from the program is shown here:

```
Here is a: 5, 6, 7
Here is b: 10, 10, 10
Here is c: 0, 0, 0

a is true.
b is true.
c is false.

Use & and |
a & b is true.
```

```
a & c is false.
a | b is true.
a | c is true.

Use short-circuit && and ||
a && b is true.
a && c is false.
a || b is true.
a || c is true.
```

Let's look closely at how the **&** and **|** are implemented. They are shown here:

```
// Overload | for short-circuit evaluation.
public static ThreeD operator |(ThreeD op1, ThreeD op2)
{
  if( ((op1.x != 0) || (op1.y != 0) || (op1.z != 0)) |
      ((op2.x != 0) || (op2.y != 0) || (op2.z != 0)) )
    return new ThreeD(1, 1, 1);
  else
    return new ThreeD(0, 0, 0);
}

// Overload & for short-circuit evaluation.
public static ThreeD operator &(ThreeD op1, ThreeD op2)
{
  if( ((op1.x != 0) && (op1.y != 0) && (op1.z != 0)) &
      ((op2.x != 0) && (op2.y != 0) && (op2.z != 0)) )
    return new ThreeD(1, 1, 1);
  else
    return new ThreeD(0, 0, 0);
}
```

Notice first that both now return an object of type **ThreeD**. Pay attention to how this object is generated. If the outcome of the operation is true, then a true **ThreeD** object (one in which at least one coordinate is non-zero) is created and returned. If the outcome is false, then a false object is created and returned. Thus, in a statement like this

```
if(a & b) Console.WriteLine("a & b is true.");
else Console.WriteLine("a & b is false.");
```

the outcome of **a & b** is a **ThreeD** object, which in this case is a true object. Since the operators **true** and **false** are defined, this resulting object is subjected to the **true** operator, and a **bool** result is returned. In this case, the result is **true** and the **if** succeeds.

Because the necessary rules have been followed, the short-circuit operators are now available for use on **ThreeD** objects. They work like this. The first operand is tested by using **operator true** (for ||) or **operator false** (for &&). If it can determine the outcome of the operation, then the corresponding **&** or **|** is not evaluated. Otherwise, the corresponding overloaded **&** or **|** is used to determine the result. Thus, using a **&&** or **||** causes the corresponding **&** or **|** to be invoked only when the first operand cannot determine the outcome of the expression. For example, consider this statement from the program:

```
if(a || c) Console.WriteLine("a || c is true.");
```

The **true** operator is first applied to **a**. Since **a** is true in this situation, there is no need to use the | operator method. However, if the statement were rewritten like this:

```
if(c || a) Console.WriteLine("c || a is true.");
```

then the **true** operator would first be applied to **c**, which in this case is false. Thus, the | operator method would be invoked to determine if **a** was true (which it is in this case).

Although you might at first think that the technique used to enable the short-circuit operators is a bit convoluted, it makes sense if you think about it a bit. By overloading **true** and **false** for a class, you enable the compiler to utilize the short-circuit operators without having to explicitly overload either. Furthermore, you gain the ability to use objects in conditional expressions. In general, unless you need a very narrow implementation of **&** and |, you are better off creating a full implementation.

Conversion Operators

In some situations, you will want to use an object of a class in an expression involving other types of data. Sometimes, overloading one or more operators can provide the means of doing this. However, in other cases, what you want is a simple type conversion from the class type to the target type. To handle these cases, C# allows you to create a special type of **operator** method called a *conversion operator*. A conversion operator converts an object of your class into another type. Conversion operators help fully integrate class types into the C# programming environment by allowing objects of a class to be freely mixed with other data types as long as a conversion to those other types is defined.

There are two forms of conversion operators, implicit and explicit. The general form for each is shown here:

> public static operator implicit *target-type(source-type v)* { return *value*; }
> public static operator explicit *target-type(source-type v)* { return *value*; }

Here, *target-type* is the target type that you are converting to; *source-type* is the type you are converting from; and *value* is the value of the class after conversion. The conversion operators return data of type *target-type*, and no other return type specifier is allowed.

If the conversion operator specifies **implicit**, then the conversion is invoked automatically, such as when an object is used in an expression with the target type. When the conversion operator specifies **explicit**, the conversion is invoked when a cast is used. You cannot define both an implicit and explicit conversion operator for the same target and source types.

To illustrate a conversion operator, we will create one for the **ThreeD** class. Suppose you want to convert an object of type **ThreeD** into an integer so it can be used in an integer expression. Further, the conversion will take place by using the product of the three dimensions. To accomplish this, you will use an implicit conversion operator that looks like this:

```
public static implicit operator int(ThreeD op1)
{
   return op1.x * op1.y * op1.z;
}
```

Here is a program that illustrates this conversion operator:

```
// An example that uses an implicit conversion operator.

using System;

// A three-dimensional coordinate class.
class ThreeD {
  int x, y, z; // 3-D coordinates

  public ThreeD() { x = y = z = 0; }
  public ThreeD(int i, int j, int k) { x = i; y = j; z = k; }

  // Overload binary +.
  public static ThreeD operator +(ThreeD op1, ThreeD op2)
  {
    ThreeD result = new ThreeD();

    result.x = op1.x + op2.x;
    result.y = op1.y + op2.y;
    result.z = op1.z + op2.z;

    return result;
  }

  // An implicit conversion from ThreeD to int.
  public static implicit operator int(ThreeD op1)
  {
    return op1.x * op1.y * op1.z;
  }

  // Show X, Y, Z coordinates.
  public void Show()
  {
    Console.WriteLine(x + ", " + y + ", " + z);
  }
}

class ThreeDDemo {
  static void Main() {
    ThreeD a = new ThreeD(1, 2, 3);
    ThreeD b = new ThreeD(10, 10, 10);
    ThreeD c = new ThreeD();
    int i;

    Console.Write("Here is a: ");
    a.Show();
    Console.WriteLine();
    Console.Write("Here is b: ");
    b.Show();
    Console.WriteLine();

    c = a + b; // add a and b together
    Console.Write("Result of a + b: ");
```

```
      c.Show();
      Console.WriteLine();

      i = a; // convert to int
      Console.WriteLine("Result of i = a: " + i);
      Console.WriteLine();

      i = a * 2 - b; // convert to int
      Console.WriteLine("result of a * 2 - b: " + i);
    }
}
```

This program displays the output:

```
Here is a: 1, 2, 3

Here is b: 10, 10, 10

Result of a + b: 11, 12, 13

Result of i = a: 6

result of a * 2 - b: -988
```

As the program illustrates, when a **ThreeD** object is used in an integer expression, such as **i = a**, the conversion is applied to the object. In this specific case, the conversion returns the value 6, which is the product of coordinates stored in **a**. However, when an expression does not require a conversion to **int**, the conversion operator is not called. This is why **c = a + b** *does not* invoke **operator int( )**.

Remember that you can create different conversion operators to meet different needs. You could define a second conversion operator that converts **ThreeD** to **double**, for example. Each conversion is applied automatically and independently.

An implicit conversion operator is applied automatically when a conversion is required in an expression, when passing an object to a method, in an assignment, and also when an explicit cast to the target type is used. Alternatively, you can create an explicit conversion operator, which is invoked only when an explicit cast is used. An explicit conversion operator is not invoked automatically. For example, here is the previous program reworked to use an explicit conversion to **int**:

```
// Use an explicit conversion.

using System;

// A three-dimensional coordinate class.
class ThreeD {
  int x, y, z; // 3-D coordinates

  public ThreeD() { x = y = z = 0; }
  public ThreeD(int i, int j, int k) { x = i; y = j; z = k; }

  // Overload binary +.
  public static ThreeD operator +(ThreeD op1, ThreeD op2)
  {
```

```
    ThreeD result = new ThreeD();

    result.x = op1.x + op2.x;
    result.y = op1.y + op2.y;
    result.z = op1.z + op2.z;

    return result;
  }

  // This is now explicit.
  public static explicit operator int(ThreeD op1)
  {
    return op1.x * op1.y * op1.z;
  }

  // Show X, Y, Z coordinates.
  public void Show()
  {
    Console.WriteLine(x + ", " + y + ", " + z);
  }
}

class ThreeDDemo {
  static void Main() {
    ThreeD a = new ThreeD(1, 2, 3);
    ThreeD b = new ThreeD(10, 10, 10);
    ThreeD c = new ThreeD();
    int i;

    Console.Write("Here is a: ");
    a.Show();
    Console.WriteLine();
    Console.Write("Here is b: ");
    b.Show();
    Console.WriteLine();

    c = a + b; // add a and b together
    Console.Write("Result of a + b: ");
    c.Show();
    Console.WriteLine();

    i = (int) a; // explicitly convert to int -- cast required
    Console.WriteLine("Result of i = a: " + i);
    Console.WriteLine();

    i = (int)a * 2 - (int)b; // casts required
    Console.WriteLine("result of a * 2 - b: " + i);

  }
}
```

Because the conversion operator is now marked as explicit, conversion to **int** must be explicitly cast. For example, in this line:

```
i = (int) a; // explicitly convert to int -- cast required
```

if you remove the cast, the program will not compile.

There are a few restrictions to conversion operators:

- Either the target type or the source type of the conversion must be the class in which the conversion is declared. You cannot, for example, redefine the conversion from **double** to **int**.
- You cannot define a conversion to or from **object**.
- You cannot define both an implicit and an explicit conversion for the same source and target types.
- You cannot define a conversion from a base class to a derived class. (See Chapter 11 for a discussion of base and derived classes.)
- You cannot define a conversion from or to an interface. (See Chapter 12 for a discussion of interfaces.)

In addition to these rules, there are suggestions that you should normally follow when choosing between implicit and explicit conversion operators. Although convenient, implicit conversions should be used only in situations in which the conversion is inherently error-free. To ensure this, implicit conversions should be created only when these two conditions are met: First, that no loss of information, such as truncation, overflow, or loss of sign, occurs. Second, that the conversion does not cause an exception. If the conversion cannot meet these two requirements, then you should use an explicit conversion.

Operator Overloading Tips and Restrictions

The action of an overloaded operator as applied to the class for which it is defined need not bear any relationship to that operator's default usage, as applied to C#'s built-in types. However, for the purposes of the structure and readability of your code, an overloaded operator should reflect, when possible, the spirit of the operator's original use. For example, the + relative to **ThreeD** is conceptually similar to the + relative to integer types. There would be little benefit in defining the + operator relative to some class in such a way that it acts more the way you would expect the / operator to perform, for instance. The central concept is that while you can give an overloaded operator any meaning you like, for clarity it is best when its new meaning is related to its original meaning.

There are some restrictions to overloading operators. You cannot alter the precedence of any operator. You cannot alter the number of operands required by the operator, although your operator method could choose to ignore an operand. There are several operators that you cannot overload. Perhaps most significantly, you cannot overload any assignment operator, including the compound assignments, such as +=. Here are the other operators that cannot be overloaded. (This list includes several operators that are discussed later in this book.)

&&	()	.	?
??	[ ]	||	=
=>	->	as	checked
default	is	new	sizeof
typeof	unchecked		

Although you cannot overload the cast operator ( ) explicitly, you can create conversion operators, as shown earlier, that perform this function.

It may seem like a serious restriction that operators such as += can't be overloaded, but it isn't. In general, if you have defined an operator, then if that operator is used in a compound assignment, your overloaded operator method is invoked. Thus, += automatically uses your version of **operator+( )**. For example, assuming the **ThreeD** class, if you use a sequence like this

```
ThreeD a = new ThreeD(1, 2, 3);
ThreeD b = new ThreeD(10, 10, 10);

b += a; // add a and b together
```

ThreeD's **operator+( )** is automatically invoked, and **b** will contain the coordinate 11, 12, 13.

One last point: Although you cannot overload the [ ] array indexing operator using an **operator** method, you can create indexers, which are described in the next chapter.

Another Example of Operator Overloading

Throughout this chapter we have been using the **ThreeD** class to demonstrate operator overloading, and in this regard it has served us well. Before concluding this chapter, however, it is useful to work through another example. Although the general principles of operator overloading are the same no matter what class is used, the following example helps show the power of operator overloading—especially where type extensibility is concerned.

This example develops a four-bit integer type and defines several operations for it. As you might know, in the early days of computing, the four-bit quantity was common because it represented half a byte. It is also large enough to hold one hexadecimal digit. Since four bits are half a byte, a four-bit quantity is sometimes referred to as a *nybble*. In the days of front-panel machines in which programmers entered code one nybble at a time, thinking in terms of nybbles was an everyday affair! Although not as common now, a four-bit type still makes an interesting addition to the other C# integers. Traditionally, a nybble is an unsigned value.

The following example uses the **Nybble** class to implement a nybble data type. It uses an **int** for its underlying storage, but it restricts the values that can be held to 0 through 15. It defines the following operators:

- Addition of a **Nybble** to a **Nybble**
- Addition of an **int** to a **Nybble**
- Addition of a **Nybble** to an **int**
- Greater than and less than
- The increment operator
- Conversion to **Nybble** from **int**
- Conversion to **int** from **Nybble**

These operations are sufficient to show how a class type can be fully integrated into the C# type system. However, for complete **Nybble** implementation, you will need to define all of the other operators. You might want to try adding others on your own.

The complete **Nybble** class is shown here along with a **NybbleDemo**, which demonstrates its use:

```
// Create a 4-bit type called Nybble.

using System;

// A 4-bit type.
class Nybble {
  int val; // underlying storage

  public Nybble() { val = 0; }

  public Nybble(int i) {
    val = i;
    val = val & 0xF; // retain lower 4 bits
  }

  // Overload binary + for Nybble + Nybble.
  public static Nybble operator +(Nybble op1, Nybble op2)
  {
    Nybble result = new Nybble();

    result.val = op1.val + op2.val;

    result.val = result.val & 0xF; // retain lower 4 bits

    return result;
  }

  // Overload binary + for Nybble + int.
  public static Nybble operator +(Nybble op1, int op2)
  {
    Nybble result = new Nybble();

    result.val = op1.val + op2;

    result.val = result.val & 0xF; // retain lower 4 bits

    return result;
  }

  // Overload binary + for int + Nybble.
  public static Nybble operator +(int op1, Nybble op2)
  {
    Nybble result = new Nybble();

    result.val = op1 + op2.val;

    result.val = result.val & 0xF; // retain lower 4 bits

    return result;
  }

  // Overload ++.
```

```
public static Nybble operator ++(Nybble op)
{
  Nybble result = new Nybble();
  result.val = op.val + 1;

  result.val = result.val & 0xF; // retain lower 4 bits

  return result;
}

// Overload >.
public static bool operator >(Nybble op1, Nybble op2)
{
  if(op1.val > op2.val) return true;
  else return false;
}

// Overload <.
public static bool operator <(Nybble op1, Nybble op2)
{
  if(op1.val < op2.val) return true;
  else return false;
}

// Convert a Nybble into an int.
public static implicit operator int (Nybble op)
{
  return op.val;
}

// Convert an int into a Nybble.
public static implicit operator Nybble (int op)
{
  return new Nybble(op);
}
}

class NybbleDemo {
  static void Main() {
    Nybble a = new Nybble(1);
    Nybble b = new Nybble(10);
    Nybble c = new Nybble();
    int t;

    Console.WriteLine("a: " + (int) a);
    Console.WriteLine("b: " + (int) b);

    // Use a Nybble in an if statement.
    if(a < b) Console.WriteLine("a is less than b\n");

    // Add two Nybbles together.
    c = a + b;
    Console.WriteLine("c after c = a + b: " + (int) c);
```

```
   // Add an int to a Nybble.
   a += 5;
   Console.WriteLine("a after a += 5: " + (int) a);

   Console.WriteLine();

   // Use a Nybble in an int expression.
   t = a * 2 + 3;
   Console.WriteLine("Result of a * 2 + 3: " + t);

   Console.WriteLine();

   // Illustrate int assignment and overflow.
   a = 19;
   Console.WriteLine("Result of a = 19: " + (int) a);

   Console.WriteLine();

   // Use a Nybble to control a loop.
   Console.WriteLine("Control a for loop with a Nybble.");
   for(a = 0; a < 10; a++)
     Console.Write((int) a + " ");

   Console.WriteLine();
   }
}
```

The output from the program is shown here:

```
a: 1
b: 10
a is less than b

c after c = a + b: 11
a after a += 5: 6

Result of a * 2 + 3: 15

Result of a = 19: 3

Control a for loop with a Nybble.
0 1 2 3 4 5 6 7 8 9
```

Although most of the operation of **Nybble** should be easy to understand, there is one important point to make: The conversion operators play a large role in the integration of **Nybble** into the C# type system. Because conversions are defined from **Nybble** to **int** and from **int** to **Nybble**, a **Nybble** object can be freely mixed in arithmetic expressions. For example, consider this expression from the program:

```
t = a * 2 + 3;
```

Here, **t** is an **int**, as are 2 and 3, but **a** is a **Nybble**. These two types are compatible in the expression because of the implicit conversion of **Nybble** to **int**. In this case, since the rest of the expression is of type **int**, **a** is converted to **int** by its conversion method.

The conversion from **int** to **Nybble** allows a **Nybble** object to be assigned an **int** value. For example, in the program, the statement

```
a = 19;
```

works like this. The conversion operator from **int** to **Nybble** is executed. This causes a new **Nybble** object to be created that contains the low-order 4 bits of the value 19 (which is 3 because 19 overflows the range of a **Nybble**). This object is then assigned to **a**. Without the conversion operators, such expressions would not be allowed.

The conversion of **Nybble** to **int** is also used by the **for** loop. Without this conversion, it would not be possible to write the **for** loop in such a straightforward way.

Indexers and Properties

This chapter examines two special types of class members that have a close relationship to each other: indexers and properties. Each expands the power of a class by enhancing its integration into C#'s type system and improving its resiliency. Indexers provide the mechanism by which an object can be indexed like an array. Properties offer a streamlined way to manage access to a class' instance data. They relate to each other because both rely upon another feature of C#: the accessor.

Indexers

As you know, array indexing is performed using the [ ] operator. It is possible to define the [ ] operator for classes that you create, but you don't use an **operator** method. Instead, you create an *indexer*. An indexer allows an object to be indexed like an array. The main use of indexers is to support the creation of specialized arrays that are subject to one or more constraints. However, you can use an indexer for any purpose for which an array-like syntax is beneficial. Indexers can have one or more dimensions. We will begin with one-dimensional indexers.

Creating One-Dimensional Indexers

A one-dimensional indexer has this general form:

```
element-type this[int index] {
   // The get accessor
   get {
      // return the value specified by index
   }

   // The set accessor
   set {
      // set the value specified by index
   }
}
```

Here, *element-type* is the element type of the indexer. Thus, each element accessed by the indexer will be of type *element-type*. This type corresponds to the element type of an array. The parameter *index* receives the index of the element being accessed. Technically, this parameter does not have to be of type **int**, but since indexers are typically used to provide array indexing, an integer type is customary.

Inside the body of the indexer two *accessors* are defined that are called **get** and **set**. An accessor is similar to a method except that it does not declare a return type or parameters. The accessors are automatically called when the indexer is used, and both accessors receive *index* as a parameter. If the indexer is on the left side of an assignment statement, then the **set** accessor is called and the element specified by *index* must be set. Otherwise, the **get** accessor is called and the value associated with *index* must be returned. The **set** method also receives an implicit parameter called **value**, which contains the value being assigned to the specified index.

One of the benefits of an indexer is that you can control precisely how an array is accessed, heading off improper access. Here is an example. In the following program, the **FailSoftArray** class implements an array that traps boundary errors, thus preventing runtime exceptions if the array is indexed out-of-bounds. This is accomplished by encapsulating the array as a private member of a class, allowing access to the array only through the indexer. With this approach, any attempt to access the array beyond its boundaries can be prevented, with such an attempt failing gracefully (resulting in a "soft landing" rather than a "crash"). Since **FailSoftArray** uses an indexer, the array can be accessed using the normal array notation.

```
// Use an indexer to create a fail-soft array.

using System;

class FailSoftArray {
  int[] a;     // reference to underlying array

  public int Length; // Length is public

  public bool ErrFlag; // indicates outcome of last operation

  // Construct array given its size.
  public FailSoftArray(int size) {
    a = new int[size];
    Length = size;
  }

  // This is the indexer for FailSoftArray.
  public int this[int index] {
    // This is the get accessor.
    get {
      if(ok(index)) {
        ErrFlag = false;
        return a[index];
      } else {
        ErrFlag = true;
        return 0;
      }
    }
  }
```

```
    // This is the set accessor.
    set {
      if(ok(index)) {
        a[index] = value;
        ErrFlag = false;
      }
      else ErrFlag = true;
    }
  }

  // Return true if index is within bounds.
  private bool ok(int index) {
   if(index >= 0 & index < Length) return true;
   return false;
  }
}

// Demonstrate the fail-soft array.
class FSDemo {
  static void Main() {
    FailSoftArray fs = new FailSoftArray(5);
    int x;

    // Show quiet failures.
    Console.WriteLine("Fail quietly.");
    for(int i=0; i < (fs.Length * 2); i++)
      fs[i] = i*10;

    for(int i=0; i < (fs.Length * 2); i++) {
      x = fs[i];
      if(x != -1) Console.Write(x + " ");
    }
    Console.WriteLine();

    // Now, display failures.
    Console.WriteLine("\nFail with error reports.");
    for(int i=0; i < (fs.Length * 2); i++) {
      fs[i] = i*10;
      if(fs.ErrFlag)
        Console.WriteLine("fs[" + i + "] out-of-bounds");
    }

    for(int i=0; i < (fs.Length * 2); i++) {
      x = fs[i];
      if(!fs.ErrFlag) Console.Write(x + " ");
      else
        Console.WriteLine("fs[" + i + "] out-of-bounds");
    }
  }
}
```

The output from the program is shown here:

```
Fail quietly.
0 10 20 30 40 0 0 0 0 0
```

```
Fail with error reports.
fs[5] out-of-bounds
fs[6] out-of-bounds
fs[7] out-of-bounds
fs[8] out-of-bounds
fs[9] out-of-bounds
0 10 20 30 40 fs[5] out-of-bounds
fs[6] out-of-bounds
fs[7] out-of-bounds
fs[8] out-of-bounds
fs[9] out-of-bounds
```

The indexer prevents the array boundaries from being overrun. Let's look closely at each part of the indexer. It begins with this line:

```
public int this[int index] {
```

This declares an indexer that operates on **int** elements. The index is passed in *index*. The indexer is public, allowing it to be used by code outside of its class.

The **get** accessor is shown here:

```
get {
  if(ok(index)) {
    ErrFlag = false;
    return a[index];
  } else {
    ErrFlag = true;
    return 0;
  }
}
```

The **get** accessor prevents array boundary errors by first confirming that the index is not out-of-bounds. This range check is performed by the **ok()** method, which returns true if the index is valid and false otherwise. If the specified index is within bounds, the element corresponding to the index is returned. If it is out of bounds, no operation takes place and no overrun occurs. In this version of **FailSoftArray**, a variable called **ErrFlag** contains the outcome of each operation. This field can be examined after each operation to assess the success or failure of the operation. (In Chapter 13, you will see a better way to handle errors by using C#'s exception subsystem, but for now, using an error flag is an acceptable approach.)

The **set** accessor is shown here. It too prevents a boundary error.

```
set {
  if(ok(index)) {
    a[index] = value;
    ErrFlag = false;
  }
  else ErrFlag = true;
}
```

Here, if **index** is within bounds, the value passed in **value** is assigned to the corresponding element. Otherwise, **ErrFlag** is set to **true**. Recall that in an accessor method, **value** is an

implicit parameter that contains the value being assigned. You do not need to (nor can you) declare it.

It is not necessary for an indexer to support both **get** and **set**. You can create a read-only indexer by implementing only the **get** accessor. You can create a write-only indexer by implementing only **set**.

Indexers Can Be Overloaded

An indexer can be overloaded. The version executed will be the one that has the closest type-match between its parameter and the argument used as an index. Here is an example that overloads the **FailSoftArray** indexer for indexes of type **double**. The **double** indexer rounds its index to the nearest integer value.

```
// Overload the FailSoftArray indexer.

using System;

class FailSoftArray {
  int[] a;     // reference to underlying array

  public int Length; // Length is public

  public bool ErrFlag; // indicates outcome of last operation

  // Construct array given its size.
  public FailSoftArray(int size) {
    a = new int[size];
    Length = size;
  }

  // This is the int indexer for FailSoftArray.
  public int this[int index] {
    // This is the get accessor.
    get {
      if(ok(index)) {
        ErrFlag = false;
        return a[index];
      } else {
        ErrFlag = true;
        return 0;
      }
    }

    // This is the set accessor.
    set {
      if(ok(index)) {
        a[index] = value;
        ErrFlag = false;
      }
      else ErrFlag = true;
    }
  }
}
```

```
/* This is another indexer for FailSoftArray.
   This index takes a double argument. It then
   rounds that argument to the nearest integer index. */
public int this[double idx] {
  // This is the get accessor.
  get {
    int index;

    // Round to nearest int.
    if( (idx - (int) idx) < 0.5) index = (int) idx;
    else index = (int) idx + 1;

    if(ok(index)) {
      ErrFlag = false;
      return a[index];
    } else {
      ErrFlag = true;
      return 0;
    }
  }

  // This is the set accessor.
  set {
    int index;

    // Round to nearest int.
    if( (idx - (int) idx) < 0.5) index = (int) idx;
    else index = (int) idx + 1;

    if(ok(index)) {
      a[index] = value;
      ErrFlag = false;
    }
    else ErrFlag = true;
  }
}

// Return true if index is within bounds.
private bool ok(int index) {
 if(index >= 0 & index < Length) return true;
 return false;
}
}

// Demonstrate the fail-soft array.
class FSDemo {
  static void Main() {
    FailSoftArray fs = new FailSoftArray(5);

    // Put some values in fs.
    for(int i=0; i < fs.Length; i++)
      fs[i] = i;

    // Now index with ints and doubles.
    Console.WriteLine("fs[1]: " + fs[1]);
```

```
      Console.WriteLine("fs[2]: " + fs[2]);

      Console.WriteLine("fs[1.1]: " + fs[1.1]);
      Console.WriteLine("fs[1.6]: " + fs[1.6]);
   }
}
```

This program produces the following output:

```
fs[1]: 1
fs[2]: 2
fs[1.1]: 1
fs[1.6]: 2
```

As the output shows, the **double** indexes are rounded to their nearest integer value. Specifically, 1.1 is rounded to 1, and 1.6 is rounded to 2.

Although overloading an indexer as shown in this program is valid, it is not common. Most often, an indexer is overloaded to enable an object of a class to be used as an index, with the index computed in some special way.

Indexers Do Not Require an Underlying Array

It is important to understand that there is no requirement that an indexer actually operate on an array. It simply must provide functionality that appears "array-like" to the user of the indexer. For example, the following program has an indexer that acts like a read-only array that contains the powers of 2 from 0 to 15. Notice, however, that no actual array exists. Instead, the indexer simply computes the proper value for a given index.

```
// Indexers don't have to operate on actual arrays.

using System;

class PwrOfTwo {

  /* Access a logical array that contains
     the powers of 2 from 0 to 15. */
  public int this[int index] {
    // Compute and return power of 2.
    get {
      if((index >= 0) && (index < 16)) return pwr(index);
      else return -1;
    }

    // There is no set accessor.
  }

  int pwr(int p) {
    int result = 1;

    for(int i=0; i < p; i++)
      result *= 2;

    return result;
  }
}
```

```
class UsePwrOfTwo {
  static void Main() {
    PwrOfTwo pwr = new PwrOfTwo();

    Console.Write("First 8 powers of 2: ");
    for(int i=0; i < 8; i++)
      Console.Write(pwr[i] + " ");
    Console.WriteLine();

    Console.Write("Here are some errors: ");
    Console.Write(pwr[-1] + " " + pwr[17]);

    Console.WriteLine();
  }
}
```

The output from the program is shown here:

```
First 8 powers of 2: 1 2 4 8 16 32 64 128
Here are some errors: -1 -1
```

Notice that the indexer for **PwrOfTwo** includes a **get** accessor, but no **set** accessor. As explained, this means that the indexer is read-only. Thus, a **PwrOfTwo** object can be used on the right side of an assignment statement, but not on the left. For example, attempting to add this statement to the preceding program won't work:

```
pwr[0] = 11; // won't compile
```

This statement will cause a compilation error because no **set** accessor is defined for the indexer.

There are two important restrictions to using indexers. First, because an indexer does not define a storage location, a value produced by an indexer cannot be passed as a **ref** or **out** parameter to a method. Second, an indexer must be an instance member of its class; it cannot be declared **static**.

Multidimensional Indexers

You can create indexers for multidimensional arrays, too. For example, here is a two-dimensional fail-soft array. Pay close attention to the way that the indexer is declared.

```
// A two-dimensional fail-soft array.

using System;

class FailSoftArray2D {
  int[,] a; // reference to underlying 2D array
  int rows, cols; // dimensions
  public int Length; // Length is public

  public bool ErrFlag; // indicates outcome of last operation

  // Construct array given its dimensions.
  public FailSoftArray2D(int r, int c) {
```

```
      rows = r;
      cols = c;
      a = new int[rows, cols];
      Length = rows * cols;
   }

   // This is the indexer for FailSoftArray2D.
   public int this[int index1, int index2] {
      // This is the get accessor.
      get {
         if(ok(index1, index2)) {
            ErrFlag = false;
            return a[index1, index2];
         } else {
            ErrFlag = true;
            return 0;
         }
      }

      // This is the set accessor.
      set {
         if(ok(index1, index2)) {
            a[index1, index2] = value;
            ErrFlag = false;
         }
         else ErrFlag = true;
      }
   }

   // Return true if indexes are within bounds.
   private bool ok(int index1, int index2) {
    if(index1 >= 0 & index1 < rows &
       index2 >= 0 & index2 < cols)
          return true;

    return false;
   }
}

// Demonstrate a 2D indexer.
class TwoDIndexerDemo {
   static void Main() {
      FailSoftArray2D fs = new FailSoftArray2D(3, 5);
      int x;

      // Show quiet failures.
      Console.WriteLine("Fail quietly.");
      for(int i=0; i < 6; i++)
         fs[i, i] = i*10;

      for(int i=0; i < 6; i++) {
         x = fs[i,i];
         if(x != -1) Console.Write(x + " ");
      }
```

```
    Console.WriteLine();

    // Now, display failures.
    Console.WriteLine("\nFail with error reports.");
    for(int i=0; i < 6; i++) {
      fs[i,i] = i*10;
      if(fs.ErrFlag)
        Console.WriteLine("fs[" + i + ", " + i + "] out-of-bounds");
    }

    for(int i=0; i < 6; i++) {
      x = fs[i,i];
      if(!fs.ErrFlag) Console.Write(x + " ");
      else
        Console.WriteLine("fs[" + i + ", " + i + "] out-of-bounds");
    }
  }
}
```

The output from this program is shown here:

```
Fail quietly.
0 10 20 0 0 0

Fail with error reports.
fs[3, 3] out-of-bounds
fs[4, 4] out-of-bounds
fs[5, 5] out-of-bounds
0 10 20 fs[3, 3] out-of-bounds
fs[4, 4] out-of-bounds
fs[5, 5] out-of-bounds
```

Properties

Another type of class member is the *property*. As a general rule, a property combines a field with the methods that access it. As some examples earlier in this book have shown, you will often want to create a field that is available to users of an object, but you want to maintain control over the operations allowed on that field. For instance, you might want to limit the range of values that can be assigned to that field. While it is possible to accomplish this goal through the use of a private variable along with methods to access its value, a property offers a better, more streamlined approach.

Properties are similar to indexers. A property consists of a name along with **get** and **set** accessors. The accessors are used to get and set the value of a variable. The key benefit of a property is that its name can be used in expressions and assignments like a normal variable, but in actuality the **get** and **set** accessors are automatically invoked. This is similar to the way that an indexer's **get** and **set** accessors are automatically used.

The general form of a property is shown here:

type name {
  get {
    // get accessor code
  }

```
      set {
        // set accessor code
      }
    }
```

Here, *type* specifies the type of the property, such as **int**, and *name* is the name of the property. Once the property has been defined, any use of *name* results in a call to its appropriate accessor. The **set** accessor automatically receives a parameter called **value** that contains the value being assigned to the property.

It is important to understand that properties do not define storage locations. Instead, a property typically manages access to a field. It does not, itself, provide that field. The field must be specified independently of the property. (The exception is the *auto-implemented* property added by C# 3.0, which is described shortly.)

Here is a simple example that defines a property called **MyProp**, which is used to access the field **prop**. In this case, the property allows only positive values to be assigned.

```
// A simple property example.

using System;

class SimpProp {
  int prop; // field being managed by MyProp

  public SimpProp() { prop = 0; }

  /* This is the property that supports access to
     the private instance variable prop. It
     allows only positive values. */
  public int MyProp {
    get {
      return prop;
    }
    set {
      if(value >= 0) prop = value;
    }
  }
}

// Demonstrate a property.
class PropertyDemo {
  static void Main() {
    SimpProp ob = new SimpProp();

    Console.WriteLine("Original value of ob.MyProp: " + ob.MyProp);

    ob.MyProp = 100; // assign value
    Console.WriteLine("Value of ob.MyProp: " + ob.MyProp);

    // Can't assign negative value to prop.
    Console.WriteLine("Attempting to assign -10 to ob.MyProp");
    ob.MyProp = -10;
    Console.WriteLine("Value of ob.MyProp: " + ob.MyProp);
  }
}
```

Output from this program is shown here:

```
Original value of ob.MyProp: 0
Value of ob.MyProp: 100
Attempting to assign -10 to ob.MyProp
Value of ob.MyProp: 100
```

Let's examine this program carefully. The program defines one private field, called **prop**, and a property called **MyProp** that manages access to **prop**. As explained, a property by itself does not define a storage location. Instead, most properties simply manage access to a field. Furthermore, because **prop** is private, it can be accessed *only* through **MyProp**.

The property **MyProp** is specified as **public** so it can be accessed by code outside of its class. This makes sense because it provides access to **prop**, which is private. The **get** accessor simply returns the value of **prop**. The **set** accessor sets the value of **prop** if and only if that value is positive. Thus, the **MyProp** property controls what values **prop** can have. This is the essence of why properties are important.

The type of property defined by **MyProp** is called a read-write property because it allows its underlying field to be read and written. It is possible, however, to create read-only and write-only properties. To create a read-only property, define only a **get** accessor. To define a write-only property, define only a **set** accessor.

You can use a property to further improve the fail-soft array class. As you know, all arrays have a **Length** property associated with them. Up to now, the **FailSoftArray** class simply used a public integer field called **Length** for this purpose. This is not good practice, though, because it allows **Length** to be set to some value other than the length of the fail-soft array. (For example, a malicious programmer could intentionally corrupt its value.) We can remedy this situation by transforming **Length** into a read-only property, as shown in the following version of **FailSoftArray**:

```
// Add Length property to FailSoftArray.

using System;

class FailSoftArray {
  int[] a; // reference to underlying array
  int len; // length of array -- underlies Length property

  public bool ErrFlag; // indicates outcome of last operation

  // Construct array given its size.
  public FailSoftArray(int size) {
    a = new int[size];
    len = size;
  }

  // Read-only Length property.
  public int Length {
    get {
      return len;
    }
  }
```

```
    // This is the indexer for FailSoftArray.
    public int this[int index] {
      // This is the get accessor.
      get {
        if(ok(index)) {
          ErrFlag = false;
          return a[index];
        } else {
          ErrFlag = true;
          return 0;
        }
      }

      // This is the set accessor.
      set {
        if(ok(index)) {
          a[index] = value;
          ErrFlag = false;
        }
        else ErrFlag = true;
      }
    }

    // Return true if index is within bounds.
    private bool ok(int index) {
     if(index >= 0 & index < Length) return true;
     return false;
    }
}

// Demonstrate the improved fail-soft array.
class ImprovedFSDemo {
  static void Main() {
    FailSoftArray fs = new FailSoftArray(5);
    int x;

    // Can read Length.
    for(int i=0; i < fs.Length; i++)
      fs[i] = i*10;

    for(int i=0; i < fs.Length; i++) {
      x = fs[i];
      if(x != -1) Console.Write(x + " ");
    }
    Console.WriteLine();

    // fs.Length = 10; // Error, illegal!
  }
}
```

Length is now a property that uses the private variable **len** for its storage. **Length** defines only a **get** accessor, which means that it is read-only. Thus, **Length** can be read, but not

changed. To prove this to yourself, try removing the comment symbol preceding this line in the program:

```
// fs.Length = 10; // Error, illegal!
```

When you try to compile, you will receive an error message stating that **Length** is read-only.

Although the addition of the **Length** property improves **FailSoftArray**, it is not the only improvement that properties can make. The **ErrFlag** member is also a prime candidate for conversion into a property since access to it should also be limited to read-only. Here is the final improvement of **FailSafeArray**. It creates a property called **Error** that uses the original **ErrFlag** variable as its storage, and **ErrFlag** is made private to **FailSoftArray**.

```
// Convert ErrFlag into a property.

using System;

class FailSoftArray {
  int[] a; // reference to underlying array
  int len; // length of array

  bool ErrFlag; // now private

  // Construct array given its size.
  public FailSoftArray(int size) {
    a = new int[size];
    len = size;
  }

  // Read-only Length property.
  public int Length {
    get {
      return len;
    }
  }

  // Read-only Error property.
  public bool Error {
    get {
      return ErrFlag;
    }
  }

  // This is the indexer for FailSoftArray.
  public int this[int index] {
    // This is the get accessor.
    get {
      if(ok(index)) {
        ErrFlag = false;
        return a[index];
      } else {
        ErrFlag = true;
        return 0;
      }
    }
```

```
    // This is the set accessor.
    set {
      if(ok(index)) {
        a[index] = value;
        ErrFlag = false;
      }
      else ErrFlag = true;
    }
  }

  // Return true if index is within bounds.
  private bool ok(int index) {
   if(index >= 0 & index < Length) return true;
   return false;
  }
}

// Demonstrate the improved fail-soft array.
class FinalFSDemo {
  static void Main() {
    FailSoftArray fs = new FailSoftArray(5);

    // Use Error property.
    for(int i=0; i < fs.Length + 1; i++) {
      fs[i] = i*10;
      if(fs.Error)
        Console.WriteLine("Error with index " + i);
    }
  }
}
```

The creation of the **Error** property has caused two changes to be made to **FailSoftArray**. First, **ErrFlag** has been made private because it is now used as the underlying storage for the **Error** property. Thus, it won't be available directly. Second, the read-only **Error** property has been added. Now, programs that need to detect errors will interrogate **Error**. This is demonstrated in **Main( )**, where a boundary error is intentionally generated, and the **Error** property is used to detect it.

Auto-Implemented Properties

Beginning with C# 3.0, it is possible to implement very simple properties without having to explicitly define the variable managed by the property. Instead, you can let the compiler automatically supply the underlying variable. This is called an *auto-implemented property*. It has the following general form:

> *type name* { get; set; }

Here, *type* specifies the type of the property and *name* specifies the name. Notice that **get** and **set** are immediately followed by a semicolon. The accessors for an auto-implemented property have no bodies. This syntax tells the compiler to automatically create a storage location (sometimes referred to as a *backing field*) that holds the value. This variable is not named and is not directly available to you. Instead, it can be accessed only through the property.

Here is how a property called **UserCount** is declared using an auto-implemented property:

```
public int UserCount { get; set; }
```

Notice that no variable is explicitly declared. As explained, the compiler automatically generates an anonymous field that holds the value. Otherwise, **UserCount** acts like and is used like any other property.

Unlike normal properties, an auto-implemented property cannot be read-only or write-only. Both the **get** and **set** must be specified in all cases. However, you can approximate the same effect by declaring either **get** or **set** as **private**, as explained in "Use Access Modifiers with Accessors" later in this chapter.

Although auto-implemented properties offer convenience, their use is limited to those cases in which you do not need control over the getting or setting of the backing field. Remember, you cannot access the backing field directly. This means that there is no way to constrain the value an auto-implemented property can have. Thus, auto-implemented properties simply let the name of the property act as a proxy for the field, itself. However, sometimes this is exactly what you want. Also, they can be very useful in cases in which properties are used to expose functionality to a third party, possibly through a design tool.

Use Object Initializers with Properties

As discussed in Chapter 8, C# 3.0 adds a new feature called an *object initializer*, which provides an alternative to explicitly calling a constructor when creating an object. When using object initializers, you specify initial values for the fields and/or properties that you want to initialize. Furthermore, the object initializer syntax is the same for both properties or fields. For example, here is the object initializer demonstration program from Chapter 8, reworked to show the use of object initializers with properties. Recall that the version shown in Chapter 8 used fields. The only difference between this version of the program and the one shown in Chapter 8 is that **Count** and **Str** have been converted from fields into properties. The object initializer syntax is unchanged.

```
// Use object initializers with properties.

using System;

class MyClass {
  // These are now properties.
  public int Count { get; set; }
  public string Str { get; set; }
}

class ObjInitDemo {
  static void Main() {
    // Construct a MyClass object by using object initializers.
    MyClass obj = new MyClass { Count = 100, Str = "Testing" };

    Console.WriteLine(obj.Count + " " + obj.Str);
  }
}
```

As you can see, the properties **Count** and **Str** are set via object initializer expressions. The output is the same as that produced by the program in Chapter 8 and is shown here:

```
100 Testing
```

As explained in Chapter 8, the object initializer syntax is most useful when working with anonymous types generated by a LINQ expression. In most other cases, you will use the normal constructor syntax.

Property Restrictions

Properties have some important restrictions. First, because a property does not define a storage location, it cannot be passed as a **ref** or **out** parameter to a method. Second, you cannot overload a property. (You *can* have two different properties that both access the same variable, but this would be unusual.) Finally, a property should not alter the state of the underlying variable when the **get** accessor is called. Although this rule is not enforced by the compiler, violating it is semantically wrong. A **get** operation should be nonintrusive.

Use Access Modifiers with Accessors

By default, the **set** and **get** accessors have the same accessibility as the indexer or property of which they are a part. For example, if the property is declared **public**, then by default the **get** and **set** accessors are also public. It is possible, however, to give **set** or **get** its own access modifier, such as **private**. In all cases, the access modifier for an accessor must be more restrictive then the access specification of its property or indexer.

There are a number of reasons why you may want to restrict the accessibility of an accessor. For example, you might want to let anyone obtain the value of a property, but allow only members of its class to set the property. To do this, declare the **set** accessor as **private**. For example, here is a property called **MyProp** that has its **set** accessor specified as **private**.

```
// Use an access modifier with an accessor.

using System;

class PropAccess {
  int prop; // field being managed by MyProp

  public PropAccess() { prop = 0; }

  /* This is the property that supports access to
     the private instance variable prop. It allows
     any code to obtain the value of prop, but only
     other class members can set the value of prop. */
  public int MyProp {
    get {
      return prop;
    }
    private set { // now, private
      prop = value;
    }
  }
```

```
   // This class member increments the value of MyProp.
   public void IncrProp() {
     MyProp++; // OK, in same class.
   }
}

// Demonstrate accessor access modifier.
class PropAccessDemo {
  static void Main() {
    PropAccess ob = new PropAccess();

    Console.WriteLine("Original value of ob.MyProp: " + ob.MyProp);

//    ob.MyProp = 100; // can't access set

    ob.IncrProp();
    Console.WriteLine("Value of ob.MyProp after increment: "
                     + ob.MyProp);
  }
}
```

In the **PropAccess** class, the **set** accessor is specified **private**. This means that it can be accessed by other class members, such as **IncrProp()**, but it cannot be accessed by code outside of **PropAccess**. This is why the attempt to assign **ob.MyProp** a value inside **PropAccessDemo** is commented out.

Perhaps the most important use of restricting an accessor's access is found when working with auto-implemented properties. As explained, it is not possible to create a read-only or write-only auto-implemented property because both the **get** and **set** accessors must be specified when the auto-implemented property is declared. However, you can gain much the same effect by declaring either **get** or **set** as **private**. For example, this declares what is effectively a read-only, auto-implemented **Length** property for the **FailSoftArray** class shown earlier.

```
public int Length { get; private set; }
```

Because **set** is **private**, **Length** can be set only by code within its class. Outside its class, an attempt to change **Length** is illegal. Thus, outside its class, **Length** is effectively read-only. The same technique can also be applied to the **Error** property, like this:

```
public bool Error { get; private set; }
```

This allows **Error** to be read, but not set, by code outside **FailSoftArray**.

To try the auto-implemented version of **Length** and **Error** with **FailSoftArray**, first remove the **len** and **ErrFlag** variables. They are no longer needed. Then, replace each use of **len** inside **FailSoftArray** with **Length** and each use of **ErrFlag** with **Error**. Here is the updated version of **FailSoftArray** along with a **Main()** method to demonstrate it:

```
// Use read-only, auto-implemented properties for Length and Error.

using System;
```

```csharp
class FailSoftArray {
  int[] a; // reference to underlying array

  // Construct array given its size.
  public FailSoftArray(int size) {
    a = new int[size];
    Length = size;
  }

  // An auto-implemented, read-only Length property.
  public int Length { get; private set; }

  // An auto-implemented, read-only Error property.
  public bool Error { get; private set; }

  // This is the indexer for FailSoftArray.
  public int this[int index] {
    // This is the get accessor.
    get {
      if(ok(index)) {
        Error = false;
        return a[index];
      } else {
        Error = true;
        return 0;
      }
    }

    // This is the set accessor.
    set {
      if(ok(index)) {
        a[index] = value;
        Error = false;
      }
      else Error = true;
    }
  }

  // Return true if index is within bounds.
  private bool ok(int index) {
   if(index >= 0 & index < Length) return true;
   return false;
  }
}

// Demonstrate the improved fail-soft array.
class FinalFSDemo {
  static void Main() {
    FailSoftArray fs = new FailSoftArray(5);

    // Use Error property.
    for(int i=0; i < fs.Length + 1; i++) {
      fs[i] = i*10;
```

```
      if(fs.Error)
        Console.WriteLine("Error with index " + i);
    }
  }
}
```

This version of **FailSoftArray** works the same as the previous version, but it does not contain the explicitly declared backing fields.

Here are some restrictions that apply to using access modifiers with accessors. First, only the **set** or **get** accessor can be modified, not both. Furthermore, the access modifier must be more restrictive than the access level of the property or indexer. Finally, an access modifier cannot be used when declaring an accessor within an interface or when implementing an accessor specified by an interface. (Interfaces are described in Chapter 12.)

Using Indexers and Properties

Although the preceding examples have demonstrated the basic mechanism of indexers and properties, they haven't displayed their full power. To conclude this chapter, a class called **RangeArray** is developed that uses indexers and properties to create an array type in which the index range of the array is determined by the programmer.

As you know, in C# all arrays begin indexing at zero. However, some applications would benefit from an array that allows indexes to begin at any arbitrary point. For example, in some situations it might be more convenient for an array to begin indexing with 1. In another situation, it might be beneficial to allow negative indexes, such as an array that runs from –5 to 5. The **RangeArray** class developed here allows these and other types of indexing.

Using **RangeArray**, you can write code like this:

```
RangeArray ra = new RangeArray(-5, 10); // array with indexes from -5 to 10

for(int i=-5; i <= 10; i++) ra[i] = i; // index from -5 to 10
```

As you can guess, the first line constructs a **RangeArray** that runs from –5 to 10, inclusive. The first argument specifies the beginning index. The second argument specifies the ending index. Once **ra** has been constructed, it can be indexed from –5 to 10.

The entire **RangeArray** class is shown here, along with **RangeArrayDemo**, which demonstrates the array. As implemented here, **RangeArray** supports arrays of **int**, but you can change the data type, if desired.

```
/* Create a specifiable range array class.
   The RangeArray class allows indexing to begin at
   some value other than 0. When you create a RangeArray,
   you specify the beginning and ending index. Negative
   indexes are also allowed. For example, you can create
   arrays that index from -5 to 5, 1 to 10, or 50 to 56.
*/

using System;

class RangeArray {
  // Private data.
  int[] a; // reference to underlying array
```

```
int lowerBound; // smallest index
int upperBound; // largest index

// An auto-implemented, read-only Length property.
public int Length { get; private set; }

// An auto-implemented, read-only Error property.
public bool Error { get; private set; }

// Construct array given its size.
public RangeArray(int low, int high) {
  high++;
  if(high <= low) {
    Console.WriteLine("Invalid Indices");
    high = 1; // create a minimal array for safety
    low = 0;
  }
  a = new int[high - low];
  Length = high - low;

  lowerBound = low;
  upperBound = --high;
}

// This is the indexer for RangeArray.
public int this[int index] {
  // This is the get accessor.
  get {
    if(ok(index)) {
      Error = false;
      return a[index - lowerBound];
    } else {
      Error = true;
      return 0;
    }
  }

  // This is the set accessor.
  set {
    if(ok(index)) {
      a[index - lowerBound] = value;
      Error = false;
    }
    else Error = true;
  }
}

// Return true if index is within bounds.
private bool ok(int index) {
  if(index >= lowerBound & index <= upperBound) return true;
  return false;
}
}
```

```
// Demonstrate the index-range array.
class RangeArrayDemo {
  static void Main() {
    RangeArray ra = new RangeArray(-5, 5);
    RangeArray ra2 = new RangeArray(1, 10);
    RangeArray ra3 = new RangeArray(-20, -12);

    // Demonstrate ra.
    Console.WriteLine("Length of ra: " + ra.Length);

    for(int i = -5; i <= 5; i++)
      ra[i] = i;

    Console.Write("Contents of ra: ");
    for(int i = -5; i <= 5; i++)
      Console.Write(ra[i] + " ");

    Console.WriteLine("\n");

    // Demonstrate ra2.
    Console.WriteLine("Length of ra2: " + ra2.Length);

    for(int i = 1; i <= 10; i++)
      ra2[i] = i;

    Console.Write("Contents of ra2: ");
    for(int i = 1; i <= 10; i++)
      Console.Write(ra2[i] + " ");

    Console.WriteLine("\n");

    // Demonstrate ra3.
    Console.WriteLine("Length of ra3: " + ra3.Length);

    for(int i = -20; i <= -12; i++)
      ra3[i] = i;

    Console.Write("Contents of ra3: ");
    for(int i = -20; i <= -12; i++)
      Console.Write(ra3[i] + " ");

    Console.WriteLine("\n");
  }
}
```

The output from the program is shown here:

```
Length of ra: 11
Contents of ra: -5 -4 -3 -2 -1 0 1 2 3 4 5

Length of ra2: 10
Contents of ra2: 1 2 3 4 5 6 7 8 9 10

Length of ra3: 9
Contents of ra3: -20 -19 -18 -17 -16 -15 -14 -13 -12
```

As the output verifies, objects of type **RangeArray** can be indexed in ways other than starting at zero. Let's look more closely at how **RangeArray** is implemented.

RangeArray begins by defining the following private instance variables:

```
// Private data.
int[] a; // reference to underlying array
int lowerBound; // smallest index
int upperBound; // largest index
```

The underlying array is referred to by **a**. This array is allocated by the **RangeArray** constructor. The index of the lower bound of the array is stored in **lowerBound**, and the index of the upper bound is stored in **upperBound**.

Next, the auto-implemented, read-only properties **Length** and **Error** are declared:

```
// An auto-implemented, read-only Length property.
public int Length { get; private set; }

// An auto-implemented, read-only Error property.
public bool Error { get; private set; }
```

Notice that for both properties, the **set** accessor is private. As explained earlier in this chapter, this results in what is effectively a read-only, auto-implemented property.

The **RangeArray** constructor is shown here:

```
// Construct array given its size.
public RangeArray(int low, int high) {
  high++;
  if(high <= low) {
    Console.WriteLine("Invalid Indices");
    high = 1; // create a minimal array for safety
    low = 0;
  }
  a = new int[high - low];
  Length = high - low;

  lowerBound = low;
  upperBound = --high;
}
```

A **RangeArray** is constructed by passing the lower bound index in **low** and the upper bound index in **high**. The value of **high** is then incremented because the indexes specified are inclusive. Next, a check is made to ensure that the upper index is greater than the lower index. If not, an error is reported and a one-element array is created. Next, storage for the array is allocated and assigned to **a**. Then the **Length** property is set equal to the number of elements in the array. Finally, **lowerBound** and **upperBound** are set.

Next, **RangeArray** implements its indexer, as shown here:

```
// This is the indexer for RangeArray.
public int this[int index] {
  // This is the get accessor.
  get {
    if(ok(index)) {
```

```
      Error = false;
      return a[index - lowerBound];
    } else {
      Error = true;
      return 0;
    }
  }

  // This is the set accessor.
  set {
    if(ok(index)) {
      a[index - lowerBound] = value;
      Error = false;
    }
    else Error = true;
  }
}
```

This indexer is similar to the one used by **FailSoftArray**, with one important exception. Notice the expression that indexes **a**. It is

```
index - lowerBound
```

This expression transforms the index passed in **index** into a zero-based index suitable for use on **a**. This expression works whether **lowerBound** is positive, negative, or zero.

The **ok( )** method is shown here:

```
// Return true if index is within bounds.
private bool ok(int index) {
  if(index >= lowerBound & index <= upperBound) return true;
  return false;
}
```

It is similar to the one used by **FailSoftArray** except that the range is checked by testing it against the values in **lowerBound** and **upperBound**.

RangeArray illustrates just one kind of custom array that you can create through the use of indexers and properties. There are, of course, several others. For example, you can create dynamic arrays, which expand and contract as needed, associative arrays, and sparse arrays. You might want to try creating one of these types of arrays as an exercise.

Inheritance

Inheritance is one of the three foundational principles of object-oriented programming because it allows the creation of hierarchical classifications. Using inheritance, you can create a general class that defines traits common to a set of related items. This class can then be inherited by other, more specific classes, each adding those things that are unique to it.

In the language of C#, a class that is inherited is called a *base class*. The class that does the inheriting is called a *derived class*. Therefore, a derived class is a specialized version of a base class. It inherits all of the variables, methods, properties, and indexers defined by the base class and adds its own unique elements.

Inheritance Basics

C# supports inheritance by allowing one class to incorporate another class into its declaration. This is done by specifying a base class when a derived class is declared. Let's begin with an example. The following class called **TwoDShape** stores the width and height of a two-dimensional object, such as a square, rectangle, triangle, and so on.

```
// A class for two-dimensional objects.
class TwoDShape {
  public double Width;
  public double Height;

  public void ShowDim() {
    Console.WriteLine("Width and height are " +
                      Width + " and " + Height);
  }
}
```

TwoDShape can be used as a base class (that is, as a starting point) for classes that describe specific types of two-dimensional objects. For example, the following program uses **TwoDShape** to derive a class called **Triangle**. Pay close attention to the way that **Triangle** is declared.

```
// A simple class hierarchy.
```

```csharp
using System;

// A class for two-dimensional objects.
class TwoDShape {
  public double Width;
  public double Height;

  public void ShowDim() {
    Console.WriteLine("Width and height are " +
                         Width + " and " + Height);
  }
}

// Triangle is derived from TwoDShape.
class Triangle : TwoDShape {
  public string Style; // style of triangle

  // Return area of triangle.
  public double Area() {
    return Width * Height / 2;
  }

  // Display a triangle's style.
  public void ShowStyle() {
    Console.WriteLine("Triangle is " + Style);
  }
}

class Shapes {
  static void Main() {
    Triangle t1 = new Triangle();
    Triangle t2 = new Triangle();

    t1.Width = 4.0;
    t1.Height = 4.0;
    t1.Style = "isosceles";

    t2.Width = 8.0;
    t2.Height = 12.0;
    t2.Style = "right";

    Console.WriteLine("Info for t1: ");
    t1.ShowStyle();
    t1.ShowDim();
    Console.WriteLine("Area is " + t1.Area());

    Console.WriteLine();

    Console.WriteLine("Info for t2: ");
    t2.ShowStyle();
    t2.ShowDim();
    Console.WriteLine("Area is " + t2.Area());
  }
}
```

The output from this program is shown here:

```
Info for t1:
Triangle is isosceles
Width and height are 4 and 4
Area is 8

Info for t2:
Triangle is right
Width and height are 8 and 12
Area is 48
```

The **Triangle** class creates a specific type of **TwoDShape**, in this case, a triangle. The **Triangle** class includes all of **TwoDShape** and adds the field **Style**, the method **Area( )**, and the method **ShowStyle( )**. A description of the type of triangle is stored in **Style**; **Area( )** computes and returns the area of the triangle; and **ShowStyle( )** displays the triangle style.

Notice the syntax that **Triangle** uses to inherit **TwoDShape**:

```
class Triangle : TwoDShape {
```

This syntax can be generalized. Whenever one class inherits another, the base class name follows the name of the derived class, separated by a colon. In C#, the syntax for inheriting a class is remarkably simple and easy to use.

Because **Triangle** includes all of the members of its base class, **TwoDShape**, it can access **Width** and **Height** inside **Area( )**. Also, inside **Main( )**, objects **t1** and **t2** can refer to **Width** and **Height** directly, as if they were part of **Triangle**. Figure 11-1 depicts conceptually how **TwoDShape** is incorporated into **Triangle**.

Even though **TwoDShape** is a base for **Triangle**, it is also a completely independent, stand-alone class. Being a base class for a derived class does not mean that the base class cannot be used by itself. For example, the following is perfectly valid:

```
TwoDShape shape = new TwoDShape();

shape.Width = 10;
shape.Height = 20;

shape.ShowDim();
```

Of course, an object of **TwoDShape** has no knowledge of or access to any classes derived from **TwoDShape**.

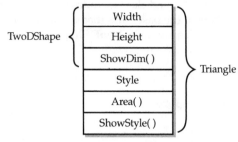

FIGURE 11-1   A conceptual depiction of the **Triangle** class

The general form of a **class** declaration that inherits a base class is shown here:

class *derived-class-name* : *base-class-name* {
  // body of class
}

You can specify only one base class for any derived class that you create. C# does not support the inheritance of multiple base classes into a single derived class. (This differs from C++, in which you can inherit multiple base classes. Be aware of this when converting C++ code to C#.) You can, however, create a hierarchy of inheritance in which a derived class becomes a base class of another derived class. (Of course, no class can be a base class of itself, either directly or indirectly.) In all cases, a derived class inherits all of the members of its base class. This includes instance variables, methods, properties, and indexers.

A major advantage of inheritance is that once you have created a base class that defines the attributes common to a set of objects, it can be used to create any number of more specific derived classes. Each derived class can precisely tailor its own classification. For example, here is another class derived from **TwoDShape** that encapsulates rectangles:

```
// A derived class of TwoDShape for rectangles.
class Rectangle : TwoDShape {
  // Return true if the rectangle is square.
  public bool IsSquare() {
    if(Width == Height) return true;
    return false;
  }

  // Return area of the rectangle.
  public double Area() {
    return Width * Height;
  }
}
```

The **Rectangle** class includes **TwoDShape** and adds the methods **IsSquare( )**, which determines if the rectangle is square, and **Area( )**, which computes the area of a rectangle.

Member Access and Inheritance

As explained in Chapter 8, members of a class are often declared private to prevent their unauthorized use or tampering. Inheriting a class *does not* overrule the private access restriction. Thus, even though a derived class includes all of the members of its base class, it cannot access those members of the base class that are private. For example, if, as shown here, **Width** and **Height** are made private in **TwoDShape**, then **Triangle** will not be able to access them:

```
// Access to private members is not inherited.

// This example will not compile.
using System;

// A class for two-dimensional objects.
class TwoDShape {
```

```
  double Width;  // now private
  double Height; // now private

  public void ShowDim() {
    Console.WriteLine("Width and height are " +
                      Width + " and " + Height);
  }
}

// Triangle is derived from TwoDShape.
class Triangle : TwoDShape {
  public string Style; // style of triangle

  // Return area of triangle.
  public double Area() {
    return Width * Height / 2; // Error, can't access private member
  }

  // Display a triangle's style.
  public void ShowStyle() {
    Console.WriteLine("Triangle is " + Style);
  }
}
```

The **Triangle** class will not compile because the use of **Width** and **Height** inside the **Area( )** method is illegal. Since **Width** and **Height** are now private, they are accessible only to other members of their own class. Derived classes have no access to them.

REMEMBER   *A private class member will remain private to its class. It is not accessible to any code outside its class, including derived classes.*

At first, you might think that it is a serious restriction that derived classes do not have access to the private members of base classes because it would prevent the use of private members in many situations. However, this is not true; C# provides various solutions. One is to use **protected** members, which is described in the next section. A second is to use public properties to provide access to private data.

As explained in the previous chapter, a property allows you to manage access to an instance variable. For example, you can enforce constraints on its values, or you can make the variable read-only. By making a property public, but declaring its underlying variable private, a derived class can still use the property, but it cannot directly access the underlying private variable.

Here is a rewrite of the **TwoDShape** class that makes **Width** and **Height** into properties. In the process, it ensures that the values of **Width** and **Height** will be positive. This would allow you, for example, to specify the **Width** and **Height** using the coordinates of the shape in any quadrant of the Cartesian plane without having to first obtain their absolute values.

```
// Use public properties to set and get private members.

using System;

// A class for two-dimensional objects.
```

```
class TwoDShape {
  double pri_width;  // now private
  double pri_height; // now private

  // Properties for width and height.
  public double Width {
     get { return pri_width; }
     set { pri_width = value < 0 ? -value : value; }
  }

  public double Height {
     get { return pri_height; }
     set { pri_height = value < 0 ? -value : value; }
  }

  public void ShowDim() {
    Console.WriteLine("Width and height are " +
                      Width + " and " + Height);
  }
}

// A derived class of TwoDShape for triangles.
class Triangle : TwoDShape {
  public string Style; // style of triangle

  // Return area of triangle.
  public double Area() {
    return Width * Height / 2;
  }

  // Display a triangle's style.
  public void ShowStyle() {
    Console.WriteLine("Triangle is " + Style);
  }
}

class Shapes2 {
  static void Main() {
    Triangle t1 = new Triangle();
    Triangle t2 = new Triangle();

    t1.Width = 4.0;
    t1.Height = 4.0;
    t1.Style = "isosceles";

    t2.Width = 8.0;
    t2.Height = 12.0;
    t2.Style = "right";

    Console.WriteLine("Info for t1: ");
    t1.ShowStyle();
    t1.ShowDim();
    Console.WriteLine("Area is " + t1.Area());
```

```
    Console.WriteLine();

    Console.WriteLine("Info for t2: ");
    t2.ShowStyle();
    t2.ShowDim();
    Console.WriteLine("Area is " + t2.Area());
  }
}
```

In this version, the properties **Width** and **Height** provide access to the private members, **pri_width** and **pri_height**, which actually store the values. Therefore, even though **pri_width** and **pri_height** are private to **TwoDShape**, their values can still be set and obtained through their corresponding public properties.

When referring to base and derived classes, sometimes the terms *superclass* and *subclass* are used. These terms come from Java programming. What Java calls a superclass, C# calls a base class. What Java calls a subclass, C# calls a derived class. You will commonly hear both sets of terms applied to a class of either language, but this book will continue to use the standard C# terms. C++ also uses the base-class/derived-class terminology.

Using Protected Access

As just explained, a private member of a base class is not accessible to a derived class. This would seem to imply that if you wanted a derived class to have access to some member in the base class, it would need to be public. Of course, making the member public also makes it available to all other code, which may not be desirable. Fortunately, this implication is untrue because C# allows you to create a *protected member*. A protected member is public within a class hierarchy, but private outside that hierarchy.

A protected member is created by using the **protected** access modifier. When a member of a class is declared as **protected**, that member is, with one important exception, private. The exception occurs when a protected member is inherited. In this case, a protected member of the base class becomes a protected member of the derived class and is, therefore, accessible to the derived class. Therefore, by using **protected**, you can create class members that are private to their class but that can still be inherited and accessed by a derived class.

Here is a simple example that uses **protected**:

```
// Demonstrate protected.

using System;

class B {
  protected int i, j; // private to B, but accessible by D

  public void Set(int a, int b) {
    i = a;
    j = b;
  }

  public void Show() {
    Console.WriteLine(i + " " + j);
  }
}
```

```
class D : B {
  int k; // private

  // D can access B's i and j
  public void Setk() {
    k = i * j;
  }

  public void Showk() {
    Console.WriteLine(k);
  }
}

class ProtectedDemo {
  static void Main() {
    D ob = new D();

    ob.Set(2, 3); // OK, known to D
    ob.Show();    // OK, known to D

    ob.Setk();  // OK, part of D
    ob.Showk(); // OK, part of D
  }
}
```

In this example, because **B** is inherited by **D** and because **i** and **j** are declared as **protected** in **B**, the **Setk( )** method can access them. If **i** and **j** had been declared as private by **B**, then **D** would not have access to them, and the program would not compile.

Like **public** and **private**, **protected** status stays with a member no matter how many layers of inheritance are involved. Therefore, when a derived class is used as a base class for another derived class, any protected member of the initial base class that is inherited by the first derived class is also inherited as protected by a second derived class.

Although **protected** access is quite useful, it doesn't apply in all situations. For example, in the case of **TwoDShape** shown in the preceding section, we specifically want the **Width** and **Height** values to be publicly accessible. It's just that we want to manage the values they are assigned. Therefore, declaring them **protected** is not an option. In this case, the use of properties supplies the proper solution by controlling, rather than preventing, access. Remember, use **protected** when you want to create a member that is accessible throughout a class hierarchy, but otherwise private. To manage access to a value, use a property.

Constructors and Inheritance

In a hierarchy, it is possible for both base classes and derived classes to have their own constructors. This raises an important question: What constructor is responsible for building an object of the derived class? The one in the base class, the one in the derived class, or both? Here is the answer: The constructor for the base class constructs the base class portion of the object, and the constructor for the derived class constructs the derived class part. This makes sense because the base class has no knowledge of or access to any element in a derived class. Thus, their construction must be separate. The preceding examples have relied upon the default constructors created automatically by C#, so this was not an issue. However, in practice, most classes will define constructors. Here you will see how to handle this situation.

When only the derived class defines a constructor, the process is straightforward: Simply construct the derived class object. The base class portion of the object is constructed automatically using its default constructor. For example, here is a reworked version of **Triangle** that defines a constructor. It also makes **Style** private since it is now set by the constructor.

```
// Add a constructor to Triangle.

using System;

// A class for two-dimensional objects.
class TwoDShape {
  double pri_width;
  double pri_height;

  // Properties for Width and Height.
  public double Width {
    get { return pri_width; }
    set { pri_width = value < 0 ? -value : value; }
  }

  public double Height {
    get { return pri_height; }
    set { pri_height = value < 0 ? -value : value; }
  }

  public void ShowDim() {
    Console.WriteLine("Width and height are " +
                       Width + " and " + Height);
  }
}

// A derived class of TwoDShape for triangles.
class Triangle : TwoDShape {
  string Style;

  // Constructor.
  public Triangle(string s, double w, double h) {
    Width = w;   // init the base class
    Height = h; // init the base class

    Style = s;   // init the derived class
  }

  // Return area of triangle.
  public double Area() {
    return Width * Height / 2;
  }

  // Display a triangle's style.
  public void ShowStyle() {
    Console.WriteLine("Triangle is " + Style);
  }
}
```

```
class Shapes3 {
  static void Main() {
    Triangle t1 = new Triangle("isosceles", 4.0, 4.0);
    Triangle t2 = new Triangle("right", 8.0, 12.0);

    Console.WriteLine("Info for t1: ");
    t1.ShowStyle();
    t1.ShowDim();
    Console.WriteLine("Area is " + t1.Area());

    Console.WriteLine();

    Console.WriteLine("Info for t2: ");
    t2.ShowStyle();
    t2.ShowDim();
    Console.WriteLine("Area is " + t2.Area());
  }
}
```

Here, **Triangle**'s constructor initializes the members of **TwoDShape** that it inherits along with its own **Style** field.

When both the base class and the derived class define constructors, the process is a bit more complicated because both the base class and derived class constructors must be executed. In this case, you must use another of C#'s keywords, **base**, which has two uses. The first use is to call a base class constructor. The second is to access a member of the base class that has been hidden by a member of a derived class. Here, we will look at its first use.

Calling Base Class Constructors

A derived class can call a constructor defined in its base class by using an expanded form of the derived class' constructor declaration and the **base** keyword. The general form of this expanded declaration is shown here:

> *derived-constructor(parameter-list)* : base(*arg-list*) {
> // body of constructor
> }

Here, *arg-list* specifies any arguments needed by the constructor in the base class. Notice the placement of the colon.

To see how **base** is used, consider the version of **TwoDShape** in the following program. It defines a constructor that initializes the **Width** and **Height** properties. This constructor is then called by the **Triangle** constructor.

```
// Add constructor to TwoDShape.

using System;

// A class for two-dimensional objects.
class TwoDShape {
  double pri_width;
  double pri_height;
```

```csharp
    // Constructor for TwoDShape.
    public TwoDShape(double w, double h) {
      Width = w;
      Height = h;
    }

    // Properties for Width and Height.
    public double Width {
       get { return pri_width; }
       set { pri_width = value < 0 ? -value : value; }
    }

    public double Height {
       get { return pri_height; }
       set { pri_height = value < 0 ? -value : value; }
    }

    public void ShowDim() {
      Console.WriteLine("Width and height are " +
                        Width + " and " + Height);
    }
}

 // A derived class of TwoDShape for triangles.
class Triangle : TwoDShape {
  string Style;

  // Call the base class constructor.
  public Triangle(string s, double w, double h) : base(w, h) {
    Style = s;
  }

  // Return area of triangle.
  public double Area() {
    return Width * Height / 2;
  }

  // Display a triangle's style.
  public void ShowStyle() {
    Console.WriteLine("Triangle is " + Style);
  }
}

class Shapes4 {
  static void Main() {
    Triangle t1 = new Triangle("isosceles", 4.0, 4.0);
    Triangle t2 = new Triangle("right", 8.0, 12.0);

    Console.WriteLine("Info for t1: ");
    t1.ShowStyle();
    t1.ShowDim();
    Console.WriteLine("Area is " + t1.Area());
```

```
    Console.WriteLine();

    Console.WriteLine("Info for t2: ");
    t2.ShowStyle();
    t2.ShowDim();
    Console.WriteLine("Area is " + t2.Area());
  }
}
```

Notice that the **Triangle** constructor is now declared as shown here.

```
public Triangle(string s, double w, double h) : base(w, h) {
```

In this version, **Triangle( )** calls **base** with the parameters **w** and **h**. This causes the
TwoDShape( ) constructor to be called, which initializes **Width** and **Height** using these
values. **Triangle** no longer initializes these values itself. It need only initialize the value
unique to it: **Style**. This leaves **TwoDShape** free to construct its subobject in any manner
that it chooses. Furthermore, **TwoDShape** can add functionality about which existing
derived classes have no knowledge, thus preventing existing code from breaking.

Any form of constructor defined by the base class can be called by **base**. The constructor
executed will be the one that matches the arguments. For example, here are expanded
versions of both **TwoDShape** and **Triangle** that include default constructors and constructors
that take one argument.

```
// Add more constructors to TwoDShape.

using System;

class TwoDShape {
  double pri_width;
  double pri_height;

  // Default constructor.
  public TwoDShape() {
    Width = Height = 0.0;
  }

  // Constructor for TwoDShape.
  public TwoDShape(double w, double h) {
    Width = w;
    Height = h;
  }

  // Construct object with equal width and height.
  public TwoDShape(double x) {
    Width = Height = x;
  }

  // Properties for Width and Height.
  public double Width {
     get { return pri_width; }
     set { pri_width = value < 0 ? -value : value; }
  }
```

```
  public double Height {
     get { return pri_height; }
     set { pri_height = value < 0 ? -value : value; }
  }

  public void ShowDim() {
    Console.WriteLine("Width and height are " +
                      Width + " and " + Height);
  }
}

// A derived class of TwoDShape for triangles.
class Triangle : TwoDShape {
  string Style;

  /* A default constructor. This automatically invokes
     the default constructor of TwoDShape. */
  public Triangle() {
    Style = "null";
  }

  // Constructor that takes three arguments.
  public Triangle(string s, double w, double h) : base(w, h) {
    Style = s;
  }

  // Construct an isosceles triangle.
  public Triangle(double x) : base(x) {
    Style = "isosceles";
  }

  // Return area of triangle.
  public double Area() {
    return Width * Height / 2;
  }

  // Display a triangle's style.
  public void ShowStyle() {
    Console.WriteLine("Triangle is " + Style);
  }
}

class Shapes5 {
  static void Main() {
    Triangle t1 = new Triangle();
    Triangle t2 = new Triangle("right", 8.0, 12.0);
    Triangle t3 = new Triangle(4.0);

    t1 = t2;

    Console.WriteLine("Info for t1: ");
    t1.ShowStyle();
    t1.ShowDim();
    Console.WriteLine("Area is " + t1.Area());
```

```
    Console.WriteLine();

    Console.WriteLine("Info for t2: ");
    t2.ShowStyle();
    t2.ShowDim();
    Console.WriteLine("Area is " + t2.Area());

    Console.WriteLine();

    Console.WriteLine("Info for t3: ");
    t3.ShowStyle();
    t3.ShowDim();
    Console.WriteLine("Area is " + t3.Area());

    Console.WriteLine();
  }
}
```

Here is the output from this version:

```
Info for t1:
Triangle is right
Width and height are 8 and 12
Area is 48

Info for t2:
Triangle is right
Width and height are 8 and 12
Area is 48

Info for t3:
Triangle is isosceles
Width and height are 4 and 4
Area is 8
```

Let's review the key concepts behind **base**. When a derived class specifies a **base** clause, it is calling the constructor of its immediate base class. Thus, **base** always refers to the base class immediately above the calling class. This is true even in a multileveled hierarchy. You pass arguments to the base constructor by specifying them as arguments to **base**. If no **base** clause is present, then the base class' default constructor is called automatically.

Inheritance and Name Hiding

It is possible for a derived class to define a member that has the same name as a member in its base class. When this happens, the member in the base class is hidden within the derived class. While this is not technically an error in C#, the compiler will issue a warning message. This warning alerts you to the fact that a name is being hidden. If your intent is to hide a base class member, then to prevent this warning, the derived class member must be preceded by the **new** keyword. Understand that this use of **new** is separate and distinct from its use when creating an object instance.

Here is an example of name hiding:

```
// An example of inheritance-related name hiding.

using System;

class A {
  public int i = 0;
}

// Create a derived class.
class B : A {
  new int i; // this i hides the i in A

  public B(int b) {
    i = b; // i in B
  }

  public void Show() {
    Console.WriteLine("i in derived class: " + i);
  }
}

class NameHiding {
  static void Main() {
    B ob = new B(2);

    ob.Show();
  }
}
```

First, notice the use of **new** in this line.

```
new int i; // this i hides the i in A
```

In essence, it tells the compiler that you know a new variable called **i** is being created that hides the **i** in the base class **A**. If you leave **new** out, a warning is generated.

The output produced by this program is shown here:

```
i in derived class: 2
```

Since **B** defines its own instance variable called **i**, it hides the **i** in **A**. Therefore, when **Show( )** is invoked on an object of type **B**, the value of **i** as defined by **B** is displayed—not the one defined in **A**.

Using base to Access a Hidden Name

There is a second form of **base** that acts somewhat like **this**, except that it always refers to the base class of the derived class in which it is used. This usage has the following general form:

base.*member*

Here, *member* can be either a method or an instance variable. This form of **base** is most applicable to situations in which member names of a derived class hide members by the

same name in the base class. Consider this version of the class hierarchy from the preceding example:

```
// Using base to overcome name hiding.

using System;

class A {
  public int i = 0;
}

// Create a derived class.
class B : A {
  new int i; // this i hides the i in A

  public B(int a, int b) {
    base.i = a; // this uncovers the i in A
    i = b; // i in B
  }

  public void Show() {
    // This displays the i in A.
    Console.WriteLine("i in base class: " + base.i);

    // This displays the i in B.
    Console.WriteLine("i in derived class: " + i);
  }
}

class UncoverName {
  static void Main() {
    B ob = new B(1, 2);

    ob.Show();
  }
}
```

This program displays the following:

```
i in base class: 1
i in derived class: 2
```

Although the instance variable **i** in **B** hides the **i** in **A**, **base** allows access to the **i** defined in the base class.

Hidden methods can also be called through the use of **base**. For example, in the following code, class **B** inherits class **A**, and both **A** and **B** declare a method called **Show()**. Inside, **B**'s **Show()**, the version of **Show()** defined by **A** is called through the use of **base**.

```
// Call a hidden method.

using System;

class A {
```

```
  public int i = 0;

  // Show() in A
  public void Show() {
    Console.WriteLine("i in base class: " + i);
  }
}

// Create a derived class.
class B : A {
  new int i; // this i hides the i in A

  public B(int a, int b) {
    base.i = a; // this uncovers the i in A
    i = b; // i in B
  }

  // This hides Show() in A. Notice the use of new.
  new public void Show() {
    base.Show(); // this calls Show() in A

    // this displays the i in B
    Console.WriteLine("i in derived class: " + i);
  }
}

class UncoverName {
  static void Main() {
    B ob = new B(1, 2);

    ob.Show();
  }
}
```

The output from the program is shown here:

```
i in base class: 1
i in derived class: 2
```

As you can see, **base.Show( )** calls the base class version of **Show( )**.

One other point: Notice that **new** is used in this program to tell the compiler that you know a new method called **Show( )** is being declared that hides the **Show( )** in **A**.

Creating a Multilevel Hierarchy

Up to this point, we have been using simple class hierarchies consisting of only a base class and a derived class. However, you can build hierarchies that contain as many layers of inheritance as you like. As mentioned, it is perfectly acceptable to use a derived class as a base class of another. For example, given three classes called **A**, **B**, and **C**, **C** can be derived from **B**, which can be derived from **A**. When this type of situation occurs, each derived class inherits all of the traits found in all of its base classes. In this case, **C** inherits all aspects of **B** and **A**.

To see how a multilevel hierarchy can be useful, consider the following program. In it, the derived class **Triangle** is used as a base class to create the derived class called **ColorTriangle**. **ColorTriangle** inherits all of the traits of **Triangle** and **TwoDShape** and adds a field called **color**, which holds the color of the triangle.

```csharp
// A multilevel hierarchy.

using System;

class TwoDShape {
  double pri_width;
  double pri_height;

  // Default constructor.
  public TwoDShape() {
    Width = Height = 0.0;
  }

  // Constructor for TwoDShape.
  public TwoDShape(double w, double h) {
    Width = w;
    Height = h;
  }

  // Construct object with equal width and height.
  public TwoDShape(double x) {
    Width = Height = x;
  }

  // Properties for Width and Height.
  public double Width {
    get { return pri_width; }
    set { pri_width = value < 0 ? -value : value; }
  }

  public double Height {
    get { return pri_height; }
    set { pri_height = value < 0 ? -value : value; }
  }

  public void ShowDim() {
    Console.WriteLine("Width and height are " +
                      Width + " and " + Height);
  }
}

// A derived class of TwoDShape for triangles.
class Triangle : TwoDShape {
  string Style; // private

  /* A default constructor. This invokes the default
     constructor of TwoDShape. */
  public Triangle() {
    Style = "null";
  }
```

```
  // Constructor.
  public Triangle(string s, double w, double h) : base(w, h) {
    Style = s;
  }

  // Construct an isosceles triangle.
  public Triangle(double x) : base(x) {
    Style = "isosceles";
  }

  // Return area of triangle.
  public double Area() {
    return Width * Height / 2;
  }

  // Display a triangle's style.
  public void ShowStyle() {
    Console.WriteLine("Triangle is " + Style);
  }
}

// Extend Triangle.
class ColorTriangle : Triangle {
  string color;

  public ColorTriangle(string c, string s,
                       double w, double h) : base(s, w, h) {
    color = c;
  }

  // Display the color.
  public void ShowColor() {
    Console.WriteLine("Color is " + color);
  }
}

class Shapes6 {
  static void Main() {
    ColorTriangle t1 =
        new ColorTriangle("Blue", "right", 8.0, 12.0);
    ColorTriangle t2 =
        new ColorTriangle("Red", "isosceles", 2.0, 2.0);

    Console.WriteLine("Info for t1: ");
    t1.ShowStyle();
    t1.ShowDim();
    t1.ShowColor();
    Console.WriteLine("Area is " + t1.Area());

    Console.WriteLine();

    Console.WriteLine("Info for t2: ");
    t2.ShowStyle();
    t2.ShowDim();
    t2.ShowColor();
```

```
    Console.WriteLine("Area is " + t2.Area());
  }
}
```

The output of this program is shown here:

```
Info for t1:
Triangle is right
Width and height are 8 and 12
Color is Blue
Area is 48

Info for t2:
Triangle is isosceles
Width and height are 2 and 2
Color is Red
Area is 2
```

Because of inheritance, **ColorTriangle** can make use of the previously defined classes of **Triangle** and **TwoDShape**, adding only the extra information it needs for its own, specific application. This is part of the value of inheritance; it allows the reuse of code.

This example illustrates one other important point: **base** always refers to the constructor in the closest base class. The **base** in **ColorTriangle** calls the constructor in **Triangle**. The **base** in **Triangle** calls the constructor in **TwoDShape**. In a class hierarchy, if a base class constructor requires parameters, then all derived classes must pass those parameters "up the line." This is true whether or not a derived class needs parameters of its own.

When Are Constructors Called?

In the foregoing discussion of inheritance and class hierarchies, an important question may have occurred to you: When a derived class object is created, whose constructor is executed first? The one in the derived class or the one defined by the base class? For example, given a derived class called **B** and a base class called **A**, is **A**'s constructor called before **B**'s, or vice versa? The answer is that in a class hierarchy, constructors are called in order of derivation, from base class to derived class. Furthermore, this order is the same whether or not **base** is used. If **base** is not used, then the default (parameterless) constructor of each base class will be executed. The following program illustrates the order of constructor execution:

```
// Demonstrate when constructors are called.

using System;

// Create a base class.
class A {
  public A() {
    Console.WriteLine("Constructing A.");
  }
}

// Create a class derived from A.
class B : A {
  public B() {
```

```
    Console.WriteLine("Constructing B.");
  }
}

// Create a class derived from B.
class C : B {
  public C() {
    Console.WriteLine("Constructing C.");
  }
}

class OrderOfConstruction {
  static void Main() {
    C c = new C();
  }
}
```

The output from this program is shown here:

```
Constructing A.
Constructing B.
Constructing C.
```

As you can see, the constructors are called in order of derivation.

If you think about it, it makes sense that constructors are executed in order of derivation. Because a base class has no knowledge of any derived class, any initialization it needs to perform is separate from and possibly prerequisite to any initialization performed by the derived class. Therefore, it must be executed first.

Base Class References and Derived Objects

As you know, C# is a strongly typed language. Aside from the standard conversions and automatic promotions that apply to its value types, type compatibility is strictly enforced. Therefore, a reference variable for one class type cannot normally refer to an object of another class type. For example, consider the following program that declares two classes that are identical in their composition:

```
// This program will not compile.

class X {
  int a;

  public X(int i) { a = i; }
}

class Y {
  int a;

  public Y(int i) { a = i; }
}

class IncompatibleRef {
  static void Main() {
```

```
   X x = new X(10);
   X x2;
   Y y = new Y(5);

   x2 = x; // OK, both of same type

   x2 = y; // Error, not of same type
 }
}
```

Here, even though class **X** and class **Y** are physically the same, it is not possible to assign a reference of type **Y** to a variable of type **X** because they have different types. Therefore, this line is incorrect because it causes a compile-time type mismatch:

```
x2 = y; // Error, not of same type
```

In general, an object reference variable can refer only to objects of its type.

There is, however, an important exception to C#'s strict type enforcement. A reference variable of a base class can be assigned a reference to an object of any class derived from that base class. This is legal because an instance of a derived type encapsulates an instance of the base type. Thus, a base class reference can refer to it. Here is an example:

```
// A base class reference can refer to a derived class object.

using System;

class X {
  public int a;

  public X(int i) {
    a = i;
  }
}

class Y : X {
  public int b;

  public Y(int i, int j) : base(j) {
    b = i;
  }
}

class BaseRef {
  static void Main() {
    X x = new X(10);
    X x2;
    Y y = new Y(5, 6);

    x2 = x; // OK, both of same type
    Console.WriteLine("x2.a: " + x2.a);

    x2 = y; // OK because Y is derived from X
    Console.WriteLine("x2.a: " + x2.a);
```

```
     // X references know only about X members
     x2.a = 19; // OK
//      x2.b = 27; // Error, X doesn't have a b member
   }
}
```

In this program, **Y** is derived from **X**. Now, the assignment

```
x2 = y; // OK because Y is derived from X
```

is permissible because a base class reference, **x2** in this case, can refer to a derived class object (which is the object referred to by **y**).

It is important to understand that it is the type of the reference variable—not the type of the object that it refers to—that determines what members can be accessed. That is, when a reference to a derived class object is assigned to a base class reference variable, you will have access only to those parts of the object defined by the base class. This is why **x2** can't access **b** even when it refers to a **Y** object. This makes sense because the base class has no knowledge of what a derived class adds to it. This is why the last line of code in the program is commented out.

Although the preceding discussion may seem a bit esoteric, it has some important practical applications. One is described here. The other is discussed later in this chapter, when virtual methods are covered.

An important place where derived class references are assigned to base class variables is when constructors are called in a class hierarchy. As you know, it is common for a class to define a constructor that takes an object of its class as a parameter. This allows the class to construct a copy of an object. Classes derived from such a class can take advantage of this feature. For example, consider the following versions of **TwoDShape** and **Triangle**. Both add constructors that take an object as a parameter.

```
// Pass a derived class reference to a base class reference.

using System;

class TwoDShape {
  double pri_width;
  double pri_height;

  // Default constructor.
  public TwoDShape() {
    Width = Height = 0.0;
  }

  // Constructor for TwoDShape.
  public TwoDShape(double w, double h) {
    Width = w;
    Height = h;
  }

  // Construct object with equal width and height.
  public TwoDShape(double x) {
    Width = Height = x;
  }
```

```csharp
    // Construct a copy of a TwoDShape object.
    public TwoDShape(TwoDShape ob) {
      Width = ob.Width;
      Height = ob.Height;
    }

    // Properties for Width and Height.
    public double Width {
       get { return pri_width; }
       set { pri_width = value < 0 ? -value : value; }
    }

    public double Height {
       get { return pri_height; }
       set { pri_height = value < 0 ? -value : value; }
    }

    public void ShowDim() {
      Console.WriteLine("Width and height are " +
                        Width + " and " + Height);
    }
}

// A derived class of TwoDShape for triangles.
class Triangle : TwoDShape {
  string Style;

  // A default constructor.
  public Triangle() {
    Style = "null";
  }

  // Constructor for Triangle.
  public Triangle(string s, double w, double h) : base(w, h) {
    Style = s;
  }

  // Construct an isosceles triangle.
  public Triangle(double x) : base(x) {
    Style = "isosceles";
  }

  // Construct a copy of a Triangle object.
  public Triangle(Triangle ob) : base(ob) {
    Style = ob.Style;
  }

  // Return area of triangle.
  public double Area() {
    return Width * Height / 2;
  }
```

```
  // Display a triangle's style.
  public void ShowStyle() {
    Console.WriteLine("Triangle is " + Style);
  }
}

class Shapes7 {
  static void Main() {
    Triangle t1 = new Triangle("right", 8.0, 12.0);

    // Make a copy of t1.
    Triangle t2 = new Triangle(t1);

    Console.WriteLine("Info for t1: ");
    t1.ShowStyle();
    t1.ShowDim();
    Console.WriteLine("Area is " + t1.Area());

    Console.WriteLine();

    Console.WriteLine("Info for t2: ");
    t2.ShowStyle();
    t2.ShowDim();
    Console.WriteLine("Area is " + t2.Area());
  }
}
```

In this program, **t2** is constructed from **t1** and is, thus, identical. The output is shown here:

```
Info for t1:
Triangle is right
Width and height are 8 and 12
Area is 48

Info for t2:
Triangle is right
Width and height are 8 and 12
Area is 48
```

Pay special attention to this **Triangle** constructor:

```
public Triangle(Triangle ob) : base(ob) {
  Style = ob.Style;
}
```

It receives an object of type **Triangle**, and it passes that object (through **base**) to this **TwoDShape** constructor:

```
public TwoDShape(TwoDShape ob) {
  Width = ob.Width;
  Height = ob.Height;
}
```

The key point is that **TwoDShape( )** is expecting a **TwoDShape** object. However, **Triangle( )** passes it a **Triangle** object. As explained, the reason this works is because a base class reference can refer to a derived class object. Thus, it is perfectly acceptable to pass **TwoDShape( )** a reference to an object of a class derived from **TwoDShape**. Because the **TwoDShape( )** constructor is initializing only those portions of the derived class object that are members of **TwoDShape**, it doesn't matter that the object might also contain other members added by derived classes.

Virtual Methods and Overriding

A *virtual method* is a method that is declared as **virtual** in a base class. The defining characteristic of a virtual method is that it can be redefined in one or more derived classes. Thus, each derived class can have its own version of a virtual method. Virtual methods are interesting because of what happens when one is called through a base class reference. In this situation, C# determines which version of the method to call based upon the *type* of the object *referred to* by the reference—and this determination is made *at runtime*. Thus, when different objects are referred to, different versions of the virtual method are executed. In other words, it is the type of the object being referred to (not the type of the reference) that determines which version of the virtual method will be executed. Therefore, if a base class contains a virtual method and classes are derived from that base class, then when different types of objects are referred to through a base class reference, different versions of the virtual method are executed.

You declare a method as virtual inside a base class by preceding its declaration with the keyword **virtual**. When a virtual method is redefined by a derived class, the **override** modifier is used. Thus, the process of redefining a virtual method inside a derived class is called *method overriding*. When overriding a method, the name, return type, and signature of the overriding method must be the same as the virtual method that is being overridden. Also, a virtual method cannot be specified as **static** or **abstract** (discussed later in this chapter).

Method overriding forms the basis for one of C#'s most powerful concepts: *dynamic method dispatch*. Dynamic method dispatch is the mechanism by which a call to an overridden method is resolved at runtime, rather than compile time. Dynamic method dispatch is important because this is how C# implements runtime polymorphism.

Here is an example that illustrates virtual methods and overriding:

```
// Demonstrate a virtual method.

using System;

class Base {
  // Create virtual method in the base class.
  public virtual void Who() {
    Console.WriteLine("Who() in Base");
  }
}

class Derived1 : Base {
  // Override Who() in a derived class.
  public override void Who() {
    Console.WriteLine("Who() in Derived1");
  }
}
```

```
class Derived2 : Base {
  // Override Who() again in another derived class.
  public override void Who() {
    Console.WriteLine("Who() in Derived2");
  }
}

class OverrideDemo {
  static void Main() {
    Base baseOb = new Base();
    Derived1 dOb1 = new Derived1();
    Derived2 dOb2 = new Derived2();

    Base baseRef; // a base class reference

    baseRef = baseOb;
    baseRef.Who();

    baseRef = dOb1;
    baseRef.Who();

    baseRef = dOb2;
    baseRef.Who();
  }
}
```

The output from the program is shown here:

```
Who() in Base
Who() in Derived1
Who() in Derived2
```

This program creates a base class called **Base** and two derived classes, called **Derived1** and **Derived2**. **Base** declares a method called **Who( )**, and the derived classes override it. Inside the **Main( )** method, objects of type **Base**, **Derived1**, and **Derived2** are declared. Also, a reference of type **Base**, called **baseRef**, is declared. The program then assigns a reference to each type of object to **baseRef** and uses that reference to call **Who( )**. As the output shows, the version of **Who( )** executed is determined by the type of object being referred to at the time of the call, not by the class type of **baseRef**.

It is not necessary to override a virtual method. If a derived class does not provide its own version of a virtual method, then the one in the base class is used. For example:

```
/* When a virtual method is not overridden,
   the base class method is used. */

using System;

class Base {
  // Create virtual method in the base class.
  public virtual void Who() {
    Console.WriteLine("Who() in Base");
  }
}
```

```
class Derived1 : Base {
  // Override Who() in a derived class.
  public override void Who() {
    Console.WriteLine("Who() in Derived1");
  }
}

class Derived2 : Base {
  // This class does not override Who().
}

class NoOverrideDemo {
  static void Main() {
    Base baseOb = new Base();
    Derived1 dOb1 = new Derived1();
    Derived2 dOb2 = new Derived2();

    Base baseRef; // a base class reference

    baseRef = baseOb;
    baseRef.Who();

    baseRef = dOb1;
    baseRef.Who();

    baseRef = dOb2;
    baseRef.Who(); // calls Base's Who()
  }
}
```

The output from this program is shown here:

```
Who() in Base
Who() in Derived1
Who() in Base
```

Here, **Derived2** does not override **Who( )**. Thus, when **Who( )** is called on a **Derived2** object, the **Who( )** in **Base** is executed.

In the case of a multilevel hierarchy, if a derived class does not override a virtual method, then, while moving up the hierarchy, the first override of the method that is encountered is the one executed. For example:

```
/* In a multilevel hierarchy, the first override of a virtual
   method that is found while moving up the hierarchy is the
   one executed. */

using System;

class Base {
  // Create virtual method in the base class.
  public virtual void Who() {
    Console.WriteLine("Who() in Base");
```

```
    }
}

class Derived1 : Base {
  // Override Who() in a derived class.
  public override void Who() {
    Console.WriteLine("Who() in Derived1");
  }
}

class Derived2 : Derived1 {
  // This class also does not override Who().
}

class Derived3 : Derived2 {
  // This class does not override Who().
}

class NoOverrideDemo2 {
  static void Main() {
    Derived3 dOb = new Derived3();
    Base baseRef; // a base class reference

    baseRef = dOb;
    baseRef.Who(); // calls Derived1's Who()
  }
}
```

The output is shown here:

```
Who() in Derived1
```

Here, **Derived3** inherits **Derived2**, which inherits **Derived1**, which inherits **Base**. As the output verifies, since **Who( )** is not overridden by either **Derived3** or **Derived2**, it is the override of **Who( )** in **Derived1** that is executed, since it is the first version of **Who( )** that is found.

One other point: Properties can also be modified by the **virtual** keyword and overridden using **override**. The same is true for indexers.

Why Overridden Methods?

Overridden methods allow C# to support runtime polymorphism. Polymorphism is essential to object-oriented programming for one reason: It allows a general class to specify methods that will be common to all of its derivatives, while allowing derived classes to define the specific implementation of some or all of those methods. Overridden methods are another way that C# implements the "one interface, multiple methods" aspect of polymorphism.

Part of the key to applying polymorphism successfully is understanding that the base classes and derived classes form a hierarchy that moves from lesser to greater specialization. Used correctly, the base class provides all elements that a derived class can use directly. Through virtual methods, it also defines those methods that the derived class can implement on its own. This allows the derived class flexibility, yet still enforces a consistent interface. Thus, by combining inheritance with overridden methods, a base class can define the general form of the methods that will be used by all of its derived classes.

Applying Virtual Methods

To better understand the power of virtual methods, we will apply them to the **TwoDShape** class. In the preceding examples, each class derived from **TwoDShape** defines a method called **Area( )**. This suggests that it might be better to make **Area( )** a virtual method of the **TwoDShape** class, allowing each derived class to override it, defining how the area is calculated for the type of shape that the class encapsulates. The following program does this. For convenience, it also adds a name property to **TwoDShape**. (This makes it easier to demonstrate the classes.)

```
// Use virtual methods and polymorphism.

using System;

class TwoDShape {
  double pri_width;
  double pri_height;

  // A default constructor.
  public TwoDShape() {
    Width = Height = 0.0;
    name = "null";
  }

  // Parameterized constructor.
  public TwoDShape(double w, double h, string n) {
    Width = w;
    Height = h;
    name = n;
  }

  // Construct object with equal width and height.
  public TwoDShape(double x, string n) {
    Width = Height = x;
    name = n;
  }

  // Construct a copy of a TwoDShape object.
  public TwoDShape(TwoDShape ob) {
    Width = ob.Width;
    Height = ob.Height;
    name = ob.name;
  }

  // Properties for Width and Height.
  public double Width {
    get { return pri_width; }
    set { pri_width = value < 0 ? -value : value; }
  }

  public double Height {
    get { return pri_height; }
    set { pri_height = value < 0 ? -value : value; }
  }
```

```
  public string name { get; set; }

  public void ShowDim() {
    Console.WriteLine("Width and height are " +
                        Width + " and " + Height);
  }

  public virtual double Area() {
    Console.WriteLine("Area() must be overridden");
    return 0.0;
  }
}

// A derived class of TwoDShape for triangles.
class Triangle : TwoDShape {
  string Style;

  // A default constructor.
  public Triangle() {
    Style = "null";
  }

  // Constructor for Triangle.
  public Triangle(string s, double w, double h) :
    base(w, h, "triangle") {
      Style = s;
  }

  // Construct an isosceles triangle.
  public Triangle(double x) : base(x, "triangle") {
    Style = "isosceles";
  }

  // Construct a copy of a Triangle object.
  public Triangle(Triangle ob) : base(ob) {
    Style = ob.Style;
  }

  // Override Area() for Triangle.
  public override double Area() {
    return Width * Height / 2;
  }

  // Display a triangle's style.
  public void ShowStyle() {
    Console.WriteLine("Triangle is " + Style);
  }
}

// A derived class of TwoDShape for rectangles.
class Rectangle : TwoDShape {

  // Constructor for Rectangle.
  public Rectangle(double w, double h) :
    base(w, h, "rectangle"){ }
```

```
  // Construct a square.
  public Rectangle(double x) :
    base(x, "rectangle") { }

  // Construct a copy of a Rectangle object.
  public Rectangle(Rectangle ob) : base(ob) { }

  // Return true if the rectangle is square.
  public bool IsSquare() {
    if(Width == Height) return true;
    return false;
  }

  // Override Area() for Rectangle.
  public override double Area() {
    return Width * Height;
  }
}

class DynShapes {
  static void Main() {
    TwoDShape[] shapes = new TwoDShape[5];

    shapes[0] = new Triangle("right", 8.0, 12.0);
    shapes[1] = new Rectangle(10);
    shapes[2] = new Rectangle(10, 4);
    shapes[3] = new Triangle(7.0);
    shapes[4] = new TwoDShape(10, 20, "generic");

    for(int i=0; i < shapes.Length; i++) {
      Console.WriteLine("object is " + shapes[i].name);
      Console.WriteLine("Area is " + shapes[i].Area());

      Console.WriteLine();
    }
  }
}
```

The output from the program is shown here:

```
object is triangle
Area is 48

object is rectangle
Area is 100

object is rectangle
Area is 40

object is triangle
Area is 24.5

object is generic
Area() must be overridden
Area is 0
```

Let's examine this program closely. First, as explained, **Area( )** is declared as **virtual** in the **TwoDShape** class and is overridden by **Triangle** and **Rectangle**. Inside **TwoDShape**, **Area( )** is given a placeholder implementation that simply informs the user that this method must be overridden by a derived class. Each override of **Area( )** supplies an implementation that is suitable for the type of object encapsulated by the derived class. Thus, if you were to implement an ellipse class, for example, then **Area( )** would need to compute the area of an ellipse.

There is one other important feature in the preceding program. Notice in **Main( )** that **shapes** is declared as an array of **TwoDShape** objects. However, the elements of this array are assigned **Triangle**, **Rectangle**, and **TwoDShape** references. This is valid because a base class reference can refer to a derived class object. The program then cycles through the array, displaying information about each object. Although quite simple, this illustrates the power of both inheritance and method overriding. The type of object stored in a base class reference variable is determined at runtime and acted on accordingly. If an object is derived from **TwoDShape**, then its area can be obtained by calling **Area( )**. The interface to this operation is the same no matter what type of shape is being used.

Using Abstract Classes

Sometimes you will want to create a base class that defines only a generalized form that will be shared by all of its derived classes, leaving it to each derived class to fill in the details. Such a class determines the nature of the methods that the derived classes must implement, but does not, itself, provide an implementation of one or more of these methods. One way this situation can occur is when a base class is unable to create a meaningful implementation for a method. This is the case with the version of **TwoDShape** used in the preceding example. The definition of **Area( )** is simply a placeholder. It will not compute and display the area of any type of object.

You will see as you create your own class libraries that it is not uncommon for a method to have no meaningful definition in the context of its base class. You can handle this situation two ways. One way, as shown in the previous example, is to simply have it report a warning message. Although this approach can be useful in certain situations—such as debugging—it is not usually appropriate. You may have methods that must be overridden by the derived class in order for the derived class to have any meaning. Consider the class **Triangle**. It is incomplete if **Area( )** is not defined. In such a case, you want some way to ensure that a derived class does, indeed, override all necessary methods. C#'s solution to this problem is the *abstract method*.

An abstract method is created by specifying the **abstract** type modifier. An abstract method contains no body and is, therefore, not implemented by the base class. Thus, a derived class must override it—it cannot simply use the version defined in the base class. As you can probably guess, an abstract method is automatically virtual, and there is no need to use the **virtual** modifier. In fact, it is an error to use **virtual** and **abstract** together.

To declare an abstract method, use this general form:

abstract *type name(parameter-list)*;

As you can see, no method body is present. The **abstract** modifier can be used only on instance methods. It cannot be applied to **static** methods. Properties and indexers can also be abstract.

A class that contains one or more abstract methods must also be declared as abstract by preceding its **class** declaration with the **abstract** specifier. Since an abstract class does not define a complete implementation, there can be no objects of an abstract class. Thus, attempting to create an object of an abstract class by using **new** will result in a compile-time error.

When a derived class inherits an abstract class, it must implement all of the abstract methods in the base class. If it doesn't, then the derived class must also be specified as **abstract**. Thus, the **abstract** attribute is inherited until such time as a complete implementation is achieved.

Using an abstract class, you can improve the **TwoDShape** class. Since there is no meaningful concept of area for an undefined two-dimensional figure, the following version of the preceding program declares **Area( )** as **abstract** inside **TwoDShape** and **TwoDShape** as **abstract**. This, of course, means that all classes derived from **TwoDShape** must override **Area( )**.

```
// Create an abstract class.

using System;

abstract class TwoDShape {
  double pri_width;
  double pri_height;

  // A default constructor.
  public TwoDShape() {
    Width = Height = 0.0;
    name = "null";
  }

  // Parameterized constructor.
  public TwoDShape(double w, double h, string n) {
    Width = w;
    Height = h;
    name = n;
  }

  // Construct object with equal width and height.
  public TwoDShape(double x, string n) {
    Width = Height = x;
    name = n;
  }

  // Construct a copy of a TwoDShape object.
  public TwoDShape(TwoDShape ob) {
    Width = ob.Width;
    Height = ob.Height;
    name = ob.name;
  }

  // Properties for Width and Height.
  public double Width {
    get { return pri_width; }
    set { pri_width = value < 0 ? -value : value; }
  }
```

```csharp
  public double Height {
    get { return pri_height; }
    set { pri_height = value < 0 ? -value : value; }
  }

  public string name { get; set; }

  public void ShowDim() {
    Console.WriteLine("Width and height are " +
                      Width + " and " + Height);
  }

  // Now, Area() is abstract.
  public abstract double Area();
}

// A derived class of TwoDShape for triangles.
class Triangle : TwoDShape {
  string Style;

  // A default constructor.
  public Triangle() {
    Style = "null";
  }

  // Constructor for Triangle.
  public Triangle(string s, double w, double h) :
    base(w, h, "triangle") {
      Style = s;
  }

  // Construct an isosceles triangle.
  public Triangle(double x) : base(x, "triangle") {
    Style = "isosceles";
  }

  // Construct a copy of a Triangle object.
  public Triangle(Triangle ob) : base(ob) {
    Style = ob.Style;
  }

  // Override Area() for Triangle.
  public override double Area() {
    return Width * Height / 2;
  }

  // Display a triangle's style.
  public void ShowStyle() {
    Console.WriteLine("Triangle is " + Style);
  }
}

// A derived class of TwoDShape for rectangles.
class Rectangle : TwoDShape {
```

```
    // Constructor for Rectangle.
    public Rectangle(double w, double h) :
      base(w, h, "rectangle"){ }

    // Construct a square.
    public Rectangle(double x) :
      base(x, "rectangle") { }

    // Construct a copy of a Rectangle object.
    public Rectangle(Rectangle ob) : base(ob) { }

    // Return true if the rectangle is square.
    public bool IsSquare() {
      if(Width == Height) return true;
      return false;
    }

    // Override Area() for Rectangle.
    public override double Area() {
      return Width * Height;
    }
}

class AbsShape {
  static void Main() {
    TwoDShape[] shapes = new TwoDShape[4];

    shapes[0] = new Triangle("right", 8.0, 12.0);
    shapes[1] = new Rectangle(10);
    shapes[2] = new Rectangle(10, 4);
    shapes[3] = new Triangle(7.0);

    for(int i=0; i < shapes.Length; i++) {
      Console.WriteLine("object is " + shapes[i].name);
      Console.WriteLine("Area is " + shapes[i].Area());

      Console.WriteLine();
    }
  }
}
```

As the program illustrates, all derived classes *must* override **Area( )** (or also be declared **abstract**). To prove this to yourself, try creating a derived class that does not override **Area( )**. You will receive a compile-time error. Of course, it is still possible to create an object reference of type **TwoDShape**, which the program does. However, it is no longer possible to declare objects of type **TwoDShape**. Because of this, in **Main( )** the **shapes** array has been shortened to 4, and a generic **TwoDShape** object is no longer created.

One other point: Notice that **TwoDShape** still includes the **ShowDim( )** method and that it is not modified by **abstract**. It is perfectly acceptable—indeed, quite common—for an abstract class to contain concrete methods that a derived class is free to use as-is. Only those methods declared as **abstract** must be overridden by derived classes.

Using sealed to Prevent Inheritance

As powerful and useful as inheritance is, sometimes you will want to prevent it. For example, you might have a class that encapsulates the initialization sequence of some specialized hardware device, such as a medical monitor. In this case, you don't want users of your class to be able to change the way the monitor is initialized, possibly setting the device incorrectly. Whatever the reason, in C# it is easy to prevent a class from being inherited by using the keyword **sealed**.

To prevent a class from being inherited, precede its declaration with **sealed**. As you might expect, it is illegal to declare a class as both **abstract** and **sealed** because an abstract class is incomplete by itself and relies upon its derived classes to provide complete implementations.

Here is an example of a **sealed** class:

```
sealed class A {
  // ...
}

// The following class is illegal.
class B : A { // ERROR! Can't derive from class A
  // ...
}
```

As the comments imply, it is illegal for **B** to inherit **A** because **A** is declared as **sealed**.

One other point: **sealed** can also be used on virtual methods to prevent further overrrides. For example, assume a base class called **B** and a derived class called **D**. A method declared **virtual** in **B** can be declared **sealed** by **D**. This would prevent any class that inherits **D** from overriding the method. This situation is illustrated by the following:

```
class B {
  public virtual void MyMethod() { /* ... */ }
}

class D : B {
  // This seals MyMethod() and prevents further overrides.
  sealed public override void MyMethod() { /* ... */ }
}

class X : D {
  // Error! MyMethod() is sealed!
  public override void MyMethod() { /* ... */ }
}
```

Because **MyMethod()** is sealed by **D**, it can't be overridden by **X**.

The object Class

C# defines one special class called **object** that is an implicit base class of all other classes and for all other types (including the value types). In other words, all other types are derived from **object**. This means that a reference variable of type **object** can refer to an object of any

other type. Also, since arrays are implemented as objects, a variable of type **object** can also refer to any array. Technically, the C# name **object** is just another name for **System.Object**, which is part of the .NET Framework class library.

The **object** class defines the methods shown in Table 11-1, which means that they are available in every object.

A few of these methods warrant some additional explanation. By default, the **Equals(object)** method determines if the invoking object refers to the same object as the one referred to by the argument. (That is, it determines if the two references are the same.) It returns **true** if the objects are the same, and **false** otherwise. You can override this method in classes that you create. Doing so allows you to define what equality means relative to a class. For example, you could define **Equals(object)** so that it compares the contents of two objects for equality. The **Equals(object, object)** method invokes **Equals(object)** to compute its result.

The **GetHashCode( )** method returns a hash code associated with the invoking object. This hash code can be used with any algorithm that employs hashing as a means of accessing stored objects.

As mentioned in Chapter 9, if you overload the = = operator, then you will usually need to override **Equals(object)** and **GetHashCode( )** because most of the time you will want the = = operator and the **Equals(object)** methods to function the same. When **Equals( )** is overridden, you should also override **GetHashCode( )**, so that the two methods are compatible.

The **ToString( )** method returns a string that contains a description of the object on which it is called. Also, this method is automatically called when an object is output using

Method	Purpose
public virtual bool Equals(object *ob*)	Determines whether the invoking object is the same as the one referred to by *ob*.
public static bool Equals(object *ob1*, object *ob2*)	Determines whether *ob1* is the same as *ob2*.
protected virtual Finalize( )	Performs shutdown actions prior to garbage collection. In C#, **Finalize( )** is accessed through a destructor.
public virtual int GetHashCode( )	Returns the hash code associated with the invoking object.
public Type GetType( )	Obtains the type of an object at runtime.
protected object MemberwiseClone( )	Makes a "shallow copy" of the object. This is one in which the members are copied, but objects referred to by members are not.
public static bool ReferenceEquals(object *ob1*, object *ob2*)	Determines whether *ob1* and *ob2* refer to the same object.
public virtual string ToString( )	Returns a string that describes the object.

TABLE 11-1   Methods of the **object** Class

WriteLine( ). Many classes override this method. Doing so allows them to tailor a description specifically for the types of objects that they create. For example:

```
// Demonstrate ToString()

using System;

class MyClass {
  static int count = 0;
  int id;

  public MyClass() {
    id = count;
    count++;
  }

  public override string ToString() {
    return "MyClass object #" + id;
  }
}

class Test {
  static void Main() {
    MyClass ob1 = new MyClass();
    MyClass ob2 = new MyClass();
    MyClass ob3 = new MyClass();

    Console.WriteLine(ob1);
    Console.WriteLine(ob2);
    Console.WriteLine(ob3);
  }
}
```

The output from the program is shown here:

```
MyClass object #0
MyClass object #1
MyClass object #2
```

Boxing and Unboxing

As explained, all C# types, including the value types, are derived from **object**. Thus, a reference of type **object** can be used to refer to any other type, including value types. When an **object** reference refers to a value type, a process known as *boxing* occurs. Boxing causes the value of a value type to be stored in an object instance. Thus, a value type is "boxed" inside an object. This object can then be used like any other object. In all cases, boxing occurs automatically. You simply assign a value to an **object** reference. C# handles the rest.

Unboxing is the process of retrieving a value from a boxed object. This action is performed using an explicit cast from the **object** reference to its corresponding value type. Attempting to unbox an object into a different type will result in a runtime error.

Here is a simple example that illustrates boxing and unboxing:

```
// A simple boxing/unboxing example.

using System;

class BoxingDemo {
  static void Main() {
    int x;
    object obj;

    x = 10;
    obj = x; // box x into an object

    int y = (int)obj; // unbox obj into an int
    Console.WriteLine(y);
  }
}
```

This program displays the value 10. Notice that the value in **x** is boxed simply by assigning it to **obj**, which is an **object** reference. The integer value in **obj** is retrieved by casting **obj** to **int**.

Here is another, more interesting example of boxing. In this case, an **int** is passed as an argument to the **Sqr( )** method, which uses an **object** parameter.

```
// Boxing also occurs when passing values.

using System;

class BoxingDemo {
  static void Main() {
    int x;

    x = 10;
    Console.WriteLine("Here is x: " + x);

    // x is automatically boxed when passed to Sqr().
    x = BoxingDemo.Sqr(x);
    Console.WriteLine("Here is x squared: " + x);
  }

  static int Sqr(object o) {
    return (int)o * (int)o;
  }
}
```

The output from the program is shown here:

```
Here is x: 10
Here is x squared: 100
```

Here, the value of **x** is automatically boxed when it is passed to **Sqr( )**.

Boxing and unboxing allow C#'s type system to be fully unified. All types derive from **object**. A reference to any type can be assigned to a variable of type **object**. Boxing and

unboxing automatically handle the details for the value types. Furthermore, because all types are derived from **object**, they all have access to **object's** methods. For example, consider the following rather surprising program:

```
// Boxing makes it possible to call methods on a value!

using System;

class MethOnValue {
  static void Main() {

    Console.WriteLine(10.ToString());

  }
}
```

This program displays 10. The reason is that the **ToString( )** method returns a string representation of the object on which it is called. In this case, the string representation of 10 is 10!

Is object a Universal Data Type?

Given that **object** is a base class for all other types and that boxing of the value types takes place automatically, it is possible to use **object** as a "universal" data type. For example, consider the following program that creates an array of **object** and then assigns various other types of data to its elements:

```
// Use object to create a "generic" array.

using System;

class GenericDemo {
  static void Main() {
    object[] ga = new object[10];

    // Store ints.
    for(int i=0; i < 3; i++)
      ga[i] = i;

    // Store doubles.
    for(int i=3; i < 6; i++)
      ga[i] = (double) i / 2;


    // Store two strings, a bool, and a char.
    ga[6] = "Hello";
    ga[7] = true;
    ga[8] = 'X';
    ga[9] = "end";

    for(int i = 0; i < ga.Length; i++)
      Console.WriteLine("ga[" + i + "]: " + ga[i] + " ");
  }
}
```

The output is shown here:

```
ga[0]: 0
ga[1]: 1
ga[2]: 2
ga[3]: 1.5
ga[4]: 2
ga[5]: 2.5
ga[6]: Hello
ga[7]: True
ga[8]: X
ga[9]: end
```

As this program illustrates, because an **object** reference can hold a reference to any other type of data, it is possible to use an **object** reference to refer to any type of data. Thus, an array of **object** as used by the program can store any type of data. Expanding on this concept, it is easy to see how you could construct a stack class, for example, that stored **object** references. This would enable the stack to store any type of data.

Although the universal-type feature of **object** is powerful and can be used quite effectively in some situations, it is a mistake to think that you should use **object** as a way around C#'s otherwise strong type checking. In general, when you need to store an **int**, use an **int** variable; when you need to store a **string**, use a **string** reference; and so on.

More importantly, since version 2.0, true generic types are available to the C# programmer. (Generics are described in Chapter 18.) The addition of generics enables you to easily define classes and algorithms that automatically work with different types of data in a type-safe manner. Because of generics, you will normally not need to use **object** as a universal type when creating new code. Today, it's best to reserve **object**'s universal nature for specialized situations.

Interfaces, Structures, and Enumerations

This chapter discusses one of C#'s most important features: the interface. An *interface* defines a set of methods that will be implemented by a class. An interface does not, itself, implement any method. Thus, an interface is a purely logical construct that describes functionality without specifying implementation.

Also discussed in this chapter are two more C# data types: structures and enumerations. *Structures* are similar to classes except that they are handled as value types rather than reference types. *Enumerations* are lists of named integer constants. Structures and enumerations contribute to the richness of the C# programming environment.

Interfaces

In object-oriented programming it is sometimes helpful to define what a class must do, but not how it will do it. You have already seen an example of this: the abstract method. An abstract method declares the return type and signature for a method, but provides no implementation. A derived class must provide its own implementation of each abstract method defined by its base class. Thus, an abstract method specifies the *interface* to the method, but not the *implementation*. Although abstract classes and methods are useful, it is possible to take this concept a step further. In C#, you can fully separate a class' interface from its implementation by using the keyword **interface**.

Interfaces are syntactically similar to abstract classes. However, in an interface, no method can include a body. That is, an interface provides no implementation whatsoever. It specifies what must be done, but not how. Once an interface is defined, any number of classes can implement it. Also, one class can implement any number of interfaces.

To implement an interface, a class must provide bodies (implementations) for the methods described by the interface. Each class is free to determine the details of its own implementation. Thus, two classes might implement the same interface in different ways, but each class still supports the same set of methods. Therefore, code that has knowledge of the interface can use objects of either class since the interface to those objects is the same. By providing the interface, C# allows you to fully utilize the "one interface, multiple methods" aspect of polymorphism.

Interfaces are declared by using the **interface** keyword. Here is a simplified form of an interface declaration:

interface *name* {
    ret-type method-name1(param-list);
    ret-type method-name2(param-list);
    // ...
    ret-type method-nameN(param-list);
}

The name of the interface is specified by *name*. Methods are declared using only their return type and signature. They are, essentially, abstract methods. As explained, in an interface, no method can have an implementation. Thus, each class that includes an interface must implement all of the methods. In an interface, methods are implicitly **public**, and no explicit access specifier is allowed.

Here is an example of an interface. It specifies the interface to a class that generates a series of numbers.

```
public interface ISeries {
  int GetNext(); // return next number in series
  void Reset(); // restart
  void SetStart(int x); // set starting value
}
```

The name of this interface is **ISeries**. Although the prefix **I** is not necessary, many programmers prefix interfaces with **I** to differentiate them from classes. **ISeries** is declared **public** so that it can be implemented by any class in any program.

In addition to methods, interfaces can specify properties, indexers, and events. Events are described in Chapter 15, and we will be concerned with only methods, properties, and indexers here. Interfaces cannot have data members. They cannot define constructors, destructors, or operator methods. Also, no member can be declared as **static**.

Implementing Interfaces

Once an interface has been defined, one or more classes can implement that interface. To implement an interface, the name of the interface is specified after the class name in just the same way that a base class is specified. The general form of a class that implements an interface is shown here:

class *class-name* : *interface-name* {
    // class-body
}

The name of the interface being implemented is specified in *interface-name*. When a class implements an interface, the class must implement the entire interface. It cannot pick and choose which parts to implement, for example.

A class can implement more than one interface. When a class implements more than one interface, specify each interface in a comma-separated list. A class can inherit a base class and also implement one or more interfaces. In this case, the name of the base class must come first in the comma-separated list.

The methods that implement an interface must be declared **public**. The reason for this is that methods are implicitly public within an interface, so their implementation must also be public. Also, the return type and signature of the implementing method must match exactly the return type and signature specified in the **interface** definition.

Here is an example that implements the **ISeries** interface shown earlier. It creates a class called **ByTwos**, which generates a series of numbers, each two greater than the previous one.

```
// Implement ISeries.
class ByTwos : ISeries {
  int start;
  int val;

  public ByTwos() {
    start = 0;
    val = 0;
  }

  public int GetNext() {
    val += 2;
    return val;
  }

  public void Reset() {
    val = start;
  }

  public void SetStart(int x) {
    start = x;
    val = start;
  }
}
```

As you can see, **ByTwos** implements all three methods defined by **ISeries**. As explained, this is necessary since a class cannot create a partial implementation of an interface.

Here is a class that demonstrates **ByTwos**:

```
// Demonstrate the ByTwos interface.

using System;

class SeriesDemo {
  static void Main() {
    ByTwos ob = new ByTwos();

    for(int i=0; i < 5; i++)
      Console.WriteLine("Next value is " +
                        ob.GetNext());

    Console.WriteLine("\nResetting");
    ob.Reset();
    for(int i=0; i < 5; i++)
      Console.WriteLine("Next value is " +
                        ob.GetNext());
```

```
      Console.WriteLine("\nStarting at 100");
      ob.SetStart(100);
      for(int i=0; i < 5; i++)
        Console.WriteLine("Next value is " +
                            ob.GetNext());

   }
}
```

To compile **SeriesDemo**, you must include the files that contain **ISeries**, **ByTwos**, and **SeriesDemo** in the compilation. The compiler will automatically compile all three files to create the final executable. For example, if you called these files **ISeries.cs**, **ByTwos.cs**, and **SeriesDemo.cs**, then the following command line will compile the program:

```
>csc SeriesDemo.cs ISeries.cs ByTwos.cs
```

If you are using the Visual C++ IDE, simply add all three files to your C# project. One other point: It is perfectly valid to put all three of these classes in the same file, too.

The output from this program is shown here:

```
Next value is 2
Next value is 4
Next value is 6
Next value is 8
Next value is 10

Resetting
Next value is 2
Next value is 4
Next value is 6
Next value is 8
Next value is 10

Starting at 100
Next value is 102
Next value is 104
Next value is 106
Next value is 108
Next value is 110
```

It is both permissible and common for classes that implement interfaces to define additional members of their own. For example, the following version of **ByTwos** adds the method **GetPrevious( )**, which returns the previous value:

```
// Implement ISeries and add GetPrevious().
 class ByTwos : ISeries {
   int start;
   int val;
   int prev;

   public ByTwos() {
     start = 0;
     val = 0;
     prev = -2;
   }
```

```
public int GetNext() {
  prev = val;
  val += 2;
  return val;
}

public void Reset() {
  val = start;
  prev = start - 2;
}

public void SetStart(int x) {
  start = x;
  val = start;
  prev = val - 2;
}

// A method not specified by ISeries.
public int GetPrevious() {
  return prev;
}
}
```

Notice that the addition of **GetPrevious( )** required a change to the implementations of the methods defined by **ISeries**. However, since the interface to those methods stays the same, the change is seamless and does not break preexisting code. This is one of the advantages of interfaces.

As explained, any number of classes can implement an **interface**. For example, here is a class called **Primes** that generates a series of prime numbers. Notice that its implementation of **ISeries** is fundamentally different than the one provided by **ByTwos**.

```
// Use ISeries to implement a series of prime numbers.
class Primes : ISeries {
  int start;
  int val;

  public Primes() {
    start = 2;
    val = 2;
  }

  public int GetNext() {
    int i, j;
    bool isprime;

    val++;
    for(i = val; i < 1000000; i++) {
      isprime = true;
      for(j = 2; j <= i/j; j++) {
        if((i%j)==0) {
          isprime = false;
          break;
        }
      }
```

```
      if(isprime) {
        val = i;
        break;
      }
    }
    return val;
  }

  public void Reset() {
    val = start;
  }

  public void SetStart(int x) {
    start = x;
    val = start;
  }
}
```

The key point is that even though **ByTwos** and **Primes** generate completely unrelated series of numbers, both implement **ISeries**. As explained, an interface says nothing about the implementation, so each class is free to implement the interface as it sees fit.

Using Interface References

You might be somewhat surprised to learn that you can declare a reference variable of an interface type. In other words, you can create an interface reference variable. Such a variable can refer to any object that implements its interface. When you call a method on an object through an interface reference, it is the version of the method implemented by the object that is executed. This process is similar to using a base class reference to access a derived class object, as described in Chapter 11.

The following example illustrates the use of an interface reference. It uses the same interface reference variable to call methods on objects of both **ByTwos** and **Primes**. For clarity, it shows all pieces of the program, assembled into a single file.

```
// Demonstrate interface references.

using System;

// Define the interface.
public interface ISeries {
  int GetNext(); // return next number in series
  void Reset(); // restart
  void SetStart(int x); // set starting value
}

// Use ISeries to implement a series in which each
// value is two greater than the previous one.
class ByTwos : ISeries {
  int start;
  int val;
```

```
    public ByTwos() {
      start = 0;
      val = 0;
    }

    public int GetNext() {
      val += 2;
      return val;
    }

    public void Reset() {
      val = start;
    }

    public void SetStart(int x) {
      start = x;
      val = start;
    }
}

// Use ISeries to implement a series of prime numbers.
class Primes : ISeries {
  int start;
  int val;

  public Primes() {
    start = 2;
    val = 2;
  }

  public int GetNext() {
    int i, j;
    bool isprime;

    val++;
    for(i = val; i < 1000000; i++) {
      isprime = true;
      for(j = 2; j <= i/j; j++) {
        if((i%j)==0) {
          isprime = false;
          break;
        }
      }
      if(isprime) {
        val = i;
        break;
      }
    }
    return val;
  }

  public void Reset() {
    val = start;
  }
```

```
    public void SetStart(int x) {
        start = x;
        val = start;
    }
}

class SeriesDemo2 {
    static void Main() {
        ByTwos twoOb = new ByTwos();
        Primes primeOb = new Primes();
        ISeries ob;

        for(int i=0; i < 5; i++) {
            ob = twoOb;
            Console.WriteLine("Next ByTwos value is " +
                                    ob.GetNext());
            ob = primeOb;
            Console.WriteLine("Next prime number is " +
                                    ob.GetNext());

        }
    }
}
```

The output from the program is shown here:

```
Next ByTwos value is 2
Next prime number is 3
Next ByTwos value is 4
Next prime number is 5
Next ByTwos value is 6
Next prime number is 7
Next ByTwos value is 8
Next prime number is 11
Next ByTwos value is 10
Next prime number is 13
```

In **Main( )**, **ob** is declared to be a reference to an **ISeries** interface. This means that it can be used to store references to any object that implements **ISeries**. In this case, it is used to refer to **twoOb** and **primeOb**, which are objects of type **ByTwos** and **Primes**, respectively, which both implement **ISeries**.

One other point: An interface reference variable has knowledge only of the methods declared by its **interface** declaration. Thus, an interface reference cannot be used to access any other variables or methods that might be supported by the object.

Interface Properties

Like methods, properties are specified in an interface without any body. Here is the general form of a property specification:

```
// interface property
type name {
    get;
    set;
}
```

Of course, only **get** or **set** will be present for read-only or write-only properties, respectively.

Although the declaration of a property in an interface looks similar to how an auto-implemented property is declared in a class, the two are not the same. The interface declaration does not cause the property to be auto-implemented. It only specifies the name and type of the property. Implementation is left to each implementing class. Also, no access modifiers are allowed on the accessors when a property is declared in an **interface**. Thus, the **set** accessor, for example, cannot be specified as private in an **interface**.

Here is a rewrite of the **ISeries** interface and the **ByTwos** class that uses a property called **Next** to obtain and set the next element in the series:

```
// Use a property in an interface.

using System;

public interface ISeries {
  // An interface property.
  int Next {
    get; // return the next number in series
    set; // set next number
  }
}

// Implement ISeries.
class ByTwos : ISeries {
  int val;

  public ByTwos() {
    val = 0;
  }

  // Get or set value.
  public int Next {
    get {
      val += 2;
      return val;
    }
    set {
      val = value;
    }
  }
}

// Demonstrate an interface property.
class SeriesDemo3 {
  static void Main() {
    ByTwos ob = new ByTwos();

    // Access series through a property.
    for(int i=0; i < 5; i++)
      Console.WriteLine("Next value is " + ob.Next);

    Console.WriteLine("\nStarting at 21");
    ob.Next = 21;
```

```
    for(int i=0; i < 5; i++)
      Console.WriteLine("Next value is " + ob.Next);
  }
}
```

The output from this program is shown here:

```
Next value is 2
Next value is 4
Next value is 6
Next value is 8
Next value is 10

Starting at 21
Next value is 23
Next value is 25
Next value is 27
Next value is 29
Next value is 31
```

Interface Indexers

An interface can specify an indexer. A one-dimensional indexer declared in an interface has this general form:

> // interface indexer
> *element-type* this[int *index*] {
>   get;
>   set;
> }

As before, only **get** or **set** will be present for read-only or write-only indexers, respectively. Also, no access modifiers are allowed on the accessors when an indexer is declared in an **interface**.

Here is another version of **ISeries** that adds a read-only indexer that returns the *i*-th element in the series.

```
// Add an indexer in an interface.

using System;

public interface ISeries {
  // An interface property.
  int Next {
    get; // return the next number in series
    set; // set next number
  }

  // An interface indexer.
  int this[int index] {
    get; // return the specified number in series
  }
}
```

```
// Implement ISeries.
class ByTwos : ISeries {
  int val;

  public ByTwos() {
    val = 0;
  }

  // Get or set value using a property.
  public int Next {
    get {
      val += 2;
      return val;
    }
    set {
      val = value;
    }
  }

  // Get a value using an index.
  public int this[int index] {
    get {
      val = 0;
      for(int i=0; i < index; i++)
        val += 2;
      return val;
    }
  }
}

// Demonstrate an interface indexer.
class SeriesDemo4 {
  static void Main() {
    ByTwos ob = new ByTwos();

    // Access series through a property.
    for(int i=0; i < 5; i++)
      Console.WriteLine("Next value is " + ob.Next);

    Console.WriteLine("\nStarting at 21");
    ob.Next = 21;
    for(int i=0; i < 5; i++)
      Console.WriteLine("Next value is " +
                          ob.Next);

    Console.WriteLine("\nResetting to 0");
    ob.Next = 0;

    // Access series through an indexer.
    for(int i=0; i < 5; i++)
      Console.WriteLine("Next value is " + ob[i]);
  }
}
```

The output from this program is shown here:

```
Next value is 2
Next value is 4
Next value is 6
Next value is 8
Next value is 10

Starting at 21
Next value is 23
Next value is 25
Next value is 27
Next value is 29
Next value is 31

Resetting to 0
Next value is 0
Next value is 2
Next value is 4
Next value is 6
Next value is 8
```

Interfaces Can Be Inherited

One interface can inherit another. The syntax is the same as for inheriting classes. When a class implements an interface that inherits another interface, it must provide implementations for all the members defined within the interface inheritance chain. Here is an example:

```csharp
// One interface can inherit another.

using System;

public interface IA {
  void Meth1();
  void Meth2();
}

// B now includes Meth1() and Meth2() -- it adds Meth3().
public interface IB : IA {
  void Meth3();
}

// This class must implement all of IA and IB.
class MyClass : IB {
  public void Meth1() {
    Console.WriteLine("Implement Meth1().");
  }

  public void Meth2() {
    Console.WriteLine("Implement Meth2().");
  }

  public void Meth3() {
    Console.WriteLine("Implement Meth3().");
```

```
    }
  }

class IFExtend {
  static void Main() {
    MyClass ob = new MyClass();

    ob.Meth1();
    ob.Meth2();
    ob.Meth3();
  }
}
```

As an experiment, you might try removing the implementation for **Meth1( )** in **MyClass**. This will cause a compile-time error. As stated earlier, any class that implements an interface must implement all methods defined by that interface, including any that are inherited from other interfaces.

Name Hiding with Interface Inheritance

When one interface inherits another, it is possible to declare a member in the derived interface that hides one defined by the base interface. This happens when a member in a derived interface has the same declaration as one in the base interface. In this case, the base interface name is hidden. This will cause a warning message unless you specify the derived interface member with **new**.

Explicit Implementations

When implementing a member of an interface, it is possible to *fully qualify* its name with its interface name. Doing this creates an *explicit interface member implementation*, or *explicit implementation*, for short. For example, given

```
interface IMyIF {
  int MyMeth(int x);
}
```

then it is legal to implement **IMyIF** as shown here:

```
class MyClass : IMyIF {
  int IMyIF.MyMeth(int x) {
    return x / 3;
  }
}
```

As you can see, when the **MyMeth( )** member of **IMyIF** is implemented, its complete name, including its interface name, is specified.

There are two reasons that you might need to create an explicit implementation of an interface method. First, when you implement an interface method using its fully qualified name, you are providing an implementation that *cannot* be accessed through an object of the class. Instead, it must be accessed via an interface reference. Thus, an explicit implementation gives you a way to implement an interface method so that it is not a public member of the

class that provides the implementation. Second, it is possible for a class to implement two interfaces, both of which declare methods by the same name and type signature. Qualifying the names with their interfaces removes the ambiguity from this situation. Let's look at an example of each.

The following program contains an interface called **IEven**, which defines two methods, **IsEven( )** and **IsOdd( )**, which determine if a number is even or odd. **MyClass** then implements **IEven**. When it does so, it implements **IsOdd( )** explicitly.

```
// Explicitly implement an interface member.

using System;

interface IEven {
  bool IsOdd(int x);
  bool IsEven(int x);
}

class MyClass : IEven {

  // Explicit implementation. Notice that this member is private
  // by default.
  bool IEven.IsOdd(int x) {
    if((x%2) != 0) return true;
    else return false;
  }

  // Normal implementation.
  public bool IsEven(int x) {
    IEven o = this; // Interface reference to the invoking object.

    return !o.IsOdd(x);
  }
}

class Demo {
  static void Main() {
    MyClass ob = new MyClass();
    bool result;

    result = ob.IsEven(4);
    if(result) Console.WriteLine("4 is even.");

    // result = ob.IsOdd(4); // Error, IsOdd not exposed.

    // But, this is OK. It creates an IEven reference to a MyClass object
    // and then calls IsOdd() through that reference.
    IEven iRef = (IEven) ob;
    result = iRef.IsOdd(3);
    if(result) Console.WriteLine("3 is odd.");

  }
}
```

Since **IsOdd()** is implemented explicitly, it is not exposed as a public member of **MyClass**. Instead, **IsOdd()** can be accessed only through an interface reference. This is why it is invoked through **o** (which is a reference variable of type **IEven**) in the implementation for **IsEven()**.

Here is an example in which two interfaces are implemented and both interfaces declare a method called **Meth( )**. Explicit implementation is used to eliminate the ambiguity inherent in this situation.

```
// Use explicit implementation to remove ambiguity.

using System;

interface IMyIF_A {
  int Meth(int x);
}

interface IMyIF_B {
  int Meth(int x);
}

// MyClass implements both interfaces.
class MyClass : IMyIF_A, IMyIF_B {

  // Explicitly implement the two Meth()s.
  int IMyIF_A.Meth(int x) {
    return x + x;
  }
  int IMyIF_B.Meth(int x) {
    return x * x;
  }

  // Call Meth() through an interface reference.
  public int MethA(int x){
    IMyIF_A a_ob;
    a_ob = this;
    return a_ob.Meth(x); // calls IMyIF_A
  }

  public int MethB(int x){
    IMyIF_B b_ob;
    b_ob = this;
    return b_ob.Meth(x); // calls IMyIF_B
  }
}

class FQIFNames {
  static void Main() {
    MyClass ob = new MyClass();

    Console.Write("Calling IMyIF_A.Meth(): ");
    Console.WriteLine(ob.MethA(3));
```

```
      Console.Write("Calling IMyIF_B.Meth(): ");
      Console.WriteLine(ob.MethB(3));
   }
}
```

The output from this program is shown here:

```
Calling IMyIF_A.Meth(): 6
Calling IMyIF_B.Meth(): 9
```

Looking at the program, first notice that **Meth( )** has the same signature in both **IMyIF_A** and **IMyIF_B**. Thus, when **MyClass** implements both of these interfaces, it explicitly implements each one separately, fully qualifying its name in the process. Since the only way that an explicitly implemented method can be called is on an interface reference, **MyClass** creates two such references, one for **IMyIF_A** and one for **IMyIF_B**. It then calls two of its own methods, which call the interface methods, thereby removing the ambiguity.

Choosing Between an Interface and an Abstract Class

One of the more challenging parts of C# programming is knowing when to create an interface and when to use an abstract class in cases in which you want to describe functionality but not implementation. The general rule is this: When you can fully describe the concept in terms of "what it does" without needing to specify any "how it does it," then you should use an interface. If you need to include some implementation details, then you will need to represent your concept in an abstract class.

The .NET Standard Interfaces

The .NET Framework defines a large number of interfaces that a C# program can use. For example, **System.IComparable** defines the **CompareTo( )** method, which allows objects to be compared when an ordering relationship is required. Interfaces also form an important part of the Collections classes, which provide various types of storage (such as stacks and queues) for groups of objects. For example, **System.Collections.ICollection** defines the functionality of a collection. **System.Collections.IEnumerator** offers a way to sequence through the elements in a collection. These and many other interfaces are described in Part II.

Structures

As you know, classes are reference types. This means that class objects are accessed through a reference. This differs from the value types, which are accessed directly. However, sometimes it would be useful to be able to access an object directly, in the way that value types are. One reason for this is efficiency. Accessing class objects through a reference adds overhead onto every access. It also consumes space. For very small objects, this extra space might be significant. To address these concerns, C# offers the structure. A *structure* is similar to a class, but is a value type, rather than a reference type.

Structures are declared using the keyword **struct** and are syntactically similar to classes. Here is the general form of a **struct**:

```
struct name : interfaces {
  // member declarations
}
```

The name of the structure is specified by *name*.

Structures cannot inherit other structures or classes or be used as a base for other structures or classes. (Of course, like all C# types, structures do inherit **object**.) However, a structure can implement one or more interfaces. These are specified after the structure name using a comma-separated list. Like classes, structure members include methods, fields, indexers, properties, operator methods, and events. Structures can also define constructors, but not destructors. However, you cannot define a default (parameterless) constructor for a structure. The reason for this is that a default constructor is automatically defined for all structures, and this default constructor can't be changed. The default constructor initializes the fields of a structure to their default value. Since structures do not support inheritance, structure members cannot be specified as **abstract**, **virtual**, or **protected**.

A structure object can be created using **new** in the same way as a class object, but it is not required. When **new** is used, the specified constructor is called. When **new** is not used, the object is still created, but it is not initialized. Thus, you will need to perform any initialization manually.

Here is an example that uses a structure to hold information about a book:

```
// Demonstrate a structure.

using System;

// Define a structure.
struct Book {
  public string Author;
  public string Title;
  public int Copyright;

  public Book(string a, string t, int c) {
    Author = a;
    Title = t;
    Copyright = c;
  }
}

// Demonstrate Book structure.
class StructDemo {
  static void Main() {
    Book book1 = new Book("Herb Schildt",
                    "C# 3.0: The Complete Reference",
                    2009); // explicit constructor

    Book book2 = new Book(); // default constructor
    Book book3; // no constructor

    Console.WriteLine(book1.Title + " by " + book1.Author +
                    ", (c) " + book1.Copyright);
    Console.WriteLine();
```

```
    if(book2.Title == null)
      Console.WriteLine("book2.Title is null.");

    // Now, give book2 some info.
    book2.Title = "Brave New World";
    book2.Author = "Aldous Huxley";
    book2.Copyright = 1932;
    Console.Write("book2 now contains: ");
    Console.WriteLine(book2.Title + " by " + book2.Author +
                      ", (c) " + book2.Copyright);

    Console.WriteLine();

// Console.WriteLine(book3.Title); // error, must initialize first
    book3.Title = "Red Storm Rising";

    Console.WriteLine(book3.Title); // now OK
  }
}
```

The output from this program is shown here:

```
C# 3.0: The Complete Reference by Herb Schildt, (c) 2009

book2.Title is null.
book2 now contains: Brave New World by Aldous Huxley, (c) 1932

Red Storm Rising
```

As the program shows, a structure can be initialized either by using **new** to invoke a constructor or by simply declaring an object. If **new** is used, then the fields of the structure will be initialized either by the default constructor, which initializes all fields to their default value, or by a user-defined constructor. If **new** is not used, as is the case with **book3**, then the object is not initialized, and its fields must be set prior to using the object.

When you assign one structure to another, a copy of the object is made. This is an important way in which **struct** differs from **class**. As explained earlier in this book, when you assign one class reference to another, you are simply making the reference on the left side of the assignment refer to the same object as that referred to by the reference on the right. When you assign one **struct** variable to another, you are making a *copy* of the object on the right. For example, consider the following program:

```
// Copy a struct.

using System;

// Define a structure.
struct MyStruct {
  public int x;
}

// Demonstrate structure assignment.
class StructAssignment {
```

```
static void Main() {
  MyStruct a;
  MyStruct b;

  a.x = 10;
  b.x = 20;

  Console.WriteLine("a.x {0}, b.x {1}", a.x, b.x);

  a = b;
  b.x = 30;

  Console.WriteLine("a.x {0}, b.x {1}", a.x, b.x);
  }
}
```

The output is shown here:

```
a.x 10, b.x 20
a.x 20, b.x 30
```

As the output shows, after the assignment

```
a = b;
```

the structure variables **a** and **b** are still separate and distinct. That is, **a** does not refer to or relate to **b** in any way other than containing a copy of **b**'s value. This would not be the case if **a** and **b** were class references. For example, here is the **class** version of the preceding program:

```
// Use a class.

using System;

// Now a class.
class MyClass {
  public int x;
}

// Now show a class object assignment.
class ClassAssignment {
  static void Main() {
    MyClass a = new MyClass();
    MyClass b = new MyClass();

    a.x = 10;
    b.x = 20;

    Console.WriteLine("a.x {0}, b.x {1}", a.x, b.x);

    a = b;
    b.x = 30;
```

```
   Console.WriteLine("a.x {0}, b.x {1}", a.x, b.x);
 }
}
```

The output from this version is shown here:

```
a.x 10, b.x 20
a.x 30, b.x 30
```

As you can see, after the assignment of **b** to **a**, both variables refer to the same object—the one originally referred to by **b**.

Why Structures?

At this point, you might be wondering why C# includes the **struct** since it seems to be a less-capable version of a **class**. The answer lies in efficiency and performance. Because structures are value types, they are operated on directly rather than through a reference. Thus, a **struct** does not require a separate reference variable. This means that less memory is used in some cases. Furthermore, because a **struct** is accessed directly, it does not suffer from the performance loss that is inherent in accessing a class object. Because classes are reference types, all access to class objects is through a reference. This indirection adds overhead to every access. Structures do not incur this overhead. In general, if you need to simply store a group of related data, but don't need inheritance and don't need to operate on that data through a reference, then a **struct** can be a more efficient choice.

Here is another example that shows how a structure might be used in practice. It simulates an e-commerce transaction record. Each transaction includes a packet header that contains the packet number and the length of the packet. This is followed by the account number and the amount of the transaction. Because the packet header is a self-contained unit of information, it is organized as a structure. This structure can then be used to create a transaction record, or any other type of information packet.

```
// Structures are good when grouping small amounts of data.

using System;

// Define a packet structure.
struct PacketHeader {
  public uint PackNum; // packet number
  public ushort PackLen; // length of packet
}

// Use PacketHeader to create an e-commerce transaction record.
class Transaction {
  static uint transacNum = 0;

  PacketHeader ph;  // incorporate PacketHeader into Transaction
  string accountNum;
  double amount;
```

```
  public Transaction(string acc, double val) {
   // create packet header
    ph.PackNum = transacNum++;
    ph.PackLen = 512;   // arbitrary length

    accountNum = acc;
    amount = val;
  }

  // Simulate a transaction.
  public void sendTransaction() {
    Console.WriteLine("Packet #: " + ph.PackNum +
                  ", Length: " + ph.PackLen +
                  ",\n     Account #: " + accountNum +
                  ", Amount: {0:C}\n", amount);
  }
}

// Demonstrate Packet.
class PacketDemo {
  static void Main() {
    Transaction t = new Transaction("31243", -100.12);
    Transaction t2 = new Transaction("AB4655", 345.25);
    Transaction t3 = new Transaction("8475-09", 9800.00);

    t.sendTransaction();
    t2.sendTransaction();
    t3.sendTransaction();
  }
}
```

The output from the program is shown here:

```
Packet #: 0, Length: 512,
    Account #: 31243, Amount: ($100.12)

Packet #: 1, Length: 512,
    Account #: AB4655, Amount: $345.25

Packet #: 2, Length: 512,
    Account #: 8475-09, Amount: $9,800.00
```

PacketHeader is a good choice for a **struct** because it contains only a small amount of data and does not use inheritance or even contain methods. As a structure, **PacketHeader** does not incur the additional overhead of a reference, as a class would. Thus, any type of transaction record can use **PacketHeader** without affecting its efficiency.

As a point of interest, C++ also has structures and uses the **struct** keyword. However, C# and C++ structures are not the same. In C++, **struct** defines a class type. Thus, in C++, **struct** and **class** are nearly equivalent. (The difference has to do with the default access of their members, which is private for **class** and public for **struct**.) In C#, a **struct** defines a value type, and a **class** defines a reference type.

Enumerations

An *enumeration* is a set of named integer constants. The keyword **enum** declares an enumerated type. The general form for an enumeration is

enum *name* { *enumeration list* };

Here, the type name of the enumeration is specified by *name*. The *enumeration list* is a comma-separated list of identifiers.

Here is an example. It defines an enumeration called **Apple** that enumerates various types of apples:

```
enum Apple { Jonathan, GoldenDel, RedDel, Winesap,
            Cortland, McIntosh };
```

A key point to understand about an enumeration is that each of the symbols stands for an integer value. However, no implicit conversions are defined between an **enum** type and the built-in integer types, so an explicit cast must be used. Also, a cast is required when converting between two enumeration types. Since enumerations represent integer values, you can use an enumeration to control a **switch** statement or as the control variable in a **for** loop, for example.

Each enumeration symbol is given a value one greater than the symbol that precedes it. By default, the value of the first enumeration symbol is 0. Therefore, in the **Apple** enumeration, **Jonathan** is 0, **GoldenDel** is 1, **RedDel** is 2, and so on.

The members of an enumeration are accessed through their type name via the dot operator. For example

```
Console.WriteLine(Apple.RedDel + " has the value " +
                  (int)Apple.RedDel);
```

displays

```
RedDel has the value 2
```

As the output shows, when an enumerated value is displayed, its name is used. To obtain its integer value, a cast to **int** must be employed.

Here is a program that illustrates the **Apple** enumeration:

```
// Demonstrate an enumeration.

using System;

class EnumDemo {
  enum Apple { Jonathan, GoldenDel, RedDel, Winesap,
               Cortland, McIntosh };

  static void Main() {
    string[] color = {
      "Red",
      "Yellow",
```

```
      "Red",
      "Red",
      "Red",
      "Reddish Green"
    };

    Apple i; // declare an enum variable

    // Use i to cycle through the enum.
    for(i = Apple.Jonathan; i <= Apple.McIntosh; i++)
      Console.WriteLine(i + " has value of " + (int)i);

    Console.WriteLine();

    // Use an enumeration to index an array.
    for(i = Apple.Jonathan; i <= Apple.McIntosh; i++)
      Console.WriteLine("Color of " + i + " is " +
                        color[(int)i]);
  }
}
```

The output from the program is shown here:

```
Jonathan has value of 0
GoldenDel has value of 1
RedDel has value of 2
Winesap has value of 3
Cortland has value of 4
McIntosh has value of 5

Color of Jonathan is Red
Color of GoldenDel is Yellow
Color of RedDel is Red
Color of Winesap is Red
Color of Cortland is Red
Color of McIntosh is Reddish Green
```

Notice how the **for** loops are controlled by a variable of type **Apple**. Because the enumerated values in **Apple** start at zero, these values can be used to index **color** to obtain the color of the apple. Notice that a cast is required when the enumeration value is used to index the **color** array. As mentioned, there are no implicit conversions defined between integers and enumeration types. An explicit cast is required.

Initialize an Enumeration

You can specify the value of one or more of the symbols by using an initializer. Do this by following the symbol with an equal sign and an integer value. Symbols that appear after initializers are assigned values greater than the previous initialization value. For example, the following code assigns the value of 10 to **RedDel**:

```
enum Apple { Jonathan, GoldenDel, RedDel = 10, Winesap,
             Cortland, McIntosh };
```

Now the values of these symbols are

Jonathan	0
GoldenDel	1
RedDel	10
Winesap	11
Cortland	12
McIntosh	13

Specify the Underlying Type of an Enumeration

By default, enumerations are based on type **int**, but you can create an enumeration of any integral type, except for type **char**. To specify a type other than **int**, put the desired type after the enumeration name, separated by a colon. For example, this statement makes **Apple** an enumeration based on **byte**:

```
enum Apple : byte { Jonathan, GoldenDel, RedDel, Winesap,
                    Cortland, McIntosh };
```

Now **Apple.Winesap**, for example, is a **byte** quantity.

Use Enumerations

At first glance you might think that enumerations are an interesting but relatively unimportant part of C#, yet this is not the case. Enumerations are very useful when your program requires one or more specialized symbols. For example, imagine that you are writing a program that controls a conveyor belt in a factory. You might create a method called **Conveyor( )** that accepts the following commands as parameters: start, stop, forward, and reverse. Instead of passing **Conveyor( )** integers, such as 1 for start, 2 for stop, and so on, which is error-prone, you can create an enumeration that assigns words to these values. Here is an example of this approach:

```
// Simulate a conveyor belt.

using System;

class ConveyorControl {
  // Enumerate the conveyor commands.
  public enum Action { Start, Stop, Forward, Reverse };

  public void Conveyor(Action com) {
    switch(com) {
      case Action.Start:
        Console.WriteLine("Starting conveyor.");
        break;
      case Action.Stop:
        Console.WriteLine("Stopping conveyor.");
        break;
```

```
      case Action.Forward:
        Console.WriteLine("Moving forward.");
        break;
      case Action.Reverse:
        Console.WriteLine("Moving backward.");
        break;
    }
  }
}

class ConveyorDemo {
  static void Main() {
    ConveyorControl c = new ConveyorControl();

    c.Conveyor(ConveyorControl.Action.Start);
    c.Conveyor(ConveyorControl.Action.Forward);
    c.Conveyor(ConveyorControl.Action.Reverse);
    c.Conveyor(ConveyorControl.Action.Stop);

  }
}
```

The output from the program is shown here:

```
Starting conveyor.
Moving forward.
Moving backward.
Stopping conveyor.
```

Because **Conveyor( )** takes an argument of type **Action**, only the values defined by **Action** can be passed to the method. For example, here an attempt is made to pass the value 22 to **Conveyor( )**:

```
c.Conveyor(22); // Error!
```

This won't compile because there is no predefined conversion from **int** to **Action**. This prevents the passing of invalid commands to **Conveyor( )**. Of course, you could use a cast to force a conversion, but this would require a premeditated act, not an accidental misuse. Also, because commands are specified by name rather than by number, it is less likely that a user of **Conveyor( )** will inadvertently pass the wrong value.

There is one other interesting thing in this example: Notice that an enumeration type is used to control the **switch** statement. As mentioned, because enumerations are integral types, they are perfectly valid for use in a **switch**.

Exception Handling

An *exception* is an error that occurs at runtime. Using C#'s exception handling subsystem, you can, in a structured and controlled manner, handle runtime errors. A principal advantage of exception handling is that it automates much of the error-handling code that previously had to be entered "by hand" into any large program. For example, in a computer language without exception handling, error codes must be returned when a method fails, and these values must be checked manually each time the method is called. This approach is both tedious and error-prone. Exception handling streamlines error-handling by allowing your program to define a block of code, called an *exception handler*, that is executed automatically when an error occurs. It is not necessary to manually check the success or failure of each specific operation or method call. If an error occurs, it will be processed by the exception handler.

Exception handling is also important because C# defines standard exceptions for common program errors, such as divide-by-zero or index-out-of-range. To respond to these errors, your program must watch for and handle these exceptions. In the final analysis, to be a successful C# programmer means that you are fully capable of navigating C#'s exception-handling subsystem.

The System.Exception Class

In C#, exceptions are represented by classes. All exception classes must be derived from the built-in exception class **Exception**, which is part of the **System** namespace. Thus, all exceptions are subclasses of **Exception**.

One very important subclass of **Exception** is **SystemException**. This is the exception class from which all exceptions generated by the C# runtime system (that is, the CLR) are derived. **SystemException** does not add anything to **Exception**. It simply defines the top of the standard exceptions hierarchy.

The .NET Framework defines several built-in exceptions that are derived from **SystemException**. For example, when a division-by-zero is attempted, a **DivideByZeroException** exception is generated. As you will see later in this chapter, you can create your own exception classes by deriving them from **Exception**.

Exception Handling Fundamentals

C# exception handling is managed via four keywords: **try, catch, throw**, and **finally**. They form an interrelated subsystem in which the use of one implies the use of another. Throughout the course of this chapter, each keyword is examined in detail. However, it is useful at the outset to have a general understanding of the role each plays in exception handling. Briefly, here is how they work.

Program statements that you want to monitor for exceptions are contained within a **try** block. If an exception occurs within the **try** block, it is *thrown*. Your code can catch this exception using **catch** and handle it in some rational manner. System-generated exceptions are automatically thrown by the runtime system. To manually throw an exception, use the keyword **throw**. Any code that absolutely must be executed upon exiting from a **try** block is put in a **finally** block.

Using try and catch

At the core of exception handling are **try** and **catch**. These keywords work together, and you can't have a **catch** without a **try**. Here is the general form of the **try/catch** exception-handling blocks:

```
try {
    // block of code to monitor for errors
}
catch (ExcepType1 exOb) {
    // handler for ExcepType1
}
catch (ExcepType2 exOb) {
    // handler for ExcepType2
}
.
.
.
```

Here, *ExcepType* is the type of exception that has occurred. When an exception is thrown, it is caught by its corresponding **catch** clause, which then processes the exception. As the general form shows, more than one **catch** clause can be associated with a **try**. The type of the exception determines which **catch** is executed. That is, if the exception type specified by a **catch** matches that of the exception, then that **catch** is executed (and all others are bypassed). When an exception is caught, the exception variable *exOb* will receive its value.

Actually, specifying *exOb* is optional. If the exception handler does not need access to the exception object (as is often the case), there is no need to specify *exOb*. The exception type alone is sufficient. For this reason, many of the examples in this chapter will not specify *exOb*.

Here is an important point: If no exception is thrown, then a **try** block ends normally, and all of its **catch** clauses are bypassed. Execution resumes with the first statement following the last **catch**. Thus, a **catch** is executed only if an exception is thrown.

A Simple Exception Example

Here is a simple example that illustrates how to watch for and catch an exception. As you know, it is an error to attempt to index an array beyond its boundaries. When this error occurs, the CLR throws an **IndexOutOfRangeException**, which is a standard exception

defined by the .NET Framework. The following program purposely generates such an exception and then catches it:

```
// Demonstrate exception handling.

using System;

class ExcDemo1 {
  static void Main() {
    int[] nums = new int[4];

    try {
      Console.WriteLine("Before exception is generated.");

      // Generate an index out-of-bounds exception.
      for(int i=0; i < 10; i++) {
        nums[i] = i;
        Console.WriteLine("nums[{0}]: {1}", i, nums[i]);
      }

      Console.WriteLine("this won't be displayed");
    }
    catch (IndexOutOfRangeException) {
      // Catch the exception.
      Console.WriteLine("Index out-of-bounds!");
    }
    Console.WriteLine("After catch block.");
  }
}
```

This program displays the following output:

```
Before exception is generated.
nums[0]: 0
nums[1]: 1
nums[2]: 2
nums[3]: 3
Index out-of-bounds!
After catch block.
```

Notice that **nums** is an **int** array of four elements. However, the **for** loop tries to index **nums** from 0 to 9, which causes an **IndexOutOfRangeException** to occur when an index value of 4 is tried.

Although quite short, the preceding program illustrates several key points about exception handling. First, the code that you want to monitor for errors is contained within a **try** block. Second, when an exception occurs (in this case, because of the attempt to index **nums** beyond its bounds inside the **for** loop), the exception is thrown out of the **try** block and caught by the **catch**. At this point, control passes to the **catch** block, and the **try** block is terminated. That is, **catch** is *not* called. Rather, program execution is transferred to it. Thus, the **WriteLine( )** statement following the out-of-bounds index will never execute. After the **catch** block executes, program control continues with the statements following the **catch**. Thus, it is the job of your exception handler to remedy the problem that caused the exception so program execution can continue normally.

Notice that no exception variable is specified in the **catch** clause. Instead, only the type of the exception (**IndexOutOfRangeException** in this case) is required. As mentioned, an exception variable is needed only when access to the exception object is required. In some cases, the value of the exception object can be used by the exception handler to obtain additional information about the error, but in many cases, it is sufficient to simply know that an exception occurred. Thus, it is not unusual for the **catch** variable to be absent in the exception handler, as is the case in the preceding program.

As explained, if no exception is thrown by a **try** block, no **catch** will be executed and program control resumes after the **catch**. To confirm this, in the preceding program, change the **for** loop from

```
for(int i=0; i < 10; i++) {
```

to

```
for(int i=0; i < nums.Length; i++) {
```

Now, the loop does not overrun **nums'** boundary. Thus, no exception is generated, and the **catch** block is not executed.

A Second Exception Example

It is important to understand that all code executed within a **try** block is monitored for exceptions. This includes exceptions that might be generated by a method called from within the **try** block. An exception thrown by a method called from within a **try** block can be caught by that **try** block, assuming, of course, that the method itself did not catch the exception.

For example, consider the following program. **Main()** establishes a **try** block from which the method **GenException()** is called. Inside **GenException()**, an **IndexOutOfRangeException** is generated. This exception is not caught by **GenException()**. However, since **GenException()** was called from within a **try** block in **Main()**, the exception is caught by the **catch** statement associated with that **try**.

```
/* An exception can be generated by one
   method and caught by another. */

using System;

class ExcTest {
  // Generate an exception.
  public static void GenException() {
    int[] nums = new int[4];

    Console.WriteLine("Before exception is generated.");

    // Generate an index out-of-bounds exception.
    for(int i=0; i < 10; i++) {
      nums[i] = i;
      Console.WriteLine("nums[{0}]: {1}", i, nums[i]);
    }
```

```
      Console.WriteLine("this won't be displayed");
    }
  }

class ExcDemo2 {
  static void Main() {

    try {
      ExcTest.GenException();
    }
    catch (IndexOutOfRangeException) {
      // Catch the exception.
      Console.WriteLine("Index out-of-bounds!");
    }
    Console.WriteLine("After catch block.");
  }
}
```

This program produces the following output, which is the same as that produced by the first version of the program shown earlier:

```
Before exception is generated.
nums[0]: 0
nums[1]: 1
nums[2]: 2
nums[3]: 3
Index out-of-bounds!
After catch block.
```

As explained, because **GenException( )** is called from within a **try** block, the exception that it generates (and does not catch) is caught by the **catch** in **Main( )**. Understand, however, that if **GenException( )** had caught the exception, then it never would have been passed back to **Main( )**.

The Consequences of an Uncaught Exception

Catching one of the standard exceptions, as the preceding program does, has a side benefit: It prevents abnormal program termination. When an exception is thrown, it must be caught by some piece of code, somewhere. In general, if your program does not catch an exception, it will be caught by the runtime system. The trouble is that the runtime system will report an error and terminate the program. For instance, in this example, the index out-of-bounds exception is not caught by the program:

```
// Let the C# runtime system handle the error.

using System;

class NotHandled {
  static void Main() {
    int[] nums = new int[4];
```

```
    Console.WriteLine("Before exception is generated.");

    // Generate an index out-of-bounds exception.
    for(int i=0; i < 10; i++) {
      nums[i] = i;
      Console.WriteLine("nums[{0}]: {1}", i, nums[i]);
    }

  }
}
```

When the array index error occurs, execution is halted and the following error message is displayed:

```
Unhandled Exception: System.IndexOutOfRangeException:
        Index was outside the bounds of the array.
   at NotHandled.Main()
```

Although such a message is useful while debugging, you would not want others to see it, to say the least! This is why it is important for your program to handle exceptions itself.

As mentioned earlier, the type of the exception must match the type specified in a **catch**. If it doesn't, the exception won't be caught. For example, the following program tries to catch an array boundary error with a **catch** for a **DivideByZeroException** (another built-in exception). When the array boundary is overrun, an **IndexOutOfRangeException** is generated, but it won't be caught by the **catch**. This results in abnormal program termination.

```
// This won't work!

using System;

class ExcTypeMismatch {
  static void Main() {
    int[] nums = new int[4];

    try {
      Console.WriteLine("Before exception is generated.");

      // Generate an index out-of-bounds exception.
      for(int i=0; i < 10; i++) {
        nums[i] = i;
        Console.WriteLine("nums[{0}]: {1}", i, nums[i]);
      }

      Console.WriteLine("this won't be displayed");
    }

    /* Can't catch an array boundary error with a
       DivideByZeroException. */
    catch (DivideByZeroException) {
      // Catch the exception.
      Console.WriteLine("Index out-of-bounds!");
    }
```

```
      Console.WriteLine("After catch block.");
  }
}
```

The output is shown here:

```
Before exception is generated.
nums[0]: 0
nums[1]: 1
nums[2]: 2
nums[3]: 3

Unhandled Exception: System.IndexOutOfRangeException:
        Index was outside the bounds of the array.
   at ExcTypeMismatch.Main()
```

As the output demonstrates, a **catch** for **DivideByZeroException** won't catch an **IndexOutOfRangeException**.

Exceptions Let You Handle Errors Gracefully

One of the key benefits of exception handling is that it enables your program to respond to an error and then continue running. For example, consider the following example that divides the elements of one array by the elements of another. If a division-by-zero occurs, a **DivideByZeroException** is generated. In the program, this exception is handled by reporting the error and then continuing with execution. Thus, attempting to divide by zero does not cause an abrupt runtime error resulting in the termination of the program. Instead, it is handled gracefully, allowing program execution to continue.

```
// Handle error gracefully and continue.

using System;

class ExcDemo3 {
  static void Main() {
    int[] numer = { 4, 8, 16, 32, 64, 128 };
    int[] denom = { 2, 0, 4, 4, 0, 8 };

    for(int i=0; i < numer.Length; i++) {
      try {
        Console.WriteLine(numer[i] + " / " +
                          denom[i] + " is " +
                          numer[i]/denom[i]);
      }
      catch (DivideByZeroException) {
        // Catch the exception.
        Console.WriteLine("Can't divide by Zero!");
      }
    }
  }
}
```

The output from the program is shown here:

```
4 / 2 is 2
Can't divide by Zero!
16 / 4 is 4
32 / 4 is 8
Can't divide by Zero!
128 / 8 is 16
```

This example makes another important point: Once an exception has been handled, it is removed from the system. Therefore, in the program, each pass through the loop enters the **try** block anew—any prior exceptions have been handled. This enables your program to handle repeated errors.

Using Multiple catch Clauses

You can associate more than one **catch** clause with a **try**. In fact, it is common to do so. However, each **catch** must catch a different type of exception. For example, the program shown here catches both array boundary and divide-by-zero errors:

```csharp
// Use multiple catch clauses.

using System;

class ExcDemo4 {
  static void Main() {
    // Here, numer is longer than denom.
    int[] numer = { 4, 8, 16, 32, 64, 128, 256, 512 };
    int[] denom = { 2, 0, 4, 4, 0, 8 };

    for(int i=0; i < numer.Length; i++) {
      try {
        Console.WriteLine(numer[i] + " / " +
                          denom[i] + " is " +
                          numer[i]/denom[i]);
      }
      catch (DivideByZeroException) {
        Console.WriteLine("Can't divide by Zero!");
      }
      catch (IndexOutOfRangeException) {
        Console.WriteLine("No matching element found.");
      }
    }
  }
}
```

This program produces the following output:

```
4 / 2 is 2
Can't divide by Zero!
16 / 4 is 4
32 / 4 is 8
Can't divide by Zero!
128 / 8 is 16
```

```
No matching element found.
No matching element found.
```

As the output confirms, each **catch** clause responds only to its own type of exception.

In general, **catch** clauses are checked in the order in which they occur in a program. Only the first matching clause is executed. All other **catch** blocks are ignored.

Catching All Exceptions

Occasionally, you might want to catch all exceptions, no matter the type. To do this, use a **catch** clause that specifies no exception type or variable. It has this general form:

```
catch {
   // handle exceptions
}
```

This creates a "catch all" handler that ensures that all exceptions are caught by your program.

Here is an example of a "catch all" exception handler. Notice that it catches both the **IndexOutOfRangeException** and the **DivideByZeroException** generated by the program:

```
// Use the "catch all" catch.

using System;

class ExcDemo5 {
  static void Main() {
    // Here, numer is longer than denom.
    int[] numer = { 4, 8, 16, 32, 64, 128, 256, 512 };
    int[] denom = { 2, 0, 4, 4, 0, 8 };

    for(int i=0; i < numer.Length; i++) {
      try {
        Console.WriteLine(numer[i] + " / " +
                          denom[i] + " is " +
                          numer[i]/denom[i]);
      }
      catch { // A "catch-all" catch.
        Console.WriteLine("Some exception occurred.");
      }
    }
  }
}
```

The output is shown here:

```
4 / 2 is 2
Some exception occurred.
16 / 4 is 4
32 / 4 is 8
Some exception occurred.
128 / 8 is 16
Some exception occurred.
Some exception occurred.
```

There is one point to remember about using a catch-all **catch**: It must be the last **catch** clause in the **catch** sequence.

NOTE *In the vast majority of cases you should not use the "catch all" handler as a means of dealing with exceptions. It is normally better to deal individually with the exceptions that your code can generate. The inappropriate use of the "catch all" handler can lead to situations in which errors that would otherwise be caught during testing are masked. It is also difficult to correctly handle all types of exceptions with a single hander. That said, a "catch all" handler might be appropriate in certain specialized circumstances, such as in a runtime code analysis tool.*

Nesting try Blocks

One **try** block can be nested within another. An exception generated within the inner **try** block that is not caught by a **catch** associated with that **try** is propagated to the outer **try** block. For example, here the **IndexOutOfRangeException** is not caught by the inner **try** block, but by the outer **try**:

```
// Use a nested try block.

using System;

class NestTrys {
  static void Main() {
    // Here, numer is longer than denom.
    int[] numer = { 4, 8, 16, 32, 64, 128, 256, 512 };
    int[] denom = { 2, 0, 4, 4, 0, 8 };

    try { // outer try
      for(int i=0; i < numer.Length; i++) {
        try { // nested try
          Console.WriteLine(numer[i] + " / " +
                            denom[i] + " is " +
                            numer[i]/denom[i]);
        }
        catch (DivideByZeroException) {
          Console.WriteLine("Can't divide by Zero!");
        }
      }
    }
    catch (IndexOutOfRangeException) {
      Console.WriteLine("No matching element found.");
      Console.WriteLine("Fatal error -- program terminated.");
    }
  }
}
```

The output from the program is shown here:

```
4 / 2 is 2
Can't divide by Zero!
16 / 4 is 4
```

```
32 / 4 is 8
Can't divide by Zero!
128 / 8 is 16
No matching element found.
Fatal error -- program terminated.
```

In this example, an exception that can be handled by the inner **try**—in this case a divide-by-zero error—allows the program to continue. However, an array boundary error is caught by the outer **try**, which causes the program to terminate.

Although certainly not the only reason for nested **try** statements, the preceding program makes an important point that can be generalized. Often, nested **try** blocks are used to allow different categories of errors to be handled in different ways. Some types of errors are catastrophic and cannot be fixed. Some are minor and can be handled immediately. Many programmers use an outer **try** block to catch the most severe errors, allowing inner **try** blocks to handle less serious ones. You can also use an outer **try** block as a "catch all" block for those errors that are not handled by the inner block.

Throwing an Exception

The preceding examples have been catching exceptions generated automatically by the runtime system. However, it is possible to throw an exception manually by using the **throw** statement. Its general form is shown here:

throw *exceptOb*;

The *exceptOb* must be an object of an exception class derived from **Exception**.

Here is an example that illustrates the **throw** statement by manually throwing a **DivideByZeroException**:

```
// Manually throw an exception.

using System;

class ThrowDemo {
  static void Main() {
    try {
      Console.WriteLine("Before throw.");
      throw new DivideByZeroException();
    }
    catch (DivideByZeroException) {
      Console.WriteLine("Exception caught.");
    }
    Console.WriteLine("After try/catch statement.");
  }
}
```

The output from the program is shown here:

```
Before throw.
Exception caught.
After try/catch statement.
```

Notice how the **DivideByZeroException** was created using **new** in the **throw** statement. Remember, **throw** throws an object. Thus, you must create an object for it to throw. That is, you can't just throw a type. In this case, the default constructor is used to create a **DivideByZeroException** object, but other constructors are available for exceptions.

Most often, exceptions that you throw will be instances of exception classes that you created. As you will see later in this chapter, creating your own exception classes allows you to handle errors in your code as part of your program's overall exception handling strategy.

Rethrowing an Exception

An exception caught by one **catch** can be rethrown so that it can be caught by an outer **catch**. The most likely reason for rethrowing an exception is to allow multiple handlers access to the exception. For example, perhaps one exception handler manages one aspect of an exception, and a second handler copes with another aspect. To rethrow an exception, you simply specify **throw**, without specifying an expression. That is, you use this form of **throw**:

throw ;

Remember, when you rethrow an exception, it will not be recaught by the same **catch** clause. Instead, it will propagate to an outer **catch**.

The following program illustrates rethrowing an exception. In this case, it rethrows an **IndexOutOfRangeException**.

```
// Rethrow an exception.

using System;

class Rethrow {
  public static void GenException() {
    // Here, numer is longer than denom.
    int[] numer = { 4, 8, 16, 32, 64, 128, 256, 512 };
    int[] denom = { 2, 0, 4, 4, 0, 8 };

    for(int i=0; i<numer.Length; i++) {
      try {
        Console.WriteLine(numer[i] + " / " +
                          denom[i] + " is " +
                          numer[i]/denom[i]);
      }
      catch (DivideByZeroException) {
        Console.WriteLine("Can't divide by Zero!");
      }
      catch (IndexOutOfRangeException) {
        Console.WriteLine("No matching element found.");
        throw; // rethrow the exception
      }
    }
  }
}

class RethrowDemo {
  static void Main() {
    try {
```

```
        Rethrow.GenException();
      }
    catch(IndexOutOfRangeException) {
      // recatch exception
      Console.WriteLine("Fatal error -- " + "program terminated.");
      }
    }
  }
}
```

In this program, divide-by-zero errors are handled locally, by **GenException( )**, but an array boundary error is rethrown. In this case, the **IndexOutOfRangeException** is handled by **Main( )**.

Using finally

Sometimes you will want to define a block of code that will execute when a **try/catch** block is left. For example, an exception might cause an error that terminates the current method, causing its premature return. However, that method may have opened a file or a network connection that needs to be closed. Such types of circumstances are common in programming, and C# provides a convenient way to handle them: **finally**.

To specify a block of code to execute when a **try/catch** block is exited, include a **finally** block at the end of a **try/catch** sequence. The general form of a **try/catch** that includes **finally** is shown here:

```
try {
   // block of code to monitor for errors
}
catch (ExcepType1 exOb) {
   // handler for ExcepType1
}
catch (ExcepType2 exOb) {
   // handler for ExcepType2
}
  .
  .
  .
finally {
   // finally code
}
```

The **finally** block will be executed whenever execution leaves a **try/catch** block, no matter what conditions cause it. That is, whether the **try** block ends normally, or because of an exception, the last code executed is that defined by **finally**. The **finally** block is also executed if any code within the **try** block or any of its **catch** blocks returns from the method.

Here is an example of **finally**:

```
// Use finally.

using System;

class UseFinally {
  public static void GenException(int what) {
```

```
      int t;
      int[] nums = new int[2];

      Console.WriteLine("Receiving " + what);
      try {
        switch(what) {
          case 0:
            t = 10 / what; // generate div-by-zero error
            break;
          case 1:
            nums[4] = 4; // generate array index error
            break;
          case 2:
            return; // return from try block
        }
      }
      catch (DivideByZeroException) {
        Console.WriteLine("Can't divide by Zero!");
        return; // return from catch
      }
      catch (IndexOutOfRangeException) {
        Console.WriteLine("No matching element found.");
      }
      finally {
        Console.WriteLine("Leaving try.");
      }
    }
}

class FinallyDemo {
  static void Main() {

    for(int i=0; i < 3; i++) {
      UseFinally.GenException(i);
      Console.WriteLine();
    }
  }
}
```

Here is the output produced by the program:

```
Receiving 0
Can't divide by Zero!
Leaving try.

Receiving 1
No matching element found.
Leaving try.

Receiving 2
Leaving try.
```

As the output shows, no matter how the **try** block is exited, the **finally** block executed.

One other point: Syntactically, when a **finally** block follows a **try** block, no **catch** clauses are technically required. Thus, you can have a **try** followed by a **finally** with no **catch** clauses. In this case, the **finally** block is executed when the **try** exits, but no exceptions are handled.

A Closer Look at the Exception Class

Up to this point, we have been catching exceptions, but we haven't been doing anything with the exception object itself. As explained earlier, a **catch** clause allows you to specify an exception type *and* a variable. The variable receives a reference to the exception object. Since all exceptions are derived from **Exception**, all exceptions support the members defined by **Exception**. Here we will examine several of its most useful members and constructors, and put the exception variable to use.

Exception defines several properties. Three of the most interesting are **Message**, **StackTrace**, and **TargetSite**. All are read-only. **Message** contains a string that describes the nature of the error. **StackTrace** contains a string that contains the stack of calls that lead to the exception. **TargetSite** obtains an object that specifies the method that generated the exception.

Exception also defines several methods. One that you will often use is **ToString( )**, which returns a string that describes the exception. **ToString( )** is automatically called when an exception is displayed via **WriteLine( )**, for example.

The following program demonstrates these properties and this method:

```
// Using Exception members.

using System;

class ExcTest {
  public static void GenException() {
    int[] nums = new int[4];

    Console.WriteLine("Before exception is generated.");

    // Generate an index out-of-bounds exception.
      for(int i=0; i < 10; i++) {
        nums[i] = i;
        Console.WriteLine("nums[{0}]: {1}", i, nums[i]);
      }

    Console.WriteLine("this won't be displayed");
  }
}

class UseExcept {
  static void Main() {

    try {
      ExcTest.GenException();
    }
    catch (IndexOutOfRangeException exc) {
```

```
        Console.WriteLine("Standard message is: ");
        Console.WriteLine(exc); // calls ToString()
        Console.WriteLine("Stack trace: " + exc.StackTrace);
        Console.WriteLine("Message: " + exc.Message);
        Console.WriteLine("TargetSite: " + exc.TargetSite);
    }
    Console.WriteLine("After catch block.");
  }
}
```

The output from this program is shown here:

```
Before exception is generated.
nums[0]: 0
nums[1]: 1
nums[2]: 2
nums[3]: 3
Standard message is:
System.IndexOutOfRangeException: Index was outside the bounds of the array.
    at ExcTest.GenException()
    at UseExcept.Main()
Stack trace:     at ExcTest.GenException()
    at UseExcept.Main()
Message: Index was outside the bounds of the array.
TargetSite: Void GenException()
After catch block.
```

Exception defines the following four constructors:

public Exception( )

public Exception(string *str*)

public Exception(string *str*, Exception *inner*)

protected Exception(System.Runtime.Serialization.SerializationInfo *si*,
                System.Runtime.Serialization.StreamingContext *sc*)

The first is the default constructor. The second specifies the string associated with the
Message property associated with the exception. The third specifies what is called an *inner
exception*. It is used when one exception gives rise to another. In this case, *inner* specifies the
first exception, which will be null if no inner exception exists. (The inner exception, if it
exists, can be obtained from the **InnerException** property defined by **Exception**.) The last
constructor handles exceptions that occur remotely and require deserialization.

One other point: In the fourth **Exception** constructor shown above, notice that the types
SerializationInfo and **StreamingContext** are contained in the **System.Runtime.Serialization**
namespace.

Commonly Used Exceptions

The **System** namespace defines several standard, built-in exceptions. All are derived from
SystemException since they are generated by the CLR when runtime errors occur. Several
of the more commonly used standard exceptions are shown in Table 13-1.

Exception	Meaning
ArrayTypeMismatchException	Type of value being stored is incompatible with the type of the array.
DivideByZeroException	Division by zero attempted.
IndexOutOfRangeException	Array index is out of bounds.
InvalidCastException	A runtime cast is invalid.
OutOfMemoryException	Insufficient free memory exists to continue program execution. For example, this exception will be thrown if there is not sufficient free memory to create an object via **new**.
OverflowException	An arithmetic overflow occurred.
NullReferenceException	An attempt was made to operate on a null reference—that is, a reference that does not refer to an object.
StackOverflowException	The stack was overrun.

TABLE 13-1   Commonly Used Exceptions Defined Within the **System** Namespace

Most of the exceptions in Table 13-1 are self-explanatory, with the possible exception of **NullReferenceException**. This exception is thrown when there is an attempt to use a null reference as if it referred to an object—for example, if you attempt to call a method on a null reference. A *null reference* is a reference that does not point to any object. One way to create a null reference is to explicitly assign it the value null by using the keyword **null**. Null references can also occur in other ways that are less obvious. Here is a program that demonstrates the **NullReferenceException**:

```
// Use the NullReferenceException.

using System;

class X {
  int x;
  public X(int a) {
    x = a;
  }

  public int Add(X o) {
    return x + o.x;
  }
}

// Demonstrate NullReferenceException.
class NREDemo {
  static void Main() {
    X p = new X(10);
    X q = null; // q is explicitly assigned null
    int val;
```

```
try {
    val = p.Add(q); // this will lead to an exception
} catch (NullReferenceException) {
    Console.WriteLine("NullReferenceException!");
    Console.WriteLine("fixing...\n");

    // Now, fix it.
    q = new X(9);
    val = p.Add(q);
}

    Console.WriteLine("val is {0}", val);
    }
}
```

The output from the program is shown here:

```
NullReferenceException!
fixing...

val is 19
```

The program creates a class called **X** that defines a member called **x** and the **Add( )** method, which adds the invoking object's **x** to the **x** in the object passed as a parameter. In **Main( )**, two **X** objects are created. The first, **p**, is initialized. The second, **q**, is not. Instead, it is explicitly assigned **null**. Then **p.Add( )** is called with **q** as an argument. Because **q** does not refer to any object, a **NullReferenceException** is generated when the attempt is made to obtain the value of **q.x**.

An interesting exception is **StackOverflowException**, which is thrown when the system stack is overrun. One situation in which this can happen is when a recursive method runs wild. Because the stack is exhausted, a **StackOverflowException** can't be caught by your program. Instead, a stack overflow results in the abnormal termination of your program.

Deriving Exception Classes

Although C#'s built-in exceptions handle most common errors, C#'s exception handling mechanism is not limited to these errors. In fact, part of the power of C#'s approach to exceptions is its ability to handle exceptions that you create. You can use custom exceptions to handle errors in your own code. Creating an exception is easy. Just define a class derived from **Exception**. Your derived classes don't need to actually implement anything—it is their existence in the type system that allows you to use them as exceptions.

NOTE *In the past, custom exceptions were derived from **ApplicationException** since this is the hierarchy that was originally reserved for application-related exceptions. However, Microsoft no longer recommends this. Instead, at the time of this writing, Microsoft recommends deriving custom exceptions from **Exception**. For this reason, this approach is used here.*

The exception classes that you create will automatically have the properties and methods defined by **Exception** available to them. Of course, you can override one or more of these members in exception classes that you create.

When creating your own exception class, you will generally want your class to support all of the constructors defined by **Exception**. For simple custom exception classes, this is easy to do because you can simply pass along the constructor's arguments to the corresponding **Exception** constructor via **base**. Of course, technically, you need to provide only those constructors actually used by your program.

Here is an example that makes use of a custom exception type. At the end of Chapter 10 an array class called **RangeArray** was developed. As you may recall, **RangeArray** supports single-dimensional **int** arrays in which the starting and ending index is specified by the user. For example, an array that ranges from –5 to 27 is perfectly legal for a **RangeArray**. In Chapter 10, if an index was out of range, a special error variable defined by **RangeArray** was set. This meant that the error variable had to be checked after each operation by the code that used **RangeArray**. Of course, such an approach is error-prone and clumsy. A far better design is to have **RangeArray** throw a custom exception when a range error occurs. This is precisely what the following version of **RangeArray** does:

```
// Use a custom Exception for RangeArray errors.

using System;

// Create a RangeArray exception.
class RangeArrayException : Exception {
  /* Implement all of the Exception constructors. Notice that
     the constructors simply execute the base class constructor.
     Because RangeArrayException adds nothing to Exception,
     there is no need for any further actions. */
  public RangeArrayException() : base() { }
  public RangeArrayException(string str) : base(str) { }
  public RangeArrayException(string str, Exception inner) :
    base(str, inner) { }
  protected RangeArrayException(
    System.Runtime.Serialization.SerializationInfo si,
    System.Runtime.Serialization.StreamingContext sc) :
      base(si, sc) { }

  // Override ToString for RangeArrayException.
  public override string ToString() {
    return Message;
  }
}

// An improved version of RangeArray.
class RangeArray {
  // Private data.
  int[] a; // reference to underlying array
  int lowerBound; // smallest index
  int upperBound; // largest index

  // An auto-implemented, read-only Length property.
  public int Length { get; private set; }
```

```csharp
    // Construct array given its size.
    public RangeArray(int low, int high) {
      high++;
      if(high <= low) {
        throw new RangeArrayException("Low index not less than high.");
      }
      a = new int[high - low];
      Length = high - low;

      lowerBound = low;
      upperBound = --high;
    }

    // This is the indexer for RangeArray.
    public int this[int index] {
      // This is the get accessor.
      get {
        if(ok(index)) {
          return a[index - lowerBound];
        } else {
          throw new RangeArrayException("Range Error.");
        }
      }

      // This is the set accessor.
      set {
        if(ok(index)) {
          a[index - lowerBound] = value;
        }
        else throw new RangeArrayException("Range Error.");
      }
    }

    // Return true if index is within bounds.
    private bool ok(int index) {
      if(index >= lowerBound & index <= upperBound) return true;
      return false;
    }
}

// Demonstrate the index-range array.
class RangeArrayDemo {
  static void Main() {
    try {
      RangeArray ra = new RangeArray(-5, 5);
      RangeArray ra2 = new RangeArray(1, 10);

      // Demonstrate ra.
      Console.WriteLine("Length of ra: " + ra.Length);

      for(int i = -5; i <= 5; i++)
        ra[i] = i;
```

```
      Console.Write("Contents of ra: ");
      for(int i = -5; i <= 5; i++)
        Console.Write(ra[i] + " ");

      Console.WriteLine("\n");

      // Demonstrate ra2.
      Console.WriteLine("Length of ra2: " + ra2.Length);

      for(int i = 1; i <= 10; i++)
        ra2[i] = i;

      Console.Write("Contents of ra2: ");
      for(int i = 1; i <= 10; i++)
        Console.Write(ra2[i] + " ");

      Console.WriteLine("\n");

    } catch (RangeArrayException exc) {
        Console.WriteLine(exc);
    }

    // Now, demonstrate some errors.
    Console.WriteLine("Now generate some range errors.");

    // Use an invalid constructor.
    try {
      RangeArray ra3 = new RangeArray(100, -10); // Error
    } catch (RangeArrayException exc) {
        Console.WriteLine(exc);
    }

    // Use an invalid index.
    try {
      RangeArray ra3 = new RangeArray(-2, 2);

      for(int i = -2; i <= 2; i++)
        ra3[i] = i;

      Console.Write("Contents of ra3: ");
      for(int i = -2; i <= 10; i++) // generate range error
        Console.Write(ra3[i] + " ");

    } catch (RangeArrayException exc) {
        Console.WriteLine(exc);
    }
  }
}
```

The output from the program is shown here:

```
Length of ra: 11
Contents of ra: -5 -4 -3 -2 -1 0 1 2 3 4 5
```

```
Length of ra2: 10
Contents of ra2: 1 2 3 4 5 6 7 8 9 10

Now generate some range errors.
Low index not less than high.
Contents of ra3: -2 -1 0 1 2 Range Error.
```

When a range error occurs, **RangeArray** throws an object of type **RangeArrayException**. Notice there are three places in **RangeArray** that this might occur: in the **get** indexer accessor, in the **set** indexer accessor, and by the **RangeArray** constructor. To catch these exceptions implies that **RangeArray** objects must be constructed and accessed from within a **try** block, as the program illustrates. By using an exception to report errors, **RangeArray** now acts like one of C#'s built-in types and can be fully integrated into a program's exception-handling mechanism.

Notice that none of the **RangeArrayException** constructors provide any statements in their body. Instead, they simply pass their arguments along to **Exception** via **base**. As explained, in cases in which your exception class does not add any functionality, you can simply let the **Exception** constructors handle the process. There is no requirement that your derived class add anything to what is inherited from **Exception**.

Before moving on, you might want to experiment with this program a bit. For example, try commenting-out the override of **ToString( )** and observe the results. Also, try creating an exception using the default constructor, and observe what C# generates as its default message.

Catching Derived Class Exceptions

You need to be careful how you order **catch** clauses when trying to catch exception types that involve base and derived classes, because a **catch** for a base class will also match any of its derived classes. For example, because the base class of all exceptions is **Exception**, catching **Exception** catches all possible exceptions. Of course, using **catch** without an exception type provides a cleaner way to catch all exceptions, as described earlier. However, the issue of catching derived class exceptions is very important in other contexts, especially when you create exceptions of your own.

If you want to catch exceptions of both a base class type and a derived class type, put the derived class first in the **catch** sequence. This is necessary because a base class **catch** will also catch all derived classes. Fortunately, this rule is self-enforcing because putting the base class first causes a compile-time error.

The following program creates two exception classes called **ExceptA** and **ExceptB**. **ExceptA** is derived from **Exception**. **ExceptB** is derived from **ExceptA**. The program then throws an exception of each type. For brevity, the custom exceptions supply only one constructor (which takes a string that describes the exception). But remember, in commercial code, your custom exception classes will normally provide all four of the constructors defined by **Exception**.

```
// Derived exceptions must appear before base class exceptions.

using System;

// Create an exception.
class ExceptA : Exception {
  public ExceptA(string str) : base(str) { }
```

```
  public override string ToString() {
    return Message;
  }
}

// Create an exception derived from ExceptA.
class ExceptB : ExceptA {
  public ExceptB(string str) : base(str) { }

  public override string ToString() {
    return Message;
  }
}

class OrderMatters {
  static void Main() {
    for(int x = 0; x < 3; x++) {
      try {
        if(x==0) throw new ExceptA("Caught an ExceptA exception");
        else if(x==1) throw new ExceptB("Caught an ExceptB exception");
        else throw new Exception();
      }
      catch (ExceptB exc) {
        Console.WriteLine(exc);
      }
      catch (ExceptA exc) {
        Console.WriteLine(exc);
      }
      catch (Exception exc) {
        Console.WriteLine(exc);
      }
    }
  }
}
```

The output from the program is shown here:

```
Caught an ExceptA exception
Caught an ExceptB exception
System.Exception: Exception of type 'System.Exception' was thrown.
  at OrderMatters.Main()
```

Notice the type and order of the **catch** clauses. This is the only order in which they can occur. Since **ExceptB** is derived from **ExceptA**, the **catch** for **ExceptB** must be before the one for **ExceptA**. Similarly, the **catch** for **Exception** (which is the base class for all exceptions) must appear last. To prove this point for yourself, try rearranging the **catch** clauses. Doing so will result in a compile-time error.

One good use of a base class **catch** clause is to catch an entire category of exceptions. For example, imagine you are creating a set of exceptions for some device. If you derive all of the exceptions from a common base class, then applications that don't need to know precisely what problem occurred could simply catch the base class exception, avoiding the unnecessary duplication of code.

Using checked and unchecked

A special feature in C# relates to the generation of overflow exceptions in arithmetic computations. As you know, it is possible for some types of arithmetic computations to produce a result that exceeds the range of the data type involved in the computation. When this occurs, the result is said to *overflow*. For example, consider the following sequence:

```
byte a, b, result;
a = 127;
b = 127;

result = (byte)(a * b);
```

Here, the product of **a** and **b** exceeds the range of a **byte** value. Thus, the result overflows the type of the result.

C# allows you to specify whether your code will raise an exception when overflow occurs by using the keywords **checked** and **unchecked**. To specify that an expression be checked for overflow, use **checked**. To specify that overflow be ignored, use **unchecked**. In this case, the result is truncated to fit into the target type of the expression.

The **checked** keyword has these two general forms. One checks a specific expression and is called the *operator form* of **checked**. The other checks a block of statements and is called the *statement form.*

> checked (*expr*)

> checked {
>   // statements to be checked
> }

Here, *expr* is the expression being checked. If a checked expression overflows, then an **OverflowException** is thrown.

The **unchecked** keyword also has two general forms. The first is the operator form, which ignores overflow for a specific expression. The second ignores overflow for a block of statements.

> unchecked (*expr*)

> unchecked {
>   // statements for which overflow is ignored
> }

Here, *expr* is the expression that is not being checked for overflow. If an unchecked expression overflows, then truncation will occur.

Here is a program that demonstrates both **checked** and **unchecked**:

```
// Using checked and unchecked.

using System;

class CheckedDemo {
  static void Main() {
    byte a, b;
```

```
  byte result;

  a = 127;
  b = 127;

  try {
    result = unchecked((byte)(a * b));
    Console.WriteLine("Unchecked result: " + result);

    result = checked((byte)(a * b)); // this causes exception
    Console.WriteLine("Checked result: " + result); // won't execute
  }
  catch (OverflowException exc) {
    Console.WriteLine(exc);
  }
  }
}
```

The output from the program is shown here:

```
Unchecked result: 1
System.OverflowException: Arithmetic operation resulted in an overflow.
   at CheckedDemo.Main()
```

As is evident, the unchecked expression resulted in a truncation. The checked expression caused an exception.

The preceding program demonstrated the use of **checked** and **unchecked** for a single expression. The following program shows how to check and uncheck a block of statements.

```
// Using checked and unchecked with statement blocks.

using System;

class CheckedBlocks {
  static void Main() {
    byte a, b;
    byte result;

    a = 127;
    b = 127;

    try {
      unchecked {
        a = 127;
        b = 127;
        result = unchecked((byte)(a * b));
        Console.WriteLine("Unchecked result: " + result);

        a = 125;
        b = 5;
        result = unchecked((byte)(a * b));
        Console.WriteLine("Unchecked result: " + result);
      }
```

```
     checked {
       a = 2;
       b = 7;
       result = checked((byte)(a * b)); // this is OK
       Console.WriteLine("Checked result: " + result);

       a = 127;
       b = 127;
       result = checked((byte)(a * b)); // this causes exception
       Console.WriteLine("Checked result: " + result); // won't execute
     }
   }
   catch (OverflowException exc) {
     Console.WriteLine(exc);
   }
 }
}
```

The output from the program is shown here:

```
Unchecked result: 1
Unchecked result: 113
Checked result: 14
System.OverflowException: Arithmetic operation resulted in an overflow.
   at CheckedBlocks.Main()
```

As you can see, the unchecked block results in the overflow being truncated. When overflow occurred in the checked block, an exception was raised.

One reason that you may need to use **checked** or **unchecked** is that the default checked/unchecked status of overflow is determined by the setting of a compiler option and the execution environment, itself. Thus, for some types of programs, it is best to specify the overflow check status explicitly.

Using I/O

The earlier chapters of this book have used parts of the C# I/O system, such as **Console.WriteLine( )**, but have done so without much formal explanation. Because the I/O system is built upon a hierarchy of classes, it was not possible to present its theory and details without first discussing classes, inheritance, and exceptions. Now it is time to examine I/O in detail. Because C# uses the I/O system and classes defined by the .NET Framework, a discussion of I/O under C# is also a discussion of the .NET I/O system, in general.

This chapter examines both console I/O and file I/O. Be forewarned that the I/O system is quite large. This chapter describes the most important and commonly used features.

C#'s I/O Is Built Upon Streams

C# programs perform I/O through streams. A *stream* is an abstraction that either produces or consumes information. A stream is linked to a physical device by the I/O system. All streams behave in the same manner, even if the actual physical devices they are linked to differ. Thus, the I/O classes and methods can be applied to many types of devices. For example, the same methods that you use to write to the console can also be used to write to a disk file.

Byte Streams and Character Streams

At the lowest level, all C# I/O operates on bytes. This makes sense because many devices are byte oriented when it comes to I/O operations. Frequently, though, we humans prefer to communicate using characters. Recall that in C#, **char** is a 16-bit type, and **byte** is an 8-bit type. If you are using the ASCII character set, then it is easy to convert between **char** and **byte**; just ignore the high-order byte of the **char** value. But this won't work for the rest of the Unicode characters, which need both bytes (and possibly more). Thus, byte streams are not perfectly suited to handling character-based I/O. To solve this problem, the .NET Framework defines several classes that convert a byte stream into a character stream, handling the translation of **byte**-to-**char** and **char**-to-**byte** automatically.

The Predefined Streams

Three predefined streams, which are exposed by the properties called **Console.In**, **Console.Out**, and **Console.Error**, are available to all programs that use the **System** namespace. **Console.Out** refers to the standard output stream. By default, this is the

console. When you call **Console.WriteLine( )**, for example, it automatically sends information to **Console.Out**. **Console.In** refers to standard input, which is, by default, the keyboard. **Console.Error** refers to the standard error stream, which is also the console by default. However, these streams can be redirected to any compatible I/O device. The standard streams are character streams. Thus, these streams read and write characters.

The Stream Classes

The .NET Framework defines both byte and character stream classes. However, the character stream classes are really just wrappers that convert an underlying byte stream to a character stream, handling any conversion automatically. Thus, the character streams, while logically separate, are built upon byte streams.

The core stream classes are defined within the **System.IO** namespace. To use these classes, you will usually include the following statement near the top of your program:

```
using System.IO;
```

The reason that you don't have to specify **System.IO** for console input and output is that the **Console** class is defined in the **System** namespace.

The Stream Class

The core stream class is **System.IO.Stream**. **Stream** represents a byte stream and is a base class for all other stream classes. It is also abstract, which means that you cannot instantiate a **Stream** object. **Stream** defines a set of standard stream operations. Table 14-1 shows several commonly used methods defined by **Stream**.

Several of the methods shown in Table 14-1 will throw an **IOException** if an I/O error occurs. If an invalid operation is attempted, such as attempting to write to a stream that is read-only, a **NotSupportedException** is thrown. Other exceptions are possible, depending on the specific method.

Method	Description
void Close( )	Closes the stream.
void Flush( )	Writes the contents of the stream to the physical device.
int ReadByte( )	Returns an integer representation of the next available byte of input. Returns −1 when the end of the file is encountered.
int Read(byte[ ] *buf*, int *offset*, int *numBytes*)	Attempts to read up to *numBytes* bytes into *buf* starting at *buf*[*offset*], returning the number of bytes successfully read.
long Seek(long *offset*, SeekOrigin *origin*)	Sets the current position in the stream to the specified *offset* from the specified *origin*. It returns the new position.
void WriteByte(byte *b*)	Writes a single byte to an output stream.
int Write(byte[ ] *buf*, int *offset*, int *numBytes*)	Writes a subrange of *numBytes* bytes from the array *buf*, beginning at *buf*[*offset*]. The number of bytes written is returned.

TABLE 14-1 Some of the Methods Defined by **Stream**

Notice that **Stream** defines methods that read and write data. However, not all streams will support both of these operations because it is possible to open read-only or write-only streams. Also, not all streams will support position requests via **Seek( )**. To determine the capabilities of a stream, you will use one or more of **Stream**'s properties. They are shown in Table 14-2. Also shown are the **Length** and **Position** properties, which contain the length of the stream and its current position.

The Byte Stream Classes

Several concrete byte streams are derived from **Stream**. Those defined in the **System.IO** namespace are shown here:

Stream Class	Description
BufferedStream	Wraps a byte stream and adds buffering. Buffering provides a performance enhancement in many cases.
FileStream	A byte stream designed for file I/O.
MemoryStream	A byte stream that uses memory for storage.
UnmanagedMemoryStream	A byte stream that uses unmanaged memory for storage.

Several other concrete stream classes are also supported by the .NET framework, which provide support for compressed files, sockets, and pipes, among others. It is also possible to derive your own stream classes. However, for the vast majority of applications, the built-in streams will be sufficient.

The Character Stream Wrapper Classes

To create a character stream, wrap a byte stream inside one of the character stream wrappers. At the top of the character stream hierarchy are the abstract classes **TextReader** and **TextWriter**. **TextReader** handles input and **TextWriter** handles output. The methods defined by these two abstract classes are available to all of their subclasses. Thus, they form a minimal set of I/O functions that all character streams will have.

Method	Description
bool CanRead	This property is true if the stream can be read. This property is read-only.
bool CanSeek	This property is true if the stream supports position requests. This property is read-only.
bool CanTimeout	This property is true if the stream can time out. This property is read-only.
bool CanWrite	This property is true if the stream can be written. This property is read-only.
long Length	This property contains the length of the stream. This property is read-only.
long Position	This property represents the current position of the stream. This property is read/write.
int ReadTimeout	This property represents the length of time before a time-out will occur for read operations. This property is read/write.
int WriteTimeout	This property represents the length of time before a time-out will occur for write operations. This property is read/write.

TABLE 14-2   The Properties Defined by **Stream**

Table 14-3 shows the input methods in **TextReader**. In general, these methods can throw an **IOException** on error. (Some can throw other types of exceptions, too.) Of particular interest is the **ReadLine( )** method, which reads an entire line of text, returning it as a **string**. This method is useful when reading input that contains embedded spaces.

TextWriter defines versions of **Write( )** and **WriteLine( )** that output all of the built-in types. For example, here are just a few of their overloaded versions:

Method	Description
void Write(int *val*)	Writes an **int**.
void Write(double *val*)	Writes a **double**.
void Write(bool *val*)	Writes a **bool**.
void WriteLine(string *val*)	Writes a **string** followed by a newline.
void WriteLine(uint *val*)	Writes a **uint** followed by a newline.
void WriteLine(char *val*)	Writes a character followed by a newline.

All throw an **IOException** if an error occurs while writing.

TextWriter also defines the **Close( )** and **Flush( )** methods shown here:

```
virtual void Close( )
virtual void Flush( )
```

Flush( ) causes any data remaining in the output buffer to be written to the physical medium. **Close( )** closes the stream.

Method	Description
int Peek( )	Obtains the next character from the input stream, but does not remove that character. Returns –1 if no character is available.
int Read( )	Returns an integer representation of the next available character from the invoking input stream. Returns –1 when the end of the stream is encountered.
int Read(char[ ] *buf*, int *offset*, int *numChars*)	Attempts to read up to *numChars* characters into *buf* starting at *buf*[*offset*], returning the number of characters successfully read.
int ReadBlock(char[ ] *buf*, int *offset*, int *numChars*)	Attempts to read up to *numChars* characters into *buf* starting at *buf*[*offset*], returning the number of characters successfully read.
string ReadLine( )	Reads the next line of text and returns it as a string. Null is returned if an attempt is made to read at end-of-file.
string ReadToEnd( )	Reads all of the remaining characters in a stream and returns them as a string.

TABLE 14-3 The Input Methods Defined by **TextReader**

The **TextReader** and **TextWriter** classes are implemented by several character-based stream classes, including those shown here. Thus, these streams provide the methods and properties specified by **TextReader** and **TextWriter**.

Stream Class	Description
StreamReader	Read characters from a byte stream. This class wraps a byte input stream.
StreamWriter	Write characters to a byte stream. This class wraps a byte output stream.
StringReader	Read characters from a string.
StringWriter	Write characters to a string.

Binary Streams

In addition to the byte and character streams, there are two binary stream classes that can be used to read and write binary data directly. These streams are called **BinaryReader** and **BinaryWriter**. We will look closely at these later in this chapter when binary file I/O is discussed.

Now that you understand the general layout of the I/O system, the rest of this chapter will examine its various pieces in detail, beginning with console I/O.

Console I/O

Console I/O is accomplished through the standard streams **Console.In**, **Console.Out**, and **Console.Error**. Console I/O has been used since Chapter 2, so you are already familiar with it. As you will see, it has some additional capabilities.

Before we begin, however, it is important to emphasize a point made earlier in this book: Most real applications of C# will not be text-based, console programs. Rather, they will be graphically oriented programs or components that rely upon a windowed interface for interaction with the user, or will be server-side code. Thus, the portion of the I/O system that relates to console input and output is not widely used. Although text-based programs are excellent as teaching examples, for short utility programs, and for some types of components, they are not suitable for most real-world applications.

Reading Console Input

Console.In is an instance of **TextReader**, and you can use the methods and properties defined by **TextReader** to access it. However, you will generally use the methods provided by **Console**, which automatically read from **Console.In**. **Console** defines three input methods. The first two, **Read( )** and **ReadLine( )**, have been available since .NET Framework 1.0. The third, **ReadKey( )**, was added by .NET Framework 2.0.

To read a single character, use the **Read( )** method:

    static int Read( )

Read( ) returns the next character read from the console. It waits until the user presses a key and then returns the result. The character is returned as an **int**, which must be cast to **char**. **Read( )** returns –1 on error. This method will throw an **IOException** on failure. When using **Read( )**, console input is line-buffered, so you must press ENTER before any character that you type will be sent to your program.

Here is a program that reads a character from the keyboard using **Read( )**:

```
// Read a character from the keyboard.

using System;

class KbIn {
  static void Main() {
    char ch;

    Console.Write("Press a key followed by ENTER: ");

    ch = (char) Console.Read(); // get a char

    Console.WriteLine("Your key is: " + ch);
  }
}
```

Here is a sample run:

```
Press a key followed by ENTER: t
Your key is: t
```

The fact that **Read( )** is line-buffered is a source of annoyance at times. When you press ENTER, a carriage-return, line-feed sequence is entered into the input stream. Furthermore, these characters are left pending in the input buffer until you read them. Thus, for some applications, you may need to remove them (by reading them) before the next input operation. (To read keystrokes from the console in a non-line-buffered manner, you can use **ReadKey( )**, described later in this section.)

To read a string of characters, use the **ReadLine( )** method. It is shown here:

static string ReadLine( )

ReadLine( ) reads characters until you press ENTER and returns them in a **string** object. This method will also throw an **IOException** on failure.

Here is a program that demonstrates reading a string from **Console.In** by using **ReadLine( )**:

```
// Input from the console using ReadLine().

using System;

class ReadString {
  static void Main() {
    string str;

    Console.WriteLine("Enter some characters.");
    str = Console.ReadLine();
    Console.WriteLine("You entered: " + str);
  }
}
```

Here is a sample run:

```
Enter some characters.
This is a test.
You entered: This is a test.
```

Although the **Console** methods are the easiest way to read from **Console.In**, you can call methods on the underlying **TextReader**. For example, here is the preceding program rewritten to use the **ReadLine( )** method defined by **TextReader**:

```
// Read a string from the keyboard, using Console.In directly.

using System;

class ReadChars2 {
  static void Main() {
    string str;

    Console.WriteLine("Enter some characters.");

    str = Console.In.ReadLine(); // call TextReader's ReadLine() method

    Console.WriteLine("You entered: " + str);
  }
}
```

Notice how **ReadLine( )** is now invoked directly on **Console.In**. The key point here is that if you need access to the methods defined by the **TextReader** that underlies **Console.In**, you will invoke those methods as shown in this example.

Using ReadKey( )

Beginning with version 2.0, the .NET Framework has included a method in **Console** that enables you to read individual keystrokes directly from the keyboard in a non-line-buffered manner. This method is called **ReadKey( )**. When it is called, it waits until a key is pressed. When a key is pressed, **ReadKey( )** returns the keystroke immediately. The user does not need to press ENTER. Thus, **ReadKey( )** allows keystrokes to be read and processed in real time.

ReadKey( ) has these two forms.

static ConsoleKeyInfo ReadKey( )

static ConsoleKeyInfo ReadKey(bool *noDisplay*)

The first form waits for a key to be pressed. When that occurs, it returns the key and also displays the key on the screen. The second form also waits for and returns a keypress. However, if *noDisplay* is true, then the key is not displayed. If *noDisplay* is false, the key is displayed.

ReadKey( ) returns information about the keypress in an object of type **ConsoleKeyInfo**, which is a structure. It contains the following read-only properties.

char KeyChar

ConsoleKey Key

ConsoleModifiers Modifiers

KeyChar contains the **char** equivalent of the character that was pressed. **Key** contains a value from the **ConsoleKey** enumeration, which is an enumeration of all the keys on the keyboard. **Modifiers** describes which, if any, of the keyboard modifiers ATL, CTRL, or SHIFT were pressed when the keystroke was generated. These modifiers are represented by the **ConsoleModifiers** enumeration, which has these values: **Control**, **Shift**, and **Alt**. More than one modifier value might be present in **Modifiers**.

The major advantage to **ReadKey( )** is that it provides a means of achieving interactive keyboard input because it is not line buffered. To see the effect of this, try the following program:

```
// Read keystrokes from the console by using ReadKey().

using System;

class ReadKeys {
  static void Main() {
    ConsoleKeyInfo keypress;

    Console.WriteLine("Enter keystrokes. Enter Q to stop.");

    do {
      keypress = Console.ReadKey(); // read keystrokes

      Console.WriteLine(" Your key is: " + keypress.KeyChar);

      // Check for modifier keys.
      if((ConsoleModifiers.Alt & keypress.Modifiers) != 0)
        Console.WriteLine("Alt key pressed.");
      if((ConsoleModifiers.Control & keypress.Modifiers) != 0)
        Console.WriteLine("Control key pressed.");
      if((ConsoleModifiers.Shift & keypress.Modifiers) != 0)
        Console.WriteLine("Shift key pressed.");

    } while(keypress.KeyChar != 'Q');
  }
}
```

A sample run is shown here:

```
Enter keystrokes. Enter Q to stop.
a Your key is: a
b Your key is: b
d Your key is: d
A Your key is: A
Shift key pressed.
B Your key is: B
Shift key pressed.
C Your key is: C
Shift key pressed.
• Your key is: •
Control key pressed.
Q Your key is: Q
Shift key pressed.
```

As the output confirms, each time a key is pressed, **ReadKey( )** immediately returns the keypress. As explained, this differs from **Read( )** and **ReadLine( )**, which use line-buffered input. Therefore, if you want to achieve interactive responses from the keyboard, use **ReadKey( )**.

Writing Console Output

Console.Out and **Console.Error** are objects of type **TextWriter**. Console output is most easily accomplished with **Write( )** and **WriteLine( )**, with which you are already familiar. Versions of these methods exist that output for each of the built-in types. **Console** defines its own versions of **Write( )** and **WriteLine( )** so they can be called directly on **Console**, as you have been doing throughout this book. However, you can invoke these (and other) methods on the **TextWriter** that underlies **Console.Out** and **Console.Error** if you choose.

Here is a program that demonstrates writing to **Console.Out** and **Console.Error**. By default, both write to the console.

```
// Write to Console.Out and Console.Error.

using System;

class ErrOut {
  static void Main() {
    int a=10, b=0;
    int result;

    Console.Out.WriteLine("This will generate an exception.");
    try {
      result = a / b; // generate an exception
    } catch(DivideByZeroException exc) {
      Console.Error.WriteLine(exc.Message);
    }
  }
}
```

The output from the program is shown here:

```
This will generate an exception.
Attempted to divide by zero.
```

Sometimes newcomers to programming are confused about when to use **Console.Error**. Since both **Console.Out** and **Console.Error** default to writing their output to the console, why are there two different streams? The answer lies in the fact that the standard streams can be redirected to other devices. For example, **Console.Error** can be redirected to write to a disk file, rather than the screen. Thus, it is possible to direct error output to a log file, for example, without affecting console output. Conversely, if console output is redirected and error output is not, then error messages will appear on the console, where they can be seen. We will examine redirection later, after file I/O has been described.

FileStream and Byte-Oriented File I/O

The .NET Framework provides classes that allow you to read and write files. Of course, the most common type of files are disk files. At the operating system level, all files are byte

oriented. As you would expect, there are methods to read and write bytes from and to a file. Thus, reading and writing files using byte streams is very common. You can also wrap a byte-oriented file stream within a character-based object. Character-based file operations are useful when text is being stored. Character streams are discussed later in this chapter. Byte-oriented I/O is described here.

To create a byte-oriented stream attached to a file, you will use the **FileStream** class. **FileStream** is derived from **Stream** and contains all of **Stream**'s functionality.

Remember, the stream classes, including **FileStream**, are defined in **System.IO**. Thus, you will usually include

```
using System.IO;
```

near the top of any program that uses them.

Opening and Closing a File

To create a byte stream linked to a file, create a **FileStream** object. **FileStream** defines several constructors. Perhaps its most commonly used is the one shown here:

FileStream(string *filename*, FileMode *mode*)

Here, *filename* specifies the name of the file to open, which can include a full path specification. The *mode* parameter specifies how the file will be opened. It must be one of the values defined by the **FileMode** enumeration. These values are shown in Table 14-4. In general, this constructor opens a file for read/write access. The exception is when the file is opened using **FileMode.Append**. In this case, the file is write-only.

If a failure occurs when attempting to open the file, an exception will be thrown. If the file cannot be opened because it does not exist, **FileNotFoundException** will be thrown. If the file cannot be opened because of some type of I/O error, **IOException** will be thrown. Other possible exceptions are **ArgumentNullException** (the filename is null), **ArgumentException** (the filename is invalid), **ArgumentOutOfRangeException** (the mode is invalid), **SecurityException** (user does not have access rights), **PathTooLongException** (the filename/path is too long), **NotSupportedException** (the filename specifies an unsupported device), and **DirectoryNotFoundException** (specified directory is invalid).

Value	Description
FileMode.Append	Output is appended to the end of file.
FileMode.Create	Creates a new output file. Any preexisting file by the same name will be destroyed.
FileMode.CreateNew	Creates a new output file. The file must not already exist.
FileMode.Open	Opens a preexisting file.
FileMode.OpenOrCreate	Opens a file if it exists, or creates the file if it does not already exist.
FileMode.Truncate	Opens a preexisting file, but reduces its length to zero.

TABLE 14-4   The **FileMode** Values

The exceptions **PathTooLongException, DirectoryNotFoundException,** and **FileNotFoundException** are subclasses of **IOException.** Thus, it is possible to catch all three by catching **IOException.**

The following shows one way to open the file **test.dat** for input:

```
FileStream fin;

try {
  fin = new FileStream("test", FileMode.Open);
}
catch(IOException exc) { // catch all I/O exceptions
  Console.WriteLine(exc.Message);
  // Handle the error.
}
catch(Exception exc { // catch any other exception.
  Console.WriteLine(exc.Message);
  // Handle the error.
}
```

Here, the first **catch** clause handles situations in which the file is not found, the path is too long, the directory does not exist, or other I/O errors occur. The second **catch,** which is a "catch all" clause for all other types of exceptions, handles the other possible errors (possibly by rethrowing the exception). You could also check for each error individually, reporting more specifically the problem that occurred and taking remedial action specific to that error.

For the sake of simplicity, the examples in this book will catch only **IOException,** but your real-world code may (probably will) need to handle the other possible exceptions, depending upon the circumstances. Also, the exception handlers in this chapter simply report the error, but in many cases, your code should take steps to correct the problem when possible. For example, you might reprompt the user for a filename if the one previously entered is not found.

REMEMBER   *To keep the code simple, the examples in this chapter catch only* **IOException,** *but your own code may need to handle other possible exceptions or handle each type of I/O exception individually.*

As mentioned, the **FileStream** constructor just described opens a file that has read/ write access. If you want to restrict access to just reading or just writing, use this constructor instead:

FileStream(string *filename,* FileMode *mode,* FileAccess *how*)

As before, *filename* specifies the name of the file to open, and *mode* specifies how the file will be opened. The value passed in *how* determines how the file can be accessed. It must be one of the values defined by the **FileAccess** enumeration, which are shown here:

FileAccess.Read	FileAccess.Write	FileAccess.ReadWrite

For example, this opens a read-only file:

```
FileStream fin = new FileStream("test.dat", FileMode.Open, FileAccess.Read);
```

When you are done with a file, you should close it by calling **Close( )**. Its general form is shown here:

void Close( )

Closing a file releases the system resources allocated to the file, allowing them to be used by another file. As a point of interest, **Close( )** works by calling **Dispose( )**, which actually frees the resources.

NOTE *The* **using** *statement, described in Chapter 20, offers a way to automatically close a file when it is no longer needed. This approach is beneficial in many file-handling situations because it provides a simple means to ensure that a file is closed when it is no longer needed. However, to clearly illustrate the fundamentals of file handling, including the point at which a file can be closed, this chapter explicitly calls* **Close( )** *in all cases.*

Reading Bytes from a FileStream

FileStream defines two methods that read bytes from a file: **ReadByte( )** and **Read( )**. To read a single byte from a file, use **ReadByte( )**, whose general form is shown here:

int ReadByte( )

Each time it is called, it reads a single byte from the file and returns it as an integer value. It returns –1 when the end of the file is encountered. Possible exceptions include **NotSupportedException** (the stream is not opened for input) and **ObjectDisposedException** (the stream is closed).

To read a block of bytes, use **Read( )**, which has this general form:

int Read(byte[ ] *buf*, int *offset*, int *numBytes*)

Read( ) attempts to read up to *numBytes* bytes into *buf* starting at *buf*[*offset*]. It returns the number of bytes successfully read. An **IOException** is thrown if an I/O error occurs. Several other types of exceptions are possible, including **NotSupportedException**, which is thrown if reading is not supported by the stream.

The following program uses **ReadByte( )** to input and display the contents of a text file, the name of which is specified as a command-line argument. Note the program handles two errors that might occur when this program is first executed: the specified file not being found or the user forgetting to include the name of the file.

```
/* Display a text file.

   To use this program, specify the name of the file that you
   want to see. For example, to see a file called TEST.CS,
   use the following command line.

   ShowFile TEST.CS
*/

using System;
using System.IO;

class ShowFile {
  static void Main(string[] args) {
```

```
int i;
FileStream fin;

if(args.Length != 1) {
  Console.WriteLine("Usage: ShowFile File");
  return;
}

try {
  fin = new FileStream(args[0], FileMode.Open);
} catch(IOException exc) {
  Console.WriteLine("Cannot Open File");
  Console.WriteLine(exc.Message);
  return;
}

// Read bytes until EOF is encountered.
do {
  try {
    i = fin.ReadByte();
  } catch(IOException exc) {
    Console.WriteLine("Error Reading File");
    Console.WriteLine(exc.Message);
    break;
  }
  if(i != -1) Console.Write((char) i);
} while(i != -1);

  fin.Close();
  }
}
```

Writing to a File

To write a byte to a file, use the **WriteByte( )** method. Its simplest form is shown here:

void WriteByte(byte *val*)

This method writes the byte specified by *val* to the file. If the underlying stream is not opened for output, a **NotSupportedException** is thrown. If the stream is closed, **ObjectDisposedException** is thrown.

You can write an array of bytes to a file by calling **Write( )**. It is shown here:

void Write(byte[ ] *buf*, int *offset*, int *numBytes*)

Write( ) writes *numBytes* bytes from the array *buf*, beginning at *buf*[*offset*], to the file. The number of bytes written is returned. If an error occurs during writing, an **IOException** is thrown. If the underlying stream is not opened for output, a **NotSupportedException** is thrown. Several other exceptions are also possible.

As you may know, when file output is performed, often that output is not immediately written to the actual physical device. Instead, output is buffered by the operating system until a sizable chunk of data can be written all at once. This improves the efficiency of the system. For example, disk files are organized by sectors, which might be anywhere from 128 bytes long, on up. Output is usually buffered until an entire sector can be written all at once.

However, if you want to cause data to be written to the physical device whether the buffer is full or not, you can call **Flush( )**, shown here:

void Flush( )

An **IOException** is thrown on failure. If the stream is closed, **ObjectDisposedException** is thrown.

Once you are done with an output file, you must remember to close it using **Close( )**. Doing so ensures that any output remaining in a disk buffer is actually written to the disk. Thus, there is no reason to call **Flush( )** before closing a file.

Here is a simple example that writes to a file:

```
// Write to a file.

using System;
using System.IO;

class WriteToFile {
  static void Main(string[] args) {
    FileStream fout;

    // Open output file.
    try {
      fout = new FileStream("test.txt", FileMode.Create);
    } catch(IOException exc) {
      Console.WriteLine("Cannot Open File");
      Console.WriteLine(exc.Message);
      return;
    }

    // Write the alphabet to the file.
    try {
      for(char c = 'A'; c <= 'Z'; c++)
        fout.WriteByte((byte) c);
    } catch(IOException exc) {
      Console.WriteLine("Error Writing File");
      Console.WriteLine(exc.Message);
    }

    fout.Close();
  }
}
```

The program first opens a file called **test.txt** for output. It then writes the uppercase alphabet to the file. Finally, it closes the file. Notice how possible I/O errors are handled by the **try/catch** blocks. After this program executes, **test.txt** will contain the following output:

ABCDEFGHIJKLMNOPQRSTUVWXYZ

Using FileStream to Copy a File

One advantage to the byte-oriented I/O used by **FileStream** is that you can use it on any type of file—not just those that contain text. For example, the following program copies any type of file, including executable files. The names of the source and destination files are specified on the command line.

```
/* Copy a file.

   To use this program, specify the name of the source
   file and the destination file. For example, to copy a
   file called FIRST.DAT to a file called SECOND.DAT, use
   the following command line:

   CopyFile FIRST.DAT SECOND.DAT
*/

using System;
using System.IO;

class CopyFile {
  static void Main(string[] args) {
    int i;
    FileStream fin;
    FileStream fout;

    if(args.Length != 2) {
      Console.WriteLine("Usage: CopyFile From To");
      return;
    }

    // Open input file.
    try {
      fin = new FileStream(args[0], FileMode.Open);
    } catch(IOException exc) {
      Console.WriteLine("Cannot Open Input File");
      Console.WriteLine(exc.Message);
      return;
    }

    // Open output file.
    try {
      fout = new FileStream(args[1], FileMode.Create);
    } catch(IOException exc) {
      Console.WriteLine("Cannot Open Output File");
      Console.WriteLine(exc.Message);
      fin.Close();
      return;
    }

    // Copy File
    try {
      do {
        i = fin.ReadByte();
        if(i != -1) fout.WriteByte((byte)i);
      } while(i != -1);
    } catch(IOException exc) {
      Console.WriteLine("Error Copying File");
      Console.WriteLine(exc.Message);
    }

    fin.Close();
```

```
      fout.Close();
   }
}
```

Character-Based File I/O

Although byte-oriented file handling is quite common, it is possible to use character-based streams for this purpose. The advantage to the character streams is that they operate directly on Unicode characters. Thus, if you want to store Unicode text, the character streams are certainly your best option. In general, to perform character-based file operations, you will wrap a **FileStream** inside either a **StreamReader** or a **StreamWriter**. These classes automatically convert a byte stream into a character stream, and vice versa.

Remember, at the operating system level, a file consists of a set of bytes. Using a **StreamReader** or **StreamWriter** does not alter this fact.

StreamWriter is derived from **TextWriter**. **StreamReader** is derived from **TextReader**. Thus, **StreamWriter** and **StreamReader** have access to the methods and properties defined by their base classes.

Using StreamWriter

To create a character-based output stream, wrap a **Stream** object (such as a **FileStream**) inside a **StreamWriter**. **StreamWriter** defines several constructors. One of its most popular is shown here:

StreamWriter(Stream *stream*)

Here, *stream* is the name of an open stream. This constructor throws an **ArgumentException** if *stream* is not opened for output and an **ArgumentNullException** if *stream* is null. Once created, a **StreamWriter** automatically handles the conversion of characters to bytes.

Here is a simple key-to-disk utility that reads lines of text entered at the keyboard and writes them to a file called "test.txt." Text is read until the user enters the word "stop". It uses a **FileStream** wrapped in a **StreamWriter** to output to the file.

```
// A simple key-to-disk utility that demonstrates a StreamWriter.

using System;
using System.IO;

class KtoD {
  static void Main() {
    string str;
    FileStream fout;

    try {
      fout = new FileStream("test.txt", FileMode.Create);
    }
    catch(IOException exc) {
      Console.WriteLine("Cannot Open File");
      Console.WriteLine(exc.Message);
      return ;
    }
    StreamWriter fstr_out = new StreamWriter(fout);
```

```
    Console.WriteLine("Enter text ('stop' to quit).");
    do {
      Console.Write(": ");
      str = Console.ReadLine();

      if(str != "stop") {
        str = str + "\r\n"; // add newline
        try {
          fstr_out.Write(str);
          } catch(IOException exc) {
            Console.WriteLine("Error Writing File");
            Console.WriteLine(exc.Message);
            break;
          }
      }
    } while(str != "stop");

    fstr_out.Close();
  }
}
```

In some cases, it might be more convenient to open a file directly using **StreamWriter**. To do so, use one of these constructors:

StreamWriter(string *filename*)
StreamWriter(string *filename*, bool *appendFlag*)

Here, *filename* specifies the name of the file to open, which can include a full path specifier. In the second form, if *appendFlag* is true, then output is appended to the end of an existing file. Otherwise, output overwrites the specified file. In both cases, if the file does not exist, it is created. Also, both throw an **IOException** if an I/O error occurs. Other exceptions are also possible.

Here is the key-to-disk program rewritten so that it uses **StreamWriter** to open the output file:

```
// Open a file using StreamWriter.

using System;
using System.IO;

class KtoD {
  static void Main() {
    string str;
    StreamWriter fstr_out;

    try {
      fstr_out = new StreamWriter("test.txt");
    }
    catch(IOException exc) {
      Console.WriteLine("Cannot Open File");
      Console.WriteLine(exc.Message);
      return ;
    }

    Console.WriteLine("Enter text ('stop' to quit).");
```

```
    do {
      Console.Write(": ");
      str = Console.ReadLine();

      if(str != "stop") {
        str = str + "\r\n"; // add newline
        try {
          fstr_out.Write(str);
        } catch(IOException exc) {
          Console.WriteLine("Error Writing File");
          Console.WriteLine(exc.Message);
          break;
        }
      }
    } while(str != "stop");

    fstr_out.Close();
  }
}
```

Using a StreamReader

To create a character-based input stream, wrap a byte stream inside a **StreamReader**. **StreamReader** defines several constructors. A frequently used one is shown here:

StreamReader(Stream *stream*)

Here, *stream* is the name of an open stream. This constructor throws an **ArgumentNullException** if *stream* is null. It throws **ArgumentException** if *stream* is not opened for input. Once created, a **StreamReader** will automatically handle the conversion of bytes to characters.

The following program creates a simple disk-to-screen utility that reads a text file called "test.txt" and displays its contents on the screen. Thus, it is the complement of the key-to-disk utility shown in the previous section:

```
// A simple disk-to-screen utility that demonstrates a StreamReader.

using System;
using System.IO;

class DtoS {
  static void Main() {
    FileStream fin;
    string s;

    try {
      fin = new FileStream("test.txt", FileMode.Open);
    }
    catch(IOException exc) {
      Console.WriteLine("Error Opening File");
      Console.WriteLine(exc.Message);
      return ;
    }

    StreamReader fstr_in = new StreamReader(fin);
```

```
    try {
      while((s = fstr_in.ReadLine()) != null) {
        Console.WriteLine(s);
      }
    } catch(IOException exc) {
      Console.WriteLine("Error Reading File");
      Console.WriteLine(exc.Message);
    }

    fstr_in.Close();
  }
}
```

In the program, notice how the end of the file is determined. When the reference returned by **ReadLine( )** is null, the end of the file has been reached. Although this approach works, **StreamReader** provides an alternative means of detecting the end of the stream: the **EndOfStream** property. This read-only property is true when the end of the stream has been reached and false otherwise. Therefore, you can use **EndOfStream** to watch for the end of a file. For example, here is another way to write the **while** loop that reads the file:

```
while(!fstr_in.EndOfStream) {
  s = fstr_in.ReadLine();
  Console.WriteLine(s);
}
```

In this case, the use of **EndOfStream** makes the code a bit easier to understand but does not change the overall structure of the sequence. There are times, however, when the use of **EndOfStream** can simplify an otherwise tricky situation, adding clarity and improving structure.

As with **StreamWriter**, in some cases, you might find it easier to open a file directly using **StreamReader**. To do so, use this constructor:

StreamReader(string *filename*)

Here, *filename* specifies the name of the file to open, which can include a full path specifier. The file must exist. If it doesn't, a **FileNotFoundException** is thrown. If *filename* is null, then an **ArgumentNullException** is thrown. If *filename* is an empty string, **ArgumentException** is thrown. **IOException** and **DirectoryNotFoundException** are also possible.

Redirecting the Standard Streams

As mentioned earlier, the standard streams, such as **Console.In**, can be redirected. By far, the most common redirection is to a file. When a standard stream is redirected, input and/or output is automatically directed to the new stream, bypassing the default devices. By redirecting the standard streams, your program can read commands from a disk file, create log files, or even read input from a network connection.

Redirection of the standard streams can be accomplished in two ways. First, when you execute a program on the command line, you can use the < and > operators to redirect **Console.In** and/or **Console.Out**, respectively. For example, given this program:

```
using System;
```

```
class Test {
  static void Main() {
    Console.WriteLine("This is a test.");
  }
}
```

executing the program like this

Test > log

will cause the line "This is a test." to be written to a file called **log**. Input can be redirected in the same way. The thing to remember when input is redirected is that you must make sure that what you specify as an input source contains sufficient input to satisfy the demands of the program. If it doesn't, the program will hang.

The < and > command-line redirection operators are not part of C#, but are provided by the operating system. Thus, if your environment supports I/O redirection (as is the case with Windows), you can redirect standard input and standard output without making any changes to your program. However, there is a second way that you can redirect the standard streams that is under program control. To do so, you will use the **SetIn( )**, **SetOut( )**, and **SetError( )** methods, shown here, which are members of **Console**:

static void SetIn(TextReader *input*)
static void SetOut(TextWriter *output*)
static void SetError(TextWriter *output*)

Thus, to redirect input, call **SetIn( )**, specifying the desired stream. You can use any input stream as long as it is derived from **TextReader**. To redirect output, call **SetOut ( )**, specifying the desired output stream, which must be derived from **TextWriter**. For example, to redirect output to a file, specify a **FileStream** that is wrapped in a **StreamWriter**. The following program shows an example:

```
// Redirect Console.Out.

using System;
using System.IO;

class Redirect {
  static void Main() {
    StreamWriter log_out;

    try {
      log_out = new StreamWriter("logfile.txt");
    }
    catch(IOException exc) {
      Console.WriteLine("Error Opening Log File");
      Console.WriteLine(exc.Message);
      return ;
    }

    // Redirect standard out to logfile.txt.
    Console.SetOut(log_out);
```

```
try {
  Console.WriteLine("This is the start of the log file.");

  for(int i=0; i<10; i++) Console.WriteLine(i);

  Console.WriteLine("This is the end of the log file.");
} catch(IOException exc) {
  Console.WriteLine("Error Writing Log File");
  Console.WriteLine(exc.Message);
}

log_out.Close();
  }
}
```

When you run this program, you won't see any of the output on the screen, but the file **logfile.txt** will contain the following:

```
This is the start of the log file.
0
1
2
3
4
5
6
7
8
9
This is the end of the log file.
```

On your own, you might want to experiment with redirecting the other built-in streams.

Reading and Writing Binary Data

So far, we have just been reading and writing bytes or characters, but it is possible—indeed, common—to read and write other types of data. For example, you might want to create a file that contains the **int**s, **double**s, or **short**s. To read and write binary values of the C# built-in types, you will use **BinaryReader** and **BinaryWriter**. When using these streams, it is important to understand that this data is read and written using its internal, binary format, not its human-readable text form.

BinaryWriter

A **BinaryWriter** is a wrapper around a byte stream that manages the writing of binary data. Its most commonly used constructor is shown here:

BinaryWriter(Stream *outputStream*)

Here, *outputStream* is the stream to which data is written. To write output to a file, you can use the object created by **FileStream** for this parameter. If *outputStream* is null, then an **ArgumentNullException** is thrown. If *outputStream* has not been opened for writing, **ArgumentException** is thrown.

BinaryWriter defines methods that can write all of C#'s built-in types. Several are shown in Table 14-5. Notice that a **string** is written using its internal format, which includes a length specifier. **BinaryWriter** also defines the standard **Close( )** and **Flush( )** methods, which work as described earlier.

BinaryReader

A **BinaryReader** is a wrapper around a byte stream that handles the reading of binary data. Its most commonly used constructor is shown here:

> BinaryReader(Stream *inputStream*)

Here, *inputStream* is the stream from which data is read. To read from a file, you can use the object created by **FileStream** for this parameter. If *inputStream* has not been opened for reading or is otherwise invalid, **ArgumentException** is thrown.

BinaryReader provides methods for reading all of C#'s simple types. Several commonly used methods are shown in Table 14-6. Notice that **ReadString( )** reads a **string** that is stored using its internal format, which includes a length specifier. These methods throw an **IOException** if an error occurs. (Other exceptions are also possible.)

Method	Description
void Write(sbyte *val*)	Writes a signed byte.
void Write(byte *val*)	Writes an unsigned byte.
void Write(byte[ ] *buf*)	Writes an array of bytes.
void Write(short *val*)	Writes a short integer.
void Write(ushort *val*)	Writes an unsigned short integer.
void Write(int *val*)	Writes an integer.
void Write(uint *val*)	Writes an unsigned integer.
void Write(long *val*)	Writes a long integer.
void Write(ulong *val*)	Writes an unsigned long integer.
void Write(float *val*)	Writes a **float**.
void Write(double *val*)	Writes a **double**.
void Write(char *val*)	Writes a character.
void Write(char[ ] *buf*)	Writes an array of characters.
void Write(string *val*)	Writes a **string** using its internal representation, which includes a length specifier.

TABLE 14-5 Commonly Used Output Methods Defined by **BinaryWriter**

BinaryReader also defines three versions of **Read( )**, which are shown here:

Method	Description
int Read( )	Returns an integer representation of the next available character from the invoking input stream. Returns −1 when attempting to read at the end of the file.
int Read(byte[ ] *buf*, int *offset*, int *num*)	Attempts to read up to *num* bytes into *buf* starting at *buf*[*offset*], returning the number of bytes successfully read.
int Read(char[ ] *buf*, int *offset*, int *num*)	Attempts to read up to *num* characters into *buf* starting at *buf*[*offset*], returning the number of characters successfully read.

These methods will throw an **IOException** on failure. Other exceptions are possible. Also defined is the standard **Close( )** method.

Method	Description
bool ReadBoolean( )	Reads a **bool**.
byte ReadByte( )	Reads a **byte**.
sbyte ReadSByte( )	Reads an **sbyte**.
byte[ ] ReadBytes(int *num*)	Reads *num* bytes and returns them as an array.
char ReadChar( )	Reads a **char**.
char[ ] ReadChars(int *num*)	Reads *num* characters and returns them as an array.
double ReadDouble( )	Reads a **double**.
float ReadSingle( )	Reads a **float**.
short ReadInt16( )	Reads a **short**.
int ReadInt32( )	Reads an **int**.
long ReadInt64( )	Reads a **long**.
ushort ReadUInt16( )	Reads a **ushort**.
uint ReadUInt32( )	Reads a **uint**.
ulong ReadUInt64( )	Reads a **ulong**.
string ReadString( )	Reads a **string** that is represented in its internal, binary format, which includes a length specifier. This method should only be used to read a string that has been written using a **BinaryWriter**.

TABLE 14-6   Commonly Used Input Methods Defined by **BinaryReader**

Demonstrating Binary I/O

Here is a program that demonstrates **BinaryReader** and **BinaryWriter**. It writes and then reads back various types of data to and from a file.

```
// Write and then read back binary data.

using System;
using System.IO;

class RWData {
  static void Main() {
    BinaryWriter dataOut;
    BinaryReader dataIn;

    int i = 10;
    double d = 1023.56;
    bool b = true;
    string str = "This is a test";
    try {
      dataOut = new
        BinaryWriter(new FileStream("testdata", FileMode.Create));
    }
    catch(IOException exc) {
      Console.WriteLine("Cannot Open File For Output");
      Console.WriteLine(exc.Message);
      return;
    }

    // Write data to a file.
    try {
      Console.WriteLine("Writing " + i);
      dataOut.Write(i);

      Console.WriteLine("Writing " + d);
      dataOut.Write(d);

      Console.WriteLine("Writing " + b);
      dataOut.Write(b);

      Console.WriteLine("Writing " + 12.2 * 7.4);
      dataOut.Write(12.2 * 7.4);

      Console.WriteLine("Writing " + str);
      dataOut.Write(str);
    }
    catch(IOException exc) {
      Console.WriteLine("Error Writing File");
      Console.WriteLine(exc.Message);
    }

    dataOut.Close();

    Console.WriteLine();
```

```
        // Now, read the data.
        try {
          dataIn = new
              BinaryReader(new FileStream("testdata", FileMode.Open));
        }
        catch(IOException exc) {
          Console.WriteLine("Cannot Open File For Input");
          Console.WriteLine(exc.Message);
          return;
        }

        try {
          i = dataIn.ReadInt32();
          Console.WriteLine("Reading " + i);

          d = dataIn.ReadDouble();
          Console.WriteLine("Reading " + d);

          b = dataIn.ReadBoolean();
          Console.WriteLine("Reading " + b);

          d = dataIn.ReadDouble();
          Console.WriteLine("Reading " + d);

          str = dataIn.ReadString();
          Console.WriteLine("Reading " + str);
        }
        catch(IOException exc) {
          Console.WriteLine("Error Reading File");
          Console.WriteLine(exc.Message);
        }

        dataIn.Close();
    }
}
```

The output from the program is shown here:

```
Writing 10
Writing 1023.56
Writing True
Writing 90.28
Writing This is a test

Reading 10
Reading 1023.56
Reading True
Reading 90.28
Reading This is a test
```

If you examine the **testdata** file produced by this program, you will find that it contains binary data, not human-readable text.

Here is a more practical example that shows how powerful binary I/O is. The following program implements a very simple inventory program. For each item in the inventory, the

program stores the item's name, the number on hand, and its cost. Next, the program prompts the user for the name of an item. It then searches the database. If the item is found, the inventory information is displayed.

```csharp
/* Use BinaryReader and BinaryWriter to implement
   a simple inventory program. */

using System;
using System.IO;

class Inventory {
  static void Main() {
    BinaryWriter dataOut;
    BinaryReader dataIn;

    string item; // name of item
    int onhand;  // number on hand
    double cost; // cost

    try {
      dataOut = new
        BinaryWriter(new FileStream("inventory.dat",
                                    FileMode.Create));
    }
    catch(IOException exc) {
      Console.WriteLine("Cannot Open Inventory File For Output");
      Console.WriteLine(exc.Message);
      return;
    }

    // Write some inventory data to the file.
    try {
      dataOut.Write("Hammers");
      dataOut.Write(10);
      dataOut.Write(3.95);

      dataOut.Write("Screwdrivers");
      dataOut.Write(18);
      dataOut.Write(1.50);

      dataOut.Write("Pliers");
      dataOut.Write(5);
      dataOut.Write(4.95);

      dataOut.Write("Saws");
      dataOut.Write(8);
      dataOut.Write(8.95);
    }
    catch(IOException exc) {
      Console.WriteLine("Error Writing Inventory File");
      Console.WriteLine(exc.Message);
    }

    dataOut.Close();
```

```
      Console.WriteLine();

      // Now, open inventory file for reading.
      try {
        dataIn = new
            BinaryReader(new FileStream("inventory.dat",
                          FileMode.Open));
      }
      catch(IOException exc) {
        Console.WriteLine("Cannot Open Inventory File For Input");
        Console.WriteLine(exc.Message);
        return;
      }

      // Lookup item entered by user.
      Console.Write("Enter item to lookup: ");
      string what = Console.ReadLine();
      Console.WriteLine();

      try {
        for(;;) {
          // Read an inventory entry.
          item = dataIn.ReadString();
          onhand = dataIn.ReadInt32();
          cost = dataIn.ReadDouble();

          // See if the item matches the one requested.
          // If so, display information.
          if(item.CompareTo(what) == 0) {
            Console.WriteLine(onhand + " " + item + " on hand. " +
                            "Cost: {0:C} each", cost);
            Console.WriteLine("Total value of {0}: {1:C}." ,
                            item, cost * onhand);
            break;
          }
        }
      }
      catch(EndOfStreamException) {
        Console.WriteLine("Item not found.");
      }
      catch(IOException exc) {
        Console.WriteLine("Error Reading Inventory File");
        Console.WriteLine(exc.Message);
      }

      dataIn.Close();
    }
  }
```

Here is a sample run:

```
Enter item to look up: Screwdrivers

18 Screwdrivers on hand. Cost: $1.50 each
Total value of Screwdrivers: $27.00.
```

In the program, notice how inventory information is stored in its binary format. Thus, the number of items on hand and the cost is stored using their binary format rather than their human-readable text-based equivalents. This makes it is possible to perform computations on the numeric data without having to convert it from its human-readable form.

There is one other point of interest in the inventory program. Notice how the end of the file is detected. Since the binary input methods throw an **EndOfStreamException** when the end of the stream is reached, the program simply reads the file until either it finds the desired item or this exception is generated. Thus, no special mechanism is needed to detect the end of the file.

Random Access Files

Up to this point, we have been using *sequential files*, which are files that are accessed in a strictly linear fashion, one byte after another. However, you can also access the contents of a file in random order. One way to do this is to use the **Seek( )** method defined by **FileStream**. This method allows you to set the *file position indicator* (also called the *file pointer* or simply the *current position*) to any point within a file.

The method **Seek( )** is shown here:

long Seek(long *newPos*, SeekOrigin *origin*)

Here, *newPos* specifies the new position, in bytes, of the file pointer from the location specified by *origin*. The origin will be one of these values, which are defined by the **SeekOrigin** enumeration:

Value	Meaning
SeekOrigin.Begin	Seek from the beginning of the file.
SeekOrigin.Current	Seek from the current location.
SeekOrigin.End	Seek from the end of the file.

After a call to **Seek( )**, the next read or write operation will occur at the new file position. The new position is returned. If an error occurs while seeking, an **IOException** is thrown. If the underlying stream does not support position requests, a **NotSupportedException** is thrown. Other exceptions are possible.

Here is an example that demonstrates random access I/O. It writes the uppercase alphabet to a file and then reads it back in nonsequential order.

```
// Demonstrate random access.

using System;
using System.IO;

class RandomAccessDemo {
  static void Main() {
    FileStream f;
    char ch;
    try {
      f = new FileStream("random.dat", FileMode.Create);
    }
```

```
    catch(IOException exc) {
      Console.WriteLine("Cannot Open File");
      Console.WriteLine(exc.Message);
      return ;
    }

    // Write the alphabet.
    for(int i=0; i < 26; i++) {
      try {
        f.WriteByte((byte)('A'+i));
      }
      catch(IOException exc) {
        Console.WriteLine("Error Writing File");
        Console.WriteLine(exc.Message);
        f.Close();
        return ;
      }
    }

    try {
      // Now, read back specific values.
      f.Seek(0, SeekOrigin.Begin); // seek to first byte
      ch = (char) f.ReadByte();
      Console.WriteLine("First value is " + ch);

      f.Seek(1, SeekOrigin.Begin); // seek to second byte
      ch = (char) f.ReadByte();
      Console.WriteLine("Second value is " + ch);

      f.Seek(4, SeekOrigin.Begin); // seek to 5th byte
      ch = (char) f.ReadByte();
      Console.WriteLine("Fifth value is " + ch);

      Console.WriteLine();

      // Now, read every other value.
      Console.WriteLine("Here is every other value: ");
      for(int i=0; i < 26; i += 2) {
        f.Seek(i, SeekOrigin.Begin); // seek to ith character
        ch = (char) f.ReadByte();
        Console.Write(ch + " ");
      }
    }
    catch(IOException exc) {
      Console.WriteLine("Error Reading or Seeking");
      Console.WriteLine(exc.Message);
    }

    Console.WriteLine();
    f.Close();
  }
}
```

The output from the program is shown here:

```
First value is A
Second value is B
Fifth value is E

Here is every other value:
A C E G I K M O Q S U W Y
```

Although **Seek( )** offers the greatest flexibility, there is another way to set the current file position. You can use the **Position** property. As shown previously in Table 14-2, **Position** is a read/write property. Therefore, you can use it to obtain the current position or to set the current position. For example, here is the code sequence from the preceding program that reads the "random.dat" file, rewritten to use the **Position** property:

```
// Use Position rather than Seek() to set the current
// file position.
try {
  f.Position = 0;
  ch = (char) f.ReadByte();
  Console.WriteLine("First value is " + ch);

  f.Position = 1;
  ch = (char) f.ReadByte();
  Console.WriteLine("Second value is " + ch);

  f.Position = 4;
  ch = (char) f.ReadByte();
  Console.WriteLine("Fifth value is " + ch);

  Console.WriteLine();

  // Now, read every other value.
  Console.WriteLine("Here is every other value: ");
  for(int i=0; i < 26; i += 2) {
    f.Position = i; // seek to ith character
    ch = (char) f.ReadByte();
    Console.Write(ch + " ");
  }
}
catch(IOException exc) {
  Console.WriteLine("Error Reading or Seeking");
  Console.WriteLine(exc.Message);
}
```

Using MemoryStream

Sometimes it is useful to read input from or to write output to an array, rather than directly from or to a device. To do this, you will use **MemoryStream**. **MemoryStream** is an implementation of **Stream** that uses an array of bytes for input and/or output. **MemoryStream** defines several constructors. Here is the one we will use:

MemoryStream(byte[ ] *buf*)

Here, *buf* is an array of bytes that will be used for the source and/or target of I/O requests. The stream created by this constructor can be written or read, and supports **Seek( )**. When using this constructor, you must remember to make *buf* large enough to hold whatever output you will be directing to it.

Here is a program that demonstrates the use of **MemoryStream**:

```
// Demonstrate MemoryStream.

using System;
using System.IO;

class MemStrDemo {
  static void Main() {
    byte[] storage = new byte[255];

    // Create a memory-based stream.
    MemoryStream memstrm = new MemoryStream(storage);

    // Wrap memstrm in a reader and a writer.
    StreamWriter memwtr = new StreamWriter(memstrm);
    StreamReader memrdr = new StreamReader(memstrm);

    // Write to storage, through memwtr.
    for(int i=0; i < 10; i++)
      memwtr.WriteLine("byte [" + i + "]: " + i);

    // Put a period at the end.
    memwtr.WriteLine(".");

    memwtr.Flush();

    Console.WriteLine("Reading from storage directly: ");

    // Display contents of storage directly.
    foreach(char ch in storage) {
      if (ch == '.') break;
      Console.Write(ch);
    }

    Console.WriteLine("\nReading through memrdr: ");

    // Read from memstrm using the stream reader.
    memstrm.Seek(0, SeekOrigin.Begin); // reset file pointer

    string str = memrdr.ReadLine();
    while(str != null) {
      str = memrdr.ReadLine();
      if(str.CompareTo(".") == 0) break;
      Console.WriteLine(str);
    }
  }
}
```

The output from the program is shown here:

```
Reading from storage directly:
byte [0]: 0
byte [1]: 1
byte [2]: 2
byte [3]: 3
byte [4]: 4
byte [5]: 5
byte [6]: 6
byte [7]: 7
byte [8]: 8
byte [9]: 9

Reading through memrdr:
byte [1]: 1
byte [2]: 2
byte [3]: 3
byte [4]: 4
byte [5]: 5
byte [6]: 6
byte [7]: 7
byte [8]: 8
byte [9]: 9
```

In the program, an array of bytes called **storage** is created. This array is then used as the underlying storage for a **MemoryStream** called **memstrm**. From **memstrm** are created a **StreamReader** called **memrdr** and a **StreamWriter** called **memwtr**. Using **memwtr**, output is written to the memory-based stream. Notice that after the output has been written, **Flush( )** is called on **memwtr**. This is necessary to ensure that the contents of **memwtr**'s buffer are actually written to the underlying array. Next, the contents of the underlying byte array are displayed manually, using a **foreach** loop. Then, using **Seek( )**, the file pointer is reset to the start of the stream, and the memory stream is read using **memrdr**.

Memory-based streams are quite useful in programming. For example, you can construct complicated output in advance, storing it in the array until it is needed. This technique is especially useful when programming for a GUI environment, such as Windows. You can also redirect a standard stream to read from an array. This might be useful for feeding test information into a program, for example.

Using StringReader and StringWriter

For some applications, it might be easier to use a **string** rather than a **byte** array for the underlying storage when performing memory-based I/O operations. When this is the case, use **StringReader** and **StringWriter**. **StringReader** inherits **TextReader**, and **StringWriter** inherits **TextWriter**. Thus, these streams have access to methods defined by those two classes. For example, you can call **ReadLine( )** on a **StringReader** and **WriteLine( )** on a **StringWriter**.

The constructor for **StringReader** is shown here:

StringReader(string *str*)

Here, *str* is the string that will be read from.

StringWriter defines several constructors. Here is the one that we will use:

StringWriter( )

This constructor creates a writer that will put its output into a string. This string (in the form of a **StringBuilder**) is automatically created by **StringWriter**. You can obtain the contents of this string by calling **ToString( )**.

Here is an example that uses **StringReader** and **StringWriter**:

```
// Demonstrate StringReader and StringWriter.

using System;
using System.IO;

class StrRdrDemo {
  static void Main() {
    // Create a StringWriter.
    StringWriter strwtr = new StringWriter();

    // Write to StringWriter.
    for(int i=0; i < 10; i++)
      strwtr.WriteLine("This is i: " + i);

    // Create a StringReader.
    StringReader strrdr = new StringReader(strwtr.ToString());

    // Now, read from StringReader.
    string str = strrdr.ReadLine();
    while(str != null) {
      str = strrdr.ReadLine();
      Console.WriteLine(str);
    }
  }
}
```

The output is shown here:

```
This is i: 1
This is i: 2
This is i: 3
This is i: 4
This is i: 5
This is i: 6
This is i: 7
This is i: 8
This is i: 9
```

The program first creates a **StringWriter** called **strwtr** and outputs to it using **WriteLine( )**. Next, it creates a **StringReader** using the string contained in **strwtr**. This string is obtained by calling **ToString( )** on **strwtr**. Finally, the contents of this string are read using **ReadLine( )**.

Converting Numeric Strings to Their Internal Representation

Before leaving the topic of I/O, we will examine a technique useful when reading numeric strings. As you know, **WriteLine( )** provides a convenient way to output various types of data to the console, including numeric values of the built-in types, such as **int** and **double**. Thus, **WriteLine( )** automatically converts numeric values into their human-readable form. However, a parallel input method that reads and converts strings containing numeric values into their internal, binary format is not provided. For example, there is no version of **Read( )** that reads from the keyboard a string such as "100" and then automatically converts it into its corresponding binary value that can be stored in an **int** variable. Instead, there are other ways to accomplish this task. Perhaps the easiest is to use a method that is defined for all of the built-in numeric types: **Parse( )**.

Before we begin, it is necessary to state an important fact: All of C#'s built-in types, such as **int** and **double**, are actually just *aliases* (that is, other names) for structures defined by the .NET framework. In fact, the C# type and .NET structure type are indistinguishable. One is just another name for the other. Because C#'s value types are supported by structures, the value types have members defined for them.

For the numeric types, the .NET structure names and their C# keyword equivalents are shown here:

.NET Structure Name	C# Name
Decimal	decimal
Double	double
Single	float
Int16	short
Int32	int
Int64	long
UInt16	ushort
UInt32	uint
UInt64	ulong
Byte	byte
SByte	sbyte

These structures are defined inside the **System** namespace. Thus, the fully qualified name for **Int32** is **System.Int32**. These structures offer a wide array of methods that help fully integrate the value types into C#'s object hierarchy. As a side benefit, the numeric structures also define a static method called **Parse( )** that converts a numeric string into its corresponding binary equivalent.

There are several overloaded forms of **Parse( )**. The simplest version for each numeric structure is shown here. It performs the conversion using the default locale and numeric style. (Other versions let you perform locale-specific conversions and specify the numeric style.) Notice that each method returns a binary value that corresponds to the string.

Structure	Conversion Method
Decimal	static decimal Parse(string *str*)
Double	static double Parse(string *str*)
Single	static float Parse(string *str*)
Int64	static long Parse(string *str*)
Int32	static int Parse(string *str*)
Int16	static short Parse(string *str*)
UInt64	static ulong Parse(string *str*)
UInt32	static uint Parse(string *str*)
UInt16	static ushort Parse(string *str*)
Byte	static byte Parse(string *str*)
SByte	static sbyte Parse(string *str*)

The **Parse( )** methods will throw a **FormatException** if *str* does not contain a valid number as defined by the invoking type. **ArgumentNullException** is thrown if *str* is null, and **OverflowException** is thrown if the value in *str* exceeds the bounds of the invoking type.

The parsing methods give you an easy way to convert a numeric value, read as a string from the keyboard or a text file, into its proper internal format. For example, the following program averages a list of numbers entered by the user. It first asks the user for the number of values to be averaged. It then reads that number using **ReadLine( )** and uses **Int32.Parse( )** to convert the string into an integer. Next, it inputs the values, using **Double.Parse( )** to convert the strings into their **double** equivalents.

```
// This program averages a list of numbers entered by the user.

using System;
using System.IO;

class AvgNums {
  static void Main() {
    string str;
    int n;
    double sum = 0.0;
    double avg, t;

    Console.Write("How many numbers will you enter: ");
    str = Console.ReadLine();
    try {
      n = Int32.Parse(str);
    } catch(FormatException exc) {
      Console.WriteLine(exc.Message);
      return;
    } catch(OverflowException exc) {
      Console.WriteLine(exc.Message);
      return;
    }
```

```
      Console.WriteLine("Enter " + n + " values.");
      for(int i=0; i < n ; i++)   {
        Console.Write(": ");
        str = Console.ReadLine();
        try {
          t = Double.Parse(str);
        } catch(FormatException exc) {
          Console.WriteLine(exc.Message);
          t = 0.0;
        } catch(OverflowException exc) {
          Console.WriteLine(exc.Message);
          t = 0;
        }
        sum += t;
      }
      avg = sum / n;
      Console.WriteLine("Average is " + avg);
  }
}
```

Here is a sample run:

```
How many numbers will you enter: 5
Enter 5 values.
 : 1.1
 : 2.2
 : 3.3
 : 4.4
 : 5.5
Average is 3.3
```

One other point: You must use the right parsing method for the type of value you are trying to convert. For example, trying to use **Int32.Parse( )** on a string that contains a floating-point value will not produce the desired result.

As explained, **Parse( )** will throw an exception on failure. You can avoid generating an exception when converting numeric strings by using the **TryParse( )** method, which is defined for all of the numeric structures. Here is an example. It shows one version of **TryParse( )** as defined by **Int32**.

static bool TryParse(string *str*, out int *result*)

The numeric string is passed in *str*. The result is returned in *result*. It performs the conversion using the default locale and numeric style. (A second version of **TryParse( )** is available that lets you specify the numeric style and locale.) If the conversion fails, such as when *str* does not contain a numeric string in the proper form, **TryParse( )** returns false. Otherwise, it returns true. Therefore, you must check the return value to confirm that a successful conversion has occurred.

Delegates, Events, and Lambda Expressions

This chapter examines three innovative C# features: delegates, events, and lambda expressions. A *delegate* provides a way to encapsulate a method. An *event* is a notification that some action has occurred. Delegates and events are related because an event is built upon a delegate. Both expand the set of programming tasks to which C# can be applied. The *lambda expression* is a new syntactic feature provided by C# 3.0. It offers a streamlined, yet powerful way to define what is, essentially, a unit of executable code. Lambda expressions are often used when working with delegates and events because a delegate can refer to a lambda expression. (Lambda expressions are also very important to LINQ, which is described in Chapter 19.) Also examined are anonymous methods, covariance, contravariance, and method group conversions.

Delegates

Let's begin by defining the term *delegate*. In straightforward language, a delegate is an object that can refer to a method. Therefore, when you create a delegate, you are creating an object that can hold a reference to a method. Furthermore, the method can be called through this reference. In other words, a delegate can invoke the method to which it refers. As you will see, this is a very powerful concept.

It is important to understand that the same delegate can be used to call different methods during the runtime of a program by simply changing the method to which the delegate refers. Thus, the method that will be invoked by a delegate is not determined at compile time, but rather at runtime. This is the principal advantage of a delegate.

NOTE *If you are familiar with C/C++, then it will help to know that a delegate in C# is similar to a function pointer in C/C++.*

A delegate type is declared using the keyword **delegate**. The general form of a delegate declaration is shown here:

delegate *ret-type name(parameter-list);*

Here, *ret-type* is the type of value returned by the methods that the delegate will be calling. The name of the delegate is specified by *name*. The parameters required by the methods called through the delegate are specified in the *parameter-list*. Once created, a delegate instance can refer to and call methods whose return type and parameter list match those specified by the delegate declaration.

A key point to understand is that a delegate can be used to call *any* method that agrees with its signature and return type. Furthermore, the method can be either an instance method associated with an object or a **static** method associated with a class. All that matters is that the return type and signature of the method agree with those of the delegate.

To see delegates in action, let's begin with the simple example shown here:

```
// A simple delegate example.

using System;

// Declare a delegate type.
delegate string StrMod(string str);

class DelegateTest {
  // Replaces spaces with hyphens.
  static string ReplaceSpaces(string s) {
    Console.WriteLine("Replacing spaces with hyphens.");
    return s.Replace(' ', '-');
  }

  // Remove spaces.
  static string RemoveSpaces(string s) {
    string temp = "";
    int i;

    Console.WriteLine("Removing spaces.");
    for(i=0; i < s.Length; i++)
      if(s[i] != ' ') temp += s[i];

    return temp;
  }

  // Reverse a string.
  static string Reverse(string s) {
    string temp = "";
    int i, j;

    Console.WriteLine("Reversing string.");
    for(j=0, i=s.Length-1; i >= 0; i--, j++)
      temp += s[i];

    return temp;
  }

  static void Main() {
    // Construct a delegate.
    StrMod strOp = new StrMod(ReplaceSpaces);
    string str;
```

```
    // Call methods through the delegate.
    str = strOp("This is a test.");
    Console.WriteLine("Resulting string: " + str);
    Console.WriteLine();

    strOp = new StrMod(RemoveSpaces);
    str = strOp("This is a test.");
    Console.WriteLine("Resulting string: " + str);
    Console.WriteLine();

    strOp = new StrMod(Reverse);
    str = strOp("This is a test.");
    Console.WriteLine("Resulting string: " + str);
  }
}
```

The output from the program is shown here:

```
Replacing spaces with hyphens.
Resulting string: This-is-a-test.

Removing spaces.
Resulting string: Thisisatest.

Reversing string.
Resulting string: .tset a si sihT
```

Let's examine this program closely. The program declares a delegate type called **StrMod**, shown here:

```
delegate string StrMod(string str);
```

Notice that **StrMod** takes one **string** parameter and returns a **string**.

Next, in **DelegateTest**, three **static** methods are declared, each with a single parameter of type **string** and a return type of **string**. Thus, they match the **StrMod** delegate. These methods perform some type of string modification. Notice that **ReplaceSpaces( )** uses one of **string**'s methods, called **Replace( )**, to replace spaces with hyphens.

In **Main( )**, a **StrMod** reference called **strOp** is created and assigned a reference to **ReplaceSpaces( )**. Pay close attention to this line:

```
StrMod strOp = new StrMod(ReplaceSpaces);
```

Notice how the method **ReplaceSpaces( )** is passed as a parameter. Only its name is used; no parameters are specified. This can be generalized. When instantiating a delegate, you specify only the name of the method to which you want the delegate to refer. Of course, the method's signature must match that of the delegate's declaration. If it doesn't, a compile-time error will result.

Next, **ReplaceSpaces( )** is called through the delegate instance **strOp**, as shown here:

```
str = strOp("This is a test.");
```

Because **strOp** refers to **ReplaceSpaces( )**, **ReplaceSpaces( )** is invoked.

Next, **strOp** is assigned a reference to **RemoveSpaces( )**, and then **strOp** is called again. This time, **RemoveSpaces( )** is invoked.

Finally, **strOp** is assigned a reference to **Reverse( )** and **strOp** is called. This results in **Reverse( )** being called.

The key point of the example is that the invocation of **strOp** results in a call to the method referred to by **strOp** at the time at which the invocation occurs. Thus, the method to call is resolved at runtime, not compile time.

Delegate Method Group Conversion

Beginning with version 2.0, C# has included an option that significantly simplifies the syntax that assigns a method to a delegate. This feature is called *method group conversion*, and it allows you to simply assign the name of a method to a delegate, without using **new** or explicitly invoking the delegate's constructor.

For example, here is the **Main( )** method of the preceding program rewritten to use method group conversions:

```
static void Main() {
  // Construct a delegate using method group conversion.
  StrMod strOp = ReplaceSpaces; // use method group conversion
  string str;

  // Call methods through the delegate.
  str = strOp("This is a test.");
  Console.WriteLine("Resulting string: " + str);
  Console.WriteLine();

  strOp = RemoveSpaces; // use method group conversion
  str = strOp("This is a test.");
  Console.WriteLine("Resulting string: " + str);
  Console.WriteLine();

  strOp = Reverse; // use method group conversion
  str = strOp("This is a test.");
  Console.WriteLine("Resulting string: " + str);
}
```

Pay special attention to the way that **strOp** is created and assigned the method **ReplaceSpaces** in this line:

```
StrMod strOp = ReplaceSpaces; // use method group conversion
```

The name of the method is assigned directly to **strOp**. C# automatically provides a conversion from the method to the delegate type. This syntax can be generalized to any situation in which a method is assigned to (or converted to) a delegate type.

Because the method group conversion syntax is simpler than the old approach, it is used throughout the remainder of this book.

Using Instance Methods as Delegates

Although the preceding example used **static** methods, a delegate can also refer to instance methods. It must do so, however, through an object reference. For example, here is a rewrite of the previous example, which encapsulates the string operations inside a class called

StringOps. Notice that the method group conversion syntax can also be applied in this situation.

```
// Delegates can refer to instance methods, too.

using System;

// Declare a delegate type.
delegate string StrMod(string str);

class StringOps {
  // Replaces spaces with hyphens.
  public string ReplaceSpaces(string s) {
    Console.WriteLine("Replacing spaces with hyphens.");
    return s.Replace(' ', '-');
  }

  // Remove spaces.
  public string RemoveSpaces(string s) {
    string temp = "";
    int i;

    Console.WriteLine("Removing spaces.");
    for(i=0; i < s.Length; i++)
      if(s[i] != ' ') temp += s[i];

    return temp;
  }

  // Reverse a string.
  public string Reverse(string s) {
    string temp = "";
    int i, j;

    Console.WriteLine("Reversing string.");
    for(j=0, i=s.Length-1; i >= 0; i--, j++)
      temp += s[i];

    return temp;
  }
}

class DelegateTest {
  static void Main() {
    StringOps so = new StringOps(); // create an instance of StringOps

    // Initialize a delegate.
    StrMod strOp = so.ReplaceSpaces;
    string str;

    // Call methods through delegates.
    str = strOp("This is a test.");
    Console.WriteLine("Resulting string: " + str);
    Console.WriteLine();
```

```
  strOp = so.RemoveSpaces;
  str = strOp("This is a test.");
  Console.WriteLine("Resulting string: " + str);
  Console.WriteLine();

  strOp = so.Reverse;
  str = strOp("This is a test.");
  Console.WriteLine("Resulting string: " + str);
  }
}
```

This program produces the same output as the first, but in this case, the delegate refers to methods on an instance of **StringOps**.

Multicasting

One of the most exciting features of a delegate is its support for *multicasting*. In simple terms, multicasting is the ability to create an *invocation list*, or chain, of methods that will be automatically called when a delegate is invoked. Such a chain is very easy to create. Simply instantiate a delegate, and then use the **+** or **+=** operator to add methods to the chain. To remove a method, use **–** or **– =**. If the delegate returns a value, then the value returned by the last method in the list becomes the return value of the entire delegate invocation. Thus, a delegate that makes use of multicasting will often have a **void** return type.

Here is an example of multicasting. Notice that it reworks the preceding examples by changing the string manipulation method's return type to **void** and using a **ref** parameter to return the altered string to the caller. This makes the methods more appropriate for multicasting.

```
// Demonstrate multicasting.

using System;

// Declare a delegate type.
delegate void StrMod(ref string str);

class MultiCastDemo {
  // Replaces spaces with hyphens.
  static void ReplaceSpaces(ref string s) {
    Console.WriteLine("Replacing spaces with hyphens.");
    s = s.Replace(' ', '-');
  }

  // Remove spaces.
  static void RemoveSpaces(ref string s) {
    string temp = "";
    int i;

    Console.WriteLine("Removing spaces.");
    for(i=0; i < s.Length; i++)
      if(s[i] != ' ') temp += s[i];

    s = temp;
  }
```

```csharp
    // Reverse a string.
    static void Reverse(ref string s) {
      string temp = "";
      int i, j;

      Console.WriteLine("Reversing string.");
      for(j=0, i=s.Length-1; i >= 0; i--, j++)
        temp += s[i];

      s = temp;
    }

    static void Main() {
      // Construct delegates.
      StrMod strOp;
      StrMod replaceSp = ReplaceSpaces;
      StrMod removeSp = RemoveSpaces;
      StrMod reverseStr = Reverse;
      string str = "This is a test";

      // Set up multicast.
      strOp = replaceSp;
      strOp += reverseStr;

      // Call multicast.
      strOp(ref str);
      Console.WriteLine("Resulting string: " + str);
      Console.WriteLine();

      // Remove replace and add remove.
      strOp -= replaceSp;
      strOp += removeSp;

      str = "This is a test."; // reset string

      // Call multicast.
      strOp(ref str);
      Console.WriteLine("Resulting string: " + str);
      Console.WriteLine();
    }
}
```

Here is the output:

```
Replacing spaces with hyphens.
Reversing string.
Resulting string: tset-a-si-sihT

Reversing string.
Removing spaces.
Resulting string: .tsetasisihT
```

In **Main( )**, four delegate instances are created. One, **strOp**, is null. The other three refer to specific string modification methods. Next, a multicast is created that calls **RemoveSpaces( )** and **Reverse( )**. This is accomplished via the following lines:

```
strOp = replaceSp;
strOp += reverseStr;
```

First, **strOp** is assigned **replaceSp**. Next, using **+=**, **reverseStr** is added. When **strOp** is invoked, both methods are invoked, replacing spaces with hyphens and reversing the string, as the output illustrates.

Next, **replaceSp** is removed from the chain, using this line:

```
strOp -= replaceSp;
```

and **removeSP** is added using this line:

```
strOp += removeSp;
```

Then, **strOp** is again invoked. This time, spaces are removed and the string is reversed.

Delegate chains are a powerful mechanism because they allow you to define a set of methods that can be executed as a unit. This can increase the structure of some types of code. Also, as you will soon see, delegate chains have a special value to events.

Covariance and Contravariance

There are two features that add flexibility to delegates: *covariance* and *contravariance*. Normally, the method that you pass to a delegate must have the same return type and signature as the delegate. However, covariance and contravariance relax this rule slightly, as it pertains to derived types. Covariance enables a method to be assigned to a delegate when the method's return type is a class derived from the class specified by the return type of the delegate. Contravariance enables a method to be assigned to a delegate when a method's parameter type is a base class of the class specified by the delegate's declaration.

Here is an example that illustrates both covariance and contravariance:

```
// Demonstrate covariance and contravariance.

using System;

class X {
  public int Val;
}

// Y is derived from X.
class Y : X { }

// This delegate returns X and takes a Y argument.
delegate X ChangeIt(Y obj);

class CoContraVariance {

  // This method returns X and has an X parameter.
```

```
static X IncrA(X obj) {
  X temp = new X();
  temp.Val = obj.Val + 1;
  return temp;
}

// This method returns Y and has a Y parameter.
static Y IncrB(Y obj) {
  Y temp = new Y();
  temp.Val = obj.Val + 1;
  return temp;
}

static void Main() {
  Y Yob = new Y();

  // In this case, the parameter to IncrA
  // is X and the parameter to ChangeIt is Y.
  // Because of contravariance, the following
  // line is OK.
  ChangeIt change = IncrA;

  X Xob = change(Yob);

  Console.WriteLine("Xob: " + Xob.Val);

  // In the next case, the return type of
  // IncrB is Y and the return type of
  // ChangeIt is X. Because of covariance,
  // the following line is OK.
  change = IncrB;

  Yob = (Y) change(Yob);

  Console.WriteLine("Yob: " + Yob.Val);
  }
}
```

The output from the program is shown here:

```
Xob: 1
Yob: 1
```

In the program, notice that class **Y** is derived from class **X**. Next, notice that the delegate **ChangeIt( )** is declared like this:

```
delegate X ChangeIt(Y obj);
```

ChangeIt( ) returns **X** and has a **Y** parameter. Next, notice that the methods **IncrA( )** and **IncrB( )** are declared as shown here:

```
static X IncrA(X obj)
static Y IncrB(Y obj)
```

The **IncrA( )** method has an **X** parameter and returns **X**. The **IncrB( )** method has a **Y** parameter and returns **Y**. Given covariance and contravariance, either of these methods can be passed to **ChangeIt**, as the program illustrates.

Therefore, this line

```
ChangeIt change = IncrA;
```

uses contravariance to enable **IncrA( )** to be passed to the delegate because **IncrA( )** has an **X** parameter, but the delegate has a **Y** parameter. This works because, with contravariance, if the parameter type of the method passed to a delegate is a base class of the parameter type used by the delegate, then the method and the delegate are compatible.

The next line is also legal, but this time it is because of covariance:

```
change = IncrB;
```

In this case, the return type of **IncrB( )** is **Y**, but the return type of **ChangeIt( )** is **X**. However, because the return type of the method is a class derived from the return type of the delegate, the two are compatible.

System.Delegate

All delegates are classes that are implicitly derived from **System.Delegate**. You don't normally need to use its members directly, and this book makes no explicit use of **System.Delegate**. However, its members may be useful in certain specialized situations.

Why Delegates

Although the preceding examples show the "how" behind delegates, they don't really illustrate the "why." In general, delegates are useful for two main reasons. First, as shown later in this chapter, delegates support events. Second, delegates give your program a way to execute methods at runtime without having to know precisely what those methods are at compile time. This ability is quite useful when you want to create a framework that allows components to be plugged in. For example, imagine a drawing program (a bit like the standard Windows Paint accessory). Using a delegate, you could allow the user to plug in special color filters or image analyzers. Furthermore, the user could create a sequence of these filters or analyzers. Such a scheme could be easily handled using a delegate.

Anonymous Functions

You will often find that the method referred to by a delegate is used only for that purpose. In other words, the only reason for the method is so it can be invoked via a delegate. The method is never called on its own. In such a case, you can avoid the need to create a separate method by using an *anonymous function*. An anonymous function is, essentially, an unnamed block of code that is passed to a delegate constructor. One advantage to using an anonymous function is simplicity. There is no need to declare a separate method whose only purpose is to be passed to a delegate.

Beginning with version 3.0, C# defines two types of anonymous functions: *anonymous methods* and *lambda expressions*. The anonymous method was added by C# 2.0. The lambda expression was added by C# 3.0. In general, the lambda expression improves on the concept

of the anonymous method and is now the preferred approach to creating an anonymous function. However, anonymous methods are widely used in existing C# code. Therefore, they are still an important part of C#. Furthermore, anonymous methods are the precursor to lambda expressions and a clear understanding of anonymous methods makes it easier to understand aspects of the lambda expression. Also, there is a narrow set of cases in which an anonymous method can be used, but a lambda expression cannot. Therefore, both anonymous methods and lambda expressions are described in this chapter.

Anonymous Methods

An anonymous method is one way to create an unnamed block of code that is associated with a specific delegate instance. An anonymous method is created by following the keyword **delegate** with a block of code. To see how this is done, let's begin with a simple example. The following program uses an anonymous method that counts from 0 to 5.

```
// Demonstrate an anonymous method.

using System;

// Declare a delegate type.
delegate void CountIt();

class AnonMethDemo {

  static void Main() {

    // Here, the code for counting is passed
    // as an anonymous method.
    CountIt count = delegate {
       // This is the block of code passed to the delegate.
      for(int i=0; i <= 5; i++)
        Console.WriteLine(i);
    }; // notice the semicolon

    count();
  }
}
```

This program first declares a delegate type called **CountIt** that has no parameters and returns **void**. Inside **Main( )**, a **CountIt** instance called **count** is created, and it is passed the block of code that follows the **delegate** keyword. This block of code is the anonymous method that will be executed when **count** is called. Notice that the block of code is followed by a semicolon, which terminates the declaration statement. The output from the program is shown here:

```
0
1
2
3
4
5
```

Pass Arguments to an Anonymous Method

It is possible to pass one or more arguments to an anonymous method. To do so, follow the **delegate** keyword with a parenthesized parameter list. Then, pass the argument(s) to the delegate instance when it is called. For example, here is the preceding program rewritten so that the ending value for the count is passed:

```
// Demonstrate an anonymous method that takes an argument.

using System;

// Notice that CountIt now has a parameter.
delegate void CountIt(int end);

class AnonMethDemo2 {

  static void Main() {

    // Here, the ending value for the count
    // is passed to the anonymous method.
    CountIt count = delegate (int end) {
      for(int i=0; i <= end; i++)
        Console.WriteLine(i);
    };

    count(3);
    Console.WriteLine();
    count(5);
  }
}
```

In this version, **CountIt** now takes an integer argument. Notice how the parameter list is specified after the **delegate** keyword when the anonymous method is created. The code inside the anonymous method has access to the parameter **end** in just the same way it would if a named method were being created. The output from this program is shown next:

```
0
1
2
3

0
1
2
3
4
5
```

Return a Value from an Anonymous Method

An anonymous method can return a value. The value is returned by use of the **return** statement, which works the same in an anonymous method as it does in a named method. As you would expect, the type of the return value must be compatible with the return type

specified by the delegate. For example, here the code that performs the count also computes the summation of the count and returns the result:

```
// Demonstrate an anonymous method that returns a value.

using System;

// This delegate returns a value.
delegate int CountIt(int end);

class AnonMethDemo3 {

  static void Main() {
    int result;

    // Here, the ending value for the count
    // is passed to the anonymous method.
    // A summation of the count is returned.
    CountIt count = delegate (int end) {
      int sum = 0;

      for(int i=0; i <= end; i++) {
        Console.WriteLine(i);
        sum += i;
      }
      return sum; // return a value from an anonymous method
    };

    result = count(3);
    Console.WriteLine("Summation of 3 is " + result);
    Console.WriteLine();

    result = count(5);
    Console.WriteLine("Summation of 5 is " + result);
  }
}
```

In this version, the value of **sum** is returned by the code block that is associated with the **count** delegate instance. Notice that the **return** statement is used in an anonymous method in just the same way that it is used in a named method. The output is shown here:

```
0
1
2
3
Summation of 3 is 6

0
1
2
3
4
5
Summation of 5 is 15
```

Use Outer Variables with Anonymous Methods

A local variable or parameter whose scope includes an anonymous method is called an *outer variable*. An anonymous method has access to and can use these outer variables. When an outer variable is used by an anonymous method, that variable is said to be *captured*. A captured variable will stay in existence at least until the delegate that captured it is subject to garbage collection. Thus, even though a local variable will normally cease to exist when its block is exited, if that local variable is being used by an anonymous method, then that variable will stay in existence at least until the delegate referring to that method is destroyed.

The capturing of a local variable can lead to unexpected results. For example, consider this version of the counting program. As in the previous version, the summation of the count is computed. However, in this version, a **CountIt** object is constructed and returned by a static method called **Counter( )**. This object uses the variable **sum**, which is declared in the enclosing scope provided by **Counter( )**, rather than in the anonymous method, itself. Thus, **sum** is captured by the anonymous method. Inside **Main( )**, **Counter( )** is called to obtain a **CountIt** object. Thus, **sum** will not be destroyed until the program finishes.

```
// Demonstrate a captured variable.

using System;

// This delegate returns int and takes an int argument.
delegate int CountIt(int end);

class VarCapture {

  static CountIt Counter() {
    int sum = 0;

    // Here, a summation of the count is stored
    // in the captured variable sum.
    CountIt ctObj = delegate (int end) {
      for(int i=0; i <= end; i++) {
        Console.WriteLine(i);
        sum += i;
      }
      return sum;
    };
    return ctObj;
  }

  static void Main() {
    // Get a counter.
    CountIt count = Counter();

    int result;

    result = count(3);
    Console.WriteLine("Summation of 3 is " + result);
    Console.WriteLine();

    result = count(5);
    Console.WriteLine("Summation of 5 is " + result);
```

```
    }
}
```

The output is shown here. Pay special attention to the summation value.

```
0
1
2
3
Summation of 3 is 6

0
1
2
3
4
5
Summation of 5 is 21
```

As you can see, the count still proceeds normally. However, notice the summation value for 5. It shows 21 instead of 15! The reason for this is that **sum** is captured by **ctObj** when it is created by the **Counter( )** method. This means it remains in existence until **count** is subject to garbage collection at the end of the program. Thus, its value is not destroyed when **Counter( )** returns or with each call to the anonymous method when **count** is called in **Main( )**.

Although captured variables can result in rather counterintuitive situations, such as the one just shown, it makes sense if you think about it a bit. The key point is that when an anonymous method captures a variable, that variable cannot go out of existence until the delegate that captures it is no longer being used. If this were not the case, then the captured variable could be undefined when it is needed by the delegate.

Lambda Expressions

Although anonymous methods are a valuable feature, they have been largely superceded by a better approach: the *lambda expression*. It is not an overstatement to say that the lambda expression is one of the two most important features added by C# 3.0 (the other being LINQ). Based on an entirely new syntactic element, the lambda expression provides a powerful alternative to the anonymous method. Although a principal use of lambda expressions is found when working with LINQ (see Chapter 19), they are also applicable to (and commonly used with) delegates and events. This use of lambda expressions is described here.

A lambda expression is the second way that an anonymous function can be created. (The other type of anonymous function is the anonymous method, described in the preceding section.) Thus, a lambda expression can be assigned to a delegate. Because a lambda expression is more streamlined than the equivalent anonymous method, lambda expressions are now the recommended approach in almost all cases.

The Lambda Operator

All lambda expressions use the new *lambda operator*, which is =>. This operator divides a lambda expression into two parts. On the left the input parameter (or parameters) is specified. On the right is the lambda body. The => operator is sometimes verbalized as "goes to" or "becomes."

C# supports two types of lambda expressions, and it is the lambda body that determines what type is being created. If the lambda body consists of a single expression, then an *expression lambda* is being created. In this case, the body is free-standing—it is not enclosed between braces. If the lambda body consists of a block of statements enclosed by braces, then a *statement lambda* is being created. A statement lambda can contain multiple statements and include such things as loops, method calls, and **if** statements. The following sections describe both kinds of lambdas.

Expression Lambdas

In an expression lambda, the expression on the right side of the **=>** acts on the parameter (or parameters) specified by the left side. The result of the expression becomes the result of the lambda operator and is returned.

Here is the general form of an expression lambda that takes only one parameter:

param => expr

When more than one parameter is required, then the following form is used:

(param-list) => expr

Therefore, when two or more parameters are needed, they must be enclosed by parentheses. If no parameters are needed, then empty parentheses must be used.

Here is a simple expression lambda:

count => count + 2

Here **count** is the parameter that is acted on by the expression **count + 2**. Thus, the result is the value of **count** increased by two. Here is another example:

n => n % 2 == 0

In this case, this expression returns true if **n** is even and false if it is odd.

To use a lambda expression involves two steps. First, declare a delegate type that is compatible with the lambda expression. Second, declare an instance of the delegate, assigning to it the lambda expression. Once this has been done, the lambda expression can be executed by calling the delegate instance. The result of the lambda expression becomes the return value.

The following program shows how to put the two expression lambdas just shown into action. It declares two delegate types. The first, called **Incr**, takes an **int** argument and returns an **int** result. The second, called **IsEven**, takes an **int** argument and returns a **bool** result. It then assigns the lambda expressions to instances of those delegates. Finally, it executes the lambda expressions through the delegate instances.

```
// Use two simple lambda expressions.

using System;

// Declare a delegate that takes an int argument
// and returns an int result.
delegate int Incr(int v);

// Declare a delegate that takes an int argument
// and returns a bool result.
```

```
delegate bool IsEven(int v);

class SimpleLambdaDemo {

  static void Main() {

    // Create an Incr delegate instance that refers to
    // a lambda expression that increases its parameter by 2.
    Incr incr = count => count + 2;

    // Now, use the incr lambda expression.
    Console.WriteLine("Use incr lambda expression: ");
    int x = -10;
    while(x <= 0) {
      Console.Write(x + " ");
      x = incr(x); // increase x by 2
    }

    Console.WriteLine("\n");

    // Create an IsEven delegate instance that refers to
    // a lambda expression that returns true if its parameter
    // is even and false otherwise.
    IsEven isEven = n => n % 2 == 0;

    // Now, use the isEven lambda expression.
    Console.WriteLine("Use isEven lambda expression: ");
    for(int i=1; i <= 10; i++)
      if(isEven(i)) Console.WriteLine(i + " is even.");

  }
}
```

The output is shown here:

```
Use incr lambda expression:
-10 -8 -6 -4 -2 0

Use isEven lambda expression:
2 is even.
4 is even.
6 is even.
8 is even.
10 is even.
```

In the program, pay special attention to these declarations:

```
Incr incr = count => count + 2;
IsEven isEven = n => n % 2 == 0;
```

The first assigns to **incr** a lambda expression that returns the result of increasing the value passed to **count** by 2. This expression can be assigned to an **Incr** delegate because it is compatible with **Incr**'s declaration. The argument used in the call to **incr** is passed to **count**. The result is returned. The second declaration assigns to **isEven** an expression that returns

true if the argument is even and false otherwise. Thus, it is compatible with the **IsEven** delegate declaration.

At this point, you might be wondering how the compiler knows the type of the data used in a lambda expression. For example, in the lambda expression assigned to **incr**, how does the compiler know that **count** is an **int**? The answer is that the compiler infers the type of the parameter and the expression's result type from the delegate type. Thus, the lambda parameters and return value must be compatible with the parameter type(s) and return type of the delegate.

Although type inference is quite useful, in some cases, you might need to explicitly specify the type of a lambda parameter. To do so, simply include the type name. For example, here is another way to declare the **incr** delegate instance:

```
Incr incr = (int count) => count + 2;
```

Notice now that **count** is explicitly declared as an **int**. Also notice the use of parentheses. They are now necessary. (Parentheses can be omitted only when exactly one parameter is specified and no type specifier is used.)

Although the preceding two lambda expressions each used one parameter, lambda expressions can use any number, including zero. When using more than one parameter you *must* enclose them within parentheses. Here is an example that uses a lambda expression to determine if a value is within a specified range:

```
(low, high, val) => val >= low && val <= high;
```

Here is a delegate type that is compatible with this lambda expression:

```
delegate bool InRange(int lower, int upper, int v);
```

Thus, you could create an **InRange** delegate instance like this:

```
InRange rangeOK = (low, high, val) => val >= low && val <= high;
```

After doing so, the lambda expression can be executed as shown here:

```
if(rangeOK(1, 5, 3)) Console.WriteLine("3 is within 1 to 5.");
```

One other point: Lambda expressions can use outer variables in the same way as anonymous methods, and they are captured in the same way.

Statement Lambdas

As mentioned, there are two basic flavors of the lambda expression. The first is the expression lambda, which was discussed in the preceding section. As explained, the body of an expression lambda consists solely of a single expression. The second type of lambda expression is the *statement lambda*. A statement lambda expands the types of operations that can be handled within a lambda expression because it allows the body of lambda to contain multiple statements. For example, using a statement lambda you can use loops, **if** statements, declare variables, and so on. A statement lambda is easy to create. Simply enclose the body within braces. Aside from allowing multiple statements, it works much like the expression lambdas just discussed.

Here is an example that uses a statement lambda to compute and return the factorial of an **int** value:

```
// Demonstrate a statement lambda.
using System;

// IntOp takes one int argument and returns an int result.
delegate int IntOp(int end);

class StatementLambdaDemo {

  static void Main() {

    // A statement lambda that returns the factorial
    // of the value it is passed.
    IntOp fact = n => {
                       int r = 1;
                       for(int i=1; i <= n; i++)
                         r = i * r;
                       return r;
                     };

    Console.WriteLine("The factorial of 3 is " + fact(3));
    Console.WriteLine("The factorial of 5 is " + fact(5));
  }
}
```

The output is shown here:

```
The factorial of 3 is 6
The factorial of 5 is 120
```

In the program, notice that the statement lambda declares a variable called **r**, uses a **for** loop, and has a **return** statement. These are legal inside a statement lambda. In essence, a statement lambda closely parallels an anonymous method. Therefore, many anonymous methods will be converted to statement lambdas when updating legacy code. (As mentioned, as of C# 3.0, lambda expressions are the preferred way of creating anonymous functions.) One other point: When a **return** statement occurs within a lambda expression, it simply causes a return from the lambda. It does not cause the enclosing method to return.

Before concluding, it is worthwhile to see another example that shows the statement lambda in action. The following program reworks the first delegate example in this chapter so it uses statement lambdas (rather than standalone methods) to accomplish various string modifications:

```
// The first delegate example rewritten to use
// statement lambdas.

using System;

// Declare a delegate type.
delegate string StrMod(string s);
```

```
class UseStatementLambdas {

  static void Main() {
    // Create delegates that refer to lambda expressions
    // that perform various string modifications.

    // Replaces spaces with hyphens.
    StrMod ReplaceSpaces = s => {
            Console.WriteLine("Replacing spaces with hyphens.");
            return s.Replace(' ', '-');
          };

    // Remove spaces.
    StrMod RemoveSpaces = s => {
            string temp = "";
            int i;

            Console.WriteLine("Removing spaces.");
            for(i=0; i < s.Length; i++)
              if(s[i] != ' ') temp += s[i];

            return temp;
          };


    // Reverse a string.
    StrMod Reverse = s => {
            string temp = "";
            int i, j;

            Console.WriteLine("Reversing string.");
            for(j=0, i=s.Length-1; i >= 0; i--, j++)
            temp += s[i];

            return temp;
          };

    string str;

    // Call methods through the delegate.
    StrMod strOp = ReplaceSpaces;
    str = strOp("This is a test.");
    Console.WriteLine("Resulting string: " + str);
    Console.WriteLine();

    strOp = RemoveSpaces;
    str = strOp("This is a test.");
    Console.WriteLine("Resulting string: " + str);
    Console.WriteLine();

    strOp = Reverse;
    str = strOp("This is a test.");
```

```
    Console.WriteLine("Resulting string: " + str);
  }
}
```

The output, which is the same as the original version, is shown here:

```
Replacing spaces with hyphens.
Resulting string: This-is-a-test.

Removing spaces.
Resulting string: Thisisatest.

Reversing string.
Resulting string: .tset a si sihT
```

Events

Another important C# feature is built upon the foundation of delegates: the *event*. An event is, essentially, an automatic notification that some action has occurred. Events work like this: An object that has an interest in an event registers an event handler for that event. When the event occurs, all registered handlers are called. Event handlers are represented by delegates.

Events are members of a class and are declared using the **event** keyword. Its most commonly used form is shown here:

event *event-delegate event-name*;

Here, *event-delegate* is the name of the delegate used to support the event, and *event-name* is the name of the specific event object being declared.

Let's begin with a very simple example:

```
// A very simple event demonstration.

using System;

// Declare a delegate type for an event.
delegate void MyEventHandler();

// Declare a class that contains an event.
class MyEvent {
  public event MyEventHandler SomeEvent;

  // This is called to fire the event.
  public void OnSomeEvent() {
    if(SomeEvent != null)
      SomeEvent();
  }
}

class EventDemo {
  // An event handler.
  static void Handler() {
    Console.WriteLine("Event occurred");
  }
```

```
static void Main() {
  MyEvent evt = new MyEvent();

  // Add Handler() to the event list.
  evt.SomeEvent += Handler;

  // Fire the event.
  evt.OnSomeEvent();
}
}
```

This program displays the following output:

```
Event occurred
```

Although simple, this program contains all the elements essential to proper event handling. Let's look at it carefully. The program begins by declaring a delegate type for the event handler, as shown here:

```
delegate void MyEventHandler();
```

All events are activated through a delegate. Thus, the event delegate type defines the return type and signature for the event. In this case, there are no parameters, but event parameters are allowed.

Next, an event class, called **MyEvent**, is created. Inside the class, an event called **SomeEvent** is declared, using this line:

```
public event MyEventHandler SomeEvent;
```

Notice the syntax. The keyword **event** tells the compiler that an event is being declared.

Also declared inside **MyEvent** is the method **OnSomeEvent( )**, which is the method a program will call to signal (or "fire") an event. (That is, this is the method called when the event occurs.) It calls an event handler through the **SomeEvent** delegate, as shown here:

```
if(SomeEvent != null)
  SomeEvent();
```

Notice that a handler is called if and only if **SomeEvent** is not **null**. Since other parts of your program must register an interest in an event in order to receive event notifications, it is possible that **OnSomeEvent( )** could be called before any event handler has been registered. To prevent calling on a **null** reference, the event delegate must be tested to ensure that it is not **null**.

Inside **EventDemo**, an event handler called **Handler( )** is created. In this simple example, the event handler simply displays a message, but other handlers could perform more meaningful actions. In **Main( )**, a **MyEvent** object is created, and **Handler( )** is registered as a handler for this event, by adding it as shown here:

```
MyEvent evt = new MyEvent();

// Add Handler() to the event list.
evt.SomeEvent += Handler;
```

Notice that the handler is added using the += operator. Events support only += and – =. In this case, **Handler( )** is a **static** method, but event handlers can also be instance methods.

Finally, the event is fired as shown here:

```
// Fire the event.
evt.OnSomeEvent();
```

Calling **OnSomeEvent( )** causes all registered event handlers to be called. In this case, there is only one registered handler, but there could be more, as the next section explains.

A Multicast Event Example

Like delegates, events can be multicast. This enables multiple objects to respond to an event notification. Here is an event multicast example:

```
// An event multicast demonstration.

using System;

// Declare a delegate type for an event.
delegate void MyEventHandler();

// Declare a class that contains an event.
class MyEvent {
  public event MyEventHandler SomeEvent;

  // This is called to fire the event.
  public void OnSomeEvent() {
    if(SomeEvent != null)
      SomeEvent();
  }
}

class X {
  public void Xhandler() {
    Console.WriteLine("Event received by X object");
  }
}

class Y {
  public void Yhandler() {
    Console.WriteLine("Event received by Y object");
  }
}

class EventDemo2 {
  static void Handler() {
    Console.WriteLine("Event received by EventDemo");
  }

  static void Main() {
    MyEvent evt = new MyEvent();
    X xOb = new X();
    Y yOb = new Y();
```

```
   // Add handlers to the event list.
   evt.SomeEvent += Handler;
   evt.SomeEvent += xOb.Xhandler;
   evt.SomeEvent += yOb.Yhandler;

   // Fire the event.
   evt.OnSomeEvent();
   Console.WriteLine();

   // Remove a handler.
   evt.SomeEvent -= xOb.Xhandler;
   evt.OnSomeEvent();
  }
}
```

The output from the program is shown here:

```
Event received by EventDemo
Event received by X object
Event received by Y object

Event received by EventDemo
Event received by Y object
```

This example creates two additional classes, called **X** and **Y**, which also define event handlers compatible with **MyEventHandler**. Thus, these handlers can also become part of the event chain. Notice that the handlers in **X** and **Y** are not **static**. This means that objects of each must be created, and the handler linked to each instance must be added to the event chain. The differences between instance and **static** handlers is examined in the next section.

Instance Methods vs. Static Methods as Event Handlers

Although both instance methods and **static** methods can be used as event handlers, they do differ in one important way. When a **static** method is used as a handler, an event notification applies to the class. When an instance method is used as an event handler, events are sent to specific object instances. Thus, each object of a class that wants to receive an event notification must register individually. In practice, most event handlers are instance methods, but, of course, this is subject to the specific application. Let's look at an example of each.

The following program creates a class called **X** that defines an instance method as an event handler. This means that each **X** object must register individually to receive events. To demonstrate this fact, the program multicasts an event to three objects of type **X**.

```
/* Individual objects receive notifications when instance
   event handlers are used. */

using System;

// Declare a delegate type for an event.
delegate void MyEventHandler();

// Declare a class that contains an event.
class MyEvent {
```

```
    public event MyEventHandler SomeEvent;

    // This is called to fire the event.
    public void OnSomeEvent() {
      if(SomeEvent != null)
        SomeEvent();
    }
}

class X {
  int id;

  public X(int x) { id = x; }

  // This is an instance method that will be used as an event handler.
  public void Xhandler() {
    Console.WriteLine("Event received by object " + id);
  }
}

class EventDemo3 {
  static void Main() {
    MyEvent evt = new MyEvent();
    X o1 = new X(1);
    X o2 = new X(2);
    X o3 = new X(3);

    evt.SomeEvent += o1.Xhandler;
    evt.SomeEvent += o2.Xhandler;
    evt.SomeEvent += o3.Xhandler;

    // Fire the event.
    evt.OnSomeEvent();
  }
}
```

The output from this program is shown here:

```
Event received by object 1
Event received by object 2
Event received by object 3
```

As the output shows, each object registers its interest in an event separately, and each receives a separate notification.

Alternatively, when a **static** method is used as an event handler, events are handled independently of any object, as the following program shows:

```
/* A class receives the notification when
   a static method is used as an event handler. */

using System;

// Declare a delegate type for an event.
```

```
delegate void MyEventHandler();

// Declare a class that contains an event.
class MyEvent {
  public event MyEventHandler SomeEvent;

  // This is called to fire the event.
  public void OnSomeEvent() {
    if(SomeEvent != null)
      SomeEvent();
  }
}

class X {

  /* This is a static method that will be used as
     an event handler. */
  public static void Xhandler() {
    Console.WriteLine("Event received by class.");
  }
}

class EventDemo4 {
  static void Main() {
    MyEvent evt = new MyEvent();

    evt.SomeEvent += X.Xhandler;

    // Fire the event.
    evt.OnSomeEvent();
  }
}
```

The output from this program is shown here:

```
Event received by class.
```

In the program, notice that no object of type **X** is ever created. However, since **Xhandler( )** is a **static** method of **X**, it can be attached to **SomeEvent** and executed when **OnSomeEvent( )** is called.

Using Event Accessors

The form of **event** used in the preceding examples created events that automatically manage the event handler invocation list, including the adding and subtracting of event handlers to and from the list. Thus, you did not need to implement any of the list management functionality yourself. Because they manage the details for you, these types of events are by far the most commonly used. It is possible, however, to provide the event handler list operations yourself, perhaps to implement some type of specialized event storage mechanism.

To take control of the event handler list, you will use an expanded form of the **event** statement, which allows the use of *event accessors*. The accessors give you control over how the event handler list is implemented. This form is shown here:

```
event event-delegate event-name {
  add {
    // code to add an event to the chain
  }

  remove {
    // code to remove an event from the chain
  }
}
```

This form includes the two event accessors **add** and **remove**. The **add** accessor is called when an event handler is added to the event chain, by using +=. The **remove** accessor is called when an event handler is removed from the chain, by using – =.

When **add** or **remove** is called, it receives the handler to add or remove as a parameter. As with other types of accessors, this parameter is called **value**. By implementing **add** and **remove**, you can define a custom event-handler storage scheme. For example, you could use an array, a stack, or a queue to store the handlers.

Here is an example that uses the accessor form of **event**. It uses an array to hold the event handlers. Because the array is only three elements long, only three event handlers can be held in the chain at any one time.

```
// Create a custom means of managing the event invocation list.

using System;

// Declare a delegate type for an event.
delegate void MyEventHandler();

// Declare a class that holds up to 3 events.
class MyEvent {
  MyEventHandler[] evnt = new MyEventHandler[3];

  public event MyEventHandler SomeEvent {
    // Add an event to the list.
    add {
      int i;

      for(i=0; i < 3; i++)
        if(evnt[i] == null) {
          evnt[i] = value;
          break;
        }
      if (i == 3) Console.WriteLine("Event list full.");
    }

    // Remove an event from the list.
    remove {
      int i;

      for(i=0; i < 3; i++)
        if(evnt[i] == value) {
```

```
            evnt[i] = null;
            break;
          }
        if (i == 3) Console.WriteLine("Event handler not found.");
      }
    }

    // This is called to fire the events.
    public void OnSomeEvent() {
      for(int i=0; i < 3; i++)
        if(evnt[i] != null) evnt[i]();
    }

}

// Create some classes that use MyEventHandler.
class W {
  public void Whandler() {
    Console.WriteLine("Event received by W object");
  }
}

class X {
  public void Xhandler() {
    Console.WriteLine("Event received by X object");
  }
}

class Y {
  public void Yhandler() {
    Console.WriteLine("Event received by Y object");
  }
}

class Z {
  public void Zhandler() {
    Console.WriteLine("Event received by Z object");
  }
}

class EventDemo5 {
  static void Main() {
    MyEvent evt = new MyEvent();
    W wOb = new W();
    X xOb = new X();
    Y yOb = new Y();
    Z zOb = new Z();

    // Add handlers to the event list.
    Console.WriteLine("Adding events.");
    evt.SomeEvent += wOb.Whandler;
    evt.SomeEvent += xOb.Xhandler;
    evt.SomeEvent += yOb.Yhandler;
```

```
    // Can't store this one -- full.
    evt.SomeEvent += zOb.Zhandler;
    Console.WriteLine();

    // Fire the events.
    evt.OnSomeEvent();
    Console.WriteLine();

    // Remove a handler.
    Console.WriteLine("Remove xOb.Xhandler.");
    evt.SomeEvent -= xOb.Xhandler;
    evt.OnSomeEvent();

    Console.WriteLine();

    // Try to remove it again.
    Console.WriteLine("Try to remove xOb.Xhandler again.");
    evt.SomeEvent -= xOb.Xhandler;
    evt.OnSomeEvent();

    Console.WriteLine();

    // Now, add Zhandler.
    Console.WriteLine("Add zOb.Zhandler.");
    evt.SomeEvent += zOb.Zhandler;
    evt.OnSomeEvent();

  }
}
```

The output from the program is shown here:

```
Adding events.
Event list full.

Event received by W object
Event received by X object
Event received by Y object

Remove xOb.Xhandler.
Event received by W object
Event received by Y object

Try to remove xOb.Xhandler again.
Event handler not found.
Event received by W object
Event received by Y object

Add zOb.Zhandler.
Event received by W object
Event received by Z object
Event received by Y object
```

Let's examine this program closely. First, an event handler delegate called **MyEventHandler** is defined. Next, the class **MyEvent** is declared. It begins by defining a three-element array of event handlers called **evnt**, as shown here:

```
MyEventHandler[] evnt = new MyEventHandler[3];
```

This array will be used to store the event handlers that are added to the event chain. The elements in **evnt** are initialized to **null** by default.

Next, the event **SomeEvent** is declared. It uses the accessor form of the **event** statement, as shown here:

```
public event MyEventHandler SomeEvent {
  // Add an event to the list.
  add {
    int i;

    for(i=0; i < 3; i++)
      if(evnt[i] == null) {
        evnt[i] = value;
        break;
      }
    if (i == 3) Console.WriteLine("Event queue full.");
  }

  // Remove an event from the list.
  remove {
    int i;

    for(i=0; i < 3; i++)
      if(evnt[i] == value) {
        evnt[i] = null;
        break;
      }
    if (i == 3) Console.WriteLine("Event handler not found.");
  }
}
```

When an event handler is added, **add** is called and a reference to the handler (contained in **value**) is put into the first unused (that is, null) element of **evnt**. If no element is free, then an error is reported. (Of course, throwing an exception when the list is full would be a better approach for real-world code.) Since **evnt** is only three elements long, only three event handlers can be stored. When an event handler is removed, **remove** is called and the **evnt** array is searched for the reference to the handler passed in **value**. If it is found, its element in the array is assigned **null**, thus removing the handler from the list.

When an event is fired, **OnSomeEvent( )** is called. It cycles through the **evnt** array, calling each event handler in turn.

As the preceding example shows, it is relatively easy to implement a custom event-handler storage mechanism if one is needed. For most applications, though, the default storage provided by the non-accessor form of **event** is better. The accessor-based form of **event** can be useful in certain specialized situations, however. For example, if you have a program in which event handlers need to be executed in order of their priority and not in the order in which they are added to the chain, then you could use a priority queue to store the handlers.

> **NOTE** *In multithreaded applications, you will usually need to synchronize access to the event accessors. For information on multithreaded programming, see Chapter 23.*

Miscellaneous Event Features

Events can be specified in interfaces. Implementing classes must supply the event.

Events can also be specified as **abstract**. A derived class must implement the event. Accessor-based events cannot, however, be **abstract**.

An event can be specified as **sealed**.

Finally, an event can be virtual, which means that it can be overridden in a derived class.

Use Anonymous Methods and Lambda Expressions with Events

Anonymous methods and lambda expressions are especially useful when working with events because often the event handler is not called by any code other than the event handling mechanism. As a result, there is usually no reason to create a standalone method. Thus, the use of lambda expressions or anonymous methods can significantly streamline event handling code.

Since lambda expressions are now the preferred approach, we will start there. Here is an example that uses a lambda expression as an event handler:

```
// Use a lambda expression as an event handler.
using System;

// Declare a delegate type for an event.
delegate void MyEventHandler(int n);

// Declare a class that contains an event.
class MyEvent {
  public event MyEventHandler SomeEvent;

  // This is called to fire the event.
  public void OnSomeEvent(int n) {
    if(SomeEvent != null)
      SomeEvent(n);
  }
}

class LambdaEventDemo {
  static void Main() {
    MyEvent evt = new MyEvent();

    // Use a lambda expression as an event handler.
    evt.SomeEvent += (n) =>
      Console.WriteLine("Event received. Value is " + n);

    // Fire the event twice.
    evt.OnSomeEvent(1);
    evt.OnSomeEvent(2);
  }
}
```

The output is shown here:

```
Event received. Value is 1
Event received. Value is 2
```

In the program, pay special attention to the way the lambda expression is used as an event handler, as shown here:

```
evt.SomeEvent += (n) =>
  Console.WriteLine("Event received. Value is " + n);
```

The syntax for using a lambda expression event handler is the same as that for using a lambda expression with any other type of delegate.

Although lambda expressions are now the preferred way to construct an anonymous function, you can still use an anonymous method as an event handler if you so choose. For example, here is the event handler from the previous example rewritten to use an anonymous method:

```
// Use an anonymous method as an event handler.
evt.SomeEvent += delegate(int n)  {
  Console.WriteLine("Event received. Value is" + n);
};
```

As you can see, the syntax for using an anonymous event handler is the same as that for any anonymous method.

.NET Event Guidelines

C# allows you to write any type of event you desire. However, for component compatibility with the .NET Framework, you will need to follow the guidelines Microsoft has established for this purpose. At the core of these guidelines is the requirement that event handlers have two parameters. The first is a reference to the object that generated the event. The second is a parameter of type **EventArgs** that contains any other information required by the handler. Thus, .NET-compatible event handlers will have this general form:

```
void handler(object source, EventArgs arg) {
  // ...
}
```

Typically, the *source* parameter is passed **this** by the calling code. The **EventArgs** parameter contains additional information and can be ignored if it is not needed.

The **EventArgs** class itself does not contain fields that you use to pass additional data to a handler. Instead, **EventArgs** is used as a base class from which you will derive a class that contains the necessary fields. **EventArgs** does include one **static** field called **Empty**, which is an **EventArgs** object that contains no data.

Here is an example that creates a .NET-compatible event:

```
// A .NET-compatible event.

using System;

// Derive a class from EventArgs.
class MyEventArgs : EventArgs {
  public int EventNum;
```

```
  }

// Declare a delegate type for an event.
delegate void MyEventHandler(object source, MyEventArgs arg);

// Declare a class that contains an event.
class MyEvent {
  static int count = 0;

  public event MyEventHandler SomeEvent;

  // This fires SomeEvent.
  public void OnSomeEvent() {
    MyEventArgs arg = new MyEventArgs();

    if(SomeEvent != null) {
      arg.EventNum = count++;
      SomeEvent(this, arg);
    }
  }
}

class X {
  public void Handler(object source, MyEventArgs arg) {
    Console.WriteLine("Event " + arg.EventNum +
                      " received by an X object.");
    Console.WriteLine("Source is " + source);
    Console.WriteLine();
  }
}

class Y {
  public void Handler(object source, MyEventArgs arg) {
    Console.WriteLine("Event " + arg.EventNum +
                      " received by a Y object.");
    Console.WriteLine("Source is " + source);
    Console.WriteLine();
  }
}

class EventDemo6 {
  static void Main() {
    X ob1 = new X();
    Y ob2 = new Y();
    MyEvent evt = new MyEvent();

    // Add Handler() to the event list.
    evt.SomeEvent += ob1.Handler;
    evt.SomeEvent += ob2.Handler;

    // Fire the event.
    evt.OnSomeEvent();
    evt.OnSomeEvent();
  }
}
```

Here is the output:

```
Event 0 received by an X object.
Source is MyEvent

Event 0 received by a Y object.
Source is MyEvent

Event 1 received by an X object.
Source is MyEvent

Event 1 received by a Y object.
Source is MyEvent
```

In this example, **MyEventArgs** is derived from **EventArgs**. **MyEventArgs** adds just one field of its own: **EventNum**. The event handler delegate **MyEventHandler** now takes the two parameters required by the .NET Framework. As explained, the first is an object reference to the generator of the event. The second is a reference to **EventArgs** or a class derived from **EventArgs**. The event handlers in the **X** and **Y** classes, **Handler( )**, also have the same types of parameters.

Inside **MyEvent**, a **MyEventHandler** called **SomeEvent** is declared. In the **OnSomeEvent( )** method, **SomeEvent** is called with the first argument being **this**, and the second argument being a **MyEventArgs** instance. Thus, the proper arguments are passed to **MyEventHandler** to fulfill the requirements for .NET compatibility.

Use EventHandler

For many events, the **EventArgs** parameter is unused. To help facilitate the creation of code in these situations, the .NET Framework includes a built-in delegate type called **EventHandler**, which can be used to declare event handlers in which no extra information is needed. Here is an example that uses **EventHandler**:

```
// Use the built-in EventHandler delegate.

using System;

// Declare a class that contains an event.
class MyEvent {
  public event EventHandler SomeEvent; // uses EventHandler delegate

  // This is called to fire SomeEvent.
  public void OnSomeEvent() {
    if(SomeEvent != null)
      SomeEvent(this, EventArgs.Empty);
  }
}

class EventDemo7 {
  static void Handler(object source, EventArgs arg) {
    Console.WriteLine("Event occurred");
    Console.WriteLine("Source is " + source);
  }
```

```
static void Main() {
  MyEvent evt = new MyEvent();

  // Add Handler() to the event list.
  evt.SomeEvent += Handler;

  // Fire the event.
  evt.OnSomeEvent();
  }
}
```

In this case, the **EventArgs** parameter is unused and is passed the placeholder object **EventArgs.Empty**. The output is shown here:

```
Event occurred
Source is MyEvent
```

Applying Events: A Case Study

Events are frequently used in message-based environments such as Windows. In such an environment, a program simply waits until it receives a message, and then it takes the appropriate action. Such an architecture is well suited for C#-style event handling because it is possible to create event handlers for various messages and then simply invoke a handler when a message is received. For example, the left-button mouse click message could be tied to an event called **LButtonClick**. When a left-button click is received, a method called **OnLButtonClick()** can be called, and all registered handlers will be notified.

Although developing a Windows program that demonstrates this approach is beyond the scope of this chapter, it is possible to give an idea of how such an approach would work. The following program creates an event handler that processes keystrokes. The event is called **KeyPress**, and each time a key is pressed, the event is fired by calling **OnKeyPress()**. Notice that .NET-compatible events are created and that lambda expressions provide the event handlers.

```
// A keypress event example.

using System;

// Derive a custom EventArgs class that holds the key.
class KeyEventArgs : EventArgs {
  public char ch;
}

// Declare a delegate type for an event.
delegate void KeyHandler(object source, KeyEventArgs arg);

// Declare a keypress event class.
class KeyEvent {
  public event KeyHandler KeyPress;

  // This is called when a key is pressed.
  public void OnKeyPress(char key) {
```

```
      KeyEventArgs k = new KeyEventArgs();

      if(KeyPress != null) {
        k.ch = key;
        KeyPress(this, k);
      }
    }
  }
}

// Demonstrate KeyEvent.
class KeyEventDemo {
  static void Main() {
    KeyEvent kevt = new KeyEvent();
    ConsoleKeyInfo key;
    int count = 0;

    // Use a lambda expression to display the keypress.
    kevt.KeyPress += (source, arg) =>
      Console.WriteLine(" Received keystroke: " + arg.ch);

    // Use a lambda expression to count keypresses.
    kevt.KeyPress += (source, arg) =>
      count++; // count is an outer variable

    Console.WriteLine("Enter some characters. " +
                      "Enter a period to stop.");
    do {
      key = Console.ReadKey();
      kevt.OnKeyPress(key.KeyChar);
    } while(key.KeyChar != '.');

    Console.WriteLine(count + " keys pressed.");
  }
}
```

Here is a sample run:

```
Enter some characters. Enter a period to stop.
t Received keystroke: t
e Received keystroke: e
s Received keystroke: s
t Received keystroke: t
. Received keystroke: .
5 keys pressed.
```

The program begins by deriving a class from **EventArgs** called **KeyEventArgs**, which is used to pass a keystroke to an event handler. Next, a delegate called **KeyHandler** defines the event handler for keystroke events. The class **KeyEvent** encapsulates the keypress event. It defines the event **KeyPress**.

In **Main( )**, a **KeyEvent** object called **kevt** is created. Next, an event handler based on a lambda expression is added to **kvet.KeyPress** that displays each key as it is entered, as shown here:

```
kevt.KeyPress += (source, arg) =>
  Console.WriteLine(" Received keystroke: " + arg.ch);
```

Next, another lambda expression–based handler is added to **kvet.KeyPress** by the following code. It counts the number of keypresses.

```
kevt.KeyPress += (source, arg) =>
  count++; // count is an outer variable
```

Notice that **count** is a local variable declared in **Main( )** that is initialized to zero.

Next, a loop is started that calls **kevt.OnKeyPress( )** when a key is pressed. This causes the registered event handlers to be notified. When the loop ends, the number of keypresses is displayed. Although quite simple, this example illustrates the essence of event handling. The same basic approach will be used for other event handling situations. Of course, in some cases, anonymous event handlers will not be appropriate and named methods will need to be employed.

Namespaces, the Preprocessor, and Assemblies

This chapter discusses three C# features that give you greater control over the organization and accessibility of a program. These are namespaces, the preprocessor, and assemblies.

Namespaces

The namespace was mentioned briefly in Chapter 2 because it is a concept fundamental to C#. In fact, every C# program makes use of a namespace in one way or another. We didn't need to examine namespaces in detail before now because C# automatically provides a default, global namespace for your program. Thus, the programs in earlier chapters simply used the global namespace. In the real world, however, many programs will need to create their own namespaces or interact with other namespaces. Here, they are examined in detail.

A *namespace* defines a declarative region that provides a way to keep one set of names separate from another. In essence, names declared in one namespace will not conflict with the same names declared in another. The namespace used by the .NET Framework library (which is the C# library) is **System**. This is why you have included

```
using System;
```

near the top of every program. As explained in Chapter 14, the I/O classes are defined within a namespace subordinate to **System** called **System.IO**. There are many other namespaces subordinate to **System** that hold other parts of the C# library.

Namespaces are important because there has been an explosion of variable, method, property, and class names over the past few years. These include library routines, third-party code, and your own code. Without namespaces, all of these names would compete for slots in the global namespace and conflicts would arise. For example, if your program defined a class called **Finder**, it could conflict with another class called **Finder** supplied by a third-party library that your program uses. Fortunately, namespaces prevent this type of problem because a namespace restricts the visibility of names declared within it.

Declaring a Namespace

A namespace is declared using the **namespace** keyword. The general form of **namespace** is shown here:

namespace *name* {
    // members
}

Here, *name* is the name of the namespace. A namespace declaration defines a scope. Anything declared immediately inside the namespace is in scope throughout the namespace. Within a namespace, you can declare classes, structures, delegates, enumerations, interfaces, or another namespace.

Here is an example of a **namespace** that creates a namespace called **Counter**. It localizes the name used to implement a simple countdown counter class called **CountDown**.

```
// Declare a namespace for counters.

namespace Counter {
  // A simple countdown counter.
  class CountDown {
    int val;

    public CountDown(int n) {
      val = n;
    }

    public void Reset(int n) {
      val = n;
    }

    public int Count() {
      if(val > 0) return val--;
      else return 0;
    }
  }
} // This is the end of the Counter namespace.
```

Notice how the class **CountDown** is declared within the scope defined by the **Counter** namespace. To follow along with the example, put this code into a file called **Counter.cs**.

Here is a program that demonstrates the use of the **Counter** namespace:

```
// Demonstrate the Counter namespace.

using System;

class NSDemo {
  static void Main() {
    // Notice how CountDown is qualified by Counter.
    Counter.CountDown cd1 = new Counter.CountDown(10);
    int i;

    do {
      i = cd1.Count();
      Console.Write(i + " ");
```

```
  } while(i > 0);
  Console.WriteLine();

  // Again, notice how CountDown is qualified by Counter.
  Counter.CountDown cd2 = new Counter.CountDown(20);

  do {
    i = cd2.Count();
    Console.Write(i + " ");
  } while(i > 0);
  Console.WriteLine();

  cd2.Reset(4);
  do {
    i = cd2.Count();
    Console.Write(i + " ");
  } while(i > 0);
  Console.WriteLine();
  }
}
```

The output from the program is shown here:

```
10 9 8 7 6 5 4 3 2 1 0
20 19 18 17 16 15 14 13 12 11 10 9 8 7 6 5 4 3 2 1 0
4 3 2 1 0
```

To compile this program, you must include both the preceding code and the code contained in the **Counter** namespace. Assuming you called the preceding code **NSDemo.cs** and put the source code for the **Counter** namespace into a file called **Counter.cs** as mentioned earlier, then you can use this command line to compile the program:

```
csc NSDemo.cs counter.cs
```

Some important aspects of this program warrant close examination. First, since **CountDown** is declared within the **Counter** namespace, when an object is created, **CountDown** must be qualified with **Counter**, as shown here:

```
Counter.CountDown cd1 = new Counter.CountDown(10);
```

This rule can be generalized. Whenever you use a member of a namespace, you must qualify it with the namespace name. If you don't, the member of the namespace won't be found by the compiler.

Second, once an object of type **Counter** has been created, it is not necessary to further qualify it or any of its members with the namespace. Thus, **cd1.Count( )** can be called directly without namespace qualification, as this line shows:

```
i = cd1.Count();
```

Third, for the sake of illustration, this example uses two separate files. One holds the **Counter** namespace and the other holds the **NSDemo** program. However, both could have been contained in the same file. Furthermore, a single file can contain two or more named namespaces, with each namespace defining its own declarative region. When a named

namespace ends, the outer namespace resumes, which in the case of the **Counter** is the global namespace. For clarity, subsequent examples will show all namespaces required by a program within the same file, but remember that separate files would be equally valid (and more commonly used in production code).

REMEMBER *For clarity, the remaining namespace examples in this chapter show all namespaces required by a program within the same file. In real-world code, however, a namespace will often be defined in its own file, as the preceding example illustrates.*

Namespaces Prevent Name Conflicts

The key point about a namespace is that names declared within it won't conflict with similar names declared outside of it. For example, the following program defines two namespaces. The first is **Counter**, shown earlier. The second is called **Counter2**. Both contain classes called **CountDown**, but because they are in separate namespaces, the two classes do not conflict. Also notice how both namespaces are specified within the same file. As just explained, a single file can contain multiple namespace declarations. Of course, separate files for each namespace could also have been used.

```
// Namespaces prevent name conflicts.

using System;

// Declare the Counter namespace.
namespace Counter {
  // A simple countdown counter.
  class CountDown {
    int val;

    public CountDown(int n) {
      val = n;
    }

    public void Reset(int n) {
      val = n;
    }

    public int Count() {
      if(val > 0) return val--;
      else return 0;
    }
  }
}

// Declare the Counter2 namespace.
namespace Counter2 {
  /* This CountDown is in the Counter2 namespace and
     does not conflict with the one in Counter. */
  class CountDown {
    public void Count() {
      Console.WriteLine("This is Count() in the " +
                        "Counter2 namespace.");
    }
```

```
    }
  }

class NSDemo2 {
  static void Main() {
    // This is CountDown in the Counter namespace.
    Counter.CountDown cd1 = new Counter.CountDown(10);

    // This is CountDown in the Counter2 namespace.
    Counter2.CountDown cd2 = new Counter2.CountDown();

    int i;

    do {
      i = cd1.Count();
      Console.Write(i + " ");
    } while(i > 0);
    Console.WriteLine();

    cd2.Count();
  }
}
```

The output is shown here:

```
10 9 8 7 6 5 4 3 2 1 0
This is Count() in the Counter2 namespace.
```

As the output confirms, the **CountDown** class inside **Counter** is separate from the **CountDown** class in the **Counter2** namespace, and no name conflicts arise. Although this example is quite simple, it is easy to see how putting classes into a namespace helps prevent name conflicts between your code and code written by others.

using

If your program includes frequent references to the members of a namespace, having to specify the namespace each time you need to refer to one quickly becomes tedious. The **using** directive alleviates this problem. Throughout this book, you have been using it to bring the C# **System** namespace into view, so you are already familiar with it. As you would expect, **using** can also be employed to bring namespaces that you create into view.

There are two forms of the **using** directive. The first is shown here:

using *name*;

Here, *name* specifies the name of the namespace you want to access. This is the form of **using** that you have already seen. All of the members defined within the specified namespace are brought into view and can be used without qualification. A **using** directive must be specified at the top of each file, prior to any other declarations, or at the start of a namespace body.

The following program reworks the counter example to show how you can employ **using** to bring a namespace that you create into view:

```
// Demonstrate the using directive.

using System;
```

```
// Bring Counter into view.
using Counter;

// Declare a namespace for counters.
namespace Counter {
  // A simple countdown counter.
  class CountDown {
    int val;

    public CountDown(int n) {
      val = n;
    }

    public void Reset(int n) {
      val = n;
    }

    public int Count() {
      if(val > 0) return val--;
      else return 0;
    }
  }
}

class NSDemo3 {
  static void Main() {
    // now, CountDown can be used directly.
    CountDown cd1 = new CountDown(10);
    int i;

    do {
      i = cd1.Count();
      Console.Write(i + " ");
    } while(i > 0);
    Console.WriteLine();

    CountDown cd2 = new CountDown(20);

    do {
      i = cd2.Count();
      Console.Write(i + " ");
    } while(i > 0);
    Console.WriteLine();

    cd2.Reset(4);
    do {
      i = cd2.Count();
      Console.Write(i + " ");
    } while(i > 0);
    Console.WriteLine();
  }
}
```

This version of the program contains two important changes. The first is this **using** statement, near the top of the program:

```
using Counter;
```

This brings the **Counter** namespace into view. The second change is that it is no longer necessary to qualify **CountDown** with **Counter**, as this statement in **Main( )** shows:

```
CountDown cd1 = new CountDown(10);
```

Because **Counter** is now in view, **CountDown** can be used directly.

The program illustrates one other important point: Using one namespace does not override another. When you bring a namespace into view, it simply lets you use its contents without qualification. Thus, in the example, both **System** and **Counter** have been brought into view.

A Second Form of using

The **using** directive has a second form that creates another name, called an alias, for a type or a namespace. This form is shown here:

    using *alias* = *name*;

Here, *alias* becomes another name for the type (such as a class type) or namespace specified by *name*. Once the alias has been created, it can be used in place of the original name.

Here the example from the preceding section has been reworked so that an alias for **Counter.CountDown** called **MyCounter** is created:

```
// Demonstrate a using alias.

using System;

// Create an alias for Counter.CountDown.
using MyCounter = Counter.CountDown;

// Declare a namespace for counters.
namespace Counter {
  // A simple countdown counter.
  class CountDown {
    int val;

    public CountDown(int n) {
      val = n;
    }

    public void Reset(int n) {
      val = n;
    }

    public int Count() {
      if(val > 0) return val--;
      else return 0;
    }
  }
}

class NSDemo4 {
```

```
static void Main() {
  // Here, MyCounter is used as a name for Counter.CountDown.
  MyCounter cd1 = new MyCounter(10);
  int i;

  do {
    i = cd1.Count();
    Console.Write(i + " ");
  } while(i > 0);
  Console.WriteLine();

  MyCounter cd2 = new MyCounter(20);

  do {
    i = cd2.Count();
    Console.Write(i + " ");
  } while(i > 0);
  Console.WriteLine();

  cd2.Reset(4);
  do {
    i = cd2.Count();
    Console.Write(i + " ");
  } while(i > 0);
  Console.WriteLine();
  }
}
```

The **MyCounter** alias is created using this statement:

```
using MyCounter = Counter.CountDown;
```

Once **MyCounter** has been specified as another name for **Counter.CountDown**, it can be used to declare objects without any further namespace qualification. For example, in the program, this line

```
MyCounter cd1 = new MyCounter(10);
```

creates a **CountDown** object.

Namespaces Are Additive

There can be more than one namespace declaration of the same name. This allows a namespace to be split over several files or even separated within the same file. For example, the following program defines two **Counter** namespaces. One contains the **CountDown** class. The other contains the **CountUp** class. When compiled, the contents of both **Counter** namespaces are added together.

```
// Namespaces are additive.

using System;

// Bring Counter into view.
using Counter;
```

PART I

```csharp
// Here is one Counter namespace.
namespace Counter {
  // A simple countdown counter.
  class CountDown {
    int val;

    public CountDown(int n) {
      val = n;
    }

    public void Reset(int n) {
      val = n;
    }

    public int Count() {
      if(val > 0) return val--;
      else return 0;
    }
  }
}

// Here is another Counter namespace.
namespace Counter {
  // A simple count-up counter.
  class CountUp {
    int val;
    int target;

    public int Target {
      get{
        return target;
      }
    }

    public CountUp(int n) {
      target = n;
      val = 0;
    }

    public void Reset(int n) {
      target = n;
      val = 0;
    }

    public int Count() {
      if(val < target) return val++;
      else return target;
    }
  }
}

class NSDemo5 {
  static void Main() {
    CountDown cd = new CountDown(10);
```

```
    CountUp cu = new CountUp(8);
    int i;

    do {
      i = cd.Count();
      Console.Write(i + " ");
    } while(i > 0);
    Console.WriteLine();

    do {
      i = cu.Count();
      Console.Write(i + " ");
    } while(i < cu.Target);

  }
}
```

This program produces the following output:

```
10 9 8 7 6 5 4 3 2 1 0
0 1 2 3 4 5 6 7 8
```

Notice one other thing: The directive

```
using Counter;
```

brings into view the entire contents of the **Counter** namespace. Thus, both **CountDown** and **CountUp** can be referred to directly, without namespace qualification. It doesn't matter that the **Counter** namespace was split into two parts.

Namespaces Can Be Nested

One namespace can be nested within another. Consider this program:

```
// Namespaces can be nested.

using System;

namespace NS1 {
  class ClassA {
    public ClassA() {
      Console.WriteLine("constructing ClassA");
    }
  }
  namespace NS2 { // a nested namespace
    class ClassB {
      public ClassB() {
        Console.WriteLine("constructing ClassB");
      }
    }
  }
}

class NestedNSDemo {
  static void Main() {
```

```
    NS1.ClassA a = new NS1.ClassA();

 // NS2.ClassB b = new NS2.ClassB(); // Error!!! NS2 is not in view

    NS1.NS2.ClassB b = new NS1.NS2.ClassB(); // this is right
  }
}
```

This program produces the following output:

```
constructing ClassA
constructing ClassB
```

In the program, the namespace **NS2** is nested within **NS1**. Thus, to refer to **ClassB**, you must qualify it with both the **NS1** and **NS2** namespaces. **NS2**, by itself, is insufficient. As shown, the namespace names are separated by a period. Therefore, to refer to **ClassB** within **Main( )**, you must use **NS1.NS2.ClassB**.

Namespaces can be nested by more than two levels. When this is the case, a member in a nested namespace must be qualified with all of the enclosing namespace names.

You can specify a nested namespace using a single **namespace** statement by separating each namespace with a period. For example,

```
namespace OuterNS {
  namespace InnerNS {
    // ...
  }
}
```

can also be specified like this:

```
namespace OuterNS.InnerNS {
  // ...
}
```

The Global Namespace

If you don't declare a namespace for your program, then the default global namespace is used. This is why you have not needed to use **namespace** for the programs in the preceding chapters. Although the global namespace is convenient for the short, sample programs found in this book, most real-world code will be contained within a declared namespace. The main reason for encapsulating your code within a declared namespace is that it prevents name conflicts. Namespaces are another tool that you have to help you organize programs and make them viable in today's complex, networked environment.

Using the :: Namespace Alias Qualifier

Although namespaces help prevent name conflicts, they do not completely eliminate them. One way that a conflict can still occur is when the same name is declared within two different namespaces, and you then try to bring both namespaces into view. For example, assume that two different namespaces contain a class called **MyClass**. If you attempt to bring these two namespaces into view via **using** statements, **MyClass** in the first namespace will conflict with **MyClass** in the second namespace, causing an ambiguity error. In this situation, you can use the **::** *namespace alias qualifier* to explicitly specify which namespace is intended.

The :: operator has this general form.

namespace-alias::identifier

Here, *namespace-alias* is the name of a namespace alias and *identifier* is the name of a member of that namespace.

To understand why the namespace alias qualifier is needed, consider the following program. It creates two namespaces, **Counter** and **AnotherCounter**, and both declare a class called **CountDown**. Furthermore, both namespaces are brought into view by **using** statements. Finally, in **Main( )**, an attempt is made to instantiate an object of type **CountDown**.

```
// Demonstrate why the :: qualifier is needed.
//
// This program will not compile.

using System;

// Use both the Counter and AnotherCounter namespace.
using Counter;
using AnotherCounter;

// Declare a namespace for counters.
namespace Counter {
  // A simple countdown counter.
  class CountDown {
    int val;

    public CountDown(int n) {
      val = n;
    }

    // ...
  }
}

// Declare another namespace for counters.
namespace AnotherCounter {
  // Declare another class called CountDown, which
  // is in the AnotherCounter namespace.
  class CountDown {
    int val;

    public CountDown(int n) {
      val = n;
    }

    // ...
  }
}

class WhyAliasQualifier {
  static void Main() {
    int i;
```

```
    // The following line is inherently ambiguous!
    // Does it refer to CountDown in Counter or
    // to CountDown in AnotherCounter?
    CountDown cd1 = new CountDown(10); // Error! ! !

    // ...
  }
}
```

If you try to compile this program, you will receive an error message stating that this line in **Main( )** is ambiguous:

```
CountDown cd1 = new CountDown(10); // Error! ! !
```

The trouble is that both namespaces, **Counter** and **AnotherCounter**, declare a class called **CountDown**, and both namespaces have been brought into view. Thus, to which version of **CountDown** does the preceding declaration refer? The **::** qualifier was designed to handle these types of problems.

To use the **::**, you must first define an alias for the namespace you want to qualify. Then, simply qualify the ambiguous element with the alias. For example, here is one way to fix the preceding program:

```
// Demonstrate the :: qualifier.

using System;

using Counter;
using AnotherCounter;

// Give Counter an alias called Ctr.
using Ctr = Counter;

// Declare a namespace for counters.
namespace Counter {
  // A simple countdown counter.
  class CountDown {
    int val;

    public CountDown(int n) {
      val = n;
    }

    // ...
  }
}

// Another counter namespace.
namespace AnotherCounter {
  // Declare another class called CountDown, which
  // is in the AnotherCounter namespace.
  class CountDown {
    int val;
```

```
    public CountDown(int n) {
      val = n;
    }

    // ...
  }
}

class AliasQualifierDemo {
  static void Main() {

    // Here, the :: operator to resolve
    // tells the compiler to use the CountDown
    // that is in the Counter namespace.
    Ctr::CountDown cd1 = new Ctr::CountDown(10);

    // ...
  }
}
```

In this version, the alias **Ctr** is specified for **Counter** by the following line:

```
using Ctr = Counter;
```

Then, inside **Main( )**, this alias is used to qualify **CountDown**, as shown here:

```
Ctr::CountDown cd1 = new Ctr::CountDown(10);
```

The use of the :: qualifier removes the ambiguity because it specifies that the **CountDown** in **Ctr** (which stands for **Counter**) is desired, and the program now compiles.

You can use the :: qualifier to refer to the global namespace by using the predefined identifier **global**. For example, in the following program, a class called **CountDown** is declared in both the **Counter** namespace and in the global namespace. To access the version of **CountDown** in the global namespace, the predefined alias **global** is used.

```
// Use the global alias.

using System;

// Give Counter an alias called Ctr.
using Ctr = Counter;

// Declare a namespace for counters.
namespace Counter {
  // A simple countdown counter.
  class CountDown {
    int val;

    public CountDown(int n) {
      val = n;
    }

    // ...
  }
```

```
  }

  // Declare another class called CountDown, which
  // is in the global namespace.
  class CountDown {
    int val;

    public CountDown(int n) {
      val = n;
    }

    // ...
  }

  class GlobalAliasQualifierDemo {
    static void Main() {

      // Here, the :: qualifier tells the compiler
      // to use the CountDown in the Counter namespace.
      Ctr::CountDown cd1 = new Ctr::CountDown(10);

      // Next, create CountDown object from global namespace.
      global::CountDown cd2 = new global::CountDown(10);

      // ...
    }
  }
```

Notice how the **global** identifier is used to access the version of **CountDown** in the default namespace:

```
global::CountDown cd2 = new global::CountDown(10);
```

This same general approach can be generalized to any situation in which you need to specify the default namespace.

One final point: You can also use the namespace alias qualifier with **extern** aliases, which are described in Chapter 20.

The Preprocessor

C# defines several *preprocessor directives,* which affect the way that your program's source file is interpreted by the compiler. These directives affect the text of the source file in which they occur, prior to the translation of the program into object code. The term *preprocessor directive* comes from the fact that these instructions were traditionally handled by a separate compilation phase called the *preprocessor.* Today's modern compiler technology no longer requires a separate preprocessing stage to handle the directives, but the name has stuck.

C# defines the following preprocessor directives:

#define	#elif	#else	#endif
#endregion	#error	#if	#line
#pragma	#region	#undef	#warning

All preprocessor directives begin with a # sign. In addition, each preprocessor directive must be on its own line.

Given C#'s modern, object-oriented architecture, there is not as much need for the preprocessor directives as there is in older languages. Nevertheless, they can be of value from time to time, especially for conditional compilation. Each directive is examined in turn.

#define

The **#define** directive defines a character sequence called a *symbol*. The existence or nonexistence of a symbol can be determined by **#if** or **#elif** and is used to control compilation. Here is the general form for **#define**:

#define *symbol*

Notice that there is no semicolon in this statement. There may be any number of spaces between the **#define** and the symbol, but once the symbol begins, it is terminated only by a newline. For example, to define the symbol **EXPERIMENTAL**, use this directive:

```
#define EXPERIMENTAL
```

NOTE *In C/C++ you can use **#define** to perform textual substitutions, such as defining a name for a value, and to create function-like macros. C# does not support these uses of **#define**. In C#, **#define** is used only to define a symbol.*

#if and #endif

The **#if** and **#endif** directives enable conditional compilation of a sequence of code based upon whether an expression involving one or more symbols evaluates to true. A symbol is true if it has been defined. It is false otherwise. Thus, if a symbol has been defined by a **#define** directive, it will evaluate as true.

The general form of **#if** is

#if *symbol-expression*
   statement sequence
#endif

If the expression following **#if** is true, the code that is between it and **#endif** is compiled. Otherwise, the intervening code is skipped. The **#endif** directive marks the end of an **#if** block.

A symbol expression can be as simple as just the name of a symbol. You can also use these operators in a symbol expression: !, = =, !=, &&, and | |. Parentheses are also allowed. Here's an example:

```
// Demonstrate #if, #endif, and #define.

#define EXPERIMENTAL

using System;

class Test {
  static void Main() {

    #if EXPERIMENTAL
      Console.WriteLine("Compiled for experimental version.");
```

```
  #endif

    Console.WriteLine("This is in all versions.");
  }
}
```

This program displays the following:

```
Compiled for experimental version.
This is in all versions.
```

The program defines the symbol **EXPERIMENTAL**. Thus, when the **#if** is encountered, the symbol expression evaluates to true, and the first **WriteLine( )** statement is compiled. If you remove the definition of **EXPERIMENTAL** and recompile the program, the first **WriteLine( )** statement will not be compiled, because the **#if** will evaluate to false. In all cases, the second **WriteLine( )** statement is compiled because it is not part of the **#if** block.

As explained, you can use a symbol expression in an **#if**. For example,

```
// Use a symbol expression.

#define EXPERIMENTAL
#define TRIAL

using System;

class Test {
  static void Main() {

    #if EXPERIMENTAL
      Console.WriteLine("Compiled for experimental version.");
    #endif

    #if EXPERIMENTAL && TRIAL
      Console.Error.WriteLine("Testing experimental trial version.");
    #endif

    Console.WriteLine("This is in all versions.");
  }
}
```

The output from this program is shown here:

```
Compiled for experimental version.
Testing experimental trial version.
This is in all versions.
```

In this example, two symbols are defined, **EXPERIMENTAL** and **TRIAL**. The second **WriteLine( )** statement is compiled only if both are defined.

You can use the ! to compile code when a symbol is not defined. For example,

```
#if !EXPERIMENTAL
  Console.WriteLine("Code is not experimental!");
#endif
```

The call to **WriteLine( )** will be compiled only if **EXPERIMENTAL** *has not* been defined.

#else and #elif

The **#else** directive works much like the **else** that is part of the C# language: It establishes an alternative if **#if** fails. The previous example can be expanded as shown here:

```
// Demonstrate #else.

#define EXPERIMENTAL

using System;

class Test {
  static void Main() {

    #if EXPERIMENTAL
      Console.WriteLine("Compiled for experimental version.");
    #else
      Console.WriteLine("Compiled for release.");
    #endif

    #if EXPERIMENTAL && TRIAL
      Console.Error.WriteLine("Testing experimental trial version.");
    #else
      Console.Error.WriteLine("Not experimental trial version.");
    #endif

    Console.WriteLine("This is in all versions.");
  }
}
```

The output is shown here:

```
Compiled for experimental version.
Not experimental trial version.
This is in all versions.
```

Since **TRIAL** is not defined, the **#else** portion of the second conditional code sequence is used.

Notice that **#else** marks both the end of the **#if** block and the beginning of the **#else** block. This is necessary because there can only be one **#endif** associated with any **#if**. Furthermore, there can be only one **#else** associated with any **#if**.

The **#elif** directive means "else if" and establishes an if-else-if chain for multiple compilation options. **#elif** is followed by a symbol expression. If the expression is true, that block of code is compiled and no other **#elif** expressions are tested. Otherwise, the next block in the series is checked. If no **#elif** succeeds, then if there is a **#else**, the code sequence associated with the **#else** is compiled. Otherwise, no code in the entire **#if** is compiled.

The general form for **#elif** is

#if *symbol-expression*
   statement sequence
#elif *symbol-expression*
   statement sequence
#elif *symbol-expression*

```
    statement sequence
  // . . .
  #endif
```

Here's an example:

```
// Demonstrate #elif.

#define RELEASE

using System;

class Test {
  static void Main() {

    #if EXPERIMENTAL
      Console.WriteLine("Compiled for experimental version.");
    #elif RELEASE
      Console.WriteLine("Compiled for release.");
    #else
      Console.WriteLine("Compiled for internal testing.");
    #endif

    #if TRIAL && !RELEASE
       Console.WriteLine("Trial version.");
    #endif

    Console.WriteLine("This is in all versions.");
  }
}
```

The output is shown here:

```
Compiled for release.
This is in all versions.
```

#undef

The **#undef** directive removes a previously defined symbol. That is, it "undefines" a symbol. The general form for **#undef** is

    #undef *symbol*

Here's an example:

```
#define SMALL

#if SMALL
  // ...
#undef SMALL
// at this point SMALL is undefined.
```

After the **#undef** directive, **SMALL** is no longer defined.

  #undef is used principally to allow symbols to be localized to only those sections of code that need them.

#error

The **#error** directive forces the compiler to stop compilation. It is used for debugging. The general form of the **#error** directive is

#error *error-message*

When the **#error** directive is encountered, the error message is displayed. For example, when the compiler encounters this line:

```
#error This is a test error!
```

compilation stops and the error message "This is a test error!" is displayed.

#warning

The **#warning** directive is similar to **#error**, except that a warning rather than an error is produced. Thus, compilation is not stopped. The general form of the **#warning** directive is

#warning *warning-message*

#line

The **#line** directive sets the line number and filename for the file that contains the **#line** directive. The number and the name are used when errors or warnings are output during compilation. The general form for **#line** is

#line *number "filename"*

where *number* is any positive integer, which becomes the new line number, and the optional *filename* is any valid file identifier, which becomes the new filename. **#line** is primarily used for debugging and special applications.

#line allows two options. The first is **default**, which returns the line numbering to its original condition. It is used like this:

```
#line default
```

The second is **hidden**. When stepping through a program, the **hidden** option allows a debugger to bypass lines between a

```
#line hidden
```

directive and the next **#line** directive that does not include the **hidden** option.

#region and #endregion

The **#region** and **#endregion** directives let you define a region that will be expanded or collapsed when using outlining in the Visual Studio IDE. The general form is shown here:

#region *text*
  // code sequence
#endregion *text*

Here, *text* is an optional string.

#pragma

The **#pragma** directive gives instructions, such as specifying an option, to the compiler. It has this general form:

#pragma *option*

Here, *option* is the instruction passed to the compiler.

In C# 3.0, there are two options supported by **#pragma**. The first is **warning**, which is used to enable or disable specific compiler warnings. It has these two forms:

#pragma warning disable *warnings*

#pragma warning restore *warnings*

Here, *warnings* is a comma-separated list of warning numbers. To disable a warning, use the **disable** option. To enable a warning, use the **restore** option.

For example, this **#pragma** statement disables warning 168, which indicates when a variable is declared but not used:

```
#pragma warning disable 168
```

The second **#pragma** option is **checksum**. It is used to generate checksums for ASP.NET projects. It has this general form.

#pragma checksum *"filename" "{GUID}" "check-sum"*

Here, *filename* is the name of the file, *GUID* is the globally unique identifier associated with *filename*, and *check-sum* is a hexadecimal number that contains the checksum. This string must contain an even number of digits.

Assemblies and the internal Access Modifier

An integral part of C# programming is the assembly. An *assembly* is a file (or files) that contains all deployment and version information for a program. Assemblies are fundamental to the .NET environment. They provide mechanisms that support safe component interaction, interlanguage operability, and versioning. An assembly also defines a scope.

An assembly is composed of four sections. The first is the assembly *manifest*. The manifest contains information about the assembly, itself. This data includes such things as the name of the assembly, its version number, type mapping information, and cultural settings. The second section is *type metadata,* which is information about the data types used by the program. Among other benefits, type metadata aids in cross-language interoperability. The third part of an assembly is the *program code,* which is stored in Microsoft Intermediate Language (MSIL) format. The fourth constituent of an assembly is the resources used by the program.

Fortunately, when using C#, assemblies are produced automatically, with little or no extra effort on your part. The reason for this is that the **exe** file created when you compile a C# program is actually an assembly that contains your program's executable code as well as other types of information. Thus, when you compile a C# program, an assembly is automatically produced.

There are many other features and topics that relate to assemblies, but a discussion of these is outside the scope of this book. (Assemblies are an integral part of .NET development,

but are not technically a feature of the C# language.) However, there is one part of C# that relates directly to the assembly: the **internal** access modifier, which is examined next.

The internal Access Modifier

In addition to the access modifiers **public**, **private**, and **protected**, which you have been using throughout this book, C# also defines **internal**. The **internal** modifier declares that a member is known throughout all files in an assembly, but unknown outside that assembly. Thus, in simplified terms, a member marked as **internal** is known throughout a program, but not elsewhere. The **internal** access modifier is particularly useful when creating software components.

The **internal** modifier can be applied to classes and members of classes and to structures and members of structures. The **internal** modifier can also be applied to interface and enumeration declarations.

You can use **protected** in conjunction with **internal** to produce the **protected internal** access modifier pair. The **protected internal** access level can be given only to class members. A member declared with **protected internal** access is accessible within its own assembly or to derived types.

Here is an example that uses **internal**:

```
// Use internal.

using System;

class InternalTest {
  internal int x;
}

class InternalDemo {
  static void Main() {
    InternalTest ob = new InternalTest();

    ob.x = 10; // can access -- in same file

    Console.WriteLine("Here is ob.x: " + ob.x);

  }
}
```

Inside **InternalTest**, the field **x** is declared **internal**. This means that it is accessible within the program, as its use in **InternalDemo** shows, but unavailable outside the program.

Runtime Type ID, Reflection, and Attributes

This chapter discusses three interrelated and powerful features: runtime type identification, reflection, and attributes. *Runtime type ID* is the mechanism that lets you identify a type during the execution of a program. *Reflection* is the feature that enables you to obtain information about a type. Using this information, you can construct and use objects at runtime. This feature is very powerful because it lets a program add functionality dynamically, during execution. An *attribute* describes a characteristic of some element of a C# program. For example, you can specify attributes for classes, methods, and fields, among others. Attributes can be interrogated at runtime, and the attribute information obtained. Attributes use both runtime type identification and reflection.

Runtime Type Identification

Runtime type identification (RTTI) allows the type of an object to be determined during program execution. RTTI is useful for many reasons. For example, you can discover precisely what type of object is being referred to by a base-class reference. Another use of RTTI is to test in advance whether a cast will succeed, preventing an invalid cast exception. Runtime type identification is also a key component of reflection.

C# includes three keywords that support runtime type identification: **is**, **as**, and **typeof**. Each is examined in turn.

Testing a Type with is

You can determine if an object is of a certain type by using the **is** operator. Its general form is shown here:

expr is *type*

Here, *expr* is an expression that describes an object whose type is being tested against *type*. If the type of *expr* is the same as, or compatible with, *type,* then the outcome of this operation is true. Otherwise, it is false. Thus, if the outcome is true, *expr* is some form of *type*. As it applies to **is**, one type is compatible with another if both are the same type, or if a reference, boxing, or unboxing conversion exists.

Here is an example that uses **is**:

```
// Demonstrate is.

using System;

class A {}
class B : A {}

class UseIs {
  static void Main() {
    A a = new A();
    B b = new B();

    if(a is A) Console.WriteLine("a is an A");
    if(b is A)
      Console.WriteLine("b is an A because it is derived from A");
    if(a is B)
      Console.WriteLine("This won't display -- a not derived from B");

    if(b is B) Console.WriteLine("B is a B");
    if(a is object) Console.WriteLine("a is an object");
  }
}
```

The output is shown here:

```
a is an A
b is an A because it is derived from A
B is a B
a is an object
```

Most of the **is** expressions are self-explanatory, but two may need a little discussion. First, notice this statement:

```
if(b is A)
  Console.WriteLine("b is an A because it is derived from A");
```

The **if** succeeds because **b** is an object of type **B**, which is derived from type **A**. Thus, **b** *is* an **A**. However, the reverse is not true. When this line is executed,

```
if(a is B)
  Console.WriteLine("This won't display -- a not derived from B");
```

the **if** does not succeed, because **a** is of type **A**, which is not derived from **B**. Thus, **a** *is not* **B**.

Using as

Sometimes you will want to try a conversion at runtime, but not throw an exception if the conversion fails (which is the case when a cast is used). To do this, use the **as** operator, which has this general form:

expr as *type*

Here, *expr* is the expression being converted to *type*. If the conversion succeeds, then a reference to *type* is returned. Otherwise, a null reference is returned. The **as** operator can be used to perform only reference, boxing, unboxing, or identity conversions.

The **as** operator offers a streamlined alternative to **is** in some cases. For example, consider the following program that uses **is** to prevent an invalid cast from occurring:

```
// Use is to avoid an invalid cast.

using System;

class A {}
class B : A {}

class CheckCast {
  static void Main() {
    A a = new A();
    B b = new B();

    // Check to see if a can be cast to B.
    if(a is B)  // if so, do the cast
      b = (B) a;
    else // if not, skip the cast
      b = null;

    if(b==null)
      Console.WriteLine("The cast in b = (B) a is NOT allowed.");
    else
      Console.WriteLine("The cast in b = (B) a is allowed");
  }
}
```

This program displays the following output:

```
The cast in b = (B) a is NOT allowed.
```

As the output shows, since **a** is not a **B**, the cast of **a** to **B** is invalid and is prevented by the **if** statement. However, this approach requires two steps. First, the validity of the cast must be confirmed. Second, the cast must be made. These two steps can be combined into one through the use of **as**, as the following program shows:

```
// Demonstrate as.

using System;

class A {}
class B : A {}

class CheckCast {
  static void Main() {
    A a = new A();
    B b = new B();

    b = a as B; // cast, if possible
```

```
    if(b==null)
      Console.WriteLine("The cast in b = (B) a is NOT allowed.");
    else
      Console.WriteLine("The cast in b = (B) a is allowed");
  }
}
```

Here is the output, which is the same as before:

```
The cast in b = (B) a is NOT allowed.
```

In this version, the **as** statement checks the validity of the cast and then, if valid, performs the cast, all in one statement.

Using typeof

Although useful in their own ways, the **as** and **is** operators simply test the compatibility of two types. Often, you will need to obtain information about a type. To do this, C# supplies the **typeof** operator. It retrieves a **System.Type** object for a given type. Using this object, you can determine the type's characteristics.

The **typeof** operator has this general form:

typeof(*type*)

Here, *type* is the type being obtained. The **Type** object returned encapsulates the information associated with *type*.

Once you have obtained a **Type** object for a given type, you can obtain information about it through the use of various properties, fields, and methods defined by **Type**. **Type** is a large class with many members, and a discussion is deferred until the next section, where reflection is examined. However, to briefly demonstrate **Type**, the following program uses three of its properties: **FullName**, **IsClass**, and **IsAbstract**. To obtain the full name of the type, use **FullName**. **IsClass** returns true if the type is a class. **IsAbstract** returns true if a class is abstract.

```
// Demonstrate typeof.

using System;
using System.IO;

class UseTypeof {
  static void Main() {
    Type t = typeof(StreamReader);

    Console.WriteLine(t.FullName);

    if(t.IsClass) Console.WriteLine("Is a class.");
    if(t.IsAbstract) Console.WriteLine("Is abstract.");
    else Console.WriteLine("Is concrete.");
  }
}
```

This program outputs the following:

```
System.IO.StreamReader
Is a class.
Is concrete.
```

This program obtains a **Type** object that describes **StreamReader**. It then displays the full name, and determines if it is a class and whether it is abstract.

Reflection

Reflection is the feature that enables you to obtain information about a type. The term *reflection* comes from the way the process works: A **Type** object mirrors the underlying type that it represents. To obtain information, you ask the **Type** object questions, and it returns (reflects) the information associated with the type back to you. Reflection is a powerful mechanism because it allows you to learn and use the capabilities of types that are known only at runtime.

Many of the classes that support reflection are part of the .NET Reflection API, which is in the **System.Reflection** namespace. Thus, you will normally include the following in programs that use reflection:

```
using System.Reflection;
```

The Reflection Core: System.Type

System.Type is at the core of the reflection subsystem because it encapsulates a type. It contains many properties and methods that you will use to obtain information about a type at runtime. **Type** is derived from an abstract class called **System.Reflection.MemberInfo**.

MemberInfo defines the following read-only properties:

Property	Description
Type DeclaringType	Obtains the type of the class or interface in which the member is declared.
MemberTypes MemberType	Obtains the kind of the member. This value indicates if the member is a field, method, property, event, or constructor.
int MetadataToken	Obtains a value associated with a specific metadata.
Module Module	Obtains a **Module** object that represents the module (an executable file) in which the reflected type resides.
string Name	The name of the type.
Type ReflectedType	The type of the object being reflected.

Notice that the return type of **MemberType** is **MemberTypes**. **MemberTypes** is an enumeration that defines values that indicate the various member types. Among others, these include

MemberTypes.Constructor
MemberTypes.Method
MemberTypes.Field
MemberTypes.Event
MemberTypes.Property

Thus, the type of a member can be determined by checking **MemberType**. For example, if **MemberType** equals **MemberTypes.Method**, then that member is a method.

MemberInfo includes two abstract methods: **GetCustomAttributes( )** and **IsDefined( )**. These both relate to attributes. The first obtains a list of the custom attributes associated with the invoking object. The second determines if an attribute is defined for the invoking object. (Attributes are described later in this chapter.)

To the methods and properties defined by **MemberInfo**, **Type** adds a great many of its own. For example, here are several commonly used methods defined by **Type**:

Method	Purpose
ConstructorInfo[ ] GetConstructors( )	Obtains a list of the constructors for the specified type.
EventInfo[ ] GetEvents( )	Obtains a list of events for the specified type.
FieldInfo[ ] GetFields( )	Obtains a list of the fields for the specified type.
Type[ ] GetGenericArguments( )	Obtains a list of the type arguments bound to a closed constructed generic type or the type parameters if the specified type is a generic type definition. For an open constructed type, the list may contain both type arguments and type parameters. (See Chapter 18 for a discussion of generics.)
MemberInfo[ ] GetMembers( )	Obtains a list of the members for the specified type.
MethodInfo[ ] GetMethods( )	Obtains a list of methods for the specified type.
PropertyInfo[ ] GetProperties( )	Obtains a list of properties for the specified type.

Here are several commonly used, read-only properties defined by **Type**:

Property	Purpose
Assembly Assembly	Obtains the assembly for the specified type.
TypeAttributes Attributes	Obtains the attributes for the specified type.
Type BaseType	Obtains the immediate base type for the specified type.
string FullName	Obtains the complete name of the specified type.
bool IsAbstract	Is true if the specified type is abstract.
bool isArray	Is true if the specified type is an array.
bool IsClass	Is true if the specified type is a class.
bool IsEnum	Is true if the specified type is an enumeration.
bool IsGenericParameter	Is true if the specified type is a generic type parameter. (See Chapter 18 for a discussion of generics.)
bool IsGenericType	Is true if the specified type is a generic type. (See Chapter 18 for a discussion of generics.)
string Namespace	Obtains the namespace of the specified type.

Using Reflection

Using **Type**'s methods and properties, it is possible to obtain detailed information about a type at runtime. This is an extremely powerful feature, because once you have obtained information about a type, you can invoke its constructors, call its methods, and use its properties. Thus, reflection enables you to use code that was not available at compile time.

The Reflection API is quite large, and it is not possible to cover the entire topic here. (Complete coverage of reflection could easily fill an entire book!) However, because the Reflection API is logically designed, once you understand how to use a part of it, the rest just falls into place. With this thought in mind, the following sections demonstrate four key reflection techniques: obtaining information about methods, invoking methods, constructing objects, and loading types from assemblies.

Obtaining Information About Methods

Once you have a **Type** object, you can obtain a list of methods supported by the type by using **GetMethods( )**. One form is shown here:

MethodInfo[ ] GetMethods( )

It returns an array of **MethodInfo** objects that describe the methods supported by the invoking type. **MethodInfo** is in the **System.Reflection** namespace.

MethodInfo is derived from the abstract class **MethodBase**, which inherits **MemberInfo**. Thus, the properties and methods defined by all three of these classes are available for your use. For example, to obtain the name of a method, use the **Name** property. Two members that are of particular interest at this time are **ReturnType** and **GetParameters( )**.

The return type of a method is found in the read-only **ReturnType** property, which is an object of **Type**.

The method **GetParameters( )** returns a list of the parameters associated with a method. It has this general form:

ParameterInfo[ ] GetParameters( );

The parameter information is held in a **ParameterInfo** object. **ParameterInfo** defines a large number of properties and methods that describe the parameter. Two properties that are of particular value are **Name**, which is a string that contains the name of the parameter, and **ParameterType**, which describes the parameter's type. The parameter's type is encapsulated within a **Type** object.

Here is a program that uses reflection to obtain the methods supported by a class called **MyClass**. For each method, it displays the return type and name of the method, and the name and type of any parameters that each method may have.

```
// Analyze methods using reflection.

using System;
using System.Reflection;

class MyClass {
  int x;
  int y;
```

```
  public MyClass(int i, int j) {
    x = i;
    y = j;
  }

  public int Sum() {
    return x+y;
  }

  public bool IsBetween(int i) {
    if(x < i && i < y) return true;
    else return false;
  }

  public void Set(int a, int b) {
    x = a;
    y = b;
  }

  public void Set(double a, double b) {
    x = (int) a;
    y = (int) b;
  }

  public void Show() {
    Console.WriteLine(" x: {0}, y: {1}", x, y);
  }
}

class ReflectDemo {
  static void Main() {
    Type t = typeof(MyClass); // get a Type object representing MyClass

    Console.WriteLine("Analyzing methods in " + t.Name);
    Console.WriteLine();

    Console.WriteLine("Methods supported: ");

    MethodInfo[] mi = t.GetMethods();

    // Display methods supported by MyClass.
    foreach(MethodInfo m in mi) {
      // Display return type and name.
      Console.Write("   " + m.ReturnType.Name +
                    " " + m.Name + "(");

      // Display parameters.
      ParameterInfo[] pi = m.GetParameters();

      for(int i=0; i < pi.Length; i++) {
        Console.Write(pi[i].ParameterType.Name +
                      " " + pi[i].Name);
        if(i+1 < pi.Length) Console.Write(", ");
      }
```

```
        Console.WriteLine(")");

        Console.WriteLine();
      }
    }
}
```

The output is shown here:

```
Analyzing methods in MyClass

Methods supported:
    Int32 Sum()

    Boolean IsBetween(Int32 i)

    Void Set(Int32 a, Int32 b)

    Void Set(Double a, Double b)

    Void Show()

    Type GetType()

    String ToString()

    Boolean Equals(Object obj)

    Int32 GetHashCode()
```

Notice that in addition to the methods defined by **MyClass**, the methods defined by **object** are also displayed. This is because all types in C# inherit **object**. Also notice that the .NET structure names are used for the type names. Observe that **Set( )** is displayed twice. This is because **Set( )** is overloaded. One version takes **int** arguments. The other takes **double** arguments.

Let's look at this program closely. First, notice that **MyClass** defines a public constructor and a number of public methods, including the overloaded **Set( )** method.

Inside **Main( )**, a **Type** object representing **MyClass** is obtained using this line of code:

```
Type t = typeof(MyClass); // get a Type object representing MyClass
```

Recall that **typeof** returns a **Type** object that represents the specified type, which in this case is **MyClass**.

Using **t** and the Reflection API, the program then displays information about the methods supported by **MyClass**. First, a list of the methods is obtained by the following statement:

```
MethodInfo[] mi = t.GetMethods();
```

Next, a **foreach** loop is established that cycles through **mi**. With each pass, the return type, name, and parameters for each method are displayed by the following code:

```
// Display return type and name.
Console.Write("   " + m.ReturnType.Name +
            " " + m.Name + "(");
```

```
// Display parameters.
ParameterInfo[] pi = m.GetParameters();

for(int i=0; i < pi.Length; i++) {
  Console.Write(pi[i].ParameterType.Name +
                " " + pi[i].Name);
  if(i+1 < pi.Length) Console.Write(", ");
}
```

In this sequence, the parameters associated with each method are obtained by calling **GetParameters( )** and stored in the **pi** array. Then a **for** loop cycles through the **pi** array, displaying the type and name of each parameter. The key point is that this information is obtained dynamically at runtime without relying on prior knowledge of **MyClass**.

A Second Form of GetMethods( )

A second form of **GetMethods( )** lets you specify various flags that filter the methods that are retrieved. It has this general form:

MethodInfo[ ] GetMethods(BindingFlags *flags*)

This version obtains only those methods that match the criteria you specify. **BindingFlags** is an enumeration. Here are several commonly used values:

Value	Meaning
DeclaredOnly	Retrieves only those methods defined by the specified class. Inherited methods are not included.
Instance	Retrieves instance methods.
NonPublic	Retrieves nonpublic methods.
Public	Retrieves public methods.
Static	Retrieves **static** methods.

You can OR together two or more flags. In fact, minimally you must include either **Instance** or **Static** with **Public** or **NonPublic**. Failure to do so will result in no methods being retrieved.

One of the main uses of the **BindingFlags** form of **GetMethods( )** is to enable you to obtain a list of the methods defined by a class without also retrieving the inherited methods. This is especially useful for preventing the methods defined by **object** from being obtained. For example, try substituting this call to **GetMethods( )** into the preceding program:

```
// Now, only methods declared by MyClass are obtained.
MethodInfo[] mi = t.GetMethods(BindingFlags.DeclaredOnly |
                      BindingFlags.Instance |
                      BindingFlags.Public) ;
```

After making this change, the program produces the following output:

```
Analyzing methods in MyClass

Methods supported:
  Int32 Sum()
```

```
Boolean IsBetween(Int32 i)

Void Set(Int32 a, Int32 b)

Void Set(Double a, Double b)

Void Show()
```

As you can see, only those methods explicitly defined by **MyClass** are displayed.

Calling Methods Using Reflection

Once you know what methods a type supports, you can call one or more of them. To do this, you will use the **Invoke( )** method that is contained in **MethodInfo**. One of its forms is shown here:

> object Invoke(object *ob*, object[ ] *args*)

Here, *ob* is a reference to the object on which the method is invoked. For **static** methods, pass **null** to *ob*. Any arguments that need to be passed to the method are specified in the array *args*. If no arguments are needed, *args* must be **null**. Also, *args* must contain exactly the same number of elements as there are arguments. Therefore, if two arguments are needed, then *args* must be two elements long. It can't, for example, be three or four elements long. The value returned by the invoked method is returned by **Invoke( )**.

To call a method, simply call **Invoke( )** on an instance of **MethodInfo** that was obtained by calling **GetMethods( )**. The following program demonstrates the procedure:

```
// Invoke methods using reflection.

using System;
using System.Reflection;

class MyClass {
  int x;
  int y;

  public MyClass(int i, int j) {
    x = i;
    y = j;
  }

  public int Sum() {
    return x+y;
  }

  public bool IsBetween(int i) {
    if((x < i) && (i < y)) return true;
    else return false;
  }

  public void Set(int a, int b) {
    Console.Write("Inside Set(int, int). ");
    x = a;
```

```
      y = b;
      Show();
    }

    // Overload set.
    public void Set(double a, double b) {
      Console.Write("Inside Set(double, double). ");
      x = (int) a;
      y = (int) b;
      Show();
    }

    public void Show() {
      Console.WriteLine("Values are x: {0}, y: {1}", x, y);
    }
  }

  class InvokeMethDemo {
    static void Main() {
      Type t = typeof(MyClass);
      MyClass reflectOb = new MyClass(10, 20);
      int val;

      Console.WriteLine("Invoking methods in " + t.Name);
      Console.WriteLine();
      MethodInfo[] mi = t.GetMethods();

      // Invoke each method.
      foreach(MethodInfo m in mi) {
        // Get the parameters.
        ParameterInfo[] pi = m.GetParameters();

        if(m.Name.CompareTo("Set")==0 &&
           pi[0].ParameterType == typeof(int)) {
          object[] args = new object[2];
          args[0] = 9;
          args[1] = 18;
          m.Invoke(reflectOb, args);
        }
        else if(m.Name.CompareTo("Set")==0 &&
                pi[0].ParameterType == typeof(double)) {
          object[] args = new object[2];
          args[0] = 1.12;
          args[1] = 23.4;
          m.Invoke(reflectOb, args);
        }
        else if(m.Name.CompareTo("Sum")==0) {
          val = (int) m.Invoke(reflectOb, null);
          Console.WriteLine("sum is " + val);
        }
        else if(m.Name.CompareTo("IsBetween")==0) {
          object[] args = new object[1];
          args[0] = 14;
          if((bool) m.Invoke(reflectOb, args))
```

```
          Console.WriteLine("14 is between x and y");
      }
      else if(m.Name.CompareTo("Show")==0) {
        m.Invoke(reflectOb, null);
      }
    }
  }
}
```

The output is shown here:

```
Invoking methods in MyClass

sum is 30
14 is between x and y
Inside Set(int, int). Values are x: 9, y: 18
Inside Set(double, double). Values are x: 1, y: 23
Values are x: 1, y: 23
```

Look closely at how the methods are invoked. First, a list of methods is obtained. Then, inside the **foreach** loop, parameter information is retrieved. Next, using a series of if/else statements, each method is executed with the proper type and number of arguments. Pay special attention to the way that the overloaded **Set( )** method is executed by the following code:

```
if(m.Name.CompareTo("Set")==0 &&
   pi[0].ParameterType == typeof(int)) {
  object[] args = new object[2];
  args[0] = 9;
  args[1] = 18;
  m.Invoke(reflectOb, args);
}
else if(m.Name.CompareTo("Set")==0 &&
   pi[0].ParameterType == typeof(double)) {
  object[] args = new object[2];
  args[0] = 1.12;
  args[1] = 23.4;
  m.Invoke(reflectOb, args);
}
```

If the name of the method is **Set**, then the type of the first parameter is tested to determine which version of the method was found. If it was **Set(int, int)**, then **int** arguments are loaded into **args**. Otherwise, **double** arguments are used.

Obtaining a Type's Constructors

In the previous example, there is no advantage to using reflection to invoke methods on **MyClass** since an object of type **MyClass** was explicitly created. It would be easier to just call its methods normally. However, the power of reflection starts to become apparent when an object is created dynamically at runtime. To do this, you will need to first obtain a list of the constructors. Then, you will create an instance of the type by invoking one of the constructors. This mechanism allows you to instantiate any type of object at runtime without naming it in a declaration statement.

To obtain the constructors for a type, call **GetConstructors( )** on a **Type** object. One commonly used form is shown here:

ConstructorInfo[ ] GetConstructors( )

It returns an array of **ConstructorInfo** objects that describe the constructors.

ConstructorInfo is derived from the abstract class **MethodBase**, which inherits **MemberInfo**. It also defines several members of its own. The one we are interested in is **GetParameters( )**, which returns a list of the parameters associated with a constructor. It works just like **GetParameters( )** defined by **MethodInfo**, described earlier.

Once an appropriate constructor has been found, an object is created by calling the **Invoke( )** method defined by **ConstructorInfo**. One form is shown here:

object Invoke(object[ ] *args*)

Any arguments that need to be passed to the method are specified in the array *args*. If no arguments are needed, pass **null** to *args*. In all cases, *args* must contain exactly the same number of elements as there are arguments and the types of arguments must be compatible with the types of the parameters. **Invoke( )** returns a reference to the object that was constructed.

The following program uses reflection to create an instance of **MyClass**:

```
// Create an object using reflection.

using System;
using System.Reflection;

class MyClass {
  int x;
  int y;

  public MyClass(int i) {
    Console.WriteLine("Constructing MyClass(int, int). ");
    x = y = i;
  }

  public MyClass(int i, int j) {
    Console.WriteLine("Constructing MyClass(int, int). ");
    x = i;
    y = j;
    Show();
  }

  public int Sum() {
    return x+y;
  }

  public bool IsBetween(int i) {
    if((x < i) && (i < y)) return true;
    else return false;
  }

  public void Set(int a, int b) {
    Console.Write("Inside Set(int, int). ");
```

```
    x = a;
    y = b;
    Show();
  }

  // Overload Set.
  public void Set(double a, double b) {
    Console.Write("Inside Set(double, double). ");
    x = (int) a;
    y = (int) b;
    Show();
  }

  public void Show() {
    Console.WriteLine("Values are x: {0}, y: {1}", x, y);
  }

}

class InvokeConsDemo {
  static void Main() {
    Type t = typeof(MyClass);
    int val;

    // Get constructor info.
    ConstructorInfo[] ci = t.GetConstructors();

    Console.WriteLine("Available constructors: ");
    foreach(ConstructorInfo c in ci) {
      // Display return type and name.
      Console.Write("    " + t.Name + "(");

      // Display parameters.
      ParameterInfo[] pi = c.GetParameters();

      for(int i=0; i < pi.Length; i++) {
        Console.Write(pi[i].ParameterType.Name +
                      " " + pi[i].Name);
        if(i+1 < pi.Length) Console.Write(", ");
      }

      Console.WriteLine(")");
    }
    Console.WriteLine();

    // Find matching constructor.
    int x;

    for(x=0; x < ci.Length; x++) {
      ParameterInfo[] pi =  ci[x].GetParameters();
      if(pi.Length == 2) break;
    }

    if(x == ci.Length) {
```

```
        Console.WriteLine("No matching constructor found.");
        return;
      }
      else
        Console.WriteLine("Two-parameter constructor found.\n");

      // Construct the object.
      object[] consargs = new object[2];
      consargs[0] = 10;
      consargs[1] = 20;
      object reflectOb = ci[x].Invoke(consargs);

      Console.WriteLine("\nInvoking methods on reflectOb.");
      Console.WriteLine();
      MethodInfo[] mi = t.GetMethods();

      // Invoke each method.
      foreach(MethodInfo m in mi) {
        // Get the parameters.
        ParameterInfo[] pi = m.GetParameters();

        if(m.Name.CompareTo("Set")==0 &&
            pi[0].ParameterType == typeof(int)) {
          // This is Set(int, int).
          object[] args = new object[2];
          args[0] = 9;
          args[1] = 18;
          m.Invoke(reflectOb, args);
        }
        else if(m.Name.CompareTo("Set")==0 &&
                  pi[0].ParameterType == typeof(double)) {
          // This is Set(double, double).
          object[] args = new object[2];
          args[0] = 1.12;
          args[1] = 23.4;
          m.Invoke(reflectOb, args);
        }
        else if(m.Name.CompareTo("Sum")==0) {
          val = (int) m.Invoke(reflectOb, null);
          Console.WriteLine("sum is " + val);
        }
        else if(m.Name.CompareTo("IsBetween")==0) {
          object[] args = new object[1];
          args[0] = 14;
          if((bool) m.Invoke(reflectOb, args))
            Console.WriteLine("14 is between x and y");
        }
        else if(m.Name.CompareTo("Show")==0) {
          m.Invoke(reflectOb, null);
        }
      }
    }
  }
}
```

The output is shown here:

```
Available constructors:
   MyClass(Int32 i)
   MyClass(Int32 i, Int32 j)

Two-parameter constructor found.

Constructing MyClass(int, int).
Values are x: 10, y: 20

Invoking methods on reflectOb.

sum is 30
14 is between x and y
Inside Set(int, int). Values are x: 9, y: 18
Inside Set(double, double). Values are x: 1, y: 23
Values are x: 1, y: 23
```

Let's look at how reflection is used to construct a **MyClass** object. First, a list of the public constructors is obtained using the following statement:

```
ConstructorInfo[] ci = t.GetConstructors();
```

Next, for the sake of illustration, the constructors are displayed. Then the list is searched for a constructor that takes two arguments, using this code:

```
for(x=0; x < ci.Length; x++) {
  ParameterInfo[] pi =  ci[x].GetParameters();
  if(pi.Length == 2) break;
}
```

If the constructor is found (as it will be in this case), an object is instantiated by the following sequence:

```
// Construct the object.
object[] consargs = new object[2];
consargs[0] = 10;
consargs[1] = 20;
object reflectOb = ci[x].Invoke(consargs);
```

After the call to **Invoke( )**, **reflectOb** will refer to an object of type **MyClass**. The program then executes methods on that instance.

One important point needs to be made. In this example, for the sake of simplicity, it was assumed that the only two-argument constructor was one that took two **int** arguments. Obviously, in real-world code this would need to be verified by checking the parameter type of each argument.

Obtaining Types from Assemblies

In the preceding example, everything about **MyClass** has been discovered using reflection except for one item: the type **MyClass**, itself. That is, although the preceding examples dynamically determined information about **MyClass**, they still relied upon the fact that the

type name **MyClass** was known in advance and used in a **typeof** statement to obtain a **Type** object upon which all of the reflection methods either directly or indirectly operated. Although this might be useful in a number of circumstances, the full power of reflection is found when the types available to a program are determined dynamically by analyzing the contents of other assemblies.

As you know from Chapter 16, an assembly carries with it type information about the classes, structures, and so on, that it contains. The Reflection API allows you to load an assembly, discover information about it, and create instances of any of its publicly available types. Using this mechanism, a program can search its environment, utilizing functionality that might be available without having to explicitly define that functionality at compile time. This is an extremely potent, and exciting, concept. For example, you can imagine a program that acts as a "type browser," displaying the types available on a system. Another application could be a design tool that lets you visually "wire together" a program that is composed of the various types supported by the system. Since all information about a type is discoverable, there is no inherent limitation to the ways reflection can be applied.

To obtain information about an assembly, you will first create an **Assembly** object. The **Assembly** class does not define a public constructor. Instead, an **Assembly** object is obtained by calling one of its methods. The one we will use is **LoadFrom( )**, which loads an assembly given its filename. The form we will use is shown here:

static Assembly LoadFrom(string *filename*)

Here, *filename* specifies the filename of the assembly.

Once you have obtained an **Assembly** object, you can discover the types that it defines by calling **GetTypes( )** on it. Here is its general form:

Type[ ] GetTypes( )

It returns an array of the types contained in the assembly.

To demonstrate the discovery of types in an assembly, you will need two files. The first will contain a set of classes that will be discovered by the second. To begin, create a file called **MyClasses.cs** that contains the following:

```csharp
// A file that contains three classes. Call this file MyClasses.cs.

using System;

class MyClass {
  int x;
  int y;

  public MyClass(int i) {
    Console.WriteLine("Constructing MyClass(int). ");
    x = y = i;
    Show();
  }

  public MyClass(int i, int j) {
    Console.WriteLine("Constructing MyClass(int, int). ");
    x = i;
    y = j;
```

```
      Show();
    }

    public int Sum() {
      return x+y;
    }

    public bool IsBetween(int i) {
      if((x < i) && (i < y)) return true;
      else return false;
    }

    public void Set(int a, int b) {
      Console.Write("Inside Set(int, int). ");
      x = a;
      y = b;
      Show();
    }

    // Overload Set.
    public void Set(double a, double b) {
      Console.Write("Inside Set(double, double). ");
      x = (int) a;
      y = (int) b;
      Show();
    }

    public void Show() {
      Console.WriteLine("Values are x: {0}, y: {1}", x, y);
    }
}

class AnotherClass {
  string msg;

  public AnotherClass(string str) {
    msg = str;
  }

  public void Show() {
    Console.WriteLine(msg);
  }
}

class Demo {
  static void Main() {
    Console.WriteLine("This is a placeholder.");
  }
}
```

This file contains **MyClass**, which we have been using in the previous examples. It also adds a second class called **AnotherClass** and a third class called **Demo**. Thus, the assembly

produced by this program will contain three classes. Next, compile this file so the file **MyClasses.exe** is produced. This is the assembly that will be interrogated.

The program that will discover information about **MyClasses.exe** is shown here. Enter it at this time.

```csharp
/* Locate an assembly, determine types, and create
   an object using reflection. */

using System;
using System.Reflection;

class ReflectAssemblyDemo {
  static void Main() {
    int val;

    // Load the MyClasses.exe assembly.
    Assembly asm = Assembly.LoadFrom("MyClasses.exe");

    // Discover what types MyClasses.exe contains.
    Type[] alltypes = asm.GetTypes();
    foreach(Type temp in alltypes)
      Console.WriteLine("Found: " + temp.Name);

    Console.WriteLine();

    // Use the first type, which is MyClass in this case.
    Type t = alltypes[0]; // use first class found
    Console.WriteLine("Using: " + t.Name);

    // Obtain constructor info.
    ConstructorInfo[] ci = t.GetConstructors();

    Console.WriteLine("Available constructors: ");
    foreach(ConstructorInfo c in ci) {
      // Display return type and name.
      Console.Write("    " + t.Name + "(");

      // Display parameters.
      ParameterInfo[] pi = c.GetParameters();

      for(int i=0; i < pi.Length; i++) {
        Console.Write(pi[i].ParameterType.Name +
                      " " + pi[i].Name);
        if(i+1 < pi.Length) Console.Write(", ");
      }

      Console.WriteLine(")");
    }
    Console.WriteLine();

    // Find matching constructor.
    int x;

    for(x=0; x < ci.Length; x++) {
```

```
    ParameterInfo[] pi =  ci[x].GetParameters();
    if(pi.Length == 2) break;
}

if(x == ci.Length) {
  Console.WriteLine("No matching constructor found.");
  return;
}
else
  Console.WriteLine("Two-parameter constructor found.\n");

// Construct the object.
object[] consargs = new object[2];
consargs[0] = 10;
consargs[1] = 20;
object reflectOb = ci[x].Invoke(consargs);

Console.WriteLine("\nInvoking methods on reflectOb.");
Console.WriteLine();
MethodInfo[] mi = t.GetMethods();

// Invoke each method.
foreach(MethodInfo m in mi) {
  // Get the parameters.
  ParameterInfo[] pi = m.GetParameters();

  if(m.Name.CompareTo("Set")==0 &&
     pi[0].ParameterType == typeof(int)) {
    // This is Set(int, int).
    object[] args = new object[2];
    args[0] = 9;
    args[1] = 18;
    m.Invoke(reflectOb, args);
  }
  else if(m.Name.CompareTo("Set")==0 &&
     pi[0].ParameterType == typeof(double)) {
    // This is Set(double, double).
    object[] args = new object[2];
    args[0] = 1.12;
    args[1] = 23.4;
    m.Invoke(reflectOb, args);
  }
  else if(m.Name.CompareTo("Sum")==0) {
    val = (int) m.Invoke(reflectOb, null);
    Console.WriteLine("sum is " + val);
  }
  else if(m.Name.CompareTo("IsBetween")==0) {
    object[] args = new object[1];
    args[0] = 14;
    if((bool) m.Invoke(reflectOb, args))
      Console.WriteLine("14 is between x and y");
  }
  else if(m.Name.CompareTo("Show")==0) {
    m.Invoke(reflectOb, null);
```

```
        }
      }

    }
}
```

The output from the program is shown here:

```
Found: MyClass
Found: AnotherClass
Found: Demo

Using: MyClass
Available constructors:
   MyClass(Int32 i)
   MyClass(Int32 i, Int32 j)

Two-parameter constructor found.

Constructing MyClass(int, int).
Values are x: 10, y: 20

Invoking methods on reflectOb.

sum is 30
14 is between x and y
Inside Set(int, int). Values are x: 9, y: 18
Inside Set(double, double). Values are x: 1, y: 23
Values are x: 1, y: 23
```

As the output shows, all three classes contained within **MyClasses.exe** were found. The first one, which in this case was **MyClass**, was then used to instantiate an object and execute methods.

The types in **MyClasses.exe** are discovered using this sequence of code, which is near the start of **Main( )**:

```
// Load the MyClasses.exe assembly.
Assembly asm = Assembly.LoadFrom("MyClasses.exe");

// Discover what types MyClasses.exe contains.
Type[] alltypes = asm.GetTypes();
foreach(Type temp in alltypes)
  Console.WriteLine("Found: " + temp.Name);
```

You can use such a sequence whenever you need to dynamically load and interrogate an assembly.

On a related point, an assembly need not be an **exe** file. Assemblies can also be contained in dynamic link library (DLL) files that use the **dll** extension. For example, if you were to compile **MyClasses.cs** using this command line,

```
csc /t:library MyClasses.cs
```

then the output file would be **MyClasses.dll**. One advantage to putting code into a DLL is that no **Main( )** method is required. All **exe** files require an entry point, such as **Main( )**, that

defines where execution begins. This is why the **Demo** class contained a placeholder **Main( )** method. Such a method is not required by a DLL. If you try making **MyClass** into a DLL, you will need to change the call to **LoadFrom( )** as shown here:

```
Assembly asm = Assembly.LoadFrom("MyClasses.dll");
```

Fully Automating Type Discovery

Before we leave the topic of reflection, one last example will be instructive. Even though the preceding program was able to fully use **MyClass** without explicitly specifying **MyClass** in the program, it still relied upon prior knowledge of the contents of **MyClass**. For example, the program knew the names of its methods, such as **Set** and **Sum**. However, using reflection it is possible to utilize a type about which you have no prior knowledge. To do this, you must discover all information necessary to construct an object and to generate method calls. Such an approach would be useful to a visual design tool, for example, because it could utilize the types available on the system.

To see how the full dynamic discovery of a type can be accomplished, consider the following example, which loads the **MyClasses.exe** assembly, constructs a **MyClass** object, and then calls all of the methods declared by **MyClass**, all without assuming any prior knowledge:

```
// Utilize MyClass without assuming any prior knowledge.

using System;
using System.Reflection;

class ReflectAssemblyDemo {
  static void Main() {
    int val;
    Assembly asm = Assembly.LoadFrom("MyClasses.exe");

    Type[] alltypes = asm.GetTypes();

    Type t = alltypes[0]; // use first class found

    Console.WriteLine("Using: " + t.Name);

    ConstructorInfo[] ci = t.GetConstructors();

    // Use first constructor found.
    ParameterInfo[] cpi = ci[0].GetParameters();
    object reflectOb;

    if(cpi.Length > 0) {
      object[] consargs = new object[cpi.Length];

      // Initialize args.
      for(int n=0; n < cpi.Length; n++)
        consargs[n] = 10 + n * 20;

      // Construct the object.
      reflectOb = ci[0].Invoke(consargs);
    } else
```

```
   reflectOb = ci[0].Invoke(null);


Console.WriteLine("\nInvoking methods on reflectOb.");
Console.WriteLine();

// Ignore inherited methods.
MethodInfo[] mi = t.GetMethods(BindingFlags.DeclaredOnly |
                               BindingFlags.Instance |
                               BindingFlags.Public) ;

// Invoke each method.
foreach(MethodInfo m in mi) {
  Console.WriteLine("Calling {0} ", m.Name);

  // Get the parameters.
  ParameterInfo[] pi = m.GetParameters();

  // Execute methods.
  switch(pi.Length) {
    case 0: // no args
      if(m.ReturnType == typeof(int)) {
        val = (int) m.Invoke(reflectOb, null);
        Console.WriteLine("Result is " + val);
      }
      else if(m.ReturnType == typeof(void)) {
        m.Invoke(reflectOb, null);
      }
      break;
    case 1: // one arg
      if(pi[0].ParameterType == typeof(int)) {
        object[] args = new object[1];
        args[0] = 14;
        if((bool) m.Invoke(reflectOb, args))
          Console.WriteLine("14 is between x and y");
        else
          Console.WriteLine("14 is not between x and y");
      }
      break;
    case 2: // two args
      if((pi[0].ParameterType == typeof(int)) &&
         (pi[1].ParameterType == typeof(int))) {
        object[] args = new object[2];
        args[0] = 9;
        args[1] = 18;
        m.Invoke(reflectOb, args);
      }
      else if((pi[0].ParameterType == typeof(double)) &&
              (pi[1].ParameterType == typeof(double))) {
        object[] args = new object[2];
        args[0] = 1.12;
        args[1] = 23.4;
        m.Invoke(reflectOb, args);
      }
      break;
```

```
        }
      Console.WriteLine();
    }

  }
}
```

Here is the output produced by the program:

```
Using: MyClass
Constructing MyClass(int).
Values are x: 10, y: 10

Invoking methods on reflectOb.

Calling Sum
Result is 20

Calling IsBetween
14 is not between x and y

Calling Set
Inside Set(int, int). Values are x: 9, y: 18

Calling Set
Inside Set(double, double). Values are x: 1, y: 23

Calling Show
Values are x: 1, y: 23
```

The operation of the program is straightforward, but a couple of points are worth mentioning. First, notice that only the methods explicitly declared by **MyClass** are obtained and used. This is accomplished by using the **BindingFlags** form of **GetMethods( )**. The reason for this is to prevent calling the methods inherited from **object**. Second, notice how the number of parameters and return type of each method are obtained dynamically. A **switch** statement determines the number of parameters. Within each **case**, the parameter type(s) and return type are checked. A method call is then constructed based on this information.

Attributes

C# allows you to add declarative information to a program in the form of an *attribute*. An attribute defines additional information (metadata) that is associated with a class, structure, method, and so on. For example, you might define an attribute that determines the type of button that a class will display. Attributes are specified between square brackets, preceding the item to which they apply. Thus, an attribute is not a member of a class. Rather, an attribute specifies supplemental information that is attached to an item.

Attribute Basics

An attribute is supported by a class that inherits **System.Attribute**. Thus, all attribute classes must be subclasses of **Attribute**. Although **Attribute** defines substantial functionality, this functionality is not always needed when working with attributes. By convention, attribute classes often use the suffix **Attribute**. For example, **ErrorAttribute** would be a name for an attribute class that described an error.

When an attribute class is declared, it is preceded by an attribute called **AttributeUsage**. This built-in attribute specifies the types of items to which the attribute can be applied. Thus, the usage of an attribute can be restricted to methods, for example.

Creating an Attribute

In an attribute class, you will define the members that support the attribute. Often attribute classes are quite simple, containing just a small number of fields or properties. For example, an attribute might define a remark that describes the item to which the attribute is being attached. Such an attribute might look like this:

```
[AttributeUsage(AttributeTargets.All)]
public class RemarkAttribute : Attribute {
  string pri_remark; // underlies Remark property

  public RemarkAttribute(string comment) {
    pri_remark = comment;
  }

  public string Remark {
    get {
      return pri_remark;
    }
  }
}
```

Let's look at this class, line by line.

The name of this attribute is **RemarkAttribute**. Its declaration is preceded by the **AttributeUsage** attribute, which specifies that **RemarkAttribute** can be applied to all types of items. Using **AttributeUsage**, it is possible to narrow the list of items to which an attribute can be attached, and we will examine its capabilities later in this chapter.

Next, **RemarkAttribute** is declared and it inherits **Attribute**. Inside **RemarkAttribute** there is one private field, **pri_remark**, which supports one public, read-only property: **Remark**. This property holds the description that will be associated with the attribute. (**Remark** could also have been declared as an auto-implemented property with a private set accessor, but a read-only property is used for the purposes of illustration.) There is one public constructor that takes a string argument and assigns it to **Remark**.

At this point, no other steps are needed, and **RemarkAttribute** is ready for use.

Attaching an Attribute

Once you have defined an attribute class, you can attach the attribute to an item. An attribute precedes the item to which it is attached and is specified by enclosing its constructor inside square brackets. For example, here is how **RemarkAttribute** can be associated with a class:

```
[RemarkAttribute("This class uses an attribute.")]
class UseAttrib {
  // ...
}
```

This constructs a **RemarkAttribute** that contains the comment, "This class uses an attribute." This attribute is then associated with **UseAttrib**.

When attaching an attribute, it is not actually necessary to specify the **Attribute** suffix. For example, the preceding class could be declared this way:

```
[Remark("This class uses an attribute.")]
class UseAttrib {
  // ...
}
```

Here, only the name **Remark** is used. Although the short form is correct, it is usually safer to use the full name when attaching attributes, because it avoids possible confusion and ambiguity.

Obtaining an Object's Attributes

Once an attribute has been attached to an item, other parts of the program can retrieve the attribute. To retrieve an attribute, you will usually use one of two methods. The first is **GetCustomAttributes( )**, which is defined by **MemberInfo** and inherited by **Type**. It retrieves a list of all attributes attached to an item. Here is one of its forms:

object[ ] GetCustomAttributes(bool *searchBases*)

If *searchBases* is true, then the attributes of all base classes through the inheritance chain will be included. Otherwise, only those classes defined by the specified type will be found.

The second method is **GetCustomAttribute( )**, which is defined by **Attribute**. One of its forms is shown here:

static Attribute GetCustomAttribute(MemberInfo *mi*, Type *attribtype*)

Here, *mi* is a **MemberInfo** object that describes the item for which the attributes are being obtained. The attribute desired is specified by *attribtype*. You will use this method when you know the name of the attribute you want to obtain, which is often the case. For example, assuming that the **UseAttrib** class has the **RemarkAttribute**, to obtain a reference to the **RemarkAttribute**, you can use a sequence like this:

```
// Get a MemberInfo instance associated with a
// class that has the RemarkAttribute.
Type t = typeof(UseAttrib);

// Retrieve the RemarkAttribute.
Type tRemAtt = typeof(RemarkAttribute);
RemarkAttribute ra = (RemarkAttribute)
      Attribute.GetCustomAttribute(t, tRemAtt);
```

This sequence works because **MemberInfo** is a base class of **Type**. Thus, **t** is a **MemberInfo** instance.

Once you have a reference to an attribute, you can access its members. This makes information associated with an attribute available to a program that uses an element to which an attribute is attached. For example, the following statement displays the **Remark** property:

```
Console.WriteLine(ra.Remark);
```

The following program puts together all of the pieces and demonstrates the use of **RemarkAttribute**:

```
// A simple attribute example.

using System;
using System.Reflection;

[AttributeUsage(AttributeTargets.All)]
public class RemarkAttribute : Attribute {
  string pri_remark; // underlies Remark property

  public RemarkAttribute(string comment) {
    pri_remark = comment;
  }

  public string Remark {
    get {
      return pri_remark;
    }
  }
}

[RemarkAttribute("This class uses an attribute.")]
class UseAttrib {
  // ...
}

class AttribDemo {
  static void Main() {
    Type t = typeof(UseAttrib);

    Console.Write("Attributes in " + t.Name + ": ");

    object[] attribs = t.GetCustomAttributes(false);
    foreach(object o in attribs) {
      Console.WriteLine(o);
    }

    Console.Write("Remark: ");

    // Retrieve the RemarkAttribute.
    Type tRemAtt = typeof(RemarkAttribute);
    RemarkAttribute ra = (RemarkAttribute)
         Attribute.GetCustomAttribute(t, tRemAtt);

    Console.WriteLine(ra.Remark);
  }
}
```

The output from the program is shown here:

```
Attributes in UseAttrib: RemarkAttribute
Remark: This class uses an attribute.
```

Positional vs. Named Parameters

In the preceding example, **RemarkAttribute** was initialized by passing the description
string to the constructor, using the normal constructor syntax. In this case, the **comment**
parameter to **RemarkAttribute( )** is called a *positional parameter*. This term relates to the fact
that the argument is linked to a parameter by its position in the argument list. This is the way
that all methods and constructors work in C#. For example, given a method called **test( )**,
declared as shown here:

```
void test(int a, double b, string c)
```

the following call to **test( )**

```
test(10, 1.1, "hello");
```

passes 10 to **a**, 1.1 to **b**, and "hello" to **c** because of the position (i.e., order) of the arguments.
However, for an attribute, you can also create *named parameters*, which can be assigned initial
values by using their name. In this case, it is the name of the parameter, not its position, that
is important.

A named parameter is supported by either a public field or property, which must be
read-write and nonstatic. Any such field or property is automatically able to be used as a
named parameter. A named parameter is given a value by an assignment statement that is
located within the argument list when the attribute's constructor is invoked. Here is the
general form of an attribute specification that includes named parameters:

[*attrib(positional-param-list, named-param1 = value, named-param2 = value, ...)*]

The positional parameters (if they exist) come first. Next, each named parameter is assigned
a value. The order of the named parameters is not important. Named parameters do not
need to be given a value. In this case, their default value will be used.

To understand how to use a named parameter, it is best to work through an example.
Here is a version of **RemarkAttribute** that adds a field called **Supplement**, which can be
used to hold a supplemental remark:

```
[AttributeUsage(AttributeTargets.All)]
public class RemarkAttribute : Attribute {
  string pri_remark; // underlies Remark property

  // This can be used as a named parameter:
  public string Supplement;

  public RemarkAttribute(string comment) {
    pri_remark = comment;
    Supplement = "None";
  }

  public string Remark {
    get {
      return pri_remark;
    }
  }
}
```

As you can see, **Supplement** is initialized to the string "None" by the constructor. There is no way of using the constructor to assign it a different initial value. However, because **Supplement** is a public field of **RemarkAttribute**, it can be used as a named parameter, as shown here:

```
[RemarkAttribute("This class uses an attribute.",
        Supplement = "This is additional info.")]
class UseAttrib {
  // ...
}
```

Pay close attention to the way **RemarkAttribute**'s constructor is called. First, the positional argument is specified as it was before. Next is a comma, followed by the named parameter, **Supplement**, which is assigned a value. Finally, the closing) ends the call to the constructor. Thus, the named parameter is initialized within the call to the constructor. This syntax can be generalized. Position parameters must be specified in the order in which they appear. Named parameters are specified by assigning values to their name.

Here is a program that demonstrates the **Supplement** field:

```
// Use a named attribute parameter.

using System;
using System.Reflection;

[AttributeUsage(AttributeTargets.All)]
public class RemarkAttribute : Attribute {
  string pri_remark; // underlies Remark property

  public string Supplement; // this is a named parameter

  public RemarkAttribute(string comment) {
    pri_remark = comment;
    Supplement = "None";
  }

  public string Remark {
    get {
      return pri_remark;
    }
  }
}

[RemarkAttribute("This class uses an attribute.",
                 Supplement = "This is additional info.")]
class UseAttrib {
  // ...
}

class NamedParamDemo {
  static void Main() {
    Type t = typeof(UseAttrib);

    Console.Write("Attributes in " + t.Name + ": ");
```

```
      object[] attribs = t.GetCustomAttributes(false);
      foreach(object o in attribs) {
        Console.WriteLine(o);
      }

      // Retrieve the RemarkAttribute.
      Type tRemAtt = typeof(RemarkAttribute);
      RemarkAttribute ra = (RemarkAttribute)
            Attribute.GetCustomAttribute(t, tRemAtt);

      Console.Write("Remark: ");
      Console.WriteLine(ra.Remark);

      Console.Write("Supplement: ");
      Console.WriteLine(ra.Supplement);
    }
  }
```

The output from the program is shown here:

```
Attributes in UseAttrib: RemarkAttribute
Remark: This class uses an attribute.
Supplement: This is additional info.
```

Before moving on, it is important to emphasize that **pri_remark** *cannot* be used as a named parameter because it is private to **RemarkAttribute**. The **Remark** property *cannot* be used as a named parameter because it is read-only. Remember that only public, read-write fields and properties can be used as named parameters.

A public, read-write property can be used as a named parameter in the same way as a field. For example, here an auto-implemented **int** property called **Priority** is added to **RemarkAttribute**:

```
// Use a property as a named attribute parameter.

using System;
using System.Reflection;

[AttributeUsage(AttributeTargets.All)]
public class RemarkAttribute : Attribute {
  string pri_remark; // underlies Remark property

  public string Supplement; // this is a named parameter

  public RemarkAttribute(string comment) {
    pri_remark = comment;
    Supplement = "None";
    Priority = 1;
  }

  public string Remark {
    get {
      return pri_remark;
    }
  }
```

```
    // Use a property as a named parameter.
    public int Priority { get; set; }
}

[RemarkAttribute("This class uses an attribute.",
                 Supplement = "This is additional info.",
                 Priority = 10)]
class UseAttrib {
  // ...
}

class NamedParamDemo {
  static void Main() {
    Type t = typeof(UseAttrib);

    Console.Write("Attributes in " + t.Name + ": ");

    object[] attribs = t.GetCustomAttributes(false);
    foreach(object o in attribs) {
      Console.WriteLine(o);
    }

    // Retrieve the RemarkAttribute.
    Type tRemAtt = typeof(RemarkAttribute);
    RemarkAttribute ra = (RemarkAttribute)
          Attribute.GetCustomAttribute(t, tRemAtt);

    Console.Write("Remark: ");
    Console.WriteLine(ra.Remark);

    Console.Write("Supplement: ");
    Console.WriteLine(ra.Supplement);

    Console.WriteLine("Priority: " + ra.Priority);
  }
}
```

The output is shown here:

```
Attributes in UseAttrib: RemarkAttribute
Remark: This class uses an attribute.
Supplement: This is additional info.
Priority: 10
```

There is one point of interest in the program. Notice the attribute specified before **UseAttrib** that is shown here:

```
[RemarkAttribute("This class uses an attribute.",
                 Supplement = "This is additional info.",
                 Priority = 10)]
```

The named attributes **Supplement** and **Priority** are *not* in any special order. These two assignments can be reversed without any change to the attribute.

One last point: For both positional and named parameters, the type of an attribute parameter must be either one of the built-in primitive types, **object**, **Type**, an enumeration, or a one-dimensional array of one of these types.

Three Built-in Attributes

C# defines several built-in attributes, but three are especially important because they apply to a wide variety of situations: **AttributeUsage**, **Conditional**, and **Obsolete**. They are examined here.

AttributeUsage

As mentioned earlier, the **AttributeUsage** attribute specifies the types of items to which an attribute can be applied. **AttributeUsage** is another name for the **System.AttributeUsageAttribute** class. **AttributeUsage** has the following constructor:

AttributeUsage(AttributeTargets *item*)

Here, *item* specifies the item or items upon which the attribute can be used. **AttributeTargets** is an enumeration that defines the following values:

All	Assembly	Class	Constructor
Delegate	Enum	Event	Field
GenericParameter	Interface	Method	Module
Parameter	Property	ReturnValue	Struct

Two or more of these value can be ORed together. For example, to specify an attribute that can be applied only to fields and properties, use

```
AttributeTargets.Field | AttributeTargets.Property
```

AttributeUsage supports two named parameters. The first is **AllowMultiple**, which is a **bool** value. If this value is true, then the attribute can be applied more than one time to a single item. The second is **Inherited**, which is also a **bool** value. If this value is true, then the attribute is inherited by derived classes. Otherwise, it is not inherited. The default setting is false for **AllowMultiple** and true for **Inherited**.

AttributeUsage also specifies a read-only property called **ValidOn**, which returns a value of type **AttributeTargets**, which specifies what types of items the attribute can be used on. The default is **AttributeTargets.All**.

The Conditional Attribute

The attribute **Conditional** is perhaps C#'s most interesting built-in attribute. It allows you to create *conditional methods.* A conditional method is invoked only when a specific symbol has been defined via **#define**. Otherwise, the method is bypassed. Thus, a conditional method offers an alternative to conditional compilation using **#if**.

Conditional is another name for **System.Diagnostics.ConditionalAttribute**. To use the **Conditional** attribute, you must include the **System.Diagnostics** namespace.

Let's begin with an example:

```
// Demonstrate the Conditional attribute.

#define TRIAL

using System;
using System.Diagnostics;

class Test {

  [Conditional("TRIAL")]
  void Trial() {
    Console.WriteLine("Trial version, not for distribution.");
  }

  [Conditional("RELEASE")]
  void Release() {
    Console.WriteLine("Final release version.");
  }

  static void Main() {
    Test t = new Test();

    t.Trial(); // called only if TRIAL is defined
    t.Release(); // called only if RELEASE is defined
  }
}
```

The output from this program is shown here:

```
Trial version, not for distribution.
```

Let's look closely at this program to understand why this output is produced. First, notice the program defines the symbol **TRIAL**. Next, notice how the methods **Trial( )** and **Release( )** are coded. They are both preceded with the **Conditional** attribute, which has this general form:

[Conditional *symbol*]

where *symbol* is the symbol that determines whether the method will be executed. This attribute can be used only on methods. If the symbol is defined, then when the method is called, it will be executed. If the symbol is not defined, then the method is not executed.

Inside **Main( )**, both **Trial( )** and **Release( )** are called. However, only **TRIAL** is defined. Thus, **Trial( )** is executed. The call to **Release( )** is ignored. If you define **RELEASE**, then **Release( )** will also be called. If you remove the definition for **TRIAL**, then **Trial( )** will not be called.

Conditional methods have a few restrictions. First, they must return **void**. Second, they must be members of a class or structure, not an interface. Third, they cannot be preceded with the **override** keyword.

The Obsolete Attribute

The **Obsolete** attribute, which is short for **System.ObsoleteAttribute**, lets you mark a program element as obsolete. It has this general form:

[Obsolete("*message*")]

Here, *message* is displayed when that program element is compiled. Here is a short example:

```
// Demonstrate the Obsolete attribute.

using System;

class Test {

  [Obsolete("Use MyMeth2, instead.")]
  public static int MyMeth(int a, int b) {
    return a / b;
  }

  // Improved version of MyMeth.
  public static int MyMeth2(int a, int b) {
    return b == 0 ? 0 : a /b;
  }

  static void Main() {
   // Warning displayed for this.
    Console.WriteLine("4 / 3 is " + Test.MyMeth(4, 3));

   // No warning here.
    Console.WriteLine("4 / 3 is " + Test.MyMeth2(4, 3));
  }
}
```

When the call to **MyMeth( )** is encountered in **Main( )** when this program is compiled, a warning will be generated that tells the user to use **MyMeth2( )** instead.

A second form of **Obsolete** is shown here:

[Obsolete("*message*", *error*)]

Here, *error* is a Boolean value. If it is true, then use of the obsolete item generates a compilation error rather than a warning. The difference is, of course, that a program containing an error cannot be compiled into an executable program.

Generics

This chapter examines one of C#'s most sophisticated and powerful features: *generics*. Interestingly, although generics are now an indispensable part of C# programming, they were not included in the original 1.0 release. Instead, they were added by C# 2.0. It is not an overstatement to say that the addition of generics fundamentally changed the character of C#. Not only did it add a new syntactic element, it also added new capabilities and resulted in many changes and upgrades to the library. Although it has been a few years since the inclusion of generics in C#, the effects still reverberate throughout the language.

The generics feature is so important because it enables the creation of classes, structures, interfaces, methods, and delegates that work in a type-safe manner with various kinds of data. As you may know, many algorithms are logically the same no matter what type of data they are being applied to. For example, the mechanism that supports a queue is the same whether the queue is storing items of type **int**, **string**, **object**, or a user-defined class. Prior to generics, you might have created several different versions of the same algorithm to handle different types of data. Through the use of generics, you can define a solution once, independently of any specific type of data, and then apply that solution to a wide variety of data types without any additional effort.

This chapter describes the syntax, theory, and use of generics. It also shows how generics provide type safety for some previously difficult cases. Once you have completed this chapter, you will want to examine Chapter 24, which covers Collections. There you will find many examples of generics at work in the generic collection classes.

What Are Generics?

At its core, the term *generics* means *parameterized types*. Parameterized types are important because they enable you to create classes, structures, interfaces, methods, and delegates in which the type of data upon which they operate is specified as a parameter. Using generics, it is possible to create a single class, for example, that automatically works with different types of data. A class, structure, interface, method, or delegate that operates on a parameterized type is called *generic*, as in *generic class* or *generic method*.

It is important to understand that C# has always given you the ability to create generalized code by operating through references of type **object**. Because **object** is the base class of all other classes, an **object** reference can refer to any type of object. Thus, in pre-generics code, generalized code used **object** references to operate on a variety of different kinds of objects.

The problem was that it could not do so with type safety because casts were needed to convert between the **object** type and the actual type of the data. This was a potential source of errors because it was possible to accidentally use an incorrect cast. Generics avoid this problem by providing the type safety that was lacking. Generics also streamline the process because it is no longer necessary to employ casts to translate between **object** and the type of data that is actually being operated upon. Thus, generics expand your ability to re-use code, and let you do so safely and easily.

> **NOTE** *A Warning to C++ and Java Programmers: Although C# generics are similar to templates in C++ and generics in Java, they are not the same as either. In fact, there are some fundamental differences among these three approaches to generics. If you have a background in C++ or Java, it is important to not jump to conclusions about how generics work in C#.*

A Simple Generics Example

Let's begin with a simple example of a generic class. The following program defines two classes. The first is the generic class **Gen**, and the second is **GenericsDemo**, which uses **Gen**.

```
// A simple generic class.

using System;

// In the following Gen class, T is a type parameter
// that will be replaced by a real type when an object
// of type Gen is created.
class Gen<T> {
  T ob; // declare a variable of type T

  // Notice that this constructor has a parameter of type T.
  public Gen(T o) {
    ob = o;
  }

  // Return ob, which is type T.
  public T GetOb() {
    return ob;
  }

  // Show type of T.
  public void ShowType() {
    Console.WriteLine("Type of T is " + typeof(T));
  }
}

// Demonstrate the generic class.
class GenericsDemo {
  static void Main() {
    // Create a Gen reference for int.
    Gen<int> iOb;

    // Create a Gen<int> object and assign its reference to iOb.
    iOb = new Gen<int>(102);
```

```
    // Show the type of data used by iOb.
    iOb.ShowType();

    // Get the value in iOb.
    int v = iOb.GetOb();
    Console.WriteLine("value: " + v);

    Console.WriteLine();

    // Create a Gen object for strings.
    Gen<string> strOb = new Gen<string>("Generics add power.");

    // Show the type of data stored in strOb.
    strOb.ShowType();

    // Get the value in strOb.
    string str = strOb.GetOb();
    Console.WriteLine("value: " + str);
  }
}
```

The output produced by the program is shown here:

```
Type of T is System.Int32
value: 102

Type of T is System.String
value: Generics add power.
```

Let's examine this program carefully.

First, notice how **Gen** is declared by the following line.

```
class Gen<T> {
```

Here, **T** is the name of a *type parameter*. This name is used as a placeholder for the actual type that will be specified when a **Gen** object is created. Thus, **T** is used within **Gen** whenever the type parameter is needed. Notice that **T** is contained within **< >**. This syntax can be generalized. Whenever a type parameter is being declared, it is specified within angle brackets. Because **Gen** uses a type parameter, **Gen** is a *generic class*.

In the declaration of **Gen**, there is no special significance to the name **T**. Any valid identifier could have been used, but **T** is traditional. Other commonly used type parameter names include **V** and **E**. Of course, you can also use descriptive names for type parameters, such as **TValue** or **TKey**. When using a descriptive name, it is common practice to use **T** as the first letter.

Next, **T** is used to declare a variable called **ob**, as shown here:

```
T ob; // declare a variable of type T
```

As explained, **T** is a placeholder for the actual type that will be specified when a **Gen** object is created. Thus, **ob** will be a variable of the type *bound to* **T** when a **Gen** object is instantiated. For example, if type **string** is specified for **T**, then in that instance, **ob** will be of type **string**.

Now consider **Gen**'s constructor:

```
public Gen(T o) {
   ob = o;
}
```

Notice that its parameter, **o**, is of type **T**. This means that the actual type of **o** is determined by the type bound to **T** when a **Gen** object is created. Also, because both the parameter **o** and the instance variable **ob** are of type **T**, they will both be of the same actual type when a **Gen** object is created.

The type parameter **T** can also be used to specify the return type of a method, as is the case with the **GetOb( )** method, shown here:

```
public T GetOb() {
   return ob;
}
```

Because **ob** is also of type **T**, its type is compatible with the return type specified by **GetOb( )**.

The **ShowType( )** method displays the type of **T** by passing **T** to the **typeof** operator. Because a real type will be substituted for **T** when an object of type **Gen** is created, **typeof** will obtain type information about the actual type.

The **GenericsDemo** class demonstrates the generic **Gen** class. It first creates a version of **Gen** for type **int**, as shown here:

```
Gen<int> iOb;
```

Look closely at this declaration. First, notice that the type **int** is specified within the angle brackets after **Gen**. In this case, **int** is a *type argument* that is bound to **Gen**'s type parameter, **T**. This creates a version of **Gen** in which all uses of **T** are replaced by **int**. Thus, for this declaration, **ob** is of type **int**, and the return type of **GetOb( )** is of type **int**.

The next line assigns to **iOb** a reference to an instance of an **int** version of the **Gen** class:

```
iOb = new Gen<int>(102);
```

Notice that when the **Gen** constructor is called, the type argument **int** is also specified. This is necessary because the type of the variable (in this case **iOb**) to which the reference is being assigned is of type **Gen<int>**. Thus, the reference returned by **new** must also be of type **Gen<int>**. If it isn't, a compile-time error will result. For example, the following assignment will cause a compile-time error:

```
iOb = new Gen<double>(118.12); // Error!
```

Because **iOb** is of type **Gen<int>**, it can't be used to refer to an object of **Gen<double>**. This type checking is one of the main benefits of generics because it ensures type safety.

The program then displays the type of **ob** within **iOb**, which is **System.Int32**. This is the .NET structure that corresponds to **int**. Next, the program obtains the value of **ob** by use of the following line:

```
int v = iOb.GetOb();
```

Because the return type of **GetOb( )** is **T**, which was replaced by **int** when **iOb** was declared, the return type of **GetOb( )** is also **int**. Thus, this value can be assigned to an **int** variable.

Next, **GenericsDemo** declares an object of type **Gen<string>**:

```
Gen<string> strOb = new Gen<string>("Generics add power.");
```

Because the type argument is **string**, **string** is substituted for **T** inside **Gen**. This creates a **string** version of **Gen**, as the remaining lines in the program demonstrate.

Before moving on, a few terms need to be defined. When you specify a type argument such as **int** or **string** for **Gen**, you are creating what is referred to in C# as a *closed constructed type*. Thus, **Gen<int>** is a closed constructed type. In essence, a generic type, such as **Gen<T>**, is an abstraction. It is only after a specific version, such as **Gen<int>**, has been constructed that a concrete type has been created. In C# terminology, a construct such as **Gen<T>** is called an *open constructed type*, because the type parameter **T** (rather than an actual type, such as **int**) is specified.

More generally, C# defines the concepts of an *open type* and a *closed type*. An open type is a type parameter or any generic type whose type argument is (or involves) a type parameter. Any type that is not an open type is a closed type. A *constructed type* is a generic type for which all type arguments have been supplied. If those type arguments are all closed types, then it is a closed constructed type. If one or more of those type arguments are open types, it is an open constructed type.

Generic Types Differ Based on Their Type Arguments

A key point to understand about generic types is that a reference of one specific version of a generic type is not type-compatible with another version of the same generic type. For example, assuming the program just shown, the following line of code is in error and will not compile:

```
iOb = strOb; // Wrong!
```

Even though both **iOb** and **strOb** are of type **Gen<T>**, they are references to different types because their type arguments differ.

How Generics Improve Type Safety

At this point, you might be asking yourself the following question. Given that the same functionality found in the generic **Gen** class can be achieved without generics, by simply specifying **object** as the data type and employing the proper casts, what is the benefit of making **Gen** generic? The answer is that generics automatically ensure the type safety of all operations involving **Gen**. In the process, generics eliminate the need for you to use casts and type-check code by hand.

To understand the benefits of generics, first consider the following program that creates a non-generic equivalent of **Gen**:

```
// NonGen is functionally equivalent to Gen but does not use generics.

using System;

class NonGen {
  object ob; // ob is now of type object

  // Pass the constructor a reference of type object.
  public NonGen(object o) {
```

```
    ob = o;
  }

  // Return type object.
  public object GetOb() {
    return ob;
  }

  // Show type of ob.
  public void ShowType() {
    Console.WriteLine("Type of ob is " + ob.GetType());
  }
}

// Demonstrate the non-generic class.
class NonGenDemo {
  static void Main() {
    NonGen iOb;

    // Create NonGen object.
    iOb = new NonGen(102);

    // Show the type of data stored in iOb.
    iOb.ShowType();

    // Get the value in iOb.
    // This time, a cast is necessary.
    int v = (int) iOb.GetOb();
    Console.WriteLine("value: " + v);

    Console.WriteLine();

    // Create another NonGen object and store a string in it.
    NonGen strOb = new NonGen("Non-Generics Test");

    // Show the type of data stored in strOb.
    strOb.ShowType();

    // Get the value of strOb.
    // Again, notice that a cast is necessary.
    String str = (string) strOb.GetOb();
    Console.WriteLine("value: " + str);

    // This compiles, but is conceptually wrong!
    iOb = strOb;

    // The following line results in a runtime exception.
    // v = (int) iOb.GetOb(); // runtime error!
  }
}
```

This program produces the following output:

```
Type of ob is System.Int32
value: 102
```

```
Type of ob is System.String
value: Non-Generics Test
```

As you can see, the output is similar to the previous version of the program.

There are several things of interest in this version. First, notice that **NonGen** replaces all uses of **T** with **object**. This makes **NonGen** able to store any type of object, as can the generic version. However, this approach is bad for two reasons. First, explicit casts must be employed to retrieve the stored data. Second, many kinds of type mismatch errors cannot be found until runtime. Let's look closely at each problem.

We will begin with this line:

```
int v = (int) iOb.GetOb();
```

Because the return type of **GetOb( )** is now **object**, the cast to **int** is necessary to enable the value returned by **GetOb( )** to be unboxed and stored in **v**. If you remove the cast, the program will not compile. In the generic version of the program, this cast was not needed because **int** was specified as a type argument when **iOb** was constructed. In the non-generic version, the cast must be employed. This is not only an inconvenience, but a potential source of error.

Now, consider the following sequence from near the end of the program:

```
// This compiles, but is conceptually wrong!
iOb = strOb;

// The following line results in a runtime exception.
// v = (int) iOb.GetOb(); // runtime error!
```

Here, **strOb** is assigned to **iOb**. However, **strOb** refers to an object that contains a string, not an integer. This assignment is syntactically valid because all **NonGen** references are the same, and any **NonGen** reference can refer to any other **NonGen** object. However, the statement is semantically wrong, as the commented-out line shows. In that line, the return type of **GetOb( )** is cast to **int** and then an attempt is made to assign this value to **v**. The trouble is that **iOb** now refers to an object that stores a **string**, not an **int**. Unfortunately, without generics, the compiler won't catch this error. Instead, a runtime exception will occur when the cast to **int** is attempted. To see this for yourself, try removing the comment symbol from the start of the line and then compiling and running the program. A runtime error will occur.

The preceding sequence can't occur when generics are used. If this sequence were attempted in the generic version of the program, the compiler would catch it and report an error, thus preventing a serious bug that results in a runtime exception. The ability to create type-safe code in which type-mismatch errors are caught at compile time is a key advantage of generics. Although using **object** references to create "generic" code has always been possible in C#, that code was not type-safe and its misuse could result in runtime exceptions. Generics prevent this from occurring. In essence, through generics, what were once runtime errors have become compile-time errors. This is a major benefit.

There is one other point of interest in the **NonGen** program. Notice how the type of the **NonGen** instance variable **ob** is obtained by **ShowType( )**:

```
Console.WriteLine("Type of ob is " + ob.GetType());
```

Recall from Chapter 11 that **object** defines several methods that are available to all data types. One of these methods is **GetType( )**, which returns a **Type** object that describes the type of

the invoking object at runtime. Thus, even though the type of **ob** is specified as **object** in the program's source code, at runtime, the actual type of object being referred to is known. This is why the CLR will generate an exception if you try an invalid cast during program execution.

A Generic Class with Two Type Parameters

You can declare more than one type parameter in a generic type. To specify two or more type parameters, simply use a comma-separated list. For example, the following **TwoGen** class is a variation of the **Gen** class that has two type parameters:

```
// A simple generic class with two type parameters: T and V.

using System;

class TwoGen<T, V> {
  T ob1;
  V ob2;

  // Notice that this constructor has parameters of type T and V.
  public TwoGen(T o1, V o2) {
    ob1 = o1;
    ob2 = o2;
  }

  // Show types of T and V.
  public void showTypes() {
    Console.WriteLine("Type of T is " + typeof(T));
    Console.WriteLine("Type of V is " + typeof(V));
  }

  public T getob1() {
    return ob1;
  }

  public V GetObj2() {
    return ob2;
  }
}

// Demonstrate two generic type parameters.
class SimpGen {
  static void Main() {

    TwoGen<int, string> tgObj =
      new TwoGen<int, string>(119, "Alpha Beta Gamma");

    // Show the types.
    tgObj.showTypes();

    // Obtain and show values.
    int v = tgObj.getob1();
    Console.WriteLine("value: " + v);
```

```
      string str = tgObj.GetObj2();
      Console.WriteLine("value: " + str);
   }
}
```

The output from this program is shown here:

```
Type of T is System.Int32
Type of V is System.String
value: 119
value: Alpha Beta Gamma
```

Notice how **TwoGen** is declared:

```
class TwoGen<T, V> {
```

It specifies two type parameters: **T** and **V**, separated by a comma. Because it has two type parameters, two type arguments must be specified when a **TwoGen** object is created, as shown here:

```
TwoGen<int, string> tgObj =
  new TwoGen<int, string>(119, "Alpha Beta Gamma");
```

In this case, **int** is substituted for **T** and **string** is substituted for **V**.

Although the two type arguments differ in this example, it is possible for both types to be the same. For example, the following line of code is valid:

```
TwoGen<string, string> x = new TwoGen<string, string>("Hello", "Goodbye");
```

In this case, both **T** and **V** would be of type **string**. Of course, if the type arguments were always the same, then two type parameters would be unnecessary.

The General Form of a Generic Class

The generics syntax shown in the preceding examples can be generalized. Here is the syntax for declaring a generic class:

   class *class-name<type-param-list>* { // ...

Here is the syntax for declaring a reference to a generics class:

   class-name<type-arg-list> var-name =
      new *class-name<type-arg-list>(cons-arg-list)*;

Constrained Types

In the preceding examples, the type parameters could be replaced by any type. For example, given this declaration

```
class Gen<T> {
```

any type can be specified for **T**. Thus, it is legal to create **Gen** objects in which **T** is replaced by **int**, **double**, **string**, **FileStream**, or any other type. Although having no restrictions on the

type argument is fine for many purposes, sometimes it is useful to limit the types that can be used as a type argument. For example, you might want to create a method that operates on the contents of a stream, including a **FileStream** or **MemoryStream**. This situation seems perfect for generics, but you need some way to ensure that only stream types are used as type arguments. You don't want to allow a type argument of **int**, for example. You also need some way to tell the compiler that the methods defined by a stream will be available for use. For example, your generic code needs some way to know that it can call the **Read( )** method.

To handle such situations, C# provides *constrained types*. When specifying a type parameter, you can specify a constraint that the type parameter must satisfy. This is accomplished through the use of a **where** clause when specifying the type parameter, as shown here:

class *class-name<type-param>* where *type-param* : *constraints* { // ...

Here, *constraints* is a comma-separated list of constraints.

C# defines the following types of constraints.

- You can require that a certain base class be present in a type argument by using a *base class constraint*. This constraint is specified by naming the desired base class. There is a variation of this constraint, called a *naked type constraint,* in which a type parameter (rather than an actual type) specifies the base class. This enables you to establish a relationship between two type parameters.

- You can require that one or more interfaces be implemented by a type argument by using an *interface constraint*. This constraint is specified by naming the desired interface.

- You can require that the type argument supply a parameterless constructor. This is called a *constructor constraint.* It is specified by **new( )**.

- You can specify that a type argument must be a reference type by specifying the *reference type constraint:* **class**.

- You can specify that the type argument be a value type by specifying the *value type constraint:* **struct**.

Of these constraints, the base class constraint and the interface constraint are probably the most often used, but all are important. Each constraint is examined in the following sections.

Using a Base Class Constraint

The base class constraint enables you to specify a base class that a type argument must inherit. A base class constraint serves two important purposes. First, it lets you use the members of the base class specified by the constraint within the generic class. For example, you can call a method or use a property of the base class. Without a base class constraint, the compiler has no way to know what type of members a type argument might have. By supplying a base class constraint, you are letting the compiler know that all type arguments will have the members defined by that base class.

The second purpose of a base class constraint is to ensure that only type arguments that support the specified base class are used. This means that for any given base class constraint, the type argument must be either the base class, itself, or a class derived from that base class. If you attempt to use a type argument that does not match or inherit the specified base class, a compile-time error will result.

The base class constraint uses this form of the **where** clause:

where *T* : *base-class-name*

Here, *T* is the name of the type parameter, and *base-class-name* is the name of the base class. Only one base class can be specified.

Here is a simple example that demonstrates the base class constraint mechanism:

```
// A simple demonstration of a base class constraint.

using System;

class A {
  public void Hello() {
    Console.WriteLine("Hello");
  }
}

// Class B inherits A.
class B : A { }

// Class C does not inherit A.
class C { }

// Because of the base class constraint, all type arguments
// passed to Test must have A as a base class.
class Test<T> where T : A {
  T obj;

  public Test(T o) {
    obj = o;
  }

  public void SayHello() {
    // OK to call Hello() because it's declared
    // by the base class A.
    obj.Hello();
  }
}

class BaseClassConstraintDemo {
  static void Main() {
    A a = new A();
    B b = new B();
    C c = new C();

    // The following is valid because A is the specified base class.
    Test<A> t1 = new Test<A>(a);

    t1.SayHello();

    // The following is valid because B inherits A.
    Test<B> t2 = new Test<B>(b);
```

```
    t2.SayHello();


    // The following is invalid because C does not inherit A.
//    Test<C> t3 = new Test<C>(c); // Error!
//    t3.SayHello(); // Error!
  }
}
```

In this program, class **A** is inherited by **B**, but not by **C**. Notice also that **A** declares a method called **Hello( )**. Next, notice that **Test** is a generic class that is declared like this:

```
class Test<T> where T : A {
```

The **where** clause stipulates that any type argument specified for **T** must have **A** as a base class.

Now notice that **Test** declares the method **SayHello( )**, shown next:

```
public void SayHello() {
  // OK to call Hello() because it's declared
  // by the base class A.
  obj.Hello();
}
```

This method calls **Hello( )** on **obj**, which is a **T** object. The key point is that the only reason that **Hello( )** can be called is because the base class constraint requires that any type argument bound to **T** must be **A** or inherit **A**, and **A** declares **Hello( )**. Thus, any valid **T** will define **Hello( )**. If the base class constraint had not been used, the compiler would have no way of knowing that a method called **Hello( )** could be called on a object of type **T**. You can prove this for yourself by removing the **where** clause. The program will no longer compile because the **Hello( )** method will be unknown.

In addition to enabling access to members of the base class, the base class constraint enforces that only types that inherit the base class can be passed as type arguments. This is why the following two lines are commented-out:

```
//    Test<C> t3 = new Test<C>(c); // Error!
//    t3.SayHello(); // Error!
```

Because **C** does not inherit **A**, it can't be used as a type argument when constructing a **Test** object. You can prove this by removing the comment symbols and trying to recompile.

Before continuing, let's review the two effects of a base class constraint: A base class constraint enables a generic class to access the members of the base class. It also ensures that only those type arguments that fulfill this constraint are valid, thus preserving type safety.

Although the preceding example shows the "how" of base class constraints, it does not show the "why." To better understand the value of base type constraints, let's work through another, more practical example. Assume you want to create a mechanism that manages lists of telephone numbers. Furthermore, assume you want to use different lists for different groupings of numbers. Specifically, you want one list for friends, another for suppliers, and so on. To accomplish this, you might start by creating a base class called **PhoneNumber** that stores a name and a phone number linked to that name. Such a class might look like this:

```
// A base class that stores a name and phone number.
class PhoneNumber {
  public PhoneNumber(string n, string num) {
    Name = n;
    Number = num;
  }

  // Auto-implemented properties that hold a name and phone number.
  public string Number { get; set; }
  public string Name { get; set; }
}
```

Next, you create two classes that inherit **PhoneNumber**: **Friend** and **Supplier**. They are shown here:

```
// A class of phone numbers for friends.
class Friend : PhoneNumber {

  public Friend(string n, string num, bool wk) :
    base(n, num)
  {
    IsWorkNumber = wk;
  }

  public bool IsWorkNumber { get; private set; }
  // ...
}

// A class of phone numbers for suppliers.
class Supplier : PhoneNumber {
  public Supplier(string n, string num) :
    base(n, num) { }

  // ...
}
```

Notice that **Friend** adds a property called **IsWorkNumber**, which returns true if the telephone number is a work number.

To manage telephone lists, you create a class called **PhoneList**. Because you want this class to manage any type of phone list, you make it generic. Furthermore, because part of the list management is looking up numbers given names, and vice versa, you add the constraint that requires that the type of objects stored in the list must be instances of a class derived from **PhoneNumber**.

```
// PhoneList can manage any type of phone list
// as long as it is derived from PhoneNumber.
class PhoneList<T> where T : PhoneNumber {
  T[] phList;
  int end;

  public PhoneList() {
    phList = new T[10];
```

```
    end = 0;
  }

  // Add an entry to the list.
  public bool Add(T newEntry) {
    if(end == 10) return false;

    phList[end] = newEntry;
    end++;

    return true;
  }

  // Given a name, find and return the phone info.
  public T FindByName(string name) {

    for(int i=0; i<end; i++) {
      // Name can be used because it is a member of
      // PhoneNumber, which is the base class constraint.
      if(phList[i].Name == name)
        return phList[i];
    }

    // Name not in list.
    throw new NotFoundException();
  }

  // Given a number, find and return the phone info.
  public T FindByNumber(string number) {

    for(int i=0; i<end; i++) {
      // Number can be used because it is also a member of
      // PhoneNumber, which is the base class constraint.
      if(phList[i].Number == number)
        return phList[i];
    }

    // Number not in list.
    throw new NotFoundException();
  }

  // ...
}
```

The base class constraint enables code inside **PhoneList** to access the properties **Name** and **Number** for any type of telephone list. It also guarantees that only valid types are used to construct a **PhoneList** object. Notice that **PhoneList** throws a **NotFoundException** if a name or number is not found. This is a custom exception that is declared as shown here:

```
class NotFoundException : Exception {
  /* Implement all of the Exception constructors. Notice that
     the constructors simply execute the base class constructor.
     Because NotFoundException adds nothing to Exception,
     there is no need for any further actions. */
```

```
  public NotFoundException() : base() { }
  public NotFoundException(string str) : base(str) { }
  public NotFoundException(string str, Exception inner) :
    base(str, inner) { }
  protected NotFoundException(
    System.Runtime.Serialization.SerializationInfo si,
    System.Runtime.Serialization.StreamingContext sc) :
      base(si, sc) { }
}
```

Although only the default constructor is used by this example, **NotFoundException**
implements all of the constructors defined by **Exception** for the sake of illustration.
Notice that these constructors simply invoke the equivalent base class constructor
defined by **Exception**. Because **NotFoundException** adds nothing to **Exception**, there
is no reason for any further action.

The following program puts together all the pieces and demonstrates **PhoneList**. Notice
that a class called **EmailFriend** is also created. This class does not inherit **PhoneNumber**.
Thus, it *cannot* be used to create a **PhoneList**.

```
// A more practical demonstration of a base class constraint.

using System;

// A custom exception that is thrown if a name or number is not found.
class NotFoundException : Exception {
  /* Implement all of the Exception constructors. Notice that
     the constructors simply execute the base class constructor.
     Because NotFoundException adds nothing to Exception,
     there is no need for any further actions. */
  public NotFoundException() : base() { }
  public NotFoundException(string str) : base(str) { }
  public NotFoundException(string str, Exception inner) :
    base(str, inner) { }
  protected NotFoundException(
    System.Runtime.Serialization.SerializationInfo si,
    System.Runtime.Serialization.StreamingContext sc) :
      base(si, sc) { }
}
// A base class that stores a name and phone number.
class PhoneNumber {

  public PhoneNumber(string n, string num) {
    Name = n;
    Number = num;
  }

  public string Number { get; set; }
  public string Name { get; set; }

}

// A class of phone numbers for friends.
class Friend : PhoneNumber {
```

```
  public Friend(string n, string num, bool wk) :
    base(n, num)
  {
    IsWorkNumber = wk;
  }

  public bool IsWorkNumber { get; private set; }

  // ...
}

// A class of phone numbers for suppliers.
class Supplier : PhoneNumber {
  public Supplier(string n, string num) :
    base(n, num) { }

  // ...
}

// Notice that this class does not inherit PhoneNumber.
class EmailFriend {
  // ...
}

// PhoneList can manage any type of phone list
// as long as it is derived from PhoneNumber.
class PhoneList<T> where T : PhoneNumber {
  T[] phList;
  int end;

  public PhoneList() {
    phList = new T[10];
    end = 0;
  }

  // Add an entry to the list.
  public bool Add(T newEntry) {
    if(end == 10) return false;

    phList[end] = newEntry;
    end++;

    return true;
  }

  // Given a name, find and return the phone info.
  public T FindByName(string name) {

    for(int i=0; i<end; i++) {
      // Name can be used because it is a member of
      // PhoneNumber, which is the base class constraint.
      if(phList[i].Name == name)
        return phList[i];
    }
```

```
        // Name not in list.
        throw new NotFoundException();
    }

    // Given a number, find and return the phone info.
    public T FindByNumber(string number) {

        for(int i=0; i<end; i++) {
            // Number can be used because it is also a member of
            // PhoneNumber, which is the base class constraint.
            if(phList[i].Number == number)
                return phList[i];
        }

        // Number not in list.
        throw new NotFoundException();
    }

    // ...
}

// Demonstrate base class constraints.
class UseBaseClassConstraint {
    static void Main() {

        // The following code is OK because Friend
        // inherits PhoneNumber.
        PhoneList<Friend> plist = new PhoneList<Friend>();
        plist.Add(new Friend("Tom", "555-1234", true));
        plist.Add(new Friend("Gary", "555-6756", true));
        plist.Add(new Friend("Matt", "555-9254", false));

        try {
            // Find the number of a friend given a name.
            Friend frnd = plist.FindByName("Gary");

            Console.Write(frnd.Name + ": " + frnd.Number);

            if(frnd.IsWorkNumber)
                Console.WriteLine(" (work)");
            else
                Console.WriteLine();
        } catch(NotFoundException) {
            Console.WriteLine("Not Found");
        }

        Console.WriteLine();

        // The following code is also OK because Supplier
        // inherits PhoneNumber.
        PhoneList<Supplier> plist2 = new PhoneList<Supplier>();
        plist2.Add(new Supplier("Global Hardware", "555-8834"));
        plist2.Add(new Supplier("Computer Warehouse", "555-9256"));
        plist2.Add(new Supplier("NetworkCity", "555-2564"));
```

```
    try {
      // Find the name of a supplier given a number.
      Supplier sp = plist2.FindByNumber("555-2564");
      Console.WriteLine(sp.Name + ": " + sp.Number);
    } catch(NotFoundException) {
        Console.WriteLine("Not Found");
    }

    // The following declaration is invalid because EmailFriend
    // does NOT inherit PhoneNumber.
//    PhoneList<EmailFriend> plist3 =
//        new PhoneList<EmailFriend>(); // Error!
  }
}
```

The output from the program is shown here:

```
Gary: 555-6756 (work)

NetworkCity: 555-2564
```

You might want to try experimenting with this program a bit. For example, try creating different types of telephone lists. Also, try using **IsWorkNumber** from within **PhoneList**. As you will see, the compiler won't let you do it. The reason is that **IsWorkNumber** is a property defined by **Friend**, not by **PhoneNumber**. Thus, **PhoneList** has no knowledge of it.

Using an Interface Constraint

The interface constraint enables you to specify an interface that a type argument must implement. The interface constraint serves the same two important purposes as the base class constraint. First, it lets you use the members of the interface within the generic class. Second, it ensures that only type arguments that implement the specified interface are used. This means that for any given interface constraint, the type argument must be either the interface or a type that implements that interface.

The interface constraint uses this form of the **where** clause:

where *T* : *interface-name*

Here, *T* is the name of the type parameter, and *interface-name* is the name of the interface. More than one interface can be specified by using a comma-separated list. If a constraint includes both a base class and interface, then the base class must be listed first.

The following program illustrates the interface constraint by reworking the telephone list example shown in the previous section. In this version, the **PhoneNumber** class has been converted into an interface called **IPhoneNumber**. This interface is then implemented by **Friend** and **Supplier**.

```
// Use an interface constraint.

using System;

// A custom exception that is thrown if a name or number is not found.
class NotFoundException : Exception {
  /* Implement all of the Exception constructors. Notice that
```

```
      the constructors simply execute the base class constructor.
      Because NotFoundException adds nothing to Exception,
      there is no need for any further actions. */
   public NotFoundException() : base() { }
   public NotFoundException(string str) : base(str) { }
   public NotFoundException(string str, Exception inner) :
     base(str, inner) { }
   protected NotFoundException(
     System.Runtime.Serialization.SerializationInfo si,
     System.Runtime.Serialization.StreamingContext sc) :
       base(si, sc) { }
}

// An interface that supports a name and phone number.
public interface IPhoneNumber {

   string Number {
     get;
     set;
   }

   string Name {
     get;
     set;
   }
}

// A class of phone numbers for friends.
// It implements IPhoneNumber.
class Friend : IPhoneNumber {

   public Friend(string n, string num, bool wk) {
     Name = n;
     Number = num;

     IsWorkNumber = wk;
   }

   public bool IsWorkNumber { get; private set; }

   // Implement IPhoneNumber.
   public string Number { get; set; }
   public string Name { get; set; }

   // ...
}

// A class of phone numbers for suppliers.
class Supplier : IPhoneNumber {

   public Supplier(string n, string num) {
     Name = n;
     Number = num;
   }
```

```
    // Implement IPhoneNumber.
    public string Number { get; set; }
    public string Name { get; set; }

    // ...
}

// Notice that this class does not implement IPhoneNumber.
class EmailFriend {
    // ...
}

// PhoneList can manage any type of phone list
// as long as it implements IPhoneNumber.
class PhoneList<T> where T : IPhoneNumber {
    T[] phList;
    int end;

    public PhoneList() {
        phList = new T[10];
        end = 0;
    }

    public bool Add(T newEntry) {
        if(end == 10) return false;

        phList[end] = newEntry;
        end++;

        return true;
    }

    // Given a name, find and return the phone info.
    public T FindByName(string name) {

        for(int i=0; i<end; i++) {
            // Name can be used because it is a member of
            // IPhoneNumber, which is the interface constraint.
            if(phList[i].Name == name)
                return phList[i];
        }

        // Name not in list.
        throw new NotFoundException();
    }

    // Given a number, find and return the phone info.
    public T FindByNumber(string number) {

        for(int i=0; i<end; i++) {
            // Number can be used because it is also a member of
            // IPhoneNumber, which is the interface constraint.
            if(phList[i].Number == number)
                return phList[i];
        }
```

```
      // Number not in list.
      throw new NotFoundException();
    }

  // ...
}

// Demonstrate interface constraints.
class UseInterfaceConstraint {
  static void Main() {

    // The following code is OK because Friend
    // implements IPhoneNumber.
    PhoneList<Friend> plist = new PhoneList<Friend>();
    plist.Add(new Friend("Tom", "555-1234", true));
    plist.Add(new Friend("Gary", "555-6756", true));
    plist.Add(new Friend("Matt", "555-9254", false));

    try {
      // Find the number of a friend given a name.
      Friend frnd = plist.FindByName("Gary");

      Console.Write(frnd.Name + ": " + frnd.Number);

      if(frnd.IsWorkNumber)
        Console.WriteLine(" (work)");
      else
        Console.WriteLine();
    } catch(NotFoundException) {
      Console.WriteLine("Not Found");
    }

    Console.WriteLine();

    // The following code is also OK because Supplier
    // implements IPhoneNumber.
    PhoneList<Supplier> plist2 = new PhoneList<Supplier>();
    plist2.Add(new Supplier("Global Hardware", "555-8834"));
    plist2.Add(new Supplier("Computer Warehouse", "555-9256"));
    plist2.Add(new Supplier("NetworkCity", "555-2564"));

    try {
      // Find the name of a supplier given a number.
      Supplier sp = plist2.FindByNumber("555-2564");
      Console.WriteLine(sp.Name + ": " + sp.Number);
    } catch(NotFoundException) {
        Console.WriteLine("Not Found");
    }

    // The following declaration is invalid because EmailFriend
    // does NOT implement IPhoneNumber.
//    PhoneList<EmailFriend> plist3 =
//         new PhoneList<EmailFriend>(); // Error!
  }
}
```

In this version of the program, the interface constraint specified by **PhoneList** requires that a type argument implement the **IPhoneList** interface. Because both **Friend** and **Supplier** implement **IPhoneList**, they are valid types to be bound to **T**. However, **EmailFriend** does not implement **IPhoneList** and cannot be bound to **T**. To prove this, remove the comment symbols from the last two lines in **Main( )**. As you will see, the program will not compile.

Using the new( ) Constructor Constraint

The **new( )** constructor constraint enables you to instantiate an object of a generic type. Normally, you cannot create an instance of a generic type parameter. However, the **new( )** constraint changes this because it requires that a type argument supply a parameterless constructor. This can be the default constructor provided automatically when no explicit constructor is declared or a parameterless constructor explicitly defined by you. With the **new( )** constraint in place, you can invoke the parameterless constructor to create an object.

Here is a simple example that illustrates the use of **new( )**:

```
// Demonstrate a new() constructor constraint.

using System;

class MyClass {

  public MyClass() {
    // ...
  }

  //...
}

class Test<T> where T : new() {
  T obj;

  public Test() {
    // This works because of the new() constraint.
    obj = new T(); // create a T object
  }

  // ...
}

class ConsConstraintDemo {
  static void Main() {

    Test<MyClass> x = new Test<MyClass>();

  }
}
```

First, notice the declaration of the **Test** class, shown here:

```
class Test<T> where T : new() {
```

Because of the **new( )** constraint, any type argument must supply a parameterless constructor.

Next, examine the **Test** constructor, shown here:

```
public Test() {
  // This works because of the new() constraint.
  obj = new T(); // create a T object
}
```

A new object of type **T** is created and a reference to it is assigned to **obj**. This statement is valid only because the **new( )** constraint ensures that a constructor will be available. To prove this, try removing the **new( )** constraint and then attempt to recompile the program. As you will see, an error will be reported.

In **Main( )**, an object of type **Test** is instantiated, as shown here:

```
Test<MyClass> x = new Test<MyClass>();
```

Notice that the type argument is **MyClass**, and that **MyClass** defines a parameterless constructor. Thus, it is valid for use as a type argument for **Test**. It must be emphasized that it was not necessary for **MyClass** to explicitly declare a parameterless constructor. Its default constructor would also satisfy the constraint. However, if a class needs other constructors in addition to a parameterless one, then it would be necessary to also explicitly declare a parameterless version, too.

There are three important points about using **new( )**. First, it can be used with other constraints, but it must be the last constraint in the list. Second, **new( )** allows you to construct an object using only the parameterless constructor, even when other constructors are available. In other words, it is not permissible to pass arguments to the constructor of a type parameter. Third, you cannot use **new( )** in conjunction with a value type constraint, described next.

The Reference Type and Value Type Constraints

The next two constraints enable you to indicate that a type argument must be either a reference type or a value type. These are useful in the few cases in which the difference between reference and value types are important to generic code. Here is the general form of the reference type constraint:

where T : class

In this form of the **where** clause, the keyword **class** specifies that T must be a reference type. Thus, an attempt to use a value type, such as **int** or **bool**, for T will result in a compilation error.

Here is the general form of the value type constraint:

where T : struct

In this case, the keyword **struct** specifies that T must be a value type. (Recall that structures are value types.) Thus, an attempt to use a reference type, such as **string**, for T will result in a compilation error. In both cases, when additional constraints are present, **class** or **struct** must be the first constraint in the list.

Here is an example that demonstrates the reference type constraint:

```
// Demonstrate a reference constraint.

using System;

class MyClass {
  //...
}

// Use a reference constraint.
class Test<T> where T : class {
  T obj;

  public Test() {
    // The following statement is legal only
    // because T is guaranteed to be a reference
    // type, which can be assigned the value null.
    obj = null;
  }

  // ...
}

class ClassConstraintDemo {
  static void Main() {

    // The following is OK because MyClass is a class.
    Test<MyClass> x = new Test<MyClass>();

    // The next line is in error because int is a value type.
//    Test<int> y = new Test<int>();
  }
}
```

First, notice how **Test** is declared:

```
class Test<T> where T : class {
```

The **class** constraint requires that any type argument for **T** be a reference type. In this program, this is necessary because of what occurs inside the **Test** constructor:

```
public Test() {
  // The following statement is legal only
  // because T is guaranteed to be a reference
  // type, which can be assigned the value null.
  obj = null;
}
```

Here, **obj** (which is of type **T**) is assigned the value **null**. This assignment is valid only for reference types. As a general rule, you cannot assign **null** to a value type. (The exception to this rule is the *nullable type,* which is a special structure type that encapsulates a value type and allows the value **null**. See Chapter 20 for details.) Therefore, without the constraint, the

assignment would not have been valid and the compile would have failed. This is one case in which the difference between value types and reference types might be important to a generic routine.

The value type constraint is the complement of the reference type constraint. It simply ensures that any type argument is a value type, including a **struct** or an **enum**. (In this context, a nullable type is not considered a value type.) Here is an example:

```
// Demonstrate a value type constraint.

using System;

struct MyStruct {
  //...
}

class MyClass {
  // ...
}

class Test<T> where T : struct {
  T obj;

  public Test(T x) {
    obj = x;
  }

  // ...
}

class ValueConstraintDemo {
  static void Main() {

    // Both of these declarations are legal.

    Test<MyStruct> x = new Test<MyStruct>(new MyStruct());

    Test<int> y = new Test<int>(10);

    // But, the following declaration is illegal!
//    Test<MyClass> z = new Test<MyClass>(new MyClass());
  }
}
```

In this program, **Test** is declared as shown here:

```
class Test<T> where T : struct {
```

Because **T** of **Test** now has the **struct** constraint, **T** can be bound only to value type arguments. This means that **Test<MyStruct>** and **Test<int>** are valid, but **Test<MyClass>** is not. To prove this, try removing the comment symbols from the start of the last line in the program and recompiling. An error will be reported.

Using a Constraint to Establish a Relationship Between Two Type Parameters

There is a variation of the base class constraint that allows you to establish a relationship between two type parameters. For example, consider the following generic class declaration:

```
class Gen<T, V> where V : T {
```

In this declaration, the **where** clause tells the compiler that the type argument bound to **V** must be identical to or inherit from the type argument bound to **T**. If this relationship is not present when an object of type **Gen** is declared, then a compile-time error will result. A constraint that uses a type parameter, such as that just shown, is called a *naked type constraint*. The following example illustrates this constraint:

```
// Create relationship between two type parameters.

using System;

class A {
  //...
}

class B : A {
  // ...
}

// Here, V must be or inherit from T.
class Gen<T, V> where V : T {
  // ...
}

class NakedConstraintDemo {
  static void Main() {

    // This declaration is OK because B inherits A.
    Gen<A, B> x = new Gen<A, B>();

    // This declaration is in error because
    // A does not inherit B.
//    Gen<B, A> y = new Gen<B, A>();

  }
}
```

First, notice that class **B** inherits class **A**. Next, examine the two **Gen** declarations in **Main()**. As the comments explain, the first declaration

```
Gen<A, B> x = new Gen<A, B>();
```

is legal because **B** inherits **A**. However, the second declaration

```
//    Gen<B, A> y = new Gen<B, A>();
```

is illegal because **A** does not inherit **B**.

Using Multiple Constraints

There can be more than one constraint associated with a type parameter. When this is the case, use a comma-separated list of constraints. In this list, the first constraint must be **class** or **struct** (if present) or the base class (if one is specified). It is illegal to specify both a **class** or **struct** constraint and a base class constraint. Next in the list must be any interface constraints. The **new( )** constraint must be last. For example, this is a valid declaration.

```
class Gen<T> where T : MyClass, IMyInterface, new() { // ...
```

In this case, **T** must be replaced by a type argument that inherits **MyClass**, implements **IMyInterface**, and has a parameterless constructor.

When using two or more type parameters, you can specify a constraint for each parameter by using a separate **where** clause. Here is an example:

```
// Use multiple where clauses.

using System;

// Gen has two type arguments and both have a where clause.
class Gen<T, V> where T : class
                where V : struct {
  T ob1;
  V ob2;

  public Gen(T t, V v) {
    ob1 = t;
    ob2 = v;
  }
}

class MultipleConstraintDemo {
  static void Main() {
    // This is OK because string is a class and
    // int is a value type.
    Gen<string, int> obj = new Gen<string, int>("test", 11);

    // The next line is wrong because bool is not
    // a reference type.
//    Gen<bool, int> obj = new Gen<bool, int>(true, 11);
  }
}
```

In this example, **Gen** takes two type arguments and both have a **where** clause. Pay special attention to its declaration:

```
class Gen<T, V> where T : class
                where V : struct {
```

Notice the only thing that separates the first **where** clause from the second is whitespace. No other punctuation is required or valid.

Creating a Default Value of a Type Parameter

When writing generic code, there will be times when the difference between value types and reference types is an issue. One such situation occurs when you want to give a variable of a type parameter a default value. For reference types, the default value is **null**. For non-**struct** value types, the default value is 0. The default value for a **struct** is an object of that **struct** with all fields set to their defaults. Thus, trouble occurs if you want to give a variable of a type parameter a default value. What value would you use: **null**, 0, or something else?

For example, given a generic class called **Test** declared like this:

```
class Test<T> {
  T obj;
  // ...
```

if you want to give **obj** a default value, would you use

```
obj = null; // works only for reference types
```

or

```
obj = 0; // works only for numeric types and enums, but not structs
```

The solution to this problem is to use another form of **default**, shown here:

default(*type*)

This is the operator form of **default**, and it produces a default value of the specified *type*, no matter what type is used. Thus, continuing with the example, to assign **obj** a default value of type **T**, you would use this statement:

```
obj = default(T);
```

This will work for all type arguments, whether they are value or reference types.

Here is a short program that demonstrates **default**:

```
// Demonstrate the default operator.

using System;

class MyClass {
  //...
}

// Construct a default value of T.
class Test<T> {
  public T obj;

  public Test() {
    // The following statement would work only for reference types.
//    obj = null; // can't use

    // The following statement will work only for numeric value types.
//    obj = 0; // can't use
```

```
    // This statement works for both reference and value types.
    obj = default(T); // Works!
  }

  // ...
}

class DefaultDemo {
  static void Main() {

    // Construct Test using a reference type.
    Test<MyClass> x = new Test<MyClass>();

    if(x.obj == null)
      Console.WriteLine("x.obj is null.");

    // Construct Test using a value type.
    Test<int> y = new Test<int>();

    if(y.obj == 0)
      Console.WriteLine("y.obj is 0.");
  }
}
```

The output is shown here:

```
x.obj is null.
y.obj is 0.
```

Generic Structures

C# allows you to create generic structures. The syntax is the same as for generic classes. For example, in the following program, the **XY** structure, which stores X, Y coordinates, is generic:

```
// Demonstrate a generic struct.
using System;

// This structure is generic.
struct XY<T> {
  T x;
  T y;

  public XY(T a, T b) {
    x = a;
    y = b;
  }

  public T X {
    get { return x; }
    set { x = value; }
  }

  public T Y {
    get { return y; }
```

```
      set { y = value; }
   }
}

class StructTest {
  static void Main() {
    XY<int> xy = new XY<int>(10, 20);
    XY<double> xy2 = new XY<double>(88.0, 99.0);

    Console.WriteLine(xy.X + ", " + xy.Y);

    Console.WriteLine(xy2.X + ", " + xy2.Y);
  }
}
```

The output is shown here:

```
10, 20
88, 99
```

Like generic classes, generic structures can have constraints. For example, this version of **XY** restricts type arguments to value types:

```
struct XY<T> where T : struct {
// ...
```

Creating a Generic Method

As the preceding examples have shown, methods inside a generic class can make use of a class' type parameter and are, therefore, automatically generic relative to the type parameter. However, it is possible to declare a generic method that uses one or more type parameters of its own. Furthermore, it is possible to create a generic method that is enclosed within a non-generic class.

Let's begin with an example. The following program declares a non-generic class called **ArrayUtils** and a static generic method within that class called **CopyInsert( )**. The **CopyInsert( )** method copies the contents of one array to another, inserting a new element at a specified location in the process. It can be used with any type of array.

```
// Demonstrate a generic method.

using System;

// A class of array utilities. Notice that this is not
// a generic class.
class ArrayUtils {

  // Copy an array, inserting a new element
  // in the process. This is a generic method.
  public static bool CopyInsert<T>(T e, uint idx,
                                   T[] src, T[] target) {

    // See if target array is big enough.
    if(target.Length < src.Length+1)
      return false;
```

```
    // Copy src to target, inserting e at idx in the process.
    for(int i=0, j=0; i < src.Length; i++, j++) {
      if(i == idx) {
        target[j] = e;
        j++;
      }
      target[j] = src[i];
    }

    return true;
  }
}

class GenMethDemo {
  static void Main() {
    int[] nums = { 1, 2, 3 };
    int[] nums2 = new int[4];

    // Display contents of nums.
    Console.Write("Contents of nums: ");
    foreach(int x in nums)
      Console.Write(x + " ");

    Console.WriteLine();

    // Operate on an int array.
    ArrayUtils.CopyInsert(99, 2, nums, nums2);

    // Display contents of nums2.
    Console.Write("Contents of nums2: ");
    foreach(int x in nums2)
      Console.Write(x + " ");

    Console.WriteLine();


    // Now, use copyInsert on an array of strings.
    string[] strs = { "Generics", "are", "powerful."};
    string[] strs2 = new string[4];

    // Display contents of strs.
    Console.Write("Contents of strs: ");
    foreach(string s in strs)
      Console.Write(s + " ");

    Console.WriteLine();

    // Insert into a string array.
    ArrayUtils.CopyInsert("in C#", 1, strs, strs2);

    // Display contents of strs2.
    Console.Write("Contents of strs2: ");
    foreach(string s in strs2)
      Console.Write(s + " ");
```

```
      Console.WriteLine();

      // This call is invalid because the first argument
      // is of type double, and the third and fourth arguments
      // have element types of int.
//    ArrayUtils.CopyInsert(0.01, 2, nums, nums2);
    }
}
```

The output from the program is shown here:

```
Contents of nums: 1 2 3
Contents of nums2: 1 2 99 3
Contents of strs: Generics are powerful.
Contents of strs2: Generics in C# are powerful.
```

Let's examine **CopyInsert( )** closely. First, notice how it is declared by this line:

```
public static bool CopyInsert<T>(T e, uint idx,
                                 T[] src, T[] target) {
```

The type parameter is declared *after* the method name, but *before* the parameter list. Also notice that **CopyInsert( )** is static, enabling it to be called independently of any object. Understand, though, that generic methods can be either static or non-static. There is no restriction in this regard.

Now, notice how **CopyInsert( )** is called within **Main( )** by use of the normal call syntax, without the need to specify type arguments. This is because the types of the arguments are automatically discerned, and the type of **T** is adjusted accordingly. This process is called *type inference*. For example, in the first call:

```
ArrayUtils.CopyInsert(99, 2, nums, nums2);
```

the type of **T** becomes **int** because 99 and the element types of **nums** and **nums2** are **int**. In the second call, **string** types are used, and **T** is replaced by **string**.

Now, notice the commented-out code, shown here:

```
//    ArrayUtils.CopyInsert(0.01, 2, nums, nums2);
```

If you remove the comments and then try to compile the program, you will receive an error. The reason is that the type of the first argument is **double**, but the element types of **nums** and **nums2** are **int**. However, all three types must be substituted for the same type parameter, **T**. This causes a type-mismatch, which results in a compile-time error. This ability to enforce type safety is one of the most important advantages of generic methods.

The syntax used to create **CopyInsert( )** can be generalized. Here is the general form of a generic method:

ret-type meth-name<type-param-list>(param-list) { // ...

In all cases, *type-param-list* is a comma-separated list of type parameters. Notice that for a generic method, the type parameter list follows the method name.

Using Explicit Type Arguments to Call a Generic Method

Although implicit type inference is adequate for most invocations of a generic method, it is possible to explicitly specify the type argument. To do so, specify the type argument after the method name when calling the method. For example, here **CopyInsert( )** is explicitly passed type **string**:

```
ArrayUtils.CopyInsert<string>("in C#", 1, strs, strs2);
```

You will need to explicitly specify the type when the compiler cannot infer the type for the **T** parameter or if you want to override the type inference.

Using a Constraint with a Generic Method

You can add constraints to the type arguments of a generic method by specifying them after the parameter list. For example, the following version of **CopyInsert( )** will work only with reference types:

```
public static bool CopyInsert<T>(T e, uint idx,
                          T[] src, T[] target) where T : class {
```

If you were to try this version in the program shown earlier, then the following call to **CopyInsert( )** would not compile because **int** is a value type, not a reference type:

```
// Now wrong because T must be reference type!
ArrayUtils.CopyInsert(99, 2, nums, nums2); // Now illegal!
```

Generic Delegates

Like methods, delegates can also be generic. To declare a generic delegate, use this general form:

> delegate *ret-type delegate-name<type-parameter-list>(arg-list)*;

Notice the placement of the type parameter list. It immediately follows the delegate's name. The advantage of generic delegates is that they let you define, in a type-safe manner, a generalized form that can then be matched to any compatible method.

The following program demonstrates a generic delegate called **SomeOp** that has one type parameter called **T**. It returns type **T** and takes an argument of type **T**.

```
// A simple generic delegate.

using System;

// Declare a generic delegate.
delegate T SomeOp<T>(T v);

class GenDelegateDemo {
  // Return the summation of the argument.
  static int Sum(int v) {
    int result = 0;
    for(int i=v; i>0; i--)
```

```
      result += i;

    return result;
  }

  // Return a string containing the reverse of the argument.
  static string Reflect(string str) {
    string result = "";

    foreach(char ch in str)
      result = ch + result;

    return result;
  }

  static void Main() {
    // Construct an int delegate.
    SomeOp<int> intDel = Sum;
    Console.WriteLine(intDel(3));

    // Construct a string delegate.
    SomeOp<string> strDel = Reflect;
    Console.WriteLine(strDel("Hello"));
  }
}
```

The output is shown here:

```
6
olleH
```

Let's look closely at this program. First, notice how the **SomeOp** delegate is declared:

```
delegate T SomeOp<T>(T v);
```

Notice that **T** can be used as the return type even though the type parameter **T** is specified after the name **SomeOp**.

Inside **GenDelegateDemo**, the methods **Sum( )** and **Reflect( )** are declared, as shown here:

```
static int Sum(int v) {
```

```
static string Reflect(string str) {
```

The **Sum( )** method returns the summation of the integer value passed as an argument. The **Reflect( )** method returns a string that is the reverse of the string passed as an argument.

Inside **Main( )**, a delegate called **intDel** is instantiated and assigned a reference to **Sum( )**:

```
SomeOp<int> intDel = Sum;
```

Because **Sum( )** takes an **int** argument and returns an **int** value, **Sum( )** is compatible with an **int** instance of **SomeOp**.

In similar fashion, the delegate **strDel** is created and assigned a reference to **Reflect( )**:

```
SomeOp<string> strDel = Reflect;
```

Because **Reflect( )** takes a **string** argument and returns a **string** result, it is compatible with the string version of **SomeOp**.

Because of the type safety inherent in generics, you cannot assign incompatible methods to delegates. For example, assuming the preceding program, the following statement would be in error:

```
SomeOp<int> intDel = Reflect; // Error!
```

Because **Reflect( )** takes a **string** argument and returns a **string** result, it cannot be assigned to an **int** version of **SomeOp**.

As explained in Chapter 15, one of the major uses of delegates occurs when handling events. Although events, themselves, cannot be generic, the delegate that supports an event can. The following program reworks an example from Chapter 15 (the .NET-compatible event demonstration) so that it uses a generic delegate:

```
// Convert event example from Chapter 15 to use generic delegate.

using System;

// Derive a class from EventArgs.
class MyEventArgs : EventArgs {
  public int EventNum;
}

// Declare a generic delegate for an event.
delegate void MyEventHandler<T, V>(T source, V args);

// Declare an event class.
class MyEvent {
  static int count = 0;

  public event MyEventHandler<MyEvent, MyEventArgs> SomeEvent;

  // This fires SomeEvent.
  public void OnSomeEvent() {
    MyEventArgs arg = new MyEventArgs();

    if(SomeEvent != null) {
      arg.EventNum = count++;
      SomeEvent(this, arg);
    }
  }
}

class X {
  public void Handler<T, V>(T source, V arg) where V : MyEventArgs {
    Console.WriteLine("Event " + arg.EventNum +
                      " received by an X object.");
```

```
      Console.WriteLine("Source is " + source);
      Console.WriteLine();
   }
}

class Y {
   public void Handler<T,V>(T source, V arg) where V : MyEventArgs {
      Console.WriteLine("Event " + arg.EventNum +
                        " received by a Y object.");
      Console.WriteLine("Source is " + source);
      Console.WriteLine();
   }
}

class UseGenericEventDelegate {
   static void Main() {
      X ob1 = new X();
      Y ob2 = new Y();
      MyEvent evt = new MyEvent();

      // Add Handler() to the event list.
      evt.SomeEvent += ob1.Handler;
      evt.SomeEvent += ob2.Handler;

      // Fire the event.
      evt.OnSomeEvent();
      evt.OnSomeEvent();
   }
}
```

The output is show here:

```
Event 0 received by an X object.
Source is MyEvent

Event 0 received by a Y object.
Source is MyEvent

Event 1 received by an X object.
Source is MyEvent

Event 1 received by a Y object.
Source is MyEvent
```

Generic Interfaces

In addition to generic classes and methods, you can also have generic interfaces. Generic interfaces are specified just like generic classes. Here is an example that reworks the **ISeries** interface developed in Chapter 12. (Recall that **ISeries** defines the interface to a class that generates a series of numbers.) The data type upon which it operates is now specified by a type parameter.

```csharp
// Demonstrate a generic interface.

using System;

public interface ISeries<T> {
  T GetNext(); // return next element in series
  void Reset(); // restart the series
  void SetStart(T v); // set the starting element
}

// Implement ISeries.
class ByTwos<T> : ISeries<T> {
  T start;
  T val;

  // This delegate defines the form of a method
  // that will be called when the next element in
  // the series is needed.
  public delegate T IncByTwo(T v);

  // This delegate reference will be assigned the
  // method passed to the ByTwos constructor.
  IncByTwo incr;

  public ByTwos(IncByTwo incrMeth) {
    start = default(T);
    val = default(T);
    incr = incrMeth;
  }

  public T GetNext() {
    val = incr(val);
    return val;
  }

  public void Reset() {
    val = start;
  }

  public void SetStart(T v) {
    start = v;
    val = start;
  }
}

class ThreeD {
  public int x, y, z;

  public ThreeD(int a, int b, int c) {
    x = a;
    y = b;
    z = c;
  }
}
```

```
class GenIntfDemo {
  // Define plus two for int.
  static int IntPlusTwo(int v) {
    return v + 2;
  }

  // Define plus two for double.
  static double DoublePlusTwo(double v) {
    return v + 2.0;
  }

  // Define plus two for ThreeD.
  static ThreeD ThreeDPlusTwo(ThreeD v) {
    if(v==null) return new ThreeD(0, 0, 0);
    else return new ThreeD(v.x + 2, v.y + 2, v.z + 2);
  }

  static void Main() {

    // Demonstrate int series.
    ByTwos<int> intBT = new ByTwos<int>(IntPlusTwo);

    for(int i=0; i < 5; i++)
      Console.Write(intBT.GetNext() + "  ");

    Console.WriteLine();


    // Demonstrate double series.
    ByTwos<double> dblBT = new ByTwos<double>(DoublePlusTwo);

    dblBT.SetStart(11.4);

    for(int i=0; i < 5; i++)
      Console.Write(dblBT.GetNext() + "  ");

    Console.WriteLine();


    // Demonstrate ThreeD series.
    ByTwos<ThreeD> ThrDBT = new ByTwos<ThreeD>(ThreeDPlusTwo);

    ThreeD coord;
    for(int i=0; i < 5; i++) {
      coord = ThrDBT.GetNext();
      Console.Write(coord.x + "," +
                    coord.y + "," +
                    coord.z + "  ");
    }

    Console.WriteLine();
  }
}
```

The output is shown here:

```
2   4   6   8   10
13.4   15.4   17.4   19.4   21.4
0,0,0   2,2,2   4,4,4   6,6,6   8,8,8
```

There are several things of interest in the preceding example. First, notice how **ISeries** is declared:

```
public interface ISeries<T> {
```

As mentioned, a generic interface uses a syntax similar to that of a generic class.

Now, notice how **ByTwos**, which implements **ISeries**, is declared:

```
class ByTwos<T> : ISeries<T> {
```

The type parameter **T** is specified by **ByTwos** and is also specified in **ISeries**. This is important. A class that implements a generic version of a generic interface must, itself, be generic. For example, the following declaration would be illegal because **T** is not defined:

```
class ByTwos : ISeries<T> { // Wrong!
```

The type argument required by the **ISeries** interface must be passed to **ByTwos**. Otherwise, there is no way for the interface to receive the type argument.

Next, the current value of the series, **val**, and the starting value, **start**, are declared to be objects of the generic type **T**. Then, a delegate called **IncByTwo** is declared. This delegate defines the form of a method that will be used to increase an object of type **T** by two. In order for **ByTwos** to work with any type of data, there must be some way to define what an increase by two means for each type of data. This is achieved by passing to the **ByTwos** constructor a reference to a method that performs an increase by two. This reference is stored in **incr**. When the next element in the series is needed, that method is called through the **incr** delegate to obtain the next value in the series.

Notice the class **ThreeD**. It encapsulates three-dimensional (X,Z,Y) coordinates. It is used to demonstrate **ByTwos** on a class type.

In **GenIntfDemo**, three increment methods are declared; one for **int**, one for **double**, and one for objects of type **ThreeD**. These are passed to the **ByTwos** constructor when objects of their respective types are created. Pay special attention to **ThreeDPlusTwo( )**, shown here:

```
// Define plus two for ThreeD.
static ThreeD ThreeDPlusTwo(ThreeD v) {
  if(v==null) return new ThreeD(0, 0, 0);
  else return new ThreeD(v.x + 2, v.y + 2, v.z + 2);
}
```

Notice that it first checks if **v** is **null**. If it is, then it returns a new **ThreeD** object in which all fields are set to zero. The reason for this is that **v** is set to **default(T)** by the **ByTwos** constructor. This value is zero for value types and **null** for object types. Thus, (unless **SetStart( )** has been called) for the first increment, **v** will contain **null** instead of a reference to an object. This means that for the first increment, a new object is required.

A type parameter for a generic interface can have constraints in the same way as it can for a generic class. For example, this version of **ISeries** restricts its use to reference types:

```
public interface ISeries<T> where T : class {
```

When this version of **ISeries** is implemented, the implementing class must also specify the same constraint for **T**, as shown here:

```
class ByTwos<T> : ISeries<T> where T : class {
```

Because of the reference constraint, this version of **ISeries** cannot be used on value types. Thus, in the preceding program, only **ByTwos<ThreeD>** would be valid. **ByTwos<int>** and **ByTwos<double>** would be invalid.

Comparing Instances of a Type Parameter

Sometimes you will want to compare two instances of a type parameter. For example, you might want to write a generic method called **IsIn( )** that returns true if some value is contained within an array. To accomplish this, you might first try something like this:

```
// This won't work!
public static bool IsIn<T>(T what, T[] obs) {
  foreach(T v in obs)
    if(v == what) // Error!
      return true;

  return false;
}
```

Unfortunately, this attempt won't work. Because **T** is a generic type, the compiler has no way to know precisely how two objects should be compared for equality. Should a bitwise comparison be done? Should only certain fields be compared? Should reference equality be used? The compiler has no way to answer these questions.

To enable two objects of a generic type parameter to be compared, you must use the **CompareTo( )** method defined by one of .NET's standard interfaces: **IComparable**. This interface is implemented by all of C#'s built-in types, including **int**, **string**, and **double**. It is also easy to implement for classes that you create.

The **IComparable** interface defines only the **CompareTo( )** method shown here:

int CompareTo(object *obj*)

CompareTo( ) compares the invoking object to *obj*. It returns zero if the two objects are equal, a positive value if the invoking object is greater than *obj*, and a negative value if the invoking object is less than *obj*.

To use **CompareTo( )**, you must specify a constraint that requires every type argument to implement the **IComparable** interface. Then, when you need to compare two instances of the type parameter, simply call **CompareTo( )**. For example, here is a corrected version of **IsIn( )**:

```
// Require IComparable interface.
public static bool IsIn<T>(T what, T[] obs) where T : IComparable {
  foreach(T v in obs)
```

```
    if(v.CompareTo(what) == 0) // now OK, uses CompareTo()
       return true;

  return false;
}
```

Notice the use of the constraint

```
where T : IComparable
```

This constraint ensures that only types that implement **IComparable** are valid type arguments for **IsIn( )**.

The following program demonstrates **IsIn( )**. It also shows how **IComparable** can be easily implemented by a class:

```
// Demonstrate IComparable.

using System;

class MyClass : IComparable {
  public int Val;

  public MyClass(int x) { Val = x; }

  // Implement IComparable.
  public int CompareTo(object obj) {
    return Val - ((MyClass) obj).Val;
  }
}

class CompareDemo {

  // Require IComparable interface.
  public static bool IsIn<T>(T what, T[] obs) where T : IComparable {
    foreach(T v in obs)
      if(v.CompareTo(what) == 0) // now OK, uses CompareTo()
        return true;

    return false;
  }

  // Demonstrate comparisons.
  static void Main() {
    // Use IsIn() with int.
    int[] nums = { 1, 2, 3, 4, 5 };

    if(IsIn(2, nums))
      Console.WriteLine("2 is found.");

    if(IsIn(99, nums))
      Console.WriteLine("This won't display.");


    // Use IsIn() with string.
```

```
    string[] strs = { "one", "two", "Three"};

    if(IsIn("two", strs))
      Console.WriteLine("two is found.");

    if(IsIn("five", strs))
      Console.WriteLine("This won't display.");


    // Use IsIn with MyClass.
    MyClass[] mcs = { new MyClass(1), new MyClass(2),
                      new MyClass(3), new MyClass(4) };

    if(IsIn(new MyClass(3), mcs))
      Console.WriteLine("MyClass(3) is found.");

    if(IsIn(new MyClass(99), mcs))
      Console.WriteLine("This won't display.");
  }
}
```

The output is shown here:

```
2 is found.
two is found.
MyClass(3) is found.
```

Although the preceding program is correct, there is still one potential trouble spot. Notice how **CompareTo( )** is implemented by **MyClass**:

```
public int CompareTo(object obj) {
  return Val - ((MyClass) obj).Val;
}
```

Because the parameter to **CompareTo( )** must be of type **object**, **obj** must be explicitly cast to **MyClass** in order for **Val** to be accessed. However, it's precisely this type of thing that generics were designed to eliminate!

To solve this problem, C# provides a generic version of **IComparable**, which is declared like this:

  public interface IComparable<T>

In this version, the type of data being compared is passed as a type argument to **T**. This causes the declaration of **CompareTo( )** to be changed, as shown next:

  int CompareTo(T *obj*)

Now, the parameter to **CompareTo( )** can be specified as the proper type and no cast from **object** is needed. **IComparable<T>** is also implemented by all built-in types.

Here is an improved version of **MyClass** that implements **IComparable<T>**:

```
// This version of MyClass implements IComparable<T>
class MyClass : IComparable<MyClass> {
  public int Val;
```

```
  public MyClass(int x) { Val = x; }

  public int CompareTo(MyClass obj) {
    return Val - obj.Val; // Now, no cast is needed.
  }
}
```

Notice that a cast is no longer required by this line in **CompareTo( )**:

```
return Val - obj.Val; // Now, no cast is needed.
```

Because the type parameter to **IComparable** is **MyClass**, the type of **obj** is now known to be
MyClass.

Here is an updated version of **IsIn( )** that requires **IComparable<T>**:

```
// Require IComparable<T> interface.
public static bool IsIn<T>(T what, T[] obs) where T : IComparable<T> {
  foreach(T v in obs)
    if(v.CompareTo(what) == 0) // now OK, uses CompareTo()
      return true;

  return false;
}
```

NOTE *If a type parameter specifies a reference or a base class constraint, then = = and ! = can be
applied to instances of that type parameter, but they only test for reference equality. To compare
values, you must implement **IComparable** or **IComparable<T>**.*

Generic Class Hierarchies

Generic classes can be part of a class hierarchy in just the same way as non-generic classes.
Thus, a generic class can act as a base class or be a derived class. The key difference between
generic and non-generic hierarchies is that in a generic hierarchy, any type arguments needed
by a generic base class must be passed up the hierarchy by all derived classes. This is similar
to the way that constructor arguments must be passed up a hierarchy.

Using a Generic Base Class

Here is a simple example of a hierarchy that uses a generic base class:

```
// A simple generic class hierarchy.
using System;

// A generic base class.
class Gen<T> {
  T ob;

  public Gen(T o) {
    ob = o;
  }

  // Return ob.
  public T GetOb() {
```

```
    return ob;
  }
}

// A class derived from Gen.
class Gen2<T> : Gen<T> {
  public Gen2(T o) : base(o) {
    // ...
  }
}

class GenHierDemo {
  static void Main() {
    Gen2<string> g2 = new Gen2<string>("Hello");

    Console.WriteLine(g2.GetOb());
  }
}
```

In this hierarchy, **Gen2** inherits the generic class **Gen**. Notice how **Gen2** is declared by the following line:

```
class Gen2<T> : Gen<T> {
```

The type parameter **T** is specified by **Gen2** and is also passed to **Gen**. This means that whatever type is passed to **Gen2** will also be passed to **Gen**. For example, this declaration

```
Gen2<string> g2 = new Gen2<string>("Hello");
```

passes **string** as the type parameter to **Gen**. Thus, the **ob** inside the **Gen** portion of **Gen2** will be of type **string**.

Notice also that **Gen2** does not use the type parameter **T** except to pass it along to the **Gen** base class. Thus, even if a derived class would otherwise not need to be generic, it still must specify the type parameter(s) required by its generic base class.

Of course, a derived class is free to add its own type parameters, if needed. For example, here is a variation on the preceding hierarchy in which **Gen2** adds a type parameter of its own:

```
// A derived class can add its own type parameters.
using System;

// A generic base class.
class Gen<T> {
  T ob; // declare a variable of type T

  // Pass the constructor a reference of type T.
  public Gen(T o) {
    ob = o;
  }

  // Return ob.
  public T GetOb() {
    return ob;
```

```
    }
}

// A derived class of Gen that defines a second
// type parameter, called V.
class Gen2<T, V> : Gen<T> {
  V ob2;

  public Gen2(T o, V o2) : base(o) {
    ob2 = o2;
  }

  public V GetObj2() {
    return ob2;
  }
}

// Create an object of type Gen2.
class GenHierDemo2 {
  static void Main() {

    // Create a Gen2 object for string and int.
    Gen2<string, int> x =
      new Gen2<string, int>("Value is: ", 99);

    Console.Write(x.GetOb());
    Console.WriteLine(x.GetObj2());
  }
}
```

Notice the declaration of this version of **Gen2**, which is shown here:

```
class Gen2<T, V> : Gen<T> {
```

Here, **T** is the type passed to **Gen**, and **V** is the type that is specific to **Gen2**. **V** is used to declare an object called **ob2** and as a return type for the method **GetObj2( )**. In **Main( )**, a **Gen2** object is created in which type parameter **T** is **string**, and type parameter **V** is **int**. The program displays the following, expected, result:

```
Value is: 99
```

A Generic Derived Class

It is perfectly acceptable for a non-generic class to be the base class of a generic derived class. For example, consider this program:

```
// A non-generic class can be the base class of a generic derived class.
using System;

// A non-generic class.
class NonGen {
  int num;

  public NonGen(int i) {
```

```
      num = i;
    }

    public int GetNum() {
      return num;
    }
}

// A generic derived class.
class Gen<T> : NonGen {
  T ob;

  public Gen(T o, int i) : base (i) {
    ob = o;
  }

  // Return ob.
  public T GetOb() {
    return ob;
  }
}

// Create a Gen object.
class HierDemo3 {
  static void Main() {

    // Create a Gen object for string.
    Gen<String> w = new Gen<String>("Hello", 47);

    Console.Write(w.GetOb() + " ");
    Console.WriteLine(w.GetNum());
  }
}
```

The output from the program is shown here:

```
Hello 47
```

In the program, notice how **Gen** inherits **NonGen** in the following declaration:

```
class Gen<T> : NonGen {
```

Because **NonGen** is not generic, no type argument is specified. Thus, even though **Gen** declares the type parameter **T**, it is not needed by (nor can it be used by) **NonGen**. Thus, **NonGen** is inherited by **Gen** in the normal way. No special conditions apply.

Overriding Virtual Methods in a Generic Class

A virtual method in a generic class can be overridden just like any other method. For example, consider this program in which the virtual method **GetOb( )** is overridden:

```
// Overriding a virtual method in a generic class.
using System;
```

```
// A generic base class.
class Gen<T> {
  protected T ob;

  public Gen(T o) {
    ob = o;
  }

  // Return ob. This method is virtual.
  public virtual T GetOb() {
    Console.Write("Gen's GetOb(): " );
    return ob;
  }
}

// A derived class of Gen that overrides GetOb().
class Gen2<T> : Gen<T> {

  public Gen2(T o) : base(o) {  }

  // Override GetOb().
  public override T GetOb() {
    Console.Write("Gen2's GetOb(): ");
    return ob;
  }
}

// Demonstrate generic method override.
class OverrideDemo {
  static void Main() {

    // Create a Gen object for int.
    Gen<int> iOb = new Gen<int>(88);

    // This calls Gen's version of GetOb().
    Console.WriteLine(iOb.GetOb());


    // Now, create a Gen2 object and assign its
    // reference to iOb (which is a Gen<int> variable).
    iOb = new Gen2<int>(99);

    // This calls Gen2's version of GetOb().
    Console.WriteLine(iOb.GetOb());
  }
}
```

The output is shown here:

```
Gen's GetOb(): 88
Gen2's GetOb(): 99
```

As the output confirms, the overridden version of **GetOb( )** is called for an object of type **Gen2**, but the base class version is called for an object of type **Gen**.

Notice one other thing: This line

```
iOb = new Gen2<int>(99);
```

is valid because **iOb** is a variable of type **Gen<int>**. Thus, it can refer to any object of type **Gen<int>** or any object of a class derived from **Gen<int>**, including **Gen2<int>**. Of course, **iOb** couldn't be used to refer to an object of type **Gen2<double>**, for example, because of the type mismatch.

Overloading Methods That Use Type Parameters

Methods that use type parameters to declare method parameters can be overloaded. However, the rules are a bit more stringent than they are for methods that don't use type parameters. In general, a method that uses a type parameter as the data type of a parameter can be overloaded as long as the signatures of the two versions differ. This means the type and/or number of their parameters must differ. However, the determination of type difference is not based on the generic type parameter, but on the type argument substituted for the type parameter when a constructed type is created. Therefore, it is possible to overload a method that uses type parameters in such a way that it "looks right," but won't work in all specific cases.

For example, consider this generic class:

```
// Ambiguity can result when overloading methods that
// use type parameters.
//
// This program will not compile.

using System;

// A generic class that contains a potentially ambiguous
// overload of the Set() method.
class Gen<T, V> {
  T ob1;
  V ob2;

  // ...

  // In some cases, these two methods
  // will not differ in their parameter types.
  public void Set(T o) {
    ob1 = o;
  }

  public void Set(V o) {
    ob2 = o;
  }
}

class AmbiguityDemo {
  static void Main() {
    Gen<int, double> ok = new Gen<int, double>();
```

```
    Gen<int, int> notOK = new Gen<int, int>();

    ok.Set(10); // is valid, type args differ

    notOK.Set(10); // ambiguous, type args are the same!
  }
}
```

Let's examine this program closely. First, notice that **Gen** declares two type parameters: **T** and **V**. Inside **Gen**, **Set( )** is overloaded based on parameters of type **T** and **V**, as shown here:

```
public void Set(T o) {
  ob1 = o;
}

public void Set(V o) {
  ob2 = o;
}
```

This looks reasonable because **T** and **V** appear to be different types. However, this overloading creates a potential ambiguity problem.

As **Gen** is written, there is no requirement that **T** and **V** actually be different types. For example, it is perfectly correct (in principle) to construct a **Gen** object as shown here:

```
Gen<int, int> notOK = new Gen<int, int>();
```

In this case, both **T** and **V** will be replaced by **int**. This makes both versions of **Set( )** identical, which is, of course, an error. Thus, when the attempt to call **Set( )** on **notOK** occurs later in **Main( )**, a compile-time ambiguity error is reported.

In general, you can overload methods that use type parameters as long as there is no constructed type that results in a conflict. It is important to understand that type constraints do not participate in overload resolution. Thus, type constraints cannot be used to eliminate ambiguity. Like methods, constructors, operators, and indexers that use type parameters can also be overloaded, and the same rules apply.

How Generic Types Are Instantiated

One question that is often raised when working with generics is whether the use of a generic class leads to code-bloat at runtime. The simple answer is no. The reason is that C# implements generics in a highly efficient manner that creates new constructed types only when they are needed. Here is how the process works.

When a generic class is compiled into MSIL, it retains all of its type parameters in their generic form. At runtime, when a specific instance of the class is required, the JIT compiler constructs a specific, executable code version of the class in which the type parameters are replaced by the type arguments. Each instance of the class that uses the same type arguments will use the same executable code version.

For example, given some generic class called **Gen<T>**, then all **Gen<int>** objects will use the same executable code. Thus, code-bloat is reduced and only those versions of the class that are actually used in the program will be created. When a different constructed type is needed, a new version of the class is compiled.

In general, a new executable version of a generic class is created for each constructed type in which the type argument is a value type, such as **int** or **double**. Thus, each object of **Gen<int>** will use one version of **Gen** and each object of type **Gen<double>** will use another version of **Gen**, with each version of **Gen** tailored to the specific value type. However, there will be *only one version* of a generic class that handles all cases in which the type argument is a reference type. This is because the size (in bytes) of all references is the same. Thus, only one version is needed to handle all types of references. This optimization also reduces code-bloat.

Some Generic Restrictions

Here are a few restrictions that you need to keep in mind when using generics:

- Properties, operators, indexers, and events cannot be generic. However, these items can be used in a generic class and can make use of the generic type parameters of that class.

- The **extern** modifier cannot be applied to a generic method.

- Pointer types cannot be used as type arguments.

- If a generic class contains a **static** field, then *each constructed type has its own copy* of that field. This means that each instance of the *same constructed type* shares the same **static** field. However, a different constructed type shares a different copy of that field. Thus, a **static** field is not shared by all constructed types.

Final Thoughts on Generics

Generics are a powerful extension to C# because they streamline the creation of type-safe, reusable code. Although the generic syntax can seem a bit overwhelming at first, it will quickly become second nature. Likewise, learning how and when to use constraints takes a bit of practice, but becomes easier over time. Generics are now an integral part of C# programming. It's worth the effort it takes to master this important feature.

LINQ

Future generations of programmers will look back on version 3.0 as a pivotal event in the evolution of C# because it fundamentally and irrevocably reshapes the core of the language. The reason for this dramatic impact can be stated in a single acronym: *LINQ*. LINQ adds to C# an entirely new syntactic element, several new keywords, and a powerful new capability. The inclusion of LINQ significantly increases the scope of the language, expanding the range of tasks to which C# can be applied. Moreover, LINQ has charted the future direction of computer language development because it offers a new way to think about and solve some of the most common, yet challenging problems that face today's programmers. Simply put, the integration of LINQ into C# sets a new standard that will affect the course of language design well into the future. LINQ *is* that important.

NOTE *LINQ in C# is essentially a language within a language. As a result, the subject of LINQ is quite large, involving many features, options, and alternatives. Although this chapter describes LINQ in significant detail, it is not possible to explore all facets, nuances, and applications of this powerful feature. To do so would require an entire book of its own. Instead, this chapter focuses on the core elements of LINQ and presents numerous examples. It is important to understand that we are just now at the beginning of the LINQ revolution. Going forward, LINQ is a subsystem that you will want to study in greater detail.*

What Is LINQ?

LINQ stands for *Language-Integrated Query*. It encompasses a set of features that let you retrieve information from a data source. As you may know, the retrieval of data constitutes an important part of many programs. For example, a program might obtain information from a customer list, look up product information in a catalog, or access an employee's record. In many cases, such data is stored in a database that is separate from the application. For example, a product catalog might be stored in a relational database. In the past, interacting with such a database would involve generating queries using Structured Query Language (SQL). Other sources of data, such as XML, required their own approach. Therefore, prior to C# 3.0, support for such queries was not built into C#. LINQ changes this.

LINQ adds to C# the ability to generate queries for any LINQ-compatible data source. Furthermore, the syntax used for the query is the same, no matter what data source is used. This means that the syntax used to query data in a relational database is the same as that

used to query data stored in an array, for example. It is no longer necessary to use SQL or any other non-C# mechanism. The query capability is fully integrated into the C# language.

In addition to using LINQ with SQL, LINQ can be used with XML files and ADO.NET Datasets. Perhaps equally important, it can also be used with C# arrays and collections (described in Chapter 24). Therefore, LINQ gives you a uniform way to access data. This is a powerful, innovative concept. It is not only changing the way that data is accessed, but it also offers a new way to think about and approach old problems. In the future, many programming solutions will be crafted in terms of LINQ. Its effects will not be limited to just database access.

LINQ is supported by a set of interrelated features, including the query syntax added to the C# language, lambda expressions, anonymous types, and extension methods. Lambda expressions are described in Chapter 15. The others are examined here.

LINQ Fundamentals

At LINQ's core is the *query*. A query specifies what data will be obtained from a data source. For example, a query on a customer mailing list might request the addresses of all customers that reside in a specific city, such as Chicago or Tokyo. A query on an inventory database might request a list of out-of-stock items. A query on a log of Internet usage could ask for a list of the websites with the highest hit counts. Although these queries differ in their specifics, all can be expressed using the same LINQ syntactic elements.

After a query has been created, it can be executed. One way this is done is by using the query in a **foreach** loop. Executing a query causes its results to be obtained. Thus, using a query involves two key steps. First, the form of the query is created. Second, the query is executed. Therefore, the query defines *what* to retrieve from a data source. Executing the query actually *obtains the results.*

In order for a source of data to be used by LINQ, it must implement the **IEnumerable** interface. There are two forms of this interface: one generic, one not. In general, it is easier if the data source implements the generic version, **IEnumerable<T>**, where **T** specifies the type of data being enumerated. The rest of the chapter assumes that a data source implements **IEnumerable<T>**. This interface is declared in **System.Collections.Generic**. A class that implements **IEnumerable<T>** supports enumeration, which means that its contents can be obtained one at a time, in sequence. All C# arrays support **IEnumerable<T>**. Thus, arrays can be used to demonstrate the central concepts of LINQ. Understand, however, that LINQ is not limited to arrays.

A Simple Query

At this point, it will be helpful to work through a simple LINQ example. The following program uses a query to obtain the positive values contained in an array of integers:

```
// Create a simple LINQ query.
using System;
using System.Linq;

class SimpQuery {
  static void Main() {

    int[] nums = { 1, -2, 3, 0, -4, 5 };
```

```
     // Create a query that obtains only positive numbers.
     var posNums = from n in nums
                   where n > 0
                   select n;

     Console.Write("The positive values in nums: ");

     // Execute the query and display the results.
     foreach(int i in posNums) Console.Write(i + " ");

     Console.WriteLine();
   }
}
```

This program produces the following output:

```
The positive values in nums: 1 3 5
```

As you can see, only the positive values in the **nums** array are displayed. Although quite simple, this program demonstrates the key features of LINQ. Let's examine it closely.

The first thing to notice in the program is the **using** directive:

```
using System.Linq;
```

To use the LINQ features, you must include the **System.Linq** namespace.

Next, an array of **int** called **nums** is declared. All arrays in C# are implicitly convertible to **IEnumerable<T>**. This makes any C# array usable as a LINQ data source.

Next, a query is declared that retrieves those elements in **nums** that are positive. It is shown here:

```
var posNums = from n in nums
              where n > 0
              select n;
```

The variable **posNums** is called the *query variable*. It refers to the set of rules defined by the query. Notice it uses **var** to implicitly declare **posNums**. As you know, this makes **posNums** an implicitly typed variable. In queries, it is often convenient to use implicitly typed variables, although you can also explicitly declare the type (which must be some form of **IEnumerable<T>**). The variable **posNums** is then assigned the query expression.

All queries begin with **from**. This clause specifies two items. The first is the *range variable*, which will receive elements obtained from the data source. In this case, the range variable is **n**. The second item is the data source, which in this case is the **nums** array. The type of the range variable is inferred from the data source. In this case, the type of **n** is **int**. Generalizing, here is the syntax of the **from** clause:

from *range-variable* in *data-source*

The next clause in the query is **where**. It specifies a condition that an element in the data source must meet in order to be obtained by the query. Its general form is shown here:

where *boolean-expression*

The *boolean-expression* must produce a **bool** result. (This expression is also called a *predicate*.) There can be more than one **where** clause in a query. In the program, this **where** clause is used:

```
where n > 0
```

It will be true only for an element whose value is greater than zero. This expression will be evaluated for every **n** in **nums** when the query executes. Only those values that satisfy this condition will be obtained. In other words, a **where** clause acts as a filter on the data source, allowing only certain items through.

All queries end with either a **select** clause or a **group** clause. This example employs the **select** clause. It specifies precisely what is obtained by the query. For simple queries, such as the one in this example, the range value is selected. Therefore, it returns those integers from **nums** that satisfy the **where** clause. In more sophisticated situations, it is possible to finely tune what is selected. For example, when querying a mailing list, you might return just the last name of each recipient, rather than the entire address. Notice that the **select** clause ends with a semicolon. Because **select** ends a query, it ends the statement and requires a semicolon. Notice, however, that the other clauses in the query do not end with a semicolon.

At this point, a query variable called **posNums** has been created, but no results have been obtained. It is important to understand that a query simply defines a set of rules. It is not until the query is executed that results are obtained. Furthermore, the same query can be executed two or more times, with the possibility of differing results if the underlying data source changes between executions. Therefore, simply declaring the query **posNums** does not mean that it contains the results of the query.

To execute the query, the program uses the **foreach** loop shown here:

```
foreach(int i in posNums) Console.WriteLine(i + " ");
```

Notice that **posNums** is specified as the collection being iterated over. When the **foreach** executes, the rules defined by the query specified by **posNums** are executed. With each pass through the loop, the next element returned by the query is obtained. The process ends when there are no more elements to retrieve. In this case, the type of the iteration variable **i** is explicitly specified as **int** because this is the type of the elements retrieved by the query. Explicitly specifying the type of the iteration variable is fine in this situation, since it is easy to know the type of the value selected by the query. However, in more complicated situations, it will be easier (or in some cases, necessary) to implicitly specify the type of the iteration variable by using **var**.

A Query Can Be Executed More Than Once

Because a query defines a set of rules that are used to retrieve data, but does not, itself, produce results, the same query can be run multiple times. If the data source changes between runs, then the results of the query may differ. Therefore, once you define a query, executing it will always produce the most current results. Here is an example. In the following version of the preceding program, the contents of the **nums** array are changed between two executions of **posNums**:

```
// Create a simple query.
using System;
using System.Linq;
using System.Collections.Generic;
```

```
class SimpQuery {
  static void Main() {

    int[] nums = { 1, -2, 3, 0, -4, 5 };

    // Create a query that obtains only positive numbers.
    var posNums = from n in nums
                  where n > 0
                  select n;

    Console.Write("The positive values in nums: ");

    // Execute the query and display the results.
    foreach(int i in posNums) Console.Write(i + " ");
    Console.WriteLine();

    // Change nums.
    Console.WriteLine("\nSetting nums[1] to 99.");
    nums[1] = 99;

    Console.Write("The positive values in nums after change: ");

    // Execute the query a second time.
    foreach(int i in posNums) Console.Write(i + " ");
    Console.WriteLine();
  }
}
```

The following output is produced:

```
The positive values in nums: 1 3 5

Setting nums[1] to 99.
The positive values in nums after change: 1 99 3 5
```

As the output confirms, after the value in **nums[1]** was changed from –2 to 99, the result of rerunning the query reflects the change. This is a key point that must be emphasized. Each execution of a query produces its own results, which are obtained by enumerating the current contents of the data source. Therefore, if the data source changes, so, too, might the results of executing a query. The benefits of this approach are quite significant. For example, if you are obtaining a list of pending orders for an online store, then you want each execution of your query to produce all orders, including those just entered.

How the Data Types in a Query Relate

As the preceding examples have shown, a query involves variables whose types relate to one another. These are the query variable, the range variable, and the data source. Because the correspondence among these types is both important and a bit confusing at first, they merit a closer look.

The type of the range variable must agree with the type of the elements stored in the data source. Thus, the type of the range variable is dependent upon the type of the data source. In many cases, C# can infer the type of the range variable. As long as the data source implements **IEnumerable<T>**, the type inference can be made because **T** describes the type

of the elements in the data source. (As mentioned, all arrays implement **IEnumerable<T>**, as do many other data sources.) However, if the data source implements the non-generic version of **IEnumerable**, then you will need to explicitly specify the type of the range variable. This is done by specifying its type in the **from** clause. For example, assuming the preceding examples, this shows how to explicitly declare **n** to be an **int**:

```
var posNums = from int n in nums
  // ...
```

Of course, the explicit type specification is not needed here because all arrays are implicitly convertible to **IEnumerable<T>**, which enables the type of the range variable to be inferred.

The type of object returned by a query is an instance of **IEnumerable<T>**, where **T** is the type of the elements. Thus, the type of the query variable must be an instance of **IEnumerable<T>**. The value of **T** is determined by the type of the value specified by the **select** clause. In the case of the preceding examples, **T** is **int** because **n** is an **int**. (As explained, **n** is an **int** because **int** is the type of elements stored in **nums**.) Therefore, the query could have been written like this, with the type explicitly specified as **IEnumerable <int>**:

```
IEnumerable<int> posNums = from n in nums
                          where n > 0
                          select n;
```

The key point is that the type of the item selected by **select** must agree with the type argument passed to **IEnumerable<T>** used to declare the query variable. Often query variables use **var** rather than explicitly specifying the type because this lets the compiler infer the proper type from the **select** clause. As you will see, this approach is particularly useful when **select** returns something other than an individual element from the data source.

When a query is executed by the **foreach** loop, the type of the iteration variable must be the same as the type of the range variable. In the preceding examples, this type was explicitly specified as **int**, but you can let the compiler infer the type by specifying this variable as **var**. As you will see, there are also some cases in which **var** must be used because the data type has no name.

The General Form of a Query

All queries share a general form, which is based on a set of contextual keywords, shown here:

ascending	descending	equals	from
group	in	into	join
let	on	orderby	select
where			

Of these, the following begin query clauses:

from	group	join	let
orderby	select	where	

A query must begin with the keyword **from** and end with either a **select** or **group** clause. The **select** clause determines what type of value is enumerated by the query. The **group**

clause returns the data by groups, with each group being able to be enumerated individually. As the preceding examples have shown, the **where** clause specifies criteria that an item must meet in order for it to be returned. The remaining clauses help you fine-tune a query. The follows sections examine each query clause.

Filter Values with where

As explained, **where** is used to filter the data returned by a query. The preceding examples have shown only its simplest form, in which a single condition is used. A key point to understand is that you can use **where** to filter data based on more than one condition. One way to do this is through the use of multiple **where** clauses. For example, consider the following program that displays only those values in the array that are both positive and less than 10:

```
// Use multiple where clauses.
using System;
using System.Linq;

class TwoWheres {
  static void Main() {

    int[] nums =  { 1, -2, 3, -3, 0, -8, 12, 19, 6, 9, 10 };

    // Create a query that obtains positive values less than 10.
    var posNums = from n in nums
                  where n > 0
                  where n < 10
                  select n;

    Console.Write("The positive values less than 10: ");

    // Execute the query and display the results.
    foreach(int i in posNums) Console.Write (i + " ");
    Console.WriteLine();
  }
}
```

The output is shown here:

```
The positive values less than 10: 1 3 6 9
```

As you can see, only positive values less than 10 are retrieved. This outcome is achieved by the use of the following two **where** clauses:

```
where n > 0
where n < 10
```

The first **where** requires that an element be greater than zero. The second requires the element to be less than 10. Thus, an element must be between 1 and 9 (inclusive) to satisfy both clauses.

Although it is not wrong to use two **where** clauses as just shown, the same effect can be achieved in a more compact manner by using a single **where** in which both tests are combined into a single expression. Here is the query rewritten to use this approach:

```
var posNums = from n in nums
              where n > 0 && n < 10
              select n;
```

In general, a **where** condition can use any valid C# expression that evaluates to a Boolean result. For example, the following program defines an array of **string**s. Several of the strings define Internet addresses. The query **netAddrs** retrieves only those strings that have more than four characters and that end with ".net". Thus, it finds those strings that contain Internet addresses that use the **.net** top-level domain name.

```
// Demonstrate another where clause.
using System;
using System.Linq;

class WhereDemo2 {

  static void Main() {

    string[] strs = { ".com", ".net", "hsNameA.com", "hsNameB.net",
                      "test", ".network", "hsNameC.net", "hsNameD.com" };

    // Create a query that obtains Internet addresses that
    // end with .net.
    var netAddrs = from addr in strs
                   where addr.Length > 4 && addr.EndsWith(".net")
                   select addr;

    // Execute the query and display the results.
    foreach(var str in netAddrs) Console.WriteLine(str);
  }
}
```

The output is shown here:

```
hsNameB.net
hsNameC.net
```

Notice that the program makes use of one of **string**'s methods called **EndsWith( )** within the **where** clause. It returns true if the invoking string ends with the character sequence specified as an argument.

Sort Results with orderby

Often you will want the results of a query to be sorted. For example, you might want to obtain a list of past-due accounts, in order of the remaining balance, from greatest to least. Or, you might want to obtain a customer list, alphabetized by name. Whatever the purpose, LINQ gives you an easy way to produce sorted results: the **orderby** clause.

You can use **orderby** to sort on one or more criteria. We will begin with the simplest case: sorting on a single item. The general form of **orderby** that sorts based on a single criterion is shown here:

orderby *sort-on how*

The item on which to sort is specified by *sort-on*. This can be as inclusive as the entire element stored in the data source or as restricted as a portion of a single field within the element. The value of *how* determines if the sort is ascending or descending, and it must be either **ascending** or **descending**. The default direction is ascending, so you won't normally specify **ascending**.

Here is an example that uses **orderby** to retrieve the values in an **int** array in ascending order:

```
// Demonstrate orderby.
using System;
using System.Linq;

class OrderbyDemo {

  static void Main() {

    int[] nums =  { 10, -19, 4, 7, 2, -5, 0 };

    // Create a query that obtains the values in sorted order.
    var posNums = from n in nums
                  orderby n
                  select n;

    Console.Write("Values in ascending order: ");

    // Execute the query and display the results.
    foreach(int i in posNums) Console.Write(i + " ");

    Console.WriteLine();
  }
}
```

The output is shown here:

```
Values in ascending order: -19 -5 0 2 4 7 10
```

To change the order to descending, simply specify the **descending** option, as shown here:

```
var posNums = from n in nums
              orderby n descending
              select n;
```

If you try this, you will see that the order of the values is reversed.

Although sorting on a single criterion is often what is needed, you can use **orderby** to sort on multiple items by using this form:

orderby *sort-onA direction, sort-onB direction, sort-onC direction,* ...

In this form, *sort-onA* is the item on which the primary sorting is done. Then, each group of equivalent items is sorted on *sort-onB*, and each of those groups is sorted on *sort-onC*, and so on. Thus, each subsequent *sort-on* specifies a "then by" item on which to sort. In all cases, *direction* is optional, defaulting to **ascending**. Here is an example that uses three sort criteria to sort bank account information by last name, then by first name, and finally by account balance:

```csharp
// Sort on multiple criteria with orderby.
using System;
using System.Linq;

class Account {
  public string FirstName { get; private set; }
  public string LastName { get; private set; }
  public double Balance { get; private set; }
  public string AccountNumber { get; private set; }

  public Account(string fn, string ln, string accnum, double b) {
    FirstName = fn;
    LastName = ln;
    AccountNumber = accnum;
    Balance = b;
  }
}

class OrderbyDemo {

  static void Main() {

    // Create some data.
    Account[] accounts = { new Account("Tom", "Smith", "132CK", 100.23),
                           new Account("Tom", "Smith", "132CD", 10000.00),
                           new Account("Ralph", "Jones", "436CD", 1923.85),
                           new Account("Ralph", "Jones", "454MM", 987.132),
                           new Account("Ted", "Krammer", "897CD", 3223.19),
                           new Account("Ralph", "Jones", "434CK", -123.32),
                           new Account("Sara", "Smith", "543MM", 5017.40),
                           new Account("Sara", "Smith", "547CD", 34955.79),
                           new Account("Sara", "Smith", "843CK", 345.00),
                           new Account("Albert", "Smith", "445CK", 213.67),
                           new Account("Betty", "Krammer","968MM",5146.67),
                           new Account("Carl", "Smith", "078CD", 15345.99),
                           new Account("Jenny", "Jones", "108CK", 10.98)
                         };

    // Create a query that obtains the accounts in sorted order.
    // Sorting first by last name, then within same last names sorting by
    // by first name, and finally by account balance.
    var accInfo = from acc in accounts
                  orderby acc.LastName, acc.FirstName, acc.Balance
                  select acc;
```

```
Console.WriteLine("Accounts in sorted order: ");

string str = "";

// Execute the query and display the results.
foreach(Account acc in accInfo) {
  if(str != acc.FirstName) {
    Console.WriteLine();
    str = acc.FirstName;
  }

  Console.WriteLine("{0}, {1}\tAcc#: {2}, {3,10:C}",
              acc.LastName, acc.FirstName,
              acc.AccountNumber, acc.Balance);
}
Console.WriteLine();
}
}
```

The output is shown here:

```
Accounts in sorted order:

Jones, Jenny      Acc#: 108CK,       $10.98

Jones, Ralph      Acc#: 434CK,     ($123.32)
Jones, Ralph      Acc#: 454MM,      $987.13
Jones, Ralph      Acc#: 436CD,    $1,923.85

Krammer, Betty    Acc#: 968MM,    $5,146.67

Krammer, Ted      Acc#: 897CD,    $3,223.19

Smith, Albert     Acc#: 445CK,     ($213.67)

Smith, Carl       Acc#: 078CD,   $15,345.99

Smith, Sara       Acc#: 843CK,      $345.00
Smith, Sara       Acc#: 543MM,    $5,017.40
Smith, Sara       Acc#: 547CD,   $34,955.79

Smith, Tom        Acc#: 132CK,      $100.23
Smith, Tom        Acc#: 132CD,   $10,000.00
```

In the query, look closely at how the **orderby** clause is written:

```
var accInfo = from acc in accounts
           orderby acc.LastName, acc.FirstName, acc.Balance
           select acc;
```

Here is how it works. First, the results are sorted by last name, and then entries with the same last name are sorted by the first name. Finally, groups of entries with the same first

and last name are sorted by the account balance. This is why the list of accounts under the name Jones is shown in this order:

```
Jones, Jenny        Acc#: 108CK,      $10.98

Jones, Ralph        Acc#: 434CK,    ($123.32)
Jones, Ralph        Acc#: 454MM,     $987.13
Jones, Ralph        Acc#: 436CD,   $1,923.85
```

As the output confirms, the list is sorted by last name, then by first name, and finally by account balance.

When using multiple criteria, you can reverse the condition of any sort by applying the **descending** option. For example, this query causes the results to be shown in order of decreasing balance:

```
var accInfo = from acc in accounts
              orderby x.LastName, x.FirstName, x.Balance descending
              select acc;
```

When using this version, the list of Jones entries will be displayed like this:

```
Jones, Jenny        Acc#: 108CK,      $10.98

Jones, Ralph        Acc#: 436CD,   $1,923.85
Jones, Ralph        Acc#: 454MM,     $987.13
Jones, Ralph        Acc#: 434CK,   ($123.32)
```

As you can see, now the accounts for Ralph Jones are displayed from greatest to least.

A Closer Look at select

The **select** clause determines what type of elements are obtained by a query. Its general form is shown here:

select *expression*

So far we have been using **select** to return the range variable. Thus, *expression* has simply named the range variable. However, **select** is not limited to this simple action. It can return a specific portion of the range variable, the result of applying some operation or transformation to the range variable, or even a new type of object that is constructed from pieces of the information retrieved from the range variable. This is called *projecting*.

To begin examining the other capabilities of **select**, consider the following program. It displays the square roots of the positive values contained in an array of **double** values.

```
// Use select to return the square root of all positive values
// in an array of doubles.
using System;
using System.Linq;

class SelectDemo {

  static void Main() {
```

```
    double[] nums =  { -10.0, 16.4, 12.125, 100.85, -2.2, 25.25, -3.5 } ;

    // Create a query that returns the square roots of the
    // positive values in nums.
    var sqrRoots = from n in nums
                   where n > 0
                   select Math.Sqrt(n);

    Console.WriteLine("The square roots of the positive values" +
                      " rounded to two decimal places:");

    // Execute the query and display the results.
    foreach(double r in sqrRoots) Console.WriteLine("{0:#.##}", r);
  }
}
```

The output is shown here:

```
The square roots of the positive values rounded to two decimal places:
4.05
3.48
10.04
5.02
```

In the query, pay special attention to the **select** clause:

```
select Math.Sqrt(n);
```

It returns the square root of the range variable. It does this by obtaining the result of passing the range variable to **Math.Sqrt( )**, which returns the square root of its argument. This means that the sequence obtained when the query is executed will contain the square roots of the positive values in **nums**. If you generalize this concept, the power of **select** becomes apparent. You can use **select** to generate any type of sequence you need, based on the values obtained from the data source.

Here is a program that shows another way to use **select**. It creates a class called **EmailAddress** that contains two properties. The first holds a person's name. The second contains an e-mail address. The program then creates an array that contains several **EmailAddress** entries. The program uses a query to obtain a list of just the e-mail addresses by themselves.

```
// Return a portion of the range variable.
using System;
using System.Linq;

class EmailAddress {
  public string Name { get; set; }
  public string Address { get; set; }

  public EmailAddress(string n, string a) {
    Name = n;
    Address = a;
  }
}
```

```
class SelectDemo2 {
  static void Main() {

    EmailAddress[] addrs = {
        new EmailAddress("Herb", "Herb@HerbSchildt.com"),
        new EmailAddress("Tom", "Tom@HerbSchildt.com"),
        new EmailAddress("Sara", "Sara@HerbSchildt.com")
    };

    // Create a query that selects e-mail addresses.
    var eAddrs = from entry in addrs
                   select entry.Address;

    Console.WriteLine("The e-mail addresses are");

    // Execute the query and display the results.
    foreach(string s in eAddrs) Console.WriteLine("  " + s);
  }
}
```

The output is shown here:

```
The e-mail addresses are
  Herb@HerbSchildt.com
  Tom@HerbSchildt.com
  Sara@HerbSchildt.com
```

Pay special attention to the **select** clause:

```
select entry.Address;
```

Instead of returning the entire range variable, it returns only the **Address** portion. This fact is evidenced by the output. This means the query returns a sequence of strings, not a sequence of **EmailAddress** objects. This is why the **foreach** loop specifies **s** as a **string**. As explained, the type of sequence returned by a query is determined by the type of value returned by the **select** clause.

One of the more powerful features of **select** is its ability to return a sequence that contains elements created during the execution of the query. For example, consider the following program. It defines a class called **ContactInfo**, which stores a name, e-mail address, and telephone number. It also defines the **EmailAddress** class used by the preceding example. Inside **Main( )**, an array of **ContactInfo** is created. Then, a query is declared in which the data source is an array of **ContactInfo**, but the sequence returned contains **EmailAddress** objects. Thus, the type of the sequence returned by **select** is not **ContactInfo**, but rather **EmailAddress**, and these objects are created during the execution of the query.

```
// Use a query to obtain a sequence of EmailAddresses
// from a list of ContactInfo.
using System;
using System.Linq;

class ContactInfo {
  public string Name { get; set; }
  public string Email { get; set; }
```

```
    public string Phone { get; set; }

    public ContactInfo(string n, string a, string p) {
      Name = n;
      Email = a;
      Phone = p;
    }
}

class EmailAddress {
  public string Name { get; set; }
  public string Address { get; set; }

  public EmailAddress(string n, string a) {
    Name = n;
    Address = a;
  }
}

class SelectDemo3 {
  static void Main() {

    ContactInfo[] contacts = {
        new ContactInfo("Herb", "Herb@HerbSchildt.com", "555-1010"),
        new ContactInfo("Tom", "Tom@HerbSchildt.com", "555-1101"),
        new ContactInfo("Sara", "Sara@HerbSchildt.com", "555-0110")
    };

    // Create a query that creates a list of EmailAddress objects.
    var emailList = from entry in contacts
                    select new EmailAddress(entry.Name, entry.Email);

    Console.WriteLine("The e-mail list is");

    // Execute the query and display the results.
    foreach(EmailAddress e in emailList)
      Console.WriteLine("  {0}: {1}", e.Name, e.Address );
  }
}
```

The output is shown here:

```
The e-mail list is
  Herb: Herb@HerbSchildt.com
  Tom: Tom@HerbSchildt.com
  Sara: Sara@HerbSchildt.com
```

In the query, pay special attention to the **select** clause :

```
select new EmailAddress(entry.Name, entry.Email);
```

It creates a new **EmailAddress** object that contains the name and e-mail address obtained from a **ContactInfo** object in the **contacts** array. The key point is that new **EmailAddress** objects are created by the query in its **select** clause, during the query's execution.

Use Nested from Clauses

A query can contain more than one **from** clause. Thus, a query can contain nested **from** clauses. One common use of a nested **from** clause is found when a query needs to obtain data from two different sources. Here is a simple example. It uses two **from** clauses to iterate over two different character arrays. It produces a sequence that contains all possible combinations of the two sets of characters.

```
// Use two from clauses to create a list of all
// possible combinations of the letters A, B, and C
// with the letters X, Y, and Z.
using System;
using System.Linq;


// This class holds the result of the query.
class ChrPair {
  public char First;
  public char Second;

  public ChrPair(char c, char c2) {
    First = c;
    Second = c2;
  }
}

class MultipleFroms {
  static void Main() {

    char[] chrs = { 'A', 'B', 'C' };
    char[] chrs2 = { 'X', 'Y', 'Z' };

    // Notice that the first from iterates over chrs and
    // the second from iterates over chrs2.
    var pairs = from ch1 in chrs
                from ch2 in chrs2
                select new ChrPair(ch1, ch2);

    Console.WriteLine("All combinations of ABC with XYZ: ");

    foreach(var p in pairs)
      Console.WriteLine("{0} {1}", p.First, p.Second);
  }
}
```

The output is shown here:

```
All combinations of ABC with XYZ:
A X
A Y
A Z
B X
B Y
```

```
B  Z
C  X
C  Y
C  Z
```

The program begins by creating a class called **ChrPair** that will hold the results of the query. It then creates two character arrays, called **chrs** and **chrs2**. It uses the following query to produce all possible combinations of the two sequences:

```
var pairs = from ch1 in chrs
            from ch2 in chrs2
            select new ChrPair(ch1, ch2);
```

The nested **from** clauses cause both **chrs** and **chrs2** to be iterated over. Here is how it works. First, a character is obtained from **chrs** and stored in **ch1**. Then, the **chrs2** array is enumerated. With each iteration of the inner **from**, a character from **chrs2** is stored in **ch2** and the **select** clause is executed. The result of the **select** clause is a new object of type **ChrPair** that contains the character pair **ch1, ch2** produced by each iteration of the inner **from**. Thus, a **ChrPair** is produced in which each possible combination of characters is obtained.

Another common use of a nested **from** is to iterate over a data source that is contained within another data source. An example of this is found in the section, "Use **let** to Create a Variable in a Query," later in this chapter.

Group Results with group

One of the most powerful query features is provided by the **group** clause because it enables you to create results that are grouped by keys. Using the sequence obtained from a group, you can easily access all of the data associated with a key. This makes **group** an easy and effective way to retrieve data that is organized into sequences of related items. The **group** clause is one of only two clauses that can end a query. (The other is **select**.)

The **group** clause has the following general form:

group *range-variable* by *key*

It returns data grouped into sequences, with each sequence sharing the key specified by *key*.

The result of **group** is a sequence that contains elements of type **IGrouping<TKey, TElement>**, which is declared in the **System.Linq** namespace. It defines a collection of objects that share a common key. The type of query variable in a query that returns a group is **IEnumerable<IGrouping<TKey, TElement>>**. **IGrouping** defines a read-only property called **Key**, which returns the key associated with each sequence.

Here is an example that illustrates the use of **group**. It declares an array that contains a list of websites. It then creates a query that groups the list by top-level domain name, such as **.org** or **.com**.

```
// Demonstrate the group clause.
using System;
using System.Linq;

class GroupDemo {

  static void Main() {
```

```
      string[] websites = { "hsNameA.com", "hsNameB.net", "hsNameC.net",
                            "hsNameD.com", "hsNameE.org", "hsNameF.org",
                            "hsNameG.tv",  "hsNameH.net", "hsNameI.tv" };

      // Create a query that groups websites by top-level domain name.
      var webAddrs = from addr in websites
                     where addr.LastIndexOf(".") != -1
                     group addr by addr.Substring(addr.LastIndexOf("."));

      // Execute the query and display the results.
      foreach(var sites in webAddrs) {
        Console.WriteLine("Web sites grouped by " + sites.Key);
        foreach(var site in sites)
          Console.WriteLine("   " + site);
        Console.WriteLine();
      }
    }
  }
}
```

The output is shown here:

```
Web sites grouped by .com
  hsNameA.com
  hsNameD.com

Web sites grouped by .net
  hsNameB.net
  hsNameC.net
  hsNameH.net

Web sites grouped by .org
  hsNameE.org
  hsNameF.org

Web sites grouped by .tv
  hsNameG.tv
  hsNameI.tv
```

As the output shows, the data is grouped based on the top-level domain name of a website. Notice how this is achieved by the **group** clause:

```
var webAddrs = from addr in websites
               where addr.LastIndexOf(".") != -1
               group addr by addr.Substring(addr.LastIndexOf("."));
```

The key is obtained by use of the **LastIndexOf( )** and **Substring( )** methods defined by **string**. (These are described in Chapter 7. The version of **Substring( )** used here returns the substring that starts at the specified index and runs to the end of the invoking string.) The index of the last period in a website name is found using **LastIndexOf( )**. Using this index, the **Substring( )** method obtains the remainder of the string, which is the part of the website name that contains the top-level domain name. One other point: Notice the use of the **where** clause to filter out any strings that don't contain a period. The **LastIndexOf( )** method returns –1 if the specified string is not contained in the invoking string.

Because the sequence obtained when **webAddrs** is executed is a list of groups, you will need to use two **foreach** loops to access the members of each group. The outer loop obtains each group. The inner loop enumerates the members within the group. The iteration variable of the outer **foreach** loop must be an **IGrouping** instance compatible with the key and element type. In the example both the keys and elements are **string**. Therefore, the type of the **sites** iteration variable of the outer loop is **IGrouping<string, string>**. The type of the iteration variable of the inner loop is **string**. For brevity, the example implicitly declares these variables, but they could have been explicitly declared as shown here:

```
foreach(IGrouping<string, string> sites in webAddrs) {
  Console.WriteLine("Web sites grouped by " + sites.Key);
  foreach(string site in sites)
    Console.WriteLine("  " + site);
  Console.WriteLine();
}
```

Use into to Create a Continuation

When using **select** or **group**, you will sometimes want to generate a temporary result that will be used by a subsequent part of the query to produce the final result. This is called a *query continuation* (or just a *continuation* for short), and it is accomplished through the use of **into** with a **select** or **group** clause. It has the following general form:

> into *name query-body*

where *name* is the name of the range variable that iterates over the temporary result and is used by the continuing query, specified by *query-body*. This is why **into** is called a query continuation when used with **select** or **group**—it continues the query. In essence, a query continuation embodies the concept of building a new query that queries the results of the preceding query.

NOTE *There is also a form of **into** that can be used with **join**, which creates a group join. This is described later in this chapter.*

Here is an example that uses **into** with **group**. The following program reworks the **GroupDemo** example shown earlier, which creates a list of websites grouped by top-level domain name. In this case, the initial results are queried by a range variable called **ws**. This result is then filtered to remove all groups that have fewer than three elements.

```
// Use into with group.
using System;
using System.Linq;

class IntoDemo {

  static void Main() {

    string[] websites = { "hsNameA.com", "hsNameB.net", "hsNameC.net",
                          "hsNameD.com", "hsNameE.org", "hsNameF.org",
                          "hsNameG.tv",  "hsNameH.net", "hsNameI.tv" };
```

```
    // Create a query that groups websites by top-level domain name,
    // but select only those groups that have more than two members.
    // Here, ws is the range variable over the set of groups
    // returned when the first half of the query is executed.
    var webAddrs = from addr in websites
                   where addr.LastIndexOf(".") != -1
                   group addr by addr.Substring(addr.LastIndexOf("."))
                        into ws
                   where ws.Count() > 2
                   select ws;

    // Execute the query and display the results.
    Console.WriteLine("Top-level domains with more than 2 members.\n");

    foreach(var sites in webAddrs) {
      Console.WriteLine("Contents of " + sites.Key + " domain:");
      foreach(var site in sites)
        Console.WriteLine("   " + site);
      Console.WriteLine();
    }
  }
}
```

The following output is produced:

```
Top-level domains with more than 2 members.

Contents of .net domain:
  hsNameB.net
  hsNameC.net
  hsNameH.net
```

As the output shows, only the **.net** group is returned because it is the only group that has more than two elements.

In the program, pay special attention to this sequence of clauses in the query:

```
group addr by addr.Substring(addr.LastIndexOf(".", addr.Length))
         into ws
where ws.Count() > 2
select ws;
```

First, the results of the **group** clause are stored (creating a temporary result) and a new query begins that operates on the stored results. The range variable of the new query is **ws**. At this point, **ws** will range over each group returned by the first query. (It ranges over groups because the first query results in a sequence of groups.) Next, the **where** clause filters the query so the final result contains only those groups that contain more than two members. This determination is made by calling **Count( )**, which is an *extension method* that is implemented for all **IEnumerable** objects. It returns the number of elements in a sequence. (You'll learn more about extension methods later in this chapter.) The resulting sequence of groups is returned by the **select** clause.

Use let to Create a Variable in a Query

In a query, you will sometimes want to retain a value temporarily. For example, you might want to create an enumerable variable that can, itself, be queried. Or, you might want to store a value that will be used later on in a **where** clause. Whatever the purpose, these types of actions can be accomplished through the use of **let**.

The **let** clause has this general form:

let *name* = *expression*

Here, *name* is an identifier that is assigned the value of *expression*. The type of *name* is inferred from the type of the expression.

Here is an example that shows how **let** can be used to create another enumerable data source. The query takes as input an array of strings. It then converts those strings into **char** arrays. This is accomplished by use of another **string** method called **ToCharArray( )**, which returns an array containing the characters in the string. The result is assigned to a variable called **chrArray**, which is then used by a nested **from** clause to obtain the individual characters in the array. The query then sorts the characters and returns the resulting sequence.

```
// Use a let clause and a nested from clause.
using System;
using System.Linq;

class LetDemo {

  static void Main() {

    string[] strs = { "alpha", "beta", "gamma" };

    // Create a query that obtains the characters in the
    // strings, returned in sorted order. Notice the use
    // of a nested from clause.
    var chrs = from str in strs
               let chrArray = str.ToCharArray()
                 from ch in chrArray
                 orderby ch
                 select ch;

    Console.WriteLine("The individual characters in sorted order:");

    // Execute the query and display the results.
    foreach(char c in chrs) Console.Write(c + " ");

    Console.WriteLine();
  }
}
```

The output is shown here:

```
The individual characters in sorted order:
a a a a a b e g h l m m p t
```

In the program, notice how the **let** clause assigns to **chrArray** a reference to the array returned by **str.ToCharArray( )**:

```
let chrArray = str.ToCharArray()
```

After the **let** clause, other clauses can make use of **chrArray**. Furthermore, because all arrays in C# are convertible to **IEnumerable<T>**, **chrArray** can be used as a data source for a second, nested **from** clause. This is what happens in the example. It uses the nested **from** to enumerate the individual characters in the array, sorting them into ascending sequence and returning the result.

You can also use a **let** clause to hold a non-enumerable value. For example, the following is a more efficient way to write the query used in the **IntoDemo** program shown in the preceding section.

```
var webAddrs = from addr in websites
            let idx = addr.LastIndexOf(".")
            where idx != -1
            group addr by addr.Substring(idx)
                    into ws
            where ws.Count() > 2
            select ws;
```

In this version, the index of the last occurrence of a period is assigned to **idx**. This value is then used by **Substring( )**. This prevents the search for the period from having to be conducted twice.

Join Two Sequences with join

When working with databases, it is common to want to create a sequence that correlates data from two different data sources. For example, an online store might have one database that associates the name of an item with its item number, and a second database that associates the item number with its in-stock status. Given this situation, you might want to generate a list that shows the in-stock status of items by name, rather than by item number. You can do this by correlating the data in the two databases. Such an action is easy to accomplish in LINQ through the use of the **join** clause.

The general form of **join** is shown here (in context with the **from**):

> from *range-varA* in *data-sourceA*
>   join *range-varB* in *data-sourceB*
>   on *range-varA.property* equals *range-varB.property*

The key to using **join** is to understand that each data source must contain data in common, and that data can be compared for equality. Thus, in the general form, *data-sourceA* and *data-sourceB* must have something in common that can be compared. The items being compared are specified by the **on** section. Thus, when *range-varA.property* is equal to *range-varB.property*, the correlation succeeds. In essence, **join** acts like a filter, allowing only those elements that share a common value to pass through.

When using **join**, often the sequence returned is a composite of portions of the two data sources. Therefore, **join** lets you generate a new list that contains elements from two different data sources. This enables you to organize data in a new way.

The following program creates a class called **Item**, which encapsulates an item's name with its number. It creates another class called **InStockStatus**, which links an item number with a Boolean property that indicates whether or not the item is in stock. It also creates a class called **Temp**, which has two fields: one **string** and one **bool**. Objects of this class will hold the result of the query. The query uses **join** to produce a list in which an item's name is associated with its in-stock status.

```
// Demonstrate join.
using System;
using System.Linq;

// A class that links an item name with its number.
class Item {
  public string Name { get; set; }
  public int ItemNumber { get; set; }

  public Item(string n, int inum) {
    Name = n;
    ItemNumber = inum;
  }
}

// A class that links an item number with its in-stock status.
class InStockStatus {
  public int ItemNumber { get; set; }
  public bool InStock { get; set; }

  public InStockStatus(int n, bool b) {
    ItemNumber = n;
    InStock = b;
  }
}

// A class that encapsulates a name with its status.
class Temp {
  public string Name { get; set; }
  public bool InStock { get; set; }

  public Temp(string n, bool b) {
    Name = n;
    InStock  = b;
  }
}

class JoinDemo {
  static void Main() {

    Item[] items = {
        new Item("Pliers", 1424),
        new Item("Hammer", 7892),
        new Item("Wrench", 8534),
        new Item("Saw", 6411)
    };
```

```
    InStockStatus[] statusList = {
        new InStockStatus(1424, true),
        new InStockStatus(7892, false),
        new InStockStatus(8534, true),
        new InStockStatus(6411, true)
    };


    // Create a query that joins Item with InStockStatus to
    // produce a list of item names and availability. Notice
    // that a sequence of Temp objects is produced.
    var inStockList = from item in items
                      join entry in statusList
                        on item.ItemNumber equals entry.ItemNumber
                      select new Temp(item.Name, entry.InStock);

    Console.WriteLine("Item\tAvailable\n");

    // Execute the query and display the results.
    foreach(Temp t in inStockList)
      Console.WriteLine("{0}\t{1}", t.Name, t.InStock);
  }
}
```

The output is shown here:

```
Item    Available

Pliers  True
Hammer  False
Wrench  True
Saw     True
```

To understand how **join** works, let's walk through each line in the query. The query begins in the normal fashion with this **from** clause:

```
var inStockList = from item in items
```

This clause specifies that **item** is the range variable for the data source specified by **items**. The **items** array contains objects of type **Item**, which encapsulate a name and a number for an inventory item.

Next comes the **join** clause shown here:

```
join entry in statusList
  on item.ItemNumber equals entry.ItemNumber
```

This clause specifies that **entry** is the range variable for the **statusList** data source. The **statusList** array contains objects of type **InStockStatus**, which link an item number with its status. Thus, **items** and **statusList** have a property in common: the item number. This is used by the **on/equals** portion of the **join** clause to describe the correlation. Thus, **join** matches items from the two data sources when their item numbers are equal.

Finally, the **select** clause returns a **Temp** object that contains an item's name along with its in-stock status:

```
select new Temp(item.Name, entry.InStock);
```

Therefore, the sequence obtained by the query consists of **Temp** objects.

Although the preceding example is fairly straightforward, **join** supports substantially more sophisticated operations. For example, you can use **into** with **join** to create a *group join*, which creates a result that consists of an element from the first sequence and a group of all matching elements from the second sequence. (You'll see an example of this a bit later in this chapter.) In general, the time and effort needed to fully master **join** is well worth the investment because it gives you the ability to reorganize data at runtime. This is a powerful capability. This capability is made even more powerful by the use of anonymous types, described in the next section.

Anonymous Types

C# 3.0 adds a new feature called the *anonymous type* that directly relates to LINQ. As the name implies, an anonymous type is a class that has no name. Its primary use is to create an object returned by the **select** clause. Often, the outcome of a query is a sequence of objects that are either a composite of two (or more) data sources (such as in the case of **join**) or include a subset of the members of one data source. In either case, often the type of the object being returned is needed only because of the query and is not used elsewhere in the program. In this case, using an anonymous type eliminates the need to declare a class that will be used simply to hold the outcome of the query.

An anonymous type is created through the use of this general form:

new { *nameA = valueA, nameB = valueB, ...* }

Here, the names specify identifiers that translate into read-only properties that are initialized by the values. For example,

```
new { Count = 10, Max = 100, Min = 0 }
```

This creates a class type that has three public read-only properties: **Count**, **Max**, and **Min**. These are given the values 10, 100, and 0, respectively. These properties can be referred to by name by other code. Notice that an anonymous type uses object initializers to initialize fields and properties. As explained in Chapter 8, object initializers provide a way to initialize an object without explicitly invoking a constructor. This is necessary in the case of anonymous types because there is no way to explicitly call a constructor. (Recall that constructors have the same name as their class. In the case of an anonymous class, there is no name. So, how would you invoke the constructor?)

Because an anonymous type has no name, you must use an implicitly typed variable to refer to it. This lets the compiler infer the proper type. For example,

```
var myOb = new { Count = 10, Max = 100, Min = 0 }
```

creates a variable called **myOb** that is assigned a reference to the object created by the anonymous type expression. This means that the following statements are legal:

```
Console.WriteLine("Count is " + myOb.Count);

if(i <= myOb.Max && i >= myOb.Min) // ...
```

Remember, when an anonymous type is created, the identifiers that you specify become read-only public properties. Thus, they can be used by other parts of your code.

Although the term *anonymous type* is used, it's not quite completely true! The type is anonymous relative to you, the programmer. However, the compiler does give it an internal name. Thus, anonymous types do not violate C#'s strong type checking rules.

To fully understand the value of anonymous types, consider this rewrite of the previous program that demonstrated **join**. Recall that in the previous version, a class called **Temp** was needed to encapsulate the result of the **join**. Through the use of an anonymous type, this "placeholder" class is no longer needed and no longer clutters the source code to the program. The output from the program is unchanged from before.

```
// Use an anonymous type to improve the join demo program.
using System;
using System.Linq;

// A class that links an item name with its number.
class Item {
  public string Name { get; set; }
  public int ItemNumber { get; set; }

  public Item(string n, int inum) {
    Name = n;
    ItemNumber = inum;
  }
}

// A class that links an item number with its in-stock status.
class InStockStatus {
  public int ItemNumber { get; set; }
  public bool InStock { get; set; }

  public InStockStatus(int n, bool b) {
    ItemNumber = n;
    InStock = b;
  }
}

class AnonTypeDemo {
  static void Main() {

    Item[] items = {
        new Item("Pliers", 1424),
        new Item("Hammer", 7892),
        new Item("Wrench", 8534),
        new Item("Saw", 6411)
    };

    InStockStatus[] statusList = {
        new InStockStatus(1424, true),
        new InStockStatus(7892, false),
        new InStockStatus(8534, true),
        new InStockStatus(6411, true)
    };
```

```
// Create a query that joins Item with InStockStatus to
// produce a list of item names and availability.
// Now, an anonymous type is used.
var inStockList = from item in items
                  join entry in statusList
                    on item.ItemNumber equals entry.ItemNumber
                  select new { Name = item.Name,
                               InStock =  entry.InStock };

Console.WriteLine("Item\tAvailable\n");

// Execute the query and display the results.
foreach(var t in inStockList)
  Console.WriteLine("{0}\t{1}", t.Name, t.InStock);
    }
}
```

Pay special attention to the **select** clause:

```
select new { Name = item.Name,
             InStock =  entry.InStock };
```

It returns an object of an anonymous type that has two read-only properties, **Name** and **InStock**. These are given the values specified by the item's name and availability. Because of the anonymous type, there is no longer any need for the **Temp** class.

One other point. Notice the **foreach** loop that executes the query. It now uses **var** to declare the iteration variable. This is necessary because the type of the object contained in **inStockList** has no name. This situation is one of the reasons that C# 3.0 added implicitly typed variables. They are needed to support anonymous types.

Before moving on, there is one more aspect of anonymous types that warrants a mention. In some cases, including the one just shown, you can simplify the syntax of the anonymous type through the use of a *projection initializer*. In this case, you simply specify the name of the initializer by itself. This name automatically becomes the name of the property. For example, here is another way to code the **select** clause used by the preceding program:

```
select new { item.Name, entry.InStock };
```

Here, the property names are still **Name** and **InStock**, just as before. The compiler automatically "projects" the identifiers **Name** and **InStock**, making them the property names of the anonymous type. Also as before, the properties are given the values specified by **item.Name** and **entry.InStock**.

Create a Group Join

As explained earlier, you can use **into** with **join** to create a *group join*, which creates a sequence in which each entry in the result consists of an entry from the first sequence and a group of all matching elements from the second sequence. No example was presented then because often a group join makes use of an anonymous type. Now that anonymous types have been covered, an example of a simple group join can be given.

The following example uses a group join to create a list in which various transports, such as cars, boats, and planes, are organized by their general transportation category, which is

land, sea, and air. The program first creates a class called **Transport** that links a transport type with its classification. Inside **Main( )**, it creates two input sequences. The first is an array of strings that contains the names of the general means by which one travels, which is land, sea, and air. The second is an array of **Transport**, which encapsulates various means of transportation. It then uses a group join to produce a list of transports that are organized by their category.

```csharp
// Demonstrate a simple group join.
using System;
using System.Linq;

// This class links the name of a transport, such as Train,
// with its general classification, such as land, sea, or air.
class Transport {
  public string Name { get; set; }
  public string How { get; set; }

  public Transport(string n, string h) {
    Name = n;
    How = h;
  }
}

class GroupJoinDemo {
  static void Main() {

    // An array of transport classifications.
    string[] travelTypes = {
        "Air",
        "Sea",
        "Land"
    };

    // An array of transports.
    Transport[] transports = {
        new Transport("Bicycle", "Land"),
        new Transport("Balloon", "Air"),
        new Transport("Boat", "Sea"),
        new Transport("Jet", "Air"),
        new Transport("Canoe", "Sea"),
        new Transport("Biplane", "Air"),
        new Transport("Car", "Land"),
        new Transport("Cargo Ship", "Sea"),
        new Transport("Train", "Land")
    };

    // Create a query that uses a group join to produce
    // a list of item names and IDs organized by category.
    var byHow = from how in travelTypes
                join trans in transports
                on how equals trans.How
                into lst
                select new { How = how, Tlist = lst };
```

```
// Execute the query and display the results.
foreach(var t in byHow) {
  Console.WriteLine("{0} transportation includes:", t.How);

    foreach(var m in t.Tlist)
      Console.WriteLine("  " + m.Name);

    Console.WriteLine();
  }
 }
}
```

The output is shown here:

```
Air transportation includes:
  Balloon
  Jet
  Biplane

Sea transportation includes:
  Boat
  Canoe
  Cargo Ship

Land transportation includes:
  Bicycle
  Car
  Train
```

The key part of the program is, of course, the query, which is shown here:

```
var byHow = from how in travelTypes
              join trans in transports
              on how equals trans.How
              into lst
              select new { How = how, Tlist = lst };
```

Here is how it works. The **from** statement uses **how** to range over the **travelTypes** array. Recall that **travelTypes** contains an array of the general travel classifications: air, land, and sea. The **join** clause joins each travel type with those transports that use that type. For example, the type Land is joined with Bicycle, Car, and Train. However, because of the **into** clause, for each travel type, the **join** produces a list of the transports that use that travel type. This list is represented by **lst**. Finally, **select** returns an anonymous type that encapsulates each value of **how** (the travel type) with a list of transports. This is why the two **foreach** loops shown here are needed to display the results of the query:

```
foreach(var t in byHow) {
  Console.WriteLine("{0} transportation includes:", t.How);

  foreach(var m in t.Tlist)
    Console.WriteLine("  " + m.Name);

  Console.WriteLine();
}
```

The outer loop obtains an object that contains the name of the travel type and the list of the transports for that type. The inner loop displays the individual transports.

The Query Methods

The query syntax described by the preceding sections is the way you will probably write most queries in C#. It is convenient, powerful, and compact. It is, however, not the only way to write a query. The other way is to use the *query methods.* These methods can be called on any enumerable object, such as an array.

The Basic Query Methods

The query methods are defined by **System.Linq.Enumerable** and are implemented as *extension methods* that extend the functionality of **IEnumerable<T>**. (Query methods are also defined by **System.Linq.Queryable**, which extends the functionality of **IQueryable<T>**, but this interface is not used in this chapter.) An extension method adds functionality to another class, but without the use of inheritance. Support for extension methods was added by C# 3.0, and we will look more closely at them later in this chapter. For now, it is sufficient to understand that query methods can be called only on an object that implements **IEnumerable<T>**.

The **Enumerable** class provides many query methods, but at the core are those that correspond to the query keywords described earlier. These methods are shown here, along with the keywords to which they relate. Understand that these methods have overloaded forms and only their simplest form is shown. However, this is also the form that you will often use.

Query Keyword	Equivalent Query Method
select	Select(*arg*)
where	Where(*arg*)
orderby	OrderBy(*arg*) or OrderByDescending(*arg*)
join	Join(*seq2, key1, key2, result*)
group	GroupBy(*arg*)

Except for **Join( )**, the other methods take one argument, *arg,* which is an object of type **Func<T, TResult>**, as a parameter. This is a delegate type defined by LINQ. It is declared like this:

delegate TResult Func<T, TResult>(T *arg*)

Here, **TResult** specifies the result of the delegate and **T** specifies the parameter type. In the query methods, *arg* determines what action the query method takes. For example, in the case of **Where( )**, *arg* determines how the query filters the data. Each of these query methods returns an enumerable object. Thus, the result of one can be used to execute a call on another, allowing the methods to be chained together.

The **Join( )** method takes four arguments. The first is a reference to the second sequence to be joined. The first sequence is the one on which **Join( )** is called. The key selector for the first sequence is passed via *key1,* and the key selector for the second sequence is passed via

key2. The result of the join is described by *result.* The type of *key1* is **Func<TOuter, TKey>**, and the type of *key2* is **Func<TInner, TKey>**. The *result* argument is of type **Func<TOuter, TInner, TResult>**. Here, **TOuter** is the element type of the invoking sequence; **TInner** is the element type of the passed sequence; and **TResult** is the type of the resulting elements. An enumerable object is returned that contains the result of the join.

Although an argument to a query method such as **Where( )** is a method compatible with the specified form of the **Func** delegate, it does not need to be an explicitly declared method. In fact, most often it won't be. Instead, you will usually use a lambda expression. As explained in Chapter 15, a lambda expression is a new syntactic feature provided by C# 3.0. It offers a streamlined, yet powerful way to define what is, essentially, an anonymous method. The C# compiler automatically converts a lambda expression into a form that can be passed to a **Func** parameter. Because of the streamlined convenience offered by lambda expressions, they are used by all of the examples in this section.

Create Queries by Using the Query Methods

By using the query methods in conjunction with lambda expressions, it is possible to create queries that do not use the C# query syntax. Instead, the query methods are called. Let's begin with a simple example. It reworks the first program in this chapter so that it uses calls to **Where( )** and **Select( )** rather than the query keywords.

```
// Use the query methods to create a simple query.
// This is a reworked version of the first program in this chapter.
using System;
using System.Linq;

class SimpQuery {
  static void Main() {

    int[] nums =  { 1, -2, 3, 0, -4, 5 };

    // Use Where() and Select() to create a simple query.
    var posNums = nums.Where(n => n > 0).Select(r => r);

    Console.Write("The positive values in nums: ");

    // Execute the query and display the results.
    foreach(int i in posNums) Console.Write(i + " ");
    Console.WriteLine();
  }
}
```

The output, shown here, is the same as the original version:

```
The positive values in nums: 1 3 5
```

In the program, pay special attention to this line:

```
var posNums = nums.Where(n => n > 0).Select(r => r);
```

This creates a query called **posNums** that creates a sequence of the positive values in **nums**. It does this by use of the **Where( )** method (to filter the values) and **Select( )** (to select the

values). The **Where( )** method can be invoked on **nums** because all arrays implement **IEnumerable<T>**, which supports the query extension methods.

Technically, the **Select( )** method in the preceding example is not necessary because in this simple case, the sequence returned by **Where( )** already contains the result. However, you can use more sophisticated selection criteria, just as you did with the query syntax. For example, this query returns the positive values in **nums** increased by an order of magnitude:

```
var posNums = nums.Where(n => n > 0).Select(r => r * 10);
```

As you might expect, you can chain together other operations. For example, this query selects the positive values, sorts them into descending order, and returns the resulting sequence:

```
var posNums = nums.Where(n => n > 0).OrderByDescending(j => j);
```

Here, the expression **j => j** specifies that the ordering is dependent on the input parameter, which is an element from the sequence obtained from **Where( )**.

Here is an example that demonstrates the **GroupBy( )** method. It reworks the **group** example shown earlier.

```
// Demonstrate the GroupBy() query method.
// This program reworks the earlier version that used
// the query syntax.
using System;
using System.Linq;

class GroupByDemo {

  static void Main() {

    string[] websites = { "hsNameA.com", "hsNameB.net", "hsNameC.net",
                          "hsNameD.com", "hsNameE.org", "hsNameF.org",
                          "hsNameG.tv",  "hsNameH.net", "hsNameI.tv" };

    // Use query methods to group websites by top-level domain name.
    var webAddrs = websites.Where(w => w.LastIndexOf(".") != 1).
        GroupBy(x => x.Substring(x.LastIndexOf(".", x.Length)));

    // Execute the query and display the results.
    foreach(var sites in webAddrs) {
      Console.WriteLine("Web sites grouped by " + sites.Key);
      foreach(var site in sites)
        Console.WriteLine("  " + site);
      Console.WriteLine();
    }
  }
}
```

This version produces the same output as the earlier version. The only difference is how the query is created. In this version, the query methods are used.

Here is another example. Recall the **join** query used in the **JoinDemo** example shown earlier:

```
var inStockList = from item in items
                  join entry in statusList
                    on item.ItemNumber equals entry.ItemNumber
                  select new Temp(item.Name, entry.InStock);
```

This query produces a sequence that contains objects that encapsulate the name and the in-stock status of an inventory item. This information is synthesized from joining the two lists **items** and **statusList**. The following version reworks this query so that it uses the **Join( )** method rather than the C# query syntax:

```
// Use Join() to produce a list of item names and status.
var inStockList = items.Join(statusList,
                  k1 => k1.ItemNumber,
                  k2 => k2.ItemNumber,
                  (k1, k2) => new Temp(k1.Name, k2.InStock) );
```

Although this version uses the named class called **Temp** to hold the resulting object, an anonymous type could have been used instead. This approach is shown next:

```
var inStockList = items.Join(statusList,
                  k1 => k1.ItemNumber,
                  k2 => k2.ItemNumber,
                  (k1, k2) => new { k1.Name, k2.InStock} );
```

Query Syntax vs. Query Methods

As the preceding section has explained, C# has two ways of creating queries: the query syntax and the query methods. What is interesting, and not readily apparent by simply looking at a program's source code, is that the two approaches are more closely related than you might at first assume. The reason is that the query syntax is compiled into calls to the query methods. Thus, when you write something like

```
where x < 10
```

the compiler translates it into

```
Where(x => x < 10)
```

Therefore, the two approaches to creating a query ultimately lead to the same place.

Given that the two approaches are ultimately equivalent, the following question naturally arises: Which approach is best for a C# program? The answer: In general, you will want to use the query syntax. It is fully integrated into the C# language, supported by keywords and syntax, and is cleaner.

More Query-Related Extension Methods

In addition to the methods that correspond to the query keywords supported by C#, the .NET Framework provides several other query-related extension methods that are often helpful in a query. These query-related methods are defined for **IEnumerable<T>** by **Enumerable**. Here is a sampling of several commonly used methods. Because many of the methods are overloaded, only their general form is shown.

Method	Description
All(*condition*)	Returns true if all elements in a sequence satisfy a specified condition.
Any(*condition*)	Returns true if any element in a sequence satisfies a specified condition.
Average( )	Returns the average of the values in a numeric sequence.
Contains(*obj*)	Returns true if the sequence contains the specified object.
Count( )	Returns the length of a sequence. This is the number of elements that it contains.
First( )	Returns the first element in a sequence.
Last( )	Returns the last element in a sequence.
Max( )	Returns the maximum value in a sequence.
Min( )	Returns the minimum value in a sequence.
Sum( )	Returns the summation of the values in a numeric sequence.

You have already seen **Count( )** in action earlier in this chapter. Here is a program that demonstrates the others:

```
// Use several of the extension methods defined by Enumerable.
using System;
using System.Linq;

class ExtMethods {
  static void Main() {

    int[] nums = { 3, 1, 2, 5, 4 };

    Console.WriteLine("The minimum value is " + nums.Min());
    Console.WriteLine("The maximum value is " + nums.Max());

    Console.WriteLine("The first value is " + nums.First());
    Console.WriteLine("The last value is " + nums.Last());

    Console.WriteLine("The sum is " + nums.Sum());
    Console.WriteLine("The average is " + nums.Average());

    if(nums.All(n => n > 0))
      Console.WriteLine("All values are greater than zero.");

    if(nums.Any(n => (n % 2) == 0))
      Console.WriteLine("At least one value is even.");

    if(nums.Contains(3))
      Console.WriteLine("The array contains 3.");
  }
}
```

The output is shown here:

```
The minimum value is 1
The maximum value is 5
The first value is 3
The last value is 4
The sum is 15
The average is 3
All values are greater than zero.
At least one value is even.
The array contains 3.
```

You can also use the query-related extension methods within a query based on the C# query syntax. In fact, it is quite common to do so. For example, this program uses **Average( )** to obtain a sequence that contains only those values that are less than the average of the values in an array.

```
// Use Average() with the query syntax.
using System;
using System.Linq;

class ExtMethods2 {
  static void Main() {

    int[] nums = { 1, 2, 4, 8, 6, 9, 10, 3, 6, 7 };

    var ltAvg = from n in nums
                let x = nums.Average()
                where n < x
                select n;

    Console.WriteLine("The average is " + nums.Average());

    Console.Write("These values are less than the average: ");

    // Execute the query and display the results.
    foreach(int i in ltAvg) Console.Write(i + " ");

    Console.WriteLine();
  }
}
```

The output is shown here:

```
The average is 5.6
These values are less than the average: 1 2 4 3
```

Pay special attention to the query:

```
    var ltAvg = from n in nums
                let x = nums.Average()
                where n < x
                select n;
```

Notice in the **let** statement, **x** is set equal to the average of the values in **nums**. This value is obtained by calling **Average( )** on **nums**.

Deferred vs. Immediate Query Execution

In LINQ, queries have two different modes of execution: immediate and deferred. As explained early in this chapter, a query defines a set of rules that are not actually executed until a **foreach** statement executes. This is called *deferred execution.*

However, if you use one of the extension methods that produces a nonsequence result, then the query must be executed to obtain that result. For example, consider the **Count( )** method. In order for **Count( )** to return the number of elements in the sequence, the query must be executed, and this is done automatically when **Count( )** is called. In this case, *immediate execution* takes place, with the query being executed automatically in order to obtain the result. Therefore, even though you don't explicitly use the query in a **foreach** loop, the query is still executed.

Here is a simple example. It obtains the number of positive elements in the sequence.

```
// Use immediate execution.
using System;
using System.Linq;

class ImmediateExec {
  static void Main() {

    int[] nums =  { 1, -2, 3, 0, -4, 5 };

    // Create a query that obtains the number of positive
    // values in nums.
    int len = (from n in nums
               where n > 0
               select n).Count();

    Console.WriteLine("The number of positive values in nums: " + len);
  }
}
```

The output is

```
The number of positive values in nums: 3
```

In the program, notice that no explicit **foreach** loop is specified. Instead, the query automatically executes because of the call to **Count( )**.

As a point of interest, the query in the preceding program could also have been written like this:

```
var posNums = from n in nums
              where n > 0
              select n;

int len = posNums.Count(); // query executes here
```

In this case, **Count( )** is called on the query variable. At that point, the query is executed to obtain the count.

Two other methods that cause immediate execution of a query are **ToArray( )** and **ToList( )**. Both are extension methods defined by **Enumerable**. **ToArray( )** returns the results

of a query in an array. **ToList( )** returns the results of a query in the form of a **List** collection. (See Chapter 24 for a discussion of collections.) In both cases, the query is executed to obtain the results. For example, the following sequence obtains an array of the results generated by the **posNums** query just shown. It then displays the results.

```
int[] pnums = posNum.ToArray(); // query executes here

foreach(int i in pnums)
  Console.Write(i + " ");
}
```

Expression Trees

Another new LINQ-related feature is the *expression tree*. An expression tree is a representation of a lambda expression as data. Thus, an expression tree, itself, cannot be executed. It can, however, be converted into an executable form. Expression trees are encapsulated by the **System.Linq.Expressions.Expression<T>** class. Expression trees are useful in situations in which a query will be executed by something outside the program, such as a database that uses SQL. By representing the query as data, the query can be converted into a format understood by the database. This process is used by the LINQ to SQL feature provided by Visual C#, for example. Thus, expression trees help C# support a variety of data sources.

You can obtain an executable form of an expression tree by calling the **Compile( )** method defined by **Expression**. It returns a reference that can be assigned to a delegate and then executed. You can declare your own delegate type or use one of the predefined **Func** delegate types defined within the **System** namespace. Two forms of the **Func** delegate were mentioned earlier, when the query methods were described. Here is a list of all its forms:

>   delegate TResult Func<TResult>( )

>   delegate TResult Func<T1, TResult>( )

>   delegate TResult Func<T1, T2, TResult>( )

>   delegate TResult Func<T1, T2, T3, TResult>( )

>   delegate TResult Func<T1, T2, T3, T4, TResult>( )

These forms represent methods that return a value and take from zero to four parameters (whose types are **T1** through **T4**). If your expression requires more than four parameters, then you will need to define your own delegate type.

Expression trees have one key restriction: Only expression lambdas can be represented by expression trees. They cannot be used to represent statement lambdas.

Here is a simple example of an expression tree in action. It creates an expression tree whose data represents a method that determines if one integer is a factor of another. It then compiles the expression tree into executable code. Finally, it demonstrates the compiled code.

```
// A simple expression tree.
using System;
using System.Linq;
using System.Linq.Expressions;
```

```
class SimpleExpTree {
  static void Main() {

    // Represent a lambda expression as data.
    Expression<Func<int, int, bool>>
      IsFactorExp = (n, d) => (d != 0) ? (n % d) == 0 : false;

    // Compile the expression data into executable code.
    Func<int, int, bool> IsFactor = IsFactorExp.Compile();

    // Execute the expression.
    if(IsFactor(10, 5))
      Console.WriteLine("5 is a factor of 10.");

    if(!IsFactor(10, 7))
      Console.WriteLine("7 is not a factor of 10.");

    Console.WriteLine();
  }
}
```

The output is shown here:

```
5 is a factor of 10.
7 is not a factor of 10.
```

The program illustrates the two key steps in using an expression tree. First, it creates an expression tree by using this statement:

```
Expression<Func<int, int, bool>>
  IsFactorExp = (n, d) => (d != 0) ? (n % d) == 0 : false;
```

This constructs a representation of a lambda expression in memory. As explained, this representation is data, not code. This representation is referred to by **IsFactorExp**. The following statement converts the expression data into executable code:

```
Func<int, int, bool> IsFactor = IsFactorExp.Compile();
```

After this statement executes, the **IsFactor** delegate can be called to determine if one value is a factor of another.

One other point: Notice that **Func<int, int, bool>** indicates the delegate type. This form of **Func** specifies two parameters of type **int** and a return type of **bool**. This is the form of **Func** that is compatible with the lambda expression used in the program because that expression requires two parameters. Other lambda expressions may require different forms of **Func**, based on the number of parameters they require. In general, the specific form of **Func** must match the requirements of the lambda expression.

Extension Methods

As mentioned earlier, extension methods provide a means by which functionality can be added to a class without using the normal inheritance mechanism. Although you won't often create your own extension methods (because the inheritance mechanism offers a

better solution in many cases), it is still important that you understand how they work because of their integral importance to LINQ.

An extension method is a static method that must be contained within a static, non-generic class. The type of its first parameter determines the type of objects on which the extension method can be called. Furthermore, the first parameter must be modified by **this**. The object on which the method is invoked is passed automatically to the first parameter. It is not explicitly passed in the argument list. A key point is that even though an extension method is declared **static**, it can still be called on an object, just as if it were an instance method.

Here is the general form of an extension method:

static *ret-type name*(this *invoked-on-type ob, param-list*)

Of course, if there are no arguments other than the one passed implicitly to *ob*, then *param-list* will be empty. Remember, the first parameter is automatically passed the object on which the method is invoked. In general, an extension method will be a public member of its class.

Here is an example that creates three simple extension methods:

```
// Create and use some extension methods.
using System;

static class MyExtMeths {

  // Return the reciprocal of a double.
  public static double Reciprocal(this double v) {
    return 1.0 / v;
  }

  // Reverse the case of letters within a string and
  // return the result.
  public static string RevCase(this string str) {
    string temp = "";

    foreach(char ch in str) {
      if(Char.IsLower(ch)) temp += Char.ToUpper(ch);
      else temp += Char.ToLower(ch);
    }
    return temp;
  }

  // Return the absolute value of n / d.
  public static double AbsDivideBy(this double n, double d) {
    return Math.Abs(n / d);
  }
}

class ExtDemo {
  static void Main() {
    double val = 8.0;
    string str = "Alpha Beta Gamma";

    // Call the Recip() extension method.
    Console.WriteLine("Reciprocal of {0} is {1}",
                      val, val.Reciprocal());
```

```
      // Call the RevCase() extension method.
      Console.WriteLine(str + " after reversing case is " +
                        str.RevCase());

      // Use AbsDivideBy();
      Console.WriteLine("Result of val.AbsDivideBy(-2): " +
                        val.AbsDivideBy(-2));
   }
}
```

The output is shown here:

```
Reciprocal of 8 is 0.125
Alpha Beta Gamma after reversing case is aLPHA bETA gAMMA
Result of val.AbsDivideBy(-2): 4
```

In the program, notice that each extension method is contained in a static class called **MyExtMeths**. As explained, an extension method must be declared within a static class. Furthermore, this class must be in scope in order for the extension methods that it contains to be used. (This is why you needed to include the **System.Linq** namespace to use the LINQ-related extension methods.) Next, notice the calls to the extension methods. They are invoked on an object, in just the same way that an instance method is called. The main difference is that the invoking object is passed to the first parameter of the extension method. Therefore, when the expression

```
val.AbsDivideBy(-2)
```

executes, **val** is passed to the **n** parameter of **AbsDivideBy( )** and –2 is passed to the **d** parameter.

As a point of interest, because the methods **Reciprocal( )** and **AbsDivideBy( )** are defined for **double**, it is legal to invoke them on a **double** literal, as shown here:

```
8.0.Reciprocal()
8.0.AbsDivideBy(-1)
```

Furthermore, **RevCase( )** can be invoked like this:

```
"AbCDe".RevCase()
```

Here, the reversed-case version of a string literal is returned.

Unsafe Code, Pointers, Nullable Types, and Miscellaneous Topics

This chapter covers a feature of C# whose name usually takes programmers by surprise: unsafe code. Unsafe code often involves the use of pointers. Together, unsafe code and pointers enable C# to be used to create applications that one might normally associate with C++: high-performance, systems code. Moreover, the inclusion of unsafe code and pointers gives C# capabilities that are lacking in Java.

Also covered in this chapter are nullable types, partial class and partial method definitions, and fixed-size buffers. The chapter concludes by discussing the few keywords that have not been covered by the preceding chapters.

Unsafe Code

C# allows you to write what is called "unsafe" code. Although this statement might seem shocking, it really isn't. Unsafe code is not code that is poorly written; it is code that does not execute under the full management of the common language runtime (CLR). As explained in Chapter 1, C# is normally used to create managed code. It is possible, however, to write code that does not execute under the full control of the CLR. This unmanaged code is not subject to the same controls and constraints as managed code, so it is called "unsafe" because it is not possible to verify that it won't perform some type of harmful action. Thus, the term *unsafe* does not mean that the code is inherently flawed. It simply means that it is possible for the code to perform actions that are not subject to the supervision of the managed context.

Given that unsafe code might cause problems, you might ask why anyone would want to create such code. The answer is that managed code prevents the use of *pointers.* If you are familiar with C or C++, then you know that pointers are variables that hold the addresses of other objects. Thus, pointers are a bit like references in C#. The main difference is that a pointer can point anywhere in memory; a reference always refers to an object of its type. Because a pointer can point anywhere in memory, it is possible to misuse a pointer. It is also

easy to introduce a coding error when using pointers. This is why C# does not support pointers when creating managed code. Pointers are, however, both useful and necessary for some types of programming (such as system-level utilities), and C# does allow you to create and use pointers. However, all pointer operations must be marked as unsafe since they execute outside the managed context.

The declaration and use of pointers in C# parallels that of C/C++—if you know how to use pointers in C/C++, then you can use them in C#. But remember, the essence of C# is the creation of managed code. Its ability to support unmanaged code allows it to be applied to a special class of problems. It is not for normal C# programming. In fact, to compile unmanaged code, you must use the **/unsafe** compiler option.

Since pointers are at the core of unsafe code, we will begin there.

Pointer Basics

A pointer is a variable that holds the address of some other object, such as another variable. For example, if **x** contains the address of **y**, then **x** is said to "point to" **y**. When a pointer points to a variable, the value of that variable can be obtained or changed through the pointer. Operations through pointers are often referred to as *indirection*.

Declaring a Pointer

Pointer variables must be declared as such. The general form of a pointer variable declaration is

   type * *var-name*;

Here, *type* is the pointer's *referent type,* which must be a nonreference type. Thus, you cannot declare a pointer to a class object. A pointer's referent type is also sometimes called its *base type.* Notice the placement of the *. It follows the type name. *var-name* is the name of the pointer variable.

Here is an example. To declare **ip** to be a pointer to an **int**, use this declaration:

```
int* ip;
```

For a **float** pointer, use

```
float* fp;
```

In general, in a declaration statement, following a type name with an * creates a pointer type.

The type of data that a pointer will point to is determined by its referent type. Thus, in the preceding examples, **ip** can be used to point to an **int**, and **fp** can be used to point to a **float**. Understand, however, that there is nothing that actually prevents a pointer from pointing elsewhere. This is why pointers are potentially unsafe.

If you come from a C/C++ background, then you need to be aware of an important difference between the way C# and C/C++ declare pointers. When you declare a pointer type in C/C++, the * is not distributive over a list of variables in a declaration. Thus, in C/C++, this statement

```
int* p, q;
```

declares an **int** pointer called **p** and an **int** called **q**. It is equivalent to the following two declarations:

```
int* p;
int q;
```

However, in C#, the * *is* distributive and the declaration

```
int* p, q;
```

creates two pointer variables. Thus, in C# it is the same as these two declarations:

```
int* p;
int* q;
```

This is an important difference to keep in mind when porting C/C++ code to C#.

The * and & Pointer Operators

Two operators are used with pointers: * and **&**. The **&** is a unary operator that returns the memory address of its operand. (Recall that a unary operator requires only one operand.) For example,

```
int* ip;
int num = 10;

ip = &num;
```

puts into **ip** the memory address of the variable **num**. This address is the location of the variable in the computer's internal memory. It has *nothing* to do with the *value* of **num**. Thus, **ip** *does not* contain the value 10 (**num**'s initial value). It contains the address at which **num** is stored. The operation of **&** can be remembered as returning "the address of" the variable it precedes. Therefore, the preceding assignment statement could be verbalized as "**ip** receives the address of **num**."

The second operator is *, and it is the complement of **&**. It is a unary operator that evaluates to the value of the variable located at the address specified by its operand. That is, it refers to the value of the variable pointed to by a pointer. Continuing with the same example, if **ip** contains the memory address of the variable **num**, then

```
int val = *ip;
```

will place into **val** the value 10, which is the value of **num**, which is pointed to by **ip**. The operation of * can be remembered as "at address." In this case, then, the statement could be read as "**val** receives the value at address **ip**."

The * can also be used on the left side of an assignment statement. In this usage, it sets the value pointed to by the pointer. For example,

```
*ip = 100;
```

This statement assigns 100 to the variable pointed to by **ip**, which is **num** in this case. Thus, this statement can be read as "at address **ip**, put the value 100."

Using unsafe

Any code that uses pointers must be marked as unsafe by using the **unsafe** keyword. You can mark types (such as classes and structures), members (such as methods and operators),

or individual blocks of code as unsafe. For example, here is a program that uses pointers inside **Main( )**, which is marked unsafe:

```
// Demonstrate pointers and unsafe.

using System;

class UnsafeCode {
  // Mark Main as unsafe.
  unsafe static void Main() {
    int count = 99;
    int* p; // create an int pointer

    p = &count; // put address of count into p

    Console.WriteLine("Initial value of count is " + *p);

    *p = 10; // assign 10 to count via p

    Console.WriteLine("New value of count is " + *p);
  }
}
```

The output of this program is shown here:

```
Initial value of count is 99
New value of count is 10
```

Using fixed

The **fixed** modifier is often used when working with pointers. It prevents a managed variable from being moved by the garbage collector. This is needed when a pointer refers to a field in a class object, for example. Because the pointer has no knowledge of the actions of the garbage collector, if the object is moved, the pointer will point to the wrong object. Here is the general form of **fixed**:

```
fixed (type* p = &fixedObj) {
  // use fixed object
}
```

Here, *p* is a pointer that is being assigned the address of an object. The object will remain at its current memory location until the block of code has executed. You can also use a single statement for the target of a **fixed** statement. The **fixed** keyword can be used only in an unsafe context. You can declare more than one fixed pointer at a time using a comma-separated list.

Here is an example of **fixed**:

```
// Demonstrate fixed.

using System;

class Test {
  public int num;
  public Test(int i) { num = i; }
}
```

```
class FixedCode {
  // Mark Main as unsafe.
  unsafe static void Main() {
    Test o = new Test(19);

    fixed (int* p = &o.num) { // use fixed to put address of o.num into p

      Console.WriteLine("Initial value of o.num is " + *p);

      *p = 10; // assign 10 to count via p

      Console.WriteLine("New value of o.num is " + *p);
    }
  }
}
```

The output from this program is shown here:

```
Initial value of o.num is 19
New value of o.num is 10
```

Here, **fixed** prevents **o** from being moved. Because **p** points to **o.num**, if **o** were moved, then **p** would point to an invalid location.

Accessing Structure Members Through a Pointer

A pointer can point to an object of a structure type as long as the structure does not contain reference types. When you access a member of a structure through a pointer, you must use the arrow operator, which is –>, rather than the dot (.) operator. For example, given this structure,

```
struct MyStruct {
  public int a;
  public int b;
  public int Sum() { return a + b; }
}
```

you would access its members through a pointer, like this:

```
MyStruct o = new MyStruct();
MyStruct* p; // declare a pointer

p = &o;
p->a = 10; // use the -> operator
p->b = 20; // use the -> operator

Console.WriteLine("Sum is " + p->Sum());
```

Pointer Arithmetic

There are only four arithmetic operators that can be used on pointers: ++, – –, +, and –. To understand what occurs in pointer arithmetic, we will begin with an example. Let **p1** be an **int** pointer with a current value of 2,000 (that is, it contains the address 2,000). After this expression,

```
p1++;
```

the contents of **p1** will be 2,004, not 2,001! The reason is that each time **p1** is incremented, it will point to the *next* **int**. Since **int** in C# is 4 bytes long, incrementing **p1** increases its value by 4. The reverse is true of decrements. Each decrement decreases **p1**'s value by 4. For example,

```
p1--;
```

will cause **p1** to have the value 1,996, assuming it previously was 2,000.

Generalizing from the preceding example, each time that a pointer is incremented, it will point to the memory location of the next element of its referent type. Each time it is decremented, it will point to the location of the previous element of its referent type.

Pointer arithmetic is not limited to only increment and decrement operations. You can also add or subtract integers to or from pointers. The expression

```
p1 = p1 + 9;
```

makes **p1** point to the ninth element of **p1**'s referent type, beyond the one it is currently pointing to.

Although you cannot add pointers, you can subtract one pointer from another (provided they are both of the same referent type). The remainder will be the number of elements of the referent type that separate the two pointers.

Other than addition and subtraction of a pointer and an integer, or the subtraction of two pointers, no other arithmetic operations can be performed on pointers. For example, you cannot add or subtract **float** or **double** values to or from pointers.

To see the effects of pointer arithmetic, execute the next short program. It prints the actual physical addresses to which an integer pointer (**ip**) and a floating-point pointer (**fp**) are pointing. Observe how each changes, relative to its referent type, each time the loop is repeated.

```
// Demonstrate the effects of pointer arithmetic.

using System;

class PtrArithDemo {
  unsafe static void Main() {
    int x;
    int i;
    double d;

    int* ip = &i;
    double* fp = &d;

    Console.WriteLine("int      double\n");

    for(x=0; x < 10; x++) {
      Console.WriteLine((uint) (ip) + " " + (uint) (fp));
      ip++;
      fp++;
    }
  }
}
```

Sample output is shown here. Your output may differ, but the intervals will be the same.

```
int      double

1243464 1243468
1243468 1243476
1243472 1243484
1243476 1243492
1243480 1243500
1243484 1243508
1243488 1243516
1243492 1243524
1243496 1243532
1243500 1243540
```

As the output shows, pointer arithmetic is performed relative to the referent type of the pointer. Since an **int** is 4 bytes and a **double** is 8 bytes, the addresses change in increments of these values.

Pointer Comparisons

Pointers can be compared using the relational operators, such as = =, <, and >. However, for the outcome of a pointer comparison to be meaningful, usually the two pointers must have some relationship to each other. For example, if **p1** and **p2** are pointers that point to two separate and unrelated variables, then any comparison between **p1** and **p2** is generally meaningless. However, if **p1** and **p2** point to variables that are related to each other, such as elements of the same array, then **p1** and **p2** can be meaningfully compared.

Pointers and Arrays

In C#, pointers and arrays are related. For example, within a **fixed** statement, the name of an array without any index generates a pointer to the start of the array. Consider the following program:

```
/* An array name without an index yields a pointer to the
   start of the array. */

using System;

class PtrArray {
  unsafe static void Main() {
    int[] nums = new int[10];

    fixed(int* p = &nums[0], p2 = nums) {
      if(p == p2)
        Console.WriteLine("p and p2 point to same address.");
    }
  }
}
```

The output is shown here:

```
p and p2 point to same address.
```

As the output shows, the expression

```
&nums[0]
```

is the same as

```
nums
```

Since the second form is shorter, most programmers use it when a pointer to the start of an array is needed.

Indexing a Pointer

When a pointer refers to an array, the pointer can be indexed as if it were an array. This syntax provides an alternative to pointer arithmetic that can be more convenient in some situations. Here is an example:

```csharp
// Index a pointer as if it were an array.

using System;

class PtrIndexDemo {
  unsafe static void Main() {
    int[] nums = new int[10];

    // Index a pointer.
    Console.WriteLine("Index pointer like array.");
    fixed (int* p = nums) {
      for(int i=0; i < 10; i++)
        p[i] = i; // index pointer like array

      for(int i=0; i < 10; i++)
        Console.WriteLine("p[{0}]: {1} ", i, p[i]);
    }

    // Use pointer arithmetic.
    Console.WriteLine("\nUse pointer arithmetic.");
    fixed (int* p = nums) {
      for(int i=0; i < 10; i++)
        *(p+i) = i; // use pointer arithmetic

      for(int i=0; i < 10; i++)
        Console.WriteLine("*(p+{0}): {1} ", i, *(p+i));
    }
  }
}
```

The output is shown here:

```
Index pointer like array.
p[0]: 0
p[1]: 1
p[2]: 2
p[3]: 3
```

```
p[4]: 4
p[5]: 5
p[6]: 6
p[7]: 7
p[8]: 8
p[9]: 9

Use pointer arithmetic.
*(p+0): 0
*(p+1): 1
*(p+2): 2
*(p+3): 3
*(p+4): 4
*(p+5): 5
*(p+6): 6
*(p+7): 7
*(p+8): 8
*(p+9): 9
```

As the program illustrates, a pointer expression with this general form

*(ptr + i)

can be rewritten using array-indexing syntax like this:

ptr[i]

There are two important things to understand about indexing a pointer: First, no boundary checking is applied. Thus, it is possible to access an element beyond the end of the array to which the pointer refers. Second, a pointer does not have a **Length** property. So, using the pointer, there is no way of knowing how long the array is.

Pointers and Strings

Although strings are implemented as objects in C#, it is possible to access the characters in a string through a pointer. To do so, you will assign a pointer to the start of the string to a **char*** pointer using a **fixed** statement like this:

fixed(char* *p* = *str*) { // ...

After the **fixed** statement executes, **p** will point to the start of the array of characters that make up the string. This array is *null-terminated*, which means that it ends with a zero. You can use this fact to test for the end of the array. Null-terminated character arrays are the way that strings are implemented in C/C++. Thus, obtaining a **char*** pointer to a **string** allows you to operate on strings in much the same way as does C/C++.

Here is a program that demonstrates accessing a string through a **char*** pointer:

```
// Use fixed to get a pointer to the start of a string.

using System;

class FixedString {
  unsafe static void Main() {
    string str = "this is a test";
```

```
// Point p to start of str.
fixed(char* p = str) {

  // Display the contents of str via p.
  for(int i=0; p[i] != 0; i++)
    Console.Write(p[i]);
}

Console.WriteLine();

  }
}
```

The output is shown here:

```
this is a test
```

Multiple Indirection

You can have a pointer point to another pointer that points to the target value. This situation is called *multiple indirection*, or *pointers to pointers*. Pointers to pointers can be confusing. Figure 20-1 helps clarify the concept of multiple indirection. As you can see, the value of a normal pointer is the address of the variable that contains the value desired. In the case of a pointer to a pointer, the first pointer contains the address of the second pointer, which points to the variable that contains the value desired.

Multiple indirection can be carried on to whatever extent desired, but more than a pointer to a pointer is rarely needed. In fact, excessive indirection is difficult to follow and prone to conceptual errors.

A variable that is a pointer to a pointer must be declared as such. You do this by placing an additional asterisk after the type name. For example, the following declaration tells the compiler that **q** is a pointer to a pointer of type **int**:

```
int** q;
```

You should understand that **q** is not a pointer to an integer, but rather a pointer to an **int** pointer.

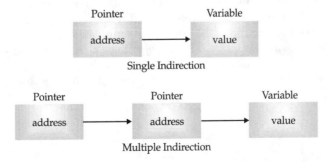

FIGURE 20-1 Single and multiple indirection

To access the target value indirectly pointed to by a pointer to a pointer, you must apply the asterisk operator twice, as in this example:

```
using System;

class MultipleIndirect {
  unsafe static void Main() {
    int x;   // holds an int value
    int* p;  // holds an int pointer
    int** q; // holds a pointer to an int pointer

    x = 10;
    p = &x; // put address of x into p
    q = &p; // put address of p into q

    Console.WriteLine(**q); // display the value of x
  }
}
```

The output is the value of **x**, which is 10. In the program, **p** is declared as a pointer to an **int** and **q** as a pointer to an **int** pointer.

One last point: Do not confuse multiple indirection with high-level data structures, such as linked lists. These are two fundamentally different concepts.

Arrays of Pointers

Pointers can be arrayed like any other data type. The declaration for an **int** pointer array of size 3 is

```
int * [] ptrs = new int * [3];
```

To assign the address of an **int** variable called **var** to the third element of the pointer array, write

```
ptrs[2] = &var;
```

To find the value of **var**, write

```
*ptrs[2]
```

sizeof

When working in an unsafe context, you might occasionally find it useful to know the size, in bytes, of one of C#'s value types. To obtain this information, use the **sizeof** operator. It has this general form:

   sizeof(*type*)

Here, type is the *type* whose size is being obtained. In general, **sizeof** is intended primarily for special-case situations, especially when working with a blend of managed and unmanaged code.

stackalloc

You can allocate memory from the stack by using **stackalloc**. It can be used only when initializing local variables and has this general form:

type *p = stackalloc *type*[*size*]

Here, *p* is a pointer that receives the address of the memory that is large enough to hold *size* number of objects of *type*. Also, *type* must be a nonreference type. If there is not room on the stack to allocate the memory, a **System.StackOverflowException** is thrown. Finally, **stackalloc** can be used only in an unsafe context.

Normally, memory for objects is allocated from the *heap*, which is a region of free memory. Allocating memory from the stack is the exception. Variables allocated on the stack are not garbage-collected. Rather, they exist only while the method in which they are declared is executing. When the method is left, the memory is freed. One advantage to using **stackalloc** is that you don't need to worry about the memory being moved about by the garbage collector.

Here is an example that uses **stackalloc**:

```
// Demonstrate stackalloc.

using System;

class UseStackAlloc {
  unsafe static void Main() {
    int* ptrs = stackalloc int[3];

    ptrs[0] = 1;
    ptrs[1] = 2;
    ptrs[2] = 3;

    for(int i=0; i < 3; i++)
      Console.WriteLine(ptrs[i]);
  }
}
```

The output is shown here:

```
1
2
3
```

Creating Fixed-Size Buffers

There is a second use of the **fixed** keyword that enables you to create fixed-sized, single-dimensional arrays. In the C# documentation, these are referred to as *fixed-size buffers*. A fixed-size buffer is always a member of a **struct**. The purpose of a fixed-size buffer is to allow the creation of a **struct** in which the array elements that make up the buffer are contained within the **struct**. Normally, when you include an array member in a **struct**, only a reference to the array is actually held within the **struct**. By using a fixed-size buffer, you cause the entire array to be contained within the **struct**. This results in a structure that can be used in situations in which the size of a **struct** is important, such as in mixed-language programming, interfacing to data not created by a C# program, or whenever a nonmanaged **struct** containing an array is required. Fixed-size buffers can be used only within an unsafe context.

To create a fixed-size buffer, use this form of **fixed**:

fixed *type buf-name*[*size*];

Here, *type* is the data type of the array; *buf-name* is the name of the fixed-size buffer; and *size* is the number of elements in the buffer. Fixed-size buffers can be specified only within a **struct**.

To understand why a fixed-size buffer might be useful, consider a situation in which you want to pass bank account information to an account management program that is written in C++. Furthermore, assume that each account record uses the following organization:

Name	An 8-bit, ASCII character string, 80 bytes long
Balance	A **double**, 8 bytes long
ID	A **long**, 8 bytes long

In C++, each structure, itself, contains the **Name** array. This differs from C#, which would normally just store a reference to the array. Thus, representing this data in a C# **struct** requires the use of a fixed-size buffer, as shown here:

```
// Use a fixed-size buffer.
unsafe struct FixedBankRecord {
  public fixed byte Name[80]; // create a fixed-size buffer
  public double Balance;
  public long ID;
}
```

By using a fixed-size buffer for **Name**, each instance of **FixedBankRecord** will contain all 80 bytes of the **Name** array, which is the way that a C++ **struct** would be organized. Thus, the overall size of **FixedBankRecord** is 96, which is the sum of its members. Here is a program that demonstrates this fact:

```
// Demonstrate a fixed-size buffer.

using System;

// Create a fixed-size buffer.
unsafe struct FixedBankRecord {
  public fixed byte Name[80]; // create a fixed-size buffer
  public double Balance;
  public long ID;
}

class FixedSizeBuffer {
  // Mark Main as unsafe.
  unsafe static void Main() {
    Console.WriteLine("Size of FixedBankRecord is " +
                      sizeof(FixedBankRecord));
  }
}
```

The output is shown here:

```
Size of FixedBankRecord is 96
```

Although the size of **FixedBankRecord** is the exact sum of its members, this may not be the case for all **struct**s that have fixed-size buffers. C# is free to pad the overall length of structure so that it aligns on an even boundary (such as a word boundary) for efficiency reasons. Therefore, the overall length of a **struct** might be a few bytes greater than the sum of its fields, even when fixed-size buffers are used. In most cases, an equivalent C++ **struct** would also use the same padding. However, be aware that a difference in this regard may be possible.

One last point: In the program, notice how the fixed-size buffer for **Name** is created:

```
public fixed byte Name[80]; // create a fixed-size buffer
```

Pay special attention to how the dimension of the array is specified. The brackets containing the array size follow the array name. This is C++-style syntax, and it differs from normal C# array declarations. This statement allocates 80 bytes of storage within each **FixedBankRecord** object.

Nullable Types

Beginning with version 2.0, C# has included a feature that provides an elegant solution to what is both a common and irritating problem. The feature is the *nullable type*. The problem is how to recognize and handle fields that do not contain values (in other words, unassigned fields). To understand the problem, consider a simple customer database that keeps a record of the customer's name, address, customer ID, invoice number, and current balance. In such a situation, it is possible to create a customer entry in which one or more of those fields would be unassigned. For example, a customer may simply request a catalog. In this case, no invoice number would be needed and the field would be unused.

In the past, handling the possibility of unused fields required the use of either placeholder values or an extra field that simply indicated whether a field was in use. Of course, placeholder values could work only if there was a value that would otherwise be invalid, which won't be the case in all situations. Adding an extra field to indicate if a field is in use works in all cases, but having to manually create and manage such a field is an annoyance. The nullable type solves both problems.

Nullable Basics

A nullable type is a special version of a value type that is represented by a structure. In addition to the values defined by the underlying type, a nullable type can also store the value **null**. Thus, a nullable type has the same range and characteristics as its underlying type. It simply adds the ability to represent a value that indicates that a variable of that type is unassigned. Nullable types are objects of **System.Nullable<T>**, where **T** must be a non-nullable value type.

REMEMBER *Only value types have nullable equivalents.*

A nullable type can be specified two different ways. First, you can explicitly declare objects of type **Nullable<T>**, which is defined in the **System** namespace. For example, this creates **int** and **bool** nullable types:

```
System.Nullable<int> count;
System.Nullable<bool> done;
```

PART I

The second way to declare a nullable type is much shorter and is more commonly used. Simply follow the type name with a **?**. For example, the following shows the more common way to declare a nullable **int** and **bool** type:

```
int? count;
bool? done;
```

When using nullable types, you will often see a nullable object created like this:

```
int? count = null;
```

This explicitly initializes **count** to **null**. This satisfies the constraint that a variable must be given a value before it is used. In this case, the value simply means undefined.

You can assign a value to a nullable variable in the normal way because a conversion from the underlying type to the nullable type is predefined. For example, this assigns the value 100 to **count**.

```
count = 100;
```

There are two ways to determine if a variable of a nullable type is **null** or contains a value. First, you can test its value against **null**. For example, using **count** declared by the preceding statement, the following determines if it has a value:

```
if(count != null) // has a value
```

If **count** is not **null**, then it contains a value.

The second way to determine if a nullable type contains a value is to use the **HasValue** read-only property defined by **Nullable<T>**. It is shown here:

```
bool HasValue
```

HasValue will return true if the instance on which it is called contains a value. It will return false otherwise. Using the **HasValue** property, here is the second way to determine if the nullable object **count** has a value:

```
if(count.HasValue) // has a value
```

Assuming that a nullable object contains a value, you can obtain its value by using the **Value** read-only property defined by **Nullable<T>**, which is shown here:

```
T Value
```

It returns the value of the nullable instance on which it is called. If you try to obtain a value from a variable that is **null**, a **System.InvalidOperationException** will be thrown. It is also possible to obtain the value of a nullable instance by casting it into its underlying type.

The following program puts together the pieces and demonstrates the basic mechanism that handles a nullable type:

```
// Demonstrate a nullable type.

using System;

class NullableDemo {
  static void Main() {
```

```
int? count = null;

if(count.HasValue)
  Console.WriteLine("count has this value: " + count.Value);
else
  Console.WriteLine("count has no value");

count = 100;

if(count.HasValue)
  Console.WriteLine("count has this value: " + count.Value);
else
  Console.WriteLine("count has no value");
  }
}
```

The output is shown here:

```
count has no value
count has this value: 100
```

Nullable Objects in Expressions

A nullable object can be used in expressions that are valid for its underlying type. Furthermore, it is possible to mix nullable objects and non-nullable objects within the same expression. This works because of the predefined conversion that exists from the underlying type to the nullable type. When non-nullable and nullable types are mixed in an operation, the outcome is a nullable value.

The following program illustrates the use of nullable types in expressions:

```
// Use nullable objects in expressions.

using System;

class NullableDemo {
  static void Main() {
    int? count = null;
    int? result = null;

    int incr = 10; // notice that incr is a non-nullable type

    // result contains null, because count is null.
    result = count + incr;

    if(result.HasValue)
      Console.WriteLine("result has this value: " + result.Value);
    else
      Console.WriteLine("result has no value");

    // Now, count is given a value and result will contain a value.
    count = 100;
    result = count + incr;
```

```
      if(result.HasValue)
        Console.WriteLine("result has this value: " + result.Value);
      else
        Console.WriteLine("result has no value");

  }
}
```

The output is shown here:

```
result has no value
result has this value: 110
```

The ?? Operator

If you attempt to use a cast to convert a nullable object to its underlying type, a **System.InvalidOperationException** will be thrown if the nullable object contains a **null** value. This can occur, for example, when you use a cast to assign the value of a nullable object to a variable of its underlying type. You can avoid the possibility of this exception being thrown by using the **??** operator, which is called the *null coalescing operator*. It lets you specify a default value that will be used when the nullable object contains **null**. It also eliminates the need for the cast.

The **??** operator has this general form:

   nullable-object **??** *default-value*

If *nullable-object* contains a value, then the value of the **??** is that value. Otherwise, the value of the **??** operation is *default-value*.

For example, in the following code **balance** is **null**. This causes **currentBalance** to be assigned the value 0.0 and no exception will be thrown.

```
double? balance = null;
double currentBalance;

currentBalance = balance ?? 0.0;
```

In the next sequence, **balance** is given the value 123.75:

```
double? balance = 123.75;
double currentBalance;

currentBalance = balance ?? 0.0;
```

Now, **currentBalance** will contain the value of **balance**, which is 123.75.

One other point: The right-hand expression of the **??** is evaluated only if the left-hand expression does not contain a value. The following program demonstrates this fact:

```
// Using ??

using System;

class NullableDemo2 {
```

```
// Return a zero balance.
static double GetZeroBal() {
  Console.WriteLine("In GetZeroBal().");
    return 0.0;
}

static void Main() {
  double? balance = 123.75;
  double currentBalance;

  // Here, GetZeroBal( ) is not called because balance
  // contains a value.
  currentBalance = balance ?? GetZeroBal();

  Console.WriteLine(currentBalance);
  }
}
```

In this program, the method **GetZeroBal( )** is not called because **balance** contains a value. As explained, when the left-hand expression of **??** contains a value, the right-hand expression is not evaluated.

Nullable Objects and the Relational and Logical Operators

Nullable objects can be used in relational expressions in just the same way as their corresponding non-nullable types. However, there is one additional rule that applies. When two nullable objects are compared using the <, >, <=, or >= operators, the result is false if either of the objects is **null**. For example, consider this sequence:

```
byte? lower = 16;
byte? upper = null;

// Here, lower is defined, but upper isn't.
if(lower < upper) // false
```

Here, the result of the test for less than is false. However, somewhat counterintuitively, so is the inverse comparison:

```
if(lower > upper) // .. also false!
```

Thus, when one (or both) of the nullable objects used in a comparison is **null**, the result of that comparison is always false. Thus, **null** does not participate in an ordering relationship.

You can test whether a nullable object contains **null**, however, by using the **==** or **!=** operators. For example, this is a valid test that will result in a true outcome:

```
if(upper == null) // ...
```

When a logical expression involves two **bool?** objects, the outcome of that expression will be one of three values: **true**, **false**, or **null** (undefined). Here are the entries that are added to the truth table for the **&** and **|** operators that apply to **bool?**.

P	Q	P | Q	P & Q
true	null	true	null
false	null	null	false
null	true	true	null
null	false	null	false
null	null	null	null

One other point: When the ! operator is applied to a **bool?** value that is **null**, the outcome is **null**.

Partial Types

Beginning with C# 2.0, a class, structure, or interface definition can be broken into two or more pieces, with each piece residing in a separate file. This is accomplished through the use of the **partial** keyword. When your program is compiled, the pieces are united.

When used to create a partial type, the **partial** modifier has this general form:

partial *type typename* { // ...

Here, *typename* is the name of the class, structure, or interface that is being split into pieces. Each part of a partial type must be modified by **partial**.

Here is an example that divides a simple XY coordinate class into three separate files. The first file is shown here:

```
partial class XY {
  public XY(int a, int b) {
    X = a;
    Y = b;
  }
}
```

The second file is shown next:

```
partial class XY {
  public int X { get; set; }
}
```

The third file is

```
partial class XY {
  public int Y { get; set; }
}
```

The following file demonstrates the use of **XY**:

```
// Demonstrate partial class definitions.
using System;
```

```
class Test {
  static void Main() {
    XY xy = new XY(1, 2);


    Console.WriteLine(xy.X + "," + xy.Y);
  }
}
```

To use **XY**, all files must be included in the compile. For example, assuming the **XY** files are called **xy1.cs**, **xy2.cs**, and **xy3.cs**, and that the **Test** class is contained in a file called **test.cs**, then to compile **Test**, use the following command line:

```
csc test.cs xy1.cs xy2.cs xy3.cs
```

One last point: It is legal to have partial generic classes. However, the type parameters of each partial declaration must match the other parts.

Partial Methods

As the preceding section described, you can use **partial** to create a partial type. Beginning with C# 3.0, there is a second use of **partial** that lets you create a *partial method* within a partial type. A partial method has its declaration in one part and its implementation in another part. Thus, in a partial class or structure, **partial** can be used to allow the declaration of a method to be separate from its implementation.

The key aspect of a partial method is that the implementation is not required! When the partial method is not implemented by another part of the class or structure, then all calls to the partial method are silently ignored. This makes it possible for a class to specify, but not require, optional functionality. If that functionality is not implemented, then it is simply ignored.

Here is an expanded version of the preceding program that creates a partial method called **Show( )**. It is called by another method called **ShowXY( )**. (For convenience, all pieces of the partial class **XY** are shown in one file, but they could have been organized into separate files, as illustrated in the preceding section.)

```
// Demonstrate a partial method.
using System;

partial class XY {
  public XY(int a, int b) {
    X = a;
    Y = b;
  }

  // Declare a partial method.
  partial void Show();
}

partial class XY {
  public int X { get; set; }
```

```
  // Implement a partial method.
  partial void Show() {
    Console.WriteLine("{0}, {1}", X, Y);
  }
}

partial class XY {
  public int Y { get; set; }

  // Call a partial method.
  public void ShowXY() {
    Show();
  }
}

class Test {
  static void Main() {
    XY xy = new XY(1, 2);

    xy.ShowXY();
  }
}
```

Notice that **Show( )** is declared in one part of **XY** and implemented by another part. The implementation displays the values of **X** and **Y**. This means that when **Show( )** is called by **ShowXY( )**, the call has effect, and it will, indeed, display **X** and **Y**. However, if you comment-out the implementation of **Show( )**, then the call to **Show( )** within **ShowXY( )** does nothing.

Partial methods have several restrictions, including these: They must return **void**. They cannot have access modifiers. They cannot be virtual. They cannot use **out** parameters.

Friend Assemblies

It is possible to make one assembly the *friend* of another. A friend has access to the private members of the assembly of which it is a friend. This feature makes it possible to share members between selected assemblies without making those members public.

To declare a friend assembly, you must specify the friend assembly's name and its public key token in an **InternalsVisibleTo** attribute.

Miscellaneous Keywords

To conclude Part I, the few remaining keywords defined by C# that have not been described elsewhere are briefly discussed.

lock

The **lock** keyword is used when creating multithreaded programs. It is examined in detail in Chapter 23, where multithreaded programming is discussed. A brief description is given here for the sake of completeness.

In C#, a program can contain more than one *thread of execution*. When this is the case, the program is said to be *multithreaded*, and pieces of the program are executed concurrently. Thus, pieces of the program execute independently and simultaneously. This raises the prospect of a special type of problem: What if two threads try to use a resource that can be used by only one thread at a time? To solve this problem, you can create a *critical code section* that will be executed by one and only one thread at a time. This is accomplished by **lock**. Its general form is shown here:

lock(*obj*) {
   // *critical section*
}

Here, *obj* is the object on which the lock is synchronized. If one thread has already entered the critical section, then a second thread will wait until the first thread exits the critical section. When the first thread leaves the critical section, the lock is released and the second thread can be granted the lock, at which point the second thread can execute the critical section.

NOTE *lock is discussed in detail in Chapter 23.*

---

readonly

You can create a read-only field in a class by declaring it as **readonly**. A **readonly** field can be given a value only by using an initializer when it is declared or by assigning it a value within a constructor. Once the value has been set, it can't be changed outside the constructor. Thus, a **readonly** field is a good way to create a fixed value that has its value set by a constructor. For example, you might use a **readonly** field to represent an array dimension that is used frequently throughout a program. Both static and non-static **readonly** fields are allowed.

NOTE *Although similar,* **readonly** *fields are not the same as* **const** *fields, which are described in the following section.*

Here is an example that creates a **readonly** field:

```
// Demonstrate readonly.

using System;

class MyClass {
  public static readonly int SIZE = 10;
}

class DemoReadOnly {
  static void Main() {
    int[] source = new int[MyClass.SIZE];
    int[] target = new int[MyClass.SIZE];

    // Give source some values.
    for(int i=0; i < MyClass.SIZE; i++)
      source[i] = i;
```

```
      foreach(int i in source)
        Console.Write(i + " ");

      Console.WriteLine();

      // Reverse copy source into target.
      for(int i = MyClass.SIZE-1, j = 0; i > 0; i--, j++)
        target[j] = source[i];

      foreach(int i in target)
        Console.Write(i + " ");

      Console.WriteLine();
//    MyClass.SIZE = 100; // Error!!! can't change
    }
}
```

Here, **MyClass.SIZE** is initialized to 10. After that, it can be used, but not changed. To prove this, try removing the comment symbol from before the last line and then compiling the program. As you will see, an error will result.

const and volatile

The **const** modifier is used to declare fields or local variables that cannot be changed. These variables must be given initial values when they are declared. Thus, a **const** variable is essentially a constant. For example,

```
const int i = 10;
```

creates a **const** variable called **i** that has the value 10. Although a **const** field is similar to a **readonly** field, the two are not the same. A **const** field cannot be set within a constructor, but a **readonly** field can.

The **volatile** modifier tells the compiler that a field's value may be changed by two or more concurrently executing threads. In this situation, one thread may not know when the field has been changed by another thread. This is important because the C# compiler will automatically perform certain optimizations that work only when a field is accessed by a single thread of execution. To prevent these optimizations from being applied to a shared field, declare it **volatile**. This tells the compiler that it must obtain the value of this field each time it is accessed.

The using Statement

In addition to the **using** *directive* discussed earlier, **using** has a second form that is called the **using** *statement*. It has these general forms:

```
using (obj) {
  // use obj
}

using (type obj = initializer) {
  // use obj
}
```

Here, *obj* is an expression that must evaluate to an object that implements the **System.IDisposable** interface. It specifies a variable that will be used inside the **using** block. In the first form, the object is declared outside the **using** statement. In the second form, the object is declared within the **using** statement. When the block concludes, the **Dispose( )** method (defined by the **System.IDisposable** interface) will be called on *obj*. **Dispose( )** is called even if the **using** block ends because of an exception. Thus, a **using** statement provides a means by which objects are automatically disposed when they are no longer needed. Remember, the **using** statement applies only to objects that implement the **System.IDisposable** interface.

Here is an example of each form of the **using** statement:

```
// Demonstrate using statement.

using System;
using System.IO;

class UsingDemo {
  static void Main() {
    try {
      StreamReader sr = new StreamReader("test.txt");

      // Use object inside using statement.
      using(sr) {
        // ...
      }
    } catch(IOException exc) {
      // ...
    }

    try {
      // Create a StreamReader inside the using statement.
      using(StreamReader sr2 = new StreamReader("test.txt")) {
        // ...
      }
    } catch(IOException exc) {
      // ...
    }
  }
}
```

The class **StreamReader** implements the **IDisposable** interface (through its base class **TextReader**). Thus, it can be used in a **using** statement. When the **using** statement ends, **Dispose( )** is automatically called on the stream variable, thus closing the stream.

As the preceding example illustrates, **using** is particularly useful when working with files because the file is automatically closed at the end of the **using** block, even if the block ends because of an exception. As a result, closing a file via **using** often simplifies file-handling code.

extern

The **extern** keyword has two uses. Each is examined here.

Declaring extern Methods

The first use of **extern** has been available since the creation of C#. It indicates that a method is provided by unmanaged code that is not part of the program. In other words, that method is supplied by external code.

To declare a method as external, simply precede its declaration with the **extern** modifier. The declaration must not include any body. Thus, the general form of an **extern** declaration is as shown here:

extern *ret-type meth-name*(*arg-list*);

Notice that no braces are used.

In this use, **extern** is often used with the **DllImport** attribute, which specifies the DLL that contains the method. **DllImport** is in the **System.Runtime.InteropServices** namespace. It supports several options, but for most uses, it is sufficient to simply specify the name of the DLL that contains the **extern** method. In general, **extern** methods should be coded in C. (If you use C++, then the name of the method within the DLL might be altered with the addition of type decorations.)

To best understand how to use **extern** methods, it is helpful to work through an example. The example consists of two files. The first is the C file shown here, which defines a method called **AbsMax( )**. Call this file **ExtMeth.c**.

```
#include <stdlib.h>

int __declspec(dllexport) AbsMax(int a, int b) {
  return abs(a) < abs(b) ? abs(b) : abs(a);
}
```

The **AbsMax( )** method compares the absolute values of its two parameters and returns the maximum. Notice the use of **__declspec(dllexport)**. This is a Microsoft-specific extension to the C language that tells the compiler to export the **AbsMax( )** method within the DLL that contains it. You must use this command line to compile **ExtMeth.c**.

```
CL /LD /MD ExtMeth.c
```

This creates a DLL file called **ExtMeth.dll**.

Next is a program that uses **AbsMax( )**:

```
using System;
using System.Runtime.InteropServices;

class ExternMeth {

  // Here an extern method is declared.
  [DllImport("ExtMeth.dll")]
  public extern static int AbsMax(int a, int b);

  static void Main() {

    // Use the extern method.
```

```
    int max = AbsMax(-10, -20);
    Console.WriteLine(max);

  }
}
```

Notice the use of the **DllImport** attribute. It tells the compiler what DLL contains the **extern** method **AbsMax( )**. In this case, the file is **ExtMeth.dll**, which is the file DLL created when the C file was compiled. When the program is run, the value 20 is displayed, as expected.

Declaring an extern Assembly Alias

A second form of **extern** (which was added by C# 2.0) provides an alias for an external assembly. It is used in cases in which a program includes two separate assemblies that both contain the same name. For example, if an assembly called **test1** contains a class called **MyClass** and **test2** also contains a class called **MyClass**, then a conflict will arise if both classes need to be used within the same program.

To solve this problem, you must create an alias for each assembly. This is a two-step process. First, you must specify the aliases using the **/r** compiler option. For example:

```
/r:Asm1=test1
/r:Asm2=test2
```

Second, you must specify **extern** statements that refer to these aliases. Here is the form of **extern** that creates an assembly alias:

extern alias *assembly-name*;

Continuing the example, these lines must appear in your program:

```
extern alias Asm1;
extern alias Asm2;
```

Now, either version of **MyClass** can be accessed by qualifying it with its alias.

Here is a complete example that demonstrates an **extern** alias. It contains three files. The first is shown here. It should be put in a file called **test1.cs**.

```
using System;

namespace MyNS {
  public class MyClass {
    public MyClass() {
      Console.WriteLine("Constructing from MyClass1.dll.");
    }
  }
}
```

The second file is called **test2.cs**. It is shown here:

```
using System;

namespace MyNS {
  public class MyClass {
    public MyClass() {
      Console.WriteLine("Constructing from MyClass2.dll.");
```

```
     }
   }
}
```

Notice that both **test1.cs** and **test2.cs** define a namespace called **MyNS**, and that within that namespace, both files define a class called **MyClass**. Thus, without an **extern** alias, no program could have access to both versions of **MyClass**.

The third file, **test3.cs**, which is shown next, uses **MyClass** from both **test1.cs** and **test2.cs**. It is able to do this because of the **extern** alias statements.

```
// extern alias statements must be at the top of the file.
extern alias Asm1;
extern alias Asm2;

using System;

class Demo {
  static void Main() {
    Asm1::MyNS.MyClass t = new Asm1::MyNS.MyClass();
    Asm2::MyNS.MyClass t2 = new Asm2::MyNS.MyClass();
  }
}
```

Start by compiling **test1.cs** and **test2.cs** into DLLs. This can be easily done from the command line by using these commands:

```
csc /t:library test1.cs
csc /t:library test2.cs
```

Next, compile **test3.cs** by using this command line:

```
csc /r:Asm1=test1.dll /r:Asm2=test2.dll test3.cs
```

Notice the use of the **/r** option, which tells the compiler to reference the metadata found in the associated file. In this case, the alias **Asm1** is linked with **test1.dll** and the alias **Asm2** is linked with **test2.dll**.

Within the program, the aliases are specified by these two **extern** statements at the top of the file:

```
extern alias Asm1;
extern alias Asm2;
```

Within **Main( )**, the aliases are used to disambiguate the references to **MyClass**. Notice how the alias is used to refer to **MyClass**:

```
Asm1::MyNS.MyClass
```

The alias is specified first, followed by the namespace resolution operator, followed by the name of the namespace that contains the ambiguous class, followed by the dot operator and the class name. This same general form works with other **extern** aliases.

The output from the program is shown here:

```
Constructing from MyClass1.dll.
Constructing from MyClass2.dll.
```

PART

II

Exploring the C# Library

Part II explores the C# library. As explained in Part I, the class library used by C# is the .NET Framework class library. As a result, the material in this section applies not only to C#, but to the .NET Framework as a whole.

The .NET Framework class library is organized into namespaces. To use a portion of the library, you will normally import its namespace by including a **using** directive. Of course, you can also fully qualify the name of the item with its namespace name, but most often, it is simply easier to import the entire namespace.

The .NET library is very large, and it is beyond the scope of this book to examine each part of it. (A complete description would easily fill a very large book!) Instead, Part II examines the core elements of the library, many of which are contained in the **System** namespace. Also discussed are the collection classes, multithreading, and networking.

NOTE *The I/O classes are discussed in Chapter 14.*

Exploring the System Namespace

This chapter explores the **System** namespace. **System** is a top-level namespace of the .NET Framework class library. It directly contains those classes, structures, interfaces, delegates, and enumerations that are most commonly used by a C# program or that are deemed otherwise integral to the .NET Framework. Thus, **System** defines the core of the library.

    System also contains many nested namespaces that support specific subsystems, such as **System.Net**. Several of these subsystems are described later in this book. This chapter is concerned only with the members of **System**, itself.

The Members of System

In addition to a large number of exception classes, **System** contains the following classes:

ActivationContext	Activator	AppDomain
AppDomainManager	AppDomainSetup	ApplicationId
ApplicationIdentity	Array	AssemblyLoadEventArgs
Attribute	AttributeUsageAttribute	BitConverter
Buffer	CharEnumerator	CLSCompliantAttribute
Console	ConsoleCancelEventArgs	ContextBoundObject
ContextStaticAttribute	Convert	DBNull
Delegate	Enum	Environment
EventArgs	Exception	FileStyleUriParser
FlagsAttribute	FtpStyleUriParser	GC
GenericUriParser	GopherStyleUriParser	HttpStyleUriParser
LdapStyleUriParser	LoaderOptimizationAttribute	LocalDataStoreSlot
MarshalByRefObject	Math	MTAThreadAttribute
MulticastDelegate	NetPipeStyleUriParser	NetTcpStyleUriParser

NewsStyleUriParser	NonSerializedAttribute	Nullable
Object	ObsoleteAttribute	OperatingSystem
ParamArrayAttribute	Random	ResolveEventArgs
SerializableAttribute	STAThreadAttribute	String
StringComparer	ThreadStaticAttribute	TimeZone
TimeZoneInfo	TimeZoneInfo.AdjustmentRule	Type
UnhandledExceptionEventArgs	Uri	UriBuilder
UriParser	UriTemplate	UriTemplateEquivalenceComparer
UriTemplateTable	UriTypeConverter	ValueType
Version	WeakReference	

System defines the following structures:

ArgIterator	ArraySegment<T>	Boolean
Byte	Char	ConsoleKeyInfo
DateTime	DateTimeOffset	Decimal
Double	Guid	Int16
Int32	Int64	IntPtr
ModuleHandle	Nullable<T>	RuntimeArgumentHandle
RuntimeFieldHandle	RuntimeMethodHandle	RuntimeTypeHandle
Sbyte	Single	TimeSpan
TimeZoneInfo.TransitionTime	TypedReference	UInt16
UInt32	UInt64	UIntPtr
Void		

System defines the following interfaces:

_AppDomain	IAppDomainSetup	IAsyncResult
ICloneable	IComparable	IComparable<T>
IConvertible	ICustomFormatter	IDisposable
IEquatable<T>	IFormatProvider	IFormattable
IServiceProvider		

System defines the following delegates:

Action	Action<T>	Action<T1, T2>
Action<T1, T2, T3>	Action<T1, T2, T3, T4>	AppDomainInitializer
AssemblyLoadEventHandler	AsyncCallback	Comparison<T>
ConsoleCancelEventHandler	Converter<T, V>	CrossAppDomainDelegate
EventHandler	EventHandler<T>	Func<TResult>
Func<T, TResult>	Func<T1, T2, TResult>	Func<T1, T2, T3, TResult>
Func<T1, T2, T3. T4, TResult>	Predicate<T>	ResolveEventHandler
UnhandledExceptionEventHandler		

System defines these enumerations:

ActivationContext.contextForm	AppDomainManagerInitializationOptions	AttributeTargets
Base64FormattingOptions	ConsoleColor	ConsoleKey
ConsoleModifiers	ConsoleSpecialKey	DateTimeKind
DayOfWeek	Environment.SpecialFolder	EnvironmentVariableTarget
GCCollectionMode	GenericUriParserOptions	LoaderOptimization
MidpointRounding	PlatformID	StringComparison
StringSplitOptions	TypeCode	UriComponents
UriFormat	UriHostNameType	UriIdnScope
UriKind	UriPartial	

As the preceding tables show, **System** is quite large. It is not possible to examine all of its constituents in detail in a single chapter. Furthermore, several of **System**'s members, such as **Nullable<T>**, **Type**, **Exception**, and **Attribute**, are discussed in Part I or elsewhere in Part II. Finally, because **System.String**, which defines the C# **string** type, is such a large and important topic, it is covered in Chapter 22 along with formatting. For these reasons, this chapter explores only those members that are most commonly used by C# programmers and that are not fully covered elsewhere.

The Math Class

Math defines several standard mathematical operations, such as square root, sine, cosine, and logarithms. The **Math** class is **static**, which means all of the methods defined by **Math** are **static** and no object of type **Math** can be constructed. It also means **Math** is implicitly sealed and cannot be inherited. The methods defined by **Math** are shown in Table 21-1. All angles are in radians.

Math also defines these two fields:

public const double E
public const double PI

E is the value of the natural logarithm base, commonly referred to as *e*. **PI** is the value of pi.

Method	Meaning
public static double Abs(double *v*)	Returns the absolute value of *v*.
public static float Abs(float *v*)	Returns the absolute value of *v*.
public static decimal Abs(decimal *v*)	Returns the absolute value of *v*.
public static int Abs(int *v*)	Returns the absolute value of *v*.
public static short Abs(short *v*)	Returns the absolute value of *v*.
public static long Abs(long *v*)	Returns the absolute value of *v*.
public static sbyte Abs(sbyte *v*)	Returns the absolute value of *v*.
public static double Acos(double *v*)	Returns the arc cosine of *v*. The value of *v* must be between –1 and 1.
public static double Asin(double *v*)	Returns the arc sine of *v*. The value of *v* must be between –1 and 1.
public static double Atan(double *v*)	Returns the arc tangent of *v*.
public static double Atan2(double *y*, double *x*)	Returns the arc tangent of *y*/*x*.
public static long BigMul(int *x*, int *y*)	Returns the result of *x* * *y* as a **long** value, thus avoiding overflow.
public static double Ceiling(double *v*)	Returns the smallest integer (represented as a floating-point value) not less than *v*. For example, given 1.02, **Ceiling( )** returns 2.0. Given –1.02, **Ceiling( )** returns –1.
public static double Ceiling(decimal *v*)	Returns the smallest integer (represented as a decimal value) not less than *v*. For example, given 1.02, **Ceiling( )** returns 2.0. Given –1.02, **Ceiling( )** returns –1.
public static double Cos(double *v*)	Returns the cosine of *v*.
public static double Cosh(double *v*)	Returns the hyperbolic cosine of *v*.
public static int DivRem(int *x*, int *y*, out int *rem*)	Return the result of *x* / *y*. The remainder is returned in *rem*.
public static long DivRem(long *x*, long *y*, out long *rem*)	Return the result of *x* / *y*. The remainder is returned in *rem*.
public static double Exp(double *v*)	Returns the natural logarithm base *e* raised to the *v* power.
public static decimal Floor(decimal *v*)	Returns the largest integer (represented as a decimal value) not greater than *v*. For example, given 1.02, **Floor( )** returns 1.0. Given –1.02, **Floor( )** returns –2.

TABLE 21-1 Methods Defined by **Math**

Method	Meaning
public static double Floor(double *v*)	Returns the largest integer (represented as a floating-point value) not greater than *v*. For example, given 1.02, **Floor( )** returns 1.0. Given –1.02, **Floor( )** returns –2.
public static double IEEERemainder(double *dividend*, double *divisor*)	Returns the remainder of *dividend / divisor*.
public static double Log(double *v*)	Returns the natural logarithm for *v*.
public static double Log(double *v*, double *base*)	Returns the logarithm for *v* using base *base*.
public static double Log10(double *v*)	Returns the base 10 logarithm for *v*.
public static double Max(double *v1*, double *v2*)	Returns the greater of *v1* and *v2*.
public static float Max(float *v1*, float *v2*)	Returns the greater of *v1* and *v2*.
public static decimal Max(decimal *v1*, decimal *v2*)	Returns the greater of *v1* and *v2*.
public static int Max(int *v1*, int *v2*)	Returns the greater of *v1* and *v2*.
public static short Max(short *v1*, short *v2*)	Returns the greater of *v1* and *v2*.
public static long Max(long *v1*, long *v2*)	Returns the greater of *v1* and *v2*.
public static uint Max(uint *v1*, uint *v2*)	Returns the greater of *v1* and *v2*.
public static ushort Max(ushort *v1*, ushort *v2*)	Returns the greater of *v1* and *v2*.
public static ulong Max(ulong *v1*, ulong *v2*)	Returns the greater of *v1* and *v2*.
public static byte Max(byte *v1*, byte *v2*)	Returns the greater of *v1* and *v2*.
public static sbyte Max(sbyte *v1*, sbyte *v2*)	Returns the greater of *v1* and *v2*.
public static double Min(double *v1*, double *v2*)	Returns the lesser of *v1* and *v2*.
public static float Min(float *v1*, float *v2*)	Returns the lesser of *v1* and *v2*.
public static decimal Min(decimal *v1*, decimal *v2*)	Returns the lesser of *v1* and *v2*.
public static int Min(int *v1*, int *v2*)	Returns the lesser of *v1* and *v2*.
public static short Min(short *v1*, short *v2*)	Returns the lesser of *v1* and *v2*.
public static long Min(long *v1*, long *v2*)	Returns the lesser of *v1* and *v2*.
public static uint Min(uint *v1*, uint *v2*)	Returns the lesser of *v1* and *v2*.
public static ushort Min(ushort *v1*, ushort *v2*)	Returns the lesser of *v1* and *v2*.

TABLE 21-1 Methods Defined by **Math** *(continued)*

Method	Meaning
public static ulong Min(ulong *v1*, ulong *v2*)	Returns the lesser of *v1* and *v2*.
public static byte Min(byte *v1*, byte *v2*)	Returns the lesser of *v1* and *v2*.
public static sbyte Min(sbyte *v1*, sbyte *v2*)	Returns the lesser of *v1* and *v2*.
public static double Pow(double *base*, double *exp*)	Returns *base* raised to the *exp* power($base^{exp}$).
public static double Round(double *v*)	Returns *v* rounded to the nearest whole number.
public static decimal Round(decimal *v*)	Returns *v* rounded to the nearest whole number.
public static double Round(double *v*, int *frac*)	Returns *v* rounded to the number of fractional digits specified by *frac*.
public static decimal Round(decimal *v*, int *frac*)	Returns *v* rounded to the number of fractional digits specified by *frac*.
public static double Round(double *v*, MidpointRounding *how*)	Returns *v* rounded to the nearest whole number using the rounding mode specified by *how*.
public static decimal Round(decimal *v*, MidpointRounding *how*)	Returns *v* rounded to the nearest whole number using the rounding mode specified by *how*.
public static double Round(double *v*, int *frac*, MidpointRounding *how*)	Returns *v* rounded to the number of fractional digits specified by *frac*. It uses the rounding mode specified by *how*.
public static decimal Round(decimal *v*, int *frac*, MidpointRounding *how*)	Returns *v* rounded to the number of fractional digits specified by *frac*. It uses the rounding mode specified by *how*.
public static int Sign(double *v*)	Returns −1 if *v* is less than zero, 0 if *v* is zero, and 1 if *v* is greater than zero.
public static int Sign(float *v*)	Returns −1 if *v* is less than zero, 0 if *v* is zero, and 1 if *v* is greater than zero.
public static int Sign(decimal *v*)	Returns −1 if *v* is less than zero, 0 if *v* is zero, and 1 if *v* is greater than zero.
public static int Sign(int *v*)	Returns −1 if *v* is less than zero, 0 if *v* is zero, and 1 if *v* is greater than zero.
public static int Sign(short *v*)	Returns −1 if *v* is less than zero, 0 if *v* is zero, and 1 if *v* is greater than zero.
public static int Sign(long *v*)	Returns −1 if *v* is less than zero, 0 if *v* is zero, and 1 if *v* is greater than zero.
public static int Sign(sbyte *v*)	Returns −1 if *v* is less than zero, 0 if *v* is zero, and 1 if *v* is greater than zero.
public static double Sin(double *v*)	Returns the sine of *v*.
public static double Sinh(double *v*)	Returns the hyperbolic sine of *v*.

TABLE 21-1 Methods Defined by **Math** *(continued)*

Method	Meaning
public static double Sqrt(double *v*)	Returns the square root of *v*.
public static double Tan(double *v*)	Returns the tangent of *v*.
public static double Tanh(double *v*)	Returns the hyperbolic tangent of *v*.
public static double Truncate(double *v*)	Returns the whole number portion of *v*.
public static decimal Truncate(decimal *v*)	Returns the whole number portion of *v*.

TABLE 21-1   Methods Defined by **Math** *(continued)*

Here is an example that uses **Sqrt( )** to help implement the Pythagorean theorem. It computes the length of the hypotenuse given the lengths of the two opposing sides of a right triangle.

```
// Implement the Pythagorean Theorem.

using System;

class Pythagorean {
  static void Main() {
    double s1;
    double s2;
    double hypot;
    string str;

    Console.WriteLine("Enter length of first side: ");
    str = Console.ReadLine();
    s1 = Double.Parse(str);

    Console.WriteLine("Enter length of second side: ");
    str = Console.ReadLine();
    s2 = Double.Parse(str);

    hypot = Math.Sqrt(s1*s1 + s2*s2);

    Console.WriteLine("Hypotenuse is " + hypot);
  }
}
```

Here is a sample run:

```
Enter length of first side: 3
Enter length of second side: 4
Hypotenuse is 5
```

Next is an example that uses the **Pow( )** method to compute the initial investment required to achieve a desired future value given the annual rate of return and the number of years. The formula to compute the initial investment is shown here:

$$InitialInvestment = FutureValue / (1 + InterestRate)^{Years}$$

Because **Pow( )** requires **double** arguments, the interest rate and the number of years are held in **double** values. The future value and initial investment use the **decimal** type.

```
/* Compute the initial investment needed to attain
   a known future value given annual rate of return
   and the time period in years. */

using System;

class InitialInvestment {
  static void Main() {
    decimal initInvest; // initial investment
    decimal futVal;     // future value

    double numYears;    // number of years
    double intRate;     // annual rate of return as a decimal

    string str;

    Console.Write("Enter future value: ");
    str = Console.ReadLine();
    try {
      futVal = Decimal.Parse(str);
    } catch(FormatException exc) {
      Console.WriteLine(exc.Message);
      return;
    }

    Console.Write("Enter interest rate (such as 0.085): ");
    str = Console.ReadLine();
    try {
      intRate = Double.Parse(str);
    } catch(FormatException exc) {
      Console.WriteLine(exc.Message);
      return;
    }

    Console.Write("Enter number of years: ");
    str = Console.ReadLine();
    try {
      numYears = Double.Parse(str);
    } catch(FormatException exc) {
      Console.WriteLine(exc.Message);
      return;
    }

    initInvest = futVal / (decimal) Math.Pow(intRate+1.0, numYears);

    Console.WriteLine("Initial investment required: {0:C}",
                      initInvest);
  }
}
```

Here is a sample run:

```
Enter future value: 10000
Enter interest rate (such as 0.085): 0.07
Enter number of years: 10
Initial investment required: $5,083.49
```

The .NET Structures Corresponding to the Built-in Value Types

The structures that correspond to C#'s built-in value types were introduced in Chapter 14 when they were used to convert strings holding human-readable numeric values into their equivalent binary values. Here these structures are examined in detail.

The .NET structure names and their C# keyword equivalents are shown in the following table:

.NET Structure Name	C# Name
System.Boolean	bool
System.Char	char
System.Decimal	decimal
System.Double	double
System.Single	float
System.Int16	short
System.Int32	int
System.Int64	long
System.UInt16	ushort
System.UInt32	uint
System.UInt64	ulong
System.Byte	byte
System.SByte	sbyte

By using the members defined by these structures, you can perform operations relating to the value types. The following sections examine each of these structures.

NOTE *Some methods defined by the structures that correspond to the built-in value types take a parameter of type **IFormatProvider** or **NumberStyles**. **IFormatProvider** is briefly described later in this chapter. **NumberStyles** is an enumeration found in the **System.Globalization** namespace. The topic of formatting is discussed in Chapter 22.*

The Integer Structures

The integer structures are

Byte	SByte	Int16	UInt16
Int32	UInt32	Int64	UInt64

Each of these structures contains the same methods. They are shown in Table 21-2. The only difference from structure to structure is the return type of **Parse( )**. For each structure, **Parse( )** returns a value of the type represented by the structure. For example, for **Int32**, **Parse( )** returns an **int** value. For **UInt16**, **Parse( )** returns a **ushort** value. For an example that demonstrates **Parse( )**, see Chapter 14.

In addition to the methods shown in Table 21-2, the integer structures also define the following **const** fields:

MaxValue
MinValue

For each structure, these fields contain the largest and smallest value that type of integer can hold.

All of the integer structures implement the following interfaces: **IComparable**, **IComparable<T>**, **IConvertible**, **IFormattable**, and **IEquatable<T>**, where **T** is replaced by the corresponding data type. For example, **T** will be replaced with **int** for **Int32**.

Method	Meaning
public int CompareTo(object *v*)	Compares the numerical value of the invoking object with that of *v*. Returns zero if the values are equal. Returns a negative value if the invoking object has a lower value. Returns a positive value if the invoking object has a greater value.
public int CompareTo(*type v*)	Compares the numerical value of the invoking object with that of *v*. Returns zero if the values are equal. Returns a negative value if the invoking object has a lower value. Returns a positive value if the invoking object has a greater value. In this version of **CompareTo( )**, *type* explicitly specifies the data type, such as in **System.Int32.CompareTo(int *v*)**.
public override bool Equals(object *v*)	Returns true if the value of the invoking object equals the value of *v*.
public bool Equals(*type v*)	Returns true if the value of the invoking object equals the value of *v*. In this version of **Equals( )**, *type* explicitly specifies the data type, such as in **System.Int32.Equals(int *v*)**.
public override int GetHashCode( )	Returns the hash code for the invoking object.
public TypeCode GetTypeCode( )	Returns the **TypeCode** enumeration value for the equivalent value type. For example, for **Int32**, the type code is **TypeCode.Int32**.
public static *retType* Parse(string *str*)	Returns the binary equivalent of the numeric string in *str*. If the string does not represent a numeric value as defined by the structure type, an exception is thrown. *retType* is a placeholder for the actual type of data returned based on which numeric structure is used. For example, for **Int32**, *retType* will be **int**.

TABLE 21-2 Methods Supported by the Integer Structures

Method	Meaning

public static *retType*
    Parse(string *str*,
        IFormatProvider *fmtpvdr*)
	Returns the binary equivalent of the numeric string in *str* using the culture-specific information provided by *fmtpvdr*. If the string does not represent a numeric value as defined by the structure type, an exception is thrown. *retType* is a placeholder for the actual type of data returned based on which numeric structure is used. For example, for **Int32**, *retType* will be **int**.

public static *retType* Parse(string *str*, NumberStyles *styles*)	Returns the binary equivalent of the numeric string in *str* using the style information provided by *styles*. If the string does not represent a numeric value as defined by the structure type, an exception is thrown. *retType* is a placeholder for the actual type of data returned based on which numeric structure is used. For example, for **Int32**, *retType* will be **int**.

public static *retType*
    Parse(string *str*, NumberStyles *styles*,
        IFormatProvider *fmtpvdr*)
	Returns the binary equivalent of the numeric string in *str* using the style information provided by *styles* and the culture-specific format information provided by *fmtpvdr*. If the string does not represent a numeric value as defined by structure type, an exception is thrown. *retType* is a placeholder for the actual type of data returned based on which numeric structure is used. For example, for **Int32**, *retType* will be **int**.

public override string ToString( )	Returns the string representation of the value of the invoking object.
public string ToString(string *format*)	Returns the string representation of the value of the invoking object as specified by the format string passed in *format*.
public string ToString(IFormatProvider *fmtpvdr*)	Returns the string representation of the value of the invoking object using the culture-specific information specified in *fmtpvdr*.

public string
    ToString(string *format*,
        IFormatProvider *fmtpvdr*)
	Returns the string representation of the value of the invoking object using the culture-specific information specified in *fmtpvdr* and the format specified by *format*.

public static bool TryParse(string *str*, out *type val*)	Attempts to convert the numeric string in *str* into a binary value. If successful, the value is stored in *val* and true is returned. If no conversion takes place, false is returned. This differs from **Parse( )**, which throws an exception on failure. In **TryParse( )**, *type* explicitly specifies the data type, such as in **System.Int32.TryParse(int v)**.

TABLE 21-2   Methods Supported by the Integer Structures *(continued)*

Method	Meaning
public static bool TryParse(string *str*, NumberStyles *styles*, IFormatProvider *fmtpvdr*, out *type val*)	Attempts to convert the numeric string in *str* into a binary value using the style information provided by *styles* and the culture-specific format information provided by *fmtpvdr*. If successful, the value is stored in *val* and true is returned. If no conversion takes place, false is returned. This differs from **Parse( )**, which throws an exception on failure. In **TryParse( )**, *type* explicitly specifies the data type, such as in **System.Int32.TryParse(int *v*)**.

TABLE 21-2   Methods Supported by the Integer Structures *(continued)*

The Floating-Point Structures

There are two floating-point structures: **Double** and **Single**. **Single** represents **float**. Its methods are shown in Table 21-3, and its fields are shown in Table 21-4. **Double** represents **double**. Its methods are shown in Table 21-5, and its fields are shown in Table 21-6. As is the case with the integer structures, you can specify culture-specific information and format information in a call to **Parse( )** or **ToString( )**.

The floating-point structures implement the following interfaces: **IComparable**, **IComparable<T>**, **IConvertible**, **IFormattable**, and **IEquatable<T>**, where **T** is replaced by either **double** for **Double** or **float** for **Single**.

Method	Meaning
public int CompareTo(object *v*)	Compares the numerical value of the invoking object with that of *v*. Returns zero if the values are equal. Returns a negative value if the invoking object has a lower value. Returns a positive value if the invoking object has a greater value.
public int CompareTo(float *v*)	Compares the numerical value of the invoking object with that of *v*. Returns zero if the values are equal. Returns a negative value if the invoking object has a lower value. Returns a positive value if the invoking object has a greater value.
public override bool Equals(object *v*)	Returns true if the value of the invoking object equals the value of *v*.
public bool Equals(float *v*)	Returns true if the value of the invoking object equals the value of *v*.
public override int GetHashCode( )	Returns the hash code for the invoking object.
public TypeCode GetTypeCode( )	Returns the **TypeCode** enumeration value for **Single**, which is **TypeCode.Single**.
public static bool IsInfinity(float *v*)	Returns true if *v* represents infinity (either positive or negative). Otherwise, returns false.
public static bool IsNaN(float *v*)	Returns true if *v* is not a number. Otherwise, returns false.

TABLE 21-3   Methods Supported by **Single**

Method	Meaning
public static bool IsPositiveInfinity(float *v*)	Returns true if *v* represents positive infinity. Otherwise, returns false.
public static bool IsNegativeInfinity(float *v*)	Returns true if *v* represents negative infinity. Otherwise, returns false.
public static float Parse(string *str*)	Returns the binary equivalent of the numeric string in *str*. If the string does not represent a **float** value, an exception is thrown.
public static float Parse(string *str*, IFormatProvider *fmtpvdr*)	Returns the binary equivalent of the numeric string in *str* using the culture-specific information provided by *fmtpvdr*. If the string does not represent a **float** value, an exception is thrown.
public static float Parse(string *str*, NumberStyles *styles*)	Returns the binary equivalent of the numeric string in *str* using the style information provided by *styles*. If the string does not represent a **float** value, an exception is thrown.
public static float Parse(string *str*, NumberStyles *styles*, IFormatProvider *fmtpvdr*)	Returns the binary equivalent of the numeric string in *str* using the style information provided by *styles* and the culture-specific format information provided by *fmtpvdr*. If the string does not represent a **float** value, an exception is thrown.
public override string ToString( )	Returns the string representation of the value of the invoking object in the default format.
public string ToString(string *format*)	Returns the string representation of the value of the invoking object as specified by the format string passed in *format*.
public string ToString(IFormatProvider *fmtpvdr*)	Returns the string representation of the value of the invoking object using the culture-specific information specified in *fmtpvdr*.
public string ToString(string *format*, IFormatProvider *fmtpvdr*)	Returns the string representation of the value of the invoking object using the culture-specific information specified in *fmtpvdr* and the format specified by *format*.
public static bool TryParse(string *str*, out float *val*)	Attempts to convert the numeric string in *str* into a **float** value. If successful, the value is stored in *val* and true is returned. If no conversion takes place, false is returned. This differs from **Parse( )**, which throws an exception on failure.
public static bool TryParse(string *str*, NumberStyles *styles*, IFormatProvider *fmtpvdr*, out float *val*)	Attempts to convert the numeric string in *str* into a **float** value using the style information provided by *styles* and the culture-specific format information provided by *fmtpvdr*. If successful, the value is stored in *val* and **true** is returned. If no conversion takes place, **false** is returned. This differs from **Parse( )**, which throws an exception on failure.

PART II

TABLE 21-3   Methods Supported by **Single** (*continued*)

Field	Meaning
public const float Epsilon	The smallest non-zero positive value.
public const float MaxValue	The largest value that a **float** can hold.
public const float MinValue	The smallest value that a **float** can hold.
public const float NaN	A value that is not a number.
public const float NegativeInfinity	A value representing negative infinity.
public const float PositiveInfinity	A value representing positive infinity.

TABLE 21-4 Fields Supported by **Single**

Method	Meaning
public int CompareTo(object v)	Compares the numerical value of the invoking object with that of v. Returns zero if the values are equal. Returns a negative value if the invoking object has a lower value. Returns a positive value if the invoking object has a greater value.
public int CompareTo(double v)	Compares the numerical value of the invoking object with that of v. Returns zero if the values are equal. Returns a negative value if the invoking object has a lower value. Returns a positive value if the invoking object has a greater value.
public override bool Equals(object v)	Returns true if the value of the invoking object equals the value of v.
public bool Equals(double v)	Returns true if the value of the invoking object equals the value of v.
public override int GetHashCode( )	Returns the hash code for the invoking object.
public TypeCode GetTypeCode( )	Returns the **TypeCode** enumeration value for **Double**, which is **TypeCode.Double**.
public static bool IsInfinity(double v)	Returns true if v represents infinity (either positive or negative). Otherwise, returns false.
public static bool IsNaN(double v)	Returns true if v is not a number. Otherwise, returns false.
public static bool IsPositiveInfinity(double v)	Returns true if v represents positive infinity. Otherwise, returns false.
public static bool IsNegativeInfinity(double v)	Returns true if v represents negative infinity. Otherwise, returns false.
public static double Parse(string str)	Returns the binary equivalent of the numeric string in str. If the string does not represent a **double** value, an exception is thrown.

TABLE 21-5 Methods Supported by **Double**

Method	Meaning

public static double
    Parse(string *str*,
        IFormatProvider *fmtpvdr*)
	Returns the binary equivalent of the numeric string in *str* using the culture-specific information provided by *fmtpvdr*. If the string does not represent a **double** value, an exception is thrown.

public static double Parse(string *str*, NumberStyles *styles*)	Returns the binary equivalent of the numeric string in *str* using the style information provided by *styles*. If the string does not represent a **double** value, an exception is thrown.

public static double
    Parse(string *str*,
        NumberStyles *styles*,
        IFormatProvider *fmtpvdr*)
	Returns the binary equivalent of the numeric string in *str* using the style information provided by *styles* and the culture-specific format information provided by *fmtpvdr*. If the string does not represent a **double** value, an exception is thrown.

public override string ToString( )	Returns the string representation of the value of the invoking object in the default format.
public string ToString(string *format*)	Returns the string representation of the value of the invoking object as specified by the format string passed in *format*.
public string ToString(IFormatProvider *fmtpvdr*)	Returns the string representation of the value of the invoking object using the culture-specific information specified in *fmtpvdr*.

public string
    ToString(string *format*,
        IFormatProvider *fmtpvdr*)
	Returns the string representation of the value of the invoking object using the culture-specific information specified in *fmtpvdr* and the format specified by *format*.

public static bool TryParse(string *str*, out double *val*)	Attempts to convert the numeric string in *str* into a **double** value. If successful, the value is stored in *val* and true is returned. If no conversion takes place, false is returned. This differs from **Parse( )**, which throws an exception on failure.

public static bool TryParse(string *str*,
            NumberStyles *styles*,
            IFormatProvider *fmtpvdr*,
            out double *val*)
	Attempts to convert the numeric string in *str* into a **double** value using the style information provided by *styles* and the culture-specific format information provided by *fmtpvdr*. If successful, the value is stored in *val* and true is returned. If no conversion takes place, false is returned. This differs from **Parse( )**, which throws an exception on failure.

TABLE 21-5   Methods Supported by **Double** *(continued)*

PART II

Field	Meaning
public const double Epsilon	The smallest non-zero positive value.
public const double MaxValue	The largest value that a **double** can hold.
public const double MinValue	The smallest value that a **double** can hold.
public const double NaN	A value that is not a number.
public const double NegativeInfinity	A value representing negative infinity.
public const double PositiveInfinity	A value representing positive infinity.

TABLE 21-6 Fields Supported by **Double**

Decimal

The **Decimal** structure is a bit more complicated than its integer and floating-point relatives. It contains many constructors, fields, methods, and operators that help integrate **decimal** with the other numeric types supported by C#. For example, several of the methods provide conversions between **decimal** and the other numeric types.

Decimal offers eight public constructors. The following six are the most commonly used:

public Decimal(int v)
public Decimal(uint v)
public Decimal(long v)
public Decimal(ulong v)
public Decimal(float v)
public Decimal(double v)

Each constructs a **Decimal** from the specified value.

You can also construct a **Decimal** by specifying its constituent parts using this constructor:

public Decimal(int *low*, int *middle*, int *high*, bool *signFlag*, byte *scaleFactor*)

A decimal value consists of three parts. The first is a 96-bit integer, the second is a sign flag, and the third is a scaling factor. The 96-bit integer is passed in 32-bit chunks through *low*, *middle*, and *high*. The sign is passed through *signFlag*, which is **false** for a positive number and **true** for a negative number. The scaling factor is passed in *scaleFactor*, which must be a value between 0 and 28. This factor specifies the power of 10 (that is, $10^{scaleFactor}$) by which the number is divided, thus yielding its fractional component.

Instead of passing each component separately, you can specify the constituents of a **Decimal** in an array of integers, using this constructor:

public Decimal(int[ ] *parts*)

The first three **int**s in *parts* contain the 96-bit integer value. In *parts*[3], bit 31 specifies the sign flag (0 for positive, 1 for negative), and bits 16 through 23 contain the scale factor.

Decimal implements the following interfaces: **IComparable**, **IComparable<decimal>**, **IConvertible**, **IFormattable**, and **IEquatable<decimal>**.

Here is an example that constructs a **decimal** value by hand:

```
// Manually create a decimal number.
```

```
using System;

class CreateDec {
  static void Main() {
    decimal d = new decimal(12345, 0, 0, false, 2);

    Console.WriteLine(d);
  }
}
```

The output is shown here:

```
123.45
```

In this example, the value of the 96-bit integer is 12345. Its sign is positive, and it has two decimal fractions.

The methods defined by **Decimal** are shown in Table 21-7. The fields defined by **Decimal** are shown in Table 21-8. **Decimal** also defines a large number of operators and conversions that allow **decimal** values to be used in expressions with other numeric types. The rules governing the use of **decimal** in expressions and assignments are described in Chapter 3.

Method	Meaning
public static decimal Add(decimal *v1*, decimal *v2*)	Returns *v1* + *v2*.
public static decimal Ceiling(decimal *v*)	Returns the smallest integer (represented as a **decimal** value) not less than *v*. For example, given 1.02, **Ceiling( )** returns 2.0. Given –1.02, **Ceiling( )** returns –1.
public static int Compare(decimal *v1*, decimal *v2*)	Compares the numerical value of *v1* with that of *v2*. Returns zero if the values are equal. Returns a negative value if *v1* is less than *v2*. Returns a positive value if *v1* is greater than *v2*.
public int CompareTo(object *v*)	Compares the numerical value of the invoking object with that of *v*. Returns zero if the values are equal. Returns a negative value if the invoking object has a lower value. Returns a positive value if the invoking object has a greater value.
public int CompareTo(decimal *v*)	Compares the numerical value of the invoking object with that of *v*. Returns zero if the values are equal. Returns a negative value if the invoking object has a lower value. Returns a positive value if the invoking object has a greater value.
public static decimal Divide(decimal *v1*, decimal *v2*)	Returns *v1* / *v2*.
public bool Equals(decimal *v*)	Returns true if the value of the invoking object equals the value of *v*.

TABLE 21-7   Methods Defined by **Decimal**

Method	Meaning
public override bool Equals(object *v*)	Returns true if the value of the invoking object equals the value of *v*.
public static bool Equals(decimal *v1*, decimal *v2*)	Returns true if *v1* equals *v2*.
public static decimal Floor(decimal *v*)	Returns the largest integer (represented as a **decimal** value) not greater than *v*. For example, given 1.02, **Floor( )** returns 1.0. Given –1.02, **Floor( )** returns –2.
public static decimal FromOACurrency(long *v*)	Converts the OLE Automation currency value in *v* into its **decimal** equivalent and returns the result.
public static int[ ] GetBits(decimal *v*)	Returns the binary representation of *v* as an array of **int**. The organization of this array is as described in the text.
public override int GetHashCode( )	Returns the hash code for the invoking object.
public TypeCode GetTypeCode( )	Returns the **TypeCode** enumeration value for **Decimal**, which is **TypeCode.Decimal**.
public static decimal Multiply(decimal *v1*, decimal *v2*)	Returns *v1* * *v2*.
public static decimal Negate(decimal *v*)	Returns –*v*.
public static decimal Parse(string *str*)	Returns the binary equivalent of the numeric string in *str*. If the string does not represent a **decimal** value, an exception is thrown.
public static decimal Parse(string *str*, IFormatProvider *fmtpvdr*)	Returns the binary equivalent of the numeric string in *str* using the culture-specific information provided by *fmtpvdr*. If the string does not represent a **decimal** value, an exception is thrown.
public static decimal Parse(string *str*, NumberStyles *styles*)	Returns the binary equivalent of the numeric string in *str*, using the style information provided by *styles*. If the string does not represent a **decimal** value, an exception is thrown.
public static decimal Parse(string *str*, NumberStyles *styles*, IFormatProvider *fmtpvdr*)	Returns the binary equivalent of the numeric string in *str* using the style information provided by *styles* and the culture-specific format information provided by *fmtpvdr*. If the string does not represent a **decimal** value, an exception is thrown.
public static decimal Remainder(decimal *v1*, decimal *v2*)	Returns the remainder of the integer division *v1* / *v2*.
public static decimal Round(decimal *v*)	Returns the value of *v* rounded to the nearest whole number.
public static decimal Round(decimal *v*, int *decPlaces*)	Returns the value of *v* rounded to the number of decimal places specified by *decPlaces*, which must be between 0 and 28.

TABLE 21-7 Methods Defined by **Decimal** (*continued*)

Method	Meaning

public static decimal
  Round(decimal *v*,
    MidPointRounding *how*)
	Returns the value of *v* rounded to the nearest whole number using the rounding mode specified by *how*. The rounding mode applies only to those conditions in which *v* is at the midpoint between two whole numbers.

public static decimal
  Round(decimal *v*, int *decPlaces*,
    MidPointRounding *how*)
	Returns the value of *v* rounded to the number of decimal places specified by *decPlaces* (which must be between 0 and 28), using the rounding mode specified by *how*. The rounding mode applies only to those conditions in which *v* is at the midpoint between two rounded values.

public static decimal Subtract(decimal *v1*, decimal *v2*)	Returns *v1 – v2*.
public static byte ToByte(decimal *v*)	Returns the **byte** equivalent of *v*. Any fractional component is truncated. An **OverflowException** occurs if *v* is not within the range of a **byte**.
public static double ToDouble(decimal *v*)	Returns the **double** equivalent of *v*. A loss of precision may occur because **double** has fewer significant digits than does **decimal**.
public static short ToInt16(decimal *v*)	Returns the **short** equivalent of *v*. Any fractional component is truncated. An **OverflowException** occurs if *v* is not within the range of a **short**.
public static int ToInt32(decimal *v*)	Returns the **int** equivalent of *v*. Any fractional component is truncated. An **OverflowException** occurs if *v* is not within the range of an **int**.
public static long ToInt64(decimal *v*)	Returns the **long** equivalent of *v*. Any fractional component is truncated. An **OverflowException** occurs if *v* is not within the range of a **long**.
public static long ToOACurrency(decimal *v*)	Converts *v* into the equivalent OLE Automation currency value and returns the result.
public static sbyte ToSByte(decimal *v*)	Returns the **sbyte** equivalent of *v*. Any fractional component is truncated. An **OverflowException** occurs if *v* is not within the range of an **sbyte**.
public static float ToSingle(decimal *v*)	Returns the **float** equivalent of *v*. A loss of precision may occur because **float** has fewer significant digits than does **decimal**.
public override string ToString( )	Returns the string representation of the value of the invoking object in the default format.
public string ToString(string *format*)	Returns the string representation of the value of the invoking object as specified by the format string passed in *format*.

TABLE 21-7   Methods Defined by **Decimal** *(continued)*

PART II

Method	Meaning
public string ToString(IFormatProvider *fmtpvdr*)	Returns the string representation of the value of the invoking object using the culture-specific information specified in *fmtpvdr*.
public string ToString(string *format*, IFormatProvider *fmtpvdr*)	Returns the string representation of the value of the invoking object using the culture-specific information specified in *fmtpvdr* and the format specified by *format*.
public static ushort ToUInt16(decimal *v*)	Returns the **ushort** equivalent of *v*. Any fractional component is truncated. An **OverflowException** occurs if *v* is not within the range of a **ushort**.
public static uint ToUInt32(decimal *v*)	Returns the **uint** equivalent of *v*. Any fractional component is truncated. An **OverflowException** occurs if *v* is not within the range of a **uint**.
public static ulong ToUInt64(decimal *v*)	Returns the **ulong** equivalent of *v*. Any fractional component is truncated. An **OverflowException** occurs if *v* is not within the range of a **ulong**.
public static decimal Truncate(decimal *v*)	Returns the whole-number portion of *v*. Thus, it truncates any fractional digits.
public static bool TryParse(string *str*, out decimal *val*)	Attempts to convert the numeric string in *str* into a **decimal** value. If successful, the value is stored in *val* and true is returned. If no conversion takes place, false is returned. This differs from **Parse( )**, which throws an exception on failure.
public static bool TryParse(string *str*, NumberStyles *styles*, IFormatProvider *fmtpvdr*, out decimal *val*)	Attempts to convert the numeric string in *str* into a **decimal** value using the style information provided by *styles* and the culture-specific format information provided by *fmtpvdr*. If successful, the value is stored in *val* and true is returned. If no conversion takes place, false is returned. This differs from **Parse( )**, which throws an exception on failure.

TABLE 21-7 Methods Defined by **Decimal** *(continued)*

Char

The structure corresponding to the **char** type is **Char**. It is quite useful because it supplies a large number of methods that allow you to process and categorize characters. For example, you can convert a lowercase character to uppercase by calling **ToUpper( )**. You can determine if a character is a digit by calling **IsDigit( )**.

The methods defined by **Char** are shown in Table 21-9. Notice that several, such as **ConvertFromUtf32( )** and **ConvertToUtf32( )**, give you the ability to work with both UTF-16 and UTF-32 Unicode characters. In the past, all Unicode characters could be represented by 16 bits, which is the size of a **char**. However, a few years ago the Unicode character set was expanded and more than 16 bits are required. Each Unicode character is represented by a *code point*. The way that a code point is encoded depends on the Unicode Transformation Format (UTF) being used. In UTF-16, the most common code points require one 16-bit value, but some need two 16-bit values. When two 16-bit values are needed, two **char**

Field	Meaning
public static readonly decimal MaxValue	The largest value that a **decimal** can hold.
public static readonly decimal MinusOne	The **decimal** representation of –1.
public static readonly decimal MinValue	The smallest value that a **decimal** can hold.
public static readonly decimal One	The **decimal** representation of 1.
public static readonly decimal Zero	The **decimal** representation of 0.

TABLE 21-8   Fields Supported by **Decimal**

values are used to represent it. The first character is called the *high surrogate* and the second is called the *low surrogate*. In UTF-32, each code point uses one 32-bit value. **Char** provides the necessary conversions between UTF-16 and UTF-32.

Char defines the following fields:

```
public const char MaxValue
public const char MinValue
```

These represent the largest and smallest values that a **char** variable can hold.

Char implements the following interfaces: **IComparable, IComparable<char>, IConvertible,** and **IEquatable<char>**.

Method	Meaning
public int CompareTo(char *v*)	Compares the character in the invoking object with that of *v*. Returns zero if the characters are equal. Returns a negative value if the invoking object has a lower value. Returns a positive value if the invoking object has a greater value.
public int CompareTo(object *v*)	Compares the character in the invoking object with that of *v*. Returns zero if the characters are equal. Returns a negative value if the invoking object has a lower value. Returns a positive value if the invoking object has a greater value.
public static string ConvertFromUtf32(int *utf32Ch*)	Converts the Unicode UTF-32 code point in *utf32Ch* into a UTF-16 string and returns the result.
pubic static int ConvertToUtf32(char *highSurrogate*, char *lowSurrogate*)	Converts the high and low UTF-16 surrogates specified by *highSurrogate* and *lowSurrogate* into a UTF-32 code point. The result is returned.
pubic static int ConvertToUtf32(string str, int *idx*)	Converts the UTF-16 surrogate pair at *str*[*idx*] into its UTF-32 code point. The result is returned.
public bool Equals(char *v*)	Returns true if the value of the invoking object equals the value of *v*.
public override bool Equals(object *v*)	Returns true if the value of the invoking object equals the value of *v*.

TABLE 21-9   Methods Defined by **Char**

PART II

Method	Meaning
public override int GetHashCode( )	Returns the hash code for the invoking object.
public static double GetNumericValue(char *ch*)	Returns the numeric value of *ch* if *ch* is a digit. Otherwise, returns –1.
public static double GetNumericValue(string *str*, int *idx*)	Returns the numeric value of *str*[*idx*] if that character is a digit. Otherwise, returns –1.
public TypeCode GetTypeCode( )	Returns the **TypeCode** enumeration value for **Char**, which is **TypeCode.Char**.
public static UnicodeCategory GetUnicodeCategory(char *ch*)	Returns the **UnicodeCategory** enumeration value for *ch*. **UnicodeCategory** is an enumeration defined by **System.Globalization** that categorizes Unicode characters.
public static UnicodeCategory GetUnicodeCategory(string *str*, int *idx*)	Returns the **UnicodeCategory** enumeration value for *str*[*idx*]. **UnicodeCategory** is an enumeration defined by **System.Globalization** that categorizes Unicode characters.
public static bool IsControl(char *ch*)	Returns true if *ch* is a control character. Otherwise, returns false.
public static bool IsControl(string *str*, int *idx*)	Returns true if *str*[*idx*] is a control character. Otherwise, returns false.
public static bool IsDigit(char *ch*)	Returns true if *ch* is a digit. Otherwise, returns false.
public static bool IsDigit(string *str*, int *idx*)	Returns true if *str*[*idx*] is a digit. Otherwise, returns false.
public static bool IsHighSurrogate(char *ch*)	Returns true if *ch* is a valid UTF-32 high surrogate. Otherwise, returns false.
public static bool IsHighSurrogate(string *str*, int *idx*)	Returns true if *str*[*idx*] is a valid UTF-32 high surrogate. Otherwise, returns false.
public static bool IsLetter(char *ch*)	Returns true if *ch* is a letter of the alphabet. Otherwise, returns false.
public static bool IsLetter(string *str*, int *idx*)	Returns true if *str*[*idx*] is a letter of the alphabet. Otherwise, returns false.
public static bool IsLetterOrDigit(char *ch*)	Returns true if *ch* is either a letter of the alphabet or a digit. Otherwise, returns false.
public static bool IsLetterOrDigit(string *str*, int *idx*)	Returns true if *str*[*idx*] is either a letter of the alphabet or a digit. Otherwise, returns false.
public static bool IsLower(char *ch*)	Returns true if *ch* is a lowercase letter of the alphabet. Otherwise, returns false.
public static bool IsLower(string *str*, int *idx*)	Returns true if *str*[*idx*] is a lowercase letter of the alphabet. Otherwise, returns false.

TABLE 21-9 Methods Defined by **Char** *(continued)*

Method	Meaning
public static bool IsLowSurrogate(char *ch*)	Returns true if *ch* is a valid UTF-32 low surrogate. Otherwise, returns false.
public static bool IsLowSurrogate(string *str*, int *idx*)	Returns true if *str*[*idx*] is a valid UTF-32 low surrogate. Otherwise, returns false.
public static bool IsNumber(char *ch*)	Returns true if *ch* is a number. Otherwise, returns false.
public static bool IsNumber(string *str*, int *idx*)	Returns true if *str*[*idx*] is a number. Otherwise, returns false.
public static bool IsPunctuation(char *ch*)	Returns true if *ch* is a punctuation character. Otherwise, returns false.
public static bool IsPunctuation(string *str*, int *idx*)	Returns true if *str*[*idx*] is a punctuation character. Otherwise, returns false.
public static bool IsSeparator(char *ch*)	Returns true if *ch* is a separator character, such as a space. Otherwise, returns false.
public static bool IsSeparator(string *str*, int *idx*)	Returns true if *str*[*idx*] is a separator character, such as a space. Otherwise, returns false.
public static bool IsSurrogate(char *ch*)	Returns true if *ch* is a Unicode surrogate character. Otherwise, returns false.
public static bool IsSurrogate(string *str*, int *idx*)	Returns true if *str*[*idx*] is a Unicode surrogate character. Otherwise, returns false.
public static bool IsSurrogatePair(char *high*, char *low*)	Returns true if *high* and *low* form a valid surrogate pair. Otherwise, returns false.
public static bool IsSurrogatePair(string *str*, int *idx*)	Returns true if the two consecutive characters starting at *idx* within *str* form a valid surrogate pair. Otherwise, returns false.
public static bool IsSymbol(char *ch*)	Returns true if *ch* is a symbolic character, such as the currency symbol. Otherwise, returns false.
public static bool IsSymbol(string *str*, int *idx*)	Returns true if *str*[*idx*] is a symbolic character, such as the currency symbol. Otherwise, returns false.
public static bool IsUpper(char *ch*)	Returns true if *ch* is an uppercase letter. Otherwise, returns false.
public static bool IsUpper(string *str*, int *idx*)	Returns true if *str*[*idx*] is an uppercase letter. Otherwise, returns false.
public static bool IsWhiteSpace(char *ch*)	Returns true if *ch* is a whitespace character, such as a space or tab. Otherwise, returns false.
public static bool IsWhiteSpace(string *str*, int *idx*)	Returns true if *str*[*idx*] is a whitespace character, such as a space or tab. Otherwise, returns false.

TABLE 21-9   Methods Defined by **Char** *(continued)*

Method	Meaning
public static char Parse(string *str*)	Returns the **char** equivalent of the character in *str*. If *str* contains more than one character, a **FormatException** is thrown.
public static char ToLower(char *ch*)	Returns the lowercase equivalent of *ch* if *ch* is an uppercase letter. Otherwise, *ch* is returned unchanged.
public static char ToLower(char *ch*, CultureInfo *c*)	Returns the lowercase equivalent of *ch* if *ch* is an uppercase letter. Otherwise, *ch* is returned unchanged. The conversion is handled in accordance with the specified cultural information. **CultureInfo** is a class defined in **System.Globalization**.
public static char ToLowerInvariant(char *ch*)	Returns the lowercase version of *ch* independently of the cultural settings.
public override string ToString( )	Returns the string representation of the value of the invoking **Char**.
public static string ToString(char *ch*)	Returns the string representation of *ch*.
public string ToString(IFormatProvider *fmtpvdr*)	Returns the string representation of the invoking **Char** using the specified cultural information.
public static char ToUpper(char *ch*)	Returns the uppercase equivalent of *ch* if *ch* is a lowercase letter. Otherwise, *ch* is returned unchanged.
public static char ToUpper(char *ch*, CultureInfo *c*)	Returns the uppercase equivalent of *ch* if *ch* is a lowercase letter. Otherwise, *ch* is returned unchanged. The conversion is handled in accordance with the specified cultural information. **CultureInfo** is a class defined in **System.Globalization**.
public static char ToUpperInvariant(char *ch*)	Returns the uppercase version of *ch* independently of the cultural settings.
public static bool TryParse(string *str*, out char *ch*)	Attempts to convert the character in *str* into its **char** equivalent. If successful, the value is stored in *ch* and true is returned. If *str* contains more than one character, false is returned. This differs from **Parse( )**, which throws an exception on failure.

TABLE 21-9 Methods Defined by **Char** *(continued)*

Here is a program that demonstrates several of the methods defined by **Char**:

```
// Demonstrate several Char methods.

using System;

class CharDemo {
```

```
static void Main() {
  string str = "This is a test. $23";
  int i;

  for(i=0; i < str.Length; i++) {
    Console.Write(str[i] + " is");
    if(Char.IsDigit(str[i]))
      Console.Write(" digit");
    if(Char.IsLetter(str[i]))
      Console.Write(" letter");
    if(Char.IsLower(str[i]))
      Console.Write(" lowercase");
    if(Char.IsUpper(str[i]))
      Console.Write(" uppercase");
    if(Char.IsSymbol(str[i]))
      Console.Write(" symbol");
    if(Char.IsSeparator(str[i]))
      Console.Write(" separator");
    if(Char.IsWhiteSpace(str[i]))
      Console.Write(" whitespace");
    if(Char.IsPunctuation(str[i]))
      Console.Write(" punctuation");

    Console.WriteLine();
  }

  Console.WriteLine("Original: " + str);

  // Convert to uppercase.
  string newstr = "";
  for(i=0; i < str.Length; i++)
    newstr += Char.ToUpper(str[i]);

  Console.WriteLine("Uppercased: " + newstr);

  }
}
```

The output is shown here:

```
T is letter uppercase
h is letter lowercase
i is letter lowercase
s is letter lowercase
  is separator whitespace
i is letter lowercase
s is letter lowercase
  is separator whitespace
a is letter lowercase
  is separator whitespace
t is letter lowercase
e is letter lowercase
s is letter lowercase
t is letter lowercase
. is punctuation
```

```
  is separator whitespace
$ is symbol
2 is digit
3 is digit
Original: This is a test. $23
Uppercased: THIS IS A TEST. $23
```

The Boolean Structure

The **Boolean** structure supports the **bool** data type. The methods defined by **Boolean** are shown in Table 21-10. It defines these fields:

public static readonly string FalseString
public static readonly string TrueString

These contain the human-readable forms of **true** and **false**. For example, if you output **FalseString** using a call to **WriteLine( )**, the string "False" is displayed.

Boolean implements the following interfaces: **IComparable**, **IComparable<bool>**, **IConvertible**, and **IEquatable<bool>**.

Method	Meaning
public int CompareTo(bool *v*)	Compares the value of the invoking object with that of *v*. Returns zero if the values are equal. Returns a negative value if the invoking object is false and *v* is true. Returns a positive value if the invoking object is true and *v* is false.
public int CompareTo(object *v*)	Compares the value of the invoking object with that of *v*. Returns zero if the values are equal. Returns a negative value if the invoking object is false and *v* is true. Returns a positive value if the invoking object is true and *v* is false.
public bool Equals(bool *v*)	Returns true if the value of the invoking object equals the value of *v*.
public override bool Equals(object *v*)	Returns true if the value of the invoking object equals the value of *v*.
public override int GetHashCode( )	Returns the hash code for the invoking object.
public TypeCode GetTypeCode( )	Returns the **TypeCode** enumeration value for **Boolean**, which is **TypeCode.Boolean**.
public static bool Parse(string *str*)	Returns the **bool** equivalent of the string in *str*. If the string is neither **Boolean.TrueString** nor **Boolean.FalseString**, a **FormatException** is thrown. However, case differences are ignored.
public override string ToString( )	Returns the string representation of the value of the invoking object, which will be either **TrueString** or **FalseString**.
public string ToString(IFormatProvider *fmtpvdr*)	Returns the string representation of the value of the invoking object, which will be either **TrueString** or **FalseString**. The *fmtpvdr* parameter is ignored.

TABLE 21-10   Methods Defined by **Boolean**

Method	Meaning
public static bool TryParse(string *str*, out bool *b*)	Attempts to convert the character in *str* into its **bool** equivalent. If successful, the value is stored in *b* and true is returned. If the string is neither **Boolean.TrueString** nor **Boolean.FalseString**, false is returned. (Case differences are ignored.) This differs from **Parse( )**, which throws an exception on failure.

TABLE 21-10   Methods Defined by **Boolean** *(continued)*

The Array Class

One very useful class in **System** is **Array**. **Array** is a base class for all arrays in C#. Thus, its methods can be applied to arrays of any of the built-in types or to arrays of types that you create. **Array** defines the properties shown in Table 21-11. It defines the methods shown in Table 21-12.

Array implements the following interfaces: **ICloneable, ICollection, IEnumerable,** and **IList. ICollection, IEnumerable,** and **IList** are defined in the **System.Collections** namespace and are described in Chapter 24.

Several methods use a parameter of type **IComparer** or **IComparer<T>**. The **IComparer** interface is in **System.Collections**. It defines a method called **Compare( )**, which compares the values of two objects. It is shown here:

int Compare(object *v1*, object *v2*)

It returns greater than zero if *v1* is greater than *v2*, less than zero if *v1* is less than *v2*, and zero if the two values are equal.

IComparer<T> is in **System.Collections.Generic**. It defines a generic form of **Compare( )**, which is shown here:

int Compare(T *v1*, T *v2*)

It works the same as its non-generic relative: returning greater than zero if *v1* is greater than *v2*, less than zero if *v1* is less than *v2*, and zero if the two values are equal. The advantage to **IComparer<T>** is type safety, because the type of data being operated upon is explicitly specified. Thus, no casts from **object** are required.

The next few sections demonstrate several commonly used array operations.

Property	Meaning
public bool IsFixedSize { get; }	A read-only property that is true if the array is of fixed size and false if the array is dynamic. This value is true for arrays.
public bool IsReadOnly { get; }	A read-only property that is true if the **Array** object is read-only and false if it is not. This value is true for arrays.
public bool IsSynchronized { get; }	A read-only property that is true if the array is safe for use in a multithreaded environment and false if it is not. This value is true for arrays.

TABLE 21-11   Properties Defined by **Array**

Property	Meaning
public int Length { get; }	An **int** read-only property that contains the number of elements in the array.
public long LongLength { get; }	A **long** read-only property that contains the number of elements in the array.
public int Rank { get; }	A read-only property that contains the number of dimensions in the array.
public object SyncRoot { get; }	A read-only property that contains the object that synchronizes access to the array.

TABLE 21-11   Properties Defined by **Array** *(continued)*

Method	Meaning
public static ReadOnlyCollection<T> AsReadOnly<T>(T[ ] a)	Returns a read-only collection that wraps the array specified by *a*.
public static int BinarySearch(Array a, object v)	Searches the array specified by *a* for the value specified by *v*. Returns the index of the first match. If *v* is not found, returns a negative value. The array must be sorted and one-dimensional.
public static int BinarySearch<T>(T[ ] a, T v)	Searches the array specified by *a* for the value specified by *v*. Returns the index of the first match. If *v* is not found, returns a negative value. The array must be sorted and one-dimensional.
public static int BinarySearch(Array a, object v, IComparer comp)	Searches the array specified by *a* for the value specified by *v*, using the comparison method specified by *comp*. Returns the index of the first match. If *v* is not found, returns a negative value. The array must be sorted and one-dimensional.
public static int BinarySearch<T>(T[ ] a, T v, IComparer<T> comp)	Searches the array specified by *a* for the value specified by *v*, using the comparison method specified by *comp*. Returns the index of the first match. If *v* is not found, returns a negative value. The array must be sorted and one-dimensional.
public static int BinarySearch(Array a, int start, int count, object v)	Searches a portion of the array specified by *a* for the value specified by *v*. The search begins at the index specified by *start* and is restricted to *count* elements. Returns the index of the first match. If *v* is not found, returns a negative value. The array must be sorted and one-dimensional.
public static int BinarySearch<T>(T[ ] a, int start, int count, T v)	Searches a portion of the array specified by *a* for the value specified by *v*. The search begins at the index specified by *start* and is restricted to *count* elements. Returns the index of the first match. If *v* is not found, returns a negative value. The array must be sorted and one-dimensional.
public static int BinarySearch(Array a, int start, int count, object v, IComparer comp)	Searches a portion of the array specified by *a* for the value specified by *v*, using the comparison method specified by *comp*. The search begins at the index specified by *start* and is restricted to *count* elements. Returns the index of the first match. If *v* is not found, returns a negative value. The array must be sorted and one-dimensional.
public static int BinarySearch<T>(T [ ] a, int start, int count, T v, IComparer<T> comp)	Searches a portion of the array specified by *a* for the value specified by *v*, using the comparison method specified by *comp*. The search begins at the index specified by *start* and is restricted to *count* elements. Returns the index of the first match. If *v* is not found, returns a negative value. The array must be sorted and one-dimensional.

TABLE 21-12   Methods Defined by **Array**

Method	Meaning
public static void Clear(Array *a*, int *start*, int *count*)	Sets the specified elements of *a* to zero, **null**, or **false**, depending on whether the element type is a value type, a reference type, or Boolean. The elements to be zeroed begin at the index specified by *start* and run for *count* elements.
public object Clone( )	Returns a copy of the invoking array. The copy refers to the same elements as does the original. This is called a "shallow copy." Thus, changes to the elements affect both arrays since they both use the same elements.
public static void ConstrainedCopy(Array *source*, int *srcIdx*, Array *dest*, int *destIdx*, int *count*)	Copies *count* elements from *source* (beginning at *srcIdx*) to *dest* (beginning at *destIdx*). If both arrays are reference types, then **ConstrainedCopy( )** makes a "shallow copy," which means that both arrays will refer to the same elements. If an error occurs during the copy, *dest* is unchanged.
public static TTo[ ] ConvertAll<TFrom, TTo>(TFrom[ ] *a*, Converter<TFrom, TTo> *conv*)	Converts *a* from type **TFrom** to **TTo** and returns the resulting array. The original array is unaffected. The conversion is performed by the specified converter.
public static void Copy(Array *source*, Array *dest*, int *count*)	Beginning at the start of each array, copies *count* elements from *source* to *dest*. When both arrays are reference types, then **Copy( )** makes a "shallow copy," which means that both arrays will refer to the same elements. If an error occurs during the copy, *dest* is undefined.
public static void Copy(Array *source*, Array *dest*, long *count*)	Beginning at the start of each array, copies *count* elements from *source* to *dest*. When both arrays are reference types, then **Copy( )** makes a "shallow copy," which means that both arrays will refer to the same elements. If an error occurs during the copy, *dest* is undefined.
public static void Copy(Array *source*, int *srcStart*, Array *dest*, int *destStart*, int *count*)	Copies *count* elements from *source*[*srcStart*] to *dest*[*destStart*]. When both arrays are reference types, then **Copy( )** makes a "shallow copy," which means that both arrays will refer to the same elements. If an error occurs during the copy, *dest* is undefined.
public static void Copy(Array *source*, long *srcStart*, Array *dest*, long *destStart*, long *count*)	Copies *count* elements from *source*[*srcStart*] to *dest*[*destStart*]. When both arrays are reference types, then **Copy( )** makes a "shallow copy," which means that both arrays will refer to the same elements. If an error occurs during the copy, *dest* is undefined.
public void CopyTo(Array *dest*, int *start*)	Copies the elements of the invoking array to *dest*, beginning at *dest*[*start*].
public void CopyTo(Array *dest*, long *start*)	Copies the elements of the invoking array to *dest*, beginning at *dest*[*start*].
public static Array CreateInstance(Type *t*, int *size*)	Returns a reference to a one-dimensional array that contains *size* elements of type *t*.
public static Array CreateInstance(Type *t*, int *size1*, int *size2*)	Returns a reference to a *size1*-by-*size2* two-dimensional array. Each element is of type *t*.
public static Array CreateInstance(Type *t*, int *size1*, int *size2*, int *size3*)	Returns a reference to a *size1*-by-*size2*-by-*size3* three-dimensional array. Each element is of type *t*.
public static Array CreateInstance(Type *t*, int[ ] *sizes*)	Returns a reference to a multi-dimensional array that has the dimensions specified in *sizes*. Each element is of type *t*.
public static Array CreateInstance(Type *t*, long[ ] *sizes*)	Returns a reference to a multi-dimensional array that has the dimensions specified in *sizes*. Each element is of type *t*.
public static Array CreateInstance(Type *t*, int[ ] *sizes*, int[ ] *startIndexes*)	Returns a reference to a multi-dimensional array that has the dimensions specified in *sizes*. Each element is of type *t*. The starting index of each dimension is specified in *startIndexes*. Thus, it is possible to create arrays that begin at some index other than zero.

TABLE 21-12 Methods Defined by **Array** *(continued)*

Method	Meaning
public override bool Equals(object v)	Returns true if the value of the invoking object equals the value of v.
public static bool Exists<T>(T[ ] a, Predicate<T> pred)	Returns true if a contains at least one element that satisfies the predicate specified by pred. Returns false if no elements satisfy pred.
public static T Find<T>(T[ ] a, Predicate<T> pred)	Returns the first element in a that satisfies the predicate specified by pred. If no element satisfies pred, then **default(T)** is returned.
public static T[ ] FindAll<T>(T[ ] a, Predicate<T> pred)	Returns an array that contains all elements in a that satisfy the predicate specified by pred. If no element satisfies pred, then a zero-length array is returned.
public static int FindIndex<T>(T[ ] a, Predicate<T> pred)	Returns the index of the first element in a that satisfies the predicate specified by pred. If no element satisfies pred, −1 is returned.
public static int FindIndex<T>(T[ ] a, int start, Predicate<T> pred)	Returns the index of the first element in a that satisfies the predicate specified by pred. The search begins at a[start]. If no element satisfies pred, −1 is returned.
public static int FindIndex<T>(T[ ] a, int start, int count, Predicate<T> pred)	Returns the index of the first element in a that satisfies the predicate specified by pred. The search begins at a[start] and runs for count elements. If no element satisfies pred, −1 is returned.
public static T FindLast<T>(T[ ] a, Predicate<T> pred)	Returns the last element in a that satisfies the predicate specified by pred. If no element satisfies pred, then **default(T)** is returned.
public static int FindLastIndex<T>(T[ ] a, Predicate<T> pred)	Returns the index of the last element in a that satisfies the predicate specified by pred. If no element satisfies pred, −1 is returned.
public static int FindLastIndex<T>(T[ ] a, int start, Predicate<T> pred)	Returns the index of the last element in a that satisfies the predicate specified by pred. The search proceeds in reverse order, beginning at a[start] and stopping at a[0]. If no element satisfies pred, −1 is returned.
public static int FindLastIndex<T>(T[ ] a, int start, int count, Predicate<T> pred)	Returns the index of the last element in a that satisfies the predicate specified by pred. The search proceeds in reverse order, beginning at a[start] and running for count elements. If no element satisfies pred, −1 is returned.
public static void ForEach<T>(T[ ] a, Action<T> act)	Applies the method specified by act to each element of a.
public IEnumerator GetEnumerator( )	Returns an enumerator object for the array. An enumerator enables you to cycle through an array. Enumerators are described in Chapter 24.
public override int GetHashCode( )	Returns the hash code for the invoking object.
public int GetLength(int dim)	Returns the length of the specified dimension. The dimension is zero-based. Thus, to get the length of the first dimension, pass 0; to obtain the length of the second dimension, pass 1; and so on.
public long GetLongLength(int dim)	Returns the length of the specified dimension as a **long**. The dimension is zero-based. Thus, to get the length of the first dimension, pass 0; to obtain the length of the second dimension, pass 1; and so on.
public int GetLowerBound(int dim)	Returns the first index of the specified dimension, which is usually zero. The parameter dim is zero-based. Thus, to get the start index of the first dimension, pass 0; to obtain the start index of the second dimension, pass 1; and so on.
public int GetUpperBound(int dim)	Returns the last index of the specified dimension. The parameter dim is zero-based. Thus, to get the last index of the first dimension, pass 0; to obtain the last index of the second dimension, pass 1; and so on.

TABLE 21-12 Methods Defined by **Array** (continued)

Method	Meaning
public object GetValue(int *idx*)	Returns the value of the element at index *idx* within the invoking array. The array must be one-dimensional.
public object GetValue(long *idx*)	Returns the value of the element at index *idx* within the invoking array. The array must be one-dimensional.
public object GetValue(int *idx1*, int *idx2*)	Returns the value of the element at [*idx1, idx2*] within the invoking array. The array must be two-dimensional.
public object GetValue(long *idx1*, long *idx2*)	Returns the value of the element at [*idx1, idx2*] within the invoking array. The array must be two-dimensional.
public object GetValue(int *idx1*, int *idx2*, int *idx3*)	Returns the value of the element at [*idx1, idx2, idx3*] within the invoking array. The array must be three-dimensional.
public object GetValue(long *idx1*, long *idx2*, long *idx3*)	Returns the value of the element at [*idx1, idx2, idx3*] within the invoking array. The array must be three-dimensional.
public object GetValue(int[ ] *idxs*)	Returns the value of the element at the specified indices within the invoking array. The array must have as many dimensions as *idxs* has elements.
public object GetValue(long[ ] *idxs*)	Returns the value of the element at the specified indices within the invoking array. The array must have as many dimensions as *idxs* has elements.
public static int IndexOf(Array *a*, object *v*)	Returns the index of the first element within the one-dimensional array *a* that has the value specified by *v*. Returns −1 if the value is not found. (If the array has a lower bound other than 0, then the failure value is the lower bound −1.)
public static int IndexOf<T>(T[ ] *a*, T *v*)	Returns the index of the first element within the one-dimensional array *a* that has the value specified by *v*. Returns −1 if the value is not found.
public static int IndexOf(Array *a*, object *v*, int *start*)	Returns the index of the first element within the one-dimensional array *a* that has the value specified by *v*. The search begins at *a*[*start*]. Returns −1 if the value is not found. (If the array has a lower bound other than 0, then the failure value is the lower bound −1.)
public static int IndexOf<T>(T[ ] *a*, T *v*, int *start*)	Returns the index of the first element within the one-dimensional array *a* that has the value specified by *v*. The search begins at *a*[*start*]. Returns −1 if the value is not found.
public static int IndexOf(Array *a*, object *v*, int *start*, int *count*)	Returns the index of the first element within the one-dimensional array *a* that has the value specified by *v*. The search begins at *a*[*start*] and runs for *count* elements. Returns −1 if the value is not found within the specified range. (If the array has a lower bound other than 0, then the failure value is the lower bound −1.)
public static int IndexOf<T>(T[ ] *a*, T *v*, int *start*, int *count*)	Returns the index of the first element within the one-dimensional array *a* that has the value specified by *v*. The search begins at *a*[*start*] and runs for *count* elements. Returns −1 if the value is not found within the specified range.
public void Initialize( )	Initializes each element in the invoking array by calling the element's default constructor. This method can be used only on arrays of value types that have constructors.
public static int LastIndexOf(Array *a*, object *v*)	Returns the index of the last element within the one-dimensional array *a* that has the value specified by *v*. Returns −1 if the value is not found. (If the array has a lower bound other than 0, then the failure value is the lower bound −1.)
public static int LastIndexOf<T>(T[ ] *a*, T *v*)	Returns the index of the last element within the one-dimensional array *a* that has the value specified by *v*. Returns −1 if the value is not found.
public static int LastIndexOf(Array *a*, object *v*, int *start*)	Returns the index of the last element within a range of the one-dimensional array *a* that has the value specified by *v*. The search proceeds in reverse order, beginning at *a*[*start*] and stopping at *a*[0]. Returns −1 if the value is not found. (If the array has a lower bound other than 0, then the failure value is the lower bound −1.)

TABLE 21-12   Methods Defined by **Array** (*continued*)

PART II

Method	Meaning
public static int LastIndexOf<T>(T[ ] *a*, T *v*, int *start*)	Returns the index of the last element within a range of the one-dimensional array *a* that has the value specified by *v*. The search proceeds in reverse order, beginning at *a*[*start*] and stopping at *a*[0]. Returns –1 if the value is not found.
public static int LastIndexOf(Array *a*, object *v*, int *start*, int *count*)	Returns the index of the last element within a range of the one-dimensional array *a* that has the value specified by *v*. The search proceeds in reverse order, beginning at *a*[*start*] and running for *count* elements. Returns –1 if the value is not found within the specified range. (If the array has a lower bound other than 0, then the failure value is the lower bound –1.)
public static int LastIndexOf<T>(T[ ] *a*, T *v*, int *start*, int *count*)	Returns the index of the last element within a range of the one-dimensional array *a* that has the value specified by *v*. The search proceeds in reverse order, beginning at *a*[*start*] and running for *count* elements. Returns –1 if the value is not found within the specified range.
public static void Resize<T>(ref T[ ] *a*, int *size*)	Sets the size of *a* to *size*.
public static void Reverse(Array *a*)	Reverses the elements in *a*.
public static void Reverse(Array *a*, int *start*, int *count*)	Reverses a range of elements in *a*. The range reversed begins at *a*[*start*] and runs for *count* elements.
public void SetValue(object *v*, int *idx*)	Sets the value of the element at index *idx* within the invoking array to *v*. The array must be one-dimensional.
public void SetValue(object *v*, long *idx*)	Sets the value of the element at index *idx* within the invoking array to *v*. The array must be one-dimensional.
public void SetValue(object *v*, int *idx1*, int *idx2*)	Sets the value of the element at indices [*idx1*, *idx2*] within the invoking array to *v*. The array must be two-dimensional.
public void SetValue(object *v*, long *idx1*, long *idx2*)	Sets the value of the element at indices [*idx1*, *idx2*] within the invoking array to *v*. The array must be two-dimensional.
public void SetValue(object *v*, int *idx1*, int *idx2*, int *idx3*)	Sets the value of the element at indices [*idx1*, *idx2*, *idx3*] within the invoking array to *v*. The array must be three-dimensional.
public void SetValue(object *v*, long *idx1*, long *idx2*, long *idx3*)	Sets the value of the element at indices [*idx1*, *idx2*, *idx3*] within the invoking array to *v*. The array must be three-dimensional.
public void SetValue(object *v*, int[ ] *idxs*)	Sets the value of the element at the specified indices within the invoking array to *v*. The array must have as many dimensions as *idxs* has elements.
public void SetValue(object *v*, long[ ] *idxs*)	Sets the value of the element at the specified indices within the invoking array to *v*. The array must have as many dimensions as *idxs* has elements.
public static void Sort(Array *a*)	Sorts *a* into ascending order. The array must be one-dimensional.
public static void Sort<T>(T[ ] *a*)	Sorts *a* into ascending order. The array must be one-dimensional.
public static void Sort(Array *a*, IComparer *comp*)	Sorts *a* into ascending order using the comparison method specified by *comp*. The array must be one-dimensional.
public static void Sort<T>(T[ ] *a*, Comparison<T> *comp*)	Sorts *a* into ascending order using the comparison method specified by *comp*. The array must be one-dimensional.
public static void Sort<T>(T[ ] *a*, IComparer<T> *comp*)	Sorts *a* into ascending order using the comparison method specified by *comp*. The array must be one-dimensional.
public static void Sort(Array *k*, Array *v*)	Sorts a pair of one-dimensional arrays into ascending order. The *k* array contains the sort keys. The *v* array contains the values linked to those keys. Thus, the two arrays contain key/value pairs. After the sort, both arrays are in ascending-key order.

TABLE 21-12 Methods Defined by **Array** (continued)

Method	Meaning
public static void Sort<TK, TV>(TK[ ] k, TV[ ] v)	Sorts a pair of one-dimensional arrays into ascending order. The k array contains the sort keys. The v array contains the values linked to those keys. Thus, the two arrays contain key/value pairs. After the sort, both arrays are in ascending-key order.
public static void Sort(Array k, Array v, IComparer comp)	Sorts a pair of one-dimensional arrays into ascending order using the comparison method specified by comp. The k array contains the sort keys. The v array contains the values linked to those keys. Thus, the two arrays contain key/value pairs. After the sort, both arrays are in ascending-key order.
public static void Sort<TK, TV>(TK[ ] k, TV[ ] v, IComparer<TK> comp)	Sorts a pair of one-dimensional arrays into ascending order using the comparison method specified by comp. The k array contains the sort keys. The v array contains the values linked to those keys. Thus, the two arrays contain key/value pairs. After the sort, both arrays are in ascending-key order.
public static void Sort(Array a, int start, int count)	Sorts a range of a into ascending order. The range begins at a[start] and runs for count elements. The array must be one-dimensional.
public static void Sort<T>(T[ ] a, int start, int count)	Sorts a range of a into ascending order. The range begins at a[start] and runs for count elements. The array must be one-dimensional.
public static void Sort(Array a, int start, int count, IComparer comp)	Sorts a range of a into ascending order using the comparison method specified by comp. The range begins at a[start] and runs for count elements. The array must be one-dimensional.
public static void Sort<T>(T[ ] a, int start, int count, IComparer<T> comp)	Sorts a range of a into ascending order using the comparison method specified by comp. The range begins at a[start] and runs for count elements. The array must be one-dimensional.
public static void Sort(Array k, Array v, int start, int count)	Sorts a range within a pair of one-dimensional arrays into ascending order. Within both arrays, the range to sort begins at the index passed in start and runs for count elements. The k array contains the sort keys. The v array contains the values linked to those keys. Thus, the two arrays contain key/value pairs. After the sort, both ranges are in ascending-key order.
public static void Sort<TK, TV>(TK[ ] k, TK[ ] v, int start, int count)	Sorts a range within a pair of one-dimensional arrays into ascending order. Within both arrays, the range to sort begins at the index passed in start and runs for count elements. The k array contains the sort keys. The v array contains the values linked to those keys. Thus, the two arrays contain key/value pairs. After the sort, both ranges are in ascending-key order.
public static void Sort(Array k, Array v, int start, int count, IComparer comp)	Sorts a range within a pair of one-dimensional arrays into ascending order using the comparison method specified by comp. Within both arrays, the range to sort begins at the index passed in start and runs for count elements. The k array contains the sort keys. The v array contains the values linked to those keys. Thus, the two arrays contain key/value pairs. After the sort, both ranges are in ascending-key order.
public static void Sort<TK, TV>(TK[ ] k, TV v, int start, int count, IComparer<TK> comp)	Sorts a range within a pair of one-dimensional arrays into ascending order using the comparison method specified by comp. Within both arrays, the range to sort begins at the index passed in start and runs for count elements. The k array contains the sort keys. The v array contains the values linked to those keys. Thus, the two arrays contain key/value pairs. After the sort, both ranges are in ascending-key order.
public static bool TrueForAll<T>(T[ ] a, Predicate<T> pred)	Returns true if the predicate specified by pred is satisfied by all elements in a. If one or more elements fail to satisfy pred, then false is returned.

TABLE 21-12 Methods Defined by **Array** (continued)

Sorting and Searching Arrays

Often you will want to sort the contents of an array. To handle this, **Array** supports a rich complement of sorting methods. Using **Sort( )**, you can sort an entire array, a range within an array or a pair of arrays that contain corresponding key/value pairs. Once an array has been sorted, you can efficiently search it using **BinarySearch( )**. Here is a program that demonstrates the **Sort( )** and **BinarySearch( )** methods by sorting an array of **int**s:

```
// Sort an array and search for a value.

using System;

class SortDemo {
  static void Main() {
    int[] nums = { 5, 4, 6, 3, 14, 9, 8, 17, 1, 24, -1, 0 };

    // Display original order.
    Console.Write("Original order: ");
    foreach(int i in nums)
      Console.Write(i + " ");
    Console.WriteLine();

    // Sort the array.
    Array.Sort(nums);

    // Display sorted order.
    Console.Write("Sorted order:   ");
    foreach(int i in nums)
      Console.Write(i + " ");
    Console.WriteLine();


    // Search for 14.
    int idx = Array.BinarySearch(nums, 14);

    Console.WriteLine("Index of 14 is " + idx);
  }
}
```

The output is shown here:

```
Original order: 5 4 6 3 14 9 8 17 1 24 -1 0
Sorted order:   -1 0 1 3 4 5 6 8 9 14 17 24
Index of 14 is 9
```

In the preceding example, the array has an element type of **int**, which is a value type. All methods defined by **Array** are automatically available to all of the built-in value types. However, this may not be the case for arrays of object references. To sort or search an array of object references, the class type of those objects must implement either the **IComparable** or **IComparable<T>** interface. If the class does not implement one of these interfaces, a runtime exception will occur when attempting to sort or search the array. Fortunately, both **IComparable** and **IComparable<T>** are easy to implement.

IComparable defines just one method:

int CompareTo(object *obj*)

This method compares the invoking object against the value in *obj*. It returns greater than zero if the invoking object is greater than *obj*, zero if the two objects are equal, and less than zero if the invoking object is less than *obj*.

IComparable<T> is the generic version of **IComparable**. It defines the generic version of **CompareTo( )**:

int CompareTo(T *obj*)

The generic version of **CompareTo( )** works like the non-generic version. It compares the invoking object against the value in *obj*. It returns greater than zero if the invoking object is greater than *obj*, zero if the two objects are equal, and less than zero if the invoking object is less than *obj*. The advantage of using **IComparable<T>** is type safety because the type of data being operated upon is explicitly specified. There is no need to cast the object being compared from **object** into the desired type. Here is an example that illustrates sorting and searching an array of user-defined class objects:

```
// Sort and search an array of objects.

using System;

class MyClass : IComparable<MyClass> {
  public int i;

  public MyClass(int x) { i = x; }

  // Implement IComparable<MyClass>.
  public int CompareTo(MyClass v) {
    return i - v.i;
  }

  public bool Equals(MyClass v) {
    return i == v.i;
  }

}

class SortDemo {
  static void Main() {
    MyClass[] nums = new MyClass[5];

    nums[0] = new MyClass(5);
    nums[1] = new MyClass(2);
    nums[2] = new MyClass(3);
    nums[3] = new MyClass(4);
    nums[4] = new MyClass(1);

    // Display original order.
    Console.Write("Original order: ");
    foreach(MyClass o in nums)
      Console.Write(o.i + " ");
    Console.WriteLine();

    // Sort the array.
    Array.Sort(nums);
```

PART II

```
      // Display sorted order.
      Console.Write("Sorted order:    ");
      foreach(MyClass o in nums)
        Console.Write(o.i + " ");
      Console.WriteLine();

      // Search for MyClass(2).
      MyClass x = new MyClass(2);
      int idx = Array.BinarySearch(nums, x);

      Console.WriteLine("Index of MyClass(2) is " + idx);
   }
}
```

The output is shown here:

```
Original order: 5 2 3 4 1
Sorted order:   1 2 3 4 5
Index of MyClass(2) is 1
```

Reversing an Array

Sometimes it is useful to reverse the contents of an array. For example, you might want to change an array that has been sorted in ascending order into one sorted in descending order. Reversing an array is easy: Simply call **Reverse( )**. Using **Reverse( )**, you can reverse all or part of an array. The following program demonstrates the process:

```
// Reverse an array.

using System;

class ReverseDemo {
  static void Main() {
    int[] nums = { 1, 2, 3, 4, 5 };

    // Display original order.
    Console.Write("Original order: ");
    foreach(int i in nums)
      Console.Write(i + " ");
    Console.WriteLine();

    // Reverse the entire array.
    Array.Reverse(nums);

    // Display reversed order.
    Console.Write("Reversed order: ");
    foreach(int i in nums)
      Console.Write(i + " ");
    Console.WriteLine();

    // Reverse a range.
    Array.Reverse(nums, 1, 3);

    // Display reversed order.
    Console.Write("Range reversed: ");
    foreach(int i in nums)
```

```
      Console.Write(i + " ");
    Console.WriteLine();
  }
}
```

The output is shown here:

```
Original order: 1 2 3 4 5
Reversed order: 5 4 3 2 1
Range reversed: 5 2 3 4 1
```

Copying an Array

Copying all or part of one array to another is another common array operation. To copy an array, use **Copy( )**. **Copy( )** can put elements at the start of the destination array or in the middle, depending upon which version of **Copy( )** you use. **Copy( )** is demonstrated by the following program:

```
// Copy an array.

using System;

class CopyDemo {
  static void Main() {
    int[] source = { 1, 2, 3, 4, 5 };
    int[] target = { 11, 12, 13, 14, 15 };
    int[] source2 = { -1, -2, -3, -4, -5 };

    // Display source.
    Console.Write("source: ");
    foreach(int i in source)
      Console.Write(i + " ");
    Console.WriteLine();

    // Display original target.
    Console.Write("Original contents of target: ");
    foreach(int i in target)
      Console.Write(i + " ");
    Console.WriteLine();

    // Copy the entire array.
    Array.Copy(source, target, source.Length);

    // Display copy.
    Console.Write("target after copy:  ");
    foreach(int i in target)
      Console.Write(i + " ");
    Console.WriteLine();

    // Copy into middle of target.
    Array.Copy(source2, 2, target, 3, 2);

    // Display copy.
    Console.Write("target after copy:  ");
    foreach(int i in target)
```

```
      Console.Write(i + " ");
    Console.WriteLine();
  }
}
```

The output is shown here:

```
source: 1 2 3 4 5
Original contents of target: 11 12 13 14 15
target after copy:  1 2 3 4 5
target after copy:  1 2 3 -3 -4
```

Using a Predicate

A *predicate* is a delegate of type **System.Predicate** that returns either true or false, based upon some condition. It is declared as shown here:

public delegate bool Predicate<T> (T *obj*)

The object to be tested against the condition is passed in *obj.* If *obj* satisfies that condition, the predicate must return true. Otherwise, it must return false. Predicates are used by several methods in **Array**, including **Exists( )**, **Find( )**, **FindIndex( )**, and **FindAll( )**.

The following program demonstrates using a predicate to determine if an array of integers contains a negative value. If a negative value is found, the program then obtains the first negative value in the array. To accomplish this, the program uses **Exists( )** and **Find( )**.

```
// Demonstrate Predicate delegate.

using System;

class PredDemo {

  // A predicate method.
  // It returns true if v is negative.
  static bool IsNeg(int v) {
    if(v < 0) return true;
    return false;
  }

  static void Main() {
    int[] nums = { 1, 4, -1, 5, -9 };

    Console.Write("Contents of nums: ");
    foreach(int i in nums)
      Console.Write(i + " ");
    Console.WriteLine();

    // First see if nums contains a negative value.
    if(Array.Exists(nums, PredDemo.IsNeg)) {
      Console.WriteLine("nums contains a negative value.");

      // Now, find first negative value.
      int x = Array.Find(nums, PredDemo.IsNeg);
      Console.WriteLine("First negative value is : " + x);
    }
```

```
      else
         Console.WriteLine("nums contains no negative values.");
   }
}
```

The output is shown here:

```
Contents of nums: 1 4 -1 5 -9
nums contains a negative value.
First negative value is : -1
```

In the program, the method passed to **Exists( )** and **Find( )** for the predicate is **IsNeg( )**. Notice that **IsNeg( )** is declared like this:

```
static bool IsNeg(int v) {
```

The methods **Exists( )** and **Find( )** will automatically pass the elements of the array (in sequence) to **v**. Thus, each time **IsNeg( )** is called, **v** will contain the next element in the array.

Using an Action

The **Action** delegate is used by **Array.ForEach( )** to perform an action on each element of an array. There are various forms of **Action**, each taking a different number of type parameters. The one used here is

public delegate void Action<T> (T *obj*)

The object to be acted upon is passed in *obj*. When used with **ForEach( )**, each element of the array is passed to *obj* in turn. Thus, through the use of **ForEach( )** and **Action**, you can, in a single statement, perform an operation over an entire array.

The following program demonstrates both **ForEach( )** and **Action**. It first creates an array of **MyClass** objects, then uses the method **Show( )** to display the values. Next, it uses **Neg( )** to negate the values. Finally, it uses **Show( )** again to display the negated values. These operations all occur through calls to **ForEach( )**.

```
// Demonstrate an Action.

using System;

class MyClass {
  public int i;

  public MyClass(int x) { i = x; }
}

class ActionDemo {

  // An Action method.
  // It displays the value it is passed.
  static void Show(MyClass o) {
    Console.Write(o.i + " ");
  }

  // Another Action method.
  // It negates the value it is passed.
```

```
static void Neg(MyClass o) {
  o.i = -o.i;
}

static void Main() {
  MyClass[] nums = new MyClass[5];

  nums[0] = new MyClass(5);
  nums[1] = new MyClass(2);
  nums[2] = new MyClass(3);
  nums[3] = new MyClass(4);
  nums[4] = new MyClass(1);

  Console.Write("Contents of nums: ");

  // Use action to show the values.
  Array.ForEach(nums, ActionDemo.Show);

  Console.WriteLine();

  // Use action to negate the values.
  Array.ForEach(nums, ActionDemo.Neg);

  Console.Write("Contents of nums negated: ");

  // Use action to show the values again.
  Array.ForEach(nums, ActionDemo.Show);

  Console.WriteLine();
  }
}
```

The output is shown here:

```
Contents of nums: 5 2 3 4 1
Contents of nums negated: -5 -2 -3 -4 -1
```

BitConverter

In programming one often needs to convert a built-in data type into an array of bytes. For example, some hardware device might require an integer value, but that value must be sent one byte at a time. The reverse situation also frequently occurs. Sometimes data will be received as an ordered sequence of bytes that needs to be converted into one of the built-in types. For example, a device might output integers, sent as a stream of bytes. Whatever your conversion needs, .NET provides the **BitConverter** class to meet them.

BitConverter is **static** class. It contains the methods shown in Table 21-13. It defines the following field:

public static readonly bool IsLittleEndian

This field is **true** if the current environment stores a word with the least significant byte first and the most significant byte last. This is called "little-endian" format. **IsLittleEndian** is **false** if the current environment stores a word with the most significant byte first and the least significant byte last. This is called "big-endian" format. Intel Pentium–based machines use little-endian format.

Method	Meaning
public static long DoubleToInt64Bits(double *v*)	Converts *v* into a **long** integer and returns the result.
public static byte[ ] GetBytes(bool *v*)	Converts *v* into a 1-byte array and returns the result.
public static byte[ ] GetBytes(char *v*)	Converts *v* into a 2-byte array and returns the result.
public static byte[ ] GetBytes(double *v*)	Converts *v* into an 8-byte array and returns the result.
public static byte[ ] GetBytes(float *v*)	Converts *v* into a 4-byte array and returns the result.
public static byte[ ] GetBytes(int *v*)	Converts *v* into a 4-byte array and returns the result.
public static byte[ ] GetBytes(long *v*)	Converts *v* into an 8-byte array and returns the result.
public static byte[ ] GetBytes(short *v*)	Converts *v* into a 2-byte array and returns the result.
public static byte[ ] GetBytes(uint *v*)	Converts *v* into a 4-byte array and returns the result.
public static byte[ ] GetBytes(ulong *v*)	Converts *v* into an 8-byte array and returns the result.
public static byte[ ] GetBytes(ushort *v*)	Converts *v* into a 2-byte array and returns the result.
public static double Int64BitsToDouble(long *v*)	Converts *v* into a **double** value and returns the result.
public static bool ToBoolean(byte[ ] *a*, int *idx*)	Converts the byte at *a*[*idx*] into its **bool** equivalent and returns the result. A non-zero value is converted to true; zero is converted to false.
public static char ToChar(byte[ ] *a*, int *start*)	Converts two bytes starting at *a*[*start*] into its **char** equivalent and returns the result.
public static double ToDouble(byte[ ] *a*, int *start*)	Converts eight bytes starting at *a*[*start*] into its **double** equivalent and returns the result.
public static short ToInt16(byte[ ] *a*, int *start*)	Converts two bytes starting at *a*[*start*] into its **short** equivalent and returns the result.
public static int ToInt32(byte[ ] *a*, int *start*)	Converts four bytes starting at *a*[*start*] into its **int** equivalent and returns the result.
public static long ToInt64(byte[ ] *a*, int *start*)	Converts eight bytes starting at *a*[*start*] into its **long** equivalent and returns the result.
public static float ToSingle(byte[ ] *a*, int *start*)	Converts four bytes starting at *a*[*start*] into its **float** equivalent and returns the result.

TABLE 21-13   Methods Defined by **BitConverter**

PART II

Method	Meaning
public static string ToString(byte[ ] *a*)	Converts the bytes in *a* into a string. The string contains the hexadecimal values associated with the bytes, separated by hyphens.
public static string ToString(byte[ ] *a*, int *start*)	Converts the bytes in *a*, beginning at *a*[*start*], into a string. The string contains the hexadecimal values associated with the bytes, separated by hyphens.
public static string ToString(byte[ ] *a*, int *start*, int *count*)	Converts the bytes in *a*, beginning at *a*[*start*] and running for *count* bytes, into a string. The string contains the hexadecimal values associated with the bytes, separated by hyphens.
public static ushort ToUInt16(byte[ ] *a*, int *start*)	Converts two bytes starting at *a*[*start*] into its **ushort** equivalent and returns the result.
public static uint ToUInt32(byte[ ] *a*, int *start*)	Converts four bytes starting at *a*[*start*] into its **uint** equivalent and returns the result.
public static ulong ToUInt64(byte[ ] *a*, int *start*)	Converts eight bytes starting at *a*[*start*] into its **ulong** equivalent and returns the result.

TABLE 21-13   Methods Defined by **BitConverter** *(continued)*

Generating Random Numbers with Random

To generate a sequence of pseudorandom numbers, you will use the **Random** class. Sequences of random numbers are useful in a variety of situations, including simulations and modeling. The starting point of the sequence is determined by a *seed* value, which can be automatically provided by **Random** or explicitly specified.

    Random defines these two constructors:

    public Random( )
    public Random(int *seed*)

The first version creates a **Random** object that uses the system time to compute the seed value. The second uses the value of *seed* as the seed value.

    Random defines the methods shown in Table 21-14.

    Here is a program that demonstrates **Random** by creating a pair of computerized dice:

```
// An automated pair of dice.

using System;

class RandDice {
  static void Main() {
    Random ran = new Random();

    Console.Write(ran.Next(1, 7) + " ");
    Console.WriteLine(ran.Next(1, 7));
  }
}
```

Method	Meaning
public virtual int Next( )	Returns the next random integer, which will be between 0 and **Int32.MaxValue**–1, inclusive.
public virtual int Next(int *upperBound*)	Returns the next random integer that is between 0 and *upperBound*–1, inclusive.
public virtual int Next(int *lowerBound*, int *upperBound*)	Returns the next random integer that is between *lowerBound* and *upperBound*–1, inclusive.
public virtual void NextBytes(byte[ ] *buf*)	Fills *buf* with a sequence of random integers. Each byte in the array will be between 0 and **Byte.MaxValue**–1, inclusive.
public virtual double NextDouble( )	Returns the next random value from the sequence represented as a floating-point number that is greater than or equal to 0.0 and less than 1.0.
protected virtual double Sample( )	Returns the next random value from the sequence represented as a floating-point number that is greater than or equal to 0.0 and less than 1.0. To create a skewed or specialized distribution, override this method in a derived class.

TABLE 21-14   Methods Defined by **Random**

Here are three sample runs:

```
5 2
4 4
1 6
```

The program works by first creating a **Random** object. Then it requests the two random values, each between 1 and 6, inclusive.

Memory Management and the GC Class

The **GC** class encapsulates the garbage-collection facility. The methods defined by **GC** are shown in Table 21-15. It defines the read-only property shown here:

    public static int MaxGeneration { get; }

MaxGeneration contains the maximum generation number available to the system. A generation number indicates the age of an allocation. Newer allocations have a lower number than older ones. Generation numbers help improve the efficiency of the garbage collector.

For most applications, you will not use any of the capabilities of **GC**. However, in specialized cases, they can be very useful. For example, you might want to use **Collect( )** to force garbage collection to occur at a time of your choosing. Normally, garbage collection occurs at times unspecified by your program. Since garbage collection takes time, you might not want it to occur during some time-critical task, or you might want to take advantage of idle time to perform garbage collection and other types of "housekeeping" chores.

There are two methods that are especially important if you have unmanaged code in your project: **AddMemoryPressure( )** and **RemoveMemoryPressure( )**. These are used to indicate that a large amount of unmanaged memory has been allocated or released by the program. They are important because the memory management system has no oversight on unmanaged memory. If a program allocates a large amount of unmanaged memory, then performance might be affected because the system has no way of knowing that free memory has been reduced. By calling **AddMemoryPressure( )** when allocating large amounts of unmanaged memory, you let the CLR know that memory has been reduced. By calling **RemoveMemoryPressure( )**, you let the CLR know the memory has been freed. Remember: **RemoveMemoryPressure( )** must be called only to indicate that memory reported by a call to **AddMemoryPressure( )** has been released.

Method	Meaning
public static void AddMemoryPressure(long *size*)	Indicates that *size* number of bytes of unmanaged memory have been allocated.
public static void Collect( )	Initiates garbage collection.
public static void Collect(int *maxGen*)	Initiates garbage collection for memory with generation numbers of 0 through *maxGen.*
public static void Collect(int *maxGen*, GCCollectionMode *GCMode*)	Initiates garbage collection for memory with generation numbers of 0 through *maxGen* as specified by *GCMode*.
public static int CollectionCount(int *gen*)	Returns the number of garbage collections that have taken place for memory having the generation number specified by *gen*.
public static int GetGeneration(object *o*)	Returns the generation number for the memory referred to by *o*.
public static int GetGeneration(WeakReference *o*)	Returns the generation number for the memory referred to by the weak reference specified by *o*. A weak reference does not prevent the object from being garbage-collected.
public static long GetTotalMemory(bool *collect*)	Returns the total number of bytes currently allocated. If *collect* is true, garbage collection occurs first.
public static void KeepAlive(object *o*)	Creates a reference to *o*, thus preventing it from being garbage collected. This reference ends when **KeepAlive( )** executes.
public static void RemoveMemoryPressure(long *size*)	Indicates that *size* number of bytes of unmanaged memory have been released.
public static void ReRegisterForFinalize(object *o*)	Causes the finalizer (i.e., the destructor) for *o* to be called. This method undoes the effects of **SuppressFinalize( )**.
public static void SuppressFinalize(object *o*)	Prevents the finalizer (i.e., the destructor) for *o* from being called.
public static void WaitForPendingFinalizers( )	Halts execution of the invoking thread until all pending finalizers (i.e., destructors) have been called.

TABLE 21-15 Methods Defined by **GC**

Object

Object is the class that underlies the C# **object** type. The members of **Object** were discussed in Chapter 11, but because of its central role in C#, its methods are repeated in Table 21-16 for your convenience. **Object** defines one constructor, which is shown here:

    public Object( )

It constructs an empty object.

The IComparable and IComparable<T> Interfaces

Many classes will need to implement either the **IComparable** or **IComparable<T>** interface because it enables one object to be compared to another by various methods defined by the .NET Framework. Chapter 18 introduced the **IComparable** and **IComparable<T>** interfaces, where they were used to enable two objects of a generic type parameter to be compared. They were also mentioned in the discussion of **Array**, earlier in this chapter. However, because of their importance and applicability to many situations, they are formally examined here.

    IComparable is especially easy to implement because it consists of just this one method:

    int CompareTo(object v)

This method compares the invoking object against the value in v. It returns greater than zero if the invoking object is greater than v, zero if the two objects are equal, and less than zero if the invoking object is less than v.

Method	Purpose
public virtual bool Equals(object *ob*)	Returns true if the invoking object is the same as the one referred to by *object*. Returns false otherwise.
public static bool Equals(object *ob1*, object *ob2*)	Returns true if *ob1* is the same as *ob2*. Returns false otherwise.
protected Finalize( )	Performs shutdown actions prior to garbage collection. In C#, **Finalize( )** is accessed through a destructor.
public virtual int GetHashCode( )	Returns the hash code associated with the invoking object.
public Type GetType( )	Obtains the type of an object at runtime.
protected object MemberwiseClone( )	Makes a "shallow copy" of the object. This is one in which the members are copied, but objects referred to by members are not.
public static bool ReferenceEquals(object *ob1*, object *ob2*)	Returns true if *ob1* and *ob2* refer to the same object. Returns false otherwise.
public virtual string ToString( )	Returns a string that describes the object.

TABLE 21-16   Methods Defined by **Object**

The generic version of **IComparable** is declared like this:

public interface IComparable<T>

In this version, the type of data being compared is passed as a type argument to **T**. This causes the declaration of **CompareTo( )** to be changed, as shown next.

int CompareTo(T *obj*)

Here, the type of data that **CompareTo( )** operates on can be explicitly specified. This makes **IComparable<T>** type-safe. For this reason, **IComparable<T>** is now preferable to **IComparable**.

The IEquatable<T> Interface

IEquatable<T>is implemented by those classes that need to define how two objects should be compared for equality. It defines only one method, **Equals( )**, which is shown here:

bool Equals(T *obj*)

The method returns **true** if *obj* is equal to the invoking object and **false** otherwise.

IEquatable<T> is implemented by several classes and structures in the .NET Framework, including the numeric structures, **Char**, **Int32**, **Boolean**, and **String**.

The IConvertible Interface

The **IConvertible** interface is implemented by all of the value-type structures, **string**, and **DateTime**. It specifies various type conversions. Normally, classes that you create will not need to implement this interface.

The ICloneable Interface

By implementing the **ICloneable** interface, you enable a copy of an object to be made. **ICloneable** defines only one method, **Clone( )**, which is shown here:

object Clone( )

This method makes a copy of the invoking object. How you implement **Clone( )** determines how the copy is made. In general, there are two types of copies: deep and shallow. When a deep copy is made, the copy and original are completely independent. Thus, if the original object contained a reference to another object *O*, then a copy of *O* will also be made. In a shallow copy, members are copied, but objects referred to by members are not. If an object refers to some other object *O*, then after a shallow copy, both the copy and the original will refer to the same *O*, and any changes to *O* affect both the copy and the original. Usually, you will implement **Clone( )** so that it performs a deep copy. Shallow copies can be made by using **MemberwiseClone( )**, which is defined by **Object**.

Here is an example that illustrates **ICloneable**. It creates a class called **Test** that contains a reference to an object of a class called **X**. **Test** uses **Clone( )** to create a deep copy.

```
// Demonstrate ICloneable.

using System;

class X {
```

```
  public int a;

  public X(int x) { a = x; }
}

class Test : ICloneable {
  public X o;
  public int b;

  public Test(int x, int y) {
    o = new X(x);
    b = y;
  }

  public void Show(string name) {
    Console.Write(name + " values are ");
    Console.WriteLine("o.a: {0}, b: {1}", o.a, b);
  }

  // Make a deep copy of the invoking object.
  public object Clone() {
    Test temp = new Test(o.a, b);
    return temp;
  }

}

class CloneDemo {
  static void Main() {
    Test ob1 = new Test(10, 20);

    ob1.Show("ob1");

    Console.WriteLine("Make ob2 a clone of ob1.");
    Test ob2 = (Test) ob1.Clone();

    ob2.Show("ob2");

    Console.WriteLine("Changing ob1.o.a to 99 and ob1.b to 88.");
    ob1.o.a = 99;
    ob1.b = 88;

    ob1.Show("ob1");
    ob2.Show("ob2");
  }
}
```

The output is shown here:

```
ob1 values are o.a: 10, b: 20
Make ob2 a clone of ob1.
ob2 values are o.a: 10, b: 20
Changing ob1.o.a to 99 and ob1.b to 88.
ob1 values are o.a: 99, b: 88
ob2 values are o.a: 10, b: 20
```

As the output shows, **ob2** is a clone of **ob1**, but **ob1** and **ob2** are completely separate objects. Changing one does not affect the other. This is accomplished by constructing a new **Test** object, which allocates a new **X** object for the copy. The new **X** instance is given the same value as the **X** object in the original.

To implement a shallow copy, simply have **Clone( )** call **MemberwiseClone( )** defined by **Object**. For example, try changing **Clone( )** in the preceding program as shown here:

```
// Make a shallow copy of the invoking object.
public object Clone() {
  Test temp = (Test) MemberwiseClone();
  return temp;
}
```

After making this change, the output of the program will look like this:

```
ob1 values are o.a: 10, b: 20
Make ob2 a clone of ob1.
ob2 values are o.a: 10, b: 20
Changing ob1.o.a to 99 and ob1.b to 88.
ob1 values are o.a: 99, b: 88
ob2 values are o.a: 99, b: 20
```

Notice that **o** in **ob1** and **o** in **ob2** both refer to the same **X** object. Changing one affects both. Of course, the **int** field **b** in each is still separate because the value types are not accessed via references.

IFormatProvider and IFormattable

The **IFormatProvider** interface defines one method called **GetFormat( )**, which returns an object that controls the formatting of data into a human-readable string. The general form of **GetFormat( )** is shown here:

object GetFormat(Type *fmt*)

Here, *fmt* specifies the format object to obtain.

The **IFormattable** interface supports the formatting of human-readable output. **IFormattable** defines this method:

string ToString(string *fmt*, IFormatProvider *fmtpvdr*)

Here, *fmt* specifies formatting instructions and *fmtpvdr* specifies the format provider.

NOTE *Formatting is described in detail in Chapter 22.*

Strings and Formatting

This chapter examines the **String** class, which underlies C#'s **string** type. As all programmers know, string handling is a part of almost any program. For this reason, the **String** class defines an extensive set of methods, properties, and fields that give you detailed control over the construction and manipulation of strings. Closely related to string handling is the formatting of data into its human-readable form. Using the formatting subsystem, you can format the C# numeric types, date and time, and enumerations.

Strings in C#

An overview of C#'s string handling was presented in Chapter 7, and that discussion is not repeated here. However, it is worthwhile to review how strings are implemented in C# before examining the **String** class.

In all computer languages, a *string* is a sequence of characters, but precisely how such a sequence is implemented varies from language to language. In some computer languages, such as C++, strings are arrays of characters, but this is not the case with C#. Instead, C# strings are objects of the built-in **string** data type. Thus, **string** is a reference type. Moreover, **string** is C#'s name for **System.String**, the standard .NET string type. Thus, a C# string has access to all of the methods, properties, fields, and operators defined by **String**.

Once a string has been created, the character sequence that comprises a string cannot be altered. This restriction allows C# to implement strings more efficiently. Though this restriction probably sounds like a serious drawback, it isn't. When you need a string that is a variation on one that already exists, simply create a new string that contains the desired changes, and discard the original string if it is no longer needed. Because unused string objects are automatically garbage-collected, you don't need to worry about what happens to the discarded strings. It must be made clear, however, that **string** reference variables may, of course, change the object to which they refer. It is just that the character sequence of a specific **string** object cannot be changed after it is created.

To create a string that can be changed, C# offers a class called **StringBuilder**, which is in the **System.Text** namespace. For most purposes, however, you will want to use **string**, not **StringBuilder**.

The String Class

String is defined in the **System** namespace. It implements the **IComparable**, **IComparable<string>**, **ICloneable**, **IConvertible**, **IEnumerable**, **IEnumerable<char>**, and **IEquatable<string>** interfaces. **String** is a sealed class, which means that it cannot be inherited. **String** provides string-handling functionality for C#. It underlies C#'s built-in **string** type and is part of the .NET Framework. The next few sections examine **String** in detail.

The String Constructors

The **String** class defines several constructors that allow you to construct a string in a variety of ways. To create a string from a character array, use one of these constructors:

public String(char[ ] *chrs*)
public String(char[ ] *chrs*, int *start*, int *count*)

The first form constructs a string that contains the characters in *chrs*. The second form uses *count* characters from *chrs*, beginning at the index specified by *start*.

You can create a string that contains a specific character repeated a number of times using this constructor:

public String(char *ch*, int *count*)

Here, *ch* specifies the character that will be repeated *count* times.

You can construct a string given a pointer to a character array using one of these constructors:

public String(char* *chrs*)
public String(char* *chrs*, int *start*, int *count*)

The first form constructs a string that contains the characters pointed to by *chrs*. It is assumed that *chrs* points to a null-terminated array, which is used in its entirety. The second form uses *count* characters from the array pointed to by *chrs*, beginning at the index specified by *start*. Because they use pointers, these constructors can be used only in unsafe code.

You can construct a string given a pointer to an array of bytes using one of these constructors:

public String(sbyte* *chrs*)
public String(sbyte* *chrs*, int *start*, int *count*)
public String(sbyte* *chrs*, int *start*, int *count*, Encoding *en*)

The first form constructs a string that contains the bytes pointed to by *chrs*. It is assumed that *chrs* points to a null-terminated array, which is used in its entirety. The second form uses *count* characters from the array pointed to by *chrs*, beginning at the index specified by *start*. The third form lets you specify how the bytes are encoded. The default encoding is **ASCIIEncoding**. The **Encoding** class is in the **System.Text** namespace. Because they use pointers, these constructors can be used only in unsafe code.

A string literal automatically creates a string object. For this reason, a **string** object is often initialized by assigning it a string literal, as shown here:

```
string str = "a new string";
```

The String Field, Indexer, and Property

The **String** class defines one field, shown here:

public static readonly string Empty

Empty specifies an empty string, which is a string that contains no characters. This differs from a null **String** reference, which simply refers to no object.

There is one read-only indexer defined for **String**, which is shown here:

public char this[int idx] { get; }

This indexer allows you to obtain the character at a specified index. Like arrays, the indexing for strings begins at zero. Since **String** objects are immutable, it makes sense that **String** supports a read-only indexer.

There is one read-only property:

public int Length { get; }

Length returns the number of characters in the string.

The String Operators

The **String** class overloads two operators: = = and !=. To test two strings for equality, use the = = operator. Normally, when the = = operator is applied to object references, it determines if both references refer to the same object. This differs for objects of type **String**. When the = = is applied to two **String** references, the contents of the strings, themselves, are compared for equality. The same is true for the != operator: When comparing **String** objects, the contents of the strings are compared. However, the other relational operators, such as < or >=, compare the references, just like they do for other types of objects. To determine if one string is greater than or less than another, use the **Compare( )** method defined by **String**.

The String Methods

The **String** class defines a large number of methods, and many of the methods have two or more overloaded forms. For this reason, it is neither practical nor useful to list them all. Instead, several of the more commonly used methods will be presented, along with examples that illustrate them.

Comparing Strings

Perhaps the most frequently used string-handling operation is the comparison of one string to another. Because of its importance, **String** provides a wide array of comparison methods. These are shown in Table 22-1. Be aware that string comparisons are sensitive to cultural differences. Comparison methods that do not pass cultural information use the currently selected cultural settings.

Method	Description
public static int Compare(string *str1*, string *str2*)	Compares the string referred to by *str1* with *str2*. Returns greater than zero if *str1* is greater than *str2*, less than zero if *str1* is less than *str2*, and zero if *str1* and *str2* are equal.

public static int
  Compare(string *str1*, string *str2*,
      bool *ignoreCase*)
	Compares the string referred to by *str1* with *str2*. Returns greater than zero if *str1* is greater than *str2*, less than zero if *str1* is less than *str2*, and zero if *str1* and *str2* are equal. If *ignoreCase* is **true**, the comparison ignores case differences. Otherwise, case differences matter.

public static int
  Compare(string *str1*, string *str2*,
      StringComparison *how*)
	Compares the string referred to by *str1* with *str2*. Returns greater than zero if *str1* is greater than *str2*, less than zero if *str1* is less than *str2*, and zero if *str1* and *str2* are equal. How the comparison is performed is specified by *how*.

public static int
  Compare(string *str1*, string *str2*,
      bool *ignoreCase*,
      CultureInfo *ci*)
	Compares the string referred to by *str1* with *str2* using the cultural information passed in *ci*. Returns greater than zero if *str1* is greater than *str2*, less than zero if *str1* is less than *str2*, and zero if *str1* and *str2* are equal. If *ignoreCase* is **true**, the comparison ignores case differences. Otherwise, case differences matter. The **CultureInfo** class is defined in the **System.Globalization** namespace.

public static int
  Compare(string *str1*, int *start1*,
      string *str2*, int *start2*,
      int *count*)
	Compares portions of the strings referred to by *str1* and *str2*. The comparison begins at *str1*[*start1*] and *str2*[*start2*] and runs for *count* characters. Returns greater than zero if *str1* is greater than *str2*, less than zero if *str1* is less than *str2*, and zero if *str1* and *str2* are equal.

public static int
  Compare(string *str1*, int *start1*,
      string *str2*, int *start2*,
      int *count*,
      bool *ignoreCase*)
	Compares portions of the strings referred to by *str1* and *str2*. The comparison begins at *str1*[*start1*] and *str2*[*start2*] and runs for *count* characters. Returns greater than zero if *str1* is greater than *str2*, less than zero if *str1* is less than *str2*, and zero if *str1* and *str2* are equal. If *ignoreCase* is **true**, the comparison ignores case differences. Otherwise, case differences matter.

public static int
  Compare(string *str1*, int *start1*,
      string *str2*, int *start2*,
      int *count*,
      StringComparison *how*)
	Compares portions of the strings referred to by *str1* and *str2*. The comparison begins at *str1*[*start1*] and *str2*[*start2*] and runs for *count* characters. Returns greater than zero if *str1* is greater than *str2*, less than zero if *str1* is less than *str2*, and zero if *str1* and *str2* are equal. How the comparison is performed is specified by *how*.

TABLE 22-1   The **String** Comparison Methods

Method	Description
public static int Compare(string *str1*, int *start1*, string *str2*, int *start2*, int *count*, bool *ignoreCase*, CultureInfo *ci*)	Compares portions of the strings referred to by *str1* and *str2* using the cultural information passed in *ci*. The comparison begins at *str1*[*start1*] and *str2*[*start2*] and runs for *count* characters. Returns greater than zero if *str1* is greater than *str2*, less than zero if *str1* is less than *str2*, and zero if *str1* and *str2* are equal. If *ignoreCase* is true, the comparison ignores case differences. Otherwise, case differences matter. The **CultureInfo** class is defined in the **System.Globalization** namespace.
public static int CompareOrdinal(string *str1*, string *str2*)	Compares the string referred to by *str1* with *str2* independently of culture, region, or language. Returns greater than zero if *str1* is greater than *str2*, less than zero if *str1* is less than *str2*, and zero if *str1* and *str2* are equal.
public static int CompareOrdinal(string *str1*, int *start1*, string *str2*, int *start2*, int *count*)	Compares portions of the strings referred to by *str1* and *str2* independently of culture, region, or language. The comparison begins at *str1*[*start1*] and *str2*[*start2*] and runs for *count* characters. Returns greater than zero if *str1* is greater than *str2*, less than zero if *str1* is less than *str2*, and zero if *str1* and *str2* are equal.
public int CompareTo(object *str*)	Compares the invoking string with *str*. Returns greater than zero if the invoking string is greater than *str*, less than zero if the invoking string is less than *str*, and zero if the two are equal.
public int CompareTo(string *str*)	Compares the invoking string with *str*. Returns greater than zero if the invoking string is greater than *str*, less than zero if the invoking string is less than *str*, and zero if the two are equal.

TABLE 22-1   The **String** Comparison Methods *(continued)*

Of the comparison methods, the **Compare( )** method is the most versatile. It can compare two strings in their entirety or in parts. It can use case-sensitive comparisons or ignore case. In general, string comparisons use dictionary order to determine whether one string is greater than, equal to, or less than another. You can also specify cultural information that governs the comparison. The following program demonstrates several versions of **Compare( )**:

```
// Compare strings.
using System;

class CompareDemo {
  static void Main() {
    string str1 = "one";
    string str2 = "one";
```

```
    string str3 = "ONE";
    string str4 = "two";
    string str5 = "one, too";


    if(String.Compare(str1, str2) == 0)
      Console.WriteLine(str1 + " and " + str2 +
                        " are equal.");
    else
      Console.WriteLine(str1 + " and " + str2 +
                        " are not equal.");

    if(String.Compare(str1, str3) == 0)
      Console.WriteLine(str1 + " and " + str3 +
                        " are equal.");
    else
      Console.WriteLine(str1 + " and " + str3 +
                        " are not equal.");

    if(String.Compare(str1, str3, true) == 0)
      Console.WriteLine(str1 + " and " + str3 +
                        " are equal ignoring case.");
    else
      Console.WriteLine(str1 + " and " + str3 +
                        " are not equal ignoring case.");

    if(String.Compare(str1, str5) == 0)
      Console.WriteLine(str1 + " and " + str5 +
                        " are equal.");
    else
      Console.WriteLine(str1 + " and " + str5 +
                        " are not equal.");

    if(String.Compare(str1, 0, str5, 0, 3) == 0)
      Console.WriteLine("First part of " + str1 + " and " +
                        str5 + " are equal.");
    else
      Console.WriteLine("First part of " + str1 + " and " +
                        str5 + " are not equal.");

    int result = String.Compare(str1, str4);
    if(result < 0)
      Console.WriteLine(str1 + " is less than " + str4);
    else if(result > 0)
      Console.WriteLine(str1 + " is greater than " + str4);
    else
      Console.WriteLine(str1 + " equals " + str4);
  }
}
```

The output is shown here:

```
one and one are equal.
one and ONE are not equal.
one and ONE are equal ignoring case.
one and one, too are not equal.
First part of one and one, too are equal.
one is less than two
```

Using The StringComparison Enumeration

In Table 22-1, notice the two **Compare( )** methods that take a parameter of type **StringComparison**. These versions are shown here:

public static int Compare(string *str1*, string *str2*, StringComparison *how*)

public static int Compare(string *str1*, int *start1*, string *str2*, int *start2*,
                 int *count*, StringComparison *how*)

For each version, the *how* parameter specifies how the comparison of *str1* with *str2* takes place. **StringComparison** is an enumeration that defines the values shown in Table 22-2. Using these values, it is possible to craft a comparison that meets the specific needs of your application. Thus, the addition of the **StringComparison** parameter expands the capabilities of **Compare( )**.

One particularly good use of the **StringComparison** form of **Compare( )** is to compare a string against an invariant file name or password. For example, imagine a situation in which the user must enter the password **we~23&blx$**. This password is the same no matter what cultural settings are in effect. Thus, you want to compare the string entered by the user to the password without cultural differences affecting the comparison. One way to do this is

Value	Description
CurrentCulture	Comparisons are performed using the currently active cultural settings.
CurrentCultureIgnoreCase	Case-insensitive comparisons are performed using the currently active cultural settings.
InvariantCulture	Comparisons are performed using an invariant (that is, universal and unchanging) culture.
InvariantCultureIngoreCase	Case-insensitive comparisons are performed using an invariant (that is, universal and unchanging) culture.
Ordinal	Comparisons are performed using the ordinal values of the characters in the string. Thus, dictionary-order may not result and cultural conventions are ignored.
OrdinalIgnoreCase	Case-insensitive comparisons are performed using the ordinal values of the characters in the string. Thus, dictionary-order may not result and cultural conventions are ignored.

TABLE 22-2   The **StringComparison** Enumeration Values

to specify **StringComparison.InvariantCulture** for the *how* parameter in which case all cultural differences are avoided. This approach is demonstrated by the following program:

```
// Compare strings using StringComparison enumeration.

using System;

class StrCompDemo {
  static void Main() {
    // Note: Never embed a password in real code.
    // This is for demonstration purposes only.
    string pswd = "we~23&blx$";

    string str;

    Console.WriteLine("Enter password: ");
    str = Console.ReadLine();

    // Compare using invariant culture.
    if(String.Compare(pswd, str,
                      StringComparison.InvariantCulture) == 0)
      Console.WriteLine("Password accepted.");
    else
      Console.WriteLine("Password invalid.");
  }
}
```

Concatenating Strings

There are two ways to concatenate (join together) two or more strings. First, you can use the + operator, as demonstrated in Chapter 7. Second, you can use one of the various concatenation methods defined by **String**. Although using + is the easiest approach in many cases, the concatenation methods give you an alternative.

The method that performs concatenation is called **Concat( )**. One of its most commonly used forms is shown here:

public static string Concat(string *str1*, string *str2*)

This method returns a string that contains *str2* concatenated to the end of *str1*. Another form of **Concat( )**, shown here, concatenates three strings:

public static string Concat(string *str1*, string *str2*, string *str3*)

In this version, a string that contains the concatenation of *str1*, *str2*, and *str3* is returned. There is also a form that concatenates four strings:

public static string Concat(string *str1*, string *str2*, string *str3*, string *str4*)

This version returns the concatenation of all four strings.

The version of **Concat( )** shown next concatenates an arbitrary number of strings:

public static string Concat(params string[ ] *strs*)

Here, *strs* refers to a variable number of arguments that are concatenated, and the result is returned. Because this version of **Concat( )** can be used to concatenate any number of strings, including two, three, or four strings, you might wonder why the other forms just shown

exist. The reason is efficiency; passing up to four arguments is more efficient than using a variable-length argument list.

The following program demonstrates the variable-length argument version of **Concat( )**:

```
// Demonstrate Concat().

using System;

class ConcatDemo {
  static void Main() {

    string result = String.Concat("This ", "is ", "a ",
                                  "test ", "of ", "the ",
                                  "String ", "class.");

    Console.WriteLine("result: " + result);

  }
}
```

The output is shown here:

```
result: This is a test of the String class.
```

There are also versions of the **Concat( )** method that take **object** references, rather than **string** references. These obtain the string representation of the objects with which they are called and return a string containing the concatenation of those strings. (The string representations are obtained by calling **ToString( )** on the objects.) These versions of **Concat( )** are shown here:

> public static string Concat(object *v1*)
> public static string Concat(object *v1*, object *v2*)
> public static string Concat(object *v1*, object *v2*, object *v3*)
> public static string Concat(object *v1*, object *v2*, object *v3*, object *v4*)
> public static string Concat(params object[ ] *v*)

The first method simply returns the string equivalent of *v1*. The other methods return a string that contains the concatenation of their arguments. The **object** forms of **Concat( )** are very convenient because they let you avoid having to manually obtain string representations prior to concatenation. To see how useful these methods can be, consider the following program:

```
// Demonstrate the object form of Concat().

using System;

class MyClass {
  public static int Count = 0;

  public MyClass() { Count++; }
}

class ConcatDemo {
  static void Main() {
```

```
    string result = String.Concat("The value is " + 19);
    Console.WriteLine("result: " + result);

    result = String.Concat("hello ", 88, " ", 20.0, " ",
                           false, " ",  23.45M);
    Console.WriteLine("result: " + result);

    MyClass mc = new MyClass();

    result = String.Concat(mc, " current count is ",
                           MyClass.Count);
    Console.WriteLine("result: " + result);
  }
}
```

The output is shown here:

```
result: The value is 19
result: hello 88 20 False 23.45
result: MyClass current count is 1
```

In this example, **Concat( )** concatenates the string representations of various types of data. For each argument, the **ToString( )** method associated with that argument is called to obtain a string representation. Thus, in this call to **Concat( )**

```
string result = String.Concat("The value is " + 19);
```

Int32.ToString( ) is invoked to obtain the string representation of the integer value 19. **Concat( )** then concatenates the strings and returns the result.

Also notice how an object of the user-defined class **MyClass** can be used in this call to **Concat( )**:

```
result = String.Concat(mc, " current count is ",
                       MyClass.Count);
```

In this case, the string representation of **mc**, which is of type **MyClass**, is returned. By default, this is simply its class name. However, if you override the **ToString( )** method, then **MyClass** can return a different string. For example, try adding this version of **ToString( )** to **MyClass** in the preceding program:

```
public override string ToString() {
  return "An object of type MyClass";
}
```

When this version is used, the last line in the output will be

```
result: An object of type MyClass current count is 1
```

Searching a String

String offers many methods that allow you to search a string. For example, you can search for either a substring or a character. You can also search for the first or last occurrence of either.

To search for the first occurrence of a character or substring, use the **IndexOf( )** method. Here are two of its forms:

public int IndexOf(char *ch*)
public int IndexOf(String *str*)

The first form returns the index of the first occurrence of the character *ch* within the invoking string. The second form returns the first occurrence of the string *str*. Both return –1 if the item is not found.

To search for the last occurrence of a character or substring, use the **LastIndexOf( )** method. Here are two of its forms:

public int LastIndexOf(char *ch*)
public int LastIndexOf(string *str*)

The first form returns the index of the last occurrence of the character *ch* within the invoking string. The second form returns the index of the last occurrence of the string *str*. Both return –1 if the item is not found.

String offers two interesting supplemental search methods: **IndexOfAny( )** and **LastIndexOfAny( )**. These search for the first or last character that matches any of a set of characters. Here are their simplest forms:

public int IndexOfAny(char[ ] *a*)
public int LastIndexOfAny(char[ ] *a*)

IndexOfAny( ) returns the index of the first occurrence of any character in *a* that is found within the invoking string. **LastIndexOfAny( )** returns the index of the last occurrence of any character in *a* that is found within the invoking string. Both return –1 if no match is found.

When working with strings, it is often useful to know if a string begins with or ends with a given substring. To accomplish these tasks, use the **StartsWith( )** and **EndsWith( )** methods. Here are their two simplest forms:

public bool StartsWith(string *str*)
public bool EndsWith(string *str*)

StartsWith( ) returns true if the invoking string begins with the string passed in *str*. **EndsWith( )** returns true if the invoking string ends with the string passed in *str*. Both return false on failure.

Here is a program that demonstrates several of the string search methods:

```
// Search strings.

using System;

class StringSearchDemo {
  static void Main() {
    string str = "C# has powerful string handling.";
    int idx;

    Console.WriteLine("str: " + str);

    idx = str.IndexOf('h');
    Console.WriteLine("Index of first 'h': " + idx);
```

```
      idx = str.LastIndexOf('h');
      Console.WriteLine("Index of last 'h': " + idx);

      idx = str.IndexOf("ing");
      Console.WriteLine("Index of first \"ing\": " + idx);

      idx = str.LastIndexOf("ing");
      Console.WriteLine("Index of last \"ing\": " + idx);

      char[] chrs = { 'a', 'b', 'c' };
      idx = str.IndexOfAny(chrs);
      Console.WriteLine("Index of first 'a', 'b', or 'c': " + idx);

      if(str.StartsWith("C# has"))
        Console.WriteLine("str begins with \"C# has\"");

      if(str.EndsWith("ling."))
        Console.WriteLine("str ends with \"ling.\"");
  }
}
```

The output from the program is shown here:

```
str: C# has powerful string handling.
Index of first 'h': 3
Index of last 'h': 23
Index of first "ing": 19
Index of last "ing": 28
Index of first 'a', 'b', or 'c': 4
str begins with "C# has"
str ends with "ling."
```

A string search method that you will find useful in many circumstances is **Contains( )**. Its general form is shown here:

public bool Contains(string *str*)

It returns true if the invoking string contains the string specified by *str* and false otherwise. This method is especially useful when all you need to know is if a specific substring exists within another string. Here is an example that demonstrates its use:

```
// Demonstrate Contains().

using System;

class ContainsDemo {
  static void Main() {
    string str = "C# combines power with performance.";

    if(str.Contains("power"))
      Console.WriteLine("The sequence power was found.");

    if(str.Contains("pow"))
      Console.WriteLine("The sequence pow was found.");
```

```
      if(!str.Contains("powerful"))
        Console.WriteLine("The sequence powerful was not found.");
    }
}
```

The output is shown here:

```
The sequence power was found.
The sequence pow was found.
The sequence powerful was not found.
```

As the output shows, **Contains( )** searches for a matching sequence, not for whole words. Thus, both "pow" and "power" are found. However, since there is no sequence that matches "powerful", it is (correctly) not found.

Several of the search methods have additional forms that allow you to begin a search at a specified index or to specify a range to search within. All versions of the **String** search methods are shown in Table 22-3.

Method	Description
public bool Contains(string *str*)	Returns true if the invoking string contains the string specified by *str*. False is returned if *str* is not found.
public bool EndsWith(string *str*)	Returns true if the invoking string ends with the string passed in *str*. Otherwise, false is returned.
public bool EndsWith(string *str*, StringComparison *how*)	Returns true if the invoking string ends with the string passed in *str*. Otherwise, false is returned. How the search is performed is specified by *how*.
public bool EndsWith(string *str*, bool *ignoreCase*, CultureInfo *ci*)	Returns true if the invoking string ends with the string passed in *str*. Otherwise, false is returned. If *ignoreCase* is **true**, the search ignores case differences. Otherwise, case differences matter. The search is conducted using the cultural information passed in *ci*.
public int IndexOf(char *ch*)	Returns the index of the first occurrence of *ch* within the invoking string. Returns –1 if *ch* is not found.
public int IndexOf(string *str*)	Returns the index of the first occurrence of *str* within the invoking string. Returns –1 if *str* is not found.
public int IndexOf(char *ch*, int *start*)	Returns the index of the first occurrence of *ch* within the invoking string. Searching begins at the index specified by *start*. Returns –1 if *ch* is not found.
public int IndexOf(string *str*, int *start*)	Returns the index of the first occurrence of *str* within the invoking string. Searching begins at the index specified by *start*. Returns –1 if *str* is not found.

TABLE 22-3 The Search Methods Offered by **String**

Method	Description
public int IndexOf(char *ch*, int *start*, int *count*)	Returns the index of the first occurrence of *ch* within the invoking string. Searching begins at the index specified by *start* and runs for *count* elements. Returns −1 if *ch* is not found.
public int IndexOf(string *str*, int *start*, int *count*)	Returns the index of the first occurrence of *str* within the invoking string. Searching begins at the index specified by *start* and runs for *count* elements. Returns −1 if *str* is not found.
public int IndexOf(string *str*, StringComparison *how*)	Returns the index of the first occurrence of *str* within the invoking string. How the search is performed is specified by *how*. Returns −1 if *str* is not found.
public int IndexOf(string *str*, int *start*, StringComparison *how*)	Returns the index of the first occurrence of *str* within the invoking string. Searching begins at the index specified by *start*. How the search is performed is specified by *how*. Returns −1 if *str* is not found.
public int IndexOf(string *str*, int *start*, int *count*, StringComparison *how*)	Returns the index of the first occurrence of *str* within the invoking string. Searching begins at the index specified by *start* and runs for *count* elements. How the search is performed is specified by *how*. Returns −1 if *ch* is not found.
public int LastIndexOf(char *ch*)	Returns the index of the last occurrence of *ch* within the invoking string. Returns −1 if *ch* is not found.
public int LastIndexOf(string *str*)	Returns the index of the last occurrence of *str* within the invoking string. Returns −1 if *str* is not found.
public int LastIndexOf(char *ch*, int *start*)	Returns the index of the last occurrence of *ch* within a range of the invoking string. The search proceeds in reverse order, beginning at the index specified by *start* and stopping at 0. Returns −1 if the *ch* is not found.
public int LastIndexOf(string *str*, int *start*)	Returns the index of the last occurrence of *str* within a range of the invoking string. The search proceeds in reverse order, beginning at the index specified by *start* and stopping at 0. Returns −1 if *str* is not found.
public int LastIndexOf(char *ch*, int *start*, int *count*)	Returns the index of the last occurrence of *ch* within the invoking string. The search proceeds in reverse order, beginning at the index specified by *start* and running for *count* elements. Returns −1 if *ch* is not found.

TABLE 22-3   The Search Methods Offered by **String** *(continued)*

Method	Description
public int LastIndexOf(string *str*, int *start*, 　　　　int *count*)	Returns the index of the last occurrence of *str* within the invoking string. The search proceeds in reverse order, beginning at the index specified by *start* and running for *count* elements. Returns –1 if *str* is not found.
public int LastIndexOf(string *str*, 　　　StringComparison *how*)	Returns the index of the last occurrence of *str* within the invoking string. How the search is performed is specified by *how*. Returns –1 if *str* is not found.
public int LastIndexOf(string *str*, int *start*, 　　　StringComparison *how*)	Returns the index of the last occurrence of *str* within a range of the invoking string. The search proceeds in reverse order, beginning at the index specified by *start* and stopping at 0. How the search is performed is specified by *how*. Returns –1 if *str* is not found.
public int LastIndexOf(string *str*, int *start*, 　　　int *count*, 　　　StringComparison *how*)	Returns the index of the last occurrence of *str* within the invoking string. The search proceeds in reverse order, beginning at the index specified by *start* and running for *count* elements. How the search is performed is specified by *how*. Returns –1 if *str* is not found.
public bool StartsWith(string *str*)	Returns true if the invoking string begins with the string passed in *str*. Otherwise, false is returned.
public bool StartsWith(string *str*, 　　　StringComparison *how*)	Returns true if the invoking string begins with the string passed in *str*. Otherwise, false is returned. How the search is performed is specified by *how*.
public bool StartsWith(string *str*, 　　　bool *ignoreCase*, 　　　CultureInfo *ci*)	Returns true if the invoking string begins with the string passed in *str*. Otherwise, false is returned. If *ignoreCase* is **true**, the search ignores case differences. Otherwise, case differences matter. The search is conducted using the cultural information passed in *ci*.

TABLE 22-3　The Search Methods Offered by **String** *(continued)*

Splitting and Joining Strings

Two fundamental string-handling operations are split and join. A *split* decomposes a string into its constituent parts. A *join* constructs a string from a set of parts. To split a string, **String** defines **Split( )**. To join a set of strings, **String** provides **Join( )**.

There are several versions of **Split( )**. Two commonly used forms, which have been available since C# 1.0, are shown here:

```
public string[ ] Split(params char[ ] seps)
public string[ ] Split(params char[ ] seps, int count)
```

The first form splits the invoking string into pieces and returns an array containing the substrings. The characters that delimit each substring are passed in *seps*. If *seps* is null or refers to an empty string, then whitespace is used as the separator. In the second form, no more than *count* substrings will be returned.

The two forms of the **Join( )** method are shown here:

public static string Join(string *sep*, string[ ] *strs*)
public static string Join(string *sep*, string[ ] *strs*, int *start*, int *count*)

The first form returns a string that contains the concatenation of the strings in *strs*. The second form returns a string that contains the concatenation of *count* strings in *strs*, beginning at *strs[start]*. For both versions, each string is separated from the next by the string specified by *sep*.

The following program demonstrates **Split( )** and **Join( )**:

```
// Split and join strings.

using System;

class SplitAndJoinDemo {
  static void Main() {
    string str = "One if by land, two if by sea.";
    char[] seps = {' ', '.', ',' };

    // Split the string into parts.
    string[] parts = str.Split(seps);
    Console.WriteLine("Pieces from split: ");
    for(int i=0; i < parts.Length; i++)
      Console.WriteLine(parts[i]);

    // Now, join the parts.
    string whole = String.Join(" | ", parts);
    Console.WriteLine("Result of join: ");
    Console.WriteLine(whole);
  }
}
```

Here is the output:

```
Pieces from split:
One
if
by
land

two
if
by
sea

Result of join:
One | if | by | land |  | two | if | by | sea |
```

There is one important thing to notice in this output: the empty string that occurs between "land" and "two". This is caused by the fact that in the original string, the word "land" is followed by a comma and a space, as in "land, two". However, both the comma and the space are specified as separators. Thus, when this string is split, the empty string that exists between the two separators (the comma and the space) is returned.

There are several additional forms of **Split( )** that take a parameter of type **StringSplitOptions**. This parameter controls whether empty strings are part of the resulting split. Here are these forms of **Split( )**:

public string[ ] Split(params char[ ] *seps,* StringSplitOptions *how*)
public string[ ] Split(string[ ] *seps,* StringSplitOptions *how*)
public string[ ] Split(params char[ ] *seps,* int *count,* StringSplitOptions *how*)
public string[ ] Split(string[ ] *seps,* int *count,* StringSplitOptions *how*)

The first two forms split the invoking string into pieces and return an array containing the substrings. The characters that delimit each substring are passed in *seps*. If *seps* is null, then whitespace is used as the separator. In the third and fourth forms, no more than *count* substrings will be returned. For all versions, the value of *how* determines how to handle empty strings that result when two separators are adjacent to each other. The **StringSplitOptions** enumeration defines only two values: **None** and **RemoveEmptyEntries**. If *how* is **None**, then empty strings are included in the result (as the previous program showed). If *how* is **RemoveEmptyEntries**, empty strings are excluded from the result.

To understand the effects of removing empty entries, try replacing this line in the preceding program:

```
string[] parts = str.Split(seps);
```

with the following:

```
string[] parts = str.Split(seps, StringSplitOptions.RemoveEmptyEntries);
```

When you run the program, the output will be as shown next:

```
Pieces from split:
One
if
by
land
two
if
by
sea
Result of join:
One | if | by | land | two | if | by | sea
```

As you can see, the empty string that previously resulted because of the combination of the comma and space after "land" has been removed.

Splitting a string is an important string-manipulation procedure because it is often used to obtain the individual *tokens* that comprise the string. For example, a database program might use **Split( )** to decompose a query such as "show me all balances greater than 100"

into its individual parts, such as "show" and "100". In the process, the separators are removed. Thus, "show" (without any leading or trailing spaces) is obtained, not " show". The following program illustrates this concept. It tokenizes strings containing binary mathematical operations, such as 10 + 5. It then performs the operation and displays the result.

```
// Tokenize strings.

using System;

class TokenizeDemo {
  static void Main() {
    string[] input = {
                       "100 + 19",
                       "100 / 3.3",
                       "-3 * 9",
                       "100 - 87"
                     };
    char[] seps = {' '};

    for(int i=0; i < input.Length; i++) {
      // split string into parts
      string[] parts = input[i].Split(seps);
      Console.Write("Command: ");
      for(int j=0; j < parts.Length; j++)
        Console.Write(parts[j] + " ");

      Console.Write(", Result: ");
      double n = Double.Parse(parts[0]);
      double n2 = Double.Parse(parts[2]);

      switch(parts[1]) {
        case "+":
          Console.WriteLine(n + n2);
          break;
        case "-":
          Console.WriteLine(n - n2);
          break;
        case "*":
          Console.WriteLine(n * n2);
          break;
        case "/":
          Console.WriteLine(n / n2);
          break;
      }
    }
  }
}
```

Here is the output:

```
Command: 100 + 19 , Result: 119
Command: 100 / 3.3 , Result: 30.3030303030303
Command: -3 * 9 , Result: -27
Command: 100 - 87 , Result: 13
```

Padding and Trimming Strings

Sometimes you will want to remove leading and trailing spaces from a string. This type of operation, called *trimming*, is often needed by command processors. For example, a database might recognize the word "print." However, a user might enter this command with one or more leading or trailing spaces. Any such spaces must be removed before the string can be recognized by the database. Conversely, sometimes you will want to pad a string with spaces so that it meets some minimal length. For example, if you are preparing formatted output, you might need to ensure that each line is of a certain length in order to maintain alignment. Fortunately, C# includes methods that make these types of operations easy.

To trim a string, use one of these **Trim( )** methods:

public string Trim( )
public string Trim(params char[ ] *chrs*)

The first form removes leading and trailing whitespace from the invoking string. The second form removes leading and trailing occurrences of the characters specified by *chrs*. In both cases, the resulting string is returned.

You can pad a string by adding characters to either the left or the right side of the string. To pad a string on the left, use one of the methods shown here:

public string PadLeft(int *len*)
public string PadLeft(int *len*, char *ch*)

The first form adds spaces on the left as needed to the invoking string so that its total length equals *len*. The second form adds the character specified by *ch* as needed to the invoking string so that its total length equals *len*. In both cases, the resulting string is returned. If *len* is less than the length of the invoking string, a copy of the invoking string is returned unaltered.

To pad a string to the right, use one of these methods:

public string PadRight(int *len*)
public string PadRight(int *len*, char *ch*)

The first form adds spaces on the right as needed to the invoking string so that its total length equals *len*. The second form adds the characters specified by *ch* as needed to the invoking string so that its total length equals *len*. In both cases, the resulting string is returned. If *len* is less than the length of the invoking string, a copy of the invoking string is returned unaltered.

The following program demonstrates trimming and padding:

```
// Trimming and padding.

using System;

class TrimPadDemo {
  static void Main() {
    string str = "test";

    Console.WriteLine("Original string: " + str);

    // Pad on left with spaces.
    str = str.PadLeft(10);
    Console.WriteLine("|" + str + "|");
```

```
// Pad on right with spaces.
str = str.PadRight(20);
Console.WriteLine("|" + str + "|");

// Trim spaces.
str = str.Trim();
Console.WriteLine("|" + str + "|");

// Pad on left with #s.
str = str.PadLeft(10, '#');
Console.WriteLine("|" + str + "|");

// Pad on right with #s.
str = str.PadRight(20, '#');
Console.WriteLine("|" + str + "|");

// Trim #s.
str = str.Trim('#');
Console.WriteLine("|" + str + "|");
  }
}
```

The output is shown here:

```
Original string: test
|        test|
|        test          |
|test|
|######test|
|######test##########|
|test|
```

Inserting, Removing, and Replacing

You can insert a string into another using the **Insert( )** method, shown here:

   public string Insert(int *start*, string *str*)

Here, *str* is inserted into the invoking string at the index specified by *start*. The resulting string is returned.

   You can remove a portion of a string using **Remove( )**, shown next:

   public string Remove(int *start*)
   public string Remove(int *start*, int *count*)

The first form begins at the index specified by *start* and removes all remaining characters in the string. The second form begins at count and removes *count* number of characters. In both cases, the resulting string is returned.

   You can replace a portion of a string by using **Replace( )**. It has these forms:

   public string Replace(char *ch1*, char *ch2*)
   public string Replace(string *str1*, string *str2*)

The first form replaces all occurrences of *ch1* in the invoking string with *ch2*. The second form replaces all occurrences of *str1* in the invoking string with *str2*. In both cases, the resulting string is returned.

Here is an example that demonstrates **Insert( )**, **Remove( )**, and **Replace( )**:

```
// Inserting, replacing, and removing.

using System;

class InsRepRevDemo {
  static void Main() {
    string str = "This test";

    Console.WriteLine("Original string: " + str);

    // Insert
    str = str.Insert(5, "is a ");
    Console.WriteLine(str);

    // Replace string
    str = str.Replace("is", "was");
    Console.WriteLine(str);

    // Replace characters
    str = str.Replace('a', 'X');
    Console.WriteLine(str);

    // Remove
    str = str.Remove(4, 5);
    Console.WriteLine(str);
  }
}
```

The output is shown here:

```
Original string: This test
This is a test
Thwas was a test
ThwXs wXs X test
ThwX X test
```

Changing Case

String offers two convenient methods that enable you to change the case of letters within a string. These are called **ToUpper( )** and **ToLower( )**. Here are their simplest forms:

> public string ToLower( )
> public string ToUpper( )

ToLower( ) lowercases all letters within the invoking string. **ToUpper( )** uppercases all letters within the invoking string. The resulting string is returned. There are also versions of these methods that allow you to specify cultural settings.

Also available are the methods **ToUpperInvariant( )** and **ToLowerInvariant( )**, shown here:

> public string ToUpperInvariant( )
> public string ToLowerInvariant( )

These work like **ToUpper( )** and **ToLower( )** except that they use the invariant culture to perform the transformations to upper- or lowercase.

Using the Substring( ) Method

You can obtain a portion of a string by using the **Substring( )** method. It has these two forms:

public string Substring(int *idx*)
public string Substring(int *idx*, int *count*)

In the first form, the substring begins at the index specified by *idx* and runs to the end of the invoking string. In the second form, the substring begins at *idx* and runs for *count* characters. In each case, the substring is returned.

The following program demonstrates the **Substring( )** method:

```
// Use Substring().

using System;

class SubstringDemo {
  static void Main() {
    string str = "ABCDEFGHIJKLMNOPQRSTUVWXYZ";

    Console.WriteLine("str: " + str);

    Console.Write("str.Substring(15): ");
    string substr = str.Substring(15);
    Console.WriteLine(substr);

    Console.Write("str.Substring(0, 15): ");
    substr = str.Substring(0, 15);
    Console.WriteLine(substr);
  }
}
```

The following output is produced:

```
str: ABCDEFGHIJKLMNOPQRSTUVWXYZ
str.Substring(15): PQRSTUVWXYZ
str.Substring(0, 15): ABCDEFGHIJKLMNO
```

The String Extension Methods

As mentioned earlier, **String** implements **IEnumerable<T>**. This means that beginning with C# 3.0, a **String** object can call the extension methods defined by **Enumerable** and **Queryable**, which are both in the **System.Linq** namespace. These extension methods primarily provide support for LINQ, but some can also be used for other purposes, such as certain types of string handling. See Chapter 19 for a discussion of extension methods.

Formatting

When a human-readable form of a built-in type, such as **int** or **double**, is needed, a string representation must be created. Although C# automatically supplies a default format for this representation, it is also possible to specify a format of your own choosing. For example, as you saw in Part I, it is possible to output numeric data using a dollars and cents format. A number

of methods format data, including **Console.WriteLine( )**, **String.Format( )**, and the **ToString( )** method defined for the numeric structure types. The same approach to formatting is used by all three; once you have learned to format data for one, you can apply it to the others.

Formatting Overview

Formatting is governed by two components: *format specifiers* and *format providers*. The form that the string representation of a value will take is controlled through the use of a format specifier. Thus, it is the format specifier that dictates how the human-readable form of the data will look. For example, to output a numeric value using scientific notation, you will use the E format specifier.

In many cases, the precise format of a value will be affected by the culture and language in which the program is running. For example, in the United States, money is represented in dollars. In Europe, money is represented in euros. To handle the cultural and language differences, C# uses format providers. A format provider defines the way that a format specifier will be interpreted. A format provider is created by implementing the **IFormatProvider** interface, which defines the **GetFormat( )** method. Format providers are predefined for the built-in numeric types and many other types in the .NET Framework. In general, you can format data without having to worry about specifying a format provider, and format providers are not examined further in this book.

To format data, include a format specifier in a call to a method that supports formatting. The use of format specifiers was introduced in Chapter 3, but is worthwhile reviewing here. The discussion that follows uses **Console.WriteLine( )**, but the same basic approach applies to other methods that support formatting.

To format data using **WriteLine( )**, use the version of **WriteLine( )** shown here:

WriteLine(*"format string"*, *arg0*, *arg1*, ... , *argN*);

In this version, the arguments to **WriteLine( )** are separated by commas and not + signs. The *format string* contains two items: regular, printing characters that are displayed as-is, and format commands.

Format commands take this general form:

{*argnum*, *width*: *fmt*}

Here, *argnum* specifies the number of the argument (starting from zero) to display. The minimum width of the field is specified by *width,* and the format specifier is represented by *fmt*. Both *width* and *fmt* are optional. Thus, in its simplest form, a format command simply indicates which argument to display. For example, {0} indicates *arg0*, {1} specifies *arg1*, and so on.

During execution, when a format command is encountered in the format string, the corresponding argument, as specified by *argnum*, is substituted and displayed. Thus, it is the position of a format specifier within the format string that determines where its matching data will be displayed. It is the argument number that determines which argument will be formatted.

If *fmt* is present, then the data is displayed using the specified format. Otherwise, the default format is used. If *width* is present, then output is padded with spaces to ensure that the minimum field width is attained. If *width* is positive, output is right-justified. If *width* is negative, output is left-justified.

The remainder of this chapter examines formatting and format specifiers in detail.

The Numeric Format Specifiers

There are several format specifiers defined for numeric data. They are shown in Table 22-4. Each format specifier can include an optional precision specifier. For example, to specify that a value be represented as a fixed-point value with two decimal places, use F2.

As explained, the precise effect of certain format specifiers depends upon the cultural settings. For example, the currency specifier, C, automatically displays a value in the monetary format of the selected culture. For most users, the default cultural information matches their locale and language. Thus, the same format specifier can be used without concern about the cultural context in which the program is executed.

Here is a program that demonstrates several of the numeric format specifiers:

```
// Demonstrate various format specifiers.

using System;

class FormatDemo {
  static void Main() {
    double v = 17688.65849;
    double v2 = 0.15;
    int x = 21;

    Console.WriteLine("{0:F2}", v);

    Console.WriteLine("{0:N5}", v);

    Console.WriteLine("{0:e}", v);

    Console.WriteLine("{0:r}", v);

    Console.WriteLine("{0:p}", v2);

    Console.WriteLine("{0:X}", x);

    Console.WriteLine("{0:D12}", x);

    Console.WriteLine("{0:C}", 189.99);
  }
}
```

The output is shown here:

```
17688.66
17,688.65849
1.768866e+004
17688.65849
15.00 %
15
000000000021
$189.99
```

Notice the effect of the precision specifier in several of the formats.

Specifier	Format	Meaning of Precision Specifier
C	Currency (that is, a monetary value).	Specifies the number of decimal places.
c	Same as C.	
D	Whole number numeric data. (Use with integers only.)	Minimum number of digits. Leading zeros will be used to pad the result, if necessary.
d	Same as D.	
E	Scientific notation (uses uppercase E).	Specifies the number of decimal places. The default is six.
e	Scientific notation (uses lowercase e).	Specifies the number of decimal places. The default is six.
F	Fixed-point notation.	Specifies the number of decimal places.
f	Same as F.	
G	Use either E or F format, whichever is shorter.	See E and F.
g	Use either e or f format, whichever is shorter.	See e and f.
N	Fixed-point notation, with comma separators.	Specifies the number of decimal places.
n	Same as N.	
P	Percentage	Specifies the number of decimal places.
p	Same as P.	
R or r	Numeric value that can be parsed, using **Parse( )**, back into its equivalent internal form. (This is called the "round-trip" format.)	Not used.
X	Hexadecimal (uses uppercase letters *A* through *F*).	Minimum number of digits. Leading zeros will be used to pad the result, if necessary.
x	Hexadecimal (uses lowercase letters *a* through *f*).	Minimum number of digits. Leading zeros will be used to pad the result if necessary.

TABLE 22-4 The Format Specifiers

Understanding Argument Numbers

It is important to understand that the argument associated with a format specifier is determined by the argument number, not the argument's position in the argument list. This means the same argument can be output more than once within the same call to **WriteLine( )**. It also

means that arguments can be displayed in a sequence different than they are specified in the argument list. For example, consider the following program:

```
using System;

class FormatDemo2 {
  static void Main() {

    // Format the same argument three different ways:
    Console.WriteLine("{0:F2}   {0:F3}   {0:e}", 10.12345);

    // Display arguments in non-sequential order.
    Console.WriteLine("{2:d} {0:d} {1:d}", 1, 2, 3);
  }
}
```

The output is shown here:

```
10.12   10.123   1.012345e+001
3 1 2
```

In the first **WriteLine( )** statement, the same argument, 10.12345, is formatted three different ways. This is possible because each format specifier refers to the first (and only) argument. In the second **WriteLine( )** statement, the three arguments are displayed in non-sequential order. Remember, there is no rule that format specifiers must use the arguments in sequence. Any format specifier can refer to any argument.

Using String.Format( ) and ToString( ) to Format Data

Although embedding format commands into **WriteLine( )** is a convenient way to format output, sometimes you will want to create a string that contains the formatted data, but not immediately display that string. Doing so lets you format data in advance, allowing you to output it later, to the device of your choosing. This is especially useful in a GUI environment, such as Windows, in which console-based I/O is rarely used, or for preparing output for a web page.

In general, there are two ways to obtain the formatted string representation of a value. One way is to use **String.Format( )**. The other is to pass a format specifier to the **ToString( )** method of the built-in numeric types. Each approach is examined here.

Using String.Format( ) to Format Values

You can obtain a formatted value by calling one of the **Format( )** methods defined by **String**. They are shown in Table 22-5. **Format( )** works much like **WriteLine( )**, except that it returns a formatted string rather than outputting it to the console.

Method	Description
public static string Format(string *str*, object *v*)	Formats *v* according to the first format command in *str*. Returns a copy of *str* in which formatted data has been substituted for the format command.
public static string Format(string *str*, object *v1*, object *v2*)	Formats *v1* according to the first format command in *str*, and *v2* according to the second format command in *str*. Returns a copy of *str* in which formatted data has been substituted for the format commands.

public static string
    Format(string *str*, object *v1*,
        object *v2*, object *v3*)
	Formats *v1*, *v2*, and *v3* according to the corresponding format commands in *str*. Returns a copy of *str* in which formatted data has been substituted for the format commands.

public static string Format(string *str*, params object[ ] *v*)	Formats the values passed in *v* according to the format commands in *str*. Returns a copy of *str* in which formatted data has been substituted for each format command.

public static string
    Format(IFormatProvider *fmtprvdr*,
        string *str*, params object[ ] *v*)
	Formats the values passed in *v* according to the format commands in *str* using the format provider specified by *fmtprvdr*. Returns a copy of *str* in which formatted data has been substituted for each format command.

TABLE 22-5   The **Format( )** Methods

Here is the previous format demonstration program rewritten to use **String.Format( )**. It produces the same output as the earlier version.

```
// Use String.Format() to format a value.

using System;

class FormatDemo {
  static void Main() {
    double v = 17688.65849;
    double v2 = 0.15;
    int x = 21;

    string str = String.Format("{0:F2}", v);
    Console.WriteLine(str);

    str = String.Format("{0:N5}", v);
    Console.WriteLine(str);
```

```
    str = String.Format("{0:e}", v);
    Console.WriteLine(str);

    str = String.Format("{0:r}", v);
    Console.WriteLine(str);

    str = String.Format("{0:p}", v2);
    Console.WriteLine(str);

    str = String.Format("{0:X}", x);
    Console.WriteLine(str);

    str = String.Format("{0:D12}", x);
    Console.WriteLine(str);

    str = String.Format("{0:C}", 189.99);
    Console.WriteLine(str);
  }
}
```

Like **WriteLine( )**, **String.Format( )** lets you embed regular text along with format specifiers, and you can use more than one format specifier and value. For example, consider this program, which displays the running sum and product of the numbers 1 through 10:

```
// A closer look at Format().

using System;

class FormatDemo2 {
  static void Main() {
    int i;
    int sum = 0;
    int prod = 1;
    string str;

    /* Display the running sum and product
       for the numbers 1 through 10. */
    for(i=1; i <= 10; i++) {
      sum += i;
      prod *= i;
      str = String.Format("Sum:{0,3:D}   Product:{1,8:D}",
                          sum, prod);
      Console.WriteLine(str);
    }
  }
}
```

The output is shown here:

```
Sum:  1  Product:        1
Sum:  3  Product:        2
Sum:  6  Product:        6
Sum: 10  Product:       24
Sum: 15  Product:      120
Sum: 21  Product:      720
Sum: 28  Product:     5040
```

```
Sum: 36   Product:    40320
Sum: 45   Product:   362880
Sum: 55   Product:  3628800
```

In the program, pay close attention to this statement:

```
str = String.Format("Sum:{0,3:D}  Product:{1,8:D}",
                    sum, prod);
```

This call to **Format( )** contains two format specifiers, one for **sum** and one for **prod**. Notice that the argument numbers are specified just as they are when using **WriteLine( )**. Also, notice that regular text, such as "Sum:" is included. This text is passed through and becomes part of the output string.

Using ToString( ) to Format Data

For all of the built-in numeric structure types, such as **Int32** or **Double**, you can use **ToString( )** to obtain a formatted string representation of the value. To do so, you will use this version of **ToString( )**:

public string ToString(string *fmt*)

It returns the string representation of the invoking object as specified by the format specifier passed in *fmt*. For example, the following statement creates a monetary representation of the value 188.99 through the use of the C format specifier:

```
string str = 189.99.ToString("C");
```

Notice how the format specifier is passed directly to **ToString( )**. Unlike embedded format commands used by **WriteLine( )** or **Format( )**, which supply an argument-number and field-width component, **ToString( )** requires only the format specifier, itself.

Here is a rewrite of the previous format program that uses **ToString( )** to obtain formatted strings. It produces the same output as the earlier versions.

```
// Use ToString() to format values.

using System;

class ToStringDemo {
  static void Main() {
    double v = 17688.65849;
    double v2 = 0.15;
    int x = 21;

    string str = v.ToString("F2");
    Console.WriteLine(str);

    str = v.ToString("N5");
    Console.WriteLine(str);

    str = v.ToString("e");
    Console.WriteLine(str);

    str = v.ToString("r");
```

```
    Console.WriteLine(str);

    str = v2.ToString("p");
    Console.WriteLine(str);

    str = x.ToString("X");
    Console.WriteLine(str);

    str = x.ToString("D12");
    Console.WriteLine(str);

    str = 189.99.ToString("C");
    Console.WriteLine(str);
  }
}
```

Creating a Custom Numeric Format

Although the predefined numeric format specifiers are quite useful, C# gives you the ability to define your own, custom format using a feature sometimes called *picture format*. The term *picture format* comes from the fact that you create a custom format by specifying an example (that is, picture) of how you want the output to look. This approach was mentioned briefly in Part I. Here it is examined in detail.

The Custom Format Placeholder Characters

When you create a custom format, you specify that format by creating an example (or picture) of what you want the data to look like. To do this, you use the characters shown in Table 22-6 as placeholders. Each is examined in turn.

The period specifies where the decimal point will be located.

The # placeholder specifies a digit position. The # can occur on the left or right side of the decimal point or by itself. When one or more #s occur on the right side of the decimal point, they specify the number of decimal digits to display. The value is rounded if necessary. When the # occurs to the left of the decimal point, it specifies the digit positions for the whole-number part of the value. Leading zeros will be added if necessary. If the whole-number portion of the value has more digits than there are #s, the entire whole-number portion will be displayed. In no cases will the whole-number portion of a value be truncated. If there is no decimal point, then the # causes the value to be rounded to its integer value. A zero value that is not significant, such as a trailing zero, will not be displayed. This causes a somewhat odd quirk, however, because a format such as #.## displays nothing at all if the value being formatted is zero. To output a zero value, use the 0 placeholder described next.

The 0 placeholder causes a leading or trailing 0 to be added to ensure that a minimum number of digits will be present. It can be used on both the right and left side of the decimal point. For example,

```
Console.WriteLine("{0:00##.#00}", 21.3);
```

displays this output:

```
0021.300
```

Values containing more digits will be displayed in full on the left side of the decimal point and rounded on the right side.

You can insert commas into large numbers by specifying a pattern that embeds a comma within a sequence of #s. For example, this:

```
Console.WriteLine("{0:#,###.#}", 3421.3);
```

displays

```
3,421.3.
```

It is not necessary to specify each comma for each position. Specifying one comma causes it to be inserted into the value every third digit from the left of the decimal point. For example,

```
Console.WriteLine("{0:#,###.#}", 8763421.3);
```

produces this output:

```
8,763,421.3.
```

Commas have a second meaning. When they occur on the immediate left of the decimal point, they act as a scaling factor. Each comma causes the value to be divided by 1,000. For example,

```
Console.WriteLine("Value in thousands: {0:#,###,.#}", 8763421.3);
```

produces this output:

```
Value in thousands: 8,763.4
```

As the output shows, the value is scaled in terms of thousands.

In addition to the placeholders, a custom format specifier can contain other characters. Any other characters are simply passed through, appearing in the formatted string exactly as they appear in the format specifier. For example, this **WriteLine( )** statement:

```
Console.WriteLine("Fuel efficiency is {0:##.# mpg}", 21.3);
```

produces this output:

```
Fuel efficiency is 21.3 mpg
```

You can also use the escape sequences, such as **\t** or **\n**, if necessary.

The *E* and *e* placeholders cause a value to be displayed in scientific notation. At least one 0, but possibly more, must follow the *E* or *e*. The 0s indicate the number of decimal digits that will be displayed. The decimal component will be rounded to fit the format. Using an uppercase *E* causes an uppercase *E* to be displayed; using a lowercase *e* causes a lowercase *e* to be displayed. To ensure that a sign character precedes the exponent, use the *E+* or *e+* forms. To display a sign character for negative values only, use *E*, *e*, *E-*, or *e-*.

The ";" is a separator that enables you to specify different formats for positive, negative, and zero values. Here is the general form of a custom format specifier that uses the ";":

positive-fmt;negative-fmt;zero-fmt

Here is an example:

```
Console.WriteLine("{0:#.##;(#.##);0.00}", num);
```

If **num** is positive, the value is displayed with two decimal places. If **num** is negative, the value is displayed with two decimal places and is between a set of parentheses. If **num** is zero, the string 0.00 is displayed. When using the separators, you don't need to supply all parts. If you just want to specify how positive and negative values will look, omit the zero format. To use the default for negative values, omit the negative format. In this case, the positive format and the zero format will be separated by two semicolons.

The following program demonstrates just a few of the many possible custom formats that you can create:

```
// Using custom formats.

using System;

class PictureFormatDemo {
  static void Main() {
    double num = 64354.2345;

    Console.WriteLine("Default format: " + num);

    // Display with 2 decimal places.
    Console.WriteLine("Value with two decimal places: " +
                      "{0:#.##}", num);

    // Display with commas and 2 decimal places.
    Console.WriteLine("Add commas: {0:#,###.##}", num);

    // Display using scientific notation.
    Console.WriteLine("Use scientific notation: " +
                      "{0:#.###e+00}", num);

    // Scale the value by 1000.
    Console.WriteLine("Value in 1,000s: " +
                      "{0:#0,}", num);

    /* Display positive, negative, and zero
       values differently. */
    Console.WriteLine("Display positive, negative, " +
                      "and zero values differently.");
    Console.WriteLine("{0:#.#;(#.##);0.00}", num);
    num = -num;
    Console.WriteLine("{0:#.##;(#.##);0.00}", num);
    num = 0.0;
    Console.WriteLine("{0:#.##;(#.##);0.00}", num);

    // Display a percentage.
    num = 0.17;
    Console.WriteLine("Display a percentage: {0:#%}", num);
  }
}
```

Placeholder	Meaning
#	Digit
.	Decimal point
,	Thousands separator
%	Percentage, which is the value being formatted multiplied by 100
0	Pads with leading and trailing zeros
;	Separates sections that describe the format for positive, negative, and zero values
E0 E+0 E-0 e0 e+0 e-0	Scientific notation

TABLE 22-6 Custom Format Placeholder Characters

The output is shown here:

```
Default format: 64354.2345
Value with two decimal places: 64354.23
Add commas: 64,354.23
Use scientific notation: 6.435e+04
Value in 1,000s: 64
Display positive, negative, and zero values differently.
64354.2
(64354.23)
0.00
Display a percentage: 17%
```

Formatting Date and Time

In addition to formatting numeric values, another data type to which formatting is often applied is **DateTime**. **DateTime** is a structure that represents date and time. Date and time values can be displayed a variety of ways. Here are just a few examples:

06/05/2006
Monday, June 5, 2006
12:59:00
12:59:00 PM

Also, the date and time representations can vary from country to country. For these reasons, the .NET Framework provides an extensive formatting subsystem for time and date values.

Date and time formatting is handled through format specifiers. The format specifiers for date and time are shown in Table 22-7. Because the specific date and time representation may vary from country to country and by language, the precise representation generated will be influenced by the cultural settings.

Specifier	Format
D	Date in long form.
d	Date in short form.
F	Date and time in long form.
f	Date and time in short form.
G	Date in short form, time in long form.
gg	Date in short form, time in short form.
M	Month and day.
m	Same as M.
O	A form of date and time that includes the time zone. The string produced by the O format can be parsed back into the equivalent date and time. This is called the "round trip" format.
o	Same as O.
R	Date and time in standard, GMT form.
r	Same as R.
s	A sortable form of date and time.
T	Time in long form.
t	Time in short form.
U	Long form, universal form of date and time. Time is displayed as UTC.
u	Short form, universal form of date and time.
Y	Month and year.
y	Same as Y.

TABLE 22-7   The Date and Time Format Specifiers

Here is a program that demonstrates the date and time format specifiers:

```
// Format time and date information.

using System;

class TimeAndDateFormatDemo {
  static void Main() {
    DateTime dt = DateTime.Now; // obtain current time

    Console.WriteLine("d format: {0:d}", dt);
    Console.WriteLine("D format: {0:D}", dt);

    Console.WriteLine("t format: {0:t}", dt);
    Console.WriteLine("T format: {0:T}", dt);

    Console.WriteLine("f format: {0:f}", dt);
    Console.WriteLine("F format: {0:F}", dt);
```

```
      Console.WriteLine("g format: {0:g}", dt);
      Console.WriteLine("G format: {0:G}", dt);

      Console.WriteLine("m format: {0:m}", dt);
      Console.WriteLine("M format: {0:M}", dt);

      Console.WriteLine("o format: {0:o}", dt);
      Console.WriteLine("O format: {0:O}", dt);

      Console.WriteLine("r format: {0:r}", dt);
      Console.WriteLine("R format: {0:R}", dt);

      Console.WriteLine("s format: {0:s}", dt);

      Console.WriteLine("u format: {0:u}", dt);
      Console.WriteLine("U format: {0:U}", dt);

      Console.WriteLine("y format: {0:y}", dt);
      Console.WriteLine("Y format: {0:Y}", dt);
  }
}
```

Sample output is shown here:

```
d format: 6/18/2008
D format: Wednesday, June 18, 2008
t format: 11:53 AM
T format: 11:53:09 AM
f format: Wednesday, June 18, 2008 11:53 AM
F format: Wednesday, June 18, 2008 11:53:09 AM
g format: 6/18/2008 11:53 AM
G format: 6/18/2008 11:53:09 AM
m format: June 18
M format: June 18
o format: 2008-06-18T11:53:09.5074933-05:00
O format: 2008-06-18T11:53:09.5074933-05:00
r format: Wed, 18 Jun 2008 11:53:09 GMT
R format: Wed, 18 Jun 2008 11:53:09 GMT
s format: 2008-06-18T11:53:09
u format: 2008-06-18 11:53:09Z
U format: Wednesday, June 18, 2008 4:53:09 PM
y format: June, 2008
Y format: June, 2008
```

The next program creates a very simple clock. The time is updated once every second. At the top of each hour, the computer's bell is sounded. It uses the **ToString( )** method of **DateTime** to obtain the formatted time prior to outputting it. If the top of the hour has been reached, then the alert character (**\a**) is appended to the formatted time, thus ringing the bell.

```
// A simple clock.

using System;

class SimpleClock {
  static void Main() {
    string t;
```

```
    int seconds;

    DateTime dt = DateTime.Now;
    seconds = dt.Second;

    for(;;) {
      dt = DateTime.Now;

      // update time if seconds change
      if(seconds != dt.Second) {
        seconds = dt.Second;

        t = dt.ToString("T");

        if(dt.Minute==0 && dt.Second==0)
          t = t + "\a"; // ring bell at top of hour

        Console.WriteLine(t);
      }
    }
  }
}
```

Creating a Custom Date and Time Format

Although the standard date and time format specifiers will apply to the vast majority of situations, you can create your own, custom formats. The process is similar to creating custom formats for the numeric types, as described earlier. In essence, you simply create an example (picture) of what you want the date and time information to look like. To create a custom date and time format, you will use one or more of the placeholders shown in Table 22-8.

If you examine Table 22-8, you will see that the placeholders *d, f, g, m, M, s,* and *t* are the same as the date and time format specifiers shown in Table 22-7. In general, if one of these characters is used by itself, it is interpreted as a format specifier. Otherwise, it is assumed to be a placeholder. If you want use one of these characters by itself but have it interpreted as a placeholder, then precede the character with a %.

The following program demonstrates several custom time and date formats:

```
// Format time and date information.

using System;

class CustomTimeAndDateFormatsDemo {
  static void Main() {
    DateTime dt = DateTime.Now;

    Console.WriteLine("Time is {0:hh:mm tt}", dt);
    Console.WriteLine("24 hour time is {0:HH:mm}", dt);
    Console.WriteLine("Date is {0:ddd MMM dd, yyyy}", dt);

    Console.WriteLine("Era: {0:gg}", dt);

    Console.WriteLine("Time with seconds: " +
                      "{0:HH:mm:ss tt}", dt);
```

```
        Console.WriteLine("Use m for day of month: {0:m}", dt);
        Console.WriteLine("use m for minutes: {0:%m}", dt);
    }
}
```

Placeholder	Replaced By
d	Day of month as a number between 1 and 31.
dd	Day of month as a number between 1 and 31. A leading 0 prefixes the values 1 through 9.
ddd	Abbreviated weekday name.
dddd	Full weekday name.
f, ff, fff, ffff, fffff, ffffff, fffffff	Fractional seconds, with the number of decimal places specified by the number of fs. (If uppercase Fs are used, trailing 0s are not displayed.)
g	Era.
h	Hour as a number between 1 and 12.
hh	Hour as a number between 1 and 12. A leading 0 prefixes the values 1 through 9.
H	Hour as a number between 0 and 23.
HH	Hour as a number between 0 and 23. A leading 0 prefixes the values 0 through 9.
K	Time zone offset in hours. It uses the value of the **DateTime.Kind** property to automatically adjust for local time and UTC time. (This specifier is now recommended over the z-based specifiers.)
m	Minutes.
mm	Minutes. A leading 0 prefixes the values 0 through 9.
M	Month as a number between 1 and 12.
MM	Month as a number between 1 and 12. A leading 0 prefixes the values 1 through 9.
MMM	Abbreviated month name.
MMMM	Full month name.
s	Seconds.
ss	Seconds. A leading 0 prefixes the values 0 through 9.
t	A or P, indicating A.M. or P.M.
tt	A.M. or P.M.
y	Year as two digits, unless only one digit is needed.
yy	Year as two digits. A leading 0 prefixes the values 0 through 9.
yyy	Year as three digits.
yyyy	Year using four digits.
yyyyy	Year using five digits.
z	Time zone offset in hours.

TABLE 22-8   The Custom Date and Time Placeholder Characters

Placeholder	Replaced By
zz	Time zone offset in hours. A leading 0 prefixes the values 0 through 9.
zzz	Time zone offset in hours and minutes.
:	Separator for time components.
/	Separator for date components.
%fmt	The standard format associated with fmt.

TABLE 22-8 The Custom Date and Time Placeholder Characters *(continued)*

The output is shown here:

```
Time is 11:55 AM
24 hour time is 11:55
Date is Wed Jun 18, 2008
Era: A.D.
Time with seconds: 11:55:52 AM
Use m for day of month: June 18
use m for minutes: 55
```

Formatting Enumerations

C# allows you to format the values defined by an enumeration. In general, enumeration values can be displayed using their name or their value. The enumeration format specifiers are shown in Table 22-9. Pay special attention to the G and F formats. Enumerations that will be used to represent bit-fields can be preceded by the **Flags** attribute. Typically, bit-fields hold values that represent individual bits and are arranged in powers of two. If the **Flags** attribute is present, then the G specifier will display the names of all of the values that comprise the value, assuming the value is valid. The F specifier will display the names of all of the values that comprise the value if the value can be constructed by ORing together two or more fields defined by the enumeration.

The following program demonstrates the enumeration specifiers:

```
// Format an enumeration.

using System;

class EnumFmtDemo {
  enum Direction { North, South, East, West }
  [Flags] enum Status { Ready=0x1, OffLine=0x2,
                        Waiting=0x4, TransmitOK=0x8,
                        ReceiveOK=0x10, OnLine=0x20 }

  static void Main() {
    Direction d = Direction.West;

    Console.WriteLine("{0:G}", d);
    Console.WriteLine("{0:F}", d);
```

```
    Console.WriteLine("{0:D}", d);
    Console.WriteLine("{0:X}", d);

    Status s = Status.Ready | Status.TransmitOK;

    Console.WriteLine("{0:G}", s);
    Console.WriteLine("{0:F}", s);
    Console.WriteLine("{0:D}", s);
    Console.WriteLine("{0:X}", s);
  }
}
```

The output is shown here:

```
West
West
3
00000003
Ready, TransmitOK
Ready, TransmitOK
9
00000009
```

Specifier	Meaning
D	Displays the value as a decimal integer.
d	Same as D.
F	Displays the name of the value. However, if the value can be created by ORing together two or more values defined by the enumeration, then the names of each part of the value will be displayed. This applies whether or not the **Flags** attribute has been specified.
f	Same as F.
G	Displays the name of the value. If the enumeration is preceded by the **Flags** attribute, then all names that are part of the value will be displayed (assuming a valid value).
g	Same as G.
X	Displays the value as a hexadecimal integer. Leading zeros will be added to ensure that at least eight digits are shown.
x	Same as X.

TABLE 22-9   The Enumeration Format Specifiers

Multithreaded Programming

A lthough C# contains many exciting features, one of its most powerful is its built-in support for *multithreaded programming*. A multithreaded program contains two or more parts that can run concurrently. Each part of such a program is called a *thread*, and each thread defines a separate path of execution. Thus, multithreading is a specialized form of multitasking.

Multithreaded programming relies on a combination of features defined by the C# language and by classes in the .NET Framework. Because support for multithreading is built into C#, many of the problems associated with multithreading in other languages are minimized or eliminated.

Multithreading Fundamentals

There are two distinct types of multitasking: process-based and thread-based. It is important to understand the difference between the two. A *process* is, in essence, a program that is executing. Thus, *process-based multitasking* is the feature that allows your computer to run two or more programs concurrently. For example, process-based multitasking allows you to run a word processor at the same time you are using a spreadsheet or browsing the Internet. In process-based multitasking, a program is the smallest unit of code that can be dispatched by the scheduler.

A *thread* is a dispatchable unit of executable code. The name comes from the concept of a "thread of execution." In a *thread-based* multitasking environment, all processes have at least one thread, but they can have more. This means that a single program can perform two or more tasks at once. For instance, a text editor can be formatting text at the same time that it is printing, as long as these two actions are being performed by two separate threads.

The differences between process-based and thread-based multitasking can be summarized like this: Process-based multitasking handles the concurrent execution of programs. Thread-based multitasking deals with the concurrent execution of pieces of the same program.

The principal advantage of multithreading is that it enables you to write very efficient programs because it lets you utilize the idle time that is present in most programs. As you probably know, most I/O devices, whether they be network ports, disk drives, or the keyboard, are much slower than the CPU. Thus, a program will often spend a majority of its execution time waiting to send or receive information to or from a device. By using multithreading, your program can execute another task during this idle time. For example,

while one part of your program is sending a file over the Internet, another part can be reading keyboard input, and still another can be buffering the next block of data to send.

A thread can be in one of several states. In general terms, it can be *running*. It can be *ready to run* as soon as it gets CPU time. A running thread can be *suspended*, which is a temporary halt to its execution. It can later be *resumed*. A thread can be *blocked* when waiting for a resource. A thread can be *terminated*, in which case its execution ends and cannot be resumed.

The .NET Framework defines two types of threads: *foreground* and *background*. By default, when you create a thread, it is a foreground thread, but you can change it to a background thread. The only difference between foreground and background threads is that a background thread will be automatically terminated when all foreground threads in its process have stopped.

Along with thread-based multitasking comes the need for a special type of feature called *synchronization*, which allows the execution of threads to be coordinated in certain well-defined ways. C# has a complete subsystem devoted to synchronization, and its key features are also described here.

All processes have at least one thread of execution, which is usually called the *main thread* because it is the one that is executed when your program begins. Thus, the main thread is the thread that all of the preceding example programs in the book have been using. From the main thread, you can create other threads.

C# and the .NET Framework support both process-based and thread-based multitasking. Thus, using C#, you can create and manage both processes and threads. However, little programming effort is required to start a new process because each process is largely separate from the next. Rather, it is C#'s support for multithreading that is important. Because support for multithreading is built in, C# makes it easier to construct high-performance, multithreaded programs than do some other languages.

The classes that support multithreaded programming are defined in the **System.Threading** namespace. Thus, you will usually include this statement at the start of any multithreaded program:

```
using System.Threading;
```

The Thread Class

The multithreading system is built upon the **Thread** class, which encapsulates a thread of execution. The **Thread** class is sealed, which means that it cannot be inherited. **Thread** defines several methods and properties that help manage threads. Throughout this chapter, several of its most commonly used members will be examined.

Creating and Starting a Thread

There are a number of ways to create and start a thread. This section describes the basic mechanism. Various options are described later in this chapter.

To create a thread, instantiate an object of type **Thread**, which is a class defined in **System.Threading**. The simplest **Thread** constructor is shown here:

public Thread(ThreadStart *entryPoint*)

Here, *entryPoint* is the name of the method that will be called to begin execution of the thread. **ThreadStart** is a delegate defined by the .NET Framework as shown here:

public delegate void ThreadStart( )

Thus, your entry point method must have a **void** return type and take no arguments.

Once created, the new thread will not start running until you call its **Start( )** method, which is defined by **Thread**. The **Start( )** method has two forms. The one used here is

public void Start( )

Once started, the thread will run until the method specified by *entryPoint* returns. Thus, when *entryPoint* returns, the thread automatically stops. If you try to call **Start( )** on a thread that has already been started, a **ThreadStateException** will be thrown.

Here is an example that creates a new thread and starts it running:

```
// Create a thread of execution.

using System;
using System.Threading;

class MyThread {
  public int Count;
  string thrdName;

  public MyThread(string name) {
    Count = 0;
    thrdName = name;
  }

  // Entry point of thread.
  public void Run() {
    Console.WriteLine(thrdName + " starting.");

    do {
      Thread.Sleep(500);
      Console.WriteLine("In " + thrdName +
                          ", Count is " + Count);
      Count++;
    } while(Count < 10);

    Console.WriteLine(thrdName + " terminating.");
  }
}

class MultiThread {
  static void Main() {
    Console.WriteLine("Main thread starting.");

    // First, construct a MyThread object.
    MyThread mt = new MyThread("Child #1");

    // Next, construct a thread from that object.
    Thread newThrd = new Thread(mt.Run);

    // Finally, start execution of the thread.
    newThrd.Start();

    do {
      Console.Write(".");
```

```
    Thread.Sleep(100);
  } while (mt.Count != 10);

  Console.WriteLine("Main thread ending.");
  }
}
```

Let's look closely at this program. **MyThread** defines a class that will be used to create a second thread of execution. Inside its **Run( )** method, a loop is established that counts from 0 to 9. Notice the call to **Sleep( )**, which is a **static** method defined by **Thread**. The **Sleep( )** method causes the thread from which it is called to suspend execution for the specified period of milliseconds. When a thread suspends, another thread can run. The form used by the program is shown here:

public static void Sleep(int *milliseconds*)

The number of milliseconds to suspend is specified in *milliseconds*. If *milliseconds* is zero, the calling thread is suspended only to allow a waiting thread to execute.

Inside **Main( )**, a new **Thread** object is created by the following sequence of statements:

```
// First, construct a MyThread object.
MyThread mt = new MyThread("Child #1");

// Next, construct a thread from that object.
Thread newThrd = new Thread(mt.Run);

// Finally, start execution of the thread.
newThrd.Start();
```

As the comments suggest, first an object of **MyThread** is created. This object is then used to construct a **Thread** object by passing the **mt.Run( )** method as the entry point. Finally, execution of the new thread is started by calling **Start( )**. This causes **mt.Run( )** to begin executing in its own thread. After calling **Start( )**, execution of the main thread returns to **Main( )**, and it enters **Main( )**'s **do** loop. Both threads continue running, sharing the CPU, until their loops finish. The output produced by this program is as follows. (The precise output that you see may vary slightly because of differences in your execution environment, operating system, and task load.)

```
Main thread starting.
Child #1 starting.
.....In Child #1, Count is 0
.....In Child #1, Count is 1
.....In Child #1, Count is 2
.....In Child #1, Count is 3
.....In Child #1, Count is 4
.....In Child #1, Count is 5
.....In Child #1, Count is 6
.....In Child #1, Count is 7
.....In Child #1, Count is 8
.....In Child #1, Count is 9
Child #1 terminating.
Main thread ending.
```

Often in a multithreaded program, you will want the main thread to be the last thread to finish running. Technically, a program continues to run until all of its foreground threads

have finished. Thus, having the main thread finish last is not a requirement. It is, however, often good practice to follow because it clearly defines your program's endpoint. The preceding program tries to ensure that the main thread will finish last, by checking the value of **Count** within **Main( )**'s **do** loop, stopping when **Count** equals 10, and through the use of calls to **Sleep( )**. However, this is an imperfect approach. Later in this chapter, you will see better ways for one thread to wait until another finishes.

Some Simple Improvements

While the preceding program is perfectly valid, some easy improvements will make it more efficient. First, it is possible to have a thread begin execution as soon as it is created. In the case of **MyThread**, this is done by instantiating a **Thread** object inside **MyThread**'s constructor. Second, there is no need for **MyThread** to store the name of the thread since **Thread** defines a property called **Name** that can be used for this purpose. **Name** is defined like this:

```
public string Name { get; set; }
```

Since **Name** is a read-write property, you can use it to set the name of a thread or to retrieve the thread's name.

Here is a version of the preceding program that makes these three improvements:

```
// An alternate way to start a thread.

using System;
using System.Threading;

class MyThread {
  public int Count;
  public Thread Thrd;

  public MyThread(string name) {
    Count = 0;
    Thrd = new Thread(this.Run);
    Thrd.Name = name; // set the name of the thread
    Thrd.Start(); // start the thread
  }

  // Entry point of thread.
  void Run() {
    Console.WriteLine(Thrd.Name + " starting.");

    do {
      Thread.Sleep(500);
      Console.WriteLine("In " + Thrd.Name +
                        ", Count is " + Count);
      Count++;
    } while(Count < 10);

    Console.WriteLine(Thrd.Name + " terminating.");
  }
}

class MultiThreadImproved {
  static void Main() {
```

```
      Console.WriteLine("Main thread starting.");

      // First, construct a MyThread object.
      MyThread mt = new MyThread("Child #1");

      do {
        Console.Write(".");
        Thread.Sleep(100);
      } while (mt.Count != 10);

      Console.WriteLine("Main thread ending.");
    }
  }
```

This version produces the same output as before. Notice that the thread object is stored in **Thrd** inside **MyThread**.

Creating Multiple Threads

The preceding examples have created only one child thread. However, your program can spawn as many threads as it needs. For example, the following program creates three child threads:

```
// Create multiple threads of execution.

using System;
using System.Threading;

class MyThread {
  public int Count;
  public Thread Thrd;

  public MyThread(string name) {
    Count = 0;
    Thrd = new Thread(this.Run);
    Thrd.Name = name;
    Thrd.Start();
  }

  // Entry point of thread.
  void Run() {
    Console.WriteLine(Thrd.Name + " starting.");

    do {
      Thread.Sleep(500);
      Console.WriteLine("In " + Thrd.Name +
                          ", Count is " + Count);
      Count++;
    } while(Count < 10);

    Console.WriteLine(Thrd.Name + " terminating.");
  }
}
```

```
class MoreThreads {
  static void Main() {
    Console.WriteLine("Main thread starting.");

    // Construct three threads.
    MyThread mt1 = new MyThread("Child #1");
    MyThread mt2 = new MyThread("Child #2");
    MyThread mt3 = new MyThread("Child #3");

    do {
      Console.Write(".");
      Thread.Sleep(100);
    } while (mt1.Count < 10 ||
             mt2.Count < 10 ||
             mt3.Count < 10);

    Console.WriteLine("Main thread ending.");
  }
}
```

Sample output from this program is shown next:

```
Main thread starting.
.Child #1 starting.
Child #2 starting.
Child #3 starting.
....In Child #1, Count is 0
In Child #2, Count is 0
In Child #3, Count is 0
.....In Child #1, Count is 1
In Child #2, Count is 1
In Child #3, Count is 1
.....In Child #1, Count is 2
In Child #2, Count is 2
In Child #3, Count is 2
.....In Child #1, Count is 3
In Child #2, Count is 3
In Child #3, Count is 3
.....In Child #1, Count is 4
In Child #2, Count is 4
In Child #3, Count is 4
.....In Child #1, Count is 5
In Child #2, Count is 5
In Child #3, Count is 5
.....In Child #1, Count is 6
In Child #2, Count is 6
In Child #3, Count is 6
.....In Child #1, Count is 7
In Child #2, Count is 7
In Child #3, Count is 7
.....In Child #1, Count is 8
In Child #2, Count is 8
In Child #3, Count is 8
.....In Child #1, Count is 9
```

PART II

```
Child #1 terminating.
In Child #2, Count is 9
Child #2 terminating.
In Child #3, Count is 9
Child #3 terminating.
Main thread ending.
```

As you can see, once started, all three child threads share the CPU. Again, because of differences among system configurations, operating systems, and other environmental factors, when you run the program, the output you see may differ slightly from that shown here.

Determining When a Thread Ends

Often it is useful to know when a thread has ended. In the preceding examples, this was attempted by watching the **Count** variable—hardly a satisfactory or generalizable solution. Fortunately, **Thread** provides two means by which you can determine whether a thread has ended. First, you can interrogate the read-only **IsAlive** property for the thread. It is defined like this:

> public bool IsAlive { get; }

IsAlive returns true if the thread upon which it is called is still running. It returns false otherwise. To try **IsAlive**, substitute this version of **MoreThreads** for the one shown in the preceding program:

```csharp
// Use IsAlive to wait for threads to end.
class MoreThreads {
  static void Main() {
    Console.WriteLine("Main thread starting.");

    // Construct three threads.
    MyThread mt1 = new MyThread("Child #1");
    MyThread mt2 = new MyThread("Child #2");
    MyThread mt3 = new MyThread("Child #3");

    do {
      Console.Write(".");
      Thread.Sleep(100);
    } while (mt1.Thrd.IsAlive &&
             mt2.Thrd.IsAlive &&
             mt3.Thrd.IsAlive);

    Console.WriteLine("Main thread ending.");
  }
}
```

This version produces the same output as before. The only difference is that it uses **IsAlive** to wait for the child threads to terminate.

Another way to wait for a thread to finish is to call **Join( )**. Its simplest form is shown here:

> public void Join( )

Join( ) waits until the thread on which it is called terminates. Its name comes from the concept of the calling thread waiting until the specified thread *joins* it. A **ThreadStateException** will be thrown if the thread has not been started. Additional forms of **Join( )** allow you to specify a maximum amount of time that you want to wait for the specified thread to terminate.

Here is a program that uses **Join( )** to ensure that the main thread is the last to stop:

```
// Use Join().

using System;
using System.Threading;

class MyThread {
  public int Count;
  public Thread Thrd;

  public MyThread(string name) {
    Count = 0;
    Thrd = new Thread(this.Run);
    Thrd.Name = name;
    Thrd.Start();
  }

  // Entry point of thread.
  void Run() {
    Console.WriteLine(Thrd.Name + " starting.");

    do {
      Thread.Sleep(500);
      Console.WriteLine("In " + Thrd.Name +
                        ", Count is " + Count);
      Count++;
    } while(Count < 10);

    Console.WriteLine(Thrd.Name + " terminating.");
  }
}

// Use Join() to wait for threads to end.
class JoinThreads {
  static void Main() {
    Console.WriteLine("Main thread starting.");

    // Construct three threads.
    MyThread mt1 = new MyThread("Child #1");
    MyThread mt2 = new MyThread("Child #2");
    MyThread mt3 = new MyThread("Child #3");

    mt1.Thrd.Join();
    Console.WriteLine("Child #1 joined.");

    mt2.Thrd.Join();
    Console.WriteLine("Child #2 joined.");
```

```
    mt3.Thrd.Join();
    Console.WriteLine("Child #3 joined.");

    Console.WriteLine("Main thread ending.");
  }
}
```

Sample output from this program is shown here. Remember when you try the program, your output may vary slightly.

```
Main thread starting.
Child #1 starting.
Child #2 starting.
Child #3 starting.
In Child #1, Count is 0
In Child #2, Count is 0
In Child #3, Count is 0
In Child #1, Count is 1
In Child #2, Count is 1
In Child #3, Count is 1
In Child #1, Count is 2
In Child #2, Count is 2
In Child #3, Count is 2
In Child #1, Count is 3
In Child #2, Count is 3
In Child #3, Count is 3
In Child #1, Count is 4
In Child #2, Count is 4
In Child #3, Count is 4
In Child #1, Count is 5
In Child #2, Count is 5
In Child #3, Count is 5
In Child #1, Count is 6
In Child #2, Count is 6
In Child #3, Count is 6
In Child #1, Count is 7
In Child #2, Count is 7
In Child #3, Count is 7
In Child #1, Count is 8
In Child #2, Count is 8
In Child #3, Count is 8
In Child #1, Count is 9
Child #1 terminating.
In Child #2, Count is 9
Child #2 terminating.
In Child #3, Count is 9
Child #3 terminating.
Child #1 joined.
Child #2 joined.
Child #3 joined.
Main thread ending.
```

As you can see, after the calls to **Join( )** return, the threads have stopped executing.

Passing an Argument to a Thread

In the early days of the .NET Framework, it was not possible to pass an argument to a thread when the thread was started because the method that serves as the entry point to a thread could not have a parameter. If information needed to be passed to a thread, various workarounds (such as using a shared variable) were required. However, this deficiency was subsequently remedied, and today it is possible to pass an argument to a thread. To do so, you must use different forms of **Start( )**, the **Thread** constructor, and the entry point method.

An argument is passed to a thread through this version of **Start( )**:

public void Start(object *arg*)

The object passed to *arg* is automatically passed to the thread's entry point method. Thus, to pass an argument to a thread, you pass it to **Start( )**.

To make use of the parameterized version of **Start( )**, you must use the following form of the **Thread** constructor:

public Thread(ParameterizedThreadStart *entryPoint*)

Here, *entryPoint* is the name of the method that will be called to begin execution of the thread. Notice in this version, the type of *entryPoint* is **ParameterizedThreadStart** rather than **ThreadStart**, as used by the preceding examples. **ParameterizedThreadStart** is a delegate that is declared as shown here:

public delegate void ParameterizedThreadStart(object *arg*)

As you can see, this delegate takes an argument of type **object**. Therefore, to use this form of the **Thread** constructor, the thread entry point method must have an **object** parameter.

Here is an example that demonstrates the passing of an argument to a thread:

```
// Passing an argument to the thread method.

using System;
using System.Threading;

class MyThread {
  public int Count;
  public Thread Thrd;

  // Notice that MyThread is also passed an int value.
  public MyThread(string name, int num) {
    Count = 0;

    // Explicitly invoke ParameterizedThreadStart constructor
    // for the sake of illustration.
    Thrd = new Thread(this.Run);

    Thrd.Name = name;

    // Here, Start() is passed num as an argument.
    Thrd.Start(num);
  }
```

```
    // Notice that this version of Run() has
    // a parameter of type object.
    void Run(object num) {
      Console.WriteLine(Thrd.Name +
                        " starting with count of " + num);

      do {
        Thread.Sleep(500);
        Console.WriteLine("In " + Thrd.Name +
                          ", Count is " + Count);
        Count++;
      } while(Count < (int) num);

      Console.WriteLine(Thrd.Name + " terminating.");
    }
}

class PassArgDemo {
  static void Main() {

    // Notice that the iteration count is passed
    // to these two MyThread objects.
    MyThread mt = new MyThread("Child #1", 5);
    MyThread mt2 = new MyThread("Child #2", 3);

    do {
      Thread.Sleep(100);
    } while (mt.Thrd.IsAlive | mt2.Thrd.IsAlive);

    Console.WriteLine("Main thread ending.");
  }
}
```

The output is shown here. (The actual output you see may vary.)

```
Child #1 starting with count of 5
Child #2 starting with count of 3
In Child #2, Count is 0
In Child #1, Count is 0
In Child #1, Count is 1
In Child #2, Count is 1
In Child #2, Count is 2
Child #2 terminating.
In Child #1, Count is 2
In Child #1, Count is 3
In Child #1, Count is 4
Child #1 terminating.
Main thread ending.
```

As the output shows, the first thread iterates five times and the second thread iterates three times. The iteration count is specified in the **MyThread** constructor and then passed to the thread entry method **Run( )** through the use of the **ParameterizedThreadStart** version of **Start( )**.

The IsBackground Property

As mentioned earlier, the .NET Framework defines two types of threads: foreground and background. The only difference between the two is that a process won't end until all of its foreground threads have ended, but background threads are terminated automatically after all foreground threads have stopped. By default, a thread is created as a foreground thread. It can be changed to a background thread by using the **IsBackground** property defined by **Thread**, as shown here:

    public bool IsBackground { get; set; }

To set a thread to background, simply assign **IsBackground** a **true** value. A value of **false** indicates a foreground thread.

Thread Priorities

Each thread has a priority setting associated with it. A thread's priority determines, in part, how frequently a thread gains access to the CPU. In general, low-priority threads gain access to the CPU less often than high-priority threads. As a result, within a given period of time, a low-priority thread will often receive less CPU time than a high-priority thread. As you might expect, how much CPU time a thread receives profoundly affects its execution characteristics and its interaction with other threads currently executing in the system.

It is important to understand that factors other than a thread's priority can also affect how frequently a thread gains access to the CPU. For example, if a high-priority thread is waiting on some resource, perhaps for keyboard input, it will be blocked, and a lower-priority thread will run. Thus, in this situation, a low-priority thread may gain greater access to the CPU than the high-priority thread over a specific period. Finally, precisely how task scheduling is implemented by the operating system affects how CPU time is allocated.

When a child thread is started, it receives a default priority setting. You can change a thread's priority through the **Priority** property, which is a member of **Thread**. This is its general form:

    public ThreadPriority Priority{ get; set; }

ThreadPriority is an enumeration that defines the following five priority settings:

    ThreadPriority.Highest
    ThreadPriority.AboveNormal
    ThreadPriority.Normal
    ThreadPriority.BelowNormal
    ThreadPriority.Lowest

The default priority setting for a thread is **ThreadPriority.Normal**.

To understand how priorities affect thread execution, we will use an example that executes two threads, one having a higher priority than the other. The threads are created as instances of the **MyThread** class. The **Run( )** method contains a loop that counts the number of iterations. The loop stops when either the count reaches 1,000,000,000 or the static variable **stop** is **true**. Initially, **stop** is set to **false**. The first thread to count to 1,000,000,000 sets **stop** to **true**. This causes the second thread to terminate with its next time slice. Each time through the loop, the string in **currentName** is checked against the name of the executing thread. If

they don't match, it means that a task-switch occurred. Each time a task-switch happens, the name of the new thread is displayed and **currentName** is given the name of the new thread. This allows you to watch how often each thread has access to the CPU. After both threads stop, the number of iterations for each loop is displayed.

```csharp
// Demonstrate thread priorities.

using System;
using System.Threading;

class MyThread {
  public int Count;
  public Thread Thrd;

  static bool stop = false;
  static string currentName;

  /* Construct a new thread. Notice that this
     constructor does not actually start the
     threads running. */
  public MyThread(string name) {
    Count = 0;
    Thrd = new Thread(this.Run);
    Thrd.Name = name;
    currentName = name;
  }

  // Begin execution of new thread.
  void Run() {
    Console.WriteLine(Thrd.Name + " starting.");
    do {
      Count++;

      if(currentName != Thrd.Name) {
        currentName = Thrd.Name;
        Console.WriteLine("In " + currentName);
      }

    } while(stop == false && Count < 1000000000);
    stop = true;

    Console.WriteLine(Thrd.Name + " terminating.");
  }
}

class PriorityDemo {
  static void Main() {
    MyThread mt1 = new MyThread("High Priority");
    MyThread mt2 = new MyThread("Low Priority");

    // Set the priorities.
    mt1.Thrd.Priority = ThreadPriority.AboveNormal;
    mt2.Thrd.Priority = ThreadPriority.BelowNormal;
```

```
// Start the threads.
mt1.Thrd.Start();
mt2.Thrd.Start();

mt1.Thrd.Join();
mt2.Thrd.Join();

Console.WriteLine();
Console.WriteLine(mt1.Thrd.Name + " thread counted to " +
                  mt1.Count);
Console.WriteLine(mt2.Thrd.Name + " thread counted to " +
                  mt2.Count);
  }
}
```

Here is sample output:

```
High Priority starting.
In High Priority
Low Priority starting.
In Low Priority
In High Priority
In Low Priority
In High Priority
In Low Priority
In High Priority
In Low Priority
In High Priority
In Low Priority
In High Priority
High Priority terminating.
Low Priority terminating.

High Priority thread counted to 1000000000
Low Priority thread counted to 23996334
```

In this run, of the CPU time allotted to the program, the high-priority thread got approximately 98 percent. Of course, the precise output you see may vary, depending on the speed of your CPU and the number of other tasks running on the system. Which version of Windows you are running will also have an effect.

Because multithreaded code can behave differently in different environments, you should never base your code on the execution characteristics of a single environment. For example, in the preceding example, it would be a mistake to assume that the low-priority thread will always execute at least a small amount of time before the high-priority thread finishes. In a different environment, the high-priority thread might complete before the low-priority thread has executed even once, for example.

Synchronization

When using multiple threads, you will sometimes need to coordinate the activities of two or more of the threads. The process by which this is achieved is called *synchronization*. The most common reason for using synchronization is when two or more threads need access to a

shared resource that can be used by only one thread at a time. For example, when one thread is writing to a file, a second thread must be prevented from doing so at the same time. Another situation in which synchronization is needed is when one thread is waiting for an event that is caused by another thread. In this case, there must be some means by which the first thread is held in a suspended state until the event has occurred. Then the waiting thread must resume execution.

The key to synchronization is the concept of a *lock*, which controls access to a block of code within an object. When an object is locked by one thread, no other thread can gain access to the locked block of code. When the thread releases the lock, the object is available for use by another thread.

The lock feature is built into the C# language. Thus, all objects can be synchronized. Synchronization is supported by the keyword **lock**. Since synchronization was designed into C# from the start, it is much easier to use than you might first expect. In fact, for many programs, the synchronization of objects is almost transparent.

The general form of **lock** is shown here:

```
lock(lockObj) {
    // statements to be synchronized
}
```

Here, *lockObj* is a reference to the object being synchronized. If you want to synchronize only a single statement, the curly braces are not needed. A **lock** statement ensures that the section of code protected by the lock for the given object can be used only by the thread that obtains the lock. All other threads are blocked until the lock is removed. The lock is released when the block is exited.

The object you lock on is an object that represents the resource being synchronized. In some cases, this will be an instance of the resource itself or simply an arbitrary instance of **object** that is being used to provide synchronization. A key point to understand about **lock** is that the lock-on object should not be publically accessible. Why? Because it is possible that another piece of code that is outside your control could lock on the object and never release it. In the past, it was common to use a construct such as **lock(this)**. However, this works only if **this** refers to a private object. Because of the potential for error and conceptual mistakes in this regard, **lock(this)** is no longer recommended for general use. Instead, it is better to simply create a private object on which to lock. This is the approach used by the examples in this chapter. Be aware that you will still find many examples of **lock(this)** in legacy C# code. In some cases, it will be safe. In others, it will need to be changed to avoid problems.

The following program demonstrates synchronization by controlling access to a method called **SumIt( )**, which sums the elements of an integer array:

```
// Use lock to synchronize access to an object.

using System;
using System.Threading;

class SumArray {
  int sum;
  object lockOn = new object(); // a private object to lock on

  public int SumIt(int[] nums) {
```

```
      lock(lockOn) { // lock the entire method
        sum = 0; // reset sum

        for(int i=0; i < nums.Length; i++) {
          sum += nums[i];
          Console.WriteLine("Running total for " +
                  Thread.CurrentThread.Name +
                  " is " + sum);
          Thread.Sleep(10); // allow task-switch
        }
        return sum;
      }
    }
  }
}

class MyThread {
  public Thread Thrd;
  int[] a;
  int answer;

  // Create one SumArray object for all instances of MyThread.
  static SumArray sa = new SumArray();

  // Construct a new thread.
  public MyThread(string name, int[] nums) {
    a = nums;
    Thrd = new Thread(this.Run);
    Thrd.Name = name;
    Thrd.Start(); // start the thread
  }

  // Begin execution of new thread.
  void Run() {
    Console.WriteLine(Thrd.Name + " starting.");

    answer = sa.SumIt(a);

    Console.WriteLine("Sum for " + Thrd.Name +
                " is " + answer);

    Console.WriteLine(Thrd.Name + " terminating.");
  }
}

class Sync {
  static void Main() {
    int[] a = {1, 2, 3, 4, 5};

    MyThread mt1 = new MyThread("Child #1", a);
    MyThread mt2 = new MyThread("Child #2", a);

    mt1.Thrd.Join();
    mt2.Thrd.Join();
  }
}
```

PART II

Here is sample output from the program. (The actual output you see may vary slightly.)

```
Child #1 starting.
Running total for Child #1 is 1
Child #2 starting.
Running total for Child #1 is 3
Running total for Child #1 is 6
Running total for Child #1 is 10
Running total for Child #1 is 15
Running total for Child #2 is 1
Sum for Child #1 is 15
Child #1 terminating.
Running total for Child #2 is 3
Running total for Child #2 is 6
Running total for Child #2 is 10
Running total for Child #2 is 15
Sum for Child #2 is 15
Child #2 terminating.
```

As the output shows, both threads compute the proper sum of 15.

Let's examine this program in detail. The program creates three classes. The first is **SumArray**. It defines the method **SumIt( )**, which sums an integer array. The second class is **MyThread**, which uses a **static** object called **sa** that is of type **SumArray**. Thus, only one object of **SumArray** is shared by all objects of type **MyThread**. This object is used to obtain the sum of an integer array. Notice that **SumArray** stores the running total in a field called **sum**. Thus, if two threads use **SumIt( )** concurrently, both will be attempting to use **sum** to hold the running total. Because this will cause errors, access to **SumIt( )** must be synchronized. Finally, the class **Sync** creates two threads and has them compute the sum of an integer array.

Inside **SumIt( )**, the **lock** statement prevents simultaneous use of the method by different threads. Notice that **lock** uses **lockOn** as the object being synchronized. This is a private object that is used solely for synchronization. **Sleep( )** is called to purposely allow a task-switch to occur, if one can—but it can't in this case. Because the code within **SumIt( )** is locked, it can be used by only one thread at a time. Thus, when the second child thread begins execution, it does not enter **SumIt( )** until after the first child thread is done with it. This ensures the correct result is produced.

To understand the effects of **lock** fully, try removing it from the body of **SumIt( )**. After doing this, **SumIt( )** is no longer synchronized, and any number of threads can use it concurrently on the same object. The problem with this is that the running total is stored in **sum**, which will be changed by each thread that calls **SumIt( )**. Thus, when two threads call **SumIt( )** at the same time on the same object, incorrect results are produced because **sum** reflects the summation of both threads, mixed together. For example, here is sample output from the program after **lock** has been removed from **SumIt( )**:

```
Child #1 starting.
Running total for Child #1 is 1
Child #2 starting.
Running total for Child #2 is 1
Running total for Child #1 is 3
Running total for Child #2 is 5
Running total for Child #1 is 8
Running total for Child #2 is 11
```

```
Running total for Child #1 is 15
Running total for Child #2 is 19
Running total for Child #1 is 24
Running total for Child #2 is 29
Sum for Child #1 is 29
Child #1 terminating.
Sum for Child #2 is 29
Child #2 terminating.
```

As the output shows, both child threads are using **SumIt( )** at the same time on the same object, and the value of **sum** is corrupted.

The effects of **lock** are summarized here:

- For any given object, once a lock has been acquired, the object is locked and no other thread can acquire the lock.

- Other threads trying to acquire the lock on the same object will enter a wait state until the code is unlocked.

- When a thread leaves the locked block, the object is unlocked.

An Alternative Approach

Although locking a method's code, as shown in the previous example, is an easy and effective means of achieving synchronization, it will not work in all cases. For example, you might want to synchronize access to a method of a class you did not create, which is itself not synchronized. This can occur if you want to use a class that was written by a third party and for which you do not have access to the source code. Thus, it is not possible for you to add a **lock** statement to the appropriate method within the class. How can access to an object of this class be synchronized? Fortunately, the solution to this problem is simple: Lock access to the object from code outside the object by specifying the object in a **lock** statement. For example, here is an alternative implementation of the preceding program. Notice that the code within **SumIt( )** is no longer locked and no longer declares the **lockOn** object. Instead, calls to **SumIt( )** are locked within **MyThread**.

```
// Another way to use lock to synchronize access to an object.

using System;
using System.Threading;

class SumArray {
  int sum;

  public int SumIt(int[] nums) {
    sum = 0; // reset sum

    for(int i=0; i < nums.Length; i++) {
      sum += nums[i];
      Console.WriteLine("Running total for " +
            Thread.CurrentThread.Name +
            " is " + sum);
      Thread.Sleep(10); // allow task-switch
    }
    return sum;
```

PART II

```
    }
  }

class MyThread {
  public Thread Thrd;
  int[] a;
  int answer;

  /* Create one SumArray object for all
     instances of MyThread. */
  static SumArray sa = new SumArray();

  // Construct a new thread.
  public MyThread(string name, int[] nums) {
    a = nums;
    Thrd = new Thread(this.Run);
    Thrd.Name = name;
    Thrd.Start(); // start the thread
  }

  // Begin execution of new thread.
  void Run() {
    Console.WriteLine(Thrd.Name + " starting.");

    // Lock calls to SumIt().
    lock(sa) answer = sa.SumIt(a);

    Console.WriteLine("Sum for " + Thrd.Name +
                        " is " + answer);

    Console.WriteLine(Thrd.Name + " terminating.");
  }
}

class Sync {
  static void Main() {
    int[] a = {1, 2, 3, 4, 5};

    MyThread mt1 = new MyThread("Child #1", a);
    MyThread mt2 = new MyThread("Child #2", a);

    mt1.Thrd.Join();
    mt2.Thrd.Join();
  }
}
```

Here, the call to **sa.SumIt( )** is locked, rather than the code inside **SumIt( )** itself. The code that accomplishes this is shown here:

```
// Lock calls to SumIt().
lock(sa) answer = sa.SumIt(a);
```

Because **sa** is a private object, it is safe to lock on. Using this approach, the program produces the same correct results as the original approach.

The Monitor Class and lock

The C# keyword **lock** is really just shorthand for using the synchronization features defined by the **Monitor** class, which is defined in the **System.Threading** namespace. **Monitor** defines several methods that control or manage synchronization. For example, to obtain a lock on an object, call **Enter( )**. To release a lock, call **Exit( )**. These methods are shown here:

```
public static void Enter(object syncOb)
public static void Exit(object syncOb)
```

Here, *syncOb* is the object being synchronized. If the object is not available when **Enter( )** is called, the calling thread will wait until it becomes available. You will seldom use **Enter( )** or **Exit( )**, however, because a **lock** block automatically provides the equivalent. For this reason, **lock** is the preferred method of obtaining a lock on an object when programming in C#.

One method in **Monitor** that you may find useful on occasion is **TryEnter( )**. One of its forms is shown here:

```
public static bool TryEnter(object syncOb)
```

It returns true if the calling thread obtains a lock on *syncOb* and false if it doesn't. In no case does the calling thread wait. You could use this method to implement an alternative if the desired object is unavailable.

Monitor also defines these three methods: **Wait( )**, **Pulse( )**, and **PulseAll( )**. They are described in the next section.

Thread Communication Using Wait( ), Pulse( ), and PulseAll( )

Consider the following situation. A thread called *T* is executing inside a **lock** block and needs access to a resource, called *R*, that is temporarily unavailable. What should *T* do? If *T* enters some form of polling loop that waits for *R*, then *T* ties up the object, blocking other threads' access to it. This is a less than optimal solution because it partially defeats the advantages of programming for a multithreaded environment. A better solution is to have *T* temporarily relinquish control of the object, allowing another thread to run. When *R* becomes available, *T* can be notified and resume execution. Such an approach relies upon some form of interthread communication in which one thread can notify another that it is blocked and be notified when it can resume execution. C# supports interthread communication with the **Wait( )**, **Pulse( )**, and **PulseAll( )** methods.

The **Wait( )**, **Pulse( )**, and **PulseAll( )** methods are defined by the **Monitor** class. These methods can be called only from within a locked block of code. Here is how they are used. When a thread is temporarily blocked from running, it calls **Wait( )**. This causes the thread to go to sleep and the lock for that object to be released, allowing another thread to use the object. At a later point, the sleeping thread is awakened when some other thread enters the same lock and calls **Pulse( )** or **PulseAll( )**. A call to **Pulse( )** resumes the first thread in the queue of threads waiting for the lock. A call to **PulseAll( )** signals the release of the lock to all waiting threads.

Here are two commonly used forms of **Wait( )**:

```
public static bool Wait(object waitOb)
public static bool Wait(object waitOb, int milliseconds)
```

The first form waits until notified. The second form waits until notified or until the specified period of milliseconds has expired. For both, *waitOb* specifies the object upon which to wait.

Here are the general forms for **Pulse( )** and **PulseAll( )**:

public static void Pulse(object *waitOb*)
public static void PulseAll(object *waitOb*)

Here, *waitOb* is the object being released.

A **SynchronizationLockException** will be thrown if **Wait( )**, **Pulse( )**, or **PulseAll( )** is called from code that is not within synchronized code, such as a **lock** block.

An Example That Uses Wait( ) and Pulse( )

To understand the need for and the application of **Wait( )** and **Pulse( )**, we will create a program that simulates the ticking of a clock by displaying the words "Tick" and "Tock" on the screen. To accomplish this, we will create a class called **TickTock** that contains two methods: **Tick( )** and **Tock( )**. The **Tick( )** method displays the word "Tick" and **Tock( )** displays "Tock". To run the clock, two threads are created, one that calls **Tick( )** and one that calls **Tock( )**. The goal is to make the two threads execute in a way that the output from the program displays a consistent "Tick Tock"—that is, a repeated pattern of one "Tick" followed by one "Tock."

```
// Use Wait() and Pulse() to create a ticking clock.

using System;
using System.Threading;

class TickTock {
  object lockOn = new object();

  public void Tick(bool running) {
    lock(lockOn) {
      if(!running) { // stop the clock
        Monitor.Pulse(lockOn); // notify any waiting threads
        return;
      }

      Console.Write("Tick ");
      Monitor.Pulse(lockOn); // let Tock() run

      Monitor.Wait(lockOn); // wait for Tock() to complete
    }
  }

  public void Tock(bool running) {
    lock(lockOn) {
      if(!running) { // stop the clock
        Monitor.Pulse(lockOn); // notify any waiting threads
        return;
      }

      Console.WriteLine("Tock");
      Monitor.Pulse(lockOn); // let Tick() run

      Monitor.Wait(lockOn); // wait for Tick() to complete
    }
  }
}
```

```
}

class MyThread {
  public Thread Thrd;
  TickTock ttOb;

  // Construct a new thread.
  public MyThread(string name, TickTock tt) {
    Thrd = new Thread(this.Run);
    ttOb = tt;
    Thrd.Name = name;
    Thrd.Start();
  }

  // Begin execution of new thread.
  void Run() {
    if(Thrd.Name == "Tick") {
      for(int i=0; i<5; i++) ttOb.Tick(true);
      ttOb.Tick(false);
    }
    else {
      for(int i=0; i<5; i++) ttOb.Tock(true);
      ttOb.Tock(false);
    }
  }
}

class TickingClock {
  static void Main() {
    TickTock tt = new TickTock();
    MyThread mt1 = new MyThread("Tick", tt);
    MyThread mt2 = new MyThread("Tock", tt);

    mt1.Thrd.Join();
    mt2.Thrd.Join();
    Console.WriteLine("Clock Stopped");
  }
}
```

Here is the output produced by the program:

```
Tick Tock
Tick Tock
Tick Tock
Tick Tock
Tick Tock
Clock Stopped
```

Let's take a close look at this program. In **Main( )**, a **TickTock** object called **tt** is created, and this object is used to start two threads of execution. Inside the **Run( )** method of **MyThread**, if the name of the thread is "Tick," calls to **Tick( )** are made. If the name of the thread is "Tock," the **Tock( )** method is called. Five calls that pass **true** as an argument are made to each method. The clock runs as long as **true** is passed. A final call that passes **false** to each method stops the clock.

The most important part of the program is found in the **Tick( )** and **Tock( )** methods. We will begin with the **Tick( )** method, which, for convenience, is shown here:

```
public void Tick(bool running) {
  lock(lockOn) {
    if(!running) { // stop the clock
      Monitor.Pulse(lockOn); // notify any waiting threads
      return;
    }

    Console.Write("Tick ");
    Monitor.Pulse(lockOn); // let Tock() run

    Monitor.Wait(lockOn); // wait for Tock() to complete
  }
}
```

First, notice that the code in **Tick( )** is contained within a **lock** block. Recall, **Wait( )** and **Pulse( )** can be used only inside synchronized blocks. The method begins by checking the value of the **running** parameter. This parameter is used to provide a clean shutdown of the clock. If it is **false**, then the clock has been stopped. If this is the case, a call to **Pulse( )** is made to enable any waiting thread to run. We will return to this point in a moment. Assuming the clock is running when **Tick( )** executes, the word "Tick" is displayed, and then a call to **Pulse( )** takes place followed by a call to **Wait( )**. The call to **Pulse( )** allows a thread waiting on the same object to run. The call to **Wait( )** causes **Tick( )** to suspend until another thread calls **Pulse( )**. Thus, when **Tick( )** is called, it displays one "Tick," lets another thread run, and then suspends.

The **Tock( )** method is an exact copy of **Tick( )**, except that it displays "Tock." Thus, when entered, it displays "Tock," calls **Pulse( )**, and then waits. When viewed as a pair, a call to **Tick( )** can be followed only by a call to **Tock( )**, which can be followed only by a call to **Tick( )**, and so on. Therefore, the two methods are mutually synchronized.

The reason for the call to **Pulse( )** when the clock is stopped is to allow a final call to **Wait( )** to succeed. Remember, both **Tick( )** and **Tock( )** execute a call to **Wait( )** after displaying their message. The problem is that when the clock is stopped, one of the methods will still be waiting. Thus, a final call to **Pulse( )** is required in order for the waiting method to run. As an experiment, try removing this call to **Pulse( )** and watch what happens. As you will see, the program will "hang," and you will need to press CTRL-C to exit. The reason for this is that when the final call to **Tock( )** calls **Wait( )**, there is no corresponding call to **Pulse( )** that lets **Tock( )** conclude. Thus, **Tock( )** just sits there, waiting forever.

Before moving on, if you have any doubt that the calls to **Wait( )** and **Pulse( )** are actually needed to make the "clock" run right, substitute this version of **TickTock** into the preceding program. It has all calls to **Wait( )** and **Pulse( )** removed.

```
// A nonfunctional version of TickTock.
class TickTock {

  object lockOn = new object();

  public void Tick(bool running) {
    lock(lockOn) {
      if(!running) { // stop the clock
        return;
```

```
        }

      Console.Write("Tick ");
    }
  }

  public void Tock(bool running) {
    lock(lockOn) {
      if(!running) { // stop the clock
        return;
      }

      Console.WriteLine("Tock");
    }
  }
}
```

After the substitution, the output produced by the program will look like this:

```
Tick Tick Tick Tick Tick Tock
Tock
Tock
Tock
Tock
Clock Stopped
```

Clearly, the **Tick( )** and **Tock( )** methods are no longer synchronized!

Deadlock and Race Conditions

When developing multithreaded programs, you must be careful to avoid deadlock and race conditions. *Deadlock* is, as the name implies, a situation in which one thread is waiting for another thread to do something, but that other thread is waiting on the first. Thus, both threads are suspended, waiting for each other, and neither executes. This situation is analogous to two overly polite people both insisting that the other step through a door first!

Avoiding deadlock seems easy, but it's not. For example, deadlock can occur in roundabout ways. Consider the **TickTock** class. As explained, if a final **Pulse( )** is not executed by **Tick( )** or **Tock( )**, then one or the other will be waiting indefinitely and the program is deadlocked. Often the cause of the deadlock is not readily understood simply by looking at the source code to the program, because concurrently executing threads can interact in complex ways at runtime. To avoid deadlock, careful programming and thorough testing is required. In general, if a multithreaded program occasionally "hangs," deadlock is the likely cause.

A *race condition* occurs when two (or more) threads attempt to access a shared resource at the same time, without proper synchronization. For example, one thread may be writing a new value to a variable while another thread is incrementing the variable's current value. Without synchronization, the outcome will depend on the order in which the threads execute. (Does the second thread increment the original value or the new value written by the first thread?) In situations like this, the two threads are said to be "racing each other," with the final outcome determined by which thread finishes first. Like deadlock, a race condition can occur in difficult-to-discover ways. The solution is prevention: careful programming that properly synchronizes access to shared resources.

Using MethodImplAttribute

It is possible to synchronize an entire method by using the **MethodImplAttribute** attribute. This approach can be used as an alternative to the **lock** statement in cases in which the entire contents of a method are to be locked. **MethodImplAttribute** is defined within the **System.Runtime.CompilerServices** namespace. The constructor that applies to synchronization is shown here:

public MethodImplAttribute(MethodImplOptions *opt*)

Here, *opt* specifies the implementation attribute. To synchronize a method, specify **MethodImplOptions.Synchronized**. This attribute causes the entire method to be locked on the instance (that is, via **this**). (In the case of **static** methods, the type is locked on.) Thus, it must not be used on a public object or with a public class.

Here is a rewrite of the **TickTock** class that uses **MethodImplAttribute** to provide synchronization:

```
// Use MethodImplAttribute to synchronize a method.

using System;
using System.Threading;
using System.Runtime.CompilerServices;

// Rewrite of TickTock to use MethodImplOptions.Synchronized.
class TickTock {

  /* The following attribute synchronizes the entire
     Tick() method. */
  [MethodImplAttribute(MethodImplOptions.Synchronized)]
  public void Tick(bool running) {
    if(!running) { // stop the clock
      Monitor.Pulse(this); // notify any waiting threads
      return;
    }

    Console.Write("Tick ");
    Monitor.Pulse(this); // let Tock() run

    Monitor.Wait(this); // wait for Tock() to complete
  }


  /* The following attribute synchronizes the entire
     Tock() method. */
  [MethodImplAttribute(MethodImplOptions.Synchronized)]
  public void Tock(bool running) {
    if(!running) { // stop the clock
      Monitor.Pulse(this); // notify any waiting threads
      return;
    }

    Console.WriteLine("Tock");
```

```
      Monitor.Pulse(this); // let Tick() run

      Monitor.Wait(this); // wait for Tick() to complete
    }
}

class MyThread {
  public Thread Thrd;
  TickTock ttOb;

  // Construct a new thread.
  public MyThread(string name, TickTock tt) {
    Thrd = new Thread(this.Run);
    ttOb = tt;
    Thrd.Name = name;
    Thrd.Start();
  }

  // Begin execution of new thread.
  void Run() {
    if(Thrd.Name == "Tick") {
      for(int i=0; i<5; i++) ttOb.Tick(true);
      ttOb.Tick(false);
    }
    else {
      for(int i=0; i<5; i++) ttOb.Tock(true);
      ttOb.Tock(false);
    }
  }
}

class TickingClock {
  static void Main() {
    TickTock tt = new TickTock();
    MyThread mt1 = new MyThread("Tick", tt);
    MyThread mt2 = new MyThread("Tock", tt);

    mt1.Thrd.Join();
    mt2.Thrd.Join();
    Console.WriteLine("Clock Stopped");
  }
}
```

The proper Tick Tock output is the same as before.

As long as the method being synchronized is not defined by a public class or called on a public object, then whether you use **lock** or **MethodImplAttribute** is your decision. Both produce the same results. Because **lock** is a keyword built into C#, that is the approach the examples in this book will use.

REMEMBER *Do not use **MethodImplAttribute** with public classes or with public instances. Instead, use **lock**, locking on a private object (as explained earlier).*

Using a Mutex and a Semaphore

Although C#'s **lock** statement is sufficient for many synchronization needs, some situations, such as restricting access to a shared resource, are sometimes more conveniently handled by other synchronization mechanisms built into the .NET Framework. The two described here are related to each other: mutexes and semaphores.

The Mutex

A *mutex* is a mutually exclusive synchronization object. This means it can be acquired by one and only one thread at a time. The mutex is designed for those situations in which a shared resource can be used by only one thread at a time. For example, imagine a log file that is shared by several processes, but only one process can write to that file at any one time. A mutex is the perfect synchronization device to handle this situation.

The mutex is supported by the **System.Threading.Mutex** class. It has several constructors. Two commonly used ones are shown here:

public Mutex( )
public Mutex(bool *owned*)

The first version creates a mutex that is initially unowned. In the second version, if *owned* is **true**, the initial state of the mutex is owned by the calling thread. Otherwise, it is unowned.

To acquire the mutex, your code will call **WaitOne( )** on the mutex. This method is inherited by **Mutex** from the **Thread.WaitHandle** class. Here is its simplest form:

public bool WaitOne( );

It waits until the mutex on which it is called can be acquired. Thus, it blocks execution of the calling thread until the specified mutex is available. It always returns true.

When your code no longer needs ownership of the mutex, it releases it by calling **ReleaseMutex( )**, shown here:

public void ReleaseMutex( )

This releases the mutex on which it is called, enabling the mutex to be acquired by another thread.

To use a mutex to synchronize access to a shared resource, you will use **WaitOne( )** and **ReleaseMutex( )**, as shown in the following sequence:

```
Mutex myMtx = new Mutex();

// ...

myMtx.WaitOne(); // wait to acquire the mutex

// Access the shared resource.

myMtx.ReleaseMutex(); // release the mutex
```

When the call to **WaitOne( )** takes place, execution of the thread will suspend until the mutex can be acquired. When the call to **ReleaseMutex( )** takes place, the mutex is released and another thread can acquire it. Using this approach, access to a shared resource can be limited to one thread at a time.

The following program puts this framework into action. It creates two threads, **IncThread** and **DecThread**, which both access a shared resource called **SharedRes.Count**. **IncThread** increments **SharedRes.Count** and **DecThread** decrements it. To prevent both threads from accessing **SharedRes.Count** at the same time, access is synchronized by the **Mtx** mutex, which is also part of the **SharedRes** class.

```
// Use a Mutex.

using System;
using System.Threading;

// This class contains a shared resource (Count),
// and a mutex (Mtx) to control access to it.
class SharedRes {
  public static int Count = 0;
  public static Mutex Mtx = new Mutex();
}

// This thread increments SharedRes.Count.
class IncThread {
  int num;
  public Thread Thrd;

  public IncThread(string name, int n) {
    Thrd = new Thread(this.Run);
    num = n;
    Thrd.Name = name;
    Thrd.Start();
  }

  // Entry point of thread.
  void Run() {

    Console.WriteLine(Thrd.Name + " is waiting for the mutex.");

    // Acquire the Mutex.
    SharedRes.Mtx.WaitOne();

    Console.WriteLine(Thrd.Name + " acquires the mutex.");

    do {
      Thread.Sleep(500);
      SharedRes.Count++;
      Console.WriteLine("In " + Thrd.Name +
                        ", SharedRes.Count is " + SharedRes.Count);
      num--;
    } while(num > 0);

    Console.WriteLine(Thrd.Name + " releases the mutex.");

    // Release the Mutex.
    SharedRes.Mtx.ReleaseMutex();
  }
}
```

```
// This thread decrements SharedRes.Count.
class DecThread {
  int num;
  public Thread Thrd;

  public DecThread(string name, int n) {
    Thrd = new Thread(new ThreadStart(this.Run));
    num = n;
    Thrd.Name = name;
    Thrd.Start();
  }

  // Entry point of thread.
  void Run() {

    Console.WriteLine(Thrd.Name + " is waiting for the mutex.");

    // Acquire the Mutex.
    SharedRes.Mtx.WaitOne();

    Console.WriteLine(Thrd.Name + " acquires the mutex.");

    do {
      Thread.Sleep(500);
      SharedRes.Count--;
      Console.WriteLine("In " + Thrd.Name +
                        ", SharedRes.Count is " + SharedRes.Count);
      num--;
    } while(num > 0);

    Console.WriteLine(Thrd.Name + " releases the mutex.");

    // Release the Mutex.
    SharedRes.Mtx.ReleaseMutex();
  }
}

class MutexDemo {
  static void Main() {

    // Construct three threads.
    IncThread mt1 = new IncThread("Increment Thread", 5);

    Thread.Sleep(1); // let the Increment thread start

    DecThread mt2 = new DecThread("Decrement Thread", 5);

    mt1.Thrd.Join();
    mt2.Thrd.Join();
  }
}
```

The output is shown here:

```
Increment Thread is waiting for the mutex.
Increment Thread acquires the mutex.
```

```
Decrement Thread is waiting for the mutex.
In Increment Thread, SharedRes.Count is 1
In Increment Thread, SharedRes.Count is 2
In Increment Thread, SharedRes.Count is 3
In Increment Thread, SharedRes.Count is 4
In Increment Thread, SharedRes.Count is 5
Increment Thread releases the mutex.
Decrement Thread acquires the mutex.
In Decrement Thread, SharedRes.Count is 4
In Decrement Thread, SharedRes.Count is 3
In Decrement Thread, SharedRes.Count is 2
In Decrement Thread, SharedRes.Count is 1
In Decrement Thread, SharedRes.Count is 0
Decrement Thread releases the mutex.
```

As the output shows, access to **SharedRes.Count** is synchronized, with only one thread at a time being able to change its value.

To prove that the **Mtx** mutex was needed to produce the preceding output, try commenting out the calls to **WaitOne( )** and **ReleaseMutex( )** in the preceding program. When you run the program, you will see the following sequence (the actual output you see may vary):

```
In Increment Thread, SharedRes.Count is 1
In Decrement Thread, SharedRes.Count is 0
In Increment Thread, SharedRes.Count is 1
In Decrement Thread, SharedRes.Count is 0
In Increment Thread, SharedRes.Count is 1
In Decrement Thread, SharedRes.Count is 0
In Increment Thread, SharedRes.Count is 1
In Decrement Thread, SharedRes.Count is 0
In Increment Thread, SharedRes.Count is 1
```

As this output shows, without the mutex, increments and decrements to **SharedRes.Count** are interspersed rather than sequenced.

The mutex created by the previous example is known only to the process that creates it. However, it is possible to create a mutex that is known systemwide. To do so, you must create a named mutex, using one of these constructors:

   public Mutex(bool *owned*, string *name*)
   public Mutex(bool *owned*, string *name*, out bool *whatHappened*)

In both forms, the name of the mutex is passed in *name*. In the first form, if *owned* is **true**, then ownership of the mutex is requested. However, because a systemwide mutex might already be owned by another process, it is better to specify **false** for this parameter. In the second form, on return, *whatHappened* will be **true** if ownership was requested and acquired. It will be **false** if ownership was denied. (There is also a third form of the **Mutex** constructor that allows you to specify a **MutexSecurity** object, which controls access.) Using a named mutex enables you to manage interprocess synchronization.

One other point: It is legal for a thread that has acquired a mutex to make one or more additional calls to **WaitOne( )** prior to calling **ReleaseMutex( )**, and these additional calls will succeed. That is, redundant calls to **WaitOne( )** will not block a thread that already owns the mutex. However, the number of calls to **WaitOne( )** must be balanced by the same number of calls to **ReleaseMutex( )** before the mutex is released.

The Semaphore

A semaphore is similar to a mutex except that it can grant more than one thread access to a shared resource at the same time. Thus, the semaphore is useful when a collection of resources is being synchronized. A semaphore controls access to a shared resource through the use of a counter. If the counter is greater than zero, then access is allowed. If it is zero, access is denied. What the counter is counting are *permits*. Thus, to access the resource, a thread must be granted a permit from the semaphore.

In general, to use a semaphore, the thread that wants access to the shared resource tries to acquire a permit. If the semaphore's counter is greater than zero, the thread acquires a permit, which causes the semaphore's count to be decremented. Otherwise, the thread will block until a permit can be acquired. When the thread no longer needs access to the shared resource, it releases the permit, which causes the semaphore's count to be incremented. If there is another thread waiting for a permit, then that thread will acquire a permit at that time. The number of simultaneous accesses permitted is specified when the semaphore is created. If you create a semaphore that allows only one access, then a semaphore acts just like a mutex.

Semaphores are especially useful in situations in which a shared resource consists of a group or *pool*. For example, a collection of network connections, any of which can be used for communication, is a resource pool. A thread needing a network connection doesn't care which one it gets. In this case, a semaphore offers a convenient mechanism to manage access to the connections.

The semaphore is implemented by **System.Threading.Semaphore**. It has several constructors. The simplest form is shown here:

public Semaphore(int *initial*, int *max*)

Here, *initial* specifies the initial value of the semaphore permit counter, which is the number of permits available. The maximum value of the counter is passed in *max*. Thus, *max* represents the maximum number of permits that can granted by the semaphore. The value in *initial* specifies how many of these permits are initially available.

Using a semaphore is similar to using a mutex, described earlier. To acquire access, your code will call **WaitOne( )** on the semaphore. This method is inherited by **Semaphore** from the **WaitHandle** class. **WaitOne( )** waits until the semaphore on which it is called can be acquired. Thus, it blocks execution of the calling thread until the specified semaphore can grant permission.

When your code no longer needs ownership of the semaphore, it releases it by calling **Release( )**, which is shown here:

public int Release( )
public int Release(int *num*)

The first form releases one permit. The second form releases the number of permits specified by *num*. Both return the permit count that existed prior to the release.

It is possible for a thread to call **WaitOne( )** more than once before calling **Release( )**. However, the number of calls to **WaitOne( )** must be balanced by the same number of calls to **Release( )** before the permit is released. Alternatively, you can call the **Release(int)** form, passing a number equal to the number of times that **WaitOne( )** was called.

Here is an example that illustrates the semaphore. In the program, the class **MyThread** uses a semaphore to allow only two **MyThread** threads to be executed at any one time. Thus, the resource being shared is the CPU.

```
// Use a Semaphore.

using System;
using System.Threading;

// This thread allows only two instances of itself
// to run at any one time.
class MyThread {
  public Thread Thrd;

  // This creates a semaphore that allows up to two
  // permits to be granted and that initially has
  // two permits available.
  static Semaphore sem = new Semaphore(2, 2);

  public MyThread(string name) {
    Thrd = new Thread(this.Run);
    Thrd.Name = name;
    Thrd.Start();
  }

  // Entry point of thread.
  void Run() {

    Console.WriteLine(Thrd.Name + " is waiting for a permit.");

    sem.WaitOne();

    Console.WriteLine(Thrd.Name + " acquires a permit.");

    for(char ch='A'; ch < 'D'; ch++) {
      Console.WriteLine(Thrd.Name + " : " + ch + " ");
      Thread.Sleep(500);
    }

    Console.WriteLine(Thrd.Name + " releases a permit.");

    // Release the semaphore.
    sem.Release();
  }
}


class SemaphoreDemo {
  static void Main() {

    // Construct three threads.
```

```
MyThread mt1 = new MyThread("Thread #1");
MyThread mt2 = new MyThread("Thread #2");
MyThread mt3 = new MyThread("Thread #3");

mt1.Thrd.Join();
mt2.Thrd.Join();
mt3.Thrd.Join();
  }
}
```

MyThread declares the semaphore **sem**, as shown here:

```
static Semaphore sem = new Semaphore(2, 2);
```

This creates a semaphore that can grant up to two permits and that initially has both permits available.

In **MyThread.Run( )**, notice that execution cannot continue until a permit is granted by the semaphore, **sem**. If no permits are available, then execution of that thread suspends. When a permit does become available, execution resumes and the thread can run. In **Main( )**, three **MyThread** threads are created. However, only the first two get to execute. The third must wait until one of the other threads terminates. The output, shown here, verifies this. (The actual output you see may vary slightly.)

```
Thread #1 is waiting for a permit.
Thread #1 acquires a permit.
Thread #1 : A
Thread #2 is waiting for a permit.
Thread #2 acquires a permit.
Thread #2 : A
Thread #3 is waiting for a permit.
Thread #1 : B
Thread #2 : B
Thread #1 : C
Thread #2 : C
Thread #1 releases a permit.
Thread #3 acquires a permit.
Thread #3 : A
Thread #2 releases a permit.
Thread #3 : B
Thread #3 : C
Thread #3 releases a permit.
```

The semaphore created by the previous example is known only to the process that creates it. However, it is possible to create a semaphore that is known systemwide. To do so, you must create a named semaphore. To do this, use one of these constructors:

public Semaphore(int *initial*, int *max*, string *name*)
public Semaphore(int *initial*, int *max*, string *name*, out bool *whatHappened*)

In both forms, the name of the semaphore is passed in *name*. In the first form, if a semaphore by the specified name does not already exist, it is created using the values of *initial* and *max*. If it does already exist, then the values of *initial* and *max* are ignored. In the second form, on return, *whatHappened* will be **true** if the semaphore was created. In this case, the values of *initial* and *max* will be used to create the semaphore. If *whatHappened* is **false**, then the

semaphore already exists and the values of *initial* and *max* are ignored. (There is also a third form of the **Semaphore** constructor that allows you to specify a **SemaphoreSecurity** object, which controls access.) Using a named semaphore enables you to manage interprocess synchronization.

Using Events

C# supports another type of synchronization object: the event. There are two types of events: manual reset and auto reset. These are supported by the classes **ManualResetEvent** and **AutoResetEvent**. These classes are derived from the top-level class **EventWaitHandle**. These classes are used in situations in which one thread is waiting for some event to occur in another thread. When the event takes place, the second thread signals the first, allowing it to resume execution.

The constructors for **ManualResetEvent** and **AutoResetEvent** are shown here:

public ManualResetEvent(bool *status*)
public AutoResetEvent(bool *status*)

Here, if *status* is **true**, the event is initially signaled. If *status* is **false**, the event is initially non-signaled.

Events are easy to use. For a **ManualResetEvent**, the procedure works like this. A thread that is waiting for some event simply calls **WaitOne( )** on the event object representing that event. **WaitOne( )** returns immediately if the event object is in a signaled state. Otherwise, it suspends execution of the calling thread until the event is signaled. After another thread performs the event, that thread sets the event object to a signaled state by calling **Set( )**. Thus, a call to **Set( )** can be understood as signaling that an event has occurred. After the event object is set to a signaled state, the call to **WaitOne( )** will return and the first thread will resume execution. The event is returned to a non-signaled state by calling **Reset( )**.

The difference between **AutoResetEvent** and **ManualResetEvent** is how the event gets reset. For **ManualResetEvent**, the event remains signaled until a call to **Reset( )** is made. For **AutoResetEvent**, the event automatically changes to a non-signaled state as soon as a thread waiting on that event receives the event notification and resumes execution. Thus, a call to **Reset( )** is not necessary when using **AutoResetEvent**.

Here is an example that illustrates **ManualResetEvent**:

```
// Use a manual event object.

using System;
using System.Threading;

// This thread signals the event passed to its constructor.
class MyThread {
  public Thread Thrd;
  ManualResetEvent mre;

  public MyThread(string name, ManualResetEvent evt) {
    Thrd = new Thread(this.Run);
    Thrd.Name = name;
    mre = evt;
    Thrd.Start();
  }
```

```
    // Entry point of thread.
    void Run() {
      Console.WriteLine("Inside thread " + Thrd.Name);

      for(int i=0; i<5; i++) {
        Console.WriteLine(Thrd.Name);
        Thread.Sleep(500);
      }

      Console.WriteLine(Thrd.Name + " Done!");

      // Signal the event.
      mre.Set();
    }
}

class ManualEventDemo {
  static void Main() {
    ManualResetEvent evtObj = new ManualResetEvent(false);

    MyThread mt1 = new MyThread("Event Thread 1", evtObj);

    Console.WriteLine("Main thread waiting for event.");

    // Wait for signaled event.
    evtObj.WaitOne();

    Console.WriteLine("Main thread received first event.");


    // Reset the event.
    evtObj.Reset();


    mt1 = new MyThread("Event Thread 2", evtObj);

    // Wait for signaled event.
    evtObj.WaitOne();

    Console.WriteLine("Main thread received second event.");
  }
}
```

The output is shown here. (The actual output you see may vary slightly.)

```
Inside thread Event Thread 1
Event Thread 1
Main thread waiting for event.
Event Thread 1
Event Thread 1
Event Thread 1
Event Thread 1
Event Thread 1 Done!
Main thread received first event.
Inside thread Event Thread 2
```

```
Event Thread 2
Event Thread 2
Event Thread 2
Event Thread 2
Event Thread 2
Event Thread 2 Done!
Main thread received second event.
```

First, notice that **MyThread** is passed a **ManualResetEvent** in its constructor. When **MyThread**'s **Run( )** method finishes, it calls **Set( )** on that event object, which puts the event object into a signaled state. Inside **Main( )**, a **ManualResetEvent** called **evtObj** is created with an initially unsignaled state. Then, a **MyThread** instance is created and passed **evtObj**. Next, the main thread waits on the event object. Because the initial state of **evtObj** is not signaled, this causes the main thread to wait until the instance of **MyThread** calls **Set( )**, which puts **evtObj** into a signaled state. This allows the main thread to run again. Then the event is reset and the process is repeated for the second thread. Without the use of the event object, all threads would have run simultaneously and their output would have been jumbled. To verify this, try commenting out the call to **WaitOne( )** inside **Main( )**.

In the preceding program, if an **AutoResetEvent** object rather than a **ManualResetEvent** object were used, then the call to **Reset( )** in **Main( )** would not be necessary. The reason is that the event is automatically set to a non-signaled state when a thread waiting on the event is resumed. To try this, simply change all references to **ManualResetEvent** to **AutoResetEvent** and remove the calls to **Reset( )**. This version will execute the same as before.

The Interlocked Class

One other class that is related to synchronization is **Interlocked**. This class offers an alternative to the other synchronization features when all you need to do is change the value of a shared variable. The methods provided by **Interlocked** guarantee that their operation is performed as a single, uninterruptable operation. Thus, no other synchronization is needed. **Interlocked** provides static methods that add two integers, increment an integer, decrement an integer, compare and set an object, exchange objects, and obtain a 64-bit value. All of these operations take place without interruption.

The following program demonstrates two **Interlocked** methods: **Increment( )** and **Decrement( )**. Here the forms of these methods that will be used:

   public static int Increment(ref int *v*)

   public static int Decrement(ref int *v*)

Here, *v* is the value to be incremented or decremented.

```
// Use Interlocked operations.

using System;
using System.Threading;

// A shared resource.
class SharedRes {
  public static int Count = 0;
}
```

```
// This thread increments SharedRes.Count.
class IncThread {
  public Thread Thrd;

  public IncThread(string name) {
    Thrd = new Thread(this.Run);
    Thrd.Name = name;
    Thrd.Start();
  }

  // Entry point of thread.
  void Run() {

    for(int i=0; i<5; i++) {
      Interlocked.Increment(ref SharedRes.Count);
      Console.WriteLine(Thrd.Name + " Count is " + SharedRes.Count);
    }
  }
}

// This thread decrements SharedRes.Count.
class DecThread {
  public Thread Thrd;

  public DecThread(string name) {
    Thrd = new Thread(this.Run);
    Thrd.Name = name;
    Thrd.Start();
  }

  // Entry point of thread.
  void Run() {

    for(int i=0; i<5; i++) {
      Interlocked.Decrement(ref SharedRes.Count);
      Console.WriteLine(Thrd.Name + " Count is " + SharedRes.Count);
    }
  }
}

class InterlockedDemo {
  static void Main() {

    // Construct two threads.
    IncThread mt1 = new IncThread("Increment Thread");
    DecThread mt2 = new DecThread("Decrement Thread");

    mt1.Thrd.Join();
    mt2.Thrd.Join();
  }
}
```

Terminating a Thread

It is sometimes useful to stop a thread prior to its normal conclusion. For example, a debugger may need to stop a thread that has run wild. Once a thread has been terminated, it is removed from the system and cannot be restarted.

To terminate a thread prior to its normal ending point, use **Thread.Abort( )**. Its simplest form is shown here:

public void Abort( )

Abort( ) causes a **ThreadAbortException** to be thrown to the thread on which **Abort( )** is called. This exception causes the thread to terminate. This exception can also be caught by your code (but is automatically rethrown in order to stop the thread). **Abort( )** may not always be able to stop a thread immediately, so if it is important that a thread be stopped before your program continues, you will need to follow a call to **Abort( )** with a call to **Join( )**. Also, in rare cases, it is possible that **Abort( )** won't be able to stop a thread. One way this could happen is if a **finally** block goes into an infinite loop.

The following example shows how to stop a thread by use of **Abort( )**:

```
// Stopping a thread by use of Abort().

using System;
using System.Threading;

class MyThread {
  public Thread Thrd;

  public MyThread(string name) {
    Thrd = new Thread(this.Run);
    Thrd.Name = name;
    Thrd.Start();
  }

  // This is the entry point for thread.
  void Run() {
    Console.WriteLine(Thrd.Name + " starting.");

    for(int i = 1; i <= 1000; i++) {
      Console.Write(i + " ");
      if((i%10)==0) {
        Console.WriteLine();
        Thread.Sleep(250);
      }
    }
    Console.WriteLine(Thrd.Name + " exiting.");
  }
}

class StopDemo {
  static void Main() {
```

```
    MyThread mt1 = new MyThread("My Thread");

    Thread.Sleep(1000); // let child thread start executing

    Console.WriteLine("Stopping thread.");
    mt1.Thrd.Abort();

    mt1.Thrd.Join(); // wait for thread to terminate

    Console.WriteLine("Main thread terminating.");
  }
}
```

The output from this program is shown here:

```
My Thread starting.
1 2 3 4 5 6 7 8 9 10
11 12 13 14 15 16 17 18 19 20
21 22 23 24 25 26 27 28 29 30
31 32 33 34 35 36 37 38 39 40
Stopping thread.
Main thread terminating.
```

NOTE *Abort( ) should not be used as the normal means of stopping a thread. It is meant for specialized situations. Usually, a thread should end because its entry point method returns.*

An Abort( ) Alternative

You might find a second form of **Abort( )** useful in some cases. Its general form is shown here:

    public void Abort(object *info*)

Here, *info* contains any information that you want to pass to the thread when it is being stopped. This information is accessible through the **ExceptionState** property of **ThreadAbortException**. You might use this to pass a termination code to a thread. The following program demonstrates this form of **Abort( )**:

```
// Using Abort(object).

using System;
using System.Threading;

class MyThread {
  public Thread Thrd;

  public MyThread(string name) {
    Thrd = new Thread(this.Run);
    Thrd.Name = name;
    Thrd.Start();
  }

  // This is the entry point for thread.
  void Run() {
    try {
```

```
        Console.WriteLine(Thrd.Name + " starting.");

        for(int i = 1; i <= 1000; i++) {
          Console.Write(i + " ");
          if((i%10)==0) {
            Console.WriteLine();
            Thread.Sleep(250);
          }
        }
        Console.WriteLine(Thrd.Name + " exiting normally.");
      } catch(ThreadAbortException exc) {
        Console.WriteLine("Thread aborting, code is " +
                          exc.ExceptionState);
      }
    }
  }
}

class UseAltAbort {
  static void Main() {
    MyThread mt1 = new MyThread("My Thread");

    Thread.Sleep(1000); // let child thread start executing

    Console.WriteLine("Stopping thread.");
    mt1.Thrd.Abort(100);

    mt1.Thrd.Join(); // wait for thread to terminate

    Console.WriteLine("Main thread terminating.");
  }
}
```

The output is shown here:

```
My Thread starting.
1 2 3 4 5 6 7 8 9 10
11 12 13 14 15 16 17 18 19 20
21 22 23 24 25 26 27 28 29 30
31 32 33 34 35 36 37 38 39 40
Stopping thread.
Thread aborting, code is 100
Main thread terminating.
```

As the output shows, the value 100 is passed to **Abort( )**. This value is then accessed through the **ExceptionState** property of the **ThreadAbortException** caught by the thread when it is terminated.

Canceling Abort( )

A thread can override a request to abort. To do so, the thread must catch the **ThreadAbortException** and then call **ResetAbort( )**. This prevents the exception from being automatically rethrown when the thread's exception handler ends. **ResetAbort( )** is declared like this:

  public static void ResetAbort( )

A call to **ResetAbort( )** can fail if the thread does not have the proper security setting to cancel the abort.

The following program demonstrates **ResetAbort( )**:

```
// Using ResetAbort().

using System;
using System.Threading;

class MyThread {
  public Thread Thrd;

  public MyThread(string name) {
    Thrd = new Thread(this.Run);
    Thrd.Name = name;
    Thrd.Start();
  }

  // This is the entry point for thread.
  void Run() {
    Console.WriteLine(Thrd.Name + " starting.");

    for(int i = 1; i <= 1000; i++) {
      try {
        Console.Write(i + " ");
        if((i%10)==0) {
          Console.WriteLine();
          Thread.Sleep(250);
        }
      } catch(ThreadAbortException exc) {
        if((int)exc.ExceptionState == 0) {
          Console.WriteLine("Abort Cancelled! Code is " +
                            exc.ExceptionState);
          Thread.ResetAbort();
        }
        else
          Console.WriteLine("Thread aborting, code is " +
                            exc.ExceptionState);
      }
    }
    Console.WriteLine(Thrd.Name + " exiting normally.");
  }
}

class ResetAbort {
  static void Main() {
    MyThread mt1 = new MyThread("My Thread");

    Thread.Sleep(1000); // let child thread start executing

    Console.WriteLine("Stopping thread.");
    mt1.Thrd.Abort(0); // this won't stop the thread
```

```
    Thread.Sleep(1000); // let child execute a bit longer

    Console.WriteLine("Stopping thread.");
    mt1.Thrd.Abort(100); // this will stop the thread

    mt1.Thrd.Join(); // wait for thread to terminate

    Console.WriteLine("Main thread terminating.");
  }
}
```

The output is shown here:

```
My Thread starting.
1 2 3 4 5 6 7 8 9 10
11 12 13 14 15 16 17 18 19 20
21 22 23 24 25 26 27 28 29 30
31 32 33 34 35 36 37 38 39 40
Stopping thread.
Abort Cancelled! Code is 0
41 42 43 44 45 46 47 48 49 50
51 52 53 54 55 56 57 58 59 60
61 62 63 64 65 66 67 68 69 70
71 72 73 74 75 76 77 78 79 80
Stopping thread.
Thread aborting, code is 100
Main thread terminating.
```

In this example, if **Abort( )** is called with an argument that equals zero, then the abort request is cancelled by the thread by calling **ResetAbort( )**, and the thread's execution continues. Any other value causes the thread to stop.

Suspending and Resuming a Thread

In early versions of the .NET Framework, a thread could be suspended by calling **Thread.Suspend( )** and resumed by calling **Thread.Resume( )**. Today, however, both of these methods are marked as obsolete and should not be used for new code. One reason is that **Suspend( )** is inherently dangerous because it can be used to suspend a thread that is currently holding a lock, thus preventing the lock from being released, resulting in deadlock. This can cause a systemwide problem. You must use C#'s other synchronization features, such as a mutex, to suspend and resume a thread.

Determining a Thread's State

The state of a thread can be obtained from the **ThreadState** property provided by **Thread**. It is shown here:

    public ThreadState ThreadState{ get; }

The state of the thread is returned as a value defined by the **ThreadState** enumeration. It defines the following values:

ThreadState.Aborted	ThreadState.AbortRequested
ThreadState.Background	ThreadState.Running
ThreadState.Stopped	ThreadState.StopRequested
ThreadState.Suspended	ThreadState.SuspendRequested
ThreadState.Unstarted	ThreadState.WaitSleepJoin

All but one of these values is self-explanatory. The one that needs some explanation is **ThreadState.WaitSleepJoin**. A thread enters this state when it is waiting because of a call to **Wait( )**, **Sleep( )**, or **Join( )**.

Using the Main Thread

As mentioned at the start of this chapter, all C# programs have at least one thread of execution, called the *main thread*, which is given to the program automatically when it begins running. The main thread can be handled just like all other threads.

To access the main thread, you must obtain a **Thread** object that refers to it. You do this through the **CurrentThread** property, which is a member of **Thread**. Its general form is shown here:

public static Thread CurrentThread{ get; }

This property returns a reference to the thread in which it is used. Therefore, if you use **CurrentThread** while execution is inside the main thread, you will obtain a reference to the main thread. Once you have this reference, you can control the main thread just like any other thread.

The following program obtains a reference to the main thread and then gets and sets the main thread's name and priority:

```
// Control the main thread.

using System;
using System.Threading;

class UseMain {
  static void Main() {
    Thread Thrd;

    // Get the main thread.
    Thrd = Thread.CurrentThread;

    // Display main thread's name.
    if(Thrd.Name == null)
      Console.WriteLine("Main thread has no name.");
    else
      Console.WriteLine("Main thread is called: " + Thrd.Name);

    // Display main thread's priority.
    Console.WriteLine("Priority: " + Thrd.Priority);
```

```
    Console.WriteLine();

    // Set the name and priority.
    Console.WriteLine("Setting name and priority.\n");
    Thrd.Name = "Main Thread";
    Thrd.Priority = ThreadPriority.AboveNormal;

    Console.WriteLine("Main thread is now called: " +
                       Thrd.Name);

    Console.WriteLine("Priority is now: " +
                       Thrd.Priority);
  }
}
```

The output from the program is shown here:

```
Main thread has no name.
Priority: Normal

Setting name and priority.

Main thread is now called: Main Thread
Priority is now: AboveNormal
```

One word of caution: You need to be careful about what operations you perform on the main thread. For example, if you add this call to **Join( )** to the end of **Main( )**,

```
Thrd.Join();
```

the program will never terminate because it will be waiting for the main thread to end!

Multithreading Tips

The key to effectively utilizing multithreading is to think concurrently rather than serially. For example, when you have two subsystems within a program that can execute concurrently, make them into individual threads. A word of caution is in order, however. If you create too many threads, you can actually degrade your program's performance rather than enhance it. Remember, there is some overhead associated with context switching. If you create too many threads, more CPU time will be spent changing contexts than in executing your program!

Starting a Separate Task

Although thread-based multitasking is what you will use most often when programming in C#, it is possible to utilize process-based multitasking where appropriate. When using process-based multitasking, instead of starting another thread within the same program, one program starts the execution of another program. In C#, you do this by using the **Process** class. **Process** is defined within the **System.Diagnostics** namespace. To conclude this chapter, a brief look at starting and managing another process is offered.

The easiest way to start another process is to use the **Start( )** method defined by **Process**. Here is one of its simplest forms:

publicstatic Process Start(string *name*)

Here, *name* specifies the name of an executable file that will be executed or a file that is associated with an executable.

When a process that you create ends, call **Close( )** to free the memory associated with that process. It is shown here:

        public void Close( )

You can terminate a process in two ways. If the process is a Windows GUI application, then to terminate the process, call **CloseMainWindow( )**, shown here:

        public bool CloseMainWindow( )

This method sends a message to the process, instructing it to stop. It returns true if the message was received. It returns false if the application was not a GUI application, or does not have a main window. Furthermore, **CloseMainWindow( )** is only a request to shut down. If the application ignores the request, the application will not be terminated.

To positively terminate a process, call **Kill( )**, as shown here:

        public void Kill( )

Use **Kill( )** carefully. It causes an uncontrolled termination of the process. Any unsaved data associated with the process will most likely be lost.

You can wait for a process to end by calling **WaitForExit( )**. Its two forms are shown here:

        public void WaitForExit( )
        public bool WaitForExit(int *milliseconds*)

The first form waits until the process terminates. The second waits for only the specified number of milliseconds. The second form returns true if the process has terminated and false if it is still running.

The following program demonstrates how to create, wait for, and close a process. It starts the standard Windows utility program **WordPad.exe**. It then waits for WordPad to end.

```
// Starting a new process.

using System;
using System.Diagnostics;

class StartProcess {
  static void Main() {
    Process newProc = Process.Start("wordpad.exe");

    Console.WriteLine("New process started.");

    newProc.WaitForExit();

    newProc.Close(); // free resources

    Console.WriteLine("New process ended.");
  }
}
```

When you run this program, WordPad will start, and you will see the message, "New process started." The program will then wait until you close WordPad. Once WordPad has been terminated, the final message "New process ended." is displayed.

Collections, Enumerators, and Iterators

This chapter discusses one of the most important parts of the .NET Framework: collections. In C#, a *collection* is a group of objects. The .NET Framework contains a large number of interfaces and classes that define and implement various types of collections. Collections simplify many programming tasks because they provide off-the-shelf solutions to several common, but sometimes tedious-to-develop, data structures. For example, there are built-in collections that support dynamic arrays, linked lists, stacks, queues, and hash tables. Collections are a state-of-the-art technology that merits close attention by all C# programmers.

Originally, there were only non-generic collection classes. However, the addition of generics in C# 2.0 coincided with the addition of many new generic classes and interfaces to the .NET Framework. The inclusion of the generic collections essentially doubled the number of collection classes and interfaces. Thus, the Collections API is now quite large. Although the generic and non-generic collections work in similar ways, there are some differences, and both are described in this chapter.

Also described in this chapter are two features that relate to collections: enumerators and iterators. Both enumerators and iterators enable the contents of a class to be cycled through via a **foreach** loop.

Collections Overview

The principal benefit of collections is that they standardize the way groups of objects are handled by your programs. All collections are designed around a set of cleanly defined interfaces. Several built-in implementations of these interfaces, such as **ArrayList**, **Hashtable**, **Stack**, and **Queue**, are provided, which you can use as-is. You can also implement your own collection, but you will seldom need to.

The .NET Framework supports four general types of collections: non-generic, specialized, bit based, and generic. The non-generic collections implement several fundamental data structures, including a dynamic array, stack, and queue. They also include *dictionaries*, in which you can store key/value pairs. An essential point to understand about the non-generic collections is that they operate on data of type **object**.

Thus, they can be used to store any type of data, and different types of data can be mixed within the same collection. Of course, because they store **object** references, they are not type-safe. The non-generic collection classes and interfaces are in **System.Collections**.

The specialized collections operate on a specific type of data or operate in a unique way. For example, there are specialized collections for strings. There are also specialized collections that use a singly linked list. The specialized collections are declared in **System.Collections.Specialized**.

The Collections API defines one bit-based collection called **BitArray**. **BitArray** supports bitwise operations on bits, such as AND and XOR. As such, it differs significantly in its capabilities from the other collections. **BitArray** is declared in **System.Collections**.

The generic collections provide generic implementations of several standard data structures, such as linked lists, stacks, queues, and dictionaries. Because these collections are generic, they are type-safe. This means that only items that are type-compatible with the type of the collection can be stored in a generic collection, thus eliminating accidental type mismatches. Generic collections are declared in **System.Collections.Generic**.

There are also several classes in the **System.Collections.ObjectModel** namespace that support programmers who want to create their own generic collections.

Fundamental to all collections is the concept of an *enumerator,* which is supported by the non-generic interfaces **IEnumerator** and **IEnumerable**, and the generic interfaces **IEnumerator<T>** and **IEnumerable<T>**. An enumerator provides a standardized way of accessing the elements within a collection, one at a time. Thus, it *enumerates* the contents of a collection. Because each collection must implement either a generic or non-generic form of **IEnumerable**, the elements of any collection class can be accessed through the methods defined by **IEnumerator** or **IEnumerator<T>**. Therefore, with only small changes, the code that cycles through one type of collection can be used to cycle through another. As a point of interest, the **foreach** loop uses the enumerator to cycle through the contents of a collection.

A feature related to an enumerator is the *iterator.* It simplifies the process of creating classes, such as custom collections, that can be cycled through by a **foreach** loop. Iterators are also described in this chapter.

One last thing: If you are familiar with C++, then you will find it helpful to know that the collection classes are similar in spirit to the Standard Template Library (STL) classes defined by C++. What a C++ programmer calls a *container,* a C# programmer calls a *collection.* The same is true of Java. If you are familiar with Java's Collections Framework, then you will have no trouble learning to use C# collections.

Because of the differences among the four types of collections—non-generic, bit-based, specialized, and generic—this chapter discusses each separately.

The Non-Generic Collections

The non-generic collections have been part of the .NET Framework since version 1.0. They are defined in the **System.Collections** namespace. The non-generic collections are general-purpose data structures that operate on **object** references. Thus, they can manage any type of object, but not in a type-safe manner. This is both their advantage and disadvantage. Because they operate on **object** references, you can mix various types of data within the same collection. This makes them useful in situations in which you need to manage a collection of different types of objects or when the type of objects being stored are not known in advance. However, if you intend a collection to store a specific type of object, then the non-generic collections do not have the type safety that is found in the generic collections.

The non-generic collections are defined by a set of interfaces and the classes that implement those interfaces. Each is described by the following sections.

The Non-Generic Interfaces

System.Collections defines a number of non-generic interfaces. It is necessary to begin with the collection interfaces because they determine the functionality common to all of the non-generic collection classes. The interfaces that underpin collections are summarized in Table 24-1. The following sections examine each interface in detail.

The ICollection Interface

The **ICollection** interface is the foundation upon which all non-generic collections are built. It declares the core methods and properties that all non-generic collections will have. It also inherits the **IEnumerable** interface.

ICollection defines the following properties:

Property	Meaning
int Count { get; }	The number of items currently held in the collection.
bool IsSynchronized { get; }	Is true if the collection is synchronized and false if it is not. By default, collections are not synchronized. It is possible, though, to obtain a synchronized version of most collections.
object SyncRoot { get; }	An object upon which the collection can be synchronized.

Count is the most often used property because it contains the number of elements currently held in a collection. If **Count** is zero, then the collection is empty.

ICollection defines the following method:

void CopyTo(Array *target*, int *startIdx*)

CopyTo( ) copies the contents of a collection to the array specified by *target*, beginning at the index specified by *startIdx*. Thus, **CopyTo( )** provides a pathway from a collection to a standard C# array.

Interface	Description
ICollection	Defines the elements that all non-generic collections must have.
IComparer	Defines the **Compare( )** method that performs a comparison on objects stored in a collection.
IDictionary	Defines a collection that consists of key/value pairs.
IDictionaryEnumerator	Defines the enumerator for a collection that implements **IDictionary**.
IEnumerable	Defines the **GetEnumerator( )** method, which supplies the enumerator for a collection class.
IEnumerator	Provides methods that enable the contents of a collection to be obtained one at a time.
IEqualityComparer	Compares two objects for equality.
IHashCodeProvider	Declared obsolete. Use **IEqualityComparer** instead.
IList	Defines a collection that can be accessed via an indexer.

TABLE 24-1 The Non-Generic Collection Interfaces

Because **ICollection** inherits **IEnumerable**, it also includes the sole method defined by **IEnumerable**: **GetEnumerator( )**, which is shown here:

IEnumerator GetEnumerator( )

It returns the enumerator for the collection.

Because **ICollection** inherits **IEnumerable**, three extension methods are defined for it. They are **AsQueryable( )**, **Cast( )**, and **OfType( )**. **AsQueryable( )** is declared in **System.Linq.Queryable**. Both **Cast( )** and **OfType( )** are declared in **System.Linq.Enumerable**. These methods are designed primarily to support LINQ, but may be useful in other contexts.

The IList Interface

The **IList** interface declares the behavior of a non-generic collection that allows elements to be accessed via a zero-based index. It inherits **ICollection** and **IEnumerable**. In addition to the methods defined by **ICollection** and **IEnumerable**, **IList** defines several of its own. These are summarized in Table 24-2. Several of these methods imply the modification of a collection. If the collection is read-only or of fixed size, then these methods will throw a **NotSupportedException**.

Objects are added to an **IList** collection by calling **Add( )**. Notice that **Add( )** takes an argument of type **object**. Since **object** is a base class for all types, any type of object can be stored in a non-generic collection. This includes the value types, because boxing and unboxing will automatically take place.

You can remove an element using **Remove( )** or **RemoveAt( )**. **Remove( )** removes the specified object. **RemoveAt( )** removes the object at a specified index. To empty the collection, call **Clear( )**.

Method	Description
int Add(object *obj*)	Adds *obj* into the invoking collection. Returns the index at which the object is stored.
void Clear( )	Deletes all elements from the invoking collection.
bool Contains(object *obj*)	Returns true if the invoking collection contains *obj*. Returns false if *obj* is not in the collection.
int IndexOf(object *obj*)	Returns the index of *obj* if *obj* is contained within the invoking collection. If *obj* is not found, –1 is returned.
void Insert(int *idx*, object *obj*)	Inserts *obj* at the index specified by *idx*. Elements at and below *idx* are moved down to make room for *obj*.
void Remove(object *obj*)	Removes the first occurrence of *obj* from the invoking collection. Elements at and below the removed element are moved up to close the gap.
void RemoveAt(int *idx*)	Removes the object at the index specified by *idx* from the invoking collection. Elements at and below *idx* are moved up to close the gap.

TABLE 24-2   The Methods Defined by **IList**

You can determine whether a collection contains a specific object by calling **Contains( )**. You can obtain the index of an object by called **IndexOf( )**. You can insert an element at a specific index by calling **Insert( )**.

IList defines the following properties:

```
bool IsFixedSize { get; }
bool IsReadOnly { get; }
```

If the collection is of fixed size, **IsFixedSize** is true. This means elements cannot be inserted or removed. If the collection is read-only, then **IsReadOnly** is true. This means the contents of the collection cannot be changed.

IList defines the following indexer:

```
object this[int idx] { get; set; }
```

You will use this indexer to get or set the value of an element. However, you cannot use it to add a new element to the collection. To add an element to a list, call **Add( )**. Once it is added, you can access the element through the indexer.

The IDictionary Interface

The **IDictionary** interface defines the behavior of a non-generic collection that maps unique keys to values. A key is an object that you use to retrieve a value at a later date. Thus, a collection that implements **IDictionary** stores key/value pairs. Once the pair is stored, you can retrieve it by using its key. **IDictionary** inherits **ICollection** and **IEnumerable**. The methods declared by **IDictionary** are summarized in Table 24-3. Several methods throw an **ArgumentNullException** if an attempt is made to specify a null key and null keys are not allowed.

To add a key/value pair to an **IDictionary** collection, use **Add( )**. Notice that the key and its value are specified separately. To remove an element, specify the key of the object in a call to **Remove( )**. To empty the collection, call **Clear( )**.

You can determine whether a collection contains a specific object by calling **Contains( )** with the key of the desired item. **GetEnumerator( )** obtains an enumerator compatible with an **IDictionary** collection. This enumerator operates on key/value pairs.

Method	Description
void Add(object *k*, object *v*)	Adds the key/value pair specified by *k* and *v* to the invoking collection. *k* must not be null.
void Clear( )	Removes all key/value pairs from the invoking collection.
bool Contains(object *k*)	Returns true if the invoking collection contains *k* as a key. Otherwise, returns false.
IDictionaryEnumerator GetEnumerator( )	Returns the enumerator for the invoking collection.
void Remove(object *k*)	Removes the entry whose key equals *k*.

TABLE 24-3 The Methods Defined by **IDictionary**

IDictionary defines the following properties:

Property	Description
bool IsFixedSize { get; }	Is true if the dictionary is of fixed size.
bool IsReadOnly { get; }	Is true if the dictionary is read-only.
ICollection Keys { get; }	Obtains a collection of the keys.
ICollection Values { get; }	Obtains a collection of the values.

Notice that the keys and values contained within the collection are available as separate lists through the **Keys** and **Values** properties.

IDictionary defines the following indexer:

object this[object *key*] { get; set; }

You can use this indexer to get or set the value of an element. You can also use it to add a new element to the collection. Notice that the "index" is not actually an index, but rather the key of the item.

IEnumerable, IEnumerator, and IDictionaryEnumerator

IEnumerable is the non-generic interface that a class must implement if it is to support enumerators. As explained, all of the non-generic collection classes implement **IEnumerable** because it is inherited by **ICollection**. The sole method defined by **IEnumerable** is **GetEnumerator( )**, which is shown here:

IEnumerator GetEnumerator( )

It returns the enumerator for the collection. Also, implementing **IEnumerable** allows the contents of a collection to be obtained by a **foreach** loop.

IEnumerator is the interface that defines the functionality of an enumerator. Using its methods, you can cycle through the contents of a collection. For collections that store key/value pairs (dictionaries), **GetEnumerator( )** returns an object of type **IDictionaryEnumerator**, rather than **IEnumerator**. **IDictionaryEnumerator** inherits **IEnumerator** and adds functionality to facilitate the enumeration of dictionaries.

IEnumerator defines the methods **MoveNext( )** and **Reset( )** and the **Current** property. The techniques needed to use them are described in detail later in this chapter. Briefly, **Current** holds the element currently being obtained. **MoveNext( )** moves to the next element. **Reset( )** restarts the enumeration from the beginning.

IComparer and IEqualityComparer

The **IComparer** interface defines a method called **Compare( )**, which defines the way two objects are compared. It is shown here:

int Compare(object *v1*, object *v2*)

It must return greater than zero if *v1* is greater than *v2*, less than zero if *v1* is less than *v2*, and zero if the two values are the same. This interface can be used to specify how the elements of a collection should be sorted.

IEqualityComparer defines these two methods:

bool Equals(object *obj1*, object *obj2*)

int GetHashCode(object *obj*)

Equals( ) must return true if **obj1** and **obj2** are equal. **GetHashCode( )** must return the hash code for *obj*.

The DictionaryEntry Structure

System.Collections defines one structure type called **DictionaryEntry**. Non-generic collections that hold key/value pairs store those pairs in a **DictionaryEntry** object. This structure defines the following two properties:

    public object Key { get; set; }
    public object Value { get; set; }

These properties are used to access the key or value associated with an entry. You can construct a **DictionaryEntry** object by using the following constructor:

    public DictionaryEntry(object *k*, object *v*)

Here, *k* is the key and *v* is the value.

The Non-Generic Collection Classes

Now that you are familiar with the non-generic collection interfaces, we can examine the standard classes that implement them. With the exception of **BitArray**, described later, the non-generic collection classes are summarized here:

Class	Description
ArrayList	A dynamic array. This is an array that can grow as needed.
Hashtable	A hash table for key/value pairs.
Queue	A first-in, first-out list.
SortedList	A sorted list of key/value pairs.
Stack	A first-in, last-out list.

The following sections examine these collection classes and illustrate their use.

ArrayList

The **ArrayList** class supports dynamic arrays, which can grow or shrink as needed. In C#, standard arrays are of a fixed length, which cannot be changed during program execution. This means you must know in advance how many elements an array will hold. But sometimes you may not know until runtime precisely how large an array you will need. To handle this situation, use **ArrayList**. An **ArrayList** is a variable-length array of object references that can dynamically increase or decrease in size. An **ArrayList** is created with an initial size. When this size is exceeded, the collection is automatically enlarged. When objects are removed, the array can be shrunk. **ArrayList** is currently in wide use in existing code. For this reason, it is examined in depth here. However, many of the same techniques that apply to **ArrayList** apply to the other collections as well, including the generic collections.

   ArrayList implements **ICollection**, **IList**, **IEnumerable**, and **ICloneable**. **ArrayList** has the constructors shown here:

    public ArrayList( )
    public ArrayList(ICollection *c*)
    public ArrayList(int *capacity*)

The first constructor builds an empty **ArrayList** with an initial capacity of zero. The second constructor builds an **ArrayList** that is initialized with the elements specified by c and has an initial capacity equal to the number of elements. The third constructor builds an array list that has the specified initial *capacity*. The capacity is the size of the underlying array that is used to store the elements. The capacity grows automatically as elements are added to an **ArrayList**.

In addition to the methods defined by the interfaces that it implements, **ArrayList** defines several methods of its own. Some of the more commonly used ones are shown in Table 24-4. An **ArrayList** can be sorted by calling **Sort( )**. Once sorted, it can be efficiently searched by **BinarySearch( )**. The contents of an **ArrayList** can be reversed by calling **Reverse( )**.

ArrayList supports several methods that operate on a range of elements within a collection. You can insert another collection into an **ArrayList** by calling **InsertRange( )**. You can remove a range by calling **RemoveRange( )**. You can overwrite a range within an **ArrayList** with the elements of another collection by calling **SetRange( )**. You can also sort or search a range rather than the entire collection.

By default, an **ArrayList** is not synchronized. To obtain a synchronized wrapper around a collection, call **Synchronized( )**.

Method	Description
public virtual void AddRange(ICollection *c*)	Adds the elements in *c* to the end of the invoking **ArrayList**.
public virtual int BinarySearch(object *v*)	Searches the invoking collection for the value passed in *v*. The index of the matching element is returned. If the value is not found, a negative value is returned. The invoking list must be sorted.
public virtual int BinarySearch(object *v*, IComparer *comp*)	Searches the invoking collection for the value passed in *v* using the comparison object specified by *comp*. The index of the matching element is returned. If the value is not found, a negative value is returned. The invoking list must be sorted.
public virtual int BinarySearch(int *startIdx*, int *count*, object *v*, IComparer *comp*)	Searches the invoking collection for the value passed in *v* using the comparison object specified by *comp*. The search begins at *startIdx* and runs for *count* elements. The index of the matching element is returned. If the value is not found, a negative value is returned. The invoking list must be sorted.
public virtual void CopyTo(Array *ar*)	Copies the contents of the invoking collection to the array specified by *ar*, which must be a one-dimensional array compatible with the type of the elements in the collection.
public virtual void CopyTo(Array *ar*, int *startIdx*)	Copies the contents of the invoking collection to the array specified by *ar*, beginning at *startIdx*. The array must be a one-dimensional array compatible with the type of the elements in the collection.

TABLE 24-4   Several Commonly Used Methods Defined by **ArrayList**

Method	Description
public virtual void CopyTo(int *srcIdx*, Array *ar*, int *destIdx*, int *count*)	Copies a portion of the invoking collection, beginning at *srcIdx* and running for *count* elements, to the array specified by *ar*, beginning at *destIdx*. *ar* must be a one-dimensional array compatible with the type of the elements in the collection.
public static ArrayList FixedSize(ArrayList *ar*)	Wraps *ar* in a fixed-size **ArrayList** and returns the result.
public virtual ArrayList GetRange(int *idx*, int *count*)	Returns a portion of the invoking **ArrayList**. The range returned begins at *idx* and runs for *count* elements. The returned object refers to the same elements as the invoking object.
public virtual int IndexOf(object *v*)	Returns the index of the first occurrence of *v* in the invoking collection. Returns –1 if *v* is not found.
public virtual void InsertRange(int *startIdx*, ICollection *c*)	Inserts the elements of *c* into the invoking collection, starting at the index specified by *startIdx*.
public virtual int LastIndexOf(object *v*)	Returns the index of the last occurrence of *v* in the invoking collection. Returns –1 if *v* is not found.
public static ArrayList ReadOnly(ArrayList *ar*)	Wraps *ar* in a read-only **ArrayList** and returns the result.
public virtual void RemoveRange(int *idx*, int *count*)	Removes *count* elements from the invoking collection, beginning at *idx*.
public virtual void Reverse( )	Reverses the contents of the invoking collection.
public virtual void Reverse(int *startIdx*, int *count*)	Reverses *count* elements of the invoking collection, beginning at *startIdx*.
public virtual void SetRange(int *startIdx*, ICollection *c*)	Replaces elements within the invoking collection, beginning at *startIdx*, with those specified by *c*.
public virtual void Sort( )	Sorts the collection into ascending order.
public virtual void Sort(IComparer *comp*)	Sorts the collection using the specified comparison object. If *comp* is null, the default comparison for each object is used.
public virtual void Sort(int *startIdx*, int *count*, IComparer *comp*)	Sorts a portion of the collection using the specified comparison object. The sort begins at *startIdx* and runs for *count* elements. If *comp* is null, the default comparison for each object is used.
public static ArrayList Synchronized(ArrayList *list*)	Returns a synchronized version of the invoking **ArrayList**.
public virtual object[ ] ToArray( )	Returns an array that contains copies of the elements of the invoking object.

TABLE 24-4   Several Commonly Used Methods Defined by **ArrayList** *(continued)*

Method	Description
public virtual Array ToArray(Type *type*)	Returns an array that contains copies of the elements of the invoking object. The type of the elements in the array are specified by *type*.
public virtual void TrimToSize( )	Sets **Capacity** to **Count**.

TABLE 24-4   Several Commonly Used Methods Defined by **ArrayList** *(continued)*

In addition to those properties defined by the interfaces that it implements, **ArrayList** adds **Capacity**, shown here:

public virtual int Capacity { get; set; }

Capacity gets or sets the capacity of the invoking **ArrayList**. The capacity is the number of elements that can be held before the **ArrayList** must be enlarged. As mentioned, an **ArrayList** grows automatically, so it is not necessary to set the capacity manually. However, for efficiency reasons, you might want to set the capacity when you know in advance how many elements the list will contain. This prevents the overhead associated with the allocation of more memory.

Conversely, if you want to reduce the size of the array that underlies an **ArrayList**, you can set **Capacity** to a smaller value. However, this value must not be less than **Count**. Recall that **Count** is a property defined by **ICollection** that holds the number of objects currently stored in a collection. Attempting to set **Capacity** to a value less than **Count** causes an **ArgumentOutOfRangeException** to be generated. To obtain an **ArrayList** that is precisely as large as the number of items that it is currently holding, set **Capacity** equal to **Count**. You can also call **TrimToSize( )**.

The following program demonstrates **ArrayList**. It creates an **ArrayList** and then adds characters to it. The list is then displayed. Some of the elements are removed, and the list is displayed again. Next, more elements are added, forcing the capacity of the list to be increased. Finally, the contents of elements are changed.

```
// Demonstrate ArrayList.

using System;
using System.Collections;

class ArrayListDemo {
  static void Main() {
    // Create an array list.
    ArrayList al = new ArrayList();

    Console.WriteLine("Initial number of elements: " +
                      al.Count);

    Console.WriteLine();

    Console.WriteLine("Adding 6 elements");
    // Add elements to the array list
    al.Add('C');
```

```
    al.Add('A');
    al.Add('E');
    al.Add('B');
    al.Add('D');
    al.Add('F');

    Console.WriteLine("Number of elements: " +
                        al.Count);

    // Display the array list using array indexing.
    Console.Write("Current contents: ");
    for(int i=0; i < al.Count; i++)
      Console.Write(al[i] + " ");
    Console.WriteLine("\n");

    Console.WriteLine("Removing 2 elements");
    // Remove elements from the array list.
    al.Remove('F');
    al.Remove('A');

    Console.WriteLine("Number of elements: " +
                        al.Count);

    // Use foreach loop to display the list.
    Console.Write("Contents: ");
    foreach(char c in al)
      Console.Write(c + " ");
    Console.WriteLine("\n");

    Console.WriteLine("Adding 20 more elements");
    // Add enough elements to force al to grow.
    for(int i=0; i < 20; i++)
      al.Add((char)('a' + i));
    Console.WriteLine("Current capacity: " +
                        al.Capacity);
    Console.WriteLine("Number of elements after adding 20: " +
                        al.Count);
    Console.Write("Contents: ");
    foreach(char c in al)
      Console.Write(c + " ");
    Console.WriteLine("\n");

    // Change contents using array indexing.
    Console.WriteLine("Change first three elements");
    al[0] = 'X';
    al[1] = 'Y';
    al[2] = 'Z';
    Console.Write("Contents: ");
    foreach(char c in al)
      Console.Write(c + " ");
    Console.WriteLine();
  }
}
```

The output from this program is shown here:

```
Initial number of elements: 0

Adding 6 elements
Number of elements: 6
Current contents: C A E B D F

Removing 2 elements
Number of elements: 4
Contents: C E B D

Adding 20 more elements
Current capacity: 32
Number of elements after adding 20: 24
Contents: C E B D a b c d e f g h i j k l m n o p q r s t

Change first three elements
Contents: X Y Z D a b c d e f g h i j k l m n o p q r s t
```

Sorting and Searching an ArrayList   An **ArrayList** can be sorted by **Sort( )**. Once sorted, it can be efficiently searched by **BinarySearch( )**. The following program demonstrates these methods:

```csharp
// Sort and search an ArrayList.

using System;
using System.Collections;

class SortSearchDemo {
  static void Main() {
    // Create an array list.
    ArrayList al = new ArrayList();

    // Add elements to the array list.
    al.Add(55);
    al.Add(43);
    al.Add(-4);
    al.Add(88);
    al.Add(3);
    al.Add(19);

    Console.Write("Original contents: ");
    foreach(int i in al)
      Console.Write(i + " ");
    Console.WriteLine("\n");

    // Sort
    al.Sort();

    // Use foreach loop to display the list.
    Console.Write("Contents after sorting: ");
    foreach(int i in al)
      Console.Write(i + " ");
    Console.WriteLine("\n");
```

```
    Console.WriteLine("Index of 43 is " +
                      al.BinarySearch(43));
  }
}
```

The output is shown here:

```
Original contents: 55 43 -4 88 3 19

Contents after sorting: -4 3 19 43 55 88

Index of 43 is 3
```

Although an **ArrayList** can store objects of any type within the same list, when sorting or searching a list, it is necessary for those objects to be comparable. For example, the preceding program would have generated an exception if the list had included a string. (It is possible to create custom comparison methods that would allow the comparison of strings and integers, however. Custom comparators are discussed later in this chapter.)

Obtaining an Array from an ArrayList   When working with **ArrayList**, you will sometimes want to obtain an actual array that contains the contents of the list. You can do this by calling **ToArray( )**. There are several reasons why you might want to convert a collection into an array. Here are two: You may want to obtain faster processing times for certain operations, or you might need to pass an array to a method that is not overloaded to accept a collection. Whatever the reason, converting an **ArrayList** to an array is a trivial matter, as the following program shows:

```
// Convert an ArrayList into an array.

using System;
using System.Collections;

class ArrayListToArray {
  static void Main() {
    ArrayList al = new ArrayList();

    // Add elements to the array list.
    al.Add(1);
    al.Add(2);
    al.Add(3);
    al.Add(4);

    Console.Write("Contents: ");
    foreach(int i in al)
      Console.Write(i + " ");
    Console.WriteLine();

    // Get the array.
    int[] ia = (int[]) al.ToArray(typeof(int));
    int sum = 0;

    // Sum the array.
    for(int i=0; i<ia.Length; i++)
      sum += ia[i];
```

```
      Console.WriteLine("Sum is: " + sum);
   }
}
```

The output from the program is shown here:

```
Contents: 1 2 3 4
Sum is: 10
```

The program begins by creating a collection of integers. Next, **ToArray( )** is called with the type specified as **int**. This causes an array of integers to be created. Since the return type of **ToArray( )** is **Array**, the contents of the array must still be cast to **int[ ]**. (Recall that **Array** is the base type of all C# arrays.) Finally, the values are summed.

Hashtable

Hashtable creates a collection that uses a hash table for storage. As most readers will know, a *hash table* stores information using a mechanism called *hashing*. In hashing, the informational content of a key is used to determine a unique value, called its *hash code*. The hash code is then used as the index at which the data associated with the key is stored in the table. The transformation of the key into its hash code is performed automatically—you never see the hash code itself. The advantage of hashing is that it allows the execution time of lookup, retrieve, and set operations to remain near constant, even for large sets. **Hashtable** implements the **IDictionary**, **ICollection**, **IEnumerable**, **ISerializable**, **IDeserializationCallback**, and **ICloneable** interfaces.

    Hashtable defines many constructors, including these frequently used ones:

    public Hashtable( )
    public Hashtable(IDictionary *c*)
    public Hashtable(int *capacity*)
    public Hashtable(int *capacity*, float *fillRatio*)

The first form constructs a default **Hashtable**. The second form initializes the **Hashtable** by using the elements of *c*. The third form initializes the capacity of the **Hashtable** to *capacity*. The fourth form initializes both the capacity and fill ratio. The fill ratio (also called the *load factor*) must be between 0.1 and 1.0, and it determines how full the hash table can be before it is resized upward. Specifically, when the number of elements is greater than the capacity of the table multiplied by its fill ratio, the table is expanded. For constructors that do not take a fill ratio, 1.0 is used.

    In addition to the methods defined by the interfaces that it implements, **Hashtable** also defines several methods of its own. Some commonly used ones are shown in Table 24-5. To determine if a **Hashtable** contains a key, call **ContainsKey( )**. To see if a specific value is stored, call **ContainsValue( )**. To enumerate the contents of a **Hashtable**, obtain an **IDictionaryEnumerator** by calling **GetEnumerator( )**. Recall that **IDictionaryEnumerator** is used to enumerate the contents of a collection that stores key/value pairs.

    The public properties available in **Hashtable** are those defined by the interfaces that it implements. Two especially important ones are **Keys** and **Values** because they let you obtain a collection of a **Hashtable**'s keys or values. They are specified by **IDictionary** and are shown here:

    public virtual ICollection Keys { get; }
    public virtual ICollection Values { get; }

Method	Description
public virtual bool ContainsKey(object *k*)	Returns true if *k* is a key in the invoking **Hashtable**. Returns false otherwise.
public virtual bool ContainsValue(object *v*)	Returns true if *v* is a value in the invoking **Hashtable**. Returns false otherwise.
public virtual IDictionaryEnumerator GetEnumerator( )	Returns an **IDictionaryEnumerator** for the invoking **Hashtable**.
public static Hashtable Synchronized(Hashtable *ht*)	Returns a synchronized version of the **Hashtable** passed in *ht*.

TABLE 24-5   Several Commonly Used Methods Defined by **Hashtable**

Because **Hashtable** does not maintain an ordered collection, there is no specific order to the collection of keys or values obtained. **Hashtable** also has two protected properties: **EqualityComparer** and **KeyComparer**. Two other properties called **hcp** and **comparer** are flagged as obsolete.

Hashtable stores key/value pairs in the form of a **DictionaryEntry** structure, but most of the time, you won't be aware of it directly because the properties and methods work with keys and values individually. For example, when you add an element to a **Hashtable**, you call **Add( )**, which takes two arguments: the key and the value.

It is important to note that **Hashtable** does not guarantee the order of its elements. This is because the process of hashing does not usually lend itself to the creation of sorted tables.

Here is an example that demonstrates **Hashtable**:

```
// Demonstrate Hashtable.

using System;
using System.Collections;

class HashtableDemo {
  static void Main() {
    // Create a hash table.
    Hashtable ht = new Hashtable();

    // Add elements to the table.
    ht.Add("house", "Dwelling");
    ht.Add("car", "Means of transport");
    ht.Add("book", "Collection of printed words");
    ht.Add("apple", "Edible fruit");

    // Can also add by using the indexer.
    ht["tractor"] = "Farm implement";

    // Get a collection of the keys.
    ICollection c = ht.Keys;

    // Use the keys to obtain the values.
    foreach(string str in c)
      Console.WriteLine(str + ": " + ht[str]);
  }
}
```

The output from this program is shown here:

```
book: Collection of printed words
tractor: Farm implement
apple: Edible fruit
house: Dwelling
car: Means of transport
```

As the output shows, the key/value pairs are not stored in sorted order. Notice how the contents of the hash table **ht** were obtained and displayed. First, a collection of the keys was retrieved by the **Keys** property. Each key was then used to index **ht**, yielding the value associated with each key. Remember, the indexer defined by **IDictionary** and implemented by **Hashtable** uses a key as the index.

SortedList

SortedList creates a collection that stores key/value pairs in sorted order, based on the value of the keys. **SortedList** implements the **IDictionary**, **ICollection**, **IEnumerable**, and **ICloneable** interfaces.

SortedList has several constructors, including those shown here:

public SortedList( )
public SortedList(IDictionary *c*)
public SortedList(int *capacity*)
public SortedList(IComparer *comp*)

The first constructor builds an empty collection with an initial capacity of zero. The second constructor builds a **SortedList** that is initialized with the elements of *c* and has an initial capacity equal to the number of elements. The third constructor builds an empty **SortedList** that has the initial capacity specified by *capacity*. The capacity is the size of the underlying array that is used to store the elements. The fourth form lets you specify a comparison method that will be used to compare the object contained in the list. This form creates an empty collection with an initial capacity of zero.

The capacity of a **SortedList** grows automatically as needed when elements are added to the list. When the current capacity is exceeded, the capacity is increased. The advantage of specifying a capacity when creating a **SortedList** is that you can prevent or minimize the overhead associated with resizing the collection. Of course, it makes sense to specify an initial capacity only if you have some idea of how many elements will be stored.

In addition to the methods defined by the interfaces that it implements, **SortedList** also defines several methods of its own. Some of the most commonly used ones are shown in Table 24-6. To determine if a **SortedList** contains a key, call **ContainsKey( )**. To see if a specific value is stored, call **ContainsValue( )**. To enumerate the contents of a **SortedList**, obtain an **IDictionaryEnumerator** by calling **GetEnumerator( )**. Recall that **IDictionaryEnumerator** is used to enumerate the contents of a collection that stores key/value pairs. You can obtain a synchronized wrapper around a **SortedList** by calling **Synchronized( )**.

There are various ways to set or obtain a value or key. To obtain the value associated with a specific index, call **GetByIndex( )**. To set a value given its index, call **SetByIndex( )**. You can retrieve the key associated with a specific index by calling **GetKey( )**. To obtain a list of all the keys, use **GetKeyList( )**. To get a list of all the values, use **GetValueList( )**. You can obtain the index of a key by calling **IndexOfKey( )** and the index of a value by calling **IndexOfValue( )**. Of course, **SortedList** also supports the indexer defined by **IDictionary** that lets you set or obtain a value given its key.

Method	Description
public virtual bool ContainsKey(object *k*)	Returns true if *k* is a key in the invoking **SortedList**. Returns false otherwise.
public virtual bool ContainsValue(object *v*)	Returns true if *v* is a value in the invoking **SortedList**. Returns false otherwise.
public virtual object GetByIndex(int *idx*)	Returns the value at the index specified by *idx*.
public virtual IDictionaryEnumerator GetEnumerator( )	Returns an **IDictionaryEnumerator** for the invoking **SortedList**.
public virtual object GetKey(int *idx*)	Returns the value of the key at the index specified by *idx*.
public virtual IList GetKeyList( )	Returns an **IList** collection of the keys in the invoking **SortedList**.
public virtual IList GetValueList( )	Returns an **IList** collection of the values in the invoking **SortedList**.
public virtual int IndexOfKey(object *k*)	Returns the index of the key specified by *k*. Returns –1 if the key is not in the list.
public virtual int IndexOfValue(object *v*)	Returns the index of the first occurrence of the value specified by *v*. Returns –1 if the value is not in the list.
public virtual void SetByIndex(int *idx*, object *v*)	Sets the value at the index specified by *idx* to the value passed in *v*.
public static SortedList Synchronized(SortedList *sl*)	Returns a synchronized version of the **SortedList** passed in *sl*.
public virtual void TrimToSize( )	Sets **Capacity** to **Count**.

TABLE 24-6   Several Commonly Used Methods Defined by **SortedList**

The public properties available in **SortedList** are those defined by the interfaces that it implements. As is the case with **Hashtable**, two especially important properties are **Keys** and **Values** because they let you obtain a read-only collection of a **SortedList**'s keys or values. They are specified by **IDictionary** and are shown here:

public virtual ICollection Keys { get; }
public virtual ICollection Values { get; }

The order of the keys and values reflects that of the **SortedList**.

Like **Hashtable**, a **SortedList** stores key/value pairs in the form of a **DictionaryEntry** structure, but you will usually access the keys and values individually using the methods and properties defined by **SortedList**.

The following program demonstrates **SortedList**. It reworks and expands the **Hashtable** demonstration program from the previous section, substituting **SortedList**. When you examine the output, you will see that the **SortedList** version is sorted by key.

```
// Demonstrate a SortedList.

using System;
using System.Collections;
```

```
class SLDemo {
  static void Main() {
    // Create a sorted SortedList.
    SortedList sl = new SortedList();

    // Add elements to the table.
    sl.Add("house", "Dwelling");
    sl.Add("car", "Means of transport");
    sl.Add("book", "Collection of printed words");
    sl.Add("apple", "Edible fruit");

    // Can also add by using the indexer.
    sl["tractor"] = "Farm implement";

    // Get a collection of the keys.
    ICollection c = sl.Keys;

    // Use the keys to obtain the values.
    Console.WriteLine("Contents of list via indexer.");
    foreach(string str in c)
      Console.WriteLine(str + ": " + sl[str]);

    Console.WriteLine();

    // Display list using integer indexes.
    Console.WriteLine("Contents by integer indexes.");
    for(int i=0; i < sl.Count; i++)
      Console.WriteLine(sl.GetByIndex(i));

    Console.WriteLine();

    // Show integer indexes of entries.
    Console.WriteLine("Integer indexes of entries.");
    foreach(string str in c)
      Console.WriteLine(str + ": " + sl.IndexOfKey(str));
  }
}
```

The output is shown here:

```
Contents of list via indexer.
apple: Edible fruit
book: Collection of printed words
car: Means of transport
house: Dwelling
tractor: Farm implement

Contents by integer indexes.
Edible fruit
Collection of printed words
Means of transport
Dwelling
Farm implement
```

```
Integer indexes of entries.
apple: 0
book: 1
car: 2
house: 3
tractor: 4
```

Stack

As most readers know, a stack is a first-in, last-out list. To visualize a stack, imagine a stack of plates on a table. The first plate put down is the last one to be picked up. The stack is one of the most important data structures in computing. It is frequently used in system software, compilers, and AI-based backtracking routines, to name just a few examples.

The collection class that supports a stack is called **Stack**. It implements the **ICollection**, **IEnumerable**, and **ICloneable** interfaces. **Stack** is a dynamic collection that grows as needed to accommodate the elements it must store. Each time the capacity must be increased, the capacity is doubled.

Stack defines the following constructors:

public Stack( )
public Stack(int *capacity*)
public Stack(ICollection *c*)

The first form creates an empty stack. The second form creates an empty stack with the initial capacity specified by *capacity*. The third form creates a stack that contains the elements of the collection specified by *c* and an initial capacity equal to the number of elements.

In addition to the methods defined by the interfaces that it implements, **Stack** defines the methods shown in Table 24-7. In general, here is how you use **Stack**. To put an object on the top of the stack, call **Push( )**. To remove and return the top element, call **Pop( )**. You can use **Peek( )** to return, but not remove, the top object. An **InvalidOperationException** is thrown if you call **Pop( )** or **Peek( )** when the invoking stack is empty.

Method	Description
public virtual void Clear( )	Sets **Count** to zero, which effectively clears the stack.
public virtual bool Contains(object *v*)	Returns true if *v* is on the invoking stack. If *v* is not found, false is returned.
public virtual object Peek( )	Returns the element on the top of the stack, but does not remove it.
public virtual object Pop( )	Returns the element on the top of the stack, removing it in the process.
public virtual void Push(object *v*)	Pushes *v* onto the stack.
public static Stack Synchronized(Stack *stk*)	Returns a synchronized version of the **Stack** passed in *stk*.
public virtual object[ ] ToArray( )	Returns an array that contains copies of the elements of the invoking stack.

TABLE 24-7   The Methods Defined by **Stack**

PART II

Here is an example that creates a stack, pushes several integers onto it, and then pops them off again:

```
// Demonstrate the Stack class.

using System;
using System.Collections;

class StackDemo {
  static void ShowPush(Stack st, int a) {
    st.Push(a);
    Console.WriteLine("Push(" + a + ")");

    Console.Write("stack: ");
    foreach(int i in st)
      Console.Write(i + " ");

    Console.WriteLine();
  }

  static void ShowPop(Stack st) {
    Console.Write("Pop -> ");
    int a = (int) st.Pop();
    Console.WriteLine(a);

    Console.Write("stack: ");
    foreach(int i in st)
      Console.Write(i + " ");

    Console.WriteLine();
  }

  static void Main() {
    Stack st = new Stack();

    foreach(int i in st)
      Console.Write(i + " ");

    Console.WriteLine();

    ShowPush(st, 22);
    ShowPush(st, 65);
    ShowPush(st, 91);
    ShowPop(st);
    ShowPop(st);
    ShowPop(st);

    try {
      ShowPop(st);
    } catch (InvalidOperationException) {
      Console.WriteLine("Stack empty.");
```

```
        }
      }
    }
```

Here's the output produced by the program. Notice how the exception handler for **InvalidOperationException** manages a stack underflow.

```
Push(22)
stack: 22
Push(65)
stack: 65 22
Push(91)
stack: 91 65 22
Pop -> 91
stack: 65 22
Pop -> 65
stack: 22
Pop -> 22
stack:
Pop -> Stack empty.
```

Queue

Another familiar data structure is the queue, which is a first-in, first-out list. That is, the first item put in a queue is the first item retrieved. Queues are common in real life. For example, lines at a bank or fast-food restaurant are queues. In programming, queues are used to hold such things as the currently executing processes in the system, a list of pending database transactions, or data packets received over the Internet. They are also often used in simulations.

The collection class that supports a queue is called **Queue**. It implements the **ICollection**, **IEnumerable**, and **ICloneable** interfaces. **Queue** is a dynamic collection that grows as needed to accommodate the elements it must store. When more room is needed, the size of the queue is increased by a growth factor, which, by default, is 2.0.

Queue defines the following constructors:

public Queue( )
public Queue (int *capacity*)
public Queue (int *capacity*, float *growFact*)
public Queue (ICollection *c*)

The first form creates an empty queue with an initial capacity of 32 and uses the default growth factor of 2.0. The second form creates an empty queue with the initial capacity specified by *capacity* and a growth factor of 2.0. The third form allows you to specify a growth factor in *growFact* (which must be between 1.0 and 10.0). The fourth form creates a queue that contains the elements of the collection specified by *c*, and an initial capacity equal to the number of elements. In this form, the default growth factor of 2.0 is used.

In addition to the methods defined by the interfaces that it implements, **Queue** defines the methods shown in Table 24-8. In general, here is how you use **Queue**. To put an object in the queue, call **Enqueue( )**. To remove and return the object at the front of the queue, call **Dequeue( )**. You can use **Peek( )** to return, but not remove, the next object. An **InvalidOperationException** is thrown if you call **Dequeue( )** or **Peek( )** when the invoking queue is empty.

Method	Description
public virtual void Clear( )	Sets **Count** to zero, which effectively clears the queue.
public virtual bool Contains(object *v*)	Returns true if *v* is in the invoking queue. If *v* is not found, false is returned.
public virtual object Dequeue( )	Returns the object at the front of the invoking queue. The object is removed in the process.
public virtual void Enqueue(object *v*)	Adds *v* to the end of the queue.
public virtual object Peek( )	Returns the object at the front of the invoking queue, but does not remove it.
public static Queue Synchronized(Queue *q*)	Returns a synchronized version of *q*.
public virtual object[ ] ToArray( )	Returns an array that contains copies of the elements of the invoking queue.
public virtual void TrimToSize( )	Sets **Capacity** to **Count**.

TABLE 24-8   The Methods Defined by **Queue**

Here is an example that demonstrates **Queue**:

```
// Demonstrate the Queue class.

using System;
using System.Collections;

class QueueDemo {
  static void ShowEnq(Queue q, int a) {
    q.Enqueue(a);
    Console.WriteLine("Enqueue(" + a + ")");

    Console.Write("queue: ");
    foreach(int i in q)
      Console.Write(i + " ");

    Console.WriteLine();
  }

  static void ShowDeq(Queue q) {
    Console.Write("Dequeue -> ");
    int a = (int) q.Dequeue();
    Console.WriteLine(a);

    Console.Write("queue: ");
    foreach(int i in q)
      Console.Write(i + " ");

    Console.WriteLine();
  }

  static void Main() {
```

```
    Queue q = new Queue();

    foreach(int i in q)
      Console.Write(i + " ");

    Console.WriteLine();

    ShowEnq(q, 22);
    ShowEnq(q, 65);
    ShowEnq(q, 91);
    ShowDeq(q);
    ShowDeq(q);
    ShowDeq(q);

    try {
      ShowDeq(q);
    } catch (InvalidOperationException) {
      Console.WriteLine("Queue empty.");
    }
  }
}
```

The output is shown here:

```
Enqueue(22)
queue: 22
Enqueue(65)
queue: 22 65
Enqueue(91)
queue: 22 65 91
Dequeue -> 22
queue: 65 91
Dequeue -> 65
queue: 91
Dequeue -> 91
queue:
Dequeue -> Queue empty.
```

Storing Bits with BitArray

The **BitArray** class supports a collection of bits. Because it stores bits rather than objects, **BitArray** has capabilities different from those of the other collections. However, it still supports the basic collection underpinning by implementing **ICollection** and **IEnumerable**. It also implements **ICloneable**.

BitArray defines several constructors. You can construct a **BitArray** from an array of Boolean values using this constructor:

public BitArray(bool[ ] *bits*)

In this case, each element of *bits* becomes a bit in the collection. Thus, each bit in the collection corresponds to an element of *bits*. Furthermore, the ordering of the elements of *bits* and the bits in the collection are the same.

You can create a **BitArray** from an array of bytes using this constructor:

public BitArray(byte[ ] *bits*)

Here, the bit pattern in *bits* becomes the bits in the collection, with *bits*[0] specifying the first 8 bits, *bits*[1] specifying the second 8 bits, and so on. In similar fashion, you can construct a **BitArray** from an array of **int**s using this constructor:

public BitArray(int[ ] *bits*)

In this case, *bits*[0] specifies the first 32 bits, *bits*[1] specifies the second 32 bits, and so on.
    You can create a **BitArray** of a specific size using this constructor:

public BitArray(int *size*)

Here, *size* specifies the number of bits. The bits in the collection are initialized to **false**. To specify a size and initial value of the bits, use the following constructor:

public BitArray(int *size*, bool *v*)

In this case, all bits in the collection will be set to the value passed in *v*.
    Finally, you can create a new **BitArray** from an existing one by using this constructor:

public BitArray(BitArray *bits*)

The new object will contain the same collection of bits as *bits*, but the two collections will be otherwise separate.
    BitArrays can be indexed. Each index specifies an individual bit, with an index of zero indicating the low-order bit.
    In addition to the methods specified by the interfaces that it implements, **BitArray** defines the methods shown in Table 24-9. Notice that **BitArray** does not supply a **Synchronized( )** method. Thus, a synchronized wrapper is not available, and the **IsSynchronized** property is always false. However, you can control access to a **BitArray** by synchronizing on the object provided by **SyncRoot**.

Method	Description
public BitArray And(BitArray *ba*)	ANDs the bits of the invoking object with those specified by *ba* and returns a **BitArray** that contains the result.
public bool Get(int *idx*)	Returns the value of the bit at the index specified by *idx*.
public BitArray Not( )	Performs a bitwise, logical NOT on the invoking collection and returns a **BitArray** that contains the result.
public BitArray Or(BitArray *ba*)	ORs the bits of the invoking object with those specified by *ba* and returns a **BitArray** that contains the result.
public void Set(int *idx*, bool *v*)	Sets the bit at the index specified by *idx* to *v*.
public void SetAll(bool *v*)	Sets all bits to *v*.
public BitArray Xor(BitArray *ba*)	XORs the bits of the invoking object with those specified by *ba* and returns a **BitArray** that contains the result.

TABLE 24-9   The Methods Defined by **BitArray**

To the properties specified by the interfaces that it implements, **BitArray** adds **Length**, which is shown here:

public int Length { get; set; }

Length sets or obtains the number of bits in the collection. Thus, **Length** gives the same value as does the standard **Count** property, which is defined for all collections. However, **Count** is read-only, but **Length** is not. Thus, **Length** can be used to change the size of a **BitArray**. If you shorten a **BitArray**, bits are truncated from the high-order end. If you lengthen a **BitArray**, false bits are added to the high-order end.

BitArray defines the following indexer:

public bool this[int *idx*] { get; set; }

You can use this indexer to get or set the value of an element.

Here is an example that demonstrates **BitArray**:

```
// Demonstrate BitArray.

using System;
using System.Collections;

class BADemo {
  public static void ShowBits(string rem,
                       BitArray bits) {
    Console.WriteLine(rem);
    for(int i=0; i < bits.Count; i++)
      Console.Write("{0, -6} ", bits[i]);
    Console.WriteLine("\n");
  }

  static void Main() {
    BitArray ba = new BitArray(8);
    byte[] b = { 67 };
    BitArray ba2 = new BitArray(b);

    ShowBits("Original contents of ba:", ba);

    ba = ba.Not();

    ShowBits("Contents of ba after Not:", ba);

    ShowBits("Contents of ba2:", ba2);

    BitArray ba3 = ba.Xor(ba2);

    ShowBits("Result of ba XOR ba2:", ba3);
  }
}
```

The output is shown here:

```
Original contents of ba:
False  False  False  False  False  False  False  False
```

```
Contents of ba after Not:
True    True    True    True    True    True    True    True

Contents of ba2:
True    True    False   False   False   False   True    False

Result of ba XOR ba2:
False   False   True    True    True    True    False   True
```

The Specialized Collections

The .NET Framework provides some specialized collections that are optimized to work on a specific type of data or in a specific way. These non-generic collection classes are defined inside the **System.Collections.Specialized** namespace. They are synopsized in the following table:

Specialized Collection	Description
CollectionsUtil	Contains factory methods that create collections.
HybridDictionary	A collection that uses a **ListDictionary** to store key/value pairs when there are few elements in the collection. When the collection grows beyond a certain size, a **Hashtable** is automatically used to store the elements.
ListDictionary	A collection that stores key/value pairs in a linked list. It is recommended only for small collections.
NameValueCollection	A sorted collection of key/value pairs in which both the key and value are of type **string**.
OrderedDictionary	A collection of key/value pairs that can be indexed.
StringCollection	A collection optimized for storing strings.
StringDictionary	A hash table of key/value pairs in which both the key and the value are of type **string**.

System.Collections also defines three abstract base classes, **CollectionBase**, **ReadOnlyCollectionBase**, and **DictionaryBase**, which can be inherited and used as a starting point for developing custom specialized collections.

The Generic Collections

The addition of generics greatly expanded the Collections API, essentially doubling the amount of collection classes and interfaces. The generic collections are declared in the **System.Collections.Generic** namespace. In many cases, the generic collection classes are simply generic equivalents of the non-generic classes discussed earlier. However, the correspondence is not one-to-one. For example, there is a generic collection called **LinkedList** that implements a doubly linked list, but no non-generic equivalent. In some cases, parallel functionality exists between the generic and non-generic classes, but the names differ. For example, the generic version of **ArrayList** is called **List**, and the generic version of **HashTable**

is called **Dictionary**. Also, the specific contents of the various interfaces and classes contain minor reorganizations, with some functionality shifting from one interface to another, for example. However, overall, if you understand the non-generic collections, then you can easily use the generic collections.

In general, the generic collections work in the same way as the non-generic collections with the exception that a generic collection is type-safe. Thus, a generic collection can store only items that are compatible with its type argument. Therefore, if you want a collection that is capable of storing unrelated, mixed types, you should use one of the non-generic classes. However, for all cases in which a collection is storing only one type of object, then a generic collection is now your best choice.

The generic collections are defined by a set of interfaces and the classes that implement those interfaces. Each is described by the following sections.

The Generic Interfaces

System.Collections.Generic defines a number of generic interfaces, all of which parallel their corresponding non-generic counterparts. The generic interfaces are summarized in Table 24-10.

The ICollection<T> Interface

The **ICollection<T>** interface defines those features that all generic collections have in common. It inherits the **IEnumerable** and **IEnumerable<T>** interfaces. **ICollection<T>** is the generic version of the non-generic **ICollection** interface. However, there are some differences between the two.

ICollection<T> defines the following properties:

int Count { get; }

bool IsReadOnly { get; }

Count contains the number of items currently held in the collection. **IsReadOnly** is true if the collection is read-only. It is false if the collection is read/write.

Interface	Description
ICollection<T>	Defines the foundational features for the generic collections.
IComparer<T>	Defines the generic **Compare( )** method that performs a comparison on objects stored in a collection.
IDictionary<TK, TV>	Defines a generic collection that consists of key/value pairs.
IEnumerable<T>	Defines the generic **GetEnumerator( )** method, which supplies the enumerator for a collection class.
IEnumerator<T>	Provides members that enable the contents of a collection to be obtained one at a time.
IEqualityComparer<T>	Compares two objects for equality.
IList<T>	Defines a generic collection that can be accessed via an indexer.

TABLE 24-10 The Generic Collection Interfaces

ICollection<T> defines the following methods. Notice it defines a few more methods than does its non-generic counterpart.

Method	Description
void Add(T *obj*)	Adds *obj* to the invoking collection. Throws a **NotSupportedException** if the collection is read-only.
void Clear( )	Deletes all elements from the invoking collection and sets **Count** to zero.
bool Contains(T *obj*)	Returns true if the invoking collection contains the object passed in *obj* and false otherwise.
void CopyTo(T[ ] *target*, int *startIdx*)	Copies the contents of the invoking collection to the array specified by *target*, beginning at the index specified by *startIdx*.
bool Remove(T *obj*)	Removes the first occurrence of *obj* from the invoking collection. Returns true if *obj* was removed and false if it was not found in the invoking collection.

Several of these methods will throw **NotSupportedException** if the collection is read-only. Because **ICollection<T>** inherits **IEnumerable** and **IEnumerable<T>**, it also includes both the generic and non-generic forms of the method **GetEnumerator( )**.

Because **ICollection<T>** inherits **IEnumerable<T>**, it supports the extension methods defined by **Enumerable**. Although the extension methods were designed mostly for LINQ, they are available for other uses, including collections.

The IList<T> Interface

The **IList<T>** interface defines the behavior of a generic collection that allows elements to be accessed via a zero-based index. It inherits **IEnumerable**, **IEnumerable<T>**, and **ICollection<T>** and is the generic version of the non-generic **IList** interface. **IList<T>** defines the methods shown in Table 24-11. Two of these methods imply the modification of a collection. If the collection is read-only or of fixed size, then the **Insert( )** and **RemoveAt( )** methods will throw a **NotSupportedException**.

IList<T> defines the following indexer:

T this[int *idx*] { get; set; }

This indexer sets or gets the value of the element at the index specified by *idx*.

Method	Description
int IndexOf(T *obj*)	Returns the index of the first occurrence of *obj* if *obj* is contained within the invoking collection. If *obj* is not found, −1 is returned.
void Insert(int *idx*, T *obj*)	Inserts *obj* at the index specified by *idx*.
void RemoveAt(int *idx*)	Removes the object at the index specified by *idx* from the invoking collection.

TABLE 24-11   The Methods Defined by **IList<T>**

The IDictionary<TK, TV> Interface

The **IDictionary<TK, TV>** interface defines the behavior of a generic collection that maps unique keys to values. That is, it defines a collection that stores key/value pairs. **IDictionary<TK, TV>** inherits **IEnumerable**, **IEnumerable<KeyValuePair<TK, TV>>**, and **ICollection< KeyValuePair<TK, TV>>** and is the generic version of the non-generic **IDictionary**. The methods declared by **IDictionary<TK, TV>** are summarized in Table 24-12. All throw an **ArgumentNullException** if an attempt is made to specify a null key.

IDictionary<TK, TV> defines the following properties:

Property	Description
ICollection Keys<TK> { get; }	Obtains a collection of the keys.
ICollection Values<TV> { get; }	Obtains a collection of the values.

Notice that the keys and values contained within the collection are available as separate lists through the **Keys** and **Values** properties.

IDictionary<TK, TV> defines the following indexer:

TV this[TK *key*] { get; set; }

You can use this indexer to get or set the value of an element. You can also use it to add a new element to the collection. Notice that the "index" is not actually an index, but rather the key of the item.

IEnumerable<T> and IEnumerator<T>

IEnumerable<T> and **IEnumerator<T>** are the generic equivalents of the non-generic **IEnumerable** and **IEnumerator** interfaces described earlier. They declare the same methods and properties, and work in the same way. Of course, the generic versions operate on data of the type specified by the type argument.

IEnumerable<T> declares the **GetEnumerator( )** method as shown here:

IEnumerator<T> GetEnumerator( )

It returns an enumerator of type **T** for the collection. Thus, it returns a type-safe enumerator.

Method	Description
void Add(TK *k*, TV *v*)	Adds the key/value pair specified by *k* and *v* to the invoking collection. An **ArgumentException** is thrown if *k* is already stored in the collection.
bool ContainsKey(TK *k*)	Returns true if the invoking collection contains *k* as a key. Otherwise, returns false.
bool Remove(TK *k*)	Removes the entry whose key equals *k*.
bool TryGetValue(TK *k*, out TV *v*)	Attempts to retrieve the value associated with *k*, putting it into *v*. Returns true if successful and false otherwise. If *k* is not found, *v* is given its default value.

TABLE 24-12   The Methods Defined by **IDictionary<TK, TV>**

IEnumerator<T> has the same two methods as does the non-generic **IEnumerator**: **MoveNext( )** and **Reset( )**. It also declares a generic version of the **Current** property, as shown here:

T Current { get; }

It returns a **T** reference to the next object. Thus, the generic version of **Current** is type-safe.

There is one other difference between **IEnumerator** and **IEnumerator<T>**: **IEnumerator<T>** inherits the **IDisposable** interface, but **IEnumerator** does not. **IDisposable** defines the **Dispose( )** method, which is used to free unmanaged resources.

NOTE *IEnumerable<T> also implements the non-generic IEnumerable interface. Thus, it supports the non-generic version of GetEnumerator( ). IEnumerator<T> also implements the non-generic IEnumerator interface, thus supporting the non-generic versions of Current.*

IComparer<T>
The **IComparer<T>** interface is the generic version of **IComparer** described earlier. The main difference between the two is that **IComparer<T>** is type-safe, declaring the generic version of **Compare( )** shown here:

int Compare(T *obj1*, T *obj2*)

This method compares *obj1* with *obj2* and returns greater than zero if *obj1* is greater than *obj2*, zero if the two objects are the same, and less than zero if *obj1* is less that *obj2*.

IEqualityComparer<T>
The **IEqualityComparer<T>** interface is the equivalent of its non-generic relative **IEqualityComparer**. It defines these two methods:

bool Equals(T *obj1*, T *obj2*)

int GetHashCode(T *obj*)

Equals( ) must return true if **obj1** and **obj2** are equal. **GetHashCode( )** must return the hash code for *obj*.

The KeyValuePair<TK, TV> Structure
System.Collections.Generic defines a structure called **KeyValuePair<TK, TV>**, which is used to store a key and its value. It is used by the generic collection classes that store key/ value pairs, such as **Dictionary<TK, TV>**. This structure defines the following two properties:

public TK Key { get; };
public TV Value { get; };

These properties hold the key or value associated with an entry. You can construct a **KeyValuePair<TK, TV>** object by using the following constructor:

public KeyValuePair(TK *k*, TV *v*)

Here, *k* is the key and *v* is the value.

The Generic Collection Classes

As mentioned at the start of this section, the generic collection classes largely parallel their non-generic relatives, although in some cases the names have been changed. Also, some differences in organization and functionality exist. The generic collections are defined in **System.Collections.Generic**. The ones described in this chapter are shown in Table 24-13. These classes form the core of the generic collections.

> **NOTE** *System.Collections.Generic also includes the following classes: SynchronizedCollection<T> is a synchronized collection based on IList<T>. SynchronizedReadOnlyCollection<T> is a read-only synchronized collection based on IList<T>. SynchronizedKeyCollection<K, V> is an abstract class used as a base class by System.ServiceModel.UriSchemeKeyedCollection. KeyedByTypeCollection<T> is a collection that uses types as keys.*

The List<T> Collection

The **List<T>** class implements a generic dynamic array and is conceptually similar to the non-generic **ArrayList** class. **List<T>** implements the **ICollection**, **ICollection<T>**, **IList**, **IList<T>**, **IEnumerable**, and **IEnumerable<T>** interfaces. **List<T>** has the constructors shown here:

```
public List( )
public List(IEnumerable<T> c)
public List(int capacity)
```

The first constructor builds an empty **List** with a default initial capacity. The second constructor builds a **List** that is initialized with the elements of the collection specified by *c* and with an initial capacity at least equal to the number of elements. The third constructor builds an array list that has the specified initial *capacity*. The capacity is the size of the underlying array that is used to store the elements. The capacity grows automatically as elements are added to a **List<T>**. Each time the list must be enlarged, its capacity is increased.

Class	Description
Dictionary<TK, TV>	Stores key/value pairs. Provides functionality similar to that found in the non-generic **Hashtable** class.
HashSet<T>	Stores a set of unique values using a hash table.
LinkedList<T>	Stores elements in a doubly linked list.
List<T>	A dynamic array. Provides functionality similar to that found in the non-generic **ArrayList** class.
Queue<T>	A first-in, first-out list. Provides functionality similar to that found in the non-generic **Queue** class.
SortedDictionary<TK, TV>	A sorted list of key/value pairs.
SortedList<TK, TV>	A sorted list of key/value pairs. Provides functionality similar to that found in the non-generic **SortedList** class.
Stack<T>	A first-in, last-out list. Provides functionality similar to that found in the non-generic **Stack** class.

TABLE 24-13   The Core Generic Collection Classes

In addition to the methods defined by the interfaces that it implements, **List<T>** defines several methods of its own. A sampling is shown in Table 24-14.

Method	Description
public void AddRange(IEnumerable<T> c)	Adds the elements in c to the end of the invoking list.
public virtual int BinarySearch(T v)	Searches the invoking collection for the value passed in v. The index of the matching element is returned. If the value is not found, a negative value is returned. The invoking list must be sorted.
public int BinarySearch(T v, IComparer<T> comp)	Searches the invoking collection for the value passed in v using the comparison object specified by comp. The index of the matching element is returned. If the value is not found, a negative value is returned. The invoking list must be sorted.
public int BinarySearch(int startIdx, int count, T v, IComparer<T> comp)	Searches the invoking collection for the value passed in v using the comparison object specified by comp. The search begins at startIdx and runs for count elements. The index of the matching element is returned. If the value is not found, a negative value is returned. The invoking list must be sorted.
public List<T> GetRange(int idx, int count)	Returns a portion of the invoking list. The range returned begins at idx and runs for count elements. The returned object refers to the same elements as the invoking object.
public int IndexOf(T v)	Returns the index of the first occurrence of v in the invoking collection. Returns −1 if v is not found.
public void InsertRange(int startIdx, IEnumerable<T> c)	Inserts the elements of c into the invoking collection, starting at the index specified by startIdx.
public int LastIndexOf(T v)	Returns the index of the last occurrence of v in the invoking collection. Returns −1 if v is not found.
public void RemoveRange(int idx, int count)	Removes count elements from the invoking collection, beginning at idx.
public void Reverse( )	Reverses the contents of the invoking collection.
public void Reverse(int startIdx, int count)	Reverses count elements of the invoking collection, beginning at startIdx.
public void Sort( )	Sorts the collection into ascending order.
public void Sort(IComparer<T> comp)	Sorts the collection using the specified comparison object. If comp is null, the default comparer for each object is used.
public void Sort(Comparison<T> comp)	Sorts the collection using the specified comparison delegate.

TABLE 24-14 A Sampling of Methods Defined by **List<T>**

Method	Description

public void
    Sort(int *startIdx*, int *count*,
        IComparer<T> *comp*)
	Sorts a portion of the collection using the specified comparison object. The sort begins at *startIdx* and runs for *count* elements. If *comp* is null, the default comparer for each object is used.

public T[ ] ToArray( )	Returns an array that contains copies of the elements of the invoking object.
public void TrimExcess( )	Reduces the capacity of the invoking list so that it is no more than 10 percent greater than the number of elements that it currently holds.

TABLE 24-14   A Sampling of Methods Defined by **List<T>** *(continued)*

PART II

In addition to the properties defined by the interfaces that it implements, **List<T>** adds **Capacity**, shown here:

public int Capacity { get; set; }

Capacity gets or sets the capacity of the invoking list. The capacity is the number of elements that can be held before the list must be enlarged. Because a list grows automatically, it is not necessary to set the capacity manually. However, for efficiency reasons, you might want to set the capacity when you know in advance how many elements the list will contain. This prevents the overhead associated with the allocation of more memory.

The following indexer, defined by **IList<T>**, is implemented by **List<T>**, as shown here:

public T this[int *idx*] { get; set; }

It sets or gets the value of the element at the index specified by *idx*.

Here is a program the demonstrates **List<T>**. It reworks the first **ArrayList** program shown earlier in this chapter. The only changes necessary are to substitute the name **List** for **ArrayList** and to use the generic type parameters.

```
// Demonstrate List<T>.

using System;
using System.Collections.Generic;

class GenListDemo {
  static void Main() {
    // Create a list.
    List<char> lst = new List<char>();

    Console.WriteLine("Initial number of elements: " +
                      lst.Count);

    Console.WriteLine();

    Console.WriteLine("Adding 6 elements");
    // Add elements to the list.
    lst.Add('C');
    lst.Add('A');
```

```
    lst.Add('E');
    lst.Add('B');
    lst.Add('D');
    lst.Add('F');

    Console.WriteLine("Number of elements: " +
                      lst.Count);

    // Display the list using array indexing.
    Console.Write("Current contents: ");
    for(int i=0; i < lst.Count; i++)
      Console.Write(lst[i] + " ");
    Console.WriteLine("\n");

    Console.WriteLine("Removing 2 elements");
    // Remove elements from the list.
    lst.Remove('F');
    lst.Remove('A');

    Console.WriteLine("Number of elements: " +
                      lst.Count);

    // Use foreach loop to display the list.
    Console.Write("Contents: ");
    foreach(char c in lst)
      Console.Write(c + " ");
    Console.WriteLine("\n");

    Console.WriteLine("Adding 20 more elements");
    // Add enough elements to force lst to grow.
    for(int i=0; i < 20; i++)
      lst.Add((char)('a' + i));
    Console.WriteLine("Current capacity: " +
                      lst.Capacity);
    Console.WriteLine("Number of elements after adding 20: " +
                      lst.Count);
    Console.Write("Contents: ");
    foreach(char c in lst)
      Console.Write(c + " ");
    Console.WriteLine("\n");

    // Change contents using array indexing.
    Console.WriteLine("Change first three elements");
    lst[0] = 'X';
    lst[1] = 'Y';
    lst[2] = 'Z';

    Console.Write("Contents: ");
    foreach(char c in lst)
      Console.Write(c + " ");
    Console.WriteLine();

    // Because of generic type-safety,
```

```
        // the following line is illegal.
//    lst.Add(99); // Error, not a char!
  }
}
```

The output, shown here, is the same as that produced by the non-generic version of the program:

```
Initial number of elements: 0

Adding 6 elements
Number of elements: 6
Current contents: C A E B D F

Removing 2 elements
Number of elements: 4
Contents: C E B D

Adding 20 more elements
Current capacity: 32
Number of elements after adding 20: 24
Contents: C E B D a b c d e f g h i j k l m n o p q r s t

Change first three elements
Contents: X Y Z D a b c d e f g h i j k l m n o p q r s t
```

LinkedList<T>

The **LinkedList<T>** class implements a generic doubly linked list. It implements **ICollection**, **ICollection<T>**, **IEnumerable**, **IEnumerable<T>**, **ISerializable**, and **IDeserializationCallback**. (The last two interfaces support the serialization of the list.) **LinkedList<T>** defines two public constructors, shown here:

> public LinkedList( )
> public LinkedList(IEnumerable<T> c)

The first creates an empty linked list. The second creates a list initialized with the elements in c.

Like most linked list implementations, **LinkedList<T>** encapsulates the values stored in the list in *nodes* that contain links to the previous and next elements in the list. These nodes are objects of type **LinkedListNode<T>**. **LinkedListNode<T>** provides the four properties shown here:

> public LinkedListNode<T> Next { get; }
>
> public LinkedListNode<T> Previous { get; }
>
> public LinkedList<T> List { get; }
>
> public T Value { get; set; }

Next and **Previous** obtain a reference to the next or previous node in the list, respectively. You can use these properties to traverse the list in either direction. A null reference is returned if no next or previous node exists. You can obtain a reference to the list itself via **List**. You can get or set the value within a node by using **Value**.

LinkedList<T> defines many methods. A sampling is shown in Table 24-15. In addition to the properties defined by the interfaces that it implements, **LinkedList<T>** defines these properties:

public LinkedListNode<T> First { get; }

public LinkedListNode<T> Last { get; }

First obtains the first node in the list. **Last** obtains the last node in the list.

Method	Description
public LinkedListNode<T> AddAfter(LinkedListNode<T> n, T v)	Adds a node with the value v to the list immediately after the node specified by n. The node passed in n must not be **null**. Returns a reference to the node containing the value v.
public void AddAfter(LinkedListNode<T> n, LinkedListNode<T> new)	Adds the node passed in new to the list immediately after the node specified by n. The node passed in n must not be **null**. Throws an **InvalidOperationException** if n is not in the list or if new is part of another list.
public LinkedListNode<T> AddBefore(LinkedListNode<T> n, T v)	Adds a node with the value v to the list immediately before the node specified by n. The node passed in n must not be **null**. Returns a reference to the node containing the value v.
public void AddBefore(LinkedListNode<T> n, LinkedListNode<T> new)	Adds the node passed in new to the list immediately before the node specified by n. The node passed in n must not be **null**. Throws an **InvalidOperationException** if n is not in the list or if new is part of another list.
public LinkedList<T> AddFirst(T v)	Adds a node with the value v to the start of the list. Returns a reference to the node containing the value v.
public void AddFirst(LinkedListNode new)	Adds new to the start of the list. Throws an **InvalidOperationException** if new is part of another list.
public LinkedList<T> AddLast(T v)	Adds a node with the value v to the end of the list. Returns a reference to the node containing the value v.
public void AddLast(LinkedListNode new)	Adds new to the end of the list. Throws an **InvalidOperationException** if new is part of another list.
public LinkedList<T> Find(T v)	Returns a reference to the first node in the list that has the value v. **null** is returned if v is not in the list.
public LinkedList<T> FindLast(T v)	Returns a reference to the last node in the list that has the value v. **null** is returned if v is not in the list.
public bool Remove(T v)	Removes the first node in the list that has the value v. Returns true if the node was removed. (That is, if a node with the value v was in the list and it was removed.) Returns false otherwise.

TABLE 24-15 A Sampling of Methods Defined by **LinkedList<T>**

Method	Description
public void Remove(LinkedList<T> n)	Removes the node that matches n. Throws an **InvalidOperationException** if n is not in the list.
public void RemoveFirst( )	Removes the first node in the list.
public void RemoveLast( )	Removes the last node in the list.

TABLE 24-15   A Sampling of Methods Defined by **LinkedList<T>** *(continued)*

Here is an example that demonstrates the **LinkedList<T>** class:

```
// Demonstrate LinkedList<T>.

using System;
using System.Collections.Generic;

class GenLinkedListDemo {
  static void Main() {
    // Create a linked list.
    LinkedList<char> ll = new LinkedList<char>();

    Console.WriteLine("Initial number of elements: " +
                      ll.Count);

    Console.WriteLine();

    Console.WriteLine("Adding 5 elements.");
    // Add elements to the linked list.
    ll.AddFirst('A');
    ll.AddFirst('B');
    ll.AddFirst('C');
    ll.AddFirst('D');
    ll.AddFirst('E');

    Console.WriteLine("Number of elements: " +
                      ll.Count);

    // Display the linked list by manually walking
    // through the list.
    LinkedListNode<char> node;

    Console.Write("Display contents by following links: ");
    for(node = ll.First; node != null; node = node.Next)
      Console.Write(node.Value + " ");

    Console.WriteLine("\n");

    //Display the linked list by use of a foreach loop.
    Console.Write("Display contents with foreach loop: ");
    foreach(char ch in ll)
      Console.Write(ch + " ");

    Console.WriteLine("\n");
```

```
    // Display the list backward by manually walking
    // from last to first.
    Console.Write("Follow links backwards: ");
      for(node = ll.Last; node != null; node = node.Previous)
      Console.Write(node.Value + " ");

    Console.WriteLine("\n");

    // Remove two elements.
    Console.WriteLine("Removing 2 elements.");
    // Remove elements from the linked list.
    ll.Remove('C');
    ll.Remove('A');

    Console.WriteLine("Number of elements: " +
                      ll.Count);

    // Use foreach loop to display the modified list.
    Console.Write("Contents after deletion: ");
    foreach(char ch in ll)
      Console.Write(ch + " ");

    Console.WriteLine("\n");

    // Add three elements to the end of the list.
    ll.AddLast('X');
    ll.AddLast('Y');
    ll.AddLast('Z');

    Console.Write("Contents after addition to end: ");
    foreach(char ch in ll)
      Console.Write(ch + " ");

    Console.WriteLine("\n");
  }
}
```

Here is the output:

```
Initial number of elements: 0

Adding 5 elements.
Number of elements: 5
Display contents by following links: E D C B A

Display contents with foreach loop: E D C B A

Follow links backwards: A B C D E

Removing 2 elements.
Number of elements: 3
Contents after deletion: E D B

Contents after addition to end: E D B X Y Z
```

Perhaps the most important thing to notice in this program is that the list is traversed in both the forward and backward direction by following the links provided by the **Next** and **Previous** properties. The bidirectional property of doubly linked lists is especially important in applications such as databases in which the ability to move efficiently through the list in both directions is often necessary.

The Dictionary<TK, TV> Class

The **Dictionary<TK, TV>** class stores key/value pairs. In a dictionary, values are accessed through their keys. In this regard, it is similar to the non-generic **Hashtable** class. **Dictionary<TK, TV>** implements **IDictionary**, **IDictionary<TV, TV>**, **ICollection**, **ICollection<KeyValuePair<TK, TV>>**, **IEnumerable**, **IEnumerable<KeyValuePair<TK, TV>>**, **ISerializable**, and **IDeserializationCallback**. (The last two interfaces support the serialization of the list.) Dictionaries are dynamic, growing as needed.

Dictionary<TK, TV> provides many constructors. Here is a sampling:

public Dictionary( )

public Dictionary(IDictionary<TK, TV> *dict*)

public Dictionary(int *capacity*)

The first constructor creates an empty dictionary with a default capacity. The second creates a dictionary that contains the same elements as those in *dict*. The third lets you specify an initial capacity. If you know in advance that you will need a dictionary of a certain size, then specifying that capacity will prevent the resizing of the dictionary at runtime, which is a costly process.

Dictionary<TK, TV> defines several methods. Some commonly used ones are shown in Table 24-16.

Method	Description
public void Add(TK *k*, TV *v*)	Adds the key/value pair specified by *k* and *v* to the dictionary. If *k* is already in the dictionary, then its value is unchanged and an **ArgumentException** is thrown.
public bool ContainsKey(TK *k*)	Returns true if *k* is a key in the invoking dictionary. Returns false otherwise.
public bool ContainsValue(TV *v*)	Returns true if *v* is a value in the invoking dictionary. Returns false otherwise.
public IDictionary.Enumerator<TK, TV> GetEnumerator( )	Returns an enumerator for the invoking dictionary.
public bool Remove(TK *k*)	Removes *k* from the dictionary. Returns true if successful. Returns false if *k* was not in the dictionary.

TABLE 24-16   Several Commonly Used Methods Defined by **Dictionary<TK, TV>**

In addition to the properties defined by the interfaces that it implements, **Dictionary<TK, TV>** defines these properties:

Property	Description
public IEqualityComparer<TK> Comparer { get; }	Obtains the comparer for the invoking dictionary.
public Dictionary<TK, TV>.KeyCollection Keys { get; }	Obtains a collection of the keys.
public Dictionary<TK, TV>.ValueCollection Values { get; }	Obtains a collection of the values.

Notice that the keys and values contained within the collection are available as separate lists through the **Keys** and **Values** properties. The types **Dictionary<TK, TV>.KeyCollection** and **Dictionary<TK, TV>.ValueCollection** are collections that implement both the generic and non-generic forms of **ICollection** and **IEnumerable**.

The following indexer, defined by **IDictionary<TK, TV>**, is implemented by **Dictionary<TK, TV>** as shown here:

public TV this[TK *key*] { get; set; }

You can use this indexer to get or set the value of an element. You can also use it to add a new element to the collection. Notice that the "index" is not actually an index, but rather the key of the item.

When enumerating the collection, **Dictionary<TK, TV>** returns key/value pairs in the form of a **KeyValuePair<TK, TV>** structure. Recall that this structure defines the following two fields:

public TK Key;
public TV Value;

These fields hold the key or value associated with an entry. Most of the time you won't need to use **KeyValuePair<TK, TV>** directly because **Dictionary<TK, TV>** allows you to work the keys and values individually. However, when enumerating a **Dictionary<TK, TV>**, such as in a **foreach** loop, the objects being enumerated are **KeyValuePair**s.

In a **Dictionary<TK, TV>**, all keys must be unique, and a key must not change while it is in use as a key. Values need not be unique. The objects in a **Dictionary<TK, TV>** are not stored in sorted order.

Here is an example that demonstrates **Dictionary<TK, TV>**:

```
// Demonstrate the generic Dictionary<TK, TV> class.

using System;
using System.Collections.Generic;

class GenDictionaryDemo {
```

```
static void Main() {
  // Create a Dictionary that holds employee
  // names and their corresponding salary.
  Dictionary<string, double> dict =
    new Dictionary<string, double>();

  // Add elements to the collection.
  dict.Add("Butler, John", 73000);
  dict.Add("Swartz, Sarah", 59000);
  dict.Add("Pyke, Thomas", 45000);
  dict.Add("Frank, Ed", 99000);

  // Get a collection of the keys (names).
  ICollection<string> c = dict.Keys;

  // Use the keys to obtain the values (salaries).
  foreach(string str in c)
    Console.WriteLine("{0}, Salary: {1:C}", str, dict[str]);
  }
}
```

Here is the output:

```
Butler, John, Salary: $73,000.00
Swartz, Sarah, Salary: $59,000.00
Pyke, Thomas, Salary: $45,000.00
Frank, Ed, Salary: $99,000.00
```

The SortedDictionary<TK, TV> Class

The **SortedDictionary<TV, TK>** class stores key/value pairs and is similar to **Dictionary<TK, TV>** except that it is sorted by key. **SortedDictionary<TK, TV>** implements **IDictionary**, **IDictionary<TK, TV>**, **ICollection**, **ICollection<KeyValuePair<TK, TV>>**, **IEnumerable**, and **IEnumerable<KeyValuePair<TK, TV>>**. **SortedDictionary<TK, TV>** provides the following constructors:

public SortedDictionary( )

public SortedDictionary(IDictionary<TK, TV> *dict*)

public SortedDictionary(IComparer<TK> *comp*)

public SortedDictionary(IDictionary<TK, TV> *dict*, IComparer<TK> *comp*)

The first constructor creates an empty dictionary. The second creates a dictionary that contains the same elements as those in *dict*. The third lets you specify the **IComparer** that the dictionary will use for sorting, and the fourth lets you initialize the dictionary and specify the **IComparer**.

SortedDictionary<TK, TV> defines several methods. A sampling is shown in Table 24-17.

Method	Description
public void Add(TK *k*, TV *v*)	Adds the key/value pair specified by *k* and *v* to the dictionary. If *k* is already in the dictionary, then its value is unchanged and an **ArgumentException** is thrown.
public bool ContainsKey(TK *k*)	Returns true if *k* is a key in the invoking dictionary. Returns false otherwise.
public bool ContainsValue(TV *v*)	Returns true if *v* is a value in the invoking dictionary. Returns false otherwise.
public SortedDictionary.Enumerator<TK, TV> GetEnumerator( )	Returns an enumerator for the invoking dictionary.
public bool Remove(TK *k*)	Removes *k* from the dictionary. Returns true if successful. Returns false if *k* was not in the dictionary.

TABLE 24-17   A Sampling of Methods Defined by **SortedDictionary<TK, TV>**

In addition to the properties defined by the interfaces that it implements, **SortedDictionary<TK, TV>** defines the following properties:

Property	Description
public IComparer<TK> Comparer { get; }	Obtains the comparer for the invoking dictionary.
public SortedDictionary<TK, TV>.KeyCollection Keys { get; }	Obtains a collection of the keys.
public SortedDictionary<TK, TV>.ValueCollection Values { get; }	Obtains a collection of the values.

Notice that the keys and values contained within the collection are available as separate lists through the **Keys** and **Values** properties. The types

SortedDictionary<TK, TV>.KeyCollection
SortedDictionary<TK, TV>.ValueCollection

are collections that implement both the generic and non-generic forms of **ICollection** and **IEnumerable**.

SortedDictionary<TK, TV> defines the following indexer (which is specified by **IDictionary<TK, TV>**):

public TV this[TK *key*] { get; set; }

You can use this indexer to get or set the value of an element. You can also use it to add a new element to the collection. Notice that the "index" is not actually an index, but rather the key of the item.

When enumerated, **SortedDictionary<TK, TV>** returns key/value pairs in the form of a **KeyValuePair<TK, TV>** structure. Recall that this structure defines the following two fields:

    public TK Key;
    public TV Value;

These fields hold the key or value associated with an entry. Most of the time you won't need to use **KeyValuePair<TK, TV>** directly because **SortedDictionary<TK, TV>** allows you to work the keys and values individually. However, when enumerating a **SortedDictionary<TK, TV>**, such as in a **foreach** loop, the objects being enumerated are **KeyValuePairs**.

In a **SortedDictionary<TK, TV>**, all keys must be unique, and a key must not change while it is in use as a key. Values need not be unique.

Here is an example that demonstrates **SortedDictionary<TK, TV>**. It reworks the **Dictionary<TK, TV>** example shown in the preceding section. In this version, the database of employees and salaries is sorted based on name (which is the key).

```
// Demonstrate the generic SortedDictionary<TK, TV> class.

using System;
using System.Collections.Generic;

class GenSortedDictionaryDemo {
  static void Main() {
    // Create a Dictionary that holds employee
    // names and their corresponding salary.
    SortedDictionary<string, double> dict =
      new SortedDictionary<string, double>();

    // Add elements to the collection.
    dict.Add("Butler, John", 73000);
    dict.Add("Swartz, Sarah", 59000);
    dict.Add("Pyke, Thomas", 45000);
    dict.Add("Frank, Ed", 99000);

    // Get a collection of the keys (names).
    ICollection<string> c = dict.Keys;

    // Use the keys to obtain the values (salaries).
    foreach(string str in c)
      Console.WriteLine("{0}, Salary: {1:C}", str, dict[str]);
  }
}
```

The output is shown here:

```
Butler, John, Salary: $73,000.00
Frank, Ed, Salary: $99,000.00
Pyke, Thomas, Salary: $45,000.00
Swartz, Sarah, Salary: $59,000.00
```

As you can see, the list is now sorted based on the key, which is the employee's name.

The SortedList<TK, TV> Class

The **SortedList<TK, TV>** class stores a sorted list of key/value pairs. It is the generic equivalent of the non-generic **SortedList** class. **SortedList<TK, TV>** implements **IDictionary**, **IDictionary<TK, TV>**, **ICollection**, **ICollection< KeyValuePair<TK, TV>>**, **IEnumerable**, and **IEnumerable< KeyValuePair<TK, TV>>**. The size of a **SortedList<TK, TV>** is dynamic and will automatically grow as needed. **SortedList<TV, TK>** is similar to **SortedDictionary<TK, TV>** but has different performance characteristics. For example, a **SortedList<TK, TV>** uses less memory, but a **SortedDictionary<TK, TV>** is faster when inserting out-of-order elements.

SortedList<TK, TV> provides many constructors. Here is a sampling:

public SortedList( )

public SortedList(IDictionary<TK, TV> *dict*)

public SortedList(int *capacity*)

public SortedList(IComparer<TK> *comp*)

The first constructor creates an empty list with a default capacity. The second creates a list that contains the same elements as those in *dict*. The third lets you specify an initial capacity. If you know in advance that you will need a list of a certain size, then specifying that capacity will prevent the resizing of the list at runtime, which is a costly process. The fourth form lets you specify a comparison method that will be used to compare the objects contained in the list.

The capacity of a **SortedList<TK, TV>** list grows automatically as needed when elements are added to a list. When the current capacity is exceeded, the capacity is increased. The advantage of specifying a capacity is that you can prevent or minimize the overhead associated with resizing the collection. Of course, it makes sense to specify an initial capacity only if you have some idea of how many elements will be stored.

In addition to the methods defined by the interfaces that it implements, **SortedList<TK, TV>** also defines several methods of its own. A sampling is shown in Table 24-18. Notice that the enumerator returned by **GetEnumerator( )** enumerates the key/value pairs stored in the list as objects of type **KeyValuePair**.

Method	Description
public void Add(TK *k*, TV *v*)	Adds the key/value pair specified by *k* and *v* to the list. If *k* is already in the list, then its value is unchanged and an **ArgumentException** is thrown.
public bool ContainsKey(TK *k*)	Returns true if *k* is a key in the invoking list. Returns false otherwise.
public bool ContainsValue(TV *v*)	Returns true if *v* is a value in the invoking list. Returns false otherwise.
public IEnumerator<KeyValuePair<TK, TV>> GetEnumerator( )	Returns an enumerator for the invoking list.
public int IndexOfKey(TK *k*)	Returns the index of the key specified by *k*. Returns −1 if the key is not in the list.

TABLE 24-18 Several Commonly Used Methods Defined by **SortedList<TK, TV>**

Method	Description
public int IndexOfValue(TV *v*)	Returns the index of the first occurrence of the value specified by *v*. Returns –1 if the value is not in the list.
public bool Remove(TK *k*)	Removes the key/value pair associated with *k* from the list. Returns true if successful. Returns false if *k* is not in the list.
public void RemoveAt(int *idx*)	Removes the key/value pair at the index specified by *idx*.
public void TrimExcess( )	Removes the excess capacity of the invoking list.

TABLE 24-18   Several Commonly Used Methods Defined by **SortedList<TK, TV>** *(continued)*

In addition to the properties defined by the interfaces that it implements, **SortedList<TK, TV>** defines the following properties:

Property	Description
public int Capacity { get; set; }	Obtains or sets the capacity of the invoking list.
public IComparer<TK> Comparer { get; }	Obtains the comparer for the invoking list.
public IList<TK> Keys { get; }	Obtains a collection of the keys.
public IList<TV> Values { get; }	Obtains a collection of the values.

SortedList<TK, TV> defines the following indexer (which is defined by **IDictionary<TK, TV>**):

    public TV this[TK *key*] { get; set; }

You can use this indexer to get or set the value of an element. You can also use it to add a new element to the collection. Notice that the "index" is not actually an index, but rather the key of the item.

Here is an example that demonstrates **SortedList<TK, TV>**. It reworks the employee database example one more time. In this version, the database is stored in a **SortedList**.

```
// Demonstrate a SortedList<TK, TV>.

using System;
using System.Collections.Generic;

class GenSLDemo {
  static void Main() {
    // Create a sorted SortedList for
    // employee names and salary.
    SortedList<string, double> sl =
      new SortedList<string, double>();
```

```
    // Add elements to the collection.
    sl.Add("Butler, John", 73000);
    sl.Add("Swartz, Sarah", 59000);
    sl.Add("Pyke, Thomas", 45000);
    sl.Add("Frank, Ed", 99000);

    // Get a collection of the keys.
    ICollection<string> c = sl.Keys;

    // Use the keys to obtain the values.
    foreach(string str in c)
      Console.WriteLine("{0}, Salary: {1:C}", str, sl[str]);

    Console.WriteLine();
  }
}
```

The output is shown here:

```
Butler, John, Salary: $73,000.00
Frank, Ed, Salary: $99,000.00
Pyke, Thomas, Salary: $45,000.00
Swartz, Sarah, Salary: $59,000.00
```

As the output shows, the list is sorted based on employee name, which is the key.

The Stack<T> Class

Stack<T> is the generic equivalent of the non-generic **Stack** class. **Stack<T>** supports a first-in, last-out stack. It implements the **ICollection**, **IEnumerable**, and **IEnumerable<T>** interfaces. **Stack<T>** directly implements the **Clear( )**, **Contains( )**, and **CopyTo( )** methods defined by **ICollection<T>**. (The **Add( )** and **Remove( )** methods are not supported, nor is the **IsReadOnly** property.) **Stack<T>** is a dynamic collection that grows as needed to accommodate the elements it must store. It defines the following constructors:

> public Stack( )
> public Stack(int *capacity*)
> public Stack(IEnumerable<T> *c*)

The first form creates an empty stack with a default initial capacity. The second form creates an empty stack with the initial capacity specified by *capacity*. The third form creates a stack that contains the elements of the collection specified by *c*.

In addition to the methods defined by the interfaces that it implements (and those methods defined by **ICollection<T>** that it implements on its own), **Stack<T>** defines the methods shown in Table 24-19. **Stack<T>** works just like its non-generic counterpart. To put an object on the top of the stack, call **Push( )**. To remove and return the top element, call **Pop( )**. You can use **Peek( )** to return, but not remove, the top object. An **InvalidOperationException** is thrown if you call **Pop( )** or **Peek( )** when the invoking stack is empty.

Method	Description
public T Peek( )	Returns the element on the top of the stack, but does not remove it.
public T Pop( )	Returns the element on the top of the stack, removing it in the process.
public void Push(T *v*)	Pushes *v* onto the stack.
public T[ ] ToArray( )	Returns an array that contains copies of the elements of the invoking stack.
public void TrimExcess( )	Removes the excess capacity of the invoking stack.

TABLE 24-19 The Methods Defined by **Stack\<T>**

The following program demonstrates **Stack\<T>**:

```
// Demonstrate the Stack<T> class.

using System;
using System.Collections.Generic;

class GenStackDemo {
  static void Main() {
    Stack<string> st = new Stack<string>();

    st.Push("One");
    st.Push("Two");
    st.Push("Three");
    st.Push("Four");
    st.Push("Five");

    while(st.Count > 0) {
      string str = st.Pop();
      Console.Write(str + " ");
    }

    Console.WriteLine();
  }
}
```

The output is shown here:

```
Five Four Three Two One
```

The Queue\<T> Class

Queue\<T> is the generic equivalent of the non-generic **Queue** class. It supports a first-in, first-out list. **Queue\<T>** implements the **ICollection**, **IEnumerable**, and **IEnumerable\<T>** interfaces. **Queue\<T>** directly implements the **Clear( )**, **Contains( )**, and **CopyTo( )** methods

defined by **ICollection<T>**. (The **Add( )** and **Remove( )** methods are not supported, nor is the **IsReadOnly** property.) **Queue<T>** is a dynamic collection that grows as needed to accommodate the elements it must store. It defines the following constructors:

public Queue( )
public Queue(int *capacity*)
public Queue(IEnumerable<T> *c*)

The first form creates an empty queue with an initial default capacity. The second form creates an empty queue with the initial capacity specified by *capacity*. The third form creates a queue that contains the elements of the collection specified by *c*.

In addition to the methods defined by the interfaces that it implements (and those methods defined by **ICollection<T>** that it implements on its own), **Queue<T>** defines the methods shown in Table 24-20. **Queue<T>** works just like its non-generic counterpart. To put an object in the queue, call **Enqueue( )**. To remove and return the object at the front of the queue, call **Dequeue( )**. You can use **Peek( )** to return, but not remove, the next object. An **InvalidOperationException** is thrown if you call **Dequeue( )** or **Peek( )** when the invoking queue is empty.

Here is an example that demonstrates **Queue<T>**:

```
// Demonstrate the Queue<T> class.

using System;
using System.Collections.Generic;

class GenQueueDemo {
  static void Main() {
    Queue<double> q = new Queue<double>();

    q.Enqueue(98.6);
    q.Enqueue(212.0);
    q.Enqueue(32.0);
    q.Enqueue(3.1416);

    double sum = 0.0;
    Console.Write("Queue contents: ");
    while(q.Count > 0) {
      double val = q.Dequeue();
      Console.Write(val + " ");
      sum += val;
    }

    Console.WriteLine("\nTotal is " + sum);
  }
}
```

The output is shown here:

```
Queue contents: 98.6 212 32 3.1416
Total is 345.7416
```

Method	Description
public T Dequeue( )	Returns the object at the front of the invoking queue. The object is removed in the process.
public void Enqueue(T *v*)	Adds *v* to the end of the queue.
public T Peek( )	Returns the object at the front of the invoking queue, but does not remove it.
public T[ ] ToArray( )	Returns an array that contains copies of the elements of the invoking queue.
public void TrimExcess( )	Removes the excess capacity of the invoking stack.

TABLE 24-20   The Methods Defined by **Queue<T>**

HashSet<T>

HashSet<T> is a new collection added to the .NET Framework by version 3.5. It supports a collection that implements a set. It uses a hash table for storage. **HashSet<T>** implements the **ICollection<T>**, **IEnumerable**, **IEnumerable<T>**, **ISerializable**, and **IDeserializationCallback** interfaces. **HashSet<T>** implements a set in which all elements are unique. In other words, duplicates are not allowed. The order of the elements is not specified. **HashSet<T>** defines a full complement of set operations, such as intersection, union, and symmetric difference. This makes **HashSet<T>** the perfect choice for working with sets of objects. **HashSet<T>** is a dynamic collection that grows as needed to accommodate the elements it must store.

Here are four commonly used constructors defined by **HashSet<T>**:

    public HashSet( )
    public HashSet(IEnumerable<T> *c*)
    public HashSet(IEqualityCompare *comp*)
    public HashSet(IEnumerable<T> *c*, IEqualityCompare *comp*)

The first form creates an empty set. The second creates a set that contains the elements of the collection specified by *c*. The third lets you specify the comparer. The fourth creates a set that contains the elements in the collection specified by *c* and uses the comparer specified by *comp*. There is also a fifth constructor that lets you initialize a set from serialized data.

In addition to the methods defined by the interfaces that it implements, **HashSet<T>** defines several of its own, most of which support various set operations. The set operation methods defined by **HashSet<T>** are shown in Table 24-21. Notice that the arguments to these methods are **IEnumerable<T>**. This means you can pass something other than another **HashSet<T>** as the second set. Most often, however, both operands will be instances of **HashSet<T>**.

In addition to the properties defined by **ICollection<T>**, **HashSet<T>** adds **Comparer**, shown here:

    public IEqualityComparer<T> Comparer { get; }

It obtains the comparer for the invoking hash set.

Method	Description
public void ExceptWith(IEnumerable<T> *set2*)	Removes the elements in *set2* from the invoking set.
public void IntersectWith(IEnumerable<T> *set2*)	Removes from the invoking set those elements not common to both the invoking set and *set2*.
public bool IsProperSubsetOf(IEnumerable<T> *set2*)	Returns true if the invoking set is a proper subset of *set2*.
public bool IsProperSupersetOf(IEnumerable<T> *set2*)	Returns true if the invoking set is a proper superset of *set2*.
public bool IsSubsetOf(IEnumerable<T> *set2*)	Returns true if the invoking set is a subset of *set2*.
public bool IsSuperSetOf(IEnumerable<T> *set2*)	Returns true if the invoking set is a superset of *set2*.
public bool SetEquals(IEnumerable<T> *set2*)	Returns true if the invoking set is equivalent to *set2*. This determination is independent of the order of the elements.
public void SymmetricExceptWith(IEnumerable<T> *set2*)	Changes the invoking set so that it contains all elements from both the invoking set and *set2*, except for those elements common to both sets. This is usually called the symmetric difference of the two sets.
public void UnionWith(IEnumerable<T> *set2*)	Adds the elements from *set2* to the invoking set. Duplicates are not included. Thus, it creates a union of the two sets.

TABLE 24-21   The Set Operations Defined by **HashSet<T>**

Here is an example that shows **HashSet<T>** in action:

```
// Demonstrate the HashSet<T> class.

using System;
using System.Collections.Generic;

class HashSetDemo {

  static void Show(string msg, HashSet<char> set) {
    Console.Write(msg);
    foreach(char ch in set)
      Console.Write(ch + " ");
    Console.WriteLine();
  }

  static void Main() {
    HashSet<char> setA = new HashSet<char>();
    HashSet<char> setB = new HashSet<char>();

    setA.Add('A');
```

```
      setA.Add('B');
      setA.Add('C');

      setB.Add('C');
      setB.Add('D');
      setB.Add('E');

      Show("Initial content of setA: ", setA);
      Show("Initial content of setB: ", setB);

      setA.SymmetricExceptWith(setB);
      Show("setA after Symmetric difference with SetB: ", setA);

      setA.UnionWith(setB);
      Show("setA after union with setB: ", setA);

      setA.ExceptWith(setB);
      Show("setA after subtracting setB: ", setA);

      Console.WriteLine();
  }
}
```

The output is shown here:

```
Initial content of setA: A B C
Initial content of setB: C D E
setA after Symmetric difference with SetB: A B D E
setA after union with setB: A B D E C
setA after subtracting setB: A B
```

Storing User-Defined Classes in Collections

For the sake of simplicity, the foregoing examples have stored built-in types, such as **int**, **string**, or **char**, in a collection. Of course, collections are not limited to the storage of built-in objects. Quite the contrary. The power of collections is that they can store any type of object, including objects of classes that you create.

Let's begin with an example that uses the non-generic class **ArrayList** to store inventory information that is encapsulated by the **Inventory** class:

```
// A simple inventory example.

using System;
using System.Collections;

class Inventory {
  string name;
  double cost;
  int onhand;

  public Inventory(string n, double c, int h) {
    name = n;
    cost = c;
    onhand = h;
```

```
    }

    public override string ToString() {
      return
        String.Format("{0,-10}Cost: {1,6:C}  On hand: {2}",
                         name, cost, onhand);
    }
  }
}

class InventoryList {
  static void Main() {
    ArrayList inv = new ArrayList();

    // Add elements to the list
    inv.Add(new Inventory("Pliers", 5.95, 3));
    inv.Add(new Inventory("Wrenches", 8.29, 2));
    inv.Add(new Inventory("Hammers", 3.50, 4));
    inv.Add(new Inventory("Drills", 19.88, 8));

    Console.WriteLine("Inventory list:");
    foreach(Inventory i in inv) {
      Console.WriteLine("    " + i);
    }
  }
}
```

The output from the program is shown here:

```
Inventory list:
    Pliers     Cost:  $5.95  On hand: 3
    Wrenches   Cost:  $8.29  On hand: 2
    Hammers    Cost:  $3.50  On hand: 4
    Drills     Cost: $19.88  On hand: 8
```

In the program, notice that no special actions were required to store objects of type
Inventory in a collection. Because all types inherit **object**, any type of object can be stored in
any non-generic collection. Thus, using a non-generic collection, it is trivially easy to store
objects of classes that you create. Of course, it also means the collection is not type-safe.

To store objects of classes that you create in a type-safe collection, you must use one of
the generic collection classes. For example, here is a version of the preceding program
rewritten to use **List<T>**. The output is the same as before.

```
// Store Inventory Objects in a List<T> collection.

using System;
using System.Collections.Generic;

class Inventory {
  string name;
  double cost;
  int onhand;

  public Inventory(string n, double c, int h) {
    name = n;
```

```
      cost = c;
      onhand = h;
    }

    public override string ToString() {
      return
        String.Format("{0,-10}Cost: {1,6:C}  On hand: {2}",
                      name, cost, onhand);
    }
}

class TypeSafeInventoryList {
  static void Main() {
    List<Inventory> inv = new List<Inventory>();

    // Add elements to the list.
    inv.Add(new Inventory("Pliers", 5.95, 3));
    inv.Add(new Inventory("Wrenches", 8.29, 2));
    inv.Add(new Inventory("Hammers", 3.50, 4));
    inv.Add(new Inventory("Drills", 19.88, 8));

    Console.WriteLine("Inventory list:");
    foreach(Inventory i in inv) {
      Console.WriteLine("    " + i);
    }
  }
}
```

In this version, notice the only real difference is the passing of the type **Inventory** as a type argument to **List<T>**. Other than that, the two programs are nearly identical. The fact that the use of a generic collection requires virtually no additional effort and adds type safety argues strongly for its use when storing a specific type of object within a collection.

In general, there is one other thing to notice about the preceding programs: Both are quite short. When you consider that each sets up a dynamic array that can store, retrieve, and process inventory information in less than 40 lines of code, the power of collections begins to become apparent. As most readers will know, if all of this functionality had to be coded by hand, the program would have been several times longer. Collections offer ready-to-use solutions to a wide variety of programming problems. You should use them whenever the situation warrants.

There is one limitation to the preceding programs that may not be immediately apparent: The collection can't be sorted. The reason for this is that neither **ArrayList** nor **List<T>** has a way to compare two **Inventory** objects. There are two ways to remedy this situation. First, **Inventory** can implement the **IComparable** interface. This interface defines how two objects of a class are compared. Second, an **IComparer** object can be specified when comparisons are required. The following sections illustrate both approaches.

Implementing IComparable

If you want to sort a collection that contains user-defined objects (or if you want to store those objects in a collection such as **SortedList**, which maintains its elements in sorted order), then the collection must know how to compare those objects. One way to do this is

for the object being stored to implement the **IComparable** interface. The **IComparable** interface comes in two forms: generic and non-generic. Although the way each is used is similar, there are some small differences. Each is examined here.

Implementing IComparable for Non-Generic Collections

If you want to sort objects that are stored in a non-generic collection, then you will implement the non-generic version of **IComparable**. This version defines only one method, **CompareTo( )**, which determines how comparisons are performed. The general form of **CompareTo( )** is shown here:

    int CompareTo(object *obj)*

CompareTo( ) compares the invoking object to *obj*. To sort in ascending order, your implementation must return zero if the objects are equal, a positive value if the invoking object is greater than *obj*, and a negative value if the invoking object is less than *obj*. You can sort in descending order by reversing the outcome of the comparison. The method can throw an **ArgumentException** if the type of *obj* is not compatible for comparison with the invoking object.

Here is an example that shows how to implement **IComparable**. It adds **IComparable** to the **Inventory** class developed in the preceding section. It implements **CompareTo( )** so that it compares the **name** field, thus enabling the inventory to be sorted by name. By implementing **IComparable**, it allows a collection of **Inventory** objects to be sorted, as the program illustrates.

```
// Implement IComparable.

using System;
using System.Collections;

// Implement the non-generic IComparable interface.
class Inventory : IComparable {
  string name;
  double cost;
  int onhand;

  public Inventory(string n, double c, int h) {
    name = n;
    cost = c;
    onhand = h;
  }

  public override string ToString() {
    return
      String.Format("{0,-10}Cost: {1,6:C}  On hand: {2}",
                    name, cost, onhand);
  }

  // Implement the IComparable interface.
  public int CompareTo(object obj) {
    Inventory b;
    b = (Inventory) obj;
```

```
        return name.CompareTo(b.name);
    }
}

class IComparableDemo {
  static void Main() {
    ArrayList inv = new ArrayList();

    // Add elements to the list.
    inv.Add(new Inventory("Pliers", 5.95, 3));
    inv.Add(new Inventory("Wrenches", 8.29, 2));
    inv.Add(new Inventory("Hammers", 3.50, 4));
    inv.Add(new Inventory("Drills", 19.88, 8));

    Console.WriteLine("Inventory list before sorting:");
    foreach(Inventory i in inv) {
      Console.WriteLine("    " + i);
    }
    Console.WriteLine();

    // Sort the list.
    inv.Sort();

    Console.WriteLine("Inventory list after sorting:");
    foreach(Inventory i in inv) {
      Console.WriteLine("    " + i);
    }
  }
}
```

Here is the output. Notice that after the call to **Sort( )**, the inventory is sorted by name.

```
Inventory list before sorting:
    Pliers    Cost:  $5.95  On hand: 3
    Wrenches  Cost:  $8.29  On hand: 2
    Hammers   Cost:  $3.50  On hand: 4
    Drills    Cost: $19.88  On hand: 8

Inventory list after sorting:
    Drills    Cost: $19.88  On hand: 8
    Hammers   Cost:  $3.50  On hand: 4
    Pliers    Cost:  $5.95  On hand: 3
    Wrenches  Cost:  $8.29  On hand: 2
```

Implementing IComparable<T> for Generic Collections

If you want to sort objects that are stored in a generic collection, then you will implement
IComparable<T>. This version defines the generic form of **CompareTo( )** shown here:

    int CompareTo(T *obj*)

CompareTo( ) compares the invoking object to *obj*. To sort in ascending order, your
implementation must return zero if the objects are equal, a positive value if the invoking
object is greater than *obj*, and a negative value if the invoking object is less than *obj*. To

sort in descending order, reverse the outcome of the comparison. When implementing **IComparable<T>**, you will usually pass the type name of the implementing class as a type argument.

The following example reworks the preceding program so that it uses **IComparable<T>**. Notice it uses the generic **List<T>** collection rather than the non-generic **ArrayList**.

```csharp
// Implement IComparable<T>.

using System;
using System.Collections.Generic;

// Implement the generic IComparable<T> interface.
class Inventory : IComparable<Inventory> {
  string name;
  double cost;
  int onhand;

  public Inventory(string n, double c, int h) {
    name = n;
    cost = c;
    onhand = h;
  }

  public override string ToString() {
    return
      String.Format("{0,-10}Cost: {1,6:C}  On hand: {2}",
                    name, cost, onhand);
  }

  // Implement the IComparable<T> interface.
  public int CompareTo(Inventory obj) {
    return name.CompareTo(obj.name);
  }
}

class GenericIComparableDemo {
  static void Main() {
    List<Inventory> inv = new List<Inventory>();

    // Add elements to the list.
    inv.Add(new Inventory("Pliers", 5.95, 3));
    inv.Add(new Inventory("Wrenches", 8.29, 2));
    inv.Add(new Inventory("Hammers", 3.50, 4));
    inv.Add(new Inventory("Drills", 19.88, 8));

    Console.WriteLine("Inventory list before sorting:");
    foreach(Inventory i in inv) {
      Console.WriteLine("   " + i);
    }
    Console.WriteLine();

    // Sort the list.
    inv.Sort();
```

```
      Console.WriteLine("Inventory list after sorting:");
      foreach(Inventory i in inv) {
        Console.WriteLine("   " + i);
      }
    }
  }
}
```

This program produces the same output as the previous, non-generic version.

Using an IComparer

Although implementing **IComparable** for classes that you create is often the easiest way to allow objects of those classes to be sorted, you can approach the problem in a different way by using **IComparer**. To use **IComparer**, first create a class that implements **IComparer**, and then specify an object of that class when comparisons are required.

There are two versions of **IComparer**: generic and non-generic. Although the way each is used is similar, there are some small differences, and each approach is examined here.

Using a Non-Generic IComparer

The non-generic **IComparer** defines only one method, **Compare( )**, which is shown here:

int Compare(object *obj1*, object *obj2*)

Compare( ) compares *obj1* to *obj2*. To sort in ascending order, your implementation must return zero if the objects are equal, a positive value if *obj1* is greater than *obj2*, and a negative value if *obj1* is less than *obj2*. You can sort in descending order by reversing the outcome of the comparison. The method can throw an **ArgumentException** if the type of *obj* is not compatible for comparison with the invoking object.

An **IComparer** can be specified when constructing a **SortedList**, when calling **ArrayList.Sort(IComparer)**, and at various other places throughout the collection classes. The main advantage of using **IComparer** is that you can sort objects of classes that do not implement **IComparable**.

The following program reworks the non-generic inventory program so that it uses an **IComparer** to sort the inventory list. It first creates a class called **CompInv** that implements **IComparer** and compares two **Inventory** objects. An object of this class is then used in a call to **Sort( )** to sort the inventory list.

```
// Use IComparer.

using System;
using System.Collections;

// Create an IComparer for Inventory objects.
class CompInv : IComparer {
  // Implement the IComparer interface.
  public int Compare(object obj1, object obj2) {
    Inventory a, b;
    a = (Inventory) obj1;
    b = (Inventory) obj2;
    return a.name.CompareTo(b.name);
  }
}
```

```
class Inventory {
  public string name;
  double cost;
  int onhand;

  public Inventory(string n, double c, int h) {
    name = n;
    cost = c;
    onhand = h;
  }

  public override string ToString() {
    return
      String.Format("{0,-10}Cost: {1,6:C}  On hand: {2}",
                     name, cost, onhand);
  }
}

class IComparerDemo {
  static void Main() {
    CompInv comp = new CompInv();
    ArrayList inv = new ArrayList();

    // Add elements to the list.
    inv.Add(new Inventory("Pliers", 5.95, 3));
    inv.Add(new Inventory("Wrenches", 8.29, 2));
    inv.Add(new Inventory("Hammers", 3.50, 4));
    inv.Add(new Inventory("Drills", 19.88, 8));

    Console.WriteLine("Inventory list before sorting:");
    foreach(Inventory i in inv) {
      Console.WriteLine("   " + i);
    }
    Console.WriteLine();

    // Sort the list using an IComparer.
    inv.Sort(comp);

    Console.WriteLine("Inventory list after sorting:");
    foreach(Inventory i in inv) {
      Console.WriteLine("   " + i);
    }
  }
}
```

The output is the same as the previous version of the program.

Using a Generic IComparer<T>

The **IComparer<T>** interface is the generic version of **IComparer**. It defines the generic version of **Compare( )**, shown here:

int Compare(T *obj1*, T *obj2*)

This method compares *obj1* with *obj2* and returns greater than zero if *obj1* is greater than *obj2*, zero if the two objects are the same, and less than zero if *obj1* is less that *obj2*.

Here is a generic version of the preceding program that uses **IComparer<T>**. It produces the same output as the previous versions of the program.

```
// Use IComparer<T>.

using System;
using System.Collections.Generic;

// Create an IComparer<T> for Inventory objects.
class CompInv<T> : IComparer<T> where T : Inventory {

  // Implement the IComparer<T> interface.
  public int Compare(T obj1, T obj2) {
    return obj1.name.CompareTo(obj2.name);
  }
}

class Inventory {
  public string name;
  double cost;
  int onhand;

  public Inventory(string n, double c, int h) {
    name = n;
    cost = c;
    onhand = h;
  }

  public override string ToString() {
    return
      String.Format("{0,-10}Cost: {1,6:C}  On hand: {2}",
                    name, cost, onhand);
  }
}

class GenericIComparerDemo {
  static void Main() {
    CompInv<Inventory> comp = new CompInv<Inventory>();
    List<Inventory> inv = new List<Inventory>();

    // Add elements to the list.
    inv.Add(new Inventory("Pliers", 5.95, 3));
    inv.Add(new Inventory("Wrenches", 8.29, 2));
    inv.Add(new Inventory("Hammers", 3.50, 4));
    inv.Add(new Inventory("Drills", 19.88, 8));

    Console.WriteLine("Inventory list before sorting:");
    foreach(Inventory i in inv) {
      Console.WriteLine("   " + i);
    }
    Console.WriteLine();
```

```
    // Sort the list using an IComparer.
    inv.Sort(comp);

    Console.WriteLine("Inventory list after sorting:");
    foreach(Inventory i in inv) {
      Console.WriteLine("   " + i);
    }
  }
}
```

Accessing a Collection via an Enumerator

Often you will want to cycle through the elements in a collection. For example, you might want to display each element. One way to do this is to use a **foreach** loop, as the preceding examples have done. Another way is to use an enumerator. An *enumerator* is an object that implements either the non-generic **IEnumerator** or the generic **IEnumerator<T>** interface.

IEnumerator defines one property called **Current**. The non-generic version is shown here:

object Current { get; }

For **IEnumerator<T>**, **Current** is declared like this:

T Current { get; }

In both cases, **Current** obtains the current element being enumerated. Since **Current** is a read-only property, an enumerator can only be used to retrieve, but not modify, the objects in a collection.

IEnumerator defines two methods. The first is **MoveNext( )**:

bool MoveNext( )

Each call to **MoveNext( )** moves the current position of the enumerator to the next element in the collection. It returns true if the next element is available, or false if the **end** of the collection has been reached. Prior to the first call to **MoveNext( )**, the value of **Current** is undefined. (Conceptually, prior to the first call to **MoveNext( )**, the enumerator refers to the nonexistent element that is just before the first element. Thus, you must call **MoveNext( )** to move to the first element.)

You can reset the enumerator to the start of the collection by calling **Reset( )**, shown here:

void Reset( )

After calling **Reset( )**, enumeration will again begin at the start of the collection. Thus, you must call **MoveNext( )** before obtaining the first element.

In **IEnumerator<T>**, the methods **MoveNext( )** and **Reset( )** work in the same way.

Two other points: First, you cannot use an enumerator to change the collection that it is enumerating. Thus, enumerators are read-only relative to the collection. Second, any change to the collection under enumeration invalidates the enumerator.

Using an Enumerator

Before you can access a collection through an enumerator, you must obtain one. Each of the collection classes provides a **GetEnumerator( )** method that returns an enumerator to the start of the collection. Using this enumerator, you can access each element in the collection, one element at a time. In general, to use an enumerator to cycle through the contents of a collection, follow these steps:

1. Obtain an enumerator to the start of the collection by calling the collection's **GetEnumerator( )** method.

2. Set up a loop that makes a call to **MoveNext( )**. Have the loop iterate as long as **MoveNext( )** returns true.

3. Within the loop, obtain each element through **Current**.

Here is an example that implements these steps. It uses an **ArrayList**, but the general principles apply to any type of collection, including the generic collections.

```
// Demonstrate an enumerator.

using System;
using System.Collections;

class EnumeratorDemo {
  static void Main() {
    ArrayList list = new ArrayList(1);

    for(int i=0; i < 10; i++)
      list.Add(i);

    // Use enumerator to access list.
    IEnumerator etr = list.GetEnumerator();
    while(etr.MoveNext())
      Console.Write(etr.Current + " ");

    Console.WriteLine();

    // Re-enumerate the list.
    etr.Reset();
    while(etr.MoveNext())
      Console.Write(etr.Current + " ");

    Console.WriteLine();
  }
}
```

The output is shown here:

```
0 1 2 3 4 5 6 7 8 9
0 1 2 3 4 5 6 7 8 9
```

In general, when you need to cycle through a collection, a **foreach** loop is more convenient to use than an enumerator. However, an enumerator gives you a little extra control by allowing you to reset the enumerator at will.

Using the IDictionaryEnumerator

When using a non-generic **IDictionary**, such as **Hashtable**, you will use an **IDictionaryEnumerator** instead of an **IEnumerator** when cycling through the collection. The **IDictionaryEnumerator** inherits **IEnumerator** and adds three properties. The first is

DictionaryEntry Entry { get; }

Entry obtains the next key/value pair from the enumerator in the form of a **DictionaryEntry** structure. Recall that **DictionaryEntry** defines two properties, called **Key** and **Value**, which can be used to access the key or value contained within the entry. The other two properties defined by **IDictionaryEnumerator** are shown here:

```
object Key { get; }
object Value { get; }
```

These allow you to access the key or value directly.

An **IDictionaryEnumerator** is used just like a regular enumerator, except that you will obtain the current value through the **Entry**, **Key**, or **Value** properties rather than **Current**. Thus, after obtaining an **IDictionaryEnumerator**, you must call **MoveNext( )** to obtain the first element. Continue to call **MoveNext( )** to obtain the rest of the elements in the collection. **MoveNext( )** returns false when there are no more elements.

Here is an example that enumerates the elements in a **Hashtable** through an **IDictionaryEnumerator**:

```
// Demonstrate IDictionaryEnumerator.

using System;
using System.Collections;

class IDicEnumDemo {
  static void Main() {
    // Create a hash table.
    Hashtable ht = new Hashtable();

    // Add elements to the table.
    ht.Add("Tom", "555-3456");
    ht.Add("Mary", "555-9876");
    ht.Add("Todd", "555-3452");
    ht.Add("Ken", "555-7756");

    // Demonstrate enumerator.
    IDictionaryEnumerator etr = ht.GetEnumerator();
    Console.WriteLine("Display info using Entry.");
    while(etr.MoveNext())
     Console.WriteLine(etr.Entry.Key + ": " +
                       etr.Entry.Value);

    Console.WriteLine();

    Console.WriteLine("Display info using Key and Value directly.");
    etr.Reset();
    while(etr.MoveNext())
     Console.WriteLine(etr.Key + ": " +
                       etr.Value);

  }
}
```

The output is shown here:

```
Display info using Entry.
Ken: 555-7756
Mary: 555-9876
Tom: 555-3456
Todd: 555-3452

Display info using Key and Value directly.
Ken: 555-7756
Mary: 555-9876
Tom: 555-3456
Todd: 555-3452
```

Implementing IEnumerable and IEnumerator

As mentioned earlier, normally it is easier (and better) to use a **foreach** loop to cycle through a collection than it is to explicitly use **IEnumerator** methods. However, understanding the operation of these interfaces is important for another reason: If you want to create a class that contains objects that can be enumerated via a **foreach** loop, then that class must implement **IEnumerator**. It must also implement **IEnumerable**. In other words, to enable an object of a class that you create to be used in a **foreach** loop, you must implement **IEnumerator** and **IEnumerable**, using either their generic or non-generic form. Fortunately, because these interfaces are so small, they are easy to implement.

NOTE   *Technically, in order for a class to be used with a* **foreach** *loop, it does not actually have to specify* **IEnumerator** *or* **IEnumerable** *as implemented interfaces. It does, however, have to provide their methods, which are* **GetEnumerator( )**, **Reset( )**, **MoveNext( )**, *and the property* **Current***. However, not specifying these interfaces reduces the usability of the class in a mixed-language environment.*

Here is an example that implements the non-generic versions of **IEnumerable** and **IEnumerator** so that the contents of the array encapsulated within **MyClass** can be enumerated:

```
// Implement IEnumerable and IEnumerator.
using System;
using System.Collections;

class MyClass : IEnumerator, IEnumerable {
  char[] chrs = { 'A', 'B', 'C', 'D' };
  int idx = -1;

  // Implement IEnumerable.
  public IEnumerator GetEnumerator() {
    return this;
  }

  // The following methods implement IEnumerator.

  // Return the current object.
  public object Current {
    get {
```

```
      return chrs[idx];
    }
  }

  // Advance to the next object.
  public bool MoveNext() {
    if(idx == chrs.Length-1) {
      Reset(); // reset enumerator at the end
      return false;
    }

    idx++;
    return true;
  }

  // Reset the enumerator to the start.
  public void Reset() { idx = -1; }
}

class EnumeratorImplDemo {
  static void Main() {
    MyClass mc = new MyClass();

    // Display the contents of mc.
    foreach(char ch in mc)
      Console.Write(ch + " ");

    Console.WriteLine();

    // Display the contents of mc, again.
    foreach(char ch in mc)
      Console.Write(ch + " ");

    Console.WriteLine();
  }
}
```

Here is the output:

```
A B C D
A B C D
```

In the program, first examine **MyClass**. It encapsulates a small **char** array that contains the characters A through D. An index into this array is stored in **idx**, which is initialized to −1. **MyClass** then implements both **IEnumerator** and **IEnumerable**. **GetEnumerator( )** returns a reference to the enumerator, which in this case is the current object. The **Current** property returns the next character in the array, which is the object at **idx**. The **MoveNext( )** method advances **idx** to the next location. It returns false if the end of the collection has been reached and true otherwise. **Reset( )** sets **idx** to −1. Recall that an enumerator is undefined until after the first call to **MoveNext( )**. Thus, in a **foreach** loop, **MoveNext( )** is automatically called before **Current**. This is why *idx* must initially be −1; it is advanced to zero when the **foreach** loop begins. A generic implementation would work in a similar fashion.

Inside **Main( )**, an object of type **MyClass** called **mc** is created and the contents of the object are twice displayed by use of a **foreach** loop.

Using Iterators

As the preceding example shows, it is not difficult to implement **IEnumerator** and **IEnumerable**. However, it can be made even easier through the use of an *iterator*. An iterator is a method, operator, or accessor that returns the members of a set of objects, one member at a time, from start to finish. For example, assuming some array that has five elements, then an iterator for that array will return those five elements, one at a time. By implementing an iterator, you make it possible for an object of a class to be used in a **foreach** loop.

Let's begin with an example of a simple iterator. The following program is a modified version of the preceding program that uses an iterator rather than explicitly implementing **IEnumerator** and **IEnumerable**.

```
// A simple example of an iterator.

using System;
using System.Collections;

class MyClass {
  char[] chrs = { 'A', 'B', 'C', 'D' };

  // This iterator returns the characters
  // in the chrs array.
  public IEnumerator GetEnumerator() {
    foreach(char ch in chrs)
      yield return ch;
  }
}

class ItrDemo {
  static void Main() {
    MyClass mc = new MyClass();

    foreach(char ch in mc)
      Console.Write(ch + " ");

    Console.WriteLine();
  }
}
```

The output is shown here:

```
A B C D
```

As you can see, the contents of **mc.chrs** were enumerated.

Let's examine this program carefully. First, notice that **MyClass** does not specify **IEnumerator** as an implemented interface. When creating an iterator, the compiler automatically implements this interface for you. Second, pay special attention to the **GetEnumerator( )** method, which is shown again here for your convenience.

PART II

```
// This iterator returns the characters
// in the chrs array.
public IEnumerator GetEnumerator() {
  foreach(char ch in chrs)
    yield return ch;
}
```

This is the iterator for **MyClass**. Notice that it implicitly implements the **GetEnumerator( )** method defined by **IEnumerable**. Now, look at the body of the method. It contains a **foreach** loop that returns the elements in **chrs**. It does this through the use of a **yield return** statement. The **yield return** statement returns the next object in the collection, which in this case is the next character in **chrs**. This feature enables **mc** (a **MyClass** object) to be used within the **foreach** loop inside **Main( )**.

The term **yield** is a *contextual keyword* in the C# language. This means that it only has special meaning inside an iterator block. Outside of an iterator, **yield** can be used like any other identifier.

One important point to understand is that an iterator does not need to backed by an array or other type of collection. It simply must return the next element in a group of elements. This means the elements can be dynamically constructed using an algorithm. For example, here is a version of the previous program that returns all uppercase letters in the alphabet. Instead of using an array, it generates the letters using a **for** loop.

```
// Iterated values can be dynamically constructed.

using System;
using System.Collections;

class MyClass {
  char ch = 'A';

  // This iterator returns the letters of the alphabet.
  public IEnumerator GetEnumerator() {
    for(int i=0; i < 26; i++)
      yield return (char) (ch + i);
  }
}

class ItrDemo2 {
  static void Main() {
    MyClass mc = new MyClass();

    foreach(char ch in mc)
      Console.Write(ch + " ");

    Console.WriteLine();
  }
}
```

The output is shown here:

```
A B C D E F G H I J K L M N O P Q R S T U V W X Y Z
```

Stopping an Iterator

You can stop an iterator early by using this form of the **yield** statement:

yield break;

When this statement executes, the iterator signals that the end of the collection has been reached, which effectively stops the iterator.

The following program modifies the preceding program so that it displays only the first ten letters in the alphabet.

```
// Use yield break.

using System;
using System.Collections;

class MyClass {
  char ch = 'A';

  // This iterator returns the first 10
  // letters of the alphabet.
  public IEnumerator GetEnumerator() {
    for(int i=0; i < 26; i++) {
      if(i == 10) yield break; // stop iterator early
      yield return (char) (ch + i);
    }
  }
}

class ItrDemo3 {
  static void Main() {
    MyClass mc = new MyClass();

    foreach(char ch in mc)
      Console.Write(ch + " ");

    Console.WriteLine();
  }
}
```

The output is shown here:

```
A B C D E F G H I J
```

Using Multiple yield Directives

You can have more than one **yield** statement in an iterator. However, each **yield** must return the next element in the collection. For example, consider this program:

```
// Multiple yield statements are allowed.

using System;
using System.Collections;
```

PART II

```
class MyClass {
  // This iterator returns the letters
  // A, B, C, D, and E.
  public IEnumerator GetEnumerator() {
    yield return 'A';
    yield return 'B';
    yield return 'C';
    yield return 'D';
    yield return 'E';
  }
}

class ItrDemo5 {
  static void Main() {
    MyClass mc = new MyClass();

    foreach(char ch in mc)
      Console.Write(ch + " ");

    Console.WriteLine();
  }
}
```

The output is shown here:

```
A  B  C  D  E
```

Inside **GetEnumerator( )**, five yield statements occur. The important thing to understand is that they are executed one at a time, in order, each time another element in the collection is obtained. Thus, each time through the **foreach** loop in **Main( )**, one character is returned.

Creating a Named Iterator

Although the preceding examples have shown the easiest way to implement an iterator, there is an alternative: the named iterator. In this approach, you create a method, operator, or accessor that returns a reference to an **IEnumerable** object. Your code will use this object to supply the iterator. A named iterator is a method with the following general form:

```
public IEnumerable itr-name(param-list) {
  // ...
  yield return obj;

}
```

Here, *itr-name* is the name of the method, *param-list* specifies zero or more parameters that will be passed to the iterator method, and *obj* is the next object returned by the iterator. Once you have created a named iterator, you can use it anywhere that an iterator is needed. For example, you can use the named iterator to control a **foreach** loop.

Named iterators are very useful in some circumstances because they allow you to pass arguments to the iterator that control what elements are obtained. For example, you might pass the iterator the beginning and ending points of a range of elements to iterate. This form of iterator can also be overloaded, further adding to its flexibility. The following program

illustrates two ways that a named iterator can be used to obtain elements. One enumerates a range of elements given the endpoints. The other enumerates the elements beginning at the start of the sequence and ending at the specified stopping point.

```
// Use named iterators.

using System;
using System.Collections;

class MyClass {
  char ch = 'A';

  // This iterator returns the letters
  // of the alphabet, beginning at A and
  // stopping at the specified stopping point.
  public IEnumerable MyItr(int end) {
    for(int i=0; i < end; i++)
      yield return (char) (ch + i);
  }

  // This iterator returns the specified
  // range of letters.
  public IEnumerable MyItr(int begin, int end) {
    for(int i=begin; i < end; i++)
      yield return (char) (ch + i);
  }
}

class ItrDemo4 {
  static void Main() {
    MyClass mc = new MyClass();

    Console.WriteLine("Iterate the first 7 letters:");
    foreach(char ch in mc.MyItr(7))
      Console.Write(ch + " ");

    Console.WriteLine("\n");


    Console.WriteLine("Iterate letters from F to L:");
    foreach(char ch in mc.MyItr(5, 12))
      Console.Write(ch + " ");

    Console.WriteLine();
  }
}
```

The output is shown here:

```
Iterate the first 7 letters:
A B C D E F G

Iterate letters from F to L:
F G H I J K L
```

Creating a Generic Iterator

The preceding examples of iterators have been non-generic, but it is, of course, also possible to create generic iterators. Doing so is quite easy: Simply return an object of the generic **IEnumerator<T>** or **IEnumerable<T>** type. Here is an example that creates a generic iterator:

```
// A simple example of a generic iterator.

using System;
using System.Collections.Generic;

class MyClass<T> {
  T[] array;

  public MyClass(T[] a) {
    array = a;
  }

  // This iterator returns the characters
  // in the chrs array.
  public IEnumerator<T> GetEnumerator() {
    foreach(T obj in array)
      yield return obj;
  }
}

class GenericItrDemo {
  static void Main() {
    int[] nums = { 4, 3, 6, 4, 7, 9 };
    MyClass<int> mc = new MyClass<int>(nums);

    foreach(int x in mc)
      Console.Write(x + " ");

    Console.WriteLine();


    bool[] bVals = { true, true, false, true };
    MyClass<bool> mc2 = new MyClass<bool>(bVals);

    foreach(bool b in mc2)
      Console.Write(b + " ");

    Console.WriteLine();
  }
}
```

The output is shown here:

```
4 3 6 4 7 9
True True False True
```

In this example, the array containing the objects to be iterated is passed to **MyClass** through its constructor. The type of the array is specified as a type argument to **MyClass**.

The **GetEnumerator( )** method operates on data of type **T** and returns an **IEnumerator<T>** enumerator. Thus, the iterator defined by **MyClass** can enumerate any type of data.

Collection Initializers

C# 3.0 includes a new feature called the *collection initializer*, which makes it easier to initialize certain collections. Instead of having to explicitly call **Add( )**, you can specify a list of initializers when a collection is created. When this is done, the compiler automatically calls **Add( )** for you, using these values. The syntax is similar to an array initialization. Here is an example. It creates a **List<char>** that is initialized by the characters C, A, E, B, D, and F.

```
List<char> lst = new List<char>() { 'C', 'A', 'E', 'B', 'D', 'F' };
```

After this statement executes, **lst.Count** will equal 6, because there are six initializers, and this **foreach** loop

```
foreach(ch in lst)
  Console.Write(ch + " ");
```

will display

```
C A E B D F
```

When using a collection such as **LinkedList<TK, TV>** that store key/value pairs, you will need to supply pairs of initializers, as shown here:

```
SortedList<int, string> lst =
  new SortedList<int, string>() { {1, "One"}, {2, "Two" }, {3, "Three"} };
```

The compiler passes each group of values as arguments to **Add( )**. Thus, the first pair of initializers is translated into a call to **Add(1, "One")** by the compiler.

Because the compiler automatically calls **Add( )** to add initializers to a collection, collection initializers can be used only with collections that support a public implementation of **Add( )**. Therefore, collection initializers cannot be used with the **Stack**, **Stack<T>**, **Queue**, or **Queue<T>** collections because they don't support **Add( )**. You also can't use a collection initializer with a collection such as **LinkedList<T>**, which provides **Add( )** as an explicit interface implementation.

Networking Through the Internet Using System.Net

C# is a language designed for the modern computing environment, of which the Internet is, obviously, an important part. A main design criteria for C# was, therefore, to include those features necessary for accessing the Internet. Although earlier languages, such as C and C++, could be used to access the Internet, support server-side operations, download files, and obtain resources, the process was not as streamlined as most programmers would like. C# remedies that situation. Using standard features of C# and the .NET Framework, it is easy to "Internet-enable" your applications and write other types of Internet-based code.

Networking support is contained in several namespaces defined by the .NET Framework. The primary namespace for networking is **System.Net**. It defines a large number of high-level, easy-to-use classes that support the various types of operations common to the Internet. Several namespaces nested under **System.Net** are also provided. For example, low-level networking control through sockets is found in **System.Net.Sockets**. Mail support is found in **System.Net.Mail**. Support for secure network streams is found in **System.Net.Security**. Several other nested namespaces provide additional functionality. Another important networking-related namespace is **System.Web**. It (and its nested namespaces) support ASP.NET-based network applications.

Although the .NET Framework offers great flexibility and many options for networking, for many applications the functionality provided by **System.Net** is a best choice. It offers both convenience and ease-of-use. For this reason, **System.Net** is the namespace we will be using in this chapter.

The System.Net Members

System.Net is a large namespace that contains many members. It is far beyond the scope of this chapter to discuss them all or to discuss all aspects related to Internet programming. (In fact, an entire book is needed to fully cover networking and C#'s support for it in detail.) However, it is worthwhile to list the members of **System.Net** so you have an idea of what is available for your use.

The classes defined by **System.Net** are shown here:

AuthenticationManager	Authorization
Cookie	CookieCollection
CookieContainer	CookieException
CredentialCache	Dns
DnsPermission	DnsPermissionAttribute
DownloadDataCompletedEventArgs	DownloadProgressChangedEventArgs
DownloadStringCompletedEventArgs	EndPoint
EndpointPermission	FileWebRequest
FileWebResponse	FtpWebRequest
FtpWebResponse	HttpListener
HttpListenerBasicIdentity	HttpListenerContext
HttpListenerException	HttpListenerPrefixCollection
HttpListenerRequest	HttpListenerResponse
HttpVersion	HttpWebRequest
HttpWebResponse	IPAddress
IPEndPoint	IPEndPointCollection
IPHostEntry	IrDAEndPoint
NetworkCredential	OpenReadCompletedEventArgs
OpenWriteCompletedEventArgs	ProtocolViolationException
ServicePoint	ServicePointManager
SocketAddress	SocketPermission
SocketPermissionAttribute	UploadDataCompletedEventArgs
UploadFileCompletedEventArgs	UploadProgressChangedEventArgs
UploadStringCompletedEventArgs	UploadValuesCompletedEventArgs
WebClient	WebException
WebHeaderCollection	WebPermission
WebPermissionAttribute	WebProxy
WebRequest	WebRequestMethods
WebRequestMethods.File	WebRequestMethods.Ftp
WebRequestMethods.Http	WebResponse

System.Net defines the following interfaces:

IAuthenticationModule	ICertificatePolicy	ICredentialPolicy
ICredentials	ICredentialsByHost	IWebProxy
IWebProxyScript	IWebRequestCreate	

It defines these enumerations:

AuthenticationSchemes	DecompressionMethods	FtpStatusCode
HttpRequestHeader	HttpResponseHeader	HttpStatusCode
NetworkAccess	SecurityProtocolType	TransportType
WebExceptionStatus		

System.Net also defines several delegates.

Although **System.Net** defines many members, only a few are needed to accomplish most common Internet programming tasks. At the core of networking are the abstract classes **WebRequest** and **WebResponse**. These classes are inherited by classes that support a specific network protocol. (A *protocol* defines the rules used to send information over a network.) For example, the derived classes that support the standard HTTP protocol are **HttpWebRequest** and **HttpWebResponse**.

Even though **WebRequest** and **WebResponse** are easy to use, for some tasks you can employ an even simpler approach based on **WebClient**. For example, if you only need to upload or download a file, then **WebClient** is often the best way to accomplish it.

Uniform Resource Identifiers

Fundamental to Internet programming is the Uniform Resource Identifier (URI). A *URI* describes the location of some resource on the network. A URI is also commonly called a *URL*, which is short for *Uniform Resource Locator.* Because Microsoft uses the term *URI* when describing the members of **System.Net**, this book will do so, too. You are no doubt familiar with URIs because you use one every time you enter an address into your Internet browser.

A URI has the following general form:

Protocol://ServerID/FilePath?Query

Protocol specifies the protocol being used, such as HTTP. *ServerID* identifies the specific server, such as mhprofessional.com or HerbSchildt.com. *FilePath* specifies the path to a specific file. If *FilePath* is not specified, the default page at the specified *ServerID* is obtained. Finally, *Query* specifies information that will be sent to the server. *Query* is optional. In C#, URIs are encapsulated by the **Uri** class, which is examined later in this chapter.

Internet Access Fundamentals

The classes contained in **System.Net** support a request/response model of Internet interaction. In this approach, your program, which is the client, requests information from the server and then waits for the response. For example, as a request, your program might send to the server the URI of some website. The response that you will receive is the hypertext associated with that URI. This request/response approach is both convenient and simple to use because most of the details are handled for you.

The hierarchy of classes topped by **WebRequest** and **WebResponse** implement what Microsoft calls *pluggable protocols*. As most readers know, there are several different types of network communication protocols. The most common for Internet use is HyperText Transfer Protocol (HTTP). Another is File Transfer Protocol (FTP). When a URI is constructed, the

prefix of the URI specifies the protocol. For example, http://www.HerbSchildt.com uses the prefix *http*, which specifies hypertext transfer protocol.

As mentioned earlier, **WebRequest** and **WebResponse** are abstract classes that define the general request/response operations that are common to all protocols. From them are derived concrete classes that implement specific protocols. Derived classes register themselves, using the static method **RegisterPrefix( )**, which is defined by **WebRequest**. When you create a **WebRequest** object, the protocol specified by the URI's prefix will automatically be used, if it is available. The advantage of this "pluggable" approach is that most of your code remains the same no matter what type of protocol you are using.

The .NET runtime automatically defines the HTTP, HTTPS, file, and FTP protocols. Thus, if you specify a URI that uses the HTTP prefix, you will automatically receive the HTTP-compatible class that supports it. If you specify a URI that uses the FTP prefix, you will automatically receive the FTP-compatible class that supports it.

Because HTTP is the most commonly used protocol, it is the only one discussed in this chapter. (The same techniques, however, will apply to all supported protocols.) The classes that support HTTP are **HttpWebRequest** and **HttpWebResponse**. These classes inherit **WebRequest** and **WebResponse** and add several members of their own, which apply to the HTTP protocol.

System.Net supports both synchronous and asynchronous communication. For many Internet uses, synchronous transactions are the best choice because they are easy to use. With synchronous communications, your program sends a request and then waits until the response is received. For some types of high-performance applications, asynchronous communication is better. Using the asynchronous approach, your program can continue processing while waiting for information to be transferred. However, asynchronous communications are more difficult to implement. Furthermore, not all programs benefit from an asynchronous approach. For example, often when information is needed from the Internet, there is nothing to do until the information is received. In cases like this, the potential gains from the asynchronous approach are not realized. Because synchronous Internet access is both easier to use and more universally applicable, it is the only type examined in this chapter.

Since **WebRequest** and **WebResponse** are at the heart of **System.Net**, they will be examined next.

WebRequest

The **WebRequest** class manages a network request. It is abstract because it does not implement a specific protocol. It does, however, define those methods and properties common to all requests. The methods defined by **WebRequest** that support synchronous communications are shown in Table 25-1. The properties defined by **WebRequest** are shown in Table 25-2. The default values for the properties are determined by derived classes. **WebRequest** defines no public constructors.

To send a request to a URI, you must first create an object of a class derived from **WebRequest** that implements the desired protocol. This is done by calling **Create( )**, which is a **static** method defined by **WebRequest**. **Create( )** returns an object of a class that inherits **WebRequest** and implements a specific protocol.

Method	Description
public static WebRequest Create(string *uri*)	Creates a **WebRequest** object for the URI specified by the string passed by *uri*. The object returned will implement the protocol specified by the prefix of the URI. Thus, the object will be an instance of a class that inherits **WebRequest**. A **NotSupportedException** is thrown if the requested protocol is not available. A **UriFormatException** is thrown if the URI format is invalid.
public static WebRequest Create(Uri *uri*)	Creates a **WebRequest** object for the URI specified by *uri*. The object returned will implement the protocol specified by the prefix of the URI. Thus, the object will be an instance of a class that inherits **WebRequest**. A **NotSupportedException** is thrown if the requested protocol is not available.
public virtual Stream GetRequestStream( )	Returns an output stream associated with the previously requested URI.
public virtual WebResponse GetResponse( )	Sends the previously created request and waits for a response. When a response is received, it is returned as a **WebReponse** object. Your program will use this object to obtain information from the specified URI.

TABLE 25-1   The Methods Defined by **WebRequest** that Support Synchronous Communications

Property	Description
public AuthenticationLevel AuthenticationLevel(get; set; }	Obtains or sets the authentication level.
public virtual RequestCachePolicy CachePolicy { get; set; }	Obtains or sets the cache policy, which controls when a response can be obtained from the cache.
public virtual string ConnectionGroupName { get; set; }	Obtains or sets the connection group name. Connection groups are a way of creating a set of requests. They are not needed for simple Internet transactions.
public virtual long ContentLength { get; set; }	Obtains or sets the length of the content.
public virtual string ContentType { get; set; }	Obtains or sets the description of the content.
public virtual ICredentials Credentials { get; set; }	Obtains or sets credentials.
public static RequestCachePolicy DefaultCachePolicy { get; set; }	Obtains or sets the default cache policy, which controls when a request can be obtained from the cache.

TABLE 25-2   The Properties Defined by **WebRequest**

Property	Description
public static IWebProxy DefaultWebProxy { get; set; }	Obtains or sets the default proxy.
public virtual WebHeaderCollection Headers{ get; set; }	Obtains or sets a collection of the headers.
public TokenImpersonationLevel ImpersonationLevel { get; set; }	Obtains or sets the impersonation level.
public virtual string Method { get; set; }	Obtains or sets the protocol.
public virtual bool PreAuthenticate { get; set; }	If true, authentication information is included when the request is sent. If false, authentication information is provided only when requested by the URI.
public virtual IWebProxy Proxy { get; set; }	Obtains or sets the proxy server. This applies only to environments in which a proxy server is used.
public virtual Uri RequestUri { get; }	Obtains the URI of the request.
public virtual int Timeout { get; set; }	Obtains or sets the number of milliseconds that a request will wait for a response. To wait forever, use **Timeout.Infinite**.
public virtual bool UseDefaultCredential { get; set; }	Obtains or sets a value that determines if default credentials are used for authentication. If true, the default credentials (i.e., those of the user) are used. They are not used if false.

TABLE 25-2   The Properties Defined by **WebRequest** *(continued)*

WebResponse

WebResponse encapsulates a response that is obtained as the result of a request. **WebResponse** is an abstract class. Inheriting classes create specific, concrete versions of it that support a protocol. A **WebResponse** object is normally obtained by calling the **GetResponse( )** method defined by **WebRequest**. This object will be an instance of a concrete class derived from **WebResponse** that implements a specific protocol. The methods defined by **WebResponse** that are most commonly used are shown in Table 25-3. The properties defined by **WebResponse** are shown in Table 25-4. The values of these properties are set based on each individual response. **WebResponse** defines no public constructors.

HttpWebRequest and HttpWebResponse

The classes **HttpWebRequest** and **HttpWebResponse** inherit the **WebRequest** and **WebResponse** classes and implement the HTTP protocol. In the process, both add several properties that give you detailed information about an HTTP transaction. Some of these

Method	Description
public virtual void Close( )	Closes the response. It also closes the response stream returned by **GetResponseStream( )**.
public virtual Stream GetResponseStream( )	Returns an input stream connected to the requested URI. Using this stream, data can be read from the URI.

TABLE 25-3   Commonly Used Methods Defined by **WebResponse**

properties are used later in this chapter. However, for simple Internet operations, you will not often need to use these extra capabilities.

A Simple First Example

Internet access centers around **WebRequest** and **WebResponse**. Before we examine the process in detail, it will be useful to see an example that illustrates the request/response approach to Internet access. After you see these classes in action, it is easier to understand why they are organized as they are.

The following program performs a simple, yet very common, Internet operation. It obtains the hypertext contained at a specific website. In this case, the content of McGraw-Hill.com is obtained, but you can substitute any other website. The program displays the

Property	Description
public virtual long ContentLength { get; set; }	Obtains or sets the length of the content being received. This will be −1 if the content length is not available.
public virtual string ContentType { get; set; }	Obtains or sets a description of the content.
public virtual WebHeaderCollection Headers { get; }	Obtains a collection of the headers associated with the URI.
public virtual bool IsFromCache { get; }	If the response came from the cache, this property is true. It is false if the response was delivered over the network.
public virtual bool IsMutuallyAuthenticated { get; }	If the client and server are both authenticated, then this property is true. It is false otherwise.
public virtual Uri ResponseUri { get; }	Obtains the URI that generated the response. This may differ from the one requested if the response was redirected to another URI.

TABLE 25-4   The Properties Defined by **WebResponse**

hypertext on the screen in chunks of 400 characters, so you can see what is being received before it scrolls off the screen.

```
// Access a website.

using System;
using System.Net;
using System.IO;

class NetDemo {
  static void Main() {
    int ch;

    // First, create a WebRequest to a URI.
    HttpWebRequest req = (HttpWebRequest)
          WebRequest.Create("http://www.McGraw-Hill.com");

    // Next, send that request and return the response.
    HttpWebResponse resp = (HttpWebResponse)
          req.GetResponse();

    // From the response, obtain an input stream.
    Stream istrm = resp.GetResponseStream();


    /* Now, read and display the html present at
       the specified URI. So you can see what is
       being displayed, the data is shown
       400 characters at a time. After each 400
       characters are displayed, you must press
       ENTER to get the next 400. */

    for(int i=1; ; i++) {
      ch =  istrm.ReadByte();
      if(ch == -1) break;
      Console.Write((char) ch);
      if((i%400)==0) {
        Console.Write("\nPress Enter.");
        Console.ReadLine();
      }
    }

    // Close the response. This also closes istrm.
    resp.Close();
  }
}
```

The first part of the output is shown here. (Of course, over time this content will differ from that shown here.)

```
<html>
<head>
<title>Home - The McGraw-Hill Companies</title>
<meta name="keywords" content="McGraw-Hill Companies,McGraw-Hill, McGraw Hill,
Aviation Week, BusinessWeek, Standard and Poor's, Standard & Poor's,CTB/Mc-
```

PART II

```
Graw-Hill,Glencoe/McGraw-Hill,The Grow Network/McGraw-Hill,Macmillan/McGraw-
Hill,McGraw-Hill Contemporary,McGraw-Hill Digital Learning,McGraw-Hill Professional
Development,SRA/McGraw-Hi
Press Enter.
ll,Wright Group/McGraw-Hill,McGraw-Hill Higher Education,McGraw-Hill/Irwin,McGraw-
Hill/Primis Custom Publishing,McGraw-Hill/Ryerson,Tata/McGraw-Hill,McGraw-Hill
Interamericana,Open University Press, Healthcare Information Group, Platts, McGraw-
Hill Construction, Information & Media Services" />
<meta name="description" content="The McGraw-Hill Companies Corporate Website." />
<meta http-equiv="Con
Press Enter.
tent-Type" content="text/html; charset=iso-8859-1">
<META HTTP-EQUIV="Refresh" CONTENT="900">
<META HTTP-EQUIV="EXPIRES" CONTENT="-1">
<META HTTP-EQUIV="Pragma" CONTENT="no-cache">
<link rel="stylesheet" href="stylesheet.css" type="text/css" media="screen,projecti
on">
<link rel="stylesheet" href="print.css" type"text/css" media="print">

<script language="JavaScript1.2" src="scripts.js"></script>

Press Enter.
```

This is part of the hypertext associated with the McGraw-Hill.com website. Because the program simply displays the content character-by-character, it is not formatted as it would be by a browser; it is displayed in its raw form.

Let's examine this program line-by-line. First, notice that the **System.Net** namespace is used. As explained, this is the namespace that contains the networking classes. Also notice that **System.IO** is included. This namespace is needed because the information from the website is read using a **Stream** object.

The program begins by creating a **WebRequest** object that contains the desired URI. Notice that the **Create( )** method, rather than a constructor, is used for this purpose. **Create( )** is a **static** member of **WebRequest**. Even though **WebRequest** is an abstract class, it is still possible to call a **static** method of that class. **Create( )** returns a **WebRequest** object that has the proper protocol "plugged in," based on the protocol prefix of the URI. In this case, the protocol is HTTP. Thus, **Create( )** returns an **HttpWebRequest** object. Of course, its return value must still be cast to **HttpWebRequest** when it is assigned to the **HttpWebRequest** reference called **req**. At this point, the request has been created, but not yet sent to the specified URI.

To send the request, the program calls **GetResponse( )** on the **WebRequest** object. After the request has been sent, **GetResponse( )** waits for a response. Once a response has been received, **GetResponse( )** returns a **WebResponse** object that encapsulates the response. This object is assigned to **resp**. Since, in this case, the response uses the HTTP protocol, the result is cast to **HttpWebResponse**. Among other things, the response contains a stream that can be used to read data from the URI.

Next, an input stream is obtained by calling **GetResponseStream( )** on **resp**. This is a standard **Stream** object, having all of the attributes and features of any other input stream. A reference to the stream is assigned to **istrm**. Using **istrm**, the data at the specified URI can be read in the same way that a file is read.

Next, the program reads the data from McGraw-Hill.com and displays it on the screen. Because there is a lot of information, the display pauses every 400 characters and waits for you to press ENTER. This way the first part of the information won't simply scroll off the

screen. Notice that the characters are read using **ReadByte( )**. Recall that this method returns the next byte from the input stream as an **int**, which must be cast to **char**. It returns –1 when the end of the stream has been reached.

Finally, the response is closed by calling **Close( )** on **resp**. Closing the response stream automatically closes the input stream, too. It is important to close the response between each request. If you don't, it is possible to exhaust the network resources and prevent the next connection.

Before leaving this example, one other important point needs to be made: It was not actually necessary to use an **HttpWebRequest** or **HttpWebResponse** object to display the hypertext received from the server. Because the preceding program did not use any HTTP-specific features, the standard methods defined by **WebRequest** and **WebResponse** were sufficient to handle this task. Thus, the calls to **Create( )** and **GetResponse( )** could have been written like this:

```
// First, create a WebRequest to a URI.
WebRequest req =  WebRequest.Create("http://www.McGraw-Hill.com");

// Next, send that request and return the response.
WebResponse resp =  req.GetResponse();
```

In cases in which you don't need to employ a cast to a specific type of protocol implementation, it is better to use **WebRequest** and **WebResponse** because it allows protocols to be changed with no impact on your code. However, since all of the examples in this chapter will be using HTTP, and a few will be using HTTP-specific features, the programs will use **HttpWebRequest** and **HttpWebResponse**.

Handling Network Errors

Although the program in the preceding section is correct, it is not resilient. Even the simplest network error will cause it to end abruptly. Although this isn't a problem for the example programs shown in this chapter, it is something that must be avoided in real-world applications. To fully handle all network exceptions that the program might generate, you must monitor calls to **Create( )**, **GetResponse( )**, and **GetResponseStream( )**. It is important to understand that the exceptions that can be generated depend upon the protocol being used. The following discussion describes the errors possible when using HTTP.

Exceptions Generated by Create( )

The **Create( )** method defined by **WebRequest** can generate four exceptions. If the protocol specified by the URI prefix is not supported, then **NotSupportedException** is thrown. If the URI format is invalid, **UriFormatException** is thrown. If the user does not have the proper authorization, a **System.Security.SecurityException** will be thrown. **Create( )** can also throw an **ArgumentNullException** if it is called with a null reference, but this is not an error generated by networking.

Exceptions Generated by GetReponse( )

A number of errors can occur when obtaining an HTTP response by calling **GetResponse( )**. These are represented by the following exceptions: **InvalidOperationException**, **ProtocolViolationException**, **NotSupportedException**, and **WebException**. Of these, the one of most interest is **WebException**.

WebException has two properties that relate to network errors: **Response** and **Status**. You can obtain a reference to the **WebResponse** object inside an exception handler through the **Response** property. For the HTTP protocol, this object describes the error. It is defined like this:

> public WebResponse Response { get; }

When an error occurs, you can use the **Status** property of **WebException** to find out what went wrong. It is defined like this:

> public WebExceptionStatus Status {get; }

WebExceptionStatus is an enumeration that contains the following values:

CacheEntryNotFound	ConnectFailure	ConnectionClosed
KeepAliveFailure	MessageLengthLimitExceeded	NameResolutionFailure
Pending	PipelineFailure	ProtocolError
ProxyNameResolutionFailure	ReceiveFailure	RequestCanceled
RequestProhibitedByCachePolicy	RequestProhibitedByProxy	SecureChannelFailure
SendFailure	ServerProtocolViolation	Success
Timeout	TrustFailure	UnknownError

Once the cause of the error has been determined, your program can take appropriate action.

Exceptions Generated by GetResponseStream( )

For the HTTP protocol, the **GetResponseStream( )** method of **WebResponse** can throw a **ProtocolViolationException**, which, in general, means that some error occurred relative to the specified protocol. As it relates to **GetResponseStream( )**, it means that no valid response stream is available. An **ObjectDisposedException** will be thrown if the response has already been disposed. Of course, an **IOException** could occur while reading the stream, depending on how input is accomplished.

Using Exception Handling

The following program adds handlers for all possible network exceptions to the example shown earlier:

```
// Handle network exceptions.

using System;
using System.Net;
using System.IO;

class NetExcDemo {
  static void Main() {
    int ch;

    try {

      // First, create a WebRequest to a URI.
      HttpWebRequest req = (HttpWebRequest)
```

```
                WebRequest.Create("http://www.McGraw-Hill.com");

        // Next, send that request and return the response.
        HttpWebResponse resp = (HttpWebResponse)
              req.GetResponse();

        // From the response, obtain an input stream.
        Stream istrm = resp.GetResponseStream();

        /* Now, read and display the html present at
           the specified URI. So you can see what is
           being displayed, the data is shown
           400 characters at a time. After each 400
           characters are displayed, you must press
           ENTER to get the next 400. */

        for(int i=1; ; i++) {
          ch =  istrm.ReadByte();
          if(ch == -1) break;
          Console.Write((char) ch);
          if((i%400)==0) {
            Console.Write("\nPress Enter.");
            Console.ReadLine();
          }
        }

        // Close the response. This also closes istrm.
        resp.Close();

    } catch(WebException exc) {
      Console.WriteLine("Network Error: " + exc.Message +
                        "\nStatus code: " + exc.Status);
    } catch(ProtocolViolationException exc) {
      Console.WriteLine("Protocol Error: " + exc.Message);
    } catch(UriFormatException exc) {
      Console.WriteLine("URI Format Error: " + exc.Message);
    } catch(NotSupportedException exc) {
      Console.WriteLine("Unknown Protocol: " + exc.Message);
    } catch(IOException exc) {
      Console.WriteLine("I/O Error: " + exc.Message);
    } catch(System.Security.SecurityException exc) {
      Console.WriteLine("Security Exception: " + exc.Message);
    } catch(InvalidOperationException exc) {
      Console.WriteLine("Invalid Operation: " + exc.Message);
    }
  }
}
```

Now the exceptions that the networking methods might generate have been caught. For example, if you change the call to **Create( )** as shown here,

```
WebRequest.Create("http://www.McGraw-Hill.com/moonrocket");
```

and then recompile and run the program, you will see this output:

```
Network Error: The remote server returned an error: (404) Not Found.
Status code: ProtocolError
```

Since the McGraw-Hill.com website does not have a directory called "moonrocket," this URI is not found, as the output confirms.

To keep the examples short and uncluttered, most of the programs in this chapter will not contain full exception handling. However, your real-world applications must.

The Uri Class

In Table 25-1, notice that **WebRequest.Create( )** has two different versions. One accepts the URI as a string. This is the version used by the preceding programs. The other takes the URI as an instance of the **Uri** class, which is defined in the **System** namespace. The **Uri** class encapsulates a URI. Using **Uri**, you can construct a URI that can be passed to **Create( )**. You can also dissect a **Uri**, obtaining its parts. Although you don't need to use **Uri** for many simple Internet operations, you may find it valuable in more sophisticated situations.

Uri defines several constructors. Two commonly used ones are shown here:

> public Uri(string *uri*)
> public Uri(Uri *base*, string *rel*)

The first form constructs a **Uri** given a URI in string form. The second constructs a **Uri** by adding a relative URI specified by *rel* to an absolute base URI specified by *base*. An absolute URI defines a complete URI. A relative URI defines only the path.

Uri defines many fields, properties, and methods that help you manage URIs or that give you access to the various parts of a URI. Of particular interest are the properties shown here:

Property	Description
public string Host { get; }	Obtains the name of the server.
public string LocalPath { get; }	Obtains the local file path.
public string PathAndQuery { get; }	Obtains the absolute path and query string.
public int Port { get; }	Obtains the port number for the specified protocol. For HTTP, the port is 80.
public string Query { get; }	Obtains the query string.
public string Scheme { get; }	Obtains the protocol.

These properties are useful for breaking a URI into its constituent parts. The following program demonstrates their use:

```
// Use Uri.

using System;
using System.Net;
```

```
class UriDemo {
  static void Main() {

    Uri sample = new Uri("http://HerbSchildt.com/somefile.txt?SomeQuery");

    Console.WriteLine("Host: " + sample.Host);
    Console.WriteLine("Port: " + sample.Port);
    Console.WriteLine("Scheme: " + sample.Scheme);
    Console.WriteLine("Local Path: " + sample.LocalPath);
    Console.WriteLine("Query: " + sample.Query);
    Console.WriteLine("Path and query: " + sample.PathAndQuery);

  }
}
```

The output is shown here:

```
Host: HerbSchildt.com
Port: 80
Scheme: http
Local Path: /somefile.txt
Query: ?SomeQuery
Path and query: /somefile.txt?SomeQuery
```

Accessing Additional HTTP Response Information

When using **HttpWebResponse**, you have access to information other than the content of
the specified resource. This information includes such things as the time the resource was
last modified and the name of the server, and is available through various properties
associated with the response. These properties, which include the six defined by
WebResponse, are shown in Table 25-5. The following sections illustrate how to use
representative samples.

Accessing the Header

You can access the header information associated with an HTTP response through the
Headers property defined by **HttpWebResponse**. It is shown here:

    public WebHeaderCollection Headers{ get; }

An HTTP header consists of pairs of names and values represented as strings. Each name/
value pair is stored in a **WebHeaderCollection**. This specialized collection stores key/value
pairs and can be used like any other collection. (See Chapter 24.) A **string** array of the names
can be obtained from the **AllKeys** property. You can obtain the values associated with a
name by calling the **GetValues( )** method. It returns an array of strings that contains the
values associated with the header passed as an argument. **GetValues( )** is overloaded to
accept a numeric index or the name of the header.

Property	Description
public string CharacterSet { get; }	Obtains the name of the character set being used.
public string ContentEncoding { get; }	Obtains the name of the encoding scheme.
public long ContentLength { get; }	Obtains the length of the content being received. This will be −1 if the content length is not available.
public string ContentType { get; }	Obtains a description of the content.
public CookieCollection Cookies { get; set; }	Obtains or sets a list of the cookies attached to the response.
public WebHeaderCollection Headers{ get; }	Obtains a collection of the headers attached to the response.
public bool IsFromCache { get; }	If the response came from the cache, this property is true. It is false if the response was delivered over the network.
public bool IsMutuallyAuthenticated { get; }	If the client and server are both authenticated, then this property is true. It is false otherwise.
public DateTime LastModified { get; }	Obtains the time at which the resource was last changed.
public string Method { get; }	Obtains a string that specifies the response method.
public Version ProtocolVersion { get; }	Obtains a **Version** object that describes the version of HTTP used in the transaction.
public Uri ReponseUri { get; }	Obtains the URI that generated the response. This may differ from the one requested if the response was redirected to another URI.
public string Server { get; }	Obtains a string that represents the name of the server.
public HttpStatusCode StatusCode { get; }	Obtains an **HttpStatusCode** object that describes the status of the transaction.
public string StatusDescription { get; }	Obtains a string that represents the status of the transaction in a human-readable form.

TABLE 25-5   The Properties Defined by **HttpWebResponse**

The following program displays headers associated with McGraw-Hill.com:

```
// Examine the headers.

using System;
using System.Net;
```

```
class HeaderDemo {
  static void Main() {

    // Create a WebRequest to a URI.
    HttpWebRequest req = (HttpWebRequest)
        WebRequest.Create("http://www.McGraw-Hill.com");

    // Send that request and return the response.
    HttpWebResponse resp = (HttpWebResponse)
        req.GetResponse();

    // Obtain a list of the names.
    string[] names = resp.Headers.AllKeys;

    // Display the header name/value pairs.
    Console.WriteLine("{0,-20}{1}\n", "Name", "Value");
    foreach(string n in names) {
      Console.Write("{0,-20}", n);
      foreach(string v in resp.Headers.GetValues(n))
        Console.WriteLine(v);
    }

    // Close the response.
    resp.Close();
  }
}
```

Here is the output that was produced. (Remember, all header information is subject to change, so the precise output that you see may differ.)

```
Name                Value

Transfer-encoding   chunked
Content-Type        text/html
Date                Fri, 27 Jun 2008 20:32:06 GMT
Server              Sun-ONE-Web-Server/6.1
```

Accessing Cookies

You can gain access to the cookies associated with an HTTP response through the **Cookies** property defined by **HttpWebResponse**. Cookies contain information that is stored by a browser. They consist of name/value pairs, and they facilitate certain types of web access. The **Cookies** property is defined like this:

public CookieCollection Cookies { get; set; }

CookieCollection implements **ICollection** and **IEnumerable** and can be used like any other collection. (See Chapter 24.) It has an indexer that allows a cookie to be obtained by specifying its index or its name.

CookieCollection stores objects of type **Cookie**. **Cookie** defines several properties that give you access to the various pieces of information associated with a cookie. The two that we will use here are **Name** and **Value**, which are defined like this:

public string Name { get; set; }
public string Value { get; set; }

The name of the cookie is contained in **Name**, and its value is found in **Value**.

To obtain a list of the cookies associated with a response, you must supply a cookie container with the request. For this purpose, **HttpWebRequest** defines the property **CookieContainer**, shown here:

public CookieContainer CookieContainer { get; set; }

CookieContainer provides various fields, properties, and methods that let you store cookies. By default, this property is null. To use cookies, you must set it equal to an instance of the **CookieContainer** class. For many applications, you won't need to work with the **CookieContainer** property directly. Instead, you will use the **CookieCollection** obtained from the response. **CookieContainer** simply provides the underlying storage mechanism for the cookies.

The following program displays the names and values of the cookies associated with the URI specified on the command line. Remember, not all websites use cookies, so you might have to try a few until you find one that does.

```
/* Examine Cookies.

   To see what cookies a website uses,
   specify its name on the command line.
   For example, if you call this program
   CookieDemo, then

      CookieDemo http://msn.com

   displays the cookies associated with msn.com.
*/

using System;
using System.Net;

class CookieDemo {
  static void Main(string[] args) {

    if(args.Length != 1) {
      Console.WriteLine("Usage: CookieDemo <uri>");
      return ;
    }

    // Create a WebRequest to the specified URI.
    HttpWebRequest req = (HttpWebRequest)
          WebRequest.Create(args[0]);

    // Get an empty cookie container.
    req.CookieContainer = new CookieContainer();

    // Send the request and return the response.
    HttpWebResponse resp = (HttpWebResponse)
          req.GetResponse();

    // Display the cookies.
    Console.WriteLine("Number of cookies: " +
                        resp.Cookies.Count);
    Console.WriteLine("{0,-20}{1}", "Name", "Value");
```

```
    for(int i=0; i < resp.Cookies.Count; i++)
      Console.WriteLine("{0, -20}{1}",
                              resp.Cookies[i].Name,
                              resp.Cookies[i].Value);

    // Close the response.
    resp.Close();
  }
}
```

Using the LastModified Property

Sometimes you will want to know when a resource was last updated. This is easy to find out when using **HttpWebResponse** because it defines the **LastModified** property. It is shown here:

    public DateTime LastModified { get; }

LastModified obtains the time that the content of the resource was last modified.

The following program displays the time and date at which the URI entered on the command line was last updated:

```
/* Use LastModified.

   To see the date on which a website was
   last modified, enter its URI on the command
   line. For example, if you call this program
   LastModifiedDemo, then to see the date of last
   modification for HerbSchildt.com enter

     LastModifiedDemo http://HerbSchildt.com
*/

using System;
using System.Net;

class LastModifiedDemo {
  static void Main(string[] args) {

    if(args.Length != 1) {
      Console.WriteLine("Usage: LastModifiedDemo <uri>");
      return ;
    }

    HttpWebRequest req = (HttpWebRequest)
          WebRequest.Create(args[0]);

    HttpWebResponse resp = (HttpWebResponse)
          req.GetResponse();

    Console.WriteLine("Last modified: " + resp.LastModified);

    resp.Close();
  }
}
```

MiniCrawler: A Case Study

To show how easy **WebRequest** and **WebReponse** make Internet programming, a skeletal web crawler called MiniCrawler will be developed. A *web crawler* is a program that moves from link to link to link. Search engines use web crawlers to catalog content. MiniCrawler is, of course, far less sophisticated than those used by search engines. It starts at the URI that you specify and then reads the content at that address, looking for a link. If a link is found, it then asks if you want to go to that link, search for another link on the existing page, or quit. Although this scheme is quite simple, it does provide an interesting example of accessing the Internet using C#.

MiniCrawler has several limitations. First, only absolute links that are specified using the **href="http** hypertext command are found. Relative links are not used. Second, there is no way to go back to an earlier link. Third, it displays only the links and no surrounding content. Despite these limitations, the skeleton is fully functional, and you will have no trouble enhancing MiniCrawler to perform other tasks. In fact, adding features to MiniCrawler is a good way to learn more about the networking classes and networking in general.

Here is the entire code for MiniCrawler:

```
/* MiniCrawler: A skeletal Web crawler.

   Usage:
     To start crawling, specify a starting
     URI on the command line. For example,
     to start at McGraw-Hill.com, use this
     command line:

       MiniCrawler http://McGraw-Hill.com

*/

using System;
using System.Net;
using System.IO;

class MiniCrawler {

  // Find a link in a content string.
  static string FindLink(string htmlstr,
                         ref int startloc) {
    int i;
    int start, end;
    string uri = null;
    string lowcasestr = htmlstr.ToLower();

    i = lowcasestr.IndexOf("href=\"http", startloc);
    if(i != -1) {
      start = htmlstr.IndexOf('"', i) + 1;
      end = htmlstr.IndexOf('"', start);
      uri = htmlstr.Substring(start, end-start);
      startloc = end;
    }
```

```
      return uri;
  }

  static void Main(string[] args) {
    string link = null;
    string str;
    string answer;

    int curloc; // holds current location in response

    if(args.Length != 1) {
      Console.WriteLine("Usage: MiniCrawler <uri>");
      return ;
    }

    string uristr = args[0]; // holds current URI

    try {

      do {
        Console.WriteLine("Linking to " + uristr);

        // Create a WebRequest to the specified URI.
        HttpWebRequest req = (HttpWebRequest)
              WebRequest.Create(uristr);

        uristr = null; // disallow further use of this URI

        // Send that request and return the response.
        HttpWebResponse resp = (HttpWebResponse)
              req.GetResponse();

        // From the response, obtain an input stream.
        Stream istrm = resp.GetResponseStream();

        // Wrap the input stream in a StreamReader.
        StreamReader rdr = new StreamReader(istrm);

        // Read in the entire page.
        str = rdr.ReadToEnd();

        curloc = 0;

        do {
          // Find the next URI to link to.
          link = FindLink(str, ref curloc);

          if(link != null) {
            Console.WriteLine("Link found: " + link);

            Console.Write("Link, More, Quit?");
            answer = Console.ReadLine();

            if(string.Compare(answer, "L", true) == 0) {
              uristr = string.Copy(link);
```

```
                  break;
            } else if(string.Compare(answer, "Q", true) == 0) {
                  break;
            } else if(string.Compare(answer, "M", true) == 0) {
                  Console.WriteLine("Searching for another link.");
            }
        } else {
            Console.WriteLine("No link found.");
            break;
        }

    } while(link.Length > 0);

    // Close the response.
    resp.Close();
  } while(uristr != null);

} catch(WebException exc) {
  Console.WriteLine("Network Error: " + exc.Message +
                    "\nStatus code: " + exc.Status);
} catch(ProtocolViolationException exc) {
  Console.WriteLine("Protocol Error: " + exc.Message);
} catch(UriFormatException exc) {
  Console.WriteLine("URI Format Error: " + exc.Message);
} catch(NotSupportedException exc) {
  Console.WriteLine("Unknown Protocol: " + exc.Message);
} catch(IOException exc) {
  Console.WriteLine("I/O Error: " + exc.Message);
}

Console.WriteLine("Terminating MiniCrawler.");
  }
}
```

Here is a short a sample session that begins crawling at McGraw-Hill.com. (Remember, the precise output will vary over time as content changes.)

```
Linking to http://mcgraw-hill.com
Link found: http://sti.mcgraw-hill.com:9000/cgi-bin/query?mss=search&pg=aq
Link, More, Quit? M
Searching for another link.
Link found: http://investor.mcgraw-hill.com/phoenix.zhtml?c=96562&p=irol-irhome
Link, More, Quit? L
Linking to http://investor.mcgraw-hill.com/phoenix.zhtml?c=96562&p=irol-irhome
Link found: http://www.mcgraw-hill.com/index.html
Link, More, Quit? L
Linking to http://www.mcgraw-hill.com/index.html
Link found: http://sti.mcgraw-hill.com:9000/cgi-bin/query?mss=search&pg=aq
Link, More, Quit? Q
Terminating MiniCrawler.
```

Let's take a close look at how MiniCrawler works. The URI at which MiniCrawler begins is specified on the command line. In **Main( )**, this URI is stored in the string called **uristr**. A request is created to this URI and then **uristr** is set to null, which indicates that this URI has already been used. Next, the request is sent and the response is obtained. The

content is then read by wrapping the stream returned by **GetResponseStream( )** inside a **StreamReader** and then calling **ReadToEnd( )**, which returns the entire contents of the stream as a string.

Using the content, the program then searches for a link. It does this by calling **FindLink( )**, which is a **static** method also defined by **MiniCrawler**. **FindLink( )** is called with the content string and the starting location at which to begin searching. The parameters that receive these values are **htmlstr** and **startloc**, respectively. Notice that **startloc** is a **ref** parameter. **FindLink( )** first creates a lowercase copy of the content string and then looks for a substring that matches **href="http**, which indicates a link. If a match is found, the URI is copied to **uri**, and the value of **startloc** is updated to the end of the link. Because **startloc** is a **ref** parameter, this causes its corresponding argument to be updated in **Main( )**, enabling the next search to begin where the previous one left off. Finally, **uri** is returned. Since **uri** was initialized to null, if no match is found, a null reference is returned, which indicates failure.

Back in **Main( )**, if the link returned by **FindLink( )** is not null, the link is displayed, and the user is asked what to do. The user can go to that link by pressing L, search the existing content for another link by pressing M, or quit the program by pressing Q. If the user presses L, the link is followed and the content of the link is obtained. The new content is then searched for a link. This process continues until all potential links are exhausted.

You might find it interesting to increase the power of MiniCrawler. For example, you might try adding the ability follow relative links. (This is not hard to do.) You might try completely automating the crawler by having it go to each link that it finds without user interaction. That is, starting at an initial page, have it go to the first link it finds. Then, in the new page, have it go to the first link and so on. Once a dead-end is reached, have it backtrack one level, find the next link, and then resume linking. To accomplish this scheme, you will need to use a stack to hold the URIs and the current location of the search within a URI. One way to do this is to use a **Stack** collection. As an extra challenge, try creating tree-like output that displays the links.

Using WebClient

Before concluding this chapter, a brief discussion of **WebClient** is warranted. As mentioned near the start of this chapter, if your application only needs to upload or download data to or from the Internet, then you can use **WebClient** instead of **WebRequest** and **WebResponse**. The advantage to **WebClient** is that it handles many of the details for you.

WebClient defines one constructor, shown here:

public WebClient( )

WebClient defines the properties shown in Table 25-6. **WebClient** defines a large number of methods that support both synchronous and asynchronous communication. Because asynchronous communication is beyond the scope of this chapter, only those methods that support synchronous requests are shown in Table 25-7. All methods throw a **WebException** if an error occurs during transmission.

The following program demonstrates how to use **WebClient** to download data into a file:

```
// Use WebClient to download information into a file.

using System;
using System.Net;
using System.IO;
```

```
class WebClientDemo {
  static void Main() {
    WebClient user = new WebClient();
    string uri = "http://www.McGraw-Hill.com";
    string fname = "data.txt";

    try {
      Console.WriteLine("Downloading data from " +
                        uri + " to " + fname);
      user.DownloadFile(uri, fname);
    } catch (WebException exc) {
      Console.WriteLine(exc);
    }

    Console.WriteLine("Download complete.");
  }
}
```

Property	Description
public string BaseAddress { get; set; }	Obtains or sets the base address of the desired URI. If this property is set, then addresses specified by the **WebClient** methods will be relative to the base address.
public RequestCachePolicy CachePolicy { get; set; }	Obtains or sets the policy that determines when the cache is used.
public ICredentials Credentials { get; set; }	Obtains or sets authentication information. This property is null by default.
public Encoding Encoding { get; set; }	Obtains or sets the character encoding used while transferring strings.
public WebHeaderCollection Headers{ get; set; }	Obtains or sets the collection of the request headers.
public bool IsBusy(get; }	If the request is still transferring information, this property is true. It is false otherwise.
public IWebProxy Proxy { get; set; }	Obtains or sets the proxy.
public NameValueCollection QueryString { get; set; }	Obtains or sets a query string consisting of name/value pairs that can be attached to a request. The query string is separated from the URI by a **?**. If more than one name/value pair exists, then an @ separates each pair.
public WebHeaderCollection ResponseHeaders{ get; }	Obtains a collection of the response headers.
public bool UseDefaultCredentials { get; set; }	Obtains or sets a value that determines if default credentials are used for authentication. If true, the default credentials (i.e., those of the user) are used. They are not used if false.

TABLE 25-6   The Properties Defined by **WebClient**

Method	Description
public byte[ ] DownloadData(string *uri*)	Downloads the information at the URI specified by *uri* and returns the result in an array of bytes.
public byte[ ] DownloadData(Uri *uri*)	Downloads the information at the URI specified by *uri* and returns the result in an array of bytes.
public void DownloadFile(string *uri*, string *fname*)	Downloads the information at the URI specified by *uri* and stores the result in the file specified by *fname*.
public void DownloadFile(Uri *uri*, string *fname*)	Downloads the information at the URI specified by *uri* and stores the result in the file specified by *fname*.
public string DownloadString(string *uri*)	Downloads the information at the URI specified by *uri* and returns the result as a **string**.
public string DownloadString(Uri *uri*)	Downloads the information at the URI specified by *uri* and returns the result as a **string**.
public Stream OpenRead(string *uri*)	Returns an input stream from which the information at the URI specified by *uri* can be read. This stream must be closed after reading is completed.
public Stream OpenRead(Uri *uri*)	Returns an input stream from which the information at the URI specified by *uri* can be read. This stream must be closed after reading is completed.
public Stream OpenWrite(string *uri*)	Returns an output stream to which information can be written to the URI specified by *uri*. This stream must be closed after writing is completed.
public Stream OpenWrite(Uri *uri*)	Returns an output stream to which information can be written to the URI specified by *uri*. This stream must be closed after writing is completed.
public Stream OpenWrite(string *uri*, string *how*)	Returns an output stream to which information can be written to the URI specified by *uri*. This stream must be closed after writing is completed. The string passed in *how* specifies how the information will be written.
public Stream OpenWrite(Uri *uri*, string *how*)	Returns an output stream to which information can be written to the URI specified by *uri*. This stream must be closed after writing is completed. The string passed in *how* specifies how the information will be written.
public byte[ ] UploadData(string *uri*, byte[ ] *info*)	Writes the information specified by *info* to the URI specified by *uri*. The response is returned.
public byte[ ] UploadData(Uri *uri*, byte[ ] *info*)	Writes the information specified by *info* to the URI specified by *uri*. The response is returned.

public byte[ ]
    UploadData(string *uri*,
        string *how*,
        byte[ ] *info*)
	Writes the information specified by *info* to the URI specified by *uri*. The response is returned. The string passed in *how* specifies how the information will be written.

TABLE 25-7   The Synchronous Methods Defined by **WebClient**

This program downloads the information at McGrawHill.com and puts it into a file called **data.txt**. Notice how few lines of code are involved. By changing the string specified by **uri**, you can download information from any URI, including specific files.

Method	Description

public byte[ ]
    UploadData(Uri *uri*,
            string *how*,
            byte[ ] *info*)
	Writes the information specified by *info* to the URI specified by *uri*. The response is returned. The string passed in *how* specifies how the information will be written.

public byte[ ] UploadFile(string *uri*, string *fname*)	Writes the information in the file specified by *fname* to the URI specified by *uri*. The response is returned.
public byte[ ] UploadFile(Uri *uri*, string *fname*)	Writes the information in the file specified by *fname* to the URI specified by *uri*. The response is returned.

public byte[ ]
    UploadFile(string *uri*,
            string *how*,
            string *fname*)
	Writes the information in the file specified by *fname* to the URI specified by *uri*. The response is returned. The string passed in *how* specifies how the information will be written.

public byte[ ]
    UploadFile(Uri *uri*,
            string *how*,
            string *fname*)
	Writes the information in the file specified by *fname* to the URI specified by *uri*. The response is returned. The string passed in *how* specifies how the information will be written.

public string UploadString(string *uri*, string *str*)	Writes *str* to the URI specified by *uri*. The response is returned.
public string UploadString(Uri *uri*, string *str*)	Writes *str* to the URI specified by *uri*. The response is returned.

public string UploadString(string *uri*,
            string *how*,
            string *str*)
	Writes *str* to the URI specified by *uri*. The response is returned. The string passed in *how* specifies how the information will be written.

public string UploadString(Uri *uri*,
            string how,
            string *str*)
	Writes *str* to the URI specified by *uri*. The response is returned. The string passed in *how* specifies how the information will be written.

public byte[ ]
    UploadValues(string *uri*,
            NameValueCollection *vals*)
	Writes the values in the collection specified by *vals* to the URI specified by *uri*. The response is returned.

public byte[ ]
    UploadValues(Uri *uri*,
            NameValueCollection *vals*)
	Writes the values in the collection specified by *vals* to the URI specified by *uri*. The response is returned.

public byte[ ]
    UploadValues(string *uri*,
            string *how*,
            NameValueCollection *vals*)
	Writes the values in the collection specified by *vals* to the URI specified by *uri*. The response is returned. The string passed in *how* specifies how the information will be written.

public byte[ ]
    UploadValues(Uri *uri*,
            string *how*,
            NameValueCollection *vals*)
	Writes the values in the collection specified by *vals* to the URI specified by *uri*. The response is returned. The string passed in *how* specifies how the information will be written.

TABLE 25-7   The Synchronous Methods Defined by **WebClient** *(continued)*

Although **WebRequest** and **WebResponse** give you greater control and access to more information, **WebClient** is all that many applications will need. It is particularly useful when all you need to do is download information from the Web. For example, you might use **WebClient** to allow an application to obtain documentation updates.

Use System.Windows.Forms to Create Form-Based Windows Applications

Most of the programs shown in this book are console applications. Console applications are good for demonstrating the elements of the C# language and are appropriate for some types of utility programs, such as file filters. Of course, most modern applications are designed for the Windows' graphical user interface (GUI) environment, and this book would seem incomplete without demonstrating how to use C# to create a Windows application. Therefore, it is the topic of this, the final chapter in the book.

In the past, creating a Windows application was a challenging endeavor. It was not uncommon for a newcomer to spend several weeks just learning the basic elements and architecture of a Windows application. Fortunately, C# and the .NET Framework changes all that. The .NET Framework contains an entire subsystem devoted to Windows programming called *Windows Forms.* The primary support for Windows Forms is contained in the **System.Windows.Forms** namespace. Through the use of Windows Forms, the creation of a GUI-based Windows program has been greatly simplified, and the entire development process has been streamlined.

Before we begin it is important to emphasize one point: Windows programming is a *very* large topic, with entire series of books devoted to it. It is not possible to describe all aspects of it in a single chapter, nor is it possible to examine the classes, interfaces, properties, structures, and events in **System.Windows.Forms** in detail. There are just far too many. Instead, this chapter provides a "jump-start" to form-based Windows programming. It explains how to create a window, create a menu, implement a button, and respond to a message. Although these topics just scratch the surface of Windows programming, they will give you a base upon which to advance to other aspects of forms-based Windows programming.

A Brief History of Windows Programming

To appreciate the benefits that C# and the .NET Framework bring to Windows programming, it is necessary for you to understand a bit of its history. When Windows was first created, programs interacted directly with the Windows Application Programming Interface (API),

which is an extensive set of methods defined by Windows that programs call to access the various functions provided by Windows. API-based programs are very long and complicated. For example, even a skeletal API-based program requires about 50 lines of code. API-based programs that perform any useful function have *at least* several hundred lines of code, and real applications have several thousand lines of code. Thus, in the early days, Windows programs were difficult to write and maintain.

In response to this problem, class libraries were created that encapsulated the functionality of the API. The most important of these is the Microsoft Foundation Classes (MFC). Many readers of this book will be familiar with MFC. MFC is written in C++, and MFC-based programs are also written in C++. Because MFC brought object-oriented benefits, the process of creating a Windows program was simplified. However, MFC programs were still fairly complicated affairs, involving separate header files, code files, and resource files. Furthermore, MFC was only a "thin wrapper" around the API, so many Windows-based activities still required a significant number of explicit program statements.

C# and the .NET Framework's Forms library offer a fully object-oriented way to approach Windows programming. Instead of providing just a wrapper around the API, the Forms library defines a streamlined, integrated, logically consistent way of managing the development of a Windows application. This level of integration is made possible by the unique features of the C# language, such as delegates and events. Furthermore, because of C#'s use of garbage collection, the especially troubling problem of "memory leaks" has been nearly eliminated.

If you have already programmed for Windows using either the API or MFC, you will find the Windows Forms approach remarkably refreshing. Windows Forms makes it nearly as easy to create a Windows application as it is to create a console application.

Two Ways to Write a Form-Based Windows Application

Before we begin, an important point needs to be made. Visual Studio includes a sophisticated set of design tools that automate much of the process of creating a Windows application. Using these tools, you can visually construct and position the various controls and menus used by your application. Visual Studio will also "rough in" the classes and methods that are needed for each feature. Frankly, using the Visual Studio design tools are a good choice for creating most real-world Windows applications. However, there is no requirement that you use those tools. You can also create a Windows program by using a text editor and then compiling it, just like you can do for console-based applications.

Because this book is about C#, not Visual Studio, and because the Windows programs contained in this chapter are quite short, all programs will be shown in a form in which they can be entered using a text editor. However, the general structure, design, and organization of the programs is the same as that created by the design tools. Thus, the material in this chapter applies to either approach.

How Windows Interacts with the User

The first thing that you must learn about Windows programming is how the user and Windows interact because this defines the architecture that all Windows programs share. This interaction is fundamentally different from the console-based programs shown in the other parts of this book. When you write a console program, it is your program that initiates interaction with the operating system. For example, it is the program that requests such

things as input and output by calling **Read( )** or **WriteLine( )**. Thus, console programs call the operating system. The operating system does not call your program. However, in large measure, Windows works in the opposite way. It is Windows that calls your program. The process works like this: A program waits until it is sent a *message* by Windows. Once a message is received, your program is expected to take an appropriate action. Your program may call a method defined by Windows when responding to a message, but it is still Windows that initiates the activity. More than anything else, it is the message-based interaction with Windows that dictates the general form of all Windows programs.

There are many different types of messages that Windows may send to your program. For example, each time the mouse is clicked on a window belonging to your program, a mouse-clicked message will be sent. Another type of message is sent when a button is pressed or when a menu item is selected. Keep one fact firmly in mind: As far as your program is concerned, messages arrive randomly. This is why Windows programs resemble interrupt-driven programs. You can't know what message will be next.

Windows Forms

At the core of a C# Windows program is the *form*. A form encapsulates the basic functionality necessary to create a window, display it on the screen, and receive messages. A form can represent any type of window, including the main window of the application, a child window, or even a dialog box.

When a form is first created, it is empty. To supply functionality, you add menus and controls, such as pushbuttons, lists, and check boxes. Thus, you can think of a form as a container for other Windows objects.

When a message is sent to the window, it is translated into an event. Therefore, to handle a Windows message, you will simply register an event handler for that message with the form. Then, whenever that message is received, your event handler is automatically called.

The Form Class

A form is created by instantiating an object of the **Form** class or of any class derived from **Form**. **Form** contains significant functionality of its own, and it inherits additional functionality. Two of its most important base classes are **System.ComponentModel.Component**, which supports the .NET component model, and **System.Windows.Forms.Control**. The **Control** class defines features common to all Windows controls. Because **Form** inherits **Control**, it, too,
is a control. This fact allows forms to be used to create controls. Several of the members of **Form** and **Control** are used in the examples that follow.

A Skeletal Form-Based Windows Program

We will begin by creating a minimal form-based Windows application. This application simply creates and displays a window. It contains no other features. However, this skeleton does show the steps necessary to construct a fully functional window. This framework is the starting point upon which most types of Windows applications will be built. The skeletal form-based Windows program is shown next.

```
// A form-based Windows Skeleton.

using System;
using System.Windows.Forms;

// WinSkel is derived from Form.
class WinSkel : Form {

  public WinSkel() {
    // Give the window a name.
    Text = "A Windows Skeleton";
  }

  // Main is used only to start the application.
  [STAThread]
  static void Main() {
    WinSkel skel = new WinSkel(); // create a form

    // Enable visual styles.
    Application.EnableVisualStyles();

    // Start the window running.
    Application.Run(skel);
  }
}
```

The window created by this program is shown in Figure 26-1. Let's examine this program line-by-line. First, notice that both **System** and **System.Windows.Forms** are included. **System** is needed because of the **STAThread** attribute that precedes **Main( )**. **System.Windows.Forms** supports the Windows Forms subsystem, as just explained.

Next, a class called **WinSkel** is created. It inherits **Form**. Thus, **WinSkel** defines a specific type of form. In this case, it is a minimal form.

Inside the **WinSkel** constructor is the following line of code:

```
Text = "A Windows Skeleton";
```

Text is the property that sets the title of the window. Thus, this assignment causes the title bar in the window to contain **A Windows Skeleton**. **Text** is defined like this:

```
public override string Text { get; set; }
```

FIGURE 26-1
The skeletal form-based window

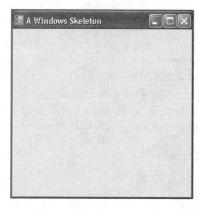

Text is inherited from **Control**.

Next is the **Main( )** method, which is declared much like the **Main( )** methods found throughout the rest of this book. It is the method at which program execution begins. Notice, however, that it is preceded by the **STAThread** attribute. As a general rule, the **Main( )** method of a Windows program should have this attribute. It sets the threading model for the program to a *single-threaded apartment* (STA). (A discussion of threading models and apartments is beyond the scope of this chapter, but briefly, a Windows application can use one of two different threading models: single-threaded apartment or multithreaded apartment.)

Inside **Main( )**, a **WinSkel** object called **skel** is created. Then, the **static** method **Application.EnableVisualStyles( )** is called. This method enables visual styles (themes) if the operating system supports it. It's not technically necessary in a Windows Forms application, but should be used because it enables better looking controls. It should be the first method called by **Main( )**. The **Application** class is defined within **System.Windows.Forms**, and it encapsulates aspects common to all Windows applications.

Next, **skel** is passed to the **Run( )** method, which is another method defined by the **Application** class, as shown here:

```
Application.Run(skel);
```

This starts the window running. The **Run( )** method used by the skeleton is shown here:

public static void Run(Form *form*)

It takes a reference to a form as a parameter. Since **WinSkel** inherits **Form**, an object of type **WinSkel** can be passed to **Run( )**.

When the program is run, it creates the window shown in Figure 26-1. The window has the default size and is fully functional. It can be resized, moved, minimized, maximized, and closed. Thus, the basic features needed by nearly all windows were achieved by writing only a few lines of form-based code. In contrast, the same program written using the C language and directly calling the Windows API would have required approximately five times as many lines of code!

The preceding skeleton defines the outline that most form-based Windows applications will take. In general, to create a form, you create a class that inherits **Form**. Initialize the form to meet your needs, create an object of your derived class, and then call **Application.Run( )** on that object.

Compiling the Windows Skeleton

You can compile a Windows program using either the command-line compiler or Visual Studio. For the very short programs shown in this chapter, the command-line compiler is the easiest way; but for real applications, you will probably want to use the IDE. (Also, as explained at the start of this chapter, you will probably want to use the design tools provided by Visual Studio, but that is not the approach described here.) Each way is shown here.

Compiling from the Command Line

Assuming that you call the skeleton **WinSkel.cs**, then to compile the skeleton from the command line, use this command:

```
csc /t:winexe WinSkel.cs
```

The **/t:winexe** switch tells the compiler to create a Windows application rather than a console program. To run the program, simply enter **WinSkel** at the command line.

Compiling from the IDE

To compile the program using the Visual Studio IDE, first create a new Windows Application project. Do this by selecting File | New Project. Then select Windows Forms Application in the New Project dialog box. Call the project **WinSkel**. Delete all C# source code files that were automatically created. Next, right-click on the WinSkel project name and select Add and then select New Item. From the Add New Item dialog box, select C# Code File, and name the file **MyWinProject.cs**. Now, enter the skeleton code exactly as shown, and then build the solution. To run the project, select Debug | Start Without Debugging.

Adding a Button

In general, the functionality of a window is expressed by two types of items: controls and menus. It is through these items that a user interacts with your program. Menus are described later in this chapter. Here you will see how to add a control to a window.

Windows defines many different types of controls, including pushbuttons, check boxes, radio buttons, and list boxes, to name just a few. Although each type of control is different, they all work in more or the less the same way. Here, we will add a pushbutton to a window, but the same basic procedure can be used to add other types of controls.

Button Basics

A pushbutton is encapsulated by the **Button** class. It inherits the abstract class **ButtonBase**, which inherits the **Control** class. **Button** defines only one constructor, which is shown here:

    public Button( )

This creates a button that has a default size and location within the window. It contains no description. Before a button can be used, it will need to be given a description by assigning a string to its **Text** property.

To specify the location of the button within the window, you must assign the coordinates of its upper-left corner to the **Location** property. The **Location** property is inherited from **Control** and defined like this:

    public Point Location { get; set; }

The coordinates are contained within a **Point** structure, which is defined in the **System.Drawing** namespace. It includes these two properties:

    public int X { get; set; }
    public int Y { get; set; }

Thus, to create a button that contains the description "Press Here" and is positioned at location 100, 200, use the following sequence:

```
Button MyButton = new Button();
MyButton.Text = "Press Here";
MyButton.Location = new Point(100, 200);
```

Adding a Button to a Form

After you have created a button, you must add it to a form. You do this by calling the **Add( )** method on the collection of controls linked to that form. This collection is available through

the **Controls** property, which is inherited from the **Control** class. The **Add( )** method is defined like this:

public virtual void Add(Control *cntl*)

Here, *cntl* is the control being added. Once a control has been added to a form, it will be displayed when the form is displayed.

A Simple Button Example

The following program adds a button to the skeleton shown earlier. At this time, the button does not do anything, but it is present in the form and can be clicked.

```
// Add a Button.

using System;
using System.Windows.Forms;
using System.Drawing;

class ButtonForm : Form {
  Button MyButton;

  public ButtonForm() {
    Text = "Using a Button";

    MyButton = new Button();
    MyButton.Text = "Press Here";
    MyButton.Location = new Point(100, 200);

    Controls.Add(MyButton);
  }

  [STAThread]
  static void Main() {
    ButtonForm skel = new ButtonForm();

    Application.EnableVisualStyles();
    Application.Run(skel);
  }
}
```

This program creates a class called **ButtonForm**, which is derived from **Form**. It contains a **Button** field called **MyButton**. Inside the constructor, the button is created, initialized, and added to the form. When run, the program displays the window shown in Figure 26-2. You can click the button, but nothing will happen. To make the button do something, you must add a message handler, as described in the next section.

Handling Messages

In order for a program to respond to a button press (or any other type of control interaction), it must handle the message that the button generates. In general, when a user interacts with a control, those interactions are passed to your program as messages. In a form-based C# program, these messages are processed by event handlers. Therefore, to receive messages,

FIGURE 26-2
Adding a button

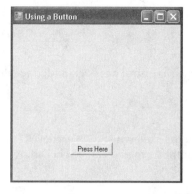

your program adds its own event handler onto the list of handlers called when a message is generated. For button-press messages, this means adding your handler to the **Click** event.

The **Click** event is specified by **Control** and defined by **Button**. It has this general form:

public Event EventHandler Click;

The **EventHandler** delegate is defined as shown here:

public delegate void EventHandler(object *who*, EventArgs *args*)

The object that generated the event is passed in *who*. Any information associated with that event is passed in *args*. For many events, *args* will be an object of a class derived from **EventArgs**. Since a button click does not require any additional information, we don't need to worry about event arguments when handling the button.

The following program adds button-response code to the preceding program. Each time the button is clicked, the location of the button is changed.

```
// Handle button messages.

using System;
using System.Windows.Forms;
using System.Drawing;

class ButtonForm : Form {
  Button MyButton;

  public ButtonForm() {
    Text = "Respond to a Button";

    MyButton = new Button();
    MyButton.Text = "Press Here";
    MyButton.Location = new Point(100, 200);

    // Add button event handler to list.
    MyButton.Click += MyButtonClick;

    Controls.Add(MyButton);
  }
```

```
[STAThread]
static void Main() {
  ButtonForm skel = new ButtonForm();

  Application.EnableVisualStyles();
  Application.Run(skel);
}

// Handler for MyButton.
void MyButtonClick(object who, EventArgs e) {

  if(MyButton.Top == 200)
    MyButton.Location = new Point(10, 10);
  else
    MyButton.Location = new Point(100, 200);
  }
}
```

Let's look closely at the event-handling code in this program. The event handler for the button click is shown here:

```
// Handler for MyButton.
void MyButtonClick(object who, EventArgs e) {

  if(MyButton.Top == 200)
    MyButton.Location = new Point(10, 10);
  else
    MyButton.Location = new Point(100, 200);
}
```

MyButtonClick( ) is compatible with the **EventHandler** delegate shown earlier, which means it can be added to the **Click** event chain. Notice it is private to **ButtonForm**. This is not technically necessary, but it is a good idea because event handlers are not intended to be called except in response to events.

Inside the handler, the location of the top of the button is determined from the **Top** property. All controls define the following properties, which specify the coordinates of the upper-left and lower-right corners:

    public int Top { get; set; }
    public int Bottom { get; }
    public int Left { get; set; }
    public int Right { get; }

Notice that the location of the control can be changed by setting **Top** and **Left**, but not by setting **Bottom** and **Right** because they are read-only. (To change the size of a control, you can use the **Width** and **Height** properties.)

When the button click event is received, if the top of the control is at its original location of 200, the location is changed to 10, 10. Otherwise, it is returned to its original location of 100, 200. Therefore, each time you click the button, the location of the button changes.

Before **MyButtonClick( )** can receive messages, it must be added to the event handler chain linked to the button's **Click** event. This is done inside the **ButtonForm** constructor, using this statement:

```
MyButton.Click += MyButtonClick;
```

After the method is added to the **Click** event, each time the button is clicked, **MyButtonClick( )** is called.

An Alternative Implementation

As a point of interest, **MyButtonClick( )** could have been written in a slightly different way. Recall that the *who* parameter of an event handler receives a reference to the object that generated the call. In the case of a button click event, this is the button that was clicked. Thus, **MyButtonClick( )** could have been written like this:

```
// An Alternative button handler.
void MyButtonClick(object who, EventArgs e) {
  Button b = (Button) who;

  if(b.Top == 200)
    b.Location = new Point(10, 10);
  else
    b.Location = new Point(100, 200);
}
```

In this version, **who** is cast to **Button**, and this reference (rather than the **MyButton** field) is used to access the button object. Although there is no advantage to this approach in this case, it is easy to imagine situations in which it would be quite valuable. For example, such an approach allows a button event handler to be written independently of any specific button.

Using a Message Box

One of the most used built-in features of Windows is the *message box*. A message box is a predefined window that lets you display a message. You can also obtain simple responses from the user, such as Yes, No, or OK. In a form-based program, a message box is supported by the **MessageBox** class. You don't create an object of that class, however. Instead, to display a message box, call the **static** method **Show( )**, which is defined by **MessageBox**.

The **Show( )** method has several forms. The one we will be using is shown here:

public static DialogResult Show(string *msg*, string *caption*,
                    MessageBoxButtons *mbb*)

The string passed through *msg* is displayed in the body of the box. The caption of the message box window is passed in *caption*. The buttons that will be displayed are specified by *mbb*. The user's response is returned.

MessageBoxButtons is an enumeration that defines the following values:

AbortRetryIgnore	OK	OKCancel
RetryCancel	YesNo	YesNoCancel

Each of these values describes the buttons that will be included in a message box. For example, if *mbb* contains **YesNo**, then the Yes and No buttons are included in the message box.

The value returned by **Show( )** indicates which button was pressed. It will be one of these values, defined by the **DialogResult** enumeration:

Abort	Cancel	Ignore	No
None	OK	Retry	Yes

Your program can examine the return value to determine the course of action the user desires. For example, if the message box prompts the user before overwriting a file, your program can prevent the overwrite if the user clicks Cancel, and it can allow the overwrite if the user clicks OK.

The following program adds a stop button and a message box to the preceding example. In the stop button handler, a message box is displayed that asks the user if he or she wants to stop the program. If the user clicks Yes, the program is stopped. If the user clicks No, the program continues running.

```
// Add a stop button.

using System;
using System.Windows.Forms;
using System.Drawing;

class ButtonForm : Form {
  Button MyButton;
  Button StopButton;

  public ButtonForm() {
    Text = "Adding a Stop Button";

    // Create the buttons.
    MyButton = new Button();
    MyButton.Text = "Press Here";
    MyButton.Location = new Point(100, 200);

    StopButton = new Button();
    StopButton.Text = "Stop";
    StopButton.Location = new Point(100, 100);

    // Add the button event handlers to the window.
    MyButton.Click += MyButtonClick;
    Controls.Add(MyButton);
    StopButton.Click += StopButtonClick;
    Controls.Add(StopButton);
  }

  [STAThread]
  static void Main() {
    ButtonForm skel = new ButtonForm();

    Application.EnableVisualStyles();
    Application.Run(skel);
  }

  // Handler for MyButton.
  void MyButtonClick(object who, EventArgs e) {

    if(MyButton.Top == 200)
      MyButton.Location = new Point(10, 10);
    else
```

```
        MyButton.Location = new Point(100, 200);
    }

    // Handler for StopButton.
    void StopButtonClick(object who, EventArgs e) {

        // If user answers Yes, terminate the program.
        DialogResult result = MessageBox.Show("Stop Program?",
                            "Terminate",
                            MessageBoxButtons.YesNo);

        if(result == DialogResult.Yes) Application.Exit();
    }
}
```

Let's look closely at how the message box is used. Inside the **ButtonForm** constructor, a second button is added. This button contains the text "Stop," and its event handler is linked to **StopButtonClick( )**.

Inside **StopButtonClick( )**, the message box is displayed by the following statement:

```
// If user answers Yes, terminate the program.
DialogResult result = MessageBox.Show("Stop Program?",
                    "Terminate",
                    MessageBoxButtons.YesNo);
```

Here, the message inside the box is "Stop Program?", the caption is "Terminate," and the buttons to be displayed are Yes and No. When **Show( )** returns, the user's response is assigned to **result**. That response is then examined by the following statement to determine the course of action:

```
if(result == DialogResult.Yes) Application.Exit();
```

If the user clicks the Yes button, the program is stopped by calling **Application.Exit( )**, which causes the immediate termination of the program. Otherwise, no action is taken, and the program continues running.

Sample output is shown in Figure 26-3.

FIGURE 26-3
Sample output
from the Stop
Button program

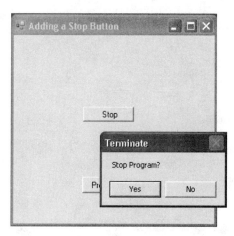

Adding a Menu

The main window of nearly all Windows applications includes a menu across the top. This is called the *main menu*. The main menu typically contains top-level categories, such as File, Edit, and Tools. From the main menu descend *drop-down menus*, which contain the actual selections associated with the categories. When a menu item is selected, a message is generated. Therefore, to process a menu selection, your program will assign an event handler to each menu item. Because menus are such a bedrock resource in Windows programming, many options are available and the topic of menus is quite large. Fortunately, it is easy to create a simple main menu.

Originally, there was only one way to create a main menu: by using the classes **MainMenu** and **MenuItem**, both of which inherit the **Menu** class. These classes create the traditional-style menus that have been used in Windows applications for years. This approach is still supported. However, version 2.0 of the .NET Framework added a second way to add menus to a window by using a set of classes based on **ToolStrip**, such as **MenuStrip** and **ToolStripMenuItem**. Menus based on **ToolStrip** have many additional capabilities and give a modern look and feel. Understand, though, that both approaches to menus are currently valid for new C# applications.

Because there are two ways to create menus, both ways are described here, beginning with the traditional approach.

Creating a Traditional-Style Main Menu

A traditional-style main menu is constructed from a combination of two classes. The first is **MainMenu**, which encapsulates the overall structure of the menu. The second is **MenuItem**, which encapsulates an individual selection. A menu selection can either represent a final action, such as Close, or activate another drop-down menu. As mentioned, both **MainMenu** and **MenuItem** inherit the **Menu** class.

When a menu item is selected, a **Click** event is generated. **Click** is defined by **MenuItem**. Therefore, to handle a menu selection, your program will add its handler to the **Click** event list for that item.

Each form has a **Menu** property, which is defined like this:

```
public MainMenu Menu { get; set; }
```

By default, no menu is assigned to this property. To display a main menu, this property must be set to the menu that you create.

Creating a main menu is straightforward, but it does involve several steps. Here is the approach we will use:

1. Create a **MainMenu** object.

2. To the **MainMenu** object, add **MenuItem**s that describe the top-level categories. This is done by calling **Add( )** on the collection referred to by the **MenuItems** property.

3. To each top-level **MenuItem**, add the list of **MenuItem**s that defines the drop-down menu associated with that top-level entry. This is also done by calling **Add( )** on the collection referred to by the **MenuItems** property.

4. Add the event handlers for each selection.

5. Assign the **MainMenu** object to the **Menu** property associated with the form.

The following sequence shows how to create a File menu that contains three selections: Open, Close, and Exit:

```
// Create a main menu object.
MainMenu MyMenu  = new MainMenu();

// Add a top-level menu item to the menu.
MenuItem m1 = new MenuItem("File");
MyMenu.MenuItems.Add(m1);

// Create File submenu.
MenuItem item1 = new MenuItem("Open");
m1.MenuItems.Add(item1);

MenuItem item2 = new MenuItem("Close");
m1.MenuItems.Add(item2);

MenuItem item3 = new MenuItem("Exit");
m1.MenuItems.Add(item3);
```

Let's examine this sequence carefully. It begins by creating a **MainMenu** object called **MyMenu**. This object will be at the top of the menu structure. This object is instantiated by use of the default constructor for **MainMenu**. This creates an empty menu.

Next, a menu item called **m1** is created. This is the File heading. It is created by using this **MenuItem** constructor:

public MenuItem(string *caption*)

Here, *caption* specifies the text that is displayed by the item. In this case, it is "File." This menu item is then added directly to **MyMenu** and is a top-level selection.

Notice that when **m1** is added to **MyMenu**, it is done through the read-only **MenuItems** property. **MenuItems** is a collection of the menu items that form a menu. It is defined by **Menu**, which means it is part of both the **MainMenu** and **MenuItem** classes. It as shown here:

public Menu.MenuItemCollection MenuItems { get; }

To add a menu item to a menu, call **Add( )** on **MenuItems**, passing in a reference to the item to add, as the example shows.

Next, the drop-down menu associated with File is created. Notice that these menu items are added to the File menu item, **m1**. When one **MenuItem** is added to another, the added item becomes part of the drop-down menu associated with the item to which it is added. Thus, after the items **item1** through **item3** have been added to **m1**, selecting File will cause a drop-down menu containing Open, Close, and Exit to be displayed.

Once the menu has been constructed, the event handlers associated with each entry must be assigned. As explained, a user making a selection generates a **Click** event. Thus, the following sequence assigns the handlers for **item1** through **item3**.

```
// Add event handlers for the menu items.
item1.Click += MMOpenClick;
item2.Click += MMCloseClick;
item3.Click += MMExitClick;
```

Therefore, if the user selects Exit, **MMExitClick( )** is executed.

Finally, the **MainMenu** object must be assigned to the **Menu** property of the form, as shown here:

```
Menu = MyMenu;
```

After this assignment takes place, the menu will be displayed when the window is created, and selections will be sent to the proper handler.

The following program puts together all the pieces and demonstrates how to create a main menu and handle menu selections.

```
// Add a Main Menu.

using System;
using System.Windows.Forms;

class MenuForm : Form {
  MainMenu MyMenu;

  public MenuForm() {
    Text = "Adding a Main Menu";

    // Create a main menu object.
    MyMenu  = new MainMenu();

    // Add top-level menu items to the menu.
    MenuItem m1 = new MenuItem("File");
    MyMenu.MenuItems.Add(m1);

    MenuItem m2 = new MenuItem("Tools");
    MyMenu.MenuItems.Add(m2);

    // Create File submenu.
    MenuItem item1 = new MenuItem("Open");
    m1.MenuItems.Add(item1);

    MenuItem item2 = new MenuItem("Close");
    m1.MenuItems.Add(item2);

    MenuItem item3 = new MenuItem("Exit");
    m1.MenuItems.Add(item3);

    // Create Tools submenu.
    MenuItem item4 = new MenuItem("Coordinates");
    m2.MenuItems.Add(item4);

    MenuItem item5 = new MenuItem("Change Size");
    m2.MenuItems.Add(item5);

    MenuItem item6 = new MenuItem("Restore");
    m2.MenuItems.Add(item6);


    // Add event handlers for the menu items.
    item1.Click += MMOpenClick;
    item2.Click += MMCloseClick;
```

```
    item3.Click += MMExitClick;
    item4.Click += MMCoordClick;
    item5.Click += MMChangeClick;
    item6.Click += MMRestoreClick;

    // Assign the menu to the form.
    Menu = MyMenu;
  }

  [STAThread]
  static void Main() {
    MenuForm skel = new MenuForm();

    Application.EnableVisualStyles();
    Application.Run(skel);
  }

  // Handler for main menu Coordinates selection.
  void MMCoordClick(object who, EventArgs e) {
    // Create a string that contains the coordinates.
    string size =
      String.Format("{0}: {1}, {2}\n{3}: {4}, {5} ",
                    "Top, Left", Top, Left,
                    "Bottom, Right", Bottom, Right);

    // Display a message box.
    MessageBox.Show(size, "Window Coordinates",
                    MessageBoxButtons.OK);
  }

  // Handler for main menu Change selection.
  void MMChangeClick(object who, EventArgs e) {
    Width = Height = 200;
  }

  // Handler for main menu Restore selection.
  void MMRestoreClick(object who, EventArgs e) {
    Width = Height = 300;
  }

  // Handler for main menu Open selection.
  void MMOpenClick(object who, EventArgs e) {

    MessageBox.Show("Inactive", "Inactive",
                    MessageBoxButtons.OK);
  }

  // Handler for main menu Close selection.
  void MMCloseClick(object who, EventArgs e) {

    MessageBox.Show("Inactive", "Inactive",
                    MessageBoxButtons.OK);
  }

  // Handler for main menu Exit selection.
```

```
    void MMExitClick(object who, EventArgs e) {

  DialogResult result = MessageBox.Show("Stop Program?",
                          "Terminate",
                            MessageBoxButtons.YesNo);

  if(result == DialogResult.Yes) Application.Exit();
  }
}
```

Sample output is shown in Figure 26-4.

This program defines two drop-down menus. The first is accessed via the File menu. It contains the Open, Close, and Exit selections. The menu handlers for Open and Close are simply placeholders that perform no function other than displaying a message box to that effect. The Close handler asks if you want to stop the program. If you answer Yes, the program is terminated.

The Tools menu has these selections: Coordinates, Change Size, and Restore. Selecting Coordinates causes the coordinates of the upper-left and lower-right corners of the window to be displayed in a message box. Try moving the window and then displaying its coordinates. Each time the window is moved to a new location, its coordinates change.

Choosing Change Size causes the window to be reduced in size so its width and height are both 200 pixels long. This is done through the **Width** and **Height** properties, shown here:

public int Width { get; set; }
public int Height { get; set; }

Selecting Restore returns the window to its default size.

Creating a New-Style Menu with MenuStrip

Although the traditional approach to creating menus described in the preceding section is still valid, the .NET Framework offers what is often a better way to manage menus that uses the **MenuStrip** control. **MenuStrip** gives your menus a modern look and additional capabilities, such as menu merging. Because of the advantages of using **MenuStrip**, its use is recommended.

The **MenuStrip** class is the modern equivalent of **MainMenu** described in the previous section. It is based on the **ToolStrip** class, which defines much of the functionality supported by the new approach to menus. **ToolStrip** is, essentially, a container for toolbar objects,

FIGURE 26-4
Sample output from the Menu program

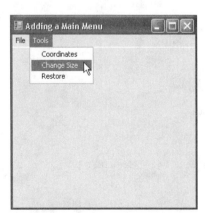

including menu items. **MenuStrip** inherits this functionality and provides specific support for menus, including the main menu. Items that are stored in a **MenuStrip** are objects of type **ToolStripMenuItem**, which is the modern equivalent of **MenuItem**, also described in the previous section.

Using **MenuStrip** and **ToolStripMenuItem** is similar to using a **MainMenu** and **MenuItem** as described in the previous section. Here is one way to create and use a **MenuStrip**:

1. Create a **MenuStrip** control.

2. To the **MenuStrip** control, add **ToolStripMenuItems** that describe the top-level categories. This is done by calling **Add( )** on the collection referred to by the **Items** property provided by **MenuStrip**.

3. To each top-level **ToolStripMenuItem**, add the list of **ToolStripMenuItems** that defines the drop-down menu associated with that top-level entry. This is done by calling **Add( )** on the collection referred to by the **DropDownItems** property.

4. Add the event handlers for each selection.

5. Add the **MenuStrip** to the list of controls for the form by calling **Add( )** on the **Controls** property.

6. Assign the **MenuStrip** control to the **MainMenuStrip** property associated with the form.

Pay special attention to Steps 2 and 3 because they differ from the parallel steps used with **MainMenu**. First, in Step 2, top-level menu items that represent submenus are added to the collection referred to by **Items**. Second, in Step 3, individual menu items are added to the collection referred to by the **DropDownItems** property. (Both **MainMenu** and **MenuItem** use the **MenuItems** property for this purpose.) Other than those differences, the two procedures are essentially the same.

The following program demonstrates **MenuStrip** by reworking the program shown in the previous section. Sample output is shown in Figure 26-5. Notice that the menu now has a modern look.

```
// Use a MenuStrip.

using System;
using System.Windows.Forms;

class MenuForm : Form {
  MenuStrip MyMenu; // use a MenuStrip

  public MenuForm() {
    Text = "Use a MenuStrip";

    // Create a main menu object.
    MyMenu  = new MenuStrip();

    // Add top-level menu items to the menu.
    ToolStripMenuItem m1 = new ToolStripMenuItem("File");
    MyMenu.Items.Add(m1);

    ToolStripMenuItem m2 = new ToolStripMenuItem("Tools");
    MyMenu.Items.Add(m2);
```

```
   // Create File submenu.
   ToolStripMenuItem item1 = new ToolStripMenuItem("Open");
   m1.DropDownItems.Add(item1);

   ToolStripMenuItem item2 = new ToolStripMenuItem("Close");
   m1.DropDownItems.Add(item2);

   ToolStripMenuItem item3 = new ToolStripMenuItem("Exit");
   m1.DropDownItems.Add(item3);

   // Create Tools submenu.
   ToolStripMenuItem item4 = new ToolStripMenuItem("Coordinates");
   m2.DropDownItems.Add(item4);

   ToolStripMenuItem item5 = new ToolStripMenuItem("Change Size");
   m2.DropDownItems.Add(item5);

   ToolStripMenuItem item6 = new ToolStripMenuItem("Restore");
   m2.DropDownItems.Add(item6);


   // Add event handlers for the menu items.
   item1.Click += MMOpenClick;
   item2.Click += MMCloseClick;
   item3.Click += MMExitClick;
   item4.Click += MMCoordClick;
   item5.Click += MMChangeClick;
   item6.Click += MMRestoreClick;

   // Add to list of controls.
   Controls.Add(MyMenu);

   // Assign the menu to the form.
   MainMenuStrip = MyMenu;
 }

 [STAThread]
 static void Main() {
   MenuForm skel = new MenuForm();

   Application.EnableVisualStyles();
   Application.Run(skel);
 }

 // Handler for main menu Coordinates selection.
 void MMCoordClick(object who, EventArgs e) {
   // Create a string that contains the coordinates.
   string size =
     String.Format("{0}: {1}, {2}\n{3}: {4}, {5} ",
                   "Top, Left", Top, Left,
                   "Bottom, Right", Bottom, Right);

   // Display a message box.
   MessageBox.Show(size, "Window Coordinates",
```

```
                                    MessageBoxButtons.OK);
      }

      // Handler for main menu Change selection.
      void MMChangeClick(object who, EventArgs e) {
        Width = Height = 200;
      }

      // Handler for main menu Restore selection.
      void MMRestoreClick(object who, EventArgs e) {
        Width = Height = 300;
      }

      // Handler for main menu Open selection.
      void MMOpenClick(object who, EventArgs e) {

        MessageBox.Show("Inactive", "Inactive",
                    MessageBoxButtons.OK);
      }

      // Handler for main menu Close selection.
      void MMCloseClick(object who, EventArgs e) {

        MessageBox.Show("Inactive", "Inactive",
                    MessageBoxButtons.OK);
      }

      // Handler for main menu Exit selection.
      void MMExitClick(object who, EventArgs e) {

        DialogResult result = MessageBox.Show("Stop Program?",
                            "Terminate",
                            MessageBoxButtons.YesNo);

        if(result == DialogResult.Yes) Application.Exit();
      }
    }
```

FIGURE 26-5
Sample output
from the **MenuStrip**
program

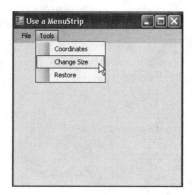

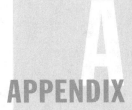

Documentation Comment
Quick Reference

C# supports three types of comments. The first two are // and /* */. The third type is based on XML tags and is called a *documentation comment*. (The term *XML comment* is also commonly used.) A single-line documentation comment begins with ///. A multiline documentation comment begins with /** and ends with */. The lines after the /** can (but are not required to) start with a single *. If all subsequent lines in the multiline comment begin with a *, the * is ignored.

Documentation comments precede the declaration of such things as classes, namespaces, methods, properties, and events. Using documentation comments, you can embed information about your program into the program itself. When you compile the program, you can have the documentation comments placed into an XML file. Documentation comments can also be utilized by the IntelliSense feature of Visual Studio.

The XML Comment Tags

C# supports the XML documentation tags shown in Table A-1. Most of the XML comment tags are readily understandable, and they work like all other XML tags with which most programmers are already familiar. However, the **<list>** tag is more complicated than the others. A list contains two components: a list header and list items. The general form of a list header is shown here:

```
<listheader>
  <term> name </term>
  <description> text </description>
</listheader>
```

Here, *text* describes *name*. For a table, *text* is not used. The general form of a list item is shown next:

```
<item>
  <term> item-name </term>
  <description> text </description>
</item>
```

Here, *text* describes *item-name*. For bulleted or numbered lists or tables, *item-name* is not used. There can be multiple **<item>** entries.

Tag	Description
<c> *code* </c>	Specifies the text specified by *code* as program code.
<code> *code* </code>	Specifies multiple lines of text specified by *code* as program code.
<example> *explanation* </example>	The text associated with *explanation* describes a code example.
<exception cref = "*name*"> *explanation* </exception>	Describes an exception. The exception is specified by *name*.
<include file = '*fname*' path = '*path* [@*tagName* "]' />	Specifies a file that contains the XML comments for the current file. The file is specified by *fname*. The path to the tag, the tag name, and the tag ID are specified by *path*, *tagName*, and *tagID*, respectively.
<list type = "*type*"> *list-header* *list-items* </list>	Specifies a list. The type of the list is specified by *type*, which must be either bullet, number, or table.
<para> *text* </para>	Specifies a paragraph of text within another tag.
<param name = '*param-name*'> *explanation* </param>	Documents the parameter specified by *param-name*. The text associated with *explanation* describes the parameter.
<paramref name = "*param-name*" />	Specifies that *param-name* is a parameter name.
<permission cref = "*identifier*"> *explanation* </permission>	Describes the permission setting associated with the class members specified by *identifier*. The text associated with *explanation* describes the permission settings.
<remarks> *explanation* </remarks>	The text specified by *explanation* is a general commentary often used to describe a type, such as a class or structure.
<returns> *explanation* </returns>	The text specified by explanation documents the return value of a method.
<see cref = "*identifier*" />	Declares a link to another element specified by *identifier*.
<seealso cref = "*identifier*" />	Declares a "see also" link to *identifier*.
<summary> *explanation* </summary>	The text specified by *explanation* is a general commentary often used to describe a method or other class member.
<typeparam name = "*param-name*"> *explanation* </typeparam>	Documents the type parameter specified by *param-name*. The text associated with *explanation* describes the type parameter.
<typeparamref name = "*param-name*" />	Specifies that *param-name* is the name of a type parameter.
<value> *explanation* </value>	The text specified by *explanation* documents a property.

TABLE A-1   The XML Comment Tags

Compiling Documentation Comments

To produce an XML file that contains the documentation comments, specify the **/doc** option. For example, to compile a file called **DocTest.cs** that contains XML comments, use this command line:

```
csc DocTest.cs /doc:DocTest.xml
```

To create an XML output file when using the Visual Studio 2008 IDE, you must activate the Properties page. Next, select Build. Then, check the XML Documentation File box and specify the name of the XML file.

An XML Documentation Example

Here is an example that demonstrates several documentation comments. It uses both the multiline and the single-line forms. As a point of interest, many programmers use a series of single-line documentation comments rather than a multiline comment even when a comment spans several lines. (Several of the comments in this example use this approach.) The advantage is that it clearly identifies each line in a longer documentation comment as being part of a documentation comment. This is, of course, a stylistic issue, but it is common practice.

```
// A documentation comment example.

using System;

/** <remark>
 This is an example of multiline XML documentation.
 The Test class demonstrates several tags.
</remark>
*/

class Test {
  /// <summary>
  /// Main is where execution begins.
  /// </summary>
  static void Main() {
    int sum;

    sum = Summation(5);
    Console.WriteLine("Summation of " + 5 + " is " + sum);
  }

  /// <summary>
  /// Summation returns the summation of its argument.
  /// <param name = "val">
  /// The value to be summed is passed in val.
  /// </param>
  /// <see cref="int"> </see>
  /// <returns>
  /// The summation is returned as an int value.
  /// </returns>
  /// </summary>
  static int Summation(int val) {
    int result = 0;

    for(int i=1; i <= val; i++)
      result += i;

    return result;
  }
}
```

Assuming the preceding program is called **XmlTest.cs**, the following line will compile the program and produce a file called **XmlTest.xml** that contains the comments:

```
csc XmlTest.cs /doc:XmlTest.xml
```

After compiling, the following XML file is produced:

```
<?xml version="1.0"?>
<doc>
    <assembly>
        <name>DocTest</name>
    </assembly>
    <members>
        <member name="T:Test">
            <remark>
             This is an example of multiline XML documentation.
             The Test class demonstrates several tags.
            </remark>
        </member>
        <member name="M:Test.Main">
            <summary>
            Main is where execution begins.
            </summary>
        </member>
        <member name="M:Test.Summation(System.Int32)">
            <summary>
            Summation returns the summation of its argument.
            <param name="val">
            The value to be summed is passed in val.
            </param>
            <see cref="T:System.Int32"> </see>
            <returns>
            The summation is returned as an int value.
            </returns>
            </summary>
        </member>
    </members>
</doc>
```

Notice that each documented element is given a unique identifier. These identifiers can be used by other programs that use the XML documentation.

Index